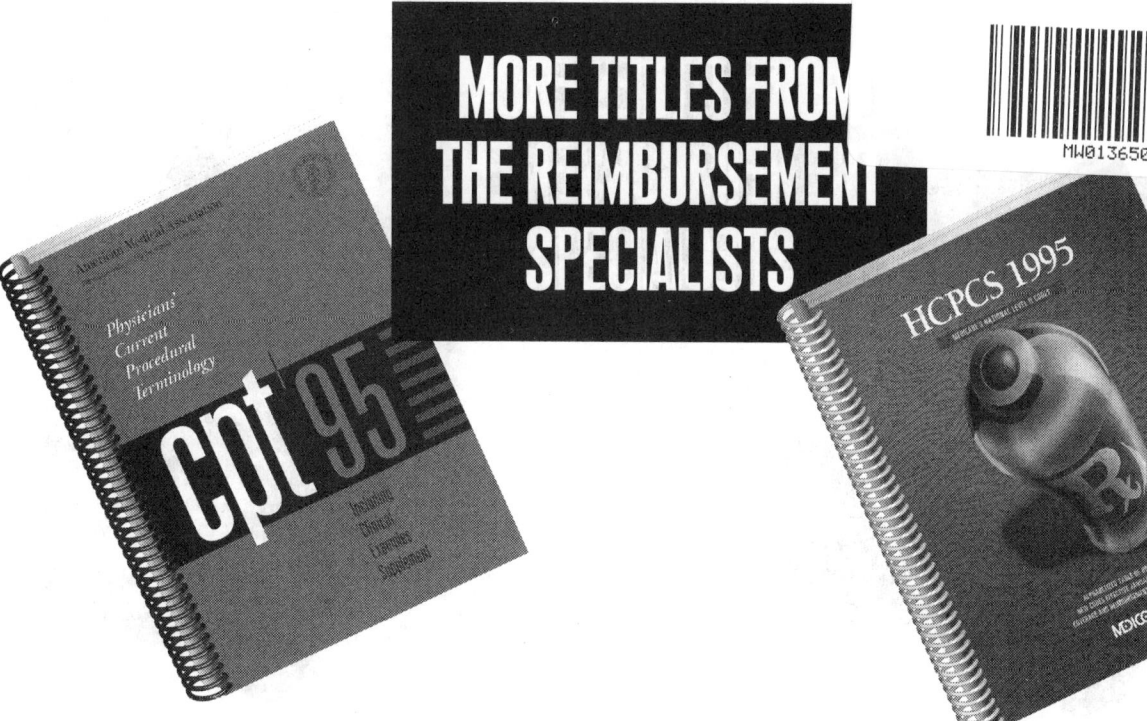

More Coding Power For Your Money

New this year, *CPT 1995* is larger (8½" x 11")to make the book easier for you to use. It has also been redesigned with these new features:

- New two-column design helps you move through the text more efficiently.
- Redesigned headings and subheadings guide you through codes easily.
- New paper stock lets you use a highlighter.
- Individual codes prominently stand out.
- Printed on recycled paper.

Medicode's New Deluxe CPT

Our new deluxe *CPT 1995* offers even more:

- Medicode's exclusive *CPT Extra* includes specialty pricing information, anatomy charts, a medical abbreviation dictionary and superbill tips — including a 20% discount coupon off customized superbills from Colwell, an industry leader in practice management tools.
- Quality spiral binding and thumb-index tabs.

Still The Easiest To Use, And Now It's Expanded

Our *HCPCS 1995* is the most user-friendly, most comprehensive coding reference available for durable medical equipment (DME), drugs and select medical services. Features include:

- An expanded, easy-to-use index that includes more product name references for supplies and DME.
- A detailed table of drugs with brand names, generic drugs, dosage, route of administration and correct J or K codes.
- Complete Medicare Carrier's Manual and Coverage Issues Manual citations wherever possible.
- Cross-referencing of generic drugs to brand names.
- Cross-referencing of deleted HCPCS codes to active HCPCS codes. An essential feature when you're completing forms.
- Instructions preceding each section to better guide you through information.
- A list of common abbreviations and their meanings.
- Specialist procedure information with applicable codes.

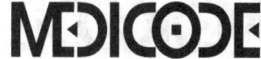

POWER TO MAKE THE RIGHT DECISIONS.™

1-800-999-4600

Medicode publications are available from your medical bookstore or call 1-800-999-4600.
For information on Medicode consulting, databases, educational programs and software, call 1-800-999-4614.

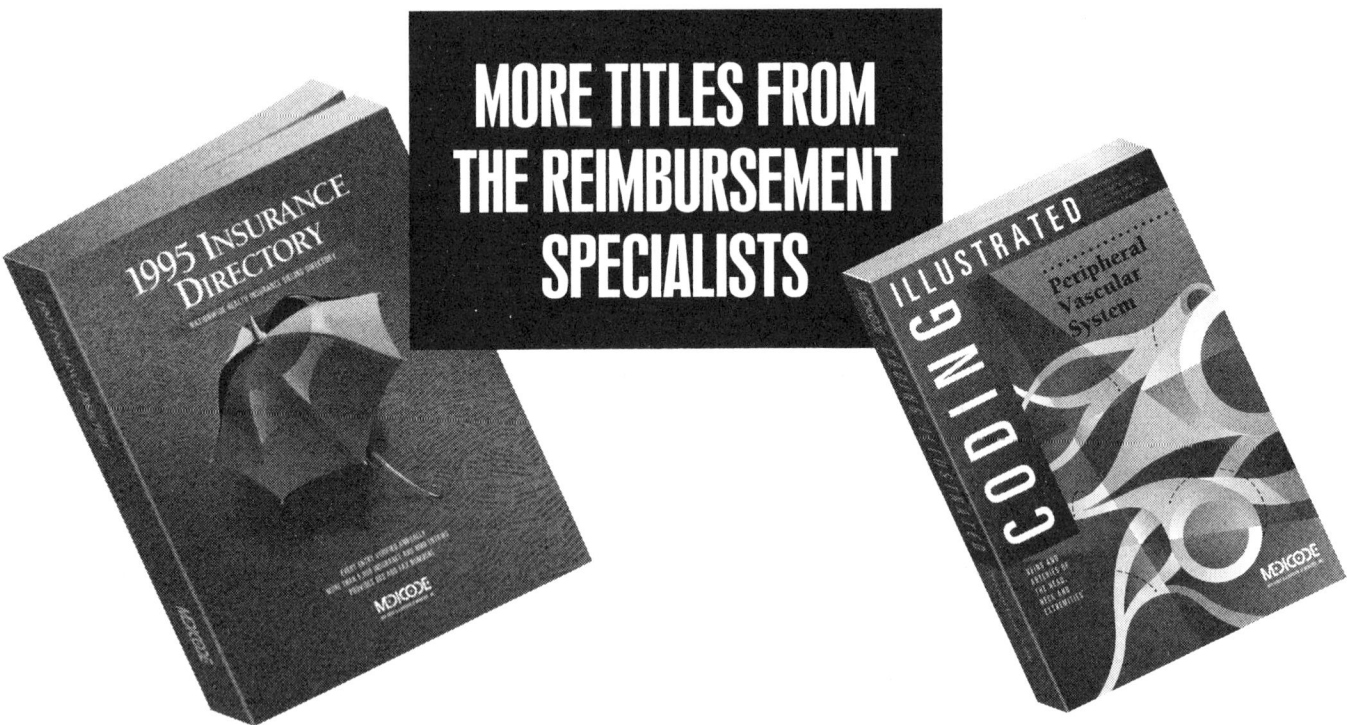

MORE TITLES FROM THE REIMBURSEMENT SPECIALISTS

We've Verified Every Entry For Accuracy

Our *1995 Insurance Directory* gives you the latest information on more than 5,000 third-party payers and self-administered corporations. We've verified the accuracy of each entry by phone — a claim no other directory can make.

Only Medicode offers you the most accurate, most up-to-date insurance listing available.

Our *Directory* includes:

- More listings than any other directory plus 800 and fax numbers make it easy for you to stay in touch.
- Symbols — not just listings — instantly identify the types of claims paid.
- Instructions help you complete HCFA-1500 forms.
- Ready-to-use claim management forms.
- Identifies companies that electronically process claims, saving you valuable time.

Quickly Cross-Reference All Major Codes

If you were to choose a single coding resource, *Coding Illustrated* would have to be the one. This essential series is the the first and only guide that uses illustration and straightforward language to effectively explain CPT codes.

We put CPT, ICD•9 and HCPCS codes together for easy cross-referencing (with ADA code cross-references when appropriate). We also offer easy-to-use tables to explain which codes can't be billed together, when assist-at-surgery is allowed, follow-up days and prior approval requirements.

And, because an illustration accompanies each CPT code, it's easier to translate operative reports into the right codes, the first time. As a complete coding resource, nothing compares to our *Coding Illustrated* series.

To make *Coding Illustrated* even better, we publish all volumes by anatomical structure and arrange them by CPT code. You buy only the volumes your practice needs, so *Coding Illustrated* is one of the smartest investments you can make.

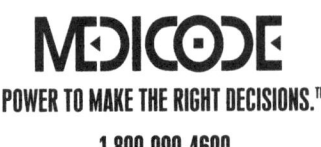

POWER TO MAKE THE RIGHT DECISIONS.™

1-800-999-4600

Medicode publications are available from your medical bookstore or call 1-800-999-4600.
For information on Medicode consulting, databases, educational programs and software, call 1-800-999-4614.

MEDICODE'S
ICD·9·CM
EXTRA

FOURTH EDITION

1995

MEDICODE

Contents

Introduction 1
   Medical Necessity 1
   Common Coding Difficulties 1

Anatomy Charts 3
   The Eye 3
   The Ear 3
   Anatomical Positions, Locations and Terms 4
   Body Planes and Movements 5
   Coding Burns 6
   Rule of Nines for Burns 6
   Skeletal System 7
   Nervous System 8
   Lymphatic Systems 8
   Digestive System 9
   Endocrine System 9
   Circulatory System 10
   Major Arteries 10
   Major Veins 10

ICD•9 for Superbills 11
   Step 1: Planning 11
   Step 2: The Codes 11
   Step 3: Insurance Processing Information 12
   Summary 12
   Dermatology 12
   Eye 13
   Family/General Practice 14
   Internal Medicine 15
   Orthopedic 16
   Obstetrics/Gynecology 16
   Otolaryngology 17
   Urology 17

CareTrends™ Demographic Charts 19

ICD•9 Self-Evaluation Tests 22
   Basic ICD•9 Test 22
   Advanced ICD•9 Test 23
   The Answers, Basic ICD•9 25
   The Answers, Advanced ICD•9 25

© Copyright 1994 Medicode, Inc.
All Rights Reserved

First Printing — August 1994

This book, or parts hereof, may not be reproduced in any form without permission.

Introduction

ICD•9 Extra is a diagnostic coding resource that augments the diagnostic coding information within this copy of ICD•9•CM. This exclusive Medicode product was developed as a response to requests from Medicode customers.

This ICD•9 supplement includes a section on anatomical charts; information on developing superbills; competency tests for beginning and advanced coders; and patient demographics data on more than 50 common diagnoses.

All these are offered as tools to make coding easier. Refer to the anatomical charts when confused by notations in the patient record. And consult the section on superbills when updating office forms for 1995 codes. Guage coding expertise in your office through the diagnostic coding tests. And gain insight into common ailments by examining the patient profile samplings gleaned from Medicode's new CareTrends product.

The introduction to Volumes 1 and 2 of ICD•9 explains the conventions for maneuvering within the ICD•9 coding hierarchy. A look at how to establish medical necessity and common coding difficulties is presented below.

MEDICAL NECESSITY
Establishing medical necessity is the first step in third-party reimbursement. Justify the care provided by presenting appropriate facts. Payers require the following information to determine the need for care:

- Knowledge of the emergent nature or severity of the patient's complaint or condition, and
- All the facts regarding signs, symptoms, complaints, or background facts describing the reason for care, such as required follow-up care.

These facts must be substantiated by the patient's medical record, and that record must be available to payers on request. Always obtain a signed release from your patient authorizing release of information to the payer.

Primary Diagnosis
The first diagnostic code referenced in item 21 on the HCFA-1500 claim form must describe the primary, or most important, reason for the service or procedure provided. Often, a single ICD•9 code adequately identifies the need for care. If additional facts are required to substantiate the care provided, list the ICD•9 codes in the order of importance.

Code only the current condition that prompted the patient's visit. Many times a patient has a long list of chronic complaints not directly associated with the specific visit. Providing nonessential information of this nature can cloud a determination of medical necessity. Code chronic complaints only when the patient has received treatment for the condition. When the record identifies an acute condition, use the code that specifies "acute" whenever it is available.

Occasionally, an unspecified code must be used until test results are confirmed. However, medical necessity may not be clearly identified if you use unspecified codes or codes with the fourth digit "9." When the diagnostic statement is general or generic, investigate further. Go back to the medical record where the documentation should give definitive information and facts. If the information is not there, go to the source — the physician — and ask questions.

COMMON CODING DIFFICULTIES
The following examples apply ICD•9 coding principles to real-life situations involving difficult or confusing coding issues. The examples present the most common coding problems Medicode professionals have encountered in years of consulting. Each scenario includes a description of the patient visit, the correct codes, and the logic for their selection.

Symptoms
A urologist sees a patient who complains of frequency of urination, abdominal pain, and occasional blood in the urine. The physician suspects a bladder tumor and schedules the patient for a diagnostic cystoscopy. The bladder tumor is often coded, but at this initial visit only the symptoms are known.

Diagnosis
599.7	Hematuria
788.41	Urinary frequency
789.0	Abdominal pain

Reason
Coding to the highest degree of certainty means coding only what you know as fact. Patients are often seen for ill-defined complaints such as "back pain." The physician may suspect the possibility of a herniated disk and order radiologic studies, but until the results are known, code only the symptom.

Codes for most symptoms are found in categories 780–789 and describe signs and complaints used as provisional diagnoses until all the facts have been examined.

Neoplasms

Past Neoplasm Not Recurrent
A patient returns for a follow-up examination six months after the surgeon removed a malignant tumor. Her treatment course of surgery (a radical mastectomy) and chemotherapy was successful with no recurrence of the tumor. The patient is symptom-free.

Diagnosis
V10.3	Personal history of malignant neoplasm of breast
V67.0	Follow-up examination, following surgery
V67.2	Follow-up examination, following chemotherapy

Reason
A neoplasm is an abnormal growth of tissue. Such growths may behave in different ways and are described as malignant,

benign, uncertain behavior, and unspecified. If the behavior is malignant, it is described as primary, secondary, or Ca in situ.

Malignant, secondary: Identifies a second cancerous neoplasm at a body site other than the original site. Use this description for all secondary cancers, even when the primary malignancy appears to have been arrested.

Malignant, Ca in situ: Identifies cancerous neoplasms that are confined, or "noninvasive," in nature.

Benign: Identifies a neoplasm that is noncancerous.

Uncertain Behavior: Identifies tissue with neoplastic characteristics, but the type of behavior cannot yet be determined. Further testing by the physician is required.

Unspecified: Used when the nature of the neoplasm is undetermined pending laboratory results.

The neoplasm entry in the Alphabetic Index provides an easy-to-read table that alphabetically lists the anatomical site of the neoplasm and six possible codes for each site based on the behavior of the neoplasm. Wait for the pathology report to code the diagnosis correctly.

Current Neoplasm
A general surgeon sees a patient requiring a breast biopsy. The biopsy results from the pathologist confirm the existence of a malignant tumor. The tumor, a primary cancer, is within the upper-outer quadrant of the right breast.

Diagnosis
174.4   Malignant neoplasm of female breast, upper-outer quadrant

Reason
For malignant neoplasms, code the location and type of cancer. Had the diagnosis been malignant carcinoma (Ca) in situ, at the same location, the code would have been 233.0.

Injuries and Complications

Injuries
An unconscious patient is brought into the emergency department with a fracture of the frontal bone resulting from an automobile accident. There is also a large laceration on the patient's shoulder. The patient (driver of the vehicle) regained consciousness within 45 minutes and did not show signs of any intracranial injury.

Diagnosis
800.02 Closed fracture of the skull without mention of intracranial injury, brief loss of consciousness
880.00 Open wound of shoulder, uncomplicated
E819.0 Motor vehicle traffic accident of unspecified nature, driver of motor vehicle other than motorcycle

Note that each of the injury codes required a fifth digit.

Reason
Codes for injuries are selected from categories 800–959. The information within these categories describes fractures, internal injuries, and open wounds.

To code injuries, determine if the injury is internal or external. Internal injuries to the chest, abdomen, and pelvis are found in 860–869.1. Codes for internal head injuries range from 850–654.19. Codes for open wounds are 870–897.7. There are separate codes for injuries to blood vessels.

Fractures are coded by the exact bone and whether the fracture is open or closed. An open fracture has an open wound. Code an open fracture only when specifically identified in the documentation. All other fractures are closed, though the physician may perform an "open" procedure to repair a closed fracture.

Complications
During a cholecystectomy for acute cholecystitis a patient suffers a cardiac arrest. The patient is successfully resuscitated, the surgical procedure completed, and the patient is placed in the coronary care unit for observation.

Diagnosis
575.0   Acute cholecystitis
997.1   Cardiac complications, postoperative
427.5   Cardiac arrest

Reason
The diagnostic code relates to the surgical procedure, while the cardiac complication code relates to care associated with the arrest. Many complications are coded to the specific body system, while others fall into the categories 996–999.

Italicized Codes

An insulin-dependent diabetic patient is seen by her ophthalmologist for proliferative diabetic retinopathy.

Diagnosis
250.51 Diabetes with ophthalmic manifestations, insulin dependent, not stated as uncontrolled
362.02   *Proliferative diabetic retinopathy*

When coding diabetes, note whether the patient is dependent on insulin, and whether the diabetes is uncontrolled.

Reason
Codes with italicized type should never be a principal diagnosis. There will always be an instructional note stating code first [name of condition] or code underlying disease. Code the cause of disease first, and the resulting problem. Together, these two codes represent the principal diagnosis.

Secondary Neoplasms

A patient with cancer of the upper and lower breast is seen for metastases to the liver.

Diagnosis
197.7   Secondary malignant neoplasm of the liver
174.8   Malignant neoplasm of other specified sites of female breast

Reason
Two codes are required when a secondary neoplasm, also known as a metastatic carcinoma, has been identified. Metastatic means that the original neoplasm has spread to a new location. As the term signifies, this growth is secondary to the original, or primary, site. If the primary malignancy was removed earlier, list the secondary neoplasm as the first diagnosis and a V code describing a personal history of malignant neoplasm as the second diagnosis. If the primary neoplasm has not been removed but the metastatic disease is being evaluated for treatment, list the metastatic site(s) first, followed by the primary site of disease. If information on the primary site is not available, use code 199.1 *Malignant neoplasm without specification of site, other*.

Anatomy Charts

Illustrations are presented here to provide coders a better understanding of the anatomical aspects of medical conditions and procedures presented in the medical record. The graphics offer a link between the technical language of the operative report or patient chart and basic human anatomy. Coders can then come to better understand the patient condition and in turn select an ICD•9 code of the highest level of specificity.

Keep in mind that the physician still holds the key to correct coding through proper documentation. Full diagnostic information must be available in the patient chart before the office staff can assign appropriate ICD•9 coding. In many cases "unspecified" codes are available if details are not; however, it is always advisable to request from the physician any additional information to make a more specific diagnosis.

The anatomy charts in this section depict major vessels of the arterial and venous systems; the major skeletal structures; major nerves; the digestive system; the lymphatic and endocrine systems; and the ear and eye.

A schematic of the planes of the body is presented on page 5 with additional information on positions and range of motion on page 4. The "Rule of Nines" for determining percentage of skin affected in burn or skin-graft coding is included with instructions on its use on page 6.

The illustrations are almost always simplified schematic presentations of complex medical systems. In some instances, proper anatomic detail is given over to a clearer depiction of the relationships within anatomical systems. However, these schematics used in combination with the ICD•9 index may help the coder more quickly and accurately determine appropriate ICD•9 codes.

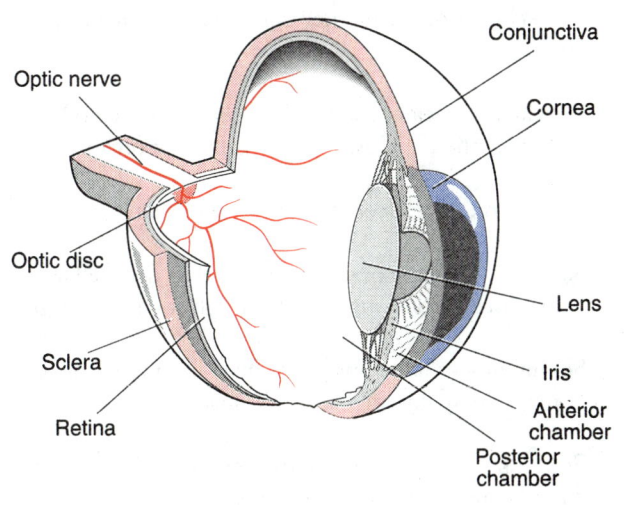

The Eye

The Ear

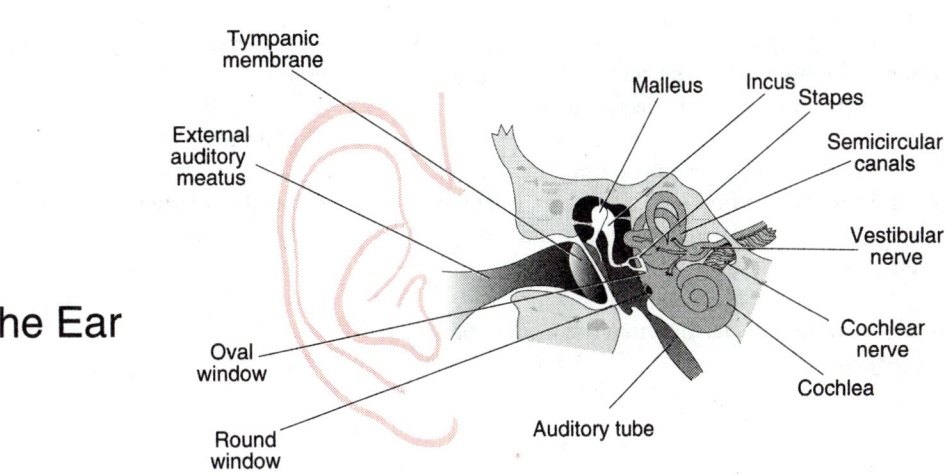

ANATOMICAL POSITIONS, LOCATIONS AND TERMS

The following is a list of medical terms denoting anatomical positions, locations, and features as commonly recorded in medical records. A more complete listing may be found in the numerous anatomy texts available to medically trained personnel as well as those directed to the lay public.

Anterior — situated on the front surface of the body; ventral

Bilateral — on both sides, having two sides

Caudal — denoting the lower half of the body; inferior

Contraction — a shortening and/or tensioning of muscle tissue

Coronal — pertaining to an imaginary longitudinal plane at right angle to the medial plane and dividing the body into ventral and dorsal components

Cranial — denoting the upper half of the body; nearer the head, relating to the head; superior

Diaphysis — the shaft portion of long bones, between the ends or extremities (epiphyses)

Distal — situated away from the center of the body, usually applied to the extremity or most distant part of a limb or organ

Dorsal — situated on the back surface of the body; back of the hand; top surface of the foot; posterior

Epiphysis — the end, or extremity, of a long bone

Fascia — the fibrous sheet enveloping the body underneath the skin

Flexion — the bending of a joint; a joint in the position of being bent

Inferior — situated below the center of the body or directly downward, nearer the feet; caudal

Joint — the junction between two or more bones of the body, and classified as fibrous (i.e., sutures of skull), cartilaginous (i.e., intervertebral discs), and synovial (i.e., elbow)

Lateral — on the side, farther from the median or midsagittal plane

Medial — relating to the middle or center, nearer the midsagittal plane

Midsagittal plane — an imaginary plane starting at the top of the head, running down through the center of the nose, etc., and dividing the body vertically into two halves, left and right

Muscle — the movement producing material of the body; consisting of three types: skeletal (voluntary control and having two attachments, an origin and an insertion); cardiac (the myocardium forming the middle of the heart, contracts spontaneously); smooth muscle (generally two-layered, circular and longitudinal, and found in walls of many visceral organs, and contracts rhythmically)

Oblique — slanting; inclined; a plane between horizontal and vertical

Palmar — referring to the palm of the hand

Plantar — referring to the sole of the foot

Posterior — denoting the back surface of the body; dorsal

Proximal — nearer the trunk or center of the body; usually applied to closest part of a limb or organ

Relaxation — a lessening of muscle tension

Sagittal — a plane or section parallel to the medial plane, usually identified as left or right of medial sagittal.

Sesamoid — small bones embedded in in tendons or joints, principally the hands and feet

Superior — situated above the center of the body or directly upwards; closer to the head; cranial

Transverse — lying across the long axis of the body or organ

Unilateral — confined to one side only

Ventral — pertaining to the belly or front surface of the body; anterior

Body Planes and Movements

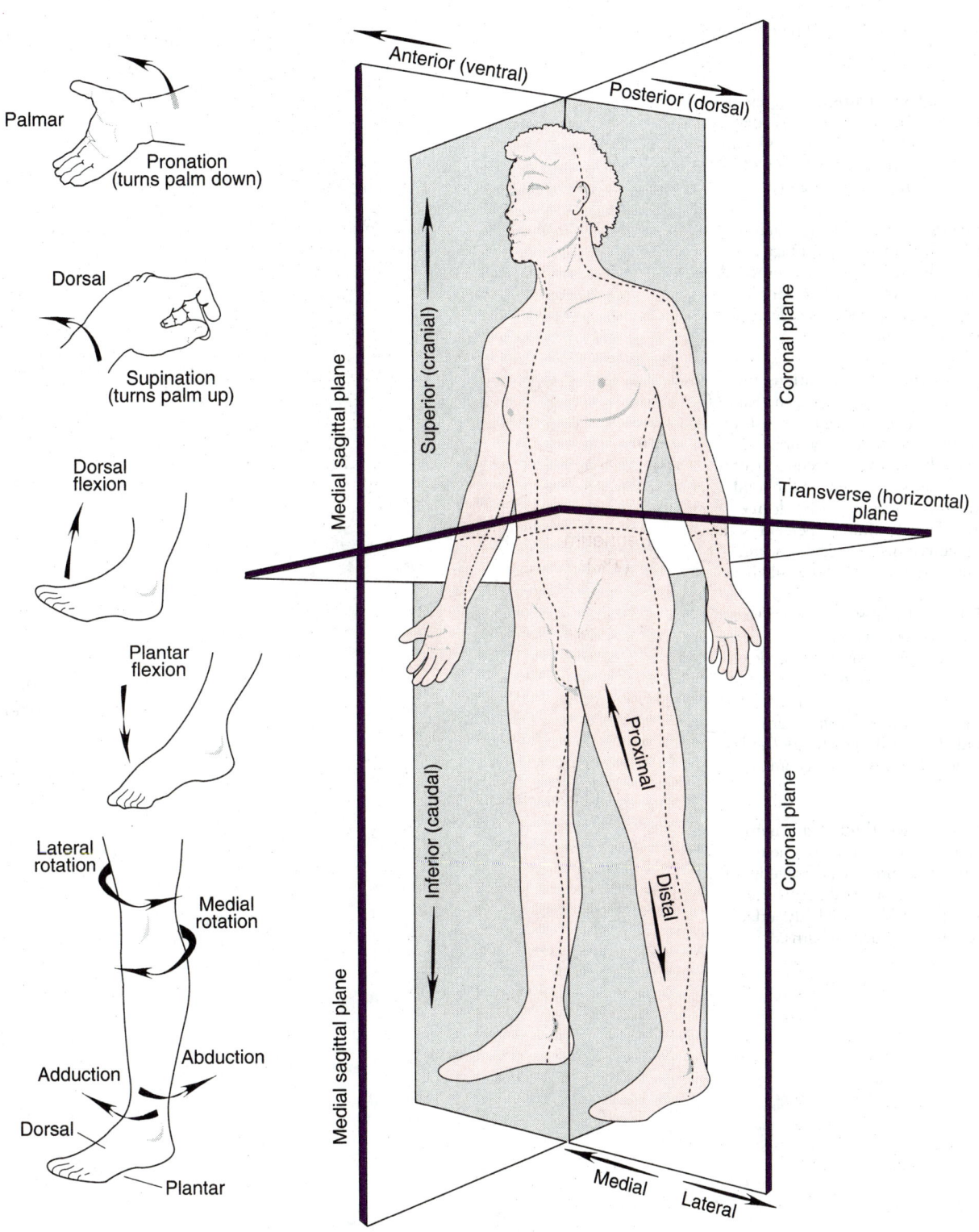

CODING BURNS

Burns present an unusual problem in that correct coding is dependent upon four factors:

- Location of the burn site
- Severity or degree of the burn
- Percentage of the total body surface burned
- Percentage of the total body surface with third-degree burns

Select codes for burns from categories 940–949. Categories 940–947 identify the burn site, the severity of the burn at that site, and often require a fifth digit to further specify the site.

Category 948 with a fourth digit is used to identify the percentage of the total body surface that was burned. A fifth digit identifies the percentage of the total body surface that received third-degree burns.

To make these determinations, use the "Rule of Nines." Using the Rule of Nines, if one entire leg is burned, 18 percent of the total body surface is burned. If half the leg received third-degree burns, 9 percent of the total body surface received third-degree burns. The remaining 9 percent of the leg received first- or second-degree burns. The correct codes would be:

945.39 Full-thickness skin loss, multiple sites of lower limb
948.10 10–19 percent of body surface, 0–10 percent third-degree burn

First and/or second degree burns should be coded using ICD•9 codes for each degree of burn according to site.

As you can see, third-degree burns require at least two codes; one to identify the burn site and severity of the burn, and one to describe the percentage of the total body surface receiving third-degree burns.

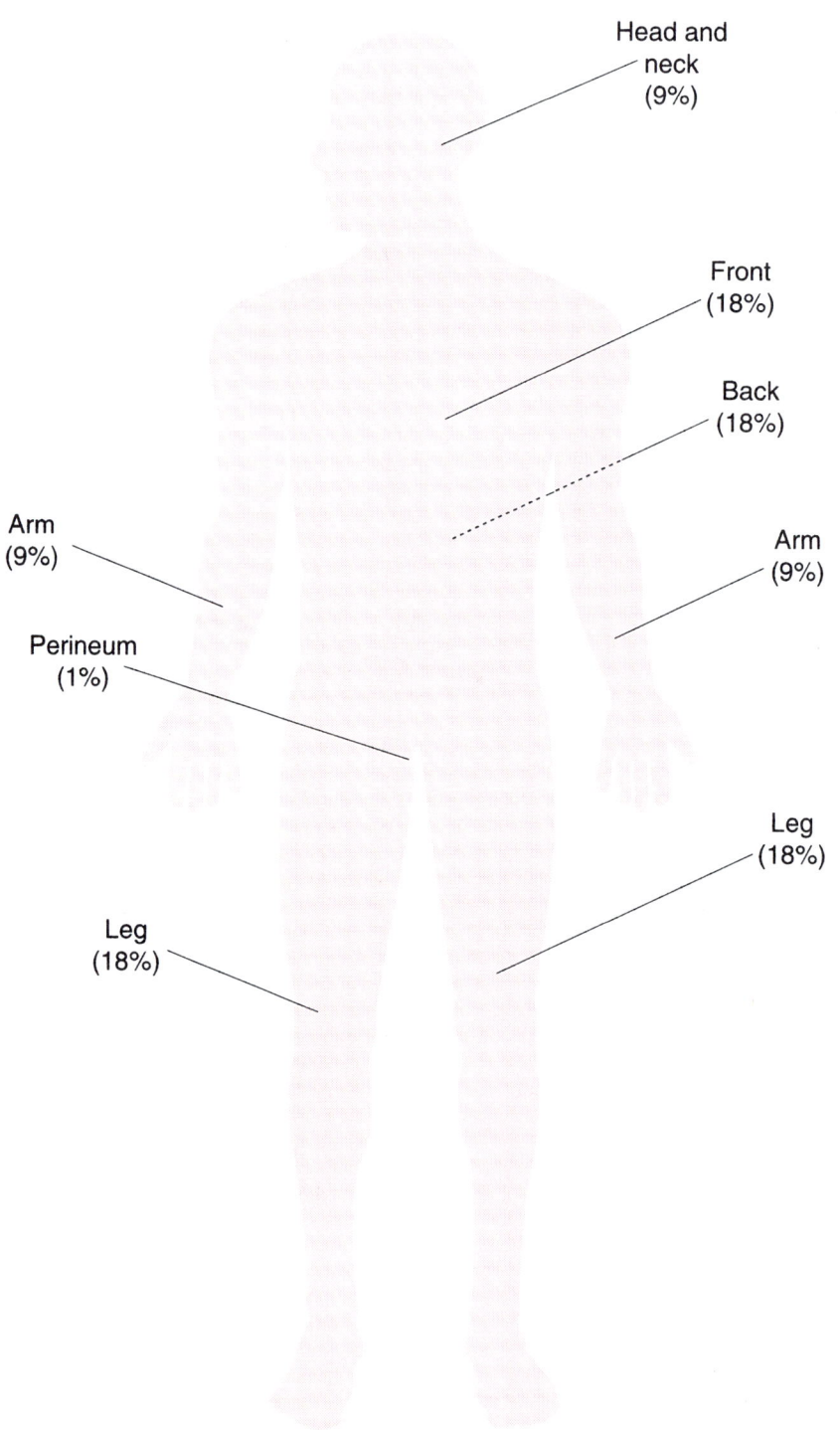

Rule of Nines for Burns

- Head and neck (9%)
- Front (18%)
- Back (18%)
- Arm (9%)
- Arm (9%)
- Perineum (1%)
- Leg (18%)
- Leg (18%)

Skeletal System

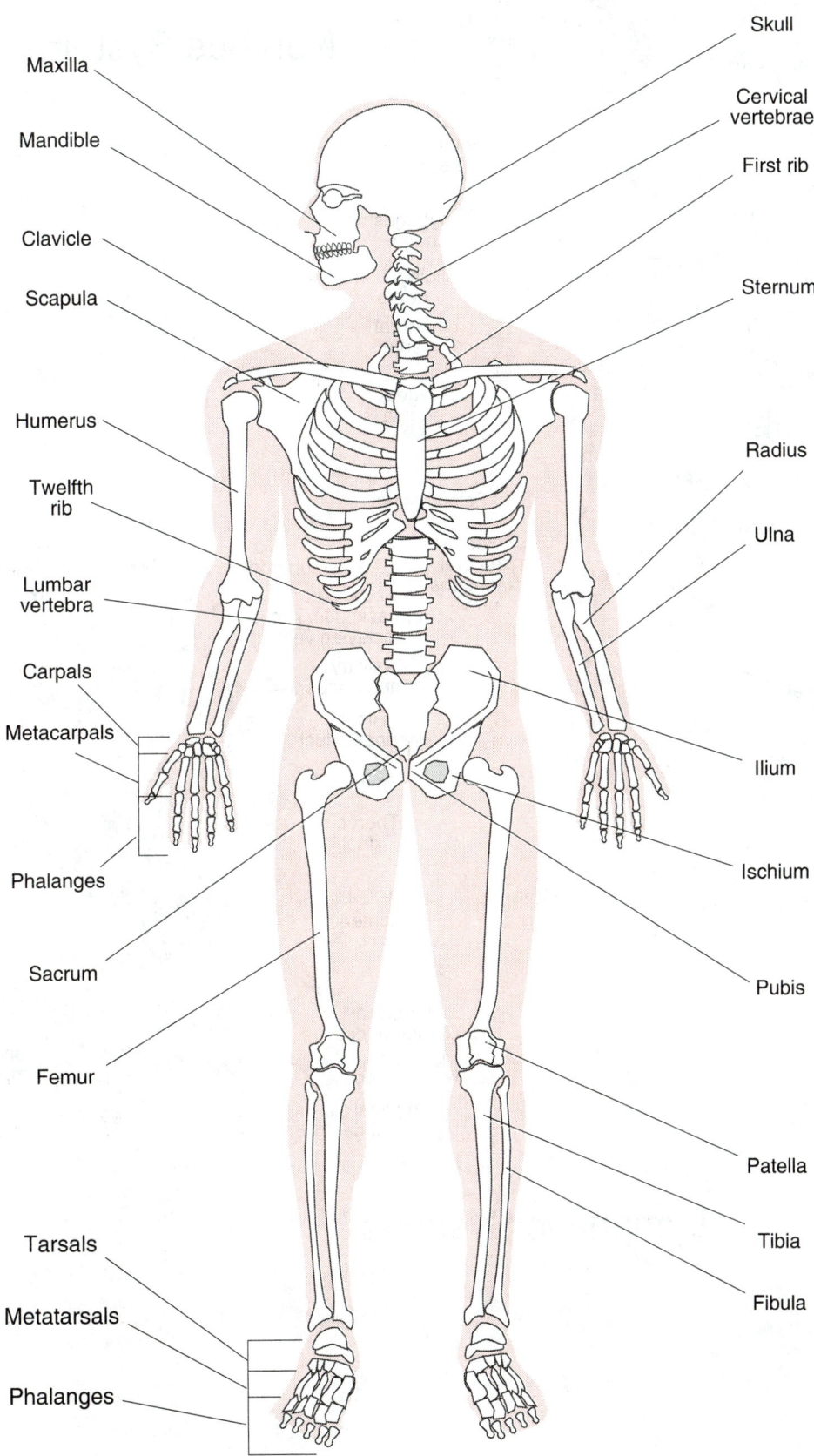

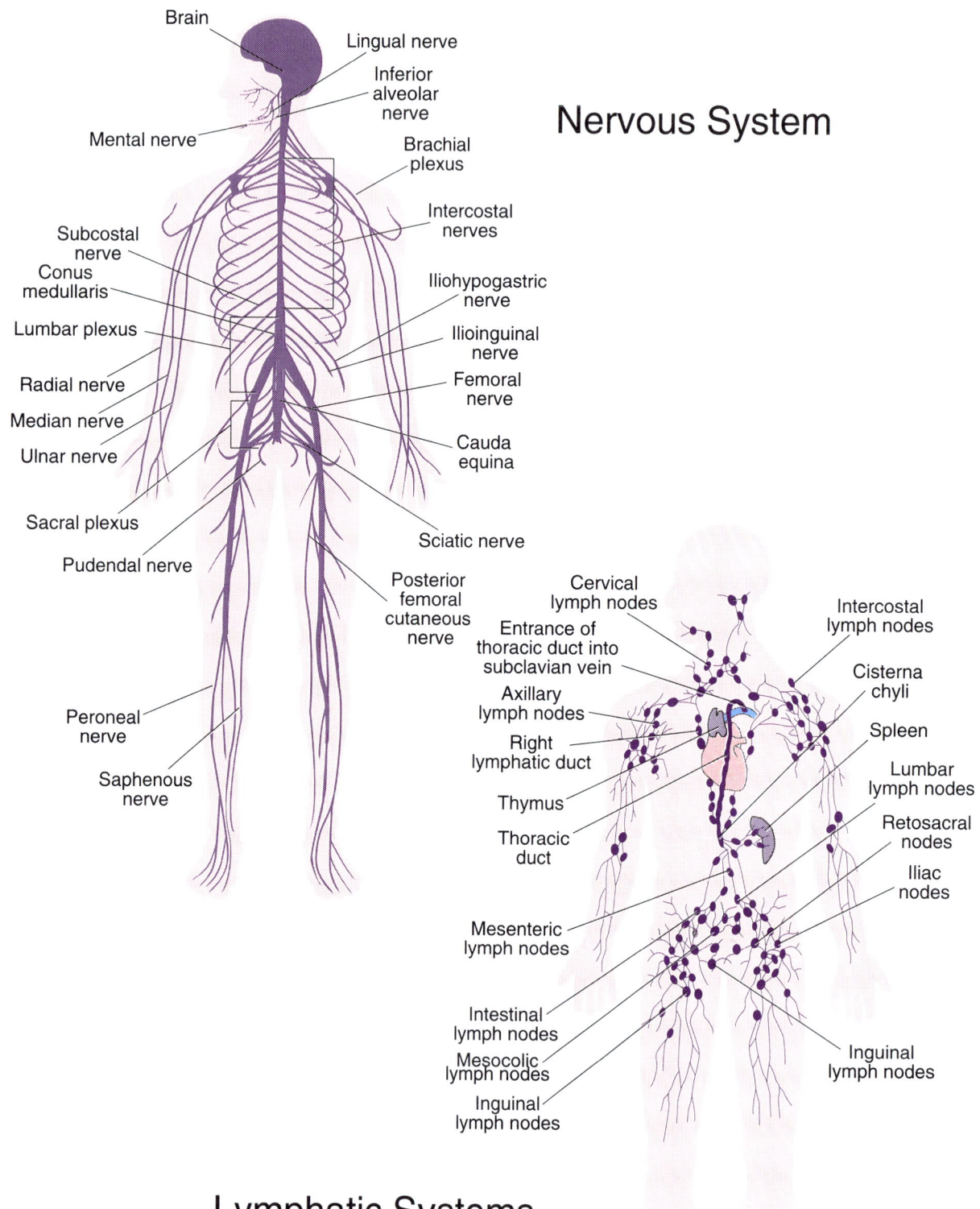

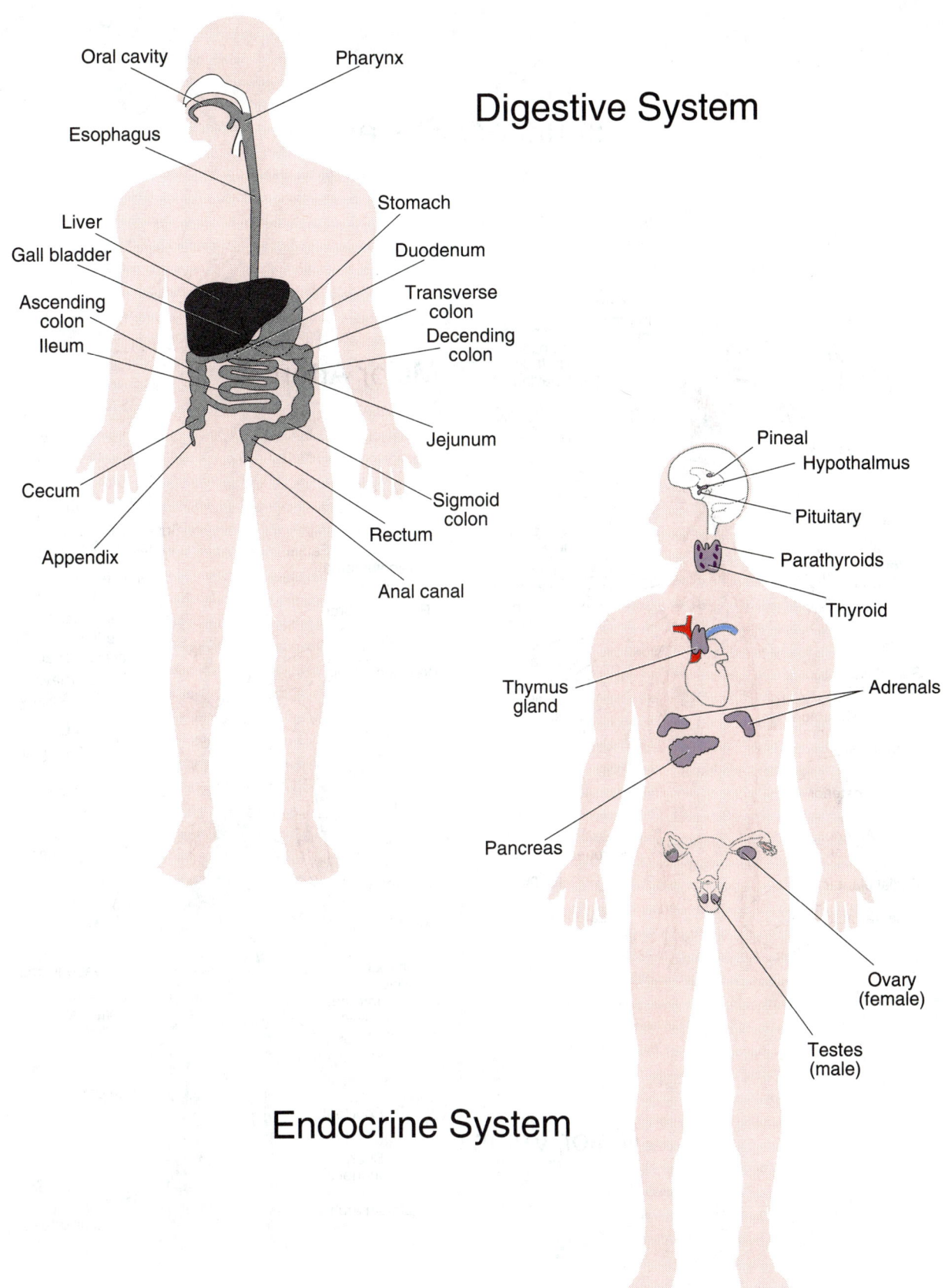

Circulatory System

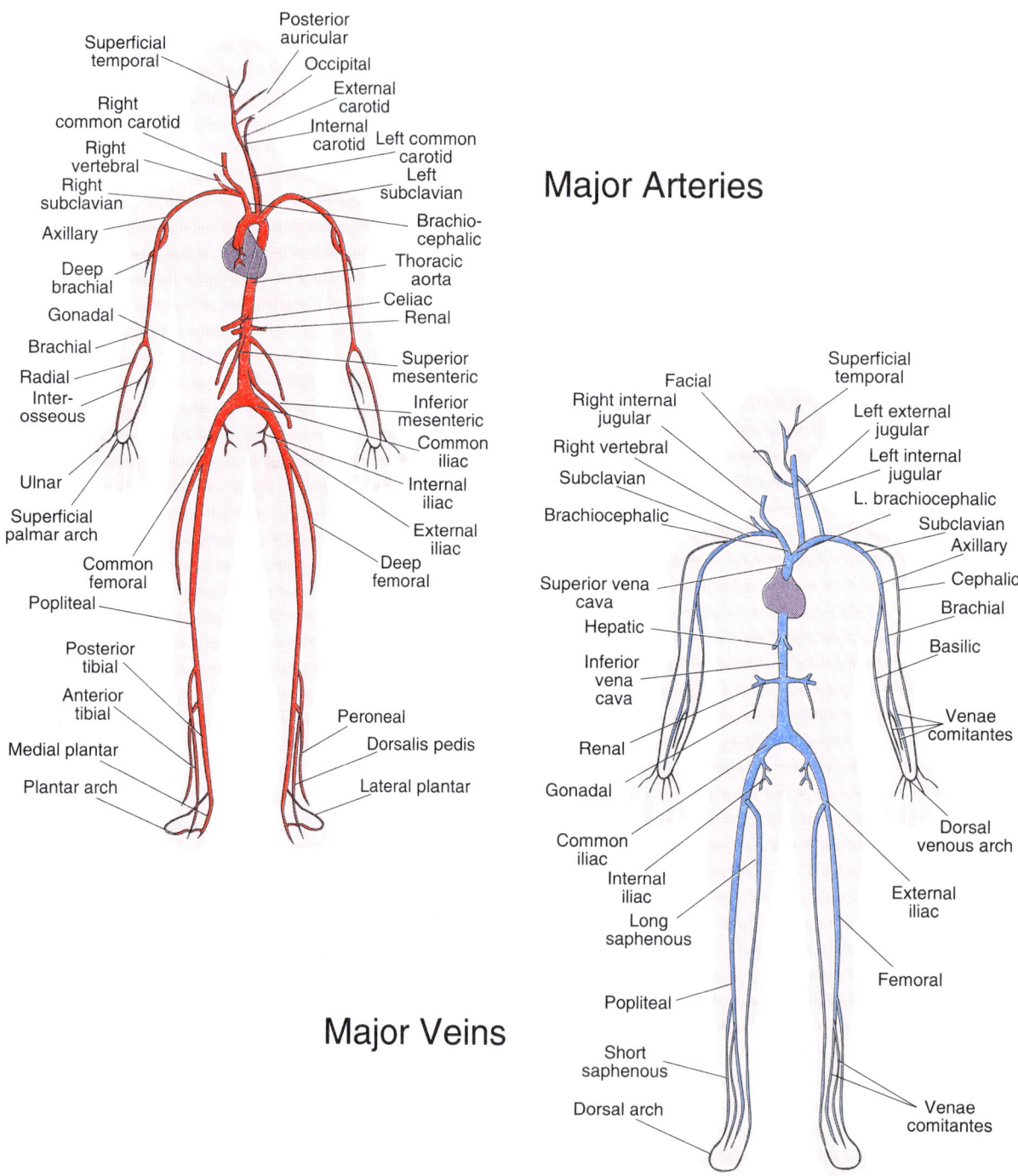

ICD-9 for Superbills

The flow of information regarding services begins with the physician and the coder, and you should already be using some type of mechanism, such as a superbill, to collect data for billing. If you are not using such a mechanism, this section offers suggestions for getting started. A well-constructed superbill not only conveys necessary facts for accurate billing, but lightens the workload.

With a superbill, physicians can easily provide information about services and procedures performed. But the superbill must be updated regularly both to fit the office needs and because CPT, ICD-9, and HCPCS codes are revised annually. If the superbill is not updated with current codes it could complicate the exchange of billing data.

STEP 1: PLANNING
Before designing a superbill, you need:

- Current CPT codes
- Current national HCPCS Level II codes
- Current state or local HCPCS Level III codes
- Current ICD-9 codes
- Any unique carrier codes, such as Blue Cross supply codes for your state
- Physician and staff input. This is the most important resource the office has. Meet several times to discuss development of the superbill.

Usage
The superbill can be used in several ways. Consider the following:

As a routing sheet. The routing sheet is used internally to "route" information to the data entry department. No duplicate is needed and it can be copied or printed on a tear-off tablet.

As an invoice to the patient. This is the most common use. It is usually printed in duplicate or triplicate to provide the patient with a billing form and a receipt at the same time. This is extremely effective for office services.

As two forms. Combining the two previous billing methods may be most effective. Print surgical or nonoffice services on the routing sheet, and the office services on the form that is given to the patient at the time of service. Having two superbills usually provides better communication of all services. Trying to combine all services on one sheet may not allow enough space for the physician to communicate adequately with the coder.

Options
Many offices need to develop superbills for different services. Here are some variations:

Office services. The superbill identifies services performed within the facility. By separating these services from out-of-office services, the number of services listed can be expanded and missed charges avoided. This type of ticket works well as an itemized statement for the patient.

Out-of-office services. Services performed away from the office might involve hospital, emergency, outpatient facility, nursing home, or house calls. Practices that provide a variety of services may want to separate them into medical and surgical services.

Surgical services. For the busy surgical practice, a separate surgical services listing provides a greater range of choices. Consider going one step further and listing services by body system — it will help avoid lost charges.

Hospital medical services. This form contains service codes for nonsurgical hospital services such as admissions, daily visits, critical care, and so on. A hospital superbill works well in a practice that codes primarily medical services, such as internal medicine or medical subspecialties.

Ancillary services (lab and x-ray). The large group practice or multispecialty clinic may want to separate ancillary services from the office services superbill. If so, here is a word of caution: Develop some type of follow-up mechanism to ensure all billing documents are accounted for and subsequently billed.

STEP 2: THE CODES
Develop checklists to assist in compiling the diagnostic, supply, and procedural codes codes needed for the superbill or routing sheet. Go through the lists carefully and check off the codes you want to include.

To help you design a customized superbill or routing sheet, Medicode has included at the end of this chapter lists of ICD-9 diagnostic codes commonly used by several specialties. Specialties with both office and hospital practices should maintain separate forms for each location. Generally, a superbill will contain between 35 and 85 codes, depending on the specialty.

Before you get started, determine how this document will be used by your practice. Only then will you be ready to develop effective and efficient superbills/routing sheets. Superbill companies like Colwell can work with your staff to develop a superbill appropriate for your practice.

Problems to Avoid
Outdated Codes
Codes are updated annually (CPT is updated each December for the following year, HCPCS is updated for January implementation, and ICD-9 is updated with new diagnostic codes each October), so try not to order more forms than the office can use before it is necessary to update.

"Created" Codes

Never "create" codes to fit your needs. Use current CPT or HCPCS Level II or Level III codes that fit the description of the service. If no appropriate code is found, use an unlisted code or one modified with an appropriate CPT modifier.

Incorrect or Misunderstood Descriptions

Stick to the descriptions that correctly identify each code. If the superbill is going to serve only as an internal routing sheet, abbreviate or use terms with which the staff and physician are familiar. When transferring this information to the HCFA-1500 form, remember to identify services correctly with standard CPT or ICD-9 nomenclature.

Oversimplification

It is better to design two or three superbills than to omit information that could result in unbilled or incorrectly billed services.

STEP 3: INSURANCE PROCESSING INFORMATION

The patient and insurance information included on the superbill must fit the needs of the office. If a superbill is being used to replace or attach to an insurance form, take a cue from the "required" fields on the HCFA-1500 form. For the computerized office using the superbill as a routing sheet, the information needed on the bill changes because the computer already has the patients' vital statistics information on file. The following information can extend a typical superbill into a replacement for the universal claim form.

Visit Information

- Physician or practice name/specialty
- Physician address
- Tax I.D. number and provider number for Medicare, Blue Cross/Blue Shield
- Place and date of service
- The day's total service fee
- Physician signature

SUMMARY

For developing a superbill appropriate to your practice, remember:

- Use only current and valid ICD-9 and CPT codes, which are updated annually.
- Choose the codes most common to your practice
- Leave adequate space for descriptions of less common procedures and diagnoses
- Design the superbill so that it can be used as an invoice to the patient as well as a routing sheet for the data entry personnel.
- Develop a separate superbill for each segment of the practice (e.g., office services and hospital medical services).
- Include laboratory information and supply codes on the superbill as appropriate to your practice.
- Consider adding Other Helpful Data:
  - Assignment of benefits and release of medical information
  - Workers' compensation information
  - Referring physician
  - Filing instructions
  - Next appointment date
- Patient Information
  - Patient's full name (following the format of the HCFA-1500 form)
  - Date of birth and sex
  - Patient's address
  - Subscriber
  - Insurance payer
  - Insurance I.D. and group number
- Final Considerations
  - Secondary insurance information
  - Social Security number
  - Date symptoms occurred
  - Reason for visit

To help you formulate superbills for your own practice, here are ICD•9 code lists for a sample of the most common specialties.

Dermatology

053.9	Herpes zoster without mention of complication
054.9	Herpes simplex without mention of complication
078.0	Molluscum contagiosum
078.10	Viral warts, unspecified
110.1	Dermatophytosis of nail
110.9	Dermatophytosis of unspecified site
111.0	Pityriasis versicolor
112.9	Candidiasis of unspecified site
133.0	Scabies
172.9	Melanoma of skin, site unspecified
173.9	Other malignant neoplasm of skin, site unspecified
216.9	Benign neoplasm of skin, site unspecified
228.01	Hemangioma of skin and subcutaneous tissue
232.9	Carcinoma in situ of skin, site unspecified
447.6	Arteritis, unspecified
448.9	Other and unspecified capillary diseases
454.1	Varicose veins of lower extremities with inflammation
454.9	Varicose veins of lower extremities without mention of ulcer or inflammation
680.9	Carbuncle and furuncle of unspecified site
681.02	Onychia and paronychia of finger
682.9	Cellulitis and abscess of unspecified sites
684	Impetigo
686.0	Pyoderma
686.1	Pyogenic granuloma of skin and subcutaneous tissue
690	Erythematosquamous dermatosis
691.8	Other atopic dermatitis and related conditions
692.79	Other dermatitis due to solar radiation
692.9	Contact dermatitis and other eczema, unspecified cause
692.9	Contact dermatitis and other eczema, unspecified cause
693.0	Dermatitis due to drugs and medicines taken internally
694.0	Dermatitis herpetiformis
695.1	Erythema multiforme
695.3	Rosacea
695.4	Lupus erythematosus
695.89	Other specified erythematous conditions
696.1	Other psoriasis and similar disorders
696.3	Pityriasis rosea
696.5	Other and unspecified pityriasis
697.0	Lichen planus
698.3	Lichenification and lichen simplex chronicus
698.3	Lichenification and lichen simplex chronicus
698.9	Unspecified pruritic disorder
700	Corns and callosities
701.1	Keratoderma, acquired
701.4	Keloid scar
701.9	Unspecified hypertrophic and atrophic conditions of skin
702.0	Actinic keratosis
702.1	Seborrheic keratosis
704.01	Alopecia areata
704.8	Other specified diseases of hair and hair follicles
705.81	Dyshidrosis
705.83	Hidradenitis
706.1	Other acne

706.2	Sebaceous cyst		**Anterior Chamber**	
706.8	Other specified diseases of sebaceous glands		364.00	Acute and subacute iridocyclitis, unspecified
707.9	Chronic ulcer of unspecified site		364.02	Recurrent iridocyclitis
708.9	Unspecified urticaria		364.10	Chronic iridocyclitis, unspecified
709.0	Dyschromia		364.3	Unspecified iridocyclitis
757.1	Ichthyosis congenita		364.41	Hyphema of iris and ciliary body
757.39	Other specified congenital anomalies of skin		364.42	Rubeosis iridis

Eye
Cornea

053.21	Herpes zoster keratoconjunctivitis		365.00	Preglaucoma, unspecified
054.40	Herpes simplex with unspecified ophthalmic complication		365.01	Open angle with borderline glaucoma findings
054.42	Dendritic keratitis		365.04	Ocular hypertension
054.43	Herpes simplex disciform keratitis		365.10	Open-angle glaucoma, unspecified
077.1	Epidemic keratoconjunctivitis		365.11	Primary open angle glaucoma
370.00	Corneal ulcer, unspecified		365.12	Low tension glaucoma
370.01	Marginal corneal ulcer		365.22	Acute angle-closure glaucoma
370.02	Ring corneal ulcer		365.60	Glaucoma associated with unspecified ocular disorder
370.03	Central corneal ulcer		365.9	Unspecified glaucoma
370.21	Punctate keratitis			
370.33	Keratoconjunctivitis sicca, not specified as sjogren's		**Lens**	
370.34	Exposure keratoconjunctivitis		366.10	Senile cataract, unspecified
370.40	Keratoconjunctivitis, unspecified		366.11	Pseudoexfoliation of lens capsule
370.60	Corneal neovascularization, unspecified		366.12	Incipient senile cataract
370.9	Unspecified keratitis		366.14	Posterior subcapsular polar senile cataract
371.00	Corneal opacity, unspecified		366.15	Cortical senile cataract
371.03	Central opacity of cornea		366.16	Senile nuclear sclerosis
371.20	Corneal edema, unspecified		366.17	Total or mature cataract
371.23	Bullous keratopathy		366.20	Traumatic cataract, unspecified
371.50	Hereditary corneal dystrophy, unspecified		366.53	After-cataract, obscuring vision
371.57	Endothelial corneal dystrophy			
371.60	Keratoconus, unspecified		**Conjunctiva/Sclera**	
375.15	Tear film insufficiency, unspecified		077.99	Unspecified diseases of conjunctiva due to viruses
375.20	Epiphora, unspecified as to cause		372.00	Acute conjunctivitis, unspecified
918.1	Superficial injury of cornea		372.02	Acute follicular conjunctivitis
930.0	Corneal foreign body		372.05	Acute atopic conjunctivitis
			372.10	Chronic conjunctivitis, unspecified

Retina

115.92	Histoplasmosis retinitis		372.14	Other chronic allergic conjunctivitis
130.2	Chorioretinitis due to toxoplasmosis		372.20	Blepharoconjunctivitis, unspecified
361.00	Retinal detachment with retinal defect, unspecified		372.30	Conjunctivitis, unspecified
361.05	Recent retinal detachment, total or subtotal		372.40	Pterygium, unspecified
361.10	Retinoschisis, unspecified		372.42	Peripheral pterygium, progressive
361.30	Retinal defect, unspecified		372.51	Pinguecula
361.31	Round hole of retina without detachment		372.72	Conjunctival hemorrhage
361.32	Horseshoe tear of retina without detachment		372.73	Conjunctival edema
361.9	Unspecified retinal detachment		372.75	Conjunctival cysts
362.01	Background diabetic retinopathy		379.00	Scleritis, unspecified
362.02	Proliferative diabetic retinopathy		930.1	Foreign body in conjunctival sac
362.11	Hypertensive retinopathy			
362.16	Retinal neovascularization nos		**Eyelids**	
362.30	Retinal vascular occlusion, unspecified		373.00	Blepharitis, unspecified
362.31	Central retinal artery occlusion		373.11	Hordeolum externum
362.32	Retinal arterial branch occlusion		373.13	Abscess of eyelid
362.34	Transient retinal arterial occlusion		373.2	Chalazion
362.35	Central retinal vein occlusion		373.32	Contact and allergic dermatitis of eyelid
362.36	Venous tributary (branch) occlusion of retina		374.00	Entropion, unspecified
362.50	Macular degeneration (senile) of retina, unspecified		374.01	Senile entropion
362.51	Nonexudative senile macular degeneration of retina		374.05	Trichiasis of eyelid without entropion
362.52	Exudative senile macular degeneration of retina		374.10	Ectropion, unspecified
362.53	Cystoid macular degeneration of retina		374.11	Senile ectropion
362.54	Macular cyst, hole, or pseudohole of retina		374.30	Ptosis of eyelid, unspecified
362.56	Macular puckering of retina		374.34	Blepharochalasis
362.57	Drusen (degenerative) of retina		374.51	Xanthelasma of eyelid
362.60	Peripheral retinal degeneration, unspecified		374.84	Cysts of eyelids
362.63	Lattice degeneration of retina			
362.74	Pigmentary retinal dystrophy		**Miscellaneous**	
362.81	Retinal hemorrhage		173.1	Other malignant neoplasm of skin of eyelid, including canthus
362.82	Retinal exudates and deposits		216.1	Benign neoplasm of eyelid, including canthus
362.83	Retinal edema		224.6	Benign neoplasm of choroid
363.20	Chorioretinitis, unspecified		242.00	Toxic diffuse goiter without mention of thyrotoxic crisis or storm
363.30	Chorioretinal scar, unspecified		250.00	Type ii or unspecified type diabetes mellitus without mention of complication, not stated as uncontrolled
			250.50	Type ii or unspecified type diabetes mellitus with ophthalmic manifestations, not stated as uncontrolled
			346.00	Classical migraine without mention of intractable migraine

346.8	Other forms of migraine
346.9	Migraine, unspecified
351.0	Bell's palsy
360.41	Blind hypotensive eye
367.0	Hypermetropia
367.1	Myopia
367.20	Astigmatism, unspecified
367.21	Regular astigmatism
367.31	Anisometropia
367.4	Presbyopia
367.53	Spasm of accommodation
367.9	Unspecified disorder of refraction and accommodation
368.00	Amblyopia, unspecified
368.01	Strabismic amblyopia
368.12	Transient visual loss
368.13	Visual discomfort
368.2	Diplopia
368.40	Visual field defect, unspecified
368.46	Homonymous bilateral field defects
368.8	Other specified visual disturbances
369.4	Legal blindness, as defined in u.S.A.
375.30	Dacryocystitis, unspecified
375.55	Obstruction of nasolacrimal duct, neonatal
375.56	Stenosis of nasolacrimal duct, acquired
376.01	Orbital cellulitis
376.30	Exophthalmos, unspecified
377.00	Papilledema, unspecified
377.10	Optic atrophy, unspecified
377.21	Drusen of optic disc
377.30	Optic neuritis, unspecified
377.41	Ischemic optic neuropathy
378.00	Esotropia, unspecified
378.10	Exotropia, unspecified
378.15	Alternating exotropia
378.35	Accommodative component in esotropia
378.35	Accommodative component in esotropia
378.41	Esophoria
378.42	Exophoria
378.51	Third or oculomotor nerve palsy, partial
378.53	Fourth or trochlear nerve palsy
378.54	Sixth or abducens nerve palsy
378.83	Convergence insufficiency or palsy
378.9	Unspecified disorder of eye movements
379.21	Vitreous degeneration
379.22	Crystalline deposits in vitreous
379.23	Vitreous hemorrhage
379.24	Other vitreous opacities
379.31	Aphakia
379.41	Anisocoria
379.50	Nystagmus, unspecified
379.91	Pain in or around eye
379.93	Redness or discharge of eye
433.10	Occlusion and stenosis of carotid artery without mention of cerebral infarction
446.5	Giant cell arteritis
706.2	Sebaceous cyst
710.2	Sicca syndrome
743.30	Congenital cataract, unspecified
743.57	Specified congenital anomalies of optic disc
780.4	Dizziness and giddiness
784.0	Headache
871.4	Unspecified laceration of eye
921.0	Black eye, not otherwise specified
921.2	Contusion of orbital tissues
921.3	Contusion of eyeball
921.9	Unspecified contusion of eye
995.3	Allergy, unspecified, not elsewhere classified
V43.1	Lens replaced by other means
V65.5	Person with feared complaint in whom no diagnosis was made
V72.0	Examination of eyes and vision
V80.2	Screening for other eye conditions

Family/General Practice

Cardiovascular

401.0	Malignant essential hypertension
401.1	Benign essential hypertension
401.9	Unspecified essential hypertension
402.10	Benign hypertensive heart disease without congestive heart failure
413.9	Other and unspecified angina pectoris
414.0	Coronary atherosclerosis
414.9	Chronic ischemic heart disease, unspecified
427.31	Atrial fibrillation
427.9	Cardiac dysrhythmia, unspecified
428.0	Congestive heart failure
429.2	Cardiovascular disease, unspecified
436	Acute, but ill-defined, cerebrovascular disease
443.9	Peripheral vascular disease, unspecified
451.9	Phlebitis and thrombophlebitis of unspecified site
785.0	Tachycardia, unspecified
785.1	Palpitations
785.2	Undiagnosed cardiac murmurs
786.09	Other dyspnea and respiratory abnormality
786.50	Unspecified chest pain

Endocrine

242.90	Thyrotoxicosis without mention of goiter or other cause, and without mention of thyrotoxic crisis or storm
244.9	Unspecified hypothyroidism
250.00	Type ii or unspecified type diabetes mellitus without mention of complication, not stated as uncontrolled
250.01	Type diabetes mellitus without mention of complication, not stated as uncontrolled
272.0	Pure hypercholesterolemia
272.1	Pure hyperglyceridemia
272.4	Other and unspecified hyperlipidemia
274.9	Gout, unspecified
276.8	Hypopotassemia

EENT

034.0	Streptococcal sore throat
372.00	Acute conjunctivitis, unspecified
372.30	Conjunctivitis, unspecified
380.10	Infective otitis externa, unspecified
380.4	Impacted cerumen
382.9	Unspecified otitis media
386.30	Labyrinthitis, unspecified
461.9	Acute sinusitis, unspecified
462	Acute pharyngitis
463	Acute tonsillitis
784.7	Epistaxis
918.1	Superficial injury of cornea

Gastrointestinal

455.6	Unspecified hemorrhoids without mention of complication
533.90	Peptic ulcer of unspecified site, unspecified as acute or chronic, without mention of hemorrhage or perforation, without mention of obstruction
535.50	Unspecified gastritis and gastroduodenitis, without mention of hemorrhage
536.9	Unspecified functional disorder of stomach
553.3	Diaphragmatic hernia without mention of obstruction or gangrene
558.9	Other and unspecified noninfectious gastroenteritis and colitis
562.11	Diverticulitis of colon (without mention of hemorrhage)
564.0	Constipation
564.1	Irritable colon

Gu/Gyn

582.9	Chronic glomerulonephritis with unspecified pathological lesion in kidney
595.0	Acute cystitis
595.9	Cystitis, unspecified
597.80	Urethritis, unspecified
599.7	Hematuria

600	Hyperplasia of prostate
601.9	Prostatitis, unspecified
610.1	Diffuse cystic mastopathy
611.71	Mastodynia
611.72	Lump or mass in breast
614.9	Unspecified inflammatory disease of female pelvic organs and tissues
616.0	Cervicitis and endocervicitis
616.10	Vaginitis and vulvovaginitis, unspecified
625.3	Dysmenorrhea
625.4	Premenstrual tension syndromes
625.9	Unspecified symptom associated with female genital organs
626.0	Absence of menstruation
626.8	Other disorders of menstruation and other abnormal bleeding from female genital tract
626.9	Unspecified disorders of menstruation and other abnormal bleeding from female genital tract
627.2	Menopausal or female climacteric states
627.3	Postmenopausal atrophic vaginitis
795.0	Nonspecific abnormal papanicolaou smear of cervix
V72.3	Gynecological examination

Musculoskeletal
354.0	Carpal tunnel syndrome
714.0	Rheumatoid arthritis
715.90	Osteoarthrosis, unspecified whether generalized or localized, involving unspecified site
719.40	Pain in joint, site unspecified
724.2	Lumbago
724.3	Sciatica
724.5	Backache, unspecified
726.10	Disorders of bursae and tendons in shoulder region, unspecified
726.90	Enthesopathy of unspecified site
727.3	Other bursitis disorders
729.1	Myalgia and myositis, unspecified
733.00	Osteoporosis, unspecified
733.99	Other disorders of bone and cartilage
845.00	Unspecified site of ankle sprain
846.0	Lumbosacral (joint) (ligament) sprain
847.0	Neck sprain
848.9	Unspecified site of sprain and strain

Neurological
332.0	Paralysis agitans
345.90	Epilepsy, unspecified, without mention of intractable epilepsy
346.90	Migraine, unspecified, without mention of intractable migraine
351.0	Bell's palsy
356.9	Unspecified idiopathic peripheral neuropathy
729.2	Neuralgia, neuritis, and radiculitis, unspecified
780.3	Convulsions
780.4	Dizziness and giddiness
784.0	Headache

Pulmonary
464.0	Acute laryngitis
464.4	Croup
465.9	Acute upper respiratory infections of unspecified site
466.0	Acute bronchitis
473.9	Unspecified sinusitis (chronic)
477.9	Allergic rhinitis, cause unspecified
486	Pneumonia, organism unspecified
487.1	Influenza with other respiratory manifestations
490	Bronchitis, not specified as acute or chronic
492.8	Other emphysema
493.90	Asthma, unspecified type, without mention of status asthmaticus
496	Chronic airway obstruction, not elsewhere classified
511.0	Pleurisy without mention of effusion or current tuberculosis
530.10	Unspecified esophagitis

Skin
053.9	Herpes zoster without mention of complication
078.10	Viral warts, unspecified
079.99	Unspecified viral infection
098.0	Gonococcal infection (acute) of lower genitourinary tract
112.1	Candidiasis of vulva and vagina
112.9	Candidiasis of unspecified site
133.0	Scabies
682.0	Cellulitis and abscess of face
682.9	Cellulitis and abscess of unspecified sites
684	Impetigo
691.0	Diaper or napkin rash
691.8	Other atopic dermatitis and related conditions
692.9	Contact dermatitis and other eczema, unspecified cause
696.1	Other psoriasis and similar disorders
702.0	Actinic keratosis
703.0	Ingrowing nail
706.1	Other acne
706.2	Sebaceous cyst
708.9	Unspecified urticaria

Miscellaneous
075	Infectious mononucleosis
276.5	Volume depletion
278.0	Obesity
281.0	Pernicious anemia
285.9	Anemia, unspecified
300.00	Anxiety state, unspecified
311	Depressive disorder, not elsewhere classified
574.20	Calculus of gallbladder without mention of cholecystitis, without mention of obstruction
780.2	Syncope and collapse
780.6	Pyrexia of unknown origin
780.7	Malaise and fatigue
782.1	Rash and other nonspecific skin eruption
782.3	Edema
783.2	Abnormal loss of weight
787.0	Nausea and vomiting
789.0	Abdominal pain
879.8	Open wound(s) (multiple) of unspecified site(s), without mention of complication
924.9	Contusion of unspecified site
995.3	Allergy, unspecified, not elsewhere classified
V20.2	Routine infant or child health check
V22.2	Pregnant state, incidental
V58.3	Attention to surgical dressings and sutures
V58.3	Attention to surgical dressings and sutures
V70.0	Routine general medical examination at health care facility
V70.3	Other general medical examination for administrative purposes
V70.5	Health examination of defined subpopulations

Internal Medicine
Cardiology
401.0	Malignant essential hypertension
401.1	Benign essential hypertension
411.1	Intermediate coronary syndrome
412	Old myocardial infarction
413.9	Other and unspecified angina pectoris
414.0	Coronary atherosclerosis
424.0	Mitral valve disorders
427.9	Cardiac dysrhythmia, unspecified
785.2	Undiagnosed cardiac murmurs
786.50	Unspecified chest pain

Dermatology
692.9	Contact dermatitis and other eczema, unspecified cause
706.1	Other acne
706.2	Sebaceous cyst
708.9	Unspecified urticaria
782.1	Rash and other nonspecific skin eruption

Endocrinology
242.90	Thyrotoxicosis without mention of goiter or other cause, and without mention of thyrotoxic crisis or storm
244.9	Unspecified hypothyroidism
250.00	Type ii or unspecified type diabetes mellitus without mention of complication, not stated as uncontrolled

250.01	Type diabetes mellitus without mention of complication, not stated as uncontrolled
272.0	Pure hypercholesterolemia
272.1	Pure hyperglyceridemia
274.9	Gout, unspecified
278.0	Obesity

Gastrointestinal
562.11	Diverticulitis of colon (without mention of hemorrhage)
564.0	Constipation
564.1	Irritable colon
569.3	Hemorrhage of rectum and anus
789.0	Abdominal pain

Genitourinary
599.0	Urinary tract infection, site not specified
625.4	Premenstrual tension syndromes
641.9	Unspecified antepartum hemorrhage

Miscellaneous
285.9	Anemia, unspecified
300.00	Anxiety state, unspecified
346.90	Migraine, unspecified, without mention of intractable migraine
372.30	Conjunctivitis, unspecified
380.10	Infective otitis externa, unspecified
380.4	Impacted cerumen
438	Late effects of cerebrovascular disease
440.9	Generalized and unspecified atherosclerosis
461.9	Acute sinusitis, unspecified
462	Acute pharyngitis
463	Acute tonsillitis
465.9	Acute upper respiratory infections of unspecified site
466.0	Acute bronchitis
473.9	Unspecified sinusitis (chronic)
477.0	Allergic rhinitis due to pollen
477.9	Allergic rhinitis, cause unspecified
482.9	Bacterial pneumonia, unspecified
486	Pneumonia, organism unspecified
487.1	Influenza with other respiratory manifestations
490	Bronchitis, not specified as acute or chronic
610.1	Diffuse cystic mastopathy
714.0	Rheumatoid arthritis
726.90	Enthesopathy of unspecified site
727.3	Other bursitis disorders
728.85	Spasm of muscle
733.99	Other disorders of bone and cartilage
780.4	Dizziness and giddiness
784.0	Headache

Orthopedic
Dislocations
832.00	Closed dislocation of elbow, unspecified site
833.00	Closed dislocation of wrist, unspecified part
833.10	Open dislocation of wrist, unspecified part
836.50	Closed dislocation of knee, unspecified part
836.60	Dislocation of knee, unspecified part, open
837.0	Closed dislocation of ankle
837.1	Open dislocation of ankle
839.79	Open dislocation, other location

Sprains/Strains
840.9	Sprain of unspecified site of shoulder and upper arm
841.9	Sprain of unspecified site of elbow and forearm
842.0	Wrist sprain
841.1	Ulnar collateral ligament sprain
844.9	Sprain of unspecified site of knee and leg
845.00	Unspecified site of ankle sprain
845.10	Unspecified site of foot sprain

Miscellaneous
927.10	Crushing injury of forearm
928.10	Crushing injury of lower leg
928.21	Crushing injury of ankle
720.0	Ankylosing spondylitis

824.8	Unspecified fracture of ankle, closed
824.9	Unspecified fracture of ankle, open

Obstetrics/Gynecology
Birth Control/Family Planning
V25.40	Contraceptive surveillance, unspecified
V25.09	Other general counseling and advice on contraceptive management
V25.1	Insertion of intrauterine contraceptive device
V25.2	Sterilization

Breast
611.72	Lump or mass in breast
610.1	Diffuse cystic mastopathy
611.6	Galactorrhea not associated with childbirth
611.0	Inflammatory disease of breast
611.71	Mastodynia
610.0	Solitary cyst of breast

Female Genital
054.10	Genital herpes, unspecified
078.10	Viral warts, unspecified

Pregnancy/Childbirth
648.80	Abnormal glucose tolerance of mother, complicating pregnancy, childbirth, or the puerperium, unspecified as to episode of care
633.9	Unspecified ectopic pregnancy
628.9	Infertility, female, of unspecified origin
632	Missed abortion
V72.4	Pregnancy examination or test, pregnancy unconfirmed
V22.2	Pregnant state, incidental
V24.2	Routine postpartum follow-up
640.00	Threatened abortion, unspecified as to episode of care
633.1	Tubal pregnancy

Vagina/Vulva
627.3	Postmenopausal atrophic vaginitis
616.2	Cyst of bartholin's gland
616.3	Abscess of bartholin's gland
112.1	Candidiasis of vulva and vagina
616.0	Cervicitis and endocervicitis
622.7	Mucous polyp of cervix
624.8	Other specified noninflammatory disorders of vulva and perineum
131.01	Trichomonal vulvovaginitis
618.0	Prolapse of vaginal walls without mention of uterine prolapse
623.5	Leukorrhea, not specified as infective
616.10	Vaginitis and vulvovaginitis, unspecified

Miscellaneous
789.0	Abdominal pain
795.0	Nonspecific abnormal papanicolaou smear of cervix
626.0	Absence of menstruation
233.1	Carcinoma in situ of cervix uteri
595.0	Acute cystitis
626.8	Other disorders of menstruation and other abnormal bleeding from female genital tract
625.3	Dysmenorrhea
625.0	Dyspareunia
622.1	Dysplasia of cervix (uteri)
617.9	Endometriosis, site unspecified
626.2	Excessive or frequent menstruation
625.9	Unspecified symptom associated with female genital organs
V72.	Special investigations and examinations
784.0	Headache
626.4	Irregular menstrual cycle
627.2	Menopausal or female climacteric states
626.9	Unspecified disorders of menstruation and other abnormal bleeding from female genital tract
626.6	Metrorrhagia
787.0	Nausea and vomiting
558.9	Other and unspecified noninfectious gastroenteritis and colitis
614.6	Pelvic peritoneal adhesions, female

614.9	Unspecified inflammatory disease of female pelvic organs and tissues
625.9	Unspecified symptom associated with female genital organs
625.4	Premenstrual tension syndromes
627.1	Postmenopausal bleeding
614.2	Salpingitis and oophoritis not specified as acute, subacute, or chronic
626.1	Scanty or infrequent menstruation
706.2	Sebaceous cyst
625.6	Stress incontinence, female
218.9	Leiomyoma of uterus, unspecified
615.9	Unspecified inflammatory disease of uterus
618.1	Uterine prolapse without mention of vaginal wall prolapse
618.4	Uterovaginal prolapse, unspecified
599.0	Urinary tract infection, site not specified

Otolaryngology
Ear
382.00	Acute suppurative otitis media without spontaneous rupture of eardrum
381.10	Chronic serous otitis media, simple or unspecified
382.2	Chronic atticoantral suppurative otitis media
382.3	Unspecified chronic suppurative otitis media
382.1	Chronic tubotympanic suppurative otitis media
389.00	Conductive hearing loss, unspecified
389.03	Conductive hearing loss, middle ear
381.81	Dysfunction of eustachian tube
931	Foreign body in ear
380.4	Impacted cerumen
386.00	Meniere's disease, unspecified
389.2	Mixed conductive and sensorineural hearing loss
872.61	Open wound of ear drum, uncomplicated
380.23	Other chronic otitis externa
380.10	Infective otitis externa, unspecified
387.9	Otosclerosis, unspecified
384.20	Perforation of tympanic membrane, unspecified
388.01	Presbyacusis
389.10	Sensorineural hearing loss, unspecified
389.11	Sensory hearing loss
388.2	Sudden hearing loss, unspecified
388.30	Tinnitus, unspecified
386.11	Benign paroxysmal positional vertigo

Nose & Sinus
738.0	Acquired deformity of nose
477.9	Allergic rhinitis, cause unspecified
470	Deviated nasal septum
932	Foreign body in nose
802.0	Nasal bones, closed fracture
478.0	Hypertrophy of nasal turbinates
471.9	Unspecified nasal polyp
478.1	Other diseases of nasal cavity and sinuses
784.7	Epistaxis
472.0	Chronic rhinitis
461.9	Acute sinusitis, unspecified
473.9	Unspecified sinusitis (chronic)
473.0	Chronic maxillary sinusitis
465.9	Acute upper respiratory infections of unspecified site

Mouth, Throat, Neck
210.2	Benign neoplasm of major salivary glands
351.0	Bell's palsy
231.0	Carcinoma in situ of larynx
787.2	Dysphagia
785.6	Enlargement of lymph nodes
682.0	Cellulitis and abscess of face
474.12	Hypertrophy of adenoids alone
474.10	Hypertrophy of tonsil with adenoids
474.11	Hypertrophy of tonsils alone
464.0	Acute laryngitis
476.0	Chronic laryngitis
161.9	Malignant neoplasm of larynx, unspecified
460	Acute nasopharyngitis (common cold)
241.0	Nontoxic uninodular goiter
475	Peritonsillar abscess
462	Acute pharyngitis
472.1	Chronic pharyngitis
478.4	Polyp of vocal cord or larynx
527.2	Sialoadenitis
528.0	Stomatitis
524.60	Temporomandibular joint disorders, unspecified
463	Acute tonsillitis
474.0	Chronic tonsillitis
478.5	Other diseases of vocal cords
478.30	Unspecified paralysis of vocal cords
784.49	Other voice disturbance

Miscellaneous
786.09	Other dyspnea and respiratory abnormality
493.90	Asthma, unspecified type, without mention of status asthmaticus
786.2	Cough
780.4	Dizziness and giddiness
784.0	Headache
780.53	Hypersomnia with sleep apnea
786.09	Other dyspnea and respiratory abnormality
784.2	Swelling, mass, or lump in head and neck

Urology
Kidney
592.0	Calculus of kidney
593.2	Cyst of kidney, acquired
753.10	Cystic kidney disease, unspecified
V10.52	Personal history of malignant neoplasm of kidney
591	Hydronephrosis
593.1	Hypertrophy of kidney
189.0	Malignant neoplasm of kidney, except pelvis
593.0	Nephroptosis
590.01	Chronic pyelonephritis with lesion of renal medullary necrosis
590.00	Chronic pyelonephritis without lesion of renal medullary necrosis
590.80	Pyelonephritis, unspecified
590.10	Acute pyelonephritis without lesion of renal medullary necrosis
590.3	Pyeloureteritis cystica
593.89	Other specified disorders of kidney and ureter
593.81	Vascular disorders of kidney
590.2	Renal and perinephric abscess
753.0	Renal agenesis and dysgenesis
593.9	Unspecified disorder of kidney and ureter
788.0	Renal colic
586	Renal failure, unspecified
589.9	Small kidney, unspecified
592.9	Urinary calculus, unspecified

Ureter
592.1	Calculus of ureter
753.2	Obstructive defects of renal pelvis and ureter, congenital
593.5	Hydroureter
593.6	Postural proteinuria
593.3	Stricture or kinking of ureter
593.82	Ureteral fistula
593.4	Other ureteric obstruction
593.7	Vesicoureteral reflux

Bladder
596.4	Atony of bladder
596.6	Rupture of bladder, nontraumatic
596.7	Hemorrhage into bladder wall
596.9	Unspecified disorder of bladder
594.1	Other calculus in bladder
596.0	Bladder neck obstruction
344.61	Cauda equina syndrome with neurogenic bladder
595.2	Other chronic cystitis
595.9	Cystitis, unspecified

595.81	Cystitis cystica	607.9	Unspecified disorder of penis
595.0	Acute cystitis	607.83	Edema of penis
596.3	Diverticulum of bladder	608.86	Edema of male genital organs
788.1	Dysuria	603.0	Encysted hydrocele
V10.51	Personal history of malignant neoplasm of bladder	603.9	Hydrocele, unspecified
596.51	Hypertonicity of bladder	607.84	Impotence of organic origin
188.9	Malignant neoplasm of bladder, part unspecified	302.72	Psychosexual dysfunction with inhibited sexual excitement
596.54	Neurogenic bladder, not otherwise specified	302.71	Psychosexual dysfunction with inhibited sexual desire
788.43	Nocturia	302.74	Psychosexual dysfunction with inhibited male orgasm
788.5	Oliguria and anuria	186.9	Malignant neoplasm of other and unspecified testis
788.61	Splitting of urinary stream	608.89	Other specified disorders of male genital organs
788.31	Urge incontinence	608.83	Vascular disorders of male genital organs
788.30	Unspecified urinary incontinence	608.4	Other inflammatory disorders of male genital organs
788.20	Retention of urine, unspecified	608.9	Unspecified disorder of male genital organs
		752.6	Hypospadias and epispadias

Urethra

		606.9	Male infertility, unspecified
599.7	Hematuria	606.1	Oligospermia
598.2	Postoperative urethral stricture	604.90	Orchitis and epididymitis, unspecified
599.1	Urethral fistula	604.0	Orchitis, epididymitis, and epididymo-orchitis, with abscess
599.2	Urethral diverticulum	604.91	Orchitis and epididymitis in diseases classified elsewhere
599.3	Urethral caruncle	302.75	Psychosexual dysfunction with premature ejaculation
788.7	Urethral discharge	607.3	Priapism
599.81	Urethral hypermobility	302.70	Psychosexual dysfunction, unspecified
598.9	Urethral stricture, unspecified	605	Redundant prepuce and phimosis
597.0	Urethral abscess	456.4	Scrotal varices
597.81	Urethral syndrome nos	608.0	Seminal vesiculitis
598.00	Urethral structure due to unspecified infection	608.1	Spermatocele
594.2	Calculus in urethra	608.85	Stricture of male genital organs
597.80	Urethritis, unspecified	608.2	Torsion of testis
597.89	Other urethritis	V26.0	Tuboplasty or vasoplasty after previous sterilization
599.6	Urinary obstruction, unspecified	752.5	Undescended testicle
599.0	Urinary tract infection, site not specified	078.10	Viral warts, unspecified

Prostate

Miscellaneous

601.2	Abscess of prostate	789.0	Abdominal pain
602.2	Atrophy of prostate	789.3	Abdominal or pelvic swelling, mass, or lump
602.0	Calculus of prostate	791.9	Other nonspecific findings on examination of urine
V10.46	Personal history of malignant neoplasm of prostate	793.5	Nonspecific abnormal findings on radiological and other examination of genitourinary organs
600	Hyperplasia of prostate		
185	Malignant neoplasm of prostate	307.6	Enuresis
602.9	Unspecified disorder of prostate	V25.09	Other general counseling and advice on contraceptive management
601.0	Acute prostatitis		
601.9	Prostatitis, unspecified	795.7	Other nonspecific immunological findings
601.1	Chronic prostatitis	596.1	Intestinovesical fistula
		724.2	Lumbago

Testis - Penis

		729.1	Myalgia and myositis, unspecified
608.3	Atrophy of testis	791.0	Proteinuria
606.0	Azoospermia	V25.2	Sterilization
607.81	Balanitis xerotica obliterans	550.90	Unilateral or unspecified inguinal hernia, without mention of obstruction or gangrene
607.1	Balanoposthitis		
607.89	Other specified disorders of penis	708.2	Urticaria due to cold and heat

CareTrends™ Demographic Charts

ICD-9 is coming full circle. First developed by the World Health Organization as a statistic-gathering tool for monitoring world health trends, ICD-9 was clinically modified in this country for standardized insurance reporting. Today, interest is returning to the statistical uses of ICD-9 – this time, by U.S. agencies planning healthcare reform, outcomes researchers, hospitals and insurance companies.

Medicode, Inc., is not only a national leader in medical reimbursement publications, but also a developer of clinical and pricing databases and software. Among Medicode's new products is CareTrends, a provider profiling software based on diagnoses.

Though most physicians agree that every patient and every treatment plan is unique, the practice of medicine is in some ways predictable. Common diagnoses are treated similarly and specific diseases are more common among certain age groups or a specific sex.

Using ICD-9 codes, CareTrends melds statistical and clinical information into a software program that provides users with benchmarks for care. CareTrends is based on more than 60 million actual episodes of care and actual treatments. The system is designed to allow payers and providers to compare their own caseloads against CareTrends statistics.

CareTrends illustrates how the significance of ICD-9 coding is growing. Diagnoses are even expected to play a part in U.S. healthcare reform payment proposals. But any plan is only as good as the information used to build it.

Physicians and their staffs can no longer tie the significance of proper ICD-9 coding to reimbursement alone. Careful coding is also necessary to ensure that future healthcare reform decisions are based on a clinically accurate picture of diagnoses and treatments in this country. Sloppy coding ultimately could lead to inequities in healthcare programs. Improper ICD-9 coding leads to incorrect diagnosis grouping, incorrect utilization patterns, and increased claim denials.

CareTrends could help physicians establish clinical guidelines for making management and treatment decisions, or help payers determine whether a treatment falls within the norm of an episode of care. The brief sampling of 50 ICD-9-driven CareTrends diagnoses presented here represents just a small portion of the CareTrends database and illustrates how ICD-9 coding is maturing. Each displayed diagnostic group is followed by information on episode of care and sex and age distribution.

Under *Length of Care*, the percentage of patients with an episode of care of a week or less is noted. Also noted is the length of the longest episode of care and what percentile of the patients were treated for that time period.

The percentage of patients treated for this diagnoses is broken out by sex in the column titled *Sex Distribution*, and the percentiles of ages of the patients are displayed under *Age Distribution*. The actual CareTrends project contains much more detail on these fields, as well as additional information on statistical treatment patterns, services, frequency, and distribution.

DIAGNOSTIC GROUP	LENGTH OF CARE		SEX DISTRIBUTION		AGE DISTRIBUTION		
Acne	Week 1 64.02%	Year 2 0.19%	Male 36.60%	Female 63.40%	00–17 46.71%	18–64 52.66%	65–99 0.63%
Airway Obstruction, Chronic	Week 1 45.71%	Year 3 0.17%	Male 51.64%	Female 48.33%	00–17 0.24%	18–64 25.89%	65–99 73.85%
Ankle and Foot, Sprain of the	Week 1 46.68%	Year 2 0.03%	Male 46.59%	Female 53.41%	00–17 33.59%	18–64 57.03%	65–99 9.38%
Atherosclerosis	Week 1 40.25%	Year 3 0.25%	Male 36.84%	Female 63.16%	18–64 11.70%	65–99 88.25%	
Arthritis, Rheumatoid	Week 1 30.29%	Year 3 1.61%	Male 24.85%	Female 75.12%	00–17 0.71%	18–64 44.61%	65–99 54.68%
Bladder, Malignant Neoplasm of the	Week 1 28.58%	Year 3 1.39%	Male 73.75%	Female 26.25%	05–17 0.14%	18–64 21.83%	65–99 78.03%
Cataract, Senile	Week 1 54.88%	Year 3 0.01%	Male 29.98%	Female 70.01%	00–17 0.06%	18–64 6.75%	65–99 93.19%

DIAGNOSTIC GROUP	LENGTH OF CARE		SEX DISTRIBUTION		AGE DISTRIBUTION		
Cellulitis or Abscess, Other	Week 1 48.99%	Year 3 0.03%	Male 45.11%	Female 54.87%	00–17 9.51%	18–64 44.55%	65–99 45.93%
Cholelithiasis	Week 1 30.04%	Year 2 0.20%	Male 29.41%	Female 70.59%	00–17 0.48%	18–64 58.47%	65–99 41.06%
Colon, Malignant Neoplasm of the	Week 1 23.40%	Year 3 1.18%	Male 44.58%	Female 55.42%	18–64 24.49%	65–99 75.51%	
Elbow, Enthesopathy of the	Week 1 32.99%	Year 3 0.08%	Male 53.95%	Female 46.05%	05–17 1.86%	18–64 77.33%	65–99 20.81%
Femur, Fracture of the Neck of the	Week 1 31.79%	Year 2 0.74%	Male 19.70%	Female 80.27%	00–17 0.59%	18–64 5.20%	65–99 94.19%
Gastroenteritis, Other Noninfectious	Week 1 39.87%	Year 3 0.05%	Male 36.98%	Female 63.01%	00–17 22.85%	18–64 46.33%	65–99 30.83%
Glaucoma, Open-angle	Week 1 71.41%	Year 2 0.07%	Male 38.69%	Female 61.30%	00–17 0.21%	18–64 20.83%	65–99 78.95%
Heart Disease, Hypertensive	Week 1 36.48%	Year 3 0.33%	Male 34.42%	Female 65.56%	00–17 0.19%	18–64 22.29%	65–99 77.53%
Heart Failure	Week 1 29.46%	Year 3 0.27%	Male 36.86%	Female 63.13%	00–17 0.50%	18–64 10.00%	65–99 89.47%
Hemorrhoids	Week 1 46.74%	Qtr 4 0.05%	Male 52.51%	Female 47.49%	00–17 0.38%	18–64 68.11%	65–99 31.51%
Hernia, Inguinal	Week 1 38.20%	Year 2 0.04%	Male 85.80%	Female 14.20%	00–17 13.47%	18–64 48.13%	65–99 38.41%
Hypertension, Essential	Week 1 58.47%	Year 3 0.03%	Male 37.15%	Female 62.83%	00–17 0.17%	18–64 47.12%	65–99 52.72%
Hypertension, Essential	Week 1 50.25%	Year 3 0.08%	Male 12.95%	Female 87.05%	00–17 1.30%	18–64 58.79%	65–99 39.90%
Hypovolemia	Week 1 59.99%	Year 2 0.02%	Male 33.36%	Female 66.64%	00–17 11.00%	18–64 19.29%	65–99 69.72%
Knee, Dislocation of the	Week 1 31.56%	Year 2 0.04%	Male 63.66%	Female 36.34%	00–17 14.16%	18–64 80.87%	65–99 4.97%
Lipoid Metabolism, Disease of	Week 1 62.44%	Year 3 0.01%	Male 37.62%	Female 62.37%	00–17 0.39%	12–17 60.92%	18–64 38.69%
Lumbar Region, Nonallopathic Lesions of	Week 1 22.00%	Year 3 0.09%	Male 46.63%	Female 53.37%	00–17 6.56%	18–64 75.75%	65–99 18.09%
Mastopathy, Diffuse Cystic	Week 1 66.53%	Year 3 0.02%	Male 0.23%	Female 99.77%	00–17 0.23%	18–64 80.58%	65–99 19.19%
Menopause, Female	Week 1 68.82%	Year 3 0.01%	Male 16.74%	Female 83.24%	02–17 11.33%	18–64 47.42%	65–9 41.23%
Menstruation, Disorder of	Week 1 47.30%	Year 3 0.01%	Male 0.00%	Female 100%	05–17 4.02%	18–64 94.53%	65–99 1.45%
Migraine	Week 1 52.27%	Year 3 0.05%	Male 21.81%	Female 78.19%	00–17 8.76%	18–64 84.19%	65–99 7.06%

DIAGNOSTIC GROUP	LENGTH OF CARE		SEX DISTRIBUTION		AGE DISTRIBUTION		
Mononeuritis of an Upper Limb	Week 1 39.71%	Year 2 0.04%	Male 30.53%	Female 69.47%	00–17 0.67%	18–64 67.92%	65–99 31.41%
Osteoporosis	Week 1 36.06%	Year 3 0.17%	Male 7.86%	Female 92.14%	00–17 0.29%	18–64 15.60%	65–99 84.11%
Peptic Ulcer of Unspecified Site	Week 1 30.15%	Year 3 0.18%	Male 41.34%	Female 58.66%	05–17 1.87%	18–64 52.28%	64–99 45.85%
Pneumonia, Organisim Unspecified	Week 1 33.63%	Year 3 0.04%	Male 43.65%	Female 56.35%	00–17 15.8%	18–64 30.19%	65–99 54.33%
Prostate, Hyperplasia of	Week 1 48.48%	Year 3 0.01%	Male 100%	Female 0.00%	18–64 23.80%	65–99 76.20%	
Refraction, Disorders of	Week 1 82.89%	Qtr 4 0.01%	Male 38.33%	Female 61.67%	00–17 29.76%	18–64 62.85%	65–99 7.39%
Renal Failure, Chronic	Week 1 19.09%	Year 3 4.57%	Male 56.61%	Female 43.39%	00–17 1.07%	18–64 37.51%	64–99 61.41%
Renal or Ureteral Calculus	Week 1 45.44%	Year 2 0.08%	Male 71.02%	Female 28.95%	00–17 1.31%	18–64 78.24%	65–99 20.45%
Sacroiliac Region, Sprain of	Week 1 34.65%	Year 3 0.05%	Male 47.26%	Female 52.71%	00–17 4.23%	18–64 76.85%	65–99 18.92%
Sinusitis, Acute	Week 1 62.66%	Year 3 0.13%	Male 31.47%	Female 68.53%	00–17 14.57%	18–64 67.30%	65–99 18.14%
Skin, Unspecified Malignant Neoplasm of	Week 1 36.09%	Year 3 0.02%	Male 54.80%	Female 45.16%	05–17 0.04%	18–64 26.19%	65–99 73.76%
Temporomandibular Joint Disorders, Unspecified	Week 1 32.01%	Year 3 0.06%	Male 16.30%	Female 83.60%	00–17 11.30%	18–64 82.60%	65–99 6.10%
Thrombophlebitis	Week 1 38.23%	Year 3 0.03%	Male 34.74%	Female 65.26%	00–17 0.29%	18–64 45.16%	65–99 54.56%
Thoracic or Lumbar Disc, Displacement of	Week 1 15.47%	Year 3 0.43%	Male 50.77%	Female 49.23%	00–17 2.07%	18–64 84.81%	65–99 13.13%
Toe, Acquired Deformities of	Week 1 45.78%	Year 2 0.06%	Male 16.70%	Female 83.30%	00–17 3.33%	18–64 61.51%	65–99 35.17%
Tonsils and Adenoids, Chronic Disease of	Week 1 41.78%	Qtr 3 0.37%	Male 40.07%	Female 59.93%	00–04 10.16%	05–17 61.12%	18–99 28.72%
Trachea or Lung, Malignant Neoplasm of	Week 1 12.09%	Year 3 0.77%	Male 56.29%	Female 43.71%	18–64 29.25%	65–99 70.75%	
Uterus, Malignant Neoplasm of the Body of	Week 1 22.34%	Year 3 0.44%	Male 0.00%	Female 100%	18–64 36.30%	65–99 63.70%	
Urinary Tract Infection, Unspecified	Week 1 50.88%	Year 3 0.01%	Male 56.53%	Female 43.47%	02–17 32.63%	18–64 58.36%	65–99 9.01%
Vaginitis	Week 1 66.78%	Year 2 0.02%	Male 0.00%	Female 100%	00–17 6.47%	18–64 82.44%	65–99 11.08%
Warts, Viral	Week 1 47.67%	Year 2 0.07%	Male 43.30%	Female 56.69%	00–17 38.48%	18–64 57.07%	65–99 4.44%

ICD•9 Self-Evaluation Tests

These self-evaluation tests, the Basic ICD•9 Test and the Advanced ICD•9 Test, have been developed to accompany your new ICD-9. Medicode is dedicated to helping you learn coding through this practical approach, which will provide you with essential hands-on experience. Good luck with the test. Answers are provided, but it is more instructive to consult them after trying a problem. You may find it helpful to check your answers after each group of 10. Space is provided here for answers, but using a separate sheet numbered from 1–50 for the Basic ICD•9 Test and 1–24 for the Advanced ICD•9 Test will be easier to check and also allows you to reuse each test.

BASIC ICD•9 TEST

The Basic ICD•9 part of the test lists diagnostic statements such as "Chronic obstructive pulmonary disease with acute respiratory failure," and "Bilateral recurrent inguinal hernia." Assign codes using each statement's information (some of these diagnoses may require up to three codes).

Diagnostic Statement	ICD-9 Code(s)
1. Headache	
2. Bronchitis	
3. Intrinsic asthma	
4. Traumatic amputation of the thumb	
5. Internal hemorrhoids	
6. Acute pericarditis due to chronic renal failure (uremic)	
7. Diabetes mellitus (Type I)	
8. Abnormal cervical Pap smear	
9. Alcohol withdrawal syndrome	
10. Old, healed myocardial infarction	
11. Perirectal abscess	
12. Acute pharyngitis	
13. Atrial flutter	
14. Ectopic tubal pregnancy	
15. Threatened abortion (not delivered)	
16. Malignant hypertension with congestive heart failure	
17. Metastatic Ca to the lung from the breast (surgery performed two years prior with no local recurrence)	
18. Ruptured berry aneurysm	

Diagnostic Statement	ICD-9 Code(s)
19. Background diabetic (Type I) retinopathy	
20. Bilateral recurrent inguinal hernia	
21. Follow-up exam after surgery	
22. Initial care of acute myocardial infarction — true posterior wall	
23. Total impairment of right eye, left eye near normal vision	
24. Laceration of scalp with concussion and moderate loss of consciousness	
25. Nasopharyngeal polyps	
26. Foreign body (steel) penetration of the eyeball and laceration of the periocular area (skin)	
27. Second-degree burns to back of hand	
28. A child trips and falls on the playground at school resulting in a Colles' fracture	
29. Painful scarring of the hands due to old third-degree burns	
30. Cancer in situ of the ovary	
31. Hodgkin's sarcoma of the intra-abdominal lymph nodes	
32. Multiple fractures/multiple sites of hand	
33. Breast mass scheduled for biopsy	

Diagnostic Statement	ICD-9 Code(s)	Diagnostic Statement	ICD-9 Code(s)
34. Acute gingivitis	_____	44. Progressive systemic sclerosis with lung involvement	_____
35. Catatonic schizophrenia	_____	45. Recurrent dislocation of shoulder	_____
36. Acute rheumatic fever with myocarditis	_____	46. Infected mosquito bite on the upper arm	_____
37. Bleeding esophageal varices due to alcoholic cirrhosis of liver	_____	47. Acute suppurative otitis media with spontaneous rupture of ear drum	_____
38. Crib death	_____	48. Urinary frequency — rule out bladder tumor	_____
39. Small intestinal diverticulosis	_____	49. Infectious gastroenteritis	_____
40. Urethral stricture due to gonococcal infection	_____	50. Whiplash injury	_____
41. Chronic obstructive pulmonary disease with acute respiratory failure	_____		
42. Abnormal thyroid scan	_____		
43. Prolonged labor (first stage) with third-degree perineal tear, delivered healthy twins	_____		

Congratulations on finishing the first of the self-evaluation tests. The answers to this Basic ICD-9 Test can be found at the end of this section.

ADVANCED ICD•9 TEST

Carefully read the diagnostic statements listed below. Determine the main term and essential modifiers, then code each statement completely. Blank lines are provided for your answers, but they do not indicate the number of codes needed.

1. Sudden blurred vision and dizziness due to a recent increased dose of digoxin.

   Code(s):

   _____ _____ _____

2. Circumferential third-degree burns to both feet, ankles, and lower and upper legs, and circumferential second-degree burns to the right forearm resulting from refueling a lawn mower. (Use the chart on page ___ to determine the percentage of total body surface area burned and the percentage of surface area with third-degree burn.)

   Code(s):

   _____ _____ _____

3. Perinatal jaundice from congenital hemolytic anemia (hereditary).

   Code(s):

   _____ _____ _____

4. Arthritis due to old dislocation of the shoulder.

   Code(s):

   _____ _____ _____

5. Cancer of the sigmoid colon removed five years ago with no recurrence.

   Code(s):

   _____ _____ _____

6. Toxic encephalitis due to lead dioxide.

   Code(s):

   _____ _____ _____

7. Acute influenzal myocarditis.

   Code(s):

   _____ _____ _____

8. Insulin dependent diabetic with gangrene of the right toe.

   Code(s):

   _____ _____ _____

9. Metastatic carcinoma of the liver originating in the stomach body.

   Code(s):

   _____ _____ _____

10. Newborn jaundice secondary to congenital bile duct obstruction.

    Code(s):

    _____ _____ _____

11. Deep laceration of the heel resulting from a power lawn mower accident in the patient's backyard.

    Code(s):

    _____ _____ _____

12. Acute respiratory distress during arthroscopy of right knee for recently torn lateral meniscus.

    Code(s): _____ _____ _____

13. Subdural hematoma in unconscious patient with fractured base of skull.

    Code(s): _____ _____ _____

14. Abnormally heavy menstruation and severe abdominal pain—possible uterine tumor.

    Code(s): _____ _____ _____

15. Glaucoma with recurrent iridocyclitis.

    Code(s): _____ _____ _____

From the following scenarios, determine all appropriate diagnoses and codes.

16. Judy falls while ice skating, fracturing the shaft of her tibia. She is taken to the emergency department where she confides to the physician on duty that she might be pregnant. A pregnancy test is performed, confirming Judy's pregnancy.

    Code(s): _____ _____ _____

17. Mrs. Hinkel is seen on Monday for severe low back pain and tingling, as well as numbness in her feet. The orthopedic surgeon suspects a herniated disk and schedules her for an MRI (magnetic resonance imaging) on Friday. The radiologist confirms the diagnosis as a displaced lumbar disk without myelopathy.

    Code(s):

    a. Orthopedic visit: _____ _____ _____

    b. Radiology visit: _____ _____ _____

18. A patient with pneumococcal meningitis has a cardiac arrest on the third day of hospitalization.

    Code(s): _____ _____ _____

    _____ _____ _____

19. A patient is seen in the emergency department with precordial chest pain. Suspecting a myocardial infarction, Dr. Dickerson, the ED physician, calls Dr. Michaels, a cardiologist. Tests confirm a posterobasalar MI and the patient is admitted to the coronary care unit. The patient does well and returns home three days later. Two weeks post-hospitalization, the patient is seen in follow-up by Dr. Michaels.

    Code(s):

    a. Dr. Dickerson's ED visit: _____ _____ _____

    b. Admission of the patient: _____ _____ _____

    c. Follow-up visit: _____ _____ _____

20. Dr. Block performs a simple cholecystectomy for her patient's acute cholecystitis. The patient develops malignant hyperthermia during the course of anesthesia.

    Code(s): _____ _____ _____

21. Dr. Brewer performs a liver transplant on a patient with hepatic failure secondary to sclerosing cholangitis. Three days postoperatively, the patient develops pulmonary insufficiency and a severe drop in blood pressure.

    Code(s): _____ _____ _____

22. A patient in the sixth month of her first pregnancy develops multiple varicose veins of her left leg with severe superficial phlebitis.

    Code(s): _____ _____ _____

23. Dr. Markin, a urologist, sees a patient for difficulty in urinating. Following a history and examination, he diagnoses a urethral stricture secondary to an undiagnosed obstetrical injury that occurred during her last delivery.

    Code(s): _____ _____ _____

24. Mrs. Smythe, a 45-year-old, sees her physician for her yearly mammogram and is found to have bilateral microcalcifications.

    Code(s): _____ _____ _____

Congratulations on finishing the second part of the self-evaluation test. The answers to this Advanced ICD-9 Test can be found at the end of this section.

THE ANSWERS, BASIC ICD•9

1. 784.0
2. 490
3. 493.10
4. 885.0
5. 455.0
6. 585
   420.0
7. 250.01
8. 795.0
9. 291.8
10. 412
11. 566
12. 462
13. 427.32
14. 633.1
15. 640.03
16. 402.01
17. 197.0
    V10.3
18. 430
19. 250.51
    362.01
20. 550.93
21. V67.0
22. 410.61
23. 369.62
24. 850.2
    873.0
25. 471.0
26. 871.5
    870.027.
    944.26
    948.00
27. 944.26
    948.00
28. 813.41
    E849.4
    E885
29. 709.2
    906.6
30. 233.3
31. 201.23
32. 817.0
33. 611.72
34. 523.0
35. 295.20
36. 391.2
37. 571.2
    456.2
38. 798.0
39. 562.00
40. 098.2
    598.01
41. 518.81
    496
42. 794.5
43. 662.01
    664.21
    V27.2
44. 710.1
    517.2
45. 718.31
46. 912.5
47. 382.01
48. 788.41
49. 009.0
50. 847.0

When you have determined your score, refer to the following rankings for an indication of your diagnostic coding expertise:

46–50	Excellent	30–35	Below average
41–45	Very Good	Below 30	Poor
36–40	Average		

THE ANSWERS, ADVANCED ICD•9

1. Option I
   - **368.8** Other specified visual disturbances
   - **780.4** Dizziness and giddiness
   - **E942.1** Cardiotonic glycosides and drugs of similar action causing adverse effects in therapeutic use

   Option II
   - **995.2** Unspecified adverse effect of drug, medicinal and biological substance, not elsewhere classified
   - **E942.0** Cardiac rhythm regulators causing adverse effects in therapeutic use
   - **386.8** Other disorders of labyrinth
   - **780.4** Dizziness and giddiness

   Rationale: This controversial question has two possible answers. Medical record coders generally prefer option I, which indicates the drug's adverse effects and then the drug type. Option II lists 995.2 *Unspecified adverse effect of drug...* as the principal diagnosis, followed by the E code indicating the drug, then the symptoms. Option II may be preferable to present the most accurate diagnosis with those payers that are able to accept only the first two diagnostic codes per claim.

2. - **945.39** Full-thickness skin loss due to burn (third degree nos) of multiple sites of lower limb(s)
   - **943.21** Blisters with epidermal loss due to burn (second degree) of forearm
   - **948.43** Burn (any degree) involving 40-49 percent of body surface with third degree burn of 30-39%
   - **E894** Ignition of highly inflammable material

   Rationale: Coding burns requires at least two diagnostic codes. The first code indicates the location and depth of the burn. The second code indicates the percentage of the total body surface area burned, plus the percentage of surface area with third-degree burn. It is often necessary to use two or more codes describing the location when multiple sites are burned.

   When possible, assign E codes describing the circumstances of the injury.

3. - **282.9** Hereditary hemolytic anemia, unspecified
   - **774.0** Perinatal jaundice from hereditary hemolytic anemias

   Rationale: The italicized code describing perinatal jaundice is followed by a note directing you to "code also the underlying disease." Jaundice is a manifestation of the disease (hereditary hemolytic anemia) and is not a principal diagnosis. The unspecified code 282.9 is correct because the diagnostic statement does not name a specific anemia.

4. - **716.91** Arthropathy, unspecified, involving shoulder region
   - **905.6** Late effect of dislocation

   Rationale: Chronic conditions resulting from injuries, poisonings, toxic effects, and other external causes that are present one year or more after the insult are coded as late effects. These conditions require at least two codes: one to identify the condition as a late effect of a specific injury (shoulder dislocation) and another to identify the specific condition (chronic arthritis).

5. **V10.05** Personal history of malignant neoplasm of large intestine

Rationale: Cancer presents a unique coding challenge. When the patient has a demonstrable malignancy, choose a code from the neoplasm section. Also use these neoplasm codes, following surgery to remove a malignancy, for services falling within the standard postsurgical follow-up period.

If no demonstrable malignancy remains after the follow-up period, the patient's diagnosis becomes, "Personal history of malignant neoplasm."

6. **984.0** Toxic effect of inorganic lead compounds
   323.7   Toxic encephalitis
   E980.9 Poisoning by other and unspecified solid and liquid substances, undetermined whether accidentally or purposely inflicted

Rationale: Poisonings and toxic effects of chemicals require three or more diagnostic codes. Code 984.0 identifies the toxic compound while 323.7 identifies the toxic effect. Finally, an E code should be assigned to describe the circumstances of the poisoning, if known (i.e., accidental, therapeutic use, suicide attempt, assault, or undetermined). The italicized code (323.7) is followed by a note directing you to "code also the underlying cause." Toxic encephalitis is a manifestation of code 984.0 and is not a principal diagnosis.

7. **487.8** Influenza with other manifestations
   422.0   Acute myocarditis in diseases classified elsewhere

Rationale: Code 422.0 is followed by a note to "code also underlying disease" which, in this case, is influenza. Properly identifying myocarditis as the main term in this diagnosis leads you to this category.

8. **785.4** Gangrene
   250.71 Type diabetes mellitus with peripheral circulatory disorders, not stated as uncontrolled

Rationale: ICD-9 gives no clear guideline regarding the importance of prioritizing diagnostic codes; however, the recognized industry standard is to list first the principal diagnosis (the medical reason for the current service). In this question, gangrene is the most pertinent diagnosis and should be listed first.

9. **197.7** Malignant neoplasm of liver, specified as secondary
   151.4   Malignant neoplasm of body of stomach

Rationale: Malignant neoplasm coding requires identifying whether the tumor is primary (site of origin) or secondary (site of distant metastasis). Next, determine which site (primary or secondary) is the focus of the service provided and code that site first.

10. **751.61** Biliary atresia, congenital
    774.5   Perinatal jaundice from other causes

Rationale: Correctly identifying jaundice as the main term in this statement should lead you to 774.5 Perinatal jaundice from other causes. This code refers you to the correct underlying cause. Code 774.5 is italicized indicating it is not a principal diagnosis. Avoid nonspecific codes, such as 576.8 Other specified disorders of biliary tract, when more specific codes are available.

11. **892.0** Open wound of foot except toe(s) alone, without mention of complication
    E920.0 Accidents caused by powered lawn mower
    E849.0 Home accidents

Rationale: This is a good example of using multiple E codes to describe an injury and its circumstances completely. Code E920.0 describes the cause of the injury, while E849.0 describes the setting.

12. **997.3** Respiratory complications, not elsewhere classified
    836.1   Tear of lateral cartilage or meniscus of knee, current

Rationale: Coding intraoperative complications requires using codes from the section titled, Complications of Surgical and Medical Care Not Elsewhere Classified (996-999). There is a code in another section describing acute respiratory distress, but the key factor in this code choice is the intraoperative occurrence of the complication.

13. **801.26** Closed fracture of base of skull with subarachnoid, subdural, and extradural hemorrhage, with loss of consciousness of unspecified duration

Rationale: Intracranial hemorrhage with skull fracture is coded from a different category than is intracranial hemorrhage without skull fracture. As with all fractures, assume a closed fracture unless otherwise specified.

The patient's state of consciousness is reported by the code's fifth digit.

14. **626.2** Excessive or frequent menstruation
    789.0   Abdominal pain

Rationale: It is incorrect to code "possible" or "rule-out" statements as a diagnosis. Until a diagnosis is confirmed, code signs or symptoms. An additional caution for this question is not to assume the abdominal pain is directly related to the heavy menstruation. Unless a diagnostic statement links the symptoms, code them separately.

15. **365.62** Glaucoma associated with ocular inflammations
    364.02 Recurrent iridocyclitis

Rationale: Conditions that are the result (sequela) of an underlying disease require two codes: one to identify the sequela (glaucoma), and another to identify the underlying disease process (recurrent iridocyclitis).

16. **823.20** Closed fracture of shaft of tibia
    V22.2   Pregnant state, incidental
    E885   Fall on same level from slipping, tripping, or stumbling

Rationale: This question demonstrates coding incidental pregnancy. When the condition being treated is not related to or complicating the pregnancy, use code V22.2.

17. a. Orthopedic visit:

    724.2   Lumbago
    782.0   Disturbance of skin sensation

   b. Radiology visit:

    722.10 Displacement of lumbar intervertebral disc without myelopathy

Rationale: As previously noted, code symptoms when no specific diagnosis has been made. Do not code a herniated disc until radiologically confirmed.

Code V72.5 Radiologic examination, not elsewhere classified is reserved for screening radiologic examinations where no diagnosis is made.

18. **427.5**   Cardiac arrest
    320.1   Pneumococcal meningitis

Rationale: When a patient has two concurrent conditions, whether related or not, both should be coded if they are managed by the same physician. However, if more than one physician is involved in the care of a patient with multiple active problems, each physician should code only those diagnoses he or she manages.

19. a: **786.51**   Precordial pain
    b: **410.61**   Acute myocardial infarction, true posterior wall infarction, initiala episode of care
    c: **410.62**   Acute myocardial infarction, true posterior wall infarction, sub- sequent episode of care

Rationale: Coding myocardial infarctions has an unusual twist. The acute phase care of each heart attack is identified with the fifth digit "1." Any follow-up care occurring after the acute phase, but within eight weeks, requires a fifth digit "2." Unfortunately, ICD-9 does not define the time frame of the acute phase. A good rule of thumb might be to define the acute phase as beginning with the onset of infarction and lasting through stabilization and discharge from the intensive care setting.

20. **575.0**   Acute cholecystitis
    995.89   Other specified adverse effects, not elsewhere classified

Rationale: In the ICD-9 index, the term hyperthermia is followed by code number 780.6. However, the qualifying parenthetical statement indicates "of unknown origin" and directs you to "see also Pyrexia." Coding from the index might cause you to choose incorrectly code 780.6 when a more specific code is available. Unfortunately, the only way to access code 995.89 through the index is under the term hyperpyrexia, but unless you know that hyperthermia and hyperpyrexia are synonymous, you cannot find the correct code without looking in the tabular listing under section Other and Unspecified Effects of External Causes (990-995).

21. **518.5**   Pulmonary insufficiency following trauma and surgery
    998.0   Postoperative shock, not elsewhere classified
    572.8   Other sequelae of chronic liver disease

Rationale: When coding postoperative complications, the complication(s) becomes the principal diagnosis, and the surgical diagnosis becomes secondary. In this question, the sclerosing cholangitis is a secondary diagnosis to liver failure. However, sclerosing cholangitis doesn't influence the care of the postoperative complication (pulmonary insufficiency) and can be omitted.

22. **671.03**   Antepartum varicose veins of legs
    671.23   Superficial thrombophlebitis, antepartum

Rationale: If you coded 454.9 Varicose veins of lower extremities, without mention of ulcer or inflammation, 451.0 Phlebitis and thrombophlebitis of superficial vessels of lower extremities, and/or V22.0 Supervision of normal first pregnancy, note that a code category exists for complications relating to pregnancy. While codes 454.9 and 451.0 identify the conditions, they do not relate it to pregnancy.

Code V22.0 indicates management of a normal pregnancy and is incorrect in this situation.

23. **598.1**   Traumatic urethral stricture

Rationale: Even though a code for urethral injury (665.52) exists in the Complications of Labor and Delivery section, this is an unrecognized injury resulting in stricture. The stricture is now the condition being treated and is reported with a specific code.

24. **793.8**   Nonspecific abnormal findings on radiological and other examination of breast

Rationale: The intent of this service is a screening mammogram; however, microcalcifications are found. This abnormal finding no longer qualifies the service as a normal mammogram.

Microcalcifications is not a diagnosis but an abnormal finding on an x-ray. This is the key to locating the correct code (Findings, abnormal).

When you have determined your score, refer to the following rankings for an indication of your diagnostic coding expertise:

22–24	Excellent	13–15	Below average
19–21	Very good	Below 13	Poor
16–18	Average		

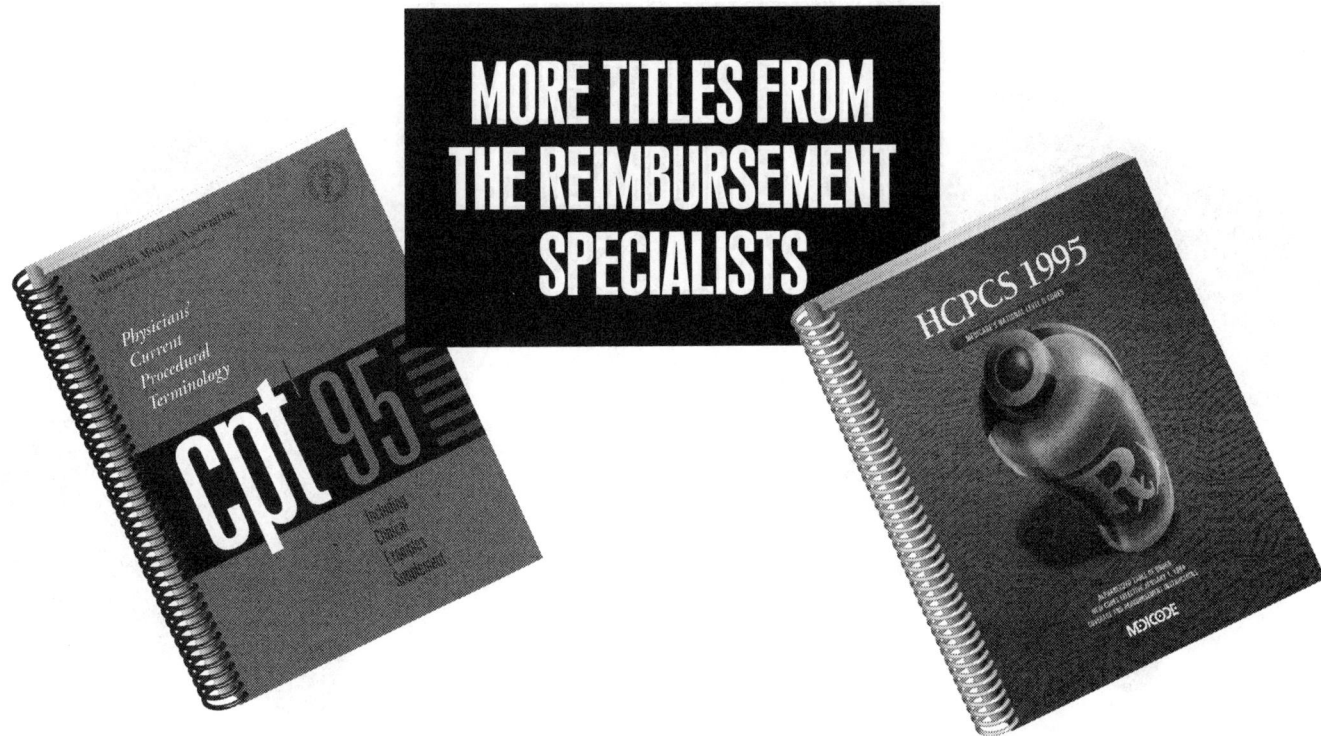

MORE TITLES FROM THE REIMBURSEMENT SPECIALISTS

More Coding Power For Your Money

New this year, *CPT 1995* is larger (8½" x 11") to make the book easier for you to use. It has also been redesigned with these new features:

- New two-column design helps you move through the text more efficiently.
- Redesigned headings and subheadings guide you through codes easily.
- New paper stock lets you use a highlighter.
- Individual codes prominently stand out.
- Printed on recycled paper.

Medicode's New Deluxe CPT

Our new deluxe *CPT 1995* offers even more:

- Medicode's exclusive *CPT Extra* includes specialty pricing information, anatomy charts, a medical abbreviation dictionary and superbill tips — including a 20% discount coupon off customized superbills from Colwell, an industry leader in practice management tools.
- Quality spiral binding and thumb-index tabs.

Still The Easiest To Use, And Now It's Expanded

Our *HCPCS 1995* is the most user-friendly, most comprehensive coding reference available for durable medical equipment (DME), drugs and select medical services. Features include:

- An expanded, easy-to-use index that includes more product name references for supplies and DME.
- A detailed table of drugs with brand names, generic drugs, dosage, route of administration and correct J or K codes.
- Complete Medicare Carrier's Manual and Coverage Issues Manual citations wherever possible.
- Cross-referencing of generic drugs to brand names.
- Cross-referencing of deleted HCPCS codes to active HCPCS codes. An essential feature when you're completing forms.
- Instructions preceding each section to better guide you through information.
- A list of common abbreviations and their meanings.
- Specialist procedure information with applicable codes.

MEDICODE
POWER TO MAKE THE RIGHT DECISIONS.™

1-800-999-4600

Medicode publications are available from your medical bookstore or call 1-800-999-4600.
For information on Medicode consulting, databases, educational programs and software, call 1-800-999-4614.

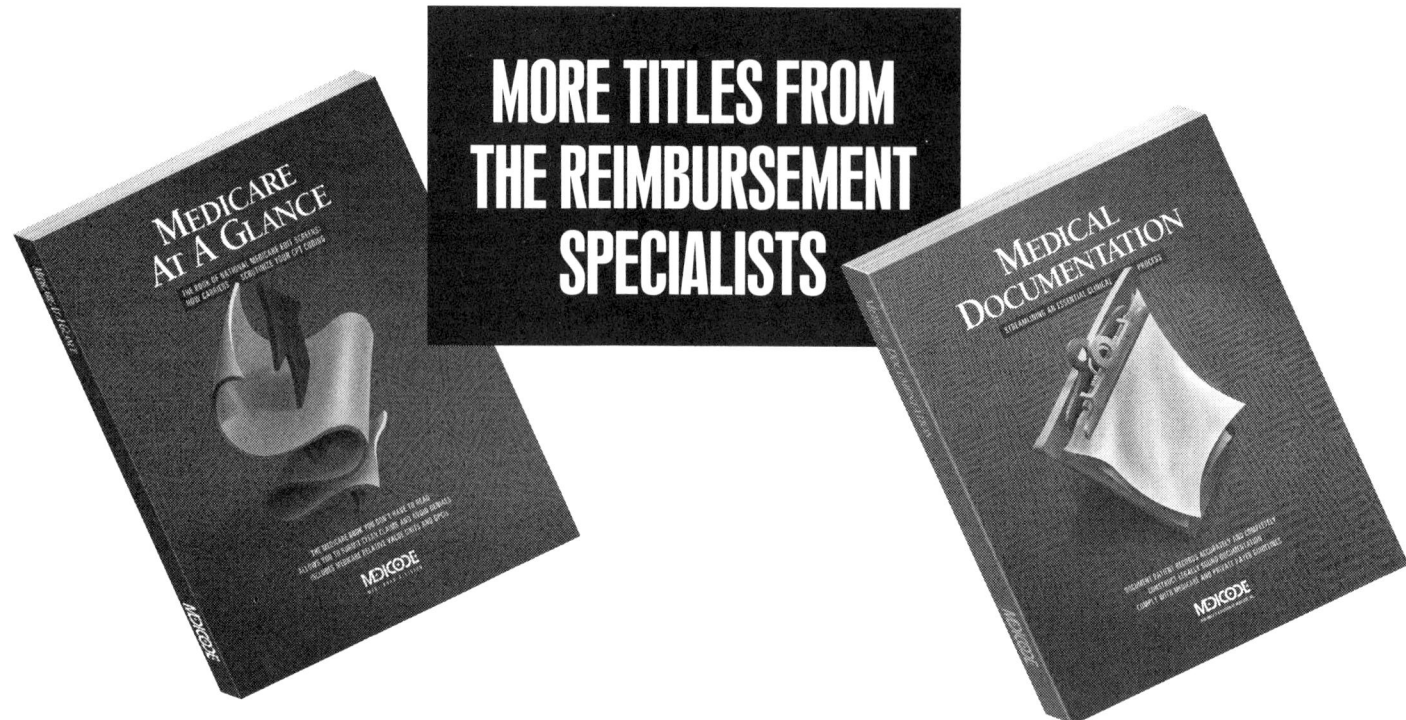

MORE TITLES FROM THE REIMBURSEMENT SPECIALISTS

Proper Medicare Claims, The First Time

Only one thing is worse that filing a Medicare claim. Filing it again. That's why we created *Medicare At A Glance* — to tell you what you most need to know about Medicare policy edits for CPT coding. Explanations written by Barbara Pappadakis, a nationally recognized Medicare policy expert, give detail when you need it.

Perhaps the best thing about this book is you don't have to read it. Unlike most Medicare books, its vital information isn't hidden in long-winded, dry recitations. Instead, it's presented in quick, organized tables for instant reference. Simply look up a CPT code to find what carriers are looking for when they examine a claim.

Appendix material offers even more help by teaching you how to translate Medicare's relative values into geographically adjusted, transition-blended fees. Other data, such as ASC groups and modifiers, ensure that all your billing meets government regulations.

Protect Yourself, Legally And Financially

You must document all cases accurately to provide quality healthcare and protect your practice from lawsuits. *Medical Documentation,* written by Jerry Seare, M.D., shows you how. You'll learn to follow Medicare and private payer guidelines while you avoid legal problems. Included in this helpful guide:

- Instructions on documenting all types of patient services, for both inpatient and outpatient settings.

- Suggestions for maintaining streamlined, yet accurate, patient records.

- Tear-out patient history and exam forms explain the fastest and most complete ways to record patient visits.

- Information on handling nursing, physician assistant and resident services.

- A pocket-sized, physician's quick-reference listing only essential documentation information.

There's even a chapter, written by a risk management attorney, that discusses documentation of legal issues and the status of medical malpractice claims nationally.

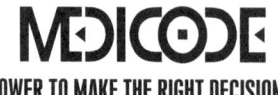

POWER TO MAKE THE RIGHT DECISIONS.™

1-800-999-4600

Medicode publications are available from your medical bookstore or call 1-800-999-4600.
For information on Medicode consulting, databases, educational programs and software, call 1-800-999-4614.

MEDICODE'S
ICD·9·CM

FOURTH EDITION
1995

International Classification of Diseases
9TH REVISION
Clinical Modification

MEDICODE

© Copyright 1994 Medicode, Inc.
All Rights Reserved

First Printing — August 1994

This book, or parts hereof, may not be reproduced in any form without permission.

Additional copies may be ordered from:

Your local bookstore
or
Medicode Publications
1-800-999-4600

ISBN 1-56337-117-0
1-56337-118-9
1-56337-116-2
1-56337-119-7

MEDICODE

Medicode Publications
5225 Wiley Post Way, Suite 500
Salt Lake City, Utah 84116-2889

International classification of diseases, 9th revision, clinical modifier: with color symbols: ICD•9•CM. — 4th ed., 1995.
    p.   cm.
  Includes index
  Contents: v. 1. Tabular list of diseases — v. 2. Alphabetic index to diseases — v. 3. Tabular and alphabetic listing of hospital inpatient procedures.
    ISBN 1-56337-116-2 (standard) — ISBN 1-56337-118-9 (deluxe: v. 1, 2 & 3) — ISBN 1-56337-117-0 (deluxe: v. 1 & 2) — ISBN 1-56337-119-7 (standard: v. 1, 2 & 3)
  1. Nosology 2. Diseases. I. Medicode (Firm) II. Title: ICD•9•CM 1995.
    [DNLM: 1. Classification. WB 15 I57 1994]
RB115.I49   1994
616'.0012—dc20
DNLM/DLC   94-30782
for Library of Congress   CIP

This publication of the *International Classification of Diseases, Ninth Revision, Clinical Modification, Fourth Edition* is designed to be an accurate and authoritative source of coding information. Every effort has been made to ensure the accuracy of the listings, and all information is believed reliable at the time of publication. Absolute accuracy cannot be guaranteed, however. This publication is made available with the understanding that the publisher is not engaged in rendering legal or other services that require a professional license.

Contents

Introduction ii

ALPHABETIC INDEX—VOLUME 2
Section 1: Index to Diseases 1
- A 1
- B 33
- C 42
- D 66
- E 103
- F 115
- G 131
- H 136
- I 156
- J 176
- K 176
- L 178
- M 187
- N 199
- O 231
- P 236
- Q 261
- R 261
- S 270
- T 295
- U 307
- V 310
- W 313
- X 316
- Y 317
- Z 317

Section 2: Table of Drugs and Chemicals 321
Section 3: Index to External Causes 385

TABULAR LIST—VOLUME 1
1. Infectious and Parasitic Diseases (001–139) 1
2. Neoplasms (140–239) 16
3. Endocrine, Nutritional and Metabolic Diseases, and Immunity Disorders (240–279) 30
4. Diseases of the Blood and Blood-forming Organs (280–289) 37
5. Mental Disorders (290–319) 40
6. Diseases of the Nervous System and Sense Organs (320–389) 50
7. Diseases of the Circulatory System (390–459) 69
8. Diseases of the Respiratory System (460–519) 79
9. Diseases of the Digestive System (520–579) 85
10. Diseases of the Genitourinary System (580–629) 95
11. Complications of Pregnancy, Childbirth, and the Puerperium (630–676) 104
12. Diseases of the Skin and Subcutaneous Tissue (680–709) 112
13. Diseases of the Musculoskeletal System and Connective Tissue (710–739) 117
14. Congenital Anomalies (740–759) 126
15. Certain Conditions Originating in the Perinatal Period (760–779) 136
16. Symptoms, Signs, and Ill-defined Conditions (780–799) 140
17. Injury and Poisoning (800–999) 147

V Codes — Supplementary Classification of Factors Influencing Health Status and Contact with Health Services (V01–V82) 173
E Codes — Supplementary Classification of External Causes of Injury and Poisoning (E800–E999) 183
Appendix A—Morphology of Neoplasms (M800–M9970/1) 207
Appendix B—Glossary of Mental Disorders 211
Appendix C—Classification of Drugs by American Hospital Formulary Service List Number and their ICD•9•CM Equivalents 221
Appendix D—Classification of Industrial Accidents According to Agency 223
Appendix E—List of Three-Digit Categories 225

Introduction

ABOUT THIS TEXT

The text you have purchased, *Medicode 1995 International Classification of Diseases, 9th Revision, Clinical Modification* (1995 ICD•9•CM), is an innovative product designed for the busy user, whether a physician writing a diagnosis, hospital staff coding a medical record, a coder preparing a claim, or a claims processor verifying an insurance form.

This introduction provides a detailed visual description of the conventions used in ICD-9. The color-coded symbols and easy-to-use format help you efficiently locate information to quickly identify variables that may affect coding. Familiarizing yourself with this Introduction will help you code diagnoses more quickly, efficiently, and accurately.

For ease of reference in this publication, ICD•9•CM is termed ICD•9 and should not be confused with the international diagnostic system by the same name used by the World Health Organization for reporting cause of death.

Medicode has reversed the order of Volume 1 and Volume 2 of ICD•9. The Alphabetic Index to Diseases (Volume 2) is presented first; the Tabular List of Diseases (Volume 1), second. This placement of the Alphabetic Index allows you to locate terms quickly for verification in the Tabular List.

New and revised codes are integrated into the Alphabetic Index and Tabular List, presenting the most current ICD•9 text available and eliminating the necessity of referring to a separate document for these codes. New and changed codes for 1995 are clearly identified. Medicode's exclusive color symbols are available to all purchasers this year. Explanation of their use is found on page iii.

DEVELOPMENT OF THE INTERNATIONAL CLASSIFICATION OF DISEASES

Diagnostic coding dates back to the seventeenth-century when statistical information was gathered through a system known as the London Bills of Mortality. By 1937 this method of tracking information had evolved into the *International List of Causes of Death*. The World Health Organization published a statistical listing in 1948 that could track both morbidity and mortality. This listing, the *International Classification of Diseases* (ICD), evolved into the current text in international use today — the *International Classification of Diseases, 9th Revision (ICD•9)*.

By 1977, when the 9th revision was published, ICD•9 had attained international recognition. Such wide acceptance prompted the U.S. National Center for Health Statistics to modify ICD•9 with clinical information. These clinical modifications provided a way to classify morbidity data for indexing of medical records, medical case reviews, and medical care programs, as well as for basic health statistics. The result was the *International Classification of Diseases, 9th Revision, Clinical Modification* (ICD•9•CM), commonly referred to as ICD•9. This version delineates the clinical picture of each patient, providing information beyond that needed for statistical groupings and analysis of healthcare trends.

In the March 4, 1994 *Federal Register*, HCFA announced all claims for physician services under Medicare Part B must include proper ICD•9 diagnostic coding on the HCFA-1500 claim form. For physician's that accept payment in an assignment related basis, failure to do so may result in denial of payment.

HCFA GUIDELINES (PART B MEDICARE)

HCFA provides specific guidelines to aid in standardizing U.S. coding practices. The guidelines for outpatient facilities, physician offices, and ancillary care are summarized below:

- Identify each service, procedure, or supply with an ICD•9 code to describe the diagnosis, symptom, complaint, condition, or problem.
- Identify services or visits for circumstances other than disease or injury, such as follow-up care after chemotherapy, with V codes provided for this purpose.
- Code the primary diagnosis first, followed by the secondary, tertiary, and so on. Code any coexisting conditions that affect the treatment of the patient for that visit or procedure as supplementary information. Do not code a diagnosis that is no longer applicable.
- Code to the highest degree of specificity. Carry the numerical code to the fourth or fifth digit when available. Remember, there are only approximately 100 valid three-digit codes; all other ICD•9 codes require additional digits.
- Code a chronic diagnosis when it is applicable to the patient's treatment.
- When only ancillary services are provided, list the appropriate V code first and the problem second. For example, if a patient is receiving only ancillary therapeutic services, such as physical therapy, use the V code first, followed by the code for the condition.
- For surgical procedures, code the diagnosis applicable to the procedure. If at the time the claim is filed the postoperative diagnosis is different from the preoperative diagnosis, use the postoperative diagnosis.

The above guidelines provide the basic knowledge necessary to apply the correct ICD•9 codes to your diagnostic statements, but you may encounter problems when faced with certain situations. The following is an illustrated discussion to help you further understand how to use ICD•9.

CONVENTIONS USED IN ICD•9

The conventions used in ICD•9 include general notes, instructional notes using specific terms, cross-references, abbreviations, punctuation marks, symbols, typeface, and format. The following pages identify and explain these conventions. Medicode has taken particular care to identify codes that require a fourth or fifth digit with an easily remembered color symbol system. Take special notice of these codes. Coding to the highest level of specificity will reduce the number of claims denied because of a missing, but essential, specifying digit.

Medicode's Color Symbol System for Volumes 1 & 2 and Standard ICD·9 Coding Conventions

● **Additional Digits Required**
The red stop sign identifies codes that require an additional fourth and/or fifth digit to be coded correctly. Either the code category or subcategory contains more specific codes, or the code choices are listed with the main category.

◆ **Nonspecific Code**
The amber caution sign indicates that a code is classified as "unspecified," "other," or "ill-defined." Codes identified by this symbol are also known as "dump" codes or "catch-all" codes. A "nonspecific" code can be a valid choice if it most closely describes your diagnosis, but use these codes only after checking all other options.

■ **Not a Primary Diagnosis**
The blue rectangle identifies codes that do not report primary diagnoses. Also known as "manifestations," these codes should only be listed as secondary diagnoses where appropriate. Simply stated, these codes are never used alone.

◆▲▼
A solid black diamond indicates a new (added) or revised code or term. Solid black triangles indicate multiple lines of additions or revisions. This convention is exclusive to Medicode's ICD·9.

● 335 **Anterior horn cell disease**
    335.0 **Werdnig-Hoffmann disease**
        Infantile spinal muscular atrophy
        Progressive muscular atrophy of infancy
● 335.1 **Spinal muscular atrophy**
    ◆ 335.10 **Spinal muscular atrophy, unspecified**
      335.11 **Kugelberg-Welander disease**
        Spinal muscular atrophy:
          familial
          juvenile
    ◆ 335.19 **Other**
        Adult spinal muscular atrophy
● 335.2 **Motor neuron disease**
    335.20 **Amyotrophic lateral sclerosis**
        Motor neuron disease (bulbar) (mixed type)
    335.21 **Progressive muscular atrophy**
        Duchenne-Aran muscular atrophy
        Progressive muscular atrophy (pure)
    335.22 **Progressive bulbar palsy**
    335.23 **Pseudobulbar palsy**
    335.24 **Primary lateral sclerosis**
    ◆ 335.29 **Other**
◆ 335.8 **Other anterior horn cell diseases**
◆ 335.9 **Anterior horn cell disease, unspecified**
● 336 **Other diseases of spinal cord**
    336.0 **Syringomyelia and syringobulbia**
    336.1 **Vascular myelopathies**
        Acute infarction of spinal cord (embolic) (nonembolic)
        Arterial thrombosis of spinal cord
        Edema of spinal cord
        Hematomyelia
        Subacute necrotic myelopathy
■ 336.2 *Subacute combined degeneration of spinal cord in diseases classified elsewhere*
    Code also underlying disease, as:
      pernicious anemia (281.0)
      other vitamin B_{12} deficiency anemia (281.1)
      vitamin B_{12} deficiency (266.2)
■ 336.3 *Myelopathy in other diseases classified elsewhere*
    Code also underlying disease, as:
      myelopathy in neoplastic disease (140.0-239.9)
    EXCLUDES myelopathy in:
        intervertebral disc disorder (722.70-722.73)
        spondylosis (721.1, 721.41-721.42, 721.91)

Absence—*continued*
  epileptic (atonic) (typical)
    (see also Epilepsy) 345.0
  erythrocyte 284.9
  erythropoiesis 284.9
    congenital 284.0
  esophagus (congenital) 750.3
  Eustachian tube (congenital) 744.24
  extremity (acquired) ◆
    congenital (see also Deformity, reduction) 755.4 ▼
      lower V49.70 ▲
      upper V49.60

NEC
As the abbreviation for "not elsewhere classifiable," NEC identifies codes and terms to be used only when you lack the information necessary to code the diagnosis to a more specific category.

SEE
See directs you to a more specific term under which the correct code can be found.

SEE ALSO
See also indicates additional information is available that may provide an additional diagnostic code.

SEE CATEGORY
See category indicates that you should review the category specified before assigning a code.

ESSENTIAL MODIFIERS
Essential modifiers are subterms which are listed below the main term in alphabetical order (with the exception of "with" and "without") and indented two spaces. An essential modifier that clarifies the previous one is indented two additional spaces to the right. If only one subterm is listed, it is separated from the main term by a comma.

NONESSENTIAL MODIFIERS
Nonessential modifiers are subterms that follow the main term and are enclosed in parentheses. They can clarify the diagnosis but are not required.

NOTES
Volume 2 notes are boxed and further define terms, clarify information, or list choices for additional digits.

Abscess—*continued*
  amebic 006.3
    bladder 006.8
    brain (with liver or lung abscess) 006.5
    liver (without mention of brain or lung
      abscess) 006.3
    with
      brain abscess (and lung abscess)
        006.5
      lung abscess 006.4
    lung (with liver abscess) 006.4
      with brain abscess 006.5
    seminal vesicle 006.8
    specified site NEC 006.8
    spleen 006.8

  Bartholin's gland 616.3
    with
      abortion — *see* Abortion, by type,
        with sepsis
      ectopic pregnancy (*see also*
        categories 633.0-633.9)
        639.0

  bowel 569.5
  brain (any part) 324.0
    amebic (with liver or lung abscess)
      006.5
    cystic 324.0
    late effect — *see* category 326

Weight
  gain (abnormal) (excessive) 783.1
    during pregnancy 646.1
      insufficient 646.8
  less than 1000 grams at birth 765.0
  loss (cause unknown) 783.2

Wound, open (by cutting or piercing instrument) (by firearms) (cut) (dissection) (incised) (laceration) (penetration) (perforating) (puncture) (with initial hemorrhage, not internal) 879.8

> Note — For fracture with open wound, see Fracture.
> For laceration, traumatic rupture, tear or penetrating wound of internal organs, such as heart, lung, liver, kidney, pelvic organs, etc., whether or not accompanied by open wound or fracture in the same region, see Injury, internal.
> For contused wound, see Contusion. For crush injury, see Crush. For abrasion, insect bite (nonvenomous), blister, or scratch, see Injury, superficial.
> Complicated includes wounds with:
>   delayed healing
>   delayed treatment
>   foreign body
>   primary infection
> For late effect of open wound, see Late, effect, wound, open, by site.

Medicode's International Classification of Diseases

NOS
As the abbreviation for "not otherwise specified," NOS indicates the code is unspecified and, if possible, the coder should continue looking for a more specific code.

EXCLUDES
Terms following the Excludes instruction are to be coded elsewhere as instructed or in addition to the code they modify.

USE ADDITIONAL CODE IF DESIRED
This note appears in categories where you must add further information (by using an additonal code) to give a more complete picture of the diagnosis or procedure.

CODE ALSO UNDERLYING DISEASE
This convention is used in categories not intended to be the principal diagnosis. The code, its title, and instructions appear in italics. The note requires that the underlying disease (etiology) be recorded first, and the particular manifestation second.

:
A colon is used after an incomplete term that needs one or more of the modifiers that follow to make it assignable to a given category.

}
Braces enclose a series of terms, each of which is modified by the statement appearing at the right of the brace.

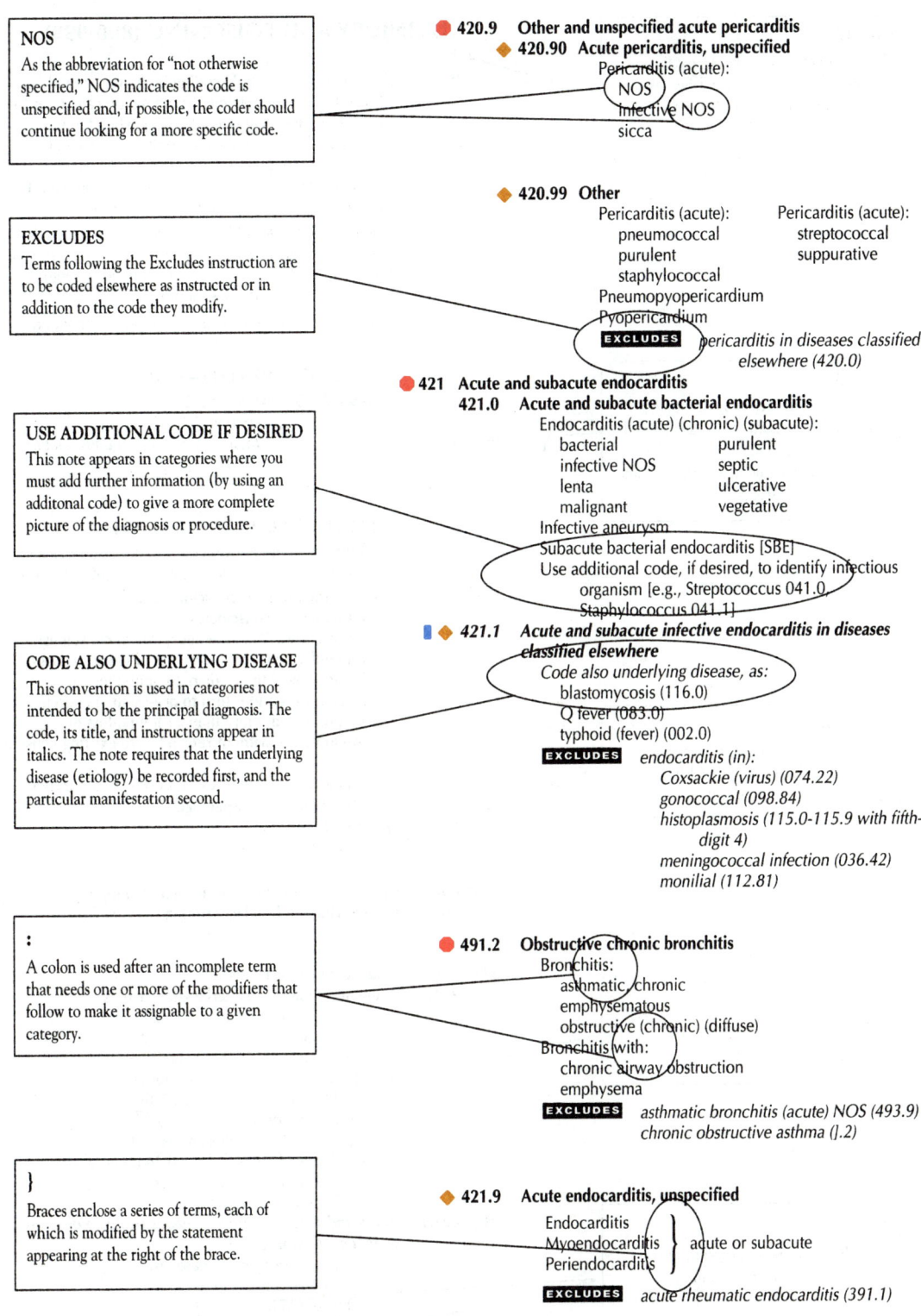

● 420.9 Other and unspecified acute pericarditis
◆ 420.90 Acute pericarditis, unspecified
Pericarditis (acute):
NOS
infective NOS
sicca

◆ 420.99 Other
Pericarditis (acute):   Pericarditis (acute):
pneumococcal   streptococcal
purulent   suppurative
staphylococcal
Pneumopyopericardium
Pyopericardium
EXCLUDES pericarditis in diseases classified elsewhere (420.0)

● 421 Acute and subacute endocarditis
421.0 Acute and subacute bacterial endocarditis
Endocarditis (acute) (chronic) (subacute):
bacterial   purulent
infective NOS   septic
lenta   ulcerative
malignant   vegetative
Infective aneurysm
Subacute bacterial endocarditis [SBE]
Use additional code, if desired, to identify infectious organism [e.g., Streptococcus 041.0, Staphylococcus 041.1]

◆ 421.1 Acute and subacute infective endocarditis in diseases classified elsewhere
Code also underlying disease, as:
blastomycosis (116.0)
Q fever (083.0)
typhoid (fever) (002.0)
EXCLUDES endocarditis (in):
Coxsackie (virus) (074.22)
gonococcal (098.84)
histoplasmosis (115.0-115.9 with fifth-digit 4)
meningococcal infection (036.42)
monilial (112.81)

● 491.2 Obstructive chronic bronchitis
Bronchitis:
asthmatic chronic
emphysematous
obstructive (chronic) (diffuse)
Bronchitis with:
chronic airway obstruction
emphysema
EXCLUDES asthmatic bronchitis (acute) NOS (493.9)
chronic obstructive asthma (].2)

◆ 421.9 Acute endocarditis, unspecified
Endocarditis
Myoendocarditis } acute or subacute
Periendocarditis
EXCLUDES acute rheumatic endocarditis (391.1)

NOTES

Volume 1 notes are not boxed, but like Volume 2 notes, they further define terms, clarify information, or list choices for additional digits.

FORMAT

Subterms are indented two spaces to the right of the term to which they are linked. If a definition requires more than one line (a carry-over line) it is printed on the next line and indented four spaces.

INCLUDES

This note appears immediately under a three-digit code title to further define or give an example of the contents of the category.

[ ]

Brackets enclose synonyms, alternate wording, or explanatory phrases.

( )

Parentheses enclose supplementary words that may be present or absent in the statement of a disease or procedure, without affecting the code number to which it is assigned.

17. INJURY AND POISONING (800-999)

Note:

1. The principle of multiple coding of injuries should be followed wherever possible. Combination categories for multiple injuries are provided for use when there is insufficient detail as to the nature of the individual conditions, or for primary tabulation purposes when it is more convenient to record a single code; otherwise, the component injuries should be coded separately.

   Where multiple sites of injury are specified in the titles, the word "with" indicates involvement of both sites, and the word "and" indicates involvement of either or both sites. The word "finger" includes thumb.

2. Categories for "late effect" of injuries are to be found at 905-909.

FRACTURES (800-829)

EXCLUDES *malunion (733.81)*
nonunion (733.82)
pathological or spontaneous fracture
(733.10-733.19)

FRACTURE OF SKULL (800-804)

The following fifth-digit subclassification is for use with the appropriate codes in categories 800, 801, 803, and 804:

◆ **0 unspecified state of consciousness**
1 with no loss of consciousness
2 with brief [less than one hour] loss of consciousness
3 with moderate [1-24 hours] loss of consciousness
4 with prolonged [more than 24 hours] loss of consciousness and return to pre-existing conscious level
5 with prolonged [more than 24 hours] loss of consciousness, without return to pre-existing conscious level
◆ **6 with loss of consciousness of unspecified duration**
◆ **9 with concussion, unspecified**

● **800 Fracture of vault of skull**
INCLUDES frontal bone
parietal bone
● **800.0 Closed without mention of intracranial injury**
● **800.1 Closed with cerebral laceration and contusion**

● **421 Acute and subacute endocarditis**
421.0 Acute and subacute bacterial endocarditis
Endocarditis (acute) (chronic) (subacute):
bacterial
infective NOS
lenta
malignant
purulent
septic
ulcerative
vegetative
Infective aneurysm
Subacute bacterial endocarditis [SBE]
Use additional code, if desired, to identify infectious organism [e.g., Streptococcus 041.0, Staphylococcus 041.1]

■ ◆ ***421.1 Acute and subacute infective endocarditis in diseases classified elsewhere***
Code also underlying disease, as:
blastomycosis (116.0)
Q fever (083.0)
typhoid (fever) (002.0)
EXCLUDES *endocarditis (in):*
Coxsackie (virus) (074.22)
gonococcal (098.84)
histoplasmosis (115.0-115.9 with fifth-digit 4)
meningococcal infection (036.42)
monilial (112.81)

ALPHABETIC INDEX TO DISEASES

VOLUME 2

SECTION 1

AAV

AAV (disease) (illness) (infection) — see Human immunodeficiency virus (disease) (illness) (infection)
Abactio — see Abortion, induced
Abactus venter — see Abortion, induced
Abarognosis 781.9
Abasia (-astasia) 307.9
   atactica 781.3
   choreic 781.3
   hysterical 300.11
   paroxysmal trepidant 781.3
   spastic 781.3
   trembling 781.3
   trepidans 781.3
Abderhalden-Kaufmann-Lignac syndrome (cystinosis) 270.0
Abdomen, abdominal — see also condition
   accordion 306.4
   acute 789.0
   angina 557.1
   burst 868.00
   convulsive equivalent (see also Epilepsy) 345.5
   heart 746.87
   muscle deficiency syndrome 756.7
   obstipum 756.7
Abdominalgia 789.0
   periodic 277.3
Abduction contracture, hip or other joint — see Contraction, joint
Abercrombie's syndrome (amyloid degeneration) 277.3
Aberrant (congenital) — see also Malposition, congenital
   adrenal gland 759.1
   blood vessel NEC 747.60
      arteriovenous NEC 747.60
      cerebrovascular 747.81
      gastrointestinal 747.61
      lower limb 747.64
      renal 747.62
      spinal 747.82
      upper limb 747.63
   breast 757.6
   endocrine gland NEC 759.2
   gastrointestinal vessel (peripheral) 747.61
   hepatic duct 751.69
   lower limb vessel (peripheral) 747.64
   pancreas 751.7
   parathyroid gland 759.2
   peripheral vascular vessel NEC 747.60
   pituitary gland (pharyngeal) 759.2
   renal blood vessel 747.62
   sebaceous glands, mucous membrane, mouth 750.26
   spinal vessel 747.82
   spleen 759.0
   testis (descent) 752.5
   thymus gland 759.2
   thyroid gland 759.2
   upper limb vessel (perpipheral) 747.63
Aberratio
   lactis 757.6
   testis 752.5
Aberration — see also Anomaly
   chromosome — see Anomaly, chromosome(s)
   distantial 368.9
   mental (see also Disorder, mental, nonpsychotic) 300.9
Abetalipoproteinemia 272.5
Abionarce 780.7
Abiotrophy 799.8
Ablatio
   placentae — see Placenta, ablatio
   retinae (see also Detachment, retina) 361.9

Ablation
   pituitary (gland) (with hypofunction) 253.7
   placenta — see Placenta, ablatio
   uterus 621.8
Ablepharia, ablepharon, ablephary 743.62
Ablepsia — see Blindness
Ablepsy — see Blindness
Ablutomania 300.3
Abnormal, abnormality, abnormalities — see also Anomaly
   acid-base balance 276.4
      fetus or newborn — see Distress, fetal
   adaptation curve, dark 368.63
   alveolar ridge 525.9
   amnion 658.9
      affecting fetus or newborn 762.9
   anatomical relationship NEC 759.9
   apertures, congenital, diaphragm 756.6
   auditory perception NEC 388.40
   autosomes NEC 758.5
      13 758.1
      18 758.2
      21 or 22 758.0
      D_1 758.1
      E_3 758.2
      G 758.0
   ballistocardiogram 794.39
   basal metabolic rate (BMR) 794.7
   biosynthesis, testicular androgen 257.2
   blood level (of)
      cobalt 790.6
      copper 790.6
      iron 790.6
      lithium 790.6
      magnesium 790.6
      mineral 790.6
      zinc 790.6
   blood pressure
      elevated (without diagnosis of hypertension) 796.2
      low (see also Hypotension) 458.9
      reading (incidental) (isolated) (nonspecific) 796.3
   bowel sounds 787.5
   breathing behavior — see Respiration
   caloric test 794.19
   cervix (acquired) NEC 622.9
      congenital 752.40
      in pregnancy or childbirth 654.6
         causing obstructed labor 660.0
            affecting fetus or newborn 763.1
   chemistry, blood NEC 790.6
   chest sounds 786.7
   chorion 658.9
      affecting fetus or newborn 762.9
   chromosomal NEC 758.9
      analysis, nonspecific result 795.2
      autosomes (see also Abnormal, autosomes NEC) 758.5
      fetal, (suspected) affecting management of pregnancy 655.1
      sex 758.8
   clinical findings NEC 796.4
   communication — see Fistula
   configuration of pupils 379.49
   coronary
      artery 746.85
      vein 746.9
   cortisol-binding globulin 255.8
   course, Eustachian tube 744.24
   dentofacial NEC 524.9
      functional 524.5
      specified type NEC 524.8

Abnormal, abnormality, abnormalities—continued
   development, developmental NEC 759.9
      bone 756.9
      central nervous system 742.9
   direction, teeth 524.3
   Dynia (see also Defect, coagulation) 286.9
   Ebstein 746.2
   echocardiogram 793.2
   echoencephalogram 794.01
   echogram NEC — see Findings, abnormal, structure
   electrocardiogram (ECG) (EKG) 794.31
   electroencephalogram (EEG) 794.02
   electromyogram (EMG) 794.17
      ocular 794.14
   electro-oculogram (EOG) 794.12
   electroretinogram (ERG) 794.11
   erythrocytes 289.9
      congenital, with perinatal jaundice 282.9 [774.0]
   Eustachian valve 746.9
   excitability under minor stress 301.9
   fat distribution 782.9
   feces 787.7
   fetal heart rate — see Distress, fetal
   fetus NEC
      affecting management of pregnancy — see Pregnancy, management affected by, fetal
      causing disproportion 653.7
         affecting fetus or newborn 763.1
         causing obstructed labor 660.1
            affecting fetus or newborn 763.1
   findings without manifest disease — see Findings, abnormal
   fluid
      amniotic 792.3
      cerebrospinal 792.0
      peritoneal 792.9
      pleural 792.9
      synovial 792.9
      vaginal 792.9
   forces of labor NEC 661.9
      affecting fetus or newborn 763.7
   form, teeth 520.2
   function studies
      auditory 794.15
      bladder 794.9
      brain 794.00
      cardiovascular 794.30
      endocrine NEC 794.6
      kidney 794.4
      liver 794.8
      nervous system
         central 794.00
         peripheral 794.19
      oculomotor 794.14
      pancreas 794.9
      placenta 794.9
      pulmonary 794.2
      retina 794.11
      special senses 794.19
      spleen 794.9
      thyroid 794.5
      vestibular 794.16
   gait 781.2
      hysterical 300.11
   gastrin secretion 251.5
   globulin
      cortisol-binding 255.8
      thyroid-binding 246.8
   glucagon secretion 251.4
   glucose tolerance test 790.2
      in pregnancy, childbirth, or puerperium 648.8
      fetus or newborn 775.0
   gravitational (G) forces or states 994.9
   hair NEC 704.2

Abnormal, abnormality, abnormalities—continued
   hard tissue formation in pulp 522.3
   head movement 781.0
   heart
      rate, fetus — see Distress, fetal
      shadow 793.2
      sounds NEC 785.3
   hemoglobin (see also Disease, hemoglobin) 282.7
      trait — see Trait, hemoglobin, abnormal
   hemorrhage, uterus — see Hemorrhage, uterus
   histology NEC 795.4
   increase
      in
         appetite 783.6
         development 783.9
   involuntary movement 781.0
   jaw closure 524.5
   karyotype 795.2
   knee jerk 796.1
   labor NEC 661.9
      affecting fetus or newborn 763.7
   laboratory findings — see Findings, abnormal
   length, organ or site, congenital — see Distortion
   loss of weight 783.2
   lung shadow 793.1
   mammogram 793.8
   Mantoux test 795.5
   membranes (fetal)
      affecting fetus or newborn 762.9
      complicating pregnancy 658.8
   menstruation — see Menstruation
   metabolism (see also condition) 783.9
   movement 781.0
      disorder NEC 333.90
      specified NEC 333.99
      head 781.0
      involuntary 781.0
      specified type NEC 333.99
   muscle contraction, localized 728.85
   myoglobin (Aberdeen) (Annapolis) 289.9
   narrowness, eyelid 743.62
   optokinetic response 379.57
   organs or tissues of pelvis NEC in pregnancy or childbirth 654.9
      affecting fetus or newborn 763.8
      causing obstructed labor 660.2
         affecting fetus or newborn 763.1
   origin — see Malposition, congenital
   palmar creases 757.2
   Papanicolaou (smear)
      cervix 795.0
      other site 795.1
   parturition
      affecting fetus or newborn 763.9
      mother — see Delivery, complicated
   pelvis (bony) — see Deformity, pelvis
   percussion, chest 786.7
   periods (grossly) (see also Menstruation) 626.9
   phonocardiogram 794.39
   placenta — see Placenta, abnormal
   plantar reflex 796.1
   plasma protein — see Deficiency, plasma, protein
   pleural folds 748.8
   position — see also Malposition
      gravid uterus 654.4
         causing obstructed labor 660.2
            affecting fetus or newborn 763.1
   posture NEC 781.9
   presentation (fetus) — see Presentation, fetus, abnormal

Abnormal, abnormality, abnormalities—continued

product of conception NEC 631
puberty — see Puberty
pulmonary
 artery 747.3
 function, newborn 770.8
 test results 794.2
 ventilation, newborn 770.8
  hyperventilation 786.01
pulsations in neck 785.1
pupil reflexes 379.40
quality of milk 676.8
radiological examination 793.9
 abdomen NEC 793.6
 biliary tract 793.3
 breast 793.8
 gastrointestinal tract 793.4
 genitourinary organs 793.5
 head 793.0
 intrathoracic organ NEC 793.2
 lung (field) 793.1
 musculoskeletal system 793.7
 retroperitoneum 793.6
 skin and subcutaneous tissue 793.9
 skull 793.0
red blood cells 790.0
 morphology 790.0
 volume 790.0
reflex NEC 796.1
renal function test 794.4
respiration signs — see Respiration
response to nerve stimulation 794.10
retinal correspondence 368.34
rhythm, heart — see also Arrhythmia
 fetus — see Distress, fetal
saliva 792.4
scan
 brain 794.09
 kidney 794.4
 liver 794.8
 lung 794.2
 thyroid 794.5
secretion
 gastrin 251.5
 glucagon 251.4
semen 792.2
serum level (of)
 acid phosphatase 790.5
 alkaline phosphatase 790.5
 amylase 790.5
 enzymes NEC 790.5
 lipase 790.5
shape
 cornea 743.41
 gallbladder 751.69
 gravid uterus 654.4
  affecting fetus or newborn 763.8
  causing obstructed labor 660.2
   affecting fetus or newborn 763.1
 head (see also Anomaly, skull) 756.0
 organ or site, congenital NEC — see Distortion
sinus venosus 747.40
size
 fetus, complicating delivery 653.5
  causing obstructed labor 660.1
 gallbladder 751.69
 head (see also Anomaly, skull) 756.0
 organ or site, congenital NEC — see Distortion
 teeth 520.2
skin and appendages, congenital NEC 757.9
soft parts of pelvis — see Abnormal, organs or tissues of pelvis
spermatozoa 792.2

Abnormal, abnormality, abnormalities—continued

sputum (amount) (color) (excessive) (odor) (purulent) 786.4
stool NEC 787.7
 bloody 578.1
  occult 792.1
 bulky 787.7
 color (dark) (light) 792.1
 content (fat) (mucus) (pus) 792.1
  occult blood 792.1
synchondrosis 756.9
test results without manifest disease — see Findings, abnormal
thebesian valve 746.9
thermography — see Findings, abnormal, structure
threshold, cones or rods (eye) 368.63
thyroid-binding globulin 246.8
thyroid product 246.8
toxicology (findings) NEC 796.0
tracheal cartilage (congenital) 748.3
transport protein 273.8
ultrasound results — see Findings, abnormal, structure
umbilical cord
 affecting fetus or newborn 762.6
 complicating delivery 663.9
 specified NEC 663.8
union
 cricoid cartilage and thyroid cartilage 748.3
 larynx and trachea 748.3
 thyroid cartilage and hyoid bone 748.3
urination NEC 788.69
 psychogenic 306.53
 stream
  intermittent 788.61
  slowing 788.62
  splitting 788.61
  weak 788.62
urine (constituents) NEC 791.9
uterine hemorrhage (see also Hemorrhage, uterus) 626.9
 climacteric 627.0
 postmenopausal 627.1
vagina (acquired) (congenital)
 in pregnancy or childbirth 654.7
  affecting fetus or newborn 763.8
  causing obstructed labor 660.2
   affecting fetus or newborn 763.1
vascular sounds 785.9
vectorcardiogram 794.39
visually evoked potential (VEP) 794.13
vulva (acquired) (congenital)
 in pregnancy or childbirth 654.8
  affecting fetus or newborn 763.8
  causing obstructed labor 660.2
   affecting fetus or newborn 763.1
weight
 gain 783.1
  of pregnancy 646.1
   with hypertension — see Toxemia, of pregnancy
 loss 783.2
x-ray examination — see Abnormal, radiological examination

Abnormally formed uterus — see Anomaly, uterus

Abnormity (any organ or part) — see Anomaly

ABO
 hemolytic disease 773.1
 incompatibility reaction 999.6

Abocclusion 524.2

Abolition, language 784.69

Aborter, habitual or recurrent NEC
 without current pregnancy 629.9
 current abortion (see also Abortion, spontaneous) 634.9
  affecting fetus or newborn 761.8
 observation in current pregnancy 646.3

Abortion (complete) (incomplete) (inevitable) (with retained products of conception) 637.9

Note — Use the following fifth-digit subclassification with categories 634-637:

 0 unspecified
 1 incomplete
 2 complete

with
 complication(s) (any) following previous abortion — see category 639
 damage to pelvic organ (laceration) (rupture) (tear) 637.2
 embolism (air) (amniotic fluid) (blood clot) (pulmonary) (pyemic) (septic) (soap) 637.6
 genital tract and pelvic infection 637.0
 hemorrhage, delayed or excessive 637.1
 metabolic disorder 637.4
 renal failure (acute) 637.3
 sepsis (genital tract) (pelvic organ) 637.0
 urinary tract 637.7
 shock (postoperative) (septic) 637.5
 specified complication NEC 637.7
 toxemia 637.3
 unspecified complication(s) 637.8
 urinary tract infection 637.7
accidental — see Abortion, spontaneous
artificial — see Abortion, induced
attempted (failed) — see Abortion, failed
criminal — see Abortion, illegal
early — see Abortion, spontaneous
elective — see Abortion, legal
failed (legal) 638.9
 with
  damage to pelvic organ (laceration) (rupture) (tear) 638.2
  embolism (air) (amniotic fluid) (blood clot) (pulmonary) (pyemic) (septic) (soap) 638.6
  genital tract and pelvic infection 638.0
  hemorrhage, delayed or excessive 638.1
  metabolic disorder 638.4
  renal failure (acute) 638.3
  sepsis (genital tract) (pelvic organ) 638.0
   urinary tract 638.7
  shock (postoperative) (septic) 638.5
  specified complication NEC 638.7
  toxemia 638.3
  unspecified complication(s) 638.8
  urinary tract infection 638.7
fetal indication — see Abortion, legal
fetus 779.6
following threatened abortion — see Abortion, by type

Abortion—continued

habitual or recurrent (care during pregnancy) 646.3
 with current abortion (see also Abortion, spontaneous) 634.9
  affecting fetus or newborn 761.8
 without current pregnancy 629.9
homicidal — see Abortion, illegal
illegal 636.9
 with
  damage to pelvic organ (laceration) (rupture) (tear) 636.2
  embolism (air) (amniotic fluid) (blood clot) (pulmonary) (pyemic) (septic) (soap) 636.6
  genital tract and pelvic infection 636.0
  hemorrhage, delayed or excessive 636.1
  metabolic disorder 636.4
  renal failure 636.3
  sepsis (genital tract) (pelvic organ) 636.0
   urinary tract 636.7
  shock (postoperative) (septic) 636.5
  specified complication NEC 636.7
  toxemia 636.3
  unspecified complication(s) 636.8
  urinary tract infection 636.7
fetus 779.6
induced 637.9
 illegal — see Abortion, illegal
 legal indications — see Abortion, legal
 medical indications — see Abortion, legal
 therapeutic — see Abortion, legal
late — see Abortion, spontaneous
legal (legal indication) (medical indication) (under medical supervision) 635.9
 with
  damage to pelvic organ (laceration) (rupture) (tear) 635.2
  embolism (air) (amniotic fluid) (blood clot) (pulmonary) (pyemic) (septic) (soap) 635.6
  genital tract and pelvic infection 635.0
  hemorrhage, delayed or excessive 635.1
  metabolic disorder 635.4
  renal failure (acute) 635.3
  sepsis (genital tract) (pelvic organ) 635.0
   urinary tract 635.7
  shock (postoperative) (septic) 635.5
  specified complication NEC 635.7
  toxemia 635.3
  unspecified complication(s) 635.8
  urinary tract infection 635.7
fetus 779.6
medical indication — see Abortion, legal
mental hygiene problem — see Abortion, legal
missed 632
operative — see Abortion, legal
psychiatric indication — see Abortion, legal
recurrent — see Abortion, spontaneous

INDEX TO DISEASES

Abortion—continued
- self-induced — see Abortion, illegal
- septic — see Abortion, by type, with sepsis
- spontaneous 634.9
  - with
    - damage to pelvic organ (laceration) (rupture) (tear) 634.2
    - embolism (air) (amniotic fluid) (blood clot) (pulmonary) (pyemic) (septic) (soap) 634.6
    - genital tract and pelvic infection 634.0
    - hemorrhage, delayed or excessive 634.1
    - metabolic disorder 634.4
    - renal failure 634.3
    - sepsis (genital tract) (pelvic organ) 634.0
    - urinary tract 634.7
    - shock (postoperative) (septic) 634.5
    - specified complication NEC 634.7
    - toxemia 634.3
    - unspecified complication(s) 634.8
    - urinary tract infection 634.7
  - fetus 761.8
  - threatened 640.0
    - affecting fetus or newborn 762.1
- surgical — see Abortion, legal
- therapeutic — see Abortion, legal
- threatened 640.0
  - affecting fetus or newborn 762.1
- tubal — see Pregnancy, tubal
- voluntary — see Abortion, legal

Abortus fever 023.9
Aboulomania 301.6
Abrachia 755.20
Abrachiatism 755.20
Abrachiocephalia 759.89
Abrachiocephalus 759.89
Abrami's disease (acquired hemolytic jaundice) 283.9
Abramov-Fiedler myocarditis (acute isolated myocarditis) 422.91
Abrasion — see also Injury, superficial, by site
- dental 521.2
- teeth, tooth (dentifrice) (habitual) (hard tissues) (occupational) (ritual) (traditional) (wedge defect) 521.2

Abrikossov's tumor (M9580/0) — see also Neoplasm, connective tissue, benign
- malignant (M9580/3) — see Neoplasm, connective tissue, malignant

Abrism 988.8
Abruption, placenta — see Placenta, abruptio
Abruptio placentae — see Placenta, abruptio

Abscess (acute) (chronic) (infectional) (lymphangitic) (metastatic) (multiple) (pyogenic) (septic) (with lymphangitis) (see also Cellulitis) 682.9
- abdomen, abdominal
  - cavity — see Abscess, peritoneum
  - wall 682.2
- abdominopelvic — see Abscess, peritoneum
- accessory sinus (chronic) (see also Sinusitis) 473.9
- adrenal (capsule) (gland) 255.8
- alveolar 522.5
  - with sinus 522.7

Abscess—continued
- amebic 006.3
  - bladder 006.8
  - brain (with liver or lung abscess) 006.5
  - liver (without mention of brain or lung abscess) 006.3
    - with
      - brain abscess (and lung abscess) 006.5
      - lung abscess 006.4
  - lung (with liver abscess) 006.4
    - with brain abscess 006.5
  - seminal vesicle 006.8
  - specified site NEC 006.8
  - spleen 006.8
- anaerobic 040.0
- ankle 682.6
- anorectal 566
- antecubital space 682.3
- antrum (chronic) (Highmore) (see also Sinusitis, maxillary) 473.0
- anus 566
- apical (tooth) 522.5
  - with sinus (alveolar) 522.7
- appendix 540.1
- areola (acute) (chronic) (nonpuerperal) 611.0
  - puerperal, postpartum 675.1
- arm (any part, above wrist) 682.3
- artery (wall) 447.2
- atheromatous 447.2
- auditory canal (external) 380.10
- auricle (ear) (staphylococcal) (streptococcal) 380.10
- axilla, axillary (region) 682.3
  - lymph gland or node 683
- back (any part) 682.2
- Bartholin's gland 616.3
  - with
    - abortion — see Abortion, by type, with sepsis
    - ectopic pregnancy (see also categories 633.0-633.9) 639.0
    - molar pregnancy (see also categories 630-632) 639.0
  - complicating pregnancy or puerperium 646.6
  - following
    - abortion 639.0
    - ectopic or molar pregnancy 639.0
- bartholinian 616.3
- Bezold's 383.01
- bile, biliary, duct or tract (see also Cholecystitis) 576.8
- bilharziasis 120.1
- bladder (wall) 595.89
  - amebic 006.8
- bone (subperiosteal) (see also Osteomyelitis) 730.0
  - accessory sinus (chronic) (see also Sinusitis) 473.9
  - acute 730.0
  - chronic or old 730.1
  - jaw (lower) (upper) 526.4
  - mastoid — see Mastoiditis, acute
  - petrous (see also Petrositis) 383.20
  - spinal (tuberculous) (see also Tuberculosis) 015.0 [730.88]
  - nontuberculous 730.08
- bowel 569.5
- brain (any part) 324.0
  - amebic (with liver or lung abscess) 006.5
  - cystic 324.0
  - late effect — see category 326
  - otogenic 324.0
  - tuberculous (see also Tuberculosis) 013.3

Abscess—continued
- breast (acute) (chronic) (nonpuerperal) 611.0
  - newborn 771.5
  - puerperal, postpartum 675.1
  - tuberculous (see also Tuberculosis) 017.9
- broad ligament (chronic) (see also Disease, pelvis, inflammatory) 614.4
  - acute 614.3
- Brodie's (chronic) (localized) (see also Osteomyelitis) 730.1
- bronchus 519.1
- buccal cavity 528.3
- bulbourethral gland 597.0
- bursa 727.89
  - pharyngeal 478.29
- buttock 682.5
- canaliculus, breast 611.0
- canthus 372.20
- cartilage 733.99
- cecum 540.1
- cerebellum, cerebellar 324.0
  - late effect — see category 326
- cerebral (embolic) 324.0
  - late effect — see category 326
- cervical (neck region) 682.1
  - lymph gland or node 683
  - stump (see also Cervicitis) 616.0
- cervix (stump) (uteri) (see also Cervicitis) 616.0
- cheek, external 682.0
  - inner 528.3
- chest 510.9
  - with fistula 510.0
  - wall 682.2
- chin 682.0
- choroid 363.00
- ciliary body 364.3
- circumtonsillar 475
- cold (tuberculous) — see also Tuberculosis, abscess
  - articular — see Tuberculosis, joint
- colon (wall) 569.5
- colostomy or enterostomy 569.6
- conjunctiva 372.00
- connective tissue NEC 682.9
- cornea 370.55
  - with ulcer 370.00
- corpus
  - cavernosum 607.2
  - luteum (see also Salpingo-oophoritis) 614.2
- Cowper's gland 597.0
- cranium 324.0
- cul-de-sac (Douglas') (posterior) (see also Disease, pelvis, inflammatory) 614.4
  - acute 614.3
- dental 522.5
  - with sinus (alveolar) 522.7
- dentoalveolar 522.5
  - with sinus (alveolar) 522.7
- diaphragm, diaphragmatic — see Abscess, peritoneum
- digit NEC 681.9
- Douglas' cul-de-sac or pouch (see also Disease, pelvis, inflammatory) 614.4
  - acute 614.3
- Dubois' 090.5
- ductless gland 259.8
- ear
  - acute 382.00
  - external 380.10
  - inner 386.30
  - middle — see Otitis media
- elbow 682.3
- endamebic — see Abscess, amebic
- entamebic — see Abscess, amebic
- enterostomy 569.6
- epididymis 604.0
- epidural 324.9
  - brain 324.0
  - late effect — see category 326

Abscess—continued
- epidural—continued
  - spinal cord 324.1
- epiglottis 478.79
- epiploon, epiploic — see Abscess, peritoneum
- erysipelatous (see also Erysipelas) 035
- esophagus 530.19
- ethmoid (bone) (chronic) (sinus) (see also Sinusitis, ethmoidal) 473.2
- external auditory canal 380.10
- extradural 324.9
  - brain 324.0
  - late effect — see category 326
  - spinal cord 324.1
- extraperitoneal — see Abscess, peritoneum
- eye 360.00
- eyelid 373.13
- face (any part, except eye) 682.0
- fallopian tube (see also Salpingo-oophoritis) 614.2
- fascia 728.89
- fauces 478.29
- fecal 569.5
- femoral (region) 682.6
- filaria, filarial (see also Infestation, filarial) 125.9
- finger (any) (intrathecal) (periosteal) (subcutaneous) (subcuticular) 681.00
- fistulous NEC 682.9
- flank 682.2
- foot (except toe) 682.7
- forearm 682.3
- forehead 682.0
- frontal (sinus) (chronic) (see also Sinusitis, frontal) 473.1
- gallbladder (see also Cholecystitis, acute) 575.0
- gastric 535.0
- genital organ or tract NEC
  - female 616.9
    - with
      - abortion — see Abortion, by type, with sepsis
      - ectopic pregnancy (see also categories 633.0-633.9) 639.0
      - molar pregnancy (see also categories 630-632) 639.0
    - following
      - abortion 639.0
      - ectopic or molar pregnancy 639.0
    - puerperal, postpartum, childbirth 670
  - male 608.4
- genitourinary system, tuberculous (see also Tuberculosis) 016.9
- gingival 523.3
- gland, glandular (lymph) (acute) NEC 683
- glottis 478.79
- gluteal (region) 682.5
- gonorrheal NEC (see also Gonococcus) 098.0
- groin 682.2
- gum 523.3
- hand (except finger or thumb) 682.4
- head (except face) 682.8
- heart 429.89
- heel 682.7
- helminthic (see also Infestation, by specific parasite) 128.9
- hepatic 572.0
  - amebic (see also Abscess, liver, amebic) 006.3
  - duct 576.8
- hip 682.6
  - tuberculous (active) (see also Tuberculosis) 015.1
- ileocecal 540.1

Abscess—*continued*
  ileostomy (bud) 569.6
  iliac (region) 682.2
    fossa 540.1
  iliopsoas (tuberculous) (*see also* Tuberculosis) 015.0 *[730.88]*
    nontuberculous 728.89
  infraclavicular (fossa) 682.3
  inguinal (region) 682.2
    lymph gland or node 683
  intersphincteric (anus) 566
  intestine, intestinal 569.5
    rectal 566
  intra-abdominal (*see also* Abscess, peritoneum) 567.2
    postoperative 998.5
  intracranial 324.0
    late effect — *see* category 326
  intramammary — *see* Abscess, breast
  intramastoid (*see also* Mastoiditis, acute) 383.00
  intraorbital 376.01
  intraperitoneal — *see* Abscess, peritoneum
  intraspinal 324.1
    late effect — *see* category 326
  intratonsillar 475
  iris 364.3
  ischiorectal 566
  jaw (bone) (lower) (upper) 526.4
    skin 682.0
  joint (*see also* Arthritis, pyogenic) 711.0
    vertebral (tuberculous) (*see also* Tuberculosis) 015.0 *[730.88]*
      nontuberculous 724.8
  kidney 590.2
    with
      abortion — *see* Abortion, by type, with urinary tract infection
      calculus 592.0
      ectopic pregnancy (*see also* categories 633.0-633.9) 639.8
      molar pregnancy (*see also* categories 630-632) 639.8
      complicating pregnancy or puerperium 646.6
        affecting fetus or newborn 760.1
      following
        abortion 639.8
        ectopic or molar pregnancy 639.8
  knee 682.6
    joint 711.06
    tuberculous (active) (*see also* Tuberculosis) 015.2
  labium (majus) (minus) 616.4
    complicating pregnancy, childbirth, or puerperium 646.6
  lacrimal (passages) (sac) (*see also* Dacryocystitis) 375.30
    caruncle 375.30
    gland (*see also* Dacryoadenitis) 375.00
  lacunar 597.0
  larynx 478.79
  lateral (alveolar) 522.5
    with sinus 522.7
  leg, except foot 682.6
  lens 360.00
  lid 373.13
  lingual 529.0
    tonsil 475
  lip 528.5
  Littre's gland 597.0
  liver 572.0
    amebic 006.3

Abscess—*continued*
  liver—*continued*
    amebic—*continued*
      with
        brain abscess (and lung abscess) 006.5
        lung abscess 006.4
      due to Entamoeba histolytica 006.3
      dysenteric (*see also* Abscess, liver, amebic) 006.3
      pyogenic 572.0
      tropical (*see also* Abscess, liver, amebic) 006.3
  loin (region) 682.2
  lumbar (tuberculous) (*see also* Tuberculosis) 015.0 *[730.88]*
    nontuberculous 682.2
  lung (miliary) (putrid) 513.0
    amebic (with liver abscess) 006.4
      with brain abscess 006.5
  lymph, lymphatic, gland or node (acute) 683
    any site, except mesenteric 683
    mesentery 289.2
  lymphangitic, acute — *see* Cellulitis
  malar 526.4
  mammary gland — *see* Abscess, breast
  marginal (anus) 566
  mastoid (process) (*see also* Mastoiditis, acute) 383.00
    subperiosteal 383.01
  maxilla, maxillary 526.4
    molar (tooth) 522.5
      with sinus 522.7
    premolar 522.5
    sinus (chronic) (*see also* Sinusitis, maxillary) 473.0
  mediastinum 513.1
  meibomian gland 373.12
  meninges (*see also* Meningitis) 320.9
  mesentery, mesenteric — *see* Abscess, peritoneum
  mesosalpinx (*see also* Salpingo-oophoritis) 614.2
  milk 675.1
  Monro's (psoriasis) 696.1
  mons pubis 682.2
  mouth (floor) 528.3
  multiple sites NEC 682.9
  mural 682.2
  muscle 728.89
  myocardium 422.92
  nabothian (follicle) (*see also* Cervicitis) 616.0
  nail (chronic) (with lymphangitis) 681.9
    finger 681.02
    toe 681.11
  nasal (fossa) (septum) 478.1
    sinus (chronic) (*see also* Sinusitis) 473.9
  nasopharyngeal 478.29
  nates 682.5
  navel 682.2
    newborn NEC 771.4
  neck (region) 682.1
    lymph gland or node 683
  nephritic (*see also* Abscess, kidney) 590.2
  nipple 611.0
    puerperal, postpartum 675.0
  nose (septum) 478.1
    external 682.0
  omentum — *see* Abscess, peritoneum
  operative wound 998.5
  orbit, orbital 376.01
  ossifluent — *see* Abscess, bone
  ovary, ovarian (corpus luteum) (*see also* Salpingo-oophoritis) 614.2

Abscess—*continued*
  oviduct (*see also* Salpingo-oophoritis) 614.2
  palate (soft) 528.3
    hard 526.4
  palmar (space) 682.4
  pancreas (duct) 577.0
  paradontal 523.3
  parafrenal 607.2
  parametric, parametrium (chronic) (*see also* Disease, pelvis, inflammatory) 614.4
    acute 614.3
  paranephric 590.2
  parapancreatic 577.0
  parapharyngeal 478.22
  pararectal 566
  parasinus (*see also* Sinusitis) 473.9
  parauterine (*see also* Disease, pelvis, inflammatory) 614.4
    acute 614.3
  paravaginal (*see also* Vaginitis) 616.10
  parietal region 682.8
  parodontal 523.3
  parotid (duct) (gland) 527.3
    region 528.3
  parumbilical 682.2
    newborn 771.4
  pectoral (region) 682.2
  pelvirectal — *see* Abscess, peritoneum
  pelvis, pelvic
    female (chronic) (*see also* Disease, pelvis, inflammatory) 614.4
      acute 614.3
    male, peritoneal (cellular tissue) — *see* Abscess, peritoneum
    tuberculous (*see also* Tuberculosis) 016.9
  penis 607.2
    gonococcal (acute) 098.0
      chronic or duration of 2 months or over 098.2
  perianal 566
  periapical 522.5
    with sinus (alveolar) 522.7
  periappendiceal 540.1
  pericardial 420.99
  pericecal 540.1
  pericemental 523.3
  pericholecystic (*see also* Cholecystitis, acute) 575.0
  pericoronal 523.3
  peridental 523.3
  perigastric 535.0
  perimetric (*see also* Disease, pelvis, inflammatory) 614.4
    acute 614.3
  perinephric, perinephritic (*see also* Abscess, kidney) 590.2
  perineum, perineal (superficial) 682.2
    deep (with urethral involvement) 597.0
    urethra 597.0
  periodontal (parietal) 523.3
    apical 522.5
  periosteum, periosteal (*see also* Periostitis) 730.3
    with osteomyelitis (*see also* Osteomyelitis) 730.2
      acute or subacute 730.0
      chronic or old 730.1
  peripleuritic 510.9
    with fistula 510.0
  periproctic 566
  periprostatic 601.2
  perirectal (staphylococcal) 566
  perirenal (tissue) (*see also* Abscess, kidney) 590.2
  perisinuous (nose) (*see also* Sinusitis) 473.9

Abscess—*continued*
  peritoneum, peritoneal (perforated) (ruptured) 567.2
    with
      abortion — *see* Abortion, by type, with sepsis
      appendicitis 540.1
      ectopic pregnancy (*see also* categories 633.0-633.9) 639.0
      molar pregnancy (*see also* categories 630-632) 639.0
    following
      abortion 639.0
      ectopic or molar pregnancy 639.0
    pelvic, female (*see also* Disease, pelvis, inflammatory) 614.4
      acute 614.3
    postoperative 998.5
    puerperal, postpartum, childbirth 670
    tuberculous (*see also* Tuberculosis) 014.0
  peritonsillar 475
  perityphlic 540.1
  periureteral 593.89
  periurethral 597.0
    gonococcal (acute) 098.0
      chronic or duration of 2 months or over 098.2
  periuterine (*see also* Disease, pelvis, inflammatory) 614.4
    acute 614.3
  perivesical 595.89
  pernicious NEC 682.9
  petrous bone — *see* Petrositis
  phagedenic NEC 682.9
    chancroid 099.0
  pharynx, pharyngeal (lateral) 478.29
  phlegmonous NEC 682.9
  pilonidal 685.0
  pituitary (gland) 253.8
  pleura 510.9
    with fistula 510.0
  popliteal 682.6
  postanal 566
  postcecal 540.1
  postlaryngeal 478.79
  postnasal 478.1
  postpharyngeal 478.24
  posttonsillar 475
  posttyphoid 002.0
  Pott's (*see also* Tuberculosis) 015.0 *[730.88]*
  pouch of Douglas (chronic) (*see also* Disease, pelvis, inflammatory) 614.4
  premammary — *see* Abscess, breast
  prepatellar 682.6
  prostate (*see also* Prostatitis) 601.2
    gonococcal (acute) 098.12
      chronic or duration of 2 months or over 098.32
  psoas (tuberculous) (*see also* Tuberculosis) 015.0 *[730.88]*
    nontuberculous 728.89
  pterygopalatine fossa 682.8
  pubis 682.2
  puerperal — Puerperal, abseess, by site
  pulmonary — *see* Abscess, lung
  pulp, pulpal (dental) 522.0
    finger 681.01
    toe 681.10
  pyemic — *see* Septicemia
  pyloric valve 535.0
  rectovaginal septum 569.5
  rectovesical 595.89
  rectum 566
  regional NEC 682.9
  renal (*see also* Abscess, kidney) 590.2

Abscess—continued
retina 363.00
retrobulbar 376.01
retrocecal — see Abscess, peritoneum
retrolaryngeal 478.79
retromammary — see Abscess, breast
retroperineal 682.2
retroperitoneal — see Abscess, peritoneum
retropharyngeal 478.24
    tuberculous (see also Tuberculosis) 012.8
retrorectal 566
retrouterine (see also Disease, pelvis, inflammatory) 614.4
    acute 614.3
retrovesical 595.89
root, tooth 522.5
    with sinus (alveolar) 522.7
round ligament (see also Disease, pelvis, inflammatory) 614.4
    acute 614.3
rupture (spontaneous) NEC 682.9
sacrum (tuberculous) (see also Tuberculosis) 015.0 [730.88]
    nontuberculous 730.08
salivary duct or gland 527.3
scalp (any part) 682.8
scapular 730.01
sclera 379.09
scrofulous (see also Tuberculosis) 017.2
scrotum 608.4
seminal vesicle 608.0
    amebic 006.8
septal, dental 522.5
    with sinus (alveolar) 522.7
septum (nasal) 478.1
serous (see also Periostitis) 730.3
shoulder 682.3
side 682.2
sigmoid 569.5
sinus (accessory) (chronic) (nasal) (see also Sinusitis) 473.9
    intracranial venous (any) 324.0
    late effect — see category 326
Skene's duct or gland 597.0
skin NEC 682.9
    tuberculous (primary) (see also Tuberculosis) 017.0
sloughing NEC 682.9
specified site NEC 682.8
    amebic 006.8
spermatic cord 608.4
sphenoidal (sinus) (see also Sinusitis, sphenoidal) 473.3
spinal
    cord (any part) (staphylococcal) 324.1
        tuberculous (see also Tuberculosis) 013.5
    epidural 324.1
spine (column) (tuberculous) (see also Tuberculosis) 015.0 [730.88]
    nontuberculous 730.08
spleen 289.59
    amebic 006.8
staphylococcal NEC 682.9
stitch 998.5
stomach (wall) 535.0
strumous (tuberculous) (see also Tuberculosis) 017.2
subarachnoid 324.9
    brain 324.0
    cerebral 324.0
    late effect — see category 326
    spinal cord 324.1
subareolar — see also Abscess, breast puerperal, postpartum 675.1
subcecal 540.1
subcutaneous NEC 682.9

Abscess—continued
subdiaphragmatic — see Abscess, peritoneum
subdorsal 682.2
subdural 324.9
    brain 324.0
    late effect — see category 326
    spinal cord 324.1
subgaleal 682.8
subhepatic — see Abscess, peritoneum
sublingual 528.3
    gland 527.3
submammary — see Abscess, breast
submandibular (region) (space) (triangle) 682.0
    gland 527.3
submaxillary (region) 682.0
    gland 527.3
submental (pyogenic) 682.0
    gland 527.3
subpectoral 682.2
subperiosteal — see Abscess, bone
subperitoneal — see Abscess, peritoneum
subphrenic — see also Abscess, peritoneum
    postoperative 998.5
subscapular 682.2
subungual 681.9
suburethral 597.0
sudoriparous 705.89
suppurative NEC 682.9
supraclavicular (fossa) 682.3
suprahepatic — see Abscess, peritoneum
suprapelvic (see also Disease, pelvis, inflammatory) 614.4
    acute 614.3
suprapubic 682.2
suprarenal (capsule) (gland) 255.8
sweat gland 705.89
syphilitic 095.8
teeth, tooth (root) 522.5
    with sinus (alveolar) 522.7
    supporting structures NEC 523.3
temple 682.0
temporal region 682.0
temporosphenoidal 324.0
    late effect — see category 326
tendon (sheath) 727.89
testicle — see Orchitis
thecal 728.89
thigh (acquired) 682.6
thorax 510.9
    with fistula 510.0
throat 478.29
thumb (intrathecal) (periosteal) (subcutaneous) (subcuticular) 681.00
thymus (gland) 254.1
thyroid (gland) 245.0
toe (any) (intrathecal) (periosteal) (subcutaneous) (subcuticular) 681.10
tongue (staphylococcal) 529.0
tonsil(s) (lingual) 475
tonsillopharyngeal 475
tooth, teeth (root) 522.5
    with sinus (alveolar) 522.7
    supporting structure NEC 523.3
trachea 478.9
trunk 682.2
tubal (see also Salpingo-oophoritis) 614.2
tuberculous — see Tuberculosis, abscess
tubo-ovarian (see also Salpingo-oophoritis) 614.2
tunica vaginalis 608.4
umbilicus NEC 682.2
    newborn 771.4
upper arm 682.3
upper respiratory 478.9
urachus 682.2
urethra (gland) 597.0

Abscess—continued
urinary 597.0
uterus, uterine (wall) (see also Endometritis) 615.9
    ligament (see also Disease, pelvis, inflammatory) 614.4
    acute 614.3
    neck (see also Cervicitis) 616.0
uvula 528.3
vagina (wall) (see also Vaginitis) 616.10
vaginorectal (see also Vaginitis) 616.10
vas deferens 608.4
vermiform appendix 540.1
vertebra (column) (tuberculous) (see also Tuberculosis) 015.0 [730.88]
    nontuberculous 730.0
vesical 595.89
vesicouterine pouch (see also Disease, pelvis, inflammatory) 614.4
vitreous (humor) (pneumococcal) 360.04
vocal cord 478.5
von Bezold's 383.01
vulva 616.4
    complicating pregnancy, childbirth, or puerperium 646.6
vulvovaginal gland (see also Vaginitis) 616.3
web-space 682.4
wrist 682.4

Absence (organ or part) (complete or partial)
acoustic nerve 742.8
adrenal (gland) (congenital) 759.1
    acquired 255.8
albumin (blood) 273.8
alimentary tract (complete) (congenital) (partial) 751.8
    lower 751.5
    upper 750.8
alpha-fucosidase 271.8
alveolar process (acquired) 525.8
    congenital 750.26
anus, anal (canal) (congenital) 751.2
aorta (congenital) 747.22
aortic valve (congenital) 746.89
appendix, congenital 751.2
arm (acquired) V49.60 ▼
    above elbow V49.66
    below elbow V49.65 ▲
    congenital (see also Deformity, reduction, upper limb) 755.20
        lower — see Absence, forearm, congenital
        upper (complete) (partial) (with absence of distal elements, incomplete) 755.24
        with
            complete absence of distal elements 755.21
            forearm (incomplete) 755.23
artery (congenital) (peripheral) NEC (see also Anomaly, peripheral vascular system) 747.60
    brain 747.81
    cerebral 747.81
    coronary 746.85
    pulmonary 747.3
    umbilical 747.5
atrial septum 745.69
auditory canal (congenital) (external) 744.01
auricle (ear) (with stenosis or atresia of auditory canal), congenital 744.01

Absence—continued
bile, biliary duct (common) or passage (congenital) 751.61
bladder (acquired) 596.8
    congenital 753.8
bone (congenital) NEC 756.9
    marrow 284.9
        acquired (secondary) 284.8
        congenital 284.0
        hereditary 284.0
        idiopathic 284.9
    skull 756.0
bowel sounds 787.5
brain 740.0
    specified part 742.2
breast(s) (acquired) 611.8
    congenital 757.6
broad ligament (congenital) 752.19
bronchus (congenital) 748.3
calvarium, calvaria (skull) 756.0
canaliculus lacrimalis, congenital 743.65
carpal(s) (congenital) (complete) (partial) (with absence of distal elements, incomplete) (see also Deformity, reduction, upper limb) 755.28
    with complete absence of distal elements 755.21
cartilage 756.9
caudal spine 756.13
cecum (acquired) (postoperative) (posttraumatic) 569.89
    congenital 751.2
cementum 520.4
cerebellum (congenital) (vermis) 742.2
cervix (acquired) (uteri) 622.8
    congenital 752.49
chin, congenital 744.89
cilia (congenital) 743.63
    acquired 374.89
circulatory system, part NEC 747.89
clavicle 755.51
clitoris (congenital) 752.49
coccyx, congenital 756.13
cold sense (see also Disturbance, sensation) 782.0
colon (acquired) (postoperative) 569.89
    congenital 751.2
congenital
    lumen — see Atresia
    organ or site NEC — see Agenesis
    septum — see Imperfect, closure
corpus callosum (congenital) 742.2
cricoid cartilage 748.3
diaphragm (congenital) (with hernia) 756.6
    with obstruction 756.6
digestive organ(s) or tract, congenital (complete) (partial) 751.8
    lower 751.5
    upper 750.8
ductus arteriosus 747.89
duodenum (acquired) (postoperative) 564.2
    congenital 751.1
ear, congenital 744.09
    acquired 388.8
    auricle 744.01
    external 744.01
    inner 744.05
    lobe, lobule 744.21
    middle, except ossicles 744.03
        ossicles 744.04
    ossicles 744.04
ejaculatory duct (congenital) 752.8
endocrine gland NEC (congenital) 759.2
epididymis (congenital) 752.8
    acquired 608.89
epiglottis, congenital 748.3

Absence—continued
   epileptic (atonic) (typical) (see also
      Epilepsy) 345.0
   erythrocyte 284.9
   erythropoiesis 284.9
      congenital 284.0
   esophagus (congenital) 750.3
   Eustachian tube (congenital) 744.24
   extremity (acquired) ◆
      congenital (see also Deformity,
         reduction) 755.4
      lower V49.70 ▼
      upper V49.60 ▲
   extrinsic muscle, eye 743.69
   eye (acquired) 360.89
      adnexa (congenital) 743.69
      congenital 743.00
      muscle (congenital) 743.69
   eyelid (fold), congenital 743.62
      acquired 374.89
   face
      bones NEC 756.0
      specified part NEC 744.89
   fallopian tube(s) (acquired) 620.8
      congenital 752.19
   femur, congenital (complete)
      (partial) (with absence of
      distal elements, incomplete)
      (see also Deformity,
      reduction, lower limb)
      755.34
      with
         complete absence of distal
            elements 755.31
         tibia and fibula (incomplete)
            755.33
   fibrin 790.92
   fibrinogen (congenital) 286.3
      acquired 286.6
   fibula, congenital (complete)
      (partial) (with absence of
      distal elements, incomplete)
      (see also Deformity,
      reduction, lower limb)
      755.37
      with
         complete absence of distal
            elements 755.31
         tibia 755.35
            with
               complete absence of
                  distal elements
                  755.31
         femur (incomplete)
            755.33
            with complete
               absence of
               distal
               elements
               755.31
   finger (acquired) V49.62 ◆
      congenital (complete) (partial)
         (see also Deformity,
         reduction, upper limb)
         755.29
         meaning all fingers
            (complete) (partial)
            755.21
         transverse 755.21
   fissures of lungs (congenital) 748.5
   foot (acquired) V49.73 ◆
      congenital (complete) 755.31
   forearm (acquired) V49.65 ◆
      congenital (complete) (partial)
         (with absence of distal
         elements, incomplete)
         (see also Deformity,
         reduction, upper limb)
         755.25
         with
            complete absence of
               distal elements
               (hand and fingers)
               755.21
            humerus (incomplete)
               755.23

Absence—continued
   fovea centralis 743.55
   fucosidase 271.8
   gallbladder (acquired) V45.89
      congenital 751.69
   gamma globulin (blood) 279.00
   genital organs, congenital
      female 752.8
         external 752.49
         internal NEC 752.8
      male 752.8
   genitourinary organs. congenital
      NEC 752.8
   glottis 748.3
   gonadal, congenital NEC 758.6
   hair (congenital) 757.4
      acquired — see Alopecia
   hand (acquired) V49.63 ◆
      congenital (complete) (see also
         Deformity, reduction,
         upper limb) 755.21
   heart (congenital) 759.89
      acquired — see Status, organ
         replacement
   heat sense (see also Disturbance,
      sensation) 782.0
   humerus, congenital (complete)
      (partial) (with absence of
      distal elements, incomplete)
      (see also Deformity,
      reduction, upper limb)
      755.24
      with
         complete absence of distal
            elements 755.21
         radius and ulna (incomplete)
            755.23
   hymen (congenital) 752.49
   ileum (acquired) (postoperative)
      (posttraumatic) 569.89
      congenital 751.1
   immunoglobulin, isolated NEC
      279.03
      IgA 279.01
      IgG 279.03
      IgM 279.02
   incus (acquired) 385.24
      congenital 744.04
   internal ear (congenital) 744.05
   intestine (acquired) (small) 569.89
      congenital 751.1
         large 751.2
      large 569.89
         congenital 751.2
   iris (congenital) 743.45
   jaw — see Absence, mandible
   jejunum (acquired) 569.89
      congenital 751.1
   joint, congenital NEC 755.8
   kidney(s) (acquired) 593.89
      congenital 753.0
   labium (congenital) (majus) (minus)
      752.49
   labyrinth, membranous 744.05
   lacrimal apparatus (congenital)
      743.65
   larynx (congenital) 748.3
   leg (acquired) V49.70 ▼
      above knee V49.76
      below knee V49.75 ▲
      congenital (partial) (unilateral)
         (see also Deformity,
         reduction, lower limb)
         755.31
         lower (complete) (partial)
            (with absence of distal
            elements, incomplete)
            755.35
            with
               complete absence of
                  distal elements
                  (foot and toes)
                  755.31
               thigh (incomplete)
                  755.33

Absence—continued
   leg—continued
      congenital—continued
         lower—continued
            with—continued
               thigh—continued
                  with complete
                     absence of
                     distal
                     elements
                     755.31
         upper — see Absence, femur
   lens (congenital) 743.35
      acquired 379.31
   ligament, broad (congenital) 752.19
   limb (acquired) ◆
      congenital (complete) (partial)
         (see also Deformity,
         reduction) 755.4
         lower 755.30
            complete 755.31
            incomplete 755.32
            longitudinal — see
               Deficiency, lower
               limb, longitudinal
            transverse 755.31
         upper 755.20
            complete 755.21
            incomplete 755.22
            longitudinal — see
               Deficiency, upper
               limb, longitudinal
            transverse 755.21
      lower NEC V49.70 ▼
      upper NEC V49.60 ▲
   lip 750.26
   liver (congenital) (lobe) 751.69
   lumbar (congenital) (vertebra)
      756.13
      isthmus 756.11
      pars articularis 756.11
   lumen — see Atresia
   lung (bilateral) (congenital) (fissure)
      (lobe) (unilateral) 748.5
      acquired (any part) 518.89
   mandible (congenital) 524.09
   maxilla (congenital) 524.09
   menstruation 626.0
   metacarpal(s), congenital
      (complete) (partial) (with
      absence of distal elements,
      incomplete) (see also
      Deformity, reduction, upper
      limb) 755.28
      with all fingers, complete
         755.21
   metatarsal(s), congenital (complete)
      (partial) (with absence of
      distal elements, incomplete)
      (see also Deformity,
      reduction, lower limb)
      755.38
      with complete absence of distal
         elements 755.31
   muscle (congenital) (pectoral)
      756.81
      ocular 743.69
   musculoskeletal system (congenital)
      NEC 756.9
   nail(s) (congenital) 757.5
   neck, part 744.89
   nerve 742.8
   nervous system, part NEC 742.8
   neutrophil 288.0
   nipple (congenital) 757.6
   nose (congenital) 748.1
      acquired 738.0
   nuclear 742.8
   ocular muscle (congenital) 743.69
   organ
      of Corti (congenital) 744.05
      or site, congenital NEC 759.89
   osseous meatus (ear) 744.03
   ovary (acquired) 620.8
      congenital 752.0
   oviduct (acquired) 620.8
      congenital 752.19

Absence—continued
   pancreas (congenital) 751.7
      acquired (postoperative)
         (posttraumatic) 577.8
   parathyroid gland (congenital)
      759.2
   parotid gland(s) (congenital) 750.21
   patella, congenital 755.64
   pelvic girdle (congenital) 755.69
   penis (congenital) 752.8
      acquired 607.89
   pericardium (congenital) 746.89
   perineal body (congenital) 756.81
   phalange(s), congenital 755.4
      lower limb (complete)
         (intercalary) (partial)
         (terminal) (see also
         Deformity, reduction,
         lower limb) 755.39
         meaning all toes (complete)
            (partial) 755.31
         transverse 755.31
      upper limb (complete)
         (intercalary) (partial)
         (terminal) (see also
         Deformity, reduction,
         upper limb) 755.29
         meaning all digits (complete)
            (partial) 755.21
         transverse 755.21
   pituitary gland (congenital) 759.2
   postoperative — see Absence, by
      site, acquired
   prostate (congenital) 752.8
      acquired 602.8
   pulmonary
      artery 747.3
      trunk 747.3
      valve (congenital) 746.01
      vein 747.49
   punctum lacrimale (congenital)
      743.65
   radius, congenital (complete)
      (partial) (with absence of
      distal elements, incomplete)
      755.26
      with
         complete absence of distal
            elements 755.21
         ulna 755.25
            with
               complete absence of
                  distal elements
                  755.21
               humerus (incomplete)
                  755.23
   ray, congenital 755.4
      lower limb (complete) (partial)
         (see also Deformity,
         reduction, lower limb)
         755.38
         meaning all rays 755.31
         transverse 755.31
      upper limb (complete) (partial)
         (see also Deformity,
         reduction, upper limb)
         755.28
         meaning all rays 755.21
         transverse 755.21
   rectum (congenital) 751.2
      acquired 569.49
   red cell 284.9
      acquired (secondary) 284.8
      congenital 284.0
      hereditary 284.0
      idiopathic 284.9
   respiratory organ (congenital) NEC
      748.9
   rib (acquired) 738.3
      congenital 756.3
   roof of orbit (congenital) 742.0
   round ligament (congenital) 752.8
   sacrum, congenital 756.13
   salivary gland(s) (congenital)
      750.21
   scapula 755.59
   scrotum, congenital 752.8

Absence—continued
  seminal tract or duct (congenital) 752.8
    acquired 608.89
  septum (congenital) — see also Imperfect, closure, septum
    atrial 745.69
      and ventricular 745.7
    between aorta and pulmonary artery 745.0
    ventricular 745.3
      and atrial 745.7
  sex chromosomes 758.8
  shoulder girdle, congenital (complete) (partial) 755.59
  skin (congenital) 757.39
  skull bone 756.0
    with
      anencephalus 740.0
      encephalocele 742.0
      hydrocephalus 742.3
        with spina bifida (see also Spina bifida) 741.0
      microcephalus 742.1
  spermatic cord (congenital) 752.8
  spinal cord 742.59
  spine, congenital 756.13
  spleen (congenital) 759.0
    acquired 289.59
  sternum, congenital 756.3
  stomach (acquired) (partial) (postoperative) 564.2
    congenital 750.7
  submaxillary gland(s) (congenital) 750.21
  superior vena cava (congenital) 747.49
  tarsal(s), congenital (complete) (partial) (with absence of distal elements, incomplete) (see also Deformity, reduction, lower limb) 755.38
  teeth, tooth (congenital) 520.0
    with abnormal spacing 524.3
    acquired 525.1
      with malocclusion 524.3
  tendon (congenital) 756.81
  testis (congenital) 752.8
    acquired 608.89
  thigh (acquired) 736.89
  thumb (acquired) V49.61 ◆
    congenital 755.29
  thymus gland (congenital) 759.2
  thyroid (gland) (surgical) 246.8
    with hypothyroidism 244.0
    cartilage, congenital 748.3
    congenital 243
  tibia, congenital (complete) (partial) (with absence of distal elements, incomplete) (see also Deformity, reduction, lower limb) 755.36
    with
      complete absence of distal elements 755.31
      fibula 755.35
        with
          complete absence of distal elements 755.31
          femur (incomplete) 755.33
            with complete absence of distal elements 755.31
  toe (acquired) V49.72 ◆
    congenital (complete) (partial) 755.39
      meaning all toes 755.31
      transverse 755.31
    great V49.71 ◆
  tongue (congenital) 750.11

Absence—continued
  tooth, teeth, (congenital) 520.0
    with abnormal spacing 524.3
    acquired 525.1
      with malocclusion 524.3
  trachea (cartilage) (congenital) (rings) 748.3
  transverse aortic arch (congenital) 747.21
  tricuspid valve 746.1
  ulna, congenital (complete) (partial) (with absence of distal elements, incomplete) (see also Deformity, reduction, upper limb) 755.27
    with
      complete absence of distal elements 755.21
      radius 755.25
        with
          complete absence of distal elements 755.21
          humerus (incomplete) 755.23
  umbilical artery (congenital) 747.5
  ureter (congenital) 753.4
    acquired 593.89
  urethra, congenital 753.8
  urinary system, part NEC 753.8
  uterus (acquired) 621.8
    congenital 752.3
  uvula (congenital) 750.26
  vagina, congenital 752.49
  vas deferens (congenital) 752.8
    acquired 608.89
  vein (congenital) (peripheral) NEC (see also Anomaly, peripheral vascular system) 747.60
    brain 747.81
    great 747.49
    portal 747.49
    pulmonary 747.49
  vena cava (congenital) (inferior) (superior) 747.49
  ventral horn cell 742.59
  ventricular septum 745.3
  vermis of cerebellum 742.2
  vertebra, congenital 756.13
  vulva, congenital 752.49
Absentia epileptica (see also Epilepsy) 345.0
Absinthemia (see also Dependence) 304.6
Absinthism (see also Dependence) 304.6
Absorbent system disease 459.89
Absorption
  alcohol, through placenta or breast milk 760.71
  antibiotics, through placenta or breast milk 760.74
  anti-infective, through placenta or breast milk 760.74
  chemical NEC 989.9
    specified chemical or substance — see Table of drugs and chemicals
    through placenta or breast milk (fetus or newborn) 760.70
      alcohol 760.71
      anti-infective agents 760.74
      cocaine 760.75
      "crack" 760.75
      diethylstilbestrol [DES] 760.76 ◆
      hallucinogenic agents 760.73
      medicinal agents NEC 760.79
      narcotics 760.72
      obstetric anesthetic or analgesic drug 763.5
      specified agent NEC 760.79

Absorption—continued
  chemical—continued
    through placenta or breast milk—continued
      suspected, affecting management of pregnancy 655.5
  cocaine, through placenta or breast milk 760.75
  drug NEC (see also Reaction, drug) 995.2
    through placenta or breast milk (fetus or newborn) 760.70
      alcohol 760.71
      anti-infective agents 760.74
      cocaine 760.75
      "crack" 760.75
      diethylstilbestrol [DES] 760.76 ◆
      hallucinogenic agents 760.73
      medicinal agents NEC 760.79
      narcotics 760.72
      obstetric anesthetic or analgesic drug 763.5
      specified agent NEC 760.79
      suspected, affecting management of pregnancy 655.5
  fat, disturbance 579.8
  hallucinogenic agents, through placenta or breast milk 760.73
  immune sera, through placenta or breast milk 760.79
  lactose defect 271.3
  medicinal agents NEC, through placenta or breast milk 760.79
  narcotics, through placenta or breast milk 760.72
  noxious substance, — see Absorption, chemical
  protein, disturbance 579.8
  pus or septic, general — see Septicemia
  quinine, through placenta or breast milk 760.74
  toxic substance, — see Absorption, chemical
  uremic — see Uremia
Abstinence symptoms or syndrome
  alcohol 291.8
  drug 292.0
Abt-Letterer-Siwe syndrome (acute histiocytosis X) (M9722/3) 202.5
Abulia 799.8
Abulomania 301.6
Abuse
  adult NEC 995.81
    as reason for
      couple seeking advice (including offender) V61.1
      non-partner seeking advice (including offender) V62.81 ▲
  alcohol (see also Alcoholism) 303.9
    non-dependent 305.0
  child NEC 995.5
    affecting parent or family (including offender) V61.21 ◆
    as reason for
      family seeking advice (including offender) V61.21
      non-family member seeking advice (including offender) V62.81 ▲

Abuse—continued
  drugs, nondependent 305.9

> Note — Use the following fifth-digit subclassification with category 305:
> 0 unspecified
> 1 continuous
> 2 episodic
> 3 in remission

  amphetamine type 305.7
  antidepressants 305.8
  barbiturates 305.4
  caffeine 305.9
  cannabis 305.2
  cocaine type 305.6
  hallucinogens 305.3
  hashish 305.2
  LSD 305.3
  marijuana 305.2
  mixed 305.9
  morphine type 305.5
  opioid type 305.5
  phencyclidine (PCP) 305.9
  specified NEC 305.9
  tranquilizers 305.4
  specified person other than child 995.81
  spouse 995.81
  tobacco 305.1
Acalcerosis 275.4
Acalcicosis 275.4
Acalculia 784.69
  developmental 315.1
Acanthocheilonemiasis 125.4
Acanthocytosis 272.5
Acanthokeratodermia 701.1
Acantholysis 701.8
  bullosa 757.39
Acanthoma (benign) (M8070/0) — see also Neoplasm, by site, benign
  malignant (M8070/3) — see Neoplasm, by site, malignant
Acanthosis (acquired) (nigricans) 701.2
  adult 701.2
  benign (congenital) 757.39
  congenital 757.39
  glycogenic
    esophagus 530.8 ▲▼
  juvenile 701.2
  tongue 529.8
Acanthrocytosis 272.5
Acapnia 276.3
Acarbia 276.2
Acardia 759.89
Acardiacus amorphus 759.89
Acardiotrophia 429.1
Acardius 759.89
Acariasis 133.9
  sarcoptic 133.0
Acaridiasis 133.9
Acarinosis 133.9
Acariosis 133.9
Acarodermatitis 133.9
  urticarioides 133.9
Acarophobia 300.29
Acatalasemia 277.8
Acatalasia 277.8
Acatamathesia 784.69
Acataphasia 784.5
Acathisia 781.0
  due to drugs 333.99 ◆
Acceleration, accelerated
  atrioventricular conduction 426.7
  idioventricular rhythm 427.89
Accessory (congenital)
  adrenal gland 759.1
  anus 751.5
  appendix 751.5
  atrioventricular conduction 426.7

Accessory—continued
  auditory ossicles 744.04
  auricle (ear) 744.1
  autosome(s) NEC 758.5
    21 or 22 758.0
  biliary duct or passage 751.69
  bladder 753.8
  blood vessels (peripheral)
      (congenital) NEC (see also
      Anomaly, peripheral vascular
      system) 747.60
    cerebral 747.81
    coronary 746.85
  bone NEC 756.9
    foot 755.67
  breast tissue, axilla 757.6
  carpal bones 755.56
  cecum 751.5
  cervix 752.49
  chromosome(s) NEC 758.9
    13-15 758.1
    16-18 758.2
    21 or 22 758.0
    autosome(s) NEC 758.5
    D₁ 758.1
    E₃ 758.2
    G 758.0
    sex 758.8
  coronary artery 746.85
  cusp(s), heart valve NEC 746.89
    pulmonary 746.09
  cystic duct 751.69
  digits 755.00
  ear (auricle) (lobe) 744.1
  endocrine gland NEC 759.2
  external os 752.49
  eyelid 743.62
  eye muscle 743.69
  face bone(s) 756.0
  fallopian tube (fimbria) (ostium)
      752.19
  fingers 755.01
  foreskin 605
  frontonasal process 756.0
  gallbladder 751.69
  genital organ(s)
    female 752.8
      external 752.49
      internal NEC 752.8
    male 752.8
  genitourinary organs NEC 752.8
  heart 746.89
    valve NEC 746.89
      pulmonary 746.09
  hepatic ducts 751.69
  hymen 752.49
  intestine (large) (small) 751.5
  kidney 753.3
  lacrimal canal 743.65
  leaflet, heart valve NEC 746.89
    pulmonary 746.09
  ligament, broad 752.19
  liver (duct) 751.69
  lobule (ear) 744.1
  lung (lobe) 748.69
  muscle 756.82
  navicular of carpus 755.56
  nervous system, part NEC 742.8
  nipple 757.6
  nose 748.1
  organ or site NEC — see Anomaly,
      specified type NEC
  ovary 752.0
  oviduct 752.19
  pancreas 751.7
  parathyroid gland 759.2
  parotid gland (and duct) 750.22
  pituitary gland 759.2
  placental lobe — see Placenta,
      abnormal
  preauricular appendage 744.1
  prepuce 605
  renal arteries (multiple) 747.62
  rib 756.3
    cervical 756.2
  roots (teeth) 520.2
  salivary gland 750.22

Accessory—continued
  sesamoids 755.8
  sinus — see condition
  skin tags 757.39
  spleen 759.0
  sternum 756.3
  submaxillary gland 750.22
  tarsal bones 755.67
  teeth, tooth 520.1
    causing crowding 524.3
  tendon 756.89
  thumb 755.01
  thymus gland 759.2
  thyroid gland 759.2
  toes 755.02
  tongue 750.13
  tragus 744.1
  ureter 753.4
  urethra 753.8
  urinary organ or tract NEC 753.8
  uterus 752.2
  vagina 752.49
  valve, heart NEC 746.89
    pulmonary 746.09
  vertebra 756.19
  vocal cords 748.3
  vulva 752.49
Accident, accidental — see also
    condition
  birth NEC 767.9
  cardiovascular (see also Disease,
      cardiovascular) 429.2
  cerebral (see also Disease,
      cerebrovascular, acute) 436
  cerebrovascular (current) (CVA) (see
      also Disease,
      cerebrovascular, acute) 436
    healed or old — see also
        category 438
      without residuals V12.5
    impending 435.9
    late effect — see category 438
  coronary (see also Infarct,
      myocardium) 410.9
  craniovascular (see also Disease,
      cerebrovascular, acute) 436
  during pregnancy, to mother
    affecting fetus or newborn 760.5
  heart, cardiac (see also Infarct,
      myocardium) 410.9
  intrauterine 779.8
  vascular — see Disease,
      cerebrovascular, acute
Accommodation
  disorder of 367.51
    drug-induced 367.89
    toxic 367.89
  insufficiency of 367.4
  paralysis of 367.51
    hysterical 300.11
  spasm of 367.53
Accouchement — see Delivery
Accreta placenta (without
    hemorrhage) 667.0
  with hemorrhage 666.0
Accretio cordis (nonrheumatic) 423.1
Accretions on teeth 523.6
Accumulation secretion, prostate
    602.8
Acephalia, acephalism, acephaly
    740.0
Acephalic monster 740.0
Acephalobrachia monster 759.89
Acephalocardia 759.89
Acephalocardius 759.89
Acephalochiria 759.89
Acephalochirus monster 759.89
Acephalogaster 759.89
Acephalostomus monster 759.89
Acephalothorax 759.89
Acephalus 740.0
Acetonemia 790.6
  diabetic 250.1
Acetonglycosuria 982.8

Acetonuria 791.6
Achalasia 530.0
  cardia 530.0
  digestive organs congenital NEC
      751.8
  esophagus 530.0
  pelvirectal 751.3
  psychogenic 306.4
  pylorus 750.5
  sphincteral NEC 564.8
Achard-Thiers syndrome
    (adrenogenital) 255.2
Ache(s) — see Pain
Acheilia 750.26
Acheiria 755.21
Achillobursitis 726.71
Achillodynia 726.71
Achlorhydria, achlorhydric 536.0
  anemia 280.9
  diarrhea 536.0
  neurogenic 536.0
  postvagotomy 564.2
  psychogenic 306.4
  secondary to vagotomy 564.2
Achloroblepsia 368.52
Achloropsia 368.52
Acholia 575.8
Acholuric jaundice (familial)
    (splenomegalic) (see also
    Spherocytosis) 282.0
  acquired 283.9
Achondroplasia 756.4
Achrestic anemia 281.8
Achroacytosis, lacrimal gland 375.00
  tuberculous (see also Tuberculosis)
      017.3
Achroma, cutis 709.00 ◆
Achromate (congenital) 368.54
Achromatopia 368.54
Achromatopsia (congenital) 368.54
Achromia
  congenital 270.2
  parasitica 111.0
  unguium 703.8
Achylia
  gastrica 536.8
    neurogenic 536.3 ◆
    psychogenic 306.4
  pancreatica 577.1
Achylosis 536.8
Acid
  burn — see also Burn, by site
    from swallowing acid — see
        Burn, internal organs
  deficiency
    amide nicotinic 265.2
    amino 270.9
    ascorbic 267
    folic 266.2
    nicotinic (amide) 265.2
    pantothenic 266.2
  intoxication 276.2
  peptic disease 536.8
  stomach 536.8
    psychogenic 306.4
Acidemia 276.2
  arginosuccinic 270.6
  fetal — see Distress, fetal
  pipecolic 270.7
Acidity, gastric (high) (low) 536.8
  psychogenic 306.4
Acidocytopenia 288.0
Acidocytosis 288.3
Acidopenia 288.0
Acidosis 276.2
  diabetic 250.1
  fetal — see also Distress, fetal
    affecting management of
        pregnancy 656.3
  intrauterine — see Distress, fetal
  kidney tubular 588.8
  lactic 276.2

Acidosis—continued
  metabolic NEC 276.2
    with respiratory acidosis 276.4
    late, of newborn 775.7
  renal
    hyperchloremic 588.8
    tubular (distal) (proximal) 588.8
  respiratory 276.2
    complicated by
      metabolic acidosis 276.4
      metabolic alkalosis 276.4
Aciduria 791.9
  arginosuccinic 270.6
  beta-aminoisobutyric (BAIB) 277.2
  glycolic 271.8
  organic 270.9
  orotic (congenital) (hereditary)
      (pyrimidine deficiency)
      281.4
Acladiosis 111.8
  skin 111.8
Aclasis
  diaphyseal 756.4
  tarsoepiphyseal 756.59
Acleistocardia 745.5
Aclusion 524.4
Acmesthesia 782.0
Acne (pustular) (vulgaris) 706.1
  agminata (see also Tuberculosis)
      017.0
  artificialis 706.1
  atrophica 706.0
  cachecticorum (Hebra) 706.1
  conglobata 706.1
  conjunctiva 706.1
  cystic 706.1
  decalvans 704.09
  erythematosa 695.3
  eyelid 706.1
  frontalis 706.0
  indurata 706.1
  keloid 706.1
  lupoid 706.0
  necrotic, necrotica 706.0
    miliaris 704.8
  nodular 706.1
  occupational 706.1
  papulosa 706.1
  rodens 706.0
  rosacea 695.3
  scorbutica 267
  scrofulosorum (Bazin) (see also
      Tuberculosis) 017.0
  summer 692.72
  tropical 706.1
  varioliformis 706.0
Acneiform drug eruptions 692.3
Acnitis (primary) (see also
    Tuberculosis) 017.0
Acomia 704.00
Acontractile bladder 344.61
Aconuresis (see also Incontinence)
    788.30
Acosta's disease 993.2
Acousma 780.1
Acoustic — see condition
Acousticophobia 300.29
Acquired — see condition
Acquired immune deficiency
    syndrome — see Human
    immunodeficiency virus
    (disease) (illness) (infection)
Acquired immunodeficiency syndrome
    — see Human
    immunodeficiency virus
    (disease) (illness) (infection)
Acragnosis 781.9
Acrania (monster) 740.0
Acroagnosis 781.9
Acroasphyxia, chronic 443.89
Acrobrachycephaly 756.0
Acrobystiolith 608.89

Acrobystitis

Acrobystitis 607.2
Acrocephalopolysyndactyly 755.55
Acrocephalosyndactyly 755.55
Acrocephaly 756.0
Acrochondrohyperplasia 759.82
Acrocyanosis 443.89
    newborn 770.8
Acrodermatitis 686.8
    atrophicans (chronica) 701.8
    continua (Hallopeau) 696.1
    enteropathica 686.8
    Hallopeau's 696.1
    perstans 696.1
    pustulosa continua 696.1
    recalcitrant pustular 696.1
Acrodynia 985.0
Acrodysplasia 755.55
Acrohyperhidrosis 780.8
Acrokeratosis verruciformis 757.39
Acromastitis 611.0
Acromegaly, acromegalia (skin) 253.0
Acromelalgia 443.89
Acromicria acromikria 756.59
Acronyx 703.0
Acropachy, thyroid (see also Thyrotoxicosis) 242.9
Acropachyderma 757.39
Acroparesthesia 443.89
    simple (Schultz's type) 443.89
    vasomotor (Nothnagel's type) 443.89
Acropathy thyroid (see also Thyrotoxicosis) 242.9
Acrophobia 300.29
Acroposthitis 607.2
Acroscleriasis (see also Scleroderma) 710.1
Acroscleroderma (see also Scleroderma) 710.1
Acrosclerosis (see also Scleroderma) 710.1
Acrosphacelus 785.4
Acrosphenosyndactylia 755.55
Acrospiroma, eccrine (M8402/0) — see Neoplasm, skin, benign
Acrostealgia 732.9
Acrosyndactyly (see also Syndactylism) 755.10
Acrotrophodynia 991.4
Actinic — see also condition
    cheilitis (due to sun) 692.72
        chronic NEC 692.74
        due to radiation, except from sun 692.82
    conjunctivitis 370.24
    dermatitis (due to sun) (see also Dermatitis, actinic 692.70
        due to
            roentgen rays or radioactive substance 692.82
            ultraviolet radiation, except from sun 692.82
            sun NEC 692.70
    elastosis solare 692.74
    granuloma 692.73
    keratitis 370.24
    ophthalmia 370.24
    reticuloid 692.73
Actinobacillosis, general 027.8
Actinobacillus
    lignieresii 027.8
    mallei 024
    muris 026.1
Actinocutitis NEC (see also Dermatitis, actinic) 692.70
Actinodermatitis NEC (see also Dermatitis, actinic) 692.70
Actinomyces
    israelii (infection) — see Actinomycosis
    muris-ratti (infection) 026.1

Actinomycosis, actinomycotic 039.9
    with
        pneumonia 039.1
    abdominal 039.2
    cervicofacial 039.3
    cutaneous 039.0
    pulmonary 039.1
    specified site NEC 039.8
    thoracic 039.1
Actinoneuritis 357.8
Action, heart
    disorder 427.9
        postoperative 997.1
    irregular 427.9
        postoperative 997.1
        psychogenic 306.2
Active — see condition
Activity decrease, functional 780.9
Acute — see also condition
    abdomen NEC 789.0
    gallbladder (see also Cholecystitis, acute) 575.0
Acyanoblepsia 368.53
Acyanopsia 368.53
Acystia 753.8
Acystinervia — see Neurogenic, bladder
Acystineuria — see Neurogenic, bladder
Adactylia, adactyly (congenital) 755.4
    lower limb (complete) (intercalary) (partial) (terminal) (see also Deformity, reduction, lower limb) 755.39
        meaning all digits (complete) (partial) 755.31
        transverse (complete) (partial) 755.31
    upper limb (complete) (intercalary) (partial) (terminal) (see also Deformity, reduction, upper limb) 755.29
        meaning all digits (complete) (partial) 755.21
        transverse (complete) (partial) 755.21
Adair-Dighton syndrome (brittle bones and blue sclera, deafness) 756.51
Adamantinoblastoma (M9310/0) — see Ameloblastoma
Adamantinoma (M9310/0) — see Ameloblastoma
Adamantoblastoma (M9310/0) — see Ameloblastoma
Adams-Stokes (-Morgagni) **disease or syndrome** (syncope with heart block) 426.9
Adaptation reaction (see also Reaction, adjustment) 309.9
Addiction — see also Dependence
    absinthe 304.6
    alcoholic (ethyl) (methyl) (wood) 303.9
        complicating pregnancy, childbirth, or puerperium 648.4
        affecting fetus or newborn 760.71
        suspected damage to fetus affecting management of pregnancy 655.4
    drug (see also Dependence) 304.9
    ethyl alcohol 303.9
    heroin 304.0
    hospital 301.51
    methyl alcohol 303.9
    methylated spirit 303.9
    morphine (-like substances) 304.0
    nicotine 305.1
    opium 304.0
    tobacco 305.1
    wine 303.9

Addison's
    anemia (pernicious) 281.0
    disease (bronze) (primary adrenal insufficiency) 255.4
        tuberculous (see also Tuberculosis) 017.6
    keloid (morphea) 701.0
    melanoderma (adrenal cortical hypofunction) 255.4
Addison-Biermer anemia (pernicious) 281.0
Addison-Gull disease — see Xanthoma
Addisonian crisis or melanosis (acute adrenocortical insufficiency) 255.4
Additional — see also Accessory
    chromosome(s) 758.9
        13-15 758.1
        16-18 758.2
        21 758.0
        autosome(s) NEC 758.5
        sex 758.8
Adduction contracture, hip or other joint — see Contraction, joint
Adenasthenia gastrica 536.0
Aden fever 061
Adenitis (see also Lymphadenitis) 289.3
    acute, unspecified site 683
        epidemic infectious 075
    axillary 289.3
        acute 683
        chronic or subacute 289.1
    Bartholin's gland 616.8
    bulbourethral gland (see also Urethritis) 597.89
    cervical 289.3
        acute 683
        chronic or subacute 289.1
    chancroid (Ducrey's bacillus) 099.0
    chronic (any lymph node, except mesenteric) 289.1
        mesenteric 289.2
    Cowper's gland (see also Urethritis) 597.89
    epidemic, acute 075
    gangrenous 683
    gonorrheal NEC 098.89
    groin 289.3
        acute 683
        chronic or subacute 289.1
    infectious 075
    inguinal (region) 289.3
        acute 683
        chronic or subacute 289.1
    lymph gland or node, except mesenteric 289.3
        acute 683
        chronic or subacute 289.1
        mesenteric (acute) (chronic) (nonspecific) (subacute) 289.2
    mesenteric (acute) (chronic) (nonspecific) (subacute) 289.2
        due to Pasteurella multocida (P. septica) 027.2
    parotid gland (suppurative) 527.2
    phlegmonous 683
    salivary duct or gland (any) (recurring) (suppurative) 527.2
    scrofulous (see also Tuberculosis) 017.2
    septic 289.3
    Skene's duct or gland (see also Urethritis) 597.89
    strumous, tuberculous (see also Tuberculosis) 017.2
    subacute, unspecified site 289.1
    sublingual gland (suppurative) 527.2
    submandibular gland (suppurative) 527.2
    submaxillary gland (suppurative) 527.2

Adenitis—continued
    suppurative 683
    tuberculous — see Tuberculosis, lymph gland
    urethral gland (see also Urethritis) 597.89
    venereal NEC 099.8
    Wharton's duct (suppurative) 527.2
Adenoacanthoma (M8570/3) — see Neoplasm, by site, malignant
Adenoameloblastoma (M9300/0) 213.1
    upper jaw (bone) 213.0
Adenocarcinoma (M8140/3) — see also Neoplasm, by site, malignant

> Note — The list of adjectival modifiers below is not exhaustive. A description of adenocarcinoma that does not appear in this list should be coded in the same manner as carcinoma with that description. Thus, "mixed acidophil-basophil adenocarcinoma," should be coded in the same manner as "mixed acidophil-basophil carcinoma," which appears in the list under "Carcinoma,"
>
> Except where otherwise indicated, the morphological varieties of adenocarcinoma in the list below should be coded by site as for "Neoplasm, malignant."

    with
        apocrine metaplasia (M8573/3)
        cartilaginous (and osseous) metaplasia (M8571/3)
        osseous (and cartilaginous) metaplasia (M8571/3)
        spindle cell metaplasia (M8572/3)
        squamous metaplasia (M8570/3)
    acidophil (M8280/3)
        specified site — see Neoplasm, by site, malignant
        unspecified site 194.3
    acinar (M8550/3)
    acinic cell (M8550/3)
    adrenal cortical (M8370/3) 194.0
    alveolar (M8251/3)
    and
        epidermoid carcinoma, mixed (M8560/3)
        squamous cell carcinoma, mixed (M8560/3)
    apocrine (M8401/3)
        breast — see Neoplasm, breast, malignant
        specified site NEC — see Neoplasm, skin, malignant
        unspecified site 173.9
    basophil (M8300/3)
        specified site — see Neoplasm, by site, malignant
        unspecified site 194.3
    bile duct type (M8160/3)
        liver 155.1
        specified site NEC — see Neoplasm, by site, malignant
        unspecified site 155.1
    bronchiolar (M8250/3) — see Neoplasm, lung, malignant
    ceruminous (M8420/3) 173.2
    chromophobe (M8270/3)
        specified site — see Neoplasm, by site, malignant
        unspecified site 194.3
    clear cell (mesonephroid type) (M8310/3)
    colloid (M8480/3)
    cylindroid type (M8200/3)

Adenocarcinoma—continued
  diffuse type (M8145/3)
    specified site — see Neoplasm, by site, malignant
    unspecified site 151.9
  duct (infiltrating) (M8500/3)
    with Paget's disease (M8541/3) — see Neoplasm, breast, malignant
    specified site — see Neoplasm, by site, malignant
    unspecified site 174.9
  embryonal (M9070/3)
  endometrioid (M8380/3) — see Neoplasm, by site, malignant
  eosinophil (M8280/3)
    specified site — see Neoplasm, by site malignant
    unspecified site 194.3
  follicular (M8330/3)
    and papillary (M8340/3) 193
    moderately differentiated type (M8332/3) 193
    pure follicle type (M8331/3) 193
    specified site — see Neoplasm, by site, malignant
    trabecular type (M8332/3) 193
    unspecified type 193
    well differentiated type (M8331/3) 193
  gelatinous (M8480/3)
  granular cell (M8320/3)
  Hürthle cell (M8290/3) 193
  in
    adenomatous
      polyp (M8210/3)
      polyposis coli (M8220/3) 153.9
    polypoid adenoma (M8210/3)
    tubular adenoma (M8210/3)
    villous adenoma (M8261/3)
  infiltrating duct (M8500/3)
    with Paget's disease (M8541/3) — see Neoplasm, breast, malignant
    specified site — see Neoplasm, by site, malignant
    unspecified site 174.9
  inflammatory (M8530/3)
    specified site — see Neoplasm, by site, malignant
    unspecified site 174.9
  in situ (M8140/2) — see Neoplasm, by site, in situ
  intestinal type (M8144/3)
    specified site — see Neoplasm, by site, malignant
    unspecified site 151.9
  intraductal (noninfiltrating) (M8500/2)
    papillary (M8503/2)
      specified site — see Neoplasm, by site, in situ
      unspecified site 233.0
    specified site — see Neoplasm, by site, in situ
    unspecified site 233.0
  islet cell (M8150/3)
    and exocrine, mixed (M8154/3)
      specified site — see Neoplasm, by site, malignant
      unspecified site 157.9
    pancreas 157.4
    specified site NEC — see Neoplasm, by site, malignant
    unspecified site 157.4
  lobular (M8520/3)
    specified site — see Neoplasm, by site, malignant
    unspecified site 174.9
  medullary (M8510/3)
  mesonephric (M9110/3)
  mixed cell (M8323/3)
  mucinous (M8480/3)

Adenocarcinoma—continued
  mucin-producing (M8481/3)
  mucoid (M8480/3) — see also Neoplasm, by site, malignant
    cell (M8300/3)
      specified site — see Neoplasm, by site, malignant
      unspecified site 194.3
  nonencapsulated sclerosing (M8350/3) 193
  oncocytic (M8290/3)
  oxyphilic (M8290/3)
  papillary (M8260/3)
    and follicular (M8340/3) 193
    intraductal (noninfiltrating) (M8503/2)
      specified site — see Neoplasm, by site, in situ
      unspecified site 233.0
    serous (M8460/3)
      specified site — see Neoplasm, by site, malignant
      unspecified site 183.0
  papillocystic (M8450/3)
    specified site — see Neoplasm, by site, malignant
    unspecified site 183.0
  pseudomucinous (M8470/3)
    specified site — see Neoplasm, by site, malignant
    unspecified site 183.0
  renal cell (M8312/3) 189.0
  sebaceous (M8410/3)
  serous (M8441/3) — see also Neoplasm, by site, malignant
    papillary
      specified site — see Neoplasm, by site malignant
      unspecified site 183.0
  signet ring cell (M8490/3)
  superficial spreading (M8143/3)
  sweat gland (M8400/3) — see Neoplasm, skin, malignant
  trabecular (M8190/3)
  tubular (M8211/3)
  villous (M8262/3)
  water-clear cell (M8322/3) 194.1

Adenofibroma (M9013/0)
  clear cell (M8313/0) — see Neoplasm, by site, benign
  endometrioid (M8381/0) 220
    borderline malignancy (M8381/1) 236.2
    malignant (M8381/3) 183.0
  mucinous (M9015/0)
    specified site — see Neoplasm, by site, benign
    unspecified site 220
  prostate 600
  serous (M9014/0)
    specified site — see Neoplasm, by site, benign
    unspecified site 220
  specified site — see Neoplasm, by site, benign
  unspecified site 220

Adenofibrosis
  breast 610.2
  endometrioid 617.0

Adenoiditis 474.0
  acute 463

Adenoids (congenital) (of nasal fossa) 474.9
  hypertrophy 474.12
  vegetations 474.2

Adenolipomatosis (symmetrical) 272.8

Adenolymphoma (M8561/0)
  specified site — see Neoplasm, by site, benign
  unspecified 210.2

Adenoma (sessile) (M8140/0) — see also Neoplasm, by site, benign

Note — Except where otherwise indicated, the morphological varieties of adenoma in the list below should be coded by site as for "Neoplasm, benign."

  acidophil (M8280/0)
    specified site — see Neoplasm, by site, benign
    unspecified site 227.3
  acinar (cell) (M8550/0)
  acinic cell (M8550/0)
  adrenal (cortex) (cortical) (functioning) (M8370/0) 227.0
    clear cell type (M8373/0) 227.0
    compact cell type (M8371/0) 227.0
    glomerulosa cell type (M8374/0) 227.0
    heavily pigmented variant (M8372/0) 227.0
    mixed cell type (M8375/0) 227.0
  alpha cell (M8152/0)
    pancreas 211.7
    specified site NEC — see Neoplasm, by site, benign
    unspecified site 211.7
  alveolar (M8251/0)
  apocrine (M8401/0)
    breast 217
    specified site NEC — see Neoplasm, skin, benign
    unspecified site 216.9
  basal cell (M8147/0)
  basophil (M8300/0)
    specified site — see Neoplasm, by site, benign
    unspecified site 227.3
  beta cell (M8151/0)
    pancreas 211.7
    specified site NEC — see Neoplasm, by site, benign
    unspecified site 211.7
  bile duct (M8160/0) 211.5
  black (M8372/0) 227.0
  bronchial (M8140/1) 235.7
    carcinoid type (M8240/0) — see Neoplasm, lung, malignant
    cylindroid type (M8200/3) — see Neoplasm, lung, malignant
  ceruminous (M8420/0) 216.2
  chief cell (M8321/0) 227.1
  chromophobe (M8270/0)
    specified site — see Neoplasm, by site, benign
    unspecified site 227.3
  clear cell (M8310/0)
  colloid (M8334/0)
    specified site — see Neoplasm, by site, benign
    unspecifited site 226
  cylindroid type, bronchus (M8200/3) — see Neoplasm, lung, malignant
  duct (M8503/0)
  embryonal (M8191/0)
  endocrine, multiple (M8360/1)
    single specified site — see Neoplasm, by site, uncertain behavior
    two or more specified sites 237.4
    unspecified site 237.4
  endometrioid (M8380/0) — see also Neoplasm, by site, benign
    borderline malignancy (M8380/1) — see Neoplasm, by site, uncertain behavior

Adenoma—continued
  eosinophil (M8280/0)
    specified site — see Neoplasm, by site, benign
    unspecified site 227.3
  fetal (M8333/0)
    specified site — see Neoplasm, by site, benign
    unspecified site 226
  follicular (M8330/0)
    specified site — see Neoplasm, by site, benign
    unspecified site 226
  hepatocellular (M8170/0) 211.5
  Hürthle cell (M8290/0) 226
  intracystic papillary (M8504/0)
  islet cell (functioning) (M8150/0)
    pancreas 211.7
    specified site NEC — see Neoplasm, by site, benign
    unspecified site 211.7
  liver cell (M8170/0) 211.5
  macrofollicular (M8334/0)
    specified site NEC — see Neoplasm, by site, benign
    unspecified site 226
  malignant, malignum (M8140/3) — see Neoplasm, by site, malignant
  mesonephric (M9110/0)
  microfollicular (M8333/0)
    specified site — see Neoplasm, by site, benign
    unspecified site 226
  mixed cell (M8323/0)
  monomorphic (M8146/0)
  mucinous (M8480/0)
  mucoid cell (M8300/0)
    specified site — see Neoplasm, by site, benign
    unspecified site 227.3
  multiple endocrine (M8360/1)
    single specified site — see Neoplasm, by site, uncertain behavior
    two or more specified sites 237.4
    unspecified site 237.4
  nipple (M8506/0) 217
  oncocytic (M8290/0)
  oxyphilic (M8290/0)
  papillary (M8260/0) — see also Neoplasm, by site, benign
    intracystic (M8504/0)
  papillotubular (M8263/0)
  Pick's tubular (M8640/0)
    specified site — see Neoplasm, by site, benign
    unspecified site
      female 220
      male 222.0
  pleomorphic (M8940/0)
  polypoid (M8210/0)
  prostate (benign) 600
  rete cell 222.0
  sebaceous, sebaceum (gland) (senile) (M8410/0) — see also Neoplasm, skin, benign
    disseminata 759.5
  Sertoli cell (M8640/0)
    specified site — see Neoplasm, by site, benign
    unspecified site
      female 220
      male 222.0
  skin appendage (M8390/0) — see Neoplasm, skin, benign
  sudoriferous gland (M8400/0) — see Neoplasm, skin, benign
  sweat gland or duct (M8400/0) — see Neoplasm, skin, benign
  testicular (M8640/0)
    specified site — see Neoplasm, by site, benign
    unspecified site
      female 220
      male 222.0

Adenoma—continued
  thyroid 226
  trabecular (M8190/0)
  tubular (M8211/0) — see also
      Neoplasm, by site, benign
    papillary (M8460/3)
    Pick's (M8640/0)
    specified site — see
        Neoplasm, by site,
        benign
    unspecified site
      female 220
      male 222.0
  tubulovillous (M8263/0)
  villoglandular (M8263/0)
  villous (M8261/1) — see Neoplasm,
      by site, uncertain behavior
  water-clear cell (M8322/0) 227.1
  wolffian duct (M9110/0)
Adenomatosis (M8220/0)
  endocrine (multiple) (M8360/1)
    single specified site — see
        Neoplasm, by site,
        uncertain behavior
    two or more specified sites
        237.4
    unspecified site 237.4
  erosive of nipple (M8506/0) 217
  pluriendocrine — see
      Adenomatosis, endocrine
  pulmonary (M8250/1) 235.7
    malignant (M8250/3) — see
        Neoplasm, lung,
        malignant
  specified site — see Neoplasm, by
      site, benign
  unspecified site 211.3
Adenomatous
  cyst, thyroid (gland) — see Goiter,
      nodular
  goiter (nontoxic) (see also Goiter,
      nodular) 241.9
    toxic or with hyperthyroidism
        242.3
Adenomyoma (M8932/0) — see also
    Neoplasm, by site, benign
  prostate 600
Adenomyometritis 617.0
Adenomyosis (uterus) (internal) 617.0
Adenopathy (lymph gland) 785.6
  inguinal 785.6
  mediastinal 785.6
  mesentery 785.6
  syphilitic (secondary) 091.4
  tracheobronchial 785.6
    tuberculous (see also
        Tuberculosis) 012.1
      primary, progressive 010.8
    tuberculous (see also Tuberculosis,
        lymph gland) 017.2
      tracheobronchial 012.1
        primary, progressive 010.8
Adenopharyngitis 462
Adenophlegmon 683
Adenosalpingitis 614.1
Adenosarcoma (M8960/3) 189.0
Adenosclerosis 289.3
Adenosis
  breast (sclerosing) 610.2
  vagina, congenital 752.49
Adentia (complete) (partial) (see also
    Absence, teeth) 520.0
Adherent
  labium (minus) 624.4
  pericardium (nonrheumatic) 423.1
    rheumatic 393
  placenta 667.0
    with hemorrhage 666.0
  prepuce 605
  scar (skin) NEC 709.2
  tendon in scar 709.2

Adhesion(s), adhesive (postinfectional)
  abdominal (wall) (see also
      Adhesions, peritoneum)
      568.0
  amnion to fetus 658.8
    affecting fetus or newborn 762.8
  appendix 543.9
  arachnoiditis — see Meningitis
  auditory tube (Eustachian) 381.89
  bands — see also Adhesions,
      peritoneum
    cervix 622.3
    uterus 621.5
  bile duct (any) 576.8
  bladder (sphincter) 596.8
  bowel (see also Adhesions,
      peritoneum) 568.0
  cardiac 423.1
    rheumatic 398.99
  cecum (see also Adhesions,
      peritoneum) 568.0
  cervicovaginal 622.3
    congenital 752.49
    postpartal 674.8
      old 622.3
  cervix 622.3
  clitoris 624.4
  colon (see also Adhesions,
      peritoneum) 568.0
  common duct 576.8
  congenital — see also Anomaly,
      specified type NEC
    fingers (see also Syndactylism,
        fingers) 755.11
    labium (majus) (minus) 752.49
    omental, anomalous 751.4
    ovary 752.0
    peritoneal 751.4
    toes (see also Syndactylism,
        toes) 755.13
    tongue (to gum or roof of
        mouth) 750.12
  conjunctiva (acquired) (localized)
      372.62
    congenital 743.63
    extensive 372.63
  cornea — see Opacity, cornea
  cystic duct 575.8
  diaphragm (see also Adhesions,
      peritoneum) 568.0
  due to foreign body — see Foreign
      body
  duodenum (see also Adhesions,
      peritoneum) 568.0
    with obstruction 537.3
  ear, middle — see Adhesions,
      middle ear
  epididymis 608.89
  epidural — see Adhesions,
      meninges
  epiglottis 478.79
  Eustachian tube 381.89
  eyelid 374.46
    postoperative 997.9
    surgically created V45.6
  gallbladder (see also Disease,
      gallbladder) 575.8
  globe 360.89
  heart 423.1
    rheumatic 398.99
  ileocecal (coil) (see also Adhesions,
      peritoneum) 568.0
  ileum (see also Adhesions,
      peritoneum) 568.0
  intestine (postoperative) (see also
      Adhesions, peritoneum)
      568.0
    with obstruction 560.81
      with hernia — see also
          Hernia, by site, with
          obstruction
        gangrenous — see
            Hernia, by site,
            with gangrene
  intra-abdominal (see also
      Adhesions, peritoneum)
      568.0

Adhesion(s)—continued
  iris 364.70
    to corneal graft 996.79
  joint (see also Ankylosis) 718.5
  kidney 593.89
  labium (majus) (minus), congenital
      752.49
  liver 572.8
  lung 511.0
  mediastinum 519.3
  meninges 349.2
    cerebral (any) 349.2
      congenital 742.4
    congenital 742.8
    spinal (any) 349.2
      congenital 742.59
    tuberculous (cerebral) (spinal)
        (see also Tuberculosis,
        meninges) 013.0
  mesenteric (see also Adhesions,
      peritoneum) 568.0
  middle ear (fibrous) 385.10
    drum head 385.19
      to
        incus 385.11
        promontorium 385.13
        stapes 385.12
    specified NEC 385.19
  nasal (septum) (to turbinates) 478.1
  nerve NEC 355.9
    spinal 355.9
      root 724.9
        cervical NEC 723.4
        lumbar NEC 724.4
        lumbosacral 724.4
        thoracic 724.4
  ocular muscle 378.60
  omentum (see also Adhesions,
      peritoneum) 568.0
  organ or site, congenital NEC —
      see Anomaly, specified type
      NEC
  ovary 614.6
    congenital (to cecum, kidney, or
        omentum) 752.0
  parauterine 614.6
  parovarian 614.6
  pelvic (peritoneal)
    female 614.6
    male (see also Adhesions,
        peritoneum) 568.0
    postpartal (old) 614.6
    tuberculous (see also
        Tuberculosis) 016.9
  penis to scrotum (congenital) 752.8
  periappendiceal (see also
      Adhesions, peritoneum)
      568.0
  pericardium (nonrheumatic) 423.1
    rheumatic 393
    tuberculous (see also
        Tuberculosis) 017.9
        [420.0]
  pericholecystic 575.8
  perigastric (see also Adhesions,
      peritoneum) 568.0
  periovarian 614.6
  periprostatic 602.8
  perirectal (see also Adhesions,
      peritoneum) 568.0
  perirenal 593.89
  peritoneum, peritoneal (fibrous)
      (postoperative) 568.0
    with obstruction (intestinal)
        560.81
      with hernia — see also
          Hernia, by site, with
          obstruction
        gangrenous — see
            Hernia, by site,
            with gangrene
        duodenum 537.3
    congenital 751.4
    pelvic, female 614.6
    postpartal, pelvic 614.6
    to uterus 614.6
  peritubal 614.6

Adhesion(s)—continued
  periureteral 593.89
  periuterine 621.5
  perivesical 596.8
  perivesicular (seminal vesicle)
      608.89
  pleura, pleuritic 511.0
    tuberculous (see also
        Tuberculosis, pleura)
        012.0
  pleuropericardial 511.0
  postoperative (gastrointestinal tract)
      (see also Adhesions,
      peritoneum) 568.0
    eyelid 997.9
    surgically created V45.6
    urethra 598.2
  postpartal, old 624.4
  preputial, prepuce 605
  pulmonary 511.0
  pylorus (see also Adhesions,
      peritoneum) 568.0
  Rosenmüller's fossa 478.29
  sciatic nerve 355.0
  seminal vesicle 608.89
  shoulder (joint) 726.0
  sigmoid flexure (see also
      Adhesions, peritoneum)
      568.0
  spermatic cord (acquired) 608.89
    congenital 752.8
  spinal canal 349.2
    nerve 355.9
      root 724.9
        cervical NEC 723.4
        lumbar NEC 724.4
        lumbosacral 724.4
        thoracic 724.4
  stomach (see also Adhesions,
      peritoneum) 568.0
  subscapular 726.2
  tendonitis 726.90
    shoulder 726.0
  testicle 608.89
  tongue (congenital) (to gum or roof
      of mouth) 750.12
    acquired 529.8
  trachea 519.1
  tubo-ovarian 614.6
  tunica vaginalis 608.89
  ureter 593.89
  uterus 621.5
    to abdominal wall 621.5
    in pregnancy or childbirth
        654.4
      affecting fetus or newborn
          763.8
  vagina (chronic) (postoperative)
      (postradiation) 623.2
  vaginitis (congenital) 752.49
  vesical 596.8
  vitreous 379.29
Adie (-Holmes) syndrome (tonic
    pupillary reaction) 379.46
Adiponecrosis neonatorum 778.1
Adiposa dolorosa 272.8
Adiposalgia 272.8
Adiposis 278.0
  cerebralis 253.8
  dolorosa 272.8
  tuberosa simplex 272.8
Adiposity 278.0
  heart (see also Degeneration,
      myocardial) 429.1
  localized 278.1
Adiposogenital dystrophy 253.8
Adjustment
  prosthesis or other device — see
      Fitting of
  reaction — see Reaction,
      adjustment
Administration, prophylactic
  antibiotics V07.39
  antitoxin, any V07.2
  antivenin V07.2

Administration, prophylactic
—*continued*
 chemotherapeutic agent NEC
  V07.39 ▼
 chemotherapy V07.39 ▲
 diphtheria antitoxin V07.2
 fluoride V07.31 ◆
 gamma globulin V07.2
 immune sera (gamma globulin)
  V07.2
 passive immunization agent V07.2
 RhoGAM V07.2

Admission (encounter)
 as organ donor — *see* Donor
 by mistake V68.9
 for
  adjustment (of)
   artificial
    arm (complete) (partial)
     V52.0
    eye V52.2
    leg (complete) (partial)
     V52.1
   brain neuropacemaker V53.0
   breast
    implant V50.1
    prosthesis V52.4
   cardiac device V53.39 ▼
    defibrillator, automatic
     implantable
      V53.32
    pacemaker V53.31
     carotid sinus V53.39 ▲
   colostomy belt V53.5
   contact lenses V53.1
   cystostomy device V53.6
   dental prosthesis V52.3
   device NEC V53.9
    abdominal V53.5
    cardiac V53.39 ▼
     defibrillator, automatic
      implantable
       V53.32
     pacemaker V53.31
      carotid sinus
       V53.39 ▲
    intrauterine contraceptive
     V25.1
    nervous system V53.0
    orthodontic V53.4
    prosthetic V52.9
     breast V52.4
     dental V52.3
     eye V52.2
     specified type NEC
      V52.8
    special senses V53.0
    substitution
     auditory V53.0
     nervous system V53.0
     visual V53.0
    urinary V53.6
   diaphragm (contraceptive)
    V25.02
   hearing aid V53.2
   ileostomy device V53.5
   intestinal appliance or
    device NEC V53.5
   intrauterine contraceptive
    device V25.1
   neuropacemaker (brain)
    (peripheral nerve)
    (spinal cord) V53.0
   orthodontic device V53.4
   orthopedic (device) V53.7
    brace V53.7
    cast V53.7
    shoes V53.7
   pacemaker
    brain V53.0
    cardiac V53.31 ▼
     carotid sinus V53.39 ▲
    peripheral nerve V53.0
    spinal cord V53.0

Admission—*continued*
 for—*continued*
  adjustment (of)—*continued*
   prosthesis V52.9
    arm (complete) (partial)
     V52.0
    breast V52.4
    dental V52.3
    eye V52.2
    leg (complete) (partial)
     V52.1
    specified type NEC V52.8
   spectacles V53.1
   wheelchair V53.8
  adoption referral or proceedings
   V68.89
  aftercare (*see also* Aftercare)
   V58.9
   cardiac pacemaker V53.31 ◆
   chemotherapy V58.1
   dialysis
    extracorporeal (renal)
     V56.0
    peritoneal V56.8
    renal V56.0
   fracture (*see also* Aftercare,
    fracture) V54.9
    specified type NEC V54.8
   medical NEC V58.8
   orthopedic V54.9
    specified type NEC V54.8
   pacemaker device
    brain V53.0
    cardiac V53.31 ▼
     carotid sinus V53.39 ▲
    nervous system V53.0
    spinal cord V53.0
   postoperative NEC V58.49 ▼
    wound closure, planned
     V58.41 ▲
   postpartum
    immediately after delivery
     V24.0
    routine follow-up V24.2
   postradiation V58.0
   radiation therapy V58.0
   specified NEC V58.89 ▼
    removal of vascular
     catheter V58.81
   surgical NEC V58.49
    wound closure, planned
     V58.41 ▲
  artificial insemination V26.1
  attention to artificial opening
   (of) V55.9
   artificial vagina V55.7
   colostomy V55.3
   cystostomy V55.5
   enterostomy V55.4
   gastrostomy V55.1
   ileostomy V55.2
   jejunostomy V55.4
   nephrostomy V55.6
   specified site NEC V55.8
    intestinal tract V55.4
    urinary tract V55.6
   tracheostomy V55.0
   ureterostomy V55.6
   urethrostomy V55.6
  battery replacement ▼
   cardiac pacemaker V53.31 ▲
  boarding V65.0
  breast ▼
   augmentation or reduction
    V50.1
   removal, prophylactic
    V50.41 ▲
  change of
   cardiac pacemaker (battery)
    V53.31 ▼
   carotid sinus pacemaker
    V53.39 ▲
   catheter in artificial opening
    — *see* Attention to,
    artificial, opening
   dressing V58.3

Admission—*continued*
 for—*continued*
  change of—*continued*
   fixation device
    external V54.8
    internal V54.0
    Kirschner wire V54.8
   neuropacemaker device
    (brain) (peripheral
    nerve) (spinal cord)
    V53.0
   pacemaker device
    brain V53.0
    cardiac V53.31 ▼
    carotid sinus V53.39 ▲
    nervous system V53.0
   plaster cast V54.8
   splint, external V54.8
   Steinmann pin V54.8
   surgical dressing V58.3
   traction device V54.8
  checkup only V70.0
  chemotherapy V58.1
  circumcision, ritual or routine
   (in absence of medical
   indication) V50.2
  clinical research investigation
   V70.7
  closure of artificial opening —
   see Attention to, artificial,
   opening
  contraceptive
   counseling V25.09
   management V25.9
    specified type NEC V25.8
  convalescence following V66.9
   chemotherapy V66.2
   psychotherapy V66.3
   radiotherapy V66.1
   surgery V66.0
   treatment (for) V66.5
    combined V66.6
    fracture V66.4
    mental disorder NEC
     V66.3
    specified condition NEC
     V66.5
  cosmetic surgery NEC V50.1
   following healed injury or
    operation V51
  counseling (*see also* Counseling)
   V65.40 ▼
   without complaint or
    sickness V65.49 ▲
   contraceptive management
    V25.09
   dietary V65.3
   excercise V65.41 ◆
   for nonattending third party
    V65.1
   genetic V26.3
   gonorrhea V65.45 ▼
   HIV V65.44
   human immunodeficiency
    virus V65.44
   injury prevention V65.43 ▲
   procreative management
    V26.4
   sexually transmitted disease
    NEC V65.45 ▼
    HIV V65.44
   specified reason NEC V65.49
   substance use and abuse
    V65.42
   syphilis V65.45 ▲
  desensitization to allergens
   V07.1
  dialysis
   extracorporeal (renal) V56.0
   peritoneal V56.8
   renal V56.0
  dietary surveillance and
   counseling V65.3
  ear piercing V50.3

Admission—*continued*
 for—*continued*
  elective surgery V50.9
   breast ▼
    augmentation or
     reduction V50.1
    removal, prophylactic
     V50.41 ▲
   circumcision, ritual or
    routine (in absence of
    medical indication)
    V50.2
   cosmetic NEC V50.1
    following healed injury or
     operation V51
   ear piercing V50.3
   face-lift V50.1
   hair transplant V50.0
   plastic
    cosmetic NEC V50.1
    following healed injury or
     operation V51
   prophylactic organ removal
    V50.49 ▼
    breast V50.41
    ovary V50.42 ▲
   repair of scarred tissue
    (following healed
    injury or operation)
    V51
   specified type NEC V50.8
  examination (*see also*
   Examination) V70.9
   administrative purpose NEC
    V70.3
   adoption V70.3
   allergy V72.7
   at health care facility V70.0
   athletic team V70.3
   camp V70.3
   cardiovascular, preoperative
    V72.81
   clinical research
    investigation V70.7
   dental V72.2
   developmental testing (child)
    (infant) V20.2
   donor (potential) V70.8
   driver's license V70.3
   ear V72.1
   employment V70.5
   eye V72.0
   follow-up (routine) — *see*
    Examination, follow-
    up
   for admission to
    old age home V70.3
    school V70.3
   general V70.9
    specified reason NEC
     V70.8
   gynecological V72.3
   health supervision (child)
    (infant) V20.2
   hearing V72.1
   immigration V70.3
   insurance certification V70.3
   laboratory V72.6
   marriage license V70.3
   medical (general) (*see also*
    Examination, medical)
    V70.9
   medicolegal reasons V70.4
   naturalization V70.3
   pelvic (annual) (periodic)
    V72.3
   postpartum checkup V24.2
   pregnancy (possible)
    (unconfirmed) V72.4
   preoperative V72.84
    cardiovascular V72.81
    respiratory V72.82
    specified NEC V72.83
   prison V70.3
   psychiatric (general) V70.2
    requested by authority
     V70.1

Admission—continued
  for—continued
    examination—continued
      radiological NEC V72.5
      respiratory, preoperative
        V72.82
      school V70.3
      screening — see Screening
      skin hypersensitivity V72.7
      specified type NEC V72.85◆
      sport competition V70.3
      vision V72.0
      well baby and child care
        V20.2
    exercise therapy V57.1
    face-lift, cosmetic reason V50.1
    fitting (of)
      artificial
        arm (complete) (partial)
          V52.0
        eye V52.2
        leg (complete) (partial)
          V52.1
      brain neuropacemaker V53.0
      breast V52.4
        implant V50.1
        prosthesis V52.4
      cardiac pacemaker V53.31◆
      colostomy belt V53.5
      contact lenses V53.1
      cystostomy device V53.6
      dental prosthesis V52.3
      device NEC V53.9
        abdominal V53.5
        intrauterine contraceptive
          V25.1
        nervous system V53.0
        orthodontic V53.4
        prosthetic V52.9
          breast V52.4
          dental V52.3
          eye V52.2
        special senses V53.0
        substitution
          auditory V53.0
          nervous system V53.0
          visual V53.0
      diaphragm (contraceptive)
        V25.02
      hearing aid V53.2
      ileostomy device V53.5
      intestinal appliance or device
        NEC V53.5
      intrauterine contraceptive
        device V25.1
      neuropacemaker (brain)
        (peripheral nerve)
        (spinal cord) V53.0
      orthodontic device V53.4
      orthopedic (device) V53.7
        brace V53.7
        cast V53.7
        shoes V53.7
      pacemaker
        brain V53.0
        cardiac V53.31 ▼
        carotid sinus V53.39 ▲
        spinal cord V53.0
      prosthesis V52.9
        arm (complete) (partial)
          V52.0
        breast V52.4
        dental V52.3
        eye V52.2
        leg (complete) (partial)
          V52.1
        specified type NEC V52.8
      spectacles V53.1
      wheelchair V53.8
    follow-up examination (routine)
      (following) V67.9
      cancer chemotherapy V67.2
      chemotherapy V67.2
      high-risk medication NEC
        V67.51
      injury NEC V67.59
      psychiatric V67.3

Admission—continued
  for—continued
    follow-up examination—
      continued
      psychotherapy V67.3
      radiotherapy V67.1
      surgery V67.0
      treatment (for) V67.9
        combined V67.6
        fracture V67.4
        involving high-risk
          medication NEC
          V67.51
        mental disorder V67.3
        specified NEC V67.59
    hair transplant, for cosmetic
      reason V50.0
    health advice, education, or
      instruction V65.4
    insertion (of)
      subdermal implantable
        contraceptive V25.5
    intrauterine device
      insertion V25.1
      management V25.42
    investigation to determine
      further disposition V63.8
    isolation V07.0
    issue of
      medical certificate NEC
        V68.0
      repeat prescription NEC
        V68.1
        contraceptive device NEC
          V25.49
    kidney dialysis V56.0
    mental health evaluation V70.2
      requested by authority V70.1
    nonmedical reason NEC V68.89
    nursing care evaluation V63.8
    observation (without need for
      further medical care) (see
      also Observation) V71.9
      accident V71.4
      alleged rape or seduction
        V71.5
      criminal assault V71.6
      following accident V71.4
        at work V71.3
      foreign body ingestion V71.8
      growth and development
        variations, childhood
        V21.0
      inflicted injury NEC V71.6
      ingestion of deleterious agent
        or foreign body V71.8
      injury V71.6
      malignant neoplasm V71.1
      mental disorder V71.09
      newborn — see Observation,
        suspected, condition,
        newborn
      rape V71.5
      specified NEC V71.8
      suspected disorder V71.9
        accident V71.4
        at work V71.3
        benign neoplasm V71.8
        cardiovascular V71.7
        heart V71.7
        inflicted injury NEC
          V71.6
        malignant neoplasm
          V71.1
        mental NEC V71.09
        specified condition NEC
          V71.8
        tuberculosis V71.2
      tuberculosis V71.2
    occupational therapy V57.21 ◆
    organ transplant, donor — see
      Donor
    ovary, ovarian removal,
      prophylactic V50.42 ◆

Admission—continued
  for—continued
    Papanicolaou smear, cervix
      V76.2
      for suspected malignant
        neoplasm V76.2
      no disease found V71.1
      routine, as part of
        gynecological
        examination V72.3
    passage of sounds or bougie in
      artificial opening — see
      Attention to, artificial,
      opening
    peritoneal dialysis V56.8
    physical therapy NEC V57.1
    plastic surgery
      cosmetic NEC V50.1
      following healed injury or
        operation V51
    postmenopausal hormone
      replacement therapy
      V07.4
    postpartum observation
      immediately after delivery
        V24.0
      routine follow-up V24.2
    poststerilization (for restoration)
      V26.0
    procreative management V26.9
      specified type NEC V26.8
    prophylactic
      administration of
        antibiotics V07.39 ◆
        antitoxin, any V07.2
        antivenin V07.2
        chemotherapeutic agent
          NEC V07.39 ▼
        chemotherapy NEC
          V07.39 ▲
        diphtheria antitoxin
          V07.2
        fluoride V07.31 ◆
        gamma globulin V07.2
        immune sera (gamma
          globulin) V07.2
        RhoGAM V07.2
        tetanus antitoxin V07.2
      breathing exercises V57.0
      chemotherapy NEC
        V07.39 ▼
        fluoride V07.31 ▲
      measure V07.9
        specified type NEC V07.8
      organ removal V50.49 ▼
        breast V50.41
        ovary V50.42 ▲
    psychiatric examination
      (general) V70.2
      requested by authority V70.1
    radiation management V58.0
    radiotherapy V58.0
    reforming of artificial opening
      — see Attention to,
      artificial, opening
    rehabilitation V57.9
      multiple types V57.89 ▼
      occupational V57.21 ▲
      orthoptic V57.4
      orthotic V57.81
      physical NEC V57.1
      specified type NEC V57.89
      speech V57.3
      vocational V57.22 ◆
    removal of
      cardiac pacemaker V53.31◆
      cast (plaster) V54.8
      catheter from artificial
        opening — see
        Attention to, artificial,
        opening
      cystostomy catheter V55.5
      device
        fixation
          external V54.8
          internal V54.0

Admission—continued
  for—continued
    removal of—continued
      device—continued
        intrauterine contraceptive
          V25.42
      traction, external V54.8
      dressing V58.3
      fixation device
        external V54.8
        internal V54.0
      intrauterine contraceptive
        device V25.42
      Kirschner wire V54.8
      neuropacemaker (brain)
        (peripheral nerve)
        (spinal cord) V53.0
      orthopedic fixation device
        external V54.8
        internal V54.0
      pacemaker device
        brain V53.0
        cardiac V53.31 ▼
        carotid sinus V53.39 ▲
        nervous system V53.0
      plaster cast V54.8
      plate (fracture) V54.0
      rod V54.0
      screw (fracture) V54.0
      splint, traction V54.8
      Steinmann pin V54.8
      subdermal implantable
        contraceptive V25.43
      surgical dressing V58.3
      sutures V58.3
      traction device, external
        V54.8
      ureteral stent V53.6 ◆
    repair of scarred tissue
      (following healed injury
      or operation) V51
    reprogramming of cardiac
      pacemaker V53.3
    restoration of organ continuity
      (poststerilization)
      (tuboplasty) (vasoplasty)
      V26.0
    sensitivity test — see also Test,
      skin
      allergy NEC V72.7
      bacterial disease NEC V74.9
      Dick V74.8
      Kveim V82.8
      Mantoux V74.1
      mycotic infection NEC V75.4
      parasitic disease NEC V75.8
      Schick V74.3
      Schultz-Charlton V74.8
    social service (agency) referral
      or evaluation V63.8
    speech therapy V57.3
    sterilization V25.2
    suspected disorder (ruled out)
      (without need for further
      care) — see Observation
    tests only — see Test
    therapy
      blood transfusion, without
        reported diagnosis
        V58.2
      breathing exercises V57.0
      chemotherapy V58.1
        prophylactic NEC
          V07.39 ▼
          fluoride V07.31 ▲
      dialysis (intermittent)
        (treatment)
        extracorporeal V56.0
        peritoneal V56.8
        renal V56.0
        specified type NEC V56.8
      exercise (remedial) NEC
        V57.1
        breathing V57.0
      occupational V57.21 ◆
      orthoptic V57.4
      physical NEC V57.1

Admission—continued
  for—continued
    therapy—continued
      radiation V58.0
      speech V57.3
      vocational V57.22 ◆
    toilet or cleaning of artificial
      opening — see Attention
      to, artificial, opening
    tubal ligation V25.2
    tuboplasty for previous
      sterilization V26.0
    vaccination, prophylactic
      (against)
      arthropod-borne virus, viral
        NEC V05.1
        disease NEC V05.1
        encephalitis V05.0
      Bacille Calmette Guérin
        (BCG) V03.2
      BCG V03.2
      chickenpox V05.4
      cholera alone V03.0
        with typhoid-paratyphoid
          (cholera + TAB)
          V06.0
      common cold V04.7
      dengue V05.1
      diphtheria alone V03.5
      diphtheria-tetanus [Td]
        without pertussis
          V06.5 ◆
      diphtheria-tetanus-pertussis
        (DTP) V06.1
        with
          poliomyelitis (DTP +
            polio) V06.3
          typhoid-paratyphoid
            (DTP + TAB)
            V06.2
      disease (single) NEC V05.9
        bacterial NEC V03.9
          specified type NEC
            V03.89 ◆
        combinations NEC V06.9
          specified type NEC
            V06.8
        specified type NEC V05.8
      encephalitis, viral,
        arthropod-borne
        V05.0
      Hemophilus infuenzae, type
        B [Hib] V03.81 ◆
      hepatitis, viral V05.3
      immune sera (gamma
        globulin) V07.2
      influenza V04.8
        with ▼
          Streptococcus
            pneumoniae
            [pneumococcus]
            V06.6 ▲
      Leishmaniasis V05.2
      measles alone V04.2
      measles-mumps-rubella
        (MMR) V06.4
      mumps alone V04.6
        with measles and rubella
          (MMR) V06.4
      not done because of
        contraindication
        V64.0
      pertussis alone V03.6
      plague V03.3
      poliomyelitis V04.0
        with diphtheria-tetanus-
          pertussis (DTP+
          polio) V06.3
      rabies V04.5
      rubella alone V04.3
        with measles and mumps
          (MMR) V06.4
      smallpox V04.1
      specified type NEC V05.8

Admission—continued
  for—continued
    vaccination, prophylactic—
      continued
      Streptococcus pneumoniae
        [pneumococcus]
        V03.82 ▼
        with
          influenza V06.6 ▲
          tetanus toxoid alone V03.7
            with diphtheria [Td]
              V06.5 ◆
              and pertussis (DTP)
                V06.1 ▲
      tuberculosis (BCG) V03.2
      tularemia V03.4
      typhoid alone V03.1
        with diphtheria-tetanus-
          pertussis (TAB +
          DTP) V06.2
      typhoid-paratyphoid alone
        (TAB) V03.1
      typhus V05.8
      varicella V05.4
      viral encephalitis, arthropod-
        borne V05.0
      viral hepatitis V05.3
      yellow fever V04.4
    vasectomy V25.2
    vasoplasty for previous
      sterilization V26.0
    vision examination V72.0
    vocational therapy V57.22 ◆
    waiting period for admission to
      other facility V63.2
    undergoing social agency
      investigation V63.8
    well baby and child care V20.2
    x-ray of chest
      for suspected tuberculosis
        V71.2
      routine V72.5
Adnexitis (suppurative) (see also
  Salpingooophoritis) 614.2
Adolescence NEC V21.2
Adoption
  agency referral V68.89
  examination V70.3
  held for V68.89
Adrenal gland — see condition
Adrenalism 255.9
  tuberculous (see also Tuberculosis)
    017.6
Adrenalitis, adrenitis 255.8
  meningococcal hemorrhagic 036.3
Adrenarche, precocious 259.1
Adrenocortical syndrome 255.2
Adrenogenital syndrome (acquired)
  (congenital) 255.2
  iatrogenic, fetus or newborn 760.79
Adventitious bursa — see Bursitis
Adynamia (episodica) (hereditary)
  (periodic) 359.3
Adynamic ileus or intestine (see also
  Ileus) 560.1
Aeration lung, imperfect, newborn
  770.5
Aerobullosis 993.3
Aerocele — see Embolism, air
Aerodermectasia
  subcutaneous (traumatic) 958.7
    surgical 998.81 ▼
    surgical 998.81 ▲
Aerodontalgia 993.2
Aeroembolism 993.3
Aerogenes capsulatus infection (see
  also Gangrene, gas) 040.0
Aero-otitis media 993.0
Aerophagy, aerophagia 306.4
  psychogenic 306.4
Aerosinusitis 993.1
Aerotitis 993.0

Affection, affections — see also
  Disease
  sacroiliac (joint), old 724.6
  shoulder region NEC 726.2
Afibrinogenemia 286.3
  acquired 286.6
  congenital 286.3
  postpartum 666.3
African
  sleeping sickness 086.5
  tick fever 087.1
  trypanosomiasis 086.5
    Gambian 086.3
    Rhodesian 086.4
Aftercare V58.9
  artificial openings — see Attention
    to, artificial, opening
  blood transfusion without reported
    diagnosis V58.2
  breathing exercise V57.0
  cardiac device V53.39 ▼
    defibrillator, automatic
      implantable V53.32
    pacemaker V53.31
      carotid sinus V53.39
  carotid sinus pacemaker V53.39 ▲
  chemotherapy session (adjunctive)
    (maintenance) V58.1
  defibrillator, automatic implantable
    cardiac V53.32 ◆
  exercise (remedial) (therapeutic)
    V57.1
    breathing V57.0
  extracorporeal dialysis (intermittent)
    (treatment) V56.0
  following surgery NEC V58.49 ▼
    wound closure, planned
      V58.41 ▲
  fracture V54.9
    removal of
      external fixation device
        V54.8
      internal fixation device
        V54.0
    specified care NEC V54.8
  gait training V57.1
    for use of artificial limb(s)
      V57.81
  involving
    dialysis (intermittent) (treatment)
      extracorporeal V56.0
      peritoneal V56.8
      renal V56.0
    gait training V57.1
      for use of artificial limb(s)
        V57.81
    orthoptic training V57.4
    orthotic training V57.81
    radiotherapy session V58.0
  removal of
    dressings V58.3
    fixation device
      external V54.8
      internal V54.0
      fracture plate V54.0
      pins V54.0
      plaster cast V54.8
      rods V54.0
      screws V54.0
    surgical dressings V58.3
    sutures V58.3
    traction device, external
      V54.8
  neuropacemaker (brain) (peripheral
    nerve) (spinal cord) V53.0
  occupational therapy V57.21 ◆
  orthodontic V58.5
  orthopedic V54.9
    change of external fixation or
      traction device V54.8
    removal of fixation device
      external V54.8
      internal V54.0
    specified care NEC V54.8
  orthoptic training V57.4
  orthotic training V57.81

Aftercare—continued
  pacemaker
    brain V53.0
    cardiac V53.31 ▼
    carotid sinus V53.39 ▲
    peripheral nerve V53.0
    spinal cord V53.0
  peritoneal dialysis (intermittent)
    (treatment) V56.8
  physical therapy NEC V57.1
    breathing exercises V57.0
  radiotherapy session V58.0
  rehabilitation procedure V57.9
    breathing exercises V57.0
    multiple types V57.89 ▼
    occupational V57.21 ▲
    orthoptic V57.4
    orthotic V57.81
    physical therapy NEC V57.1
    remedial exercises V57.1
    specified type NEC V57.89
    speech V57.3
    therapeutic exercises V57.1
    vocational V57.22 ◆
  renal dialysis (intermittent)
    (treatment) V56.0
  specified type NEC V58.89 ▼
    removal of vascular catheter
      V58.81 ▲
  speech therapy V57.3
  vocational rehabilitation V57.22 ◆
After-cataract 366.50
  obscuring vision 366.53
  specified type, not obscuring vision
    366.52
Agalactia 676.4
Agammaglobulinemia 279.00
  with lymphopenia 279.2
  acquired (primary) (secondary)
    279.06
  Bruton's X-linked 279.04
  infantile sex-linked (Bruton's)
    (congenital) 279.04
  Swiss-type 279.2
Aganglionosis (bowel) (colon) 751.3
Age (old) (see also Senile) 797
Agenesis — see also Absence, by site,
  congenital
  acoustic nerve 742.8
  adrenal (gland) 759.1
  alimentary tract (complete) (partial)
    NEC 751.8
    lower 751.2
    upper 750.8
  anus, anal (canal) 751.2
  aorta 747.22
  appendix 751.2
  arm (complete) (partial) (see also
    Deformity, reduction, upper
    limb) 755.20
  artery (peripheral) NEC (see also
    Anomaly, peripheral vascular
    system) 747.60
    brain 747.81
    coronary 746.85
    pulmonary 747.3
    umbilical 747.5
  auditory (canal) (external) 744.01
  auricle (ear) 744.01
  bile, biliary duct or passage 751.61
  bone NEC 756.9
  brain 740.0
    specified part 742.2
  breast 757.6
  bronchus 748.3
  canaliculus lacrimalis 743.65
  carpus NEC (see also Deformity,
    reduction, upper limb)
    755.28
  cartilage 756.9
  cecum 751.2
  cerebellum 742.2
  cervix 752.49
  chin 744.89
  cilia 743.63

Agenesis—continued
  circulatory system, part NEC 747.89
  clavicle 755.51
  clitoris 752.49
  coccyx 756.13
  colon 751.2
  corpus callosum 742.2
  cricoid cartilage 748.3
  diaphragm (with hernia) 756.6
  digestive organ(s), or tract (complete) (partial) NEC 751.8
    lower 751.2
    upper 750.8
  ductus arteriosus 747.89
  duodenum 751.1
  ear NEC 744.09
    auricle 744.01
    lobe 744.21
  ejaculatory duct 752.8
  endocrine (gland) NEC 759.2
  epiglottis 748.3
  esophagus 750.3
  Eustachian tube 744.24
  extrinsic muscle, eye 743.69
  eye 743.00
    adnexa 743.69
  eyelid (fold) 743.62
  face
    bones NEC 756.0
    specified part NEC 744.89
  fallopian tube 752.19
  femur NEC (see also Absence, femur, congenital) 755.34
  fibula NEC (see also Absence, fibula, congenital) 755.37
  finger NEC (see also Absence, finger, congenital) 755.29
  foot (complete) (see also Deformity, reduction, lower limb) 755.31
  gallbladder 751.69
  gastric 750.8
  genitalia, genital (organ)
    female 752.8
      external 752.49
      internal NEC 752.8
    male 752.8
  glottis 748.3
  gonadal 758.6
  hair 757.4
  hand (complete) (see also Deformity, reduction, upper limb) 755.21
  heart 746.89
    valve NEC 746.89
      aortic 746.89
      mitral 746.89
      pulmonary 746.01
  hepatic 751.69
  humerus NEC (see also Absence, humerus, congenital) 755.24
  hymen 752.49
  ileum 751.1
  incus 744.04
  intestine (small) 751.1
    large 751.2
  iris (dilator fibers) 743.45
  jaw 524.09
  jejunum 751.1
  kidney(s) (partial) (unilateral) 753.0
  labium (majus) (minus) 752.49
  labyrinth, membranous 744.05
  lacrimal apparatus (congenital) 743.65
  larynx 748.3
  leg NEC (see also Deformity, reduction, lower limb) 755.30
  lens 743.35
  limb (complete) (partial) (see also Deformity, reduction) 755.4
    lower NEC 755.30
    upper 755.20
  lip 750.26
  liver 751.69

Agenesis—continued
  lung (bilateral) (fissures) (lobe) (unilateral) 748.5
  mandible 524.09
  maxilla 524.09
  metacarpus NEC 755.28
  metatarsus NEC 755.38
  muscle (any) 756.81
  musculoskeletal system NEC 756.9
  nail(s) 757.5
  neck, part 744.89
  nerve 742.8
  nervous system, part NEC 742.8
  nipple 757.6
  nose 748.1
  nuclear 742.8
  organ
    of Corti 744.05
    or site not listed — see Anomaly, specified type NEC
  osseous meatus (ear) 744.03
  ovary 752.0
  oviduct 752.19
  pancreas 751.7
  parathyroid (gland) 759.2
  patella 755.64
  pelvic girdle (complete) (partial) 755.69
  penis 752.8
  pericardium 746.89
  perineal body 756.81
  pituitary (gland) 759.2
  prostate 752.8
  pulmonary
    artery 747.3
    trunk 747.3
    vein 747.49
  punctum lacrimale 743.65
  radioulnar NEC (see also Absence, forearm, congenital) 755.25
  radius NEC (see also Absence, radius, congenital) 755.26
  rectum 751.2
  renal 753.0
  respiratory organ NEC 748.9
  rib 756.3
  roof of orbit 742.0
  round ligament 752.8
  sacrum 756.13
  salivary gland 750.21
  scapula 755.59
  scrotum 752.8
  seminal duct or tract 752.8
  septum
    atrial 745.69
    between aorta and pulmonary artery 745.0
    ventricular 745.3
  shoulder girdle (complete) (partial) 755.59
  skull (bone) 756.0
    with
      anencephalus 740.0
      encephalocele 742.0
      hydrocephalus 742.3
        with spina bifida (see also Spina bifida) 741.0
      microcephalus 742.1
  spermatic cord 752.8
  spinal cord 742.59
  spine 756.13
    lumbar 756.13
      isthmus 756.11
      pars articularis 756.11
  spleen 759.0
  sternum 756.3
  stomach 750.7
  tarsus NEC 755.38
  tendon 756.81
  testicular 752.8
  testis 752.8
  thymus (gland) 759.2
  thyroid (gland) 243
    cartilage 748.3
  tibia NEC (see also Absence, tibia, congenital) 755.36

Agenesis—continued
  tibiofibular NEC 755.35
  toe (complete) (partial) (see also Absence, toe, congenital) 755.39
  tongue 750.11
  trachea (cartilage) 748.3
  ulna NEC (see also Absence, ulna, congenital) 755.27
  ureter 753.4
  urethra 753.8
  urinary tract NEC 753.8
  uterus 752.3
  uvula 750.26
  vagina 752.49
  vas deferens 752.8
  vein(s) (peripheral) NEC (see also Anomaly, peripheral vascular system) 747.60
    brain 747.81
    great 747.49
    portal 747.49
    pulmonary 747.49
    vena cava (inferior) (superior) 747.49
  vermis of cerebellum 742.2
  vertebra 756.13
    lumbar 756.13
      isthmus 756.11
      pars articularis 756.11
  vulva 752.49
Ageusia (see also Disturbance, sensation) 781.1
Aggressiveness 301.3
Aggressive outburst (see also Disturbance, conduct) 312.0
  in children and adolescents 313.9
Aging skin 701.8
Agitated — see condition
Agitation 307.9
  catatonic (see also Schizophrenia) 295.2
Aglossia (congenital) 750.11
Aglycogenosis 271.0
Agnail (finger) (with lymphangitis) 681.02
Agnosia (body image) (tactile) 784.69
  verbal 784.69
    auditory 784.69
      secondary to organic lesion 784.69
    developmental 315.8
    secondary to organic lesion 784.69
  visual 784.69
    developmental 315.8
    secondary to organic lesion 784.69
  visual 368.16
    developmental 315.31
Agoraphobia 300.22
  with panic attacks 300.21
Agrammatism 784.69
Agranulocytopenia 288.0
Agranulocytosis (angina) (chronic) (cyclical) (genetic) (infantile) (periodic) (pernicious) 288.0
Agraphia (absolute) 784.69
  with alexia 784.61
  developmental 315.39
Agrypnia (see also Insomnia) 780.52
Ague (see also Malaria) 084.6
  brass-founders' 985.8
  dumb 084.6
  tertian 084.1
Agyria 742.2
Ahumada-del Castillo syndrome (nonpuerperal galactorrhea and amenorrhea) 253.1
AIDS 042

AIDS-associated retrovirus (disease) (illness) 042
  infection — see Human immunodeficiency virus, infection
AIDS-associated virus (disease) (illness) 042
  infection — see Human immunodeficiency virus, infection
AIDS-like disease (illness) (syndrome) 042
AIDS-related complex 042
AIDS-related conditions 042
AIDS-related virus (disease) (illness) 042
  infection — see Human immunodeficiency virus, infection
AIDS virus (disease) (illness) 042
  infection — see Human immunodeficiency virus, infection
Ailment, heart — see Disease, heart
Ailurophobia 300.29
Ainhum (disease) 136.0
Air
  anterior mediastinum 518.1
  compressed, disease 993.3
  embolism (any site) (artery) (cerebral) 958.0
    with
      abortion — see Abortion, by type, with embolism
      ectopic pregnancy (see also categories 633.0-633.9) 639.6
      molar pregnancy (see also categories 630-632) 639.6
    due to implanted device — see Complications, due to (presence of) any device, implant, or graft classified to 996.0–996.5 NEC
    following
      abortion 639.6
      ectopic or molar pregnancy 639.6
    infusion, perfusion, or transfusion 999.1
    in pregnancy, childbirth, or puerperium 673.0
    traumatic 958.0
  hunger 786.09
    psychogenic 306.1
  leak (lung) (pulmonary) (thorax) 512.8
    iatrogenic 512.1
    postoperative 512.1
  rarefied, effects of — see Effect, adverse, high altitude
  sickness 994.6
Airplane sickness 994.6
Akathisia, acathisia 781.0
  due to drugs 333.99
Akinesia algeria 352.6
Akiyami 100.89
Akureyri disease (epidemic neuromyasthenia) 049.8
Alacrima (congenital) 743.65
Alactasia (hereditary) 271.3
Alalia 784.3
  developmental 315.31
  secondary to organic lesion 784.3
Alaninemia 270.8
Alastrim 050.1
Albarrán's disease (colibacilluria) 599.0
Albers-Schönberg's disease (marble bones) 756.52
Albert's disease 726.71

Albinism, albino (choroid) (cutaneous) (eye) (generalized) (isolated) (ocular) (oculocutaneous) (partial) 270.2
Albinismus 270.2
Albright (-Martin) (-Bantam) disease (pseudohypoparathyroidism) 275.4
Albright (-McCune) (-Sternberg) syndrome (osteitis fibrosa disseminata) 756.59
Albuminous — *see* condition
Albuminuria, albuminuric (acute) (chronic) (subacute) 791.0
    Bence-Jones 791.0
    cardiac 785.9
    complicating pregnancy, childbirth, or puerperium 646.2
        with hypertension — *see* Toxemia, of pregnancy
        affecting fetus or newborn 760.1
    cyclic 593.6
    gestational 646.2
    gravidarum 646.2
        with hypertension — *see* Toxemia, of pregnancy
        affecting fetus or newborn 760.1
    heart 785.9
    idiopathic 593.6
    orthostatic 593.6
    postural 593.6
    pre-eclamptic (mild) 642.4
        affecting fetus or newborn 760.0
        severe 642.5
            affecting fetus or newborn 760.0
    recurrent physiologic 593.6
    scarlatinal 034.1
Albumosuria 791.0
    Bence-Jones 791.0
    myelopathic (M9730/3) 203.0
Alcaptonuria 270.2
Alcohol, alcoholic
    acute intoxication 305.0
        with dependence 303.0
    addiction (*see also* Alcoholism) 303.9
        maternal
            with suspected fetal damage affecting management of pregnancy 655.4
            affecting fetus or newborn 760.71
    amnestic disorder, persisting 291.1 ▼
    anxiety 291.8 ▲
    brain syndrome, chronic 291.2
    cardiopathy 425.5
    chronic (*see also* Alcoholism) 303.9
    cirrhosis (liver) 571.2
    delirium 291.0
        acute 291.0
        chronic 291.1
        tremens 291.0
        withdrawal 291.0
    dementia NEC 291.2
    deterioration 291.2
    drunkenness (simple) 305.0
    hallucinosis (acute) 291.3
    insanity 291.9
    intoxication (acute) 305.0
        with dependence 303.0
        pathological 291.4
    jealousy 291.5
    Korsakoff's, Korsakov's, Korsakow's 291.1
    liver NEC 571.3
        acute 571.1
        chronic 571.2
    mania (acute) (chronic) 291.9
    mood 291.8 ◆
    paranoia 291.5
    paranoid (type) psychosis 291.5
    pellagra 265.2

Alcohol, alcoholic—*continued*
    poisoning, accidental (acute) NEC 980.9
        specified type of alcohol — *see* Table of drugs and chemicals
    psychosis (*see also* Psychosis, alcoholic) 291.9
        Korsakoff's, Korsakov's, Korsakow's 291.1
        polyneuritic 291.1
            with ▼
                delusions 291.5
                hallucinations 291.3 ▲
    withdrawal symptoms, syndrome NEC 291.8
        delirium 291.0
        hallucinosis 291.3
Alcoholism 303.9

> *Note* — Use the following fifth-digit subclassification with category 303:
>
> 0   unspecified
> 1   continuous
> 2   episodic
> 3   in remission

    with psychosis (*see also* Psychosis, alcoholic) 291.9
    acute 303.0
    chronic 303.9
        with psychosis 291.9
    complicating pregnancy, childbirth, or puerperium 648.4
        affecting fetus or newborn 760.71
    history V11.3
    Korsakoff's, Korsakov's, Korsakow's 291.1
    suspected damage to fetus affecting management of pregnancy 655.4
Alder's anomaly or syndrome (leukocyte granulation anomaly) 288.2
Alder-Reilly anomaly (leukocyte granulation) 288.2
Aldosteronism (primary) (secondary) 255.1
    congenital 255.1
Aldosteronoma (M8370/1) 237.2
Aldrich (-Wiskott) syndrome (eczema-thrombocytopenia) 279.12
Aleppo boil 085.1
Aleukemic — *see* condition
Aleukia
    congenital 288.0
    hemorrhagica 284.9
        acquired (secondary) 284.8
        congenital 284.0
        idiopathic 284.9
    splenica 289.4
Alexia (congenital) (developmental) 315.01
    secondary to organic lesion 784.61
Algoneurodystrophy 733.7
Algophobia 300.29
Alibert's disease (mycosis fungoides) (M9700/3) 202.1
Alibert-Bazin disease (M9700/3) 202.1
Alice in Wonderland syndrome 293.89
Alienation, mental (*see also* Psychosis) 298.9
Alkalemia 276.3
Alkalosis 276.3
    metabolic 276.3
        with respiratory acidosis 276.4
    respiratory 276.3
Alkaptonuria 270.2
Allen-Masters syndrome 620.6

Allergy, allergic (reaction) 995.3
    air-borne substance (*see also* Fever, hay) 477.9
        specified allergen NEC 477.8
    alveolitis (extrinsic) 495.9
        due to
            Aspergillus clavatus 495.4
            cryptostroma corticale 495.6
            organisms (fungal, thermophilic actinomycete, other) growing in ventilation (air conditioning systems) 495.7
        specified type NEC 495.8
    anaphylactic shock 999.4
        due to
            food — (*see* Anaphylactic shock, due to, food
    angioneurotic edema 995.1
    animal (dander) (epidermal) (hair) 477.8
    arthritis (*see also* Arthritis, allergic) 716.2
    asthma — *see* Asthma
    bee sting (anaphylactic shock) 989.5
    biological — *see* Allergy, drug
    bronchial asthma — *see* Asthma
    conjunctivitis (eczematous) 372.14
    dander (animal) 477.8
    dandruff 477.8
    dermatitis (venenata) — *see* Dermatitis
    diathesis V15.0
    drug, medicinal substance, and biological (any) (correct medicinal substance properly administered) (external) (internal) 995.2
        wrong substance given or taken NEC 977.9
        specified drug or substance — *see* Table of drugs and chemicals
    dust (house) (stock) 477.8
    eczema — *see* Eczema
    endophthalmitis 360.19
    epidermal (animal) 477.8
    feathers 477.8
    food (any) (ingested) 693.1
        atopic 691.8
        in contact with skin 692.5
    gastritis 535.4
    gastroenteritis 558.9
    gastrointestinal 558.9
    grain 477.0
    grass (pollen) 477.0
        asthma (*see also* Asthma) 493.0
        hay fever 477.0
    hair (animal) 477.8
    hay fever (grass) (pollen) (ragweed) (tree) (*see also* Fever, hay) 477.9
    history (of) V15.0
    horse serum — *see* Allergy, serum
    inhalant 477.9
        dust 477.8
        pollen 477.0
        specified allergen other than pollen 477.8
    kapok 477.8
    medicine — *see* Allergy, drug
    migraine 346.2
    pannus 370.62
    pneumonia 518.3
    pollen (any) (hay fever) 477.0
        asthma (*see also* Asthma) 493.0
    primrose 477.0
    primula 477.0
    purpura 287.0
    ragweed (pollen) (Senecio jacobae) 477.0
        asthma (*see also* Asthma) 493.0
        hay fever 477.0

Allergy, allergic—*continued*
    respiratory (*see also* Allergy, inhalant) 477.9
        due to
            drug — *see* Allergy, drug
            food — *see* Allergy, food
    rhinitis (*see also* Fever, hay) 477.9
    rose 477.0
    Senecio jacobae 477.0
    serum (prophylactic) (therapeutic) 999.5
        anaphylactic shock 999.4
    shock (anaphylactic) (due to adverse effect of correct medicinal substance properly administered) 995.0
        food — (*see* Anaphylactic shock, due to, food
        from serum or immunization 999.5
        anaphylactic 999.4
    sinusitis (*see also* Fever, hay) 477.9
    skin reaction 692.9
        specified substance — *see* Dermatitis, due to
    tree (any) (hay fever) (pollen) 477.0
        asthma (*see also* Asthma) 493.0
    upper respiratory (*see also* Fever, hay) 477.9
    urethritis 597.89
    urticaria 708.0
    vaccine — *see* Allergy, serum
Allescheriosis 117.6
Alligator skin disease (ichthyosis congenita) 757.1
    acquired 701.1
Allocheiria, allochiria (*see also* Disturbance, sensation) 782.0
Almeida's disease (Brazilian blastomycosis) 116.1
Alopecia (atrophicans) (pregnancy) (premature) (senile) 704.00
    adnata 757.4
    areata 704.01
    celsi 704.01
    cicatrisata 704.09
    circumscripta 704.01
    congenital, congenitalis 757.4
    disseminata 704.01
    effluvium (telogen) 704.02
    febrile 704.09
    generalisata 704.09
    hereditaria 704.09
    marginalis 704.01
    mucinosa 704.09
    postinfectional 704.09
    seborrheica 704.09
    specific 091.82
    syphilitic (secondary) 091.82
    telogen effluvium 704.02
    totalis 704.09
    toxica 704.09
    universalis 704.09
    x-ray 704.09
Alpers' disease 330.8
Alpha-lipoproteinemia 272.4
Alpha thalassemia 282.4
Alphos 696.1
Alpine sickness 993.2
Alport's syndrome (hereditary hematurianephropathy-deafness) 759.89
Alteration (of), altered ◆
    awareness 780.09
        transient 780.02
    consciousness 780.09
        persistent vegetative state 780.03
        transient 780.02 ◆
    mental status 780.9 ◆
Alternaria (infection) 118
Alternating-*see* condition
Altitude, high (effects) — *see* Effect, adverse, high altitude

Aluminosis (of lung) 503
Alvarez syndrome (transient cerebral ischemia) 435.9
Alveolar capillary block syndrome 516.3
Alveolitis
  allergic (extrinsic) 495.9
    due to organisms (fungal, thermophilic actinomycete, other) growing in ventilation (air conditioning systems) 495.7
    specified type NEC 495.8
  due to
    Aspergillus clavatus 495.4
    Cryptostroma corticale 495.6
  fibrosing (chronic) (cryptogenic) (lung) 516.3
    idiopathic 516.3
    rheumatoid 714.81
  jaw 526.5
  sicca dolorosa 526.5
Alveolus, alveolar — see condition
Alymphocytosis (pure) 279.2
Alymphoplasia, thymic 279.2
Alzheimer's
  dementia (senile) 290.0
    with
      delirium 290.3
      delusional features 290.20
      depressive features 290.21
  disease or sclerosis 331.0
    with dementia (see Alzheimer's, dementia
  presenile 290.10
    with
      delirium 290.11
      delusional features 290.12
      depressive features 290.13
Amastia (see also Absence, breast) 611.8
Amaurosis (acquired) (congenital) (see also Blindness) 369.00
  fugax 362.34
  hysterical 300.11
  Leber's (congenital) 362.76
  tobacco 377.34
  uremic — see Uremia
Amaurotic familial idiocy (infantile) (juvenile) (late) 330.1
Ambisexual 752.7
Amblyopia (acquired) (congenital) (partial) 368.00
  color 368.59
    acquired 368.55
  deprivation 368.02
  ex anopsia 368.00
  hysterical 300.11
  nocturnal 368.60
    vitamin A deficiency 264.5
  refractive 368.03
  strabismic 368.01
  suppression 368.01
  tobacco 377.34
  toxic NEC 377.34
  uremic — see Uremia
Ameba, amebic (histolytica) — see also Amebiasis
  abscess 006.3
    bladder 006.8
    brain (with liver and lung abscess) 006.5
    liver 006.3
      with
        brain abscess (and lung abscess) 006.5
        lung abscess 006.4
    lung (with liver abscess) 006.4
      with brain abscess 006.5
    seminal vesicle 006.8
    spleen 006.8
  carrier (suspected of) V02.2

Ameba, amebic—continued
  meningoencephalitis
    due to Naegleria (gruberi) 136.2
    primary 136.2
Amebiasis NEC 006.9
  with
    brain abscess (with liver or lung abscess) 006.5
    liver abscess (without mention of brain or lung abscess) 006.3
    lung abscess (with liver abscess) 006.4
      with brain abscess 006.5
  acute 006.0
  bladder 006.8
  chronic 006.1
  cutaneous 006.6
  cutis 006.6
  due to organism other than Entamoeba histolytica 007.8
  hepatic (see also Abscess, liver, amebic) 006.3
  nondysenteric 006.2
  seminal vesicle 006.8
  specified
    organism NEC 007.8
    site NEC 006.8
Ameboma 006.8
Amelia 755.4
  lower limb 755.31
  upper limb 755.21
Ameloblastoma (M9310/0) 213.1
  jaw (bone) (lower) 213.1
    upper 213.0
  long bones (M9261/3) — see Neoplasm, bone, malignant
  malignant (M9310/3) 170.1
    jaw (bone) (lower) 170.1
      upper 170.0
  mandible 213.1
  tibial (M9261/3) 170.7
Amelogenesis imperfecta 520.5
  nonhereditaria (segmentalis) 520.4
Amenorrhea (primary) (secondary) 626.0
  due to ovarian dysfunction 256.8
  hyperhormonal 256.8
Amentia (see also Retardation, mental) 319
  Meynert's (nonalcoholic) 294.0
    alcoholic 291.1
  nevoid 759.6
American
  leishmaniasis 085.5
  mountain tick fever 066.1
  trypanosomiasis — see Trypanosomiasis, American
Ametropia (see also Disorder, accommodation) 367.9
Amianthosis 501
Amimia 784.69
Amino acid
  deficiency 270.9
    anemia 281.4
  metabolic disorder (see also Disorder, amino acid) 270.9
Aminoaciduria 270.9
  imidazole 270.5
Amnesia (retrograde) 780.9
  auditory 784.69
    developmental 315.31
    secondary to organic lesion 784.69
  hysterical or dissociative type 300.12
  psychogenic 300.12
  transient global 437.7
Amnestic (confabulatory) syndrome 294.8
  alcohol induced 291.1
  drug-induced 292.83
  posttraumatic 294.0

Amniocentesis screening (for) V28.2
  alpha-fetoprotein level, raised V28.1
  chromosomal anomalies V28.0
Amnion, amniotic — see also condition
  nodosum 658.8
Amnionitis (complicating pregnancy) 658.4
  affecting fetus or newborn 762.7
Amoral trends 301.7
Amotio retinae (see also Detachment, retina) 361.9
Ampulla
  lower esophagus 530.89
  phrenic 530.89
Amputation
  any part of fetus, to facilitate delivery 763.8
  cervix (supravaginal) (uteri) 622.8
    in pregnancy or childbirth 654.6
      affecting fetus or newborn 763.8
  clitoris — see Wound, open, clitoris
  congenital
    lower limb 755.31
    upper limb 755.21
  neuroma (traumatic) — see also Injury, nerve, by site
  surgical complication (late) 997.61
  penis — see Amputation, traumatic, penis
  status (without complication) — see Absence, by site, acquired
  stump (surgical)
    abnormal, painful, or with complication (late) 997.60
    healed or old NEC — see also Absence, by site, acquired ▼
      lower V49.70
      upper V49.60 ▲
  traumatic (complete) (partial)

Note — "Complicated" includes traumatic amputation with delayed healing, delayed treatment, foreign body, or major infection.

  arm 887.4
    at or above elbow 887.2
      complicated 887.3
    below elbow 887.0
      complicated 887.1
    both (bilateral) (any level(s)) 887.6
      complicated 887.7
    complicated 887.5
  finger(s) (one or both hands) 886.0
    with thumb(s) 885.0
      complicated 885.1
    complicated 886.1
  foot (except toe(s) only) 896.0
    and other leg 897.6
      complicated 897.7
    both (bilateral) 896.2
      complicated 896.3
    complicated 896.1
  toe(s) only (one or both feet) 895.0
    complicated 895.1
  genital organ(s) (external) NEC 878.8
    complicated 878.9
  hand (except finger(s) only) 887.0
    and other arm 887.6
      complicated 887.7
    both (bilateral) 887.6
      complicated 887.7
    complicated 887.1

Amputation—continued
  traumatic—continued
    hand—continued
      finger(s) (one or both hands) 886.0
        with thumb(s) 885.0
          complicated 885.1
        complicated 886.1
      thumb(s) (with fingers of either hand) 885.0
        complicated 885.1
    head 874.9
    late effect — see Late, effects (of), amputation
    leg 897.4
      and other foot 897.6
        complicated 897.7
      at or above knee 897.2
        complicated 897.3
      below knee 897.0
        complicated 897.1
      both (bilateral) 897.6
        complicated 897.7
      complicated 897.5
    lower limb(s) except toe(s) — see Amputation, traumatic, leg
    nose — see Wound, open, nose
    penis 878.0
      complicated 878.1
    sites other than limbs — see Wound, open, by site
    thumb(s) (with finger(s) of eitherhand) 885.0
      complicated 885.1
    toe(s) (one or both feet) 895.0
      complicated 895.1
    upper limb(s) — see Amputation, traumatic, arm
Amputee (bilateral) (old) — see Absence, by site, acquired ◆
Amusia 784.69
  developmental 315.39
  secondary to organic lesion 784.69
Amyelencephalus 740.0
Amyelia 742.59
Amygdalitis — see Tonsillitis
Amygdalolith 474.8
Amyloid disease or degeneration 277.3
  heart 277.3 [425.7]
Amyloidosis (familial) (general) (generalized) (genetic) (primary) (secondary) 277.3
  with lung involvement 277.3 [517.8]
  heart 277.3 [425.7]
  nephropathic 277.3 [583.81]
  neuropathic (Portuguese) (Swiss) 277.3 [357.4]
  pulmonary 277.3 [517.8]
  systemic, inherited 277.3
Amylopectinosis (brancher enzyme deficiency) 271.0
Amylophagia 307.52
Amyoplasia, congenita 756.89
Amyotonia 728.2
  congenita 358.8
Amyotrophia, amyotrophy, amyotrophic 728.2
  congenita 756.89
  diabetic 250.6 [358.1]
  lateral sclerosis (syndrome) 335.20
  neuralgic 353.5
  sclerosis (lateral) 335.20
  spinal progressive 335.21
Anacidity, gastric 536.0
  psychogenic 306.4
Anaerosis of newborn 770.8
Analbuminemia 273.8
Analgesia (see also Anesthesia) 782.0
Analphalipoproteinemia 272.5

Anaphylactic shock or reaction
(correct substance properly administered) 995.0
due to
food 995.60
additives 995.66
crustaceans 995.62
eggs 995.68
fish 995.65
fruits 995.63
milk products 995.67
nuts (tree) 995.64
peanuts 995.61
seeds 995.64
specified NEC 995.69
tree nuts 995.64
vegetables 995.63
immunization 999.4
overdose or wrong substance given or taken 977.9
specified drug — see Table of drugs and chemicals
serum 999.4
following sting(s) 989.5
purpura 287.0
serum 999.4

Anaphylactoid shock or reaction — see Anaphylactic shock

Anaphylaxis — see Anaphylactic shock

Anaplasia, cervix 622.1

Anarthria 784.5

Anarthritic rheumatoid disease 446.5

Anasarca 782.3
cardiac (see also Failure, heart, congestive) 428.0
fetus or newborn 778.0
lung 514
nutritional 262
pulmonary 514
renal (see also Nephrosis) 581.9

Anaspadias 752.6

Anastomosis
aneurysmal — see Aneurysm
arteriovenous, congenital NEC (see also Anomaly, arteriovenous) 747.60
ruptured, of brain (see also Hemorrhage, subarachnoid) 430
intestinal 569.89
complicated NEC 997.4
involving urinary tract 997.5
retinal and choroidal vessels 743.58
acquired 362.17

Anatomical narrow angle (glaucoma) 365.02

Ancylostoma (infection) (infestation) 126.9
americanus 126.1
braziliense 126.2
caninum 126.8
ceylanicum 126.3
duodenale 126.0
Necator americanus 126.1

Ancylostomiasis (intestinal) 126.9
Ancylostoma
americanus 126.1
caninum 126.8
ceylanicum 126.3
duodenale 126.0
braziliense 126.2
Necator americanus 126.1

Anders' disease or syndrome (adiposis tuberosa simplex) 272.8

Andersen's glycogen storage disease 271.0

Anderson's disease 272.7

Andes disease 993.2

Andrews' disease (bacterid) 686.8

Androblastoma (M8630/1)
benign (M8630/0)
specified site — see Neoplasm, by site, benign
unspecified site
female 220
male 222.0
malignant (M8630/3)
specified site — see Neoplasm, by site, malignant
unspecified site
female 183.0
male 186.9
specified site — see Neoplasm, by site, uncertain behavior
tubular (M8640/0)
with lipid storage (M8641/0)
specified site — see Neoplasm, by site, benign
unspecified site
female 220
male 222.0
specified site — see Neoplasm, by site, benign
unspecified site
female 220
male 222.0
unspecified site
female 236.2
male 236.4

Android pelvis 755.69
with disproportion (fetopelvic) 653.3
affecting fetus or newborn 763.1
causing obstructed labor 660.1
affecting fetus or newborn 763.1

Anectasis, pulmonary (newborn or fetus) 770.5

Anemia 285.9
with
disorder of
anaerobic glycolysis 282.3
pentose phosphate pathway 282.2
koilonychia 280.9
6-phosphogluconic dehydrogenase deficiency 282.2
achlorhydric 280.9
achrestic 281.8
Addison's (pernicious) 281.0
Addison-Biermer (pernicious) 281.0
agranulocytic 288.0
amino acid deficiency 281.4
aplastic 284.9
acquired (secondary) 284.8
congenital 284.0
constitutional 284.0
due to
chronic systemic disease 284.8
drugs 284.8
infection 284.8
radiation 284.8
idiopathic 284.9
myxedema 244.9
of or complicating pregnancy 648.2
red cell (acquired) (adult) (pure) (with thymoma) 284.8
congenital 284.0
specified type NEC 284.8
toxic (paralytic) 284.8
aregenerative 284.9
congenital 284.0
asiderotic 280.9
atypical (primary) 285.9
autohemolysis of Selwyn and Dacie (type I) 282.2
autoimmune hemolytic 283.0
Baghdad Spring 282.2
Balantidium coli 007.0
Biermer's (pernicious) 281.0
blood loss (chronic) 280.0
acute 285.1
bothriocephalus 123.4

Anemia—continued
brickmakers' (see also Ancylostomiasis) 126.9
cerebral 437.8
childhood 285.9
chlorotic 280.9
chronica congenita aregenerativa 284.0
chronic simple 281.9
combined system disease NEC 281.0 [336.2]
due to dietary deficiency 281.1 [336.2]
complicating pregnancy or childbirth 648.2
congenital (following fetal blood loss) 776.5
aplastic 284.0
due to isoimmunization NEC 773.2
Heinz-body 282.7
hereditary hemolytic NEC 282.9
nonspherocytic
Type I 282.2
Type II 282.3
pernicious 281.0
spherocytic (see also Spherocytosis) 282.0
Cooley's (erythroblastic) 282.4
crescent — see Disease, sickle-cell
cytogenic 281.9
Dacie's (nonspherocytic)
Type I 282.2
Type II 282.3
Davidson's (refractory) 284.9
deficiency 281.9
2, 3 diphosphoglycurate mutase 282.3
2, 3 PG 282.3
6-PGD 282.2
6-phosphogluronic dehydrogenase 282.2
amino acid 281.4
combined B_{12} and folate 281.3
enzyme, drug-induced (hemolytic) 282.2
erythrocytic glutathione 282.2
folate 281.2
dietary 281.2
drug-induced 281.2
folic acid 281.2
dietary 281.2
drug-induced 281.2
G-6-PD 282.2
GGS-R 282.2
glucose-6-phosphate dehydrogenase (G-6-PD) 282.2
glucose-phosphate isomerase 282.3
glutathione peroxidase 282.2
glutathione reductase 282.2
glyceraldehyde phosphate dehydrogenase 282.3
GPI 282.3
G SH 282.2
hexokinase 282.3
iron (Fe) 280.9
specified NEC 280.8
nutritional 281.9
with
poor iron absorption 280.9
specified deficiency NEC 281.8
due to inadequate dietary iron intake 280.1
specified type NEC 281.8
of or complicating pregnancy 648.2
pentose phosphate pathway 282.2
PFK 282.3
phosphofructo-aldolase 282.3
phosphofructokinase 282.3
phosphoglycerate kinase 282.3
PK 282.3

Anemia—continued
deficiency—continued
protein 281.4
pyruvate kinase (PK) 282.3
TPI 282.3
triosephosphate isomerase 282.3
vitamin B_{12} NEC 281.1
dietary 281.1
pernicious 281.0
Diamond-Blackfan (congenital hypoplastic) 284.0
dibothriocephalus 123.4
dimorphic 281.9
diphasic 281.8
diphtheritic 032.89
Diphyllobothrium 123.4
drepanocytic (see also Disease, sickle-cell) 282.60
due to
blood loss (chronic) 280.0
acute 285.1
defect of Embden-Meyerhof pathway glycolysis 282.3
disorder of glutathione metabolism 282.2
fetal blood loss 776.5
fish tapeworm (D. latum) infestation 123.4
glutathione metabolism disorder 282.2
hemorrhage (chronic) 280.0
acute 285.1
hexose monophosphate (HMP) shunt deficiency 282.2
impaired absorption 280.9
loss of blood (chronic) 280.0
acute 285.1
myxedema 244.9
Necator americanus 126.1
prematurity 776.6
selective vitamin B_{12} malabsorption with proteinuria 281.1
Dyke-Young type (secondary) (symptomatic) 283.9
dyserythropoietic (congenital) (types I, II, III) 285.8
dyshemopoietic (congenital) 285.8
Egypt (see also Ancylostomiasis) 126.9
elliptocytosis (see also Elliptocytosis) 282.1
enzyme deficiency, drug-induced 282.2
epidemic (see also Ancylostomiasis) 126.9
erythroblastic
familial 282.4
fetus or newborn (see also Disease, hemolytic) 773.2
late 773.5
erythrocytic glutathione deficiency 282.2
essential 285.9
Faber's (achlorhydric anemia) 280.9
factitious (self-induced blood letting) 280.0
familial erythroblastic (microcytic) 282.4
Fanconi's (congenital pancytopenia) 284.0
favism 282.2
fetal, following blood loss 776.5
fetus or newborn
due to
ABO
antibodies 773.1
incompatibility, maternal/fetal 773.1
isoimmunization 773.1

Anemia—continued
  fetus or newborn—continued
    due to—continued
      Rh
        antibodies 773.0
        incompatibility, maternal/fetal 773.0
        isoimmunization 773.0
    following fetal blood loss 776.5
  fish tapeworm (D. latum) infestation 123.4
  folate (folic acid) deficiency 281.2
    dietary 281.2
    drug-induced 281.2
  folate malabsorption, congenital 281.2
  folic acid deficiency 281.2
    dietary 281.2
    drug-induced 281.2
  G-6-PD 282.2
  general 285.9
  glucose-6-phosphate dehydrogenase deficiency 282.2
  glutathione-reductase deficiency 282.2
  goat's milk 281.2
  granulocytic 288.0
  Heinz-body, congenital 282.7
  hemoglobin deficiency 285.9
  hemolytic 282.9
    acquired 283.9
      with hemoglobinuria NEC 283.2
      autoimmune (cold type) (idiopathic) (primary) (secondary) (symptomatic) (warm type) 283.0
      due to
        cold reactive antibodies 283.0
        drug exposure 283.0
        warm reactive antibodies 283.0
      fragmentation 283.19
      idiopathic (chronic) 283.9
      infectious 283.19
        autoimmune 283.0
        non-autoimmune NEC 283.10
      toxic 283.19
      traumatic cardiac 283.19
    acute 283.9
      due to enzyme deficiency NEC 282.3
      fetus or newborn (see also Disease, hemolytic) 773.2
      late 773.5
      Lederer's (acquired infectious hemolytic anemia) 283.19
    autoimmune (acquired) 283.0
    chronic 282.9
      idiopathic 283.9
    cold type (secondary) (symptomatic) 283.0
    congenital (spherocytic) (see also Spherocytosis) 282.0
      nonspherocytic — see Anemia, hemolytic, nonspherocytic, congenital
    drug-induced 283.0
      enzyme deficiency 282.2
    due to
      cardiac conditions 283.19
      drugs 283.0
      enzyme deficiency NEC 282.3
        drug-induced 282.2
      presence of shunt or other internal prosthetic device 283.19

Anemia—continued
  hemolytic—continued
    due to—continued
      thrombotic thrombocytopenic purpura 446.6
    elliptocytotic (see also Elliptocytosis) 282.1
    familial 282.9
    hereditary 282.9
      due to enzyme deficiency NEC 282.3
      specified NEC 282.8
    idiopathic (chronic) 283.9
    infectious (acquired) 283.19
    mechanical 283.19
    microangiopathic 283.19
    non-autoimmune NEC 283.10
    nonspherocytic
      congenital or hereditary NEC 282.3
        glucose-6-phosphate dehydrogenase deficiency 282.2
        pyruvate kinase (PK) deficiency 282.3
        type I 282.2
        type II 282.3
        type I 282.2
        type II 282.3
    of or complicating pregnancy 648.2
    resulting from presence of shunt or other internal prosthetic device 283.19
    secondary 283.19
      autoimmune 283.0
    sickle-cell — see Disease, sickle-cell
    Stransky-Regala type (Hb-E) (see also Disease, hemoglobin) 282.7
    symptomatic 283.19
      autoimmune 283.0
    toxic (acquired) 283.19
    uremic (adult) (child) 283.11
    warm type (secondary) (symptomatic) 283.0
  hemorrhagic (chronic) 280.0
    acute 285.1
  HEMPAS 285.8
  hereditary erythroblast multinuclearity-positive acidified serum test 285.8
  Herrick's (hemoglobin S disease) 282.61
  hexokinase deficiency 282.3
  high A_2 282.4
  hookworm (see also Ancylostomiasis) 126.9
  hypochromic (idiopathic) (microcytic) (normoblastic) 280.9
    with iron loading 285.0
    due to blood loss (chronic) 280.0
      acute 285.1
    familial sex linked 285.0
    pyridoxine-responsive 285.0
  hypoplasia, red blood cells 284.8
    congenital or familial 284.0
  hypoplastic (idiopathic) 284.9
    congenital 284.0
    familial 284.0
    of childhood 284.0
  idiopathic 285.9
    hemolytic, chronic 283.9
  infantile 285.9
  infective, infectional 285.9
  intertropical (see also Ancylostomiasis) 126.9
  iron (Fe) deficiency 289.0
    due to blood loss (chronic) 280.0
      acute 285.1
    of or complicating pregnancy 648.2

Anemia—continued
  iron (Fe) deficiency—continued
    specified NEC 280.8
  Jaksch's (pseudoleukemia infantum) 285.8
  Joseph-Diamond-Blackfan (congenital hypoplastic) 284.0
  labyrinth 386.50
  Lederer's (acquired infectious hemolytic anemia) 283.19
  leptocytosis (hereditary) 282.4
  leukoerythroblastic 285.8
  macrocytic 281.9
    nutritional 281.2
    of or complicating pregnancy 648.2
    tropical 281.2
  malabsorption (familial), selective B_{12} with proteinuria 281.1
  malarial (see also Malaria) 084.6
  malignant (progressive) 281.0
  malnutrition 281.9
  marsh (see also Malaria) 084.6
  Mediterranean (with hemoglobinopathy) 282.4
  megaloblastic 281.9
    combined B_{12} and folate deficiency 281.3
    nutritional (of infancy) 281.2
    of infancy 281.2
    of or complicating pregnancy 648.2
    refractory 281.3
    specified NEC 281.3
  megalocytic 281.9
  microangiopathic hemolytic 283.19
  microcytic (hypochromic) 280.9
    due to blood loss (chronic) 280.0
      acute 285.1
    familial 282.4
    hypochromic 280.9
  microdrepanocytosis 282.4
  miners' (see also Ancylostomiasis) 126.9
  myelopathic 285.8
  myelophthisic (normocytic) 285.8
  newborn (see also Disease, hemolytic) 773.2
    due to isoimmunization (see also Disease, hemolytic) 773.2
    late, due to isoimmunization 773.5
    posthemorrhagic 776.5
  nonregenerative 284.9
  nonspherocytic hemolytic — see Anemia, hemolytic, nonspherocytic
  normocytic (infectional) (not due to blood loss) 285.9
    due to blood loss (chronic) 280.0
      acute 285.1
    myelophthisic 284.8
  nutritional (deficiency) 281.9
    with
      poor iron absorption 280.9
      specified deficiency NEC 281.8
    due to inadequate dietary iron intake 280.1
    megaloblastic (of infancy) 281.2
  of childhood (see also Thalassemia) 282.4
  of or complicating pregnancy 648.2
    affecting fetus or newborn 760.8
  of prematurity 776.6
  orotic aciduric (congenital) (hereditary) 281.4
  osteosclerotic 289.8
  ovalocytosis (hereditary) (see also Elliptocytosis) 282.1
  paludal (see also Malaria) 084.6
  pentose phosphate pathway deficiency 282.2

Anemia—continued
  pernicious (combined system disease) (congenital) (dorsolateral spinal degeneration) (juvenile) (myelopathy) (neuropathy) (posterior sclerosis) (primary) (progressive) (spleen) 281.0
    of or complicating pregnancy 648.2
  pleochromic 285.9
  of sprue 281.8
  portal 285.8
  posthemorrhagic (chronic) 280.0
    acute 285.1
    newborn 776.5
  pressure 285.9
  primary 285.9
  profound 285.9
  progressive 285.9
    malignant 281.0
    pernicious 281.0
  protein-deficiency 281.4
  pseudoleukemica infantum 285.8
  puerperal 648.2
  pure red cell 284.8
    congenital 284.0
  pyridoxine-responsive (hypochromic) 285.0
  pyruvate kinase (PK) deficiency 282.3
  refractoria sideroblastica 285.0
  refractory (primary) 284.9
    with hemochromatosis 285.0
    megaloblastic 281.3
    sideroblastic 285.0
    sideropenic 280.9
  Rietti-Greppi-Micheli (thalassemia minor) 282.4
  scorbutic 281.8
  secondary (to) 285.9
    blood loss (chronic) 280.0
      acute 285.1
    hemorrhage 280.0
      acute 285.1
    inadequate dietary iron intake 280.1
  semiplastic 284.9
  septic 285.9
  sickle-cell (see also Disease, sickle-cell) 282.60
  sideroachrestic 285.0
  sideroblastic (acquired) (any type) (congenital) (drug-induced) (due to disease) (hereditary) (primary) (refractory) (secondary) (sex-linked hypochromic) (vitamin B_6 responsive) 285.0
  sideropenic (refractory) 280.9
    due to blood loss (chronic) 280.0
      acute 285.1
  simple chronic 281.9
  specified type NEC 285.8
  spherocytic (hereditary) (see also Spherocytosis) 282.0
  splenic 285.8
    familial (Gaucher's) 272.7
  splenomegalic 285.8
  stomatocytosis 282.8
  syphilitic 095.8
  target cell (oval) 282.4
  thalassemia 282.4
  thrombocytopenic (see also Thrombocytopenia) 287.5
  toxic 284.8
  triosephosphate isomerase deficiency 282.3
  tropical, macrocytic 281.2
  tuberculous (see also Tuberculosis) 017.9
  vegan's 281.1
  vitamin
    B_6-responsive 285.0
    B_{12} deficiency (dietary) 281.1
      pernicious 281.0

Anemia

Anemia—*continued*
    von Jaksch's (pseudoleukemia infantum) 285.8
    Witts' (achlorhydric anemia) 280.9
    Zuelzer (-Ogden) (nutritional megaloblastic anemia) 281.2

Anencephalus, anencephaly 740.0
    fetal, affecting management of pregnancy 655.0

Anergasia (*see also* Psychosis, organic) 294.9
    senile 290.0

Anesthesia, anesthetic 782.0
    complication or reaction NEC 995.2
    due to
        correct substance properly administered 995.2
        overdose or wrong substance given 968.4
        specified anesthetic — *see* Table of drugs and chemicals
    cornea 371.81
    death from
        correct substance properly administered 995.4
        during delivery 668.9
        overdose or wrong substance given 968.4
        specified anesthetic — *see* Table of drugs and chemicals
    eye 371.81
    functional 300.11
    hyperesthetic, thalamic 348.8
    hysterical 300.11
    local skin lesion 782.0
    olfactory 781.1
    sexual (psychogenic) 302.72
    shock
        due to
            correct substance properly administered 995.4
            overdose or wrong substance given 968.4
            specified anesthetic — *see* Table of drugs and chemicals
    skin 782.0
    tactile 782.0
    testicular 608.9
    thermal 782.0

Anetoderma (maculosum) 701.3

Aneuploidy NEC 758.5

Aneurin deficiency 265.1

Aneurysm (anastomotic) (artery) (cirsoid) (diffuse) (false) (fusiform) (multiple) (ruptured) (saccular) (varicose) 442.9
    abdominal (aorta) 441.4
        ruptured 441.3
        syphilitic 093.0
    aorta, aortic (nonsyphilitic) 441.9
        abdominal 441.4
            dissecting 441.02 ◆
            ruptured 441.3
            syphilitic 093.0
        arch 441.2
            ruptured 441.1
        arteriosclerotic NEC 441.9
            ruptured 441.5
        ascending 441.2
            ruptured 441.1
        congenital 747.29
        descending 441.9
            abdominal 441.4
                ruptured 441.3
            ruptured 441.5
            thoracic 441.2
                ruptured 441.1
        dissecting 441.00 ▼
            abdominal 441.02
            thoracic 441.01
                thoracoabdominal 441.03 ▲
        due to coarctation (aorta) 747.10

Aneurysm—*continued*
    aorta, aortic—*continued*
        ruptured 441.5
        sinus, right 747.29
        syphilitic 093.0
        thoracoabdominal 441.7
            ruptured 441.6
        thorax, thoracic (arch) (nonsyphilitic) 441.2
            dissecting 441.01 ◆
            ruptured 441.1
            syphilitic 093.0
        transverse 441.2
            ruptured 441.1
        valve (heart) (*see also* Endocarditis, aortic) 424.1
    arteriosclerotic NEC 442.9
        cerebral 437.3
            ruptured (*see also* Hemorrhage, subarachnoid) 430
    arteriovenous (congenital) (peripheral) NEC (*see also* Anomaly, arteriovenous) 747.60
        acquired NEC 447.0
        brain 437.3
            ruptured (*see also* Hemorrhage subarachnoid) 430
        coronary 414.11
        pulmonary 417.0
        brain (cerebral) 747.81
            ruptured (*see also* Hemorrhage, subarachnoid) 430
        coronary 746.85
        pulmonary 747.3
        retina 743.58
        specified site NEC 747.89
            acquired 447.0
        traumatic (*see also* Injury, blood vessel, by site) 904.9
    basal — *see* Aneurysm, brain
    berry (congenital) (ruptured) (*see also* Hemorrhage, subarachnoid) 430
    brain 437.3
        arteriosclerotic 437.3
            ruptured (*see also* Hemorrhage, subarachnoid) 430
        arteriovenous 747.81
            acquired 437.3
            ruptured (*see also* Hemorrhage, subarachnoid) 430
            ruptured (*see also* Hemorrhage, subarachnoid) 430
        berry (congenital) (ruptured) (*see also* Hemorrhage, subarachnoid) 430
        congenital 747.81
            ruptured (*see also* Hemorrhage, subarachnoid) 430
        meninges 437.3
            ruptured (*see also* Hemorrhage, subarachnoid) 430
        miliary (congenital) (ruptured) (*see also* Hemorrhage, subarachnoid) 430
        mycotic 421.0
            ruptured (*see also* Hemorrhage, subarachnoid) 430
        nonruptured 437.3
        ruptured (*See also* Hemorrhage, subarachnoid) 430
        syphilitic 094.87
        syphilitic (hemorrhage) 094.87
        traumatic — *see* Injury, intracranial

Aneurysm—*continued*
    cardiac (false) (*see also* Aneurysm, heart) 414.10
    carotid artery (common) (external) 442.81
        internal 442.81
            ruptured into brain (*see also* Hemorrhage, subarachnoid) 430
            syphilitic 093.89
            intracranial 094.87
    cavernous sinus (*see also* Aneurysm, brain) 437.3
        arteriovenous 747.81
            ruptured (*see also* Hemorrhage, subarachnoid) 430
        congenital 747.81
            ruptured (*see also* Hemorrhage, subarachnoid) 430
    celiac 442.84
    central nervous system, syphilitic 094.89
    cerebral — *see* Aneurysm, brain
    chest — *see* Aneurysm, thorax
    circle of Willis (*see also* Aneurysm, brain) 437.3
        congenital 747.81
            ruptured (*see also* Hemorrhage, subarachnoid) 430
        ruptured (*see also* Hemorrhage, subarachnoid) 430
    common iliac artery 442.2
    congenital (peripheral) NEC 747.60
        brain 747.81
            ruptured (*see also* Hemorrhage, subarachnoid) 430
            cerebral — *see* Aneurysm, brain, congenital
        coronary 746.85
        gastrointestinal 747.61
        lower limb 747.64
        pulmonary 747.3
        renal 747.62
        retina 743.58
        specified site NEC 747.89
        spinal 747.82
        upper limb 747.63
    conjunctiva 372.74
    conus arteriosus (*see also* Aneurysm, heart) 414.10
    coronary (arteriosclerotic) (artery) (vein) (*see also* Aneurysm, heart) 414.11
        arteriovenous 746.85
        congenital 746.85
        syphilitic 093.89
    cylindrical 441.9
        ruptured 441.5
        syphilitic 093.9
    dissecting 442.9
        aorta (any part) 441.00 ▼
            abdominal 441.02
            thoracic 441.01
            thoracoabdominal 441.03 ▲
        syphilitic 093.9
    ductus arteriosus 747.0
    embolic — *see* Embolism, artery
    endocardial, infective (any valve) 421.0
    femoral 442.3
    gastroduodenal 442.84
    gastroepiploic 442.84
    heart (chronic or with a stated duration of over 8 weeks) (infectional) (wall) 414.10
        acute or with a stated duration of 8 weeks or less (*see also* Infarct, myocardium) 410.9
        congenital 746.89
        valve — *see* Endocarditis
    hepatic 442.84
    iliac (common) 442.2

Aneurysm—*continued*
    infective (any valve) 421.0
    innominate (nonsyphilitic) 442.89
        syphilitic 093.89
    interauricular septum (*see also* Aneurysm, heart) 414.10
    interventricular septum (*see also* Aneurysm, heart) 414.10
    intracranial — *see* Aneurysm, brain
    intrathoracic (nonsyphilitic) 441.2
        ruptured 441.1
        syphilitic 093.0
    jugular vein 453.8
    lower extremity 442.3
    lung (pulmonary artery) 417.1
    malignant 093.9
    mediastinal (nonsyphilitic) 442.89
        syphilitic 093.89
    miliary (congenital) (ruptured) (*see also* Hemorrhage, subarachnoid) 430
    mitral (heart) (valve) 424.0
    mural (arteriovenous) (heart) (*see also* Aneurysm, heart) 414.10
    mycotic, any site 421.0
        ruptured, brain (*see also* Hemorrhage, subarachnoid) 430
    myocardium (*see also* Aneurysm, heart) 414.10
    neck 442.81
    pancreaticoduodenal 442.84
    patent ductus arteriosus 747.0
    peripheral NEC 442.89
        congenital NEC (*see also* Aneurysm, congenital) 747.60
    popliteal 442.3
    pulmonary 417.1
        arteriovenous 747.3
            acquired 417.0
        syphilitic 093.89
        valve (heart) (*see also* Endocarditis, pulmonary) 424.3
    racemose 442.9
        congenital (peripheral) NEC 747.60
    radial 442.0
    Rasmussen's (*see also* Tuberculosis) 011.2
    renal 442.1
    retinal (acquired) 362.17
        congenital 743.58
        diabetic 250.5 [362.01]
    sinus, aortic (of Valsalva) 747.29
    specified site NEC 442.89
    spinal (cord) 442.89
        congenital 747.82
        syphilitic (hemorrhage) 094.89
    spleen, splenic 442.83
    subclavian 442.82
        syphilitic 093.89
    superior mesenteric 442.84
    syphilitic 093.9
        aorta 093.0
        central nervous system 094.89
        congenital 090.5
        spine, spinal 094.89
    thoracoabdominal 441.7
        ruptured 441.6
    thorax, thoracic (arch) (nonsyphilitic) 441.2
        dissecting 441.0
        ruptured 441.1
        syphilitic 093.0
    traumatic (complication) (early) — *see* Injury, blood vessel, by site
    tricuspid (heart) (valve) — *see* Endocarditis, tricuspid
    ulnar 442.0
    upper extremity 442.0
    valve, valvular — *see* Endocarditis

Aneurysm—continued
- venous 456.8
  - congenital NEC (see also Aneurysm, congenital) 747.60
- ventricle (arteriovenous) (see also Aneurysm, heart) 414.10
- visceral artery NEC 442.84

Angiectasis 459.89

Angiectopia 459.9

Angiitis 447.6
- allergic granulomatous 446.4
- hypersensitivity 446.20
  - Goodpasture's syndrome 446.21
  - specified NEC 446.29
- necrotizing 446.0
- Wegener's (necrotizing respiratory granulomatosis) 446.4

Angina (attack) (cardiac) (chest) (effort) (heart) (pectoris) (syndrome) (vasomotor) 413.9
- abdominal 557.1
- agranulocytic 288.0
- aphthous 074.0
- catarrhal 462
- crescendo 411.1
- croupous 464.4
- cruris 443.9
  - due to atherosclerosis NEC (see also Arteriosclerosis, extremities) 440.20
- decubitus 413.0
- diphtheritic (membranous) 032.0
- erysipelatous 034.0
- erythematous 462
- exudative, chronic 476.0
- faucium 478.29
- gangrenous 462
  - diphtheritic 032.0
- infectious 462
- initial 411.1
- intestinal 557.1
- ludovici 528.3
- Ludwig's 528.3
- malignant 462
  - diphtheritic 032.0
- membranous 464.4
  - diphtheritic 032.0
- mesenteric 557.1
- monocytic 075
- nocturnal 413.0
- phlegmonous 475
  - diphtheritic 032.0
- preinfarctional 411.1
- Prinzmetal's 413.1
- progressive 411.1
- pseudomembranous 101
- psychogenic 306.2
- pultaceous, diphtheritic 032.0
- scarlatinal 034.1
- septic 034.0
- simple 462
- stable NEC 413.9
- staphylococcal 462
- streptococcal 034.0
- stridulous, diphtheritic 032.3
- syphilitic 093.9
  - congenital 090.5
- tonsil 475
- trachealis 464.4
- unstable 411.1
- variant 413.1
- Vincent's 101

Angioblastoma (M9161/1) — see Neoplasm, connective tissue, uncertain behavior

Angiocholecystitis (see also Cholecystitis, acute) 575.0

Angiocholitis (see also Cholecystitis, acute) 576.1

Angiodysgensis spinalis 336.1

Angiodysplasia (intestinalis) (intestine) 569.84
- with hemorrhage 569.85

Angiodysplasia—continued
- duodenum 537.82
  - with hemorrhage 537.83
- stomach 537.82
  - with hemorrhage 537.83

Angioedema (allergic) (any site) (with urticaria) 995.1
- hereditary 277.6

Angioendothelioma (M9130/1) — see also Neoplasm, by site, uncertain behavior
- benign (M9130/0) (see also Hemangioma, by site) 228.00
- bone (M9260/3) — see Neoplasm, bone, malignant
- Ewing's (M9260/3) — see Neoplasm, bone, malignant
- nervous system (M9130/0) 228.09

Angiofibroma (M9160/0) — see also Neoplasm, by site, benign
- juvenile (M9160/0) 210.7
- specified site — see Neoplasm, by site, benign
- unspecified site 210.7

Angiohemophilia (A) (B) 286.4

Angioid streaks (choroid) (retina) 363.43

Angiokeratoma (M9141/0) — see also Neoplasm, skin, benign
- corporis diffusum 272.7

Angiokeratosis
- diffuse 272.7

Angioleiomyoma (M8894/0) — see Neoplasm, connective tissue, benign

Angioleucitis 683

Angiolipoma (M8861/0) (see also Lipoma, by site) 214.9
- infiltrating (M8861/1) — see Neoplasm, connective tissue, uncertain behavior

Angioma (M9120/0) (see also Hemangioma, by site) 228.00
- capillary 448.1
- hemorrhagicum hereditaria 448.0
- malignant (M9120/3) — see Neoplasm, connective tissue, malignant
- pigmentosum et atrophicum 757.33
- placenta — see Placenta, abnormal
- plexiform (M9131/0) — see Hemangioma, by site
- senile 448.1
- serpiginosum 709.1
- spider 448.1
- stellate 448.1

Angiomatosis 757.32
- corporis diffusum universale 272.7
- cutaneocerebral 759.6
- encephalocutaneous 759.6
- encephalofacial 759.6
- encephalotrigeminal 759.6
- hemorrhagic familial 448.0
- hereditary familial 448.0
- heredofamilial 448.0
- meningo-oculofacial 759.6
- multiple sites 228.09
- neuro-oculocutaneous 759.6
- retina (Hippel's disease) 759.6
- retinocerebellosa 759.6
- retinocerebral 759.6
- systemic 228.09

Angiomyolipoma (M8860/0)
- specified site — see Neoplasm, connective tissue, benign
- unspecified site 223.0

Angiomyoliposarcoma (M8860/3) — see Neoplasm, connective tissue, malignant

Angiomyoma (M8894/0) — see Neoplasm, connective tissue, benign

Angiomyosarcoma (M8894/3) — see Neoplasm, connective tissue, malignant

Angioneurosis 306.2

Angioneurotic edema (allergic) (any site) (with urticaria) 995.1
- hereditary 277.6

Angiopathia, angiopathy 459.9
- diabetic (peripheral) 250.7 [443.81]
- peripheral 443.9
  - diabetic 250.7 [443.81]
  - specified type NEC 443.89
- retinae syphilitica 093.89
- retinalis (juvenilis) 362.18
  - background 362.10
  - diabetic 250.5 [362.01]
  - proliferative 362.29
  - tuberculous (see also Tuberculosis) 017.3 [362.18]

Angiosarcoma (M9120/3) — see Neoplasm, connective tissue, malignant

Angiosclerosis — see Arteriosclerosis

Angioscotoma, enlarged 368.42

Angiospasm 443.9
- brachial plexus 353.0
- cerebral 435.9
- cervical plexus 353.2
- nerve
  - arm 354.9
    - axillary 353.0
    - median 354.1
    - ulnar 354.2
  - autonomic (see also Neuropathy, peripheral, autonomic) 337.9
  - axillary 353.0
  - leg 355.8
    - plantar 355.6
  - lower extremity — see Angiospasm, nerve, leg
  - median 354.1
  - peripheral NEC 355.9
  - spinal NEC 355.9
  - sympathetic (see also Neuropathy, peripheral, autonomic) 337.9
  - ulnar 354.2
  - upper extremity — see Angiospasm, nerve, arm
- peripheral NEC 443.9
- traumatic 443.9
  - foot 443.9
  - leg 443.9
- vessel 443.9

Angiospastic disease or edema 443.9

Anguillulosis 127.2

Angulation
- cecum (see also Obstruction, intestine) 560.9
- coccyx (acquired) 738.6
  - congenital 756.19
- femur (acquired) 736.39
  - congenital 755.69
- intestine (large) (small) (see also Obstruction, intestine) 560.9
- sacrum (acquired) 738.5
  - congenital 756.19
- sigmoid (flexure) (see also Obstruction, intestine) 560.9
- spine (see also Curvature, spine) 737.9
- tibia (acquired) 736.89
  - congenital 755.69
- ureter 593.3
- wrist (acquired) 736.09
  - congenital 755.59

Angulus infectiosus 686.8

Anhedonia 302.72

Anhidrosis (lid) (neurogenic) (thermogenic) 705.0

Anhydration 276.5
- with
  - hypernatremia 276.0
  - hyponatremia 276.1

Anhydremia 276.5
- with
  - hypernatremia 276.0
  - hyponatremia 276.1

Anidrosis 705.0

Aniridia (congenital) 743.45

Anisakiasis (infection) (infestation) 127.1

Anisakis larva infestation 127.1

Aniseikonia 367.32

Anisocoria (pupil) 379.41
- congenital 743.46

Anisocytosis 790.0

Anisometropia (congenital) 367.31

Ankle — see condition

Ankyloblepharon (acquired) (eyelid) 374.46
- filiforme (adnatum) (congenital) 743.62
- total 743.62

Ankylodactly (see also Syndactylism) 755.10

Ankyloglossia 750.0

Ankylosis (fibrous) (osseous) 718.50
- ankle 718.57
- any joint, produced by surgical fusion V45.4
- cricoarytenoid (cartilage) (joint) (larynx) 478.79
- dental 521.6
- ear ossicle NEC 385.22
  - malleus 385.21
- elbow 718.52
- finger 718.54
- hip 718.55
- incostapedial joint (infectional) 385.22
- joint, produced by surgical fusion NEC V45.4
- knee 718.56
- lumbosacral (joint) 724.6
- malleus 385.21
- multiple sites 718.59
- postoperative (status) V45.4
- sacroiliac (joint) 724.6
- shoulder 718.51
- specified site NEC 718.58
- spine NEC 724.9
- surgical V45.4
- teeth, tooth (hard tissues) 521.6
- temporomandibular joint 524.61
- wrist 718.53

Ankylostoma — see Ancylostoma

Ankylostomiasis (intestinal) — see Ancylostomiasis

Ankylurethria (see also Stricture, urethra) 598.9

Annular — see also condition
- detachment, cervix 622.8
- organ or site, congenital NEC — see Distortion
- pancreas (congenital) 751.7

Anodontia (complete) (partial) (vera) 520.0
- with abnormal spacing 524.3
- acquired 525.1
- causing malocclusion 524.3

Anomaly, anomalous (congenital) (unspecified type) 759.9
- abdomen 759.9
- abdominal wall 756.7
- acoustic nerve 742.9
- adrenal (gland) 759.1
- Alder (-Reilly) (leukocyte granulation) 288.2
- alimentary tract 751.9
  - lower 751.5
  - specified type NEC 751.8

Anomaly, anomalous—*continued*
  alimentary tract—*continued*
    upper (any part, except tongue)
      750.9
      tongue 750.10
        specified type NEC
          750.19
  alveolar ridge (process) 525.8
  ankle (joint) 755.69
  anus, anal (canal) 751.5
  aorta, aortic 747.20
    arch 747.21
    coarctation (postductal)
      (preductal) 747.10
    cusp or valve NEC 746.9
    septum 745.0
    specified type NEC 747.29
  aorticopulmonary septum 745.0
  apertures, diaphragm 756.6
  appendix 751.5
  aqueduct of Sylvius 742.3
    with spina bifida (see also Spina
      bifida) 741.0
  arm 755.50
    reduction (see also Deformity,
      reduction, upper limb)
      755.20
  arteriovenous (congenital)
    (peripheral) NEC 747.60
    brain 747.81
    cerebral 747.81
    coronary 746.85
    gastrointestinal 747.61
    lower limb 747.64
    renal 747.62
    specified site NEC 747.69
    spinal 747.82
    upper limb 747.63
  artery (see also Anomaly, peripheral
    vascular system) NEC 747.60
    brain 747.81
    cerebral 747.81
    coronary 746.85
    eye 743.9
    pulmonary 747.3
    renal 747.62
    retina 743.9
    umbilical 747.5
  arytenoepiglottic folds 748.3
  atrial
    bands 746.9
    folds 746.9
    septa 745.5
  atrioventricular
    canal 745.69
    common 745.69
    conduction 426.7
    excitation 426.7
    septum 745.4
  atrium — *see* Anomaly, atrial
  auditory canal 744.3
    specified type NEC 744.29
      with hearing impairment
        744.02
  auricle
    ear 744.3
      causing impairment of
        hearing 744.02
    heart 746.9
      septum 745.5
  autosomes, autosomal NEC 758.5
  Axenfeld's 743.44
  back 759.9
  band
    atrial 746.9
    heart 746.9
    ventricular 746.9
  Bartholin's duct 750.9
  biliary duct or passage 751.60
    atresia 751.61
  bladder (neck) (sphincter) (trigone)
    753.9
    specified type NEC 753.8
  blood vessel 747.9
    artery — *see* Anomaly, artery

Anomaly, anomalous—*continued*
  blood vessel—*continued*
    peripheral vascular — *see*
      Anomaly, peripheral
      vascular system
    vein — *see* Anomaly, vein
  bone NEC 756.9
    ankle 755.69
    arm 755.50
    chest 756.3
    cranium 756.0
    face 756.0
    finger 755.50
    foot 755.67
    forearm 755.50
    frontal 756.0
    head 756.0
    hip 755.63
    leg 755.60
    lumbosacral 756.10
    nose 748.1
    pelvic girdle 755.60
    rachitic 756.4
    rib 756.3
    shoulder girdle 755.50
    skull 756.0
      with
        anencephalus 740.0
        encephalocele 742.0
        hydrocephalus 742.3
          with spina bifida (see
            also Spina
            bifida) 741.0
        microcephalus 742.1
    toe 755.66
  brain 742.9
    multiple 742.4
    reduction 742.2
    specified type NEC 742.4
    vessel 747.81
  branchial cleft NEC 744.49
    cyst 744.42
    fistula 744.41
    persistent 744.41
    sinus (external) (internal) 744.41
  breast 757.9
  broad ligament 752.10
    specified type NEC 752.19
  bronchus 748.3
  bulbar septum 745.0
  bulbus cordis 745.9
    persistent (in left ventricle)
      745.8
  bursa 756.9
  canal of Nuck 752.9
  canthus 743.9
  capillary NEC (see also Anomaly,
    peripheral vascular system)
    747.60
  cardiac 746.9
    septal closure 745.9
      acquired 429.71
    valve NEC 746.9
      pulmonary 746.00
      specified type NEC 746.89
  cardiovascular system 746.9
    complicating pregnancy,
      childbirth, or puerperium
      648.5
  carpus 755.59
  cartilage, trachea 748.3
  cartilaginous 756.9
  caruncle, lacrimal, lachrymal 743.9
  cascade stomach 750.7
  cauda equina 742.59
  cecum 751.5
  cerebral — *see also* Anomaly, brain
    vessels 747.81
  cerebrovascular system 747.81
  cervix (uterus) 752.40
    with doubling of vagina and
      uterus 752.2

Anomaly, anomalous—*continued*
  cervix—*continued*
    in pregnancy or childbirth 654.6
      affecting fetus or newborn
        763.8
      causing obstructed labor
        660.2
        affecting fetus or newborn
          763.1
  Chédiak-Higashi (-Steinbrinck)
    (congenital gigantism of
    peroxidase granules) 288.2
  cheek 744.9
  chest (wall) 756.3
  chin 744.9
    specified type NEC 744.89
  chordae tendineae 746.9
  choroid 743.9
    plexus 742.9
  chromosomes, chromosomal 758.9
    13 (13-15) 758.1
    18 (16-18) 758.2
    21 or 22 758.0
    autosomes NEC (see also
      Abnormality, autosomes)
      758.5
      deletion 758.3
    Christchurch 758.3
    D_1 758.1
    E_3 758.2
    G 758.0
    mosaics 758.9
    sex 758.8
      complement, XO 758.6
      complement, XXX 758.8
      complement, XXY 758.7
      complement, XYY 758.8
      gonadal dysgenesis 758.6
      Klinefelter's 758.7
      Turner's 758.6
    trisomy 21 758.0
  cilia 743.9
  circulatory system 747.9
    specified type NEC 747.89
  clavicle 755.51
  clitoris 752.40
  coccyx 756.10
  colon 751.5
  common duct 751.60
  communication
    coronary artery 746.85
    left ventricle with right atrium
      745.4
  concha (ear) 744.3
  connection
    renal vessels with kidney
      747.62
    total pulmonary venous 747.41
  connective tissue 756.9
    specified type NEC 756.89
  cornea 743.9
    shape 743.41
    size 743.41
    specified type NEC 743.49
  coronary
    artery 746.85
    vein 746.89
  cranium — *see* Anomaly, skull
  cricoid cartilage 748.3
  cushion, endocardial 745.60
    specified type NEC 745.69
  cystic duct 751.60
  dental arch relationship 524.2
  dentition 520.6
  dentofacial NEC 524.9
    functional 524.5
    specified type NEC 524.8
  dermatoglyphic 757.2
  Descemet's membrane 743.9
    specified type NEC 743.49
  development
    cervix 752.40
    vagina 752.40
    vulva 752.40
  diaphragm, diaphragmatic
    (apertures) NEC 756.6

Anomaly, anomalous—*continued*
  digestive organ(s) or system 751.9
    lower 751.5
    specified type NEC 751.8
    upper 750.9
  distribution, coronary artery 746.85
  ductus
    arteriosus 747.0
    Botalli 747.0
  duodenum 751.5
  dura 742.9
    brain 742.4
    spinal cord 742.59
  ear 744.3
    causing impairment of hearing
      744.00
      specified type NEC 744.09
    external 744.3
      causing impairment of
        hearing 744.02
        specified type NEC 744.29
    inner (causing impairment of
      hearing) 744.05
    middle, except ossicles (causing
      impairment of hearing)
      744.03
      ossicles 744.04
    ossicles 744.04
    prominent auricle 744.29
    specified type NEC 744.29
      with hearing impairment
        744.09
  Ebstein's (heart) 746.2
    tricuspid valve 746.2
  ectodermal 757.9
  Eisenmenger's (ventricular septal
    defect) 745.4
  ejaculatory duct 752.9
    specified type NEC 752.8
  elbow (joint) 755.50
  endocardial cushion 745.60
    specified type NEC 745.69
  endocrine gland NEC 759.2
  epididymis 752.9
  epiglottis 748.3
  esophagus 750.9
    specified type NEC 750.4
  Eustachian tube 744.3
    specified type NEC 744.24
  eye (any part) 743.9
    adnexa 743.9
      specified type NEC 743.69
    anophthalmos 743.00
    anterior
      chamber and related
        structures 743.9
        angle 743.9
          specified type NEC
            743.44
        specified type NEC
          743.44
      segment 743.9
        combined 743.48
        multiple 743.48
        specified type NEC
          743.49
    cataract (see also Cataract)
      743.30
    glaucoma (see also
      Buphthalmia) 743.20
    lid 743.9
      specified type NEC 743.63
    microphthalmos (see also
      Microphthalmos) 743.10
    posterior segment 743.9
      specified type NEC 743.59
      vascular 743.58
      vitreous 743.9
        specified type NEC
          743.51
    ptosis (eyelid) 743.61
    retina 743.9
      specified type NEC 743.59
    sclera 743.9
      specified type NEC 743.47
    specified type NEC 743.8
  eyebrow 744.89

Anomaly, anomalous—continued
  eyelid 743.9
    specified type NEC 743.63
  face (any part) 744.9
    bone(s) 756.0
    specified type NEC 744.89
  fallopian tube 752.10
    specified type NEC 752.19
  fascia 756.9
    specified type NEC 756.89
  femur 755.60
  fibula 755.60
  finger 755.50
    supernumerary 755.01
    webbed (see also Syndactylism, fingers) 755.11
  fixation, intestine 751.4
  flexion (joint) 755.9
    hip or thigh (see also Dislocation, hip, congenital) 754.30
  folds, heart 746.9
  foot 755.67
  foramen
    Botalli 745.5
    ovale 745.5
  forearm 755.50
  forehead (see also Anomaly, skull) 756.0
  form, teeth 520.2
  fovea centralis 743.9
  frontal bone (see also Anomaly, skull) 756.0
  gallbladder 751.60
  Gartner's duct 752.11
  gastrointestinal tract 751.9
    specified type NEC 751.8
    vessel 747.61
  genitalia, genital organ(s) or system
    female 752.9
      external 752.40
        specified type NEC 752.49
      internal NEC 752.9
    male (external and internal) 752.9
      epispadias 752.6
      hydrocele, congenital 778.6
      hypospadias 752.6
      testis, undescended 752.5
      specified type NEC 752.8
  genitourinary NEC 752.9
  Gerbode 745.4
  globe (eye) 743.9
  glottis 748.3
  granulation or granulocyte, genetic 288.2
    constitutional 288.2
    leukocyte 288.2
  gum 750.9
  gyri 742.9
  hair 757.9
    specified type NEC 757.4
  hand 755.50
  hard tissue formation in pulp 522.3
  head (see also Anomaly, skull) 756.0
  heart 746.9
    auricle 746.9
    bands 746.9
    fibroelastosis cordis 425.3
    folds 746.9
    malposition 746.87
    maternal, affecting fetus or newborn 760.3
    obstructive NEC 746.84
    patent ductus arteriosus (Botalli) 747.0
    septum 745.9
      acquired 429.71
      aortic 745.0
      aorticopulmonary 745.0
      atrial 745.5
      auricular 745.5
      between aorta and pulmonary artery 745.0

Anomaly, anomalous—continued
  heart—continued
    septum—continued
      endocardial cushion type 745.60
        specified type NEC 745.69
      interatrial 745.5
      interventricular 745.4
        with pulmonary stenosis or atresia, dextraposition of aorta, and hypertrophy of right ventricle 745.2
        acquired 429.71
      specified type NEC 745.8
      ventricular 745.4
        with pulmonary stenosis or atresia, dextraposition of aorta, and hypertrophy of right ventricle 745.2
        acquired 429.71
    specified type NEC 746.89
    tetralogy of Fallot 745.2
    valve NEC 746.9
      aortic 746.9
        atresia 746.89
        bicuspid valve 746.4
        insufficiency 746.4
        specified type NEC 746.89
        stenosis 746.3
          subaortic 746.81
          supravalvular 747.22
      mitral 746.9
        atresia 746.89
        insufficiency 746.6
        specified type NEC 746.89
        stenosis 746.5
      pulmonary 746.00
        atresia 746.01
        insufficiency 746.09
        stenosis 746.02
          infundibular 746.83
          subvalvular 746.83
      tricuspid 746.9
        atresia 746.1
        stenosis 746.1
    ventricle 746.9
  heel 755.67
  Hegglin's 288.2
  hemianencephaly 740.0
  hemicephaly 740.0
  hemicrania 740.0
  hepatic duct 751.60
  hip (joint) 755.63
  hourglass
    bladder 753.8
    gallbladder 751.69
    stomach 750.7
  humerus 755.50
  hymen 752.40
  hypersegmentation of neutrophils, hereditary 288.2
  hypophyseal 759.2
  ileocecal (coil) (valve) 751.5
  ileum (intestine) 751.5
  ilium 755.60
  integument 757.9
    specified type NEC 757.8
  intervertebral cartilage or disc 756.10
  intestine (large) (small) 751.5
    fixational type 751.4
  iris 743.9
    specified type NEC 743.46
  ischium 755.60
  jaw NEC 524.9
    closure 524.5
    size (major) NEC 524.00
    specified type NEC 524.8

Anomaly, anomalous—continued
  jaw-cranial base relationship 524.10
    specified NEC 524.19
  jejunum 751.5
  joint 755.9
    hip
      dislocation (see also Dislocation, hip, congenital) 754.30
      predislocation (see also Subluxation, congenital, hip) 754.32
      preluxation (see also Subluxation, congenital, hip) 754.32
      subluxation (see also Subluxation, congenital, hip) 754.32
    lumbosacral 756.10
      spondylolisthesis 756.12
      spondylosis 756.11
    multiple arthrogryposis 754.89
    sacroiliac 755.69
  Jordan's 288.2
  kidney(s) (calyx) (pelvis) 753.9
    vessel 747.62
  Klippel-Feil (brevicollis) 756.16
  knee (joint) 755.64
  labium (majus) (minus) 752.40
  labyrinth, membranous (causing impairment of hearing) 744.05
  lacrimal
    apparatus, duct or passage 743.9
      specified type NEC 743.65
    gland 743.9
      specified type NEC 743.64
  Langdon Down (mongolism) 758.0
  larynx, laryngeal (muscle) 748.3
    web, webbed 748.2
  leg (lower) (upper) 755.60
    reduction NEC (see also Deformity, reduction, lower limb) 755.30
  lens 743.9
    shape 743.36
    specified type NEC 743.39
  leukocytes, genetic 288.2
    granulation (constitutional) 288.2
  lid (fold) 743.9
  ligament 756.9
    broad 752.10
    round 752.9
  limb, except reduction deformity 755.9
    lower 755.60
      reduction deformity (see also Deformity, reduction, lower limb) 755.30
      specified type NEC 755.69
    upper 755.50
      reduction deformity (see also Deformity, reduction, upper limb) 755.20
      specified type NEC 755.59
  lip 750.9
    harelip (see also Cleft, lip) 749.10
    specified type NEC 750.26
  liver (duct) 751.60
    atresia 751.69
  lower extremity 755.60
    vessel 747.64
  lumbosacral (joint) (region) 756.10
  lung (fissure) (lobe) NEC 748.60
    agenesis 748.5
    specified type NEC 748.69
  lymphatic system 759.9
  Madelung's (radius) 755.54
  mandible 524.9
    size NEC 524.00

Anomaly, anomalous—continued
  maxilla 524.9
    size NEC 524.00
  May (-Hegglin) 288.2
  meatus urinarius 753.9
    specified type NEC 753.8
  meningeal bands or folds, constriction of 742.8
  meninges 742.9
    brain 742.4
    spinal 742.59
  meningocele (see also Spina bifida) 741.9
  mesentery 751.9
  metacarpus 755.50
  metatarsus 755.67
  middle ear, except ossicles (causing impairment of hearing) 744.03
    ossicles 744.04
  mitral (leaflets) (valve) 746.9
    atresia 746.89
    insufficiency 746.6
    specified type NEC 746.89
    stenosis 746.5
  mouth 750.9
    specified type NEC 750.26
  multiple NEC 759.7
    specified type NEC 759.89
  muscle 756.9
    eye 743.9
      specified type NEC 743.69
    specified type NEC 756.89
  musculoskeletal system, except limbs 756.9
    specified type NEC 756.9
  nail 757.9
    specified type NEC 757.5
  narrowness, eyelid 743.62
  nasal sinus or septum 748.1
  neck (any part) 744.9
    specified type NEC 744.89
  nerve 742.9
    acoustic 742.9
      specified type NEC 742.8
    optic 742.9
      specified type NEC 742.8
    specified type NEC 742.8
  nervous system NEC 742.9
    brain 742.9
      specified type NEC 742.4
    specified type NEC 742.8
  neurological 742.9
  nipple 757.9
  nonteratogenic NEC 754.89
  nose, nasal (bone) (cartilage) (septum) (sinus) 748.1
  ocular muscle 743.9
  omphalomesenteric duct 751.0
  opening, pulmonary veins 747.49
  optic
    disc 743.9
      specified type NEC 743.57
    nerve 742.9
  opticociliary vessels 743.9
  orbit (eye) 743.9
    specified type NEC 743.66
  organ
    of Corti (causing impairment of hearing) 744.05
    or site 759.9
      specified type NEC 759.89
  origin
    both great arteries from same ventricle 745.11
    coronary artery 746.85
    innominate artery 747.69
    left coronary artery from pulmonary artery 746.85
    pulmonary artery 747.3
    renal vessels 747.62
    subclavian artery (left) (right) 747.21
  osseous meatus (ear) 744.03
  ovary 752.0
  oviduct 752.10

Anomaly, anomalous—continued
  palate (hard) (soft) 750.9
    cleft (see also Cleft, palate) 749.00
  pancreas (duct) 751.7
  papillary muscles 746.9
  parathyroid gland 759.2
  paraurethral ducts 753.9
  parotid (gland) 750.9
  patella 755.64
  Pelger-Huët (hereditary hyposegmentation) 288.2
  pelvic girdle 755.60
    specified type NEC 755.69
  pelvis (bony) 755.60
    complicating delivery 653.0
    rachitic 268.1
    fetal 756.4
  penis (glans) 752.9
  pericardium 746.89
  peripheral vascular system NEC 747.60
    gastrointestinal 747.61
    lower limb 747.64
    renal 747.62
    specified site NEC 747.69
    spinal 747.82
    upper limb 747.63
  Peter's 743.44
  pharynx 750.9
    branchial cleft 744.41
    specified type NEC 750.29
  Pierre Robin 756.0
  pigmentation NEC 709.00 ◆
    congenital 757.33
  pituitary (gland) 759.2
  pleural folds 748.8
  portal vein 747.40
  position tooth, teeth 524.3
  preauricular sinus 744.46
  prepuce 752.9
  prostate 752.9
  pulmonary 748.60
    artery 747.3
    circulation 747.3
    specified type NEC 748.69
    valve 746.00
      atresia 746.01
      insufficiency 746.09
      specified type NEC 746.09
      stenosis 746.02
        infundibular 746.83
        subvalvular 746.83
    vein 747.40
    venous
      connection 747.49
        partial 747.42
        total 747.41
      return 747.49
        partial 747.42
        total (TAPVR) (complete) (subdiaphragmatic) (supradiaphragmatic) 747.41
  pupil 743.9
  pylorus 750.9
    hypertrophy 750.5
    stenosis 750.5
  rachitic, fetal 756.4
  radius 755.50
  rectovaginal (septum) 752.40
  rectum 751.5
  refraction 367.9
  renal 753.9
    vessel 747.62
  respiratory system 748.9
    specified type NEC 748.8
  rib 756.3
    cervical 756.2
  Rieger's 743.44
  rings, trachea 748.3
  rotation — see also Malrotation
    hip or thigh (see also Subluxation, congenital, hip) 754.32
  round ligament 752.9
  sacroiliac (joint) 755.69

Anomaly, anomalous—continued
  sacrum 756.10
  saddle
    back 754.2
    nose 754.0
      syphilitic 090.5
  salivary gland or duct 750.9
    specified type NEC 750.26
  scapula 755.50
  sclera 743.9
    specified type NEC 743.47
  scrotum 752.9
  sebaceous gland 757.9
  seminal duct or tract 752.9
  sense organs 742.9
    specified type NEC 742.8
  septum
    heart — see Anomaly, heart, septum
    nasal 748.1
  sex chromosomes NEC (see also Anomaly, chromosomes) 758.8
  shoulder (girdle) (joint) 755.50
    specified type NEC 755.59
  sigmoid (flexure) 751.5
  sinus of Valsalva 747.29
  site NEC 759.9
  skeleton generalized NEC 756.50
  skin (appendage) 757.9
    specified type NEC 757.39
  skull (bone) 756.0
    with
      anencephalus 740.0
      encephalocele 742.0
      hydrocephalus 742.3
        with spina bifida (see also Spina bifida) 741.0
      microcephalus 742.1
  specified type NEC
    adrenal (gland) 759.1
    alimentary tract (complete) (partial) 751.8
      lower 751.5
      upper 750.8
    ankle 755.69
    anus, anal (canal) 751.5
    aorta, aortic 747.29
      arch 747.21
    appendix 751.5
    arm 755.59
    artery (peripheral) NEC (see also Anomaly, peripheral vascular system) 747.60
      brain 747.81
      coronary 746.85
      eye 743.58
      pulmonary 747.3
      retinal 743.58
      umbilical 747.5
    auditory canal 744.29
      causing impairment of hearing 744.02
    bile duct or passage 751.69
    bladder 753.8
      neck 753.8
    bone(s) 756.9
      arm 755.59
      face 756.0
      leg 755.69
      pelvic girdle 755.69
      shoulder girdle 755.59
      skull 756.0
        with
          anencephalus 740.0
          encephalocele 742.0
          hydrocephalus 742.3
            with spina bifida (see also Spina bifida) 741.0
          microcephalus 742.1
    brain 742.4
    breast 757.6
    broad ligament 752.19
    bronchus 748.3
    canal of Nuck 752.8

Anomaly, anomalous—continued
  specified type NEC—continued
    cardiac septal closure 745.8
    carpus 755.59
    cartilaginous 756.9
    cecum 751.5
    cervix 752.49
    chest (wall) 756.3
    chin 744.89
    ciliary body 743.46
    circulatory system 747.89
    clavicle 755.51
    clitoris 752.49
    coccyx 756.19
    colon 751.5
    common duct 751.69
    connective tissue 756.89
    cricoid cartilage 748.3
    cystic duct 751.69
    diaphragm 756.6
    digestive organ(s) or tract 751.8
      lower 751.5
      upper 750.8
    duodenum 751.5
    ear 744.29
      auricle 744.29
        causing impairment of hearing 744.02
      causing impairment of hearing 744.09
      inner (causing impairment of hearing) 744.05
      middle, except ossicles 744.03
      ossicles 744.04
    ejaculatory duct 752.8
    endocrine 759.2
    epiglottis 748.3
    esophagus 750.4
    Eustachian tube 744.24
    eye 743.8
      lid 743.63
      muscle 743.69
    face 744.89
      bone(s) 756.0
    fallopian tube 752.19
    fascia 756.89
    femur 755.69
    fibula 755.69
    finger 755.59
    foot 755.67
    fovea centralis 743.55
    gallbladder 751.69
    Gartner's duct 752.8
    gastrointestinal tract 751.8
    genitalia, genital organ(s)
      female 752.8
        external 752.49
        internal NEC 752.8
      male 752.8
    genitourinary tract NEC 752.8
    glottis 748.3
    hair 757.4
    hand 755.59
    heart 746.89
      valve NEC 746.89
        pulmonary 746.09
    hepatic duct 751.69
    hydatid of Morgagni 752.8
    hymen 752.49
    integument 757.8
    intestine (large) (small) 751.5
      fixational type 751.4
    iris 743.46
    jejunum 751.5
    joint 755.8
    kidney 753.3
    knee 755.64
    labium (majus) (minus) 752.49
    labyrinth, membranous 744.05
    larynx 748.3
    leg 755.69
    lens 743.39

Anomaly, anomalous—continued
  specified type NEC—continued
    limb, except reduction deformity 755.8
      lower 755.69
        reduction deformity (see also Deformity, reduction, lower limb) 755.30
      upper 755.59
        reduction deformity (see also Deformity, reduction, upper limb) 755.20
    lip 750.26
    liver 751.69
    lung (fissure) (lobe) 748.69
    meatus urinarius 753.8
    metacarpus 755.59
    mouth 750.26
    muscle 756.89
      eye 743.69
    musculoskeletal system, except limbs 756.9
    nail 757.5
    neck 744.89
    nerve 742.8
      acoustic 742.8
      optic 742.8
    nervous system 742.8
    nipple 757.6
    nose 748.1
    organ NEC 759.89
      of Corti 744.05
    osseous meatus (ear) 744.03
    ovary 752.0
    oviduct 752.19
    pancreas 751.7
    parathyroid 759.2
    patella 755.64
    pelvic girdle 755.69
    penis 752.8
    pericardium 746.89
    peripheral vascular system NEC (see also Anomaly, peripheral vascular system) 747.60
    pharynx 750.29
    pituitary 759.2
    prostate 752.8
    radius 755.59
    rectum 751.5
    respiratory system 748.8
    rib 756.3
    round ligament 752.8
    sacrum 756.19
    salivary duct or gland 750.26
    scapula 755.59
    sclera 743.47
    scrotum 752.8
    seminal duct or tract 752.8
    shoulder girdle 755.59
    site NEC 759.89
    skin 757.39
    skull (bone(s)) 756.0
      with
        anencephalus 740.0
        encephalocele 742.0
        hydrocephalus 742.3
          with spina bifida (see also Spina bifida) 741.0
        microcephalus 742.1
    specified organ or site NEC 759.89
    spermatic cord 752.8
    spinal cord 742.59
    spine 756.19
    spleen 759.0
    sternum 756.3
    stomach 750.7
    tarsus 755.67
    tendon 756.89
    testis 752.8
    thorax (wall) 756.3
    thymus 759.2

Anomaly, anomalous—*continued*
  specified type NEC—*continued*
    thyroid (gland) 759.2
      cartilage 748.3
    tibia 755.69
    toe 755.66
    tongue 750.19
    trachea (cartilage) 748.3
    ulna 755.59
    urachus 753.7
    ureter 753.4
      obstructive 753.2
    urethra 753.8
      obstructive 753.6
    urinary tract 753.8
    uterus 752.3
    uvula 750.26
    vagina 752.49
    vascular NEC (*see also* Anomaly, peripheral vascular system) 747.60
      brain 747.81
    vas deferens 752.8
    vein(s) (peripheral) NEC (*see also* Anomaly, peripheral vascular system) 747.60
      brain 747.81
      great 747.49
      portal 747.49
      pulmonary 747.49
      vena cava (inferior) (superior) 747.49
    vertebra 756.19
    vulva 752.49
  spermatic cord 752.9
  spine, spinal 756.10
    column 756.10
    cord 742.9
      meningocele (*see also* Spina bifida) 741.9
      specified type NEC 742.59
      spina bifida (*see also* Spina bifida) 741.9
      vessel 747.82
    meninges 742.59
    nerve root 742.9
  spleen 759.0
  Sprengel's 755.52
  sternum 756.3
  stomach 750.9
    specified type NEC 750.7
  submaxillary gland 750.9
  superior vena cava 747.40
  talipes — *see* Talipes
  tarsus 755.67
    with complete absence of distal elements 755.31
  teeth, tooth NEC 520.9
    position 524.3
    spacing 524.3
  tendon 756.9
    specified type NEC 756.89
  termination
    coronary artery 746.85
  testis 752.9
  thebesian valve 746.9
  thigh 755.60
    flexion (*see also* Subluxation, congenital, hip) 754.32
  thorax (wall) 756.3
  throat 750.9
  thumb 755.50
    supernumerary 755.01
  thymus gland 759.2
  thyroid (gland) 759.2
    cartilage 748.3
  tibia 755.60
    saber 090.5
  toe 755.66
    supernumerary 755.02
    webbed (*see also* Syndactylism, toes) 755.13
  tongue 750.10
    specified type NEC 750.19
  trachea, tracheal 748.3
    cartilage 748.3
    rings 748.3

Anomaly, anomalous—*continued*
  tragus 744.3
  transverse aortic arch 747.21
  trichromata 368.59
  trichromatopsia 368.59
  tricuspid (leaflet) (valve) 746.9
    atresia 746.1
    Ebstein's 746.2
    specified type NEC 746.89
    stenosis 746.1
  trunk 759.9
  Uhl's (hypoplasia of myocardium, right ventricle) 746.84
  ulna 755.50
  umbilicus 759.9
    artery 747.5
  union, trachea with larynx 748.3
  unspecified site 759.9
  upper extremity 755.50
    vessel 747.63
  urachus 753.7
    specified type NEC 753.7
  ureter 753.9
    obstructive 753.2
    specified type NEC 753.4
  urethra (valve) 753.9
    obstructive 753.6
    specified type NEC 753.8
  urinary tract or system (any part, except urachus) 753.9
    specified type NEC 753.8
    urachus 753.7
  uterus 752.3
    with only one functioning horn 752.3
    in pregnancy or childbirth 654.0
      affecting fetus or newborn 763.8
      causing obstructed labor 660.2
        affecting fetus or newborn 763.1
  uvula 750.9
  vagina 752.40
  valleculae 748.3
  valve (heart) NEC 746.9
    formation, ureter 753.2
    pulmonary 746.00
    specified type NEC 746.89
  vascular NEC (*see also* Anomaly, peripheral vascular system) 747.60
    ring 747.21
  vas deferens 752.9
  vein(s) (peripheral) NEC (*see also* Anomaly, peripheral vascular system) 747.60
    brain 747.81
    cerebral 747.81
    coronary 746.89
    great 747.40
      specified type NEC 747.49
    portal 747.40
    pulmonary 747.40
    retina 743.9
    vena cava (inferior) (superior) 747.40
    venous return (pulmonary) 747.49
      partial 747.42
      total 747.41
  ventricle, ventricular (heart) 746.9
    bands 746.9
    folds 746.9
    septa 745.4
  vertebra 756.10
  vesicourethral orifice 753.9
  vessels NEC (*see also* Anomaly, peripheral vascular system) 747.60
    optic papilla 743.9
  vitelline duct 751.0
  vitreous humor 743.9
    specified type NEC 743.51
  vulva 752.40
  wrist (joint) 755.50
Anomia 784.69

Anonychia 757.5
  acquired 703.8
Anophthalmos, anophthalmus (clinical) (congenital) (globe) 743.00
  acquired 360.89
Anopsia (altitudinal) (quadrant) 368.46
Anorchia 752.8
Anorchism, anorchidism 752.8
Anorexia 783.0
  hysterical 300.11
  nervosa 307.1
Anosmia (*see also* Disturbance, sensation) 781.1
  hysterical 300.11
  postinfectional 478.9
  psychogenic 306.7
  traumatic 951.8
Anosognosia 780.9
Anosphrasia 781.1
Anosteoplasia 756.50
Anotia 744.09
Anovulatory cycle 628.0
Anoxemia 799.0
  newborn 770.8
Anoxia 799.0
  altitude 993.2
  cerebral 348.1
    with
      abortion — *see* Abortion, by type, with specified complication NEC
      ectopic pregnancy (*see also* categories 633.0-633.9) 639.8
      molar pregnancy (*see also* categories 630-632) 639.8
    complicating
      delivery (cesarean) (instrumental) 669.4
      ectopic or molar pregnancy 639.8
      obstetric anesthesia or sedation 668.2
      during or resulting from a procedure 997.0
    following
      abortion 639.8
      ectopic or molar pregnancy 639.8
    newborn (*see also* Distress, fetal, liveborn infant) 768.9
  due to drowning 994.1
  heart — *see* Insufficiency, coronary
  high altitude 993.2
  intrauterine
    fetal death (before onset of labor) 768.0
    during labor 768.1
    liveborn infant — *see* Distress, fetal, liveborn infant
  myocardial — *see* Insufficiency, coronary
  newborn 768.9
    mild or moderate 768.6
    severe 768.5
  pathological 799.0
Anteflexion — *see* Anteversion
Antenatal
  care, normal pregnancy V22.1
    first V22.0
  screening (for) V28.9
    based on amniocentesis NEC V28.2
      chromosomal anomalies V28.0
      raised alphafetoprotein levels V28.1
    chromosomal anomalies V28.0
    fetal growth retardation using ultrasonics V28.4
    isoimmunization V28.5

Antenatal—*continued*
  screening (for)—*continued*
    malformations using ultrasonics V28.3
    raised alphafetoprotein levels in amniotic fluid V28.1
    specified condition NEC V28.8
Antepartum — *see* condition
Anterior — *see also* condition
  spinal artery compression syndrome 721.1
Antero-occlusion 524.2
Anteversion
  cervix (*see also* Anteversion, uterus) 621.6
  femur (neck), congenital 755.63
  uterus, uterine (cervix) (postinfectional) (postpartal, old) 621.6
    congenital 752.3
    in pregnancy or childbirth 654.4
      affecting fetus or newborn 763.8
      causing obstructed labor 660.2
        affecting fetus or newborn 763.1
Anthracosilicosis (occupational) 500
Anthracosis (lung) (occupational) 500
  lingua 529.3
Anthrax 022.9
  with pneumonia 022.1 [484.5]
  colitis 022.2
  cutaneous 022.0
  gastrointestinal 022.2
  intestinal 022.2
  pulmonary 022.1
  respiratory 022.1
  septicemia 022.3
  specified manifestation NEC 022.8
Anthropoid pelvis 755.69
  with disproportion (fetopelvic) 653.2
    affecting fetus or newborn 763.1
    causing obstructed labor 660.1
      affecting fetus or newborn 763.1
Anthropophobia 300.29
Antibioma, breast 611.0
Antibodies
  maternal (blood group) (*see also* Incompatibility) 656.2
    anti-D, cord blood 656.1
      fetus or newborn 773.0
Antibody deficiency syndrome
  agammaglobulinemic 279.00
  congenital 279.04
  hypogammaglobulinemic 279.00
Anticoagulant, circulating (*see also* Circulating anticoagulants) 286.5
Antimongolism syndrome 758.3
Antimonial cholera 985.4
Antisocial personality 301.7
Antithrombinemia (*see also* Circulating anticoagulants) 286.5
Antithromboplastinemia (*see also* Circulating anticoagulants) 286.5
Antithromboplastinogenemia (*see also* Circulating anticoagulants) 286.5
Antitoxin complication or reaction — *see* Complications, vaccination
Anton (-Babinski) **syndrome** (hemiasomatognosia) 307.9
Antritis (chronic) 473.0
  acute 461.0

Antrum, antral — see condition
Anuria 788.5
  with
    abortion — see Abortion, by type, with renal failure
    ectopic pregnancy (see also categories 633.0-633.9) 639.3
    molar pregnancy (see also categories 630-632) 639.3
  calculus (impacted) (recurrent) 592.9
    kidney 592.0
    ureter 592.1
  congenital 753.3
  due to a procedure 997.5
  following
    abortion 639.3
    ectopic or molar pregnancy 639.3
  newborn 753.3
  postrenal 593.4
  puerperal, postpartum, childbirth 669.3
  specified as due to a procedure 997.5
  sulfonamide
    correct substance properly administered 788.5
    overdose or wrong substance given or taken 961.0
  traumatic (following crushing) 958.5
Anus, anal — see condition
Anusitis 569.49
Anxiety (neurosis) (reaction) (state) 300.00
  alcohol-induced 291.8 ◆
  depression 300.4
  drug-induced 292.89 ◆
  generalized 300.02
  hysteria 300.20
  in
    acute stress reaction 308.0
    transient adjustment reaction 309.24
  panic type 300.01
  separation, abnormal 309.21
Aorta, aortic — see condition
Aortectasia 441.9
Aortitis (nonsyphilitic) 447.6
  arteriosclerotic 440.0
  calcific 447.6
  Döhle-Heller 093.1
  luetic 093.1
  rheumatic (see also Endocarditis, acute, rheumatic) 391.1
  rheumatoid — see Arthritis, rheumatoid
  specific 093.1
  syphilitic 093.1
    congenital 090.5
Apethetic thyroid storm (see also Thyrotoxicosis) 242.9
Apepsia 536.8
  achlorhydric 536.0
  psychogenic 306.4
Aperistalsis, esophagus 530.0
Apert's syndrome (acrocephalosyndactyly) 755.55
Apert-Gallais syndrome (adrenogenital) 255.2
Apertognathia 524.2
Aphagia 783.0
  psychogenic 307.1
Aphakia (acquired) (bilateral) (postoperative) (unilateral) 379.31
  congenital 743.35
Aphalangia (congenital) 755.4
  lower limb (complete) (intercalary) (partial) (terminal) 755.39

Aphalangia—continued
  lower limb—continued
    meaning all digits (complete) (partial) 755.31
    transverse 755.31
  upper limb (complete) (intercalary) (partial) (terminal) 755.29
    meaning all digits (complete) (partial) 755.21
    transverse 755.21
Aphasia (amnestic) (ataxic) (auditory) (Broca's) (choreatic) (classic) (expressive) (global) (ideational) (ideokinetic) (ideomotor) (jargon) (motor) (nominal) (receptive) (semantic) (sensory) (syntactic) (verbal) (visual) (Wernicke's) 784.3
  developmental 315.31
  syphilis, tertiary 094.89
  uremic — see Uremia
Aphemia 784.3
  uremic — see Uremia
Aphonia 784.41
  clericorum 784.49
  hysterical 300.11
  organic 784.41
  psychogenic 306.1
Aphthae, aphthous — see also condition
  Bednar's 528.2
  cachectic 529.0
  epizootic 078.4
  fever 078.4
  oral 528.2
  stomatitis 528.2
  thrush 112.0
  ulcer (oral) (recurrent) 528.2
    genital organ(s) NEC
      female 629.8
      male 608.89
    larynx 478.79
Apical — see condition
Aplasia — see also Agenesis
  alveolar process (acquired) 525.8
    congenital 750.26
  aorta (congenital) 747.22
  aortic valve (congenital) 746.89
  axialis extracorticalis (congenital) 330.0
  bone marrow (myeloid) 284.9
    acquired (secondary) 284.8
    congenital 284.0
    idiopathic 284.9
  brain 740.0
    specified part 742.2
  breast 757.6
  bronchus 748.3
  cementum 520.4
  cerebellar 742.2
  congenital pure red cell 284.0
  corpus callosum 742.2
  erythrocyte 284.8
    congenital 284.0
  extracortical axial 330.0
  eye (congenital) 743.00
  fovea centralis (congenital) 743.55
  germinal (cell) 606.0
  iris 743.45
  labyrinth, membranous 744.05
  limb (congenital) 755.4
    lower NEC 755.30
    upper NEC 755.20
  lung (bilateral) (congenital) (unilateral) 748.5
  nervous system NEC 742.8
  nuclear 742.8
  ovary 752.0
  Pelizaeus-Merzbacher 330.0
  prostate (congenital) 752.8
  red cell (pure) (with thymoma) 284.8
    acquired (adult) (secondary) 284.8
    congenital 284.0
    hereditary 284.0

Aplasia—continued
  red cell—continued
    of infants 284.0
    primary 284.0
  round ligament (congenital) 752.8
  salivary gland 750.21
  skin (congenital) 757.39
  spinal cord 742.59
  spleen 759.0
  testis (congenital) 752.8
  thymic, with immunodeficiency 279.2
  thyroid 243
  uterus 752.3
  ventral horn cell 742.59
Apleuria 756.3
Apnea, apneic (spells) 786.09
  newborn, neonatorum 770.8
  psychogenic 306.1
  sleep NEC 780.57
    with
      hypersomnia 780.53
      hyposomnia 780.51
      insomnia 780.51
      sleep disturbance NEC 780.57
Apneumatosis newborn 770.4
Apodia 755.31
Apophysitis (bone) (see also Osteochondrosis) 732.9
  calcaneus 732.5
  juvenile 732.6
Apoplectiform convulsions (see also Disease, cerebrovascular, acute) 436
Apoplexia, apoplexy, apoplectic (see also Disease, cerebrovascular, acute) 436
  abdominal 569.89
  adrenal 036.3
  attack 436
  basilar (see also Disease, cerebrovascular, acute) 436
  brain (see also Disease, cerebrovascular, acute) 436
  bulbar (see also Disease, cerebrovascular, acute) 436
  capillary (see also Disease, cerebrovascular, acute) 436
  cardiac (see also Infarct, myocardium) 410.9
  cerebral (see also Disease, cerebrovascular acute) 436
  chorea (see also Disease, cerebrovascular, acute) 436
  congestive (see also Disease, cerebrovascular, acute) 436
    newborn 767.4
  embolic (see also Embolism, brain) 434.1
  fetus 767.0
  fit (see also Disease, cerebrovascular, acute) 436
  healed or old — see also category 438
    without residuals V12.5
  heart (auricle) (ventricle) (see also Infarct, myocardium) 410.9
  heat 992.0
  hemiplegia (see also Disease, cerebrovascular, acute) 436
  hemorrhagic (stroke) (see also Hemorrhage, brain) 432.9
  ingravescent (see also Disease, cerebrovascular, acute) 436
  late effect — see category 438
  lung — see Embolism, pulmonary
  meninges, hemorrhagic (see also Hemorrhage subarachnoid) 430
  neonatorum 767.0
  newborn 767.0
  pancreatitis 577.0
  placenta 641.2
  progressive (see also Disease, cerebrovascular, acute) 436

Apoplexia, apoplexy, apoplectic—continued
  pulmonary (artery) (vein) — see Embolism, pulmonary
  sanguineous (see also Disease, cerebrovascular, acute) 436
  seizure (see also Disease, cerebrovascular, acute) 436
  serous (see also Disease, cerebrovascular, acute) 436
  spleen 289.59
  stroke (see also Disease, cerebrovascular, acute) 436
  thrombotic (see also Thrombosis, brain) 434.0
  uremic — see Uremia
  uteroplacental 641.2
Appendage
  fallopian tube (cyst of Morgagni) 752.11
  intestine (epiploic) 751.5
  preauricular 744.1
  testicular (organ of Morgagni) 752.8
Appendicitis 541
  with
    perforation, peritonitis (generalized), or rupture 540.0
      with peritoneal abscess 540.1 ◆
    peritoneal abscess 540.1
  acute (catarrhal) (fulminating) (gangrenous) (inflammatory) (obstructive) (retrocecal) (suppurative) 540.9
    with
      perforation, peritonitis, or rupture 540.0
        with peritoneal abscess 540.1 ◆
      peritoneal abscess 540.1
  amebic 006.8
  chronic (recurrent) 542
  exacerbation — see Appendicitis, acute
  fulminating — see Appendicitis, acute
  gangrenous — see Appendicitis, acute
  healed (obliterative) 542
  interval 542
  neurogenic 542
  obstructive 542
  pneumococcal 541
  recurrent 542
  relapsing 542
  retrocecal 541
  subacute (adhesive) 542
  subsiding 542
  suppurative — see Appendicitis, acute
  tuberculous (see also Tuberculosis) 014.8
Appendiclausis 543.9
Appendicolithiasis 543.9
Appendicopathia oxyurica 127.4
Appendix, appendicular — see also condition
  Morgagni (male) 752.8
    fallopian tube 752.11
Appetite
  depraved 307.52
  excessive 783.6
    psychogenic 307.51
  lack or loss (see also Anorexia) 783.0
    nonorganic origin 307.59
  perverted 307.52
    hysterical 300.11
Apprehension, apprehensiveness (abnormal) (state) 300.00
  specified type NEC 300.09
Approximal wear 521.1

Apraxia (classic) (ideational)
(ideokinetic) (ideomotor) (motor)
784.69
- oculomotor, congenital 379.51
- verbal 784.69

Aptyalism 527.7

Arabicum elephantiasis (see also Infestation, filarial) 125.9

Arachnidism 989.5

Arachnitis — see Meningitis

Arachnodactyly 759.82

Arachnoidism 989.5

Arachnoiditis (acute) (adhesive) (basic) (brain) (cerebrospinal) (chiasmal) (chronic) (spinal) (see also Meningitis) 322.9
- meningococcal (chronic) 036.0
- syphilitic 094.2
- tuberculous (see also Tuberculosis, meninges) 013.0

Araneism 989.5

Arboencephalitis, Australian 062.4

Arborization block (heart) 426.6

Arbor virus, arbovirus (infection) NEC 066.9

ARC 042 ◆

Arches — see condition

Arcuatus uterus 752.3

Arcus (cornea)
- juvenilis 743.43
  - interfering with vision 743.42
- senilis 371.41

Arc-welders' lung 503

Arc-welders' syndrome (photokeratitis) 370.24

Areflexia 796.1

Areola — see condition

Argentaffinoma (M8241/1) — see also Neoplasm, by site, uncertain behavior
- benign (M8241/0) — see Neoplasm, by site, benign
- malignant (M8241/3) — see Neoplasm, by site, malignant
- syndrome 259.2

Argentinian hemorrhagic fever 078.7

Arginosuccinicaciduria 270.6

Argonz-Del Castillo syndrome (nonpuerperal galactorrhea and amenorrhea) 253.1

Argyll-Robertson phenomenon, pupil, or syndrome (syphilitic) 094.89
- atypical 379.45
- nonluetic 379.45
- nonsyphilitic 379.45
- reversed 379.45

Argyria, argyriasis NEC 985.8
- conjunctiva 372.55
- cornea 371.16
- from drug or medicinal agent
  - correct substance properly administered 709.09 ◆
  - overdose or wrong substance given or taken 961.2

Arhinencephaly 742.2

Arias-Stella phenomenon 621.3

Ariboflavinosis 266.0

Arizona enteritis 008.1

Arm — see condition

Armenian disease 277.3

Arnold-Chiari obstruction or syndrome (see also Spina bifida) 741.0
- type I 348.4 ▼
- type II (see also Spina bifida) 741.0
- type III 742.0
- type IV 742.2 ▲

Arrest, arrested
- active phase of labor 661.1
  - affecting fetus or newborn 763.7

Arrest, arrested—continued
- any plane in pelvis
  - complicating delivery 660.1
    - affecting fetus or newborn 763.1
- bone marrow (see also Anemia, aplastic) 284.9
- cardiac 427.5
  - with
    - abortion — see Abortion, by type, with specified complication NEC
    - ectopic pregnancy (see also categories 633.0-633.9) 639.8
    - molar pregnancy (see also categories 630-632) 639.8
  - complicating
    - anesthesia
      - correct substance properly administered 427.5
      - obstetric 668.1
      - overdose or wrong substance given 968.4
      - specified anesthetic — see Table of drugs and chemicals
    - delivery (cesarean) (instrumental) 669.4
    - ectopic or molar pregnancy 639.8
    - surgery (nontherapeutic) (therapeutic) 997.1
  - fetus or newborn 779.8
  - following
    - abortion 639.8
    - ectopic or molar pregnancy 639.8
  - postoperative (immediate) 997.1
    - long-term effect of cardiac surgery 429.4
- cardiorespiratory (see also Arrest, cardiac) 427.5
- deep transverse 660.3
  - affecting fetus or newborn 763.1
- development or growth
  - bone 733.91
  - child 783.4
  - fetus 764.9
    - affecting management of pregnancy 656.5
  - tracheal rings 748.3
- epiphyseal 733.91
- granulopoiesis 288.0
- heart — see Arrest, cardiac
- respiratory 799.1
  - newborn 770.8
- sinus 426.6
- transverse (deep) 660.3
  - affecting fetus or newborn 763.1

Arrhenoblastoma (M8630/1)
- benign (M8630/0)
  - specified site — see Neoplasm, by site, benign
  - unspecified site
    - female 220
    - male 222.0
- malignant (M8630/3)
  - specified site — see Neoplasm, by site, malignant
  - unspecified site
    - female 183.0
    - male 186.9
- specified site — see Neoplasm, by site, uncertain behavior
- unspecified site
  - female 236.2
  - male 236.4

Arrhinencephaly 742.2
- due to
  - trisomy 13 (13-15) 758.1
  - trisomy 18 (16-18) 758.2

Arrhythmia (auricle) (cardiac) (cordis) (gallop rhythm) (juvenile) (nodal) (reflex) (sinus) (supraventricular) (transitory) (ventricle) 427.9
- bigeminal rhythm 427.89
- block 426.9
- bradycardia 427.89
- contractions, premature 427.60
- coronary sinus 427.89
- ectopic 427.89
- extrasystolic 427.60
- postoperative 997.1
- psychogenic 306.2
- vagal 780.2

Arrillaga-Ayerza syndrome (pulmonary artery sclerosis with pulmonary hypertension) 416.0

Arsenical
- dermatitis 692.4
- keratosis 692.4
- pigmentation 985.1
  - from drug or medicinal agent
    - correct substance properly administered 709.09 ◆
    - overdose or wrong substance given or taken 961.1

Arsenism 985.1
- from drug or medicinal agent
  - correct substance properly administered 692.4
  - overdose or wrong substance given or taken 961.1

Arterial — see condition

Arteriectasis 447.8

Arteriofibrosis — see Arteriosclerosis

Arteriolar sclerosis — see Arteriosclerosis

Arteriolith — see Arteriosclerosis

Arteriolitis 447.6
- necrotizing, kidney 447.5
- renal — see Hypertension, kidney

Arteriolosclerosis — see Arteriosclerosis

Arterionephrosclerosis (see also Hypertension, kidney) 403.90

Arteriopathy 447.9

Arteriosclerosis, arteriosclerotic (artery) (deformans) (diffuse) (disease) (endarteritis) (general) (obliterans) (obliterative) (occlusive) (senile) (with calcification) 440.9
- with
  - gangrene 440.24
  - psychosis (see also Psychosis, arteriosclerotic) 290.40
- aorta 440.0
- arteries of extremities — see Arteriosclerosis, extremities ◆
- basilar (artery) (see also Occlusion, artery, basilar) 433.0
- brain 437.0
- bypass graft ▼
  - coronary artery 414.02
    - autologous vein 414.02
    - nonautologous biological 414.03
  - extremity 440.30
    - autologous vein 440.31
    - nonautologous biological 440.32
- cardiac — see Arteriosclerosis, coronary
- cardiopathy — see Arteriosclerosis, coronary ▲
- cardiorenal (see also Hypertension, cardiorenal) 404.90
- cardiovascular (see also Disease, cardiovascular) 429.2
- carotid (artery) (common) (internal) (see also Occlusion, artery, carotid) 433.1
- central nervous system 437.0
- cerebral 437.0
  - late effect — see category 438

Arteriosclerosis, arteriosclerotic—continued
- cerebrospinal 437.0
- cerebrovascular 437.0
- coronary (artery) 414.00 ▼
  - graft — see Arteriosclerosis, bypass graft
  - native artery 414.01
- extremities (native artery) NEC 440.20
  - bypass graft 440.30
    - autologous vein 440.31
    - nonautologous biological 440.32 ▲
  - claudication (intermittent) 440.21
    - and
      - gangrene 440.24
      - rest pain 440.22
        - and
          - gangrene 440.24
          - ulceration 440.23
            - and gangrene 440.24
      - ulceration 440.23
        - and gangrene 440.24
  - gangrene 440.24
  - rest pain 440.22
    - and
      - gangrene 440.24
      - ulceration 440.23
        - and gangrene 440.24
  - specified site NEC 440.29
  - ulceration 440.23
    - and gangrene 440.24
- heart (disease) — see also Arteriosclerosis, coronary ◆
  - valve 424.99
    - aortic 424.1
    - mitral 424.0
    - pulmonary 424.3
    - tricuspid 424.2
- kidney (see also Hypertension, kidney) 403.90
- labyrinth, labyrinthine 388.00
- medial NEC 440.20
- mesentery (artery) 557.1
- Mönckeberg's 440.20
- myocarditis 429.0
- nephrosclerosis (see also Hypertension, kidney) 403.90
- peripheral (of extremities) — see Arteriosclerosis, extremities ◆
- precerebral 433.9
  - specified artery NEC 433.8
- pulmonary (idiopathic) 416.0
- renal (see also Hypertension, kidney) 403.90
  - arterioles (see also Hypertension, kidney) 403.90
  - artery 440.1
- retinal (vascular) 440.8 [362.13]
- specified artery NEC 440.8
  - with gangrene 440.8 [785.4]
- spinal (cord) 437.0
- vertebral (artery) (see also Occlusion, artery, vertebral) 433.2

Arteriospasm 443.9

Arteriovenous — see condition

Arteritis 447.6
- allergic (see also Angiitis, hypersensitivity) 446.20
- aorta (nonsyphilitic) 447.6
  - syphilitic 093.1
- aortic arch 446.7
- brachiocephalica 446.7
- brain 437.4
  - syphilitic 094.89
- branchial 446.7
- cerebral 437.4
  - late effect — see category 438
  - syphilitic 094.89

Arteritis—continued
　coronary (artery) — *see also*
　　　Arteriosclerosis, coronary
　　rheumatic 391.9
　　　chronic 398.99
　　syphilitic 093.89
　cranial (left) (right) 446.5
　deformans — *see* Arteriosclerosis
　giant cell 446.5
　necrosing or necrotizing 446.0
　nodosa 446.0
　obliterans — *see also*
　　　Arteriosclerosis
　　subclaviocarotica 446.7
　pulmonary 417.8
　retina 362.18
　rheumatic — *see* Fever, rheumatic
　senile — *see* Arteriosclerosis
　suppurative 447.2
　syphilitic (general) 093.89
　　brain 094.89
　　coronary 093.89
　　spinal 094.89
　temporal 446.5
　young female, syndrome 446.7
Artery, arterial — *see* condition
Arthralgia (*see also* Pain, joint) 719.4
　allergic (*see also* Pain, joint) 719.4
　in caisson disease 993.3
　psychogenic 307.89
　rubella 056.71
　Salmonella 003.23
　temporomandibular joint 524.62
Arthritis, arthritic (acute) (chronic)
　　(subacute) 716.9

> Note — Use the following fifth-digit subclassification with categories 711-712, 715-716:
>
> 　0　site unspecified
> 　1　shoulder region
> 　2　upper arm
> 　3　forearm
> 　4　hand
> 　5　pelvic region and thigh
> 　6　lower leg
> 　7　ankle and foot
> 　8　other specified sites
> 　9　multiple sites

　allergic 716.2
　ankylosing (crippling) (spine) 720.0
　　sites other than spine 716.9
　atrophic 714.0
　　spine 720.9
　back (*see also* Arthritis, spine)
　　　721.90
　Bechterew's (ankylosing spondylitis)
　　　720.0
　blennorrhagic 098.50
　cervical, cervicodorsal (*see also*
　　　Spondylosis, cervical) 721.0
　Charcot's 094.0 *[713.5]*
　　diabetic 250.6 *[713.5]*
　　syringomyelic 336.0 *[713.5]*
　　tabetic 094.0 *[713.5]*
　chylous (*see also* Filariasis) 125.9
　　　[711.7]
　climacteric NEC 716.3
　coccyx 721.8
　cricoarytenoid 478.79
　crystal (-induced) — *see* Arthritis,
　　　due to crystals
　deformans (*see also* Osteoarthrosis)
　　　715.9
　　spine 721.90
　　　with myelopathy 721.91
　degenerative (*see also*
　　　Osteoarthrosis) 715.9
　　idiopathic 715.09
　　polyarticular 715.09
　　spine 721.90
　　　with myelopathy 721.91
　dermatoarthritis, lipoid 272.8
　　　[713.0]

Arthritis, arthritic—continued
　due to or associated with
　　acromegaly 253.0 *[713.0]*
　　actinomycosis 039.8 *[711.4]*
　　amyloidosis 277.3 *[713.7]*
　　bacterial disease NEC 040.89
　　　[711.4]
　　Behçet's syndrome 136.1
　　　[711.2]
　　blastomycosis 116.0 *[711.6]*
　　brucellosis (*see also* Brucellosis)
　　　023.9 *[711.4]*
　　caisson disease 993.3
　　coccidioidomycosis 114.3
　　　[711.6]
　　coliform (Escherichia coli) 711.0
　　colitis, ulcerative (*see also*
　　　Colitis, ulcerative) 556.9
　　　[713.1]
　　cowpox 051.0 *[711.5]*
　　crystals NEC 275.4 *[712.9]*
　　　dicalcium phosphate 275.4
　　　　[712.1]
　　　pyrophosphate 275.4 *[712.2]*
　　　specified NEC 275.4 *[712.8]*
　　dermatoarthritis, lipoid 272.8
　　　[713.0]
　　dermatological disorder NEC
　　　709.9 *[713.3]*
　　diabetes 250.6 *[713.5]*
　　diphtheria 032.89 *[711.4]*
　　dracontiasis 125.7 *[711.7]*
　　dysentery 009.0 *[711.3]*
　　endocrine disorder NEC 259.9
　　　[713.0]
　　enteritis NEC 009.1 *[711.3]*
　　　infectious (*see also* Enteritis,
　　　　infectious) 009.0
　　　　[711.3]
　　　specified organism NEC
　　　　008.8 *[711.3]*
　　　regional (*see also* Enteritis,
　　　　regional) 555.9
　　　　[713.1]
　　　specified organism NEC
　　　　008.8 *[711.3]*
　　epiphyseal slip, nontraumatic
　　　(old) 716.8
　　erysipelas 035 *[711.4]*
　　erythema
　　　epidemic 026.1
　　　multiforme 695.1 *[713.3]*
　　　nodosum 695.2 *[713.3]*
　　Escherichia coli 711.0
　　filariasis NEC 125.9 *[711.7]*
　　gastrointestinal condition NEC
　　　569.9 *[713.1]*
　　glanders 024 *[711.4]*
　　Gonococcus 098.50
　　gout 274.0
　　H. influenzae 711.0
　　helminthiasis NEC 128.9 *[711.7]*
　　hematological disorder NEC
　　　289.9 *[713.2]*
　　hemochromatosis 275.0 *[713.0]*
　　hemoglobinopathy NEC (*see
　　　also* Disease,
　　　hemoglobin) 282.7
　　　[713.2]
　　hemophilia (*see also*
　　　Hemophilia) 286.0
　　　[713.2]
　　Hemophilus influenzae (H.
　　　influenzae) 711.0
　　Henoch (-Schönlein) purpura
　　　287.0 *[713.6]*
　　histoplasmosis NEC (*see also*
　　　Histoplasmosis) 115.99
　　　[711.6]
　　hyperparathyroidism 252.0
　　　[713.0]
　　hypersensitivity reaction NEC
　　　995.3 *[713.6]*

Arthritis, arthritic—continued
　due to or associated with—
　　continued
　　hypogammaglobulinemia (*see
　　　also* Hypogamma-
　　　globulinemia) 279.00
　　　[713.0]
　　hypothyroidism NEC 244.9
　　　[713.0]
　　infection (*see also* Arthritis,
　　　infectious) 711.9
　　infectious disease NEC 136.9
　　　[711.8]
　　leprosy (*see also* Leprosy) 030.9
　　　[711.4]
　　leukemia NEC (M9800/3) 208.9
　　　[713.2]
　　lipoid dermatoarthritis 272.8
　　　[713.0]
　　Lyme disease 088.81 *[711.8]*
　　Mediterranean fever, familial
　　　277.3 *[713.7]*
　　meningococcal infection 036.82
　　metabolic disorder NEC 277.9
　　　[713.0]
　　multiple myelomatosis
　　　(M9730/3) 203.0 *[713.2]*
　　mumps 072.79 *[711.5]*
　　mycobacteria 031.8 *[711.4]*
　　mycosis NEC 117.9 *[711.6]*
　　neurological disorder NEC
　　　349.9 *[713.5]*
　　ochronosis 270.2 *[713.0]*
　　O'Nyong Nyong 066.3 *[711.5]*
　　parasitic disease NEC 136.9
　　　[711.8]
　　paratyphoid fever (*see also*
　　　Fever, paratyphoid) 002.9
　　　[711.3]
　　Pneumococcus 711.0
　　poliomyelitis (*see also*
　　　Poliomyelitis) 045.9
　　　[711.5]
　　Pseudomonas 711.0
　　psoriasis 696.0
　　pyogenic organism (E. coli) (H.
　　　influenzae)
　　　(Pseudomonas)
　　　(Streptococcus) 711.0
　　rat-bite fever 026.1 *[711.4]*
　　regional enteritis (*see also*
　　　Enteritis, regional) 555.9
　　　[713.1]
　　Reiter's disease 099.3 *[711.1]*
　　respiratory disorder NEC 519.9
　　　[713.4]
　　reticulosis, malignant (M9720/3)
　　　202.3 *[713.2]*
　　rubella 056.71
　　salmonellosis 003.23
　　sarcoidosis 135 *[713.7]*
　　serum sickness 999.5 *[713.6]*
　　Staphylococcus 711.0
　　Streptococcus 711.0
　　syphilis (*see also* Syphilis) 094.0
　　　[711.4]
　　syringomyelia 336.0 *[713.5]*
　　thalassemia 282.4 *[713.2]*
　　tuberculosis (*see also*
　　　Tuberculosis, arthritis)
　　　015.9 *[711.4]*
　　typhoid fever 002.0 *[711.3]*
　　ulcerative colitis (*see also*
　　　Colitis, ulcerative) 556.9
　　　[713.1]
　　urethritis
　　　nongonococcal (*see also*
　　　　Urethritis,
　　　　nongonococcal)
　　　　099.40 *[711.1]*
　　　nonspecific (*see also*
　　　　Urethritis,
　　　　nongonococcal)
　　　　099.40 *[711.1]*
　　　Reiter's 099.3 *[711.1]*
　　viral disease NEC 079.99
　　　[711.5]

Arthritis, arthritic—continued
　erythema epidemic 026.1
　gonococcal 098.50
　gouty (acute) 274.0
　hypertrophic (*see also*
　　　Osteoarthrosis) 715.9
　　spine 721.90
　　　with myelopathy 721.91
　idiopathic, blennorrheal 099.3
　in caisson disease 993.3 *[713.8]*
　infectious or infective (acute)
　　　(chronic) (subacute) NEC
　　　711.9
　　nonpyogenic 711.9
　　spine 720.9
　inflammatory NEC 714.9
　juvenile rheumatoid (chronic)
　　　(polyarticular) 714.30
　　acute 714.31
　　monoarticular 714.33
　　pauciarticular 714.32
　lumbar (*see also* Spondylosis,
　　　lumbar) 721.3
　meningococcal 036.82
　menopausal NEC 716.3
　migratory — *see* Fever, rheumatic
　neuropathic (Charcot's) 094.0
　　　[713.5]
　　diabetic 250.6 *[713.5]*
　　nonsyphilitic NEC 349.9 *[713.5]*
　　syringomyelic 336.0 *[713.5]*
　　tabetic 094.0 *[713.5]*
　nodosa (*see also* Osteoarthrosis)
　　　715.9
　　spine 721.90
　　　with myelopathy 721.91
　nonpyogenic NEC 716.9
　　spine 721.90
　　　with myelopathy 721.91
　ochronotic 270.2 *[713.0]*
　palindromic (*see also* Rheumatism,
　　　palindromic) 719.3
　pneumococcal 711.0
　postdysenteric 009.0 *[711.3]*
　postrheumatic, chronic (Jaccoud's)
　　　714.4
　primary progressive 714.0
　　spine 720.9
　proliferative 714.0
　　spine 720.0
　psoriatic 696.0
　purulent 711.0
　pyogenic or pyemic 711.0
　rheumatic 714.0
　　acute or subacute — *see* Fever,
　　　rheumatic
　　chronic 714.0
　　spine 720.9
　rheumatoid (nodular) 714.0
　　with
　　　splenoadenomegaly and
　　　　leukopenia 714.1
　　　visceral or systemic
　　　　involvement 714.2
　　aortitis 714.89
　　carditis 714.2
　　heart disease 714.2
　　juvenile (chronic) (polyarticular)
　　　714.30
　　　acute 714.31
　　　monoarticular 714.33
　　　pauciarticular 714.32
　　spine 720.0
　rubella 056.71
　sacral, sacroiliac, sacrococcygeal
　　　(*see also* Spondylosis, sacral)
　　　721.3
　scorbutic 267
　senile or senescent (*see also*
　　　Osteoarthrosis) 715.9
　　spine 721.90
　　　with myelopathy 721.91
　septic 711.0
　serum (nontherapeutic)
　　　(therapeutic) 999.5 *[713.6]*
　specified form NEC 716.8

Arthritis, arthritic—continued
spine 721.90
  with myelopathy 721.91
atrophic 720.9
degenerative 721.90
  with myelopathy 721.91
hypertrophic (with deformity) 721.90
  with myelopathy 721.91
infectious or infective NEC 720.9
Marie-Strümpell 720.0
nonpyogenic 721.90
  with myelopathy 721.91
pyogenic 720.9
rheumatoid 720.0
traumatic (old) 721.7
tuberculous (see also Tuberculosis) 015.0 [720.81]
staphylococcal 711.0
streptococcal 711.0
suppurative 711.0
syphilitic 094.0 [713.5]
  congenital 090.49 [713.5]
syphilitica deformans (Charcot) 094.0 [713.5]
thoracic (see also Spondylosis, thoracic) 721.2
toxic of menopause 716.3
transient 716.4
traumatic (chronic) (old) (post) 716.1
  current injury — see nature of injury
tuberculous (see also Tuberculosis, arthritis) 015.9 [711.4]
urethritica 099.3 [711.1]
urica, uratic 274.0
venereal 099.3 [711.1]
vertebral (see also Arthritis, spine) 721.90
villous 716.8
von Bechterew's 720.0

Arthrocele (see also Effusion, joint) 719.0
Arthrochondritis — see Arthritis
Arthrodesis status V45.4
Arthrodynia (see also Pain, joint) 719.4
  psychogenic 307.89
Arthrodysplasia 755.9
Arthrofibrosis, joint (see also Ankylosis) 718.5
Arthrogryposis 728.3
  multiplex, congenita 754.89
Arthrokatadysis 715.35
Arthrolithiasis 274.0
Arthro-onychodysplasia 756.89
Arthro-osteo-onychodysplasia 756.89
Arthropathy (see also Arthritis) 716.9

Note — Use the following fifth-digit subclassification with categories 711-712, 716:

  0 site unspecified
  1 shoulder region
  2 upper arm
  3 forearm
  4 hand
  5 pelvic region and thigh
  6 lower leg
  7 ankle and foot
  8 other specified sites
  9 multiple sites

Behçets 711.2 [136.1]
Charcot's 094.0 [713.5]
  diabetic 250.6 [713.5]
  syringomyelic 336.0 [713.5]
  tabetic 094.0 [713.5]
crystal (-induced)–see Arthritis, due to crystals

Arthropathy—continued
gouty 274.0
neurogenic, neuropathic (Charcot's) (tabetic) 094.0 [713.5]
  diabetic 250.6 [713.5]
  nonsyphilitic NEC 349.9 [713.5]
  syringomyelic 336.0 [713.5]
postdysenteric NEC 009.0 [711.3]
postrheumatic, chronic (Jaccoud's) 714.4
psoriatic 696.0
pulmonary 731.2
specified NEC 716.8
syringomyelia 336.0 [713.5]
tabes dorsalis 094.0 [713.5]
tabetic 094.0 [713.5]
transient 716.4
traumatic 716.1
uric acid 274.0

Arthophyte (see also Loose, body, joint) 718.1
Arthrophytis 719.80
  ankle 719.87
  elbow 719.82
  foot 719.87
  hand 719.84
  hip 719.85
  knee 719.86
  multiple sites 719.89
  pelvic region 719.85
  shoulder (region) 719.81
  specified site NEC 719.88
  wrist 719.83
Arthropyosis (see also Arthritis, pyogenic) 711.0
Arthrosis (deformans) (degenerative) (see also Osteoarthrosis) 715.9
  Charcot's 094.0 [713.5]
  polyarticular 715.09
  spine (see also Spondylosis) 721.90
Arthus' phenomenon 995.2
  due to
    correct substance properly administered 995.2
    overdose or wrong substance given or taken 977.9
    specified drug–see Table of drugs and chemicals
  serum 999.5
Articular–see also condition
  disc disorder (reducing or nonreducing) 524.63
  spondylolisthesis 756.12
Artificial
  device (prosthetic)–see Fitting, device
  insemination V26.1
  menopause (states) (symptoms) (syndrome) 627.4
  opening status (functioning) (without complication) V55.9
    anus (colostomy) V44.3
    colostomy V44.3
    cystostomy V44.5
    enterostomy V44.4
    gastrostomy V44.1
    ileostomy V44.2
    intestinal tract NEC V44.4
    jejunostomy V44.4
    nephrostomy V44.6
    specified site NEC V44.8
    tracheostomy V44.0
    ureterostomy V44.6
    urethrostomy V44.6
    urinary tract NEC V44.6
    vagina V44.7
  vagina status V44.7
ARV (disease) (illness) (infection)–see Human immunodeficiency virus (disease) (illness) (infection)
Arytenoid–see condition
Asbestosis (occupational) 501
Asboe-Hansen's disease (incontinentia pigmenti) 757.33

Ascariasis (intestinal) (lung) 127.0
Ascaridiasis 127.0
Ascaris 127.0
  lumbricoides (infestation) 127.0
  pneumonia 127.0
Ascending–see condition
Aschoff's bodies (see also Myocarditis, rheumatic) 398.0
Ascites 789.5
  abdominal NEC 789.5
  cancerous (M80000/6) 197.6
  cardiac 428.0
  chylous (nonfilarial) 457.8
    filarial (see also Infestation, filarial) 125.9
  congenital 778.0
  due to S. japonicum 120.2
  fetal, casuing fetopelvic disproportion 653.7
  heart 428.0
  joint (see also Effusion, joint) 719.0
  malignant (M8000/6) 197.6
  pseudochylous 789.5
  syphilitic 095.2
  tuberculous (see also Tuberculosis) 014.0
Ascorbic acid (vitamin C) deficiency (scurvy) 267
ASCVD (arteriosclerotic cardiovascular disease) 429.2
Aseptic–see condition
Asherman's syndrome 621.5
Asialia 527.7
Asiatic cholera (see also Cholera) 001.9
Asocial personality or trends 301.7
Aspergillosis 117.3
  with pneumonia 117.3 [484.6]
  nonsyphilitic NEC 117.3
Aspergillus (flavus) (fumigatus) (infection) (terreus) 117.3
Aspermatogenesis 606.0
Aspermia (testis) 606.0
Asphyxia, asphyxiation (by) 799.0
  with neurologic involvement 768.5
  antenatal–see Distress, fetal
  bedclothes 994.7
  birth (see also Ashpyxia, newborn) 768.9
  bunny bag 994.7
  carbon monoxide 986
  caul (see also Asphyxia, newborn)
  cave-in 994.7
    crushing–see Injury, internal, intrathoracic organs
  constriction 994.7
  crushing–see Injury, internal, intrathoracic organs
  drowning 994.1
  fetal–see Asphyxia, intrauterine
  food or foreign body (in larynx) 933.1
    bronchioles 934.8
    bronchus (main) 934.1
    lung 934.8
    nasopharynx 933.0
    nose, nasal passages 932
    pharynx 933.0
    respiratory tract 934.9
      specified part NEC 934.8
    throat 933.0
    trachea 934.0
  gas, fumes, or vapor NEC 987.9
    specified–see Table of drugs and chemicals
  gravitational changes 994.7
  hanging 994.7
  inhalation–see Inhalation
  intrauterine
    fetal death (before onset of labor) 768.0
    during labor 768.1
    liveborn infant–see Distress, fetal, liveborn infant

Asphyxia, asphyxiation—continued
local 443.0
mechanical 994.7
  during birth (see also Distress, fetal) 768.4
mucus 933.1
  bronchus (main) 934.1
  larynx 933.1
  lung 934.8
  nasal passages 932
  newborn 770.1
  pharynx 933.0
  respiratory tract 934.9
    specfied part NEC 934.8
  throat 933.0
  trachea 934.0
  vaginal (fetus or newborn) 770.1
newborn 768.9
  blue 768.6
  livida 768.6
  mild or moderate 768.6
  pallida 768.5
  severe 768.5
  white 768.5
pathological 799.0
plastic bag 994.7
postnatal (see also Asphyxia, newborn) 768.9
  mechanical 994.7
pressure 994.7
reticularis 782.61
strangulation 994.7
submersion 994.1
traumatic NEC–see Injury, internal, intrathoracic organs
vomiting, vomitus–see Asphyxia, food or foreign body

Aspiration
acid pulmonary (syndrome) 997.3
  obstetric 668.0
amniotic fluid 770.1
bronchitis 507.0
contents of birth canal 770.1
fetal pneumonitis 770.1
food, foreign body, or gasoline (with asphyxiation)–see Asphyxia, food or foreign body
meconium 770.1
mucus 933.1
  into
    bronchus (main) 934.1
    lung 934.8
    respiratory tract 934.9
      specified part NEC 934.8
    trachea 934.0
  newborn 770.1
  vaginal (fetus or newborn) 770.1
newborn 770.1
pneumonia 507.0
pneumonitis 507.0
  fetus or newborn 770.1
  obstetric 668.0
syndrome of newborn (massive) (meconium) 770.1
vernix caseosa 770.1
Asplenia 759.0
  with mesocardia 746.87
Assam fever 085.0
Assimilation, pelvis
  with disproportion 653.2
    affecting fetus or newborn 763.1
    causing obstructed labor 660.1
      affecting fetus or newborn 763.1
Assmann's focus (see also Tuberculosis) 011.0
Astasia (-asbasia) 307.9
  hysterical 300.11
Asteatosis 706.8
  cutis 706.8
Astereognosis 780.9
Asterixis 781.3
  in liver disease 572.8
Asteroid hyalitis 379.22

Asthenia, asthenic 780.7
    cardiac (see also Failure, heart) 428.9
        psychogenic 306.2
    cardiovascular (see also Failure, heart) 428.9
        psychogenic 306.2
    heart (see also Failure, heart) 428.9
        psychogenic 306.2
    hysterical 300.11
    myocardial (see also Failure, heart) 428.9
        psychogenic 306.2
    nervous 300.5
    neurocirculatory 306.2
    neurotic 300.5
    psychogenic 300.5
    psychoneurotic 300.5
    psychophysiologic 300.5
    reaction, psychoneurotic 300.5
    senile 797
    Stiller's 780.7
    tropical anhidrotic 705.1

Asthenopia 368.13
    accommodative 367.4
    hysterical (muscular) 300.11
    psychogenic 306.7

Asthenospermia 792.2

Asthma, asthmatic (bronchial) (catarrh) (spasmodic) 493.9

> Note — Use the following fifth-digit subclassification with category 493:
>
> 0 without mention of status asthmaticus
> 1 with status asthmaticus

    with
        chronic obstructive pulmonary disease (COPD) 493.2
        hay fever 493.0
        rhinitis, allergic 493.0
    allergic 493.9
        stated cause (external allergen) 493.0
    atopic 493.0
    cardiac (see also Failure, ventricular, left) 428.1
    cardiobronchial (see also Failure, ventricular, left) 428.1
    cardiorenal (see also Hypertension, cardiorenal) 404.90
    childhood 493.0
    colliers' 500
    croup 493.9
    detergent 507.8
    due to
        detergent 507.8
        inhalation of fumes 506.3
        internal immunological process 493.0
    endogenous (intrinsic) 493.1
    eosinophilic 518.3
    exogenous (cosmetics) (dander or dust) (drugs) (dust) (feathers) (food) (hay) (platinum) (pollen) 493.0
    extrinsic 493.0
    grinders' 502
    hay 493.0
    heart (see also Failure, ventricular, left) 428.1
    IgE 493.0
    infective 493.1
    intrinsic 493.1
    Kopp's 254.8
    late-onset 493.1
    meat-wrappers' 506.9
    Millar's (laryngismus stridulus) 478.75
    millstone makers' 502
    miners' 500
    Monday morning 504
    New Orleans (epidemic) 493.0
    platinum 493.0

Asthma, asthmatic—continued
    pneumoconiotic (occupational) NEC 505
    potters' 502
    psychogenic 316 [493.9]
    pulmonary eosinophilic 518.3
    red cedar 495.8
    Rostan's (see also Failure, ventricular, left) 428.1
    sandblasters' 502
    sequoiosis 495.8
    stonemasons' 502
    thymic 254.8
    tuberculous (see also Tuberculosis, pulmonary) 011.9
    Wichmann's (laryngismus stridulus) 478.75
    wood 495.8

Asomatognosia 781.8

Astigmatism (compound) (congenital) 367.20
    irregular 367.22
    regular 367.21

Astroblastoma (M9430/3)
    nose 748.1
    specified site — see Neoplasm, by site, malignant
    unspecified site 191.9

Astrocytoma (cystic) (M9400/3)
    anaplastic type (M9401/3)
        specified site — see Neoplasm, by site, malignant
        unspecified site 191.9
    fibrillary (M9420/3)
        specified site — see Neoplasm, by site, malignant
        unspecified site 191.9
    fibrous (M9420/3)
        specified site — see Neoplasm, by site, malignant
        unspecified site 191.9
    gemistocytic (M9411/3)
        specified site — see Neoplasm, by site, malignant
        unspecified site 191.9
    juvenile (M9421/3)
        specified site — see Neoplasm, by site, malignant
        unspecified site 191.9
    nose 748.1
    pilocytic (M9421/3)
        specified site — see Neoplasm, by site, malignant
        unspecified site 191.9
    piloid (M9421/3)
        specified site — see Neoplasm, by site, malignant
        unspecified site 191.9
    protoplasmic (M9410/3)
        specified site — see Neoplasm, by site, malignant
        unspecified site 191.9
    specified site — see Neoplasm, by site, malignant
    subependymal (M9383/1) 237.5
        giant cell (M9384/1) 237.5
    unspecified site 191.9

Astroglioma (M9400/3)
    nose 748.1
    specified site — see Neoplasm, by site, malignant
    unspecified site 191.9

Asymbolia 784.60

Asymmetrical breathing 786.09

Asymmetry — see also Distortion
    chest 786.9
    face 754.0
    jaw NEC 524.12
        maxillary 524.11
    pelvis with disproportion 653.0
        affecting fetus or newborn 763.1
        causing obstructed labor 660.1
            affecting fetus or newborn 763.1

Asynergia 781.3

Asynergy 781.3
    ventricular 429.89

Asystole (heart) (see also Arrest, cardiac) 427.5

Ataxia, ataxy, ataxic 781.3
    acute 781.3
    brain 331.89
    cerebellar 334.3
        hereditary (Marie's) 334.2
        in
            alcoholism 303.9 [334.4]
            myxedema (see also Myxedema) 244.9 [334.4]
            neoplastic disease NEC 239.9 [334.4]
    cerebral 331.89
    family, familial 334.2
        cerebral (Marie's) 334.2
        spinal (Friedreich's) 334.0
    Friedreich's (heredofamilial) (spinal) 334.0
    frontal lobe 781.3
    gait 781.2
        hysterical 300.11
    general 781.3
    hereditary NEC 334.2
        cerebellar 334.2
        spastic 334.1
        spinal 334.0
    heredofamilial (Marie's) 334.2
    hysterical 300.11
    locomotor (progressive) 094.0
        diabetic 250.6 [337.1]
    Marie's (cerebellar) (heredofamilial) 334.2
    nonorganic origin 307.9
    partial 094.0
    postchickenpox 052.7
    progressive 094.0
    psychogenic 307.9
    Sanger-Brown's 334.2
    spastic 094.0
        hereditary 334.1
        syphilitic 094.0
    spinal
        hereditary 334.0
        progressive 094.0
    telangiectasia 334.8

Ataxia-telangiectasia 334.8

Atelectasis (absorption collapse) (complete) (compression) (massive) (partial) (postinfective) (pressure collapse) (pulmonary) (relaxation) 518.0
    newborn (congenital) (partial) 770.5
        primary 770.4
    primary 770.4
    tuberculous (see also Tuberculosis, pulmonary) 011.9

Ateleiosis, ateliosis 253.3

Atelia — see Distortion

Ateliosis 253.3

Atelocardia 746.9

Atelomyelia 742.59

Athelia 757.6

Atheroembolism — see Atherosclerosis

Atheroma, atheromatous (see also Arteriosclerosis) 440.9
    aorta, aortic 440.0
        valve (see also Endocarditis, aortic) 424.1
    artery — see Arteriosclerosis
    basilar (artery) (see also Occlusion, artery, basilar) 433.0
    carotid (artery) (common) (internal) (see also Occlusion, artery, carotid) 433.1
    cerebral (arteries) 437.0
    coronary (artery) — see Arteriosclerosis, coronary
    degeneration — see Arteriosclerosis
    heart, cardiac — see Arteriosclerosis, coronary

Atheroma, atheromatous—continued
    mitral (valve) 424.0
    myocardium, myocardial — see Arteriosclerosis, coronary
    pulmonary valve (heart) (see also Endocarditis, pulmonary) 424.3
    skin 706.2
    tricuspid (heart) (valve) 424.2
    valve, valvular — see Endocarditis
    vertebral (artery) (see also Occlusion, artery, vertebral) 433.2

Atheromatosis — see also Arteriosclerosis
    arterial, congenital 272.8

Atherosclerosis — see Arteriosclerosis

Athetosis (acquired) 781.0
    bilateral 333.7
    congenital (bilateral) 333.7
    double 333.7
    unilateral 781.0

Athlete's
    foot 110.4
    heart 429.3

Athletic team examination V70.3

Athrepsia 261

Athyrea (acquired) (see also Hypothyroidism) 244.9
    congenital 243

Athyreosis (congenital) 243
    acquired — see Hypothyroidism

Athyroidism (acquired) (see also Hypothyroidism) 244.9
    congenital 243

Atmospheric pyrexia 992.0

Atonia, atony, atonic
    abdominal wall 728.2
    bladder (sphincter) 596.4
        neurogenic NEC 596.54
            with cauda equina syndrome 344.61
    capillary 448.9
    cecum 564.8
        psychogenic 306.4
    colon 564.8
        psychogenic 306.4
    congenital 779.8
    dyspepsia 536.3
        psychogenic 306.4
    intestine 564.8
        psychogenic 306.4
    stomach 536.3
        neurotic or psychogenic 306.4
        psychogenic 306.4
    uterus 661.2
        affecting fetus or newborn 763.7
    vesical 596.4

Atopy NEC V15.0

Atransferrinemia, congenital 273.8

Atresia, atretic (congenital) 759.89
    alimentary organ or tract NEC 751.8
        lower 751.2
        upper 750.8
    ani, anus, anal (canal) 751.2
    aorta 747.22
        with hypoplasia of ascending aorta and defective development of left ventricle (with mitral valve atresia) 746.7
        arch 747.11
        ring 747.21
    aortic (orifice) (valve) 746.89
        arch 747.11
    aqueduct of Sylvius 742.3
        with spina bifida (see also Spina bifida) 741.0
    artery NEC (see also Atresia, blood vessel) 747.60
        cerebral 747.81
        coronary 746.85
        eye 743.58

Atresia, atretic—continued
artery—continued
 pulmonary 747.3
 umbilical 747.5
auditory canal (external) 744.02
bile, biliary duct (common) or
  passage 751.61
 acquired (see also Obstruction,
  biliary) 576.2
bladder (neck) 753.6
blood vessel (peripheral) NEC
  747.60
 cerebral 747.81
 gastrointestinal 747.61
 lower limb 747.64
 pulmonary artery 747.3
 renal 747.62
 spinal 747.82
 upper limb 747.63
bronchus 748.3
canal, ear 744.02
cardiac
 valve 746.89
  aortic 746.89
  mitral 746.89
  pulmonary 746.01
  tricuspid 746.1
cecum 751.2
cervix (acquired) 622.4
 congenital 752.49
 in pregnancy or childbirth 654.6
  affecting fetus or newborn
   763.8
  causing obstructed labor
   660.2
   affecting fetus or newborn
    763.1
choana 748.0
colon 751.2
cystic duct 751.61
 acquired 575.8
  with obstruction (see also
   Obstruction,
   gallbladder) 575.2
digestive organs NEC 751.8
duodenum 751.1
ear canal 744.02
ejaculatory duct 752.8
epiglottis 748.3
esophagus 750.3
Eustachian tube 744.24
fallopian tube (acquired) 628.2
 congenital 752.19
follicular cyst 620.0
foramen of
 Luschka 742.3
  with spina bifida (see also
   Spina bifida) 741.0
 Magendie 742.3
  with spina bifida (see also
   Spina bifida) 741.0
gallbladder 751.69
genital organ
 external
  female 752.49
  male 752.8
 internal
  female 752.8
  male 752.8
glottis 748.3
gullet 750.3
heart
 valve NEC 746.89
  aortic 746.89
  mitral 746.89
  pulmonary 746.01
  tricuspid 746.1
hymen 752.42
 acquired 623.3
 postinfective 623.3
ileum 751.1
intestine (small) 751.1
 large 751.2
iris, filtration angle (see also
 Buphthalmia) 743.20
jejunum 751.1
kidney 753.3

Atresia, atretic—continued
lacrimal, apparatus 743.65
 acquired — see Stenosis,
  lacrimal
larynx 748.3
ligament, broad 752.19
lung 748.5
meatus urinarius 753.6
mitral valve 746.89
 with atresia or hypoplasia of
  aortic orifice or valve,
  with hypoplasia of
  ascending aorta and
  defective development of
  left ventricle 746.7
nares (anterior) (posterior) 748.0
nasolacrimal duct 743.65
nasopharynx 748.8
nose, nostril 748.0
 acquired 738.0
organ or site NEC — see Anomaly,
 specified type NEC
osseous meatus (ear) 744.03
oviduct (acquired) 628.2
 congenital 752.19
parotid duct 750.23
 acquired 527.8
pulmonary (artery) 747.3
 valve 746.01
 vein 747.49
pulmonic 746.01
pupil 743.46
rectum 751.2
salivary duct or gland 750.23
 acquired 527.8
sublingual duct 750.23
 acquired 527.8
submaxillary duct or gland 750.23
 acquired 527.8
trachea 748.3
tricuspid valve 746.1
ureter 753.2
ureteropelvic junction 753.2
ureterovesical orifice 753.2
urethra (valvular) 753.6
urinary tract NEC 753.2
uterus 752.3
 acquired 621.8
vagina (acquired) 623.2
 congenital 752.49
 postgonococcal (old) 098.2
 postinfectional 623.2
 senile 623.2
vascular NEC (see also Atresia,
 blood vessel) 747.60
 cerebral 747.81
vas deferens 752.8
vein NEC (see also Atresia, blood
 vessel) 747.60
 cardiac 746.89
 great 747.49
 portal 747.49
 pulmonary 747.49
 vena cava (inferior) (superior)
  747.49
vesicourethral orifice 753.6
vulva 752.49
 acquired 624.8
Atrichia, atrichosis 704.00
 congenital (universal) 757.4
Atrioventricularis commune 745.69
Atrophia — see also Atrophy
 alba 709.09
 cutis 701.8
  idiopathica progressiva 701.8
  senilis 701.8
 dermatological, diffuse (idiopathic)
  701.8
 flava hepatis (acuta) (subacuta) (see
  also Necrosis, liver) 570
 gyrata of choroid and retina
  (central) 363.54
  generalized 363.57
 senilis 797
  dermatological 701.8
 unguium 703.8
  congenita 757.5

Atrophoderma, atrophodermia 701.9
diffusum (idiopathic) 701.8
maculatum 701.3
 et striatum 701.3
  due to syphilis 095.8
 syphilitic 091.3
neuriticum 701.8
pigmentosum 757.33
reticulatum symmetricum faciei
 701.8
senile 701.8
symmetrical 701.8
vermiculata 701.8

Atrophy, atrophic
adrenal (autoimmune) (capsule)
 (cortex) (gland) 255.4
 with hypofunction 255.4
alveolar process or ridge
 (edentulous) 525.2
appendix 543.9
Aran-Duchenne muscular 335.21
arm 728.2
arteriosclerotic — see
 Arteriosclerosis
arthritis 714.0
 spine 720.9
bile duct (any) 576.8
bladder 596.8
blanche (of Milian) 701.3
bone (senile) 733.99
 due to
  disuse 733.7
  infection 733.99
  tabes dorsalis (neurogenic)
   094.0
 posttraumatic 733.99
brain (cortex) (progressive) 331.9
 with dementia 290.10
  Alzheimer's 331.0
   with dementia — see
    Alzheimer's, dementia
 circumscribed (Pick's) 331.1
  with dementia 290.10
 congenital 742.4
 hereditary 331.9
 senile 331.2
breast 611.4
 puerperal, postpartum 676.3
buccal cavity 528.9
cardiac (brown) (senile) (see also
 Degeneration, myocardial)
 429.1
cartilage (infectional) (joint) 733.99
cast, plaster of Paris 728.2
cerebellar — see Atrophy, brain
cerebral — see Atrophy, brain
cervix (endometrium) (mucosa)
 (myometrium) (senile) (uteri)
 622.8
 menopausal 627.8
Charcôt-Marie-Tooth 356.1
choroid 363.40
 diffuse secondary 363.42
 hereditary (see also Dystrophy,
  choroid) 363.50
 gyrate
  central 363.54
  diffuse 363.57
  generalized 363.57
 senile 363.41
ciliary body 364.57
colloid, degenerative 701.3
conjunctiva (senile) 372.8
corpus cavernosum 607.89
cortical (see also Atrophy, brain)
 331.9
Cruveilhier's 335.21
cystic duct 576.8
dacryosialadenopathy 710.2
degenerative
 colloid 701.3
 senile 701.3
Déjérine-Thomas 333.0
diffuse idiopathic, dermatological
 701.8

Atrophy, atrophic—continued
disuse
 bone 733.7
 muscle 728.2
Duchenne-Aran 335.21
ear 388.9
edentulous alveolar ridge 525.2
emphysema, lung 492.8
endometrium (senile) 621.8
 cervix 622.8
enteric 569.89
epididymis 608.3
eyeball, cause unknown 360.41
eyelid (senile) 374.50
facial (skin) 701.9
facioscapulohumeral (Landouzy-
 Déjérine) 359.1
fallopian tube (senile), acquired
 620.3
fatty, thymus (gland) 254.8
gallbladder 575.8
gastric 537.89
gastritis (chronic) 535.1
gastrointestinal 569.89
genital organ, male 608.89
glandular 289.3
globe (phthisis bulbi) 360.41
gum 523.2
hair 704.2
heart (brown) (senile) (see also
 Degeneration, myocardial)
 429.1
hemifacial 754.0
 Romberg 349.89
hydronephrosis 591
infantile 261
 paralysis, acute (see also
  Poliomyelits, with
  paralysis) 045.1
intestine 569.89
iris (generalized) (postinfectional)
 (sector shaped) 364.59
 essential 364.51
 progressive 364.51
 sphincter 364.54
kidney (senile) (see also Sclerosis,
 renal) 587
 with hypertension (see also
  Hypertension, kidney)
  403.90
 congenital 753.0
 hydronephrotic 591
 infantile 753.0
lacrimal apparatus (primary) 375.13
 secondary 375.14
Landouzy-Déjérine 359.1
laryngitis, infection 476.0
larynx 478.79
Leber's optic 377.16
lip 528.5
liver (acute) (subacute) (see also
 Necrosis, liver) 570
 chronic (yellow) 571.8
 yellow (congenital) 570
  with
   abortion — see Abortion,
    by type, with
    specified
    complication NEC
   ectopic pregnancy (see
    also categories
    633.0-633.9) 639.8
   molar pregnancy (see also
    categories 630-
    632) 639.8
  chronic 571.8
  complicating pregnancy
   646.7
  following
   abortion 639.8
   ectopic or molar
    pregnancy 639.8
  from injection, inoculation or
   transfusion (onset
   within 8 months after
   administration) — see
   Hepatitis, viral

Atrophy, atrophic—*continued*
    liver—*continued*
        yellow—*continued*
            healed 571.5
            obstetric 646.7
            postabortal 639.8
            postimmunization — *see*
                Hepatitis, viral
            posttransfusion — *see*
                Hepatitis, viral
            puerperal, postpartum 674.8
    lung (senile) 518.89
        congenital 748.69
    macular (dermatological) 701.3
        syphilitic, skin 091.3
        striated 095.8
    muscle, muscular 728.2
        disuse 728.2
        Duchenne-Aran 335.21
        extremity (lower) (upper) 728.2
        familial spinal 335.11
        general 728.2
        idiopathic 728.2
        infantile spinal 335.0
        myelopathic (progressive)
            335.10
        myotonic 359.2
        neuritic 356.1
        neuropathic (peroneal)
            (progressive) 356.1
        peroneal 356.1
        primary (idiopathic) 728.2
        progressive (familial) (hereditary)
            (pure) 335.21
            adult (spinal) 335.19
            infantile (spinal) 335.0
            juvenile (spinal) 335.11
            spinal 335.10
                adult 335.19
                hereditary or familial
                    335.11
                infantile 335.0
        pseudohypertrophic 359.1
        spinal (progressive) 335.10
            adult 335.19
            Aran-Duchenne 335.10
            familial 335.11
            hereditary 335.11
            infantile 335.0
            juvenile 335.11
        syphilitic 095.6
    myocardium (*see also*
        Degeneration, myocardial)
        429.1
    myometrium (senile) 621.8
        cervix 622.8
    myotatic 728.2
    myotonia 359.2
    nail 703.8
        congenital 757.5
    nasopharynx 472.2
    nerve — *see also* Disorder, nerve
        abducens 378.54
        accessory 352.4
        acoustic or auditory 388.5
        cranial 352.9
            first (olfactory) 352.0
            second (optic) (*see also*
                Atrophy, optic nerve)
                377.10
            third (oculomotor)(partial)
                378.51
                total 378.52
            fourth (trochlear) 378.53
            fifth (trigeminal) 350.8
            sixth (abducens) 378.54
            seventh (facial) 351.8
            eighth (auditory) 388.5
            ninth (glossopharyngeal)
                352.2
            tenth (pneumogastric) (vagus)
                352.3
            eleventh (accessory) 352.4
            twelfth (hypoglossal) 352.5
        facial 351.8
        glossopharyngeal 352.2
        hypoglossal 352.5

Atrophy, atrophic—*continued*
    nerve—*continued*
        oculomotor (partial) 378.51
        total 378.52
        olfactory 352.0
        peripheral 355.9
        pneumogastric 352.3
        trigeminal 350.8
        trochlear 378.53
        vagus (pneumogastric) 352.3
    nervous system, congenital 742.8
    neuritic (*see also* Disorder, nerve)
        355.9
    neurogenic NEC 355.9
        bone
            tabetic 094.0
    nutritional 261
    old age 797
    olivopontocerebellar 333.0
    optic nerve (ascending)
        (descending) (infectional)
        (nonfamilial) (papillomacular
        bundle) (postretinal)
        (secondary NEC) (simple)
        377.10
        associated with retinal
            dystrophy 377.13
        dominant hereditary 377.16
        glaucomatous 377.14
        hereditary (dominant) (Leber's)
            377.16
        Leber's (hereditary) 377.16
        partial 377.15
        postinflammatory 377.12
        primary 377.11
        syphilitic 094.84
            congenital 090.49
            tabes dorsalis 094.0
    orbit 376.45
    ovary (senile), acquired 620.3
    oviduct (senile), acquired 620.3
    palsy, diffuse 335.20
    pancreas (duct) (senile) 577.8
    papillary muscle 429.81
    paralysis 355.9
    parotid gland 527.0
    patches skin 701.3
        senile 701.8
    penis 607.89
    pharyngitis 472.1
    pharynx 478.29
    pluriglandular 258.8
    polyarthritis 714.0
    prostate 602.2
    pseudohypertrophic 359.1
    renal (*see also* Sclerosis, renal) 587
    reticulata 701.8
    retina (*see also* Degeneration,
        retina) 362.60
        hereditary (*see also* Dystrophy,
            retina) 362.70
    rhinitis 472.0
    salivary duct or gland 527.0
    scar NEC 709.2
    sclerosis, lobar (of brain) 331.0
        with dementia 290.10
    scrotum 608.89
    seminal vesicle 608.89
    senile 797
        degenerative, of skin 701.3
    skin (patches) (senile) 701.8
    spermatic cord 608.89
    spinal (cord) 336.8
        acute 336.8
        muscular (chronic) 335.10
            adult 335.19
            familial 335.11
            juvenile 335.10
        paralysis 335.10
            acute (*see also* Poliomyelitis,
                with paralysis) 045.1
    spine (column) 733.99
    spleen (senile) 289.59
    spots (skin) 701.3
        senile 701.8
    stomach 537.89

Atrophy, atrophic—*continued*
    striate and macular 701.3
        syphilitic 095.8
    subcutaneous 701.9
        due to injection 999.9
    sublingual gland 527.0
    submaxillary gland 527.0
    Sudeck's 733.7
    suprarenal (autoimmune) (capsule)
        (gland) 255.4
        with hypofunction 255.4
    tarso-orbital fascia, congenital
        743.66
    testis 608.3
    thenar, partial 354.0
    throat 478.29
    thymus (fat) 254.8
    thyroid (gland) 246.8
        with
            cretinism 243
            myxedema 244.9
        congenital 243
    tongue (senile) 529.8
        papillae 529.4
        smooth 529.4
    trachea 519.1
    tunica vaginalis 608.89
    turbinate 733.99
    tympanic membrane (nonflaccid)
        384.82
        flaccid 384.81
    ulcer (*see also* Ulcer, skin) 707.9
    upper respiratory tract 478.9
    uterus, uterine (acquired) (senile)
        621.8
        cervix 622.8
        due to radiation (intended
            effect) 621.8
    vagina (senile) 627.3
    vascular 459.89
    vas deferens 608.89
    vertebra (senile) 733.99
    vulva (primary) (senile) 624.1
    Werdnig-Hoffmann 335.0
    yellow (acute) (congenital) (liver)
        (subacute) (*see also* Necrosis,
        liver) 570
        chronic 571.8
        resulting from administration of
            blood, plasma, serum, or
            other biological
            substance (within 8
            months of administration)
            — *see* Hepatitis, viral

Attack
    akinetic (*see also* Epilepsy) 345.0
    angina — *see* Angina
    apoplectic (*see also* Disease,
        cerebrovascular, acute) 436
    benign shuddering 333.93 ▼
    bilious — *see* Vomiting ▲
    cataleptic 300.11
    cerebral (*see also* Disease,
        cerebrovascular, acute) 436
    coronary (*see also* Infarct,
        myocardium) 410.9
    cyanotic, newborn 770.84
    epileptic (*see also* Epilepsy) 345.9
    epileptiform 780.3
    heart (*see also* Infarct, myocardium)
        410.9
    hemiplegia (*see also* Disease,
        cerebrovascular, acute) 436
    hysterical 300.11
    jacksonian (*see also* Epilepsy) 345.5
    myocardium, myocardial (*see also*
        Infarct, myocardium) 410.9
    myoclonic (*see also* Epilepsy) 345.1
    panic 300.01
    paralysis (*see also* Disease,
        cerebrovascular, acute) 436
    paroxysmal 780.3
    psychomotor (*see also* Epilepsy)
        345.4
    salaam (*see also* Epilepsy) 345.6
    schizophreniform (*see also*
        Schizophrenia) 295.4

Attack—*continued*
    sensory and motor 780.3
    syncope 780.2
    toxic, cerebral 780.3
    transient ischemic (TIA) 435.9
    unconsciousness 780.2
        hysterical 300.11
    vasomotor 780.2
    vasovagal (idiopathic) (paroxysmal)
        780.2

Attention to
    artificial opening (of) V55.9
        digestive tract NEC V55.4
        specified site NEC V55.8
        urinary tract NEC V55.6
        vagina V55.7
    colostomy V55.3
    cystostomy V55.5
    gastrostomy V55.1
    ileostomy V55.2
    jejunostomy V55.4
    nephrostomy V55.6
    surgical dressings V58.3
    sutures V58.3
    tracheostomy V55.0
    ureterostomy V55.6
    urethrostomy V55.6

Attrition
    gum 523.2
    teeth (excessive) (hard tissues)
        521.1

Atypical — *see also* condition
    distribution, vessel (congenital)
        (peripheral) NEC 747.60
    endometrium 621.9
    kidney 593.89

Atypism, cervix 622.1

Audible tinnitus (*see also* Tinnitus)
    388.30

Auditory — *see* condition

Audry's syndrome (acropachyderma)
    757.39

Aujeszky's disease 078.89

Aura, jacksonian (*see also* Epilepsy)
    345.5

Aurantiasis, cutis 278.3

Auricle, auricular — *see* condition

Auriculotemporal syndrome 350.8

Australian
    Q fever 083.0
    X disease 062.4

Autism, autistic (child) (infantile)
    299.0

Autodigestion 799.8

Autoerythrocyte sensitization 287.2

Autographism 708.3

Autoimmune
    cold sensitivity 283.0
    disease NEC 279.4
    hemolytic anemia 283.0
    thyroiditis 245.2

Autoinfection, septic — *see*
    Septicemia

Autointoxication 799.8

Automatism 348.8
    epileptic (*see also* Epilepsy) 345.4
    paroxysmal, idiopathic (*see also*
        Epilepsy) 345.4

Autonomic, autonomous
    bladder 596.54
        neurogenic NEC 596.54
            with cauda equina 344.61
    faciocephalgia (*see also*
        Neuropathy, peripheral,
        autonomic) 337.9
    hysterical seizure 300.11
    imbalance (*see also* Neuropathy,
        peripheral, autonomic) 337.9

Autophony 388.40

Autosensitivity, erythrocyte 287.2

Autotopagnosia 780.9

Autotoxemia 799.8

Autumn — see condition
Avellis' syndrome 344.89
Aviators
  disease or sickness (see also Effect, adverse, high altitude) 993.2
    ear 993.0
  effort syndrome 306.2
Avitaminosis (multiple NEC) (see also Deficiency, vitamin) 269.2
  A 264.9
  B 266.9
    with
      beriberi 265.0
      pellagra 265.2
  B_1 265.1
  B_2 266.0
  B_6 266.1
  B_{12} 266.2
  C (with scurvy) 267
  D 268.9
    with
      osteomalacia 268.2
      rickets 268.0
  E 269.1
  G 266.0
  H 269.1
  K 269.0
  multiple 269.2
  nicotinic acid 265.2
  P 269.1
Avulsion (traumatic) 879.8
  blood vessel — see Injury, blood vessel, by site
  cartilage — see also Dislocation, by site
    knee, current (see also Tear, meniscus) 836.2
    symphyseal (inner), complicating delivery 665.6
  complicated 879.9
  diaphragm — see Injury, internal, diaphragm
  ear — see Wound, open, ear
  epiphysis of bone — see Fracture, by site
  external site other than limb — see Wound, open, by site
  eye 871.3
  fingernail — see Wound, open, finger
  fracture — see Fracture, by site
  genital organs, external — see Wound, open, genital organs
  head (intracranial) NEC — see also Injury, intracranial, with open intracranial wound
    complete 874.9
    external site NEC 873.8
      complicated 873.9
  internal organ or site — see Injury, internal, by site
  joint — see also Dislocation, by site
    capsule — see Sprain, by site
    ligament — see Sprain, by site
  limb — see also Amputation, traumatic, by site
    skin and subcutaneous tissue — see Wound, open, by site
  muscle — see Sprain, by site
  nerve (root) — see Injury, nerve, by site
  scalp — see Wound, open, scalp
  skin and subcutaneous tissue — see Wound, open, by site
  symphyseal cartilage (inner), complicating delivery 665.6
  tendon — see also Sprain, by site
    with open wound — see Wound, open, by site
  toenail — see Wound, open, toe(s)
  tooth 873.63
    complicated 873.73
Awareness of heart beat 785.1
Axe grinders' disease 502

Axenfeld's anomaly or syndrome 743.44
Axilla, axillary — see also condition
  breast 757.6
Axonotmesis — see Injury, nerve, by site
Ayala's disease 756.89
Ayerza's disease or syndrome (pulmonary artery sclerosis with pulmonary hypertension) 416.0
Azoospermia 606.0
Azotemia 790.6
  meaning uremia (see also Uremia) 586
Aztec ear 744.29
Azygos lobe, lung (fissure) 748.69

B

Baader's syndrome (erythema multiforme exudativum) 695.1
Baastrup's syndrome 721.5
Babesiasis 088.82
Babesiosis 088.82
Babington's disease (familial hemorrhagic telangiectasia) 448.0
Babinski's syndrome (cardiovascular syphilis) 093.89
Babinski-Fröhlich syndrome (adiposogenital dystrophy) 253.8
Babinski-Nageotte syndrome 344.89
Bacillary — see condition
Bacilluria 599.0
  asymptomatic, in pregnancy or puerperium 646.5
  tuberculous (see also Tuberculosis) 016.9
Bacillus — see also Infection, bacillus
  abortus infection 023.1
  anthracis infection 022.9
  coli
    infection 041.4
      generalized 038.42
      intestinal 008.00
    pyemia 038.42
    septicemia 038.42
  Flexner's 004.1
  fusiformis infestation 101
  mallei infection 024
  Shiga's 004.0
  suipestifer infection (see also Infection, Salmonella) 003.9
Back — see condition
Backache (postural) 724.5
  psychogenic 307.89
  sacroiliac 724.6
Backflow (pyelovenous) (see also Disease, renal) 593.9
Backknee (see also Genu, recurvatum) 736.5
Bacteremia 790.7
  with
    sepsis — see Septicemia
  during
    labor 659.3
    pregnancy 647.8
  newborn 771.8
Bacteria
  in blood (see also Bacteremia) 790.7
  in urine (see also Bacteriuiria) 599.0
Bacterial — see condition
Bactericholia (see also Cholecystitis, acute) 575.0
Bacterid, bacteride (Andrews' pustular) 686.8

Bacteriuria, bacteruria 791.9
  with
    urinary tract infection 599.0
  asymptomatic 791.9
    in pregnancy or puerperium 646.5
      affecting fetus or newborn 760.1
Bad
  breath 784.9
  heart — see Disease, heart
  trip (see also Abuse, drugs, nondependent) 305.3
Baehr-Schiffrin disease (thrombotic thrombocytopenic purpura) 446.6
Baelz's disease (cheilitis glandularis apostematosa) 528.5
Baerensprung's disease (eczema marginatum) 110.3
Bagassosis (occupational) 495.1
Baghdad boil 085.1
Bagratuni's syndrome (temporal arteritis) 446.5
Baker's
  cyst (knee) 727.51
    tuberculous (see also Tuberculosis) 015.2
  itch 692.82
Bakwin-Krida syndrome (craniometaphyseal dysplasia) 756.89
Balanitis (circinata) (gangraenosa) (infectious) (vulgaris) 607.1
  amebic 006.8
  candidal 112.2
  chlamydial 099.53
  due to Ducrey's bacillus 099.0
  erosiva circinata et gangraenosa 607.1
  gangrenous 607.1
  gonococcal (acute) 098.0
    chronic or duration of 2 months or over 098.2
  nongonococcal 607.1
  phagedenic 607.1
  venereal NEC 099.8
  xerotica obliterans 607.81
Balanoposthitis 607.1
  chlamydial 099.53
  gonococcal (acute) 098.0
    chronic or duration of 2 months or over 098.2
  ulcerative NEC 099.8
Balanorrhagia — see Balanitis
Balantidiasis 007.0
Balantidiosis 007.0
Balbuties, balbutio 307.0
Bald
  patches on scalp 704.00
  tongue 529.4
Baldness (see also Alopecia) 704.00
Balfour's disease (chloroma) 205.3
Balint's syndrome (psychic paralysis of visual fixation) 368.16
Balkan grippe 083.0
Ball
  food 938
  hair 938
Ballantyne (-Runge) syndrome (postmaturity) 766.2
Balloon disease (see also Effect, adverse, high altitude) 993.2
Ballooning posterior leaflet syndrome 424.0
Baló's disease or concentric sclerosis 341.1
Bamberger's disease (hypertrophic pulmonary osteoarthropathy) 731.2

Bamberger-Marie disease (hypertrophic pulmonary osteoarthropathy) 731.2
Bamboo spine 720.0
Bancroft's filariasis 125.0
Band(s)
  adhesive (see also Adhesions, peritoneum) 568.0
  amniotic 658.8
    affecting fetus or newborn 762.8
  anomalous or congenital — see also Anomaly, specified type NEC
    atrial 746.9
    heart 746.9
    intestine 751.4
    omentum 751.4
    ventricular 746.9
  cervix 622.3
  gallbladder (congenital) 751.69
  intestinal (adhesive) (see also Adhesions, peritoneum) 568.0
    congenital 751.4
    obstructive (see also Obstruction, intestine) 560.81
    periappendiceal (congenital) 751.4
  peritoneal (adhesive) (see also Adhesions, peritoneum) 568.0
    with intestinal obstruction 560.81
    congenital 751.4
  uterus 621.5
  vagina 623.2
Bandl's ring (contraction)
  complicating delivery 661.4
    affecting fetus or newborn 763.7
Bang's disease (Brucella abortus) 023.1
Bangkok hemorrhagic fever 065.4
Bannister's disease 995.1
Bantam-Albright-Martin disease (pseudohypoparathyroidism) 275.4
Banti's disease or syndrome (with cirrhosis) (with portal hypertension) — see Cirrhosis, liver
Bar
  calcaneocuboid 755.67
  calcaneonavicular 755.67
  cubonavicular 755.67
  prostate 600
  talocalcaneal 755.67
Baragnosis 780.9
Barasheh, barashek 266.2
Barcoo disease or rot (see also Ulcer, skin) 707.9
Bard-Pic syndrome (carcinoma, head of pancreas) 157.0
Bärensprung's disease (eczema marginatum) 110.3
Baritosis 503
Barium lung disease 503
Barlow's syndrome (meaning mitral valve prolapse) 424.0
Barlow (-Möller) disease or syndrome (meaning infantile scurvy) 267
Barodontalgia 993.2
Baron Münchausen syndrome 301.51
Barosinusitis 993.1
Barotitis 993.0
Barotrauma 993.2
  odontalgia 993.2
  otitic 993.0
  sinus 993.1
Barraquer's disease or syndrome (progressive lipodystrophy) 272.6
Barré-Guillain syndrome 357.0
Barré-Liéou syndrome (posterior cervical sympathetic) 723.2

Barrel chest 738.3
Barrett's syndrome or ulcer (chronic peptic ulcer of esophagus) 530.2
Bársony-Polgár syndrome (corkscrew esophagus) 530.5
Bársony-Teschendorf syndrome (corkscrew esophagus) 530.5
Bartholin's
  adenitis (see also Bartholinitis) 616.8
  gland — see condition
Bartholinitis (suppurating) 616.8
  gonococcal (acute) 098.0
    chronic or duration of 2 months or over 098.2
Bartonellosis 088.0
Bartter's syndrome (secondary hyperaldosteronism with juxtaglomerular hyperplasia) 255.1
Basal — see condition
Basan's (hidrotic) ectodermal dysplasia 757.31
Baseball finger 842.13
Basedow's disease or syndrome (exophthalmic goiter) 242.0
Basic — see condition
Basilar — see condition
Bason's (hidrotic) ectodermal dysplasia 757.31
Basopenia 288.0
Basophilia 288.8
Basophilism (corticoadrenal) (Cushing's) (pituitary) (thymic) 255.0
Bassen-Kornzweig syndrome (abetalipoproteinemia) 272.5
Bat ear 744.29
Bateman's
  disease 078.0
  purpura (senile) 287.2
Bathing cramp 994.1
Bathophobia 300.23
Batten's disease, retina 330.1 [362.71]
Batten-Mayou disease 330.1 [362.71]
Batten-Steinert syndrome 359.2
Battered
  adult (syndrome) 995.81
  baby or child (syndrome) 995.5
    affecting parent or family V61.21
    as reason for family seeking advice V61.21
    specified person other than child 995.81
  spouse (syndrome) 995.81
Battey mycobacterium infection 031.0
Battledore placenta — see Placenta, abnormal
Battle exhaustion (see also Reaction, stress, acute) 308.9
Baumgarten-Cruveilhier (cirrhosis) disease, or syndrome 571.5
Bauxite
  fibrosis (of lung) 503
  workers' disease 503
Bayle's disease (dementia paralytica) 094.1
Bazin's disease (primary) (see also Tuberculosis) 017.1
Beach ear 380.12
Beaded hair (congenital) 757.4
Beard's disease (neurasthenia) 300.5
Bearn-Kunkel (-Slater) syndrome (lupoid hepatitis) 571.49
Beat
  elbow 727.2
  hand 727.2
  knee 727.2

Beats
  ectopic 427.60
  escaped, heart 427.60
    postoperative 997.1
  premature (nodal) 427.60
    atrial 427.61
    auricular 427.61
    postoperative 997.1
    specified type NEC 427.69
    supraventricular 427.61
    ventricular 427.69
Beau's
  disease or syndrome (see also Degeneration, myocardial) 429.1
  lines (transverse furrows on fingernails) 703.8
Bechterew's disease (ankylosing spondylitis) 720.0
Bechterew-Strümpell-Marie syndrome (ankylosing spondylitis) 720.0
Beck's syndrome (anterior spinal artery occlusion) 433.8
Becker's
  disease (idiopathic mural endomyocardial disease) 425.2
  dystrophy 359.1
Beckwith (-Wiedemann) syndrome 759.89
Bedclothes, asphyxiation or suffocation by 994.7
Bednar's aphthae 528.2
Bedsore 707.0
  with gangrene 707.0 [785.4]
Bedwetting (see also Enuresis) 788.36
Beer-drinkers' heart (disease) 425.5
Bee sting (with allergic or anaphylactic shock) 989.5
Begbie's disease (exophthalmic goiter) 242.0
Behavior disorder, disturbance — see also Disturbance, conduct
  antisocial, without manifest psychiatric disorder
    adolescent V71.02
    adult V71.01
    child V71.02
  dyssocial, without manifest psychiatric disorder
    adolescent V71.02
    adult V71.01
    child V71.02
Behçet's syndrome 136.1
Behr's disease 362.50
Beigel's disease or morbus (white piedra) 111.2
Bejel 104.0
Bekhterev's disease (ankylosing spondylitis) 720.0
Bekhterev-Strümpell-Marie syndrome (ankylosing spondylitis) 720.0
Belching (see also Eructation) 787.3
Bell's
  disease (see also Psychosis, affective) 296.0
  mania (see also Psychosis, affective) 296.0
  palsy, paralysis 351.0
    infant 767.5
    newborn 767.5
    syphilitic 094.89
  spasm 351.0
Bence-Jones albuminuria, albuminosuria, or proteinuria 791.0
Bends 993.3
Benedikt's syndrome (paralysis) 344.89
Benign — see also condition
  prostate
    hyperplasia 600
    neoplasm 222.2

Bennett's
  disease (leukemia) 208.9
  fracture (closed) 815.01
    open 815.11
Benson's disease 379.22
Bent
  back (hysterical) 300.11
  nose 738.0
    congenital 754.0
Bereavement V62.82
  as adjustment reaction 309.0
Berger's paresthesia (lower limb) 782.0
Bergeron's disease (hysteroepilepsy) 300.11
Beriberi (acute) (atrophic) (chronic) (dry) (subacute) (wet) 265.0
  with polyneuropathy 265.0 [357.4]
  heart (disease) 265.0 [425.7]
  leprosy 030.1
  neuritis 265.0 [357.4]
Berlin's disease or edema (traumatic) 921.3
Berloque dermatitis 692.72
Bernard-Horner syndrome (see also Neuropathy, peripheral, autonomic) 337.9
Bernard-Sergent syndrome (acute adrenocortical insufficiency) 255.4
Bernard-Soulier disease or thrombopathy 287.1
Bernhardt's disease or paresthesia 355.1
Bernhardt-Roth disease or syndrome (paresthesia) 355.1
Bernheim's syndrome (see also Failure, heart, congestive) 428.0
Bertielliasis 123.8
Bertolotti's syndrome (sacralization of fifth lumbar vertebra) 756.15
Berylliosis (acute) (chronic) (lung) (occupational) 503
Besnier's
  lupus pernio 135
  prurigo (atopic dermatitis) (infantile eczema) 691.8
Besnier-Boeck disease or sarcoid 135
Besnier-Boeck-Schaumann disease (sarcoidosis) 135
Best's disease 362.76
Bestiality 302.1
Beta-adrenergic hyperdynamic circulatory state 429.82
Beta-aminoisobutyric aciduria 277.2
Beta-mercaptolactate-cysteine disulfiduria 270.0
Beta thalassemia (major) (minor) (mixed) 282.4
Beurmann's disease (sporotrichosis) 117.1
Bezoar 938
  intestine 936
  stomach 935.2
Bezold's abscess (see also Mastoiditis) 383.01
Bianchi's syndrome (aphasia-apraxia-alexia) 784.69
Bicornuate or bicornis uterus 752.3
  in pregnancy or childbirth 654.0
    with obstructed labor 660.2
      affecting fetus or newborn 763.1
    affecting fetus or newborn 763.8
Bicuspid aortic valve 746.4
Biedl-Bardet syndrome 759.89
Bielschowsky's disease 330.1
Bielschowsky-Jansky
  amaurotic familial idiocy 330.1
  disease 330.1

Biemond's syndrome (obesity, polydactyly, and mental retardation) 759.89
Biermer's anemia or disease (pernicious anemia) 281.0
Biett's disease 695.4
Bifid (congenital) — see also Imperfect, closure
  apex, heart 746.89
  clitoris 752.49
  epiglottis 748.3
  kidney 753.3
  nose 748.1
  patella 755.64
  scrotum 752.8
  toe 755.66
  tongue 750.13
  ureter 753.4
  uterus 752.3
  uvula 749.02
    with cleft lip (see also Cleft, palate, with cleft lip) 749.20
Biforis uterus (suprasimplex) 752.3
Bifurcation (congenital) — see also Imperfect, closure
  gallbladder 751.69
  kidney pelvis 753.3
  renal pelvis 753.3
  rib 756.3
  tongue 750.13
  trachea 748.3
  ureter 753.4
  urethra 753.8
  uvula 749.02
    with cleft lip (see also Cleft, palate, with cleft lip) 749.20
  vertebra 756.19
Bigeminal pulse 427.89
Bigeminy 427.89
Big spleen syndrome 289.4
Bilateral — see condition
Bile duct — see condition
Bile pigments in urine 791.4
Bilharziasis (see also Schistosomiasis) 120.9
  chyluria 120.0
  cutaneous 120.3
  galacturia 120.0
  hematochyluria 120.0
  intestinal 120.1
  lipemia 120.9
  lipuria 120.0
  Oriental 120.2
  piarhemia 120.9
  pulmonary 120.2
  tropical hematuria 120.0
  vesical 120.0
Biliary — see condition
Bilious (attack) — see also Vomiting ◆
  fever, hemoglobinuric 084.8
Bilirubinuria 791.4
Biliuria 791.4
Billroth's disease
  meningocele (see also Spina bifida) 741.9
Bilobate placenta — see Placenta, abnormal
Bilocular
  heart 745.7
  stomach 536.8
Bing-Horton syndrome (histamine cephalgia) 346.2
Binswanger's disease or dementia 290.12
Biörck (-Thorson) syndrome (malignant carcinoid) 259.2
Biparta, bipartite — see also Imperfect, closure
  carpal scaphoid 755.59
  patella 755.64
  placenta — see Placenta, abnormal

Biparta, bipartite—*continued*
   vagina 752.49
Bird
   face 756.0
   fanciers' lung or disease 495.2
Bird's disease (oxaluria) 271.8
Birth
   abnormal fetus or newborn 763.9
   accident, fetus or newborn — *see* Birth, injury
   complications in mother — *see* Delivery, complicated
   compression during NEC 767.9
   defect — *see* Anomaly
   delayed, fetus 763.9
   difficult NEC, affecting fetus or newborn 763.9
   dry, affecting fetus or newborn 761.1
   forced, NEC, affecting fetus or newborn 763.8
   forceps, affecting fetus or newborn 763.2
   hematoma of sternomastoid 767.8
   immature 765.1
      extremely 765.0
   inattention, after or at 995.5
      affecting parent or family V61.21
   induced, affecting fetus or newborn 763.8
   infant — *see* Newborn
   injury NEC 767.9
      adrenal gland 767.8
      basal ganglia 767.0
      brachial plexus (paralysis) 767.6
      brain (compression) (pressure) 767.0
      cerebellum 767.0
      cerebral hemorrhage 767.0
      conjunctiva 767.8
      eye 767.8
      fracture
         bone, any except clavicle or spine 767.3
         clavicle 767.2
         femur 767.3
         humerus 767.3
         long bone 767.3
         radius and ulna 767.3
         skeleton NEC 767.3
         skull 767.3
         spine 767.4
         tibia and fibula 767.3
      hematoma 767.8
         liver (subcapsular) 767.8
         mastoid 767.8
         skull 767.1
         sternomastoid 767.8
         testes 767.8
         vulva 767.8
      intracranial (edema) 767.0
      laceration
         brain 767.0
         by scalpel 767.8
         peripheral nerve 767.7
      liver 767.8
      meninges
         brain 767.0
         spinal cord 767.4
      nerves (cranial, peripheral) 767.7
         brachial plexus 767.6
         facial 767.5
      paralysis 767.7
         brachial plexus 767.6
         Erb (-Duchenne) 767.6
         facial nerve 767.5
         Klumpke (-Déjérine) 767.6
         radial nerve 767.6
      spinal (cord) (hemorrhage) (laceration) (rupture) 767.4
      rupture
         intracranial 767.0
         liver 767.8
         spinal cord 767.4

Birth—*continued*
   injury—*continued*
      rupture—*continued*
         spleen 767.8
         viscera 767.8
      scalp 767.1
      scalpel wound 767.8
      skeleton NEC 767.3
      specified NEC 767.8
      spinal cord 767.4
      spleen 767.8
      subdural hemorrhage 767.0
      tentorial, tear 767.0
      testes 767.8
      vulva 767.8
   instrumental, NEC, affecting fetus or newborn 763.2
   lack of care, after or at 995.5
      affecting parent or family V61.21
   multiple
      affected by maternal complications of pregnancy 761.5
      healthy liveborn — *see* Newborn, multiple
   neglect, after or at 995.5
      affecting parent or family V61.21
   newborn — *see* Newborn
   palsy or paralysis NEC 767.7
   precipitate, fetus or newborn 763.6
   premature (infant) 765.1
   prolonged, affecting fetus or newborn 763.9
   retarded, fetus or newborn 763.9
   shock, newborn 779.8
   strangulation or suffocation due to aspiration of amniotic fluid 770.1
      mechanical 767.8
   trauma NEC 767.9
   triplet
      affected by maternal complications of pregnancy 761.5
      healthy liveborn — *see* Newborn, multiple
   twin
      affected by maternal complications of pregnancy 761.5
      healthy liveborn — *see* Newborn, twin
   ventouse, affecting fetus or newborn 763.3
Birthmark 757.32
Bisalbuminemia 273.8
Biskra button 085.1
Bite(s)
   with intact skin surface — *see* Contusion
   animal — *see* Wound, open, by site
      intact skin surface — *see* Contusion
   centipede 989.5
   chigger 133.8
   fire ant 989.5
   flea — *see* Injury, superficial, by site
   human (open wound) — *see also* Wound, open, by site
      intact skin surface — *see* Contusion
   insect
      nonvenomous — *see* Injury, superficial, by site
      venomous 989.5
   mad dog (death from) 071
   poisonous 989.5
   red bug 133.8
   reptile 989.5
      nonvenomous — *see* Wound, open, by site

Bite(s)—*continued*
   snake 989.5
      nonvenomous — *see* Wound, open, by site
   spider (venomous) 989.5
      nonvenomous — *see* Injury, superficial, by site
   venomous 989.5
Biting
   cheek or lip 528.9
   nail 307.9
Black
   death 020.9
   eye NEC 921.0
   hairy tongue 529.3
   lung disease 500
Blackfan-Diamond anemia or syndrome (congenital hypoplastic anemia) 284.0
Blackhead 706.1
Blackout 780.2
Blackwater fever 084.8
Bladder — *see* condition
Blast
   blindness 921.3
   concussion — *see* Blast, injury
   injury 869.0
      with open wound into cavity 869.1
      abdomen or thorax — *see* Injury, internal, by site
      brain (*see also* Concussion, brain) 850.9
         with skull fracture — *see* Fracture, skull
      ear (acoustic nerve trauma) 951.5
         with perforation, tympanic membrane — *see* Wound, open, ear, drum
      lung (*see also* Injury, internal, lung) 861.20
      otitic (explosive) 388.11
Blastomycosis, blastomycotic (chronic) (cutaneous) (disseminated) (lung) (pulmonary) (systemic) 116.0
   Brazilian 116.1
   European 117.5
   keloidal 116.2
   North American 116.0
   primary pulmonary 116.0
   South American 116.1
Bleb(s) 709.8
   emphysematous (bullous) (diffuse) (lung) (ruptured) (solitary) 492.0
   filtering, eye (postglaucoma) (status) V45.6
      with complication 997.9
      postcataract extraction (complication) 997.9
   lung (ruptured) 492.0
      congenital 770.5
   subpleural (emphysematous) 492.0
Bleeder (familial) (hereditary) (*see also* Defect, coagulation) 286.9
   nonfamilial 286.9
Bleeding (*see also* Hemorrhage) 459.0
   anal 569.3
   anovulatory 628.0
   atonic, following delivery 666.1
   capillary 448.9
   due to subinvolution 621.1
      puerperal 666.2
   ear 388.69
   excessive, associated with menopausal onset 627.0
   familial (*see also* Defect, coagulation) 286.9
   following intercourse 626.7
   gastrointestinal 578.9
   gums 523.8
   hemorrhoids — *see* Hemorrhoids, bleeding

Bleeding—*continued*
   intermenstrual
      irregular 626.6
      regular 626.5
   intraoperative 998.1
   irregular NEC 626.4
   menopausal 627.0
   mouth 528.9
   nipple 611.79
   nose 784.7
   ovulation 626.5
   postclimacteric 627.1
   postcoital 626.7
   postmenopausal 627.1
      following induced menopause 627.4
   postoperative 998.1
   preclimacteric 627.0
   puberty 626.3
      excessive, with onset of menstrual periods 626.3
   rectum, rectal 569.3
   tendencies (*see also* Defect, coagulation) 286.9
   throat 784.8
   umbilical stump 772.3
   umbilicus 789.9
   unrelated to menstrual cycle 626.6
   uterus, uterine 626.9
      climacteric 627.0
      dysfunctional 626.8
      functional 626.8
      unrelated to menstrual cycle 626.6
   vagina, vaginal 623.8
      functional 626.8
   vicarious 625.8
Blennorrhagia, blennorrhagic — *see* Blennorrhea
Blennorrhea (acute) 098.0
   adultorum 098.40
   alveolaris 523.4
   chronic or duration of 2 months or over 098.2
   gonococcal (neonatorum) 098.40
   inclusion (neonatal) (newborn) 771.6
   neonatorum 098.40
Blepharelosis (*see also* Entropion) 374.00
Blepharitis (eyelid) 373.00
   angularis 373.01
   ciliaris 373.00
      with ulcer 373.01
   marginal 373.00
      with ulcer 373.01
   scrofulous (*see also* Tuberculosis) 017.3 *[373.00]*
   squamous 373.02
   ulcerative 373.01
Blepharochalasis 374.34
   congenital 743.62
Blepharoclonus 333.81
Blepharoconjunctivitis (*see also* Conjunctivitis) 372.20
   angular 372.21
   contact 372.22
Blepharophimosis (eyelid) 374.46
   congenital 743.62
Blepharoplegia 374.89
Blepharoptosis 374.30
   congenital 743.61
Blepharopyorrhea 098.49
Blepharospasm 333.81
Blessig's cyst 362.62
Blighted ovum 631
Blind
   bronchus (congenital) 748.3
   eye — *see also* Blindness
      hypertensive 360.42
      hypotensive 360.41
   loop syndrome (postoperative) 579.2

Blind—*continued*
   sac, fallopian tube (congenital) 752.19
   spot, enlarged 368.42
   tract or tube (congenital) NEC — *see* Atresia

Blindness (acquired) (congenital) (both eyes) 369.00
   blast 921.3
      with nerve injury — *see* Injury, nerve, optic
   Bright's — *see* Uremia
   color (congenital) 368.59
      acquired 368.55
      blue 368.53
      green 368.52
      red 368.51
      total 368.54
   concussion 950.9
   cortical 377.75
   day 368.60
      acquired 368.62
      congenital 368.61
      hereditary 368.61
      specified type NEC 368.69
   due to
      injury NEC 950.9
      refractive error — *see* Error, refractive
   eclipse (total) 363.31
   emotional 300.11
   hysterical 300.11
   legal (both eyes) (USA definition) 369.4
   with impairment of better (less impaired) eye
      near-total 369.02
      with
         lesser eye impairment 369.02
         near-total 369.04
         total 369.03
      profound 369.05
      with
         lesser eye impairment 369.05
         near-total 369.07
         profound 369.08
         total 369.06
      severe 369.21
      with
         lesser eye impairment 369.21
         blind 369.11
         near-total 369.13
         profound 369.14
         severe 369.22
         total 369.12
      total
         with lesser eye impairment
            total 369.01
   mind 784.69
   moderate
      both eyes 369.25
         with impairment of lesser eye (specified as)
            blind, not further specified 369.15
            low vision, not further specified 369.23
            near-total 369.17
            profound 369.18
            severe 369.24
            total 369.16
      one eye 369.74
         with vision of other eye (specified as)
            near-normal 369.75
            normal 369.76
   near-total
      both eyes 369.04
         with impairment of lesser eye (specified as)
            blind, not further specified 369.02
            total 369.03

Blindness—*continued*
   near total—*continued*
      one eye 369.64
         with vision of other eye (specified as)
            near-normal 369.65
            normal 369.66
   night 368.60
      acquired 368.62
      congenital (Japanese) 368.61
      hereditary 368.61
      specified type NEC 368.69
      vitamin A deficiency 264.5
   nocturnal — *see* Blindness, night
   one eye 369.60
      with low vision of other eye 369.10
   profound
      both eyes 369.08
         with impairment of lesser eye (specified as)
            blind, not further specified 369.05
            near-total 369.07
            total 369.06
      one eye 369.67
         with vision of other eye (specified as)
            near-normal 369.68
            normal 369.69
   psychic 784.69
   severe
      both eyes 369.22
         with impairment of lesser eye (specified as)
            blind, not further specified 369.11
            low vision, not further specified 369.21
            near-total 369.13
            profound 369.14
            total 369.12
      one eye 369.71
         with vision of other eye (specified as)
            near-normal 369.72
            normal 369.73
   snow 370.24
   sun 363.31
   temporary 368.12
   total
      both eyes 369.01
      one eye 369.61
         with vision of other eye (specified as)
            near-normal 369.62
            normal 369.63
   transient 368.12
   traumatic NEC 950.9
   word (developmental) 315.01
      acquired 784.61
      secondary to organic lesion 784.61

Blister — *see also* Injury, superficial, by site
   beetle dermatitis 692.89
   due to burn — *see* Burn, by site, second degree
   fever 054.9
   multiple, skin, nontraumatic 709.8

Bloating 787.3

Bloch-Siemens syndrome (incontinentia pigmenti) 757.33

Bloch-Stauffer dyshormonal dermatosis 757.33

Bloch-Sulzberger disease or syndrome (incontinentia pigmenti) (melanoblastosis) 757.33

Block
   alveolar capillary 516.3
   arborization (heart) 426.6
   arrhythmic 426.9
   atrioventricular (AV) (incomplete) (partial) 426.10

Block—*continued*
   atrioventricular—*continued*
      with
         2:1 atrioventricular response block 426.13
         atrioventricular dissociation 426.0
      first degree (incomplete) 426.11
      second degree (Mobitz type I) 426.13
      Mobitz (type) II 426.12
      third degree 426.0
      complete 426.0
         congenital 746.86
      congenital 746.86
      Mobitz (incomplete)
         type I (Wenckebach's) 426.13
         type II 426.12
      partial 426.13
   auriculoventricular (*see also* Block, atrioventricular) 426.10
      complete 426.0
      congenital 746.86
      congenital 746.86
   bifascicular (cardiac) 426.53
   bundle branch (complete) (false) (incomplete) 426.50
      bilateral 426.53
      left (complete) (main stem) 426.3
         with right bundle branch block 426.53
         anterior fascicular 426.2
         with
            posterior fascicular block 426.3
            right bundle branch block 426.52
         hemiblock 426.2
         incomplete 426.2
            with right bundle branch block 426.53
         posterior fascicular 426.2
         with
            anterior fascicular block 426.3
            right bundle branch block 426.51
      right 426.4
         with
            left bundle branch block (incomplete) (main stem) 426.53
            left fascicular block 426.53
               anterior 426.52
               posterior 426.51
      Wilson's type 426.4
   cardiac 426.9
   conduction 426.9
      complete 426.0
   Eustachian tube (*see also* Obstruction, Eustachian tube) 381.60
   fascicular (left anterior) (left posterior) 426.2
   foramen Magendie (acquired) 331.3
      congenital 742.3
         with spina bifida (*see also* Spina bifida) 741.0
   heart 426.9
      first degree (atrioventricular) 426.11
      second degree (atrioventricular) 426.13
      third degree (atrioventricular) 426.0
      bundle branch (complete) (false) (incomplete) 426.50
         bilateral 426.53
         left (*see also* Block, bundle branch, left) 426.3
         right (*see also* Block, bundle branch, right) 426.4
      complete (atrioventricular) 426.0

Block—*continued*
   heart—*continued*
      congenital 746.86
      incomplete 426.13
      intra-atrial 426.6
      intraventricular NEC 426.6
      sinoatrial 426.6
      specified type NEC 426.6
   hepatic vein 453.0
   intraventricular (diffuse) (myofibrillar) 426.6
      bundle branch (complete) (false) (incomplete) 426.50
         bilateral 426.53
         left (*see also* Block, bundle branch, left) 426.3
         right (*see also* Block, bundle branch, right) 426.4
   kidney (*see also* Disease, renal) 593.9
      postcystoscopic 997.5
   myocardial (*see also* Block, heart) 426.9
   nodal 426.10
   optic nerve 377.49
   organ or site (congenital) NEC — *see* Atresia
   parietal 426.6
   peri-infarction 426.6
   portal (vein) 452
   sinoatrial 426.6
   sinoauricular 426.6
   spinal cord 336.9
   trifascicular 426.54
   tubal 628.2
   vein NEC 453.9

Blocq's disease or syndrome (astasia-abasia) 307.9

Blood
   constituents, abnormal NEC 790.6
   disease 289.9
      specified NEC 289.8
   donor V59.0
   dyscrasia 289.9
      with
         abortion — *see* Abortion, by type, with hemorrhage, delayed or excessive
         ectopic pregnancy (*see also* categories 633.0-633.9) 639.1
         molar pregnancy (*see also* categories 630-632) 639.1
      fetus or newborn NEC 776.9
      following
         abortion 639.1
         ectopic or molar pregnancy 639.1
      puerperal, postpartum 666.3
   flukes NEC (*see also* Infestation, Schistosoma) 120.9
   in
      feces (*see also* Melena) 578.1
         occult 792.1
      urine (*see also* Hematuria) 599.7
   mole 631
   occult 792.1
   poisoning (*see also* Septicemia) 038.9
   pressure
      decreased, due to shock following injury 958.4
      fluctuating 796.4
      high (*see also* Hypertension) 401.9
         incidental reading (isolated) (nonspecific), without diagnosis of hypertension 796.2

Blood—continued
    pressure—continued
        low (see also Hypotension) 458.9
            incidental reading (isolated) (nonspecific), without diagnosis of hypotension 796.3
    spitting (see also Hemoptysis) 786.3
    staining cornea 371.12
    transfusion
        without reported diagnosis V58.2
        donor V59.0
        reaction or complication — see Complications, transfusion
    tumor — see Hematoma
    vessel rupture — see Hemorrhage
    vomiting (see also Hematemesis) 578.0
Blood-forming organ disease 289.9
Bloodgood's disease 610.1
Bloodshot eye 379.93
Bloom (-Machacek) (-Torre) **syndrome** 757.39
Blotch, palpebral 372.55
Blount's disease (tibia vara) 732.4
Blount-Barber syndrome (tibia vara) 732.4
Blue
    baby 746.9
    bloater 491.20
        with acute bronchitis or exacerbation 491.21
    diaper syndrome 270.0
    disease 746.9
    dome cyst 610.0
    drum syndrome 381.02
    sclera 743.47
        with fragility of bone and deafness 756.51
    toe syndrome — see Atherosclerosis
Blueness (see also Cyanosis) 782.5
Blurring, visual 368.8
Blushing (abnormal) (excessive) 782.62
Boarder, hospital V65.0
    infant V65.0
Bockhart's impetigo (superficial folliculitis) 704.8
Bodechtel-Guttmann disease (subacute sclerosing panencephalitis) 046.2
Boder-Sedgwick syndrome (ataxia-telangiectasia) 334.8
Body, bodies
    Aschoff (see also Myocarditis, rheumatic) 398.0
    asteroid, vitreous 379.22
    choroid, colloid (degenerative) 362.57
        hereditary 362.77
    cytoid (retina) 362.82
    drusen (retina) (see also Drusen) 362.57
        optic disc 377.21
    fibrin, pleura 511.0
    foreign — see Foreign body
    Hassall-Henle 371.41
    loose
        joint (see also Loose, body, joint) 718.1
            knee 717.6
        knee 717.6
        sheath, tendon 727.82
    Mallory's 034.1
    Mooser 081.0
    Negri 071
    rice (joint) (see also Loose, body, joint) 718.1
        knee 717.6
    rocking 307.3

Boeck's
    disease (sarcoidosis) 135
    lupoid (miliary) 135
    sarcoid 135
Boerhaave's syndrome (spontaneous esophageal rupture) 530.4
Boggy
    cervix 622.8
    uterus 621.8
Boil (see also Carbuncle) 680.9
    abdominal wall 680.2
    Aleppo 085.1
    ankle 680.6
    anus 680.5
    arm (any part, above wrist) 680.3
    auditory canal, external 680.0
    axilla 680.3
    back (any part) 680.2
    Baghdad 085.1
    breast 680.2
    buttock 680.5
    chest wall 680.2
    corpus cavernosum 607.2
    Delhi 085.1
    ear (any part) 680.0
    eyelid 373.13
    face (any part, except eye) 680.0
    finger (any) 680.4
    flank 680.2
    foot (any part) 680.7
    forearm 680.3
    Gafsa 085.1
    genital organ, male 608.4
    gluteal (region) 680.5
    groin 680.2
    hand (any part) 680.4
    head (any part, except face) 680.8
    heel 680.7
    hip 680.6
    knee 680.6
    labia 616.4
    lacrimal (see also Dacryocystitis) 375.30
        gland (see also Dacryoadenitis) 375.00
        passages (duct) (sac) (see also Dacryocystitis) 375.30
    leg, any part except foot 680.6
    multiple sites 680.9
    Natal 085.1
    neck 680.1
    nose (external) (septum) 680.0
    orbit, orbital 376.01
    partes posteriores 680.5
    pectoral region 680.2
    penis 607.2
    perineum 680.2
    pinna 680.0
    scalp (any part) 680.8
    scrotum 608.4
    seminal vesicle 608.0
    shoulder 680.3
    skin NEC 680.9
    specified site NEC 680.8
    spermatic cord 608.4
    temple (region) 680.0
    testis 608.4
    thigh 680.6
    thumb 680.4
    toe (any) 680.7
    tropical 085.1
    trunk 680.2
    tunica vaginalis 608.4
    umbilicus 680.2
    upper arm 680.3
    vas deferens 608.4
    vulva 616.4
    wrist 680.4
Bold hives (see also Urticaria) 708.9
Bolivian hemorrhagic fever 078.7
Bombé, iris 364.74
Bomford-Rhoads anemia (refractory) 284.9
Bone — see condition
Bonnevie-Ullrich syndrome 758.6

Bonnier's syndrome 386.19
Bonvale Dam fever 780.7
Bony block of joint 718.80
    ankle 718.87
    elbow 718.82
    foot 718.87
    hand 718.84
    hip 718.85
    knee 718.86
    multiple sites 718.89
    pelvic region 718.85
    shoulder (region) 718.81
    specified site NEC 718.88
    wrist 718.83
Borderline
    intellectual functioning V62.89
    pelvis 653.1
        with obstruction during labor 660.1
            affecting fetus or newborn 763.1
    psychosis (see also Schizophrenia) 295.5
        of childhood (see also Psychosis, childhood) 299.8
    schizophrenia (see also Schizophrenia) 295.5
Borna disease 062.9
Bornholm disease (epidemic pleurodynia) 074.1
Borrelia vincentii (mouth) (pharynx) (tonsils) 101
Bostock's catarrh (see also Fever, hay) 477.9
Boston exanthem 048
Botalli, ductus (patent) (persistent) 747.0
Bothriocephalus latus infestation 123.4
Botulism 005.1
Bouba (see also Yaws) 102.9
Bouffée délirante 298.3
Bouillaud's disease or syndrome (rheumatic heart disease) 391.9
Bourneville's disease (tuberous sclerosis) 759.5
Boutonneuse fever 082.1
Boutonniere
    deformity (finger) 736.21
    hand (intrinsic) 736.21
Bouveret (-Hoffmann) **disease or syndrome** (paroxysmal tachycardia) 427.2
Bovine heart — see Hypertrophy, cardiac
Bowel — see condition
Bowen's
    dermatosis (precancerous) (M8081/2) — see Neoplasm, skin, in situ
    disease (M8081/2) — see Neoplasm, skin, in situ
    epithelioma (M8081/2) — see Neoplasm, skin, in situ
    type
        epidermoid carcinoma in situ (M8081/2) — see Neoplasm, skin, in situ
        intraepidermal squamous cell carcinoma (M8081/2) — see Neoplasm, skin, in situ
Bowing
    femur 736.89
        congenital 754.42
    fibula 736.89
        congenital 754.43
    forearm 736.09
        away from midline (cubitus valgus) 736.01
        toward midline (cubitus varus) 736.02

Bowing—continued
    leg(s), long bones, congenital 754.44
    radius 736.09
        away from midline (cubitus valgus) 736.01
        toward midline (cubitus varus) 736.02
    tibia 736.89
        congenital 754.43
Bowleg(s) 736.42
    congenital 754.44
    rachitic 268.1
Boyd's dysentery 004.2
Brachial — see condition
Brachman-de Lange syndrome (Amsterdam dwarf, mental retardation, and brachycephaly) 759.89
Brachycardia 427.89
Brachycephaly 756.0
Brachymorphism and ectopia lentis 759.89
Bradley's disease (epidemic vomiting) 078.82
Bradycardia 427.89
    chronic (sinus) 427.81
    newborn 770.8 ◆
    nodal 427.89
    postoperative 997.1
    reflex 337.0
    sinoatrial 427.89
        with paroxysmal tachyarrhythmia or tachycardia 427.81
        chronic 427.81
    sinus 427.89
        with paroxysmal tachyarrhythmia or tachycardia 427.81
        chronic 427.81
        persistent 427.81
        severe 427.81
    tachycardia syndrome 427.81
    vagal 427.89
Bradypnea 786.09
Brailsford's disease 732.3
    radial head 732.3
    tarsal scaphoid 732.5
Brailsford-Morquio disease or syndrome (mucopolysaccharidosis IV) 277.5
Brain — see also condition
    death 348.8
    syndrome (acute) (chronic) (nonpsychotic) (organic) (with neurotic reaction) (with behavioral reaction) (see also Syndrome, brain) 310.9
        with
            presenile brain disease 290.10
            psychosis, psychotic reaction (see also Psychosis, organic) 294.9
        congenital (see also Retardation, mental) 319
Branched-chain amino-acid disease 270.3
Branchial — see condition
Brandt's syndrome (acrodermatitis enteropathica) 686.8
Brash (water) 787.1
Brass-founders', ague 985.8
Bravais-Jacksonian epilepsy (see also Epilepsy) 345.5
Braxton Hicks contractions 644.1
Braziers' disease 985.8
Brazilian
    blastomycosis 116.1
    leishmaniasis 085.5

Break
- cardiorenal — *see* Hypertension, cardiorenal
- retina (*see also* Defect, retina) 361.30

Breakbone fever 061

Breakdown
- device, implant, or graft — *see* Complications, mechanical
- nervous (*see also* Disorder, mental, nonpsychotic) 300.9
- perineum 674.2

Breast — *see* condition

Breath
- foul 784.9
- holder, child 312.81
- holding spells 786.9
- shortness 786.09

Breathing
- asymmetrical 786.09
- bronchial 786.09
- exercises V57.0
- labored 786.09
- mouth 784.9
- periodic 786.09
- tic 307.20

Breathlessness 786.09

Breda's disease (*see also* Yaws) 102.9

Breech
- delivery, affecting fetus or newborn 763.0
- extraction, affecting fetus or newborn 763.0
- presentation 652.2
  - with successful version 652.1
  - before labor, affecting fetus or newborn 761.7
  - causing obstructed labor 660.0
  - during labor, affecting fetus or newborn 763.0

Breisky's disease (kraurosis vulvae) 624.0

Brennemann's syndrome (acute mesenteric lymphadenitis) 289.2

Brenner's
- tumor (benign) (M9000/0) 220
  - borderline malignancy (M9000/1) 236.2
  - malignant (M9000/3) 183.0
  - proliferating (M9000/1) 236.2

Bretonneau's disease (diphtheritic malignant angina) 032.0

Breus' mole 631

Brevicollis 756.16

Bricklayers' itch 692.89

Brickmakers' anemia 126.9

Bridge
- myocardial 746.85

Bright's
- blindness — *see* Uremia
- disease (*see also* Nephritis) 583.9
  - arteriosclerotic (*see also* Hypertension, kidney) 403.90

Brill's disease (recrudescent typhus) 081.1
- flea-borne 081.0
- louse-borne 081.1

Brill-Symmers disease (follicular lymphoma) (M9690/3) 202.0

Brill-Zinsser disease (recrudescent typhus) 081.1

Brinton's disease (linitis plastica) (M8142/3) 151.9

Brion-Kayser disease (*see also* Fever, paratyphoid) 002.9

Briquet's disorder or syndrome 300.81

Brissaud's
- infantilism (infantile myxedema) 244.9
- motor-verbal tic 307.23

Brissaud-Meige syndrome (infantile myxedema) 244.9

Brittle
- bones (congenital) 756.51
- nails 703.8
  - congenital 757.5

Broad — *see also* condition
- beta disease 272.2
- ligament laceration syndrome 620.6

Brock's syndrome (atelectasis due to enlarged lymph nodes) 518.0

Brocq's disease 691.8
- atopic (diffuse) neurodermatitis 691.8
- lichen simplex chronicus 698.3
- parakeratosis psoriasiformis 696.2
- parapsoriasis 696.2

Brocq-Duhring disease (dermatitis herpetiformis) 694.0

Brodie's
- abscess (localized) (chronic) (*see also* Osteomyelitis) 730.1
- disease (joint) (*see also* Osteomyelitis) 730.1

Broken
- arches 734
  - congenital 755.67
- back — *see* Fracture, vertebra, by site
- bone — *see* Fracture, by site
- compensation — *see* Disease, heart
- implant or internal device — *see* listing under Complications, mechanical
- neck — *see* Fracture, vertebra, cervical
- nose 802.0
  - open 802.1
- tooth, teeth 873.63
  - complicated 873.73

Bromhidrosis 705.89

Bromidism, bromism
- acute 967.3
  - correct substance properly administered 349.82
  - overdose or wrong substance given or taken 967.3
- chronic (*see also* Dependence) 304.1

Bromidrosiphobia 300.23

Bromidrosis 705.89

Bronchi, bronchial — *see* condition

Bronchiectasis (cylindrical) (diffuse) (fusiform) (localized) (moniliform) (postinfectious) (recurrent) (saccular) 494
- congenital 748.61
- tuberculosis (*see also* Tuberculosis) 011.5

Bronchiolectasis — *see* Bronchiectasis

Bronchiolitis (acute) (infectious) (subacute) 466.1
- with
  - bronchospasm or obstruction 466.1
  - influenza, flu, or grippe 487.1
- catarrhal (acute) (subacute) 466.1
- chemical 506.0
  - chronic 506.4
- chronic (obliterative) 491.8
- due to external agent — *see* Bronchitis, acute, due to
- fibrosa obliterans 491.8
- influenzal 487.1
- obliterans 491.8
  - with organizing pneumonia (B.O.O.P.) 516.8
- obliterative (chronic) (diffuse) (subacute) 491.8
  - due to fumes or vapors 506.4
- vesicular — *see* Pneumonia, broncho-

Bronchitis (diffuse) (hypostatic) (infectious) (inflammatory) (simple) 490
- with
  - emphysema — *see* Emphysema
  - influenza, flu, or grippe 487.1
  - obstruction airway, chronic 491.20
    - with acute exacerbation 491.21
  - tracheitis 490
    - acute or subacute 466.0
      - with bronchospasm or obstruction 466.0
    - chronic 491.8
- acute or subacute 466.0
  - with
    - bronchospasm 466.0
    - chronic
      - bronchitis (obstructive) 491.21
      - obstructive pulmonary disease (COPD) 491.21
    - obstruction 466.0
    - tracheitis 466.0
  - chemical (due to fumes or vapors) 506.0
  - due to
    - fumes or vapors 506.0
    - radiation 508.8
- allergic (acute) (*see also* Asthma) 493.9
- arachidic 934.1
- aspiration 507.0
  - due to fumes or vapors 506.0
- asthmatic (acute) (*see also* Asthma) 493.9
  - chronic 491.20
    - with acute bronchitis or acute exacerbation 491.21
- capillary 466.1
  - with bronchospasm or obstruction 466.1
  - chronic 491.8
- caseous (*see also* Tuberculosis) 011.3
- Castellani's 104.8
- catarrhal 490
  - acute — *see* Bronchitis, acute
  - chronic 491.0
- chemical (acute) (subacute) 506.0
  - chronic 506.4
  - due to fumes or vapors (acute) (subacute) 506.0
    - chronic 506.4
- chronic 491.9
  - with
    - tracheitis (chronic) 491.8
  - asthmatic 491.20
    - with acute bronchitis or acute exacerbation 491.21
  - catarrhal 491.0
  - chemical (due to fumes and vapors) 506.4
  - due to
    - fumes or vapors (chemical) (inhalation) 506.4
    - radiation 508.8
    - tobacco smoking 491.0
  - mucopurulent 491.1
  - obstructive 491.20
    - with acute bronchitis or acute exacerbation 491.21
  - purulent 491.1
  - simple 491.0
  - specified type NEC 491.8
- croupous 466.0
  - with bronchospasm or obstruction 466.0
  - due to fumes or vapors 506.0

Bronchitis—*continued*
- emphysematous 491.20
  - with
    - acute bronchitis or acute exacerbation 491.21
- exudative 466.0
- fetid (chronic) (recurrent) 491.1
- fibrinous, acute or subacute 466.0
  - with bronchospasm or obstruction 466.0
- grippal 487.1
- influenzal 487.1
- membranous, acute or subacute 466.0
  - with bronchospasm or obstruction 466.0
- moulders' 502
- mucopurulent (chronic) (recurrent) 491.1
  - acute or subacute 466.0
- non-obstructive 491.0
- obliterans 491.8
- obstructive (chronic) 491.20
  - with
    - acute bronchitis or acute exacerbation 491.21
  - acute 466.0
- pituitous 491.1
- plastic (inflammatory) 466.0
- pneumococcal, acute or subacute 466.0
  - with bronchospasm or obstruction 466.0
- pseudomembranous 466.0
- purulent (chronic) (recurrent) 491.1
  - acute or subacute 466.0
    - with bronchospasm or obstruction 466.0
- putrid 491.1
- scrofulous (*see also* Tuberculosis) 011.3
- senile 491.9
- septic, acute or subacute 466.0
  - with bronchospasm or obstruction 466.0
- smokers' 491.0
- spirochetal 104.8
- suffocative, acute or subacute 466.0
- summer (*see also* Asthma) 493.9
- suppurative (chronic) 491.1
  - acute or subacute 466.0
- tuberculous (*see also* Tuberculosis) 011.3
- ulcerative 491.8
- Vincent's 101
- Vincent's 101
- viral, acute or subacute 466.0
  - with bronchospasm or obstruction 466.0

Bronchoalveolitis 485

Bronchoaspergillosis 117.3

Bronchocele
- meaning
  - dilatation of bronchus 519.1
  - goiter 240.9

Bronchogenic carcinoma 162.9

Bronchohemisporosis 117.9

Broncholithiasis 518.89
- tuberculous (*see also* Tuberculosis) 011.3

Bronchomoniliasis 112.89

Bronchomycosis 112.89

Bronchonocardiosis 039.1

Bronchopleuropneumonia — *see* Pneumonia, broncho-

Bronchopneumonia — *see* Pneumonia, broncho-

Bronchopneumonitis — *see* Pneumonia, broncho-

Bronchopulmonary — *see* condition

Branchopulmonitis — *see* Pneumonia, broncho-

Bronchorrhagia 786.3
  newborn 770.3
  tuberculous (see also Tuberculosis) 011.3
Bronchorrhea (chronic) (purulent) 491.0
  acute 466.0
Bronchospasm 519.1
  with
    asthma — see Asthma
    bronchiolitis, acute 466.1
    bronchitis — see Bronchitis
    COPD 496
    emphysema — see Emphysema
  due to external agent — see Condition, respiratory, acute, due to
Bronchospirochetosis 104.8
Bronchostenosis 519.1
Bronchus — see condition
Bronze, bronzed
  diabetes 275.0
  disease (Addison's) (skin) 255.4
    tuberculous (see also Tuberculosis) 017.6
Brooke's disease or tumor (M8100/0) — see Neoplasm, skin, benign
Brown's tendon sheath syndrome 378.61
Brown enamel of teeth (hereditary) 520.5
Brown-Séquard's paralysis (syndrome) 344.89
Brow presentation complicating delivery 652.4
  causing obstructed labor 660.0
Brucella, brucellosis (infection) 023.9
  abortus 023.1
  canis 023.3
  dermatitis, skin 023.9
  melitensis 023.0
  mixed 023.8
  suis 023.2
Bruck's disease 733.99
Bruck-de Lange disease or syndrome (Amsterdam dwarf, mental retardation, and brachycephaly) 759.89
Brug's filariasis 125.1
Brugsch's syndrome (acropachyderma) 757.39
Bruhl's disease (splenic anemia with fever) 285.8
Bruise (skin surface intact) — see also Contusion
  with
    fracture — see Fracture, by site
    open wound — see Wound, open, by site
    internal organ (abdomen, chest, or pelvis) — see Injury, internal, by site
  umbilical cord 663.6
    affecting fetus or newborn 762.6
Bruit 785.9
  arterial (abdominal) (carotid) 785.9
  supraclavicular 785.9
Brushburn — see Injury, superficial, by site
Bruton's X-linked agammaglobulinemia 279.04
Bruxism 306.8
Bubbly lung syndrome 770.7
Bubo 289.3
  blennorrhagic 098.89
  chancroidal 099.0
  climatic 099.1
  due to Hemophilus ducreyi 099.0
  gonococcal 098.89
  indolent NEC 099.8
  inguinal NEC 099.8
    chancroidal 099.0
    climatic 099.1

Bubo — continued
  inguinal — continued
    due to H. ducreyi 099.0
    scrofulous (see also Tuberculosis) 017.2
  soft chancre 099.0
  suppurating 683
  syphilitic 091.0
    congenital 090.0
  tropical 099.1
  venereal NEC 099.8
  virulent 099.0
Bubonic plague 020.0
Bubonocele — see Hernia, inguinal
Buccal — see condition
Buchanan's disease (juvenile osteochondrosis of iliac crest) 732.1
Buchem's syndrome (hyperostosis corticalis) 733.3
Buchman's disease (osteochondrosis, juvenile) 732.1
Bucket handle fracture (semilunar cartilage) (see also Tear, meniscus) 836.2
Budd-Chiari syndrome (hepatic vein thrombosis) 453.0
Budgerigar-fanciers' disease or lung 495.2
Büdinger-Ludloff-Läwen disease 717.89
Buerger's disease (thromboangiitis obliterans) 443.1
Bulbar — see condition
Bulbus cordis 745.9
  persistent (in left ventricle) 745.8
Bulging fontanels (congenital) 756.0
Bulimia 783.6
  nonorganic origin 307.51
Bulky uterus 621.2
Bulla(e) 709.8
  lung (emphysematous) (solitary) 492.0
Bullet wound — see also Wound, open, by site
  fracture — see Fracture, by site, open
  internal organ (abdomen, chest, or pelvis) — see Injury, internal, by site, with open wound
  intracranial — see Laceration, brain, with open wound
Bullis fever 082.8
Bullying (see also Disturbance, conduct) 312.0
Bundle
  branch block (complete) (false) (incomplete) 426.50
    bilateral 426.53
    left (see also Block, bundle branch, left) 426.3
      hemiblock 426.2
    right (see also Block, bundle branch, right) 426.4
  of His — see condition
  of Kent syndrome (anomalous atrioventricular excitation) 426.7
Bungpagga 040.81
Bunion 727.1
Bunionette 727.1
Bunyamwera fever 066.3
Buphthalmia, buphthalmos (congenital) 743.20
  associated with
    keratoglobus, congenital 743.22
    megalocornea 743.22
    ocular anomalies NEC 743.22
  isolated 743.21
  simple 743.21

Bürger-Grütz disease or syndrome (essential familial hyperlipemia) 272.3
Buried roots 525.3
Burke's syndrome 577.8
Burkitt's
  tumor (M9750/3) 200.2
  type malignant, lymphoma, lymphoblastic, or undifferentiated (M9750/3) 200.2
Burn (acid) (cathode ray) (caustic) (chemical) (electric heating appliance) (electricity) (fire) (flame) (hot liquid or object) (irradiation) (lime) (radiation) (steam) (thermal) (x-ray) 949.0

> Note — Use the following fifth-digit subclassification with category 948 to indicate the percent of body surface with third degree burn:
>
> 0 Less than 10% or unspecified
> 1 10–19%
> 2 20–29%
> 3 30–39%
> 4 40–49%
> 5 50–59%
> 6 60–69%
> 7 70–79%
> 8 80–89%
> 9 90% or more of body surface

  with
    blisters — see Burn, by site, second degree
    erythema — see Burn, by site, first degree
    skin loss (epidermal) — see also Burn, by site, second degree
    full thickness — see also Burn, by site, third degree
      with necrosis of underlying tissues — see Burn, by site, third degree, deep
    first degree — see Burn, by site, first degree
    second degree — see Burn, by site, second degree
    third degree — see Burn, by site, third degree
      deep — see Burn, by site, third degree, deep
  abdomen, abdominal (muscle) (wall) 942.03
    with
      other site(s), except trunk — see Burn, multiple, specified sites
      trunk — see Burn, trunk, multiple sites
    first degree 942.13
    second degree 942.23
    third degree 942.33
      deep 942.43
        with loss of body part 942.53
  ankle 945.03
    with
      lower limb(s) — see Burn, leg, multiple sites
      other site(s), except lower limb(s) — see Burn, multiple, specified sites
    first degree 945.13
    second degree 945.23

Burn — continued
  ankle — continued
    third degree 945.33
      deep 945.43
        with loss of body part 945.53
  anus — see Burn, trunk, specified site NEC
  arm(s) 943.00
    with other site(s) (classifiable to more than one category in 940-945) — see Burn, multiple, specified sites
    first degree 943.10
    second degree 943.20
    third degree 943.30
      deep 943.40
        with loss of body part 943.50
    lower — see Burn, forearm(s)
    multiple sites, except hand(s) or wrist(s) 943.09
      first degree 943.19
      second degree 943.29
      third degree 943.39
        deep 943.49
          with loss of body part 943.59
    upper 943.03
      with other site(s) of upper limb(s), except hand(s) or wrist(s) — see Burn, arm(s), multiple sites
      first degree 943.13
      second degree 943.23
      third degree 943.33
        deep 943.43
          with loss of body part 943.53
  auditory canal (external) — see Burn, ear
  auricle (ear) — see Burn, ear
  axilla 943.04
    with
      hand(s) and wrist(s) — see Burn, multiple, specified sites
      other site(s), except upper limb(s) — see Burn, multiple, specified sites
      upper limb(s) except hand(s) or wrist(s) — see Burn, arm(s), multiple sites
    first degree 943.14
    second degree 943.24
    third degree 943.34
      deep 943.44
        with loss of body part 943.54
  back 942.04
    with
      other site(s), except trunk — see Burn, multiple, specified sites
      trunk — see Burn, trunk, multiple sites
    first degree 942.14
    second degree 942.24
    third degree 942.34
      deep 942.44
        with loss of body part 942.54
  biceps
    brachii — see Burn, arm(s), upper
    femoris — see Burn, thigh
  breast(s) 942.01
    with
      other site(s), except trunk — see Burn, multiple, specified sites
      trunk — see Burn, trunk, multiple sites
    first degree 942.11
    second degree 942.21

Burn—continued
   breast(s)—continued
      third degree 942.31
         deep 942.41
           with loss of body part 942.51
   brow — see Burn, forehead
   buttock(s) — see Burn, back
   canthus (eye) 940.1
      chemical 940.0
   cervix (uteri) 947.4
   cheek (cutaneous) 941.07
      with
         face or head — see Burn, head, multiple sites
         other site(s), except face or head — see Burn, multiple, specified sites
      first degree 941.17
      second degree 941.27
      third degree 941.37
         deep 941.47
           with loss of body part 941.57
   chest wall (anterior) 942.02
      with
         other site(s), except trunk — see Burn, multiple, specified sites
         trunk — see Burn, trunk, multiple sites
      first degree 942.12
      second degree 942.22
      third degree 942.32
         deep 942.42
           with loss of body part 942.52
   chin 941.04
      with
         face or head — see Burn, head, multiple sites
         other site(s), except face or head — see Burn, multiple, specified sites
      first degree 941.14
      second degree 941.24
      third degree 941.34
         deep 941.44
           with loss of body part 941.54
   clitoris — see Burn, genitourinary organs, external
   colon 947.3
   conjunctiva (and cornea) 940.4
      chemical
         acid 940.3
         alkaline 940.2
   cornea (and conjunctiva) 940.4
      chemical
         acid 940.3
         alkaline 940.2
   costal region — see Burn, chest wall
   due to ingested chemical agent — see Burn, internal organs
   ear (auricle) (canal) (drum) (external) 941.01
      with
         face or head — see Burn, head, multiple sites
         other site(s), except face or head — see Burn, multiple, specified sites
      first degree 941.11
      second degree 941.21
      third degree 941.31
         deep 941.41
           with loss of a body part 941.51
   elbow 943.02
      with
         hand(s) and wrist(s) — see Burn, multiple specified sites

Burn—continued
   elbow—continued
      with—continued
         other site(s), except upper limb(s) — see Burn, multiple, specified sites
         upper limb(s) except hand(s) or wrist(s) — see also Burn, arm(s), multiple sites
      first degree 943.12
      second degree 943.22
      third degree 943.32
         deep 943.42
           with loss of body part 943.52
   electricity, electric current — See Burn, by site
   entire body — see Burn, multiple, specified sites
   epididymis — see Burn, genitourinary organs, external
   epigastric region — see Burn, abdomen
   epiglottis 947.1
   esophagus 947.2
   extent (percent of body surface)
      less than 10 percent 948.0
      10-19 percent 948.1
      20-29 percent 948.2
      30-39 percent 948.3
      40-49 percent 948.4
      50-59 percent 948.5
      60-69 percent 948.6
      70-79 percent 948.7
      80-89 percent 948.8
      90 percent or more 948.9
   extremity
      lower — see Burn, leg
      upper — see Burn, arm(s)
   eye(s) (and adnexa) (only) 940.9
      with
         face, head, or neck 941.02
           first degree 941.12
           second degree 941.22
           third degree 941.32
              deep 941.42
                 with loss of body part 941.52
         other sites (classifiable to more than one category in 940-945) — see Burn, multiple, specified sites
         resulting rupture and destruction of eyeball 940.5
      specified part — see Burn, by site
   eyeball — see also Burn, eye with resulting rupture and destruction of eyeball 940.5
   eyelid(s) 940.1
      chemical 940.0
   face — see Burn, head
   finger (nail) (subungual) 944.01
      with
         hand(s) — see Burn, hand(s), multiple sites
         other sites — see Burn, multiple, specified sites
         thumb 944.04
           first degree 944.14
           second degree 944.24
           third degree 944.34
              deep 944.44
                 with loss of body part 944.54
      first degree 944.11
      second degree 944.21
      third degree 944.31
         deep 944.41
           with loss of body part 944.51

Burn—continued
   finger—continued
      multiple (digits) 944.03
         with thumb — see Burn, finger, with thumb
         first degree 944.13
         second degree 944.23
         third degree 944.33
           deep 944.43
              with loss of body part 944.53
   flank — see Burn, abdomen
   foot 945.02
      with
         lower limb(s) — see Burn, leg, multiple sites
         other site(s), except lower limb(s) — see Burn, multiple, specified sites
      first degree 945.12
      second degree 945.22
      third degree 945.32
         deep 945.42
           with loss of body part 945.52
   forearm(s) 943.01
      with
         hand(s) and wrist(s) — see Burn, multiple, specified sites
         other site(s), except upper limb(s) — see Burn, multiple, specified sites
         upper limb(s) except hand(s) or wrist(s) — see Burn, arm(s), multiple sites
      first degree 943.11
      second degree 943.21
      third degree 943.31
         deep 943.41
           with loss of body part 943.51
   forehead 941.07
      with
         face or head — see Burn, head, multiple sites
         other site(s), except face or head — see Burn, multiple, specified sites
      first degree 941.17
      second degree 941.27
      third degree 941.37
         deep 941.47
           with loss of body part 941.57
   fourth degree — see Burn, by site, third degree, deep
   friction — see Injury, superficial, by site
   from swallowing caustic or corrosive substance NEC — see Burn, internal organs
   full thickness — see Burn, by site, third degree
   gastrointestinal tract 947.3
   genitourinary organs
      external 942.05
         with
           other site(s), except trunk — see Burn multiple, specified sites
           trunk — see Burn, trunk, multiple sites
         first degree 942.15
         second degree 942.25
         third degree 942.35
           deep 942.45
              with loss of body part 942.55
      internal 947.8
   globe (eye) — see Burn, eyeball
   groin — see Burn, abdomen
   gum 947.0

Burn—continued
   hand(s) (phalanges) (and wrist) 944.00
      with other site(s) (classifiable to more than one category in 940-945) — see Burn, multiple, specified sites
      first degree 944.10
      second degree 944.20
      third degree 944.30
         deep 944.40
           with loss of body part 944.50
      back (dorsal surface) 944.06
         first degree 944.16
         second degree 944.26
         third degree 944.36
           deep 944.46
              with loss of body part 944.56
      multiple sites 944.08
         first degree 944.18
         second degree 944.28
         third degree 944.38
           deep 944.48
              with loss of body part 944.58
   head (and face) 941.00
      with other site(s) except face or neck — see Burn, multiple, specified sites
      eye(s) only 940.9
         specified part — see Burn, by site
      first degree 941.10
      second degree 941.20
      third degree 941.30
         deep 941.40
           with loss of body part 941.50
      multiple sites 941.09
         with eyes — see Burn, eyes, with face, head, or neck
         first degree 941.19
         second degree 941.29
         third degree 941.39
           deep 941.49
              with loss of body part 941.59
   heel — see Burn, foot
   hip — see Burn, trunk, specified site NEC
   iliac region — see Burn, trunk, specified site NEC
   inhalation (see also Burn, internal organs) 947.9
   internal organs 947.9
      from caustic or corrosive substance (swallowing) NEC 947.9
      specified NEC (see also Burn, by site) 947.8
   interscapular region — see Burn, back
   intestine (large) (small) 947.3
   iris — see Burn, eyeball
   knee 945.05
      with
         lower limb(s) — see Burn, leg, multiple sites
         other site(s), except lower limb(s) — see Burn, multiple, specified sites
      first degree 945.15
      second degree 945.25
      third degree 945.35
         deep 945.45
           with loss of body part 945.55
   labium (majus) (minus) — see Burn, genitourinary organs, external
   lacrimal apparatus, duct, gland, or sac 940.1
      chemical 940.0

Burn—*continued*
  larynx 947.1
  late effect — *see* Late, effects (of), burn
  leg 945.00
    with other site(s) (classifiable to more than one category in 940-945) — *see* Burn, multiple, specified sites
    first degree 945.10
    second degree 945.20
    third degree 945.30
      deep 945.40
        with loss of body part 945.50
    lower 945.04
      with other part(s) of lower limb(s) — *see* Burn, leg, multiple sites
      first degree 945.14
      second degree 945.24
      third degree 945.34
        deep 945.44
          with loss of body part 945.54
    multiple sites 945.09
      first degree 945.19
      second degree 945.29
      third degree 945.39
        deep 945.49
          with loss of body part 945.59
    upper — *see* Burn, thigh
  lightning — *see* Burn, by site
  limb(s)
    lower (including foot or toe(s)) — *see* Burn, leg
    upper (except wrist and hand) — *see* Burn, arm(s)
  lip(s) 941.03
    with
      face or head — *see* Burn, head, multiple sites
      other site(s), except face or head — *see* Burn, multiple, specified sites
    first degree 941.13
    second degree 941.23
    third degree 941.33
      deep 941.43
        with loss of body part 941.53
  lumbar region — *see* Burn, back
  lung 947.1
  malar region — *see* Burn, cheek
  mastoid region — *see* Burn, scalp
  membrane, tympanic — *see* Burn, ear
  midthoracic region — *see* Burn, chest wall
  mouth 947.0
  multiple (*see also* Burn, unspecified) 949.0
    specified sites classifiable to more than one category in 940-945 946.0
    first degree 946.1
    second degree 946.2
    third degree 946.3
      deep 946.4
        with loss of body part 946.5
  muscle, abdominal — *see* Burn, abdomen
  nasal (septum) — *see* Burn, nose
  neck 941.08
    with
      face or head — *see* Burn, head, multiple sites
      other site(s), except face or head — *see* Burn, multiple, specified sites
    first degree 941.18
    second degree 941.28

Burn—*continued*
  neck—*continued*
    third degree 941.38
      deep 941.48
        with loss of body part 941.58
  nose (septum) 941.05
    with
      face or head — *see* Burn, head, multiple sites
      other site(s), except face or head — *see* Burn, multiple, specified sites
    first degree 941.15
    second degree 941.25
    third degree 941.35
      deep 941.45
        with loss of body part 941.55
  occipital region — *see* Burn, scalp
  orbit region 940.1
    chemical 940.0
  oronasopharynx 947.0
  palate 947.0
  palm(s) 944.05
    with
      hand(s) and wrist(s) — *see* Burn, hand(s), multiple sites
      other site(s), except hand(s) or wrist(s) — *see* Burn, multiple, specified sites
    first degree 944.15
    second degree 944.25
    third degree 944.35
      deep 944.45
        with loss of a body part 944.55
  parietal region — *see* Burn, scalp
  penis — *see* Burn, genitourinary organs, external
  perineum — *see* Burn, genitourinary organs, external
  periocular area 940.1
    chemical 940.0
  pharynx 947.0
  pleura 947.1
  popliteal space — *see* Burn, knee
  prepuce — *see* Burn, genitourinary organs, external
  pubic region — *see* Burn, genitourinary organs, external
  pudenda — *see* Burn, genitourinary organs, external
  rectum 947.3
  sac, lacrimal 940.1
    chemical 940.0
  sacral region — *see* Burn, back
  salivary (ducts) (glands) 947.0
  scalp 941.06
    with
      face or neck — *see* Burn, head, multiple sites
      other site(s), except face or neck — *see* Burn, multiple, specified sites
    first degree 941.16
    second degree 941.26
    third degree 941.36
      deep 941.46
        with loss of body part 941.56
  scapular region 943.06
    with
      other site(s), except upper limb(s) — *see* Burn, multiple, specified sites
      upper limb(s), except hand(s) or wrist(s) — *see* Burn, arm(s), multiple sites
    first degree 943.16

Burn—*continued*
  scapular region—*continued*
    second degree 943.26
    third degree 943.36
      deep 943.46
        with loss of body part 943.56
  sclera — *see* Burn, eyeball
  scrotum — *see* Burn, genitourinary organs, external
  septum, nasal — *see* Burn, nose
  shoulder(s) 943.05
    with
      hand(s) and wrist(s) — *see* Burn, multiple, specified sites
      other site(s), except upper limb(s) — *see* Burn, multiple, specified sites
      upper limb(s), except hand(s) or wrist(s) — *see* Burn, arm(s), multiple sites
    first degree 943.15
    second degree 943.25
    third degree 943.35
      deep 943.45
        with loss of body part 943.55
  skin NEC (*see also* Burn, unspecified) 949.0
  skull — *see* Burn, head
  small intestine 947.3
  sternal region — *see* Burn, chest wall
  stomach 947.3
  subconjunctival — *see* Burn, conjunctiva
  subcutaneous — *see* Burn, by site, third degree
  submaxillary region — *see* Burn, head
  submental region — *see* Burn, chin
  supraclavicular fossa — *see* Burn, neck
  supraorbital — *see* Burn, forehead
  temple — *see* Burn, scalp
  temporal region — *see* Burn, scalp
  testicle — *see* Burn, genitourinary organs, external
  testis — *see* Burn, genitourinary organs, external
  thigh 945.06
    with
      lower limb(s) — *see* Burn, leg, multiple sites
      other site(s), except lower limb(s) — *see* Burn, multiple, specified sites
    first degree 945.16
    second degree 945.26
    third degree 945.36
      deep 945.46
        with loss of body part 945.56
  thorax (external) — *see* Burn, chest wall
  throat 947.0
  thumb(s) (nail) (subungual) 944.02
    with
      finger(s) — *see* Burn, finger, with other sites, thumb
      hand(s) and wrist(s) — *see* Burn, hand(s), multiple sites
      other site(s), except hand(s) or wrist(s) — *see* Burn, multiple, specified sites
    first degree 944.12
    second degree 944.22
    third degree 944.32
      deep 944.42
        with loss of body part 944.52

Burn—*continued*
  toe (nail) (subungual) 945.01
    with
      lower limb(s) — *see* Burn, leg, multiple sites
      other site(s), except lower limb(s) — *see* Burn, multiple, specified sites
    first degree 945.11
    second degree 945.21
    third degree 945.31
      deep 945.41
        with loss of body part 945.51
  tongue 947.0
  tonsil 947.0
  trachea 947.1
  trunk 942.00
    with other site(s) (classifiable to more than one category in 940-945) — *see* Burn, multiple, specified sites
    first degree 942.10
    second degree 942.20
    third degree 942.30
      deep 942.40
        with loss of body part 942.50
    multiple sites 942.09
      first degree 942.19
      second degree 942.29
      third degree 942.39
        deep 942.49
          with loss of body part 942.59
    specified site NEC 942.09
      first degree 942.19
      second degree 942.29
      third degree 942.39
        deep 942.49
          with loss of body part 942.59
  tunica vaginalis — *see* Burn, genitourinary organs, external
  tympanic membrane — *see* Burn, ear
  tympanum — *see* Burn, ear
  unspecified site (multiple) 949.0
    with extent of body surface involved specified
      less than 10 percent 948.0
      10-19 percent 948.1
      20-29 percent 948.2
      30-39 percent 948.3
      40-49 percent 948.4
      50-59 percent 948.5
      60-69 percent 948.6
      70-79 percent 948.7
      80-89 percent 948.8
      90 percent or more 948.9
    first degree 949.1
    second degree 949.2
    third degree 949.3
      deep 949.4
        with loss of body part 949.5
  uterus 947.4
  uvula 947.0
  vagina 947.4
  vulva — *see* Burn, genitourinary organs, external
  wrist(s) 944.07
    with
      hand(s) — *see* Burn, hand(s), multiple sites
      other site(s), except hand(s) — *see* Burn, multiple, specified sites
    first degree 944.17
    second degree 944.27
    third degree 944.37
      deep 944.47
        with loss of body part 944.57

Burnett's syndrome (milk-alkali) 999.9

Burnier's syndrome (hypophyseal dwarfism) 253.3
Burning
  feet syndrome 266.2
  sensation (see also Disturbance, sensation) 782.0
    tongue 529.6
Burns' disease (osteochondrosis, lower ulna) 732.3
Bursa — see also condition
  pharynx 478.29
Bursitis NEC 727.3
  Achilles tendon 726.71
  adhesive 726.90
    shoulder 726.0
  ankle 726.79
  buttock 726.5
  calcaneal 726.79
  collateral ligament
    fibular 726.63
    tibial 726.62
  Duplay's 726.2
  elbow 726.33
  finger 726.8
  foot 726.79
  gonococcal 098.52
  hand 726.4
  hip 726.5
  infrapatellar 726.69
  ischiogluteal 726.5
  knee 726.60
  occupational NEC 727.2
  olecranon 726.33
  pes anserinus 726.61
  pharyngeal 478.29
  popliteal 727.51
  prepatellar 726.65
  radiohumeral 727.3
  scapulohumeral 726.19
    adhesive 726.0
  shoulder 726.10
    adhesive 726.0
  subacromial 726.19
    adhesive 726.0
  subcoracoid 726.19
  subdeltoid 726.19
    adhesive 726.0
  subpatellar 726.69
  syphilitic 095.7
  Thornwaldt's, Tornwaldt's (pharyngeal) 478.29
  toe 726.79
  trochanteric area 726.5
  wrist 726.4
Burst stitches or sutures (complication of surgery) 998.3
Buruli ulcer 031.1
Bury's disease (erythema elevatum diutinum) 695.89
Buschke's disease or scleredema (adultorum) 710.1
Busquet's disease (osteoperiostitis) (see also Osteomyelitis) 730.1
Busse-Buschke disease (cryptococcosis) 117.5
Buttock — see condition
Button
  Biskra 085.1
  Delhi 085.1
  oriental 085.1
Buttonhole hand (intrinsic) 736.21
Bwamba fever (encephalitis) 066.3
Byssinosis (occupational) 504
Bywaters' syndrome 958.5

C

Cacergasia 300.9
Cachexia 799.4
  cancerous (M8000/3) 199.1
  cardiac — see Disease, heart

Calcification—continued
  dehydration 276.5
    with
      hypernatremia 276.0
      hyponatremia 276.1
    due to malnutrition 261
  exophthalmic 242.0
  heart — see Disease, heart
  hypophyseal 253.2
  hypopituitary 253.2
  lead 984.9
    specified type of lead — see Table of drugs and chemicals
  malaria 084.9
  malignant (M8000/3) 199.1
  marsh 084.9
  nervous 300.5
  old age 797
  pachydermic — see Hypothyroidism
  paludal 084.9
  pituitary (postpartum) 253.2
  renal (see also Disease, renal) 593.9
  saturnine 984.9
    specified type of lead — see Table of drugs and chemicals
  senile 797
  Simmonds' (pituitary cachexia) 253.2
  splenica 289.59
  strumipriva (see also Hypothyroidism) 244.9
  tuberculous NEC (see also Tuberculosis) 011.9
Café au lait spots 709.09 ◆
Caffey's disease or syndrome (infantile cortical hyperostosis) 756.59
Caisson disease 993.3
Caked breast (puerperal, postpartum) 676.2
Cake kidney 753.3
Calabar swelling 125.2
Calcaneal spur 726.73
Calcaneoapophysitis 732.5
Calcaneonavicular bar 755.67
Calcareous — see condition
Calcicosis (occupational) 502
Calciferol (vitamin D) deficiency 268.9
  with
    osteomalacia 268.2
    rickets (see also Rickets) 268.0
Calcification
  adrenal (capsule) (gland) 255.4
    tuberculous (see also Tuberculosis) 017.6
  aorta 440.0
  artery (annular) — see Arteriosclerosis
  auricle (ear) 380.89
  bladder 596.8
    due to S. hematobium 120.0
  brain (cortex) — see Calcification, cerebral
  bronchus 519.1
  bursa 727.82
  cardiac (see also Degeneration, myocardial) 429.1
  cartilage (postinfectional) 733.99
  cerebral (cortex) 348.8
    artery 437.0
  cervix (uteri) 622.8
  choroid plexus 349.2
  conjunctiva 372.54
  corpora cavernosa (penis) 607.89
  cortex (brain) — see Calcification, cerebral
  dental pulp (nodular) 522.2
  dentinal papilla 520.4
  disc, intervertebral 722.90
    cervical, cervicothoracic 722.91
    lumbar, lumbosacral 722.93
    thoracic, thoracolumbar 722.92

Calcification—continued
  fallopian tube 620.8
  falx cerebri — see Calcification, cerebral
  fascia 728.89
  gallbladder 575.8
  general 275.4
  heart (see also Degeneration, myocardial) 429.1
    valve — see Endocarditis
  intervertebral cartilage or disc (postinfectional) 722.90
    cervical, cervicothoracic 722.91
    lumbar, lumbosacral 722.93
    thoracic, thoracolumbar 722.92
  intracranial — see Calcification, cerebral
  intraspinal ligament 728.89
  joint 719.80
    ankle 719.87
    elbow 719.82
    foot 719.87
    hand 719.84
    hip 719.85
    knee 719.86
    multiple sites 719.89
    pelvic region 719.85
    shoulder (region) 719.81
    specified site NEC 719.88
    wrist 719.83
  kidney 593.89
    tuberculous (see also Tuberculosis) 016.0
  larynx (senile) 478.79
  lens 366.8
  ligament 728.89
    intraspinal 728.89
    knee (medial collateral) 717.89
  lung 518.89
    active 518.89
    postinfectional 518.89
    tuberculous (see also Tuberculosis, pulmonary) 011.9
  lymph gland or node (postinfectional) 289.3
    tuberculous (see also Tuberculosis, lymph gland) 017.2
  massive (paraplegic) 728.10
  medial NEC (see also Arteriosclerosis, extremities) 440.20
  meninges (cerebral) 349.2
  metastatic 275.4
  Mönckeberg's — see Arteriosclerosis
  muscle 728.10
    heterotopic, postoperative 728.13
  myocardium, myocardial (see also Degeneration, myocardial) 429.1
  ovary 620.8
  pancreas 577.8
  penis 607.99
  periarticular 728.89
  pericardium (see also Pericarditis) 423.8
  pineal gland 259.8
  pleura 511.0
    postinfectional 518.89
    tuberculous (see also Tuberculosis, pleura) 012.0
  pulp (dental) (nodular) 522.2
  renal 593.89
  rider's bone 733.99
  sclera 379.16
  semilunar cartilage 717.89
  spleen 289.59
  subcutaneous 709.3
  suprarenal (capsule) (gland) 255.4
  tendon (sheath) 727.82
    with bursitis, synovitis or tenosynovitis 727.82
  trachea 519.1

Calcification—continued
  ureter 593.89
  uterus 621.8
  vitreous 379.29
Calcified — see also Calcification
  hematoma NEC 959.9
Calcinosis (generalized) (interstitial) (tumoral) (universalis) 275.4
  circumscripta 709.3
  cutis 709.3
  intervertebralis 275.4 [722.90]
  Raynaud's phenomenonsclerodactylytelangiectasis (CRST) 710.1
Calcium
  blood
    high (see also Hypercalcemia) 275.4
    low (see also Hypocalcemia) 275.4
  deposits — see also Calcification, by site
    in bursa 727.82
    in tendon (sheath) 727.82
      with bursitis, synovitis or tenosynovitis 727.82
  salts or soaps in vitreous 379.22
Calciuria 791.9
Calculi — see Calculus
Calculosis, intrahepatic — see Choledocholithiasis
Calculus, calculi, calculous 592.9
  ampulla of Vater — see Choledocholithiasis
  anuria (impacted) (recurrent) 592.0
  appendix 543.9
  bile duct (any) — see Choledocholithiasis
  biliary — see Cholelithiasis
  bilirubin, multiple — see Cholelithiasis
  bladder (encysted) (impacted) (urinary) 594.1
    diverticulum 594.0
  bronchus 518.89
  calyx (kidney) (renal) 592.0
    congenital 753.3
  cholesterol (pure) (solitary) — see Cholelithiasis
  common duct (bile) — see Choledocholithiasis
  conjunctiva 372.54
  cystic 594.1
    duct — see Cholelithiasis
  dental 523.6
    subgingival 523.6
    supragingival 523.6
  epididymis 608.89
  gallbladder — see also Cholelithiasis
    congenital 751.69
  hepatic (duct) — see Choledocholithiasis
  intestine (impaction) (obstruction) 560.39
  kidney (impacted) (multiple) (pelvis) (recurrent) (staghorn) 592.0
    congenital 753.3
  lacrimal (passages) 375.57
  liver (impacted) — see Choledocholithiasis
  lung 518.89
  nephritic (impacted) (recurrent) 592.0
  nose 478.1
  pancreas (duct) 577.8
  parotid gland 527.5
  pelvis, encysted 592.0
  prostate 602.0
  pulmonary 518.89
  pyelitis (impacted) (recurrent) 592.9
  pyelonephritis (impacted) (recurrent) 592.9
  pyonephrosis (impacted) (recurrent) 592.9

Calculus, calculi, calculous—continued
renal (impacted) (recurrent) 592.0
    congenital 753.3
salivary (duct) (gland) 527.5
seminal vesicle 608.89
staghorn 592.0
Stensen's duct 527.5
sublingual duct or gland 527.5
    congenital 750.26
submaxillary duct, gland, or region 527.5
suburethral 594.8
tonsil 474.8
tooth, teeth 523.6
tunica vaginalis 608.89
ureter (impacted) (recurrent) 592.1
urethra (impacted) 594.2
urinary (duct) (impacted) (passage) (tract) 592.9
    lower tract NEC 594.9
        specified site 594.8
vagina 623.8
vesical (impacted) 594.1
Wharton's duct 527.5

Caliectasis 593.89
California
    disease 114.0
    encephalitis 062.5
Caligo cornea 371.03
Callositas, callosity (infected) 700
Callus (infected) 700
    bone 726.91
    excessive, following fracture — see also Late, effect (of), fracture
Calvé (- Perthes) disease (osteochondrosis, femoral capital) 732.1
Calvities (see also Alopecia) 704.00
Cameroon fever (see also Malaria) 084.6
Camptocormia 300.11
Camptodactyly (congenital) 755.59
Camurati-Engelmann disease (diaphyseal sclerosis) 756.59
Canal — see condition
Canaliculitis (lacrimal) (acute) 375.31
    Actinomyces 039.8
    chronic 375.41
Canavan's disease 330.0
Cancer (M8000/3) — see also Neoplasm, by site, malignant

> Note — The term "cancer" when modified by an adjective or adjectival phrase indicating a morphological type should be coded in the same manner as "carcinoma" with that adjective or phrase. Thus, "squamous-cell cancer" should be coded in the same manner as "squamous-cell carcinoma," which appears in the list under "Carcinoma."

    bile duct type (M8160/3), liver 155.1
    hepatocellular (M8170/3) 155.0
Cancerous (M8000/3) — see Neoplasm, by site, malignant
Cancerphobia 300.29
Cancrum oris 528.1
Candidiasis, candidal 112.9
    with pneumonia 112.4
    balanitis 112.2
    congenital 771.7
    disseminated 112.5
    endocarditis 112.81
    esophagus 112.84
    intertrigo 112.3
    intestine 112.85
    lung 112.4
    meningitis 112.83
    mouth 112.0

Candidiasis, candidal—continued
nails 112.3
neonatal 771.7
onychia 112.3
otitis externa 112.82
otomycosis 112.82
paronychia 112.3
perionyxis 112.3
pneumonia 112.4
pneumonitis 112.4
skin 112.3
specified site NEC 112.89
systemic 112.5
urogenital site NEC 112.2
vagina 112.1
vulva 112.1
vulvovaginitis 112.1

Candidiosis — see Candidiasis
Candiru infection or infestation 136.8
Canities (premature) 704.3
    congenital 757.4
Canker (mouth) (sore) 528.2
    rash 034.1
Cannabinosis 504
Canton fever 081.9
Cap
    cradle 691.8
Capillariasis 127.5
Capillary — see condition
Caplan's syndrome 714.81
Caplan-Colinet syndrome 714.81
Capsule — see condition
Capsulitis (joint) 726.90
    adhesive (shoulder) 726.0
    labyrinthine 387.8
    thyroid 245.9
Caput
    crepitus 756.0
    medusae 456.8
    succedaneum 767.1
Carapata disease 087.1
Carate — see Pinta
Carboxyhemoglobinemia 986
Carbuncle 680.9
    abdominal wall 680.2
    ankle 680.6
    anus 680.5
    arm (any part, above wrist) 680.3
    auditory canal, external 680.0
    axilla 680.3
    back (any part) 680.2
    breast 680.2
    buttock 680.5
    chest wall 680.2
    corpus cavernosum 607.2
    ear (any part) (external) 680.0
    eyelid 373.13
    face (any part except eye) 680.0
    finger (any) 680.4
    flank 680.2
    foot (any part) 680.7
    forearm 680.3
    genital organ (male) 608.4
    gluteal (region) 680.5
    groin 680.2
    hand (any part) 680.4
    head (any part except face) 680.8
    heel 680.7
    hip 680.6
    kidney (see also Abscess, kidney) 590.2
    knee 680.6
    labia 616.4
    lacrimal
        gland (see also Dacryoadenitis) 375.00
        passages (duct) (sac) (see also Dacryocystitis) 375.30
    leg, any part except foot 680.6
    lower extremity, any part except foot 680.6
    malignant 022.0
    multiple sites 680.9
    neck 680.1

Carbuncle—continued
nose (external) (septum) 680.0
orbit, orbital 376.01
partes posteriores 680.5
pectoral region 680.2
penis 607.2
perineum 680.2
pinna 680.0
scalp (any part) 680.8
scrotum 608.4
seminal vesicle 608.0
shoulder 680.3
skin NEC 680.9
specified site NEC 680.8
spermatic cord 608.4
temple (region) 680.0
testis 608.4
thigh 680.6
thumb 680.4
toe (any) 680.7
trunk 680.2
tunica vaginalis 608.4
umbilicus 680.2
upper arm 680.3
urethra 597.0
vas deferens 608.4
vulva 616.4
wrist 680.4

Carbunculus (see also Carbuncle) 680.9
Carcinoid (tumor) (M8240/1) — see also Neoplasm, by site, uncertain behavior
    and struma ovarii (M9091/1) 236.2
    argentaffin (M8241/1) — see Neoplasm, by site, uncertain behavior
        malignant (M8241/3) — see Neoplasm, by site, malignant
    benign (9091/0) 220
    composite (M8244/3) — see Neoplasm, by site, malignant
    goblet cell (M8243/3) — see Neoplasm, by site, malignant
    malignant (M8240/3) — see Neoplasm, by site, malignant
    nonargentaffin (M8242/1) — see also Neoplasm, by site, uncertain behavior
        malignant (M8242/3) — see Neoplasm, by site, malignant
    strumal (M9091/1) 236.2
    syndrome (intestinal) (metastatic) 259.2
    type bronchial adenoma (M8240/3) — see Neoplasm, lung, malignant
Carcinoidosis 259.2
Carcinoma (M8010/3) — see also Neoplasm, by site, malignant

> Note — Except where otherwise indicated, the morphological varieties of carcinoma in the list below should be coded by site as for "Neoplasm, malignant."

    with
        apocrine metaplasia (M8573/3)
        cartilaginous (and osseous) metaplasia (M8571/3)
        osseous (and cartilaginous) metaplasia (M8571/3)
        productive fibrosis (M8141/3)
        spindle cell metaplasia (M8572/3)
        squamous metaplasia (M8570/3)
    acidophil (M8280/3)
        specified site — see Neoplasm, by site, malignant
        unspecified site 194.3

Carcinoma—continued
acidophil-basophil, mixed (M8281/3)
    specified site — see Neoplasm, by site, malignant
    unspecified site 194.3
acinar (cell) (M8550/3)
acinic cell (M8550/3)
adenocystic (M8200/3)
adenoid
    cystic (M8200/3)
    squamous cell (M8075/3)
adenosquamous (M8560/3)
adnexal (skin) (M8390/3) — see Neoplasm, skin, malignant
adrenal cortical (M8370/3) 194.0
alveolar (M8251/3)
    cell (M8250/3) — see Neoplasm, lung, malignant
anaplastic type (M8021/3)
apocrine (8401/3)
    breast — see Neoplasm, breast, malignant
    specified site NEC — see Neoplasm, skin, malignant
    unspecified site 173.9
basal cell (pigmented) (M8090/3) — see also Neoplasm, skin, malignant
    fibro-epithelial type (M8093/3) — see Neoplasm, skin, malignant
    morphea type (M8092/3) — see Neoplasm, skin, malignant
    multicentric (M8091/3) — see Neoplasm, skin, malignant
basaloid (M8123/3)
basal-squamous cell, mixed (M8094/3) — see Neoplasm, skin, malignant
basophil (M8300/3)
    specified site — see Neoplasm, by site, malignant
    unspecified site 194.3
basophil-acidophil, mixed (M8281/3)
    specified site — see Neoplasm, by site, malignant
    unspecified site 194.3
basosquamous (M8094/3) — see Neoplasm, skin, malignant
bile duct type (M8160/3)
    and hepatocellular, mixed (M8180/3) 155.0
    liver 155.1
    specified site NEC — see Neoplasm, by site, malignant
    unspecified site 155.1
branchial or branchiogenic 146.8
bronchial or bronchogenic — see Neoplasm, lung, malignant
bronchiolar (terminal) (M8250/3) — see Neoplasm, lung, malignant
bronchiolo-alveolar (M8250/3) — see Neoplasm, lung, malignant
bronchogenic (epidermoid) 162.9
C cell (M8510/3)
    specified site — see Neoplasm, by site, mailignant
    unspecified site 193
ceruminous (M8420/3) 173.2
chorionic (M9100/3)
    specified site — see Neoplasm, by site, malignant
    unspecified site
        female 181
        male 186.9
chromophobe (M8270/3)
    specified site — see Neoplasm, by site, malignant

Carcinoma—*continued*
  chromophobe—*continued*
    unspecified site 194.3
  clear cell (mesonephroid type) (M8310/3)
  cloacogenic (M8124/3)
    specified site — see Neoplasm, by site, malignant
    unspecified site 154.8
  colloid (M8480/3)
  cribriform (M8201/3)
  cylindroid type (M8200/3)
  diffuse type (M8145/3)
    specified site — see Neoplasm, by site, malignant
    unspecified site 151.9
  duct (cell) (M8500/3)
    with Paget's disease (M8541/3) — see Neoplasm, breast, malignant
    infiltrating (M8500/3)
      specified site — see Neoplasm, by site, malignant
      unspecified site 174.9
  ductal (M8500/3)
  ductular, infiltrating (M8521/3)
  embryonal (M9070/3)
    and teratoma, mixed (M9081/3)
    combined with choriocarcinoma (M9101/3) — see Neoplasm, by site, malignant
    infantile type (M9071/3)
    liver 155.0
    polyembryonal type (M9072/3)
  endometrioid (M8380/3)
  eosinophil (M8280/3)
    specified site — see Neoplasm, by site, malignant
    unspecified site 194.3
  epidermoid (M8070/3) — see also Carcinoma, squamous cell
    and adenocarcinoma, mixed (M8560/3)
    in situ, Bowen's type (M8081/2) — see Neoplasm, skin, in situ
    intradermal — see Neoplasm, skin, in situ
  fibroepithelial type basal cell (M8093/3) — see Neoplasm, skin, malignant
  follicular (M8330/3)
    and papillary (mixed) (M8340/3) 193
    moderately differentiated type (M8332/3) 193
    pure follicle type (M8331/3) 193
    specified site — see Neoplasm, by site, malignant
    trabecular type (M8332/3) 193
    unspecified site 193
    well differentiated type (M8331/3) 193
  gelatinous (M8480/3)
  giant cell (M8031/3)
    and spindle cell (M8030/3)
  granular cell (M8320/3)
  granulosa cell (M8620/3) 183.0
  hepatic cell (M8170/3) 155.0
  hepatocellular (M8170/3) 155.0
    and bile duct, mixed (M8180/3) 155.0
  hepatocholangiolitic (M8180/3) 155.0
  Hurthle cell (thyroid) 193
  hypernephroid (M8311/3)
  in
    adenomatous
      polyp (M82l0/3)
      polyposis coli (M8220/3) 153.9
    pleomorphic adenoma (M8940/3)
    polypoid adenoma (M8210/3)
  situ (M8010/3) — see Carcinoma, in situ

Carcinoma—*continued*
  in—*continued*
    tubular adenoma (M8210/3)
    villous adenoma (M8261/3)
  infiltrating duct (M8500/3)
    with Paget's disease (M8541/3) — see Neoplasm, breast, malignant
    specified site — see Neoplasm, by site, malignant
    unspecified site 174.9
  inflammatory (M8530/3)
    specified site — see Neoplasm, by site, malignant
    unspecified site 174.9
  in situ (M8010/2) — see also Neoplasm, by site, in situ
    epidermoid (M8070/2) — see also Neoplasm, by site, in situ
      with questionable stromal invasion (M8076/2)
      specified site — see Neoplasm, by site, in situ
      unspecified site 233.1
    Bowen's type (M8081/2) — see Neoplasm, skin, in situ
  intestinal type (M8144/3)
    specified site — see Neoplasm, by site, malignant
    unspecified site 151.9
  intraductal (M8500/2)
    specified site — see Neoplasm, by site, in situ
    unspecified site 233.0
    lobular (M8520/2)
      specified site — see Neoplasm, by site, in situ
      unspecified site 233.0
    papillary (M8050/2) — see Neoplasm, by site, in situ
    squamous cell (M8070/2) — see also Neoplasm, by site, in situ
      with questionable stromal invasion (M8076/2)
      specified site — see Neoplasm, by site, in situ
      unspecified site 233.1
    transitional cell (M8120/2) — see Neoplasm, by site, in situ
  intraductal (noninfiltrating) (M8500/2)
    papillary (M8503/2)
      specified site — see Neoplasm, by site, in situ
      unspecified site 233.0
    specified site — see Neoplasm, by site, in situ
    unspecified site 233.0
  intraepidermal (M8070/2) — see also Neoplasm, skin, in situ
    squamous cell, Bowen's type (M8081/2) — see Neoplasm, skin, in situ
  intraepithelial (M8010/2) — see also Neoplasm, by site, in situ
    squamous cell (M8072/2) — see Neoplasm, by site, in situ
  intraosseous (M9270/3) 170.1
    upper jaw (bone) 170.0
  islet cell (M8150/3)
    and exocrine, mixed (M8154/3)
    specified site — see Neoplasm, by site, malignant
    unspecified site 157.9
  pancreas 157.4

Carcinoma—*continued*
  islet cell—*continued*
    specified site NEC — see Neoplasm, by site, malignant
    unspecified site 157.4
  juvenile, breast (M8502/3) — see Neoplasm, breast, malignant
  Kulchitsky's cell (carcinoid tumor of intestine) 259.2
  large cell (M8012/3)
    squamous cell, nonkeratinizing type (M8072/3)
  Leydig cell (testis) (M8650/3)
    specified site — see Neoplasm, by site, malignant
    unspecified site 186.9
    female 183.0
    male 186.9
  liver cell (M8170/3) 155.0
  lobular (infiltrating) (M8520/3)
    non-infiltrating (M8520/3)
      specified site — see Neoplasm, by site, in situ
      unspecified site 233.0.
    specified site — see Neoplasm, by site, malignant
    unspecified site 174.9
  lymphoepithelial (M8082/3)
  medullary (M8510/3)
    with
      amyloid stroma (M8511/3)
        specified site — see Neoplasm, by site, malignant
        unspecified site 193
      lymphoid stroma (M8512/3)
        specified site — see Neoplasm, by site, malignant
        unspecified site 174.9
  mesometanephric (M9110/3)
  mesonephric (M9110/3)
  metastatic (M8010/6) — see Metastasis, cancer
  metatypical (M8095/3) — see Neoplasm, skin, malignant
  morphea type basal cell (M8092/3) — see Neoplasm, skin, malignant
  mucinous (M8480/3)
  mucin-producing (M8481/3)
  mucin-secreting (M8481/3)
  mucoepidermoid (M8430/3)
  mucoid (M8480/3)
    cell (M8300/3)
      specified site — see Neoplasm, by site, malignant
      unspecified site 194.3
  mucous (M8480/3)
  nonencapsulated sclerosing (M8350/3) 193
  noninfiltrating
    intracystic (M8504/2) — see Neoplasm, by site, in situ
    intraductal (M8500/2)
      papillary (M8503/2)
        specified site — see Neoplasm, by site, in situ
        unspecified site 233.0
      specified site — see Neoplasm, by site, in situ
      unspecified site 233.0
    lobular (M8520/2)
      specified site — see Neoplasm, by site, in situ
      unspecified site 233.0
  oat cell (M8042/3)
    specified site — see Neoplasm, by site, malignant
    unspecified site 162.9

Carcinoma—*continued*
  odontogenic (M9270/3) 170.1
    upper jaw (bone) 170.0
  onocytic (M8290/3)
  oxyphilic (M8290/3)
  papillary (M8050/3)
    and follicular (mixed) (M8340/3) 193
    epidermoid (M8052/3)
    intraductal (noninfiltrating) (M8503/2)
      specified site — see Neoplasm, by site, in situ
      unspecified site 233.0
    serous (M8460/3)
      specified site — see Neoplasm, by site, malignant
      surface (M8461/3)
        specified site — see Neoplasm, by site, malignant
        unspecified site 183.0
      unspecified site 183.0
    squamous cell (M8052/3)
    transitional cell (M8130/3)
  papillocystic (M8450/3)
    specified site — see Neoplasm, by site, malignant
    unspecified site 183.0
  parafollicular cell (M8510/3)
    specified site — see Neoplasm, by site, malignant
    unspecified site 193
  pleomorphic (M8022/3)
  polygonal cell (M8034/3)
  prickle cell (M8070/3)
  pseudoglandular, squamous cell (M8075/3)
  pseudomucinous (M8470/3)
    specified site — see Neoplasm, by site, malignant
    unspecified site 183.0
  pseudosarcomatous (M8033/3)
  regaud type (M8082/3) — see Neoplasm, nasopharynx, malignant
  renal cell (M8312/3) 189.0
  reserve cell (M8041/3)
  round cell (M8041/3)
  Schmincke (M8082/3) — see Neoplasm, nasopharynx, malignant
  Schneiderian (M8121/3)
    specified site — see Neoplasm, by site, malignant
    unspecified site 160.0
  scirrhous (M8141/3)
  sebaceous (M8410/3) — see Neoplasm, skin, malignant
  secondary (M8010/6) — see Neoplasm, by site, malignant, secondary
  secretory, breast (M8502/3) — see Neoplasm, breast, malignant
  serous (M8441/3)
    papillary (M8460/3)
      specified site — see Neoplasm, by site, malignant
      unspecified site 183.0
    surface, papillary (M8461/3)
      specified site — see Neoplasm, by site, malignant
      unspecified site 183.0
  Sertoli cell (M8640/3)
    specified site — see Neoplasm, by site, malignant
    unspecified site 186.9
  signet ring cell (M8490/3)
    metastatic (M8490/6) — see Neoplasm, by site, secondary
  simplex (M8231/3)

Carcinoma—*continued*
- skin appendage (M8390/3) — *see* Neoplasm, skin, malignant
- small cell (M8041/3)
  - fusiform cell type (M8043/3)
  - squamous cell, non-keratinizing type (M8073/3)
- solid (M8230/3)
  - with amyloid stroma (M8511/3)
    - specified site — *see* Neoplasm, by site, malignant
    - unspecified site 193
- spheroidal cell (M8035/3)
- spindle cell (M8032/3)
  - and giant cell (M8030/3)
- spinous cell (M8070/3)
- squamous (cell) (M8070/3)
  - adenoid type (M8075/3)
  - and adenocarcinoma, mixed (M8560/3)
  - intraepidermal, Bowen's type — *see* Neoplasm, skin, in situ
  - keratinizing type (large cell) (M8071/3)
  - large cell, non-keratinizing type (M8072/3)
  - microinvasive (M8076/3)
    - specified site — *see* Neoplasm, by site, malignant
    - unspecified site 180.9
  - non-keratinizing type (M8072/3)
  - papillary (M8052/3)
  - pseudoglandular (M8075/3)
  - small cell, non-keratinizing type (M8073/3)
  - spindle cell type (M8074/3)
  - verrucous (M805l/3)
- superficial spreading (M8143/3)
- sweat gland (M8400/3) — *see* Neoplasm, skin, malignant
- theca cell (M8600/3) 183.0
- thymic (M8580/3) 164.0
- trabecular (M8190/3)
- transitional (cell) (M8120/3)
  - papillary (M8130/3)
  - spindle cell type (M8122/3)
- tubular (M8211/3)
- undifferentiated type (M8020/3)
- urothelial (M8120/3)
- ventriculi 151.9
- verrucous (epidermoid) (squamous cell) (M8051/3)
- villous (M8262/3)
- water-clear cell (M8322/3) 194.1
- wolffian duct (M9110/3)

Carcinomaphobia 300.29

Carcinomatosis
- peritonei (M8010/6) 197.6
- specified site NEC (M8010/3) — *see* Neoplasm, by site, malignant
- unspecified site (M8010/6) 199.0

Carcinosarcoma (M8980/3) — *see also* Neoplasm, by site, malignant
- embryonal type (M8981/3) — *see* Neoplasm, by site, malignant

Cardia, cardial — *see* condition

Cardiac — *see also* condition
- death — *see* Disease, heart
- device
  - defibrillator, automatic implantable V45.02
    - in situ NEC V45.00
  - pacemaker
    - cardiac
      - fitting or adjustment V53.31
      - in situ V45.01
    - carotid sinus
      - fitting or adjustment V53.39
      - in situ V45.09

Cardiac—*continued*
- pacemaker — *see* Cardiac, device, pacemaker
- tamponade 423.9

Cardialgia (*see also* Pain, precordial) 786.51

Cardiectasis — *see* Hypertrophy, cardiac

Cardiochalasia 530.81

Cardiomalacia (*see also* Degeneration, myocardial) 429.1

Cardiomegalia glycogenica diffusa 271.0

Cardiomegaly (*see also* Hypertrophy, cardiac) 429.3
- congenital 746.89
- glycogen 271.0
- hypertensive (*see also* Hypertension, heart) 402.90
- idiopathic 429.3

Cardiomyoliposis (*see also* Degeneration, myocardial) 429.1

Cardiomyopathy (congestive) (constrictive) (familial) (infiltrative) (obstructive) (restrictive) (sporadic) 425.4
- alcoholic 425.5
- amyloid 277.3 [425.7]
- beriberi 265.0 [425.7]
- cobalt-beer 425.5
- congenital 425.3
- due to
  - amyloidosis 277.3 [425.71]
  - beriberi 265.0 [425.7]
  - cardiac glycogenosis 271.0 [425.7]
  - Chagas' disease 086.0
  - Friedreich's ataxia 334.0 [425.8]
  - hypertension —*see* Hypertension, with, heart involvement
  - mucopolysaccharidosis 277.5 [425.7]
  - myotonia atrophica 359.2 [425.8]
  - progressive muscular dystrophy 359.1 [425.8]
  - sarcoidosis 135 [425.8]
- glycogen storage 271.0 [425.7]
- hypertensive — *see* Hypertension, with, heart involvement
- hypertrophic
  - nonobstructive 425.4
  - obstructive 425.1
    - congenital 746.84
- idiopathic (concentric) 425.4
- in
  - Chagas' disease 086.0
  - sarcoidosis 135 [425.8]
- ischemic 414.8
- metabolic NEC 277.9 [425.7]
  - amyloid 277.3 [425.7]
  - thyrotoxic (*see also* Thyrotoxicosis) 242.9 [425.7]
  - thyrotoxicosis (*see also* Thyrotoxicosis) 242.9 [425.7]
- nutritional 269.9 [425.7]
  - beriberi 265.0 [425.7]
- obscure of Africa 425.2
- postpartum 674.8
- primary 425.4
- secondary 425.9
- thyrotoxic (*see also* Thyrotoxicosis) 242.9 [425.7]
- toxic NEC 425.9
- tuberculous (*see also* Tuberculosis) 017.9 [425.8]

Cardionephritis — *see* Hypertension, cardiorenal

Cardionephropathy — *see* Hypertension, cardiorenal

Cardionephrosis — *see* Hypertension, cardiorenal

Cardioneurosis 306.2

Cardiopathia nigra 416.0

Cardiopathy (*see also* Disease, heart) 429.9
- hypertensive (*see also* Hypertension, heart) 402.90
- idiopathic 425.4
- mucopolysaccharidosis 277.5 [425.7]

Cardiopericarditis (*see also* Pericarditis) 423.9

Cardiophobia 300.29

Cardioptosis 746.87

Cardiorenal — *see* condition

Cardiorrhexis (*see also* Infarct, myocardium) 410.9

Cardiosclerosis — *see* Arteriosclerosis, coronary

Cardiosis — *see* Disease, heart

Cardiospasm (esophagus) (reflex) (stomach) 530.0
- congenital 750.7

Cardiostenosis — *see* Disease, heart

Cardiosymphysis 423.1

Cardiothyrotoxicosis — *see* Hyperthyroidism

Cardiovascular — *see* condition

Carditis (acute) (bacterial) (chronic) (subacute) 429.89
- Coxsackie 074.20
- hypertensive (*see also* Hypertension, heart) 402.90
- meningococcal 036.40
- rheumatic — *see* Disease, heart, rheumatic
- rheumatoid 714.2

Care (of)
- child (routine) V20.1
- convalescent following V66.9
  - chemotherapy V66.2
  - medical NEC V66.5
  - psychotherapy V66.3
  - radiotherapy V66.1
  - surgery V66.0
  - surgical NEC V66.0
  - treatment (for) V66.5
    - combined V66.6
    - fracture V66.4
    - mental disorder NEC V66.3
    - specified type NEC V66.5
- family member (handicapped) (sick) creating problem for family V61.49
- provided away from home for holiday relief V60.5
- unavailable, due to
  - absence (person rendering care) (sufferer) V60.4
  - inability (any reason) of person rendering care V60.4
- holiday relief V60.5
- improper (at or after birth) (infant) (child) 995.5
  - affecting parent or family V61.21
  - as reason for family seeking advice V61.21
  - specified person other than child 995.81
- lack of (at or after birth) (infant) (child) 995.5
  - affecting parent or family V61.21
  - as reason for family seeking advice V61.21
  - specified person other than child 995.81
- lactation of mother V24.1
- postpartum
  - immediately after delivery V24.0
  - routine follow-up V24.2

Care (of)—*continued*
- prenatal V22.1
  - first pregnancy V22.0
  - high risk pregnancy V23.9
    - specified problem NEC V23.8
- unavailable, due to
  - absence of person rendering care V60.4
  - inability (any reason) of person rendering care V60.4
- well baby V20.1

Caries (bone) (*see also* Tuberculosis, bone) 015.9 [730.8]
- arrested 521.0
- cementum 521.0
- cerebrospinal (tuberculous) 015.0 [730.88]
- dental (acute) (chronic) (incipient) (infected) (with pulp exposure) 521.0
- dentin (acute) (chronic) 521.0
- enamel (acute) (chronic) (incipient) 521.0
- external meatus 380.89
- hip (*see also* Tuberculosis) 015.1 [730.85]
- knee 015.2 [730.86]
- labyrinth 386.8
- limb NEC 015.7 [730.88]
- mastoid (chronic) (process) 383.1
- middle ear 385.89
- nose 015.7 [730.88]
- orbit 015.7 [730.88]
- ossicle 385.24
- petrous bone 383.20
- sacrum (tuberculous) 015.0 [730.88]
- spine, spinal (column) (tuberculous) 015.0 [730.88]
- syphilitic 095.5
  - congenital 090.0 [730.8]
- teeth (internal) 521.0
- vertebra (column) (tuberculous) 015.0 [730.88]

Carini's syndrome (ichthyosis congenita) 757.1

Carious teeth 521.0

Carneous mole 631

Carnosinemia 270.5

Carotid body or sinus syndrome 337.0

Carotidynia 337.0

Carotinemia (dietary) 278.3

Carotinosis (cutis) (skin) 278.3

Carpal tunnel syndrome 354.0

Carpenter's syndrome 759.89

Carpopedal spasm (*see also* Tetany) 781.7

Carpoptosis 736.05

Carrier (suspected) of
- AIDS virus V02.9
- amebiasis V02.2
- bacterial discase (meningococcal, staphylococcal, streptococcal) NEC V02.5
- cholera V02.0
- defective gene V19.8
- diphtheria V02.4
- dysentery (bacillary) V02.3
  - amebic V02.2
- Endamoeba histolytica V02.2
- gastrointestinal pathogens NEC V02.3
- genetic defect V19.8
- gonorrhea V02.7
- HAA (hepatitis Australian-antigen) V02.6
- hepatitis V02.6
  - Australian-antigen (HAA) V02.6
  - serum V02.6
  - viral V02.6
- HIV V02.9
- human immunodeficiency virus V02.9
- infective organism NEC V02.9

Carrier—continued
malaria V02.9
paratyphoid V02.3
Salmonella V02.3
typhosa V02.1
serum hepatitis V02.6
Shigella V02.3
staphylococcus NEC V02.5
typhoid V02.1
venereal disease NEC V02.8

Carrión's disease (Bartonellosis) 088.0

Car sickness 994.6

Carter's
relapsing fever (Asiatic) 087.0

Cartilage — see condition

Caruncle (inflamed)
abscess, lacrimal (see also Dacryocystitis) 375.30
conjunctiva 372.00
acute 372.00
eyelid 373.00
labium (majus) (minus) 616.8
lacrimal 375.30
urethra (benign) 599.3
vagina (wall) 616.8

Cascade stomach 537.6

Caseation lymphatic gland (see also Tuberculosis) 017.2

Caseous
bronchitis — see Tuberculosis, pulmonary
meningitis 013.0
pneumonia — see Tuberculosis, pulmonary

Cassidy (-Scholte) **syndrome** (malignant carcinoid) 259.2

Castellani's bronchitis 104.8

Castleman's tumor or lymphoma (mediastinal lymph node hyperplasia) 785.6

Castration, traumatic 878.2
complicated 878.3

Casts in urine 791.7

Cat's ear 744.29

Catalepsy 300.11
catatonic (acute) (see also Schizophrenia) 295.2
hysterical 300.11
schizophrenic (see also Schizophrenia) 295.2

Cataphasia 307.0

Cataplexy (idiopathic) 347

Cataract (anterior cortical) (anterior polar) (black) (capsular) (central) (cortical) (hypermature) (immature) (incipient) (mature) (nuclear) 366.9
anterior
and posterior axial embryonal 743.33
pyramidal 743.31
subcapsular polar
infantile, juvenile, or presenile 366.01
senile 366.13
associated with
calcinosis 275.4 [366.42]
craniofacial dysostosis 756.0 [366.44]
galactosemia 271.1 [366.44]
hypoparathyroidism 252.1 [366.42]
myotonic disorders 359.2 [366.43]
neovascularization 366.33
blue dot 743.39
cerulean 743.39
complicated NEC 366.30
congenital 743.30
capsular or subcapsular 743.31
cortical 743.32
nuclear 743.33
specified type NEC 743.39
total or subtotal 743.34

Cataract—continued
congenital—continued
zonular 743.32
coronary (congenital) 743.39
acquired 366.12
cupuliform 366.14
diabetic 250.5 [366.41]
drug-induced 366.45
due to
chalcosis 366.34 [360.24]
chronic choroiditis (see also Choroiditis) 366.32 [363.20]
degenerative myopia 366.34 [360.21]
glaucoma (see also Glaucoma) 366.31 [365.9]
infection, intraocular NEC 366.32
inflammatory ocular disorder NEC 366.32
iridocyclitis, chronic 366.33 [364.10]
pigmentary retinal dystrophy 366.34 [362.74]
radiation 366.46
electric 366.46
glassblowers' 366.46
heat ray 366.46
heterochromic 366.33
in eye disease NEC 366.30
infantile (see also Cataract, juvenile) 366.00
intumescent 366.12
irradiational 366.46
juvenile 366.00
anterior subcapsular polar 366.01
combined forms 366.09
cortical 366.03
lamellar 366.03
nuclear 366.04
posterior subcapsular polar 366.02
specified NEC 366.09
zonular 366.03
lamellar 743.32
infantile, juvenile, or presenile 366.03
morgagnian 366.18
myotonic 359.2 [366.43]
myxedema 244.9 [366.44]
posterior, polar (capsular) 743.31
infantile, juvenile, or presenile 366.02
senile 366.14
presenile (see also Cataract, juvenile) 366.00
punctate
acquired 366.12
congenital 743.39
secondary (membrane) 366.50
obscuring vision 366.53
specified type, not obscuring vision 366.52
senile 366.10
anterior subcapsular polar 366.13
combined forms 366.19
cortical 366.15
hypermature 366.18
immature 366.12
incipient 366.12
mature 366.17
nuclear 366.16
posterior subcapsular polar 366.14
specified NEC 366.19
total or subtotal 366.17
snowflake 250.5 [366.41]
specified NEC 366.8
subtotal (senile) 366.17
congenital 743.34
sunflower 360.24 [366.34]
tetanic NEC 252.1 [366.42]
total (mature) (senile) 366.17
congenital 743.34

Cataract—continued
total—continued
localized 366.21
traumatic 366.22
toxic 366.45
traumatic 366.20
partially resolved 366.23
total 366.22
zonular (perinuclear) 743.32
infantile, juvenile, or presenile 366.03

Cataracta 366.10
brunescens 366.16
cerulea 743.39
complicata 366.30
congenita 743.30
coralliformis 743.39
coronaria (congenital) 743.39
acquired 366.12
diabetic 250.5 [366.41]
floriformis 360.24 [366.34]
membranacea
accreta 366.50
congenita 743.39
nigra 366.16

Catarrh, catarrhal (inflammation) (see also condition) 460
acute 460
asthma, asthmatic (see also Asthma) 493.9
Bostock's (see also Fever, hay) 477.9
bowel — see Enteritis
bronchial 490
acute 466.0
chronic 491.0
subacute 466.0
cervix, cervical (canal) (uteri) — see Cervicitis
chest (see also Bronchitis) 490
chronic 472.0
congestion 472.0
conjunctivitis 372.03
due to syphilis 095.9
congenital 090.0
enteric — see Enteritis
epidemic 487.1
Eustachian 381.50
eye (acute) (vernal) 372.03
fauces (see also Pharyngitis) 462
febrile 460
fibrinous acute 466.0
gastroenteric — see Enteritis
gastrointestinal — see Enteritis
gingivitis 523.0
hay (see also Fever, hay) 477.9
infectious 460
intestinal — see Enteritis
larynx (see also Laryngitis, chronic) 476.0
liver 070.1
with hepatic coma 070.0
lung (see also Bronchitis) 490
acute 466.0
chronic 491.0
middle ear (chronic) — see Otitis media, chronic
mouth 528.0
nasal (chronic) (see also Rhinitis) 472.0
acute 460
nasobronchial 472.2
nasopharyngeal (chronic) 472.2
acute 460
nose — see Catarrh, nasal
ophthalmia 372.03
pneumococcal, acute 466.0
pulmonary (see also Bronchitis) 490
acute 466.0
chronic 491.0
spring (eye) 372.13
suffocating (see also Asthma) 493.9
summer (hay) (see also Fever, hay) 477.9
throat 472.1
tracheitis 464.10
with obstruction 464.11

Catarrh, catarrhal—continued
tubotympanal 381.4
acute (see also Otitis media, acute, nonsuppurative) 381.00
chronic 381.10
vasomotor (see also Fever, hay) 477.9
vesical (bladder) — see Cystitis

Catarrhus aestivus (see also Fever, hay) 477.9

Catastrophe, cerebral (see also Disease, cerebrovascular, acute) 436

Catatonia, catatonic (acute) 781.9 ▼
with
affective psychosis — see Psychosis, affective ▲
agitation 295.2
dementia (praecox) 295.2
excitation 295.2
excited type 295.2
schizophrenia 295.2
stupor 295.2

Cat-scratch — see also Injury, superficial disease or fever 078.3

Cauda equina — see also condition
syndrome 344.60

Cauliflower ear 738.7

Caul over face 768.9

Causalgia 355.9
lower limb 355.71
upper limb 354.4

Cause
external, general effects NEC 994.9
not stated 799.9
unknown 799.9

Caustic burn — see also Burn, by site
from swallowing caustic or corrosive substance — see Burn, internal organs

Cavare's disease (familial periodic paralysis) 359.3

Cave-in, injury
crushing (severe) (see also Crush, by site) 869.1
suffocation 994.7

Cavernitis (penis) 607.2
lymph vessel — see Lymphangioma

Cavernositis 607.2

Cavernous — see condition

Cavitation of lung (see also Tuberculosis) 011.2
nontuberculous 518.89
primary, progressive 010.8

Cavity
lung — see Cavitation of lung
optic papilla 743.57
pulmonary — see Cavitation of lung
teeth 521.0
vitreous (humor) 379.21

Cavovarus foot, congenital 754.59

Cavus foot (congenital) 754.71
acquired 736.73

Cazenave's
disease (pemphigus) NEC 694.4
lupus (erythematosus) 695.4

Cecitis — see Appendicitis ◆

Cecocele — see Hernia

Cecum — see condition

Celiac
artery compression syndrome 447.4
disease 579.0
infantilism 579.0

Cell, cellular — see also condition
anterior chamber (eye) (positive aqueous ray) 364.04

Cellulitis (diffuse) (with lymphangitis) (see also Abscess) 682.9
abdominal wall 682.2

Cellulitis—continued
anaerobic (see also Gas gangrene) 040.0
ankle 682.6
anus 566
areola 611.0
arm (any part, above wrist) 682.3
artificial opening (external) 998.5
auditory canal (external) 380.10
axilla 682.3
back (any part) 682.2
breast 611.0
    postpartum 675.1
broad ligament (see also Disease, pelvis, inflammatory) 614.4
    acute 614.3
buttock 682.5
cervical (neck region) 682.1
cervix (uteri) (see also Cervicitis) 616.0
cheek, external 682.0
    internal 528.3
chest wall 682.2
chronic NEC 682.9
corpus cavernosum 607.2
digit 681.9
Douglas' cul-de-sac or pouch (chronic) (see also Disease, pelvis, inflammatory) 614.4
    acute 614.3
drainage site (following operation) 998.5
ear, external 380.10
erysipelar (see also Erysipelas) 035
eyelid 373.13
face (any part, except eye) 682.0
finger (intrathecal) (periosteal) (subcutaneous) (subcuticular) 681.00
flank 682.2
foot (except toe) 682.7
forearm 682.3
gangrenous (see also Gangrene) 785.4
genital organ NEC
    female — see Abscess, genital organ, female
    male 608.4
glottis 478.71
gluteal (region) 682.5
gonococcal NEC 098.0
groin 682.2
hand (except finger or thumb) 682.4
head (except face) NEC 682.8
heel 682.7
hip 682.6
jaw (region) 682.0
knee 682.6
labium (majus) (minus) (see also Vulvitis) 616.10
larynx 478.71
leg, except foot 682.6
lip 528.5
mammary gland 611.0
mouth (floor) 528.3
multiple sites NEC 682.9
nasopharynx 478.21
navel 682.2
    newborn NEC 771.4
neck (region) 682.1
nipple 611.0
nose 478.1
    external 682.0
orbit, orbital 376.01
palate (soft) 528.3
pectoral (region) 682.2
pelvis, pelvic
    with
        abortion — see Abortion, by type, with sepsis
        ectopic pregnancy (see also categories 633.0—633.9) 639.0
        molar pregnancy (see also categories 630—632) 639.0

Cellulitis—continued
pelvis, pelvic—continued
    female (see also Disease, pelvis, inflammatory) 614.4
        acute 614.3
        following
            abortion 639.0
            ectopic or molar pregnancy 639.0
    male (see also Abscess, peritoneum) 567.2
    puerperal, postpartum, childbirth 670
penis 607.2
perineal, perineum 682.2
perirectal 566
peritonsillar 475
periurethral 597.0
periuterine (see also Disease, pelvis, inflammatory) 614.4
    acute 614.3
pharynx 478.21
phlegmonous NEC 682.9
rectum 566
retromammary 611.0
retroperitoneal (see also Peritonitis) 567.2
round ligament (see also Disease, pelvis, inflammatory) 614.4
    acute 614.3
scalp (any part) 682.8
    dissecting 704.8
scrotum 608.4
seminal vesicle 608.0
septic NEC 682.9
shoulder 682.3
specified sites NEC 682.8
spermatic cord 608.4
submandibular (region) (space) (triangle) 682.0
    gland 527.3
submaxillary 528.3
    gland 527.3
submental (pyogenic) 682.0
    gland 527.3
suppurative NEC 682.9
testis 608.4
thigh 682.6
thumb (intrathecal) (periosteal) (subcutaneous) (subcuticular) 681.00
toe (intrathecal) (periosteal) (subcutaneous) (subcuticular) 681.10
tonsil 475
trunk 682.2
tuberculous (primary) (see also Tuberculosis) 017.0
tunica vaginalis 608.4
umbilical 682.2
    newborn NEC 771.4
vaccinal 999.3
vagina — see Vaginitis
vas deferens 608.4
vocal cords 478.5
vulva (see also Vulvitis) 616.10
wrist 682.4

Cementoblastoma, benign (M9273/0) 213.1
    upper jaw (bone) 213.0
Cementoma (M9273/0) 213.1
    gigantiform (M9276/0) 213.1
        upper jaw (bone) 213.0
    upper jaw (bone) 213.0
Cementoperiostitis 523.4
Cephalgia, cephalagia (see also Headache) 784.0
    histamine 346.2
    nonorganic origin 307.81
    psychogenic 307.81
    tension 307.81
Cephalhematocele, cephalematocele
    due to birth injury 767.1
    fetus or newborn 767.1
    traumatic (see also Contusion, head) 920

Cephalhematoma, cephalematoma (calcified)
    due to birth injury 767.1
    fetus or newborn 767.1
    traumatic (see also Contusion, head) 920
Cephalic — see condition
Cephalitis — see Encephalitis
Cephalocele 742.0
Cephaloma — see Neoplasm, by site, malignant
Cephalomenia 625.8
Cephalopelvic — see condition
Cercomoniasis 007.3
Cerebellitis — see Encephalitis
Cerebellum (cerebellar) — see condition
Cerebral — see condition
Cerebritis — see Encephalitis
Cerebrohepatorenal syndrome 759.89
Cerebromacular degeneration 330.1
Cerebromalacia (see also Softening, brain) 434.9
Cerebrosidosis 272.7
Cerebrospasticity — see Palsy, cerebral
Cerebrospinal — see condition
Cerebrum — see condition
Ceroid storage disease 272.7
Cerumen (accumulation) (impacted) 380.4
Cervical — see also condition
    auricle 744.43
    rib 756.2
Cervicalgia 723.1
Cervicitis (acute) (chronic) (nonvenereal) (subacute) (with erosion or ectropion) 616.0
    with
        abortion — see Abortion, by type, with sepsis
        ectopic pregnancy (see also categories 633.0— 633.9) 639.0
        molar pregnancy (see also categories 630— 632) 639.0
        ulceration 616.0
    chlamydial 099.53
    complicating pregnancy or puerperium 646.6
        affecting fetus or newborn 760.8
    following
        abortion 639.0
        ectopic or molar pregnancy 639.0
    gonococcal (acute) 098.15
        chronic or duration of 2 months or more 098.35
    senile (atrophic) 616.0
    syphilitic 095.8
    trichomonal 131.09
    tuberculous (see also Tuberculosis) 016.7
Cervicoaural fistula 744.49
Cervicocolpitis (emphysematosa) (see also Cervicitis) 616.0
Cervix — see condition
Cesarean delivery, operation or section NEC 669.7
    affecting fetus or newborn 763.4
    post mortem, affecting fetus or newborn 761.6
    previous, affecting management of pregnancy 654.2
Céstan's syndrome 344.89
Céstan-Chenais paralysis 344.89
Céstan-Raymond syndrome 433.8
Cestode infestation NEC 123.9
    specified type NEC 123.8
Cestodiasis 123.9

Chabert's disease 022.9
Chacaleh 266.2
Chafing 709.8
Chagas' disease (see also Trypanosomiasis, American) 086.2
    with heart involvement 086.0
Chagres fever 084.0
Chalasia (cardiac sphincter) 530.81
Chalazion 373.2
Chalazoderma 757.39
Chalcosis 360.24
    cornea 371.15
    crystalline lens 366.34 [360.24]
    retina 360.24
Chalicosis (occupational) (pulmonum) 502
Chancre (any genital site) (hard) (indurated) (infecting) (primary) (recurrent) 091.0
    congenital 090.0
    conjunctiva 091.2
    Ducrey's 099.0
    extragenital 091.2
    eyelid 091.2
    Hunterian 091.0
    lip (syphilis) 091.2
    mixed 099.8
    nipple 091.2
    Nisbet's 099.0
    of
        carate 103.0
        pinta 103.0
        yaws 102.0
    palate, soft 091.2
    phagedenic 099.0
    Ricord's 091.0
    Rollet's (syphilitic) 091.0
    seronegative 091.0
    seropositive 091.0
    simple 099.0
    soft 099.0
        bubo 099.0
    urethra 091.0
    yaws 102.0
Chancriform syndrome 114.1
Chancroid 099.0
    anus 099.0
    penis (Ducrey's bacillus) 099.0
    perineum 099.0
    rectum 099.0
    scrotum 099.0
    urethra 099.0
    vulva 099.0
Chandipura fever 066.8
Chandler's disease (osteochondritis dissecans, hip) 732.7
Change(s) (of) — see also Removal of
arteriosclerotic — see Arteriosclerosis
    battery ▼
        cardiac pacemaker V53.31 ▲
    bone 733.90
        diabetic 250.8 [731.8]
        in disease, unknown cause 733.90
    bowel habits 787.9
    cardiorenal (vascular) (see also Hypertension, cardiorenal) 404.90
    cardiovascular — see Disease, cardiovascular
    circulatory 459.9
    cognitive or personality change of other type, nonpsychotic 310.1
    color, teeth, tooth
        during formation 520.8
        posteruptive 521.7
    contraceptive device V25.42
    cornea, corneal
        degenerative NEC 371.40
        membrane NEC 371.30
        senile 371.41

Change—continued
  coronary (see also Ischemia, heart) 414.9
  degenerative
    chamber angle (anterior) (iris) 364.56
    ciliary body 364.57
    spine or vertebra (see also Spondylosis) 721.90
    dental pulp, regressive 522.2
    dressing V58.3
    fixation device V54.8
      external V54.8
      internal V54.0
    heart — see also Disease, heart
    hip joint 718.95
    hyperplastic larynx 478.79
    hypertrophic
      nasal sinus (see also Sinusitis) 473.9
      turbinate, nasal 478.0
      upper respiratory tract 478.9
    inflammatory — see Inflammation
    joint (see also Derangement, joint) 718.90
      sacroiliac 724.6
    Kirschner wire V54.8
    knee 717.9
    macular, congenital 743.55
    malignant (M———/3) — see also Neoplasm, by site, malignant

Note — for malignant change occurring in a neoplasm, use the appropriate M code with behavior digit /3 e.g., malignant change in uterine fibroid — M8890/3. For malignant change occurring in a nonneoplastic condition (e.g., gastric ulcer) use the M code M8000/3.

    mental (status) NEC 780.9 ◆
      due to or associated with physical condition — see Syndrome, brain
    myocardium, myocardial — see Degeneration, myocardial
    of life (see also Menopause) 627.2
    pacemaker battery (cardiac) V53.31 ◆
    peripheral nerve 355.9
    personality (nonpsychotic) NEC 310.1
    plaster cast V54.8
    refractive, transient 367.81
    regressive, dental pulp 522.2
    retina 362.9
      myopic (degenerative) (malignant) 360.21
      vascular appearance 362.13
    sacroiliac joint 724.6
    scleral 379.19
      degenerative 379.16
    senile (see also Senility) 797
    sensory (see also Disturbance, sensation) 782.0
    skin texture 782.8
    spinal cord 336.9
    splint, external V54.8
    subdermal implantable contraceptive V25.5
    suture V58.3
    traction device V54.8
    trophic 355.9
      arm NEC 354.9
      leg NEC 355.8
      lower extremity NEC 355.8
      upper extremity NEC 354.9
    vascular 459.9
    vasomotor 443.9
    voice 784.49
      psychogenic 306.1
Changing sleep-work schedule, affecting sleep 307.45
Changuinola fever 066.0
Chapping skin 709.8

Character
  depressive 301.12
Charcot's
  arthropathy 094.0 [713.5]
  cirrhosis — see Cirrhosis, biliary
  disease 094.0
    spinal cord 094.0
  fever (biliary) (hepatic) (intermittent) — see Choledocholithiasis
  joint (disease) 094.0 [713.5]
    diabetic 250.6 [713.5]
    syringomyelic 336.0 [713.5]
  syndrome (intermittent claudication) 443.9
    due to atherosclerosis 440.21
Charcot-Marie-Tooth disease, paralysis, or syndrome 356.1
Charleyhorse (quadriceps) 843.8
  muscle, except quadriceps — see Sprain, by site
Charlouis' disease (see also Yaws) 102.9
Chauffeur's fracture — see Fracture, ulna, lower end
Cheadle (-Möller) (-Barlow) disease or syndrome (infantile scurvy) 267
Checking (of)
  contraceptive device (intrauterine) V25.42
  device
    fixation V54.8
      external V54.8
      internal V54.0
    traction V54.8
    Kirschner wire V54.8
    plaster cast V54.8
    splint, external V54.8
Checkup
  following treatment — see Examination
  health V70.0
  infant (not sick) V20.2
  pregnancy (normal) V22.1
    first V22.0
    high risk pregnancy V23.9
    specified problem NEC V23.8
Chédiak-Higashi (-Steinbrinck) anomaly, disease, or syndrome (congenital gigantism of peroxidase granules) 288.2
Cheek — see also condition
  biting 528.9
Cheese itch 133.8
Cheese washers' lung 495.8
Cheilitis 528.5
  actinic (due to sun) 692.72
    chronic NEC 692.72
      due to radiation, except from sun 692.82
    due to radiation, except from sun 692.82
  acute 528.5
  angular 528.5
  catarrhal 528.5
  chronic 528.5
  exfoliative 528.5
  gangrenous 528.5
  glandularis apostematosa 528.5
  granulomatosa 351.8
  infectional 528.5
  membranous 528.5
  Miescher's 351.8
  suppurative 528.5
  ulcerative 528.5
  vesicular 528.5
Cheilodynia 528.5
Cheilopalatoschisis (see also Cleft, palate, with cleft lip) 749.20
Cheilophagia 528.5
Cheiloschisis (see also Cleft, lip) 749.10
Cheilosis 528.5
  with pellagra 265.2

Cheilosis—continued
  angular 528.5
  due to
    dietary deficiency 266.0
    vitamin deficiency 266.0
Cheiromegaly 729.89
Cheiropompholyx 705.81
Cheloid (see also Keloid) 701.4
Chemical burn — see also Burn, by site
  from swallowing chemical — see Burn, internal organs
Chemodectoma (M8693/1) — see Paraganglioma, nonchromaffin
Chemoprophylaxis NEC V07.39 ◆
Chemosis, conjunctiva 372.73
Chemotherapy
  convalescence V66.2
  encounter (for) V58.1
  maintenance V58.1
  prophylactic NEC V07.39 ▼
    fluoride V07.31 ▲
Cherubism 526.89
Chest — see condition
Cheyne-Stokes respiration (periodic) 786.09
Chiari's
  disease or syndrome (hepatic vein thrombosis) 453.0
  malformation ▼
    type I 348.4
    type II (see also Spina bifida) 741.0
    type III 742.0
    type IV 742.2 ▲
  network 746.89
Chiari-Frommel syndrome 676.6
Chicago disease (North American blastomycosis) 116.0
Chickenpox (see also Varicella) 052.9
  vaccination and inoculation (prophylactic) V05.4
Chiclero ulcer 085.4
Chiggers 133.8
Chignon 111.2
  fetus or newborn (from vacuum extraction) 767.1
Chigoe disease 134.1
Chikungunya fever 066.3
Chilaiditi's syndrome (subphrenic displacement, colon) 751.4
Chilblains 991.5
  lupus 991.5
Child
  behavior causing concern V61.20
Childbed fever 670
Childbirth — see also Delivery
  puerperal complications — see Puerperal
Childhood, period of rapid growth V21.0
Chill(s) 780.9
  with fever 780.6
  congestive 780.9
    in malarial regions 084.6
  septic — see Septicemia
  urethral 599.84
Chilomastigiasis 007.8
Chin — see condition
Chinese dysentery 004.9
Chiropractic dislocation (see also Lesion, nonallopathic, by site) 739.9
Chitral fever 066.0
Chlamydia, chlamydial — see condition
Chloasma 709.09
  cachecticorum 709.09 ▲
  eyelid 374.52
    congenital 757.33
    hyperthyroid 242.0

Chloasma—continued
  gravidarum 646.8
  idiopathic 709.09 ▼
  skin 709.09
  symptomatic 709.09 ▲
Chloroma (M9930/3) 205.3
Chlorosis 280.9
  Egyptian (see also Ancylostomiasis) 126.9
  miners' (see also Ancylostomiasis) 126.9
Chlorotic anemia 280.9
Chocolate cyst (ovary) 617.1
Choked
  disk or disc — see Papilledema
  on food, phlegm, or vomitus NEC (see also Asphyxia, food) 933.1
  phlegm 933.1
  while vomiting NEC (see also Asphyxia, food) 933.1
Chokes (resulting from bends) 993.3
Choking sensation 784.9
Cholangiectasis (see also Disease, gallbladder) 575.8
Cholangiocarcinoma (M8160/3)
  and hepatocellular carcinoma, combined (M8180/3) 155.0
  liver 155.1
  specified site NEC — see Neoplasm, by site, malignant
  unspecified site 155.1
Cholangiohepatitis 575.8
  due to fluke infestation 121.1
Cholangiohepatoma (M8180/3) 155.0
Cholangiolitis (acute) (chronic) (extrahepatic) (gangrenous) 576.1
  intrahepatic 575.8
  paratyphoidal (see also Fever, paratyphoid) 002.9
  typhoidal 002.0
Cholangioma (M8160/0) 211.5
  malignant — see Cholangiocarcinoma
Cholangitis (acute) (ascending) (catarrhal) (chronic) (infective) (malignant) (primary) (recurrent) (sclerosing) (secondary) (stenosing) (suppurative) 576.1
  chronic nonsuppurative destructive 571.6
  nonsuppurative destructive (chronic) 571.6
Cholecystdocholithiasis — see Choledocholithiasis
Cholecystitis 575.1 ◆

Note — Use the following fifth-digit subclassification with category 574:

  0 without mention of obstruction
  1 with obstruction

  with
    calculus, stones in
      bile duct (common) (hepatic) 574.4
      gallbladder 574.1
    choledocholithiasis 574.4
    cholelithiasis 574.1
  acute 575.0
    with
      calculus, stones in
        bile duct (common) (hepatic) 574.3
        gallbladder 574.0
      choledocholithiasis 574.3
      cholelithiasis 574.0

Cholecystitis—continued
  chronic 575.1
    with
      calculus, stones in
        bile duct (common)
          (hepatic) 574.4
        gallbladder 574.1
        choledocholithiasis 574.4
        cholelithiasis 574.1
  emphysematous (acute) (see also
    Cholecystitis, acute) 575.0
  gangrenous (see also Cholecystitis,
    acute) 575.0
  paratyphoidal, current (see also
    Fever, paratyphoid) 002.9
  suppurative (see also cholecystitis,
    acute) 575.0
  typhoidal 002.0
Choledochitis (suppurative) 576.1
Choledocholith — see
  Choledocholithiasis
Choledocholithiasis 574.5

Note — Use the following fifth-
digit subclassification with category
574:

  0 without mention of
     obstruction
  1 with obstruction

  with cholecystitis (chronic) 574.4
    acute 574.3
Cholelithiasis (impacted) (multiple)
  574.2

Note — Use the following fifth-
digit subclassification with category
574:

  0 without mention of
     obstruction
  1 with obstruction

  with cholecystitis (chronic) 574.1
    acute 574.0
Cholemia (see also Jaundice) 782.4
  familial 277.4
  Gilbert's (familial nonhemolytic)
    277.4
Cholemic gallstone — see
  Cholelithiasis
Choleperitoneum, choleperitonitis (see
  also Disease, gallbladder) 567.8
Cholera (algid) (Asiatic) (asphyctic)
  (epidemic) (gravis) (Indian)
  (malignant) (morbus)
  (pestilential) (spasmodic) 001.9
  antimonial 985.4
  carrier (suspected) of V02.0
  classical 001.0
  contact V01.0
  due to
    Vibrio
      cholerae (Inaba, Ogawa,
        Hikojima serotypes)
        001.0
      El Tor 001.1
  El Tor 001.1
  exposure to V01.0
  vaccination, prophylactic (against)
    V03.0
Cholerine (see also Cholera) 001.9
Cholestasis 576.8
Cholesteatoma (ear) 385.30
  attic (primary) 385.31
  diffuse 385.35
  external ear (canal) 380.21
  marginal (middle ear) 385.32
    with involvement of mastoid
      cavity 385.33
    secondary (with middle ear
      involvement) 385.33
  mastoid cavity 385.30

Cholesteatoma—continued
  middle ear (secondary) 385.32
    with involvement of mastoid
      cavity 385.33
  postmastoidectomy cavity
    (recurrent) 383.32
  primary 385.31
  recurrent, postmastoidectomy
    cavity 383.32
  secondary (middle ear) 385.32
    with involvement of mastoid
      cavity 385.33
Cholesteatosis (middle ear) (see also
  Cholesteatoma) 385.30
  diffuse 385.35
Cholesteremia 272.0
Cholesterin
  granuloma, middle ear 385.82
  in vitreous 379.22
Cholesterol
  deposit
    retina 362.82
    vitreous 379.22
  imbibition of gallbladder (see also
    Disease, gallbladder) 575.6
Cholesterolemia 272.0
  essential 272.0
  familial 272.0
  hereditary 272.0
Cholesterosis, cholesterolosis
  (gallbladder) 575.6
  with
    cholecystitis — see Cholecystitis
    cholelithiasis — see
      Cholelithiasis
  middle ear (see also Cholesteatoma)
    385.30
Cholocolic fistula (see also Fistula,
  gallbladder) 575.5
Choluria 791.4
Chondritis (purulent) 733.99
  costal 733.99
    Tietze's 733.6
  patella, posttraumatic 717.7
  posttraumatica patellae 717.7
  tuberculous (active) (see also
    Tuberculosis) 015.9
    intervertebral 015.0 [730.88]
**Chondroangiopathia calcarea seu
  punctata** 756.59
Chondroblastoma (M9230/0) — see
  also Neoplasm, bone, benign
  malignant (M9230/3) — see
    Neoplasm, bone, malignant
Chondrocalcinosis (articular) (crystal
  deposition) (dihydrate) (see also
  Arthritis, due to, crystals) 275.4
  [712.3]
  due to
    calcium pyrophosphate 275.4
      [712.2]
    dicalcium phosphate crystals
      275.4 [712.1]
    pyrophosphate crystals 275.4
      [712.2]
Chondrodermatitis nodularis helicis
  380.00
Chondrodysplasia 756.4
  angiomatose 756.4
  calcificans congenita 756.59
  epiphysialis punctata 756.59
  hereditary deforming 756.4
Chondrodystrophia (fetalis) 756.4
  calcarea 756.4
  calcificans congenita 756.59
  fetalis hypoplastica 756.59
  hypoplastica calcinosa 756.59
  punctata 756.59
  tarda 277.5
Chondrodystrophy (familial)
  (hypoplastic) 756.4
Chondroectodermal dysplasia 756.55
Chondrolysis 733.99

Chondroma (M9220/0) — see also
  Neoplasm cartilage, benign
  juxtacortical (M9221/0) — see
    Neoplasm, bone, benign
  periosteal (M9221/0) — see
    Neoplasm, bone, benign
Chondromalacia 733.92
  epiglottis (congenital) 748.3
  generalized 733.92
  knee 717.7
  larynx (congenital) 748.3
  localized, except patella 733.92
  patella, patellae 717.7
  systemic 733.92
  tibial plateau 733.92
  trachea (congenital) 748.3
Chondromatosis (M9220/1) — see
  Neoplasm, cartilage, uncertain
  behavior
Chondromyxosarcoma (M9220/3) —
  see Neoplasm, cartilage,
  malignant
Chondro-osteodysplasia (Morquio-
  Brailsford type) 277.5
Chondro-osteodystrophy 277.5
Chondro-osteoma (M9210/0) — see
  Neoplasm, bone, benign
Chondropathia tuberosa 733.6
Chondrosarcoma (M9220/3) — see
  also Neoplasm, cartilage,
  malignant
  juxtacortical (M9221/3) — see
    Neoplasm, bone, malignant
  mesenchymal (M9240/3) — see
    Neoplasm, connective tissue,
    malignant
Chordae tendineae rupture (chronic)
  429.5
Chordee (nonvenereal) 607.89
  congenital 752.6
  gonococcal 098.2
Chorditis (fibrinous) (nodosa)
  (tuberosa) 478.5
Chordoma (M9370/3) — see
  Neoplasm, by site, malignant
Chorea (gravis) (minor) (spasmodic)
  333.5
  with
    heart involvement — see
      Chorea with rheumatic
      heart disease
    rheumatic heart disease
      (chronic, inactive, or
      quiescent) (conditions
      classifiable to 393-398)
      — see also Rheumatic
      heart condition involved
      active or acute (conditions
        classifiable to 391)
        392.0
  acute — see Chorea, Sydenham's
  apoplectic (see also Disease,
    cerebrovascular, acute) 436
  chronic 333.4
  electric 049.8
  gravidarum — see Eclampsia,
    pregnancy
  habit 307.22
  hereditary 333.4
  Huntington's 333.4
  posthemiplegic 344.89
  pregnancy — see Eclampsia,
    pregnancy
  progressive 333.4
    chronic 333.4
    hereditary 333.4
  rheumatic (chronic) 392.9
    with heart disease or
      involvement — see
      Chorea, with rheumatic
      heart disease
  senile 333.5

Chorea—continued
  Sydenham's 392.9
    with heart involvement — see
      Chorea, with rheumatic
      heart disease
    nonrheumatic 333.5
  variabilis 307.23
Choreoathetosis (paroxysmal) 333.5
Chorioadenoma (destruens) (M9100/1)
  236.1
Chorioamnionitis 658.4
  affecting fetus or newborn 762.7
Chorioangioma (M9120/0) 219.8
Choriocarcinoma (M9100/3)
  combined with
    embryonal carcinoma
      (M9101/3) — see
      Neoplasm, by site,
      malignant
    teratoma (M9101/3) — see
      Neoplasm, by site,
      malignant
  specified site — see Neoplasm, by
    site, malignant
  unspecified site
    female 181
    male 186.9
Chorioencephalitis, lymphocytic
  (acute) (serous) 049.0
Chorioepithelioma (M9100/3) — see
  Choriocarcinoma
Choriomeningitis (acute) (benign)
  (lymphocytic) (serous) 049.0
Chorionepithelioma (M9100/3) — see
  Choriocarcinoma
Chorionitis (see also Scleroderma)
  710.1
Chorioretinitis 363.20
  disseminated 363.10
    generalized 363.13
    in
      neurosyphilis 094.83
      secondary syphilis 091.51
    peripheral 363.12
    posterior pole 363.11
    tuberculous (see also
      Tuberculosis) 017.3
      [363.13]
  due to
    histoplasmosis (see also
      Histoplasmosis) 115.92
    toxoplasmosis (acquired) 130.2
      congenital (active) 771.2
  focal 363.00
    juxtapapillary 363.01
    peripheral 363.04
    posterior pole NEC 363.03
  juxtapapillaris, juxtapapillary
    363.01
  progressive myopia (degeneration)
    360.21
  syphilitic (secondary) 091.51
    congenital (early) 090.0
      [363.13]
    late 090.5 [363.13]
    late 095.8 [363.13]
  tuberculous (see also Tuberculosis)
    017.3 [363.13]
Choristoma — see Neoplasm, by site,
  benign
Choroid — see condition
Choroideremia, choroidermia (initial
  stage) (late stage) (partial or total
  atrophy) 363.55
Choroiditis (see also Chorioretinitis)
  363.20
  leprous 030.9 [363.13]
  senile guttate 363.41
  sympathetic 360.11
  syphilitic (secondary) 091.51
    congenital (early) 090.0
      [363.13]
    late 090.5 [363.13]
    late 095.8 [363.13]

Choroiditis—continued
Tay's 363.41
tuberculous (see also Tuberculosis) 017.3 [363.13]
Choroidopathy NEC 363.9
degenerative (see also Degeneration, choroid) 363.40
hereditary (see also Dystrophy, choroid) 363.50
specified type NEC 363.8
Choroidoretinitis — see Chorioretinitis
Choroidosis, central serous 362.41
Choroidretinopathy, serous 362.41
Christian's syndrome (chronic histiocytosis X) 277.8
Christian-Weber disease (nodular nonsuppurative panniculitis) 729.30
Christmas disease 286.1
Chromaffinoma (M8700/0) — see also Neoplasm, by site, benign
malignant (M8700/3) — see Neoplasm, by site, malignant
Chromatopsia 368.59
Chromhidrosis, chromidrosis 705.89
Chromoblastomycosis 117.2
Chromomycosis 117.2
Chromophytosis 111.0
Chromotrichomycosis 111.8
Chronic — see condition
Chyle cyst, mesentery 457.8
Chylocele (nonfilarial) 457.8
filarial (see also Infestation, filarial) 125.9
tunica vaginalis (nonfilarial) 608.84
filarial (see also Infestation, filarial) 125.9
Chylomicronemia (fasting) (with hyperprebetalipoproteinemia) 272.3
Chylopericardium (acute) 420.90
Chylothorax (nonfilarial) 457.8
filarial (see also Infestation, filarial) 125.9
Chylous
ascites 457.8
cyst of peritoneum 457.8
hydrocele 603.9
hydrothorax (nonfilarial) 457.8
filarial (see also Infestation, filarial) 125.9
Chyluria 791.1
bilharziasis 120.0
due to
Brugia (malayi) 125.1
Wuchereria (bancrofti) 125.0
malayi 125.1
filarial (see also Infestation, filarial) 125.9
filariasis (see also Infestation, filarial) 125.9
nonfilarial 791.1
Cicatricial (deformity) — see Cicatrix
Cicatrix (adherent) (contracted) (painful) (vicious) 709.2
adenoid 474.8
alveolar process 525.8
anus 569.49
auricle 380.89
bile duct (see also Disease, biliary) 576.8
bladder 596.8
bone 733.99
brain 348.8
cervix (postoperative) (postpartal) 622.3
in pregnancy or childbirth 654.6
causing obstructed labor 660.2
chorioretinal 363.30
disseminated 363.35
macular 363.32

Cicatrix—continued
chorioretinal—continued
peripheral 363.34
posterior pole NEC 363.33
choroid — see Cicatrix, chorioretinal
common duct (see also Disease, biliary) 576.8
congenital 757.39
conjunctiva 372.64
cornea 371.00
tuberculous (see also Tuberculosis) 017.3 [371.05]
duodenum (bulb) 537.3
esophagus 530.3
eyelid 374.46
with
ectropion — see Ectropion
entropion — see Entropion
hypopharynx 478.29
knee, semilunar cartilage 717.5
lacrimal
canaliculi 375.53
duct
acquired 375.56
neonatal 375.55
punctum 375.52
sac 375.54
larynx 478.79
limbus (cystoid) 372.64
lung 518.89
macular 363.32
disseminated 363.35
peripheral 363.34
middle ear 385.89
mouth 528.9
muscle 728.89
nasolacrimal duct
acquired 375.56
neonatal 375.55
nasopharynx 478.29
palate (soft) 528.9
penis 607.89
prostate 602.8
rectum 569.49
retina 363.30
disseminated 363.35
macular 363.32
peripheral 363.34
posterior pole NEC 363.33
semilunar cartilage — see Derangement, meniscus
seminal vesicle 608.89
skin 709.2
infected 686.8
postinfectional 709.2
tuberculous (see also Tuberculosis) 017.0
specified site NEC 709.2
throat 478.29
tongue 529.8
tonsil (and adenoid) 474.8
trachea 478.9
tuberculous NEC (see also Tuberculosis) 011.9
ureter 593.89
urethra 599.84
uterus 621.8
vagina 623.4
in pregnancy or childbirth 654.7
causing obstructed labor 660.2
vocal cord 478.5
wrist, constricting (annular) 709.2
Cinchonism
correct substance properly administered 386.9
overdose or wrong substance given or taken 961.4
Circine herpes 110.5
Circle of Willis — see condition
Circular — see also condition
hymen 752.49
Circulating anticoagulants 286.5
following childbirth 666.3

Circulating anticoagulants—continued
postpartum 666.3
Circulation
collateral (venous), any site 459.89
defective 459.9
congenital 747.9
lower extremity 459.89
embryonic 747.9
failure 799.8
fetus or newborn 779.8
peripheral 785.59
fetal, persistence 747.9
heart, incomplete 747.9
Circulatory system — see condition
Circulus senilis 371.41
Circumcision
in absence of medical indication V50.2
ritual V50.2
routine V50.2
Circumscribed — see condition
Circumvallata placenta — see Placenta, abnormal
Cirrhosis, cirrhotic 571.5
with alcoholism 571.2
alcoholic (liver) 571.2
atrophic (of liver) — see Cirrhosis, portal
Baumgarten— Cruveilhier 571.5
biliary (cholangiolitic) (cholangitic) (cholestatic) (extrahepatic) (hypertrophic) (intrahepatic) (nonobstructive) (obstructive) (pericholangiolitic) (posthepatic) (primary) (secondary) (xanthomatous) 571.6
due to
clonorchiasis 121.1
flukes 121.3
brain 331.9
capsular — see Cirrhosis, portal
cardiac 571.5
alcoholic 571.2
central (liver) — see Cirrhosis, liver
Charcot's 571.6
cholangiolitic — see Cirrhosis, biliary
cholangitic — see Cirrhosis, biliary
cholestatic — see Cirrhosis, biliary
clitoris (hypertrophic) 624.2
coarsely nodular 571.5
congestive (liver) — see Cirrhosis, cardiac
Cruveilhier— Baumgarten 571.5
cryptogenic (of liver) 571.5
alcoholic 571.2
dietary (see also Cirrhosis, portal) 571.5
due to
bronzed diabetes 275.0
congestive hepatomegaly — see Cirrhosis, cardiac
cystic fibrosis 277.00
hemochromatosis 275.0
hepatolenticular degeneration 275.1
passive congestion (chronic) — see Cirrhosis, cardiac
Wilson's disease 275.1
xanthomatosis 272.2
extrahepatic (obstructive) — see Cirrhosis, biliary
fatty 571.8
alcoholic 571.0
florid 571.2
Glisson's — see Cirrhosis, portal
Hanot's (hypertrophic) — see Cirrhosis, biliary
hepatic — see Cirrhosis, liver
hepatolienal — see Cirrhosis, liver
hobnail — see Cirrhosis, portal
hypertrophic — see also Cirrhosis, liver
biliary — see Cirrhosis, biliary
Hanot's — see Cirrhosis, biliary

Cirrhosis, cirrhotic—continued
infectious NEC — see Cirrhosis, portal
insular — see Cirrhosis, portal
intrahepatic (obstructive) (primary) (secondary) — see Cirrhosis, biliary
juvenile (see also Cirrhosis, portal) 571.5
kidney (see also Sclerosis, renal) 587
Laennec's (of liver) 571.2
nonalcoholic 571.5
liver (chronic) (hepatolienal) (hypertrophic) (nodular) (splenomegalic) (unilobar) 571.5
with alcoholism 571.2
alcoholic 571.2
congenital (due to failure of obliteration of umbilical vein) 777.8
cryptogenic 571.5
alcoholic 571.2
fatty 571.8
alcoholic 571.0
macronodular 571.5
alcoholic 571.2
micronodular 571.5
alcoholic 571.2
nodular, diffuse 571.5
alcoholic 571.2
pigmentary 275.0
portal 571.5
alcoholic 571.2
postnecrotic 571.5
alcoholic 571.2
syphilitic 095.3
lung (chronic) (see also Fibrosis, lung) 515
macronodular (of liver) 571.5
alcoholic 571.2
malarial 084.9
metabolic NEC 571.5
micronodular (of liver) 571.5
alcoholic 571.2
monolobular — see Cirrhosis, portal
multilobular — see Cirrhosis, portal
nephritis (see also Sclerosis, renal) 587
nodular — see Cirrhosis, liver
nutritional (fatty) 571.5
obstructive (biliary) (extrahepatic) (intrahepatic) — see Cirrhosis, biliary
ovarian 620.8
paludal 084.9
pancreas (duct) 577.8
pericholangiolitic — see Cirrhosis, biliary
periportal — see Cirrhosis, portal
pigment, pigmentary (of liver) 275.0
portal (of liver) 571.5
alcoholic 571.2
posthepatitic (see also Cirrhosis, postnecrotic) 571.5
postnecrotic (of liver) 571.5
alcoholic 571.2
primary (intrahepatic) — see Cirrhosis, biliary
pulmonary (see also Fibrosis, lung) 515
renal (see also Sclerosis, renal) 587
septal (see also Cirrhosis, postnecrotic) 571.5
spleen 289.51
splenomegalic (of liver) — see Cirrhosis, liver
stasis (liver) — see Cirrhosis, liver
stomach 535.4
Todd's (see also Cirrhosis, biliary) 571.6
toxic (nodular) — see Cirrhosis, postnecrotic

Cirrhosis, cirrhotic — continued
  trabecular — see Cirrhosis, postnecrotic
  unilobar — see Cirrhosis, liver
  vascular (of liver) — see Cirrhosis, liver
  xanthomatous (biliary) (see also Cirrhosis, biliary) 571.6
    due to xanthomatosis (familial) (metabolic) (primary) 272.2
Cistern, subarachnoid 793.0
Citrullinemia 270.6
Citrullinuria 270.6
Ciuffini-Pancoast tumor (M8010/3) (carcinoma, pulmonary apex) 162.3
Civatte's disease or poikiloderma 709.09 ◆
Clam diggers' itch 120.3
Clap — see Gonorrhea
Clark's paralysis 343.9
Clarke-Hadfield syndrome (pancreatic infantilism) 577.8
Clastothrix 704.2
Claude's syndrome 352.6
Claude Bernard-Horner syndrome (see also Neuropathy, peripheral, autonomic) 337.9
Claudication, intermittent 443.9
  cerebral (artery) (see also Ischemia, cerebral, transient) 435.9
  due to atherosclerosis 440.21
  spinal cord (arteriosclerotic) 435.1
    syphilitic 094.89
  spinalis 435.1
  venous (axillary) 453.8
Claudicatio venosa intermittens 453.8
Claustrophobia 300.29
Clavus (infected) 700
Clawfoot (congenital) 754.71
  acquired 736.74
Clawhand (acquired) 736.06
  congenital 755.59
Clawtoe (congenital) 754.71
  acquired 735.5
Clay eating 307.52
Clay shovelers' fracture — see Fracture, vertebra, cervical
Cleansing of artificial opening (see also Attention to artificial opening) V55.9
Cleft (congenital) — see also Imperfect, closure
  alveolar process 525.8
  branchial (persistent) 744.41
    cyst 744.42
  clitoris 752.49
  cricoid cartilage, posterior 748.3
  facial (see also Cleft, lip) 749.10
  lip 749.10
    with cleft palate 749.20
      bilateral (lip and palate) 749.24
        with unilateral lip or palate 749.25
        complete 749.23
        incomplete 749.24
      unilateral (lip and palate) 749.22
        with bilateral lip or palate 749.25
        complete 749.21
        incomplete 749.22
    bilateral 749.14
      with cleft palate, unilateral 749.25
      complete 749.13
      incomplete 749.14
    unilateral 749.12
      with cleft palate, bilateral 749.25
      complete 749.11
      incomplete 749.12

Cleft — continued
  nose 748.1
  palate 749.00
    with cleft lip 749.20
      bilateral (lip and palate) 749.24
        with unilateral lip or palate 749.25
        complete 749.23
        incomplete 749.24
      unilateral (lip and palate) 749.22
        with bilateral lip or palate 749.25
        complete 749.21
        incomplete 749.22
    bilateral 749.04
      with cleft lip, unilateral 749.25
      complete 749.03
      incomplete 749.04
    unilateral 749.02
      with cleft lip, bilateral 749.25
      complete 749.01
      incomplete 749.02
  penis 752.8
  posterior, cricoid cartilage 748.3
  scrotum 752.8
  sternum (congenital) 756.3
  thyroid cartilage (congenital) 748.3
  tongue 750.13
  uvula 749.02
    with cleft lip (see also Cleft, lip, with cleft palate) 749.20
  water 366.12
Cleft hand (congenital) 755.58
Cleidocranial dysostosis 755.59
Cleidotomy, fetal 763.8
Cleptomania 312.32
Clérambault's syndrome 297.8
  erotomania 302.89
Clergyman's sore throat 784.49
Click, clicking
  systolic syndrome 785.2
Clifford's syndrome (postmaturity) 766.2
Climacteric (see also Menopause) 627.2
  arthritis NEC (see also Arthritis, climacteric) 716.3
  depression (see also Psychosis, affective) 296.2
  disease 627.2
    recurrent episode 296.3
    single episode 296.2
  female (symptoms) 627.2
  male (symptoms) (syndrome) 608.89
  melancholia (see also Psychosis, affective) 296.2
    recurrent episode 296.3
    single episode 296.2
  paranoid state 297.2
  paraphrenia 297.2
  polyarthritis NEC 716.39
    male 608.89
  symptoms (female) 627.2
Clinical research investigation V70.7
Clinodactyly 755.59
Clitoris — see condition
Cloaca, persistent 751.5
Clonorchiasis 121.1
Clonorchiosis 121.1
Clonorchis infection, liver 121.1
Clonus 781.0
Closed bite 524.2
Closure
  artificial opening (see also Attention to artificial opening) V55.9
  congenital, nose 748.0
  cranial sutures, premature 756.0
  defective or imperfect NEC — see Imperfect, closure

Closure — continued
  fistula, delayed — see Fistula
  fontanelle, delayed 756.0
  foramen ovale, imperfect 745.5
  hymen 623.3
  interauricular septum, defective 745.5
  interventricular septum, defective 745.4
  lacrimal duct 375.56
    congenital 743.65
    neonatal 375.55
  nose (congenital) 748.0
    acquired 738.0
  vagina 623.2
  valve — see Endocarditis
  vulva 624.8
Clot (blood)
  artery (obstruction) (occlusion) (see also Embolism) 444.9
  bladder 596.7
  brain (extradural or intradural) (see also Thrombosis, brain) 434.0
    late effects — see category 438
  circulation 444.9
  heart (see also Infarct, myocardium) 410.9
  vein (see also Thrombosis) 453.9
Clotting defect NEC (see also Defect, coagulation) 286.9
Clouded state 780.09
  epileptic (see also Epilepsy) 345.9
  paroxysmal (idiopathic) (see also Epilepsy) 345.9
Clouding
  corneal graft 996.51
Cloudy antrum, antra 473.0
Clouston's (hidrotic) ectodermal dysplasia 757.31
Clubbing of fingers 781.5
Clubfinger 736.29
  acquired 736.29
  congenital 754.89
Clubfoot (congenital) 754.70
  acquired 736.71
  equinovarus 754.51
  paralytic 736.71
Club hand (congenital) 754.89
  acquired 736.07
Clubnail (acquired) 703.8
  congenital 757.5
Clump kidney 753.3
Clumsiness 781.3
  syndrome 315.4
Cluttering 307.0
Clutton's joints 090.5
Coagulation, intravascular (diffuse) (disseminated) (see also Fibrinolysis) 286.6
  newborn 776.2
Coagulopathy (see also Defect, coagulation) 286.9
  consumption 286.6
  intravascular (disseminated) NEC 286.6
  newborn 776.2
Coalition
  calcaneoscaphoid 755.67
  calcaneus 755.67
  tarsal 755.67
Coal miners'
  elbow 727.2
  lung 500
Coal workers' lung or pneumoconiosis 500
Coarctation
  aorta (postductal) (preductal) 747.10
  pulmonary artery 747.3
Coated tongue 529.3
Coats' disease 362.12

Cocainism (see also Dependence) 304.2
Coccidioidal granuloma 114.3
Coccidioidomycosis 114.9
  with pneumonia 114.0
  cutaneous (primary) 114.1
  disseminated 114.3
  extrapulmonary (primary) 114.1
  lung 114.5
    acute 114.0
    chronic 114.4
    primary 114.0
  meninges 114.2
  primary (pulmonary) 114.0
    acute 114.0
  prostate 114.3
  pulmonary 114.5
    acute 114.0
    chronic 114.4
    primary 114.0
  specified site NEC 114.3
Coccidioidosis 114.9
  lung 114.5
    acute 114.0
    chronic 114.4
    primary 114.0
  meninges 114.2
Coccidiosis (colitis) (diarrhea) (dysentery) 007.2
Cocciuria 599.0
Coccus in urine 599.0
Coccydynia 724.79
Coccygodynia 724.79
Coccyx — see condition
Cochin-China
  diarrhea 579.1
    anguilluliasis 127.2
  ulcer 085.1
Cock's peculiar tumor 706.2
Cockayne's disease or syndrome (microcephaly and dwarfism) 759.89
Cockayne-Weber syndrome (epidermolysis bullosa) 757.39
Cocked-up toe 735.2
Codman's tumor (benign chondroblastoma) (M9230/0) — see Neoplasm, bone, benign
Coenurosis 123.8
Coffee workers' lung 495.8
Cogan's syndrome 370.52
  congenital oculomotor apraxia 379.51
  nonsyphilitic interstitial keratitis 370.52
Coiling, umbilical cord — see Complications, umbilical cord
Coitus, painful (female) 625.0
  male 608.89
  psychogenic 302.76
Cold 460
  with influenza, flu, or grippe 487.1
  abscess — see also Tuberculosis, abscess
    articular — see Tuberculosis, joint
  agglutinin
    disease (chronic) or syndrome 283.0
    hemoglobinuria 283.0
      paroxysmal (cold) (nocturnal) 283.2
  allergic (see also Fever, hay) 477.9
  bronchus or chest — see Bronchitis
    with grippe or influenza 487.1
  common (head) 460
    vaccination, prophylactic (against) V04.7
  deep 464.10
  effects of 991.9
    specified effect NEC 991.8
  excessive 991.9
    specified effect NEC 991.8

Cold—*continued*
  exhaustion from 991.8
  exposure to 991.9
    specified effect NEC 991.8
  grippy 487.1
  head 460
  injury syndrome (newborn) 778.2
  on lung — *see* Bronchitis
  rose 477.0
  sensitivity, autoimmune 283.0
  virus 460
Coldsore (*see also* Herpes, simplex) 054.9
Colibacillosis 041.4
  generalized 038.42
Colibacilluria 599.0
Colic (recurrent) 789.0
  abdomen 789.0
    psychogenic 307.89
  appendicular 543.9
  appendix 543.9
  bile duct — *see* Choledocholithiasis
  biliary — *see* Cholelithiasis
  bilious — *see* Cholelithiasis
  common duct — *see* Choledocholithiasis
  Devonshire NEC 984.9
    specified type of lead — *see* Table of drugs and chemicals
  flatulent 787.3
  gallbladder or gallstone — *see* Cholelithiasis
  gastric 536.8
  hepatic (duct) — *see* Choledocholithiasis
  hysterical 300.11
  infantile 789.0
  intestinal 789.0
  kidney 788.0
  lead NEC 984.9
    specified type of lead — *see* Table of drugs and chemicals
  liver (duct) — *see* Choledocholithiasis
  mucous 564.1
    psychogenic 316 [564.1]
  nephritic 788.0
  painter's NEC 984.9
  pancreas 577.8
  psychogenic 306.4
  renal 788.0
  saturnine NEC 984.9
    specified type of lead — *see* Table of drugs and chemicals
  spasmodic 789.0
  ureter 788.0
  urethral 599.84
    due to calculus 594.2
  uterus 625.8
    menstrual 625.3
  vermicular 543.9
  virus 460
  worm NEC 128.9
Colicystitis (*see also* Cystitis) 595.9
Colitis (acute) (catarrhal) (croupous) (cystica superficialis) (exudative) (hemorrhagic) (noninfectious) (phlegmonous) (presumed noninfectious) 558.9
  adaptive 564.1
  allergic 558.9
  amebic (*see also* Amebiasis) 006.9
    nondysenteric 006.2
  anthrax 022.2
  bacillary (*see also* Infection, Shigella) 004.9
  balantidial 007.0
  chronic 558.9
    ulcerative (*see also* Colitis, ulcerative) 556.9 ◆
  coccidial 007.2
  dietetic 558.9

Colitis—*continued*
  due to radiation 558.1
  functional 558.9
  gangrenous 009.0
  giardial 007.1
  granulomatous 555.1
  gravis (*see also* Colitis, ulcerative) 556.9 ◆
  infectious (*see also* Enteritis, due to, specific organism) 009.0
    presumed 009.1
  ischemic 557.9
    acute 557.0
    chronic 557.1
    due to mesenteric artery insufficiency 557.1
  membranous 564.1
    psychogenic 316 [564.1]
  mucous 564.1
    psychogenic 316 [564.1]
  necrotic 009.0
  polyposa (*see also* Colitis, ulcerative) 556.9 ◆
  protozoal NEC 007.9
  pseudomembranous 008.45
  pseudomucinous 564.1
  regional 555.1
  segmental 555.1
  septic (*see also* Enteritis, due to, specific organism) 009.0
  spastic 564.1
    psychogenic 316 [564.1]
  staphylococcus 008.41
    food 005.0
  thromboulcerative 557.0
  toxic 558.2
  transmural 555.1
  trichomonal 007.3
  tuberculous (ulcerative) 014.8
  ulcerative (chronic) (idiopathic) (nonspecific) 556.9 ▼
    entero- 556.0 ▲
    fulminant 557.0
    Ileo- 556.1 ▼
    left-sided 556.5
    procto- 556.2
    proctosigmoid 556.3 ▲
    psychogenic 316 [556]
    specified NEC 556.8 ▼
    universal 556.6 ▲
Collagen disease NEC 710.9
  nonvascular 710.9
  vascular (allergic) (*see also* Angiitis, hypersensitivity) 446.20
Collagenosis (*see also* Collagen disease) 710.9
  cardiovascular 425.4
  mediastinal 519.3
Collapse 780.2
  adrenal 255.8
  cardiorenal (*see also* Hypertension, cardiorenal) 404.90
  cardiorespiratory 785.51
    fetus or newborn 779.8
  cardiovascular (*see also* Disease, heart) 785.51
    fetus or newborn 779.8
  circulatory (peripheral) 785.59
    with
      abortion — *see* Abortion, by type, with shock
      ectopic pregnancy (*see also* categories 633.0-633.9) 639.5
      molar pregnancy (*see also* categories 630-632) 639.5
    during or after labor and delivery 669.1
    fetus or newborn 779.8
    following
      abortion 639.5
      ectopic or molar pregnancy 639.5
    during or after labor and delivery 669.1
    fetus or newborn 779.8

Collapse—*continued*
  external ear canal 380.50
    secondary to
      inflammation 380.53
      surgery 380.52
      trauma 380.51
  general 780.2
  heart — *see* Disease, heart
  heat 992.1
  hysterical 300.11
  labyrinth, membranous (congenital) 744.05
  lung (massive) (*see also* Atelectasis) 518.0
    pressure, during labor 668.0
  myocardial — *see* Disease, heart
  nervous (*see also* Disorder, mental, nonpsychotic) 300.9
  neurocirculatory 306.2
  nose 738.0
  postoperative (cardiovascular) 998.0
  pulmonary (*see also* Atelectasis) 518.0
    fetus or newborn 770.5
      partial 770.5
      primary 770.4
  thorax 512.8
    iatrogenic 512.1 ▼
    postoperative 512.1 ▲
  trachea 519.1
  valvular — *see* Endocarditis
  vascular (peripheral) 785.59
    with
      abortion — *see* Abortion, by type, with shock
      ectopic pregnancy (*see also* categories 633.0-633.9) 639.5
      molar pregnancy (*see also* categories 630-632) 639.5
    cerebral (*see also* Disease, cerebrovascular, acute) 436
    during or after labor and delivery 669.1
    fetus or newborn 779.8
    following
      abortion 639.5
      ectopic or molar pregnancy 639.5
  vasomotor 785.59
  vertebra 733.13
Collateral — *see also* condition
  circulation (venous) 459.89
  dilation, veins 459.89
Colles' fracture (closed) (reversed) (separation) 813.41
  open 813.51
Collet's syndrome 352.6
Collet-Sicard syndrome 352.6
Colliculitis urethralis (*see also* Urethritis) 597.89
Colliers'
  asthma 500
  lung 500
  phthisis (*see also* Tuberculosis) 011.4
Collodion baby (ichthyosis congenita) 757.1
Colloid milium 709.3
Coloboma NEC 743.49
  choroid 743.59
  fundus 743.52
  iris 743.46
  lens 743.36
  lids 743.62
  optic disc (congenital) 743.57
    acquired 377.23
  retina 743.56
  sclera 743.47
Coloenteritis — *see* Enteritis
Colon — *see* condition
Coloptosis 569.89

Color
  amblyopia NEC 368.59
    acquired 368.55
  blindness NEC (congenital) 368.59
    acquired 368.55
Colostomy
  attention to V55.3
  fitting or adjustment V53.5
  malfunctioning 569.6
  status V44.3
Colpitis (*see also* Vaginitis) 616.10
Colpocele 618.6
Colpocystitis (*see also* Vaginitis) 616.10
Colporrhexis 665.4
Colpospasm 625.1
Column, spinal, vertebral — *see* condition
Coma 780.01
  apoplectic (*see also* Disease, cerebrovascular, acute) 436
  diabetic (with ketoacidosis) 250.3
    hyperosmolar 250.2
  eclamptic (*see also* Eclampsia) 780.3
  epileptic 345.3
  hepatic 572.2
  hyperglycemic 250.2
  hyperosmolar (diabetic) (nonketotic) 250.2
  hypoglycemic 251.0
    diabetic 250.3
  insulin 251.3
    non-diabetic 251.0
    organic hyperinsulinism 251.0
  Kussmaul's (diabetic) 250.3
  liver 572.2
  newborn 779.2
  prediabetic 250.2
  uremic — *see* Uremia
Combat fatigue (*see also* Reaction, stress, acute) 308.9
Combined — *see* condition
Comedo 706.1
Comedocarcinoma (M8501/3) — *see also* Neoplasm, breast, malignant
  noninfiltrating (M8501/2)
    specified site — *see* Neoplasm, by site, in situ
    unspecified site 233.0
Comedomastitis 610.4
Comedones 706.1
  lanugo 757.4
Comma bacillus, carrier (suspected) of V02.3
Comminuted fracture — *see* Fracture, by site
Common
  aortopulmonary trunk 745.0
  atrioventricular canal (defect) 745.69
  atrium 745.69
  cold (head) 460
    vaccination, prophylactic (against) V04.7
  truncus (arteriosus) 745.0
  ventricle 745.3
Commotio (current)
  cerebri (*see also* Concussion, brain) 850.9
    with skull fracture — *see* Fracture, skull, by site
  retinae 921.3
  spinalis — *see* Injury, spinal, by site
Commotion (current)
  brain (without skull fracture) (*see also* Concussion, brain) 850.9
    with skull fracture — *see* Fracture, skull, by site
  spinal cord — *see* Injury, spinal, by site

Communication

Communication
- abnormal — *see also* Fistula
  - between
    - base of aorta and pulmonary artery 745.0
    - left ventricle and right atrium 745.4
    - pericardial sac and pleural sac 748.8
    - pulmonary artery and pulmonary vein 747.3
    - congenital, between uterus and anterior abdominal wall 752.3
      - bladder 752.3
      - intestine 752.3
      - rectum 752.3
  - left ventricular— right atrial 745.4
  - pulmonary artery— pulmonary vein 747.3

Compensation
- broken — *see* Failure, heart, congestive
- failure — *see* Failure, heart, congestive
- neurosis, psychoneurosis 300.11

Complaint — *see also* Disease
- bowel, functional 564.9
  - psychogenic 306.4
- intestine, functional 564.9
  - psychogenic 306.4
- kidney (*see also* Disease, renal) 593.9
- liver 573.9
- miners' 500

Complete — *see* condition

Complex
- cardiorenal (*see also* Hypertension, cardiorenal) 404.90
- castration 300.9
- Costen's 524.60
- ego-dystonic homosexuality 302.0
- Eisenmenger's (ventricular septal defect) 745.4
- homosexual, ego-dystonic 302.0
- hypersexual 302.89
- inferiority 301.9
- jumped process
  - spine — *see* Dislocation, vertebra
- primary, tuberculosis (*see also* Tuberculosis) 010.0
- Taussig-Bing (transposition, aorta and overriding pulmonary artery) 745.11

Complications
- abortion NEC — *see* categories 634-639
- accidental puncture or laceration during a procedure 998.2
- amputation stump (late) (surgical) 997.60
  - traumatic — *see* Amputation, traumatic
- anastomosis (and bypass) NEC — *see also* Complications, due to (presence of) any device, implant, or graft classified to 996.0-996.5 NEC
  - hemorrhage NEC 998.1
  - intestinal (internal) NEC 997.4
    - involving urinary tract 997.5
  - mechanical — *see* Complications, mechanical, graft
  - urinary tract (involving intestinal tract) 997.5
- anesthesia, anesthetic NEC (*see also* Anesthesia, complication) 995.2
  - in labor and delivery 668.9
    - affecting fetus or newborn 763.5
    - cardiac 668.1
    - central nervous system 668.2
    - pulmonary 668.0
    - specified type NEC 668.8

INDEX TO DISEASES

Complications—*continued*
- aortocoronary (bypass) graft 996.03
  - atherosclerosis — *see* Arteriosclerosis, coronary ▼
  - embolism 996.72
  - occlusion NEC 996.72
  - thrombus 996.72 ▲
- arthroplasty 996.4
- artificial opening
  - cecostomy 569.6
  - colostomy 569.6
  - cystostomy 997.5
  - enterostomy 569.6
  - gastrostomy 997.4
  - ileostomy 569.6
  - jejunostomy 569.6
  - nephrostomy 997.5
  - tracheostomy 519.0
  - ureterostomy 997.5
  - urethrostomy 997.5
- bile duct implant (prosthetic) NEC 996.79
  - infection or inflammation 996.69
  - mechanical 996.59
- bleeding (intraoperative) (postoperative) 998.1
- blood vessel graft 996.1
  - aortocoronary 996.03
    - atherosclerosis — *see* Arteriosclerosis, coronary ▼
    - embolism 996.72
    - occlusion NEC 996.72
    - thrombus 996.72
  - atherosclerosis — *see* Arteriosclerosis, extremities
  - embolism 996.74
  - occlusion NEC 996.74
  - thrombus 996.74 ▲
- bone growth stimulator 996.78
  - infection or inflammation 996.67
- bone marrow transplant 996.85
- breast implant (prosthetic) NEC 996.79
  - infection or inflammation 996.69
  - mechanical 996.54
- bypass — *see also* Complications, anastomosis
  - aortocoronary 996.03
    - atherosclerosis — *see* Arteriosclerosis, coronary ▼
    - embolism 996.72
    - occlusion NEC 996.72
    - thrombus 996.72 ▲
  - carotid artery 996.1
    - atherosclerosis — *see* Arteriosclerosis, extremities ▼
    - embolism 996.74
    - occlusion NEC 996.74
    - thrombus 996.74 ▲
- cardiac (*see also* Disease, heart) 429.9
  - device, implant, or graft NEC 996.72
    - infection or inflammation 996.61
    - long-term effect 429.4
    - mechanical (*see also* Complications, mechanical, by type) 996.00
    - valve prosthesis 996.71
      - infection or inflammation 996.61
  - postoperative NEC 997.1
    - long-term effect 429.4
- cardiorenal (*see also* Hypertension, cardiorenal) 404.90

Complications—*continued*
- carotid artery bypass graft 996.1
  - atherosclerosis — *see* Arteriosclerosis, extremities ▼
  - embolism 996.74
  - occlusion NEC 996.74
  - thrombus 996.74
- cataract fragments in eye 998.82 ▲
- catheter device NEC — *see also* Complications, due to (presence of) any device, implant, or graft classified to 996.0-996.5 NEC
  - mechanical — *see* Complications, mechanical, catheter
- cecostomy 569.6
- cesarean section wound 674.3
- chin implant (prosthetic) NEC 996.79
  - infection or inflammation 996.69
  - mechanical 996.59
- colostomy (enterostomy) 569.6
- contraceptive device, intrauterine NEC 996.76
  - infection 996.65
  - inflammation 996.65
  - mechanical 996.32
- cord (umbilical) — *see* Complications, umbilical cord
- cornea ▼
  - due to
    - contact lens 371.82 ▲
- coronary (artery) bypass (graft) NEC 996.03
  - atherosclerosis — *see* Arteriosclerosis, coronary ▼
  - embolism 996.72 ▲
  - infection or inflammation 996.61
  - mechanical 996.03
  - occlusion NEC 996.72 ◆
  - specified type NEC 996.72
  - thrombus 996.72
- cystostomy 997.5
- delivery 669.9
  - procedure (instrumental) (manual) (surgical) 669.4
  - specified type NEC 669.8
- dialysis (hemodialysis) (peritoneal) (renal) 999.9
  - catheter NEC — *see also* Complications, due to (presence of) any device, implant or graft classified to 996.0-996.5 NEC
    - infection or inflammation 996.62
    - peritoneal 996.69 ◆
    - mechanical 996.1
    - peritoneal 996.69 ◆
- due to (presence of) any device, implant, or graft classified to 996.0-996.5 NEC 996.70
  - with infection or inflammation — *see* Complications, infection or inflammation, due to (presence of) any device, implant, or graft classified to 996.0-996.5 NEC
  - arterial NEC 996.74
    - coronary NEC 996.03
      - atherosclerosis — *see* Arteriosclerosis, coronary ▼
      - embolism 996.72
      - occlusion NEC 996.72 ▲
      - specified type NEC 996.72
      - thrombus 996.72
      - renal dialysis 996.73
    - arteriovenous fistula or shunt NEC 996.74

Complications

Complications—*continued*
- due to—*continued*
  - bone growth stimulator 996.78
  - breast NEC 996.70
  - cardiac NEC 996.72
    - defibrillator 996.72
    - pacemaker 996.72
    - valve prosthesis 996.71
  - catheter NEC 996.79
    - spinal 996.75
    - urinary, indwelling 996.76
    - vascular NEC 996.74
      - renal dialysis 996.73
    - ventricular shunt 996.75
  - coronary (artery) bypass (graft) NEC 996.03
    - atherosclerosis — *see* Arteriosclerosis, coronary ▼
    - embolism 996.72
    - occlusion NEC 996.72 ▲
    - thrombus 996.72
  - electrodes
    - brain 996.75
    - heart 996.72
  - gastrointestinal NEC 996.79
  - genitourinary NEC 996.76
  - heart valve prosthesis NEC 996.71
  - infusion pump 996.74
  - internal
    - joint prosthesis 996.77
    - orthopedic NEC 996.78
    - specified type NEC 996.79
  - intrauterine contraceptive device NEC 996.76
  - joint prosthesis, internal NEC 996.77
  - mechanical — *see* Complications, mechanical
  - nervous system NEC 996.75
  - ocular lens NEC 996.79
  - orbital NEC 996.79
  - orthopedic NEC 996.78
    - joint, internal 996.77
  - renal dialysis 996.73
  - specified type NEC 996.79
  - urinary catheter, indwelling 996.76
  - vascular NEC 996.74
  - ventricular shunt 996.75
- during dialysis NEC 999.9
- ectopic or molar pregnancy NEC 639.9
- electroshock therapy NEC 999.9
- enterostomy 569.6
- external (fixation) device with internal component(s) NEC 996.78
  - infection or inflammation 996.67
  - mechanical 996.4
- extracorporeal circulation NEC 999.9
- eye implant (prosthetic) NEC 996.79
  - infection or inflammation 996.69
  - mechanical
    - ocular lens 996.53
    - orbital globe 996.59
- gastrointestinal, postoperative NEC (*see also* Complications, surgical procedures) 997.4
- gastrostomy 997.4
- genitourinary device, implant or graft NEC 996.76
  - infection or inflammation 996.65
  - urinary catheter, indwelling 996.64
  - mechanical (*see also* Complications, mechanical, by type) 996.30
  - specified NEC 996.39

Complications—continued
  graft (bypass) (patch) NEC — see also Complications, due to (presence of) any device, implant, or graft classified to 996.0-996.5 NEC
    bone marrow 996.85
    corneal NEC 996.79
      infection or inflammation 996.69
      rejection or reaction 996.51
      mechanical — see Complications, mechanical, graft
    organ (immune or nonimmune cause) (partial) (total) 996.80
      bone marrow 996.85
      heart 996.83
      intestines 996.89
      kidney 996.81
      liver 996.82
      lung 996.84
      pancreas 996.86
      specified NEC 996.89
    skin NEC 996.79
      infection or inflammation 996.69
      rejection 996.52
    heart — see also Disease, heart transplant (immune or nonimmune cause) 996.83
  hemorrhage (intraoperative) (postoperative) 998.1
  hyperalimentation therapy NEC 999.9
  immunization (procedure) — see Complications, vaccination
  implant NEC — see also Complications, due to (presence of) any device, implant, or graft classified to 996.0-996.5 NEC
    mechanical — see Complications, mechanical, implant
  infection and inflammation due to (presence of) any device, implant or graft classified to 996.0-996.5 NEC 996.60
    arterial NEC 996.62
      coronary 996.61
      renal dialysis 996.62
    arteriovenous fistula or shunt 996.62
    bone growth stimulator 996.67
    breast 996.69
    cardiac 996.61
    catheter NEC 996.69
      peritoneal 996.69
      spinal 996.63
      urinary, indwelling 996.64
      vascular NEC 996.62
      ventricular shunt 996.63
    coronary artery bypass 996.61
    electrodes
      brain 996.63
      heart 996.61
    gastrointestinal NEC 996.69
    genitourinary NEC 996.65
      indwelling urinary catheter 996.64
    heart valve 996.61
    infusion pump 996.62
    intrauterine contraceptive device 996.65
    joint prosthesis, internal 996.66
    ocular lens 996.69
    orbital (implant) 996.69
    orthopedic NEC 996.67
      joint, internal 996.66
    specified type NEC 996.69

Complications—continued
  infection and inflammation—continued
    due to any device, implant or graft classified to 996.0-996.5—continued
      urinary catheter, indwelling 996.64
      ventricular shunt 996.63
  infusion (procedure) 999.9
    blood — see Complications, transfusion
    infection NEC 999.3
    sepsis NEC 999.3
  inhalation therapy NEC 999.9
  injection (procedure) 999.9
    drug reaction (see also Reaction, drug) 995.2
    infection NEC 999.3
    sepsis NEC 999.3
    serum (prophylactic) (therapeutic) — see Complications, vaccination
    vaccine (any) — see Complications, vaccination
  inoculation (any) — see Complications, vaccination
  internal device (catheter) (electronic) (fixation) (prosthetic) NEC — see also Complications, due to (presence of) any device, implant, or graft classified to 996.0-996.5 NEC
    mechanical — see Complications, mechanical
  intestinal transplant (immune or nonimmune cause) 996.89
  intraoperative bleeding or hemorrhage 998.1
  intrauterine contraceptive device 996.76 — see also Complications, contraceptive device
    with fetal damage affecting management of pregnancy 655.8
    infection or inflammation 996.65
  jejunostomy 569.6
  kidney transplant (immune or nonimmune cause) 996.81
  labor 669.9
    specified condition NEC 669.8
  liver transplant (immune or nonimmune cause) 996.82
  lumbar puncture 349.0
  mechanical
    anastomosis — see Complications, mechanical, graft
    bypass — see Complications, mechanical, graft
    catheter NEC 996.59
      cardiac 996.09
      cystostomy 996.39
      dialysis 996.1
      during a procedure 998.2
      urethral, indwelling 996.31
    device NEC 996.59
      balloon (counterpulsation), intra-aortic 996.1
      cardiac 996.00
        long-term effect 429.4
        specified NEC 996.09
      contraceptive, intrauterine 996.32
      counterpulsation, intra-aortic 996.1
      fixation, external, with internal components 996.4
      fixation, internal (nail, rod, plate) 996.4

Complications—continued
  mechanical—continued
    device—continued
      genitourinary 996.30
        specified NEC 996.39
      nervous system 996.2
      orthopedic, internal 996.4
      prosthetic NEC 996.59
      umbrella, vena cava 996.1
      vascular 996.1
    dorsal column stimulator 996.2
    electrode NEC 996.59
      brain 996.2
      cardiac 996.01
      spinal column 996.2
    fistula, arteriovenous, surgically created 996.1
    graft NEC 996.52
      aortic (bifurcation) 996.1
      aortocoronary bypass 996.03
      blood vessel NEC 996.1
      bone 996.4
      cardiac 996.00
      carotid artery bypass 996.1
      cartilage 996.4
      corneal 996.51
      coronary bypass 996.03
      genitourinary 996.30
        specified NEC 996.39
      muscle 996.4
      nervous system 996.2
      organ (immune or nonimmune cause) 996.80
        heart 996.83
        intestines 996.89
        kidney 996.81
        liver 996.82
        lung 996.84
        pancreas 996.86
        specified NEC 996.89
      orthopedic, internal 996.4
      peripheral nerve 996.2
      prosthetic NEC 996.59
      skin 996.52
      specified NEC 996.59
      tendon 996.4
      tissue NEC 996.52
      tooth 996.59
      ureter, without mention of resection 996.39
      vascular 996.1
    heart valve prosthesis 996.02
      long-term effect 429.4
    implant NEC 996.59
      cardiac 996.00
        long-term effect 429.4
        specified NEC 996.09
      electrode NEC 996.59
        brain 996.2
        cardiac 996.01
        spinal column 996.2
      genitourinary 996.30
      nervous system 996.2
      orthopedic, internal 996.4
      prosthetic NEC 996.59
      in
        bile duct 996.59
        breast 996.54
        chin 996.59
        eye
          ocular lens 996.53
          orbital globe 996.59
      vascular 996.1
    nonabsorbable surgical material 996.59
    pacemaker NEC 996.59
      brain 996.2
      cardiac 996.01
      nerve (phrenic) 996.2
    patch — see Complications, mechanical, graft
    prosthesis NEC 996.59
      bile duct 996.59
      breast 996.54
      chin 996.59

Complications—continued
  mechanical—continued
    prosthesis—continued
      ocular lens 996.53
      reconstruction, vas deferens 996.39
      reimplant NEC 996.59
        extremity (see also Complications, reattached, extremity) 996.90
        organ (see also Complications, transplant, organ, by site) 996.80
      repair — see Complications, mechanical, graft
      shunt NEC 996.59
        arteriovenous, surgically created 996.1
        ventricular (communicating) 996.2
      stent NEC 996.59
      vas deferens reconstruction 996.39
    medical care NEC 999.9
      cardiac NEC 997.1
      gastrointestinal NEC 997.4
      nervous system NEC 997.0
      peripheral vascular NEC 997.2
      respiratory NEC 997.3
      urinary NEC 997.5
    nephrostomy 997.5
    nervous system
      device, implant, or graft NEC 349.1
      mechanical 996.2
      postoperative NEC 997.0
    obstetric 669.9
      procedure (instrumental) (manual) (surgical) 669.4
      specified NEC 669.8
      surgical wound 674.3
    ocular lens implant NEC 996.79
      infection or inflammation 996.69
      mechanical 996.53
    organ transplant — see Complications, transplant, organ, by site
    orthopedic device, implant, or graft
      internal (fixation) (nail) (plate) (rod) NEC 996.78
        infection or inflammation 996.67
        joint prosthesis 996.77
          infection or inflammation 996.66
        mechanical 996.4
    pacemaker (cardiac) 996.72
      infection or inflammation 996.61
      mechanical 996.01
    pancreas transplant (immune or nonimmune cause) 996.86
    perfusion NEC 999.9
    perineal repair (obstetrical) 674.3
      disruption 674.2
    pessary (uterus) (vagina) — see Complications, contraceptive device
    phototherapy 990
    postcystoscopic 997.5
    postmastoidectomy NEC 383.30
    postoperative — see Complications, surgical procedures
    pregnancy NEC 646.9
      affecting fetus or newborn 761.9
    prosthetic device, internal NEC — see also Complications, due to (presence of) any device, implant or graft classified to 996.0-996.5 NEC
      mechanical NEC (see also Complications, mechanical) 996.59

Complications—*continued*
  puerperium NEC (*see also*
       Puerperal) 674.9
  puncture, spinal 349.0
  pyelogram 997.5
  radiation 990
  radiotherapy 990
  reattached
    body part, except extremity
         996.99
    extremity (infection) (rejection)
         996.90
      arm(s) 996.94
      digit(s) (hand) 996.93
         foot 996.95
      finger(s) 996.93
      foot 996.95
      forearm 996.91
      hand 996.92
      leg 996.96
      lower NEC 996.96
      toe(s) 996.95
      upper NEC 996.94
  reimplant NEC — *see also*
       Complications, to (presence
       of) any device, implant, or
       graft classified to 996.0-
       996.5 NEC
    bone marrow 996.85
    extremity (*see also*
         Complications,
         reattached, extremity)
         996.90
      due to infection 996.90
    mechanical — *see*
         Complications,
         mechanical, reimplant
    organ (immune or nonimmune
         cause) (partial) (total) (*see
         also* Complications,
         transplant, organ, by site)
         996.80
    renal allograft 996.81
  renal dialysis — *see* Complications,
       dialysis
  respiratory 519.9
    device, implant or graft NEC
         996.79
      infection or inflammation
           996.69
      mechanical 996.59
    distress syndrome, adult,
         following trauma or
         surgery 518.5
    insufficiency, acute,
         postoperative 518.5
    postoperative NEC 997.3
    therapy NEC 999.9
  sedation during labor and delivery
       668.9
    affecting fetus or newborn 763.5
    cardiac 668.1
    central nervous system 668.2
    pulmonary 668.0
    specified type NEC 668.8
  shunt NEC — *see also*
       Complications, due to
       (presence of) any device,
       implant, or graft classified to
       996.0-996.5 NEC
    mechanical — *see*
         Complications,
         mechanical, shunt
  specified body system NEC
    device, implant, or graft NEC —
         see Complications, due to
         (presence of) any device,
         implant, or graft classified
         to 996.0-996.5 NEC
    postoperative NEC 997.9
  spinal puncture or tap 349.0
  stoma, external
    gastrointestinal tract NEC 997.4
    urinary tract 997.5
  surgical procedures 998.9
    accidental puncture or
         laceration 998.2

Complications—*continued*
  surgical procedures—*continued*
    amputation stump (late) 997.60
    anastomosis — *see*
         Complications,
         anastomosis
    burst stitches or sutures 998.3
    cardiac 997.1
      long-term effect following
           cardiac surgery 429.4
    cataract fragments in eye
         998.82 ◆
    catheter device — *see*
         Complications, catheter
         device
    cecostomy malfunction 569.6
    colostomy malfunction 569.6
    cystostomy malfunction 997.5
    dehiscence (of incision) 998.3
    dialysis NEC (*see also*
         Complications, dialysis)
         999.9
    disruption
      anastomosis (internal) — *see*
           Complications,
           mechanical, graft
      internal suture (line) 998.3
      wound 998.3
    dumping syndrome
         (postgastrectomy) 564.2
    elephantiasis or lymphedema
         997.9
      postmastectomy 457.0
    emphysema (surgical) 998.81 ◆
    enterostomy malfunction 569.6
    evisceration 998.3
    fistula (persistent postoperative)
         998.6
    foreign body inadvertently left in
         wound (sponge) (suture)
         (swab) 998.4
      from nonabsorbable surgical
           material (Dacron) (mesh)
           (permanent suture)
           (reinforcing) (Teflon) —
           see Complications, due to
           (presence of) any device,
           implant, or graft classified
           to 996.0-996.5 NEC
    gastrointestinal NEC 997.4
    gastrostomy malfunction 997.4
    hemorrhage or hematoma 998.1
    ileostomy malfunction 569.6
    internal prosthetic device NEC
         (*see also* Complications,
         internal device) 996.70
      hemolytic anemia 283.19
      infection or inflammation
           996.60
      malfunction — *see*
           Complications,
           mechanical
      mechanical complication —
           see Complications,
           mechanical
      thrombus 996.70
    jejunostomy malfunction 569.6
    malfunction of colostomy or
         enterostomy 569.6
    nervous system NEC 997.0
    obstruction, internal
      anastomosis — *see*
           Complications,
           mechanical, graft
    other body system NEC 997.9
    peripheral vascular NEC 997.2
    postcardiotomy syndrome 429.4
    postcholecystectomy syndrome
         576.0
    postcommissurotomy syndrome
         429.4
    postgastrectomy dumping
         syndrome 564.2
    postmastectomy lymphedema
         syndrome 457.0

Complications—*continued*
  surgical procedures—*continued*
    postmastoidectomy 383.30
      cholesteatoma, recurrent
           383.32
      cyst, mucosal 383.31
      granulation 383.33
      inflammation, chronic
           383.33
    postvagotomy syndrome 564.2
    postvalvulotomy syndrome
         429.4
    reattached extremity (infection)
         (rejection) (*see also*
         Complications,
         reattached, extremity)
         996.90
    respiratory NEC 997.3
    shock (endotoxic) (hypovolemic)
         (septic) 998.0
    shunt, prosthetic (thrombus) —
         see also Complications,
         due to (presence of) any
         device, implant, or graft
         classified to 996.0-996.5
         NEC
      hemolytic anemia 283.19
    specified complication NEC
         998.89 ◆
    stitch abscess 998.5
    transplant — *see* Complications,
         graft
    ureterostomy malfunction 997.5
    urethrostomy malfunction 997.5
    urinary NEC 997.5
    wound infection 998.5
  therapeutic misadventure NEC
       999.9
    surgical treatment 998.9
  tracheostomy 519.0
  transfusion (blood) (lymphocytes)
       (plasma) NEC 999.8
    atrophy, liver, yellow, subacute
         (within 8 months of
         administration) — *see*
         Hepatitis, viral
    bone marrow 996.85
    embolism
      air 999.1
      thrombus 999.2
    hemolysis NEC 999.8
      bone marrow 996.85
    hepatitis (serum) (type B) (within
         8 months after
         administration) — *see*
         Hepatitis, viral
    incompatibility reaction (ABO)
         (blood group) 999.6
      Rh (factor) 999.7
    infection 999.3
    jaundice (serum) (within 8
         months after
         administration) — *see*
         Hepatitis, viral
    sepsis 999.3
    shock or reaction NEC 999.8
      bone marrow 996.85
    subacute yellow atrophy of liver
         (within 8 months after
         administration) — *see*
         Hepatitis, viral
    thromboembolism 999.2
  transplant NEC — *see also*
       Complications, due to
       (presence of) any device,
       implant, or graft classified to
       996.0-996.5 NEC
    bone marrow 996.85
    organ (immune or nonimmune
         cause) (partial) (total)
         996.80
      bone marrow 996.85
      heart 996.83
      intestines 996.89
      kidney 996.81
      liver 996.82
      lung 996.84

Complications—*continued*
  transplant—*continued*
    organ—*continued*
      pancreas 996.86
      specified NEC 996.89
    trauma NEC (early) 958.8
    ultrasound therapy NEC 999.9
  umbilical cord
    affecting fetus or newborn 762.6
    complicating delivery 663.9
      affecting fetus or newborn
           762.6
    specified type NEC 663.8
  urethral catheter NEC 996.76
    infection or inflammation
         996.64
    mechanical 996.31
  urinary, postoperative NEC 997.5
  vaccination 999.9
    anaphylaxis NEC 999.4
    cellulitis 999.3
    encephalitis or
         encephalomyelitis 323.5
    hepatitis (serum) (type B) (within
         8 months after
         administration) — *see*
         Hepatitis, viral
    infection (general) (local) NEC
         999.3
    jaundice (serum) (within 8
         months after
         administration) — *see*
         Hepatitis, viral
    meningitis 997.0 *[321.8]*
    myelitis 323.5
    protein sickness 999.5
    reaction (allergic) 999.5
      Herxheimer's 995.0
    serum 999.5
    sepsis 999.3
    serum intoxication, sickness,
         rash, or other serum
         reaction NEC 999.5
    shock (allergic) (anaphylactic)
         999.4
    subacute yellow atrophy of liver
         (within 8 months after
         administration) — *see*
         Hepatitis, viral
    vaccinia (generalized) 999.0
      localized 999.3
  vascular
    device, implant, or graft NEC
         996.74
      infection or inflammation
           996.62
      mechanical NEC 996.1
         cardiac (*see also*
              Complications,
              mechanical, by
              type) 996.00
    following infusion, perfusion, or
         transfusion 999.2
    postoperative NEC 997.2
  ventilation therapy NEC 999.9

**Compound presentation, complicating
  delivery** 652.8
  causing obstructed labor 660.0
Compressed air disease 993.3
Compression
  with injury — *see* specific injury
  arm NEC 354.9
  artery 447.1
    celiac, syndrome 447.4
  brachial plexus 353.0
  brain (stem) 348.4
    due to
      contusion, brain — *see*
           Contusion, brain
      injury NEC — *see also*
           Hemorrhage, brain,
           traumatic
         birth — *see* Birth, injury,
              brain
      laceration, brain — *see*
           Laceration, brain
    osteopathic 739.0

Compression—continued
  bronchus 519.1
  by cicatrix — see Cicatrix
  cardiac 423.9
  cauda equina 344.60
    with neurogenic bladder 344.61
  celiac (artery) (axis) 447.4
  cerebral — see Compression, brain
  cervical plexus 353.2
  cord (umbilical) — see
      Compression, umbilical cord
  cranial nerve 352.9
    second 377.49
    third (partial) 378.51
      total 378.52
    fourth 378.53
    fifth 350.8
    sixth 378.54
    seventh 351.8
  divers' squeeze 993.3
  duodenum (external) (see also
      Obstruction, duodenum)
      537.3
  during birth 767.9
  esophagus 530.3
    congenital, external 750.3
  Eustachian tube 381.63
  facies (congenital) 754.0
  fracture — see Fracture, by site
  heart — see Disease, heart
  intestine (see also Obstruction,
      intestine) 560.9
    with hernia — see Hernia, by
        site, with obstruction
  laryngeal nerve, recurrent 478.79
  leg NEC 355.8
  lower extremity NEC 355.8
  lumbosacral plexus 353.1
  lung 518.89
  lymphatic vessel 457.1
  medulla — see Compression, brain
  nerve NEC — see also Disorder,
      nerve
    arm NEC 354.9
    autonomic nervous system (see
        also Neuropathy,
        peripheral, autonomic)
        337.9
    axillary 353.0
    cranial NEC 352.9
    due to displacement of
        intervertebral disc 722.2
      with myelopathy 722.70
        cervical 722.0
          with myelopathy 722.71
        lumbar, lumbosacral 722.10
          with myelopathy 722.73
        thoracic, thoracolumbar
            722.11
          with myelopathy 722.72
    iliohypogastric 355.79
    ilioinguinal 355.79
    leg NEC 355.8
    lower extremity NEC 355.8
    median (in carpal tunnel) 354.0
    obturator 355.79
    optic 377.49
    plantar 355.6
    posterior tibial (in tarsal tunnel)
        355.5
    root (by scar tissue) NEC 724.9
      cervical NEC 723.4
      lumbar NEC 724.4
      lumbosacral 724.4
      thoracic 724.4
    saphenous 355.79
    sciatic (acute) 355.0
    sympathetic 337.9
    traumatic — see Injury, nerve
    ulnar 354.2
    upper extremity NEC 354.9
  peripheral — see Compression,
      nerve
  spinal (cord) (old or nontraumatic)
      336.9

Compression—continued
  spinal—continued
    by displacement of
        intervertebral disc — see
        Displacement,
        intervertebral disc
    nerve
      root NEC 724.9
        postoperative 722.80
          cervical region 722.81
          lumbar region 722.83
          thoracic region
              722.82
        traumatic — see Injury,
            nerve, spinal
      traumatic — see Injury,
          nerve, spinal
    spondylogenic 721.91
      cervical 721.1
      lumbar, lumbosacral 721.42
      thoracic 721.41
    traumatic — see also Injury,
        spinal, by site
      with fracture, vertebra — see
          Fracture, vertebra, by
          site, with spinal cord
          injury
  spondylogenic — see Compression,
      spinal cord, spondylogenic
  subcostal nerve (syndrome) 354.8
  sympathetic nerve NEC 337.9
  syndrome 958.5
  thorax 512.8
    iatrogenic 512.1   ▼
    postoperative 512.1   ▲
  trachea 519.1
    congenital 748.3
  ulnar nerve (by scar tissue) 354.2
  umbilical cord
    affecting fetus or newborn 762.5
      cord prolapsed 762.4
    complicating delivery 663.2
      cord around neck 663.1
      cord prolapsed 663.0
  upper extremity NEC 354.9
  ureter 593.3
  urethra — see Stricture, urethra
  vein 459.2
  vena cava (inferior) (superior) 459.2
  vertebral NEC — see Compression,
      spinal (cord)

Compulsion, compulsive
  eating 307.51
  neurosis (obsessive) 300.3
  personality 301.4
  states (mixed) 300.3
  swearing 300.3
    in Gilles de la Tourette's
        syndrome 307.23
  tics and spasms 307.22
  water drinking NEC (syndrome)
      307.9

Concato's disease (pericardial
    polyserositis) 423.2
  peritoneal 568.82
  pleural — see Pleurisy

Concavity, chest wall 738.3

Concealed
  hemorrhage NEC 459.0
  penis 752.8

Concentric fading 368.12

Concern (normal) about sick person in
    family V61.49

Concrescence (teeth) 520.2

Concretio cordis 423.1
  rheumatic 393

Concretion — see also Calculus
  appendicular 543.9
  canaliculus 375.57
  clitoris 624.8
  conjunctiva 372.54
  eyelid 374.56
  intestine (impaction) (obstruction)
      560.39
  lacrimal (passages) 375.57

Concretion—continued
  prepuce (male) 605
    female (clitoris) 624.8
  salivary gland (any) 527.5
  seminal vesicle 608.89
  stomach 537.89
  tonsil 474.8

Concussion (current) 850.9
  with
    loss of consciousness 850.5
      brief (less than one hour)
          850.1
      moderate (1-24 hours) 850.2
      prolonged (more than 24
          hours) (with complete
          recovery) (with return
          to pre-existing
          conscious level) 850.3
        without return to pre-
            existing conscious
            level 850.4
    mental confusion or
        disorientation (without
        loss of consciousness)
        850.0
      with loss of consciousness —
          see Concussion, with,
          loss of consciousness
  without loss of consciousness 850.0
  blast (air) (hydraulic) (immersion)
      (underwater) 869.0
    with open wound into cavity
        869.1
    abdomen or thorax — see
        Injury, internal, by site
    brain — see Concussion, brain
    ear (acoustic nerve trauma)
        951.5
      with perforation, tympanic
          membrane — see
          Wound, open, ear
          drum
    thorax — see Injury, internal,
        intrathoracic organs NEC
  brain or cerebral (without skull
      fracture) 850.9
    with
      loss of consciousness 850.5
        brief (less than one hour)
            850.1
        moderate (1-24 hours)
            850.2
        prolonged (more than 24
            hours) (with
            complete recovery)
            (with return to pre-
            existing conscious
            level) 850.3
          without return to pre-
              existing
              conscious level
              850.4
      mental confusion or
          disorientation (without
          loss of consciousness)
          850.0
        with loss of
            consciousness —
            see Concussion,
            brain, with, loss of
            consciousness
      skull fracture — see Fracture,
          skull, by site
    without loss of consciousness
        850.0
  cauda equina 952.4
  cerebral — see Concussion, brain
  conus medullaris (spine) 952.4
  hydraulic — see Concussion, blast
  internal organs — see Injury,
      internal, by site
  labyrinth — see Injury, intracranial
  ocular 921.3
  osseous labyrinth — see Injury,
      intracranial

Concussion—continued
  spinal (cord) — see also Injury,
      spinal, by site
    due to
      broken
        back — see Fracture,
            vertebra, by site,
            with spinal cord
            injury
        neck — see Fracture,
            vertebra, cervical,
            with spinal cord
            injury
      fracture, fracture dislocation,
          or compression
          fracture of spine or
          vertebra — see
          Fracture, vertebra, by
          site, with spinal cord
          injury
  syndrome 310.2
  underwater blast — see
      Concussion, blast

Condition — see also Disease
  psychiatric 298.9
  respiratory NEC 519.9
    acute or subacute NEC 519.9
      due to
        external agent 508.9
          specified type NEC
              508.8
        fumes or vapors
            (chemical)
            (inhalation) 506.3
        radiation 508.0
    chronic NEC 519.9
      due to
        external agent 508.9
          specified type NEC
              508.8
        fumes or vapors
            (chemical)
            (inhalation) 506.4
        radiation 508.1
      due to
        external agent 508.9
          specified type NEC 508.8
        fumes or vapors (chemical)
            (inhalation) 506.9

Conduct disturbance (see also
    Disturbance, conduct) 312.9
  adjustment reaction 309.3
  hyperkinetic 314.2

Condyloma NEC 078.10
  acuminatum 078.11
  gonorrheal 098.0
  latum 091.3
  syphilitic 091.3
    congenital 090.0
  venereal, syphilitic 091.3

Confinement — see Delivery

Conflagration — see also Burn, by site
  asphyxia (by inhalation of smoke,
      gases, fumes, or vapors)
      987.9
    specified agent — see Table of
        drugs and chemicals

Conflict
  family V61.9
    specified circumstance NEC
        V61.8
  interpersonal NEC V62.81
  marital V61.1
    involving divorce or
        estrangement V61.0
  parent-child V61.20

Confluent — see condition

Confusion, confused (mental) (state)
    (see also State, confusional)
    298.9
  acute 293.0
  epileptic 293.0
  postoperative 293.9
  psychogenic 298.2
  reactive (from emotional stress,
      psychological trauma) 298.2

Confusion, confused—continued
subacute 293.1
Congelation 991.9
Congenital — see also condition
aortic septum 747.29
intrinsic factor deficiency 281.0
malformation — see Anomaly
Congestion, congestive (chronic) (passive)
asphyxia, newborn 768.9
bladder 596.8
bowel 569.89
brain (see also Disease, cerebrovascular NEC) 437.8
    malarial 084.9
breast 611.79
bronchi 519.1
bronchial tube 519.1
catarrhal 472.0
cerebral — see Congestion, brain
cerebrospinal — see Congestion, brain
chest 514
chill 780.9
    malarial (see also Malaria) 084.6
circulatory NEC 459.9
conjunctiva 372.71
due to disturbance of circulation 459.9
duodenum 537.3
enteritis — see Enteritis
eye 372.71
fibrosis syndrome (pelvic) 625.5
gastroenteritis — see Enteritis
general 799.8
glottis 476.0
heart (see also Failure, heart, congestive) 428.0
hepatic 573.0
hypostatic (lung) 514
intestine 569.89
intracranial — see Congestion, brain
kidney 593.89
labyrinth 386.50
larynx 476.0
liver 573.0
lung 514
    active or acute (see also Pneumonia) 486
    congenital 770.0
    chronic 514
    hypostatic 514
    idiopathic, acute 518.5
    passive 514
malaria, malarial (brain) (fever) (see also Malaria) 084.6
medulla — see Congestion, brain
nasal 478.1
orbit, orbital 376.33
    inflammatory (chronic) 376.10
        acute 376.00
ovary 620.8
pancreas 577.8
pelvic, female 625.5
pleural 511.0
prostate (active) 602.1
pulmonary — see Congestion, lung
renal 593.89
retina 362.89
seminal vesicle 608.89
spinal cord 336.1
spleen 289.51
    chronic 289.51
stomach 537.89
trachea 464.11
urethra 599.84
uterus 625.5
    with subinvolution 621.1
viscera 799.8
Congestive — see Congestion
Conical
cervix 622.6
cornea 371.60
teeth 520.2

Conjoined twins 759.4
causing disproportion (fetopelvic) 653.7
Conjugal maladjustment V61.1
involving divorce or estrangement V61.0
Conjunctiva — see condition
Conjunctivitis (exposure) (infectious) (nondiphtheritic) (pneumococcal) (pustular) (staphylococcal) (streptococcal) NEC 372.30
actinic 370.24
acute 372.00
    atopic 372.05
    contagious 372.03
    follicular 372.02
    hemorrhagic (viral) 077.4
adenoviral (acute) 077.3
allergic (chronic) 372.14
    with hay fever 372.05
anaphylactic 372.05
angular 372.03
Apollo (viral) 077.4
atopic 372.05
blennorrhagic (neonatorum) 098.40
catarrhal 372.03
chemical 372.05
chlamydial 077.98
    due to
        Chlamydia trachomatis — see Trachoma
    paratrachoma 077.0
chronic 372.10
    allergic 372.14
    follicular 372.12
    simple 372.11
    specified type NEC 372.14
    vernal 372.13
diphtheritic 032.81
due to
    dust 372.05
    enterovirus type 70 077.4
    erythema multiforme 695.1 [372.33]
    filiariasis (see also Filiariasis) 125.9 [372.15]
    mucocutaneous
        disease NEC 372.33
        leishmaniasis 085.5 [372.15]
    Reiter's disease 099.3 [372.33]
    syphilis 095.8 [372.10]
    toxoplasmosis (acquired) 130.1
        congenital (active) 771.2
    trachoma — see Trachoma
dust 372.05
eczematous 370.31
epidemic 077.1
    hemorrhagic 077.4
follicular (acute) 372.02
    adenoviral (acute) 077.3
    chronic 372.12
glare 370.24
gonococcal (neonatorum) 098.40
granular (trachomatous) 076.1
    late effect 139.1
hemorrhagic (acute) (epidemic) 077.4
herpetic (simplex) 054.43
    zoster 053.21
inclusion 077.0
infantile 771.6
influenzal 372.03
Koch-Weeks 372.03
light 372.05
medicamentosa 372.05
membranous 372.04
meningococcic 036.89
Morax-Axenfeld 372.02
mucopurulent NEC 372.03
neonatal 771.6
    gonococcal 098.40
Newcastle's 077.8
nodosa 360.14
of Beal 077.3

Conjunctivitis—continued
parasitic 372.15
    filiariasis (see also Filiariasis) 125.9 [372.15]
    mucocutaneous leishmaniasis 085.5 [372.15]
Parinaud's 372.02
petrificans 372.39
phlyctenular 370.31
pseudomembranous 372.04
    diphtheritic 032.81
purulent 372.03
Reiter's 099.3 [372.33]
rosacea 695.3 [372.31]
serous 372.01
    viral 077.99
simple chronic 372.11
specified NEC 372.39
sunlamp 372.04
swimming pool 077.0
trachomatous (follicular) 076.1
    acute 076.0
    late effect 139.1
traumatic NEC 372.39
tuberculous (see also Tuberculosis) 017.3 [370.31]
tularemic 021.3
tularensis 021.3
vernal 372.13
    limbar 372.13 [370.32]
viral 077.99
    acute hemorrhagic 077.4
    specified NEC 077.8
Conjunctoblepharitis — see Conjunctivitis
Conn (-Louis) syndrome (primary aldosteronism) 255.1
Connective tissue — see condition
Conradi (-Hünermann) syndrome or disease (chondrodysplasia calcificans congenita) 756.59
Consanguinity V19.7
Consecutive — see condition
Consolidated lung (base) — see Pneumonia, lobar
Constipation (atonic) (neurogenic) (simple) (spastic) 564.0
drug induced
    correct substance properly administered 564.0
    overdose or wrong substance given or taken 977.9
    specified drug — see Table of drugs and chemicals
neurogenic 564.0
psychogenic 306.4
Constitutional — see also condition
arterial hypotension (see also Hypotension) 458.9
obesity 278.0
psychopathic state 301.9
short stature 783.4
state, developmental V21.9
    specified development NEC V21.8
substandard 301.6
Constitutionally substandard 301.6
Constriction
anomalous, meningeal bands or folds 742.8
aortic arch (congenital) 747.10
asphyxiation or suffocation by 994.7
bronchus 519.1
canal, ear (see also Stricture, ear canal, acquired) 380.50
duodenum 537.3
gallbladder (see also Obstruction, gallbladder) 575.2
    congenital 751.69
intestine (see also Obstruction, intestine) 560.9
larynx 478.74
    congenital 748.3

Constriction—continued
meningeal bands or folds, anomalous 742.8
organ or site, congenital NEC — see Atresia
prepuce (congenital) 605
pylorus 537.0
    adult hypertrophic 537.0
    congenital or infantile 750.5
    newborn 750.5
ring (uterus) 661.4
    affecting fetus or newborn 763.7
spastic — see also Spasm
    ureter 593.3
    urethra — see Stricture, urethra
stomach 537.89
ureter 593.3
urethra — see Stricture, urethra
visual field (functional) (peripheral) 368.45
Constrictive — see condition
Consultation
medical — see also Counseling, medical
    specified reason NEC V65.8 ◆
without complaint or sickness V65.9
    feared complaint unfounded V65.5
    specified reason NEC V65.8
Consumption — see Tuberculosis
Contact
with
    AIDS virus V01.7
    cholera V01.0
    communicable disease V01.9
        specified type NEC V01.8
        viral NEC V01.7
    German measles V01.4
    gonorrhea V01.6
    HIV V01.7
    human immunodeficiency virus V01.7
    parasitic disease NEC V01.8
    poliomyelitis V01.2
    rabies V01.5
    rubella V01.4
    smallpox V01.3
    syphilis V01.6
    tuberculosis V01.1
    venereal disease V01.6
    viral disease NEC V01.7
dermatitis — see Dermatitis
Contamination, food (see also Poisoning, food) 005.9
Contraception, contraceptive
advice NEC V25.09
    family planning V25.09
    fitting of diaphragm V25.02
    prescribing or use of
        oral contraceptive agent V25.01
        specified agent NEC V25.02
counseling NEC V25.09
    family planning V25.09
    fitting of diaphragm V25.02
    prescribing or use of
        oral contraceptive agent V25.01
        specified agent NEC V25.02
device (in situ) V45.59 ◆
    causing menorrhagia 996.76
    checking V25.42
    complications 996.32
    insertion V25.1
    intrauterine V45.51 ◆
    reinsertion V25.42
    removal V25.42
    subdermal V45.52 ◆
fitting of diaphragm V25.02
insertion
    intrauterine contraceptive device V25.1
    subdermal implantable V25.5

Contraception, contraceptive—continued
maintenance V25.40
  examination V25.40
    subdermal implantable V25.43
    intrauterine device V25.42
    oral contraceptive V25.41
    specified method NEC V25.49
  intrauterine device V25.42
  oral contraceptive V25.41
  specified method NEC V25.49
  subdermal implantable V25.43
management NEC V25.49
prescription
  oral contraceptive agent V25.01
    repeat V25.41
  specified agent NEC V25.02
    repeat V25.49
sterilization V25.2
surveillance V25.40
  intrauterine device V25.42
  oral contraceptive agent V25.41
  subdermal implantable V25.43
  specified method NEC V25.49

Contraction, contracture, contracted
Achilles tendon (see also Short, tendon, Achilles) 727.81
anus 564.8
axilla 729.9
bile duct (see also Disease, biliary) 576.8
bladder 596.8
  neck or sphincter 596.0
bowel (see also Obstruction, intestine) 560.9
Braxton Hicks 644.1
bronchus 519.1
burn (old) — see Cicatrix
cecum (see also Obstruction, intestine) 560.9
cervix (see also Stricture, cervix) 622.4
  congenital 752.49
cicatricial — see Cicatrix
colon (see also Obstruction, intestine) 560.9
conjunctiva trachomatous, active 076.1
  late effect 139.1
Dupuytren's 728.6
eyelid 374.41
eye socket (after enucleation) 372.64
face 729.9
fascia (lata) (postural) 728.89
  Dupuytren's 728.6
  palmar 728.6
  plantar 728.71
finger NEC 736.29
  congenital 755.59
  joint (see also Contraction, joint) 718.44
flaccid, paralytic
  joint (see also Contraction, joint) 718.4
  muscle 728.85
    ocular 378.50
gallbladder (see also Obstruction, gallbladder) 575.2
hamstring 728.89
  tendon 727.81
heart valve — see Endocarditis
Hicks' 644.1
hip (see also Contraction, joint) 718.4
hourglass
  bladder 596.8
    congenital 753.8
  gallbladder (see also Obstruction, gallbladder) 575.2
    congenital 751.69

Contraction, contracture, contracted—continued
hourglass—continued
  stomach 536.8
    congenital 750.7
    psychogenic 306.4
  uterus 661.4
    affecting fetus or newborn 763.7
hysterical 300.11
infantile (see also Epilepsy) 345.6
internal os (see also Stricture, cervix) 622.4
intestine (see also Obstruction, intestine) 560.9
joint (abduction) (acquired) (adduction) (flexion) (rotation) 718.40
  ankle 718.47
  congenital NEC 755.8
    generalized or multiple 754.89
      lower limb joints 754.89
    hip (see also Subluxation, congenital, hip) 754.32
    lower limb (including pelvic girdle) not involving hip 754.89
    upper limb (including shoulder girdle) 755.59
  elbow 718.42
  foot 718.47
  hand 718.44
  hip 718.45
  hysterical 300.11
  knee 718.46
  multiple sites 718.49
  pelvic region 718.45
  shoulder (region) 718.41
  specified site NEC 718.48
  wrist 718.43
kidney (granular) (secondary) (see also Sclerosis, renal) 587
  congenital 753.3
  hydronephritic 591
  pyelonephritic (see also Pyelitis, chronic) 590.00
  tuberculous (see also Tuberculosis) 016.0
ligament 728.89
  congenital 756.89
liver — see Cirrhosis, liver
muscle (postinfectional) (postural) NEC 728.85
  congenital 756.89
    sternocleidomastoid 754.1
  extraocular 378.60
  eye (extrinsic) (see also Strabismus) 378.9
    paralytic (see also Strabismus, paralytic) 378.50
  flaccid 728.85
  hysterical 300.11
  ischemic (Volkmann's) 958.6
  paralytic 728.85
  posttraumatic 958.6
  psychogenic 306.0
    specified as conversion reaction 300.11
myotonic 728.85
neck (see also Torticollis) 723.5
  congenital 754.1
  psychogenic 306.0
ocular muscle (see also Strabismus) 378.9
  paralytic (see also Strabismus, paralytic) 378.50
organ or site, congenital NEC — see Atresia
outlet (pelvis) — see Contraction, pelvis
palmar fascia 728.6

Contraction, contracture, contracted—continued
paralytic
  joint (see also Contraction, joint) 718.4
  muscle 728.85
    ocular (see also Strabismus, paralytic) 378.50
pelvis (acquired) (general) 738.6
  affecting fetus or newborn 763.1
  complicating delivery 653.1
    causing obstructed labor 660.1
  generally contracted 653.1
    causing obstructed labor 660.1
  inlet 653.2
    causing obstructed labor 660.1
  midpelvic 653.8
    causing obstructed labor 660.1
  midplane 653.8
    causing obstructed labor 660.1
  outlet 653.3
    causing obstructed labor 660.1
plantar fascia 728.71
premature
  atrial 427.61
  auricular 427.61
  auriculoventricular 427.61
  heart (junctional) (nodal) 427.60
  supraventricular 427.61
  ventricular 427.69
prostate 602.8
pylorus (see also Pylorospasm) 537.81
rectosigmoid (see also Obstruction, intestine) 560.9
rectum, rectal (sphincter) 564.8
  psychogenic 306.4
ring (Bandl's) 661.4
  affecting fetus or newborn 763.7
scar — see Cicatrix
sigmoid (see also Obstruction, intestine) 560.9
socket, eye 372.64
spine (see also Curvature, spine) 737.9
stomach 536.8
  hourglass 536.8
    congenital 750.7
    psychogenic 306.4
  psychogenic 306.4
tendon (sheath) (see also Short, tendon) 727.81
toe 735.8
ureterovesical orifice (postinfectional) 593.3
urethra 599.84
uterus 621.8
  abnormal 661.9
    affecting fetus or newborn 763.7
  clonic, hourglass or tetanic 661.4
    affecting fetus or newborn 763.7
  dyscoordinate 661.4
    affecting fetus or newborn 763.7
  hourglass 661.4
    affecting fetus or newborn 763.7
  hypotonic NEC 661.2
    affecting fetus or newborn 763.7
  incoordinate 661.4
    affecting fetus or newborn 763.7
  inefficient or poor 661.2
    affecting fetus or newborn 763.7

Contraction, contracture, contracted—continued
uterus—continued
  irregular 661.2
    affecting fetus or newborn 763.7
  tetanic 661.4
    affecting fetus or newborn 763.7
vagina (outlet) 623.2
vesical 596.8
  neck or urethral orifice 596.0
visual field, generalized 368.45
Volkmann's (ischemic) 958.6

Contusion (skin surface intact) 924.9
with
  crush injury — see Crush
  dislocation — see Dislocation, by site
  fracture — see Fracture, by site
  internal injury — see also Injury, internal, by site
    heart — see Contusion, cardiac
    kidney — see Contusion, kidney
    liver — see Contusion, liver
    lung — see Contusion, lung
    spleen — see Contusion, spleen
  intracranial injury — see Injury, intracranial
  nerve injury — see Injury, nerve
  open wound — see Wound, open, by site
abdomen, abdominal (muscle) (wall) 922.2
  organ(s) NEC 868.00
adnexa, eye NEC 921.9
ankle 924.21
  with other parts of foot 924.20
arm 923.9
  lower (with elbow) 923.10
  upper 923.03
    with shoulder or axillary region 923.09
auditory canal (external) (meatus) (and other part(s) of neck, scalp, or face, except eye) 920
auricle, ear (and other part(s) of neck, scalp, or face except eye) 920
axilla 923.02
  with shoulder or upper arm 923.09
back 922.3
bone NEC 924.9

Contusion—continued
　brain (cerebral) (membrane) (with hemorrhage) 851.8

> Note — Use the following fifth-digit subclassification with categories 851-854:
>
> 0　unspecified state of consciousness
> 1　with no loss of consciousness
> 2　with brief [less than one hour] loss of consciousness
> 3　with moderate [1-24 hours] loss of consciousness
> 4　with prolonged [more than 24 hours] loss of consciousness and return to pre-existing conscious level
> 5　with prolonged [more than 24 hours] loss of consciousness, without return to pre-existing conscious level
> 6　with loss of consciousness of unspecified duration
> 9　with concussion, unspecified

　　with
　　　open intracranial wound 851.9
　　　　skull fracture — see Fracture, skull, by site
　　cerebellum 851.4
　　　with open intracranial wound 851.5
　　cortex 851.0
　　　with open intracranial wound 851.1
　　occipital lobe 851.4
　　　with open intracranial wound 851.5
　　stem 851.4
　　　with open intracranial wound 851.5
　breast 922.0
　brow (and other part(s) of neck, scalp, or face, except eye) 920
　buttock 922.3
　canthus 921.1
　cardiac 861.01
　　with open wound into thorax 861.11
　cauda equina (spine) 952.4
　cerebellum — see Contusion, brain, cerebellum
　cerebral — see Contusion, brain
　cheek(s) (and other part(s) of neck, scalp, or face, except eye) 920
　chest (wall) 922.1
　chin (and other part(s) of neck, scalp, or face, except eye) 920
　clitoris 922.4
　conjunctiva 921.1
　conus medullaris (spine) 952.4
　cornea 921.3
　corpus cavernosum 922.4
　cortex (brain) (cerebral) — see Contusion, brain, cortex
　costal region 922.1
　ear (and other part(s) of neck, scalp, or face except eye) 920
　elbow 923.11
　　with forearm 923.10
　epididymis 922.4
　epigastric region 922.2
　eye NEC 921.9

Contusion—continued
　eyeball 921.3
　eyelid(s) (and periocular area) 921.1
　face (and neck, or scalp, any part except eye) 920
　femoral triangle 922.2
　fetus or newborn 772.6
　finger(s) (nail) (subungual) 923.3
　flank 922.2
　foot (with ankle) (excluding toe(s)) 924.20
　forearm (and elbow) 923.10
　forehead (and other part(s) of neck, scalp, or face, except eye) 920
　genital organs, external 922.4
　globe (eye) 921.3
　groin 922.2
　gum(s) (and other part(s) of neck, scalp, or face, except eye) 920
　hand(s) (except fingers alone) 923.20
　head (any part, except eye) (and face) (and neck) 920
　heart — see Contusion, cardiac
　heel 924.20
　hip 924.01
　　with thigh 924.00
　iliac region 922.2
　inguinal region 922.2
　internal organs (abdomen, chest, or pelvis) NEC — see Injury, internal, by site
　interscapular region 922.3
　iris (eye) 921.3
　kidney 866.01
　　with open wound into cavity 866.11
　knee 924.11
　　with lower leg 924.10
　labium (majus) (minus) 922.4
　lacrimal apparatus, gland, or sac 921.1
　larynx (and other part(s) of neck, scalp, or face, except eye) 920
　late effect — see Late, effects (of), contusion
　leg 924.5
　　lower (with knee) 924.10
　lens 921.3
　lingual (and other part(s) of neck, scalp, or face, except eye) 920
　lip(s) (and other part(s) of neck, scalp, or face, except eye) 920
　liver 864.01
　　with
　　　laceration — see Laceration, liver
　　　open wound into cavity 864.11
　lower extremity 924.5
　　multiple sites 924.4
　lumbar region 922.3
　lung 861.21
　　with open wound into thorax 861.31
　malar region (and other part(s) of neck, scalp, or face, except eye) 920
　mandibular joint (and other part(s) of neck, scalp, or face, except eye) 920
　mastoid region (and other part(s) of neck, scalp, or face, except eye) 920
　membrane, brain — see Contusion, brain
　midthoracic region 922.1
　mouth (and other part(s) of neck, scalp, or face, except eye) 920

Contusion—continued
　multiple sites (not classifiable to same three-digit category) 924.8
　　lower limb 924.4
　　trunk 922.8
　　upper limb 923.8
　muscle NEC 924.9
　myocardium — see Contusion, cardiac
　nasal (septum) (and other part(s) of neck, scalp, or face, except eye) 920
　neck (and scalp, or face any part, except eye) 920
　nerve — see Injury, nerve, by site
　nose (and other part(s) of neck, scalp, or face, except eye) 920
　occipital region (scalp) (and neck or face, except eye) 920
　　lobe — see Contusion, brain, occipital lobe
　orbit (region) (tissues) 921.2
　palate (soft) (and other part(s) of neck, scalp, or face, except eye) 920
　parietal region (scalp) (and neck, or face, except eye) 920
　　lobe — see Contusion, brain
　penis 922.4
　pericardium — see Contusion, cardiac
　perineum 922.4
　periocular area 921.1
　pharynx (and other part(s) of neck, scalp, or face, except eye) 920
　popliteal space (see also Contusion, knee) 924.11
　prepuce 922.4
　pubic region 922.4
　pudenda 922.4
　pulmonary — see Contusion, lung
　quadriceps femoralis 924.00
　rib cage 922.1
　sacral region 922.3
　salivary ducts or glands (and other part(s) of neck, scalp, or face, except eye) 920
　scalp (and neck, or face any part, except eye) 920
　scapular region 923.01
　　with shoulder or upper arm 923.09
　sclera (eye) 921.3
　scrotum 922.4
　shoulder 923.00
　　with upper arm or axillar regions 923.09
　skin NEC 924.9
　skull 920
　spermatic cord 922.4
　spinal cord — see also Injury, spinal, by site
　　cauda equina 952.4
　　conus medullaris 952.4
　spleen 865.01
　　with open wound into cavity 865.11
　sternal region 922.1
　stomach — see Injury, internal, stomach
　subconjunctival 921.1
　subcutaneous NEC 924.9
　submaxillary region (and other part(s) of neck, scalp, or face, except eye) 920
　submental region (and other part(s) of neck, scalp, or face, except eye) 920
　subperiosteal NEC 924.9
　supraclavicular fossa (and other part(s) of neck, scalp, or face, except eye) 920

Contusion—continued
　supraorbital (and other part(s) of neck, scalp, or face, except eye) 920
　temple (region) (and other part(s) of neck, scalp, or face, except eye) 920
　testis 922.4
　thigh (and hip) 924.00
　thorax 922.1
　　organ — see Injury, internal, intrathoracic
　throat (and other part(s) of neck, scalp, or face, except eye) 920
　thumb(s) (nail) (subungual) 923.3
　toe(s) (nail) (subungual) 924.3
　tongue (and other part(s) of neck, scalp, or face, except eye) 920
　trunk 922.9
　　multiple sites 922.8
　　specified site — see Contusion, by site
　tunica vaginalis 922.4
　tympanum (membrane) (and other part(s) of neck, scalp, or face, except eye) 920
　upper extremity 923.9
　　multiple sites 923.8
　uvula (and other part(s) of neck, scalp, or face, except eye) 920
　vagina 922.4
　vocal cord(s) (and other part(s) of neck, scalp, or face, except eye) 920
　vulva 922.4
　wrist 923.21
　　with hand(s), except finger(s) alone 923.20

Conus (any type) (congenital) 743.57
　acquired 371.60
　medullaris syndrome 336.8

Convalescence (following) V66.9
　chemotherapy V66.2
　medical NEC V66.5
　psychotherapy V66.3
　radiotherapy V66.1
　surgery NEC V66.0
　treatment (for) NEC V66.5
　　combined V66.6
　　fracture V66.4
　　mental disorder NEC V66.3
　　specified disorder NEC V66.5

Conversion
　hysteria, hysterical, any type 300.11
　neurosis, any 300.11
　reaction, any 300.11

Converter, tuberculosis (test reaction) 795.5

Convulsions (idiopathic) 780.3
　apoplectiform (see also Disease, cerebrovascular, acute) 436
　brain 780.3
　cerebral 780.3
　cerebrospinal 780.3
　due to trauma NEC — see Injury, intracranial
　eclamptic (see also Eclampsia) 780.3
　epileptic (see also Epilepsy) 345.9
　epileptiform (see also Seizure, epileptiform) 780.3
　epileptoid (see also Seizure, epileptiform) 780.3
　ether
　　anesthetic
　　　correct substance properly administered 780.3
　　　overdose or wrong substance given 968.2
　　other specified type — see Table of drugs and chemicals
　febrile 780.3
　generalized 780.3

Convulsions—continued
  hysterical 300.11
  infantile 780.3
    epilepsy — see Epilepsy
  internal 780.3
  jacksonian (see also Epilepsy) 345.5
  myoclonic 333.2
  newborn 779.0
  paretic 094.1
  pregnancy (nephritic) (uremic) —
    see Eclampsia, pregnancy
  psychomotor (see also Epilepsy)
    345.4
  puerperal, postpartum — see
    Eclampsia, pregnancy
  recurrent 780.3
    epileptic — see Epilepsy
  reflex 781.0
  repetitive 780.3
    epileptic — see Epilepsy
  salaam (see also Epilepsy) 345.6
  scarlatinal 034.1
  spasmodic 780.3
  tetanus, tetanic (see also Tetanus)
    037
  thymic 254.8
  uncinate 780.3
  uremic 586
Convulsive — see also Convulsions
  disorder or state 780.3
    epileptic — see Epilepsy
  equivalent, abdominal (see also
    Epilepsy) 345.5
Cooke-Apert-Gallais syndrome
  (adrenogenital) 255.2
Cooley's anemia (erythroblastic) 282.4
Coolie itch 126.9
Cooper's
  disease 610.1
  hernia — see Hernia, Cooper's
Coordination disturbance 781.3
Copper wire arteries, retina 362.13
Copra itch 133.8
Coprolith 560.39
Coprophilia 302.89
Coproporphyria, hereditary 277.1
Coprostasis 560.39
  with hernia — see also Hernia, by
    site, with obstruction
    gangrenous — see Hernia, by
      site, with gangrene
Cor
  biloculare 745.7
  bovinum — see Hypertrophy,
    cardiac
  bovis — see also Hypertrophy,
    cardiac
  pulmonale (chronic) 416.9
    acute 415.0
  triatriatum, triatrium 746.82
  triloculare 745.8
    biatriatum 745.3
    biventriculare 745.69
Corbus' disease 607.1
Cord — see also condition
  around neck (tightly) (with
    compression) affecting fetus
    or newborn 762.5
  complicating delivery 663.1
    without compression 663.3
      affecting fetus or newborn
        762.6
  bladder NEC 344.61
    tabetic 094.0
  prolapse
    affecting fetus or newborn 762.4
    complicating delivery 663.0
Cord's angiopathy (see also
  Tuberculosis) 017.3 [362.18]
Cordis ectopia 746.87
Corditis (spermatic) 608.4
Corectopia 743.46
Cori type glycogen storage disease —
  see Disease, glycogen storage

Cork-handlers' disease or lung 495.3
Corkscrew esophagus 530.5
Corlett's pyosis (impetigo) 684
Corn (infected) 700
Cornea — see also condition
  donor V59.5
  guttata (dystrophy) 371.57
  plana 743.41
Cornelia de Lange's syndrome
  (Amsterdam dwarf, mental
  retardation, and brachycephaly)
  759.89
Cornual gestation or pregnancy — see
  Pregnancy, cornual
Cornu cutaneum 702.8
Coronary (artery) — see also condition
  arising from aorta or pulmonary
    trunk 746.85
Corpora — see also condition
  amylacea (prostate) 602.8
  cavernosa — see condition
Corpulence (see also Obesity) 278.0
Corpus — see condition
Corrigan's disease — see Insufficiency,
  aortic
Corrosive burn — see Burn, by site
Corsican fever (see also Malaria) 084.6
Cortical — see also condition
  blindness 377.75
  necrosis, kidney (acute) (bilateral)
    583.6
Corticoadrenal — see condition
Corticosexual syndrome 255.2
Coryza (acute) 460
  with grippe or influenza 487.1
  syphilitic 095.8
    congenital (chronic) 090.0
Costen's syndrome or complex 524.60
Costiveness (see also Constipation)
  564.0
Costochondritis 733.6
Cotard's syndrome (paranoia) 297.1
Cot death 798.0
Cotungo's disease 724.3
Cough 786.2
  with hemorrhage (see also
    Hemoptysis) 786.3
  affected 786.2
  bronchial 786.2
    with grippe or influenza 487.1
  chronic 786.2
  epidemic 786.2
  functional 306.1
  hemorrhagic 786.3
  hysterical 300.11
  laryngeal, spasmodic 786.2
  nervous 786.2
  psychogenic 306.1
  smokers' 491.0
  tea tasters' 112.89
Counseling NEC V65.40
  without complaint or sickness
    V65.49
  child abuse, maltreatment, or
    neglect V61.21
  contraceptive NEC V25.09
    device (intrauterine) V25.02
    maintenance V25.40
      intrauterine contraceptive
        device V25.42
      oral contraceptive (pill)
        V25.41
      specified type NEC V25.49
    subdermal implantable V25.43
    management NEC V25.9
    oral contraceptive (pill) V25.01
    prescription NEC V25.02
      oral contraceptive (pill)
        V25.01
      repeat prescription
        V25.41
      repeat prescription V25.40

Counseling—continued
  contraceptive—continued
    subdermal implantable V25.43
    surveillance NEC V25.40
  dietary V65.3
  excercise V65.41
  explanation of
    investigation finding NEC
      V65.49
    medication NEC V65.49
  family planning V25.09
  for nonattending third party V65.1
  genetic V26.3
  gonorrhea V65.45
  health (advice) (education)
    (instruction) NEC V65.49
  HIV V65.44
  human immunodeficiency virus
    V65.44
  injury prevention V65.43
  medical (for) V65.9
    boarding school resident V60.6
    condition not demonstrated
      V65.5
    feared complaint and no disease
      found V65.5
    institutional resident V60.1
    on behalf of another V65.1
    person living alone V60.3
    parent-child conflict V61.20
    specified problem NEC V61.29
  procreative V65.49
  sex NEC V65.49
    transmitted disease NEC V65.45
      HIV V65.44
  specified reason NEC V65.49
  substance use and abuse V65.42
  syphilis V65.45
Coupled rhythm 427.89
Couvelaire uterus (complicating
  delivery) — see Placenta,
  separation
Cowper's gland — see condition
Cowperitis (see also Urethritis) 597.89
  gonorrheal (acute) 098.0
    chronic or duration of 2 months
      or over 098.2
Cowpox (abortive) 051.0
  due to vaccination 999.0
  eyelid 051.0 [373.5]
  postvaccination 999.0 [373.5]
Coxa
  plana 732.1
  valga (acquired) 736.31
    congenital 755.61
    late effect of rickets 268.1
  vara (acquired) 736.32
    congenital 755.62
    late effect of rickets 268.1
Coxae malum senilis 715.25
Coxalgia (nontuberculous) 719.45
  tuberculous (see also Tuberculosis)
    015.1 [730.85]
Coxalgic pelvis 736.30
Coxitis 716.65
Coxsackie (infection) (virus) 079.2
  central nervous system NEC 048
  endocarditis 074.22
  enteritis 008.67
  meningitis (aseptic) 047.0
  myocarditis 074.23
  pericarditis 074.21
  pharyngitis 074.0
  pleurodynia 074.1
  specific disease NEC 074.8
Crabs, meaning pubic lice 132.2
Cracked nipple 611.2
  puerperal, postpartum 676.1
Cradle cap 691.8
Craft neurosis 300.89
Craigiasis 007.8
Cramp(s) 729.82
  abdominal 789.0
  bathing 994.1

Cramps—continued
  colic 789.0
    psychogenic 306.4
  due to immersion 994.1
  extremity (lower) (upper) NEC
    729.82
  fireman 992.2
  heat 992.2
  hysterical 300.11
  immersion 994.1
  intestinal 789.0
    psychogenic 306.4
  linotypist's 300.89
    organic 333.84
  muscle (extremity) (general) 729.82
    due to immersion 994.1
    hysterical 300.11
  occupational (hand) 300.89
    organic 333.84
  psychogenic 307.89
  salt depletion 276.1
  stoker 992.2
  stomach 789.0
  telegraphers' 300.89
    organic 333.84
  typists' 300.89
    organic 333.84
  uterus 625.8
    menstrual 625.3
  writers' 300.89
    organic 333.84
Cranial — see condition
Cranioclasis, fetal 763.8
Craniocleidodysostosis 755.59
Craniofenestria (skull) 756.0
Craniolacunia (skull) 756.0
Craniopagus 759.4
Craniopathy, metabolic 733.3
Craniopharyngeal — see condition
Craniopharyngioma (M9350/1) 237.0
Craniorachischisis (totalis) 740.1
Cranioschisis 756.0
Craniostenosis 756.0
Craniosynostosis 756.0
Craniotabes (cause unknown) 733.3
  rachitic 268.1
  syphilitic 090.5
Craniotomy, fetal 763.8
Cranium — see condition
Craw-craw 125.3
Creaking joint 719.60
  ankle 719.67
  elbow 719.62
  foot 719.67
  hand 719.64
  hip 719.65
  knee 719.66
  multiple sites 719.69
  pelvic region 719.65
  shoulder (region) 719.61
  specified site NEC 719.68
  wrist 719.63
Creeping
  eruption 126.9
  palsy 335.21
  paralysis 335.21
Crenated tongue 529.8
Creotoxism 005.9
Crepitus
  caput 756.0
  joint 719.60
    ankle 719.67
    elbow 719.62
    foot 719.67
    hand 719.64
    hip 719.65
    knee 719.66
    multiple sites 719.69
    pelvic region 719.65
    shoulder (region) 719.61
    specified site NEC 719.68
    wrist 719.63

Crescent or conus choroid, congenital 743.57
Cretin, cretinism (athyrotic) (congenital) (endemic) (metabolic) (nongoitrous) (sporadic) 243
  goitrous (sporadic) 246.1
  pelvis (dwarf type) (male type) 243
    with disproportion (fetopelvic) 653.1
      affecting fetus or newborn 763.1
      causing obstructed labor 660.1
        affecting fetus or newborn 763.1
  pituitary 253.3
Cretinoid degeneration 243
Creutzfeldt-Jakob disease (syndrome) 046.1
  with dementia 290.10
Crib death 798.0
Cribriform hymen 752.49
Cri-du-chat syndrome 758.3
Crigler-Najjar disease or syndrome (congenital hyperbilirubinemia) 277.4
Crimean hemorrhagic fever 065.0
Criminalism 301.7
Crisis
  abdomen 789.0
  addisonian (acute adrenocortical insufficiency) 255.4
  adrenal (cortical) 255.4
  asthmatic — see Asthma
  brain, cerebral (see also Disease, cerebrovascular, acute) 436
  celiac 579.0
  Dietl's 593.4
  emotional NEC 309.29
    acute reaction to stress 308.0
    adjustment reaction 309.9
    specific to childhood and adolescence 313.9
  gastric (tabetic) 094.0
  glaucomatocyclitic 364.22
  heart (see also Failure, heart) 428.9
  hypertensive — see Hypertension
  nitritoid
    correct substance properly administered 458.9
    overdose or wrong substance given or taken 961.1
  oculogyric 378.87
    psychogenic 306.7
  Pel's 094.0
  psychosexual identity 302.6
  rectum 094.0
  renal 593.81
  sickle cell 282.62
  stomach (tabetic) 094.0
  tabetic 094.0
  thyroid (see also Thyrotoxicosis) 242.9
  thyrotoxic (see also Thyrotoxicosis) 242.9
  vascular — see Disease, cerebrovascular, acute
Crocq's disease (acrocyanosis) 443.89
Crohn's disease (see also Enteritis, regional) 555.9
Cronkhite-Canada syndrome 211.3
Crooked septum, nasal 470
Cross
  birth (of fetus) complicating delivery 652.3
    with successful version 652.1
    causing obstructed labor 660.0
  bite, anterior or posterior 524.2
  eye (see also Esotropia) 378.00
Crossed ectopia of kidney 753.3
Crossfoot 754.50

Croup, croupous (acute) (angina) (catarrhal) (infective) (inflammatory) (laryngeal) (membranous) (nondiphtheritic) (pseudomembranous) 464.4
  asthmatic (see also Asthma) 493.9
  bronchial 466.0
  diphtheritic (membranous) 032.3
  false 478.75
  spasmodic 478.75
    diphtheritic 032.3
  stridulous 478.75
    diphtheritic 032.3
Crouzon's disease (craniofacial dysostosis) 756.0
Crowding, teeth 524.3
CRST syndrome (cutaneous systemic sclerosis) 710.1
Cruchet's disease (encephalitis lethargica) 049.8
Cruelty in children (see also Disturbance, conduct) 312.9
Crural ulcer (see also Ulcer, lower extremity) 707.1
Crush, crushed, crushing (injury) 929.9
  with
    fracture — see Fracture, by site
  abdomen 926.19
    internal — see Injury, internal, abdomen
  ankle 928.21
    with other parts of foot 928.20
  arm 927.9
    lower (and elbow) 927.10
    upper 927.03
      with shoulder or axillary region 927.09
  axilla 927.02
    with shoulder or upper arm 927.09
  back 926.11
  breast 926.19
  buttock 926.12
  cheek 925.1
  chest — see Injury, internal, chest
  ear 925.1
  elbow 927.11
    with forearm 927.10
  face 925.1
  finger(s) 927.3
    with hand(s) 927.20
      and wrist(s) 927.21
  flank 926.19
  foot, excluding toe(s) alone (with ankle) 928.20
  forearm (and elbow) 927.10
  genitalia, external (female) (male) 926.0
    internal — see Injury, internal, genital organ NEC
  hand, except finger(s) alone (and wrist) 927.20
  head — see Fracture, skull, by site
  heel 928.20
  hip 928.01
    with thigh 928.00
  internal organ (abdomen, chest, or pelvis) — see Injury, internal, by site
  knee 928.11
    with leg, lower 928.10
  labium (majus) (minus) 926.0
  larynx 925.2
  late effect — see Late, effects (of), crushing
  leg 928.9
    lower 928.10
      and knee 928.11
    upper 928.00
  limb
    lower 928.9
      multiple sites 928.8
    upper 927.9
      multiple sites 927.8
  multiple sites NEC 929.0
  neck 925.2

Crush, crushed, crushing—continued
  nerve — see Injury, nerve, by site
  nose 802.0
    open 802.1
  penis 926.0
  pharynx 925.2
  scalp 925.1
  scapular region 927.01
    with shoulder or upper arm 927.09
  scrotum 926.0
  shoulder 927.00
    with upper arm or axillary region 927.09
  skull or cranium — see Fracture, skull, by site
  spinal cord — see Injury, spinal, by site
  syndrome (complication of trauma) 958.5
  testis 926.0
  thigh (with hip) 928.00
  throat 925.2
  thumb(s) (and fingers) 927.3
  toe(s) 928.3
    with foot 928.20
      and ankle 928.21
  tonsil 925.2
  trunk 926.9
    chest — see Injury, internal, intrathoracic organs NEC
    internal organ — see Injury, internal, by site
    multiple sites 926.8
    specified site NEC 926.19
  vulva 926.0
  wrist 927.21
    with hand(s), except fingers alone 927.20
Crusta lactea 691.8
Crusts 782.8
Crutch paralysis 953.4
Cruveilhier's disease 335.21
Cruveilhier-Baumgarten cirrhosis, disease, or syndrome 571.5
Cruz-Chagas disease (see also Trypanosomiasis) 086.2
Cryoglobulinemia (mixed) 273.2
Crypt (anal) (rectal) 569.49
Cryptitis (anal) (rectal) 569.49
Cryptococcosis (European) (pulmonary) (systemic) 117.5
Cryptococcus 117.5
  epidermicus 117.5
  neoformans, infection by 117.5
Cryptopapillitis (anus) 569.49
Cryptophthalmos (eyelid) 743.06
Cryptorchid, cryptorchism, cryptorchidism 752.5
Cryptotia 744.29
Crystallopathy
  calcium pyrophosphate (see also Arthritis) 275.4 [712.2]
  dicalcium phosphate (see also Arthritis) 275.4 [712.1]
  gouty 274.0
  pyrophosphate NEC (see also Arthritis) 275.4 [712.2]
  uric acid 274.0
Crystalluria 791.9
Csillag's disease (lichen sclerosus or atrophicus) 701.0
Cuban itch 050.1
Cubitus
  valgus (acquired) 736.01
    congenital 755.59
    late effect of rickets 268.1
  varus (acquired) 736.02
    congenital 755.59
    late effect of rickets 268.1
Cultural deprivation V62.4
Cupping of optic disc 377.14

Curling's ulcer — see Ulcer, duodenum
Curling esophagus 530.5
Curschmann (-Batten) (-Steinert) disease or syndrome 359.2
Curvature
  organ or site, congenital NEC — see Distortion
  penis (lateral) 752.8
  Pott's (spinal) (see also Tuberculosis) 015.0 [737.43]
  radius, idiopathic, progressive (congenital) 755.54
  spine (acquired) (angular) (idiopathic) (incorrect) (postural) 737.9
    congenital 754.2
    due to or associated with
      Charcot-Marie-Tooth disease 356.1 [737.40]
      mucopolysaccharidosis 277.5 [737.40]
      neurofibromatosis 237.71 [737.40]
      osteitis
        deformans 731.0 [737.40]
        fibrosa cystica 252.0 [737.40]
      osteoporosis (see also Osteoporosis) 733.00 [737.40]
      poliomyelitis (see also Poliomyelitis) 138 [737.40]
      tuberculosis (Pott's curvature) (see also Tuberculosis) 015.0 [737.43]
    kyphoscoliotic (see also Kyphoscoliosis) 737.30
    kyphotic (see also Kyphosis) 737.10
    late effect of rickets 268.1 [737.40]
    Pott's 015.0 [737.40]
    scoliotic (see also Scoliosis) 737.30
    specified NEC 737.8
    tuberculous 015.0 [737.40]
Cushing's
  basophilism, disease, or syndrome (iatrogenic) (idiopathic) (pituitary basophilism) (pituitary dependent) 255.0
  ulcer — see Ulcer, peptic
Cushingoid due to steroid therapy
  correct substance properly administered 255.0
  overdose or wrong substance given or taken 962.0
Cut (external) — see Wound, open, by site
Cutaneous — see also condition
  hemorrhage 782.7
  horn (cheek) (eyelid) (mouth) 702.8
  larva migrans 126.9
Cutis — see also condition
  hyperelastic 756.83
    acquired 701.8
  laxa 756.83
    senilis 701.8
  marmorata 782.61
  osteosis 709.3
  pendula 756.83
    acquired 701.8
  rhomboidalis nuchae 701.8
  verticis gyrata 757.39
    acquired 701.8
Cyanopathy, newborn 770.8
Cyanosis 782.5
  autotoxic 289.7
  common atrioventricular canal 745.69
  congenital 770.8
  conjunctiva 372.71

Cyanosis—continued
due to
endocardial cushion defect 745.60
nonclosure, foramen botalli 745.5
patent foramen botalli 745.5
persistent foramen ovale 745.5
enterogenous 289.7
fetus or newborn 770.8
ostium primum defect 745.61
paroxysmal digital 443.0
retina, retinal 362.10

Cycle
anovulatory 628.0
menstrual, irregular 626.4

Cyclencephaly 759.89
Cyclical vomiting 536.2
psychogenic 306.4
Cyclitic membrane 364.74
Cyclitis (see also Iridocyclitis) 364.3
acute 364.00
primary 364.01
recurrent 364.02
chronic 364.10
in
sarcoidosis 135 [364.11]
tuberculosis (see also Tuberculosis) 017.3 [364.11]
Fuchs' heterochromic 364.21
granulomatous 364.10
lens induced 364.23
nongranulomatous 364.00
posterior 363.21
primary 364.01
recurrent 364.02
secondary (noninfectious) 364.04
infectious 364.03
subacute 364.00
primary 364.01
recurrent 364.02

Cyclokeratitis — see Keratitis
Cyclophoria 378.44
Cyclopia, cyclops 759.89
Cycloplegia 367.51
Cyclospasm 367.53
Cyclothymia 301.13
Cyclothymic personality 301.13
Cyclotropia 378.33
Cyesis — see Pregnancy
Cylindroma (M8200/3) — see also Neoplasm, by site, malignant
eccrine dermal (M8200/0) — see Neoplasm, skin, benign
skin (M8200/0) — see Neoplasm, skin, benign
Cylindruria 791.7
Cyllosoma 759.89
Cynanche
diphtheritic 032.3
tonsillaris 475
Cynorexia 783.6
Cyphosis — see Kyphosis
Cyprus fever (see also Brucellosis) 023.9
Cyriax's syndrome (slipping rib) 733.99

Cyst (mucus) (retention) (serous) (simple)

Note — In general, cysts are not neoplastic and are classified to the approriate category for disease of the specified anatomical site. This generalization does not apply to certain types of cysts which are neoplastic in nature, for example, dermoid, nor does it apply to cysts of certain structures, for example, branchial cleft, which are classified as developmental anomalies.

The following listing includes some of the most frequently reported sites of cysts as well as qualifiers which indicate the type of cyst. The latter qualifiers usually are not repeated under the anatomical sites. Since the code assignment for a given site may vary depending upon the type of cyst, the coder should refer to the listings under the specified type of cyst before consideration is given to the site.

accessory, fallopian tube 752.11
adenoid (infected) 474.8
adrenal gland 255.8
congenital 759.1
air, lung 518.89
allantoic 753.7
alveolar process (jaw bone) 526.2
amnion, amniotic 658.8
anterior chamber (eye) 364.60
exudative 364.62
implantation (surgical) (traumatic) 364.61
parasitic 360.13
anterior nasopalatine 526.1
antrum 478.1
anus 569.49
apical (periodontal) (tooth) 522.8
appendix 543.9
arachnoid, brain 348.0
arytenoid 478.79
auricle 706.2
Baker's (knee) 727.51
tuberculous (see also Tuberculosis) 015.2
Bartholin's gland or duct 616.2
bile duct (see also Disease, biliary) 576.8
bladder (multiple) (trigone) 596.8
Blessig's 362.62
blood, endocardial (see also Endocarditis) 424.90
blue dome 610.0
bone (local) 733.20
aneurysmal 733.22
jaw 526.2
developmental (odontogenic) 526.0
fissural 526.1
latent 526.89
solitary 733.21
unicameral 733.21
brain 348.0
congenital 742.4
hydatid (see also Echinococcus) 122.9
third ventricle (colloid) 742.4
branchial (cleft) 744.42
branchiogenic 744.42
breast (benign) (blue dome) (pedunculated) (solitary) (traumatic) 610.0
involution 610.4
sebaceous 610.8
broad ligament (benign) 620.8
embryonic 752.11
bronchogenic (mediastinal) (sequestration) 518.89
congenital 748.4
buccal 528.4

Cyst—continued
bulbourethral gland (Cowper's) 599.89
bursa, bursal 727.49
pharyngeal 478.26
calcifying odontogenic (M9301/0) 213.1
upper jaw (bone) 213.0
canal of Nuck (acquired) (serous) 629.1
congenital 752.41
canthus 372.75
carcinomatous (M8010/3) — see Neoplasm, by site, malignant
cartilage (joint) — see Derangement, joint
cauda equina 336.8
cavum septi pellucidi NEC 348.0
celomic (pericardium) 746.89
cerebellopontine (angle) — see Cyst, brain
cerebellum — see Cyst, brain
cerebral — see Cyst, brain
cervical lateral 744.42
cervix 622.8
embryonal 752.41
nabothian (gland) 616.0
chamber, anterior (eye) 364.60
exudative 364.62
implantation (surgical) (traumatic) 364.61
parasitic 360.13
chiasmal, optic NEC (see also Lesion, chiasmal) 377.54
chocolate (ovary) 617.1
choledochal (congenital) 751.69
acquired 576.8
choledochus 751.69
chorion 658.8
choroid plexus 348.0
chyle, mesentery 457.8
ciliary body 364.60
exudative 364.64
implantation 364.61
primary 364.63
clitoris 624.8
coccyx (see also Cyst, bone) 733.20
colloid
third ventricle (brain) 742.4
thyroid gland — see Goiter
colon 569.89
common (bile) duct (see also Disease, biliary) 576.8
congenital NEC 759.89
adrenal glands 759.1
epiglottis 748.3
esophagus 750.4
fallopian tube 752.11
kidney 753.10
multiple 753.19
single 753.11
larynx 748.3
liver 751.62
lung 748.4
mediastinum 748.8
ovary 752.0
oviduct 752.11
pancreas 751.7
periurethral (tissue) 753.8
prepuce 752.8
sublingual 750.26
submaxillary gland 750.26
thymus (gland) 759.2
tongue 750.19
ureterovesical orifice 753.4
vulva 752.41
conjunctiva 372.75
cornea 371.23
corpora quadrigemina 348.0
corpus
albicans (ovary) 620.2
luteum (ruptured) 620.1
Cowper's gland (benign) (infected) 599.89
cranial meninges 348.0
craniobuccal pouch 253.8
craniopharyngeal pouch 253.8

Cyst—continued
cystic duct (see also Disease, gallbladder) 575.8
Cysticercus (any site) 123.1
Dandy-Walker 742.3
with spina bifida (see also Spina bifida) 741.0
dental 522.8
developmental 526.0
eruption 526.0
lateral periodontal 526.0
primordial (keratocyst) 526.0
root 522.8
dentigerous 526.0
mandible 526.0
maxilla 526.0
dermoid (M9084/0) — see also Neoplasm, by site, benign
with malignant transformation (M9084/3) 183.0
implantation
external area or site (skin) NEC 709.8
iris 364.61
skin 709.8
vagina 623.8
vulva 624.8
mouth 528.4
oral soft tissue 528.4
sacrococcygeal 685.1
with abscess 685.0
developmental of ovary, ovarian 752.0
dura (cerebral) 348.0
spinal 349.2
ear (external) 706.2
echinococcal (see also Echinococcus) 122.9
embryonal
cervix uteri 752.41
genitalia, female external 752.41
uterus 752.3
vagina 752.41
endometrial 621.8
ectopic 617.9
endometrium (uterus) 621.8
ectopic — see Endometriosis
enteric 751.5
enterogenous 751.5
epidermal (inclusion) (see also Cyst, skin) 706.2
epidermoid (inclusion) (see also Cyst, skin) 706.2
mouth 528.4
not of skin — see Cyst, by site
oral soft tissue 528.4
epididymis 608.89
epiglottis 478.79
epiphysis cerebri 259.8
epithelial (inclusion) (see also Cyst, skin) 706.2
epoophoron 752.11
eruption 526.0
esophagus 530.89
ethmoid sinus 478.1
eye (retention) 379.8
congenital 743.03
posterior segment, congenital 743.54
eyebrow 706.2
eyelid (sebaceous) 374.84
infected 373.13
sweat glands or ducts 374.84
falciform ligament (inflammatory) 573.8
fallopian tube 620.8
female genital organs NEC 629.8
fimbrial (congenital) 752.11
fissural (oral region) 526.1
follicle (atretic) (graafian) (ovarian) 620.0
nabothian (gland) 616.0
follicular (atretic) (ovarian) 620.0
dentigerous 526.0
frontal sinus 478.1
gallbladder or duct 575.8

Cyst—continued
ganglion 727.43
Gartner's duct 752.11
gas, of mesentery 568.89
gingiva 523.8
gland of moll 374.84
globulomaxillary 526.1
graafian follicle 620.0
granulosal lutein 620.2
hemangiomatous (M9121/0) (see also Hemangioma) 228.00
hydatid (see also Echinococcus) 122.9
   fallopian tube (Morgagni) 752.11
   liver NEC 122.8
   lung NEC 122.9
   Morgagni 752.8
      fallopian tube 752.11
   specified site NEC 122.9
hymen 623.8
   embryonal 752.41
hypopharynx 478.26
hypophysis, hypophyseal (duct) (recurrent) 253.8
   cerebri 253.8
implantation (dermoid)
   anterior chamber (eye) 364.61
   external area or site (skin) NEC 709.8
   iris 364.61
   vagina 623.8
   vulva 624.8
incisor, incisive canal 526.1
inclusion (epidermal) (epithelial) (epidermoid) (mucous) (squamous) (see also Cyst, skin) 706.2
   not of skin — see Neoplasm, by site, benign
intestine (large) (small) 569.89
intracranial — see Cyst, brain
intraligamentous 728.89
   knee 717.89
intrasellar 253.8
iris (idiopathic) 364.60
   exudative 364.62
   implantation (surgical) (traumatic) 364.61
   miotic pupillary 364.55
   parasitic 360.13
Iwanoff's 362.62
jaw (bone) (aneurysmal) (extravasation) (hemorrhagic) (traumatic) 526.2
   developmental (odontogenic) 526.0
   fissural 526.1
keratin 706.2
kidney (congenital) 753.10
   acquired 593.2
   calyceal (see also Hydronephrosis) 591
   multiple 753.19
   pyelogenic (see also Hydronephrosis) 591
   simple 593.2
   single 753.11
   solitary (not congenital) 593.2
labium (majus) (minus) 624.8
   sebaceous 624.8
lacrimal
   apparatus 375.43
   gland or sac 375.12
larynx 478.79
lens 379.39
   congenital 743.39
lip (gland) 528.5
liver 573.8
   congenital 751.62
   hydatid (see also Echinococcus) 122.8
      granulosis 122.0
      multilocularis 122.5
lung 518.89
   congenital 748.4
   giant bullous 492.0

Cyst—continued
lutein 620.1
lymphangiomatous (M9173/0) 228.1
lymphoepithelial
   mouth 528.4
   oral soft tissue 528.4
macula 362.54
malignant (M8000/3) — see Neoplasm, by site, malignant
mammary gland (sweat gland) (see also Cyst, breast) 610.0
mandible 526.2
   dentigerous 526.0
   radicular 522.8
maxilla 526.2
   dentigerous 526.0
   radicular 522.8
median
   anterior maxillary 526.1
   palatal 526.1
mediastinum (congenital) 748.8
meibomian (gland) (retention) 373.2
   infected 373.12
membrane, brain 348.0
meninges (cerebral) 348.0
   spinal 349.2
meniscus knee 717.5
mesentery, mesenteric (gas) 568.89
   chyle 457.8
   gas 568.89
mesonephric duct 752.8
mesothelial
   peritoneum 568.89
   pleura (peritoneal) 569.89
milk 611.5
miotic pupillary (iris) 364.55
Morgagni (hydatid) 752.8
   fallopian tube 752.11
mouth 528.4
mullerian duct 752.8
multilocular (ovary) (M8000/1) 239.5
myometrium 621.8
nabothian (follicle) (ruptured) 616.0
nasal sinus 478.1
nasoalveolar 528.4
nasolabial 528.4
nasopalatine (duct) 526.1
   anterior 526.1
nasopharynx 478.26
neoplastic (M8000/1) — see also Neoplasm, by site, unspecified nature
   benign (M8000/0) — see Neoplasm, by site, benign
   uterus 621.8
nervous system — see Cyst, brain
neuroenteric 742.59
neuroepithelial ventricle 348.0
nipple 610.0
nose 478.1
   skin of 706.2
odontogenic, developmental 526.0
omentum (lesser) 568.89
   congenital 751.8
oral soft tissue (dermoid) (epidermoid) (lymphoepithelial) 528.4
ora serrata 361.19
orbit 376.81
ovary, ovarian (twisted) 620.2
   adherent 620.2
   chocolate 617.1
   corpus
      albicans 620.2
      luteum 620.1
   dermoid (M9084/0) 220
   developmental 752.0
   due to failure of involution NEC 620.2
   endometrial 617.1
   follicular (atretic) (graafian) (hemorrhagic) 620.0
   hemorrhagic 620.2

Cyst—continued
ovary, ovarian—continued
   in pregnancy or childbirth 654.4
      affecting fetus or newborn 763.8
      causing obstructed labor 660.2
         affecting fetus or newborn 763.1
   multilocular (M8000/1) 239.5
   pseudomucinous (M8470/0) 220
   retention 620.2
   serous 620.2
   theca lutein 620.2
   tuberculous (see also Tuberculosis) 016.6
   unspecified 620.2
oviduct 620.8
palatal papilla (jaw) 526.1
palate 526.1
   fissural 526.1
   median (fissural) 526.1
palatine, of papilla 526.1
pancreas, pancreatic 577.2
   congenital 751.7
   false 577.2
   hemorrhagic 577.2
   true 577.2
paranephric 593.2
para ovarian 752.11
paraphysis, cerebri 742.4
parasitic NEC 136.9
parathyroid (gland) 252.8
paratubal (fallopian) 620.8
paraurethral duct 599.89
paroophoron 752.11
parotid gland 527.6
   mucous extravasation or retention 527.6
parovarian 752.11
pars planus 364.60
   exudative 364.64
   primary 364.63
pelvis, female
   in pregnancy or childbirth 654.4
      affecting fetus or newborn 763.8
      causing obstructed labor 660.2
         affecting fetus or newborn 763.1
penis (sebaceous) 607.89
periapical 522.8
pericardial (congenital) 746.89
   acquired (secondary) 423.8
pericoronal 526.0
perineural (Tarlov's) 355.9
periodontal 522.8
   lateral 526.0
peripancreatic 577.2
peripelvic (lymphatic) 593.2
peritoneum 568.89
   chylous 457.8
pharynx (wall) 478.26
pilonidal (infected) (rectum) 685.1
   with abscess 685.0
   malignant (M9084/3) 173.5
pituitary (duct) (gland) 253.8
placenta (amniotic) — see Placenta, abnormal
pleura 519.8
popliteal 727.51
porencephalic 742.4
   acquired 348.0
postanal (infected) 685.1
   with abscess 685.0
posterior segment of eye, congenital 743.54
postmastoidectomy cavity 383.31
preauricular 744.47
prepuce 607.89
   congenital 752.8
primordial (jaw) 526.0
prostate 600
pseudomucinous (ovary) (M8470/0) 220

Cyst—continued
pudenda (sweat glands) 624.8
pupillary, miotic 364.55
   sebaceous 624.8
radicular (residual) 522.8
radiculodental 522.8
ranular 527.6
Rathke's pouch 253.8
rectum (epithelium) (mucous) 569.49
renal — see Cyst, kidney
residual (radicular) 522.8
retention (ovary) 620.2
retina 361.19
   macular 362.54
   parasitic 360.13
   primary 361.13
   secondary 361.14
retroperitoneal 568.89
sacrococcygeal (dermoid) 685.1
   with abscess 685.0
salivary gland or duct 527.6
   mucous extravasation or retention 527.6
Sampson's 617.1
sclera 379.19
scrotum (sebaceous) 706.2
   sweat glands 706.2
sebaceous (duct) (gland) 706.2
   breast 610.8
   eyelid 374.84
   genital organ NEC
      female 629.8
      male 608.89
   scrotum 706.2
semilunar cartilage (knee) (multiple) 717.5
seminal vesicle 608.89
serous (ovary) 620.2
sinus (antral) (ethmoidal) (frontal) (maxillary) (nasal) (sphenoidal) 478.1
Skene's gland 599.89
skin (epidermal) (epidermoid, inclusion) (epithelial) (inclusion) (retention) (sebaceous) 706.2
   breast 610.8
   eyelid 374.84
   genital organ NEC
      female 629.8
      male 608.89
   neoplastic 216.3
   scrotum 706.2
   sweat gland or duct 705.89
solitary
   bone 733.21
   kidney 593.2
spermatic cord 608.89
sphenoid sinus 478.1
spinal meninges 349.2
spine (see also Cyst, bone) 733.20
spleen NEC 289.59
   congenital 759.0
   hydatid (see also Echinococcus) 122.9
spring water (pericardium) 746.89
subarachnoid 348.0
   intrasellar 793.0
subdural (cerebral) 348.0
   spinal cord 349.2
sublingual gland 527.6
   mucous extravasation or retention 527.6
submaxillary gland 527.6
   mucous extravasation or retention 527.6
suburethral 599.89
suprarenal gland 255.8
suprasellar — see Cyst, brain
sweat gland or duct 705.89
sympathetic nervous system 337.9
synovial 727.40
   popliteal space 727.51
Tarlov's 355.9
tarsal 373.2
tendon (sheath) 727.42

Cyst—continued
  testis 608.89
  theca-lutein (ovary) 620.2
  Thornwaldt's, Tornwaldt's 478.26
  thymus (gland) 254.8
  thyroglossal (duct) (infected)
      (persistent) 759.2
  thyroid (gland) 246.2
    adenomatous — see Goiter,
        nodular
    colloid (see also Goiter) 240.9
  thyrolingual duct (infected)
      (persistent) 759.2
  tongue (mucous) 529.8
  tonsil 474.8
  tooth (dental root) 522.8
  tubo-ovarian 620.8
    inflammatory 614.1
  tunica vaginalis 608.89
  turbinate (nose) (see also Cyst,
      bone) 733.20
  Tyson's gland (benign) (infected)
      607.89
  umbilicus 759.89
  urachus 753.7
  ureter 593.89
  ureterovesical orifice 593.89
    congenital 753.4
  urethra 599.84
  urethral gland (Cowper's) 599.89
  uterine
    ligament 620.8
      embryonic 752.11
    tube 620.8
  uterus (body) (corpus) (recurrent)
      621.8
    embryonal 752.3
  utricle (ear) 386.8
    prostatic 599.89
  utriculus masculinus 599.89
  vagina, vaginal (squamous cell)
      (wall) 623.8
    embryonal 752.41
    implantation 623.8
    inclusion 623.8
  vallecula, vallecular 478.79
  ventricle, neuroepithelial 348.0
  verumontanum 599.89
  vesical (orifice) 596.8
  vitreous humor 379.29
  vulva (sweat glands) 624.8
    congenital 752.41
    implantation 624.8
    inclusion 624.8
    sebaceous gland 624.8
  vulvovaginal gland 624.8
  wolffian 752.8
Cystadenocarcinoma (M8440/3) — see
    also Neoplasm, by site,
    malignant
  bile duct type (M8161/3) 155.1
  endometrioid (M8380/3) — see
      Neoplasm, by site, malignant
  mucinous (M8470/3)
    papillary (M8471/3)
      specified site — see
          Neoplasm, by site,
          malignant
      unspecified site 183.0
    specified site — see Neoplasm,
        by site, malignant
    unspecified site 183.0
  papillary (M8450/3)
    mucinous (M8471/3)
      specified site — see
          Neoplasm, by site,
          malignant
      unspecified site 183.0
    pseudomucinous (M8471/3)
      specified site — see
          Neoplasm, by site,
          malignant
      unspecified site 183.0
    serous (M8460/3)
      specified site — see
          Neoplasm, by site,
          malignant

Cystadenocarcinoma—continued
  papillary—continued
    serous—continued
      unspecified site 183.0
    specified site — see Neoplasm,
        by site, malignant
    unspecified site 183.0
  pseudomucinous (M8470/3)
    papillary (M8471/3)
      specified site — see
          Neoplasm, by site,
          malignant
      unspecified site 183.0
    specified site — see Neoplasm,
        by site, malignant
    unspecified site 183.0
  serous (M8441/3)
    papillary (M8460/3)
      specified site — see
          Neoplasm, by site,
          malignant
      unspecified site 183.0
    specified site — see Neoplasm,
        by site, malignant
    unspecified site 183.0
Cystadenofibroma (M9013/0)
  clear cell (M8313/0) —see
      Neoplasm, by site, benign
  endometrioid (M8381/0) 220
    borderline malignancy
        (M8381/1) 236.2
    malignant (M8381/3) 183.0
  mucinous (M9015/0)
    specified site — see Neoplasm,
        by site, benign
    unspecified site 220
  serous (M9014/0)
    specified site — see Neoplasm,
        by site, benign
    unspecified site 220
  specified site — see Neoplasm, by
      site, benign
  unspecified site 220
Cystadenoma (M8440/0) — see also
    Neoplasm, by site, benign
  bile duct (M8161/0) 211.5
  endometrioid (M8380/0) — see
      also Neoplasm, by site,
      benign
    borderline malignancy
        (M8380/1) — see
        Neoplasm, by site,
        uncertain behavior
    malignant (M8440/3) — see
        Neoplasm, by site, malignant
  mucinous (M8470/0)
    borderline malignancy
        (M8470/1)
      specified site — see
          Neoplasm, uncertain
          behavior
      unspecified site 236.2
    papillary (M8471/0)
      borderline malignancy
          (M8471/1)
        specified site — see
            Neoplasm, by site,
            uncertain behavior
        unspecified site 236.2
      specified site — see
          Neoplasm, by site,
          benign
      unspecified site 220
    specified site — see Neoplasm,
        by site, benign
    unspecified site 220
  papillary (M8450/0)
    borderline malignancy
        (M8450/1)
      specified site — see
          Neoplasm, by site,
          uncertain behavior
      unspecified site 236.2
    lymphomatosum (M8561/0)
        210.2

Cystadenoma—continued
  papillary—continued
    mucinous (M8471/0)
      borderline malignancy
          (M8471/1)
        specified site — see
            Neoplasm, by site,
            uncertain behavior
        unspecified site 236.2
      specified site — see
          Neoplasm, by site,
          benign
      unspecified site 220
    pseudomucinous (M8471/0)
      borderline malignancy
          (M8471/1)
        specified site — see
            Neoplasm, by site,
            uncertain behavior
        unspecified site 236.2
      specified site — see
          Neoplasm, by site,
          benign
      unspecified site 220
    serous (M8460/0)
      borderline malignancy
          (M8460/1)
        specified site — see
            Neoplasm, by site,
            uncertain behavior
        unspecified site 236.2
      specified site — see
          Neoplasm, by site,
          benign
      unspecified site 220
    specified site — see Neoplasm,
        by site, benign
    unspecified site 220
  pseudomucinous (M8470/0)
    borderline malignancy
        (M8470/1)
      specified site — see
          Neoplasm, by site,
          uncertain behavior
      unspecified site 236.2
    papillary (M8471/0)
      borderline malignancy
          (M8471/1)
        specified site — see
            Neoplasm, by site,
            uncertain behavior
        unspecified site 236.2
      specified site — see
          Neoplasm, by site,
          benign
      unspecified site 220
    specified site — see Neoplasm,
        by site, benign
    unspecified site 220
  serous (M8441/0)
    borderline malignancy
        (M8441/1)
      specified site — see
          Neoplasm, by site,
          uncertain behavior
      unspecified site 236.2
    papillary (M8460/0)
      borderline malignancy
          (M8460/1)
        specified site — see
            Neoplasm, by site,
            uncertain behavior
        unspecified site 236.2
      specified site — see
          Neoplasm, by site,
          benign
      unspecified site 220
    specified site — see Neoplasm,
        by site, benign
    unspecified site 220
  thyroid 226
Cystathioninemia 270.4
Cystathioninuria 270.4
Cystic — see also condition
  breast, chronic 610.1
  corpora lutea 620.1

Cystic—continued
  degeneration, congenital
    brain 742.4
    kidney 753.10
  disease
    breast, chronic 610.1
    kidney, congenital 753.10
      medullary 753.16
      multiple 753.19
      polycystic — see Polycystic,
          kidney
      single 753.11
      specified NEC 753.19
    liver, congenital 751.62
    lung 518.89
      congenital 748.4
    pancreas, congenital 751.7
    semilunar cartilage 717.5
  duct — see condition
  eyeball, congenital 743.03
  fibrosis (pancreas) 277.00
  hygroma (M9173/0) 228.1
  kidney, congenital 753.10
    medullary 753.16
    multiple 753.19
    polycystic — see Polycystic,
        kidney
    single 753.11
    specified NEC 753.19
  liver, congenital 751.62
  lung 518.89
    congenital 748.4
  mass — see Cyst
  mastitis, chronic 610.1
  ovary 620.2
  pancreas, congenital 751.7
Cysticerciasis 123.1
Cysticercosis (mammary) (subretinal)
    123.1
Cysticercus 123.1
  cellulosae infestation 123.1
Cystinosis (malignant) 270.0
Cystinuria 270.0
Cystitis (bacillary) (colli) (diffuse)
    (exudative) (hemorrhagic)
    (purulent) (recurrent) (septic)
    (suppurative) (ulcerative) 595.9
  with
    abortion — see Abortion, by
        type, with urinary tract
        infection
    ectopic pregnancy (see also
        categories 633.0-633.9)
        639.8
    fibrosis 595.1
    leukoplakia 595.1
    malakoplakia 595.1
    metaplasia 595.1
    molar pregnancy (see also
        categories 630-632)
        639.8
  actinomycotic 039.8 [595.4]
  acute 595.0
    of trigone 595.3
  allergic 595.89
  amebic 006.8 [595.4]
  bilharzial 120.9 [595.4]
  blennorrhagic (acute) 098.11
    chronic or duration of 2 months
        or more 098.31
  bullous 595.89
  calculous 594.1
    chlamydial 099.53
  chronic 595.2
    interstitial 595.1
    of trigone 595.3
  complicating pregnancy, childbirth,
      or puerperium 646.6
    affecting fetus or newborn 760.1
  cystic(a) 595.81
  diphtheritic 032.84
  echinococcal
    granulosus 122.3 [595.4]
    multilocularis 122.6 [595.4]
  emphysematous 595.89
  encysted 595.81

Cystitis—continued
  follicular 595.3
  following
    abortion 639.8
    ectopic or molar pregnancy 639.8
  gangrenous 595.89
  glandularis 595.89
  gonococcal (acute) 098.11
    chronic or duration of 2 months or more 098.31
  incrusted 595.89
  interstitial 595.1
  irradiation 595.82
  irritation 595.89
  malignant 595.89
  monilial 112.2
  of trigone 595.3
  panmural 595.1
  polyposa 595.89
  prostatic 601.3
  radiation 595.82
  Reiter's (abacterial) 099.3
  specified NEC 595.89
  subacute 595.2
  submucous 595.1
  syphilitic 095.8
  trichomoniasis 131.09
  tuberculous (see also Tuberculosis) 016.1
  ulcerative 595.1
Cystocele (-rectocele)
  female (without uterine prolapse) 618.0
    with uterine prolapse 618.4
      complete 618.3
      incomplete 618.2
  in pregnancy or childbirth 654.4
    affecting fetus or newborn 763.8
    causing obstructed labor 660.2
      affecting fetus or newborn 763.1
  male 596.8
Cystoid
  cicatrix limbus 372.64
  degeneration macula 362.53
Cystolithiasis 594.1
Cystoma (M8440/0) — see also Neoplasm, by site, benign
  endometrial, ovary 617.1
  mucinous (M8470/0)
    specified site — see Neoplasm, by site, benign
    unspecified site 220
  serous (M8441/0)
    specified site — see Neoplasm, by site, benign
    unspecified site 220
  simple (ovary) 620.2
Cystoplegia 596.53
Cystoptosis 596.8
Cystopyelitis (see also Pyelitis) 590.80
Cystorrhagia 596.8
Cystosarcoma phyllodes (M9020/1) 238.3
  benign (M9020/0) 217
  malignant (M9020/3) — see Neoplasm, breast, malignant
Cystostomy status V44.5
  with complication 997.5
Cystourethritis (see also Urethritis) 597.89
Cystourethrocele (see also Cystocele)
  female (without uterine prolapse) 618.0
    with uterine prolapse 618.4
      complete 618.3
      incomplete 618.2
  male 596.8
Cytomegalic inclusion disease 078.5
  congenital 771.1
Cytomycosis, reticuloendothelial (see also Histoplasmosis, American) 115.00

Czerny's disease (periodic hydrarthrosis of the knee) 719.06

Daae (-Finsen) disease (epidemic pleurodynia) 074.1
Dabney's grip 074.1
Da Costa's syndrome (neurocirculatory asthenia) 306.2
Dacryoadenitis, dacryadenitis 375.00
 acute 375.01
 chronic 375.02
Dacryocystitis 375.30
 acute 375.32
 chronic 375.42
 neonatal 771.6
 phlegmonous 375.33
 syphilitic 095.8
  congenital 090.0
 trachomatous, active 076.1
  late effect 139.1
 tuberculous (see also Tuberculosis) 017.3
Dacryocystoblenorrhea 375.42
Dacryocystocele 375.43
Dacryolith, dacryolithiasis 375.57
Dacryoma 375.43
Dacryopericystitis (acute) (subacute) 375.32
 chronic 375.42
Dacryops 375.11
Dacryosialadenopathy, atrophic 710.2
Dacryostenosis 375.56
 congenital 743.65
Dactylitis 686.9
 bone (see also Osteomyelitis) 730.2
 sickle cell 282.61
 syphilitic 095.5
 tuberculous (see also Tuberculosis) 015.5
Dactylolysis opontaned 136.0
Dactylosymphysis (see also Syndactylism) 755.10
Damage
 arteriosclerotic — see Arteriosclerosis
 brain 348.9
  anoxic, hypoxic 348.1
   during or resulting from a procedure 997.0
  child NEC 343.9
  due to birth injury 767.0
  minimal (child) (see also Hyperkinesia) 314.9
  newborn 767.0
 cardiac — see also Disease, heart
 cardiorenal (vascular) (see also Hypertension, cardiorenal) 404.90
 central nervous system — see Damage, brain
 cerebral NEC — see Damage, brain
 coccyx, complicating delivery 665.6
 coronary (see also Ischemia, heart) 414.9
 eye, birth injury 767.8
 heart — see also Disease, heart
  valve — see Endocarditis
 hypothalamus NEC 348.9
 liver 571.9
  alcoholic 571.3
 myocardium (see also Degeneration, myocardial) 429.1
 pelvic
  joint or ligament, during delivery 665.6
  organ NEC
   with
    abortion — see Abortion, by type, with damage to pelvic organs
    ectopic pregnancy (see also categories 633.0-633.9) 639.2

Damage—continued
 pelvic—continued
  organ—continued
   with—continued
    molar pregnancy (see also categories 630-632) 639.2
    during delivery 665.5
    following
     abortion 639.2
     ectopic or molar pregnancy 639.2
 renal (see also Disease, renal) 593.9
 skin, solar 692.79
  acute 692.72
  chronic 692.74
 subendocardium, subendocardial (see also Degeneration, myocardial) 429.1
 vascular 459.9
Dameshek's syndrome (erythroblastic anemia) 282.4
Dana-Putnam syndrome (subacute combined sclerosis with pernicious anemia) 281.0 [336.2]
Danbolt (-Closs) syndrome (acrodermatitis enteropathica) 686.8
Dandruff 690
Dandy fever 061
Dandy-Walker deformity or syndrome (atresia, foramen of Magendie) 742.3
 with spina bifida (see also Spina bifida) 741.0
Dangle foot 736.79
Danielssen's disease (anesthetic leprosy) 030.1
Danlos' syndrome 756.83
Darier's disease (congenital) (keratosis follicularis) 757.39
 due to vitamin A deficiency 264.8
 meaning erythema annulare centrifugum 695.0
Darier-Roussy sarcoid 135
Darling's
 disease (see also Histoplasmosis, American) 115.00
 histoplasmosis (see also Histoplasmosis, American) 115.00
Dartre 054.9
Darwin's tubercle 744.29
Davidson's anemia (refractory) 284.9
Davies' disease 425.0
Davies-Colley syndrome (slipping rib) 733.99
Dawson's encephalitis 046.2
Day blindness (see also Blindness, day) 368.60
Dead
 fetus
  retained (in utero) 656.4
   early pregnancy (death before 22 completed weeks gestation) 632
   late (death after 22 completed weeks gestation) 656.4
  syndrome 641.3
 labyrinth 386.50
 ovum, retained 631
Deaf and dumb NEC 389.7
Deaf mutism (acquired) (congenital) NEC 389.7
 endemic 243
 hysterical 300.11
 syphilitic, congenital 090.0

Deafness (acquired) (bilateral) (both ears) (complete) (congenital) (hereditary) (middle ear) (partial) (unilateral) 389.9
 with blue sclera and fragility of bone 756.51
 auditory fatigue 389.9
 aviation 993.0
  nerve injury 951.5
 boilermakers' 951.5
 central 389.14
  with conductive hearing loss 389.2
 conductive (air) 389.00
  with sensorineural hearing loss 389.2
  combined types 389.08
  external ear 389.01
  inner ear 389.04
  middle ear 389.03
  multiple types 389.08
  tympanic membrane 389.02
 emotional (complete) 300.11
 functional (complete) 300.11
 high frequency 389.8
 hysterical (complete) 300.11
 injury 951.5
 low frequency 389.8
 mental 784.69
 mixed conductive and sensorineural 389.2
 nerve 389.12
  with conductive hearing loss 389.2
 neural 389.12
  with conductive hearing loss 389.2
 noise-induced 388.12
  nerve injury 951.5
 nonspeaking 389.7
 perceptive 389.10
  with conductive hearing loss 389.2
  central 389.14
  combined types 389.18
  multiple types 389.18
  neural 389.12
  sensory 389.11
 psychogenic (complete) 306.7
 sensorineural (see also Deafness, perceptive) 389.10
 sensory 389.11
  with conductive hearing loss 389.2
 specified type NEC 389.8
 sudden NEC 388.2
 syphilitic 094.89
 transient ischemic 388.02
 transmission — see Deafness, conductive
 traumatic 951.5
 word (secondary to organic lesion) 784.69
  developmental 315.31
Death
 after delivery (cause not stated) (sudden) 674.9
 anesthetic
  due to
   correct substance properly administered 995.4
   overdose or wrong substance given 968.4
   specified anesthetic — see Table of drugs and chemicals
  during delivery 668.9
 brain 348.8
 cardiac — see Disease, heart
 cause unknown 798.2
 cot (infant) 798.0
 crib (infant) 798.0
 fetus, fetal (cause not stated) (intrauterine) 779.9
  early, with retention (before 22 completed weeks gestation) 632

Death—continued
 fetus, fetal—continued
  from asphyxia or anoxia (before labor) 768.0
  during labor 768.1
  late, affecting management of pregnancy (after 22 completed weeks gestation) 656.4
 from pregnancy NEC 646.9
 instantaneous 798.1
 intrauterine (see also Death, fetus) 779.9
  complicating pregnancy 656.4
 maternal, affecting fetus or newborn 761.6
 neonatal NEC 779.9
 sudden (cause unknown) 798.1
  during delivery 669.9
   under anesthesia NEC 668.9
  infant, syndrome (SIDS) 798.0
  puerperal, during puerperium 674.9
 unattended (cause unknown) 798.9
 under anesthesia NEC
  due to
   correct substance properly administered 995.4
   overdose or wrong substance given 968.4
   specified anesthetic — see Table of drugs and chemicals
   during delivery 668.9
 violent 798.1
de Beurmann-Gougerot disease (sporotrichosis) 117.1
Debility (general) (infantile) (postinfectional) 799.3
 with nutritional difficulty 269.9
 congenital or neonatal NEC 779.9
 nervous 300.5
 old age 797
 senile 797
Débove's disease (splenomegaly) 789.2
Decalcification
 bone (see also Osteoporosis) 733.00
 teeth 521.8
Decapitation 874.9
 fetal (to facilitate delivery) 763.8
Decapsulation, kidney 593.89
Decay
 dental 521.0
 senile 797
 tooth, teeth 521.0
Decensus, uterus — see Prolapse, uterus
Deciduitis (acute)
 with
  abortion — see Abortion, by type, with sepsis
  ectopic pregnancy (see also categories 633.0-633.9) 639.0
  molar pregnancy (see also categories 630-632) 639.0
 affecting fetus or newborn 760.8
 following
  abortion 639.0
  ectopic or molar pregnancy 639.0
 in pregnancy 646.6
 puerperal, postpartum 670
Deciduoma malignum (M9100/3) 181
Deciduous tooth (retained) 520.6
Decline (general) (see also Debility) 799.3
Decompensation
 cardiac (acute) (chronic) (see also Disease, heart) 429.9
  failure — see Failure, heart, congestive

Decompensation—continued
  cardiorenal (see also Hypertension, cardiorenal) 404.90
  cardiovascular (see also Disease, cardiovascular) 429.2
  heart (see also Disease, heart) 429.9
    failure — see Failure, heart, congestive
  hepatic 572.2
  myocardial (acute) (chronic) (see also Disease, heart) 429.9
    failure — see Failure, heart, congestive
  respiratory 519.9
Decompression sickness 993.3
Decrease, decreased
  blood
    platelets (see also Thrombocytopenia) 287.5
    pressure 796.3
      due to shock following injury 958.4
        operation 998.0
  cardiac reserve — see Disease, heart
  estrogen 256.3
    postablative 256.2
  fragility of erythrocytes 289.8
  function
    adrenal (cortex) 255.4
      medulla 255.5
    ovary in hypopituitarism 253.4
    parenchyma of pancreas 577.8
    pituitary (gland) (lobe) (anterior) 253.2
      posterior (lobe) 253.8
  functional activity 780.9
  glucose 790.2
  haptoglobin (serum) NEC 273.8
  platelets (see also Thrombocytopenia) 287.5
  pulse pressure 785.9
  respiration due to shock following injury 958.4
  tear secretion NEC 375.15
  tolerance
    fat 579.8
    glucose 790.2
    salt and water 276.9
  vision NEC 369.9
Decubital gangrene 707.0 [785.4]
Decubiti (see also Decubitus) 707.0
Decubitus (ulcer) 707.0
  with gangrene 707.0 [785.4]
Deepening acetabulum 718.85
Defect, defective 759.9
  3-beta-hydroxysteroid dehydrogenase 255.2
  11-hydroxylase 255.2
  21-hydroxylase 255.2
  abdominal wall, congenital 756.7
  aorticopulmonary septum 745.0
  aortic septal 745.0
  atrial septal (ostium secundum type) 745.5
    acquired 429.71
    ostium primum type 745.61
  atrioventricular
    canal 745.69
    septum 745.4
      acquired 429.71
  atrium secundum 745.5
    acquired 429.71
  auricular septal 745.5
    acquired 429.71
  bilirubin excretion 277.4
  biosynthesis, testicular androgen 257.2
  bulbar septum 745.0
  butanol-insoluble iodide 246.1
  chromosome — see Anomaly, chromosome
  circulation (acquired) 459.9
    congenital 747.9
    newborn 747.9

Defect, defective—continued
  clotting NEC (see also Defect, coagulation) 286.9
  coagulation (factor) (see also Deficiency, coagulation factor) 286.9
    with
      abortion — see Abortion, by type, with hemorrhage
      ectopic pregnancy (see also categories 634-638) 639.1
      molar pregnancy (see also categories 630-632) 639.1
    acquired (any) 286.7
    antepartum or intrapartum 641.3
      affecting fetus or newborn 762.1
      causing hemorrhage of pregnancy or delivery 641.3
    due to
      liver disease 286.7
      vitamin K deficiency 286.7
    newborn, transient 776.3
    postpartum 666.3
    specified type NEC 286.3
  conduction (heart) 426.9
    bone (see also Deafness, conductive) 389.00
  congenital, organ or site NEC — see also Anomaly
  circulation 747.9
  Descemet's membrane 743.9
    specified type NEC 743.49
  diaphragm 756.6
  ectodermal 757.9
  esophagus 750.9
  pulmonic cusps — see Anomaly, heart valve
  respiratory system 748.9
    specified type NEC 748.8
  cushion endocardial 745.60
  dentin (hereditary) 520.5
  Descemet's membrane (congenital) 743.9
    acquired 371.30
    specific type NEC 743.49
  deutan 368.52
  developmental — see also Anomaly, by site
    cauda equina 742.59
    left ventricle 746.9
      with atresia or hypoplasia of aortic orifice or valve, with hypoplasia of ascending aorta 746.7
      in hypoplastic left heart syndrome 746.7
    testis 752.9
    vessel 747.9
  diaphragm
    with elevation, eventration, or hernia — see Hernia, diaphragm
    congenital 756.6
      with elevation, eventration, or hernia 756.6
        gross (with elevation, eventration, or hernia) 756.6
  ectodermal, congenital 757.9
  Eisenmenger's (ventricular septal defect) 745.4
  endocardial cushion 745.60
    specified type NEC 745.69
  esophagus, congenital 750.9
  extensor retinaculum 728.9
  fibrin polymerization (see also Defect, coagulation) 286.3
  filling
    biliary tract 793.3
    bladder 793.5
    gallbladder 793.3
    kidney 793.5
    stomach 793.4

Defect, defective—continued
  filling—continued
    ureter 793.5
  fossa ovalis 745.5
  gene, carrier (suspected) of V19.8
  Gerbode 745.4
  glaucomatous, without elevated tension 365.89
  Hageman (factor) (see also Defect, coagulation) 286.3
  hearing (see also Deafness) 389.9
  high grade 317
  homogentisic acid 270.2
  interatrial septal 745.5
    acquired 429.71
  interauricular septal 745.5
    acquired 429.71
  interventricular septal 745.4
    with pulmonary stenosis or atresia, dextraposition of aorta, and hypertrophy of right ventricle 745.2
    acquired 429.71
    in tetralogy of Fallot 745.2
  iodide trapping 246.1
  iodotyrosine dehalogenase 246.1
  kynureninase 270.2
  learning, specific 315.2
  mental (see also Retardation, mental) 319
  osteochondral NEC 738.8
  ostium
    primum 745.61
    secundum 745.5
  pericardium 746.89
  peroxidase-binding 246.1
  placental blood supply — see Placenta, insufficiency
  platelet (qualitative) 287.1
    constitutional 286.4
  postural, spine 737.9
  protan 368.51
  pulmonic cusps, congenital 746.00
  renal pelvis 753.9
    obstructive 753.2
    specified type NEC 753.3
  respiratory system, congenital 748.9
    specified type NEC 748.8
  retina, retinal 361.30
    with detachment (see also Detachment, retina, with retinal defect) 361.00
      multiple 361.33
        with detachment 361.02
      nerve fiber bundle 362.85
      single 361.30
        with detachment 361.01
  septal (closure) (heart) NEC 745.9
    acquired 429.71
    atrial 745.5
    specified type NEC 745.8
  speech NEC 784.5
    developmental 315.39
    secondary to organic lesion 784.5
  Taussig-Bing (transposition, aorta and overriding pulmonary artery) 745.11
  teeth, wedge 521.2
  thyroid hormone synthesis 246.1
  tritan 368.53
  ureter 753.9
    obstructive 753.2
  vascular (acquired) (local) 459.9
    congenital (peripheral) NEC 747.60
      gastrointestinal 747.61
      lower limb 747.64
      renal 747.62
      specified NEC 747.69
      spinal 747.82
      upper limb 747.63

Defect, defective—continued
  ventricular septal 745.4
    with pulmonary stenosis or atresia, dextraposition of aorta, and hypertrophy of right ventricle 745.2
    acquired 429.71
    atrioventricular canal type 745.69
    between infundibulum and anterior portion 745.4
    in tetralogy of Fallot 745.2
    isolated anterior 745.4
  vision NEC 369.9
  visual field 368.40
    arcuate 368.43
    heteronymous, bilateral 368.47
    homonymous, bilateral 368.46
    localized NEC 368.44
    nasal step 368.44
    peripheral 368.44
    sector 368.43
  voice 784.40
  wedge, teeth (abrasion) 521.2
Defeminization syndrome 255.2
Deferentitis 608.4
  gonorrheal (acute) 098.14
    chronic or duration of 2 months or over 098.34
Defibrination syndrome (see also Fibrinolysis) 286.6
Deficiency, deficient
  3-beta-hydroxysteroid dehydrogenase 255.2
  6-phosphogluconic dehydrogenase (anemia) 282.2
  11-beta-hydroxylase 255.2
  17-alpha-hydroxylase 255.2
  18-hydroxysteroid dehydrogenase 255.2
  20-alpha-hydroxylase 255.2
  21-hydroxylase 255.2
  abdominal muscle syndrome 756.7
  accelerator globulin (Ac G) (blood) (see also Defect, coagulation) 286.3
  AC globulin (congenital) (see also Defect, coagulation) 286.3
    acquired 286.7
  activating factor (blood) (see also, Defect, coagulation) 286.3
  adenohypophyseal 253.2
  adenosine deaminase 277.2
  aldolase (hereditary) 271.2
  alpha-1-antitrypsin 277.6
  alpha-1-trypsin inhibitor 277.6
  alpha-fucosidase 271.8
  alpha-lipoprotein 272.5
  alpha-mannosidase 271.8
  amino acid 270.9
  anemia — see Anemia, deficiency
  aneurin 265.1
    with beriberi 265.0
  antibody NEC 279.00
  antidiuretic hormone 253.5
  antihemophilic
    factor (A) 286.0
    B 286.1
    C 286.2
    globulin (AHG) NEC 286.0
  antitrypsin 277.6
  argininosuccinate synthetase or lyase 270.6
  ascorbic acid (with scurvy) 267
  autoprothrombin
    I (see also Defect, coagulation) 286.3
    II 286.1
    C (see also Defect, coagulation) 286.3
  bile salt 579.8
  biotin 266.2
  bradykinase-1 277.6
  brancher enzyme (amylopectinosis) 271.0

Deficiency, deficient—continued
   calciferol 268.9
     with
       osteomalacia 268.2
       rickets (see also Rickets)
         268.0
   calcium 275.4
     dietary 269.3
   calorie, severe 261
   carbamyl phosphate synthetase 270.6
   cardiac (see also Insufficiency, myocardial) 428.0
   carnitine palmityl transferase 791.3
   carotene 264.9
   Carr factor (see also Defect, coagulation) 286.9
   central nervous system 349.9
   ceruloplasmin 275.1
   cevitamic acid (with scurvy) 267
   choline 266.2
   Christmas factor 286.1
   chromium 269.3
   citrin 269.1
   clotting (blood) (see also Defect, coagulation) 286.9
   coagulation factor NEC 286.9
     with
       abortion — see Abortion, by type, with hemorrhage
       ectopic pregnancy (see also categories 634-638) 639.1
       molar pregnancy (see also categories 630-632) 639.1
     acquired (any) 286.7
     antepartum or intrapartum 641.3
       affecting fetus or newborn 762.1
     due to
       liver disease 286.7
       vitamin K deficiency 286.7
     newborn, transient 776.3
     postpartum 666.3
     specified type NEC 286.3
   color vision (congenital) 368.59
     acquired 368.55
   combined, two or more coagulation factors (see also Defect, coagulation) 286.9
   complement factor NEC 279.8
   contact factor (see also Defect, coagulation) 286.3
   copper NEC 275.1
   corticoadrenal 255.4
   craniofacial axis 756.0
   cyanocobalamin (vitamin B_{12}) 266.2
   debrancher enzyme (limit dextrinosis) 271.0
   desmolase 255.2
   diet 269.9
   dihydrofolate reductase 281.2
   dihydropteridine reductase 270.1
   disaccharidase (intestinal) 271.3
   disease NEC 269.9
   ear(s) V48.8
   edema 262
   endocrine 259.9
   enzymes, circulating NEC (see also Deficiency, by specific enzyme) 277.6
   ergosterol 268.9
     with
       osteomalacia 268.2
       rickets (see also Rickets) 268.0
   erythrocytic glutathione (anemia) 282.2
   eyelid(s) V48.8
   factor (See also Defect, coagulation) 286.9

Deficiency, deficient—continued
   factor—continued
     I (congenital) (fibrinogen) 286.3
       antepartum or intrapartum 641.3
         affecting fetus or newborn 762.1
       newborn, transient 776.3
       postpartum 666.3
     II (congenital) (prothrombin) 286.3
     V (congenital) (labile) 286.3
     VII (congenital) (stable) 286.3
     VIII (congenital) (functional) 286.0
       with
         functional defect 286.0
         vascular defect 286.4
     IX (Christmas) (congenital) (functional) 286.1
     X (congenital) (Stuart-Prower) 286.3
     XI (congenital) (plasma thromboplastin antecedent) 286.2
     XII (congenital) (Hageman) 286.3
     XIII (congenital) (fibrin stabilizing) 286.3
     Hageman 286.3
     multiple (congenital) 286.9
       acquired 286.7
     fibrin stabilizing factor (congenital) (see also Defect, coagulation) 286.3
       acquired 286.7
     fibrinase (see also Defect, coagulation) 286.3
     fibrinogen (congenital) (see also Defect, coagulation) 286.3
       acquired 286.6
     finger — see Absence, finger
     Fletcher factor (see also Defect, coagulation) 286.9
   fluorine 269.3
   folate, anemia 281.2
   folic acid (vitamin B_6) 266.2
     anemia 281.2
   follicle-stimulating hormone (FSH) 253.4
   fructokinase 271.2
   fructose-1, 6-diphosphate 271.2
   fructose-1-phosphate aldolase 271.2
   FSH (follicle-stimulating hormone) 253.4
   fucosidase 271.8
   galactokinase 271.1
   galactose-1-phosphate uridyl transferase 271.1
   gamma globulin in blood 279.00
   glass factor (see also Defect, coagulation) 286.3
   glucocorticoid 255.4
   glucose-6-phosphatase 271.0
   glucose-6-phosphate dehydrogenase anemia 282.2
   glucuronyl transferase 277.4
   glutathione-reductase (anemia) 282.2
   glycogen synthetase 271.0
   growth hormone 253.3
   Hageman factor (congenital) (see also Defect, coagulation) 286.3
   head V48.0
   hemoglobin (see also Anemia) 285.9
   hepatophosphorylase 271.0
   hexose monophosphate (HMP) shunt 282.2
   HGH (human growth hormone) 253.3
   HG-PRT 277.2
   homogentisic acid oxidase 270.2

Deficiency, deficient—continued
   hormone — see also Deficiency, by specific hormone
     anterior pituitary (isolated) (partial) NEC 253.4
       growth (human) 253.3
     follicle-stimulating 253.4
     growth (human) (isolated) 253.3
     human growth 253.3
     interstitial cell-stimulating 253.4
     luteinizing 253.4
     melanocyte-stimulating 253.4
     testicular 257.2
   human growth hormone 253.3
   humoral 279.00
     with
       hyper-IgM 279.05
         autosomal recessive 279.05
         X-linked 279.05
       increased IgM 279.05
     congenital hypogammaglobulinemia 279.04
     non-sex-linked 279.06
     selective immunoglobulin NEC 279.03
       IgA 279.01
       IgG 279.03
       IgM 279.02
         increased 279.05
     specified NEC 279.09
   hydroxylase 255.2
   hypoxanthine-guanine phosphoribosyltransferase (HG-PRT) 277.2
   ICSH (interstitial cell-stimulating hormone) 253.4
   immunity NEC 279.3
     cell-mediated 279.10
       with
         hyperimmunoglob- ulinemia 279.2
         thrombocytopenia and eczema 279.12
       specified NEC 279.19
     combined (severe) 279.2
       syndrome 279.2
     common variable 279.06
     humoral NEC 279.00
     IgA (secretory) 279.01
     IgG 279.03
     IgM 279.02
   immunoglobulin, selective NEC 279.03
     IgA 279.01
     IgG 279.03
     IgM 279.02
   inositol (B complex) 266.2
   interferon 279.4
   internal organ V47.0
   interstitial cell-stimulating hormone (ICSH) 253.4
   intrinsic factor (Castle's) (congenital) 281.0
   intrinsic (urethral) sphincter (ISD) 599.82
   invertase 271.3
   iodine 269.3
   iron, anemia 280.9
   labile factor (congenital) (see also Defect, coagulation) 286.3
     acquired 286.7
   lacrimal fluid (acquired) 375.15
     congenital 743.64
   lactase 271.3
   Laki-Lorand factor (see also Defect, coagulation) 286.3
   lecithin-cholesterol acyltranferase 272.5
   LH (luteinizing hormone) 253.4
   limb V49.0
     lower V49.0
       congenital (see also Deficiency, lower limb, congenital) 755.30

Deficiency, deficient—continued
   limb—continued
     upper V49.0
       congenital (see also Deficiency, upper limb, congenital) 755.20
   lipocaic 577.8
   lipoid (high-density) 272.5
   lipoprotein (familial) (high density) 272.5
   liver phosphorylase 271.0
   lower limb V49.0
     congenital 755.30
       with complete absence of distal elements 755.31
       longitudinal (complete) (partial) (with distal deficiencies, incomplete) 755.32
         with complete absence of distal elements 755.31
         combined femoral, tibial, fibular (incomplete) 755.33
         femoral 755.34
         fibular 755.37
         metatarsal(s) 755.38
         phalange(s) 755.39
           meaning all digits 755.31
         tarsal(s) 755.38
         tibia 755.36
         tibiofibular 755.35
       transverse 755.31
   luteinizing hormone (LH) 253.4
   lysosomal alpha-1, 4 glucosidase 271.0
   magnesium 275.2
   mannosidase 271.8
   melanocyte-stimulating hormone (MSH) 253.4
   menadione (vitamin K) 269.0
     newborn 776.0
   mental (familial) (hereditary) (see also Retardation, mental) 319
   mineral NEC 269.3
   molybdenum 269.3
   moral 301.7
   multiple, syndrome 260
   myocardial (see also Insufficiency, myocardial) 428.0
   myophosphorylase 271.0
   NADH (DPNH)-methemoglobin- reductase (congenital) 289.7
   NADH-diaphorase or reductase (congenital) 289.7
   neck V48.1
   niacin (amide) (-tryptophan) 265.2
   nicotinamide 265.2
   nicotinic acid (amide) 265.2
   nose V48.8
   number of teeth (see also Anodontia) 520.0
   nutrition, nutritional 269.9
     specified NEC 269.8
   ornithine transcarbamylase 270.6
   ovarian 256.3
   oxygen (see also Anoxia) 799.0
   pantothenic acid 266.2
   parathyroid (gland) 252.1
   phenylalanine hydroxylase 270.1
   phosphofructokinase 271.2
   phosphoglucomutase 271.0
   phosphohexosisomerase 271.0
   phosphorylase kinase, liver 271.0
   pituitary (anterior) 253.2
     posterior 253.5
   placenta — see Placenta, insufficiency
   plasma
     cell 279.00

Deficiency, deficient—continued
  plasma—continued
    protein (paraproteinemia)
      (pyroglobulinemia) 273.8
      gamma globulin 279.00
    thromboplastin
      antecedent (PTA) 286.2
      component (PTC) 286.1
  platelet NEC 287.1
    constitutional 286.4
  polyglandular 258.9
  potassium (K) 276.8
  proaccelerin (congenital) (see also
    Defect, congenital) 286.3
    acquired 286.7
  proconvertin factor (congenital) (see
    also Defect, coagulation)
    286.3
    acquired 286.7
  prolactin 253.4
  protein 260
    anemia 281.4
    plasma — see Deficiency,
      plasma protein
  prothrombin (congenital) (see also
    Defect coagulation) 286.3
    acquired 286.7
  Prower factor (see also Defect,
    coagulation) 286.3
  PRT 277.2
  pseudocholinesterase 289.8
  psychobiological 301.6
  PTA 286.2
  PTC 286.1
  purine nucleoside phosphorylase
    277.2
  pyracin (alpha) (Beta) 266.1
  pyridoxal 266.1
  pyridoxamine 266.1
  pyridoxine (derivatives) 266.1
  pyruvate kinase (PK) 282.3
  riboflavin (vitamin B_2) 266.0
  saccadic eye movements 379.57
  salivation 527.7
  salt 276.1
  secretion
    ovary 256.3
    salivary gland (any) 527.7
    urine 788.5
  selenium 269.3
  serum
    antitrypsin, familial 277.6
    protein (congenital) 273.8
  smooth pursuit movements (eye)
    379.58
  sodium (Na) 276.1
  SPCA (see also Defect, coagulation)
    286.3
  specified NEC 269.8
  stable factor (congenital) (see also
    Defect, coagulation) 286.3
    acquired 286.7
  Stuart (-Prower) factor (see also
    Defect, coagulation) 286.3
  sucrase 271.3
  sucrase-isomaltase 271.3
  sulfite oxidase 270.0
  syndrome, multiple 260
  thiamine, thiaminic (chloride)
    265.1
  thrombokinase (see also Defect,
    coagulation) 286.3
    newborn 776.0
  thrombopoieten 287.3
  thymolymphatic 279.2
  thyroid (gland) 244.9
  tocopherol 269.1
  toe — see Absence, toe
  tooth bud (see also Anodontia)
    520.0
  trunk V48
  UDPG-glycogen transferase 271.0
  upper limb V49.0
    congenital 755.20
      with complete absence of
        distal elements 755.21

Deficiency, deficient—continued
  upper limb—continued
    congenital—continued
      longitudinal (complete)
        (partial) (with distal
        deficiencies,
        incomplete) 755.22
      carpal(s) 755.28
      combined humeral,
        radial, ulnar
        (incomplete)
        755.23
      humeral 755.24
      metacarpal(s) 755.28
      phalange(s) 755.29
        meaning all digits
          755.21
      radial 755.26
      radioulnar 755.25
      ulnar 755.27
      transverse (complete) (partial)
        755.21
  vascular 459.9
  vasopressin 253.5
  viosterol (see also Deficiency,
    calciferol) 268.9
  vitamin (multiple) NEC 269.2
    A 264.9
      with
        Bitôt's spot 264.1
        corneal 264.2
          with corneal
            ulceration
            264.3
        keratomalacia 264.4
        keratosis, follicular 264.8
        night blindness 264.5
        scar of cornea,
          xerophthalmic
          264.6
        specified manifestation
          NEC 264.8
        ocular 264.7
        xeroderma 264.8
        xerophthalmia 264.7
        xerosis
          conjunctival 264.0
            with Bitôt's spot
              264.1
          corneal 264.2
            with corneal
              ulceraton
              264.3
    B (complex) NEC 266.9
      with
        beriberi 265.0
        pellagra 265.2
        specified type NEC 266.2
    B_1 NEC 265.1
      beriberi 265.0
    B_2 266.0
    B_6 266.1
    B_{12} 266.2
    B_9 (folic acid) 266.2
    C (ascorbic acid) (with scurvy)
      267
    D (calciferol) (ergosterol) 268.9
      with
        osteomalacia 268.2
        rickets (see also Rickets)
          268.0
    E 269.1
    folic acid 266.2
    G 266.0
    H 266.1
    K 269.0
      of newborn 776.0
    nicotinic acid 265.2
    P 269.1
    PP 265.2
    specified NEC 269.1
  zinc 269.3
Deficient — see also Deficiency
  blink reflex 374.45
  craniofacial axis 756.0
  number of teeth (see also
    Anodontia) 520.0

Deficient—continued
  secretion of urine 788.5
Deficit
  neurologic NEC 781.9
    due to
      cerebrovascular lesion (see
        also Disease,
        cerebrovascular,
        acute) 436
        late effect — see category
          438
      transient ischemic attack
        435.9
  oxygen 799.0
Deflection
  radius 736.09
  septum (acquired) (nasal) (nose)
    470
  spine — see Curvature, spine
  turbinate (nose) 470
Defluvium
  capillorum (see also Alopecia)
    704.00
  ciliorum 374.55
  unguium 703.8
Deformity 759.9
  abdomen, congenital 759.9
  abdominal wall
    acquired 738.8
    congenital 756.7
    muscle deficiency syndrome
      756.7
  acquired (unspecified site) 738.9
    specified site NEC 738.8
  adrenal gland (congenital) 759.1
  alimentary tract, congenital 751.9
    lower 751.5
    specified type NEC 751.8
    upper (any part, except tongue)
      750.9
      specified type NEC 750.8
      tongue 750.10
        specified type NEC
          750.19
  ankle (joint) (acquired) 736.70
    abduction 718.47
    congenital 755.69
    contraction 718.47
  anus (congenital) 751.5
    acquired 569.49
  aorta (congenital) 747.20
    acquired 447.8
    arch 747.21
      acquired 447.8
    coarctation 747.10
  aortic
    arch 747.21
      acquired 447.8
    cusp or valve (congenital) 746.9
      acquired (see also
        Endocarditis,
        aortic) 424.1
    ring 747.21
  appendix 751.5
  arm (acquired) 736.89
    congenital 755.50
  arteriovenous (congenital)
    (peripheral) NEC 747.60
    gastrointestinal 747.61
    lower limb 747.64
    renal 747.62
    specified NEC 747.69
    spinal 747.82
    upper limb 747.63
  artery (congenital) (peripheral) NEC
    (see also Deformity, vascular)
    747.60
    acquired 447.8
    cerebral 747.81
    coronary (congenital) 746.85
      acquired (see also Ischemia,
        heart) 414.9
    retinal 743.9
    umbilical 747.5
  atrial septal (congenital) (heart)
    745.5

Deformity—continued
  auditory canal (congenital)
    (external) (see also
    Deformity, ear) 744.3
    acquired 380.50
  auricle
    ear (congenital) (see also
      Deformity, ear) 744.3
      acquired 380.32
    heart (congenital) 746.9
  back (acquired) — see Deformity,
    spine
  Bartholin's duct (congenital) 750.9
  bile duct (congenital) 751.60
    acquired 576.8
      with calculus,
        choledocholithiasis, or
        stones — see
        Choledocholithiasis
  biliary duct or passage (congenital)
    751.60
    acquired 576.8
      with calculus,
        choledocholithiasis, or
        stones — see
        Choledocholithiasis
  bladder (neck) (spincter) (trigone)
    (acquired) 596.8
    congenital 753.9
  bone (acquired) NEC 738.9
    congenital 756.9
    turbinate 738.0
  boutonniere (finger) 736.21
  brain (congenital) 742.9
    acquired 348.8
    multiple 742.4
    reduction 742.2
    vessel (congenital) 747.81
  breast (acquired) 611.8
    congenital 757.9
  bronchus (congenital) 748.3
    acquired 519.1
  bursa, congenital 756.9
  canal of Nuck 752.9
  canthus (congenital) 743.9
    acquired 374.89
  capillary (acquired) 448.9
    congenital NEC (see also
      Deformity, vascular)
      747.60
  cardiac — see Deformity, heart
  cardiovascular system (congenital)
    746.9
  caruncle, lacrimal (congenital)
    743.9
    acquired 375.69
  cascade, stomach 537.6
  cecum (congenital) 751.5
    acquired 569.89
  cerebral (congenital) 742.9
    acquired 348.8
  cervix (acquired) (uterus) 622.8
    congenital 752.40
  cheek (acquired) 738.19
    congenital 744.9
  chest (wall) (acquired) 738.3
    congenital 754.89
    late effect of rickets 268.1
  chin (acquired) 738.19
    congenital 744.9
  choroid (congenital) 743.9
    acquired 363.8
    plexus (congenital) 742.9
      acquired 349.2
  cicatricial — see Cicatrix
  cilia (congenital) 743.9
    acquired 374.89
  circulatory system (congenital)
    747.9
  clavicle (acquired) 738.8
    congenital 755.51
  clitoris (congenital) 752.40
    acquired 624.8
  clubfoot — see Clubfoot
  coccyx (acquired) 738.6
    congenital 756.10

Deformity—continued
  colon (congenital) 751.5
    acquired 569.89
  concha (ear) (congenital) (see also
      Deformity, ear) 744.3
    acquired 380.32
  congenital, organ or site not listed
      (see also Anomaly) 759.9
  cornea (congenital) 743.9
    acquired 371.70
  coronary artery (congenital) 746.85
    acquired (see also Ischemia,
        heart) 414.9
  cranium (acquired) 738.19
    congenital (see also Deformity,
        skull, congenital) 756.0
  cricoid cartilage (congenital) 748.3
    acquired 478.79
  cystic duct (congenital) 751.60
    acquired 575.8
  Dandy-Walker 742.3
    with spina bifida (see also Spina
        bifida) 741.0
  diaphragm (congenital) 756.6
    acquired 738.8
  digestive organ(s) or system
      (congenital) NEC 751.9
    specified type NEC 751.8
  ductus arteriosus 747.0
  duodenal bulb 537.89
  duodenum (congenital) 751.5
    acquired 537.89
  dura (congenital) 742.9
    brain 742.4
      acquired 349.2
    spinal 742.59
      acquired 349.2
  ear (congenital) 744.3
    acquired 380.32
    auricle 744.3
      causing impairment of
          hearing 744.02
    causing impairment of hearing
        744.00
    external 744.3
      causing impairment of
          hearing 744.02
    internal 744.05
    lobule 744.3
    middle 744.03
      ossicles 744.04
    ossicles 744.04
  ectodermal (congenital) NEC 757.9
    specified type NEC 757.8
  ejaculatory duct (congenital) 752.9
    acquired 608.89
  elbow (joint) (acquired) 736.00
    congenital 755.50
    contraction 718.42
  endocrine gland NEC 759.2
  epididymis (congenital) 752.9
    acquired 608.89
    torsion 608.2
  epiglottis (congenital) 748.3
    acquired 478.79
  esophagus (congenital) 750.9
    acquired 530.89
  Eustachian tube (congenital) NEC
      744.3
    specified type NEC 744.24
  extremity (acquired) 736.9
    congenital, except reduction
        deformity 755.9
      lower 755.60
      upper 755.50
      reduction — see Deformity,
          reduction
  eye (congenital) 743.9
    acquired 379.8
    muscle 743.9
  eyebrow (congenital) 744.89
  eyelid (congenital) 743.9
    acquired 374.89
    specified type NEC 743.62

Deformity—continued
  face (acquired) 738.19
    congenital (any part) 744.9
      due to intrauterine
          malposition and
          pressure 754.0
  fallopian tube (congenital) 752.10
    acquired 620.8
  femur (acquired) 736.89
    congenital 755.60
  fetal
    with fetopelvic disproportion
        653.7
      affecting fetus or newborn
          763.1
    causing obstructed labor 660.1
      affecting fetus or newborn
          763.1
    known or suspected, affecting
        management of
        pregnancy 655.9
  finger (acquired) 736.20
    boutonniere type 736.21
    congenital 755.50
    flexion contracture 718.44
    swan neck 736.22
  flexion (joint) (acquired) 736.9
    congenital NEC 755.9
    hip or thigh (acquired) 736.39
      congenital (see also
          Subluxation,
          congenital, hip)
          754.32
  foot (acquired) 736.70
    cavovarus 736.75
      congenital 754.59
    congenital NEC 754.70
      specified type NEC 754.79
    valgus (acquired) 736.79
      congenital 754.60
        specified type NEC
            754.69
    varus (acquired) 736.79
      congenital 754.50
        specified type NEC
            754.59
  forearm (acquired) 736.00
    congenital 755.50
  forehead (acquired) 738.19
    congenital (see also Deformity,
        skull, congenital) 756.0
  frontal bone (acquired) 738.19
    congenital (see also Deformity,
        skull, congenital) 756.0
  gallbladder (congenital) 751.60
    acquired 575.8
  gastrointestinal tract (congenital)
      NEC 751.9
    acquired 569.89
    specified type NEC 751.8
  genitalia, genital organ(s) or system
      NEC
    congenital 752.9
    female (congenital) 752.9
      acquired 629.8
      external 752.40
      internal 752.9
    male (congenital) 752.9
      acquired 608.89
  globe (eye) (congenital) 743.9
    acquired 360.89
  gum (congenital) 750.9
    acquired 523.9
  gunstock 736.02
  hand (acquired) 736.00
    claw 736.06
    congenital 755.50
    minus (and plus) (intrinsic)
        736.09
    pill roller (intrinsic) 736.09
    plus (and minus) (intrinsic)
        736.09
    swan neck (intrinsic) 736.09
  head (acquired) 738.10
    congenital (see also Deformity,
        skull congenital) 756.0
    specified NEC 738.19

Deformity—continued
  heart (congenital) 746.9
    auricle (congenital) 746.9
    septum 745.9
      auricular 745.5
      specified type NEC 745.8
      ventricular 745.4
    valve (congenital) NEC 746.9
      acquired — see Endocarditis
      pulmonary (congenital)
          746.00
        specified type NEC 746.89
    ventricle (congenital) 746.9
  heel (acquired) 736.76
    congenital 755.67
  hepatic duct (congenital) 751.60
    acquired 576.8
      with calculus,
          choledocholithiasis, or
          stones — see
          Choledocholithiasis
  hip (joint) (acquired) 736.30
    congenital NEC 755.63
    flexion 718.45
      congenital (see also
          Subluxation,
          congenital, hip)
          754.32
  hourglass — see Contraction,
      hourglass
  humerus (acquired) 736.89
    congenital 755.50
  hymen (congenital) 752.40
  hypophyseal (congenital) 759.2
  ileocecal (coil) (valve) (congenital)
      751.5
    acquired 569.89
  ileum (intestine) (congenital) 751.5
    acquired 569.89
  ilium (acquired) 738.6
    congenital 755.60
  integument (congenital) 757.9
  intervertebral cartilage or disc
      (acquired) — see also
      Displacement, intervertebral
      disc
    congenital 756.10
  intestine (large) (small) (congenital)
      751.5
    acquired 569.89
  iris (acquired) 364.75
    congenital 743.9
    prolapse 364.8
  ischium (acquired) 738.6
    congenital 755.60
  jaw (acquired) (congenital) NEC
      524.9
    due to intrauterine malposition
        and pressure 754.0
  joint (acquired) NEC 738.8
    congenital 755.9
    contraction (abduction)
        (adduction) (extension)
        (flexion) — see
        Contraction, joint
  kidney(s) (calyx) (pelvis)
      (congenital) 753.9
    acquired 593.89
    vessel 747.62
      acquired 459.9
  Klippel-Feil (brevicollis) 756.16
  knee (acquired) NEC 736.6
    congenital 755.64
  labium (majus) (minus) (congenital)
      752.40
    acquired 624.8
  lacrimal apparatus or duct
      (congenital) 743.9
    acquired 375.69
  larynx (muscle) (congenital) 748.3
    acquired 478.79
    web (glottic) (subglottic) 748.2
  leg (lower) (upper) (acquired) NEC
      736.89
    congenital 755.60
      reduction — see Deformity,
          reduction, lower limb

Deformity—continued
  lens (congenital) 743.9
    acquired 379.39
  lid (fold) (congenital) 743.9
    acquired 374.89
  ligament (acquired) 728.9
    congenital 756.9
  limb (acquired) 736.9
    congenital, except reduction
        deformity 755.9
      lower 755.60
        reduction (see also
            Deformity,
            reduction, lower
            limb) 755.30
      upper 755.50
        reduction (see also
            Deformity,
            reduction, upper
            limb) 755.20
    specified NEC 736.89
  lip (congenital) NEC 750.9
    acquired 528.5
    specified type NEC 750.26
  liver (congenital) 751.60
    acquired 573.8
    duct (congenital) 751.60
      acquired 576.8
        with calculus, choledo-
            cholithiasis, or
            stones — see
            Choledocholithi-
            asis
  lower extremity — see Deformity,
      leg
  lumbosacral (joint) (region)
      (congenital) 756.10
    acquired 738.5
  lung (congenital) 748.60
    acquired 518.89
    specified type NEC 748.69
  lymphatic system, congenital 759.9
  Madelung's (radius) 755.54
  maxilla (acquired) (congenital)
      524.9
  meninges or membrane (congenital)
      742.9
    brain 742.4
      acquired 349.2
    spinal (cord) 742.59
      acquired 349.2
  mesentery (congenitial) 751.9
    acquired 568.89
  metacarpus (acquired) 736.00
    congenital 755.50
  metatarsus (acquired) 736.70
    congenital 754.70
  middle ear, except ossicles
      (congenital) 744.03
    ossicles 744.04
  mitral (leaflets) (valve) (congenital)
      746.9
    acquired — see Endocarditis,
        mitral
    Ebstein's 746.89
    parachute 746.5
    specified type NEC 746.89
    stenosis, congenital 746.5
  mouth (acquired) 528.9
    congenital NEC 750.9
      specified type NEC 750.26
  multiple, congenital NEC 759.7
    specified type NEC 759.89
  muscle (acquired) 728.9
    congenital 756.9
      specified type NEC 756.89
      sternocleidomastoid (due to
          intrauterine
          malposition and
          pressure) 754.1
  musculoskeletal system, congenital
      NEC 756.9
    specified type NEC 756.9
  nail (acquired) 703.9
    congenital 757.9
  nasal — see Deformity, nose

Deformity—continued
- neck (acquired) NEC 738.2
  - congenital (any part) 744.9
    - sternocleidomastoid 754.1
- nervous system (congenital) 742.9
- nipple (congenital) 757.9
  - acquired 611.8
- nose, nasal (cartilage) (acquired) 738.0
  - bone (turbinate) 738.0
  - congenital 748.1
    - bent 754.0
    - squashed 754.0
  - saddle 738.0
    - syphilitic 090.5
  - septum 470
    - congenital 748.1
  - sinus (wall) (congenital) 748.1
    - acquired 738.0
  - syphilitic (congenital) 090.5
    - late 095.8
- ocular muscle (congenital) 743.9
  - acquired 378.60
- opticociliary vessels (congenital) 743.9
- orbit (congenital) (eye) 743.9
  - acquired NEC 376.40
    - associated with craniofacial deformities 376.44
    - due to
      - bone disease 376.43
      - surgery 376.47
      - trauma 376.47
- organ of Corti (congenital) 744.05
- ovary (congenital) 752.0
  - acquired 620.8
- oviduct (congenital) 752.10
  - acquired 620.8
- palate (congenital) 750.9
  - acquired 526.89
  - cleft (congenital) (see also Cleft, palate) 749.00
  - hard, acquired 526.89
  - soft, acquired 528.9
- pancreas (congenital) 751.7
  - acquired 577.8
- parachute, mitral valve 746.5
- parathyroid (gland) 759.2
- parotid (gland) (congenital) 750.9
  - acquired 527.8
- patella (acquired) 736.6
  - congenital 755.64
- pelvis, pelvic (acquired) (bony) 738.6
  - with disproportion (fetopelvic) 653.0
    - affecting fetus or newborn 763.1
    - causing obstructed labor 660.1
      - affecting fetus or newborn 763.1
  - congenital 755.60
  - rachitic (late effect) 268.1
- penis (glans) (congenital) 752.9
  - acquired 607.89
- pericardium (congenital) 746.9
  - acquired — see Pericarditis
- pharynx (congenital) 750.9
  - acquired 478.29
- Pierre Robin (congenital) 756.0
- pinna (acquired) 380.32
  - congenital 744.3
- pituitary (congenital) 759.2
- pleural folds (congenital) 748.8
- portal vein (congenital) 747.40
- posture see Curvature, spine
- prepuce (congenital) 752.9
  - acquired 607.89
- prostate (congenital) 752.9
  - acquired 602.8
- pulmonary valve — see Endocarditis, pulmonary
- pupil (congenital) 743.9
  - acquired 364.75
- pylorus (congenital) 750.9
  - acquired 537.89

Deformity—continued
- rachitic (acquired), healed or old 268.1
- radius (acquired) 736.00
  - congenital 755.50
  - reduction — see Deformity, reduction, upper limb
- rectovaginal septum (congenital) 752.40
  - acquired 623.8
- rectum (congenital) 751.5
  - acquired 569.49
- reduction (extremity) (limb) 755.4
  - brain 742.2
  - lower limb 755.30
    - with complete absence of distal elements 755.31
    - longitudinal (complete) (partial) (with distal deficiencies, incomplete) 755.32
      - with complete absence of distal elements 755.31
      - combined femoral, tibial, fibular (incomplete) 755.33
      - femoral 755.34
      - fibular 755.37
      - metatarsal(s) 755.38
      - phalange(s) 755.39
        - meaning all digits 755.31
      - tarsal(s) 755.38
      - tibia 755.36
      - tibiofibular 755.35
    - transverse 755.31
  - upper limb 755.20
    - with complete absence of distal elements 755.21
    - longitudinal (complete) (partial) (with distal deficiencies, incomplete) 755.22
      - with complete absence of distal elements 755.21
      - carpal(s) 755.28
      - combined humeral, radial, ulnar (incomplete) 755.23
      - humeral 755.24
      - metacarpal(s) 755.28
      - phalange(s) 755.29
        - meaning all digits 755.21
      - radial 755.26
      - radioulnar 755.25
      - ulnar 755.27
    - transverse (complete) (partial) 755.21
- renal — see Deformity, kidney
- respiratory system (congenital) 748.9
  - specified type NEC 748.8
- rib (acquired) 738.3
  - congenital 756.3
  - cervical 756.2
- rotation (joint) (acquired) 736.9
  - congenital 755.9
  - hip or thigh 736.39
    - congenital (see also Subluxation, congenital, hip) 754.32
- sacroiliac joint (congenital) 755.69
  - acquired 738.5
- sacrum (acquired) 738.5
  - congenital 756.10
- saddle
  - back 737.8
  - nose 738.0
    - syphilitic 090.5
- salivary gland or duct (congenital) 750.9
  - acquired 527.8

Deformity—continued
- scapula (acquired) 736.89
  - congenital 755.50
- scrotum (congenital) 752.9
  - acquired 608.89
- sebaceous gland, acquired 706.8
- seminal tract or duct (congenital) 752.9
  - acquired 608.89
- septum (nasal) (acquired) 470
  - congenital 748.1
- shoulder (joint) (acquired) 736.89
  - congenital 755.50
    - specified type NEC 755.59
  - contraction 718.41
- sigmoid (flexure) (congenital) 751.5
  - acquired 569.89
- sinus of Valsalva 747.29
- skin (congenital) 757.9
  - acquired NEC 709.8
- skull (acquired) 738.19
  - congenital 756.0
    - with
      - anencephalus 740.0
      - encephalocele 742.0
      - hydrocephalus 742.3
        - with spina bifida (see also Spina bifida) 741.0
      - microcephalus 742.1
    - due to intrauterine malposition and pressure 754.0
- soft parts, organs or tissues (of pelvis)
  - in pregnancy or childbirth NEC 654.9
    - affecting fetus or newborn 763.8
    - causing obstructed labor 660.2
      - affecting fetus or newborn 763.1
- spermatic cord (congenital) 752.9
  - acquired 608.89
  - torsion 608.2
- spinal
  - column — see Deformity, spine
  - cord (congenital) 742.9
    - acquired 336.8
  - vessel (congenital) 747.82
- nerve root (congenital) 742.9
  - acquired 724.9
- spine (acquired) NEC 738.5
  - congenital 756.10
    - due to intrauterine malposition and pressure 754.2
  - kyphoscoliotic (see also Kyphoscoliosis) 737.30
  - kyphotic (see also Kyphosis) 737.10
  - lordotic (see also Lordosis) 737.20
  - rachitic 268.1
  - scoliotic (see also Scoliosis) 737.30
- spleen
  - acquired 289.59
  - congenital 759.0
- Sprengel's (congenital) 755.52
- sternum (acquired) 738.3
  - congenital 756.3
- stomach (congenital) 750.9
  - acquired 537.89
- submaxillary gland (congenital) 750.9
  - acquired 527.8
- swan neck (acquired)
  - finger 736.22
  - hand 736.09
- talipes — see Talipes
- teeth, tooth NEC 520.9
- testis (congenital) 752.9
  - acquired 608.89
  - torsion 608.2

Deformity—continued
- thigh (acquired) 736.89
  - congenital 755.60
- thorax (acquired) (wall) 738.3
  - congenital 754.89
  - late effect of rickets 268.1
- thumb (acquired) 736.20
  - congenital 755.50
- thymus (tissue) (congenital) 759.2
- thyroid (gland) (congenital) 759.2
  - cartilage 748.3
    - acquired 478.79
- tibia (acquired) 736.89
  - congenital 755.60
  - saber 090.5
- toe (acquired) 735.9
  - congenital 755.66
  - specified NEC 735.8
- tongue (congenital) 750.10
  - acquired 529.8
- tooth, teeth NEC 520.9
- trachea (rings) (congenital) 748.3
  - acquired 519.1
- transverse aortic arch (congenital) 747.21
- tricuspid (leaflets) (valve) (congenital) 746.9
  - acquired — see Endocarditis, tricuspid
  - atresia or stenosis 746.1
  - specified type NEC 746.89
- trunk (acquired) 738.3
  - congenital 759.9
- ulna (acquired) 736.00
  - congenital 755.50
- upper extremity — see Deformity, arm
- urachus (congenital) 753.7
- ureter (opening) (congenital) 753.9
  - acquired 593.89
- urethra (valve) (congenital) 753.9
  - acquired 599.84
- urinary tract or system (congenital) 753.9
  - urachus 753.7
- uterus (congenital) 752.3
  - acquired 621.8
- uvula (congenital) 750.9
  - acquired 528.9
- vagina (congenital) 752.40
  - acquired 623.8
- valve, valvular (heart) (congenital) 746.9
  - acquired — see Endocarditis
  - pulmonary 746.00
  - specified type NEC 746.89
- vascular (congenital) NEC 747.6
  - acquired 459.9
- vas deferens (congenital) 752.9
  - acquired 608.89
- vein (congenital) NEC (see also Deformity, vascular) 747.60
  - brain 747.81
  - coronary 746.9
  - great 747.40
- vena cava (inferior) (superior) (congenital) 747.40
- vertebra — see Deformity, spine
- vesicourethral orifice (acquired) 596.8
  - congenital NEC 753.9
    - specified type NEC 753.8
- vessels of optic papilla (congenital) 743.9
- visual field (contraction) 368.45
- vitreous humor (congenital) 743.9
  - acquired 379.29
- vulva (congenital) 752.40
  - acquired 624.8
- wrist (joint) (acquired) 736.00
  - congenital 755.50
  - contraction 718.43
  - valgus 736.03
    - congenital 755.59
  - varus 736.04
    - congenital 755.59

Degeneration, degenerative
- adrenal (capsule) (gland) 255.8
    - with hypofunction 255.4
    - fatty 255.8
    - hyaline 255.8
    - infectional 255.8
    - lardaceous 277.3
- amyloid (any site) (general) 277.3
- anterior cornua, spinal cord 336.8
- aorta, aortic 440.0
    - fatty 447.8
    - valve (heart) (see also Endocarditis, aortic) 424.1
- arteriovascular — see Arteriosclerosis
- artery, arterial (atheromatous) (calcareous) — see also Arteriosclerosis
    - amyloid 277.3
    - lardaceous 277.3
    - medial NEC (see also Arteriosclerosis, extremities) 440.20
- articular cartilage NEC (see also Disorder, cartilage, articular) 718.0
    - elbow 718.02
    - knee 717.5
    - patella 717.7
    - shoulder 718.01
    - spine (see also Spondylosis) 721.90
- atheromatous — see Arteriosclerosis
- bacony (any site) 277.3
- basal nuclei or ganglia NEC 333.0
- bone 733.90
- brachial plexus 353.0
- brain (cortical) (progressive) 331.9
    - arteriosclerotic 437.0
    - childhood 330.9
        - specified type NEC 330.8
    - congenital 742.4
    - cystic 348.0
        - congenital 742.4
    - familial NEC 331.89
    - grey matter 330.8
    - heredofamilial NEC 331.89
    - in
        - alcoholism 303.9 [331.7]
        - beriberi 265.0 [331.7]
        - cerebrovascular disease 437.9 [331.7]
        - congenital hydrocephalus 742.3 [331.7]
            - with spina bifida (see also Spina bifida) 741.0 [331.7]
        - Fabry's disease 272.7 [330.2]
        - Gaucher's disease 272.7 [330.2]
        - Hunter's disease or syndrome 277.5 [330.3]
        - lipidosis
            - cerebral 330.1
            - generalized 272.7 [330.2]
        - mucopolysaccharidosis 277.5 [330.3]
        - myxedema (see also Myxedema) 244.9 [331.7]
        - neoplastic disease NEC (M8000/1) 239.9 [331.7]
        - Niemann-Pick disease 272.7 [330.2]
        - sphingolipidosis 272.7 [330.2]
        - vitamin B₁₂ deficiency 266.2 [331.7]
    - motor centers 331.89
    - senile 331.2
    - specified type NEC 331.89
- breast — see Disease, breast
- Bruch's membrane 363.40

Degeneration, degenerative—continued
- bundle of His 426.50
    - left 426.3
    - right 426.4
- calcereous NEC 275.4
- capillaries 448.9
    - amyloid 277.3
    - fatty 448.9
    - lardaceous 277.3
- cardiac (brown) (calcareous) (fatty) (fibrous) (hyaline) (mural) (muscular) (pigmentary) (senile) (with arteriosclerosis) (see also Degeneration, myocardial) 429.1
    - valve, valvular — see Endocarditis
- cardiorenal (see also Hypertension, cardiorenal) 404.90
- cardiovascular (see also Disease, cardiovascular) 429.2
    - renal (see also Hypertension, cardiorenal) 404.90
- cartilage (joint) — see Derangement, joint
- cerebellar NEC 334.9
    - primary (hereditary) (sporadic) 334.2
- cerebral — see Degeneration, brain
- cerebromacular 330.1
- cerebrovascular 437.1
    - due to hypertension 437.2
    - late effect — see category 438
- cervical plexus 353.2
- cervix 622.8
    - due to radiation (intended effect) 622.8
        - adverse effect or misadventure 622.8
- changes, spine or vertebra (see also Spondylosis) 721.90
- chitinous 277.3
- chorioretinal 363.40
    - congenital 743.53
    - hereditary 363.50
- choroid (colloid) (drusen) 363.40
    - hereditary 363.50
    - senile 363.41
        - diffuse secondary 363.42
- cochlear 386.8
- collateral ligament (knee) (medial) 717.82
    - lateral 717.81
- combined (spinal cord) (subacute) 266.2 [336.2]
    - with anemia (pernicious) 281.0 [336.2]
        - due to dietary deficiency 281.1 [336.2]
        - due to vitamin B₁₂ deficiency anemia (dietary) 281.1 [336.2]
- conjunctiva 372.50
    - amyloid 277.3 [372.50]
- cornea 371.40
    - calcerous 371.44
    - familial (hereditary) (see also Dystrophy, cornea) 371.50
        - macular 371.55
        - reticular 371.54
    - hyaline (of old scars) 371.41
    - marginal (Terrien's) 371.48
    - mosaic (shagreen) 371.41
    - nodular 371.46
    - peripheral 371.48
    - senile 371.41
- cortical (cerebellar) (parenchymatous) 334.2
    - alcoholic 303.9 [334.4]
    - diffuse, due to arteriopathy 437.0
- corticostriatal-spinal 334.8
- cretinoid 243
- cruciate ligament (knee) (posterior) 717.84

Degeneration, degenerative—continued
- cruciate ligament—continued
    - anterior 717.83
- cutis 709.3
    - amyloid 277.3
- dental pulp 522.2
- disc disease — see Degeneration, intervertebral disc
- dorsolateral (spinal cord) — see Degeration, combined
- endocardial 424.90
- extrapyramidal NEC 333.90
- eye NEC 360.40
    - macular (see also Degeneration, macula) 362.50
    - congenital 362.75
    - hereditary 362.76
- fatty (diffuse) (general) 272.8
    - liver 571.8
        - alcoholic 571.0
    - localized site — see Degeneration, by site, fatty
    - placenta — see Placenta, abnormal
- globe (eye) NEC 360.40
    - macular — see Degeneration, macula
- grey matter 330.8
- heart (brown) (calcareous) (fatty) (fibrous) (hyaline) (mural) (muscular) (pigmentary) (senile) (with arteriosclerosis) (see also Degeneration, myocardial) 429.1
    - amyloid 277.3 [425.7]
    - atheromatous — see Arteriosclerosis, coronary
    - gouty 274.82
    - hypertensive (see also Hypertension, heart) 402.90
    - ischemic 414.9
    - valve, valvular — see Endocarditis
- hepatolenticular (Wilson's) 275.1
- hepatorenal 572.4
- heredofamilial
    - brain NEC 331.89
    - spinal cord NEC 336.8
- hyaline (diffuse) (generalized) 728.9
    - localized — see also Degeneration, by site
        - cornea 371.41
        - keratitis 371.41
- hypertensive vascular — see Hypertension
- infrapatellar fat pad 729.31
- internal semilunar cartilage 717.3
- intervertebral disc 722.6
    - with myelopathy 722.70
    - cervical, cervicothoracic 722.4
        - with myelopathy 722.71
    - lumbar, lumbosacral 722.52
        - with myelopathy 722.73
    - thoracic, thoracolumbar 722.51
        - with myelopathy 722.72
- intestine 569.89
    - amyloid 277.3
    - lardaceous 277.3
- iris (generalized) (see also Atrophy, iris) 364.59
    - pigmentary 364.53
    - pupillary margin 364.54
- ischemic — see Ischemia
- joint disease (see also Osteoarthrosis) 715.9
    - multiple sites 715.09
    - spine (see also Spondylosis) 721.90
- kidney (see also Sclerosis, renal) 587
    - amyloid 277.3 [583.81]

Degeneration, degenerative—continued
- kidney—continued
    - cyst, cystic (multiple) (solitary) 593.2
        - congenital (see also Cystic, disease, kidney) 753.10
    - fatty 593.89
    - fibrocystic (congenital) 753.19
    - lardaceous 277.3 [583.81]
    - polycystic (congenital) 753.12
        - adult type (APKD) 753.13
        - autosomal dominant 753.13
        - autosomal recessive 753.14
        - childhood type (CPKD) 753.14
        - infantile type 753.14
    - waxy 277.3 [583.81]
- Kuhnt-Junius (retina) 362.52
- labyrinth, osseous 386.8
- lacrimal passages, cystic 375.12
- lardaceous (any site) 277.3
- lateral column (posterior), spinal cord (see also Degeneration, combined) 266.2 [336.2]
- lattice 362.63
- lens 366.9
    - infantile, juvenile, or presenile 366.00
    - senile 366.10
- lenticular (familial) (progressive) (Wilson's) (with cirrhosis of liver) 275.1
    - striate artery 437.0
- lethal ball, prosthetic heart valve 996.02
- ligament
    - collateral (knee) (medial) 717.82
        - lateral 717.81
    - cruciate (knee) (posterior) 717.84
        - anterior 717.83
- liver (diffuse) 572.8
    - amyloid 277.3
    - congenital (cystic) 751.62
    - cystic 572.8
        - congenital 751.62
    - fatty 571.8
        - alcoholic 571.0
    - hypertrophic 572.8
    - lardaceous 277.3
    - parenchymatous, acute or subacute (see also Necrosis, liver) 570
    - pigmentary 572.8
    - toxic (acute) 573.8
    - waxy 277.3
- lung 518.89
- lymph gland 289.3
    - hyaline 289.3
    - lardaceous 277.3
- macula (acquired) (senile) 362.50
    - atrophic 362.51
    - Best's 362.76
    - congenital 362.75
    - cystic 362.54
    - cystoid 362.53
    - disciform 362.52
    - dry 362.51
    - exudative 362.52
    - familial pseudoinflammatory 362.77
    - hereditary 362.76
    - hole 362.54
    - juvenile (Stargardt's) 362.75
    - nonexudative 362.51
    - pseudohole 362.54
    - wet 362.52
- medullary — see Degeneration, brain
- membranous labyrinth, congenital (causing impairment of hearing) 744.05
- meniscus — see Derangement, joint
- microcystoid 362.62

Degeneration, degenerative—
  continued
  mitral — *see* Insufficiency, mitral
  Mönckeberg's (*see also*
      Arteriosclerosis, extremities)
      440.20
  moral 301.7
  motor centers, senile 331.2
  mural (*see also* Degeneration,
      myocardial) 429.1
    heart, cardiac (*see also*
        Degeneration,
        myocardial) 429.1
    myocardium, myocardial (*see
        also* Degeneration,
        myocardial) 429.1
  muscle 728.9
    fatty 728.9
    fibrous 728.9
    heart (*see also* Degeneration,
        myocardial) 429.1
    hyaline 728.9
  muscular progressive 728.2
  myelin, central nervous system NEC
      341.9
  myocardium, myocardial (brown)
      (calcareous) (fatty) (fibrous)
      (hyaline) (mural) (muscular)
      (pigmentary) (senile) (with
      arteriosclerosis) 429.1
    with rheumatic fever (conditions
        classifiable to 390) 398.0
      active, acute, or subacute
          391.2
        with chorea 392.0
      inactive or quiescent (with
          chorea) 398.0
    amyloid 277.3 [425.7]
    congenital 746.89
    fetus or newborn 779.8
    gouty 274.82
    hypertensive (*see also*
        Hypertension, heart)
        402.90
    ischemic 414.8
    rheumatic (*see also*
        Degeneration,
        myocardium, with
        rheumatic fever) 398.0
    syphilitic 093.82
  nasal sinus (mucosa) (*see also*
      Sinusitis) 473.9
    frontal 473.1
    maxillary 473.0
  nerve — *see* Disorder, nerve
  nervous system 349.89
    amyloid 277.3 [357.4]
    autonomic (*see also*
        Neuropathy, peripheral,
        autonomic) 337.9
    fatty 349.89
    peripheral autonomic NEC (*see
        also* Neuropathy,
        peripheral, autonomic)
        337.9
  nipple 611.9
  nose 478.1
  oculoacousticocerebral, congenital
      (progressive) 743.8
  olivopontocerebellar (familial)
      (hereditary) 333.0
  osseous labyrinth 386.8
  ovary 620.8
    cystic 620.2
    microcystic 620.2
  pallidal, pigmentary (progressive)
      333.0
  pancreas 577.8
    tuberculous (*see also*
        Tuberculosis) 017.9
  papillary muscle 429.81
  paving stone 362.61
  penis 607.89
  peritoneum 568.89
  pigmentary (diffuse) (general)
    localized — *see* Degeneration,
        by site

Degeneration, degenerative—
  continued
  pigmentary—*continued*
    pallidal (progressive) 333.0
    secondary 362.65
  pineal gland 259.8
  pituitary (gland) 253.8
  placenta (fatty) (fibrinoid) (fibroid)
      — *see* Placenta, abnormal
  popliteal fat pad 729.31
  posterolateral (spinal cord) (*see also*
      Degeneration, combined)
      266.2 [336.2]
  pulmonary valve (heart) (*see also*
      Endocarditis, pulmonary)
      424.3
  pulp (tooth) 522.2
  pupillary margin 364.54
  renal (*see also* Sclerosis, renal) 587
    fibrocystic 753.19
    polycystic 753.12
      adult type (APKD) 753.13
      autosomal dominant 753.13
      autosomal recessive 753.14
      childhood type (CPKD)
          753.14
      infantile type 753.14
  reticuloendothelial system 289.8
  retina (peripheral) 362.60
    with retinal defect (*see also*
        Detachment, retina, with
        retinal defect) 361.00
    cystic (senile) 362.50
    cystoid 362.53
    hereditary (*see also* Dystrophy,
        retina) 362.70
      cerebroretinal 362.71
      congenital 362.75
      juvenile (Stargardt's) 362.75
      macula 362.76
      Kuhnt-Junius 362.52
    lattice 362.63
    macular (*see also* Degeneration,
        macula) 362.50
    microcystoid 362.62
    palisade 362.63
    paving stone 362.61
    pigmentary (primary) 362.74
      secondary 362.65
    posterior pole (*see also*
        Degeneration, macula)
        362.50
    secondary 362.66
    senile 362.60
      cystic 362.53
      reticular 362.64
  saccule, congenital (causing
      impairment of hearing)
      744.05
  sacculocochlear 386.8
  senile 797
    brain 331.2
    cardiac, heart, or myocardium
        (*see also* Degeneration,
        myocardial) 429.1
    motor centers 331.2
    reticule 362.64
    retina, cystic 362.50
    vascular — *see* Arteriosclerosis
  silicone rubber poppet (prosthetic
      valve) 996.02
  sinus (cystic) (*see also* Sinusitis)
      473.9
    polypoid 471.1
  skin 709.3
    amyloid 277.3
    colloid 709.3
  spinal (cord) 336.8
    amyloid 277.3
    column 733.90
    combined (subacute) (*see also*
        Degeneration, combined)
        266.2 [336.2]
      with anemia (pernicious)
          281.0 [336.2]

Degeneration, degenerative—
  continued
  spinal—*continued*
    dorsolateral (*see also*
        Degeneration, combined)
        266.2 [336.2]
    familial NEC 336.8
    fatty 336.8
    funicular (*see also*
        Degeneration, combined)
        266.2 [336.2]
    heredofamilial NEC 336.8
    posterolateral (*see also*
        Degeneration, combined)
        266.2 [336.2]
    subacute combined — *see*
        Degeneration, combined
    tuberculous (*see also*
        Tuberculosis) 013.8
  spine 733.90
  spleen 289.59
    amyloid 277.3
    lardaceous 277.3
  stomach 537.89
    lardaceous 277.3
  strionigral 333.0
  sudoriparous (cystic) 705.89
  suprarenal (capsule) (gland) 255.8
    with hypofunction 255.4
  sweat gland 705.89
  synovial membrane (pulpy) 727.9
  tapetoretinal 362.74
    adult or presenile form 362.50
  testis (postinfectional) 608.89
  thymus (gland) 254.8
    fatty 254.8
    lardaceous 277.3
  thyroid (gland) 246.8
  tricuspid (heart) (valve) *see*
      Endocarditis, tricuspid
  tuberculous NEC (*see also*
      Tuberculosis) 011.9
  turbinate 733.90
  uterus 621.8
    cystic 621.8
  vascular (senile) — *see also*
      Arteriosclerosis
    hypertensive — *see*
        Hypertension
  vitreoretinal (primary) 362.73
    secondary 362.66
  vitreous humor (with infiltration)
      379.21
  wallerian NEC — *see* Disorder,
      nerve
  waxy (any site) 277.3
  Wilson's hepatolenticular 275.1
Deglutition
  paralysis 784.9
    hysterical 300.11
  pneumonia 507.0
Degos' disease or syndrome 447.8
**Degradation disorder, branched-chain
      amino acid** 270.3
Dehiscence
  anastomosis — *see* Complications,
      anastomosis
  cesarean wound 674.1
  episiotomy 674.2
  operation wound 998.3
  perineal wound (postpartum) 674.2
  postoperative 998.3
    abdomen 998.3
  uterine wound 674.1
Dehydration (cachexia) 276.5
  hypertonic 276.0
  hypotonic 276.1
  newborn 775.5
Deiters' nucleus syndrome 386.19
Déjérine's disease 356.0
Déjérine-Klumpke paralysis 767.6
Déjérine-Roussy syndrome 348.8
Déjérine-Sottas disease or neuropathy
  (hypertrophic) 356.0

Déjérine-Thomas atrophy or syndrome
  333.0
de Lange's syndrome (Amsterdam
    dwarf, mental retardation, and
    brachycephaly) 759.89
Delay, delayed
  adaptation, cones or rods 368.63
  any plane in pelvis
    affecting fetus or newborn 763.1
    complicating delivery 660.1
  birth or delivery NEC 662.1
    affecting fetus or newborn 763.8
    second twin, triplet, or multiple
        mate 662.3
  closure — *see also* Fistula
    cranial suture 756.0
    fontanel 756.0
  coagulation NEC 790.92
  conduction (cardiac) (ventricular)
      426.9
  delivery NEC 662.1
    second twin, triplet, etc. 662.3
    affecting fetus or newborn
        763.8
  development 783.4
    intellectual NEC 315.9
    learning NEC 315.2
    physiological 783.4
    reading 315.00
    sexual 259.0
    speech 315.39
      associated with hyperkinesis
          314.1
    spelling 315.09
  gastric emptying 536.8
  menarche 256.3
    due to pituitary hypofunction
        253.4
  menstruation (cause unknown)
      626.8
  milestone 783.4
  motility — *see* Hypomotility
  passage of meconium (newborn)
      777.1
  primary respiration 768.9
  puberty 259.0
  sexual maturation, female 259.0
Del Castillo's syndrome (germinal
    aplasia) 606.0
Deleage's disease 359.8
Delhi (boil) (button) (sore) 085.1
Delinquency (juvenile) 312.9
  group (*see also* Disturbance,
      conduct) 312.2
  neurotic 312.4
Delirium, delirious 780.09
  acute (psychotic) 293.0
  alcoholic 291.0
    acute 291.0
    chronic 291.1
  alcoholicum 291.0
  chronic (*see also* Psychosis) 293.89
    due to or associated with
        physical condition — *see*
        Psychosis, organic
  drug-induced 292.81
  eclamptic (*see also* Eclampsia)
      780.3
  exhaustion (*see also* Reaction,
      stress, acute) 308.9
  hysterical 300.11
  in
    presenile dementia 290.11
    senile dementia 290.3
  induced by drug 292.81
  manic, maniacal (acute) (*see also*
      Psychosis, affective) 296.0
    recurrent episode 296.1
    single episode 296.0
  puerperal 293.9
  senile 290.3
  subacute (psychotic) 293.1
  thyroid (*see also* Thyrotoxicosis)
      242.9
  traumatic — *see also* Injury,
      intracranial

Delirium, delirious

Delirium, delirious—continued
  traumatic—continued
    with
      lesion, spinal cord — see Injury, spinal, by site
      shock, spinal — see Injury, spinal, by site
  tremens (impending) 291.0
  uremic — see Uremia
  withdrawal
    alcoholic (acute) 291.0
      chronic 291.1
    drug 292.0

Delivery

Note — Use the following fifth-digit subclassification with categories 640-648, 651-676:

  0 unspecified as to episode of care
  1 delivered, with or without mention of antepartum condition
  2 delivered, with mention of postpartum complication
  3 antepartum condition or complication
  4 postpartum condition or complication

breech (assisted) (spontaneous) 652.2
  affecting fetus or newborn 763.0
  extraction NEC 669.6
cesarean (for) 669.7
  abnormal
    cervix 654.6
    pelvic organs or tissues 654.9
    pelvis (bony) (major) NEC 653.0
    presentation or position 652.9
      in multiple gestation 652.6
    size, fetus 653.5
    soft parts (of pelvis) 654.9
    uterus, congenital 654.0
    vagina 654.7
    vulva 654.8
  abruptio placentae 641.2
  acromion presentation 652.8
  affecting fetus or newborn 763.4
  anteversion, cervix or uterus 654.4
  atony, uterus 661.2
  bicornis or bicornuate uterus 654.0
  breech presentation 652.2
  brow presentation 652.4
  cephalopelvic disproportion (normally formed fetus) 653.4
  chin presentation 652.4
  cicatrix of cervix 654.6
  contracted pelvis (general) 653.1
    inlet 653.2
    outlet 653.3
  cord presentation or prolapse 663.0
  cystocele 654.4
  deformity (acquired) (congenital)
    pelvic organs or tissues NEC 654.9
    pelvis (bony) NEC 653.0
  displacement, uterus NEC 654.4
  disproportion NEC 653.9
  distress
    fetal 656.3
    maternal 669.0
  eclampsia 642.6
  face presentation 652.4

Delivery—continued
  cesarean—continued
    failed
      forceps 660.7
      trial of labor NEC 660.6
      vacuum extraction 660.7
      ventouse 660.7
    fetal deformity 653.7
    fetal-maternal hemorrhage 656.0
    fetus, fetal
      distress 656.3
      prematurity 656.8
    fibroid (tumor) (uterus) 654.1
    hemorrhage (antepartum) (intrapartum) NEC 641.9
    hydrocephalic fetus 653.6
    incarceration of uterus 654.3
    incoordinate uterine action 661.4
    inertia, uterus 661.2
      primary 661.0
      secondary 661.1
    lateroversion, uterus or cervix 654.4
    mal lie 652.9
    malposition
      fetus 652.9
        in multiple gestation 652.6
      pelvic organs or tissues NEC 654.9
      uterus NEC or cervix 654.4
    malpresentation NEC 652.9
      in multiple gestation 652.6
    maternal
      diabetes mellitus 648.0
      heart disease NEC 648.6
    meconium in liquor 656.3
      without mention of fetal distress — omit code
      staining only 792.3
    oblique presentation 652.3
    oversize fetus 653.5
    pelvic tumor NEC 654.9
    placental insufficiency 656.5
    placenta previa 641.0
      with hemorrhage 641.1
    poor dilation, cervix 661.0
    preeclampsia 642.4
      severe 642.5
    previous
      cesarean delivery 654.2
      surgery (to)
        cervix 654.6
        gynecological NEC 654.9
        uterus NEC 654.9
          previous cesarean delivery 654.2
        vagina 654.7
    prolapse
      arm or hand 652.7
      uterus 654.4
    prolonged labor 662.1
    rectocele 654.4
    retroversion, uterus or cervix 654.3
    rigid
      cervix 654.6
      pelvic floor 654.4
      perineum 654.8
      vagina 654.7
      vulva 654.8
    sacculation, pregnant uterus 654.4
    scar(s)
      cervix 654.6
      cesarean delivery 654.2
      uterus NEC 654.9
        due to previous cesarean delivery 654.2
    Shirodkar suture in situ 654.5
    shoulder presentation 652.8
    stenosis or stricture, cervix 654.6
    transverse presentation or lie 652.3

Delivery—continued
  cesarean—continued
    tumor, pelvic organs or tissues NEC 654.4
    umbilical cord presentation or prolapse 663.0
  completely normal case — see category 650
  complicated (by) NEC 669.9
    abdominal tumor, fetal 653.7
      causing obstructed labor 660.1
    abnormal, abnormality of
      cervix 654.6
        causing obstructed labor 660.2
      forces of labor 661.9
      formation of uterus 654.0
      pelvic organs or tissues 654.9
        causing obstructed labor 660.2
      pelvis (bony) (major) NEC 653.0
        causing obstructed labor 660.1
      presentation or position NEC 652.9
        causing obstructed labor 660.0
      size, fetus 653.5
        causing obstructed labor 660.1
      soft parts (of pelvis) 654.9
        causing obstructed labor 660.2
      uterine contractions NEC 661.9
      uterus (formation) 654.0
        causing obstructed labor 660.2
      vagina 654.7
        causing obstructed labor 660.2
    abnormally formed uterus (any type) (congenital) 654.0
      causing obstructed labor 660.2
    acromion presentation 652.8
      causing obstructed labor 660.0
    adherent placenta 667.0
      with hemorrhage 666.0
    adhesions, uterus (to abdominal wall) 654.4
    advanced maternal age NEC 659.6
      primigravida 659.5
    air embolism 673.0
    amnionitis 658.4
    amniotic fluid embolism 673.1
    anesthetic death 668.9
    annular detachment, cervix 665.3
    antepartum hemorrhage — see Delivery, complicated, hemorrhage
    anteversion, cervix or uterus 654.4
      causing obstructed labor 660.2
    apoplexy 674.0
      placenta 641.2
    arrested active phase 661.1
    asymmetrical pelvis bone 653.0
      causing obstructed labor 660.1
    atony, uterus (hypotonic) (inertia) 661.2
      hypertonic 661.4
    Bandl's ring 661.4
    battledore placenta — see Placenta, abnormal
    bicornis or bicornuate uterus 654.0
      causing obstructed labor 660.2

Delivery—continued
  complicated (by)—continued
    birth injury to mother NEC 665.9
    bleeding (see also Delivery, complicated, hemorrhage) 641.9
    breech presentation (assisted) (spontaneous) 652.2
      with successful version 652.1
      causing obstructed labor 660.0
    brow presentation 652.4
      causing obstructed labor 660.0
    cephalopelvic disproportion (normally formed fetus) 653.4
      causing obstructed labor 660.1
    cerebral hemorrhage 674.0
    cervical dystocia 661.0
    chin presentation 652.4
      causing obstructed labor 660.0
    cicatrix
      cervix 654.6
        causing obstructed labor 660.2
      vagina 654.7
        causing obstructed labor 660.2
    colporrhexis 665.4
      with perineal laceration 664.0
    compound presentation 652.8
      causing obstructed labor 660.0
    compression of cord (umbilical) 663.2
      around neck 663.1
      cord prolapsed 663.0
    contraction, contracted pelvis 653.1
      causing obstructed labor 660.1
      general 653.1
        causing obstructed labor 660.1
      inlet 653.2
        causing obstructed labor 660.1
      midpelvic 653.8
        causing obstructed labor 660.1
      midplane 653.8
        causing obstructed labor 660.1
      outlet 653.3
        causing obstructed labor 660.1
    contraction ring 661.4
    cord (umbilical) 663.9
      around neck, tightly or with compression 663.1
        without compression 663.3
      bruising 663.6
      complication NEC 663.9
        specified type NEC 663.8
      compression NEC 663.2
      entanglement NEC 663.3
        with compression 663.2
      forelying 663.0
      hematoma 663.6
      marginal attachment 663.8
      presentation 663.0
      prolapse (complete) (occult) (partial) 663.0
      short 663.4
      specified complication NEC 663.8
      thrombosis (vessels) 663.6
      vascular lesion 663.6
      velamentous insertion 663.5
    Couvelaire uterus 641.2

Delivery—continued
  complicated (by)—continued
    cretin pelvis (dwarf type) (male type) 653.1
      causing obstructed labor 660.1
    crossbirth 652.3
      with successful version 652.1
      causing obstructed labor 660.0
    cyst (Gartner's duct) 654.7
    cystocele 654.4
      causing obstructed labor 660.2
    death of fetus (near term) 656.4
      early (before 22 completed weeks gestation) 632
    deformity (acquired) (congenital)
      fetus 653.7
        causing obstructed labor 660.1
      pelvic organs or tissues NEC 654.9
        causing obstructed labor 660.2
      pelvis (bony) NEC 653.0
        causing obstructed labor 660.1
    delay, delayed
      delivery in multiple pregnancy 662.3
      due to locked mates 660.5
      following rupture of membranes (spontaneous) 658.2
        artificial 658.3
    depressed fetal heart tones 656.3
    diastasis recti 665.8
    dilation
      bladder 654.4
        causing obstructed labor 660.2
      cervix, incomplete, poor or slow 661.0
    diseased placenta 656.7
    displacement uterus NEC 654.4
      causing obstructed labor 660.2
    disproportion NEC 653.9
      causing obstructed labor 660.1
    disruptio uteri — see Delivery, complicated, rupture, uterus
    distress
      fetal 656.3
      maternal 669.0
    double uterus (congenital) 654.0
      causing obstructed labor 660.2
    dropsy amnion 657
    dysfunction, uterus 661.9
      hypertonic 661.4
      hypotonic 661.2
        primary 661.0
        secondary 661.1
      incoordinate 661.4
    dystocia
      cervical 661.0
      fetal — see Delivery, complicated, abnormal presentation
      maternal — see Delivery, complicated, prolonged labor
      pelvic — see Delivery, complicated, contraction pelvis
      positional 652.8
      shoulder girdle 660.4
    eclampsia 642.6
    ectopic kidney 654.4
      causing obstructed labor 660.2

Delivery—continued
  complicated (by)—continued
    edema, cervix 654.6
      causing obstructed labor 660.2
    effusion, amniotic fluid 658.1
    elderly primigravida 659.5
    embolism (pulmonary) 673.2
      air 673.0
      amniotic fluid 673.1
      blood clot 673.2
      cerebral 674.0
      fat 673.8
      pyemic 673.3
      septic 673.3
    entanglement, umbilical cord 663.3
      with compression 663.2
      around neck (with compression) 663.1
    eversion, cervix or uterus 665.2
    excessive
      fetal growth 653.5
        causing obstructed labor 660.1
      size of fetus 653.5
        causing obstructed labor 660.1
    face presentation 652.4
      causing obstructed labor 660.0
      to pubes 660.3
    failure, fetal head to enter pelvic brim 652.5
      causing obstructed labor 660.0
    fetal
      acid-base balance 656.3
      death (near term) NEC 656.4
        early (before 22 completed weeks gestation) 632
      deformity 653.7
        causing obstructed labor 660.1
      distress 656.3
      heart rate or rhythm 656.3
    fetopelvic disproportion 653.4
      causing obstructed labor 660.1
    fever during labor 659.2
    fibroid (tumor) (uterus) 654.1
      causing obstructed labor 660.2
    fibromyomata 654.1
      causing obstructed labor 660.2
    forelying umbilical cord 663.0
    fracture of coccyx 665.6
    hematoma 664.5
      broad ligament 665.7
      ischial spine 665.7
      pelvic 665.7
      perineum 664.5
      soft tissues 665.7
      subdural 674.0
      umbilical cord 663.6
      vagina 665.7
      vulva or perineum 664.5
    hemorrhage (uterine) (antepartum) (intrapartum) (pregnancy) 641.9
      accidental 641.2
      associated with
        afibrinogenemia 641.3
        coagulation defect 641.3
          hyperfibrinolysis 641.3
          hypofibrinogenemia 641.3
      cerebral 674.0
      due to
        low-lying placenta 641.1
        placenta previa 641.1
        premature separation of placenta (normally implanted) 641.2
        retained placenta 666.0

Delivery—continued
  complicated (by)—continued
    hemorrhage—continued
      due to—continued
        trauma 641.8
        uterine leiomyoma 641.8
      marginal sinus rupture 641.2
      placenta NEC 641.9
      postpartum (atonic) (immediate) (within 24 hours) 666.1
        with retained or trapped placenta 666.0
        delayed 666.2
        secondary 666.2
        third stage 666.0
    hourglass contraction, uterus 661.4
    hydramnios 657
    hydrocephalic fetus 653.6
      causing obstructed labor 660.1
    hydrops fetalis 653.7
      causing obstructed labor 660.1
    hypertension — see Hypertension, complicating pregnancy
    hypertonic uterine dysfunction 661.4
    hypotonic uterine dysfunction 661.2
    impacted shoulders 660.4
    incarceration, uterus 654.3
      causing obstructed labor 660.2
    incomplete dilation (cervix) 661.0
    incoordinate uterus 661.4
    indication NEC 659.9
      specified type 659.8
    inertia, uterus 661.2
      hypertonic 661.4
      hypotonic 661.2
      primary 661.0
      secondary 661.1
    infantile
      genitalia 654.4
        causing obstructed labor 660.2
      uterus (os) 654.4
        causing obstructed labor 660.2
    injury (to mother) NEC 665.9
    intrauterine fetal death (near term) NEC 656.4
      early (before 22 completed weeks gestation) 632
    inversion, uterus 665.2
    kidney, ectopic 654.4
      causing obstructed labor 660.2
    knot (true), umbilical cord 663.2
    labor, premature (before 37 completed weeks gestation) 644.2
    laceration 664.9
      anus (spincter) 664.2
        with mucosa 664.3
      bladder (urinary) 665.5
      bowel 665.5
      central 664.4
      cervix (uteri) 665.3
      fourchette 664.0
      hymen 664.0
      labia (majora) (minora) 664.0
      pelvic
        floor 664.1
        organ NEC 665.5
      perineum, perineal 664.4
        first degree 664.0
        second degree 664.1
        third degree 664.2
        fourth degree 664.3
        central 664.4
        extensive NEC 664.4
        muscles 664.1

Delivery—continued
  complicated (by)—continued
    laceration—continued
      perineum, perineal—continued
        skin 664.0
        slight 664.0
      peritoneum 665.5
      periurethral tissue 665.5
      rectovaginal (septum) (without perineal laceration) 665.4
        with perineum 664.2
          with anal rectal mucosa 664.3
      skin (perineum) 664.0
      specified site or type NEC 664.8
      sphincter ani 664.2
        with mucosa 664.3
      urethra 665.5
      uterus 665.1
        before labor 665.0
      vagina, vaginal (deep) (high) (sulcus) (wall) (without perineal laceration) 665.4
        with perineum 664.0
        muscles, with perineum 664.1
      vulva 664.0
    lateroversion, uterus or cervix 654.4
      causing obstructed labor 660.2
    locked mates 660.5
    low implantation of placenta — see Delivery, complicated, placenta, previa
    mal lie 652.9
      causing obstructed labor 660.0
    malposition
      fetus NEC 652.9
        causing obstructed labor 660.0
      pelvic organs or tissues NEC 654.9
        causing obstructed labor 660.2
      placenta 641.1
        without hemorrhage 641.0
      uterus NEC or cervix 654.4
        causing obstructed labor 660.2
    malpresentation 652.9
      causing obstructed labor 660.0
    marginal sinus (bleeding) (rupture) 641.2
    maternal hypotension syndrome 669.2
    meconium in liquor 656.3
    membranes, retained — see Delivery, complicated, placenta, retained
    mentum presentation 652.4
      causing obstructed labor 660.0
    metrorrhagia (myopathia) — see Delivery, complicated, hemorrhage
    metrorrhexis — see Delivery, complicated, rupture, uterus
    monster 653.7
      causing obstructed labor 660.1
    multiparity (grand) 659.4
    myelomeningocele, fetus 653.7
      causing obstructed labor 660.1
    Nögele's pelvis 653.0
      causing obstructed labor 660.1

Delivery—*continued*
  complicated (by)—*continued*
    nonengagement, fetal head
        652.5
      causing obstructed labor
          660.0
    oblique presentation 652.3
      causing obstructed labor
          660.0
    obstetric
      shock 669.1
      trauma NEC 665.9
    obstructed labor 660.9
      due to
        abnormality pelvic organs
            or tissues
            (conditions
            classifiable to
            654.0-654.9) 660.2
        deep transverse arrest
            660.3
        impacted shoulders 660.4
        locked twins 660.5
        malposition and
            malpresentation of
            fetus (conditions
            classifiable to
            652.0-652.9) 660.0
        persistent
            occipitoposterior
            660.3
        shoulder dystocia 660.4
    occult prolapse of umbilical
        cord 663.0
    oversize fetus 653.5
      causing obstructed labor
          660.1
    pathological retraction ring,
        uterus 661.4
    pelvic
      arrest (deep) (high) (of fetal
          head) (transverse)
          660.3
      deformity (bone) — *see also*
          Deformity, pelvis, with
          disproportion
        soft tissue 654.9
          causing obstructed
              labor 660.2
      tumor NEC 654.9
        causing obstructed labor
            660.2
    penetration, pregnant uterus by
        instrument 665.1
    perforation — *see* Delivery,
        complicated, laceration
    persistent
      hymen 654.8
        causing obstructed labor
            660.2
      occipitoposterior 660.3
    placenta, placental
      ablatio 641.2
      abnormality 656.7
        with hemorrhage 641.2
      abruptio 641.2
      accreta 667.0
        with hemorrhage 666.0
      adherent (without
          hemorrhage) 667.0
        with hemorrhage 666.0
      apoplexy 641.2
      battledore 663.8
      detachment (premature)
          641.2
      disease 656.7
      hemorrhage NEC 641.9
      increta (without hemorrhage)
          667.0
        with hemorrhage 666.0
      low (implantation) 641.0
        without hemorrhage
            641.0
      malformation 656.7
        with hemorrhage 641.2

Delivery—*continued*
  complicated (by)—*continued*
    placenta, placental—*continued*
      malposition 641.1
        without hemorrhage
            641.0
      marginal sinus rupture 641.2
      percreta 667.0
        with hemorrhage 666.0
      premature separation 641.2
      previa (central) (lateral)
          (marginal) partial)
          641.1
        without hemorrhage
            641.0
      retained (with hemorrhage)
          666.0
        without hemorrhage
            667.0
      rupture of marginal sinus
          641.2
      separation (premature) 641.2
      trapped 666.0
        without hemorrhage
            667.0
      vicious insertion 641.1
    polyhydramnios 657
    polyp, cervix 654.6
      causing obstructed labor
          660.2
    precipitate labor 661.3
    premature
      labor (before 37 completed
          weeks gestation)
          644.2
      rupture, membranes 658.1
        delayed delivery
            following 658.2
    presenting umbilical cord 663.0
    previous
      cesarean delivery 654.2
      surgery
        cervix 654.6
          causing obstructed
              labor 660.2
        gynecological NEC 654.9
          causing obstructed
              labor 660.2
        perineum 654.8
        uterus 654.9
          due to previous
              cesarean
              delivery 654.2
        vagina 654.7
          causing obstructed
              labor 660.2
        vulva 654.8
    primary uterine inertia 661.0
    primipara, elderly or old 659.5
    prolapse
      arm or hand 652.7
        causing obstructed labor
            660.0
      cord (umbilical) 663.0
      fetal extremity 652.8
      foot or leg 652.8
        causing obstructed labor
            660.0
      umbilical cord (complete)
          (occult) (partial) 663.0
      uterus 654.4
        causing obstructed labor
            660.2
    prolonged labor 662.1
      first stage 662.0
      second stage 662.2
      active phase 661.2
      due to
        cervical dystocia 661.0
        contraction ring 661.4
        tetanic uterus 661.4
        uterine inertia 661.2
          primary 661.0
          secondary 661.1
      latent phase 661.0
    pyrexia during labor 659.2

Delivery—*continued*
  complicated (by)—*continued*
    rachitic pelvis 653.2
      causing obstructed labor
          660.1
    rectocele 654.4
      causing obstructed labor
          660.2
    retained membranes or portions
        of placenta 666.2
      without hemorrhage 667.1
    retarded (prolonged) birth 662.1
    retention secundines (with
        hemorrhage) 666.2
      without hemorrhage 667.1
    retroversion, uterus or cervix
        654.3
      causing obstructed labor
          660.2
    rigid
      cervix 654.6
        causing obstructed labor
            660.2
      pelvic floor 654.4
        causing obstructed labor
            660.2
      perineum or vulva 654.8
        causing obstructed labor
            660.2
      vagina 654.7
        causing obstructed labor
            660.2
    Robert's pelvis 653.0
      causing obstructed labor
          660.1
    rupture — *see also* Delivery,
        complicated, laceration
      bladder (urinary) 665.5
      cervix 665.3
      marginal sinus 641.2
      membranes, premature
          658.1
      pelvic organ NEC 665.5
      perineum (without mention
          of other laceration) —
          see Delivery,
          complicated,
          laceration, perineum
      peritoneum 665.5
      urethra 665.5
      uterus (during labor) 665.1
        before labor 665.0
      sacculation, pregnant uterus
          654.4
      sacral teratomas, fetal 653.7
        causing obstructed labor
            660.1
      scar(s)
        cervix 654.6
          causing obstructed labor
              660.2
        cesarean delivery 654.2
          causing obstructed labor
              660.2
        perineum 654.8
          causing obstructed labor
              660.2
        uterus NEC 654.9
          causing obstructed labor
              660.2
          due to previous cesarean
              delivery 654.2
        vagina 654.7
          causing obstructed labor
              660.2
        vulva 654.8
          causing obstructed labor
              660.2
      scoliotic pelvis 653.0
        causing obstructed labor
            660.1
      secondary uterine inertia 661.1
      secundines, retained — *see*
          Delivery, complicated,
          placenta, retained

Delivery—*continued*
  complicated (by)—*continued*
    separation
      placenta (premature) 641.2
      pubic bone 665.6
      symphysis pubis 665.6
    septate vagina 654.7
      causing obstructed labor
          660.2
    shock (birth) (obstetric)
        (puerperal) 669.1
    short cord syndrome 663.4
    shoulder
      girdle dystocia 660.4
      presentation 652.8
        causing obstructed labor
            660.0
    Siamese twins 653.7
      causing obstructed labor
          660.1
    slow slope active phase 661.2
    spasm
      cervix 661.4
      uterus 661.4
    spondylolisthesis, pelvis 653.3
      causing obstructed labor
          660.1
    spondylolysis (lumbosacral)
        653.3
      causing obstructed labor
          660.1
    spondylosis 653.0
      causing obstructed labor
          660.1
    stenosis or stricture
      cervix 654.6
        causing obstructed labor
            660.2
      vagina 654.7
        causing obstructed labor
            660.2
    sudden death, unknown cause
        669.9
    tear (pelvic organ) (*see also*
        Delivery, complicated,
        laceration) 664.9
    teratomas, sacral, fetal 653.7
      causing obstructed labor
          660.1
    tetanic uterus 661.4
    tipping pelvis 653.0
      causing obstructed labor
          660.1
    transverse
      arrest (deep) 660.3
      presentation or lie 652.3
        with successful version
            652.1
        causing obstructed labor
            660.0
    trauma (obstetrical) NEC 665.9
    tumor
      abdominal, fetal 653.7
        causing obstructed labor
            660.1
      pelvic organs or tissues NEC
          654.9
        causing obstructed labor
            660.2
    umbilical cord (*see also*
        Delivery, complicated,
        cord) 663.9
      around neck tightly, or with
          compression 663.1
      entanglement NEC 663.3
        with compression 663.2
      prolapse (complete) (occult)
          (partial) 663.0
    unstable lie 652.0
      causing obstructed labor
          660.0
    uterine
      inertia (*see also* Delivery,
          complicated, inertia,
          uterus) 661.2
      spasm 661.4
    vasa previa 663.5

Delivery—continued
　complicated (by)—continued
　　velamentous insertion of cord 663.5
　　delayed NEC 662.1
　　　following rupture of membranes
　　　　(spontaneous) 658.2
　　　　artificial 658.3
　　　second twin, triplet, etc. 662.3
　　difficult NEC 669.9
　　　previous, affecting management of pregnancy or childbirth V23.4
　　specified type NEC 669.8
　　early onset (spontaneous) 644.2
　　forceps NEC 669.5
　　　affecting fetus or newborn 763.2
　　missed (at or near term) 656.4
　　multiple gestation NEC 651.9
　　　with fetal loss and retention of one or more fetus(es) 651.6
　　　specified type NEC 651.8
　　　　with fetal loss and retention of one or more fetus(es) 651.6
　　nonviable infant 656.4
　　normal — see category 650
　　precipitate 661.3
　　　affecting fetus or newborn 763.6
　　premature NEC (before 37 completed weeks gestation) 644.2
　　　previous, affecting management of pregnancy V23.4
　　quadruplet NEC 651.2
　　　with fetal loss and retention of one or more fetus(es) 651.5
　　quintuplet NEC 651.8
　　　with fetal loss and retention of one or more fetus(es) 651.6
　　sextuplet NEC 651.8
　　　with fetal loss and retention of one or more fetus(es) 651.6
　　specified complication NEC 669.8
　　stillbirth (near term) NEC 656.4
　　　early (before 22 completed weeks gestation) 632
　　term pregnancy (live birth) NEC — see category 650
　　　stillbirth NEC 656.4
　　threatened premature 644.2
　　triplets NEC 651.1
　　　with fetal loss and retention of one or more fetus(es) 651.4
　　　delayed delivery (one or more mates) 662.3
　　　locked mates 660.5
　　twins NEC 651.0
　　　with fetal loss and retention of one fetus 651.3
　　　delayed delivery (one or more mates) 662.3
　　　locked mates 660.5
　　uncomplicated — see category 650
　　vacuum extractor NEC 669.5
　　　affecting fetus or newborn 763.3
　　ventouse NEC 669.5
　　　affecting fetus or newborn 763.3

Dellen, cornea 371.41
Delusions (paranoid) 297.9
　grandiose 297.1
　parasitosis 300.29
　systematized 297.1
Dementia 294.8 ◆
　alcoholic (see also Psychosis, alcoholic) 291.2
　Alzheimer's — see Alzheimer's dementia
　arteriosclerotic (simple type) (uncomplicated) 290.40

Dementia—continued
　arteriosclerotic—continued
　　with—continued
　　　acute confusional state 290.41
　　　delirium 290.41
　　　delusional features 290.42
　　　depressive features 290.43
　　　depressed type 290.43
　　　paranoid type 290.42
　Binswanger's 290.12
　catatonic (acute) (see also Schizophrenia) 295.2
　congenital (see also Retardation, mental) 319
　degenerative 290.9
　　presenile-onset — see Dementia, presenile
　　senile-onset — see Dementia, senile
　developmental (see also Schizophrenia) 295.9
　dialysis 294.8
　　transient 293.9
　due to or associated with condition(s) classified elsewhere 294.1
　　multiple sclerosis 294.1
　　polyarteritis nodosa 294.1
　hebephrenic (acute) 295.1
　Heller's (infantile psychosis) (see also Psychosis, childhood) 299.1
　idiopathic 290.9
　　presenile-onset — see Dementia, presenile
　　senile-onset — see Dementia, senile
　in
　　Alzheimer's disease — see Alzheimer's dementia
　　arteriosclerotic brain disease 290.40
　　cerebral lipidoses 294.1
　　epilepsy 294.1
　　general paralysis of the insane 294.1
　　hepatolenticular degeneration 294.1
　　Huntington's chorea 294.1
　　Jakob-Creutzfeldt disease 290.10
　　multiple sclerosis 294.1
　　neurosyphilis 294.1
　　Pelizaeus-Merzbacher disease 294.1
　　Pick's disease 290.10
　　polyarteritis nodosa 294.1
　　senility 290.0
　　Wilson's disease 294.1
　induced by drug 292.82
　infantile, infantilia (see also Psychosis, childhood) 299.0
　multi-infarct (cerebrovascular) (see also Dementia, arteriosclerotic) 290.40
　old age 290.0
　paralytica, paralytic 094.1
　　juvenilis 090.40
　　syphilitic 094.1
　　　congenital 090.40
　　tabetic form 094.1
　paranoid (see also Schizophrenia) 295.3
　paraphrenic (see also Schizophrenia) 295.3
　paretic 094.1
　praecox (see also Schizophrenia) 295.3
　presenile 290.10
　　with
　　　acute confusional state 290.11
　　　delirium 290.11
　　　delusional features 290.12
　　　depressive features 290.13
　　　depressed type 290.13

Dementia—continued
　presenile—continued
　　paranoid type 290.12
　　simple type 290.10
　　uncomplicated 290.10
　primary (acute) (see also Schizophrenia) 295.0
　progressive, syphilitic 094.1
　puerperal — see Psychosis, puerperal
　schizophrenic (see also Schizophrenia) 295.9
　senile 290.0
　　with
　　　acute confusional state 290.3
　　　delirium 290.3
　　　delusional features 290.20
　　　depressive features 290.21
　　　depressed type 290.21
　　　exhaustion 290.0
　　　paranoid type 290.20
　　simple type (acute) (see also Schizophrenia) 295.0
　　simplex (acute) (see also Schizophrenia) 295.0
　syphilitic 094.1
　uremic — see Uremia
Demerol dependence (see also Dependence) 304.0
Demineralization, ankle (see also Osteoporosis) 733.00
Demodex folliculorum (infestation) 133.8
de Morgan's spots (senile angiomas) 448.1
Demyelination, demyelinization
　central nervous system 341.9
　　specified NEC 341.8
　corpus callosum (central) 341.8
　global 340
Dengue (fever) 061
　sandfly 061
　vaccination, prophylactic (against) V05.1
　virus hemorrhagic fever 065.4
Dens
　evaginatus 520.2
　in dente 520.2
　invaginatus 520.2
Density
　increased, bone (disseminated) (generalized) (spotted) 733.99
　lung (nodular) 518.89
Dental — see also condition
　examination only V72.2
Dentia praecox 520.6
Denticles (in pulp) 522.2
Dentigerous cyst 526.0
Dentin
　irregular (in pulp) 522.3
　opalescent 520.5
　secondary (in pulp) 522.3
　sensitive 521.8
Dentinogenesis imperfecta 520.5
Dentinoma (M9271/0) 213.1
　upper jaw (bone) 213.0
Dentition 520.7
　abnormal 520.6
　anomaly 520.6
　delayed 520.6
　difficult 520.7
　disorder of 520.6
　precocious 520.6
　retarded 520.6
Denture sore (mouth) 528.9

Dependence

> Note — Use the following fifth-digit subclassification with category 304:
>
> 　0　unspecified
> 　1　continuous
> 　2　episodic
> 　3　in remission

　with
　　withdrawal symptoms
　　　alcohol 291.8
　　　drug 292.0
　14-hydroxy-dihydromorphinone 304.0
　absinthe 304.6
　acemorphan 304.0
　acetanilid(e) 304.6
　acetophenetidin 304.6
　acetorphine 304.0
　acetyldihydrocodeine 304.0
　acetyldihydrocodeinone 304.0
　Adalin 304.1
　Afghanistan black 304.3
　agrypnal 304.1
　alcohol, alcoholic (ethyl) (methyl) (wood) 303.9
　　maternal, with suspected fetal damage affecting management of pregnancy 655.4
　allobarbitone 304.1
　allonal 304.1
　allylisopropylacetylurea 304.1
　alphaprodine (hydrochloride) 304.0
　Alurate 304.1
　Alvodine 304.0
　amethocaine 304.6
　amidone 304.0
　amidopyrine 304.6
　aminopyrine 304.6
　amobarbital 304.1
　amphetamine(s) (type) (drugs classifiable to 969.7) 304.4
　amylene hydrate 304.6
　amylobarbitone 304.1
　amylocaine 304.6
　Amytal (sodium) 304.1
　analgesic (drug) NEC 304.6
　　synthetic with morphine-like effect 304.0
　anesthetic (agent) (drug) (gas) (general) (local) NEC 304.6
　Angel dust 304.6
　anileridine 304.0
　antipyrine 304.6
　aprobarbital 304.1
　aprobarbitone 304.1
　atropine 304.6
　Avertin (bromide) 304.6
　barbenyl 304.1
　barbital(s) 304.1
　barbitone 304.1
　barbiturate(s) (compounds) (drugs classifiable to 967.0) 304.1
　barbituric acid (and compounds) 304.1
　benzedrine 304.4
　benzylmorphine 304.0
　Beta-chlor 304.1
　bhang 304.3
　blue velvet 304.0
　Brevital 304.1
　bromal (hydrate) 304.1
　bromide(s) NEC 304.1
　bromine compounds NEC 304.1
　bromisovalum 304.1
　bromoform 304.1
　Bromo-seltzer 304.1
　bromural 304.1
　butabarbital (sodium) 304.1
　butabarpal 304.1
　butallylonal 304.1
　butethal 304.1
　buthalitone (sodium) 304.1

Dependence—continued
  Butisol 304.1
  butobarbitone 304.1
  butyl chloral (hydrate) 304.1
  caffeine 304.4
  cannabis (indica) (sativa) (resin)
      (derivatives) (type) 304.3
  carbamazepine 304.6
  Carbrital 304.1
  carbromal 304.1
  carisoprodol 304.6
  Catha (edulis) 304.4
  chloral (betaine) (hydrate) 304.1
  chloralamide 304.1
  chloralformamide 304.1
  chloralose 304.1
  chlordiazepoxide 304.1
  Chloretone 304.1
  chlorobutanol 304.1
  chlorodyne 304.1
  chloroform 304.6
  Cliradon 304.0
  coca (leaf) and derivatives 304.2
  cocaine 304.2
    hydrochloride 304.2
    salt (any) 304.2
  codeine 304.0
  combination of drugs (excluding
      morphine or opioid type
      drug) NEC 304.8
    morphine or opioid type drug
        with any other drug
        304.7
  croton-chloral 304.1
  cyclobarbital 304.1
  cyclobarbitone 304.1
  dagga 304.3
  Delvinal 304.1
  Demerol 304.0
  desocodeine 304.0
  desomorphine 304.0
  desoxyephedrine 304.4
  DET 304.5
  dexamphetamine 304.4
  dexedrine 304.4
  dextromethorphan 304.0
  dextromoramide 304.0
  dextronorpseudoephedrine 304.4
  dextrorphan 304.0
  diacetylmorphine 304.0
  Dial 304.1
  diallylbarbituric acid 304.1
  diamorphine 304.0
  diazepam 304.1
  dibucaine 304.6
  dichloroethane 304.6
  diethyl barbituric acid 304.1
  diethylsulfone-diethylmethane
      304.1
  difencloxazine 304.0
  dihydrocodeine 304.0
  dihydrocodeinone 304.0
  dihydrohydroxycodeinone 304.0
  dihydroisocodeine 304.0
  dihydromorphine 304.0
  dihydromorphinone 304.0
  dihydroxycodeinone 304.0
  Dilaudid 304.0
  dimenhydrinate 304.6
  dimethylmeperidine 304.0
  dimethyltriptamine 304.5
  Dionin 304.0
  diphenoxylate 304.6
  dipipanone 304.0
  d-lysergic acid diethylamide 304.5
  DMT 304.5
  Dolophine 304.0
  DOM 304.2
  Doriden 304.1
  dormiral 304.1
  Dormison 304.1
  Dromoran 304.0
  drug NEC 304.9
    analgesic NEC 304.6

Dependence—continued
  drug—continued
    combination (excluding
        morphine or opioid type
        drug) NEC 304.8
      morphine or opioid type
          drug with any other
          drug 304.7
    complicating pregnancy,
        childbirth, or puerperium
        648.3
      affecting fetus or newborn
          779.5
    hallucinogenic 304.5
    hypnotic NEC 304.1
    narcotic NEC 304.9
    psychostimulant NEC 304.4
    sedative 304.1
    soporific NEC 304.1
    specified type NEC 304.6
    suspected damage to fetus
        affecting management of
        pregnancy 655.5
    synthetic, with morphine-like
        effect 304.0
    tranquilizing 304.1
  duboisine 304.6
  ectylurea 304.1
  Endocaine 304.6
  Equanil 304.1
  Eskabarb 304.1
  ethchlorvynol 304.1
  ether (ethyl) (liquid) (vapor) (vinyl)
      304.6
  ethidene 304.6
  ethinamate 304.1
  ethoheptazine 304.6
  ethyl
    alcohol 303.9
    bromide 304.6
    carbamate 304.6
    chloride 304.6
    morphine 304.0
  ethylene (gas) 304.6
    dichloride 304.6
  ethylidene chloride 304.6
  etilfen 304.1
  etorphine 304.0
  etoval 304.1
  eucodal 304.0
  euneryl 304.1
  Evipal 304.1
  Evipan 304.1
  fentanyl 304.0
  ganja 304.3
  gardenal 304.1
  gardenpanyl 304.1
  gelsemine 304.6
  Gelsemium 304.6
  Gemonil 304.1
  glucochloral 304.1
  glue (airplane) (sniffing) 304.6
  glutethimide 304.1
  hallucinogenics 304.5
  hashish 304.3
  headache powder NEC 304.6
  Heavenly Blue 304.5
  hedonal 304.1
  hemp 304.3
  heptabarbital 304.1
  Heptalgin 304.0
  heptobarbitone 304.1
  heroin 304.0
    salt (any) 304.0
  hexethal (sodium) 304.1
  hexobarbital 304.1
  Hycodan 304.0
  hydrocodone 304.0
  hydromorphinol 304.0
  hydromorphinone 304.0
  hydromorphone 304.0
  hydroxycodeine 304.0
  hypnotic NEC 304.1
  Indian hemp 304.3
  intranarcon 304.1
  Kemithal 304.1
  ketobemidone 304.0

Dependence—continued
  khat 304.4
  kif 304.3
  Lactuca (virosa) extract 304.1
  lactucarium 304.1
  laudanum 304.0
  Lebanese red 304.3
  Leritine 304.0
  lettuce opium 304.1
  Levanil 304.1
  Levo-Dromoran 304.0
  levo-iso-methadone 304.0
  levorphanol 304.0
  Librium 304.1
  Lomotil 304.6
  Lotusate 304.1
  LSD (-25) (and derivatives) 304.5
  Luminal 304.1
  lysergic acid 304.5
    amide 304.5
  maconha 304.3
  magic mushroom 304.5
  marihuana 304.3
  MDA (methylene
      dioxyamphetamine) 304.4
  Mebaral 304.1
  Medinal 304.1
  Medomin 304.1
  megahallucinogenics 304.5
  meperidine 304.0
  mephobarbital 304.1
  meprobamate 304.1
  mescaline 304.5
  methadone 304.0
  methamphetamine(s) 304.4
  methaqualone 304.1
  metharbital 304.1
  methitural 304.1
  methobarbitone 304.1
  methohexital 304.1
  methopholine 304.6
  methyl
    alcohol 303.9
    bromide 304.6
    morphine 304.0
    sulfonal 304.1
  methylated spirit 303.9
  methylbutinol 304.6
  methyldihydromorphinone 304.0
  methylene
    chloride 304.6
    dichloride 304.6
    dioxyamphetamine (MDA)
        304.4
  methylaparafynol 304.1
  methylphenidate 304.4
  methyprylone 304.1
  metopon 304.0
  Miltown 304.1
  morning glory seeds 304.5
  morphinan(s) 304.0
  morphine (sulfate) (sulfite) (type)
      (drugs classifiable to 965.00-
      965.09) 304.0
    or opioid type drug
        (drugs classifiable to 965.00-
        965.09) with any other drug
        304.7
  morphinol(s) 304.0
  morphinon 304.0
  morpholinylethylmorphine 304.0
  mylomid 304.1
  myristicin 304.5
  narcotic (drug) NEC 304.9
  nealbarbital 304.1
  nealbarbitone 304.1
  Nembutal 304.1
  Neonal 304.1
  Neraval 304.1
  Neravan 304.1
  neurobarb 304.1
  nicotine 305.1
  Nisentil 304.0
  nitrous oxide 304.6
  Noctec 304.1
  Noludar 304.1

Dependence—continued
  nonbarbiturate sedatives and
      tranquilizers with similar
      effect 304.1
  noptil 304.1
  normorphine 304.0
  noscapine 304.0
  Novocaine 304.6
  Numorphan 304.0
  nunol 304.1
  Nupercaine 304.6
  Oblivon 304.1
  on
    aspirator V46.0
    hyperbaric chamber V46.8
    iron lung V46.1
    machine (enabling) V46.9
      specified type NEC V46.8
    Possum (Patient-Operated-
        Selector-Mechanism)
        V46.8
    renal dialysis machine V45.1
    respirator V46.1
  opiate 304.0
  opioids 304.0
  opioid type drug 304.0
    with any other drug 304.7
  opium (alkaloids) (derivatives)
      (tincture) 304.0
  ortal 304.1
  Oxazepam 304.1
  oxycodone 304.0
  oxymorphone 304.0
  Palfium 304.0
  Panadol 304.6
  pantopium 304.0
  pantopon 304.0
  papaverine 304.0
  paracetamol 304.6
  paracodin 304.0
  paraldehyde 304.1
  paregoric 304.0
  Parzone 304.0
  PCP (phencyclidine) 304.6
  Pearly Gates 304.5
  pentazocine 304.0
  pentobarbital 304.1
  pentobarbitone (sodium) 304.1
  Pentothal 304.1
  Percaine 304.6
  Percodan 304.0
  Perichlor 304.1
  Pernocton 304.1
  Pernoston 304.1
  peronine 304.0
  pethidine (hydrochloride) 304.0
  petrichloral 304.1
  peyote 304.5
  Phanodron 304.1
  phenacetin 304.6
  phenadoxone 304.0
  phenaglycodol 304.1
  phenazocine 304.0
  phencyclidine 304.6
  phenmetrazine 304.4
  phenobal 304.1
  phenobarbital 304.1
  phenobarbitone 304.1
  phenomorphan 304.0
  phenonyl 304.1
  phenoperidine 304.0
  pholcodine 304.0
  piminodine 304.0
  Pipadone 304.0
  Pitkin's solution 304.6
  Placidyl 304.1
  polysubstance 304.8 ◆
  Pontocaine 304.6
  pot 304.3
  potassium bromide 304.1
  Preludin 304.4
  Prinadol 304.0
  probarbital 304.1
  procaine 304.6
  propanal 304.1
  propoxyphene 304.6
  psilocibin 304.5

Dependence—continued
   psilocin 304.5
   psilocybin 304.5
   psilocyline 304.5
   psilocyn 304.5
   psychedelic agents 304.5
   psychostimulant NEC 304.4
   psychotomimetic agents 304.5
   pyrahexyl 304.3
   Pyramidon 304.6
   quinalbarbitone 304.1
   racemoramide 304.0
   racemorphan 304.0
   Rela 304.6
   scopolamine 304.6
   secobarbital 304.1
   Seconal 304.1
   sedative NEC 304.1
      nonbarbiturate with barbiturate effect 304.1
   Sedormid 304.1
   sernyl 304.1
   sodium bromide 304.1
   Soma 304.6
   Somnal 304.1
   Somnos 304.1
   Soneryl 304.1
   soporific (drug) NEC 304.1
   specified drug NEC 304.6
   speed 304.4
   spinocaine 304.6
   Stovaine 304.6
   STP 304.5
   stramonium 304.6
   Sulfonal 304.1
   sulfonethylmethane 304.1
   sulfonmethane 304.1
   Surital 304.1
   synthetic drug with morphine-like effect 304.0
   talbutal 304.1
   tetracaine 304.6
   tetrahydrocannabinol 304.3
   tetronal 304.1
   THC 304.3
   thebacon 304.0
   thebaine 304.0
   thiamil 304.1
   thiamylal 304.1
   thiopental 304.1
   tobacco 305.1
   toluene, toluol 304.6
   tranquilizer NEC 304.1
      nonbarbiturate with barbiturate effect 304.1
   tribromacetaldehyde 304.6
   tribromethanol 304.6
   tribromomethane 304.6
   trichloroethanol 304.6
   trichoroethyl phosphate 304.1
   triclofos 304.1
   Trional 304.1
   Tuinal 304.1
   Turkish Green 304.3
   urethan(e) 304.6
   Valium 304.1
   Valmid 304.1
   veganin 304.0
   veramon 304.1
   Veronal 304.1
   versidyne 304.6
   vinbarbital 304.1
   vinbarbitone 304.1
   vinyl bitone 304.1
   vitamin B_6 266.1
   wine 303.9
   Zactane 304.6

Dependency
   passive 301.6
   reactions 301.6

Depersonalization (episode, in neurotic state) (neurotic) (syndrome) 300.6

Depletion
   carbohydrates 271.9
   complement factor 279.8
   extracellular fluid 276.5

Depletion—continued
   plasma 276.5
   potassium 276.8
      nephropathy 588.8
   salt or sodium 276.1
      causing heat exhaustion or prostration 992.4
      nephropathy 593.9
   volume 276.5
      extracellular fluid 276.5
      plasma 276.5

Deposit
   argentous, cornea 371.16
   bone, in Boeck's sarcoid 135
   calcareous, calcium — see Calcification
   cholesterol
      retina 362.82
      skin 709.3
      vitreous (humor) 379.22
   conjunctival 372.56
   cornea, corneal NEC 371.10
      argentous 371.16
      in
         cystinosis 270.0 [371.15]
         mucopolysaccharidosis 277.5 [371.15]
   crystalline, vitreous (humor) 379.22
   hemosiderin, in old scars of cornea 371.11
   metallic, in lens 366.45
   skin 709.3
   teeth, tooth (betel) (black) (green) (materia alba) (orange) (soft) (tobacco) 523.6
   urate, in kidney (see also Disease, renal) 593.9

Depraved appetite 307.52

Depression 311
   acute (see also Psychosis, affective) 296.2
      recurrent episode 296.3
      single episode 296.2
   agitated (see also Psychosis, affective) 296.2
      recurrent episode 296.3
      single episode 296.2
   anaclitic 309.21
   anxiety 300.4
   arches 734
      congenital 754.61
   autogenous (see also Psychosis, affective) 296.2
      recurrent episode 296.3
      single episode 296.2
   basal metabolic rate (BMR) 794.7
   bone marrow 289.9
   central nervous system 799.1
      newborn 779.2
   cerebral 331.9
      newborn 779.2
   cerebrovascular 437.8
      newborn 779.2
   chest wall 738.3
   endogenous (see also Psychosis, affective) 296.2
      recurrent episode 296.3
      single episode 296.2
   functional activity 780.9
   hysterical 300.11
   involutional, climacteric, or menopausal (see also Psychosis, affective) 296.2
      recurrent episode 296.3
      single episode 296.2
   manic (see also Psychosis, affective) 296.80
   medullary 348.8
      newborn 779.2
   mental 300.4
   metatarsal heads — see Depression, arches
   metatarsus — see Depression, arches
   monopolar (see also Psychosis, affective) 296.2
      recurrent episode 296.3

Depression—continued
   monopolar—continued
      single episode 296.2
   nervous 300.4
   neurotic 300.4
   nose 738.0
   psychogenic 300.4
      reactive 298.0
   psychoneurotic 300.4
   psychotic (see also Psychosis, affective) 296.2
      reactive 298.0
      recurrent episode 296.3
      single episode 296.2
   reactive 300.4
      neurotic 300.4
      psychogenic 298.0
      psychoneurotic 300.4
      psychotic 298.0
   recurrent 296.3
   respiratory center 348.8
      newborn 770.8
   scapula 736.89
   senile 290.21
   situational (acute) (brief) 309.0
      prolonged 309.1
   skull 754.0
   sternum 738.3
   visual field 368.40

Depressive reaction — see also Reaction, depressive
   acute (transient) 309.0
      with anxiety 309.28
   prolonged 309.1
   situational (acute) 309.0
      prolonged 309.1

Deprivation
   cultural V62.4
   emotional V62.89
      affecting infant or child 995.5
      as reason for family seeking advice V61.21
   food 994.2
      specific substance NEC 269.8
   protein (familial) (kwashiorkor) 260
   social V62.4
      affecting infant or child 995.5
      as reason for family seeking advice V61.21
   symptoms, syndrome
      alcohol 291.8
      drug 292.0
   vitamins (see also Deficiency, vitamin) 269.2
   water 994.3

de Quervain's
   disease (tendon sheath) 727.04
   thyroiditis (subacute granulomatous thyroiditis) 245.1

Derangement
   ankle (internal) 718.97
      current injury (see also Dislocation, ankle) 837.0
      recurrent 718.37
   cartilage (articular) NEC (see also Disorder, cartilage, articular) 718.0
      knee 717.9
         recurrent 718.36
      recurrent 718.3
   collateral ligament (knee) (medial) (tibial) 717.82
      current injury 844.1
         lateral (fibular) 844.0
      lateral (fibular) 717.81
         current injury 844.0
   cruciate ligament (knee) (posterior) 717.84
      anterior 717.83
         current injury 844.2
      current injury 844.2
   elbow (internal) 718.92
      current injury (see also Dislocation, elbow) 832.00
      recurrent 718.32

Derangement—continued
   gastrointestinal 536.9
   heart — see Disease, heart
   hip (joint) (internal) (old) 718.95
      current injury (see also Dislocation, hip) 835.00
      recurrent 718.35
   intervertebral disc — see Displacement, intervertebral disc
   joint (internal) 718.90
      ankle 718.97
      current injury — see also Dislocation, by site
      knee, meniscus or cartilage (see also Tear, meniscus) 836.2
      elbow 718.92
      foot 718.97
      hand 718.94
      hip 718.95
      knee 717.9
      multiple sites 718.99
      pelvic region 718.95
      recurrent 718.30
         ankle 718.37
         elbow 718.32
         foot 718.37
         hand 718.34
         hip 718.35
         knee 718.36
         multiple sites 718.39
         pelvic region 718.35
         shoulder (region) 718.31
         specified site NEC 718.38
         temporomandibular (old) 524.69
         wrist 718.33
      shoulder (region) 718.91
      specified site NEC 718.98
      spine NEC 724.9
      temporomandibular 524.69
      wrist 718.93
   knee (cartilage) (internal) 717.9
      current injury (see also Tear, meniscus) 836.2
      ligament 717.89
         capsular 717.85
         collateral — see Derangement, collateral ligament
         cruciate — see Derangement, cruciate ligament
         specified NEC 717.85
      recurrent 718.36
   low back NEC 724.9
   meniscus NEC (knee) 717.5
      current injury (see also Tear, meniscus) 836.2
      lateral 717.40
         anterior horn 717.42
         posterior horn 717.43
         specified NEC 717.49
      medial 717.3
         anterior horn 717.1
         posterior horn 717.2
      recurrent 718.3
      site other than knee — see Disorder, cartilage, articular
   mental (see also Psychosis) 298.9
   rotator cuff (recurrent) (tear) 726.10
      current 840.4
   sacroiliac (old) 724.6
      current — see Dislocation, sacroiliac
   semilunar cartilage (knee) 717.5
      current injury 836.2
         lateral 836.1
         medial 836.0
      recurrent 718.3
   shoulder (internal) 718.91
      current injury (see also Dislocation, shoulder) 831.00
      recurrent 718.31

Derangement—continued
 spine (recurrent) NEC 724.9
  current — see Dislocation,
   spine
  temporomandibular (internal) (joint)
   (old) 524.69
  current — see Dislocation, jaw
Dercum's disease or syndrome
 (adiposis dolorosa) 272.8
Derealization (neurotic) 300.6
Dermal — see condition
Dermaphytid — see Dermatophytosis
Dermatergosis — see Dermatitis
Dermatitis (allergic) (contact)
 (occupational) (venata) 692.9
 ab igne 692.82
 acneiform 692.9
 actinic (due to sun) 692.70
  acute 692.72
  chronic NEC 692.74
  other than from sun NEC 692.82
 ambustionis
  due to
   burn or scald — see Burn, by
    site
   sunburn 692.71
 amebic 006.6
 ammonia 691.0
 anaphylactoid NEC 692.9
 arsenical 692.4
 artefacta 698.4
  psychogenic 316 [698.4]
 asthmatic 691.8
 atopic (allergic) (infantile) (intrinsic)
  691.8
  psychogenic 316 [691.8]
 atrophicans 701.8
  diffusa 701.8
  maculosa 701.3
 berlock, berloque 692.72
 blastomycetic 116.0
 blister beetle 692.89
 Brucella NEC 023.9
 bullosa 694.9
  striata pratensis 692.6
 bullous 694.9
  mucosynechial, atrophic 694.60
   with ocular involvement
    694.61
  seasonal 694.8
 calorica
  due to
   burn or scald — see Burn,
    by site
   cold 692.89
   sunburn 692.71
 caterpillar 692.89
 cercarial 120.3
 combustionis
  due to
   burn or scald — see Burn, by
    site
   sunburn 692.71
 congelationis 991.5
 contusiformis 695.2
 diabetic 250.8
 diaper 691.0
 diphtheritica 032.85
 due to
  acetone 692.2
  acids 692.4
  adhesive plaster 692.4
  alcohol (skin contact)
   (substances classifiable to
   980.0-980.9) 692.4
   taken internally 693.8
  alkalis 692.4
  allergy NEC 692.9
  ammonia (household) (liquid)
   692.4
  arnica 692.3
  arsenic 692.4
   taken internally 693.8
  blister beetle 692.89
  cantharides 692.3
  carbon disulphide 692.2

Dermatitis—continued
 due to—continued
  caterpillar 692.89
  caustics 692.4
  cereal (ingested) 693.1
   contact with skin 692.5
  chemical(s) NEC 692.4
   internal 693.8
   irritant NEC 692.4
   taken internally 693.8
  chlorocompounds 692.2
  coffee (ingested) 693.1
   contact with skin 692.5
  cold weather 692.89
  cosmetics 692.81
  cyclohexanes 692.2
  deodorant 692.81
  detergents 692.0
  dichromate 692.4
  drugs and medicinals (correct
   substance properly
   administered) (internal
   use) 693.0
   external (in contact with
    skin) 692.3
   wrong substance given or
    taken 976.9
    specified substance —
     see Table of
     drugs and
     chemicals
   wrong substance given or
    taken 977.9
    specified substance —
     see Table of drugs
     and chemicals
  dyes 692.89
   hair 692.89
  epidermophytosis — see
   Dermatophytosis
  esters 692.2
  external irritant NEC 692.9
   specified agent NEC 692.89
  eye shadow 692.81
  fish (ingested) 693.1
   contact with skin 692.5
  flour (ingested) 693.1
   contact with skin 692.5
  food (ingested) 693.1
   in contact with skin 692.5
  fruit (ingested) 693.1
   contact with skin 692.5
  fungicides 692.3
  furs 692.89
  glycols 692.2
  greases NEC 692.1
  hair dyes 692.89
  hot
   objects and materials — see
    Burn, by site
   weather or places 692.89
  hydrocarbons 692.2
  infrared rays, except from sun
   692.82
  solar NEC (see also
   Dermatitis, due to,
   sun) 692.70
  ingested substance 693.9
   drugs and medicinals (see
    also Dermatitis, due
    to, drugs and
    medicinals) 693.0
   food 693.1
   specified substance NEC
    693.8
  ingestion or injection of
   chemical 693.8
  drug (correct substance
   properly administered)
   693.0
   wrong substance given or
    taken 977.9
    specified substance —
     see Table of
     drugs and
     chemicals
  insecticides 692.4

Dermatitis—continued
 due to—continued
  internal agent 693.9
   drugs and medicinals (see
    also Dermatitis, due
    to, drugs and
    medicinals) 693.0
   food (ingested) 693.1
    in contact with skin
     692.5
   specified agent NEC 693.8
  iodine 692.3
  iodoform 692.3
  irradiation 692.82
  jewelry 692.83
  keratolytics 692.3
  ketones 692.2
  lacquer tree (Rhus verniciflua)
   692.6
  light NEC (see also Dermatitis,
   due to, sun) 692.70
   other 692.82
  low temperature 692.89
  mascara 692.81
  meat (ingested) 693.1
   contact with skin 692.5
  mercury, mercurials 692.3
  metals 692.83
  milk (ingested) 693.1
   contact with skin 692.5
  Neomycin 692.3
  nylon 692.4
  oils NEC 692.1
  paint solvent 692.2
  pediculocides 692.3
  petroleum products (substances
   classifiable to 981) 692.4
  phenol 692.3
  photosensitiveness,
   photosensitivity (sun)
   692.72
   other light 692.82
  plants NEC 692.6
  plasters, medicated (any) 692.3
  plastic 692.4
  poison
   ivy (Rhus toxicodendron)
    692.6
   oak (Rhus diversiloba) 692.6
   plant or vine 692.6
   sumac (Rhus venenata)
    692.6
   vine (Rhus radicans) 692.6
  preservatives 692.89
  primrose (primula) 692.6
  primula 692.6
  radiation 692.82
   sun NEC (see also
    Dermatitis, due to,
    sun) 692.70
  radioactive substance 692.82
  radium 692.82
  ragweed (Senecio jacobae)
   692.6
  Rhus (diversiloba) (radicans)
   (toxicodendron)
   (venenata) (verniciflua)
   692.6
  rubber 692.4
  scabicides 692.3
  Senecio jacobae 692.6
  solar radiation — see
   Dermatitis, due to, sun
  solvents (any) (substances
   classifiable to 982.0-
   982.8) 692.2
   chlorocompound group
    692.2
   cyclohexane group 692.2
   ester group 692.2
   glycol group 692.2
   hydrocarbon group 692.2
   ketone group 692.2
   paint 692.2
  specified agent NEC 692.89
  sun 692.70
   acute 692.72

Dermatitis—continued
 due to—continued
  sun—continued
   chronic NEC 692.74
   specified NEC 692.79
  sunburn 692.71
  sunshine NEC (see also
   Dermatitis, due to, sun)
   692.70
  tetrachlorethylene 692.2
  toluene 692.2
  topical medications 692.3
  turpentine 692.2
  ultraviolet rays, except from sun
   692.82
   sun NEC (see also
    Dermatitis, due to,
    sun) 692.82
  vaccine or vaccination (correct
   substance properly
   administered) 693.0
   wrong substance given or
    taken
    bacterial vaccine 978.8
    specified — see Table
     of drugs and
     chemicals
    other vaccines NEC 979.9
     specified — see Table
      of drugs and
      chemicals
  varicose veins (see also
   Varicose, vein, inflamed
   or infected) 454.1
  x-rays 692.82
 dyshydrotic 705.81
 dysmenorrheica 625.8
 eczematoid NEC 692.9
  infectious 690
 eczematous NEC 692.9
 epidemica 695.89
 erysipelatosa 695.81
 escharotica — see Burn, by site
 exfoliativa, exfoliative 695.89
  generalized 695.89
  infantum 695.81
  neonatorum 695.81
 eyelid 373.31
  allergic 373.32
  contact 373.32
  eczematous 373.31
  herpes (zoster) 053.20
   simplex 054.41
  infective 373.5
   due to
    actinomycosis 039.3
     [373.5]
    herpes
     simplex 054.41 ◆
     zoster 053.20
    impetigo 684 [373.5]
    leprosy (see also Leprosy)
     030.0 [373.4]
    lupus vulgaris
     (tuberculous) (see
     also Tuberculosis)
     017.0 [373.4]
    mycotic dermatitis (see
     also
     Dermatomycosis)
     111.9 [373.5]
    vaccinia 051.0 [373.5]
     postvaccination 999.0
      [373.5]
    yaws (see also Yaws)
     102.9 [373.4]
 facta, factitia 698.4
  psychogenic 316 [698.4]
 ficta 698.4
  psychogenic 316 [698.4]
 flexural 691.8
 follicularis 704.8
 friction 709.8
 fungus 111.9
  specified type NEC 111.8
 gangrenosa, gangrenous (infantum)
  (see also Gangrene) 785.4

Dermatitis—continued
gestationis 646.8
gonococcal 098.89
gouty 274.89
harvest mite 133.8
heat 692.89
herpetiformis (bullous)
  (erythematous) (pustular)
  (vesicular) 694.0
  juvenile 694.2
  senile 694.5
hiemalis 692.89
hypostatic, hypostatica 454.1
  with ulcer 454.2
impetiginous 684
infantile (acute) (chronic)
  (intertriginous) (intrinsic)
  (seborrheic) 691.8
infectiosa eczematoides 690
infectious (staphylococcal)
  (streptococcal) 686.9
  eczematoid 690
infective eczematoid 690
Jacquet's (diaper dermatitis) 691.0
leptus 133.8
lichenified NEC 692.9
lichenoid, chronic 701.0
lichenoides purpurica pigmentosa 709.1
meadow 692.6
medicamentosa (correct substance
  properly administered)
  (internal use) (see also
  Dermatitis, due to, drugs, or
  medicinals) 693.0
  due to contact with skin 692.3
mite 133.8
multiformis 694.0
  juvenile 694.2
  senile 694.5
napkin 691.0
neuro 698.3
neurotica 694.0
nummular NEC 692.9
osteatosis, osteatotic 706.8
papillaris capillitii 706.1
pellagrous 265.2
perioral 695.3
perstans 696.1
photosensitivity (sun) 692.72
  other light 692.82
pigmented purpuric lichenoid 709.1
polymorpha dolorosa 694.0
primary irritant 692.9
pruriginosa 694.0
pruritic NEC 692.9
psoriasiform nodularis 696.2
psychogenic 316
purulent 686.0
pustular contagious 051.2
pyococcal 686.0
pyocyaneus 686.0
pyogenica 686.0
radiation 692.82
repens 696.1
Ritter's (exfoliativa) 695.81
Schamberg's (progressive
  pigmentary dermatosis) 709.09 ◆
schistosome 120.3
seasonal bullous 694.8
seborrheic 690
  infantile 691.8
sensitization NEC 692.9
septic 686.0
  gonococcal 098.89
solar, solare NEC (see also
  Dermatitis, due to, sun) 692.70
stasis 459.81
  due to
    postphlebitic syndrome 459.1
    varicose veins — see Varicose

Dermatitis—continued
stasis—continued
  ulcerated or with ulcer
    (varicose) 454.2
sunburn 692.71
suppurative 686.0
traumatic NEC 709.8
trophoneurotica 694.0
ultraviolet, except from sun 692.82
  due to sun NEC (see also
    Dermatitis, due to, sun) 692.70
varicose 454.1
  with ulcer 454.2
vegetans 686.8
verrucosa 117.2
xerotic 706.8
Dermatoarthritis, lipoid 272.8 [713.0]
Dermatochalasia, dermatochalasis 374.87
Dermatofibroma (lenticulare)
  (M8832/0) — see also
  Neoplasm, skin, benign
  protuberans (M8832/1) — see
    Neoplasm, skin, uncertain
    behavior
Dermatofibrosarcoma (protuberans)
  (M8832/3) — see Neoplasm,
  skin, malignant
Dermatographia 708.3
Dermatolysis (congenital) (exfoliativa) 757.39
  acquired 701.8
  eyelids 374.34
  palpebrarum 374.34
  senile 701.8
Dermatomegaly NEC 701.8
Dermatomucomyositis 710.3
Dermatomycosis 111.9
  furfuracea 111.0
  specified type NEC 111.8
Dermatomyositis (acute) (chronic) 710.3
Dermatoneuritis of children 985.0
Dermatophiliasis 134.1
Dermatophytide — see
  Dermatophytosis
Dermatophytosis (Epidermophyton)
  (infection) (microsporum) (tinea)
  (Trichophyton) 110.9
  beard 110.0
  body 110.5
  deep seated 110.6
  fingernails 110.1
  foot 110.4
  groin 110.3
  hand 110.2
  nail 110.1
  perianal (area) 110.3
  scalp 110.0
  scrotal 110.8
  specified site NEC 110.8
  toenails 110.1
  vulva 110.8
Dermatopolyneuritis 985.0
Dermatorrhexis 756.83
  acquired 701.8
Dermatosclerosis (see also
  Scleroderma) 710.1
  localized 701.0
Dermatosis 709.9
  Andrews' 686.8
  atopic 691.8
  Bowen's (M8081/2) — see
    Neoplasm, skin, in situ
  bullous 694.9
    specified type NEC 694.8
  erythematosquamous 690
  exfoliativa 695.89
  factitial 698.4
  gonococcal 098.89
  herpetiformis 694.0
    juvenile 694.2
    senile 694.5

Dermatosis—continued
hysterical 300.11
menstrual NEC 709.8
neutrophilic, acute febrile 695.89
occupational (see also Dermatitis) 692.9
papulosa nigra 709.8
pigmentary NEC 709.00 ▼
  progressive 709.09
  Schamberg's 709.09 ▲
  Siemens-Bloch 757.33
progressive pigmentary 709.09 ◆
psychogenic 316
pustular subcorneal 694.1
Schamberg's (progressive
  pigmentary) 709.09 ◆
senile NEC 709.3
Unna's (seborrheic dermatitis) 690
Dermographia 708.3
Dermographism 708.3
Dermoid (cyst) (M9084/0) — see also
  Neoplasm, by site, benign
  with malignant transformation
    (M9084/3) 183.0
Dermopathy
  infiltrative, with throtoxicosis 242.0
  senile NEC 709.3
Dermophytosis — see
  Dermatophytosis
Descemet's membrane — see
  condition
Descemetocele 371.72
Descending — see condition
Descensus uteri (complete)
  (incomplete) (partial) (without
  vaginal wall prolapse) 618.1
  with mention of vaginal wall
    proplapse — see Prolapse,
    uterovaginal
Desensitization to allergens V07.1
Desert
  rheumatism 114.0
  sore (see also Ulcer, skin) 707.9
Desertion (child) (newborn) 995.5
  specified person NEC 995.81
Desmoid (extra-abdominal) (tumor)
  (M8821/1) — see also
  Neoplasm, connective tissue,
  uncertain behavior
  abdominal (M8822/1) — see
    Neoplasm, connective tissue,
    uncertain behavior
Despondency 300.4
Desquamative dermatitis NEC 695.89
Destruction
  articular facet (see also
    Derangement, joint) 718.9
    vertebra 724.9
  bone 733.90
    syphilitic 095.5
  joint (see also Derangement, joint) 718.9
    sacroiliac 724.6
  kidney 593.89
  live fetus to facilitate birth NEC 763.8
  ossicles (ear) 385.24
  rectal sphincter 569.49
  septum (nasal) 478.1
  tuberculous NEC (see also
    Tuberculosis) 011.9
  tympanic membrane 384.82
  tympanum 385.89
  vertebral disc — see Degeneration,
    intervertebral disc
Destructiveness (see also Disturbance,
  conduct) 312.9
  adjustment reaction 309.3
Detachment
  cartilage — see also Sprain, by site
    knee — see Tear, meniscus
  cervix, annular 622.8
    complicating delivery 665.3

Detachment—continued
choroid (old) (postinfectional)
  (simple) (spontaneous) 363.70
  hemorrhagic 363.72
  serous 363.71
knee, medial meniscus (old) 717.3
  current injury 836.0
ligament — see Sprain, by site
placenta (premature) — see
  Placenta, separation
retina (recent) 361.9
  with retinal defect
    (rhegmatogenous) 361.00
    giant tear 361.03
    multiple 361.02
    partial
      with
        giant tear 361.03
        multiple defects 361.02
        retinal dialysis
          (juvenile) 361.04
        single defect 361.01
      retinal dialysis (juvenile) 361.04
      single 361.01
      subtotal 361.05
      total 361.05
  delimited (old) (partial) 361.06
  old
    delimited 361.06
    partial 361.06
    total or subtotal 361.07
  pigment epithelium (RPE)
    (serous) 362.42
    exudative 362.42
    hemorrhagic 362.43
  rhegmatogenous (see also
    Detachment, retina, with
    retinal defect) 361.00
  serous (without retinal defect) 361.2
  specified type NEC 361.89
  traction (with vitreoretinal
    organization) 361.81
vitreous humor 379.21
Detergent asthma 507.8
Deterioration
  epileptic 294.1
  heart, cardiac (see also
    Degeneration, myocardial) 429.1
  mental (see also Psychosis) 298.9
  myocardium, myocardial (see also
    Degeneration, myocardial) 429.1
  senile (simple) 797
  transplanted organ — see
    Complications, transplant,
    organ, by site
de Toni-Fanconi syndrome (cystinosis) 270.0
Deuteranomaly 368.52
Deuteranopia (anomalous trichromat)
  (complete) (incomplete) 368.52
Deutschländer's disease — see
  Fracture, foot
Development
  abnormal, bone 756.9
  arrested 783.4
    bone 733.91
    child 783.4
    due to malnutrition (protein-
      calorie) 263.2
    fetus or newborn 764.9
    tracheal rings (congenital) 748.3
  defective, congenital — see also
    Anomaly
    cauda equina 742.59
    left ventricle 746.9
      with atresia or hypoplasia of
        aortic orifice or valve
        with hypoplasia of
          ascending aorta 746.7

Development—continued
defective, congenital—continued
left ventricle—continued
in hypoplastic left heart syndrome 746.7
delayed (see also Delay, development) 783.4
arithmetical skills 315.1
language (skills) 315.31
expressive 315.31 ▼
mixed receptive-expressive 315.31 ▲
learning skill, specified NEC 315.2
mixed skills 315.5
motor coordination 315.4
reading 315.00
specified
learning skill NEC 315.2
type NEC, except learning 315.8
speech 315.39
associated with hyperkinesia 314.1
phonological 315.39 ◆
spelling 315.09
imperfect, congenital — see also Anomaly
heart 746.9
lungs 748.60
improper (fetus or newborn) 764.9
incomplete (fetus or newborn) 764.9
affecting management of pregnancy 656.5
bronchial tree 748.3
organ or site not listed — see Hypoplasia
respiratory system 748.9
sexual, precocious NEC 259.1
tardy, mental (see also Retardation, mental) 319
written expression 315.2 ◆

Developmental — see condition

Devergie's disease (pityriasis rubra pilaris) 696.4

Deviation
conjugate (eye) 378.87
palsy 378.81
spasm, spastic 378.82
esophagus 530.89
eye, skew 378.87
midline (jaw) (teeth) 524.2
specified site NEC — see Malposition
organ or site, congenital NEC — see Malposition, congenital
septum (acquired) (nasal) 470
congenital 754.0
sexual 302.9
bestiality 302.9
coprophilia 302.89
ego-dystonic
homosexuality 302.0
lesbianism 302.0
erotomania 302.89
Clérambault's 297.8
exhibitionism (sexual) 302.4
fetishism 302.81
transvestic 302.3 ▼
frotteurism 302.89 ▲
homosexuality, ego-dystonic 302.0
pedophilic 302.2
lesbianism, ego-dystonic 302.0
masochism 302.83
narcissism 302.89
necrophilia 302.89
nymphomania 302.89
pederosis 302.2
pedophilia 302.2
sadism 302.84
sadomasochism 302.84
satyriasis 302.89
specified type NEC 302.89
transvestic fetishism, 302.3 ◆
transvestism 302.3

Deviation—continued
sexual—continued
voyeurism 302.82
zoophilia (erotica) 302.1
teeth, midline 524.2
trachea 519.1
ureter (congenital) 753.4

Devic's disease 341.0

Device
cerebral ventricle (communicating) in situ V45.2
contraceptive — see Contraceptive, device ◆
drainage, cerebrospinal fluid V45.2

Devil's
grip 074.1
pinches (purpura simplex) 287.2

Devitalized tooth 522.9

Devonshire colic 984.9
specified type of lead — see Table of drugs and chemicals

Dextraposition, aorta 747.21
with ventricular septal defect, pulmonary stenosis or atresia, and hypertrophy of right ventricle 745.2
in tetralogy of Fallot 745.2

Dextratransposition, aorta 745.11

Dextrinosis, limit (debrancher enzyme deficiency) 271.0

Dextrocardia (corrected) (false) (isolated) (secondary) (true) 746.87
with
complete transposition of viscera 759.3
situs inversus 759.3

Dextroversion, kidney (left) 753.3

Dhobie itch 110.3

Diabetes, diabetic (brittle) (congenital) (familial) (mellitus) (severe) (slight) (without complication) 250.0 ◆

> Note — Use the following fifth-digit subclassification with category 250:
>
> 0 type II [non-insulin dependent type] [NIDDM type] [adult-onset type] or unspecified type, not stated as uncontrolled
>
> 1 type I [insulin dependent type] [IDDM type] [juvenile type], not stated as uncontrolled
>
> 2 type II [non-insulin dependent type] [NIDDM type] [adult-onset type] or unspecified type, uncontrolled
>
> 3 type I [insulin dependent type] [IDDM] [juvenile type], uncontrolled

with
coma (with ketoacidosis) 250.3
hyperosmolar (nonketotic) 250.2
complication NEC 250.9
specified NEC 250.8
gangrene 250.7 [785.4]
hyperosmolarity 250.2
ketosis, ketoacidosis 250.1
specified manifestations NEC 250.8
acetonemia 250.1
acidosis 250.1
amyotrophy 250.6 [358.1]
angiopathy, peripheral 250.7 [443.81]
asymptomatic 790.2
autonomic neuropathy (peripheral) 250.6 [337.1]

Diabetes, diabetic—continued
bone change 250.8 [731.8]
bronze, bronzed 275.0
cataract 250.5 [366.41]
chemical 790.2
complicating pregnancy, childbirth, or puerperium 648.8
coma (with ketoacidosis) 250.3
hyperglycemic 250.3
hyperosmolar (nonketotic) 250.2
hypoglycemic 250.3
insulin 250.3
complicating pregnancy, childbirth, or puerperium (maternal) 648.8
affecting fetus or newborn 775.0
complication NEC 250.9
specified NEC 250.8
dorsal sclerosis 250.6 [340]
dwarfism-obesity syndrome 258.1
gangrene 250.7 [785.4]
gestational 648.8
complicating pregnancy, childbirth, or puerperium 648.8
glaucoma 250.5 [365.44]
glomerulosclerosis (intercapillary) 250.4 [581.81]
glycogenosis, secondary 250.8 [259.8]
hemochromatosis 275.0
hyperosmolar coma 250.2
hyperosmolarity 250.2
hypertension-nephrosis syndrome 250.4 [581.81]
hypoglycemia 250.8
hypoglycemic shock 250.8
insipidus 253.5
nephrogenic 588.1
pituitary 253.5
vasopressin-resistant 588.1
intercapillary glomerulosclerosis 250.4 [581.81]
iritis 250.5 [364.42]
ketosis, ketoacidosis 250.1
Kimmelstiel (-Wilson) disease or syndrome (intercapillary glomerulosclerosis) 250.4 [581.81]
Lancereaux's (diabetes mellitus with marked emaciation) 250.8 [261]
latent (chemical) 790.2
complicating pregnancy, childbirth, or puerperium 648.8
lipoidosis 250.8 [272.7]
macular edema 250.5 [362.83] ◆
maternal
with manifest disease in the infant 775.1
affecting fetus or newborn 775.0
microaneurysms, retinal 250.5 [362.01]
mononeuropathy 250.6 [355.9]
neonatal, transient 775.1
nephropathy 250.4 [583.81]
nephrosis (syndrome) 250.4 [581.81]
neuralgia 250.6 [357.2]
neuritis 250.6 [357.2]
neurogenic arthropathy 250.6 [713.5]
neuropathy 250.6 [357.2]
nonclinical 790.2
peripheral autonomic neuropathy 250.6 [337.1]
phosphate 275.3
polyneuropathy 250.6 [357.2]
renal (true) 271.4
retinal
edema 250.5 [362.83]
hemorrhage 250.5 [362.01]
microaneurysms 250.5 [362.01]
retinitis 250.5 [362.01]
retinopathy 250.5 [362.01]
background 250.5 [362.01]

Diabetes, diabetic—continued
retinopathy—continued
proliferative 250.5 [362.02]
steroid induced
correct substance properly administered 251.8
overdose or wrong substance given or taken 962.0
stress 790.2
subclinical 790.2
subliminal 790.2
sugar 250.0
ulcer (skin) 250.8 [707.9]
lower extremity 250.8 [707.1]
specified site NEC 250.8 [707.8]
xanthoma 250.8 [272.2]

Diacyclothrombopathia 287.1

Diagnosis deferred 799.9

Dialysis (intermittent) (treatment)
anterior retinal (juvenile) (with detachment) 361.04
extracorporeal V56.0
peritoneal V56.8
renal V56.0
status only V45.1
specified type NEC V56.8

Diamond-Blackfan anemia or syndrome (congenital hypoplastic anemia) 284.0

Diamond-Gardener syndrome (autoerythrocyte sensitization) 287.2

Diaper rash 691.0

Diaphoresis (excessive) NEC 780.8

Diaphragm — see condition

Diaphragmalgia 786.52

Diaphragmitis 519.4

Diaphyseal aclasis 756.4

Diaphysitis 733.99

Diarrhea, diarrheal (acute) (autumn) (bilious) (bloody) (catarrhal) (choleraic) (chronic) (gravis) (green) (infantile) (lienteric) (noninfectious) (presumed noninfectious) (putrefactive) (secondary) (sporadic) (summer) (symptomatic) (thermic) 558.9
achlorhydric 536.0
allergic 558.9
amebic (see also Amebiasis) 006.9
with abscess — see Abscess, amebic
acute 006.0
chronic 006.1
nondysenteric 006.2
bacillary — see Dysentery, bacillary
bacterial NEC 008.5
balantidial — 007.0
bile salt-induced 579.8
cachectic NEC 558.9
chilomastix 007.8
choleriformis 001.1
chronic 558.9
ulcerative (see also Colitis, ulcerative) 556.9 ◆
coccidial 007.2
Cochin-China 579.1
anguilluliasis 127.2
psilosis 579.1
Dientamoeba 007.8
dietetic 558.9
due to
achylia gastrica 536.8
Aerobacter aerogenes 008.2
Bacillus coli — see Enteritis, E. coli
bacteria NEC 008.5
bile salts 579.8
Capillaria
hepatica 128.8
philippinensis 127.5
Clostridium perfringens (C) (F) 008.46
Enterobacter aerogenes 008.2
enterococci 008.49

Diarrhea, diarrheal—continued
due to—continued
Escherichia coli — see Enteritis, E. coli
Giardia lamblia 007.1
Heterophyes heterophyes 121.6
irritating foods 558.9
Metagonimus yokogawai 121.5
Necator americanus 126.1
Paracolobactrum arizonae 008.1
Paracolon bacillus NEC 008.47
Arizona 008.1
Proteus (bacillus) (mirabilis) (Morganii) 008.3
Pseudomonas aeruginosa 008.42
S. japonicum 120.2
specified organism NEC 008.8
bacterial 008.49
gouty 274.9
viral NEC 008.69
Staphylococcus 008.41
Streptococcus 008.49
anaerobic 008.46
Strongyloides stercoralis 127.2
Trichuris trichiuria 127.3
virus NEC (see also Enteritis, viral) 008.69
dysenteric 009.2
due to specified organism NEC 008.8
dyspeptic 558.9
endemic 009.3
due to specified organism NEC 008.8
epidemic 009.2
due to specified organism NEC 008.8
fermentative 558.9
flagellate 007.9
Flexner's (ulcerative) 004.1
functional 564.5
following gastrointestinal surgery 564.4
psychogenic 306.4
giardial 007.1
Giardia lamblia 007.1
hill 579.1
hyperperistalsis (nervous) 306.4
infectious 009.2
due to specified organism NEC 008.8
presumed 009.3
inflammatory 558.9
due to specified organism NEC 008.8
malarial (see also Malaria) 084.6
mite 133.8
mycotic 117.9
nervous 306.4
neurogenic 564.5
parenteral NEC 009.2
postgastrectomy 564.4
postvagotomy 564.4
prostaglandin induced 579.8
protozoal NEC 007.9
psychogenic 306.4
septic 009.2
due to specified organism NEC 008.8
specified organism NEC 008.8
bacterial 008.49
viral NEC 008.69
Staphylococcus 008.41
Streptococcus 008.49
anaerobic 008.46
toxic 558.2
travelers' 009.2
due to specified organism NEC 008.8
trichomonal 007.3
tropical 579.1
tuberculous 014.8
ulcerative (chronic) (see also Colitis, ulcerative) 556.9 ◆
viral (see also Enteritis, viral) 008.8
zymotic NEC 009.2

Diastasis
cranial bones 733.99
congenital 756.0
joint (traumatic) — see Dislocation, by site
muscle 728.84
congenital 756.89
recti (abdomen) 728.84
complicating delivery 665.8
congenital 756.7

Diastema, teeth, tooth 524.3
Diastematomyelia 742.51
Diataxia, cerebral, infantile 343.0

Diathesis
allergic V15.0
bleeding (familial) 287.9
cystine (familial) 270.0
gouty 274.9
hemorrhagic (familial) 287.9
newborn NEC 776.0
oxalic 271.8
scrofulous (see also Tuberculosis) 017.2
spasmophilic (see also Tetany) 781.7
ulcer 536.9
uric acid 274.9

Diaz's disease or osteochondrosis 732.5

Dibothriocephaliasis 123.4
larval 123.5

Dibothriocephalus (infection) (infestation) (latus) 123.4
larval 123.5

Dicephalus 759.4
Dichotomy, teeth 520.2
Dichromat, dichromata (congenital) 368.59
Dichromatopsia (congenital) 368.59
Dichuchwa 104.0
Dicroceliasis 121.8
Didelphys, didelphic (see also Double uterus) 752.2
Didymitis (see also Epididymitis) 604.90
Died — see also Death
without
medical attention (cause unknown) 798.9
sign of disease 798.2
Dientamoeba diarrhea 007.8

Dietary
inadequacy or deficiency 269.9
surveillance and counseling V65.3

Dietl's crisis 593.4
Dieulafoy's ulcer — see Ulcer, stomach

Difficult
birth, affecting fetus or newborn 763.9
delivery NEC 669.9

Difficulty
feeding 783.3
newborn 779.3
nonorganic (infant) NEC 307.59
mechanical, gastroduodenal stoma 537.89
reading 315.00
specific, spelling 315.09
swallowing (see also Dysphagia) 787.2
walking 719.7

Diffuse — see condition
Diffused ganglion 727.42
DiGeorge's syndrome (thymic hypoplasia) 279.11
Digestive — see condition
Di Guglielmo's disease or syndrome (M9841/3) 207.0
Diktyoma (M9051/3) — see Neoplasm, by site, malignant
Dilaceration, tooth 520.4

Dilatation
anus 564.8
venule — see Hemorrhoids
aorta (focal) (general) (see also Aneurysm, aorta) 441.9
congenital 747.29
infectional 093.0
ruptured 441.5
syphilitic 093.0
appendix (cystic) 543.9
artery 447.8
bile duct (common) (cystic) (congenital) 751.69
acquired 576.8
bladder (sphincter) 596.8
congenital 753.8
in pregnancy or childbirth 654.4
causing obstructed labor 660.2
affecting fetus or newborn 763.1
blood vessel 459.89
bronchus, bronchi 494
calyx (due to obstruction) 593.89
capillaries 448.9
cardiac (acute) (chronic) (see also Hypertrophy, cardiac) 429.3
congenital 746.89
valve NEC 746.89
pulmonary 746.09
hypertensive (see also Hypertension, heart) 402.90
cavum septi pellucidi 742.4
cecum 564.8
psychogenic 306.4
cervix (uteri) — see also Incompetency, cervix
incomplete, poor, slow
affecting fetus or newborn 763.7
complicating delivery 661.0
affecting fetus or newborn 763.7
colon 564.7
congenital 751.3
due to mechanical obstruction 560.89
psychogenic 306.4
common bile duct (congenital) 751.69
acquired 576.8
with calculus, choledocholithiasis, or stones — see Choledocholithiasis
cystic duct 751.69
acquired (any bile duct) 575.8
duct, mammary 610.4
duodenum 564.8
esophagus 530.89
congenital 750.4
due to
achalasia 530.0
cardiospasm 530.0
Eustachian tube, congenital 744.24
fontanel 756.0
gallbladder 575.8
congenital 751.69
gastric 536.8
acute 536.1
psychogenic 306.4
heart (acute) (chronic) (see also Hypertrophy, cardiac) 429.3
congenital 746.89
hypertensive (see also Hypertension, heart) 402.90
valve — see also Endocarditis
congenital 746.89
ileum 564.8
psychogenic 306.4
inguinal rings — see Hernia, inguinal
jejunum 564.8
psychogenic 306.4

Dilatation—continued
kidney (calyx) (collecting structures) (cystic) (parenchyma) (pelvis) 593.89
lacrimal passages 375.69
lymphatic vessel 457.1
mammary duct 610.4
Meckel's diverticulum (congenital) 751.0
meningeal vessels, congenital 742.8
myocardium (acute) (chronic) (see also Hypertrophy, cardiac) 429.3
organ or site, congenital NEC — see Distortion
pancreatic duct 577.8
pelvis, kidney 593.89
pericardium — see Pericarditis
pharynx 478.29
prostate 602.8
pulmonary
artery (idiopathic) 417.8
congenital 747.3
valve, congenital 746.09
pupil 379.43
rectum 564.8
renal 593.89
saccule vestibularis, congenital 744.05
salivary gland (duct) 527.8
sphincter ani 564.8
stomach 536.8
acute 536.1
psychogenic 306.4
submaxillary duct 527.8
trachea, congenital 748.3
ureter (idiopathic) 593.89
congenital 753.2
due to obstruction 593.5
urethra (acquired) 599.84
vasomotor 443.9
vein 459.89
ventricular, ventricle (acute) (chronic) (see also Hypertrophy, cardiac) 429.3
cerebral, congenital 742.4
hypertensive (see also Hypertension, heart) 402.90
venule 459.89
anus — see Hemorrhoids
vesical orifice 596.8

Dilated, dilation — see Dilatation

Diminished
hearing (acuity) (see also Deafness) 389.9
pulse pressure 785.9
vision NEC 369.9
vital capacity 794.2

Diminuta taenia 123.6

Diminution, sense or sensation (cold) (heat) (tactile) (vibratory) (see also Disturbance, sensation) 782.0

Dimitri-Sturge-Weber disease (encephalocutaneous angiomatosis) 759.6

Dimple
parasacral 685.1
with abscess 685.0
pilonidal 685.1
with abscess 685.0
postanal 685.1
with abscess 685.0

Dioctophyma renale (infection) (infestation) 128.8
Dipetalonemiasis 125.4
Diphallus 752.8
Diphtheria, diphtheritic (gangrenous) (hemorrhagic) 032.9
carrier (suspected) of V02.4
cutaneous 032.85
cystitis 032.84
faucial 032.0
infection of wound 032.85

Diphtheria, diphtheritic—continued
    inoculation (anti) (not sick) V03.5
    laryngeal 032.3
    myocarditis 032.82
    nasal anterior 032.2
    nasopharyngeal 032.1
    neurological complication 032.89
    peritonitis 032.83
    specified site NEC 032.89
Diphyllobothriasis (intestine) 123.4
    larval 123.5
Diplacusis 388.41
Diplegia (upper limbs) 344.2
    brain or cerebral 437.8
    congenital 343.0
    facial 351.0
        congenital 352.6
    infantile or congenital (cerebral) (spastic) (spinal) 343.0
    lower limbs 344.1
    syphilitic, congenital 090.49
Diplococcus, diplococcal — see condition
Diplomyelia 742.59
Diplopia 368.2
    refractive 368.15
Dipsomania (see also Alcoholism) 303.9
    with psychosis (see also Psychosis, alcoholic) 291.9
Dipylidiasis 123.8
    intestine 123.8
Direction, teeth, abnormal 524.3
Dirt-eating child 307.52
Disability
    heart — see Disease, heart
    learning NEC 315.2
    special spelling 315.09
Disarticulation (see also Derangement, joint) 718.9
    meaning
        amputation ▼
            status — see Absence, by site
            traumatic — see Amputation, traumatic ▲
        dislocation, traumatic or congenital — see Dislocation
Disaster, cerebrovascular (see also Disease, cerebrovascular, acute) 436
Discharge
    anal NEC 787.9
    breast (female) (male) 611.79
    conjunctiva 372.8
    continued locomotor idiopathic (see also Epilepsy) 345.5
    diencephalic autonomic idiopathic (see also Epilepsy) 345.5
    ear 388.60
        blood 388.69
        cerebrospinal fluid 388.61
    excessive urine 788.42
    eye 379.93
    nasal 478.1
    nipple 611.79
    patterned motor idiopathic (see also Epilepsy) 345.5
    penile 788.7
    postnasal — see Sinusitis
    sinus, from mediastinum 510.0
    umbilicus 789.9
    urethral 788.7
        bloody 599.84
    vaginal 623.5
Discitis 722.90
    cervical, cervicothoracic 722.91
    lumbar, lumbosacral 722.93
    thoracic, thoracolumbar 722.92
Discogenic syndrome — see Displacement, intervertebral disc
Discoid
    kidney 753.3

Discoid—continued
    meniscus, congenital 717.5
    semilunar cartilage 717.5
Discoloration
    mouth 528.9
    nails 703.8
    teeth 521.7
        due to
            drugs 521.7
            metals (copper) (silver) 521.7
            pulpal bleeding 521.7
        during formation 520.8
        posteruptive 521.7
Discomfort
    chest 786.59
    visual 368.13
Discomycosis — see Actinomycosis
Discontinuity, ossicles, ossicular chain 385.23
Discrepancy, leg length (acquired) 736.81
    congenital 755.30
Discrimination
    political V62.4
    racial V62.4
    religious V62.4
    sex V62.4
Disease, diseased — see also Syndrome
    Abrami's (acquired hemolytic jaundice) 283.9
    absorbent system 459.89
    accumulation — see Thesaurismosis
    acid-peptic 536.8
    Acosta's 993.2
    Adams-Stokes (-Morgagni) (syncope with heart block) 426.9
    Addison's (bronze) (primary adrenal insufficiency) 255.4
        anemia (pernicious) 281.0
        tuberculous (see also Tuberculosis) 017.6
    Addison-Gull — see Xanthoma
    adenoids (and tonsils) (chronic) 474.9
    adrenal (gland) (capsule) (cortex) 255.9
        hyperfunction 255.3
        hypofunction 255.4
        specified type NEC 255.8
    ainhum (dactylolysis spontanea) 136.0
    akamushi (scrub typhus) 081.2
    Akureyri (epidemic neuromyasthenia) 049.8
    Albarrán's (colibacilluria) 599.0
    Albers-Schönberg's (marble bones) 756.52
    Albert's 726.71
    Albright (-Martin) (-Bantam) 275.4
    Alibert's (mycosis fungoides) (M9700/3) 202.1
    Alibert-Bazin (M9700/3) 202.1
    alimentary canal 569.9
    alligator skin (ichthyosis congenita) 757.1
        acquired 701.1
    Almeida's (Brazilian blastomycosis) 116.1
    Alpers' 330.8
    alpine 993.2
    altitude 993.2
    alveoli, teeth 525.9
    Alzheimer's — see Alzheimer's
    amyloid (any site) 277.3
    anarthritic rheumatoid 446.5
    Anders' (adiposis tuberosa simplex) 272.8
    Andersen's (glycogenosis IV) 271.0
    Anderson's (angiokeratoma corporis diffusum) 272.7
    Andes 993.2
    Andrews' (bacterid) 686.8

Disease, diseased—continued
    angiospastic, angiospasmodic 443.9
        cerebral 435.9
            with transient neurologic deficit 435.9
        vein 459.89
    anterior
        chamber 364.9
        horn cell 335.9
            specified type NEC 335.8
    antral (chronic) 473.0
        acute 461.0
    anus NEC 569.49
    aorta (nonsyphilitic) 447.9
        syphilitic NEC 093.89
    aortic (heart) (valve) (see also Endocarditis, aortic) 424.1
    apollo 077.4
    aponeurosis 726.90
    appendix 543.9
    aqueous (chamber) 364.9
    arc-welders' lung 503
    Armenian 277.3
    Arnold-Chiari (see also Spina bifida) 741.0
    arterial 447.9
        occlusive (see also Occlusion, by site) 444.22
            with embolus or thrombus — see Occlusion, by site
            due to stricture or stenosis 447.1
        specified type NEC 447.8
    arteriocardiorenal (see also Hypertension, cardiorenal) 404.90
    arteriolar (generalized) (obliterative) 447.9
        specified type NEC 447.8
    arteriorenal — see Hypertension, kidney
    arteriosclerotic — see also Arteriosclerosis
        cardiovascular 429.2
        coronary — see Arteriosclerosis, coronary ▼
        heart — see Arteriosclerosis, coronary ▲
        vascular — see Arteriosclerosis
    artery 447.9
        cerebral 437.9
        coronary — see Arteriosclerosis, coronary ♦
        specified type NEC 447.8
    arthropod-borne NEC 088.9
        specified type NEC 088.89
    Asboe-Hansen's (incontinentia pigmenti) 757.33
    atticoantral, chronic (with posterior or superior marginal perforation of ear drum) 382.2
    auditory canal, ear 380.9
    Aujeszky's 078.89
    auricle, ear NEC 380.30
    Australian X 062.4
    autoimmune NEC 279.4
        hemolytic (cold type) (warm type) 283.0
        parathyroid 252.1
        thyroid 245.2
    aviators' (see also Effect, adverse, high altitude) 993.2
    ax(e)-grinders' 502
    Ayala's 756.89
    Ayerza's (pulmonary artery sclerosis with pulmonary hypertension) 416.0
    Babington's (familial hemorrhagic telangiectasia) 448.0
    back bone NEC 733.90
    bacterial NEC 040.89
        zoonotic NEC 027.9
            specified type NEC 027.8

Disease, diseased—continued
    Baehr-Schiffrin (thrombotic thrombocytopenic purpura) 446.6
    Baelz's (cheilitis glandularis apostematosa) 528.5
    Baerensprung's (eczema marginatum) 110.3
    Balfour's (chloroma) 205.3
    balloon (see also Effect, adverse, high altitude) 993.2
    Baló's 341.1
    Bamberger (-Marie) (hypertrophic pulmonary osteoarthropathy) 731.2
    Bang's (Brucella abortus) 023.1
    Bannister's 995.1
    Banti's (with cirrhosis) (with portal hypertension) — see Cirrhosis, liver
    Barcoo (see also Ulcer, skin) 707.9
    barium lung 503
    Barlow (-Möller) (infantile scurvy) 267
    barometer makers' 985.0
    Barraquer (-Simons) (progressive lipodystrophy) 272.6
    basal ganglia 333.90
        degenerative NEC 333.0
        specified NEC 333.89
    Basedow's (exophthalmic goiter) 242.0
    basement membrane NEC 583.89
        with
            pulmonary hemorrhage (Goodpasture's syndrome) 446.21 [583.81]
    Bateman's 078.0
        purpura (senile) 287.2
    Batten's 330.1 [362.71]
    Batten-Mayou (retina) 330.1 [362.71]
    Batten-Steinert 359.2
    Battey 031.0
    Baumgarten-Cruveilhier (cirrhosis of liver) 571.5
    bauxite-workers' 503
    Bayle's (dementia paralytica) 094.1
    Bazin's (primary) (see also Tuberculosis) 017.1
    Beard's (neurasthenia) 300.5
    Beau's (see also Degeneration, myocardial) 429.1
    Bechterew's (ankylosing spondylitis) 720.0
    Becker's (idiopathic mural endomyocardial disease) 425.2
    Begbie's (exophthalmic goiter) 242.0
    Behr's 362.50
    Beigel's (white piedra) 111.2
    Bekhterev's (ankylosing spondylitis) 720.0
    Bell's (see also Psychosis, affective) 296.0
    Bennett's (leukemia) 208.9
    Benson's 379.22
    Bergeron's (hysteroepilepsy) 300.11
    Berlin's 921.3
    Bernard-Soulier (thrombopathy) 287.1
    Bernhardt (-Roth) 355.1
    beryllium 503
    Besnier-Boeck (-Schaumann) (sarcoidosis) 135
    Best's 362.76
    Beurmann's (sporotrichosis) 117.1
    Bielschowsky (-Jansky) 330.1
    Biermer's (pernicious anemia) 281.0
    Biett's (discoid lupus erythematosus) 695.4
    bile duct (see also Disease, biliary) 576.9

Disease, diseased—continued
- biliary (duct) (tract) 576.9
  - with calculus, choledocholithiasis, or stones — see Choledocholithiasis
- Billroth's (meningocele) (see also Spina bifida) 741.9
- Binswanger's 290.12
- Bird's (oxaluria) 271.8
- bird fanciers' 495.2
- black lung 500
- bladder 596.9
  - specified NEC 596.8
- bleeder's 286.0
- Bloch-Sulzberger (incontinentia pigmenti) 757.33
- Blocq's (astasia-abasia) 307.9
- blood (-forming organs) 289.9
  - specified NEC 289.8
  - vessel 459.9
- Bloodgood's 610.1
- Blount's (tibia vara) 732.4
- blue 746.9
- Bodechtel-Guttmann (subacute sclerosing panencephalitis) 046.2
- Boeck's (sarcoidosis) 135
- bone 733.90
  - fibrocystic NEC 733.29
    - jaw 526.2
  - marrow 289.9
  - Paget's (osteitis deformans) 731.0
  - specified type NEC 733.99
  - von Recklinghausen's (osteitis fibrosa cystica) 252.0
- Bonfils' — see Disease, Hodgkin's
- Borna 062.9
- Bornholm (epidemic pleurodynia) 074.1
- Bostock's (see also Fever, hay) 477.9
- Bouchard's (myopathic dilatation of the stomach) 536.1
- Bouillaud's (rheumatic heart disease) 391.9
- Bourneville (-Brissaud) (tuberous sclerosis) 759.5
- Bouveret (-Hoffmann) (paroxysmal tachycardia) 427.2
- bowel 569.9
  - functional 564.9
    - psychogenic 306.4
- Bowen's (M8081/2) — see Neoplasm, skin, in situ
- Bozzolo's (multiple myeloma) (M9732/3) 203.0
- Bradley's (epidemic vomiting) 078.82
- Brailsford's 732.3
  - radius, head 732.3
  - tarsal, scaphoid 732.5
- Brailsford-Morquio (mucopolysaccharidosis IV) 277.5
- brain 348.9
  - Alzheimer's 331.0
    - with dementia — see Alzheimer's, dementia
  - arterial, artery 437.9
  - arteriosclerotic 437.0
  - congenital 742.9
  - degenerative — see Degeneration, brain
  - inflammatory — see also Encephalitis
    - late effect — see category 326
  - organic 348.9
    - arteriosclerotic 437.0
  - parasitic NEC 123.9
  - Pick's 331.1
    - with dementia 290.10
  - senile 331.2
- brazier's 985.8

Disease, diseased—continued
- breast 611.9
  - cystic (chronic) 610.1
  - fibrocystic 610.1
  - inflammatory 611.0
  - Paget's (M8540/3) 174.0
  - puerperal, postpartum NEC 676.3
  - specified NEC 611.8
- Breda's (see also Yaws) 102.9
- Breisky's (kraurosis vulvae) 624.0
- Bretonneau's (diphtheritic malignant angina) 032.0
- Bright's (see also Nephritis) 583.9
  - arteriosclerotic (see also Hypertension, kidney) 403.90
- Brill's (recrudescent typhus) 081.1
  - flea-borne 081.0
  - louse-borne 081.1
- Brill-Symmers (follicular lymphoma) (M9690/3) 202.0
- Brill-Zinsser (recrudescent typhus) 081.1
- Brinton's (leather bottle stomach) (M8142/3) 151.9
- Brion-Kayser (see also Fever, paratyphoid) 002.9
- broad
  - beta 272.2
  - ligament, noninflammatory 620.9
  - specified NEC 620.8
- Brocq's 691.8
  - meaning
    - atopic (diffuse) neurodermatitis 691.8
    - dermatitis herpetiformis 694.0
    - lichen simplex chronicus 698.3
    - parapsoriasis 696.2
    - prurigo 698.2
- Brocq-Duhring (dermatitis herpetiformis) 694.0
- Brodie's (joint) (see also Osteomyelitis) 730.1
- bronchi 519.1
- bronchopulmonary 519.1
- bronze (Addison's) 255.4
  - tuberculous (see also Tuberculosis) 017.6
- Brown-Séquard 344.89
- Bruck's 733.99
- Bruck-de Lange (Amsterdam dwarf, mental retardation and brachycephaly) 759.89
- Bruhl's (splenic anemia with fever) 285.8
- Bruton's (X-linked agammaglobulinemia) 279.04
- buccal cavity 528.9
- Buchanan's (juvenile osteochondrosis, iliac crest) 732.1
- Buchman's (osteochondrosis juvenile) 732.1
- Budgerigar-fanciers' 495.2
- Büdinger-Ludloff-Läwen 717.89
- Buerger's (thromboangiitis obliterans) 443.1
- Bürger-Grütz (essential familial hyperlipemia) 272.3
- Burns' (lower ulna) 732.3
- bursa 727.9
- Bury's (erythema elevatum diutinum) 695.89
- Buschke's 710.1
- Busquet's (see also Osteomyelitis) 730.1
- Busse-Buschke (cryptococcosis) 117.5
- C₂ (see also Alcoholism) 303.9
- Caffey's (infantile cortical hyperostosis) 756.59
- caisson 993.3

Disease, diseased—continued
- calculous 592.9
- California 114.0
- Calvé (-Perthes) (osteochondrosis, femoral capital) 732.1
- Camurati-Engelmann (diaphyseal sclerosis) 756.59
- Canavan's 330.0
- capillaries 448.9
- Carapata 087.1
- cardiac — see Disease, heart
- cardiopulmonary, chronic 416.9
- cardiorenal (arteriosclerotic) (hepatic) (hypertensive) (vascular) (see also Hypertension, cardiorenal) 404.90
- cardiovascular (arteriosclerotic) 429.2
  - congenital 746.9
  - hypertensive (see also Hypertension, heart) 402.90
    - benign 402.10
    - malignant 402.00
  - renal (see also Hypertension, cardiorenal) 404.90
  - syphilitic (asymptomatic) 093.9
- carotid gland 259.8
- Carrión's (Bartonellosis) 088.0
- cartilage NEC 733.90
  - specified NEC 733.99
- Castellani's 104.8
- cat-scratch 078.3
- Cavare's (familial periodic paralysis) 359.3
- Cazenave's (pemphigus) 694.4
- cecum 569.9
- celiac (adult) 579.0
  - infantile 579.0
- cellular tissue NEC 709.9
- central core 359.0
- cerebellar, cerebellum — see Disease, brain
- cerebral (see also Disease, brain) 348.9
  - arterial, artery 437.9
  - degenerative — see Degeneration, brain
- cerebrospinal 349.9
- cerebrovascular NEC 437.9
  - acute 436
    - embolic — see Embolism, brain
    - late effect — see category 438
    - puerperal, postpartum, childbirth 674.0
    - thrombotic — see Thrombosis, brain
  - arteriosclerotic 437.0
  - embolic — see Embolism, brain
  - ischemic, generalized NEC 437.1
  - late effect or sequela — see category 438
  - occlusive 437.1
  - puerperal, postpartum, childbirth 674.0
  - specified type NEC 437.8
  - thrombotic — see Thrombosis, brain
- ceroid storage 272.7
- cervix (uteri)
  - inflammatory 616.9
    - specified NEC 616.8
  - noninflammatory 622.9
    - specified NEC 622.8
- Chabert's 022.9
- Chagas' (see also Trypanosomiasis, American) 086.2
- Chandler's (osteochondritis dissecans, hip) 732.7
- Charcot's (joint) 094.0 [713.5]
  - spinal cord 094.0
- Charcot-Marie-Tooth 356.1
- Charlouis' (see also Yaws) 102.9

Disease, diseased—continued
- Cheadle (-Möller) (-Barlow) (infantile scurvy) 267
- Chédiak-Steinbrinck (-Higashi) (congenital gigantism of peroxidase granules) 288.2
- cheek, inner 528.9
- chest 519.9
- Chiari's (hepatic vein thrombosis) 453.0
- Chicago (North American blastomycosis) 116.0
- chignon (white piedra) 111.2
- chigoe, chigo (jigger) 134.1
- childhood granulomatous 288.1
- Chinese liver fluke 121.1
- chlamydial NEC 078.88
- cholecystic (see also Disease, gallbladder) 575.9
- choroid 363.9
  - degenerative (see also Degeneration, choroid) 363.40
  - hereditary (see also Dystrophy, choroid) 363.50
  - specified type NEC 363.8
- Christian's (chronic histiocytosis X) 277.8
- Christian-Weber (nodular nonsuppurative panniculitis) 729.30
- Christmas 286.1
- ciliary body 364.9
- circulatory (system) NEC 459.9
  - chronic, maternal, affecting fetus or newborn 760.3
  - specified NEC 459.89
  - syphilitic 093.9
    - congenital 090.5
- Civatte's (poikiloderma) 709.09 ◆
- climacteric 627.2
  - male 608.89
- coagulation factor deficiency (congenital) (see also Defect, coagulation) 286.9
- Coats' 362.12
- coccidioidal pulmonary 114.5
  - acute 114.0
  - chronic 114.4
  - primary 114.0
  - residual 114.4
- Cockayne's (microcephaly and dwarfism) 759.89
- Cogan's 370.52
- cold
  - agglutinin 283.0
    - or hemoglobinuria 283.0
    - paroxysmal (cold) (nocturnal) 283.2
  - hemagglutinin (chronic) 283.0
- collagen NEC 710.9
  - nonvascular 710.9
  - specified NEC 710.8
  - vascular (allergic) (see also Angiitis, hypersensitivity) 446.20
- colon 569.9
  - functional 564.9
    - congenital 751.3
  - ischemic 557.0
- combined system (of spinal cord) 266.2 [336.2]
  - with anemia (pernicious) 281.0 [336.2]
- compressed air 993.3
- Concato's (pericardial polyserositis) 423.2
  - peritoneal 568.82
  - pleural — see Pleurisy
- congenital NEC 799.8
- conjunctiva 372.9
  - chlamydial 077.98
  - specified NEC 077.8
  - specified type NEC 372.8
  - viral 077.99
    - specified NEC 077.8

Disease, diseased—continued
   connective tissue, diffuse (see also Disease, collagen) 710.9
   Conor and Bruch's (boutonneuse fever) 082.1
   Conradi (-Hünermann) 756.59
   Cooley's (erythroblastic anemia) 282.4
   Cooper's 610.1
   Corbus' 607.1
   cork-handlers' 495.3
   cornea (see also Keratopathy) 371.9
   coronary (see also Ischemia, heart) 414.9
      congenital 746.85
      ostial, syphilitic 093.20
         aortic 093.22
         mitral 093.21
         pulmonary 093.24
         tricuspid 093.23
   Corrigan's — see Insufficiency, aortic
   Cotugno's 724.3
   Coxsackie (virus) NEC 074.8
   cranial nerve NEC 352.9
   Creutzfeldt-Jakob 046.1
      with dementia 290.10
   Crigler-Najjar (congenital hyperbilirubinemia) 277.4
   Crocq's (acrocyanosis) 443.89
   Crohn's (intestine) (see also Enteritis, regional) 555.9
   Crouzon's (craniofacial dysostosis) 756.0
   Cruchet's (encephalitis lethargica) 049.8
   Cruveilhier's 335.21
   Cruz-Chagas (see also Trypanosomiasis, American) 086.2
   crystal deposition (see also Arthritis, due to, crystals) 712.9
   Csillag's (lichen sclerosus et atrophicus) 701.0
   Curschmann's 359.2
   Cushing's (pituitary basophilism) 255.0
   cystic
      breast (chronic) 610.1
      kidney, congenital (see also Cystic, disease, kidney) 753.10
      liver, congenital 751.62
      lung 518.89
         congenital 748.4
      pancreas 577.2
         congenital 751.7
      renal, congenital (see also Cystic, disease, kidney) 753.10
      semilunar cartilage 717.5
   cysticercus 123.1
   cystine storage (with renal sclerosis) 270.0
   cytomegalic inclusion (generalized) 078.5
      with
         pneumonia 078.5 [484.1]
      congenital 771.1
   Czerny's (periodic hydrarthrosis of the knee) 719.06
   Daae (-Finsen) (epidemic pleurodynia) 074.1
   dancing 297.8
   Danielssen's (anesthetic leprosy) 030.1
   Darier's (congenital) (keratosis follicularis) 757.39
      erythema annulare centrifugum 695.0
      vitamin A deficiency 264.8
   Darling's (histoplasmosis) (see also Histoplasmosis, American) 115.00
   Davies' 425.0
   de Beurmann-Gougerot (sporotrichosis) 117.1

Disease, diseased—continued
   Débove's (splenomegaly) 789.2
   deer fly (see also Tularemia) 021.9
   deficiency 269.9
   degenerative — see also Degeneration
      disc — see Degeneration, intervertebral disc
   Degos' 447.8
   Déjérine (-Sottas) 356.0
   Deleage's 359.8
   demyelinating, demyelinizating (brain stem) (central nervous system) 341.9
      multiple sclerosis 340
      specified NEC 341.8
   de Quervain's (tendon sheath) 727.04
      thyroid (subacute granulomatous thyroiditis) 245.1
   Dercum's (adiposis dolorosa) 272.8
   Deutschländer's — see Fracture, foot
   Devergie's (pityriasis rubra pilaris) 696.4
   Devic's 341.0
   diaphorase deficiency 289.7
   diaphragm 519.4
   diarrheal, infectious 009.2
   diatomaceous earth 502
   Diaz's (osteochondrosis astragalus) 732.5
   digestive system 569.9
   Di Guglielmo's (erythemic myelosis) (M9841/3) 207.0
   Dimitri-Sturge-Weber (encephalocutaneous angiomatosis) 759.6
   disc, degenerative — see Degeneration, intervertebral disc
   discogenic (see also Disease, intervertebral disc) 722.90
   diverticular — see Diverticula
   Down's (mongolism) 758.0
   Dubini's (electric chorea) 049.8
   Dubois' (thymus gland) 090.5
   Duchenne's 094.0
      locomotor ataxia 094.0
      muscular dystrophy 359.1
      paralysis 335.22
      pseudohypertrophy, muscles 359.1
   Duchenne-Griesinger 359.1
   ductless glands 259.9
   Duhring's (dermatitis herpetiformis) 694.0
   Dukes (-Filatov) 057.8
   duodenum NEC 537.9
      specified NEC 537.89
   Duplay's 726.2
   Dupré's (meningism) 781.6
   Dupuytren's (muscle contracture) 728.6
   Durand-Nicolas-Favre (climatic bubo) 099.1
   Duroziez's (congenital mitral stenosis) 746.5
   Dutton's (trypanosomiasis) 086.9
   Eales' 362.18
   ear (chronic) (inner) NEC 388.9
      middle 385.9
         adhesive (see also Adhesions, middle ear) 385.10
         specified NEC 385.89
   Eberth's (typhoid fever) 002.0
   Ebstein's
      heart 746.2
      meaning diabetes 250.4 [581.81]
   Echinococcus (see also Echinococcus) 122.9
   ECHO virus NEC 078.89
   Economo's (encephalitis lethargica) 049.8

Disease, diseased—continued
   Eddowes' (brittle bones and blue sclera) 756.51
   Edsall's 992.2
   Eichstedt's (pityriasis versicolor) 111.0
   Ellis-van Creveld (chondroectodermal dysplasia) 756.55
   endocardium — see Endocarditis
   endocrine glands or system NEC 259.9
      specified NEC 259.8
   endomyocardial, idiopathic mural 425.2
   Engel-von Recklinghausen (osteitis fibrosa cystica) 252.0
   Engelmann's (diaphyseal sclerosis) 756.59
   English (rickets) 268.0
   Engman's (infectious eczematoid dermatitis) 690
   enteroviral, enterovirus NEC 078.89
      central nervous system NEC 048
   epidemic NEC 136.9
   epididymis 608.9
   epigastric, functional 536.9
      psychogenic 306.4
   Erb (-Landouzy) 359.1
   Erb-Goldflam 358.0
   Erichsen's (railway spine) 300.16
   esophagus 530.9
      functional 530.5
      psychogenic 306.4
   Eulenburg's (congenital paramyotonia) 359.2
   Eustachian tube 381.9
   Evans' (thrombocytopenic purpura) 287.3
   external auditory canal 380.9
   extrapyramidal NEC 333.90
   eye 379.90
      anterior chamber 364.9
      inflammatory NEC 364.3
      muscle 378.9
   eyeball 360.9
   eyelid 374.9
   eyeworm of Africa 125.2
   Fabry's (angiokeratoma corporis diffusum) 272.7
   facial nerve (seventh) 351.9
      newborn 767.5
   Fahr-Volhard (malignant nephrosclerosis) 403.00
   fallopian tube, noninflammatory 620.9
      specified NEC 620.8
   familial periodic 277.3
      paralysis 359.3
   Fanconi's (congenital pancytopenia) 284.0
   Farber's (disseminated lipogranulomatosis) 272.8
   fascia 728.9
      inflammatory 728.9
   Fauchard's (periodontitis) 523.4
   Favre-Durand-Nicolas (climatic bubo) 099.1
   Favre-Racouchot (elastoidosis cutanea nodularis) 701.8
   Fede's 529.0
   Feer's 985.0
   Felix's (juvenile osteochondrosis, hip) 732.1
   Fenwick's (gastric atrophy) 537.89
   Fernels' (aortic aneurysm) 441.9
   fibrocaseous, of lung (see also Tuberculosis, pulmonary) 011.9
   fibrocystic — see also Fibrocystic, disease newborn 277.01
   Fiedler's (leptospiral jaundice) 100.00
   fifth 057.8
   Filatoff's (infectious mononucleosis) 075

Disease, diseased—continued
   Filatov's (infectious mononucleosis) 075
   file-cutters' 984.9
      specified type of lead — see Table of drugs and chemicals
   filterable virus NEC 078.89
   fish skin 757.1
      acquired 701.1
   Flajani (-Basedow) (exophthalmic goiter) 242.0
   Flatau-Schilder 341.1
   flax-dressers' 504
   Fleischner's 732.3
   flint 502
   fluke — see Infestation, fluke
   Følling's (phenylketonuria) 270.1
   foot and mouth 078.4
   foot process 581.3
   Forbes' (glycogenosis III) 271.0
   Fordyce's (ectopic sebaceous glands) (mouth) 750.26
   Fordyce-Fox (apocrine miliaria) 705.82
   Fothergill's
      meaning scarlatina anginosa 034.1
      neuralgia (see also Neuralgia, trigeminal) 350.1
   Fournier's 608.83
   fourth 057.8
   Fox (-Fordyce) (apocrine miliaria) 705.82
   Francis' (see also Tularemia) 021.9
   Franklin's (heavy chain) 273.2
   Frei's (climatic bubo) 099.1
   Freiberg's (flattening metatarsal) 732.5
   Friedländer's (endarteritis obliterans) — see Arteriosclerosis
   Friedreich's
      combined systemic or ataxia 334.0
      facial hemihypertrophy 756.0
      myoclonia 333.2
   Fröhlich's (adiposogenital dystrophy) 253.8
   Frommel's 676.6
   frontal sinus (chronic) 473.1
      acute 461.1
   Fuller's earth 502
   fungus, fungous NEC 117.9
   Gaisböck's (polycythemia hypertonica) 289.0
   gallbladder 575.9
      congenital 751.60
   Gamna's (siderotic splenomegaly) 289.51
   Gamstorp's (adynamia episodica hereditaria) 359.3
   Gandy-Nanta (siderotic splenomegaly) 289.51
   gannister (occupational) 502
   Garré's (see also Osteomyelitis) 730.1
   gastric (see also Disease, stomach) 537.9
   gastrointestinal (tract) 569.9
      amyloid 277.3
      functional 536.9
         psychogenic 306.4
   Gaucher's (adult) (cerebroside lipidosis) (infantile) 272.7
   Gayet's (superior hemorrhagic polioencephalitis) 265.1
   Gee (-Herter) (-Heubner) (-Thaysen) (nontropical sprue) 579.0
   generalized neoplastic (M8000/6) 199.0
   genital organs NEC
      female 629.9
         specified NEC 629.8
      male 608.9
   Gerhardt's (erythromelalgia) 443.89
   Gerlier's (epidemic vertigo) 078.81

Disease, diseased—continued
  Gibert's (pityriasis rosea) 696.3
  Gibney's (perispondylitis) 720.9
  Gierke's (glycogenosis I) 271.0
  Gilbert's (familial nonhemolytic jaundice) 277.4
  Gilchrist's (North American blastomycosis) 116.0
  Gilford (-Hutchinson) (progeria) 259.8
  Gilles de la Tourette's (motor-verbal tic) 307.23
  Giovannini's 117.9
  gland (lymph) 289.9
  Glanzmann's (hereditary hemorrhagic thrombasthenia) 287.1
  glassblowers' 527.1
  Glénard's (enteroptosis) 569.89
  Glisson's (see also Rickets) 268.0
  glomerular
    membranous, idiopathic 581.1
    minimal change 581.3
  glycogen storage (Andersen's) (Cori types 1-7) (Forbes') (McArdle-Schmid-Pearson) (Pompe's) (types I-VII) 271.0
    cardiac 271.0 [425.7]
    generalized 271.0
    glucose-6-phosphatase deficiency 271.0
    heart 271.0 [425.7]
    hepatorenal 271.0
    liver and kidneys 271.0
    myocardium 271.0 [425.7]
    von Gierke's (glycogenosis I) 271.0
  Goldflam-Erb 358.0
  Goldscheider's (epidermolysis bullosa) 757.39
  Goldstein's (familial hemorrhagic telangiectasia) 448.0
  gonococcal NEC 098.0
  Goodall's (epidemic vomiting) 078.82
  Gordon's (exudative enteropathy) 579.8
  Gougerot's (trisymptomatic) 709.1
  Gougerot-Carteaud (confluent reticulate papillomatosis) 701.8
  Gougerot-Hailey-Hailey (benign familial chronic pemphigus) 757.39
  graft-versus-host (bone marrow) 996.85
    due to organ transplant NEC — see Complications, transplant, organ
  grain-handlers' 495.8
  Grancher's (splenopneumonia) — see Pneumonia
  granulomatous (childhood) (chronic) 288.1
  graphite lung 503
  Graves' (exophthalmic goiter) 242.0
  Greenfield's 330.0
  green monkey 078.89
  Griesinger's (see also Ancylostomiasis) 126.9
  grinders' 502
  Grisel's 723.5
  Gruby's (tinea tonsurans) 110.0
  Guertin's (electric chorea) 049.8
  Guillain-Barré 357.0
  Guinon's (motor-verbal tic) 307.23
  Gull's (thyroid atrophy with myxedema) 244.8
  Gull and Sutton's — see Hypertension, kidney
  gum NEC 523.9
  Günther's (congenital erythropoietic porphyria) 277.1
  gynecological 629.9
    specified NEC 629.8
  H 270.0
  Haas' 732.3
  Habermann's (acute parapsoriasis varioliformis) 696.2
  Haff 985.1
  Hageman (congenital factor XII deficiency) (see also Defect, congenital) 286.3
  Haglund's (osteochondrosis os tibiale externum) 732.5
  Hagner's (hypertrophic pulmonary osteoarthropathy) 731.2
  Hailey-Hailey (benign familial chronic pemphigus) 757.39
  hair (follicles) NEC 704.9
    specified type NEC 704.8
  Hallervorden-Spatz 333.0
  Hallopeau's (lichen sclerosus et atrophicus) 701.0
  Hamman's (spontaneous mediastinal emphysema) 518.1
  hand, foot, and mouth 074.3
  Hand-Schüller-Christian (chronic histiocytosis X) 277.8
  Hanot's — see Cirrhosis, biliary
  Hansen's (leprosy) 030.9
    benign form 030.1
    malignant form 030.0
  Harada's 363.22
  Harley's (intermittent hemoglobinuria) 283.2
  Hart's (pellagra-cerebellar ataxia renal aminoaciduria) 270.0
  Hartnup (pellagra-cerebellar ataxia renal aminoaciduria) 270.00
  Hashimoto's (struma lymphomatosa) 245.2
  Hb — see Disease, hemoglobin
  heart (organic) 429.9
    with
      acute pulmonary edema (see also Failure, ventricular, left) 428.1
        hypertensive 402.91
          with renal failure 404.91
          benign 402.11
            with renal failure 404.11
          malignant 402.01
            with renal failure 404.01
      kidney disease — see Hypertension, cardiorenal
      rheumatic fever (conditions classifiable to 390)
        active 391.9
          with chorea 392.0
        inactive or quiescent (with chorea) 398.90
    amyloid 277.3 [425.7]
    aortic (valve) (see also Endocarditis, aortic) 424.1
    arteriosclerotic or sclerotic (minimal) (senile) — see Arteriosclerosis, coronary ▼
    artery — see Arteriosclerosis, coronary
    atherosclerotic — see Arteriosclerosis, coronary ▲
    beer drinkers' 425.5
    beriberi 265.0 [425.7]
    black 416.0
    congenital NEC 746.9
      cyanotic 746.9
      maternal, affecting fetus or newborn 760.3
      specified type NEC 746.89
    congestive (see also Failure, heart, congestive) 428.0
    coronary 414.9
    cryptogenic 429.9

Disease, diseased—continued
  heart—continued
    due to
      amyloidosis 277.3 [425.7]
      beriberi 265.0 [425.7]
      cardiac glycogenosis 271.0 [425.7]
      Friedreich's ataxia 334.0 [425.8]
      gout 274.82
      mucopolysaccharidosis 277.5 [425.7]
      myotonia atrophica 359.2 [425.8]
      progressive muscular dystrophy 359.1 [425.8]
      sarcoidosis 135 [425.8]
    fetal 746.9
      inflammatory 746.89
    fibroid (see also Myocarditis) 429.0
    functional 427.9
      postoperative 997.1
      psychogenic 306.2
    glycogen storage 271.0 [425.7]
    gonococcal NEC 098.85
    gouty 274.82
    hypertensive (see also Hypertension, heart) 402.90
      benign 402.10
      malignant 402.00
    hyperthyroid (see also Hyperthyroidism) 242.9 [425.7]
    incompletely diagnosed — see Disease, heart
    ischemic (chronic) (see also Ischemia, heart) 414.9
      acute (see also Infarct, myocardium)
        without myocardial infarction 411.89
          with coronary (artery) occlusion 411.81
      asymptomatic 412
      diagnosed on ECG or other special investigation but currently presenting no symptoms 412
    kyphoscoliotic 416.1
    mitral (see also Endocarditis, mitral) 394.9
    muscular (see also Degeneration, myocardial) 429.1
    postpartum 674.8
    psychogenic (functional) 306.2
    pulmonary (chronic) 416.9
      acute 415.0
      specified NEC 416.8
    rheumatic (chronic) (inactive) (old) (quiescent) (with chorea) 398.90
      active or acute 391.9
        with chorea (active) (rheumatic) (Sydenham's) 392.0
      specified type NEC 391.8
    maternal, affecting fetus or newborn 760.3
    rheumatoid — see Arthritis, rheumatoid
    sclerotic — see Arteriosclersis, coronary ◆
    senile (see also Myocarditis) 429.0
    specified type NEC 429.89
    syphilitic 093.89
      aortic 093.1
        aneurysm 093.0
      asymptomatic 093.89
      congenital 090.5
    thyroid (gland) (see also Hyperthyroidism) 242.9 [425.7]

Disease, diseased—continued
  heart—continued
    thyrotoxic (see also Thyrotoxicosis) 242.9 [425.7]
    tuberculous (see also Tuberculosis) 017.9 [425.8]
    valve, valvular (obstructive) (regurgitant) — see also Endocarditis
      congenital NEC (see also Anomaly, heart, valve) 746.9
        pulmonary 746.00
        specified type NEC 746.89
    vascular — see Disease, cardiovascular
  heavy-chain (gamma G) 273.2
  Heberden's 715.04
  Hebra's
    dermatitis exfoliativa 695.89
    erythema multiforme exudativum 695.1
    pityriasis
      maculata et circinata 696.3
      rubra 695.89
        pilaris 696.4
    prurigo 698.2
  Heerfordt's (uveoparotitis) 135
  Heidenhain's 290.10
    with dementia 290.10
  Heilmeyer-Schöner (M9842/3) 207.1
  Heine-Medin (see also Poliomyelitis) 045.9
  Heller's (see also Psychosis, childhood) 299.1
  Heller-Döhle (syphilitic aortitis) 093.1
  hematopoietic organs 289.9
  hemoglobin (Hb) 282.7
    with thalassemia 282.4
    abnormal (mixed) NEC 282.7
      with thalassemia 282.4
    AS genotype 282.5
    Bart's 282.7
    C (Hb-C) 282.7
      with other abnormal hemoglobin NEC 282.7
      elliptocytosis 282.7
      Hb-S 282.63
      sickle-cell 282.63
      thalassemia 282.4
    constant spring 282.7
    D (Hb-D) 282.7
      with other abnormal hemoglobin NEC 282.7
      Hb-S 282.69
      sickle-cell 282.69
      thalassemia 282.4
    E (Hb-E) 282.7
      with other abnormal hemoglobin NEC 282.7
      Hb-S 282.69
      sickle-cell 282.69
      thalassemia 282.4
    elliptocytosis 282.7
    F (Hb-F) 282.7
    G (Hb-G) 282.7
    H (Hb-H) 282.4
    hereditary persistence, fetal (HPFH) ("Swiss variety") 282.7
    high fetal gene 282.7
    I thalassemia 282.4
    M 289.7
    S — see Disease, sickle-cell, Hb-S
    spherocytosis 282.7
    unstable, hemolytic 282.7
    Zurich (Hb-Zurich) 282.7

Disease, diseased—continued
   hemolytic (fetus) (newborn) 773.2
      autoimmune (cold type) (warm type) 283.0
      due to or with incompatibility
         ABO (blood group) 773.1
         blood (group) (Duffy) (Kell) (Kidd) (Lewis) (M) (S) NEC 773.2
         Rh (blood group) (factor) 773.0
      Rh negative mother 773.0
      unstable hemoglobin 282.7
   hemorrhagic 287.9
      newborn 776.0
   Henoch (-Schönlein) (purpura nervosa) 287.0
   hepatic — see Disease, liver
   hepatolenticular 275.1
   heredodegenerative NEC
      brain 331.89
      spinal cord 336.8
   Hers' (glycogenosis VI) 271.0
   Herter (-Gee) (-Heubner) (nontropical sprue) 579.0
   Herxheimer's (diffuse idiopathic cutaneous atrophy) 701.8
   Heubner's 094.89
   Heubner-Herter (nontropical sprue) 579.0
   high fetal gene or hemoglobin thalassemia 282.4
   Hildenbrand's (typhus) 081.9
   hip (joint) NEC 719.95
      congenital 755.63
      suppurative 711.05
      tuberculous (see also Tuberculosis) 015.1 [730.85]
   Hippel's (retinocerebral angiomatosis) 759.6
   Hirschfeld's (acute diabetes mellitus) (see also Diabetes) 250.0
   Hirschsprung's (congenital megacolon) 751.3
   His (-Werner) (trench fever) 083.1
   HIV 042 ◆
   Hodgkin's (M9650/3) 201.9

Note — Use the following fifth-digit subclassification with category 201:

   0 unspecifed site
   1 lymph nodes of head, face, and neck
   2 intrathoracic lymp nodes
   3 intra-abdominal lymph nodes
   4 lymph nodes of axilla and upper limb
   5 lymph nodes of inguinal region and lower limb
   6 intrapelvic lymph nodes
   7 spleen
   8 lymph nodes of multiple sites

      lymphocytic
         depletion (M9653/3) 201.7
            diffuse fibrosis (M9654/3) 201.7
            reticular type (M9655/3) 201.7
         predominance (M9651/3) 201.4
      lymphocytic-histiocytic predominance (M9651/3) 201.4
      mixed cellularity (M9652/3) 201.6

Disease, diseased—continued
   Hodgkin's—continued
      nodular sclerosis (M9656/3) 201.5
         cellular phase (M9657/3) 201.5
   Hodgson's 441.9
      ruptured 441.5
   Hoffa (-Kastert) (liposynovitis prepatellaris) 272.8
   Holla (see also Spherocytosis) 282.0
   homozygous-Hb-S 282.61
   hoof and mouth 078.4
   hookworm (see also Ancylostomiasis) 126.9
   Horton's (temporal arteritis) 446.5
   host-versus-graft (immune or nonimmune cause) 996.80
      bone marrow 996.85
      heart 996.83
      intestines 996.89
      kidney 996.81
      liver 996.82
      lung 996.84
      pancreas 996.86
      specified NEC 996.89
   HPFH (hereditary persistence of fetal hemoglobin) ("Swiss variety") 282.7
   Huchard's (continued arterial hypertension) 401.9
   Huguier's (uterine fibroma) 218.9
   human immunodeficiency (virus) 042 ◆
   hunger 251.1
   Hunt's
      dyssynergia cerebellaris myoclonica 334.2
      herpetic geniculate ganglionitis 053.11
   Huntington's 333.4
   Huppert's (multiple myeloma) (M9730/3) 203.0
   Hurler's (mucopolysaccharidosis I) 277.5
   Hutchinson's, meaning
      angioma serpiginosum 709.1
      cheiropompholyx 705.81
      prurigo estivalis 692.72
   Hutchinson-Boeck (sarcoidosis) 135
   Hutchinson-Gilford (progeria) 259.8
   hyaline (diffuse) (generalized) 728.9
      membrane (lung) (newborn) 769
   hydatid (see also Echinococcus) 122.9
   Hyde's (prurigo nodularis) 698.3
   hyperkinetic (see also Hyperkinesia) 314.9
      heart 429.82
   hypertensive (see also Hypertension) 401.9
   hypophysis 253.9
      hyperfunction 253.1
      hypofunction 253.2
   Iceland (epidemic neuromyasthenia) 049.8
   I cell 272.7
   ill-defined 799.8
   immunologic NEC 279.9
   immunoproliferative 203.8
   inclusion 078.5
      salivary gland 078.5
   infancy, early NEC 779.9
   infective NEC 136.9
   inguinal gland 289.9
   internal semilunar cartilage, cystic 717.5
   intervertebral disc 722.90
      with myelopathy 722.70
      cervical, cervicothoracic 722.91
         with myelopathy 722.71
      lumbar, lumbosacral 722.93
         with myelopathy 722.73
      thoracic, thoracolumbar 722.92
         with myelopathy 722.72

Disease, diseased—continued
   intestine 569.9
      functional 564.9
         congenital 751.3
         psychogenic 306.4
      lardaceous 277.3
      organic 569.9
      protozoal NEC 007.9
   iris 364.9
   iron
      metabolism 275.0
      storage 275.0
   Isambert's (see also Tuberculosis, larynx) 012.3
   Iselin's (osteochondrosis, fifth metatarsal) 732.5
   Island (scrub typhus) 081.2
   itai-itai 985.5
   Jadassohn's (maculopapular erythroderma) 696.2
   Jadassohn-Pellizari's (anetoderma) 701.3
   Jakob-Creutzfeldt 046.1
      with dementia 290.10
   Jaksch (-Luzet) (pseudoleukemia infantum) 285.8
   Janet's 300.89
   Jansky-Bielschowsky 330.1
   jaw NEC 526.9
      fibrocystic 526.2
   Jensen's 363.05
   Jeune's (asphyxiating thoracic dystrophy) 756.4
   jigger 134.1
   Johnson-Stevens (erythema multiforme exudativum) 695.1
   joint NEC 719.9
      ankle 719.97
      Charcot 094.0 [713.5]
      degenerative (see also Osteoarthrosis) 715.9
         multiple 715.09
         spine (see also Spondylosis) 721.90
      elbow 719.92
      foot 719.97
      hand 719.94
      hip 719.95
      hypertrophic (chronic) (degenerative) (see also Osteoarthrosis) 715.9
         spine (see also Spondylosis) 721.90
      knee 719.96
      Luschka 721.90
      multiple sites 719.99
      pelvic region 719.95
      sacroiliac 724.6
      shoulder (region) 719.91
      specified site NEC 719.98
      spine NEC 724.9
         pseudarthrosis following fusion 733.82
         sacroiliac 724.6
      wrist 719.93
   Jourdain's (acute gingivitis) 523.0
   Jüngling's (sarcoidosis) 135
   Kahler (-Bozzolo) (multiple myeloma) (M9730/3) 203.0
   Kalischer's 759.6
   Kaposi's 757.33
      lichen ruber 697.8
         acuminatus 696.4
         moniliformis 697.8
      xeroderma pigmentosum 757.33
   Kaschin-Beck (endemic polyarthritis) 716.00
      ankle 716.07
      arm 716.02
         lower (and wrist) 716.03
         upper (and elbow) 716.02
      foot (and ankle) 716.07
      forearm (and wrist) 716.03
      hand 716.04

Disease, diseased—continued
   Kaschin-Beck—continued
      leg 716.06
         lower 716.06
         upper 716.05
      multiple sites 716.09
      pelvic region (hip) (thigh) 716.05
      shoulder region 716.01
      specified site NEC 716.08
   Katayama 120.2
   Kawasaki 446.1
   Kedani (scrub typhus) 081.2
   kidney (functional) (pelvis) (see also Disease, renal) 593.9
      cystic (congenital) 753.10
         multiple 753.19
         single 753.11
         specified NEC 753.19
      fibrocystic (congenital) 753.19
      in gout 274.10
      polycystic (congenital) 753.12
         adult type (APKD) 753.13
         autosomal dominant 753.13
         autosomal recessive 753.14
         childhood type (CPKD) 753.14
         infantile type 753.14
   Kienböck's (carpal lunate) (wrist) 732.3
   Kimmelstiel (-Wilson) (intercapillary glomerulosclerosis) 250.4 [581.81]
   Kinnier Wilson's (hepatolenticular degeneration) 275.1
   kissing 075
   Kleb's (see also Nephritis) 583.9
   Klinger's 446.4
   Klippel's 723.8
   Klippel-Feil (brevicollis) 756.16
   knight's 911.1
   Köbner's (epidermolysis bullosa) 757.39
   Koenig-Wichmann (pemphigus) 694.4
   Köhler's
      first (osteoarthrosis juvenilis) 732.5
      second (Freiberg's infraction, metatarsal head) 732.5
      patellar 732.4
      tarsal navicular (bone) (osteoarthrosis juvenilis) 732.5
   Köhler-Freiberg (infraction, metatarsal head) 732.5
   Köhler-Mouchet (osteoarthrosis juvenilis) 732.5
   Köhler-Pellegrini-Stieda (calcification, knee joint) 726.62
   König's (osteochondritis dissecans) 732.7
   Korsakoff's (nonalcoholic) 294.0
      alcoholic 291.1
   Kostmann's (infantile genetic agranulocytosis) 288.0
   Krabbe's 330.0
   Kraepelin-Morel (see also Schizophrenia) 295.9
   Kraft-Weber-Dimitri 759.6
   Kufs' 330.1
   Kugelberg-Welander 335.11
   Kuhnt-Junius 362.52
   Kümmell's (-Verneuil) (spondylitis) 721.7
   Kundrat's (lymphosarcoma) 200.1
   kuru 046.0
   Kussmaul (-Meier) (polyarteritis nodosa) 446.0
   Kyasanur Forest 065.2
   Kyrle's (hyperkeratosis follicularis in cutem penetrans) 701.1
   labia
      inflammatory 616.9
         specified NEC 616.8

Disease, diseased—*continued*
　labia—*continued*
　　noninflammatory 624.9
　　　specified NEC 624.8
　labyrinth, ear 386.8
　lacrimal system (apparatus) (passages) 375.9
　　gland 375.00
　　　specified NEC 375.89
　Lafora's 333.2
　Lagleyze-von Hippel (retinocerebral angiomatosis) 759.6
　Lancereaux-Mathieu (leptospiral jaundice) 100.0
　Landry's 357.0
　Lane's 569.89
　lardaceous (any site) 277.3
　Larrey-Weil (leptospiral jaundice) 100.00
　Larsen (-Johansson) (juvenile osteopathia patellae) 732.4
　larynx 478.70
　Lasègue's (persecution mania) 297.9
　Leber's 377.16
　Lederer's (acquired infectious hemolytic anemia) 283.19
　Legg's (capital femoral osteochondrosis) 732.1
　Legg-Calvé-Perthes (capital femoral osteochondrosis) 732.1
　Legg-Calvé-Waldenström (femoral capital osteochondrosis) 732.1
　Legg-Perthes (femoral capital osteochrondosis) 732.1
　Legionnaires' 482.83
　Leigh's 330.8
　Leiner's (exfoliative dermatitis) 695.89
　Leloir's (lupus erythematosus) 695.4
　Lenegre's 426.0
　lens (eye) 379.39
　Leriche's (osteoporosis, post-traumatic) 733.7
　Letterer-Siwe (acute histiocytosis X) (M9722/3) 202.5
　Lev's (acquired complete heart block) 426.0
　Lewandowski's (*see also* Tuberculosis) 017.0
　Lewandowski-Lutz (epidermodysplasia verruciformis) 078.19
　Leyden's (periodic vomiting) 536.2
　Libman-Sacks (verrucous endocarditis) 710.0 *[424.91]*
　Lichtheim's (subacute combined sclerosis with pernicious anemia) 281.0 *[336.2]*
　ligament 728.9
　light chain 203.0
　Lightwood's (renal tubular acidosis) 588.8
　Lignac's (cystinosis) 270.0
　Lindau's (retinocerebral angiomatosis) 759.6
　Lindau-von Hippel (angiomatosis retinocerebellosa) 759.6
　lip NEC 528.5
　lipidosis 272.7
　lipoid storage NEC 272.7
　Lipschütz's 616.50
　Little's — *see* Palsy, cerebral
　liver 573.9
　　alcoholic 571.3
　　　acute 571.1
　　　chronic 571.3
　　chronic 571.9
　　　alcoholic 571.3
　　cystic, congenital 751.62
　　drug-induced 573.3
　　due to
　　　chemicals 573.3
　　　fluorinated agents 573.3
　　　hypersensitivity drugs 573.3
　　　isoniazids 573.3

Disease, diseased—*continued*
　liver—*continued*
　　fibrocystic (congenital) 751.62
　　glycogen storage 271.0
　　organic 573.9
　　polycystic (congenital) 751.62
　Lobo's (keloid blastomycosis) 116.2
　Lobstein's (brittle bones and blue sclera) 756.51
　locomotor system 334.9
　Lorain's (pituitary dwarfism) 253.3
　Lucas-Championnière (fibrinous bronchitis) 466.0
　Ludwig's (submaxillary cellulitis) 528.3
　luetic — *see* Syphilis
　lumbosacral region 724.6
　lung NEC 518.89
　　black 500
　　congenital 748.60
　　cystic 518.89
　　　congenital 748.4
　　fibroid (chronic) (*see also* Fibrosis, lung) 515
　　fluke 121.2
　　　Oriental 121.2
　　in
　　　amyloidosis 277.3 *[517.8]*
　　　polymyositis 710.4 *[517.8]*
　　　sarcoidosis 135 *[517.8]*
　　　Sjögren's syndrome 710.2 *[517.8]*
　　　syphilis 095.1
　　　systemic lupus erythematosus 710.0 *[517.8]*
　　　systemic sclerosis 710.1 *[517.2]*
　　interstitial (chronic) 515
　　　acute 136.3
　　nonspecific, chronic 496
　　obstructive (chronic) (COPD) 496
　　　with
　　　　acute exacerbation NEC 491.21 ◆
　　　　alveolitis, allergic (*see also* Alveolitis, allergic) 495.9
　　　　asthma (chronic) (obstructive) 493.2
　　　　bronchiectasis 494
　　　　bronchitis (chronic) 491.2
　　　　emphysema NEC 492.8
　　　diffuse (with fibrosis) 496
　　polycystic 518.89
　　　asthma (chronic) (obstructive) 493.2
　　　congenital 748.4
　　　purulent (cavitary) 513.0
　　　restrictive 518.89
　　rheumatoid 714.81
　　　diffuse interstitial 714.81
　　specified NEC 518.89
　Lutembacher's (atrial septal defect with mitral stenosis) 745.5
　Lutz-Miescher (elastosis perforans serpiginosa) 701.1
　Lutz-Splendore-de Almeida (Brazilian blastomycosis) 116.1
　Lyell's (toxic epidermal necrolysis) 695.1
　　due to drug
　　　correct substance properly administered 695.1
　　　overdose or wrong substance given or taken 977.9
　　　specific drug — *see* Table of drugs and chemicals
　Lyme 088.81
　lymphatic (gland) (system) 289.9
　　channel (noninfective) 457.9
　　vessel (noninfective) 457.9
　　specified NEC 457.8

Disease, diseased—*continued*
　lymphoproliferative (chronic) (M9970/1) 238.7
　Madelung's (lipomatosis) 272.8
　Madura (actinomycotic) 039.9
　　mycotic 117.4
　Magitot's 526.4
　Majocchi's (purpura annularis telangiectodes) 709.1
　malarial (*see also* Malaria) 084.6
　Malassez's (cystic) 608.89
　Malibu 919.8
　　infected 919.9
　malignant (M8000/3) — *see also* Neoplasm, by site, malignant
　　previous, affecting management of pregnancy V23.8
　Manson's 120.1
　maple bark 495.6
　maple syrup (urine) 270.3
　Marburg (virus) 078.89
　Marchiafava (-Bignami) 341.8
　Marfan's 090.49
　　congenital syphilis 090.49
　　meaning Marfan's syndrome 759.82
　Marie-Bamberger (hypertrophic pulmonary osteoarthropathy) (secondary) 731.2
　　primary or idiopathic (acropachyderma) 757.39
　　pulmonary (hypertrophic osteoarthropathy) 731.2
　Marie-Strümpell (ankylosing spondylitis) 720.0
　Marion's (bladder neck obstruction) 596.0
　Marsh's (exophthalmic goiter) 242.0
　Martin's 715.27
　mast cell 757.33
　　systemic (M9741/3) 202.6
　mastoid (*see also* Mastoiditis) 383.9
　　process 385.9
　maternal, unrelated to pregnancy NEC, affecting fetus or newborn 760.9
　Mathieu's (leptospiral jaundice) 100.00
　Mauclaire's 732.3
　Mauriac's (erythema nodosum syphiliticum) 091.3
　Maxcy's 081.0
　McArdle (-Schmid-Pearson) (glycogenosis V) 271.0
　mediastinum NEC 519.3
　Medin's (*see also* Poliomyelitis) 045.9
　Mediterranean (with hemoglobinopathy) 282.4
　medullary center (idiopathic) (respiratory) 348.8
　Meige's (chronic hereditary edema) 757.0
　Meleda 757.39
　Ménétrier's (hypertrophic gastritis) 535.2
　Ménière's (active) 386.00
　　cochlear 386.02
　　cochleovestibular 386.01
　　inactive 386.04
　　in remission 386.04
　　vestibular 386.03
　meningeal — *see* Meningitis
　mental (*see also* Psychosis) 298.9
　Merzbacher-Pelizaeus 330.0
　mesenchymal 710.9
　mesenteric embolic 557.0
　metabolic NEC 277.9
　metal polishers' 502
　metastatic — *see* Metastasis
　Mibelli's 757.39
　microdrepanocytic 282.4
　Miescher's 709.3
　Mikulicz's (dryness of mouth, absent or decreased lacrimation) 527.1

Disease, diseased—*continued*
　Milkman (-Looser) (osteomalacia with pseudofractures) 268.2
　Miller's (osteomalacia) 268.2
　Mills' 335.29
　Milroy's (chronic hereditary edema) 757.0
　Minamata 985.0
　Minor's 336.1
　Minot's (hemorrhagic disease, newborn) 776.0
　Minot-von Willebrand-Jürgens (angiohemophilia) 286.4
　Mitchell's (erythromelalgia) 443.89
　mitral — *see* Endocarditis, mitral
　Mljet (mal de Meleda) 757.39
　Möbius', Moebius' 346.8
　Moeller's 267
　Möller (-Barlow) (infantile scurvy) 267
　Mönckeberg's (*see also* Arteriosclerosis, extremities) 440.20
　Mondor's (thrombophlebitis of breast) 451.89
　Monge's 993.2
　Morel-Kraepelin (*see also* Schizophrenia) 295.9
　Morgagni's (syndrome) (hyperostosis frontalis interna) 733.3
　Morgagni-Adams-Stokes (syncope with heart block) 426.9
　Morquio (-Brailsford) (-Ullrich) (mucopolysaccharidosis IV) 277.5
　Morton's (with metatarsalgia) 355.6
　Morvan's 336.0
　motor neuron (bulbar) (mixed type) 335.20
　Mouchet's (juvenile osteochondrosis, foot) 732.5
　mouth 528.9
　Moyamoya 437.5
　Mucha's (acute parapsoriasis varioliformis) 696.2
　mu-chain 273.2
　mucolipidosis (I) (II) (III) 272.7
　Münchmeyer's (exostosis luxurians) 728.11
　Murri's (intermittent hemoglobinuria) 283.2
　muscle 359.9
　　inflammatory 728.9
　　ocular 378.9
　musculoskeletal system 729.9
　mushroom workers' 495.5
　Myà's (congenital dilation, colon) 751.3
　mycotic 117.9
　myeloproliferative (chronic) (M9960/1) 238.7
　myocardium, myocardial (*see also* Degeneration, myocardial) 429.1
　　hypertensive (*see also* Hypertension, heart) 402.90
　　primary (idiopathic) 425.4
　myoneural 358.9
　Naegeli's 287.1
　nail 703.9
　　specified type NEC 703.8
　Nairobi sheep 066.1
　nasal 478.1
　　cavity NEC 478.1
　　sinus (chronic) — *see* Sinusitis
　navel (newborn) NEC 779.8
　nemaline body 359.0
　neoplastic, generalized (M8000/6) 199.0
　nerve — *see* Disorder, nerve
　nervous system (central) 349.9
　　autonomic, peripheral (*see also* Neuropathy, peripheral, autonomic) 337.9
　　congenital 742.9

Disease, diseased—continued
  nervous system—continued
    inflammatory — see
      Encephalitis
    parasympathetic (see also
      Neuropathy, peripheral,
      autonomic) 337.9
    peripheral NEC 355.9
    specified NEC 349.89
    sympathetic (see also
      Neuropathy, peripheral,
      autonomic) 337.9
    vegetative (see also Neuropathy,
      peripheral, autonomic)
      337.9
  Nettleship's (urticaria pigmentosa)
    757.33
  Neumann's (pemphigus vegetans)
    694.4
  neurologic (central) NEC (see also
    Disease, nervous system)
    349.9
  neuromuscular peripheral NEC 355.9
  neuromuscular system NEC 358.9
  Newcastle 077.8
  Nicolas (-Durand) — Favre
    (climatic bubo) 099.1
  Niemann-Pick (lipid histiocytosis)
    272.7
  nipple 611.9
    Paget's (M8540/3) 174.0
  Nishimoto (-Takeuchi) 437.5
  nonarthropod-borne NEC 078.89
    central nervous system NEC
      049.9
    enterovirus NEC 078.89
  non-autoimmune hemolytic NEC
    283.10
  Nonne-Milroy-Meige (chronic
    hereditary edema) 757.0
  Norrie's (congenital progressive
    oculoacousticocerebral
    degeneration) 743.8
  nose 478.1
  nucleus pulposus — see Disease,
    intervertebral disc
  nutritional 269.9
    maternal, affecting fetus or
      newborn 760.4
  oasthouse, urine 270.2
  obliterative vascular 447.1
  Odelberg's (juvenile
    osteochondrosis) 732.1
  Oguchi's (retina) 368.61
  Ohara's (see also Tularemia) 021.9
  Ollier's (chondrodysplasia) 756.4
  Opitz's (congestive splenomegaly)
    289.51
  Oppenheim's 358.8
  Oppenheim-Urbach (necrobiosis
    lipoidica diabeticorum)
    250.8 [709.3]
  optic nerve NEC 377.49
  orbit 376.9
    specified NEC 376.89
  Oriental liver fluke 121.1
  Oriental lung fluke 121.2
  Ormond's 593.4
  Osgood's tibia (tubercle) 732.4
  Osgood-Schlatter 732.4
  Osler (-Vaquez) (polycythemia vera)
    (M9950/1) 238.4
  Osler-Rendu (familial hemorrhagic
    telangiectasia) 448.0
  osteofibrocystic 252.0
  Otto's 715.35
  outer ear 380.9
  ovary (noninflammatory) NEC
    620.9
    cystic 620.2
    polycystic 256.4
    specified NEC 620.8
  Owren's (congenital) (see also
    Defect, coagulation) 286.3
  Paas' 756.59

Disease, diseased—continued
  Paget's (osteitis deformans) 731.0
    with infiltrating duct carcinoma
      of the breast (M8541/3)
      — see Neoplasm, breast,
      malignant
    bone 731.0
      osteosarcoma in (M9184/3)
        — see Neoplasm,
        bone, malignant
    breast (M8540/3) 174.0
    extramammary (M8542/3) —
      see also Neoplasm, skin,
      malignant
      anus 154.3
      skin 173.5
    malignant (M8540/3)
      breast 174.0
      specified site NEC (M8542/3)
        — see Neoplasm,
        skin, malignant
      unspecified site 174.0
    mammary (M8540/3) 174.0
    nipple (M8540/3) 174.0
  palate (soft) 528.9
  Paltauf-Sternberg 201.9
  pancreas 577.9
    cystic 577.2
      congenital 751.7
    fibrocystic 277.00
  Panner's 732.3
    capitellum humeri 732.3
    head of humerus 732.3
    tarsal navicular (bone)
      (osteochondrosis) 732.5
  panvalvular — see Endocarditis,
    mitral
  parametrium 629.9
  parasitic NEC 136.9
    cerebral NEC 123.9
    intestinal NEC 129
    mouth 112.0
    skin NEC 134.9
    specified type — see Infestation
    tongue 112.0
  parathyroid (gland) 252.9
    specified NEC 252.8
  Parkinson's 332.0
  parodontal 523.9
  Parrot's (syphilitic osteochondritis)
    090.0
  Parry's (exophthalmic goiter) 242.0
  Parson's (exophthalmic goiter)
    242.0
  Pavy's 593.6
  Paxton's (white piedra) 111.2
  Payr's (splenic flexure syndrome)
    569.89
  pearl-workers' (chronic
    osteomyelitis) (see also
    Osteomyelitis) 730.1
  Pel-Ebstein — see Disease,
    Hodgkin's
  Pelizaeus-Merzbacher 330.0
    with dementia 294.1
  Pellegrini-Stieda (calcification, knee
    joint) 726.62
  pelvis, pelvic
    female NEC 629.9
      specified NEC 629.8
    gonococcal (acute) 098.19
      chronic or duration of 2
        months or over
        098.39
    infection (see also Disease,
      pelvis, inflammatory)
      614.9
    inflammatory (female) (PID)
      614.9
      with
        abortion — see Abortion,
          by type, with
          sepsis
        ectopic pregnancy (see
          also categories
          (633.0-633.9)
          639.0

Disease, diseased—continued
  pelvis, pelvic—continued
    inflammatory—continued
      with—continued
        molar pregnancy (see also
          categories 630-
          632) 639.0
      acute 614.3
      chronic 614.4
      complicating pregnancy
        646.6
        affecting fetus or newborn
          760.8
      following
        abortion 639.0
        ectopic or molar
          pregnancy 639.0
      peritonitis (acute) 614.5
        chronic NEC 614.7
      puerperal, postpartum,
        childbirth 670
      specified NEC 614.8
      organ, female NEC 629.9
        specified NEC 629.8
      peritoneum, female NEC 629.9
        specified NEC 629.8
  penis 607.9
    inflammatory 607.2
  peptic NEC 536.9
    acid 536.8
  periapical tissues NEC 522.9
  pericardium 423.9
    specified type NEC 423.8
  perineum
    female
      inflammatory 616.9
        specified NEC 616.8
      noninflammatory 624.9
        specified NEC 624.8
    male (inflammatory) 682.2
  periodic (familial) (Reimann's) NEC
    277.3
    paralysis 359.3
  periodontal NEC 523.9
    specified NEC 523.8
  periosteum 733.90
  peripheral
    arterial 443.9
    autonomic nervous system (see
      also Neuropathy,
      autonomic) 337.9
    nerve NEC (see also
      Neuropathy) 356.9
      multiple — see
        Polyneuropathy
    vascular 443.9
      specified type NEC 443.89
  peritoneum 568.9
    pelvic, female 629.9
      specified NEC 629.8
  Perrin-Ferraton (snapping hip)
    719.65
  persistent mucosal (middle ear)
    (with posterior or superior
    marginal perforation of ear
    drum) 382.2
  Perthes' (capital femoral
    osteochondrosis) 732.1
  Petit's (see also Hernia, lumbar)
    553.8
  Peutz-Jeghers 759.6
  Peyronie's 607.89
  Pfeiffer's (infectious mononucleosis)
    075
  pharynx 478.20
  Phocas' 610.1
  photochromogenic (acid-fast
    bacilli) (pulmonary) 031.0
    nonpulmonary 031.9
  Pick's
    brain 331.1
      with dementia 290.10
    cerebral atrophy 331.1
      with dementia 290.10
    lipid histiocytosis 272.7
    liver (pericardial pseudocirrhosis
      of liver) 423.2

Disease, diseased—continued
  Pick's—continued
    pericardium (pericardial
      pseudocirrhosis of liver)
      423.2
    polyserositis (pericardial
      pseudocirrhosis of liver)
      423.2
  Pierson's (osteochondrosis)
    732.1
  pigeon fanciers' or breeders'
    495.2
  pineal gland 259.8
  pink 985.0
  Pinkus' (lichen nitidus) 697.1
  pinworm 127.4
  pituitary (gland) 253.9
    hyperfunction 253.1
    hypofunction 253.2
  pituitary snuff-takers' 495.8
  placenta
    affecting fetus or newborn
      762.2
    complicating pregnancy or
      childbirth 656.7
  pleura (cavity) (see also Pleurisy)
    511.0
  Plummer's (toxic nodular goiter)
    242.3
  pneumatic
    drill 994.9
    hammer 994.9
  policeman's 729.2
  Pollitzer's (hidradenitis
    suppurativa) 705.83
  polycystic (congenital) 759.89
    kidney or renal 753.12
      adult type (APKD) 753.13
        autosomal dominant
          753.13
        autosomal recessive
          753.14
      childhood type (CPKD)
        753.14
      infantile type 753.14
    liver or hepatic 751.62
    lung or pulmonary 518.89
      congenital 748.4
    ovary, ovaries 256.4
    spleen 759.0
  Pompe's (glycogenosis II) 271.0
  Poncet's (tuberculous rheumatism)
    (see also Tuberculosis) 015.9
  Posada-Wernicke 114.9
  Potain's (pulmonary edema) 514
  Pott's (see also Tuberculosis) 015.0
    [730.88]
    osteomyelitis 015.0 [730.88]
    paraplegia 015.0 [730.88]
    spinal curvature 015.0 [737.43]
    spondylitis 015.0 [720.81]
  Potter's 753.0
  Poulet's 714.2
  pregnancy NEC (see also
    Pregnancy) 646.9
  Preiser's (osteoporosis) 733.09
  Pringle's (tuberous sclerosis) 759.5
  Profichet's 729.9
  prostate 602.9
    specified type NEC 602.8
  protozoal NEC 136.8
    intestine, intestinal NEC 007.9
  pseudo-Hurler's (mucolipidosis III)
    272.7
  psychiatric (see also Psychosis)
    298.9
  psychotic (see also Psychosis)
    298.9
  Puente's (simple glandular cheilitis)
    528.5
  puerperal NEC (see also Puerperal)
    674.9
  pulmonary — see also Disease,
    lung
    amyloid 277.3 [517.8]
    artery 417.9

Disease, diseased—*continued*
  pulmonary—*continued*
    circulation, circulatory 417.9
      specified NEC 417.8
    diffuse obstructive (chronic) 496
      with
        asthma (chronic)
          (obstructive) 493.2
    heart (chronic) 416.9
      specified NEC 416.8
    hypertensive (vascular) 416.0
      cardiovascular 416.0
    obstructive diffuse (chronic) 496
      with
        acute exacerbation NEC 496
        asthma (chronic)
          (obstructive) 493.2
    valve (*see also* Endocarditis, pulmonary) 424.3
  pulp (dental) NEC 522.9
  pulseless 446.7
  Putnam's (subacute combined sclerosis with pernicious anemia) 281.0 *[336.2]*
  Pyle (-Cohn) (craniometaphyseal dysplasia) 756.89
  pyramidal tract 333.90
  Quervain's
    tendon sheath 727.04
    thyroid (subacute granulomatous thyroiditis) 245.1
  Quincke's — *see* Edema, angioneurotic
  Quinquaud (acne decalvans) 704.09
  rag sorters' 022.1
  Raynaud's (paroxysmal digital cyanosis) 443.0
  reactive airway — *see* Asthma
  Recklinghausen's (M9540/1) 237.71
    bone (osteitis fibrosa cystica) 252.0
  Recklinghausen-Applebaum (hemochromatosis) 275.0
  Reclus' (cystic) 610.1
  rectum NEC 569.49
  Refsum's (heredopathia atactica polyneuritiformis) 356.3
  Reichmann's (gastrosuccorrhea) 536.8
  Reimann's (periodic) 277.3
  Reiter's 099.3
  renal (functional) (pelvis) 593.9
    with
      edema (*see also* Nephrosis) 581.9
      exudative nephritis 583.89
      lesion of interstitial nephritis 583.89
      stated generalized cause — *see* Nephritis
    acute — *see* Nephritis, acute
    basement membrane NEC 583.89
      with
        pulmonary hemorrhage (Goodpasture's syndrome) 446.21 *[583.81]*
    chronic — *see* Nephritis, chronic
    complicating pregnancy or puerperium NEC 646.2
      with hypertension — *see* Toxemia, of pregnancy
    affecting fetus or newborn 760.1
    cystic, congenital (*see also* Cystic, disease, kidney) 753.10
    diabetic 250.4 *[583.81]*
    due to
      amyloidosis 277.3 *[583.81]*
      diabetes mellitus 250.4 *[583.81]*

Disease, diseased—*continued*
  renal—*continued*
    due to—*continued*
      systemic lupus erythematosis 710.0 *[583.81]*
    end-stage 585
    exudative 583.89
    fibrocystic (congenital) 753.19
    gonococcal 098.19 *[583.81]*
    gouty 274.10
    hypertensive (*see also* Hypertension, kidney) 403.90
    immune complex NEC 583.89
    interstitial (diffuse) (focal) 583.89
    lupus 710.0 *[583.81]*
    maternal, affecting fetus or newborn 760.1
      hypertensive 760.0
    phosphate-losing (tubular) 588.0
    polycystic (congenital) 753.12
      adult type (APKD) 753.13
      autosomal dominant 753.13
      autosomal recessive 753.14
      childhood type (CPKD) 753.14
      infantile type 753.14
    specified lesion or cause NEC (*see also* Glomerulonephritis) 583.89
    subacute 581.9
    syphilitic 095.4
    tuberculous (*see also* Tuberculosis) 016.0 *[583.81]*
    tubular (*see also* Nephrosis, tubular) 584.5
  Rendu-Osler-Weber (familial hemorrhagic telangiectasia) 448.0
  renovascular (arteriosclerotic) (*see also* Hypertension, kidney) 403.90
  respiratory (tract) 519.9
    acute or subacute (upper) NEC 465.9
      due to fumes or vapors 506.3
      multiple sites NEC 465.8
      noninfectious 478.9
      streptococcal 034.0
    chronic 519.9
      arising in the perinatal period 770.7
      due to fumes or vapors 506.4
    due to
      aspiration of liquids or solids 508.9
      external agents NEC 508.9
        specified NEC 508.8
      fumes or vapors 506.9
        acute or subacute NEC 506.3
        chronic 506.4
    fetus or newborn NEC 770.9
    obstructive 496
    specified type NEC 519.8
    upper (acute) (infectious) NEC 465.9
      multiple sites NEC 465.8
      noninfectious NEC 478.9
      streptococcal 034.0
  retina, retinal NEC 362.9
    Batten's or Batten-Mayou 330.1 *[362.71]*
    degeneration 362.89
    vascular lesion 362.17
  rheumatic (*see also* Arthritis) 716.8
    heart — *see* Disease, heart, rheumatic
  rheumatoid (heart) — *see* Arthritis, rheumatoid
  rickettsial NEC 083.9
    specified type NEC 083.8
  Riedel's (ligneous thyroiditis) 245.3

Disease, diseased—*continued*
  Riga (-Fede) (cachectic aphthae) 529.0
  Riggs' (compound periodontitis) 523.4
  Ritter's 695.81
  Rivalta's (cervicofacial actinomycosis) 039.3
  Robles' (onchocerciasis) 125.3 *[360.13]*
  Roger's (congenital interventricular septal defect) 745.4
  Rokitansky's (*see also* Necrosis, liver) 570
  Romberg's 349.89
  Rosenthal's (factor XI deficiency) 286.2
  Rossbach's (hyperchlorhydria) 536.8
    psychogenic 306.4
  Roth (-Bernhardt) 355.1
  Runeberg's (progressive pernicious anemia) 281.0
  Rust's (tuberculous spondylitis) (*see also* Tuberculosis) 015.0 *[720.81]*
  Rustitskii's (multiple myeloma) (M9730/3) 203.0
  Ruysch's (Hirschsprung's disease) 751.3
  Sachs (-Tay) 330.1
  sacroiliac NEC 724.6
  salivary gland or duct NEC 527.9
    inclusion 078.5
      streptococcal 034.0
    virus 078.5
  Sander's (paranoia) 297.1
  Sandhoff's 330.1
  sandworm 126.9
  Savill's (epidemic exfoliative dermatitis) 695.89
  Schamberg's (progressive pigmentary dermatosis) 709.09
  Schaumann's (sarcoidosis) 135
  Schenck's (sporotrichosis) 117.1
  Scheuermann's (osteochondrosis) 732.0
  Schilder (-Flatau) 341.1
  Schimmelbusch's 610.1
  Schlatter's tibia (tubercle) 732.4
  Schlatter-Osgood 732.4
  Schmorl's 722.30
    cervical 722.39
    lumbar, lumbosacral 722.32
    specified region NEC 722.39
    thoracic, thoracolumbar 722.31
  Scholz's 330.0
  Schönlein (-Henoch) (purpura rheumatica) 287.0
  Schottmüller's (*see also* Fever, paratyphoid) 002.9
  Schüller-Christian (chronic histiocytosis X) 277.8
  Schultz's (agranulocytosis) 288.0
  Schwalbe-Ziehen-Oppenheimer 333.6
  Schweninger-Buzzi (macular atrophy) 701.3
  sclera 379.19
  scrofulous (*see also* Tuberculosis) 017.2
  scrotum 608.9
  sebaceous glands NEC 706.9
  Secretan's (posttraumatic edema) 782.3
  semilunar cartilage, cystic 717.5
  seminal vesicle 608.9
  Senear-Usher (pemphigus erythematosus) 694.4
  serum NEC 999.5
  Sever's (osteochondrosis calcaneum) 732.5
  Sézary's (reticulosis) (M9701/3) 202.2
  Shaver's (bauxite pneumoconiosis) 503

Disease, diseased—*continued*
  Sheehan's (postpartum pituitary necrosis) 253.2
  shimamushi (scrub typus) 081.2
  shipyard 077.1
  sickle cell 282.60
    with
      crisis 282.62
      Hb-S disease 282.61
      other abnormal hemoglobin (Hb-D) (Hb-E) (Hb-G) (Hb-J) (Hb-K) (Hb-O) (Hb-P) (high fetal gene) 282.69
    elliptocytosis 282.60
    Hb-C 282.63
    Hb-S 282.61
      with
        crisis 282.62
        Hb-C 282.63
        other abnormal hemoglobin (Hb-D) (Hb-E) (Hb-G) (Hb-J) (Hb-K) (Hb-O) (Hb-P) (high fetal gene) 282.69
    spherocytosis 282.60
    thalassemia 282.4
  Siegal-Cattan-Mamou (periodic) 277.3
  silo fillers' 506.9
  Simian B 054.3
  Simmonds' (pituitary cachexia) 253.2
  Simons' (progressive lipodystrophy) 272.6
  Sinding-Larsen (juvenile osteopathia patellae) 732.4
  sinus — *see also* Sinusitis
    brain 437.9
    specified NEC 478.1
  Sirkari's 085.0
  sixth 057.8
  Sjögren (-Gougerot) 710.2
    with lung involvement 710.2 *[517.8]*
  Skevas-Zerfus 989.5
  skin NEC 709.9
    due to metabolic disorder 277.9
    specified type NEC 709.8
  sleeping 347
    meaning sleeping sickness (*see also* Trypanosomiasis) 086.5
  small vessel 443.9
  Smith-Strang (oasthouse urine) 270.2
  Sneddon-Wilkinson (subcorneal pustular dermatosis) 694.1
  South African creeping 133.8
  specific NEC (*see also* Syphilis) 097.9
  Spencer's (epidemic vomiting) 078.82
  Spielmeyer-Stock 330.1
  Spielmeyer-Vogt 330.1
  spine, spinal 733.90
    combined system (*see also* Degeneration, combined) 266.2 *[336.2]*
      with pernicious anemia 281.0 *[336.2]*
    cord NEC 336.9
      congenital 742.9
    demyelinating NEC 341.8
    joint (*see also* Disease, joint, spine) 724.9
    tuberculous 015.0 *[730.8]*
  spinocerebellar 334.9
    specified NEC 334.8
  spleen (organic) (postinfectional) 289.50
    amyloid 277.3
    lardaceous 277.3
    polycystic 759.0
    specified NEC 289.59
  sponge divers' 989.5

Disease, diseased—continued
- Stanton's (melioidosis) 025
- Stargardt's 362.75
- Steinert's 359.2
- Sternberg's — see Disease, Hodgkin's
- Stevens-Johnson (erythema multiforme exudativum) 695.1
- Sticker's (erythema infectiosum) 057.0
- Stieda's (calcification, knee joint) 726.62
- Still's (juvenile rheumatoid arthritis) 714.30
- Stiller's (asthenia) 780.7
- Stokes' (exophthalmic goiter) 242.0
- Stokes-Adams (syncope with heart block) 426.9
- Stokvis (-Talma) (enterogenous cyanosis) 289.7
- stomach NEC (organic) 537.9
  - functional 536.9
    - psychogenic 306.4
  - lardaceous 277.3
- stonemasons' 502
- storage
  - glycogen (see also Disease, glycogen storage) 271.0
  - lipid 272.7
  - mucopolysaccharide 277.5
- striatopallidal system 333.90
  - specified NEC 333.89
- Strümpell-Marie (ankylosing spondylitis) 720.0
- Stuart's (congenital factor X deficiency) (see also Defect, coagulation) 286.3
- Stuart-Prower (congenital factor X deficiency) (see also Defect, coagulation) 286.3
- Sturge (-Weber) (-Dimitri) (encephalocutaneous angiomatosis) 759.6
- Stuttgart 100.89
- Sudeck's 733.7
- supporting structures of teeth NEC 525.9
- suprarenal (gland) (capsule) 255.9
  - hyperfunction 255.3
  - hypofunction 255.4
- Sutton's 709.09 ◆
- Sutton and Gull's — see Hypertension, kidney
- sweat glands NEC 705.9
  - specified type NEC 705.89
- sweating 078.2
- Sweeley-Klionsky 272.4
- Swift (-Feer) 985.0
- swimming pool (bacillus) 031.1
- swineherd's 100.89
- Sylvest's (epidemic pleurodynia) 074.1
- Symmers (follicular lymphoma) (M9690/3) 202.0
- sympathetic nervous system (see also Neuropathy, peripheral, autonomic) 337.9
- synovium 727.9
- syphilitic — see Syphilis
- systemic tissue mast cell (M9741/3) 202.6
- Taenzer's 757.4
- Takayasu's (pulseless) 446.7
- Talma's 728.85
- Tangier (familial high-density lipoprotein deficiency) 272.5
- Tarral-Besnier (pityriasis rubra pilaris) 696.4
- Tay-Sachs 330.1
- Taylor's 701.8
- tear duct 375.69
- teeth, tooth 525.9
  - hard tissues NEC 521.9
  - pulp NEC 522.9
- tendon 727.9
  - inflammatory NEC 727.9

Disease, diseased—continued
- terminal vessel 443.9
- testis 608.9
- Thaysen-Gee (nontropical sprue) 579.0
- Thomsen's 359.2
- Thomson's (congenital poikiloderma) 757.33
- Thornwaldt's, Tornwaldt's (pharyngeal bursitis) 478.29
- throat 478.20
  - septic 034.0
- thromboembolic (see also Embolism) 444.9
- thymus (gland) 254.9
  - specified NEC 254.8
- thyroid (gland) NEC 246.9
  - heart (see also Hyperthyroidism) 242.9 [425.7]
  - lardaceous 277.3
  - specified NEC 246.8
- Tietze's 733.6
- Tommaselli's
  - correct substance properly administered 599.7
  - overdose or wrong substance given or taken 961.4
- tongue 529.9
- tonsils, tonsillar (and adenoids) (chronic) 474.9
  - specified NEC 474.8
- tooth, teeth 525.9
  - hard tissues NEC 521.9
  - pulp NEC 522.9
- Tornwaldt's (pharyngeal bursitis) 478.29
- Tourette's 307.23
- trachea 519.1
- tricuspid — see Endocarditis, tricuspid
- triglyceride-storage, type I, II, III 272.7
- triple vessel (coronary arteries) — see Arteriosclerosis, coronary ◆
- trisymptomatic, Gourgerot's 709.1
- trophoblastic (see also Hydatidiform mole) 630
  - previous, affecting management of pregnancy V23.1
- tsutsugamushi (scrub typhus) 081.2
- tube (fallopian), noninflammatory 620.9
  - specified NEC 620.8
- tuberculous NEC (see also Tuberculosis) 011.9
- tubo-ovarian
  - inflammatory (see also Salpingo-oophoritis) 614.2
  - noninflammatory 620.9
    - specified NEC 620.8
- tubotympanic, chronic (with anterior perforation of ear drum) 382.1
- tympanum 385.9
- Uhl's 746.84
- umbilicus (newborn) NEC 779.8
- Underwood's (sclerema neonatorum) 778.1
- undiagnosed 799.9
- Unna's (seborrheic dermatitis) 690
- unstable hemoglobin hemolytic 282.7
- Unverricht (-Lundborg) 333.2
- Urbach-Oppenheim (necrobiosis lipoidica diabeticorum) 250.8 [709.3]
- Urbach-Wiethe (lipoid proteinosis) 272.8
- ureter 593.9
- urethra 599.9
  - specified type NEC 599.84
- urinary (tract) 599.9
  - bladder 596.9
    - specified NEC 596.8
  - maternal, affecting fetus or newborn 760.1

Disease, diseased—continued
- Usher-Senear (pemphigus erythematosus) 694.4
- uterus (organic) 621.9
  - infective (see also Endometritis) 615.9
  - inflammatory (see also Endometritis) 615.9
  - noninflammatory 621.9
    - specified type NEC 621.8
- uveal tract
  - anterior 364.9
  - posterior 363.9
- vagabonds' 132.1
- vagina, vaginal
  - inflammatory 616.9
    - specified NEC 616.8
  - noninflammatory 623.9
    - specified NEC 623.8
- Valsuani's (progressive pernicious anemia, puerperal) 648.2
  - complicating pregnancy or puerperium 648.2
- valve, valvular — see Endocarditis
- van Bogaert-Nijssen (-Peiffer) 330.0
- van Creveld-von Gierke (glycogenosis I) 271.0
- van den Bergh's (enterogenous cyanosis) 289.7
- van Neck's (juvenile osteochondrosis) 732.1
- Vaquez (-Osler) (polycythemia vera) (M9950/1) 238.4
- vascular 459.9
  - arteriosclerotic — see Arteriosclerosis
  - hypertensive — see Hypertension
  - obliterative 447.1
    - peripheral 443.9
  - occlusive 459.9
  - peripheral (occlusive) 443.9
    - in diabetes mellitus 250.7 [443.81]
  - specified type NEC 443.89
- vas deferens 608.9
- vasomotor 443.9
- vasospastic 443.9
- vein 459.9
- venereal 099.9
  - chlamydial NEC 099.50
    - anus 099.52
    - bladder 099.53
    - cervix 099.53
    - epididymis 099.54
    - genitourinary NEC 099.55
      - lower 099.53
      - specified NEC 099.54
    - pelvic inflammatory disease 099.54
    - perihepatic 099.56
    - peritoneum 099.56
    - pharynx 099.51
    - rectum 099.52
    - specified site NEC 099.54
    - testis 099.54
    - vagina 099.53
    - vulva 099.53
  - fifth 099.1
  - sixth 099.1
  - complicating pregnancy, childbirth, or puerperium 647.2
  - specified nature or type NEC 099.8
    - chlamydial — see Disease, venereal, chlamydial
- Verneuil's (syphilitic bursitis) 095.7
- Verse's (calcinosis intervertebralis) 275.4 [722.90]
- vertebra, vertebral NEC 733.90
  - disc — see Disease, Intervertebral disc
- vibration NEC 994.9
- Vidal's (lichen simplex chronicus) 698.3
- Vincent's (trench mouth) 101

Disease, diseased—continued
- Virchow's 733.99
- virus (filterable) NEC 078.89
  - arbovirus NEC 066.9
  - arthropod-borne NEC 066.9
  - central nervous system NEC 049.9
    - specified type NEC 049.8
  - complicating pregnancy, childbirth, or puerperium 647.6
  - contact (with) V01.7
  - exposure to V01.7
  - Marburg 078.89
  - maternal
    - with fetal damage affecting management of pregnancy 655.3
  - nonarthropod-borne NEC 078.89
    - central nervous sytem NEC 049.9
      - specified NEC 049.8
- vitreous 379.29
- vocal cords NEC 478.5
- Vogt's (Cecile) 333.7
- Vogt-Spielmeyer 330.1
- Volhard-Fahr (malignant nephrosclerosis) 403.00
- Volkmann's
  - acquired 958.6
- von Bechterew's (ankylosing spondylitis) 720.0
- von Economo's (encephalitis lethargica) 049.8
- von Eulenburg's (congenital paramyotonia) 359.2
- von Gierke's (glycogenosis I) 271.0
- von Graefe's 378.72
- von Hippel's (retinocerebral angiomatosis) 759.6
- von Hippel-Lindau (angiomatosis retinocerebellosa) 759.6
- von Jaksch's (pseudoleukemia infantum) 285.8
- von Recklinghausen's (M9540/1) 237.71
  - bone (osteitis fibrosa cystica) 252.0
- von Recklinghausen-Applebaum (hemochromatosis) 275.0
- von Willebrand (-Jürgens) (angiohemophilia) 286.4
- von Zambusch's (lichen sclerosus et atrophicus) 701.0
- Voorhoeve's (dyschondroplasia) 756.4
- Vrolik's (osteogenesis imperfecta) 756.51
- vulva
  - noninflammatory 624.9
    - specified NEC 624.8
- Wagner's (colloid milium) 709.3
- Waldenström's (osteochondrosis capital femoral) 732.1
- Wallgren's (obstruction of splenic vein with collateral circulation) 459.89
- Wardrop's (with lymphangitis) 681.9
  - finger 681.02
  - toe 681.11
- Wassilieff's (leptospiral jaundice) 100.00
- wasting NEC 799.4
  - due to malnutrition 261
  - paralysis 335.21
- Waterhouse-Friderichsen 036.3
- waxy (any site) 277.3
- Weber-Christian (nodular nonsuppurative panniculitis) 729.30
- Wegner's (syphilitic osteochondritis) 090.0
- Weil's (leptospral jaundice) 100.0
  - of lung 100.0

Disease, diseased — continued

Weir Mitchell's (erythromelalgia) 443.89
Werdnig-Hoffmann 335.0
Werlhof's (see also Purpura, thrombocytopenic) 287.3
Wermer's 258.0
Werner's (progeria adultorum) 259.8
Werner-His (trench fever) 083.1
Werner-Schultz (agranulocytosis) 288.0
Wernicke's (superior hemorrhagic polioencephalitis) 265.1
Wernicke-Posadas 114.9
Whipple's (intestinal lipodystrophy) 040.2
whipworm 127.3
white
 blood cell 288.9
  specified NEC 288.8
 spot 701.0
White's (congenital) (keratosis follicularis) 757.39
Whitmore's (melioidosis) 025
Widal-Abrami (acquired hemolytic jaundice) 283.9
Wilkie's 557.1
Wilkinson-Sneddon (subcorneal pustular dermatosis) 694.1
Willis' (diabetes mellitus) (see also Diabetes) 250.0
Wilson's (hepatolenticular degeneration) 275.1
Wilson-Brocq (dermatitis exfoliativa) 695.89
winter vomiting 078.82
Wise's 696.2
Wohlfart-Kugelberg-Welander 335.11
Woillez's (acute idiopathic pulmonary congestion) 518.5
Wolman's (primary familial xanthomatosis) 272.7
wool-sorters' 022.1
Zagari's (xerostomia) 527.7
Zahorsky's (exanthem subitum) 057.8
Ziehen-Oppenheim 333.6
zoonotic, bacterial NEC 027.9
 specified type NEC 027.8

Disfigurement (due to scar) 709.2
 head V48.6
 limb V49.4
 neck V48.7
 trunk V48.7

Disgerminoma — see Dysgerminoma

Disinsertion, retina 361.04

Disintegration, complete, of the body 799.8
 traumatic 869.1

Disk kidney 753.3

Dislocatable hip, congenital (see also Dislocation, hip, congenital) 754.30

Dislocation (articulation) (closed) (displacement) (simple) (subluxation) 839.8

Note — "Closed" includes simple, complete, partial, uncomplicated, and unspecified dislocation.

"Open" includes dislocation specified as infected or compound and dislocation with foreign body.

"Chronic," "habitual," "old," or "recurrent" dislocations should be coded as indicated under the entry "Dislocation, recurrent," and "pathological" as indicated under the entry "Dislocation, pathological."

For late effect of dislocation see Late, effect, dislocation.

Dislocation — continued

with fracture — see Fracture, by site
acromioclavicular (joint) (closed) 831.04
 open 831.14
anatomical site (closed)
 specified NEC 839.69
  open 839.79
 unspecified or ill-defined 839.8
  open 839.9
ankle (scaphoid bone) (closed) 837.0
 open 837.1
arm (closed) 839.8
 open 839.9
astragalus (closed) 837.0
 open 837.1
atlanto-axial (closed) 839.01
 open 839.11
atlas (closed) 839.01
 open 839.11
axis (closed) 839.02
 open 839.12
back (closed) 839.8
 open 839.9
Bell-Daly 723.8
breast bone (closed) 839.61
 open 839.71
capsule, joint — see Dislocation, by site
carpal (bone) — see Dislocation, wrist
carpometacarpal (joint) (closed) 833.04
 open 833.14
cartilage (joint) — see also Dislocation, by site
 knee — see Tear, meniscus
cervical, cervicodorsal, or cervicothoracic (spine) (vertebra) — see Dislocation, vertebra, cervical
chiropractic (see also Lesion, nonallopathic) 739.9
chondrocostal — see Dislocation, costochondral
chronic — see Dislocation, recurrent
clavicle (closed) 831.04
 open 831.14
coccyx (closed) 839.41
 open 839.51
collar bone (closed) 831.04
 open 831.14
compound (open) NEC 839.9
congenital NEC 755.8
 hip (see also Dislocation, hip, congenital) 754.30
 lens 743.37
 rib 756.3
 sacroiliac 755.69
 spine NEC 756.19
 vertebra 756.19
coracoid (closed) 831.09
 open 831.19
costal cartilage (closed) 839.69
 open 839.79
costochondral (closed) 839.69
 open 839.79
cricoarytenoid articulation (closed) 839.69
 open 839.79
cricothyroid (cartilage) articulation (closed) 839.69
 open 839.79
dorsal vertebrae (closed) 839.21
 open 839.31
ear ossicle 385.23
elbow (closed) 832.00
 anterior (closed) 832.01
  open 832.11
 congenital 754.89
 divergent (closed) 832.09
  open 832.19
 lateral (closed) 832.04
  open 832.14

Dislocation — continued

elbow — continued
 medial (closed) 832.03
  open 832.13
 open 832.10
 posterior (closed) 832.02
  open 832.12
 recurrent 718.32
 specified type NEC 832.09
  open 832.19
eye 360.81
 lateral 376.36
eyeball 360.81
 lateral 376.36
femur
 distal end (closed) 836.50
  anterior 836.52
   open 836.62
  lateral 836.53
   open 836.63
  medial 836.54
   open 836.64
  open 836.60
  posterior 836.51
   open 836.61
 proximal end (closed) 835.00
  anterior (pubic) 835.03
   open 835.13
  obturator 835.02
   open 835.12
  open 835.10
  posterior 835.01
   open 835.11
fibula
 distal end (closed) 837.0
  open 837.1
 proximal end (closed) 836.59
  open 836.69
finger(s) (phalanx) (thumb) (closed) 834.00
 interphalangeal (joint) 834.02
  open 834.12
 metacarpal (bone), distal end 834.01
  open 834.11
 metacarpophalangeal (joint) 834.01
  open 834.11
 open 834.10
 recurrent 718.34
foot (closed) 838.00
 open 838.10
 recurrent 718.37
forearm (closed) 839.8
 open 839.9
fracture — see Fracture, by site
glenoid (closed) 831.09
 open 831.19
habitual — see Dislocation, recurrent
hand (closed) 839.8
 open 839.9
hip (closed) 835.00
 anterior 835.03
 obturator 835.02
  open 835.12
 open 835.13
 congenital (unilateral) 754.30
  with subluxation of other hip 754.35
  bilateral 754.31
 open 835.10
 posterior 835.01
  open 835.11
 recurrent 718.35
humerus (closed) 831.00
 distal end (see also Dislocation, elbow) 832.00
 open 831.10
 proximal end (closed) 831.00
  anterior (subclavicular) (subcoracoid) (subglenoid) (closed) 831.01
   open 831.11
  inferior (closed) 831.03
   open 831.13

Dislocation — continued

humerus — continued
 proximal end — continued
  open 831.10
  posterior (closed) 831.02
   open 831.12
 implant — see Complications, mechanical
incus 385.23
infracoracoid (closed) 831.01
 open 831.11
innominate (pubic juntion) (sacral junction) (closed) 839.69
 acetabulum (see also Dislocation, hip) 835.00
 open 839.79
interphalangeal (joint)
 finger or hand (closed) 834.02
  open 834.12
 foot or toe (closed) 838.06
  open 838.16
jaw (cartilage) (meniscus) (closed) 830.0
 open 830.1
 recurrent 524.69
joint NEC (closed) 839.8
 open 839.9
 pathological — see Dislocation, pathological
 recurrent — see Dislocation, recurrent
knee (closed) 836.50
 anterior 836.51
  open 836.61
 congenital (with genu recurvatum) 754.41
 habitual 718.36
 lateral 836.54
  open 836.64
 medial 836.53
  open 836.63
 old 718.36
 open 836.60
 posterior 836.52
  open 836.62
 recurrent 718.36
 rotatory 836.59
  open 836.69
lacrimal gland 375.16
leg (closed) 839.8
 open 839.9
lens (crystalline) (complete) (partial) 379.32
 anterior 379.33
 congenital 743.37
 ocular implant 996.53
 posterior 379.34
 traumatic 921.3
ligament — see Dislocation, by site
lumbar (vertebrae) (closed) 839.20
 open 839.30
lumbosacral (vertebrae) (closed) 839.20
 congenital 756.19
 open 839.30
mandible (closed) 830.0
 open 830.1
maxilla (inferior) (closed) 830.0
 open 830.1
meniscus (knee) — see also Tear, meniscus
 other sites — see Dislocation, by site
metacarpal (bone)
 distal end (closed) 834.01
  open 834.11
 proximal end (closed) 833.05
  open 833.15
metacarpophalangeal (joint) (closed) 834.01
 open 834.11
metatarsal (bone) (closed) 838.04
 open 838.14
metatarsophalangeal (joint) (closed) 838.05
 open 838.15

Dislocation INDEX TO DISEASES Disorder

Dislocation—*continued*
　midcarpal (joint) (closed) 833.03
　　open 833.13
　midtarsal (joint) (closed) 838.02
　　open 838.12
　Monteggia's — *see* Dislocation, hip
　multiple locations (except fingers only or toes only) (closed) 839.8
　　open 839.9
　navicular (bone) foot (closed) 837.0
　　open 837.1
　neck (*see also* Dislocation, vertebra, cervical) 839.00
　Nélaton's — *see* Dislocation, ankle
　nontraumatic (joint) — *see* Dislocation, pathological
　nose (closed) 839.69
　　open 839.79
　not recurrent, not current injury — *see* Dislocation, pathological
　occiput from atlas (closed) 839.01
　　open 839.11
　old — *see* Dislocation, recurrent
　open (compound) NEC 839.9
　ossicle, ear 385.23
　paralytic (flaccid) (spastic) — *see* Dislocation, pathological
　patella (closed) 836.3
　　congenital 755.64
　　open 836.4
　pathological NEC 718.20
　　ankle 718.27
　　elbow 718.22
　　foot 718.27
　　hand 718.24
　　hip 718.25
　　knee 718.26
　　lumbosacral joint 724.6
　　multiple sites 718.29
　　pelvic region 718.25
　　sacroiliac 724.6
　　shoulder (region) 718.21
　　specified site NEC 718.28
　　spine 724.8
　　　sacroiliac 724.6
　　wrist 718.23
　pelvis (closed) 839.69
　　acetabulum (*see also* Dislocation, hip) 835.00
　　open 839.79
　phalanx
　　foot or toe (closed) 838.09
　　　open 838.19
　　hand or finger (*see also* Dislocation, finger) 834.00
　postpoliomyelitic — *see* Dislocation, pathological
　prosthesis, internal — *see* Complications, mechanical
　radiocarpal (joint) (closed) 833.02
　　open 833.12
　radioulnar (joint)
　　distal end (closed) 833.01
　　　open 833.11
　　proximal end (*see also* Dislocation, elbow) 832.00
　radius
　　distal end (closed) 833.00
　　　open 833.10
　　proximal end (closed) 832.01
　　　open 832.11
　recurrent (*see also* Derangement, joint, recurrent) 718.3
　　elbow 718.32
　　hip 718.35
　　joint NEC 718.38
　　knee 718.36
　　lumbosacral (joint) 724.6
　　patella 718.36
　　sacroiliac 724.6
　　shoulder 718.31
　　temporomandibular 524.69

Dislocation—*continued*
　rib (cartilage) (closed) 839.69
　　congenital 756.3
　　open 839.79
　sacrococcygeal (closed) 839.42
　　open 839.52
　sacroiliac (joint) (ligament) (closed) 839.42
　　congenital 755.69
　　open 839.52
　　recurrent 724.6
　sacrum (closed) 839.42
　　open 839.52
　scaphoid (bone)
　　ankle or foot (closed) 837.0
　　　open 837.1
　　wrist (closed) (*see also* Dislocation, wrist) 833.00
　　　open 833.10
　scapula (closed) 831.09
　　open 831.19
　semilunar cartilage, knee — *see* Tear, meniscus
　septal cartilage (nose) (closed) 839.69
　　open 839.79
　septum (nasal) (old) 470
　sesamoid bone — *see* Dislocation, by site
　shoulder (blade) (ligament) (closed) 831.00
　　anterior (subclavicular) (subcoracoid) (subglenoid) (closed) 831.01
　　　open 831.11
　　chronic 718.31
　　inferior 831.03
　　　open 831.13
　　open 831.10
　　posterior (closed) 831.02
　　　open 831.12
　　recurrent 718.31
　skull — *see* Injury, intracranial
　Smith's — *see* Dislocation, foot
　spine (articular process) (*see also* Dislocation, vertebra) (closed) 839.40
　　atlanto-axial (closed) 839.01
　　　open 839.11
　　　recurrent 723.8
　　cervical, cervicodorsal, cervicothoracic (closed) (*see also* Dislocation, vertebrae, cervical) 839.00
　　　open 839.10
　　　recurrent 723.8
　　coccyx 839.41
　　　open 839.51
　　congenital 756.19
　　due to birth trauma 767.4
　　open 839.50
　　recurrent 724.9
　　sacroiliac 839.42
　　　recurrent 724.6
　　sacrum (sacrococcygeal) (sacroiliac) 839.42
　　　open 839.52
　spontaneous — *see* Dislocation, pathological
　sternoclavicular (joint) (closed) 839.61
　　open 839.71
　sternum (closed) 839.61
　　open 839.71
　subastragalar — *see* Dislocation, foot
　subglenoid (closed) 831.01
　　open 831.11
　symphysis
　　jaw (closed) 830.0
　　　open 830.1
　　mandibular (closed) 830.0
　　　open 830.1
　　pubis (closed) 839.69
　　　open 839.79

Dislocation—*continued*
　tarsal (bone) (joint) 838.01
　　open 838.11
　tarsometatarsal (joint) 838.03
　　open 838.13
　temporomandibular (joint) (closed) 830.0
　　open 830.1
　　recurrent 524.69
　thigh
　　distal end (*see also* Dislocation, femur, distal end) 836.50
　　proximal end (*see also* Dislocation, hip) 835.00
　thoracic (vertebrae) (closed) 839.21
　　open 839.31
　thumb(s) (*see also* Dislocation, finger) 834.00
　thyroid cartilage (closed) 839.69
　　open 839.79
　tibia
　　distal end (closed) 837.0
　　　open 837.1
　　proximal end (closed) 836.50
　　　anterior 836.51
　　　　open 836.61
　　　lateral 836.54
　　　　open 836.64
　　　medial 836.53
　　　　open 836.63
　　　open 836.60
　　　posterior 836.52
　　　　open 836.62
　　　rotatory 836.59
　　　　open 836.69
　tibiofibular
　　distal (closed) 837.0
　　　open 837.1
　　superior (closed) 836.59
　　　open 836.69
　toe(s) (closed) 838.09
　　open 838.19
　trachea (closed) 839.69
　　open 839.79
　ulna
　　distal end (closed) 833.09
　　　open 833.19
　　proximal end — *see* Dislocation, elbow
　vertebra (articular process) (body) (closed) 839.40
　　cervical, cervicodorsal or cervicothoracic (closed) 839.00
　　　first (atlas) 839.01
　　　　open 839.11
　　　second (axis) 839.02
　　　　open 839.12
　　　third 839.03
　　　　open 839.13
　　　fourth 839.04
　　　　open 839.14
　　　fifth 839.05
　　　　open 839.15
　　　sixth 839.06
　　　　open 839.16
　　　seventh 839.07
　　　　open 839.17
　　　congenital 756.19
　　　multiple sites 839.08
　　　　open 839.18
　　　open 839.10
　　congenital 756.19
　　dorsal 839.21
　　　open 839.31
　　　recurrent 724.9
　　lumbar, lumbosacral 839.20
　　　open 839.30
　　open NEC 839.50
　　recurrent 724.9
　　specified region NEC 839.49
　　　open 839.59
　　thoracic 839.21
　　　open 839.31
　wrist (carpal bone) (scaphoid) (semilunar) (closed) 833.00

Dislocation—*continued*
　wrist—*continued*
　　carpometacarpal (joint) 833.04
　　　open 833.14
　　metacarpal bone, proximal end 833.05
　　　open 833.15
　　midcarpal (joint) 833.03
　　　open 833.13
　　open 833.10
　　radiocarpal (joint) 833.02
　　　open 833.12
　　radioulnar (joint) 833.01
　　　open 833.11
　　recurrent 718.33
　　specified site NEC 833.09
　　　open 833.19
　　xiphoid cartilage (closed) 839.61
　　　open 839.71

Disobedience, hostile (covert) (overt) (*see also* Disturbance, conduct) 312.0

Disorder — *see also* Disease
　academic underachievement, childhood and adolescence 313.83
　accommodation 367.51
　　drug-induced 367.89
　　toxic 367.89
　adjustment (*see also* Reaction, adjustment) 309.9
　adrenal (capsule) (cortex) (gland) 255.9
　　specified type NEC 255.8
　adrenogenital 255.2
　affective (*see also* Psychosis, affective) 296.90
　　atypical 296.81
　aggressive, unsocialized (*see also* Disturbance, conduct) 312.0
　alcohol, alcoholic (*see also* Alcohol) 291.9 ◆
　allergic — *see* Allergy
　amnestic (*see also* Amnestic syndrome) 294.8 ◆
　amino acid (metabolic) (*see also* Disturbance, metabolism, amino acid) 270.9
　　albinism 270.2
　　alkaptonuria 270.2
　　argininosuccinicaciduria 270.6
　　beta-amino-isobutyricaciduria 277.2
　　cystathioninuria 270.4
　　cystinosis 270.0
　　cystinuria 270.0
　　glycinuria 270.0
　　homocystinuria 270.4
　　imidazole 270.5
　　maple syrup (urine) disease 270.3
　　neonatal, transitory 775.8
　　oasthouse urine disease 270.2
　　ochronosis 270.2
　　phenylketonuria 270.1
　　phenylpyruvic oligophrenia 270.1
　　purine NEC 277.2
　　pyrimidine NEC 277.2
　　renal transport NEC 270.0
　　specified type NEC 270.8
　　transport NEC 270.0
　　　renal 270.0
　　xanthinuria 277.2
　anaerobic glycolysis with anemia 282.3
　anxiety (*see also* Anxiety) 300.00 ◆
　arteriole 447.9
　　specified type NEC 447.8
　artery 447.9
　　specified type NEC 447.8
　articulation — *see* Disorder, joint
　Asperger's 299.8 ◆
　attachment of infancy 313.89
　attention deficit 314.00
　　with hyperactivity 314.01

Disorder—continued
- attention deficit—continued
  - predominantly
    - combined
      - hyperactive/inattentive 314.01
    - hyperactive/impulsive 314.01
    - inattentive 314.00
  - residual type 314.8
- autoimmune NEC 279.4
  - hemolytic (cold type) (warm type) 283.0
  - parathyroid 252.1
  - thyroid 245.2
- autistic 299.0
- avoidant, childhood or adolescence 313.21
- balance
  - acid-base 276.9
    - mixed (with hypercapnia) 276.4
  - electrolyte 276.9
  - fluid 276.9
- behavior NEC (see also Disturbance, conduct) 312.9
- bilirubin excretion 277.4
- bipolar (affective) (alternating) (type I) (see also Psychosis, affective) 296.7
  - atypical 296.7
  - currently
    - depressed 296.5
    - hypomanic 296.4
    - manic 296.4
  - mixed 296.6
  - type II (recurrent major depressive episodes with hypomania) 296.89
- bladder 596.9
  - functional NEC 596.59
  - specified NEC 596.8
- bone NEC 733.90
  - specified NEC 733.99
- brachial plexus 353.0
- branched-chain amino-acid degradation 270.3
- breast 611.9
  - puerperal, postpartum 676.3
  - specified NEC 611.8
- Briquet's 300.81
- bursa 727.9
  - shoulder region 726.10
- carbohydrate metabolism, congenital 271.9
- cardiac, functional 427.9
  - postoperative 997.1
  - psychogenic 306.2
- cardiovascular, psychogenic 306.2
- cartilage NEC 733.90
  - articular 718.00
    - ankle 718.07
    - elbow 718.02
    - foot 718.07
    - hand 718.04
    - hip 718.05
    - knee 717.9
    - multiple sites 718.09
    - pelvic region 718.05
    - shoulder region 718.01
    - specified
      - site NEC 718.08
      - type NEC 733.99
    - wrist 718.03
- cervical region NEC 723.9
- cervical root (nerve) NEC 353.2
- character NEC (see also Disorder, personality) 301.9
- coagulation (factor) (see also Defect, coagulation) 286.9
  - factor VIII (congenital) (functional) 286.0
  - factor IX (congenital) (functional) 286.1
  - neonatal, transitory 776.3
- coccyx 724.70
  - specified NEC 724.79

Disorder—continued
- colon 569.9
  - functional 564.9
  - congenital 751.3
- cognitive 294.9
- conduct (see also Disturbance, conduct) 312.9
  - adjustment reaction 309.3
  - adolescent onset type 312.82
  - childhood onset type 312.81
  - compulsive 312.30
    - specified type NEC 312.39
  - hyperkinetic 314.2
  - socialized (type) 312.20
    - aggressive 312.23
    - unaggressive 312.21
  - specified NEC 312.89
- conduction, heart 426.9
  - specified NEC 426.89
- convulsive (secondary) (see also Convulsions) 780.3
  - due to injury at birth 767.0
  - idiopathic 780.3
- coordination 781.3
- cornea NEC 371.89
  - due to contact lens 371.82
- corticosteroid metabolism NEC 255.2
- cranial nerve — see Disorder, nerve, cranial
- cyclothymic 301.13
- degradation, branched-chain amino acid 270.3
- dentition 520.6
- depressive NEC 311
  - atypical 296.82
  - major (see also Psychosis, affective) 296.2
    - recurrent episode 296.3
    - single episode 296.2
- development, specific 315.9
  - associated with hyperkinesia 314.1
  - language 315.31
  - learning 315.2
    - arithmetical 315.1
    - reading 315.00
  - mixed 315.5
  - motor coordination 315.4
  - specified type NEC 315.8
  - speech 315.39
- diaphragm 519.4
- digestive 536.9
  - fetus or newborn 777.9
    - specified NEC 777.8
  - psychogenic 306.4
- disintegrative (childhood) 299.1
- dissociative 300.14
  - identity 300.14
- dysmorphic body 300.7
- dysthymic 300.4
- ear 388.9
  - degenerative NEC 388.00
  - external 380.9
    - specified 380.89
  - pinna 380.30
  - specified type NEC 388.8
  - vascular NEC 388.00
- eating NEC 307.50
- electrolyte NEC 276.9
  - with
    - abortion — see Abortion, by type, with metabolic disorder
    - ectopic pregnancy (see also categories 633.0-633.9) 639.4
    - molar pregnancy (see also categories 630-632) 639.4
  - acidosis 276.2
    - metabolic 276.2
    - respiratory 276.2
  - alkalosis 276.3
    - metabolic 276.3
    - respiratory 276.3

Disorder—continued
- electrolyte—continued
  - following
    - abortion 639.4
    - ectopic or molar pregnancy 639.4
  - neonatal, transitory NEC 775.5
- emancipation as adjustment reaction 309.22
- emotional (see also Disorder, mental, nonpsychotic) V40.9
- endocrine 259.9
  - specified type NEC 259.8
- esophagus 530.9
  - functional 530.5
  - psychogenic 306.4
- explosive
  - intermittent 312.34
  - isolated 312.35
- eye 379.90
  - globe — see Disorder, globe
  - ill-defined NEC 379.99
  - limited duction NEC 378.63
  - specified NEC 379.8
- eyelid 374.9
  - degenerative 374.50
  - sensory 374.44
  - specified type NEC 374.89
  - vascular 374.85
- factitious — see Illness, factitious
- factor, coagulation (see also Defect, coagulation) 286.9
  - VIII (congenital) (functional) 286.0
  - IX (congenital) (funcitonal) 286.1
- fascia 728.9
- feeding — see Feeding
- female sexual arousal 302.72
- fluid NEC 276.9
- gastric (functional) 536.9
  - motility 536.8
  - psychogenic 306.4
  - secretion 536.8
- gastrointestinal (functional) NEC 536.9
  - newborn (neonatal) 777.9
    - specified NEC 777.8
  - psychogenic 306.4
- gender (child) 302.6
  - adult 302.85
- gender identity (childhood) 302.6
  - adult-life 302.85
- genitourinary system, psychogenic 306.50
- globe 360.9
  - degenerative 360.20
    - specified NEC 360.29
  - specified type NEC 360.89
- hearing — see also Deafness
  - conductive type (air) (see also Deafness, conductive) 389.00
  - mixed conductive and sensorineural 389.2
  - nerve 389.12
  - perceptive (see also Deafness, perceptive) 389.10
  - sensorineural type NEC (see also Deafness, perceptive) 389.10
- heart action 427.9
  - postoperative 997.1
- hematological, transient neonatal 776.9
  - specified type NEC 776.8
- hematopoietic organs 289.9
- hemorrhagic NEC 287.9
  - due to circulating anticoagulants 286.5
  - specified type NEC 287.8
- hemostasis (see also Defect, coagulation) 286.9
- homosexual conflict 302.0
- hypomanic (chronic) 301.11

Disorder—continued
- identity
  - childhood and adolescence 313.82
  - gender 302.6
- gender 302.6
- immune mechanism (immunity) 279.9
  - single complement (C-C) 279.8
  - specified type NEC 279.8
- impulse control (see also Disturbance, conduct, compulsive) 312.30
- integument, fetus or newborn 778.9
  - specified type NEC 778.8
- interactional psychotic (childhood) (see also Psychosis, childhood) 299.1
- intermittent explosive 312.34
- intervertebral disc 722.90
  - cervical, cervicothoracic 722.91
  - lumbar, lumbosacral 722.93
  - thoracic, thoracolumbar 722.92
- intestinal 569.9
  - functional NEC 564.9
    - congenital 751.3
    - postoperative 564.4
  - psychogenic 306.4
- introverted, of childhood and adolescence 313.22
- iron, metabolism 275.0
- isolated explosive 312.35
- joint NEC 719.90
  - ankle 719.97
  - elbow 719.92
  - foot 719.97
  - hand 719.94
  - hip 719.95
  - knee 719.96
  - multiple sites 719.99
  - pelvic region 719.95
  - psychogenic 306.0
  - shoulder (region) 719.91
  - specified site NEC 719.98
  - temporomandibular 524.60
    - specified NEC 524.69
  - wrist 719.93
- kidney 593.9
  - functional 588.9
    - specified NEC 588.8
- labyrinth, labyrinthine 386.9
  - specified type NEC 386.8
- lactation 676.9
- ligament 728.9
- ligamentous attachments, peripheral — see also Enthesopathy
  - spine 720.1
- limb NEC 729.9
  - psychogenic 306.0
- lipid
  - metabolism, congenital 272.9
  - storage 272.7
- lipoprotein deficiency (familial) 272.5
- low back NEC 724.9
  - psychogenic 306.0
- lumbosacral
  - plexus 353.1
  - root (nerve) NEC 353.4
- lymphoproliferative (chronic) NEC (M9970/1) 238.7
- male erectile 302.72
  - organic origin 607.84
- major depressive (see also Psychosis, affective) 296.2
  - recurrent episode 296.3
  - single episode 296.2
- manic (see also Psychosis, affective) 296.0
  - atypical 296.81
- meniscus NEC (see also Disorder, cartilage, articular) 718.0
- menopausal 627.9
  - specified NEC 627.8
- menstrual 626.9
  - psychogenic 306.52

Disorder—*continued*
  menstrual—*continued*
    specified NEC 626.8
  mental (nonpsychotic) 300.9
    affecting management of
        pregnancy, childbirth, or
        puerperium 648.4
    drug-induced 292.9
      hallucinogen persisting
          perception 292.89 ◆
      specified type NEC 292.89
    due to or associated with
        alcoholism 291.9
      drug consumption NEC
          292.9
        specified type NEC
            292.89
    induced by drug 292.9
      specified type NEC 292.89
    neurotic (*see also* Neurosis)
        300.9
    presenile 310.1
      psychotic NEC 290.10
    previous, affecting management
        of pregnancy V23.8
    psychoneurotic (*see also*
        Neurosis) 300.9
    psychotic (*see also* Psychosis)
        298.9
      senile 290.20
    specific, following organic brain
        damage 310.9
      cognitive or personality
          change of other type
          310.1
      frontal lobe syndrome 310.0
      postconcussional syndrome
          310.2
      specified type NEC 310.8
  metabolism NEC 277.9
    with
      abortion — *see* Abortion, by
          type with metabolic
          disorder
      ectopic pregnancy (*see also*
          categories 633.0-
          633.9) 639.4
      molar pregnancy (*see also*
          categories 630-632)
          639.4
    alkaptonuria 270.2
    amino acid (*see also* Disorder,
        amino acid) 270.9
      specified type NEC 270.8
    ammonia 270.6
    arginine 270.6
    argininosuccinic acid 270.6
    basal 794.7
    bilirubin 277.4
    calcium 275.4
    carbohydrate 271.9
      specified type NEC 271.8
    cholesterol 272.9
    citrulline 270.6
    copper 275.1
    corticosteroid 255.2
    cystine storage 270.0
    cystinuria 270.0
    fat 272.9
    following
      abortion 639.4
      ectopic or molar pregnancy
          639.4
    fructosemia 271.2
    fructosuria 271.2
    fucosidosis 271.8
    galactose-1-phosphate uridyl
        transferase 271.1
    glutamine 270.7
    glycine 270.7
    glycogen storage NEC 271.0
      hepatorenal 271.0
    hemochromatosis 275.0
    in labor and delivery 669.0
    iron 275.0
    lactose 271.3

Disorder—*continued*
  metabolism—*continued*
    lipid 272.9
      specified type NEC 272.8
      storage 272.7
    lipoprotein — *see also*
        Hyperlipemia deficiency
        (familial) 272.5
    lysine 270.7
    magnesium 275.2
    mannosidosis 271.8
    mineral 275.9
      specified type NEC 275.8
    mucopolysaccharide 277.5
    nitrogen 270.9
    ornithine 270.6
    oxalosis 271.8
    pentosuria 271.8
    phenylketonuria 270.1
    phosphate 275.3
    phosphorous 275.3
    plasma protein 273.9
      specified type NEC 273.8
    porphyrin 277.1
    purine 277.2
    pyrimidine 277.2
    serine 270.7
    sodium 276.9
    specified type NEC 277.8
    steroid 255.2
    threonine 270.7
    urea cycle 270.6
    xylose 271.8
  micturition NEC 788.69
    psychogenic 306.53
  misery and unhappiness, of
      childhood and adolescence
      313.1
  motor tic 307.20
    chronic 307.22
    transient, childhood 307.21
  movement NEC 333.90
    hysterical 300.11
    specified type NEC 333.99
    stereotypic 307.3 ◆
  mucopolysaccharide 277.5
  muscle 728.9
    psychogenic 306.0
    specified type NEC 728.3
  muscular attachments, peripheral
      — *see also* Enthesopathy
      spine 720.1
  musculoskeletal system NEC 729.9
    psychogenic 306.0
  myeloproliferative (chronic) NEC
      (M9960/1) 238.7
  myoneural 358.9
    due to lead 358.2
    specified type NEC 358.8
    toxic 358.2
  myotonic 359.2
  neck region NEC 723.9
  nerve 349.9
    abducens NEC 378.54
    accessory 352.4
    acoustic 388.5
    auditory 388.5
    auriculotemporal 350.8
    axillary 353.0
    cerebral — *see* Disorder, nerve,
        cranial
    cranial 352.9
      first 352.0
      second 377.49
      third
        partial 378.51
        total 378.52
      fourth 378.53
      fifth 350.9
      sixth 378.54
      seventh NEC 351.9
      eighth 388.5
      ninth 352.2
      tenth 352.3
      eleventh 352.4
      twelfth 352.5
      multiple 352.6

Disorder—*continued*
  nerve—*continued*
    entrapment — *see* Neuropathy,
        entrapment
    facial 351.9
      specified NEC 351.8
    femoral 355.2
    glossopharyngeal NEC 352.2
    hypoglossal 352.5
    iliohypogastric 355.79
    ilioinguinal 355.79
    intercostal 353.8
    lateral
      cutaneous of thigh 355.1
      popliteal 355.3
    lower limb NEC 355.8
    medial, popliteal 355.4
    median NEC 354.1
    obturator 355.79
    oculomotor
      partial 378.51
      total 378.52
    olfactory 352.0
    optic 377.49
      ischemic 377.41
      nutritional 377.33
      toxic 377.34
    peroneal 355.3
    phrenic 354.8
    plantar 355.6
    pneumogastric 352.3
    posterior tibial 355.5
    radial 354.3
    recurrent laryngeal 352.3
    root 353.9
      specified NEC 353.8
    saphenous 355.79
    sciatic NEC 355.0
    specified NEC 355.9
      lower limb 355.79
      upper limb 354.8
    spinal 355.9
    sympathetic NEC 337.9
    trigeminal 350.9
      specified NEC 350.8
    trochlear 378.53
    ulnar 354.2
    upper limb NEC 354.9
    vagus 352.3
  nervous system NEC 349.9
    autonomic (peripheral) (*see also*
        Neuropathy, peripheral,
        autonomic) 337.9
    cranial 352.9
    parasympathetic (*see also*
        Neuropathy, peripheral,
        autonomic) 337.9
    specified type NEC 349.89
    sympathetic (*see also*
        Neuropathy, peripheral,
        autonomic) 337.9
    vegetative (*see also* Neuropathy,
        peripheral, autonomic)
        337.9
  neurohypophysis NEC 253.6
  neurological NEC 781.9
    peripheral NEC 355.9
  neuromuscular NEC 358.9
    hereditary NEC 359.1
    specified NEC 358.8
    toxic 358.2
  neurotic 300.9
    specified type NEC 300.89
  neutrophil, polymorphonuclear
      (functional) 288.1
  obsessive-compulsive 300.3
  oppositional, childhood and
      adolescence 313.81
  optic
    chiasm 377.54
      associated with
        inflammatory disorders
            377.54
        neoplasm NEC 377.52
        pituitary 377.51
        pituitary disorders 377.51
        vascular disorders 377.53

Disorder—*continued*
  optic—*continued*
    nerve 377.49
    radiations 377.63
    tracts 377.63
  orbit 376.9
    specified NEC 376.89
  overanxious, of childhood and
      adolescence 313.0
  pancreas, internal secretion (other
      than diabetes mellitus) 251.9
    specified type NEC 251.8
  panic 300.01
    with agoraphobia 300.21 ◆
  papillary muscle NEC 429.81
  paranoid 297.9
    induced 297.3
    shared 297.3
  parathyroid 252.9
    specified type NEC 252.8
  paroxysmal, mixed 780.3
  pentose phosphate pathway with
      anemia 282.2
  personality 301.9
    affective 301.10
    aggressive 301.3
    amoral 301.7
    anancastic, anankastic 301.4
    antisocial 301.7
    asocial 301.7
    asthenic 301.6
    boderline 301.83 ◆
    compulsive 301.4
    cyclothymic 301.13
    dependent-passive 301.6
    dyssocial 301.7
    emotional instability 301.59
    epileptoid 301.3
    explosive 301.3
    following organic brain damage
        310.1
    histrionic 301.50
    hyperthymic 301.11
    hypomanic (chronic) 301.11
    hypothymic 301.12
    hysterical 301.50
    immature 301.89
    inadequate 301.6
    introverted 301.21
    labile 301.59
    moral deficiency 301.7
    obsessional 301.4
    obsessive (-compulsive) 301.4
    overconscientious 301.4
    paranoid 301.0
    passive (-dependent) 301.6
    passive-aggressive 301.84
    pathological NEC 301.9
    pseudosocial 301.7
    psychopathic 301.9
    schizoid 301.20
      introverted 301.21
      schizotypal 301.22
    schizotypal 301.22
    seductive 301.59
    type A 301.4
    unstable 301.59
  pervasive developmental,
      childhood-onset 299.8
  pigmentation, choroid (congenital)
      743.53
  pinna 380.30
    specified type NEC 380.39
  pituitary, thalamic 253.9
    anterior NEC 253.4
    iatrogenic 253.7
    postablative 253.7
    specified NEC 253.8
  pityriasis-like NEC 696.8
  platelets (blood) 287.1
  polymorphonuclear neutrophils
      (functional) 288.1
  porphyrin metabolism 277.1
  postmenopausal 627.9
    specified type NEC 627.8
  posttraumatic stress 309.81 ◆
    acute 308.3

Disorder—continued
  posttraumatic stress—continued
    brief 308.3
    chronic 309.81
  psoriatic-like NEC 696.8
  psychic, with diseases classified elsewhere 316
  psychogenic NEC (see also condition) 300.9
    allergic NEC
      respiratory 306.1
    anxiety 300.00
      atypical 300.00
      generalized 300.02
    appetite 307.50
    articulation, joint 306.0
    asthenic 300.5
    blood 306.8
    cardiovascular (system) 306.2
    compulsive 300.3
    cutaneous 306.3
    depressive 300.4
    digestive (system) 306.4
    dysmenorrheic 306.52
    dyspneic 306.1
    eczematous 306.3
    endocrine (system) 306.6
    eye 306.7
    feeding 307.59
    functional NEC 306.9
    gastric 306.4
    gastrointestinal (system) 306.4
    genitourinary (system) 306.50
    heart (function) (rhythm) 306.2
    hemic 306.8
    hyperventilatory 306.1
    hypochondriacal 300.7
    hysterical 300.10
    intestinal 306.4
    joint 306.0
    learning 315.2
    limb 306.0
    lymphatic (system) 306.8
    menstrual 306.52
    micturition 306.53
    monoplegic NEC 306.0
    motor 307.9
    muscle 306.0
    musculoskeletal 306.0
    neurocirculatory 306.2
    obsessive 300.3
    occupational 300.89
    organ or part of body NEC 306.9
    organs of special sense 306.7
    paralytic NEC 306.0
    phobic 300.20
    physical NEC 306.9
    pruritic 306.3
    rectal 306.4
    respiratory (system) 306.1
    rheumatic 306.0
    sexual (function) 302.70
      specified type NEC 302.79
    skin (allergic) (eczematous) (pruritic) 306.3
    sleep 307.40
      initiation or maintenance 307.41
        persistent 307.42
        transient 307.41
      specified type NEC 307.49
    specified part of body NEC 306.8
    stomach 306.4
  psychomotor NEC 307.9
    hysterical 300.11
  psychoneurotic (see also Neurosis) 300.9
    mixed NEC 300.89
  psychophysiologic (see also Disorder, psychosomatic) 306.9
  psychosexual identity (childhood) 302.6
    adult-life 302.85

Disorder—continued
  psychosomatic NEC 306.9
    allergic NEC
      respiratory 306.1
    articulation, joint 306.0
    cardiovascular (system) 306.2
    cutaneous 306.3
    digestive (system) 306.4
    dysmenorrheic 306.52
    dyspneic 306.1
    endocrine (system) 306.6
    eye 306.7
    gastric 306.4
    gastrointestinal (system) 306.4
    genitourinary (system) 306.50
    heart (functional) (rhythm) 306.2
    hyperventilatory 306.1
    intestinal 306.4
    joint 306.0
    limb 306.0
    lymphatic (system) 306.8
    menstrual 306.52
    micturition 306.53
    monoplegic NEC 306.0
    muscle 306.0
    musculoskeletal 306.0
    neurocirculatory 306.2
    organs of special sense 306.7
    paralytic NEC 306.0
    pruritic 306.3
    rectal 306.4
    respiratory (system) 306.1
    rheumatic 306.0
    sexual (function) 302.70
      specified type NEC 302.79
    skin 306.3
    specified part of body NEC 306.8
    stomach 306.4
  purine metabolism NEC 277.2
  pyrimidine metabolism NEC 277.2
  reactive attachment (of infancy or early childhood) 313.89 ◆
  reading, developmental 315.00
  reflex 796.1
  renal function, impaired 588.9
    specified type NEC 588.8
  renal transport NEC 588.8
  respiration, respiratory NEC 519.9
    due to
      aspiration of liquids or solids 508.9
      inhalation of fumes or vapors 506.9
    psychogenic 306.1
  retina 362.9
    specified type NEC 362.89
  sacroiliac joint NEC 724.6
  sacrum 724.6
  schizo-affective (see also Schizophrenia) 295.7
  schizoid, childhood or adolescence 313.22
  schizophreniform 295.4 ◆
  schizotypal personality 301.22
  secretion, thyrocalcitonin 246.0
  seizure 780.39
    recurrent 780.3
      epileptic — see Epilepsy
  sense of smell 781.1
    psychogenic 306.7
  separation anxiety 309.21 ◆
  sexual (see also Deviation, sexual) 302.9
    function, psychogenic 302.70
  shyness, of childhood and adolescence 313.21
  single complement (C-C) 279.8
  skin NEC 709.9
    fetus or newborn 778.9
      specified type 778.8
    psychogenic (allergic) (eczematous) (pruritic) 306.3
    specified type NEC 709.8
  vascular 709.1

Disorder—continued
  sleep 780.50
    with apnea — see Apnea, sleep
    circadian rhythm 307.45 ◆
    initiation or maintenance (see also Insomnia) 780.52
      nonorganic origin (transient) 307.41
      persistent 307.42
    nonorganic origin 307.40
      specified type NEC 307.49
    specified NEC 780.59
    social, of childhood and adolescence 313.22
    specified NEC 780.59
  soft tissue 729.9
  somatization 300.81
  somatoform 300.81
    atypical 300.7
  speech NEC 784.5
    nonorganic origin 307.9
  spine NEC 724.9
    ligamentous or muscular attachments, peripheral 720.1
  steroid metabolism NEC 255.2
  stomach (functional) (see also Disorder, gastric) 536.9
    psychogenic 306.4
  storage, iron 275.0
  stress (see also Reaction, stress, acute) 308.9
    posttraumatic
      acute 308.3
      brief 308.3
      chronic 309.81
  substitution 300.11
  suspected — see Observation
  synovium 727.9
  temperature regulation, fetus or newborn 778.4
  temporomandibular joint NEC 524.60
    specified NEC 524.69
  tendon 727.9
    shoulder region 726.10
  thoracic root (nerve) NEC 353.3
  thyrocalcitonin secretion 246.0
  thyroid (gland) NEC 246.9
    specified type NEC 246.8
  tic 307.20
    chronic (motor or vocal) 307.22 ◆
    motor-verbal 307.23
    organic origin 333.1
    transient of childhood 307.21
  tooth NEC 525.9
    development NEC 520.9
      specified type NEC 520.8
    eruption 520.6
      with abnormal position 524.3
    specified type NEC 525.8
  transport, carbohydrate 271.9
    specified type NEC 271.8
  tubular, phosphate-losing 588.0
  tympanic membrane 384.9
  unaggressive, unsocialized (see also Disturbance, conduct) 312.1
  undersocialized, unsocialized (see also Disturbance, conduct)
    aggressive (type) 312.0
    unaggressive (type) 312.1
  vision, visual NEC 368.9
    binocular NEC 368.30
    cortex 377.73
      associated with
        inflammatory disorders 377.73
        neoplasms 377.71
        vascular disorders 377.72
    pathway NEC 377.63
      associated with
        inflammatory disorders 377.63
        neoplasms 377.61
        vascular disorders 377.62

Disorder—continued
  wakefulness (see also Hypersomnia) 780.54
    nonorganic origin (transient) 307.43
    persistent 307.44
Disorganized globe 360.29
Displacement, displaced

> Note — For acquired displacement of bones, cartilage, joints, tendons, due to injury, see also Dislocation.
>
> Displacements at ages under one year should be considered congenital, provided there is no indication the condition was acquired after birth.

  acquired traumatic of bone, cartilage, joint, tendon NEC (without fracture) (see also Dislocation) 839.8
    with fracture — see Fracture, by site
  adrenal gland (congenital) 759.1
  appendix, retrocecal (congenital) 751.5
  auricle (congenital) 744.29
  bladder (acquired) 596.8
    congenital 753.8
  brachial plexus (congenital) 742.8
  brain stem, caudal 742.4
  canaliculus lacrimalis 743.65
  cardia, through esophageal hiatus 750.6
  cerebellum, caudal 742.4
  cervix (see also Malposition, uterus) 621.6
  colon (congenital) 751.4
  device, implant, or graft — see Complications, mechanical
  epithelium
    columnar of cervix 622.1
    cuboidal, beyond limits of external os (uterus) 752.49
  esophageal mucosa into cardia of stomach, congenital 750.4
  esophagus (acquired) 530.89
    congenital 750.4
  eyeball (acquired) (old) 376.36
    congenital 743.8
    current injury 871.3
    lateral 376.36
  fallopian tube (acquired) 620.4
    congenital 752.19
    opening (congenital) 752.19
  gallbladder (congenital) 751.69
  gastric mucosa 750.7
  into
    duodenum 750.7
    esophagus 750.7
    Meckel's diverticulum, congenital 750.7
  globe (acquired) (lateral) (old) 376.36
    current injury 871.3
  heart (congenital) 746.87
    acquired 429.89
  hymen (congenital) (upward) 752.49
  internal prothesis NEC — see Complications, mechanical
  intervertebral disc (with neuritis, radiculitis, sciatica, or other pain) 722.2
    with myelopathy 722.70
    cervical, cervicodorsal, cervicothoracic 722.0
      with myelopathy 722.71
    due to major trauma — see Dislocation, vertebra, cervical
    due to major trauma — see Dislocation, vertebra

Displacement, displaced—continued
intervertebral disc
lumbar, lumbosacral 722.10
with myelopathy 722.73
due to major trauma — see Dislocation, vertebra, lumbar
thoracic, thoracolumbar 722.11
with myelopathy 722.72
due to major trauma — see Dislocation, vertebra, thoracic
intrauterine device 996.32
kidney (acquired) 593.0
congenital 753.3
lacrimal apparatus or duct (congenital) 743.65
macula (congenital) 743.55
Meckel's diverticulum (congenital) 751.0
nail (congenital) 757.5
acquired 703.8
opening of Wharton's duct in mouth 750.26
organ or site, congenital NEC — see Malposition, congenital
ovary (acquired) 620.4
congenital 752.0
free in peritoneal cavity (congenital) 752.0
into hernial sac 620.4
oviduct (acquired) 620.4
congenital 752.19
parathyroid (gland) 252.8
parotid gland (congenital) 750.26
punctum lacrimale (congenital) 743.65
sacroiliac (congenital) (joint) 755.69
current injury — see Dislocation, sacroiliac
old 724.6
spine (congenital) 756.19
spleen, congenital 759.0
stomach (congenital) 750.7
acquired 537.89
subglenoid (closed) 831.01
sublingual duct (congenital) 750.26
teeth, tooth 524.3
tongue (congenital) (downward) 750.19
trachea (congenital) 748.3
ureter or ureteric opening or orifice (congenital) 753.4
uterine opening of oviducts or fallopian tubes 752.19
uterus, uterine (see also Malposition, uterus) 621.6
congenital 752.3
ventricular septum 746.89
with rudimentary ventricle 746.89
xyphoid bone (process) 738.3

Disproportion 653.9
affecting fetus or newborn 763.1
caused by
conjoined twins 653.7
contraction, pelvis (general) 653.1
inlet 653.2
midpelvic 653.8
midplane 653.8
outlet 653.3
fetal
ascites 653.7
hydrocephalus 653.6
hydrops 653.7
meningomyelocele 653.7
sacral teratoma 653.7
tumor 653.7
hydrocephalic fetus 653.6
pelvis, pelvic, abnormality (bony) NEC 653.0
unusually large fetus 653.5
causing obstructed labor 660.1

Disproportion—continued
cephalopelvic, normally formed fetus 653.4
causing obstructed labor 660.1
fetal NEC 653.5
causing obstructed labor 660.1
fetopelvic, normally formed fetus 653.4
causing obstructed labor 660.1
mixed maternal and fetal origin, normally formed fetus 653.4
pelvis, pelvic (bony) NEC 653.1
causing obstructed labor 660.1
specified type NEC 653.8

Disruption
cesarean wound 674.1
family V61.0
gastrointestinal anastomosis 997.4
ligament(s) — see also Sprain
knee
current injury — see Dislocation knee
old 717.89
capsular 717.85
collateral (medial) 717.82
lateral 717.81
cruciate (posterior) 717.84
anterior 717.83
specified site NEC 717.85
marital V61.1
involving divorce or estrangement V61.0
operation wound 998.3
organ transplant, anastomosis site — see Complications, transplant, organ, by site
ossicles, ossicular chain 385.23
traumatic — see Fracture, skull, base
parenchyma
liver (hepatic) — see Laceration, liver, major
spleen — see Laceration, spleen, parenchyma, massive
phase-shift, of 24-hour sleep-wake cycle 780.55
nonorganic origin 307.45
sleep-wake cycle (24-hour) 780.55
circadian rhythm 307.45 ◆
nonorganic origin 307.45
suture line (external) 998.3
internal 998.3
wound
cesarean operation 674.1
episiotomy 674.2
operation 998.3
cesarean 674.1
perineal (obstetric) 674.2
uterine 674.1

Disruptio uteri — see also Rupture, uterus
complicating delivery — see Delivery, complicated, rupture, uterus

Dissatisfaction with
employment V62.2
school environment V62.3

Dissecting — see condition

Dissection
aorta 441.00 ▼
abdominal 441.02
thoracic 441.01
thoracoabdominal 441.03 ▲
vascular 459.9
wound — see Wound, open, by site

Disseminated — see condition
Dissociated personality NEC 300.15

Dissociation
auriculoventricular or atrioventricular (any degree) (AV) 426.89
with heart block 426.0
interference 426.89

Dissociation—continued
isorhythmic 426.89
rhythm
atrioventricular (AV) 426.89
interference 426.89

Dissociative ▼
identity disorder 300.14
reaction NEC 300.14 ▲

Dissolution, vertebra (see also Osteoporosis) 733.00

Distention
abdomen (gaseous) 787.3
bladder 596.8
cecum 569.89
colon 569.89
gallbladder 575.8
gaseous (abdomen) 787.3
intestine 569.89
kidney 593.89
liver 573.9
seminal vesicle 608.89
stomach 536.8
acute 536.1
psychogenic 306.4
ureter 593.5
uterus 621.8

Distichia, distichiasis (eyelid) 743.63
Distoma hepaticum infestation 121.3

Distomiasis 121.9
bile passages 121.3
due to Clonorchis sinensis 121.1
hemic 120.9
hepatic (liver) 121.3
due to Clonorchis sinensis (clonorchiasis) 121.1
intestinal 121.4
liver 121.3
due to Clonorchis sinensis 121.1
lung 121.2
pulmonary 121.2

Distomolar (fourth molar) 520.1
causing crowding 524.3

Disto-occlusion 524.2

Distortion (congenital)
adrenal (gland) 759.1
ankle (joint) 755.69
anus 751.5
aorta 747.29
appendix 751.5
arm 755.59
artery (peripheral) NEC (see also Distortion, peripheral vascular system) 747.60
cerebral 747.81
coronary 746.85
pulmonary 747.3
retinal 743.58
umbilical 747.5
auditory canal 744.29
causing impairment of hearing 744.02
bile duct or passage 751.69
bladder 753.8
brain 742.4
bronchus 748.3
cecum 751.5
cervix (uteri) 752.49
chest (wall) 756.3
clavicle 755.51
clitoris 752.49
coccyx 756.19
colon 751.5
common duct 751.69
cornea 743.41
cricoid cartilage 748.3
cystic duct 751.69
duodenum 751.5
ear 744.29
auricle 744.29
causing impairment of hearing 744.02
causing impairment of hearing 744.09

Distortion—continued
ear—continued
external 744.29
causing impairment of hearing 744.02
inner 744.05
middle, except ossicles 744.03
ossicles 744.04
ossicles 744.04
endocrine (gland) NEC 759.2
epiglottis 748.3
Eustachian tube 744.24
eye 743.8
adnexa 743.69
face bone(s) 756.0
fallopian tube 752.19
femur 755.69
fibula 755.69
finger(s) 755.59
foot 755.67
gallbladder 751.69
genitalia, genital organ(s)
female 752.8
external 752.49
internal NEC 752.8
male 752.8
glottis 748.3
gyri 742.4
hand bone(s) 755.59
heart (auricle) (ventricle) 746.89
valve (cusp) 746.89
hepatic duct 751.69
humerus 755.59
hymen 752.49
ileum 751.5
intestine (large) (small) 751.5
with anomalous adhesions, fixation or malrotation 751.4
jaw NEC 524.8
jejunum 751.5
kidney 753.3
knee (joint) 755.64
labium (majus) (minus) 752.49
larynx 748.3
leg 755.69
lens 743.36
liver 751.69
lumbar spine 756.19
with disproportion (fetopelvic) 653.0
affecting fetus or newborn 763.1
causing obstructed labor 660.1
lumbosacral (joint) (region) 756.19
lung (fissures) (lobe) 748.69
nerve 742.8
nose 748.1
organ
of Corti 744.05
or site not listed — see Anomaly, specified type NEC
ossicles, ear 744.04
ovary 752.0
oviduct 752.19
pancreas 751.7
parathyroid (gland) 759.2
patella 755.64
peripheral vascular system NEC 747.60
gastrointestinal 747.61
lower limb 747.64
renal 747.62
spinal 747.82
upper limb 747.63
pituitary (gland) 759.2
radius 755.59
rectum 751.5
rib 756.3
sacroiliac joint 755.69
sacrum 756.19
scapula 755.59
shoulder girdle 755.59
site not listed — see Anomaly, specified type NEC

Distortion—continued
  skull bone(s) 756.0
    with
      anencephalus 740.0
      encephalocele 742.0
      hydrocephalus 742.3
        with spina bifida (see also
            Spina bifida) 741.0
      microcephalus 742.1
  spinal cord 742.59
  spine 756.19
  spleen 759.0
  sternum 756.3
  thorax (wall) 756.3
  thymus (gland) 759.2
  thyroid (gland) 759.2
    cartilage 748.3
  tibia 755.69
  toe(s) 755.66
  tongue 750.19
  trachea (cartilage) 748.3
  ulna 755.59
  ureter 753.4
    causing obstruction 753.2
  urethra 753.8
    causing obstruction 753.6
  uterus 752.3
  vagina 752.49
  vein (peripheral) NEC (see also
        Distortion, peripheral
        vascular system) 747.60
    great 747.49
    portal 747.49
    pulmonary 747.49
    vena cava (inferior) (superior)
        747.49
  vertebra 756.19
  visual NEC 368.15
    shape or size 368.14
  vulva 752.49
  wrist (bones) (joint) 755.59
Distress
  abdomen 789.0
  colon 789.0
  emotional V40.9
  epigastric 789.0
  fetal (syndrome) 768.4
    affecting management of
        pregnancy or childbirth
        656.3
    liveborn infant 768.4
      first noted
        before onset of labor
            768.2
        during labor or delivery
            768.3
    stillborn infant (death before
        onset of labor) 768.0
      death during labor 768.1
  gastrointestinal (functional) 536.9
    psychogenic 306.4
  intestinal (functional) NEC 564.9
    psychogenic 306.4
  intrauterine (see also Distress, fetal)
      768.4
  leg 729.5
  maternal 669.0
  mental V40.9
  respiratory 786.09
    acute (adult) 518.82
    adult syndrome (following
        shock, surgery, or trauma)
        518.5
      specified NEC 518.82
    fetus or newborn 770.8
    syndrome (idiopathic) (newborn)
        769
  stomach 536.9
    psychogenic 306.4
Distribution vessel, atypical NEC
    747.60
  coronary artery 746.85
  spinal 747.82
Districhiasis 704.2

Disturbance — see also Disease
  absorption NEC 579.9
    calcium 269.3
    carbohydrate 579.8
    fat 579.8
    protein 579.8
    specified type NEC 579.8
    vitamin (see also Deficiency,
        vitamin) 269.2
  acid-base equilibrium 276.9
  activity and attention, simple, with
      hyperkinesis 314.01
  amino acid (metabolic) (see also
        Disorder, amino acid) 270.9
    imidazole 270.5
    maple syrup (urine) disease
        270.3
    transport 270.0
  assimilation, food 579.9
  attention, simple 314.00
    with hyperactivity 314.01
  auditory, nerve, except deafness
      388.5
  behavior (see also Disturbance,
      conduct) 312.9
  blood clotting (hypoproteinemia)
      (mechanism) (see also
      Defect, coagulation) 286.9
  central nervous system NEC 349.9
  cerebral nerve NEC 352.9
  circulatory 459.9
  conduct 312.9

Note — Use the following fifth-
digit subclassification with
categories 312.0–312.2:

  0 unspecified
  1 mild
  2 moderate
  3 severe

    adjustment reaction 309.3
    adolescent onset type 312.82 ▼
    childhood onset type 312.81 ▲
    compulsive 312.30
      intermittent explosive
          disorder 312.34
      isolated explosive disorder
          312.35
      kleptomania 312.32
      pathological gambling
          312.31
      pyromania 312.33
    hyperkinetic 314.2
    intermittent explosive 312.34
    isolated explosive 312.35
    mixed with emotions 312.4
    socialized (type) 312.20
      aggressive 312.23
      unaggressive 312.21
    specified type NEC 312.89 ◆
    undersocialized, unsocialized
      aggressive (type) 312.0
      unaggressive (type) 312.1
  coordination 781.3
  cranial nerve NEC 352.9
  deep sensibility — see Disturbance,
      sensation
  digestive 536.9
    psychogenic 306.4
  electrolyte — see Imbalance,
      electrolyte
  emotions specific to childhood and
      adolescence 313.9
    with
      academic underachievement
          313.83
      anxiety and fearfulness 313.0
      elective mutism 313.23
      identity disorder 313.82
      jealousy 313.3
      misery and unhappiness
          313.1
      oppositional disorder 313.81
      overanxiousness 313.0
      sensitivity 313.21

Disturbance—continued
  emotions specific to childhood and
      adolescence—continued
    with—continued
      shyness 313.21
      social withdrawal 313.22
      withdrawal reaction 313.22
    involving relationship problems
        313.3
    mixed 313.89
    specified type NEC 313.89
  endocrine (gland) 259.9
    neonatal, transitory 775.9
      specified NEC 775.8
  equilibrium 780.4
  feeding (elderly) (infant) 783.3
    newborn 779.3
    nonorganic origin NEC 307.59
    psychogenic NEC 307.59
  fructose metabolism 271.2
  gait 781.2
    hysterical 300.11
  gastric (functional) 536.9
    motility 536.8
    psychogenic 306.4
    secretion 536.8
  gastrointestinal (functional) 536.9
    psychogenic 306.4
  habit, child 307.9
  hearing, except deafness 388.40
  heart, functional (conditions
      classifiable to 426, 427, 428)
    due to presence of (cardiac)
        prosthesis 429.4
    postoperative (immediate) 997.1
      long-term effect of cardiac
          surgery 429.4
    psychogenic 306.2
  hormone 259.9
  innervation uterus, sympathetic,
      parasympathetic 621.8
  keratinization NEC
    gingiva 523.1
    lip 528.5
    oral (mucosa) (soft tissue) 528.7
    tongue 528.7
  labyrinth, labyrinthine (vestibule)
      386.9
  learning, specific NEC 315.2
  memory (see also Amnesia) 780.9
    mild, following organic brain
        damage 310.1
  mental (see also Disorder, mental)
      300.9
    associated with diseases
        classified elsewhere 316
  metabolism (acquired) (congenital)
      (see also Disorder,
      metabolism) 277.9
    with
      abortion — see Abortion, by
          type, with metabolic
          disorder
      ectopic pregnancy (see also
          categories 633.0-
          633.9) 639.4
      molar pregnancy (see also
          categories 630-632)
          639.4
    amino acid (see also Disorder,
        amino acid) 270.9
      aromatic NEC 270.2
      branched-chain 270.3
      specified type NEC 270.8
      straight-chain NEC 270.7
      sulfur-bearing 270.4
      transport 270.0
    ammonia 270.6
    arginine 270.6
    argininosuccinic acid 270.6
    carbohydrate NEC 271.9
    cholesterol 272.7
    citrulline 270.6
    cystathionine 270.4
    fat 272.9
    following
      abortion 639.4

Disturbance—continued
  metabolism—continued
    following—continued
      ectopic or molar pregnancy
          639.4
    general 277.9
      carbohydrate 271.9
      iron 275.0
      phosphate 275.3
      sodium 276.9
    glutamine 270.7
    glycine 270.7
    histidine 270.5
    homocystine 270.4
    in labor or delivery 669.0
    iron 275.0
    isoleucine 270.3
    leucine 270.3
    lipoid 272.9
      specified type NEC 272.8
    lysine 270.7
    methionine 270.4
    neonatal, transitory 775.9
      specified type NEC 775.8
    nitrogen 788.9
    ornithine 270.6
    phosphate 275.3
    phosphatides 272.7
    serine 270.7
    sodium NEC 276.9
    threonine 270.7
    tryptophan 270.2
    tyrosine 270.2
    urea cycle 270.6
    valine 270.3
  motor 796.1
  nervous functional 799.2
  neuromuscular mechanism (eye)
      due to syphilis 094.84
  nutritional 269.9
    nail 703.8
  ocular motion 378.87
    psychogenic 306.7
  oculogyric 378.87
    psychogenic 306.7
  oculomotor NEC 378.87
    psychogenic 306.7
  olfactory nerve 781.1
  optic nerve NEC 377.49
  oral epithelium, including tongue
      528.7
  personality (pattern) (trait) (see also
      Disorder, personality) 301.9
    following organic brain damage
        310.1
  polyglandular 258.9
  psychomotor 307.9
  pupillary 379.49
  reflex 796.1
  rhythm, heart 427.9
    postoperative (immediate) 997.1
      long-term effect of cardiac
          surgery 429.4
    psychogenic 306.2
  salivary secretion 527.7
  sensation (cold) (heat) (localization)
      (tactile discrimination
      localization) (texture)
      (vibratory) NEC 782.0
    hysterical 300.11
    skin 782.0
    smell 781.1
    taste 781.1
  sensory (see also Disturbance,
      sensation) 782.0
    innervation 782.0
  situational (transient) (see also
      Reaction, adjustment) 309.9
    acute 308.3
  sleep 780.50
    with apnea — see Apnea, sleep
    initiation or maintenance (see
        also Insomnia) 780.52
      nonorganic origin 307.41
    nonorganic origin 307.40
      specified type NEC 307.49

Disturbance—continued
  sleep—continued
    specified NEC 780.59
      nonorganic origin 307.49
    wakefulness (see also
        Hypersomnia) 780.54
      nonorganic origin 307.43
  sociopathic 301.7
  speech NEC 784.5
    developmental 315.39
      associated with hyperkinesis
        314.1
    secondary to organic lesion
      784.5
  stomach (functional) (see also
      Disturbance, gastric) 536.9
  sympathetic (nerve) (see also
      Neuropathy, peripheral,
      autonomic) 337.9
  temperature sense 782.0
    hysterical 300.11
  tooth
    eruption 520.6
    formation 520.4
    structure, hereditary NEC 520.5
  touch (see also Disturbance,
      sensation) 782.0
  vascular 459.9
    arteriosclerotic — see
      Arteriosclerosis
  vasomotor 443.9
  vasospastic 443.9
  vestibular labyrinth 386.9
  vision, visual NEC 368.9
    psychophysical 368.16
    specified NEC 368.8
    subjective 368.10
  voice 784.40
  wakefulness (initiation or
      maintenance) (see also
      Hypersomnia) 780.54
    nonorganic origin 307.43
Disulfiduria, beta-mercaptolactate-cysteine 270.0
Disuse atrophy, bone 733.7
Ditthomska syndrome 307.81
Diuresis 788.42
Divers'
  palsy or paralysis 993.3
  squeeze 993.3
**Diverticula, diverticulosis,
    diverticulum** (acute) (multiple)
    (perforated) (ruptured) 562.10
  with diverticulitis 562.11
  aorta (Kommerell's) 747.21
  appendix (noninflammatory) 543.9
  bladder (acquired) (sphincter) 596.3
    congenital 753.8
  broad ligament 620.8
  bronchus (congenital) 748.3
    acquired 494
  calyx, calyceal (kidney) 593.89
  cardia (stomach) 537.1
  cecum 562.10
    with
      diverticulitis 562.11
        with hemorrhage 562.13
      hemorrhage 562.12
    congenital 751.5
  colon (acquired) 562.10
    with
      diverticulitis 562.11
        with hemorrhage 562.13
      hemorrhage 562.12
    congenital 751.5
  duodenum 562.00
    with
      diverticulitis 562.01
        with hemorrhage 562.03
      hemorrhage 562.02
    congenital 751.5
  epiphrenic (esophagus) 530.6
  esophagus (congenital) 750.4
    acquired 530.6
    epiphrenic 530.6
    pulsion 530.6

**Diverticula, diverticulosis,
    diverticulum**—continued
  esophagus—continued
    traction 530.6
    Zenker's 530.6
  Eustachian tube 381.89
  fallopian tube 620.8
  gallbladder (congenital) 751.69
  gastric 537.1
  heart (congenital) 746.89
  ileum 562.00
    with
      diverticulitis 562.01
        with hemorrhage 562.03
      hemorrhage 562.02
  intestine (large) 562.10
    with
      diverticulitis 562.11
        with hemorrhage 562.13
      hemorrhage 562.12
    congenital 751.5
    small 562.00
      with
        diverticulitis 562.01
          with hemorrhage
            562.03
        hemorrhage 562.02
      congenital 751.5
  jejunum 562.00
    with
      diverticulitis 562.01
        with hemorrhage 562.03
      hemorrhage 562.02
  kidney (calyx) (pelvis) 593.89
    with calculus 592.0
  Kommerell's 747.21
  laryngeal ventricle (congenital)
    748.3
  Meckel's (displaced) (hypertrophic)
    751.0
  midthoracic 530.6
  organ or site, congenital NEC —
    see Distortion
  pericardium (congenital) (cyst)
    746.89
    acquired (true) 423.8
  pharyngoesophageal (pulsion)
    530.6
  pharynx (congenital) 750.27
  pulsion (esophagus) 530.6
  rectosigmoid 562.10
    with
      diverticulitis 562.11
        with hemorrhage 562.13
      hemorrhage 562.12
    congenital 751.5
  rectum 562.10
    with
      diverticulitis 562.11
        with hemorrhage 562.13
      hemorrhage 562.12
  renal (calyces) (pelvis) 593.89
    with calculus 592.0
  Rokitansky's 530.6
  seminal vesicle 608.0
  sigmoid 562.10
    with
      diverticulitis 562.11
        with hemorrhage 562.13
      hemorrhage 562.12
    congenital 751.5
  small intestine 562.00
    with
      diverticulitis 562.01
        with hemorrhage 562.03
      hemorrhage 562.02
  stomach (cardia) (juxtacardia)
      (juxtapyloric) (acquired)
      537.1
    congenital 750.7
  subdiaphragmatic 530.6
  trachea (congenital) 748.3
    acquired 519.1
  traction (esophagus) 530.6
  ureter (acquired) 593.89
    congenital 753.4
  ureterovesical orifice 593.89

**Diverticula, diverticulosis,
    diverticulum**—continued
  urethra (acquired) 599.2
    congenital 753.8
  ventricle, left (congenital) 746.89
  vesical (urinary) 596.3
    congenital 753.8
  Zenker's (esophagus) 530.6
Diverticulitis (acute) (see also
    Diverticula) 562.11
  with hemorrhage 562.13
  bladder (urinary) 596.3
  cecum (perforated) 562.11
    with hemorrhage 562.13
  colon (perforated) 562.11
    with hemorrhage 562.13
  duodenum 562.01
    with hemorrhage 562.03
  esophagus 530.6
  ileum (perforated) 562.01
    with hemorrhage 562.03
  intestine (large) (perforated) 562.11
    with hemorrhage 562.13
    small 562.01
      with hemorrhage 562.03
  jejunum (perforated) 562.01
    with hemorrhage 562.03
  Meckel's (perforated) 751.0
  pharyngoesophageal 530.6
  rectosigmoid (perforated) 562.11
    with hemorrhage 562.13
  rectum 562.11
    with hemorrhage 562.13
  sigmoid (old) (perforated) 562.11
    with hemorrhage 562.13
  small intestine (perforated) 562.01
    with hemorrhage 562.03
  vesical (urinary) 596.3
Diverticulosis — see Diverticula
Division
  cervix uteri 622.8
    external os into two openings by
      frenum 752.49
    external (cervical) into two
      openings by frenum
      752.49
  glans penis 752.8
  hymen 752.49
  labia minora (congenital) 752.49
  ligament (partial or complete)
      (current) — see also Sprain,
      by site
    with open wound — see
      Wound, open, by site
  muscle (partial or complete)
      (current) — see also Sprain,
      by site
    with open wound — see
      Wound, open, by site
  nerve — see Injury, nerve, by site
  penis glans 752.8
  spinal cord — see Injury, spinal, by
    site
  vein 459.9
    traumatic — see Injury, vascular,
      by site
Divorce V61.0
Dix-Hallpike neurolabyrinthitis 386.12
Dizziness 780.4
  hysterical 300.11
  psychogenic 306.9
Doan-Wiseman syndrome (primary
  splenic neutropenia) 288.0
Dog bite — see Wound, open, by site
Döhle-Heller aortitis 093.1
**Döhle body-panmyelopathic
    syndrome** 288.2
Dolichocephaly, dolichocephalus
  754.0
Dolichocolon 751.5
Dolichostenomelia 759.82
Donohue's syndrome (leprechaunism)
  259.8

Donor
  blood V59.0
  bone V59.2
    marrow V59.3
  cornea V59.5
  heart V59.8
  kidney V59.4
  liver V59.8
  lung V59.8
  lymphocyte V59.8
  organ V59.9
    specified NEC V59.8
  potential, examination of V70.8
  skin V59.1
  specified organ or tissue NEC
    V59.8
  tissue V59.9
    specified type NEC V59.8
Donovanosis (granuloma venereum)
  099.2
DOPS (diffuse obstructive pulmonary
    syndrome) 496
Double
  albumin 273.8
  aortic arch 747.21
  auditory canal 744.29
  auricle (heart) 746.82
  bladder 753.8
  external (cervical) os 752.49
  kidney with double pelvis (renal)
    753.3
  larynx 748.3
  meatus urinarius 753.8
  monster 759.4
  organ or site NEC — see Accessory
  orifice
    heart valve NEC 746.89
    pulmonary 746.09
  outlet, right ventricle 745.11
  pelvis (renal) with double ureter
    753.4
  penis 752.8
  tongue 750.13
  ureter (one or both sides) 753.4
    with double pelvis (renal) 753.4
  urethra 753.8
  urinary meatus 753.8
  uterus (any degree) 752.2
    with doubling of cervix and
      vagina 752.2
    in pregnancy or childbirth 654.0
      affecting fetus or newborn
        763.8
  vagina 752.49
    with doubling of cervix and
      uterus 752.2
  vision 368.2
  vocal cords 748.3
  vulva 752.49
  whammy (syndrome) 360.81
Douglas' pouch, cul-de-sac — see
  condition
Down's disease or syndrome
  (mongolism) 758.0
Down-growth, epithelial (anterior
  chamber) 364.61
Dracontiasis 125.7
Dracunculiasis 125.7
Drancunculosis 125.7
Drainage
  abscess (spontaneous) — see
    Abscess
  anomalous pulmonary veins to
    hepatic veins or right atrium
    747.41
  stump (amputation) (surgical)
    997.62
  suprapubic, bladder 596.8
Dream state, hysterical 300.13
Drepanocytic anemia (see also
  Disease, sickle cell) 282.60
Dresbach's syndrome (elliptocytosis)
  282.1
Dreschlera (infection) 118
  hawaiiensis 117.8

Dressler's syndrome (postmyocardial infarction) 411.0
Dribbling (post-void) 788.35
Drift, ulnar 736.09
Drinking (alcohol) — *see also* Alcoholism
  excessive, to excess NEC (*see also* Abuse, drugs, nondependent) 305.0
    bouts, periodic 305.0
    continual 303.9
    episodic 305.0
    habitual 303.9
    periodic 305.0
Drip, postnasal (chronic) — *see* Sinusitis
Drivers' license examination V70.3
Droop, Cooper's 611.8
Drop
  finger 736.29
  foot 736.79
  toe 735.8
  wrist 736.05
Dropped
  dead 798.1
  heart beats 426.6
Dropsy, dropsical (*see also* Edema) 782.3
  abdomen 789.5
  amnion (*see also* Hydramnios) 657
  brain — *see* Hydrocephalus
  cardiac (*see also* Failure, heart, congestive) 428.0
  cardiorenal (*see also* Hypertension, cardiorenal) 404.90
  chest 511.9
  fetus or newborn 778.0
    due to isoimmunization 773.3
  gangrenous (*see also* Gangrene) 785.4
  heart (*see also* Failure, heart, congestive) 428.0
  hepatic — *see* Cirrhosis, liver
  infantile — *see* Hydrops, fetalis
  kidney (*see also* Nephrosis) 581.9
  liver — *see* Cirrhosis, liver
  lung 514
  malarial (*see also* Malaria) 084.9
  neonatorum — *see* Hydrops, fetalis
  nephritic 581.9
  newborn — *see* Hydrops, fetalis
  nutritional 269.9
  ovary 620.8
  pericardium (*see also* Pericarditis) 423.9
  renal (*see also* Nephrosis) 581.9
  uremic — *see* Uremia
Drowned, drowning 994.1
  lung 518.5
Drowsiness 780.09
Drug — *see also* condition
  addiction (*see also* listing under Dependence) 304.9
  adverse effect NEC, correct substance properly administered 995.2
  dependence (*see also* listing under Dependence) 304.9
  habit (*see also* listing under Dependence) 304.9
  overdose — *see* Table of drugs and chemicals
  poisoning — *see* Table of drugs and chemicals
  therapy (maintenance) status NEC V58.1
  wrong substance given or taken in error — *see* Table of drugs and chemicals
Drunkenness (*see also* Abuse, drugs, nondependent) 305.0
  acute in alcoholism (*see also* Alcoholism) 303.0
  chronic (*see also* Alcoholism) 303.9
  pathologic 291.4

Drunkenness—*continued*
  simple (acute) 305.0
    in alcoholism 303.0
  sleep 307.47
Drusen
  optic disc or papilla 377.21
  retina (colloid) (hyaloid degeneration) 362.57
    hereditary 362.77
Drusenfieber 075
Dry, dryness — *see also* condition
  eye 375.15
    syndrome 375.15
  larynx 478.79
  mouth 527.7
  nose 478.1
  skin syndrome 701.1
  socket (teeth) 526.5
  throat 478.29
Duane's retraction syndrome 378.71
Duane-Stilling-Türk syndrome (ocular retraction syndrome) 378.71
Dubin-Johnson disease or syndrome 277.4
Dubini's disease (electric chorea) 049.8
Dubois' abscess or disease 090.5
Duchenne's
  disease 094.0
    locomotor ataxia 094.0
    muscular dystrophy 359.1
    pseudohypertrophy, muscles 359.1
  paralysis 335.22
  syndrome 335.22
Duchenne-Aran myelopathic, muscular atrophy (nonprogressive) (progressive) 335.21
Duchenne-Griesinger disease 359.1
Ducrey's
  bacillus 099.0
  chancre 099.0
  disease (chancroid) 099.0
Duct, ductus — *see* condition
Duengero 061
Duhring's disease (dermatitis herpetiformis) 694.0
Dukes (-Filatov) **disease** 057.8
Dullness
  cardiac (decreased) (increased) 785.3
Dumb ague (*see also* Malaria) 084.6
Dumbness (*see also* Aphasia) 784.3
Dumdum fever 085.0
Dumping syndrome (postgastrectomy) 564.2
  nonsurgical 536.8
Duodenitis (nonspecific) (peptic) 535.60
  with hemorrhage 535.61
  due to
    Strongyloides stercoralis 127.2
Duodenocholangitis 575.8
Duodenum, duodenal — *see* condition
Duplay's disease, periarthritis, or syndrome 726.2
Duplex — *see also* Accessory
  kidney 753.3
  placenta — *see* Placenta, abnormal
  uterus 752.2
Duplication — *see also* Accessory
  anus 751.5
  aortic arch 747.21
  appendix 751.5
  biliary duct (any) 751.69
  bladder 753.8
  cecum 751.5
    and appendix 751.5
  clitoris 752.49
  cystic duct 751.69
  digestive organs 751.8

Duplication—*continued*
  duodenum 751.5
  esophagus 750.4
  fallopian tube 752.19
  frontonasal process 756.0
  gallbladder 751.69
  ileum 751.5
  intestine (large) (small) 751.5
  jejunum 751.5
  kidney 753.3
  liver 751.69
  nose 748.1
  pancreas 751.7
  penis 752.8
  respiratory organs NEC 748.9
  salivary duct 750.22
  spinal cord (incomplete) 742.51
  stomach 750.7
  ureter 753.4
  vagina 752.49
  vas deferens 752.8
  vocal cords 748.3
Dupré's disease or syndrome (meningism) 781.6
Dupuytren's
  contraction 728.6
  disease (muscle contracture) 728.6
  fracture (closed) 824.4
    ankle (closed) 824.4
      open 824.5
    fibula (closed) 824.4
      open 824.5
    radius (closed) 813.42
      open 813.52
  muscle contracture 728.6
Durand-Nicolas-Favre disease (climatic bubo) 099.1
Duroziez's disease (congenital mitral stenosis) 746.5
Dust
  conjunctivitis 372.05
  reticulation (occupational) 504
Dutton's
  disease (trypanosomiasis) 086.9
  relapsing fever (West African) 087.1
Dwarf, dwarfism 259.4
  with infantilism (hypophyseal) 253.3
  achondroplastic 756.4
  Amsterdam 759.89
  bird-headed 759.89
  congenital 259.4
  constitutional 259.4
  hypophyseal 253.3
  infantile 259.4
  Levi type 253.3
  Lorain-Levi (pituitary) 253.3
  Lorain type (pituitary) 253.3
  metatropic 756.4
  nephrotic-glycosuric, with hypophosphatemic rickets 270.0
  nutritional 263.2
  ovarian 758.6
  pancreatic 577.8
  pituitary 253.3
  polydystrophic 277.5
  primordial 253.3
  psychosocial 259.4
  renal 588.0
    with hypertension — *see* Hypertension, kidney
  Russell's (uterine dwarfism and craniofacial dysostosis) 759.89
Dyke-Young anemia or syndrome (acquired macrocytic hemolytic anemia) (secondary) (symptomatic) 283.9
Dynia abnormality (*see also* Defect, coagulation) 286.9
Dysacousis 388.40
Dysadrenocortism 255.9
  hyperfunction 255.3

Dysadrenocortism—*continued*
  hypofunction 255.4
Dysarthria 784.5
Dysautonomia (*see also* Neuropathy, peripheral, autonomic) 337.9
  familial 742.8
Dysbarism 993.3
Dysbasia 719.7
  angiosclerotica intermittens 443.9
    due to atherosclerosis 440.21
  hysterical 300.11
  lordotica (progressiva) 333.6
  nonorganic origin 307.9
  psychogenic 307.9
Dysbetalipoproteinemia (familial) 272.2
Dyscalculia 315.1
Dyschezia (*see also* Constipation) 564.0
Dyschondroplasia (with hemangiomata) 756.4
  Voorhoeve's 756.4
Dyschondrosteosis 756.59
Dyschromia 709.00
Dyscollagenosis 710.9
Dyscoria 743.41
Dyscraniopyophalangy 759.89
Dyscrasia
  blood 289.9
    with antepartum hemorrhage 641.3
    fetus or newborn NEC 776.9
    hemorrhage, subungual 287.8
    puerperal, postpartum 666.3
  ovary 256.8
  plasma cell 273.9
  pluriglandular 258.9
  polyglandular 258.9
Dysdiadochokinesia 781.3
Dysectasia, vesical neck 596.8
Dysendocrinism 259.9
Dysentery, dysenteric (bilious) (catarrhal) (diarrhea) (epidemic) (gangrenous) (hemorrhagic) (infectious) (sporadic) (tropical) (ulcerative) 009.0
  abscess, liver (*see also* Abscess, amebic) 006.3
  amebic (*see also* Amebiasis) 006.9
    with abscess — *see* Abscess, amebic
    acute 006.0
    carrier (suspected) of V02.2
    chronic 006.1
  arthritis (*see also* Arthritis, due to, dysentery) 009.0 [711.3]
    bacillary 004.9 [711.3]
  asylum 004.9
  bacillary 004.9
    arthritis 004.9 [711.3]
    Boyd 004.2
    Flexner 004.1
    Schmitz (-Stutzer) 004.0
    Shiga 004.0
    Shigella 004.9
      group A 004.0
      group B 004.1
      group C 004.2
      group D 004.3
      specified type NEC 004.8
    Sonne 004.3
    specified type NEC 004.8
  bacterium 004.9
  balantidial 007.0
  Balantidium coli 007.0
  Boyd's 004.2
  Chilomastix 007.8
  Chinese 004.9
  choleriform 001.1
  coccidial 007.2
  Dientamoeba fragilis 007.8
  due to specified organism NEC — *see* Enteritis, due to, by organism

Dysentery, dysenteric—continued
    Embadomonas 007.8
    Endolimax nana — see Dysentery, amebic
    Entamoba, entamebic — see Dysentery, amebic
    Flexner's 004.1
    Flexner-Boyd 004.2
    giardial 007.1
    Giardia lamblia 007.1
    Hiss-Russell 004.1
    lamblia 007.1
    leishmanial 085.0
    malarial (see also Malaria) 084.6
    metazoal 127.9
    Monilia 112.89
    protozoal NEC 007.9
    Russell's 004.8
    salmonella 003.0
    schistosomal 120.1
    Schmitz (-Stutzer) 004.0
    Shiga 004.0
    Shigella NEC (see also Dysentery, bacillary) 004.9
        boydii 004.2
        dysenteriae 004.0
            Schmitz 004.0
            Shiga 004.0
        flexneri 004.1
        Group A 004.0
        Group B 004.1
        Group C 004.2
        Group D 004.3
        Schmitz 004.0
        Shiga 004.0
        Sonnei 004.3
    Sonne 004.3
    strongyloidiasis 127.2
    trichomonal 007.3
    tuberculous (see also Tuberculosis) 014.8
    viral (see also Enteritis, viral) 008.8

Dysequilibrium 780.4

Dysesthesia 782.0
    hysterical 300.11

Dysfibrinogenemia (congenital) (see also Defect, coagulation) 286.3

Dysfunction
    adrenal (cortical) 255.9
        hyperfunction 255.3
        hypofunction 255.4
    associated with sleep stages or arousal from sleep 780.56
        nonorganic origin 307.47
    bladder NEC 596.59
    bleeding, uterus 626.8
    brain, minimal (see also Hyperkinesia) 314.9
    cerebral 348.3
    colon 564.9
        psychogenic 306.4
    colostomy or enterostomy 569.6
    cystic duct 575.8
    diastolic 429.9
        with heart failure — see Failure, heart
        due to
            cardiomyopathy — see Cardiomyopathy
            hypertension — see Hypertension, heart
    endocrine NEC 259.9
    endometrium 621.8
    enteric stoma 569.6
    enterostomy 569.6
    Eustachian tube 381.81
    gallbladder 575.8
    gastrointestinal 536.9
    gland, glandular NEC 259.9
    heart 427.9
        postoperative (immediate) 997.1
            long-term effect of cardiac surgery 429.4
    hemoglobin 288.8
    hepatic 573.9
    hepatocellular NEC 573.9

Dysfunction—continued
    hypophysis 253.9
        hyperfunction 253.1
        hypofunction 253.2
        posterior lobe 253.6
            hypofunction 253.5
    kidney (see also Disease, renal) 593.9
    labyrinthine 386.50
        specified NEC 386.58
    liver 573.9
        constitutional 277.4
    minimal brain (child) (see also Hyperkinesia) 314.9
    ovary, ovarian 256.9
        hyperfunction 256.1
            estrogen 256.0
        hypofunction 256.3
            postablative 256.2
        postablative 256.2
        specified NEC 256.8
    papillary muscle 429.81
        with myocardial infarction 410.8
    parathyroid 252.8
        hyperfunction 252.0
        hypofunction 252.1
    pineal gland 259.8
    pituitary (gland) 253.9
        hyperfunction 253.1
        hypofunction 253.2
        posterior 253.6
            hypofunction 253.5
    placental — see Placenta, insufficiency
    platelets (blood) 287.1
    polyglandular 258.9
        specified NEC 258.8
    psychosexual 302.70
        with
            dyspareunia (functional) (psychogenic) 302.76
            frigidity 302.72
            impotence 302.72 ◆
            inhibition
                orgasm
                    female 302.73
                    male 302.74
                sexual
                    desire 302.71
                    excitement 302.72
            premature ejaculation 302.75
            sexual aversion 302.79 ◆
            specified disorder NEC 302.79
            vaginismus 306.51 ◆
    pylorus 537.9
    rectum 564.9
        psychogenic 306.4
    segmental (see also Dysfunction, somatic) 739.9
    senile 797
    sinoatrial node 427.81
    somatic 739.9
        abdomen 739.9
        acromioclavicular 739.7
        cervical 739.1
        cervicothoracic 739.1
        costochondral 739.8
        costovertebral 739.8
        extremities
            lower 739.6
            upper 739.7
        head 739.0
        hip 739.5
        lumbar, lumbosacral 739.3
        occipitocervical 739.0
        pelvic 739.5
        pubic 739.5
        rib cage 739.8
        sacral 739.4
        sacrococcygeal 739.4
        sacroiliac 739.4
        specified site NEC 739.9
        sternochondral 739.8
        sternoclavicular 739.7

Dysfunction—continued
    somatic—continued
        temporomandibular 739.0
        thoracic, thoracolumbar 739.2
    stomach 536.9
        psychogenic 306.4
    suprarenal 255.9
        hyperfunction 255.3
        hypofunction 255.4
    symbolic NEC 784.60
        specified type NEC 784.69
    temporomandibular (joint) (joint-pain-syndrome) NEC 524.60
        specified NEC 524.69
    testicular 257.9
        hyperfunction 257.0
        hypofunction 257.2
        specified type NEC 257.8
    thymus 254.9
    thyroid 246.9
        complicating pregnancy, childbirth or puerperium 648.1
        hyperfunction — see Hyperthyroidism
        hypofunction — see Hypothyroidism
    uterus, complicating delivery 661.9
        affecting fetus or newborn 763.7
        hypertonic 661.4
        hypotonic 661.2
            primary 661.0
            secondary 661.1
    velopharyngeal (acquired) 528.9
        congenital 750.29
    ventricular 429.9
        with congestive heart failure (see also Failure, heart, congestive) 428.0
        due to
            cardiomyopathy — see Cardiomyopathy
            hypertension — see Hypertension, heart
    vesicourethral NEC 596.59
    vestibular 386.50
        specified type NEC 386.58

Dysgammaglobulinemia 279.06

Dysgenesis
    gonadal (due to chromosomal anomaly) 758.6
        pure 752.7
    kidney(s) 753.0
    ovarian 758.6
    renal 753.0
    reticular 279.2
    seminiferous tubules 758.6
    tidal platelet 287.3

Dysgerminoma (M9060/3)
    specified site — see Neoplasm, by site, malignant
    unspecified site
        female 183.0
        male 186.9

Dysgeusia 781.1

Dysgraphia 781.3

Dyshidrosis 705.81

Dysidrosis 705.81

Dysinsulinism 251.8

Dyskaryotic cervical smear 795.0

Dyskeratosis (see also Keratosis) 701.1
    bullosa hereditaria 757.39
    cervix 622.1
    congenital 757.39
    follicularis 757.39
        vitamin A deficiency 264.8
    gingiva 523.8
    oral soft tissue NEC 528.7
    tongue 528.7
    uterus NEC 621.8

Dyskinesia 781.3
    biliary 575.8
    esophagus 530.5
    hysterical 300.11
    intestinal 564.8

Dyskinesia—continued
    nonorganic origin 307.9
    orofacial 333.82
    psychogenic 307.9
    tardive (oral) 333.82

Dyslalia 784.5
    developmental 315.39

Dyslexia 784.61
    developmental 315.02
    secondary to organic lesion 784.61

Dysmaturity (see also Immaturity) 765.1
    lung 770.4
    pulmonary 770.4

Dysmenorrhea (essential) (exfoliative) (functional) (intrinsic) (membranous) (primary) (secondary) 625.3
    psychogenic 306.52

Dysmetria 781.3

Dysmorodystrophia mesodermalis congenita 759.82

Dysnomia 784.3

Dysorexia 783.0
    hysterical 300.11

Dysostosis
    cleidocranial, cleidocranialis 755.59
    craniofacial 756.0
    Fairbank's (idiopathic familial generalized osteophytosis) 756.50
    mandibularis 756.0
    mandibulofacial, incomplete 756.0
    multiplex 277.5
    orodigitofacial 759.89

Dyspareunia (female) 625.0
    male 608.89
    psychogenic 302.76

Dyspepsia (allergic) (congenital) (fermentative) (flatulent) (functional) (gastric) (gastrointestinal) (neurogenic) (occupational) (reflex) 536.8
    acid 536.8
    atonic 536.3 ◆
        psychogenic 306.4
    diarrhea 558.9
        psychogenic 306.4
    intestinal 564.8
        psychogenic 306.4
    nervous 306.4
    neurotic 306.4
    psychogenic 306.4

Dysphagia 787.2
    functional 300.11
    hysterical 300.11
    nervous 300.11
    psychogenic 306.4
    sideropenic 280.8
    spastica 530.5

Dysphagocytosis, congenital 288.1

Dysphasia 784.5

Dysphonia 784.49
    clericorum 784.49
    functional 300.11
    hysterical 300.11
    psychogenic 306.1
    spastica 478.79

Dyspigmentation — see also Pigmentation
    eyelid (acquired) 374.52

Dyspituitarism 253.9
    hyperfunction 253.1
    hypofunction 253.2
    posterior lobe 253.6

Dysplasia — see also Anomaly
    artery
        fibromuscular NEC 447.8
            carotid 447.8
            renal 447.3
    bladder 596.8
    bone (fibrous) NEC 733.29
        diaphyseal, progressive 756.59

Dysplasia — INDEX TO DISEASES — Eberth's disease

Dysplasia—continued
  bone—continued
    jaw 526.89
    monostotic 733.29
    polyostotic 756.54
    solitary 733.29
  brain 742.9
  bronchopulmonary, fetus or newborn 770.7
  cervix (uteri) 622.1
    cervical intraepithelial neoplasia III [CIN III] 233.1
    CIN III 233.1
  chondroectodermal 756.55
  chondromatose 756.4
  craniocarpotarsal 759.89
  craniometaphyseal 756.89
  dentinal 520.5
  diaphyseal, progressive 756.59
  ectodermal (anhidrotic) (Bason) (Clouston's) (congenital) (Feinmesser) (hereditary) (hidrotic) (Marshall) (Robinson's) 757.31
  epiphysealis 756.9
    multiplex 756.56
    punctata 756.59
  epiphysis 756.9
    multiple 756.56
  epithelial
    epiglottis 478.79
    uterine cervix 622.1
  erythroid NEC 289.8
  eye (see also Microphthalmos) 743.10
  familial metaphyseal 756.89
  fibromuscular, artery NEC 447.8
    carotid 447.8
    renal 447.3
  fibrous
    bone NEC 733.29
    diaphyseal, progressive 756.59
    jaw 526.89
    monostotic 733.29
    polyostotic 756.54
    solitary 733.29
  hip (congenital) 755.63
    with dislocation (see also Dislocation, hip, congenital) 754.30
  hypohidrotic ectodermal 757.31
  joint 755.8
  kidney 753.15
  leg 755.69
  linguofacialis 759.89
  lung 748.5
  macular 743.55
  mammary (benign) (gland) 610.9
    cystic 610.1
    specified type NEC 610.8
  metaphyseal 756.9
    familial 756.89
  monostotic fibrous 733.29
  muscle 756.89
  myeloid NEC 289.8
  nervous system (general) 742.9
  neuroectodermal 759.6
  oculoauriculovertebral 756.0
  oculodentodigital 759.89
  olfactogenital 253.4
  osteo-onycho-arthro (hereditary) 756.89
  periosteum 733.99
  polyostotic fibrous 756.54
  progressive diaphyseal 756.59
  renal 753.15
  renofacialis 753.0
  retinal NEC 743.56
  retrolental 362.21
  spinal cord 742.9
  thymic, with immunodeficiency 279.2
  vagina 623.0
  vocal cord 478.5
Dyspnea (nocturnal) (paroxysmal) 786.09

Dyspnea—continued
  asthmatic (bronchial) (see also Asthma) 493.9
    with bronchitis (see also Asthma) 493.9
      chronic 491.20
        with acute exacerbation 491.21
  cardiac (see also Failure, ventricular, left) 428.1
  cardiac (see also Failure, ventricular, left) 428.1
  functional 300.11
  hyperventilation 786.01
  hysterical 300.11
  Monday morning 504
  newborn 770.8
  psychogenic 306.1
  uremic — see Uremia
Dyspraxia 781.3
  syndrome 315.4
Dysproteinemia 273.8
  transient with copper deficiency 281.4
Dysprothrombinemia (constitutional) (see also Defect, coagulation) 286.3
Dysrhythmia
  cardiac 427.9
    postoperative (immediate) 997.1
      long-term effect of cardiac surgery 429.4
    specified type NEC 427.89
  cerebral or cortical 348.3
Dyssecretosis, mucoserous 710.2
Dyssocial reaction, without manifest psychiatric disorder
  adolescent V71.02
  adult V71.01
  child V71.02
Dyssomnia NEC 780.56
  nonorganic origin 307.47
Dyssplenism 289.4
Dyssynergia
  biliary (see also Disease, biliary) 576.8
  cerebellaris myoclonica 334.2
  detrusor sphincter (bladder) 596.55
  ventricular 429.89
Dystasia, hereditary areflexic 334.3
Dysthymia 300.4
Dysthymic disorder 300.4
Dysthyroidism 246.9
Dystocia 660.9
  affecting fetus or newborn 763.1
  cervical 661.0
    affecting fetus or newborn 763.7
  contraction ring 661.4
    affecting fetus or newborn 763.7
  fetal 660.9
    abnormal size 653.5
      affecting fetus or newborn 763.1
    deformity 653.7
  maternal 660.9
    affecting fetus or newborn 763.1
  positional 660.0
    affecting fetus or newborn 763.1
  shoulder (girdle) 660.4
    affecting fetus or newborn 763.1
  uterine NEC 661.4
    affecting fetus or newborn 763.7
Dystonia
  deformans progressiva 333.6
  due to drugs 333.7 ◆
  lenticularis 333.6
  musculorum deformans 333.6
  torsion (idiopathic) 333.6
    fragments (of) 333.89
    symptomatic 333.7
Dystonic
  movements 781.0
Dystopia kidney 753.3
Dystrophy, dystrophia 783.9
  adiposogenital 253.8

Dystrophy, dystrophic—continued
  asphyxiating thoracic 756.4
  Becker's type 359.1
  brevicollis 756.16
  Bruch's membrane 362.77
  cervical (sympathetic) NEC 337.0
  chondro-osseous with punctate epiphyseal dysplasia 756.59
  choroid (hereditary) 363.50
    central (areolar) (partial) 363.53
      total (gyrate) 363.54
    circinate 363.53
    circumpapillary (partial) 363.51
      total 363.52
    diffuse
      partial 363.56
      total 363.57
    generalized
      partial 363.56
      total 363.57
    gyrate
      central 363.54
      generalized 363.57
    helicoid 363.52
    peripapillary — see Dystrophy, choroid, circumpapillary
    serpiginous 363.54
  cornea (hereditary) 371.50
    anterior NEC 371.52
    Cogan's 371.52
    combined 371.57
    crystalline 371.56
    endothelial (Fuchs') 371.57
    epithelial 371.50
      juvenile 371.51
      microscopic cystic 371.52
    granular 371.53
    lattice 371.54
    macular 371.55
    marginal (Terrien's) 371.48
    Meesman's 371.51
    microscopic cystic (epithelial) 371.52
    nodular, Salzmann's 371.46
    polymorphous 371.58
    posterior NEC 371.58
    ring-like 371.52
    Salzmann's nodular 371.46
    stromal NEC 371.56
  dermatochondrocorneal 371.50
  Duchenne's 359.1
  due to malnutrition 263.9
  Erb's 359.1
  familial
    hyperplastic periosteal 756.59
    osseous 277.5
  foveal 362.77
  Fuchs', cornea 371.57
  Gowers' muscular 359.1
  hair 704.2
  hereditary, progressive muscular 359.1
  hypogenital, with diabetic tendency 759.81
  Landouzy-Déjérine 359.1
  Leyden-Möbius 359.1
  mesodermalis congenita 759.82
  muscular 359.1
    congenital (hereditary) 359.0
      myotonic 359.2
    distal 359.1
    Duchenne's 359.1
    Erb's 359.1
    fascioscapulohumeral 359.1
    Gowers' 359.1
    hereditary (progressive) 359.1
    Landouzy-Déjérine 359.1
    limb-girdle 359.1
    myotonic 359.2
    progressive (hereditary) 359.1
      Charcot-Marie-Tooth 356.1
    pseudohypertrophic (infantile) 359.1
  myocardium, myocardial (see also Degeneration, myocardial) 429.1
  myotonic 359.2

Dystrophy, dystrophic—continued
  myotonica 359.2
  nail 703.8
    congenital 757.5
  neurovascular (traumatic) (see also Neuropathy, peripheral, autonomic) 337.9
  nutritional 263.9
  ocular 359.1
  oculocerebrorenal 270.8
  oculopharyngeal 359.1
  ovarian 620.8
  papillary (and pigmentary) 701.1
  pelvicrural atrophic 359.1
  pigmentary (see also Acanthosis) 701.2
  pituitary (gland) 253.8
  polyglandular 258.8
  posttraumatic sympathetic — see Dystrophy, sympathetic
  progressive ophthalmoplegic 359.1
  retina, retinal (hereditary) 362.70
    albipunctate 362.74
    Bruch's membrane 362.77
    cone, progressive 362.75
    hyaline 362.77
    in
      Bassen-Kornzweig syndrome 272.5 [362.72]
      cerebroretinal lipidosis 330.1 [362.71]
      Refsum's disease 356.3 [362.72]
      systemic lipidosis 272.7 [362.71]
    juvenile (Stargardt's) 362.75
    pigmentary 362.74
    pigment epithelium 362.76
    progressive cone (-rod) 362.75
    pseudoinflammatory foveal 362.77
    rod, progressive 362.75
    sensory 362.75
    vitelliform 362.76
  Salzmann's nodular 371.46
  scapuloperoneal 359.1
  skin NEC 709.9
  sympathetic (posttraumatic) (reflex) 337.20
    lower limb 337.22
    specified NEC 337.29
    upper limb 337.21
  tapetoretinal NEC 362.74
  thoracic asphyxiating 756.4
  unguium 703.8
    congenital 757.5
  vitreoretinal (primary) 362.73
    secondary 362.66
  vulva 624.0
Dysuria 788.1
  psychogenic 306.53

E

Eales' disease (syndrome) 362.18
Ear — see also condition
  ache 388.70
    otogenic 388.71
    referred 388.72
  lop 744.29
  piercing V50.3
  swimmers' acute 380.12
  tank 380.12
  tropical 111.8 [380.15]
  wax 380.4
Earache 388.70
  otogenic 388.71
  referred 388.72
Eaton-Lambert syndrome (see also Neoplasm, by site, malignant) 199.1 [358.1]
Eberth's disease (typhoid fever) 002.0

Ebstein's
  anomaly or syndrome (downward displacement, tricuspid valve into right ventricle) 746.2
  disease (diabetes) 250.4 [581.81]
Eccentro-osteochondrodysplasia 277.5
Ecchondroma (M9210/0) — see Neoplasm, bone, benign
Ecchondrosis (M9210/1) 238.0
Ecchordosis physaliphora 756.0
Ecchymosis (multiple) 459.89
  conjunctiva 372.72
  eye (traumatic) 921.0
  eyelids (traumatic) 921.1
  newborn 772.6
  spontaneous 782.7
  traumatic — see Contusion
Echinococciasis — see Echinococcus
Echinococcosis — see Echinococcus
Echinococcus (infection) 122.9
  granulosus 122.4
    liver 122.0
    lung 122.1
    orbit 122.3 [376.13]
    specified site NEC 122.3
    thyroid 122.2
  liver NEC 122.8
    granulosus 122.0
    multilocularis 122.5
  lung NEC 122.9
    granulosus 122.1
    multilocularis 122.6
  multilocularis 122.7
    liver 122.5
    specified site NEC 122.6
  orbit 122.9 [376.13]
    granulosus 122.3 [376.13]
    multilocularis 122.6 [376.13]
  specified site NEC 122.9
    granulosus 122.3
    multilocularis 122.6 [376.13]
  thyroid NEC 122.9
    granulosus 122.2
    multilocularis 122.6
Echinorhynchiasis 127.7
Echinostomiasis 121.8
Echolalia 784.69
ECHO virus infection NEC 079.1
Eclampsia, eclamptic (coma) (convulsions) (delirium) 780.3
  female, child-bearing age NEC — see Eclampsia, pregnancy
  gravidarum — see Eclampsia, pregnancy
  male 780.3
  not associated with pregnancy or childbirth 780.3
  pregnancy, childbirth, or puerperium 642.6
    with pre-existing hypertension 642.7
    affecting fetus or newborn 760.0
  uremic 586
Eclipse blindness (total) 363.31
Economic circumstance affecting care V60.9
  specified type NEC V60.8
Economo's disease (encephalitis lethargica) 049.8
Ectasia, ectasis
  aorta (see also Aneurysm, aorta) 441.9
    ruptured 441.5
  breast 610.4
  capillary 448.9
  cornea (marginal) (postinfectional) 371.71
  duct (mammary) 610.4
  kidney 593.89
  mammary duct (gland) 610.4
  papillary 448.9

Ectasia, ectasis—continued
  renal 593.89
  salivary gland (duct) 527.8
  scar, cornea 371.71
  sclera 379.11
Ecthyma 686.8
  contagiosum 051.2
  gangrenosum 686.0
  infectiosum 051.2
Ectocardia 746.87
Ectodermal dysplasia, congenital 757.31
Ectodermosis erosiva pluriorificialis 695.1
Ectopic, ectopia (congenital) 759.89
  abdominal viscera 751.8
    due to defect in anterior abdominal wall 756.7
  ACTH syndrome 255.0
  adrenal gland 759.1
  anus 751.5
  auricular beats 427.61
  beats 427.60
  bladder 753.5
  bone and cartilage in lung 748.69
  brain 742.4
  breast tissue 757.6
  cardiac 746.87
  cerebral 742.4
  cordis 746.87
  endometrium 617.9
  gallbladder 751.69
  gastric mucosa 750.7
  gestation — see Pregnancy, ectopic
  heart 746.87
  hormone secretion NEC 259.3
  hyperparathyroidism 259.3
  kidney (crossed) (intrathoracic) (pelvis) 753.3
    in pregnancy or childbirth 654.4
      causing obstructed labor 660.2
  lens 743.37
  lentis 743.37
  mole — see Pregnancy, ectopic
  organ or site NEC — see Malposition, congenital
  ovary 752.0
  pancreas, pancreatic tissue 751.7
  pregnancy — see Pregnancy, ectopic
  pupil 364.75
  renal 753.3
  sebaceous glands of mouth 750.26
  secretion
    ACTH 255.0
    adrenal hormone 259.3
    adrenalin 259.3
    adrenocorticotropin 255.0
    antidiuretic hormone (ADH) 259.3
    epinephrine 259.3
    hormone NEC 259.3
    norepinephrine 259.3
    pituitary (posterior) 259.3
  spleen 759.0
  testis 752.5
  thyroid 759.2
  ureter 753.4
  ventricular beats 427.69
  vesicae 753.5
Ectrodactyly 755.4
  finger (see also Absence, finger, congenital) 755.29
  toe (see also Absence, toe, congenital) 755.39
Ectromelia 755.4
  lower limb 755.30
  upper limb 755.20

Ectropion 374.10
  anus 569.49
  cervix 622.0
    with mention of cervicitis 616.0
  cicatricial 374.14
  congenital 743.62
  eyelid 374.10
    cicatricial 374.14
    congenital 743.62
    mechanical 374.12
    paralytic 374.12
    senile 374.11
    spastic 374.13
  iris (pigment epithelium) 364.54
  lip (congenital) 750.26
    acquired 528.5
  mechanical 374.12
  paralytic 374.12
  rectum 569.49
  senile 374.11
  spastic 374.13
  urethra 599.84
  uvea 364.54
Eczema (acute) (allergic) (chronic) (erythematous) (fissum) (occupational) (rubrum) (squamous) 692.9
  asteatotic 706.8
  atopic 691.8
  contact NEC 692.9
  dermatitis NEC 692.9
  due to specified cause — see Dermatitis, due to
  dyshidrotic 705.81
  external ear 380.22
  flexural 691.8
  gouty 274.89
  herpeticum 054.0
  hypertrophicum 701.8
  hypostatic — see Varicose, vein
  impetiginous 684
  infantile (acute) (chronic) (due to any substance) (intertriginous) (seborrheic) 691.8
  intertriginous NEC 692.9
    infantile 691.8
  intrinsic 691.8
  lichenified NEC 692.9
  marginatum 110.3
  nummular 692.9
  pustular 686.8
  seborrheic 690
    infantile 691.8
  solare 692.72
  stasis (lower extremity) 454.1
    ulcerated 454.2
  vaccination, vaccinatum 999.0
  varicose (lower extremity) — see Varicose, vein
  verrucosum callosum 698.3
Eczematoid, exudative 691.8
Eddowes' syndrome (brittle bone and blue sclera) 756.51
Edema, edematous 782.3
  with nephritis (see also Nephrosis) 581.9
  allergic 995.1
  angioneurotic (allergic) (any site) (with urticaria) 995.1
    hereditary 277.6
  angiospastic 443.9
  Berlin's (traumatic) 921.3
  brain 348.5
    due to birth injury 767.8
    fetus or newborn 767.8
  cardiac (see also Failure, heart, congestive) 428.0
  cardiovascular (see also Failure, heart, congestive) 428.0
  cerebral — see Edema, brain
  cerebrospinal vessel — see Edema, brain
  cervix (acute) (uteri) 622.8
    puerperal, postpartum 674.8

Edema, edematous—continued
  chronic hereditary 757.0
  circumscribed, acute 995.1
    hereditary 277.6
  complicating pregnancy (gestational) 646.1
    with hypertension — see Toxemia, of pregnancy
  conjunctiva 372.73
  connective tissue 782.3
  cornea 371.20
    due to contact lenses 371.24
    idiopathic 371.21
    secondary 371.22
  due to
    lymphatic obstruction — see Edema, lymphatic
    salt retention 276.0
  epiglottis — see Edema, glottis
  essential, acute 995.1
    hereditary 277.6
  extremities, lower — see Edema, legs
  eyelid NEC 374.82
  familial, hereditary (legs) 757.0
  famine 262
  fetus or newborn 778.5
  genital organs
    female 629.8
    male 608.86
  gestational 646.1
    with hypertension — see Toxemia, of pregnancy
  glottis, glottic, glottides (obstructive) (passive) 478.6
    allergic 995.1
      hereditary 277.6
    due to external agent — see Condition, respiratory, acute, due to specified agent
  heart (see also Failure, heart, congestive) 428.0
    newborn 779.8
  heat 992.7
  hereditary (legs) 757.0
  inanition 262
  infectious 782.3
  intracranial 348.5
    due to injury at birth 767.8
  iris 364.8
  joint (see also Effusion, joint) 719.0
  larynx (see also Edema, glottis) 478.6
  legs 782.3
    due to venous obstruction 459.2
    hereditary 757.0
  localized 782.3
    due to venous obstruction 459.2
    lower extremity 459.2
  lower extremities — see Edema, legs
  lung 514
    acute 518.4
      with heart disease or failure (see also Failure, ventricular, left) 428.1
      congestive 428.0
    chemical (due to fumes or vapors) 506.1
    due to
      external agent(s) NEC 508.9
      specified NEC 508.8
    fumes and vapors (chemical) (inhalation) 506.1
    radiation 508.0
    chemical (acute) 506.1
      chronic 506.4

Edema, edematous—continued
  lung—continued
    chronic 514
      chemical (due to fumes or vapors) 506.4
      due to
        external agent(s) NEC 508.9
          specified NEC 508.8
        fumes or vapors (chemical) (inhalation) 506.4
        radiation 508.1
    due to
      external agent 508.9
        specified NEC 508.8
      high altitude 993.2
      near drowning 994.1
    postoperative 518.4
    terminal 514
  lymphatic 457.1
    due to mastectomy operation 457.0
  macula 362.83
    diabetic 250.5 [362.83] ◆
  malignant (see also Gangrene, gas) 040.0
  Milroy's 757.0
  nasopharynx 478.25
  neonatorum 778.5
  nutritional (newborn) 262
    with dyspigmentation, skin and hair 260
  optic disc or nerve — see Papilledema
  orbit 376.33
    circulatory 459.89
  palate (soft) (hard) 528.9
  pancrease 577.8
  penis 607.83
  periodic 995.1
    hereditary 277.6
  pharynx 478.25
  pitting 782.3
  pulmonary — see Edema, lung
  Quincke's 995.1
    hereditary 277.6
  renal (see also Nephrosis) 581.9
  retina (localized) (macular) (perepheral) 362.83
    diabetic 250.5 [362.83] ◆
  salt 276.0
  scrotum 608.86
  seminal vesicle 608.86
  spermatic cord 608.86
  spinal cord 336.1
  starvation 262
  subconjunctival 372.73
  subglottic (see also Edema, glottis) 478.6
  supraglottic (see also Edema, glottis) 478.6
  testis 608.86
  toxic NEC 782.3
  traumatic NEC 782.3
  tunica vaginalis 608.86
  vas deferens 608.86
  vocal cord — see Edema, glottis
  vulva (acute) 624.8
Edentia (complete) (partial) (see also Absence, tooth) 520.0
  causing malocclusion 524.3
  congenital (deficiency of tooth buds) 520.0
  due to accident, extraction, or local periodontal disease 525.1
Edsall's disease 992.2
Educational handicap V62.3
Edwards' syndrome 758.2
Effect, adverse NEC
  abnormal gravitation (G) forces or states 994.9
  air pressure — see Effect, adverse, atmospheric pressure

Effect, adverse—continued
  altitude (high) — see Effect, adverse, high altitude
  anesthetic
    in labor and delivery NEC 668.9
      affecting fetus or newborn 763.5
  antitoxin — see Complications, vaccination
  atmospheric pressure 993.9
    due to explosion 993.4
    high 993.3
    low — see Effect, adverse, high altitude
    specified effect NEC 993.8
  biological, correct substance properly administered (see also Effect, adverse, drug) 995.2
  blood (derivatives) (serum) (transfusion) — see Complications, transfusion
  chemical substance NEC 989.9
    specified — see Table of drugs and chemicals
  cobalt, radioactive (see also Effect, adverse, radioactive substance) 990
  cold (temperature) (weather) 991.9
    chilblains 991.5
    frostbite — see Frostbite
    specified effect NEC 991.8
  drugs and medicinals NEC 995.2
    correct substance properly administered 995.2
    overdose or wrong substance given or taken 977.9
    specified drug — see Table of drugs and chemicals
  electric current (shock) 994.8
    burn — see Burn, by site
  electricity (electrocution) (shock) 994.8
    burn — see Burn, by site
  exertion (excessive) 994.5
  exposure 994.9
    exhaustion 994.4
  external cause NEC 994.9
  fallout (radioactive) NEC 990
  fluoroscopy NEC 990
  foodstuffs
    allergic reaction (see also Allergy, food) 693.1
    anaphylactic shock due to food NEC 995.60
    noxious 988.9
      specified type NEC (see also Poisoning, by name of noxious foodstuff) 988.8
  gases, fumes, or vapors — see Table of drugs and chemicals
  glue (airplane) sniffing 304.6
  heat — see Heat
  high altitude NEC 993.2
    anoxia 993.2
    on
      ears 993.0
      sinuses 993.1
    polycythemia 289.0
  hot weather — see Heat
  hunger 994.2
  immersion, foot 991.4
  immunization — see Complications, vaccination
  immunological agents — see Complications, vaccination
  implantation (removable) of isotope or radium NEC 990
  infrared (radiation) (rays) NEC 990
    burn — see Burn, by site
    dermatitis or eczema 692.82

Effect, adverse—continued
  infusion — see Complications, infusion
  ingestion or injection of isotope (therapeutic) NEC 990
  irradiation NEC (see also Effect, adverse, radiation) 990
  isotope (radioactive) NEC 990
  lack of care (child) (infant) (newborn) 995.5
    specified person NEC 995.81
  lightning 994.0
    burn — see Burn, by site
  Lirugin — see Complications, vaccination
  medicinal substance, correct, properly administered (see also Effect, adverse, drugs) 995.2
  mesothorium NEC 990
  motion 994.6
  noise, inner ear 388.10
  overheated places — see Heat
  polonium NEC 990
  psychosocial, of work environment V62.1
  radiation (diagnostic) (fallout) (infrared) (natural source) (therapeutic) (tracer) (ultraviolet) (x-ray) NEC 990
    with pulmonary manifestations
      acute 508.0
      chronic 508.1
    dermatitis or eczema 692.82
      due to sun NEC (see also Dermatitis, due to, sun) 692.70
    fibrosis of lungs 508.1
    maternal with suspected damage to fetus affecting management of pregnancy 655.6
    pneumonitis 508.0
  radioactive substance NEC 990
    dermatitis or eczema 692.82
  radioactivity NEC 990
  radiotherapy NEC 990
    dermatitis or eczema 692.82
  radium NEC 990
  reduced temperature 991.9
    frostbite — see Frostbite
    immersion, foot (hand) 991.4
    specified effect NEC 991.8
  roentgenography NEC 990
  roentgenoscopy NEC 990
  roentgen rays NEC 990
  serum (prophylactic) (therapeutic) NEC 999.5
  specified NEC 995.89
    external cause NEC 994.9
  strangulation 994.7
  submersion 994.1
  teletherapy NEC 990
  thirst 994.3
  transfusion — see Complications, transfusion
  ultraviolet (radiation) (rays) NEC 990
    burn — see also Burn, by site from sun 692.71
    dermatitis or eczema 692.82
      due to sun NEC (see also Dermatitis, due to, sun) 692.70
  uranium NEC 990
  vaccine (any) — see Complications, vaccination
  weightlessness 994.9
  whole blood — see also Complications, transfusion
    overdose or wrong substance given (see also Table of drugs and chemicals) 964.7
  working environment V62.1
  x-rays NEC 990
    dermatitis or eczema 692.82

Effects, late — see Late, effect (of)
Effluvium, telogen 704.02
Effort
  intolerance 306.2
  syndrome (aviators) (psychogenic) 306.2
Effusion
  amniotic fluid (see also Rupture, membranes, premature) 658.1
  brain (serous) 348.5
  bronchial (see also Bronchitis) 490
  cerebral 348.5
  cerebrospinal (see also Meningitis) 322.9
    vessel 348.5
  chest — see Effusion, pleura
  intracranial 348.5
  joint 719.00
    ankle 719.07
    elbow 719.02
    foot 719.07
    hand 719.04
    hip 719.05
    knee 719.06
    multiple sites 719.09
    pelvic region 719.05
    shoulder (region) 719.01
    specified site NEC 719.08
    wrist 719.03
  meninges (see also Meningitis) 322.9
  pericardium, pericardial (see also Pericarditis) 423.9
    acute 420.90
  peritoneal (chronic) 568.82
  pleura, pleurisy, pleuritic, pleuropericardial 511.9
    bacterial, nontuberculous 511.1
    fetus or newborn 511.9
    malignant 197.2
    nontuberculous 511.9
      bacterial 511.1
      pneumococcal 511.1
      staphylococcal 511.1
      streptococcal 511.1
    tuberculous (see also Tuberculosis, pleura) 012.0
      primary progressive 010.1
  pulmonary — see Effusion, pleura
  spinal (see also Meningitis) 322.9
  thorax, thoracic — see Effusion, pleura
Eggshell nails 703.8
  congenital 757.5
Ego-dystonic
  homosexuality 302.0
  lesbianism 302.0
Egyptian splenomegaly 120.1
Ehlers-Danlos syndrome 756.83
Eichstedt's disease (pityriasis versicolor) 111.0
Eisenmenger's complex or syndrome (ventricular septal defect) 745.4
Ejaculation, semen
  painful 608.89
    psychogenic 306.59
  premature 302.75
Ekbom syndrome (restless legs) 333.99
Ekman's syndrome (brittle bones and blue sclera) 756.51
Elastic skin 756.83
  acquired 701.8
Elastofibroma (M8820/0) — see Neoplasm, connective tissue, benign
Elastoidosis
  cutanea nodularis 701.8
  cutis cystica et comedonica 701.8

Elastoma 757.39
- juvenile 757.39
- Miescher's (elastosis perforans serpiginosa) 701.1

Elastomyofibrosis 425.3

Elastosis 701.8
- atrophicans 701.8
- perforans serpiginosa 701.1
- reactive perforating 701.1
- senilis 701.8
- solar (actinic) 692.74

Elbow — see condition

Electric
- current, electricity, effects (concussion) (fatal) (nonfatal) (shock) 994.8
  - burn — see Burn, by site
- feet (foot) syndrome 266.2

Electrocution 994.8

Electrolyte imbalance 276.9
- with
  - abortion — see Abortion, by type with metabolic disorder
  - ectopic pregnancy (see also categories 633.0-633.9) 639.4
  - hyperemesis gravidarum (before 22 completed weeks gestation) 643.1
  - molar pregnancy (see also categories 630-632) 639.4
- following
  - abortion 639.4
  - ectopic or molar pregnancy 639.4

Elephantiasis (nonfilarial) 457.1
- arabicum (see also Infestation, filarial) 125.9
- congenita hereditaria 757.0
- congenital (any site) 757.0
- due to
  - Brugia (malayi) 125.1
  - mastectomy operation 457.0
  - Wuchereria (bancrofti) 125.0
    - malayi 125.1
- eyelid 374.83
- filarial (see also Infestation, filarial) 125.9
- filariensis (see also Infestation, filarial) 125.9
- gingival 523.8
- glandular 457.1
- graecorum 030.9
- lymphangiectatic 457.1
- lymphatic vessel 457.1
  - due to mastectomy operation 457.0
- neuromatosa 237.71
- postmastectomy 457.0
- scrotum 457.1
- streptococcal 457.1
- surgical 997.9
  - postmastectomy 457.0
- telangiectodes 457.1
- vulva (nonfilarial) 624.8

Elevated — see Elevation

Elevation
- 17-ketosteroids 791.9
- acid phosphatase 790.5
- alkaline phosphatase 790.5
- amylase 790.5
- antibody titers 795.79 ◆
- basal metabolic rate (BMR) 794.7
- blood pressure (see also Hypertension) 401.9
  - reading (incidental) (isolated) (nonspecific), no diagnosis or hypertension 796.2
- body temperature (of unknown origin) (see also Pyrexia) 780.6
- conjugate, eye 378.81

Elevation—continued
- diaphragm, congenital 756.6
- immunoglobulin level 795.79 ◆
- indolacetic acid 791.9
- lactic acid dehydrogenase (LDH) level 790.4
- lipase 790.5
- prostate specific antigen (PSA) 790.93
- renin 790.99
  - in hypertension (see also Hypertension, renovascular) 405.91
- Rh titer 999.7
- scapula, congenital 755.52
- sedimentation rate 790.1
- SGOT 790.4
- SGPT 790.4
- transaminase 790.4
- vanillylmandelic acid 791.9
- venous pressure 459.89
- VMA 791.9

Elliptocytosis (congenital) (hereditary) 282.1
- Hb-C (disease) 282.7
- hemoglobin disease 282.7
- sickle-cell (disease) 282.60
- trait 282.5

Ellis-van Creveld disease or syndrome (chondroectodermal dysplasia) 756.55

Ellison-Zollinger syndrome (gastric hypersecretion with pancreatic islet cell tumor) 251.5

Elongation, elongated (congenital) — see also Distortion
- bone 756.9
- cervix (uteri) 752.49
  - acquired 622.6
  - hypertrophic 622.6
- colon 751.5
- common bile duct 751.69
- cystic duct 751.69
- frenulum, penis 752.8
- labia minora, acquired 624.8
- ligamentum patellae 756.89
- petiolus (epiglottidis) 748.3
- styloid bone (process) 733.99
- tooth, teeth 520.2
- uvula 750.26
  - acquired 528.9

Elschnig bodies or pearls 366.51

El Tor cholera 001.1

Emaciation (due to malnutrition) 261

Emancipation disorder 309.22

Embadomoniasis 007.8

Embarrassment heart, cardiac — see Disease, heart

Embedded tooth, teeth 520.6
- with abnormal position (same or adjacent tooth) 524.3
- root only 525.3

Embolic — see conditon

Embolism (septic) 444.9
- with
  - abortion — see Abortion, by type, with embolism
  - ectopic pregnancy (see also categories 633.0-633.9) 639.6
  - molar pregnancy (see also categories 630-632) 639.6
- air (any site) 958.0
  - with
    - abortion — see Abortion, by type, with embolism
    - ectopic pregnancy (see also categories 633.0-633.9) 639.6
    - molar pregnancy (see also categories 630-632) 639.6

Embolism—continued
- air—continued
  - due to implanted device — see Complications, due to (presence of) any device, implant, or graft classified to 996.0-996.5 NEC
  - following
    - abortion 639.6
    - ectopic or molar pregnancy 639.6
  - infusion, perfusion, or transfusion 999.1
  - in pregnancy, childbirth, or puerperium 673.0
  - traumatic 958.0
- amniotic fluid (pulmonary) 673.1
  - with
    - abortion — see Abortion, by type, with embolism
    - ectopic pregnancy (see also categories 633.0-633.9) 639.6
    - molar pregnancy (see also categories 630-632) 639.6
  - following
    - abortion 639.6
    - ectopic or molar pregnancy 639.6
- aorta, aortic 444.1
  - abdominal 444.0
  - bifurcation 444.0
  - saddle 444.0
  - thoracic 444.1
- artery 444.9
  - auditory, internal 433.8
  - basilar (see also Occlusion, artery, basilar) 433.0
  - bladder 444.89
  - carotid (common) (internal) (see also Occlusion, artery, carotid) 433.1
  - cerebellar (anterior inferior) (posterior inferior) (superior) 433.8
  - cerebral (see also Embolism, brain) 434.1
  - choroidal (anterior) 433.8
  - communicating posterior 433.8
  - coronary (see also Infarct, myocardium) 410.9
    - without myocardial infarction 411.81
  - extremity 444.22
    - lower 444.22
    - upper 444.21
  - hypophyseal 433.8
  - mesenteric (with gangrene) 557.0
  - ophthalmic (see also Occlusion, retina) 362.30
  - peripheral 444.22
  - pontine 433.8
  - precerebral NEC — see Occlusion, artery, precerebral
  - pulmonary — see Embolism, pulmonary
  - renal 593.81
  - retinal (see also Occlusion, retina) 362.30
  - specified site NEC 444.89
  - vertebral (see also Occlusion, artery, vertebral) 433.2
- auditory, internal 433.8
- basilar (artery) (see also Occlusion, artery, basilar) 433.0
- birth, mother — see Embolism, obstetrical

Embolism—continued
- blood-clot
  - with
    - abortion — see Abortion, by type, with embolism
    - ectopic pregnancy (see also categories 633.0-633.9) 639.6
    - molar pregnancy (see also categories 630-632) 639.6
  - following
    - abortion 639.6
    - ectopic or molar pregnancy 639.6
  - in pregnancy, childbirth, or puerperium 673.2
- brain 434.1
  - with
    - abortion — see Abortion, by type, with embolism
    - ectopic pregnancy (see also categories 633.0-633.9) 639.6
    - molar pregnancy (see also categories 630-632) 639.6
  - following
    - abortion 639.6
    - ectopic or molar pregnancy 639.6
  - late effect — see category 438
  - puerperal, postpartum, childbirth 674.0
- capillary 448.9
- cardiac (see also Infarct, myocardium) 410.9
- carotid (artery) (common) (internal) (see also Occlusion, artery, carotid) 433.1
- cavernous sinus (venous) — see Embolism, intracranial venous sinus
- cerebral (see also Embolism, brain) 434.1
- choroidal (anterior) (artery) 433.8
- coronary (artery or vein) (systemic) (see also Infarct, myocardium) 410.9
  - without myocardial infarction 411.81
- due to (presence of) any device, implant, or graft classifiable to 996.0-996.5 — see Complications, due to (presence of) any device, implant, or graft classified to 996.0-996.5 NEC
- encephalomalacia (see also Embolism, brain) 434.1
- extremities 444.22
  - lower 444.22
  - upper 444.21
- eye 362.30
- fat (cerebral) (pulmonary) (systemic) 958.1
  - with
    - abortion — see Abortion, by type, with embolism
    - ectopic pregnancy (see also categories 633.0-633.9) 639.6
    - molar pregnancy (see also categories 630-632) 639.6
  - complicating delivery or puerperium 673.8
  - following
    - abortion 639.6
    - ectopic or molar pregnancy 639.6
  - in pregnancy, childbirth, or the puerperium 673.8

Embolism—*continued*
  femoral (artery) 444.22
    vein 453.8
  following
    abortion 639.6
    ectopic or molar pregnancy 639.6
    infusion, perfusion, or transfusion
      air 999.1
      thrombus 999.2
  heart (fatty) (*see also* Infarct, myocardium) 410.9
  hepatic (vein) 453.0
  iliac (artery) 444.81
  iliofemoral 444.81
  in pregnancy, childbirth, or puerperium (pulmonary) — *see* Embolism, obstetrical
  intestine (artery) (vein) (with gangrene) 557.0
  intracranial (*see also* Embolism, brain) 434.1
    venous sinus (any) 325
      late effect — *see* category 326
      nonpyogenic 437.6
      in pregnancy or puerperium 671.5
  kidney (artery) 593.81
  lateral sinus (venous) — *see* Embolism, intracranial venous sinus
  longitudinal sinus (venous) — *see* Embolism, intracranial venous sinus
  lower extremity 444.22
  lung (massive) — *see* Embolism, pulmonary
  meninges (*see also* Embolism, brain) 434.1
  mesenteric (artery) (with gangrene) 557.0
  multiple NEC 444.9
  obstetrical (pulmonary) 673.2
    air 673.0
    amniotic fluid (pulmonary) 673.1
    blood-clot 673.2
    cardiac 674.8
    fat 673.8
    heart 674.8
    pyemic 673.3
    septic 673.3
    specified NEC 674.8
  ophthalmic (*see also* Occlusion, retina) 362.30
  paradoxical NEC 444.9
  penis 607.82
  peripheral arteries NEC 444.22
    lower 444.22
    upper 444.21
  pituitary 253.8
  popliteal (artery) 444.22
  portal (vein) 452
  postoperative NEC 997.2
    cerebral 997.0
    peripheral vascular 997.2
    pulmonary 997.3
  precerebral artery (*see also* Occlusion, artery, precerebral) 433.9
  puerperal — *see* Embolism, obstetrical
  pulmonary (artery) (vein) 415.1
    with
      abortion — *see* Abortion, by type, with embolism
      ectopic pregnancy (*see also* categories 633.0-633.9) 639.6
      molar pregnancy (*see also* categories 630-632) 639.6

Embolism—*continued*
  pulmonary—*continued*
    following
      abortion 639.6
      ectopic or molar pregnancy 639.6
    in pregnancy, childbirth, or puerperium — *see* Embolism, obstetrical
  pyemic (multiple) 038.9
    with
      abortion — *see* Abortion, by type, with embolism
      ectopic pregnancy (*see also* categories 633.0-633.9) 639.6
      molar pregnancy (*see also* categories 630-632) 639.6
    Aerobacter aerogenes 038.49
    enteric gram-negative bacilli 038.40
    Enterobacter aerogenes 038.49
    Escherichia coli 038.42
    following
      abortion 639.6
      ectopic or molar pregnancy 639.6
    Hemophilus influenzae 038.41
    pneumococcal 038.2
    Proteus vulgaris 038.49
    Pseudomonas (aeruginosa) 038.43
    puerperal, postpartum, childbirth (any organism) 673.3
    Serratia 038.44
    specified organism NEC 038.8
    staphylococcal 038.1
    streptococcal 038.0
  renal (artery) 593.81
    vein 453.3
  retina, retinal (*see also* Occlusion, retina) 362.30
  saddle (aorta) 444.0
  septicemic — *see* Embolism, pyemic
  sinus — *see* Embolism, intracranial venous sinus
  soap
    with
      abortion — *see* Abortion, by type, with embolism
      ectopic pregnancy (*see also* categories 633.0-633.9) 639.6
      molar pregnancy (*see also* categories 630-632) 639.6
    following
      abortion 639.6
      ectopic or molar pregnancy 639.6
  spinal cord (nonpyogenic) 336.1
    in pregnancy or puerperium 671.5
    pyogenic origin 324.1
    late effect — *see* category 326
  spleen, splenic (artery) 444.89
  thrombus (thromboembolism) following infusion, perfusion, or transfusion 999.2
  upper extremity 444.21
  vein 453.9
    with inflammation or phlebitis — *see* Thrombophlebitis
    cerebral (*see also* Embolism, brain) 434.1
    coronary (*see also* Infarct, myocardium) 410.9
      without myocardial infarction 411.81
    hepatic 453.0

Embolism—*continued*
  vein—*continued*
    mesenteric (with gangrene) 557.0
    portal 452
    pulmonary — *see* Embolism, pulmonary
    renal 453.3
    specified NEC 453.8
      with inflammation or phlebitis — *see* Thrombophlebitis
    vena cava (inferior) (superior) 453.2
    vessels of brain (*see also* Embolism, brain) 434.1
Embolization — *see* Embolism ◆
Embolus — *see* Embolism
Embryoma (M9080/1) — *see also* Neoplasm, by site, uncertain behavior
  benign (M9080/0 — *see* Neoplasm, by site, benign
  kidney (M8960/3) 189.0
  liver (M8970/3) 155.0
  malignant (M9080/3) — *see also* Neoplasm, by site, malignant
    kidney (M8960/3) 189.0
    liver (M8970/3) 155.0
    testis (M9070/3) 186.9
      undescended 186.0
  testis (M9070/3) 186.9
    undescended 186.0
Embryonic
  circulation 747.9
  heart 747.9
  vas deferens 752.8
Embryopathia NEC 759.9
Embryotomy, fetal 763.8
Embryotoxon 743.43
  interfering with vision 743.42
Emesis — *see also* Vomiting ◆
  gravidarum — *see* Hyperemesis, gravidarum
Emissions, nocturnal (semen) 608.89
Emotional
  crisis — *see* Crisis, emotional
  disorder (*see also* Disorder, mental) 300.9
  instability (excessive) 301.3
  overlay — *see* Reaction, adjustment
  upset 300.9
Emotionality, pathological 301.3
Emotogenic disease (*see also* Disorder, psychogenic) 306.9
Emphysema (atrophic) (centriacinar) (centrilobular) (chronic) (diffuse) (essential) (hypertrophic) (interlobular) (lung) (obstructive) (panlobular) (paracicatricial) (paracinar) (postural) (pulmonary) (senile) (subpleural) (traction) (unilateral) (unilobular) (vesicular) 492.8
  with
    bronchitis
      acute and chronic 491.21
      chronic 491.20
        with acute bronchitis or acute exacerbation 491.21
  bullous (giant) 492.0
  cellular tissue 958.7
    surgical 998.81 ◆
  compensatory 518.2
  congenital 770.2
  conjunctiva 372.8
  connective tissue 958.7
    surgical 998.81 ◆
  due to fumes or vapors 506.4

Emphysema—*continued*
  eye 376.89
  eyelid 374.85
    surgical 998.81 ◆
    traumatic 958.7
  fetus or newborn (interstitial) (mediastinal) (unilobular) 770.2
  heart 416.9
  interstitial 518.1
    congenital 770.2
    fetus or newborn 770.2
  laminated tissue 958.7
    surgical 998.81 ◆
  mediastinal 518.1
    fetus or newborn 770.2
  newborn (interstitial) (mediastinal) (unilobular) 770.2
  obstructive diffuse with fibrosis 492.8
  orbit 376.89
  subcutaneous 958.7
    due to trauma 958.7
    nontraumatic 518.1
    surgical 998.81 ▼
  surgical 998.81 ▲
  thymus (gland) (congenital) 254.8
  traumatic 958.7
  tuberculous (*see also* Tuberculosis, pulmonary) 011.9
Employment examination (certification) V70.5
Empty sella (turcica) syndrome 253.8
Empyema (chest) (diaphragmatic) (double) (encapsulated) (general) (interlobar) (lung) (medial) (necessitatis) (perforating chest wall) (pleura) (pneumococcal) (residual) (sacculated) (streptococcal) (supradiaphragmatic) 510.9
  with fistula 510.0
  accessory sinus (chronic) (*see also* Sinusitis) 473.9
  acute 510.9
    with fistula 510.0
  antrum (chronic) (*see also* Sinusitis, maxillary) 473.0
  brain (any part) (*see also* Abcess, brain) 324.0
  ethmoidal (sinus) (chronic) (*see also* Sinusitis, ethmoidal) 473.2
  extradural (*see also* Abscess, extradural) 324.9
  frontal (sinus) (chronic) (*see also* Sinusitis, frontal) 473.1
  gallbladder (*see also* Cholecystitis, acute) 575.0
  mastoid (process) (acute) (*see also* Mastoiditis, acute) 383.00
  maxilla, maxillary 526.4
    sinus (chronic) (*see also* Sinusitis, maxillary) 473.0
  nasal sinus (chronic) (*see also* Sinusitis) 473.9
  sinus (accessory) (nasal) (*see also* Sinusitis) 473.9
  sphenoidal (chronic) (sinus) (*see also* Sinusitis, sphenoidal) 473.3
  subarachnoid (*see also* Abscess, extradural) 324.9
  subdural (*see also* Abscess, extradural) 324.9
  tuberculous (*see also* Tuberculosis, pleura) 012.0
  ureter (*see also* Ureteritis) 593.89
  ventricular (*see also* Abscess, brain) 324.0
Enameloma 520.2

Encephalitis (bacterial) (chronic) (hemorrhagic) (idiopathic) (nonepidemic) (spurious) (subacute) 323.9
acute — see also Encephalitis, viral
  disseminated (postinfectious) NEC 136.9 [323.6]
    postimmunization or postvaccination 323.5
  inclusional 049.8
  inclusion body 049.8
  necrotizing 049.8
arboviral, arbovirus NEC 064
arthropod-borne (see also Encephalitis, viral, arthropod-borne) 064
Australian X 062.4
Bwamba fever 066.3
California (virus) 062.5
Central European 063.2
Czechoslovakian 063.2
Dawson's (inclusion body) 046.2
diffuse sclerosing 046.2
due to
  actinomycosis 039.8 [323.4]
  cat-scratch disease 078.3 [323.0]
  infectious mononucleosis 075 [323.0]
  malaria (see also Malaria) 084.6 [323.2]
  Negishi virus 064
  ornithosis 073.7 [323.0]
  prophylactic inoculation against smallpox 323.5
  rickettsiosis (see also Rickettsiosis) 083.9 [323.1]
  rubella 056.01
  toxoplasmosis (acquired) 130.0
    congenital (active) 771.2 [323.4]
  typhus (fever) (see also Typhus) 081.9 [323.1]
  vaccination (smallpox) 323.5
Eastern equine 062.2
endemic 049.8
epidemic 049.8
equine (acute) (infectious) (viral) 062.9
  Eastern 062.2
  Venezuelan 066.2
  Western 062.1
Far Eastern 063.0
following vaccination or other immunization procedure 323.5
herpes 054.3
Ilheus (virus) 062.8
inclusion body 046.2
infectious (acute) (virus) NEC 049.8
influenzal 487.8 [323.4]
  lethargic 049.8
Japanese (B type) 062.0
La Crosse 062.5
Langat 063.8
late effect — see Late, effect, encephalitis
lead 984.9 [323.7]
lethargic (acute) (infectious) (influenzal) 049.8
lethargica 049.8
louping ill 063.1
lupus 710.0
lymphatica 049.0
Mengo 049.8
meningococcal 036.1
mumps 072.2
Murray Valley 062.4
myoclonic 049.8
Negishi virus 064
otitic NEC 382.4 [323.4]
parasitic NEC 123.9 [323.4]

Encephalitis—continued
periaxialis (concentrica) (diffusa) 341.1
postchickenpox 052.0
postexanthematous NEC 057.9 [323.6]
postimmunization 323.5
postinfectious NEC 136.9 [323.6]
postmeasles 055.0
posttraumatic 323.8
postvaccinal (smallpox) 323.5
postvaricella 052.0
postviral NEC 079.99 [323.6]
  postexanthematous 057.9 [323.6]
  specified NEC 057.8 [323.6]
Powassan 063.8
progressive subcortical (Binswanger's) 290.12
Rio Bravo 049.8
rubella 056.01
Russian
  autumnal 062.0
  spring-summer type (taiga) 063.0
saturnine 984.9 [323.7]
Semliki Forest 062.8
serous 048
slow-acting virus NEC 046.8
specified cause NEC 323.8
St. Louis type 062.3
subacute sclerosing 046.2
subcorticalis chronica 290.12
summer 062.0
suppurative 324.0
syphilitic 094.81
  congenital 090.41
tick-borne 063.9
torula, torular 117.5 [323.4]
toxic NEC 989.9 [323.7]
toxoplasmic (acquired) 130.0
  congenital (active) 771.2 [323.4]
trichinosis 124 [323.4]
Trypanosomiasis (see also Trypanosomiasis) 086.9 [323.2]
tuberculous (see also Tuberculosis) 013.6
type B (Japanese) 062.0
type C 062.3
van Bogaert's 046.2
Venezuelan 066.2
Vienna type 049.8
viral, virus 049.9
  arthropod-borne NEC 064
  mosquito-borne 062.9
    Australian X disease 062.4
    California virus 062.5
    Eastern equine 062.2
    Ilheus virus 062.8
    Japanese (B type) 062.0
    Murray Valley 062.4
    specified type NEC 062.8
    St. Louis 062.3
    type B 062.0
    type C 062.3
    Western equine 062.1
  tick-borne 063.9
    biundulant 063.2
    Central European 063.2
    Czechoslovakian 063.2
    diphasic meningoencephalitis 063.2
    Far Eastern 063.0
    Langat 063.8
    louping ill 063.1
    Powassan 063.8
    Russian spring-summer (taiga) 063.0
    specified type NEC 063.8
  vector unknown 064

Encephalitis—continued
viral, virus—continued
  slow acting NEC 046.8
  specified type NEC 049.8
  vaccination, prophylactic (against) V05.0
von Economo's 049.8
Western equine 062.1
West Nile type 066.3
Encephalocele 742.0
orbit 376.81
Encephalocystocele 742.0
Encephalomalacia (brain) (cerebellar) (cerebral) (cerebrospinal) (see also Softening, brain) 434.9
due to
  hemorrhage (see also Hemorrhage, brain) 431
  recurrent spasm of artery 435.9
embolic (cerebral) (see also Embolism, brain) 434.1
subcorticalis chronicus arteriosclerotica 290.12
thrombotic (see also thrombosis, brain) 434.0
Encephalomeningitis — see Meningoencephalitis
Encephalomeningocele 742.0
Encephalomeningomyelitis — see Meningoencephalitis
Encephalomeningopathy (see also Meningoencephalitis) 349.9
Encephalomyelitis (chronic) (granulomatous) (hemorrhagic necrotizing, acute) (myalgic, benign) (see also Encephalitis) 323.9
abortive disseminated 049.8
acute disseminated (postinfectious) 136.9 [323.6]
  postimmunization 323.5
due to or resulting from vaccination (any) 323.5
equine (acute) (infectious) 062.9
  Eastern 062.2
  Venezuelan 066.2
  Western 062.1
funicularis infectiosa 049.8
late effect — see Late, effect, encephalitis
Munch-Peterson's 049.8
postchickenpox 052.0
postimmunization 323.5
postmeasles 055.0
postvaccinal (smallpox) 323.5
rubella 056.01
specified cause NEC 323.8
syphilitic 094.81
Encephalomyelocele 742.0
Encephalomyelomeningitis — see Meningoencephalitis
Encephalomyeloneuropathy 349.9
Encephalomyelopathy 349.9
subacute necrotizing (infantile) 330.8
Encephalomyeloradiculitis (acute) 357.0
Encephalomyeloradiculoneuritis (acute) 357.0
Encephalomyeloradiculopathy 349.9
Encephalomyocarditis 074.23
Encephalopathia hyperbilirubinemica, newborn 774.7
due to isoimmunization (conditions classifiable to 773.0-773.2) 773.4
Encephalopathy (acute) 348.3
alcoholic 291.2
anoxic — see Damage, brain, anoxic

Encephalopathy—continued
arteriosclerotic 437.0
  late effect — see category 438
bilirubin, newborn 774.7
  due to isoimmunization 773.4
congenital 742.9
demyelinating (callosal) 341.8
due to
  birth injury (intracranial) 767.8
  dialysis 294.8
    transient 293.9
  hyperinsulinism — see Hyperinsulinism
  influenza (virus) 487.8
  lack of vitamin (see also Deficiency, vitamin) 269.2
  nicotinic acid deficiency 291.2
  serum (nontherapeutic) (therapeutic) 999.5
  syphilis 094.81
  trauma (postconcussional) 310.2
    current (see also Concussion, brain) 850.9
    with skull fracture — see Fracture, skull, by site, with intracranial injury
  vaccination 323.5
hepatic 572.2
hyperbilirubinemic, newborn 774.7
  due to isoimmunization (conditions classifiable to 773.0-773.2) 773.4
hypertensive 437.2
hypoglycemic 251.2
hypoxic — see Damage, brain, anoxic
infantile cystic necrotizing (congenital) 341.8
lead 984.9 [323.7]
leukopolio 330.0
metabolic (toxic) — see Delirium
necrotizing, subacute 330.8
pellagrous 265.2
portal-systemic 572.2
postcontusional 310.2
posttraumatic 310.2
saturnine 984.9 [323.7]
spongioform, subacute (viral) 046.1
subacute
  necrotizing 330.8
  spongioform 046.1
  viral, spongioform 046.1
subcortical progressive (Schilder) 341.1
  chronic (Binswanger's) 290.12
toxic 349.82
  metabolic — see Delirium
traumatic (postconcussional) 310.2
  current (see also Concussion, brain) 850.9
  with skull fracture — see Fracture, skull, by site, with intracranial injury
vitamin B deficiency NEC 266.9
Wernicke's (superior hemorrhagic polioencephalitis) 265.1
Encephalorrhagia (see also Hemorrhage, brain) 432.9
healed or old — see also category 438 without residuals V12.5
late effect — see category 483
Encephalosis, posttraumatic 310.2
Enchondroma (M9220/0) — see also Neoplasm, bone, benign
multiple, congenital 756.4

Enchondromatosis (cartilaginous) (congenital) (multiple) 756.4
Enchondroses, multiple (cartilaginous) (congenital) 756.4
Encopresis (see also Incontinence, feces) 787.6
 nonorganic origin 307.7
Encounter for — see also Admission for
 administrative purpose only V68.9
  referral of patient without examination or treatment V68.81
  specified purpose NEC V68.89
 chemotherapy V58.1
 radiotherapy V58.0
Encystment — see Cyst
Endamebiasis — see Amebiasis
Endamoeba — see Amebiasis
Endarteritis (bacterial, subacute) (infective) (septic) 447.6
 brain, cerebral or cerebrospinal 437.4
  late effect — see category 438
 coronary (artery) — see Arteriosclerosis, coronary ◆
 deformans — see Arteriosclerosis
 embolic (see also Embolism) 444.9
 obliterans — see also Arteriosclerosis
  pulmonary 417.8
 pulmonary 417.8
 retina 362.18
 senile — see Arteriosclerosis
 syphilitic 093.89
  brain or cerebral 094.89
  congenital 090.5
  spinal 094.89
 tuberculous (see also Tuberculosis) 017.9
Endemic — see condition
Endocarditis (chronic) (indeterminate) (interstitial) (marantis) (nonbacterial thrombotic) (residual) (sclerotic) (sclerous) (senile) (valvular) 424.90
 with
  rheumatic fever (conditions classifiable to 390)
   active — see Endocarditis, acute, rheumatic
   inactive or quiescent (with chorea) 397.9
 acute or subacute 421.9
  rheumatic (aortic) (mitral) (pulmonary) (tricuspid) 391.1
   with chorea (acute) (rheumatic) (Sydenham's) 392.0
 aortic (heart) (nonrheumatic) (valve) 424.1
  with
   mitral (valve) disease 396.9
    active or acute 391.1
     with chorea (acute) (rheumatic) (Sydenham's) 392.0
   rheumatic fever (conditions classifiable to 390)
    active — see Endocarditis, acute, rheumatic
    inactive or quiescent (with chorea) 395.9
     with mitral disease 396.9
  acute or subacute 421.9
  arteriosclerotic 424.1

Endocarditis—continued
 aortic—continued
  congenital 746.89
  hypertensive 424.1
  rheumatic (chronic) (inactive) 395.9
   with mitral (valve) disease 396.9
    active or acute 391.1
     with chorea (acute) (rheumatic) (Sydenham's) 392.0
    active or acute 391.1
     with chorea (acute) (rheumatic) (Sydenham's) 392.0
   specified cause, except rheumatic 424.1
  syphilitic 093.22
 arteriosclerotic or due to arteriosclerosis 424.99
 atypical verrucous (Libman-Sacks) 710.0 [424.91]
 bacterial (any valve) (chronic) (subacute) 421.0
 blastomycotic 116.0 [421.1]
 candidal 112.81
 congenital 425.3
 constrictive 421.0
 Coxsackie 074.22
 due to
  blastomycosis 116.0 [421.1]
  candidiasis 112.81
  Coxsackie (virus) 074.22
  disseminated lupus erythematosus 710.0 [424.91]
  histoplasmosis (see also Histoplasmosis) 115.94
  hypertension (benign) 424.99
  moniliasis 112.81
  prosthetic cardiac valve 996.61
  Q fever 083.0 [421.1]
  serratia marcescens 421.0
  typhoid (fever) 002.0 [421.1]
 fetal 425.3
 gonococcal 098.84
 hypertensive 424.99
 infectious or infective (acute) (any valve) (chronic) (subacute) 421.0
 lenta (acute) (any valve) (chronic) (subacute) 421.0
 Libman-Sacks 710.0 [424.91]
 Loeffler's (parietal fibroplastic) 421.0
 malignant (acute) (any valve) (chronic) (subacute) 421.0
 meningococcal 036.42
 mitral (chronic) (double) (fibroid) (heart) (inactive) (valve) (with chorea) 394.9
  with
   aortic (valve) disease 396.9
    active or acute 391.1
     with chorea (acute) (rheumatic) (Sydenham's) 392.0
   rheumatic fever (conditions classifiable to 390)
    active — see Endocarditis, acute, rheumatic
    inactive or quiescent (with chorea) 394.9
     with aortic valve disease 396.9
  active or acute 391.1
   with chorea (acute) (rheumatic) (Sydenham's) 392.0
   bacterial 421.0 ◆

Endocarditis—continued
 mitral—continued
  arteriosclerotic 424.0
  congenital 746.89
  hypertensive 424.0
  nonrheumatic 424.0
   acute or subacute 421.9
  syphilitic 093.21
  monilial 112.81
 mycotic (acute) (any valve) (chronic) (subacute) 421.0
 pneumococcic (acute) (any valve) (chronic) (subacute) 421.0
 pulmonary (chronic) (heart) (valve) 424.3
  with
   rheumatic fever (conditions classifiable to 390)
    active — see Endocarditis, acute, rheumatic
    inactive or quiescent (with chorea) 397.1
  acute or subacute 421.9
   rheumatic 391.1
    with chorea (acute) (rheumatic) (Sydenham's) 392.0
  arteriosclerotic or due to arteriosclerosis 424.3
  congenital 746.09
  hypertensive or due to hypertension (benign) 424.3
  rheumatic (chronic) (inactive) (with chorea) 397.1
   active or acute 391.1
    with chorea (acute) (rheumatic) (Sydenham's) 392.0
  syphilitic 093.24
 purulent (acute) (any valve) (chronic) (subacute) 421.0
 rheumatic (chronic) (inactive) (with chorea) 397.9
  active or acute (aortic) (mitral) (pulmonary) (tricuspid) 391.1
   with chorea (acute) (rheumatic) (Sydenham's) 392.0
 septic (acute) (any valve) (chronic) (subacute) 421.0
 specified cause, except rheumatic 424.99
 streptococcal (acute) (any valve) (chronic) (subacute) 421.0
 subacute — see Endocarditis, acute
 suppurative (any valve) (acute) (chronic) (subacute) 421.0
 syphilitic NEC 093.20
 toxic (see also Endocarditis, acute) 421.9
 tricuspid (chronic) (heart) (inactive) (rheumatic) (valve) (with chorea) 397.0
  with
   rheumatic fever (conditions classifiable to 390)
    active — see Endocarditis, acute, rheumatic
    inactive or quiescent (with chorea) 397.0
  active or acute 391.1
   with chorea (acute) (rheumatic) (Sydenham's) 392.0
  arteriosclerotic 424.2
  congenital 746.89
  hypertensive 424.2

Endocarditis—continued
 tricuspid—continued
  nonrheumatic 424.2
   acute or subacute 421.9
   specified cause, except rheumatic 424.2
  syphilitic 093.23
  tuberculous (see also Tuberculosis) 017.9 [424.91]
  typhoid 002.0 [421.1]
  ulcerative (acute) (any valve) (chronic) (subacute) 421.0
  vegetative (acute) (any valve) (chronic) (subacute) 421.0
  verrucous (acute) (any valve) (chronic) (subacute) NEC 710.0 [424.91]
   nonbacterial 710.0 [424.91]
   nonrheumatic 710.0 [424.91]
Endocardium, endocardial — see also condition
 cushion defect 745.60
 specified type NEC 745.69
Endocervicitis (see also Cervicitis) 616.0
 due to
  intrauterine (contraceptive) device 996.65
 gonorrheal (acute) 098.15
  chronic or duration of 2 months or over 098.35
 hyperplastic 616.0
 syphilitic 095.8
 trichomonal 131.09
 tuberculous (see also Tuberculosis) 016.7
Endocrine — see condition
Endocrinopathy, pluriglandular 258.9
Endodontitis 522.0
Endomastoiditis (see also Mastoiditis) 383.9
Endometrioma 617.9
Endometriosis 617.9
 appendix 617.5
 bladder 617.8
 bowel 617.5
 broad ligament 617.3
 cervix 617.0
 colon 617.5
 cul-de-sac (Douglas') 617.3
 exocervix 617.0
 fallopian tube 617.2
 female genital organ NEC 617.8
 gallbladder 617.8
 in scar of skin 617.6
 internal 617.0
 intestine 617.5
 lung 617.8
 myometrium 617.0
 ovary 617.1
 parametrium 617.3
 pelvic peritoneum 617.3
 peritoneal (pelvic) 617.3
 rectovaginal septum 617.4
 rectum 617.5
 round ligament 617.3
 skin 617.6
 specified site NEC 617.8
 stromal (M8931/1) 236.0
 umbilicus 617.8
 uterus 617.0
  internal 617.0
 vagina 617.4
 vulva 617.8
Endometritis (nonspecific) (purulent) (septic) (suppurative) 615.9
 with
  abortion — see Abortion, by type, with sepsis
  ectopic pregnancy (see also categories 633.0-633.9) 639.0

Endometritis—continued
　with—continued
　　molar pregnancy (see also
　　　　categories 630-632)
　　　　639.0
　　acute 615.0
　　blennorrhagic 098.16
　　　acute 098.16
　　　chronic or duration of 2
　　　　months or over 098.36
　　cervix, cervical (see also
　　　　Cervicitis) 616.0
　　　hyperplastic 616.0
　　chronic 615.1
　　complicating pregnancy 646.6
　　　affecting fetus or newborn
　　　　760.8
　　decidual 615.9
　　following
　　　abortion 639.0
　　　ectopic or molar pregnancy
　　　　639.0
　　gonorrheal (acute) 098.16
　　　chronic or duration of 2
　　　　months or over 098.36
　　hyperplastic 621.3
　　　cervix 616.0
　　polypoid — see Endometritis,
　　　hyperplastic
　　puerperal, postpartum, childbirth
　　　670
　　senile (atrophic) 615.9
　　subacute 615.0
　　tuberculous (see also
　　　Tuberculosis) 016.7
Endometrium — see condition
Endomyocardiopathy, South African
　425.2
Endomyocarditis — see Endocarditis
Endomyofibrosis 425.0
Endomyometritis (see also
　Endometritis) 615.9
Endopericarditis — see Endocarditis
Endoperineuritis — see Disorder,
　nerve
Endophlebitis (see also Phlebitis)
　451.9
　leg 451.2
　　deep (vessels) 451.19
　　superficial (vessels) 451.0
　portal (vein) 572.1
　retina 362.18
　specified site NEC 451.89
　syphilitic 093.89
Endophthalmia (see also
　Endophthalmitis) 360.00
　gonorrheal 098.42
Endophthalmitis (globe) (infective)
　(metastatic) (purulent)
　(subacute) 360.00
　acute 360.01
　chronic 360.03
　parasitis 360.13
　phacoanaphylactic 360.19
　specified type NEC 360.19
　sympathetic 360.11
Endosalpingioma (M9111/1) 236.2
Endosteitis — see Osteomyelitis
Endothelioma, bone (M9260/3) —
　see Neoplasm, bone,
　malignant
Endotheliosis 287.8
　hemorrhagic infectional 287.8
Endotoxic shock 785.59
Endotrachelitis (see also Cervicitis)
　616.0
Enema rash 692.89
Engel-von Recklinghausen disease or
　syndrome (osteitis fibrosa
　cystica) 252.0
Engelmann's disease (diaphyseal
　sclerosis) 756.9
English disease (see also Rickets)
　268.0

Engman's disease (infectious
　eczematoid dermatitis) 690
Engorgement
　breast 611.79
　　newborn 778.7
　　puerperal, postpartum 676.2
　liver 573.9
　lung 514
　pulmonary 514
　retina, venous 362.37
　stomach 536.8
　venous, retina 362.37
Enlargement, enlarged — see also
　Hypertrophy
　abdomen 789.3
　adenoids 474.12
　　and tonsils 474.10
　alveolar process or ridge 525.8
　apertures of diaphragm
　　(congenital) 756.6
　blind spot, visual field 368.42
　gingival 523.8
　heart, cardiac (see also
　　Hypertrophy, cardiac)
　　429.3
　lacrimal gland, chronic 375.03
　liver (see also Hypertrophy, liver)
　　789.1
　lymph gland or node 785.6
　orbit 376.46
　organ or site, congenital NEC —
　　see Anomaly, specified type
　　NEC
　parathyroid (gland) 252.0
　pituitary fossa 793.0
　prostate, simple 600
　sella turcica 793.0
　spleen (see also Splenomegaly)
　　789.2
　　congenital 759.0
　thymus (congenital) (gland) 254.0
　thyroid (gland) (see also Goiter)
　　240.9
　tongue 529.8
　tonsils 474.11
　　and adenoids 474.10
　uterus 621.2
Enophthalmos 376.50
　due to
　　atrophy of orbital tissue
　　　376.51
　　surgery 376.52
　　trauma 376.52
Enostosis 526.89
Entamebiasis — see Amebiasis
Entamebic — see Amebiasis
Entanglement, umbilical cord(s)
　663.3
　with compression 663.2
　affecting fetus or newborn 762.5
　around neck with compression
　　663.1
　twins in monoamniotic sac 663.2
Enteralgia 789.0
Enteric — see condition
Enteritis (acute) (catarrhal)
　(choleraic) (chronic)
　(congestive) (diarrheal)
　(exudative) (follicular)
　(hemorrhagic) (infantile)
　(lienteric) (noninfectious)
　(perforative) (phlegmonous)
　(presumed noninfectious)
　(pseudomembranous) 558.9
　adaptive 564.1
　aertrycke infection 003.0
　allergic 558.9
　amebic (see also Amebiasis)
　　006.9
　　with abscess — see Abscess,
　　　amebic
　　acute 006.0
　　　with abscess — see
　　　　Abscess, amebic
　　nondysenteric 006.2

Enteritis—continued
　amebic—continued
　　chronic 006.1
　　　with abscess — see
　　　　Abscess, amebic
　　　nondysenteric 006.2
　　nondysenteric 006.2
　anaerobic (cocci) (gram-negative)
　　(gram-positive) (mixed)
　　NEC 008.46
　bacillary NEC 004.9
　bacterial NEC 008.5
　　specified NEC 008.49
　Bacteroides (fragilis)
　　(melaninogeniscus) (oralis)
　　008.46
　Butyrivibrio (fibriosolvens) 008.46
　Campylobacter 008.43
　Candida 112.85
　Chilomastix 007.8
　choleriformis 001.1
　chronic 558.9
　　ulcerative (see also Colitis,
　　　ulcerative) 556.9
　cicatrizing (chronic) 555.0
　Clostridium
　　botulinum 005.1
　　difficile 008.45
　　haemolyticum 008.46
　　novyi 008.46
　　perfringens (C) (F) 008.46
　　specified type NEC 008.46
　coccidial 007.2
　dietetic 558.9
　due to
　　achylia gastrica 536.8
　　adenovirus 008.62
　　Aerobacter aerogenes 008.2
　　anaerobes — see Enteritis,
　　　anaerobic
　　Arizona (bacillus) 008.1
　　astrovirus 008.66
　　Bacillus coli — see Enteritis, E.
　　　coli 008.0
　　bacteria NEC 008.5
　　　specified NEC 008.49
　　Bacteroides 008.46
　　Butyrivibrio (fibriosolvens)
　　Calcivirus 008.65
　　Camplyobacter 008.43
　　Clostridium — see Enteritis,
　　　Clostridium
　　Cockle agent 008.64
　　Coxsackie (virus) 008.67
　　Ditchling agent 008.64
　　ECHO virus 008.67
　　Enterobacter aerogenes 008.2
　　enterococci 008.49
　　enterovirus NEC 008.67
　　Escherichia coli — see
　　　Enteritis, E. coli 008.0
　　Eubacterium 008.46
　　Fusobacterium (nucleatum)
　　　008.46
　　gram-negative bacteria NEC
　　　008.47
　　　anaerobic NEC 008.46
　　Hawaii agent 008.63
　　irritating foods 558.9
　　Klebsiella aerogenes 008.47
　　Marin County agent 008.66
　　Montgomery County agent
　　　008.63
　　Norwalk-like agent 008.63
　　Norwalk virus 008.63
　　Otofuke agent 008.63
　　Paracolobactrum arizonae
　　　008.1
　　paracolon bacillus NEC
　　　008.47
　　　Arizona 008.1
　　Paramatta agent 008.64
　　Peptococcus 008.46
　　Peptostreptococcus 008.46
　　Proprionibacterium 008.46
　　Proteus (bacillus) (mirabilis)
　　　(morganii) 008.3

Enteritis—continued
　due to—continued
　　Pseudomonas aeruginosa
　　　008.42
　　Rotavirus 008.61
　　Sapporo agent 008.63
　　small round virus (SRV) NEC
　　　008.64
　　　featureless NEC 008.63
　　　structured NEC 008.63
　　Snow Mountain (SM) agent
　　　008.63
　　specified
　　　bacteria NEC 008.49
　　　organism, nonbacterial
　　　　NEC 008.8
　　　virus (NEC) 008.69
　　Staphylococcus 008.41
　　Streptococcus 008.49
　　　anaerobic 008.46
　　Taunton agent 008.63
　　Torovirus 008.69
　　Treponema 008.46
　　Veillonella 008.46
　　virus 008.8
　　　specified type NEC 008.69
　　Wollan (W) agent 008.64
　　Yersinia enterocolitica 008.44
　dysentery — see Dysentery
　E. coli 008.00
　　enterohemorrhagic 008.04
　　enteroinvasive 008.03
　　enteropathogenic 008.01
　　enterotoxigenic 008.02
　　specified type NEC 008.09
　el tor 001.1
　embadomonial 007.8
　epidemic 009.0
　Eubacterium 008.46
　fermentative 558.9
　fulminant 557.0
　Fusobacterium (nucleatum)
　　008.46
　gangrenous (see also Enteritis,
　　due to, by organism) 009.0
　giardial 007.1
　gram-negative bacteria NEC
　　008.47
　　anaerobic NEC 008.46
　infectious NEC (see also Enteritis,
　　due to, by organism) 009.0
　　presumed 009.1
　influenzal 487.8
　ischemic 557.9
　　acute 557.0
　　chronic 557.1
　　due to mesenteric artery
　　　insufficiency 557.1
　membranous 564.1
　mucous 564.1
　myxomembranous 564.1
　necrotic (see also Enteritis, due
　　to, by organism) 009.0
　necroticans 005.2
　necrotizing of fetus or newborn
　　777.5
　neurogenic 564.1
　newborn 777.8
　　necrotizing 777.5
　parasitic NEC 129
　paratyphoid (fever) (see also
　　Fever, paratyphoid) 002.9
　Peptococcus 008.46
　Peptostreptococcus 008.46
　Proprionibacterium 008.46
　protozoal NEC 007.9
　regional (of) 555.9
　　intestine
　　　large (bowel, colon, or
　　　　rectum) 555.1
　　　　with small intestine
　　　　　555.2
　　　small (duodenum, ileum, or
　　　　jejunum) 555.0
　　　　with large intestine
　　　　　555.2
　Salmonella infection 003.0

Enteritis—continued
salmonellosis 003.0
segmental (see also Enteritis, regional) 555.9
septic (see also Enteritis, due to, by organism) 009.0
Shigella 004.9
simple 558.9
spasmodic 564.1
spastic 564.1
staphylococcal 008.41
 due to food 005.0
streptococcal 008.49
 anaerobic 008.46
toxic 558.2
Treponema (denticola) (macrodentium) 008.46
trichomonal 007.3
tuberculous (see also Tuberculosis) 014.8
typhosa 002.0
ulcerative (chronic) (see also Colitis, ulcerative) 556.9 ◆
Veillonella 008.46
viral 008.8
 adenovirus 008.62
 enterovirus 008.67
 specified virus NEC 008.69
Yersinia enterocolitica 008.44
zymotic 009.0

Enteroarticular syndrome 099.3
Enterobiasis 127.4
Enterobius vermicularis 127.4
Enterocele (see also Hernia) 553.9
 pelvis, pelvic (acquired) (congenital) 618.6
 vagina, vaginal (acquired) (congenital) 618.6
Enterocolitis — see also Enteritis
 fetus or newborn 777.5
 fulminant 557.0
 granulomatous 555.2
 hemorrhagic (acute) 557.0
  chronic 557.1
 necrotizing (acute) membranous) 557.0
 primary necrotizing 777.5
 pseudomembranous 008.45
 radiation 558.1
  newborn 777.5
 ulcerative 556.0 ◆
Enterocystoma 751.5
Enterogastritis — see Enteritis
Enterogenous cyanosis 289.7
Enterolith, enterolithiasis (impaction) 560.39
 with hernia — see also Hernia, by site, with obstruction
 gangrenous — see Hernia, by site, with gangrene
Enteropathy 569.9
 exudative (of Gordon) 579.8
 gluten 579.0
 hemorrhagic, terminal 557.0
 protein-losing 579.8
Enteroperitonitis (see also Peritonitis) 567.9
Enteroptosis 569.89
Enterorrhagia 578.9
Enterospasm 564.1
 psychogenic 306.4
Enterostenosis (see also Obstruction, intestine) 560.9
Enterostomy status V44.4
 with complication 569.6
Enthesopathy 726.39
 ankle and tarsus 726.70
 elbow region 726.30
  specified NEC 726.39
 hip 726.5
 knee 726.60
 peripheral NEC 726.8
 shoulder region 726.10
  adhesive 726.0

Enthesopathy—continued
spinal 720.1
wrist and carpus 726.4
Entrance, air into vein — see Embolism, air
Entrapment, nerve — see Neuropathy, entrapment
Entropion (eyelid) 374.00
 cicatricial 374.04
 congenital 743.62
 late effect of trachoma (healed) 139.1
 mechanical 374.02
 paralytic 374.02
 senile 374.01
 spastic 374.03
Enucleation of eye (current) (traumatic) 871.3
Enuresis 788.30
 habit disturbance 307.6
 nocturnal 788.36
  psychogenic 307.6
 nonorganic origin 307.6
 psychogenic 307.6
Enzymopathy 277.9
Eosinopenia 288.0
Eosinophilia 288.3
 allergic 288.3
 hereditary 288.3
 idiopathic 288.3
 infiltrative 518.3
 Loeffler's 518.3
 myalgia syndrome 710.5
 pulmonary (tropical) 518.3
 secondary 288.3
 tropical 518.3
Eosinophilic — see also condition
 fasciitis 728.89
 granuloma (bone) 277.8
 infiltration lung 518.3
Ependymitis (acute) (cerebral) (chronic) (granular) (see also Meningitis) 322.9
Ependymoblastoma (M9392/3)
 specified site — see Neoplasm, by site, malignant
 unspecified site 191.9
Ependymoma (epithelial) (malignant) (M9391/3)
 anaplastic type (M9392/3)
  specified site — see Neoplasm, by site, malignant
  unspecified site 191.9
 benign (M9391/0)
  specified site — see Neoplasm, by site, benign
  unspecified site 225.0
 myxopapillary (M9394/1) 237.5
 papillary (M9393/1) 237.5
 specified site — see Neoplasm, by site, malignant
 unspecified site 191.9
Ependymopathy 349.2
 spinal cord 349.2
Ephelides, ephelis 709.09 ◆
Ephemeral fever (see also Pyrexia) 780.6
Epiblepharon (congenital) 743.62
Epicanthus, epicanthic fold (congenital) (eyelid) 743.63
Epicondylitis (elbow) (lateral) 726.32
 medial 726.31
Epicystitis (see also Cystitis) 595.9
Epidemic — see condition
Epidermidalization, cervix — see condition
Epidermidization, cervix — see condition
Epidermis, epidermal — see condition

Epidermization, cervix — see condition
Epidermodysplasia verruciformis 078.19
Epidermoid
 cholesteatoma — see Cholesteatoma
 inclusion (see also Cyst, skin) 706.2
Epidermolysis
 acuta (combustiformis) (toxica) 695.1
 bullosa 757.39
 necroticans combustiformis 695.1
  due to drug
   correct substance properly administered 695.1
   overdose or wrong substance given or taken 977.9
  specified drug — see Table of drugs and chemicals
Epidermophytid — see Dermatophytosis
Epidermophytosis (infected) — see Dermatophytosis
Epidermosis, ear (middle) (see also Cholesteatoma) 385.30
Epididymis — see condition
Epididymitis (nonvenereal) 604.90
 with abscess 604.0
 acute 604.99
 blennorrhagic (acute) 098.0
  chronic or duration of 2 months or over 098.2
 caseous (see also Tuberculosis) 016.4
 chlamydial 099.54
 diphtheritic 032.89 [604.91]
 filarial 125.9 [604.91]
 gonococcal (acute) 098.0
  chronic or duration of 2 months or over 098.2
 recurrent 604.99
 residual 604.99
 syphilitic 095.8 [604.91]
 tuberculous (see also Tuberculosis) 016.4
Epididymo-orchitis (see also Epididymitis) 604.90
 with abscess 604.0
 chlamydial 099.54
 gonococcal (acute) 098.13
  chronic or duration of 2 months or over 098.33
Epidural — see condition
Epigastritis (see also Gastritis) 535.5
Epigastrium, epigastric — see condition
Epigastrocele (see also Hernia, epigastric) 553.29
Epiglottiditis (acute) 464.30
 with obstruction 464.31
 chronic 476.1
 viral 464.30
  with obstruction 464.31
Epiglottis — see condition
Epiglottitis (acute) 464.30
 with obstruction 464.31
 chronic 476.1
 viral 464.30
  with obstruction 464.31
Epignathus 759.4
Epilepsia
 partialis continua (see also Epilepsy) 345.7
 procursiva (see also Epilepsy) 345.8

Epilepsy, epileptic (idiopathic) 345.9

> Note — use the following fifth-digit subclassification with categories 345.0, 345.1, 345.4–345.9:
> 0 without mention of intractable epilepsy
> 1 with intractable epilepsy

abdominal 345.5
absence (attack) 345.0
akinetic 345.0
 psychomotor 345.4
automatism 345.4
autonomic diencephalic 345.5
brain 345.9
Bravais-Jacksonian 345.5
cerebral 345.9
climacteric 345.9
clonic 345.1
clouded state 345.9
coma 345.3
communicating 345.4
congenital 345.9
convulsions 345.9
cortical (focal) (motor) 345.5
cursive (running) 345.8
cysticercosis 123.1
deterioration 294.1
due to syphilis 094.89
equivalent 345.5
fit 345.9
focal (motor) 345.5
gelastic 345.8
generalized 345.9
 convulsive 345.1
 flexion 345.1
 nonconvulsive 345.0
grand mal (idiopathic) 345.1
Jacksonian (motor) (sensory) 345.5
Kojevnikoff's, Kojevnikov's, Kojewnikoff's 345.7
laryngeal 786.2
limbic system 345.4
major (motor) 345.1
minor 345.0
mixed (type) 345.9
motor partial 345.5
musicogenic 345.1
myoclonus, myoclonic 345.1
 progressive (familial) 333.2
nonconvulsive, generalized 345.0
parasitic NEC 123.9
partial (focalized) 345.5
 with
  impairment of consciousness 345.4
  memory and ideational disturbances 345.4
 abdominal type 345.5
 motor type 345.5
 psychomotor type 345.4
 psychosensory type 345.4
 secondarily generalized 345.4
 sensory type 345.5
 somatomotor type 345.5
 somatosensory type 345.5
 temporal lobe type 345.4
 visceral type 345.5
 visual type 345.5
peripheral 345.9
petit mal 345.0
photokinetic 345.8
progresive myoclonic (familial) 333.2
psychic equivalent 345.5
psychomotor 345.4
psychosensory 345.4
reflex 345.1
seizure 345.9
senile 345.9
sensory-induced 345.5
sleep 347
somatomotor type 345.5
somatosensory 345.5

Epilepsy, epileptic—continued
 specified type NEC 345.8
 status (grand mal) 345.3
  focal motor 345.7
  petit mal 345.2
  psychomotor 345.7
  temporal lobe 345.7
 symptomatic 345.9
 temporal lobe 345.4
 tonic (-clonic) 345.1
 traumatic (injury unspecified) 907.0
  injury specified — see Late, effect (of) specified injury
 twilight 293.0
 uncinate (gyrus) 345.4
 Unverricht (-Lundborg) (familial myoclonic) 333.2
 visceral 345.5
 visual 345.5
Epileptiform
 convulsions 780.3
 seizure 780.3
Epiloia 759.5
Epimenorrhea 626.2
Epipharyngitis (see also Nasopharyngitis) 460
Epiphora 375.20
 due to
  excess lacrimation 375.21
  insufficient drainage 375.22
Epiphyseal arrest 733.91
 femoral head 732.2
Epiphyseolysis, epiphysiolysis (see also Osteochondrosis) 732.9
Epiphysitis (see also Osteochondrosis) 732.9
 juvenile 732.6
 marginal (Scheuermann's) 732.0
 os calcis 732.5
 syphilitic (congenital) 090.0
 vertebral (Scheuermann's) 732.0
Epiplocele (see also Hernia) 553.9
Epiploitis (see also Peritonitis) 567.9
Epiplosarcomphalocele (see also Hernia, umbilicus) 553.1
Episcleritis 379.00
 gouty 274.89 [379.09]
 nodular 379.02
 periodica fugax 379.01
  angioneurotic — see Edema, angioneurotic
 specified NEC 379.09
 staphylococcal 379.00
 suppurative 379.00
 syphilitic 095.0
 tuberculous (see also Tuberculosis) 017.3 [379.09]
Episode
 brain (see also Disease, cerebrovascular, acute) 436
 cerebral (see also Disease, cerebrovascular, acute) 436
 depersonalization (in neurotic state) 300.6
 psychotic (see also Psychosis) 298.9
  organic, transient 293.9
 schizophrenic (acute) NEC (see also Schizophrenia) 295.4
Epispadias
 female 753.8
 male 752.6
Episplenitis 289.59
Epistaxis (multiple) 784.7
 hereditary 448.0
 vicarious menstruation 625.8
Epithelioma (malignant) (M8011/3) — see also Neoplasm, by site, malignant
 adenoides cysticum (M8100/0) — see Neoplasm, skin, benign

Epithelioma—continued
 basal cell (M8090/3) — see Neoplasm, skin, malignant
 benign (M8011/0) — see Neoplasm, by site, benign
 Bowen's (M8081/2) — see Neoplasm, skin, in situ
 calcifying (benign) (Malherbe's) (M8110/0) — see Neoplasm, skin, benign
 external site — see Neoplasm, skin, malignant
 intraepidermal, Jadassohn (M8096/0) — see Neoplasm, skin, benign
 squamous cell (M8070/3) — see Neoplasm, by site, malignant
Epitheliopathy
 pigment, retina 363.15
 posterior multifocal placoid (acute) 363.15
Epithelium, epithelial — see condition
Epituberculosis (allergic) (with atelectasis) (see also Tuberculosis) 010.8
Eponychia 757.5
Epstein's
 nephrosis or syndrome (see also Nephrosis) 581.9
 pearl (mouth) 528.4
Epstein-Barr infection (viral) 075
Epulis (giant cell) (gingiva) 523.8
Equinia 024
Equinovarus (congenital) 754.51
 acquired 736.71
Equivalent
 convulsive (abdominal) (see also Epilepsy) 345.5
 epileptic (psychic) (see also Epilepsy) 345.5
Erb's
 disease 359.1
 palsy, paralysis (birth) (brachial) (newborn) 767.6
  spinal (spastic) syphilitic 094.89
 pseudohypertrophic muscular dystrophy 359.1
Erb (-Duchenne) paralysis (birth injury) (newborn) 767.6
Erb-Goldflam disease or syndrome 358.0
Erdheim's syndrome (acromegalic macrospondylitis) 253.0
Erection, painful (persistent) 607.3
Ergosterol deficiency (vitamin D) 268.9
 with
  osteomalacia 268.2
  rickets (see also Rickets) 268.0
Ergotism (ergotized grain) 988.2
 from ergot used as drug (migraine therapy)
  correct substance properly administered 349.82
  overdose or wrong substance given or taken 975.0
Erichsen's disease (railway spine) 300.16
Erlacher-Blount syndrome (tibia vara) 732.4
Erosio interdigitalis blastomycetica 112.3
Erosion
 artery NEC 447.2
  without rupture 447.8
  arteriosclerotic plaque — see Arteriosclerosis, by site
 bone 733.99
 bronchus 519.1
 cartilage (joint) 733.99

Erosion—continued
 cervix (uteri) (acquired) (chronic) (congenital) 622.0
  with mention of cervicitis 616.0
 cornea (recurrent) (see also Keratitis) 371.42
  traumatic 918.1
 dental (idiopathic) (occupational) 521.3
 duodenum, postpyloric — see Ulcer, duodenum
 esophagus 530.89
 gastric 535.4
 intestine 569.89
 lymphatic vessel 457.8
 pylorus, pyloric (ulcer) 535.4
 sclera 379.16
 spine, aneurysmal 094.89
 spleen 289.59
 stomach 535.4
 teeth (idiopathic) (occupational) 521.3
  due to
   medicine 521.3
   persistent vomiting 521.3
 urethra 599.84
 uterus 621.8
 vertebra 733.99
Erotomania 302.89
 Clérambault's 297.8
Error
 in diet 269.9
 refractive 367.9
  astigmatism (see also Astigmatism) 367.20
  drug-induced 367.89
  hypermetropia 367.0
  hyperopia 367.0
  myopia 367.1
  presbyopia 367.4
  toxic 367.89
Eructation 787.3
 nervous 306.4
 psychogenic 306.4
Eruption
 creeping 126.9
 drug — see Dermatitis, due to, drug
 Hutchinson, summer 692.72
 Kaposi's varicelliform 054.0
 napkin (psoriasiform) 691.0
 polymorphous
  light (sun) 692.72
  other source 692.82
 psoriasiform, napkin 691.0
 recalcitrant pustular 694.8
 ringed 695.89
 skin (see also Dermatitis) 782.1
  creeping (meaning hookworm) 126.9
  due to
   chemical(s) NEC 692.4
    internal use 693.8
   drug — see Dermatitis, due to, drug
   prophylactic inoculation or vaccination against disease — see Dermatitis, due to, vaccine
   smallpox vaccination NEC — see Dermatitis, due to, vaccine
  erysipeloid 027.1
  feigned 698.4
  Hutchinson, summer 692.72
  Kaposi's, varicelliform 054.0
   vaccinia 999.0
  lichenoid, axilla 698.3
  polymorphous, due to light 692.72
  toxic NEC 695.0
  vesicular 709.8

Eruption—continued
 teeth, tooth
  accelerated 520.6
  delayed 520.6
  difficult 520.6
  disturbance of 520.6
  in abnormal sequence 520.6
  incomplete 520.6
  late 520.6
  natal 520.6
  neonatal 520.6
  obstructed 520.6
  partial 520.6
  persistent primary 520.6
  premature 520.6
 vesicular 709.8
Erysipelas (gangrenous) (infantile) (newborn) (phlegmonous) (suppurative) 035
 external ear 035 [380.13]
 puerperal, postpartum, childbirth 670
Erysipelatoid (Rosenbach's) 027.1
Erysipeloid (Rosenbach's) 027.1
Erythema, erythematous (generalized) 695.9
 ab igne — see Burn, by site, first degree
 annulare (centrifugum) (rheumaticum) 695.0
 arthriticum epidemicum 026.1
 brucellum (see also Brucellosis) 023.9
 bullosum 695.1
 caloricum — see Burn, by site, first degree
 chronicum migrans 088.81
  chronicum 088.81
 circinatum 695.1
 diaper 691.0
 due to
  chemical (contact) NEC 692.4
   internal 693.8
  drug (internal use) 693.0
   contact 692.3
 elevatum diutinum 695.89
 endemic 265.2
 epidemic, arthritic 026.1
 figuratum perstans 695.0
 gluteal 691.0
 gyratum (perstans) (repens) 695.1
 heat — see Burn, by site, first degree
 ichthyosiforme congenitum 757.1
 induratum (primary) (scrofulosorum) (see also Tuberculosis) 017.1
  nontuberculous 695.2
 infantum febrile 057.8
 infectional NEC 695.9
 infectiosum 057.0
 inflammation NEC 695.9
 intertrigo 695.89
 iris 695.1
 lupus (discoid) (localized) (see also Lupus erythematosus) 695.4
 marginatum 695.0
  rheumaticum — see Fever, rheumatic
 medicamentosum — see Dermatitis, due to, drug
 migrans 529.1
 multiforme 695.1
  bullosum 695.1
  conjunctiva 695.1
  exudativum (Hebra) 695.1
  pemphigoides 694.5
 napkin 691.0
 neonatorum 778.8
 nodosum 695.2
  tuberculous (see also Tuberculosis) 017.1
 nummular, nummulare 695.1
 palmar 695.0
 palmaris hereditarium 695.0

Erythema, erythematous—continued
  pernio 991.5
  perstans solare 692.72
  rash, newborn 778.8
  scarlatiniform (exfoliative) (recurrent) 695.0
  simplex marginatum 057.8
  solare 692.71
  streptogenes 696.5
  toxic, toxicum NEC 695.0
    newborn 778.8
  tuberculous (primary) (see also Tuberculosis) 017.0
  venenatum 695.0
Erythematosus — see condition
Erythematous — see condition
Erythermalgia (primary) 443.89
Erythralgia 443.89
Erythrasma 039.0
Erythredema 985.0
  polyneuritica 985.0
  polyneuropathy 985.0
Erythremia (acute) (M9841/3) 207.0
  chronic (M9842/3) 207.1
  secondary 289.0
Erythroblastopenia (acquired) 284.8
  congenital 284.0
Erythroblastophthisis 284.0
Erythroblastosis (fetalis) (newborn) 773.2
  due to
    ABO
      antibodies 773.1
      incompatibility, maternal/fetal 773.1
      isoimmunization 773.1
    Rh
      antibodies 773.0
      incompatibility, maternal/fetal 773.0
      isoimmunization 773.0
Erythrocyanosis (crurum) 443.89
Erythrocythemia — see Erythremia
Erythrocytosis (megalosplenic)
  familial 289.6
  oval, hereditary (see also Elliptocytosis) 282.1
  secondary 289.0
  stress 289.0
Erythroderma (see also Erythema) 695.9
  desquamativa (in infants) 695.89
  exfoliative 695.89
  ichthyosiform, congenital 757.1
  infantum 695.89
  maculopapular 696.2
  neonatorum 778.8
  psoriaticum 696.1
  secondary 695.9
Erythrogenesis imperfecta 284.0
Erythroleukemia (M9840/3) 207.0
Erythromelalgia 443.89
Erythromelia 701.8
Erythrophagocytosis 289.9
Erythrophobia 300.23
Erythroplakia
  oral mucosa 528.7
  tongue 528.7
Erythroplasia (Queyrat) (M8080/2)
  specified site — see Neoplasm, skin, in situ
  unspecified site 233.5
Erythropoiesis, idiopathic ineffective 285.0
Escaped beats, heart 427.60
  postoperative 997.1
Esoenteritis — see Enteritis
Esophagalgia 530.89
Esophagectasis 530.89
  due to cardiospasm 530.0
Esophagismus 530.5

Esophagitis (acute) (alkaline) (chemical) (chronic) (infectional) (necrotic) (peptic) (postoperative) (regurgitant) 530.10
  candidal 112.84
  reflux 530.11
  specified NEC 530.19
  tuberculous (see also Tuberculosis) 017.8
Esophagocele 530.6
Esophagodynia 530.89
Esophagomalacia 530.89
Esophagoptosis 530.89
Esophagospasm 530.5
Esophagostenosis 530.3
Esophagostomiasis 127.7
Esophagotracheal — see condition
Esophagus — see condition
Esophoria 378.41
  convergence, excess 378.84
  divergence, insufficiency 378.85
Esotropia (nonaccommodative) 378.00
  accommodative 378.35
  alternating 378.05
    with
      A pattern 378.06
      specified noncomitancy NEC 378.08
      V pattern 378.07
      X pattern 378.08
      Y pattern 378.08
    intermittent 378.22
  intermittent 378.20
    alternating 378.22
    monocular 378.21
  monocular 378.01
    with
      A pattern 378.02
      specified noncomitancy NEC 378.04
      V pattern 378.03
      X pattern 378.04
      Y pattern 378.04
    intermittent 378.21
Espundia 085.5
Essential — see condition
Esterapenia 289.8
Esthesioneuroblastoma (M9522/3) 160.0
Esthesioneurocytoma (M9521/3) 160.0
Esthesioneuroepithelioma (M9523/3) 160.0
Esthiomene 099.1
Estivo-autumnal
  fever 084.0
  malaria 084.0
Estrangement V61.0
Estriasis 134.0
Ethanolaminuria 270.8
Ethanolism (see also Alcoholism) 303.9
Ether dependence, dependency (see also Dependence) 304.6
Etherism (see also Dependence) 304.6
Ethmoid, ethmoidal — see condition
Ethmoiditis (chronic) (nonpurulent) (purulent) (see also Sinusitis, ethmoidal) 473.2
  influenzal 487.1
  Woakes' 471.1
Ethylism (see also Alcoholism) 303.9
Eulenburg's disease (congenital paramyotonia) 359.2
Eunuchism 257.2
Eunuchoidism 257.2
  hypogonadotropic 257.2
European blastomycosis 117.5

Eustachian — see condition
Euthyroidism 244.9
Evaluation
  for suspected condition (see also Observation) V71.9
    newborn — see Observation, suspected, condition, newborn
    specified condition NEC V71.8
  mental health V70.2
    requested by authority V70.1
  nursing care V63.8
  social service V63.8
Evan's syndrome (thrombocytopenic purpura) 287.3
Eventration
  colon into chest — see Hernia, diaphragm
  diaphragm (congenital) 756.6
Eversion
  bladder 596.8
  cervix (uteri) 622.0
    with mention of cervicitis 616.0
  foot NEC 736.79
    congenital 755.67
  lacrimal punctum 375.51
  punctum lacrimale (postinfectional) (senile) 375.51
  ureter (meatus) 593.89
  urethra (meatus) 599.84
  uterus 618.1
    complicating delivery 665.2
      affecting fetus or newborn 763.8
    puerperal, postpartum 674.8
Evisceration
  birth injury 767.8
  bowel (congenital) — see Hernia, ventral
  congenital (see also Hernia, ventral) 553.29
  operative wound 998.3
  traumatic NEC 869.1
    eye 871.3
Evulsion — see Avulsion
Ewing's
  angioendothelioma (M9260/3) — see Neoplasm, bone, malignant
  sarcoma (M9260/3) — see Neoplasm, bone, malignant
  tumor (M9260/3) — see Neoplasm, bone, malignant
Exaggerated lumbosacral angle (with impinging spine) 756.12
Examination (general) (routine) (of) (for) V70.9
  allergy V72.7
  annual V70.0
  cardiovascular preoperative V72.81
  cervical Papanicolaou smear V76.2
    as a part of routine gynecological examination V72.3
  child care (routine) V20.2
  clinical research investigation (normal control patient) V70.7
  dental V72.2
  developmental testing (child) (infant) V20.2
  donor (potential) V70.8
  ear V72.1
  eye V72.0
  following
    accident (motor vehicle) V71.4
    alleged rape or seduction (victim or culprit) V71.5
    inflicted injury (victim or culprit) NEC V71.6

Examination—continued
  following—continued
    rape or seduction, alleged (victim or culprit) V71.5
    treatment (for) V67.9
      combined V67.6
      fracture V67.4
      involving high-risk medication NEC V67.51
      mental disorder V67.3
      specified condition NEC V67.59
  follow-up (routine) (following) V67.9
    cancer chemotherapy V67.2
    chemotherapy V67.2
    disease NEC V67.59
    high-risk medication NEC V67.51
    injury NEC V67.59
    population survey V70.6
    postpartum V24.2
    psychiatric V67.3
    psychotherapy V67.3
    radiotherapy V67.1
    surgery V67.0
  gynecological V72.3
    for contraceptive maintenance V25.40
      intrauterine device V25.42
      pill V25.41
      specified method NEC V25.49
  health (of)
    armed forces personnel V70.5
    checkup V70.0
    child, routine V20.2
    defined subpopulation NEC V70.5
    inhabitants of institutions V70.5
    occupational V70.5
    pre-employment screening V70.5
    preschool children V70.5
      for admission to school V70.3
    prisoners V70.5
      for entrance into prison V70.3
    prostitutes V70.5
    refugees V70.5
    school children V70.5
    students V70.5
  hearing V72.1
  infant V20.2
  laboratory V72.6
  lactating mother V24.1
  medical (for) (of) V70.9
    administrative purpose NEC V70.3
    admission to
      old age home V70.3
      prison V70.3
      school V70.3
    adoption V70.3
    armed forces personnel V70.5
    at health care facility V70.0
    camp V70.3
    child, routine V20.2
    clinical research, normal comparison in V70.7
    control subject in clinical research V70.7
    defined subpopulation NEC V70.5
    donor (potential) V70.8
    driving license V70.3
    general V70.9
      routine V70.0
      specified reason NEC V70.8
    immigration V70.3
    inhabitants of institutions V70.5
    insurance certification V70.3

Examination—continued
  medical—continued
    marriage V70.3
    medicolegal reasons V70.4
    naturalization V70.3
    occupational V70.5
    population survey V70.6
    pre-employment V70.5
    preschool children V70.5
      for admission to school V70.3
    prison V70.3
    prisoners V70.5
      for entrance into prison V70.3
    prostitutes V70.5
    refugees V70.5
    school children V70.5
    specified reason NEC V70.8
    sport competition V70.3
    students V70.5
  medicolegal reason V70.4
  pelvic (annual) (periodic) V72.3
  periodic (annual) (routine) V70.0
  postpartum
    immediately after delivery V24.0
    routine follow-up V24.2
  pregnancy (unconfirmed) (possible) V72.4
  prenatal V22.1
    first pregnancy V22.0
    high-risk pregnancy V23.9
      specified problem NEC V23.8
  preoperative V72.84
    cardiovascular V72.81
    respiratory V72.82
    specified NEC V72.83
  psychiatric V70.2
    follow-up not needing further care V67.3
    requested by authority V70.1
  radiological NEC V72.5
  respiratory preoperative V72.82
  screening — see Screening
  sensitization V72.7
  skin V72.7
    hypersensitivity V72.7
  special V72.9
  specified type or reason NEC V72.85
    preoperative V72.83
      specified NEC V72.83
  teeth V72.2
  victim or culprit following alleged rape or seduction V71.5
    inflicted injury NEC V71.6
  vision V72.0
  well baby V20.2

Exanthem, exanthema (see also Rash) 782.1
  Boston 048
  epidemic, with meningitis 048
  lichenoid psoriasiform 696.2
  subitum 057.8
  viral, virus NEC 057.9
    specified type NEC 057.8

Excess, excessive, excessively
  alcohol level in blood 790.3
  carbohydrate tissue, localized 278.1
  carotene (dietary) 278.3
  cold 991.9
    specified effect NEC 991.8
  convergence 378.84
  development, breast 611.1
  diaphoresis 780.8
  divergence 378.85
  drinking (alcohol) NEC (see also Abuse, drugs, nondependent) 305.0
    continual (see also Alcoholism) 303.9
    habitual (see also Alcoholism) 303.9

Excess, excessive, excessively—continued
  eating 783.6
  eyelid fold (congenital) 743.62
  fat 278.0
    in heart (see also Degeneration, myocardial) 429.1
    tissue, localized 278.1
  foreskin 605
  gas 787.3
  gastrin 251.5
  glucagon 251.4
  heat (see also Heat) 992.9
  large
    colon 564.7
      congenital 751.3
    fetus or infant 766.0
      with obstructed labor 660.1
        affecting management of pregnancy 656.6
      causing disproportion 653.5
    newborn (weight of 4500 grams or more) 766.0
    organ or site, congenital NEC — see Anomaly, specified type NEC
  lid fold (congenital) 743.62
  long
    colon 751.5
    organ or site, congenital NEC — see Anomaly, specified type NEC
    umbilical cord (entangled)
      affecting fetus or newborn 762.5
      in pregnancy or childbirth 663.3
        with compression 663.2
  menstruation 626.2
  number of teeth 520.1
    causing crowding 524.3
  nutrients (dietary) NEC 783.6
  potassium (K) 276.7
  salivation (see also Ptyalism) 527.7
  secretion — see also Hypersecretion
    milk 676.6
    sputum 786.4
    sweat 780.8
  short
    organ or site, congenital NEC — see Anomaly, specified type NEC
    umbilical cord
      affecting fetus or newborn 762.6
      in pregnancy or childbirth 663.4
  skin NEC 701.9
    eyelid 743.62
      acquired 374.30
  sodium (Na) 276.0
  sputum 786.4
  sweating 780.8
  tearing (ducts) (eye) (see also Epiphora) 375.20
  thirst 783.5
    due to deprivation of water 994.3
  vitamin
    A (dietary) 278.2
      administered as drug (chronic) (prolonged excessive intake) 278.2
      reaction to sudden overdose 963.5
    D (dietary) 278.4
      administered as drug (chronic) (prolonged excessive intake) 278.4
      reaction to sudden overdose 963.5

Excess, excessive, excessively—continued
  weight 278.0
    gain 783.1
      of pregnancy 646.1
    loss 783.2

Excitability, abnormal, under minor stress 309.29

Excitation
  catatonic (see also Schizophrenia) 295.2
  psychogenic 298.1
  reactive (from emotional stress, psychological trauma) 298.1

Excitement
  manic (see also Psychosis, affective) 296.0
    recurrent episode 296.1
    single episode 296.0
  mental, reactive (from emotional stress, psychological trauma) 298.1
  state, reactive (from emotional stress, psychological trauma) 298.1

Excluded pupils 364.76

Excoriation (traumatic) (see also Injury, superficial, by site) 919.8
  neurotic 698.4

Excyclophoria 378.44

Excyclotropia 378.33

Exencephalus, exencephaly 742.0

Exercise
  breathing V57.0
  remedial NEC V57.1
  therapeutic NEC V57.1

Exfoliation, teeth due to systemic causes 525.0

Exfoliative — see also condition
  dermatitis 695.89

Exhaustion, exhaustive (physical NEC) 780.7
  battle (see also Reaction, stress, acute) 308.9
  cardiac (see also Failure, heart) 428.9
  delirium (see also Reaction, stress, acute) 308.9
  due to
    cold 991.8
    excessive exertion 994.5
    exposure 994.4
  fetus or newborn 779.8
  heart (see also Failure, heart) 428.9
  heat 992.5
    due to
      salt depletion 992.4
      water depletion 992.3
  manic (see also Psychosis, affective) 296.0
    recurrent episode 296.1
    single episode 296.0
  maternal, complicating delivery 669.8
    affecting fetus or newborn 763.8
  mental 300.5
  myocardium, myocardial (see also Failure, heart) 428.9
  nervous 300.5
  old age 797
  postinfectional NEC 780.7
  psychogenic 300.5
  psychosis (see also Reaction, stress, acute) 308.9
  senile 797
    dementia 290.0

Exhibitionism (sexual) 302.4

Exomphalos 756.7

Exophoria 378.42
  convergence, insufficiency 378.83
  divergence, excess 378.85

Exophthalmic
  cachexia 242.0
  goiter 242.0
  ophthalmoplegia 242.0 [376.22]

Exophthalmos 376.30
  congenital 743.66
  constant 376.31
  endocrine NEC 259.9 [376.22]
  hyperthyroidism 242.0 [376.21]
  intermittent NEC 376.34
  malignant 242.0 [376.21]
  pulsating 376.35
    endocrine NEC 259.9 [376.22]
  thyrotoxic 242.0 [376.21]

Exostosis 726.91
  cartilaginous (M9210/0) — see Neoplasm, bone, benign
  congenital 756.4
  ear canal, external 380.81
  gonococcal 098.89
  hip 726.5
  intracranial 733.3
  jaw (bone) 526.81
  luxurians 728.11
  multiple (cancellous) (congenital) (hereditary) 756.4
  nasal bones 726.91
  orbit, orbital 376.42
  osteocartilaginous (M9210/0) — see Neoplasm, bone, benign
  spine 721.8
    with spondylosis — see Spondylosis
  syphilitic 095.5
  wrist 726.4

Exotropia 378.10
  alternating 378.15
    with
      A pattern 378.16
      specified noncomitancy NEC 378.18
      V pattern 378.17
      X pattern 378.18
      Y pattern 378.18
    intermittent 378.24
  intermittent 378.20
    alternating 378.24
    monocular 378.23
  monocular 378.11
    with
      A pattern 378.12
      specified noncomitancy NEC 378.14
      V pattern 378.13
      X pattern 378.14
      Y pattern 378.14
    intermittent 378.23

Explanation of
  investigation finding V65.4
  medication V65.4

Exposure 994.9
  cold 991.9
    specified effect NEC 991.8
  effects of 994.9
  exhaustion due to 994.4
  to
    AIDS virus V01.7
    cholera V01.0
    communicable disease V01.9
      specified type NEC V01.8
    German measles V01.4
    gonorrhea V01.6
    HIV V01.7
    human immunodeficiency virus V01.7
    parasitic disease V01.8
    poliomyelitis V01.2
    rabies V01.5
    rubella V01.4
    smallpox V01.3
    syphilis V01.6

Exposure—continued
to—continued
tuberculosis V01.1
venereal disease V01.6
viral disease NEC V01.7
Exsanguination, fetal 772.0
Exstrophy
abdominal content 751.8
bladder (urinary) 753.5
Extensive — *see* condition
Extra — *see also* Accessory
rib 756.3
cervical 756.2
Extraction
with hook 763.8
breech NEC 669.6
affecting fetus or newborn 763.0
cataract postsurgical V45.6
manual NEC 669.8
affecting fetus or newborn 763.8
Extrasystole 427.60
atrial 427.61
postoperative 997.1
ventricular 427.69
Extrauterine gestation or pregnancy — *see* Pregnancy, ectopic
Extravasation
blood 459.0
lower extremity 459.0
chyle into mesentery 457.8
pelvicalyceal 593.4
pyelosinus 593.4
urine 788.8
from ureter 788.8
Extremity — *see* condition
Extrophy — *see* Exstrophy
Extroversion
bladder 753.5
uterus 618.1
complicating delivery 665.2
affecting fetus or newborn 763.8
postpartal (old) 618.1
Extrusion
breast implant (prosthetic) 996.54
device, implant, or graft — *see* Complications, mechanical
eye implant (ball) (globe) 996.59
intervertebral disc — *see* Displacement, intervertebral disc
lacrimal gland 375.43
mesh (reinforcing) 996.59
ocular lens implant 996.53
prosthetic device NEC — *see* Complications, mechanical
vitreous 379.26
Exudate, pleura — *see* Effusion, pleura
Exudates, retina 362.82
Exudative — *see* condition
Eye, eyeball, eyelid — *see* condition
Eyestrain 368.13
Eyeworm disease of Africa 125.2

F

Faber's anemia or syndrome (achlorhydric anemia) 280.9
Fabry's disease (angiokeratoma corporis diffusum) 272.7
Face, facial — *see* condition
Facet of cornea 371.44
Faciocephalgia, autonomic (*see also* Neuropathy, peripheral, autonomic) 337.9
Facioscapulohumeral myopathy 359.1
Factitious disorder, illness — *see* Illness, factitious

Factor
deficiency — *see* Deficiency, factor
psychic, associated with diseases classified elsewhere 316
Fahr-Volhard disease (malignant nephrosclerosis) 403.00
Failure, failed
adenohypophyseal 253.2
attempted abortion (legal) (*see also* Abortion, failed) 638.9
bone marrow (anemia) 284.9
acquired (secondary) 284.8
congenital 284.0
idiopathic 284.9
cardiac (*see also* Failure, heart) 428.9
newborn 779.8
cardiorenal (chronic) 428.9
hypertensive (*see also* Hypertension, cardiorenal) 404.93
cardiorespiratory 799.1
specified during or due to a procedure 997.1
long-term effect of cardiac surgery 429.4
cardiovascular (chronic) 428.9
cerebrovascular 437.8
cervical dilatation in labor 661.0
affecting fetus or newborn 763.7
circulation, circulatory 799.8
fetus or newborn 779.8
peripheral 785.50
compensation — *see* Disease, heart
congestive (*see also* Failure, heart, congestive) 428.0
coronary (*see also* Insufficiency, coronary) 411.89
descent of head (at term) 652.5
affecting fetus or newborn 763.1
in labor 660.0
affecting fetus or newborn 763.1
device, implant, or graft — *see* Complications, mechanical
engagement of head NEC 652.5
in labor 660.0
extrarenal 788.9
fetal head to enter pelvic brim 652.5
affecting fetus or newborn 763.1
in labor 660.0
affecting fetus or newborn 763.1
forceps NEC 660.7
affecting fetus or newborn 763.1
fusion (joint) (spinal) 996.4
growth 783.4
heart (acute) (sudden) 428.9
with
abortion — *see* Abortion, by type, with specified complication NEC
acute pulmonary edema (*see also* Failure, ventricular, left) 428.1
with congestion 428.0
decompensation (*see also* Failure, heart, congestive) 428.0
dilation — *see* Disease, heart
ectopic pregnancy (*see also* categories 633.0-633.9) 639.8
molar pregnancy (*see also* categories 630-632) 639.8
arteriosclerotic 440.9

Failure, failed—*continued*
heart—*continued*
combined left-right sided 428.0
compensated (*see also* Failure, heart, congestive) 428.0
complicating
abortion — *see* Abortion, by type, with specified complication NEC
delivery (cesarean) (instrumental) 669.4
ectopic pregnancy (*see also* categories 633.0-633.9) 639.8
molar pregnancy (*see also* categories 630-632) 639.8
obstetric anesthesia or sedation 668.1
surgery 997.1
congestive (compensated) (decompensated) 428.0
with rheumatic fever (conditions classifiable to 390)
active 391.8
inactive or quiescent (with chorea) 398.91
fetus or newborn 779.8
hypertensive (*see also* Hypertension, heart) 402.90
with renal disease (*see also* Hypertension, cardiorenal) 404.91
with renal failure 404.93
benign 402.11
malignant 402.01
rheumatic (chronic) (inactive) (with chorea) 398.91
active or acute 391.8
with chorea (Sydenham's) 392.0
decompensated (*see also* Failure, heart, congestive) 428.0
degenerative (*see also* Degeneration, myocardial) 429.1
due to presence of (cardiac) prosthesis 429.4
fetus or newborn 779.8
following
abortion 639.8
cardiac surgery 429.4
ectopic or molar pregnancy 639.8
high output NEC 428.9
hypertensive (*see also* Hypertension, heart) 402.91
with renal disease (*see also* Hypertension, cardiorenal) 404.91
with renal failure 404.93
benign 402.11
malignant 402.01
left (ventricular) (*see also* Failure, ventricular, left) 428.1
with right-sided failure 428.0
low output (syndrome) NEC 428.9
organic — *see* Disease, heart

Failure, failed—*continued*
heart—*continued*
postoperative (immediate) 997.1
long term effect of cardiac surgery 429.4
rheumatic (chronic) (congestive) (inactive) 398.91
right (secondary to left heart failure, conditions classifiable to 428.1) (ventricular) (*see also* Failure, heart, congestive) 428.0
senile 797
specified during or due to a procedure 997.1
long-term effect of cardiac surgery 429.4
thyrotoxic (*see also* Thyrotoxicosis) 242.9 [425.7]
valvular — *see* Endocarditis
hepatic 572.8
acute 570
due to a procedure 997.4
hepatorenal 572.4
hypertensive heart (*see also* Hypertension, heart) 402.91
benign 402.11
malignant 402.01
induction (of labor) 659.1
abortion (legal) (*see also* Abortion, failed) 638.9
affecting fetus or newborn 763.8
by oxytocic drugs 659.1
instrumental 659.0
mechanical 659.0
medical 659.1
surgical 659.0
initial alveolar expansion, newborn 770.4
involution, thymus (gland) 254.8
kidney — *see* Failure, renal
lactation 676.4
Leydig's cell, adult 257.2
liver 572.8
acute 570
medullary 799.8
mitral — *see* Endocarditis, mitral
myocardium, myocardial (*see also* Failure, heart) 428.9
chronic (*see also* Failure, heart, congestive) 428.0
congestive (*see also* Failure, heart, congestive) 428.0
ovarian (primary) 256.3
iatrogenic 256.2
postablative 256.2
postirradiation 256.2
postsurgical 256.2
ovulation 628.0
prerenal 788.9
renal 586
with
abortion — *see* Abortion, by type, with renal failure
ectopic pregnancy (*see also* categories 633.0-633.9) 639.3
edema (*see also* Nephrosis) 581.9
hypertension (*see also* Hypertension, kidney) 403.91
hypertensive heart disease (conditions classifiable to 402) 404.92
with heart failure 404.93

Failure, failed—continued
  renal—continued
    with—continued
      hypertensive heart
        disease—continued
          benign 404.12
            with heart failure 404.13
          malignant 404.02
            with heart failure 404.03
      molar pregnancy (see also categories 630-632) 639.3
      tubular necrosis (acute) 584.5
    acute 584.9
      with lesion of
        necrosis
          cortical (renal) 584.6
          medullary (renal) (papillary) 584.7
        tubular 584.5
      specified pathology NEC 584.8
    chronic 585
      hypertensive or with hypertension (see also Hypertension, kidney) 403.91
    due to a procedure 997.5
    following
      abortion 639.3
      crushing 958.5
      ectopic or molar pregnancy 639.3
      labor and delivery (acute) 669.3
    hypertensive (see also Hypertension, kidney) 403.91
    puerperal, postpartum 669.3
  respiration, respiratory 518.81
    acute (acute-on-chronic) 518.81
    center 348.8
      newborn 770.8
    chronic 518.81
    due to trauma, surgery or shock 518.5
    newborn 770.8
  rotation
    cecum 751.4
    colon 751.4
    intestine 751.4
    kidney 753.3
  segmentation — see also Fusion
    fingers (see also Syndactylism, fingers) 755.11
    toes (see also Syndactylism, toes) 755.13
  seminiferous tubule, adult 257.2
  senile (general) 797
    with psychosis 290.20
  testis, primary (seminal) 257.2
  to thrive 783.4
  transplant 996.80
    bone marrow 996.85
    organ (immune or nonimmune cause) 996.80
      bone marrow 996.85
      heart 996.83
      intestines 996.89
      kidney 996.81
      liver 996.82
      lung 996.84
      pancreas 996.86
      specified NEC 996.89
    skin 996.52
      temporary allograft or pigskin graft — omit code
  trial of labor NEC 660.6
    affecting fetus or newborn 763.1
  urinary 586

Failure, failed—continued
  vacuum extraction
    abortion — see Abortion, failed
    delivery NEC 660.7
      affecting fetus or newborn 763.1
    ventouse NEC 660.7
      affecting fetus or newborn 763.1
  ventricular (see also Failure, heart) 428.9
    left 428.1
      with rheumatic fever (conditions classifiable to 390)
        active 391.8
          with chorea 392.0
        inactive or quiescent (with chorea) 398.91
      hypertensive (see also Hypertension, heart) 402.91
        benign 402.11
        malignant 402.01
      rheumatic (chronic) (inactive) (with chorea) 398.91
        active or acute 391.8
          with chorea 392.0
    right (see also Failure, heart, congestive) 428.0
  vital centers, fetus or newborn 779.8
  weight gain 783.4
Fainting (fit) (spell) 780.2
Falciform hymen 752.49
Fall, maternal, affecting fetus or newborn 760.5
Fallen arches 734
Falling, any organ or part — see Prolapse
Fallopian
  insufflation V26.2
  tube — see condition
Fallot's
  pentalogy 745.2
  tetrad or tetralogy 745.2
  triad or trilogy 746.09
Fallout, radioactive (adverse effect) NEC 990
False — see also condition
  bundle branch block 426.50
  bursa 727.89
  croup 478.75
  joint 733.82
  labor (pains) 644.1
  opening, urinary 752.8
  passage, urethra (prostatic) 599.4
  positive
    serological test for syphilis 795.6
    Wassermann reaction 795.6
  pregnancy 300.11
Family, familial — see also condition
  disruption V61.0
  planning advice V25.09
  problem V61.9
    specified circumstance NEC V61.8
Famine 994.2
  edema 262
Fanconi's anemia (congenital pancytopenia) 284.0
Fanconi (-de Toni) (-Debré) syndrome (cystinosis) 270.0
Farber (-Uzman) syndrome or disease (disseminated lipogranulomatosis) 272.8
Farcin 024
Farcy 024

Farmers'
  lung 495.0
  skin 692.74
Farsightedness 367.0
Fascia — see condition
Fasciculation 781.0
Fasciculitis optica 377.32
Fasciitis 729.4
  eosinophilic 728.89
  necrotizing 729.4 ◆
  nodular 728.79
  perirenal 593.4
  plantar 728.71
  pseudosarcomatous 728.79
  traumatic (old) NEC 728.79
    current — see Sprain, by site
Fasciola hepatica infestation 121.3
Fascioliasis 121.3
Fasciolopsiasis (small intestine) 121.4
Fasciolopsis (small intestine) 121.4
Fast pulse 785.0
Fat
  embolism (cerebral) (pulmonary) (systemic) 958.1
    with
      abortion — see Abortion, by type, with embolism
      ectopic pregnancy (see also categories 633.0-633.9) 639.6
      molar pregnancy (see also categories 630-632) 639.6
    complicating delivery or puerperium 673.8
    following
      abortion 639.6
      ectopic or molar pregnancy 639.6
    in pregnancy, childbirth, or the puerperium 673.8
  excessive 278.0
    in heart (see also Degeneration, myocardial) 429.1
  general 278.0
  hernia, herniation 729.30
    eyelid 374.34
    knee 729.31
    orbit 374.34
    retro-orbital 374.34
    retropatellar 729.31
    specified site NEC 729.39
  indigestion 579.8
  in stool 792.1
  localized (pad) 278.1
    heart (see also Degeneration, myocardial) 429.1
    knee 729.31
    retropatellar 729.31
  necrosis — see also Fatty, degeneration breast (aseptic) (segmental) 611.3
    mesentery 567.8
    omentum 567.8
  pad 278.1
Fatal syncope 798.1
Fatigue 780.7
  auditory deafness (see also Deafness) 389.9
  chronic, syndrome 780.7
  chronic 780.7
  combat (see also Reaction, stress, acute) 308.9
  during pregnancy 646.8
  general 780.7
    psychogenic 300.5
  heat (transient) 992.6
  muscle 729.89
  myocardium (see also Failure, heart) 428.9
  nervous 300.5

Fatigue—continued
  neurosis 300.5
  operational 300.89
  postural 729.89
  posture 729.89
  psychogenic (general) 300.5
  senile 797
  syndrome NEC 300.5
  undue 780.7
  voice 784.49
Fatness 278.0
Fatty — see also condition
  apron 278.1
  degeneration (diffuse) (general) NEC 272.8
    localized — see Degeneration, by site, fatty
    placenta — see Placenta, abnormal
  heart (enlarged) (see also Degeneration, myocardial) 429.1
  infiltration (diffuse) (general) (see also Degeneration, by site, fatty) 272.8
    heart (enlarged) (see also Degeneration, myocardial) 429.1
  liver 571.8
    alcoholic 571.0
  necrosis — see Degeneration, fatty
  phanerosis 272.8
Fauces — see condition
Fauchard's disease (periodontitis) 523.4
Faucitis 478.29
Faulty — see also condition
  position of teeth 524.3
Favism (anemia) 282.2
Favre-Racouchot disease (elastoidosis cutanea nodularis) 701.8
Favus 110.9
  beard 110.0
  capitis 110.0
  corporis 110.5
  eyelid 110.8
  foot 110.4
  hand 110.2
  scalp 110.0
  specified site NEC 110.8
Fear, fearfullness (complex) (reaction) 300.20
  child 313.0
  of
    animals 300.29
    closed spaces 300.29
    crowds 300.29
    eating in public 300.23
    heights 300.29
    open spaces 300.22
      with panic attacks 300.21
    public speaking 300.23
    streets 300.22
      with panic attacks 300.21
    travel 300.22
      with panic attacks 300.21
    washing in public 300.23
  transient 308.0
Feared complaint unfounded V65.5
Febricula (continued) (simple) (see also Pyrexia) 780.6
Febrile (see also Pyrexia) 780.6
Febris (see also Fever) 780.6
  aestiva (see also Fever, hay) 477.9
  flava (see also Fever, yellow) 060.9
  melitensis 023.0
  pestis (see also Plague) 020.9
  puerperalis 670
  recurrens (see also Fever, relapsing) 087.9
    pediculo vestimenti 087.0
  rubra 034.1

Febris — continued
- typhoidea 002.0
- typhosa 002.0

Fecal — *see* condition

Fecalith (impaction) 560.39
- with hernia — *see also* Hernia, by site, with obstruction
- gangrenous — *see* Hernia, by site, with gangrene
- appendix 543.9
- congenital 777.1

Fede's disease 529.0

Feeble-minded 317

Feeble rapid pulse due to shock following injury 958.4

Feeding
- faulty (elderly) (infant) 783.3
  - newborn 779.3
- formula check V20.2
- improper (elderly) (infant) 783.3
  - newborn 779.3
- problem (elderly) (infant) 783.3
  - newborn 779.3
  - nonorganic origin 307.59

Feer's disease 985.0

Feet — *see* condition

Feigned illness V65.2

Feil-Klippel syndrome (brevicollis) 756.16

Feinmesser's (hidrotic) ectodermal dysplasia 757.31

Felix's disease (juvenile osteochondrosis, hip) 732.1

Felon (any digit) (with lymphangitis) 681.01
- herpetic 054.6

Felty's syndrome (rheumatoid arthritis with splenomegaly and leukopenia) 714.1

Feminism in boys 302.6

Feminization, testicular 257.8
- with pseudohermaphroditism, male 257.8

Femoral hernia — *see* Hernia, femoral

Femora vara 736.32

Femur, femoral — *see* condition

Fenestrata placenta — *see* Placenta, abnormal

Fenestration, fenestrated — *see also* Imperfect, closure
- aorta-pulmonary 745.0
- aorticopulmonary 745.0
- aortopulmonary 745.0
- cusps, heart valve NEC 746.89
  - pulmonary 746.09
- hymen 752.49
- pulmonic cusps 746.09

Fenwick's disease 537.89

Fermentation (gastric) (gastrointestinal) (stomach) 536.8
- intestine 564.8
  - psychogenic 306.4
- psychogenic 306.4

Fernell's disease (aortic aneurysm) 441.9

Fertile eunuch syndrome 257.2

Fertility, meaning multiparity — *see* Multiparity

Fetal alcohol syndrome 760.71

Fetalis uterus 752.3

Fetid
- breath 784.9
- sweat 705.89

Fetishism 302.81
- transvestic 302.3 ◆

Fetomaternal hemorrhage
- affecting management of pregnancy 656.0
- fetus or newborn 772.0

Fetus, fetal — *see also* condition
- papyraceous 779.8
- type lung tissue 770.4

Fever 780.6
- with chills 780.6
  - in malarial regions (*see also* Malaria) 084.6
- abortus NEC 023.9
- Aden 061
- African tick-borne 087.1
- American
  - mountain tick 066.1
  - spotted 082.0
- and ague (*see also* Malaria) 084.6
- aphthous 078.4
- arbovirus hemorrhagic 065.9
- Assam 085.0
- Australian A or Q 083.0
- Bangkok hemorrhagic 065.4
- biliary, Charcot's intermittent — *see* Choledocholithiasis
- bilious, hemoglobinuric 084.8
- blackwater 084.8
- blister 054.9
- Bonvale Dam 780.7
- boutonneuse 082.1
- brain 323.9
  - late effect — *see* category 326
- breakbone 061
- Bullis 082.8
- Bunyamwera 066.3
- Burdwan 085.0
- Bwamba (encephalitis) 066.3
- Cameroon (*see also* Malaria) 084.6
- Canton 081.9
- catarrhal (acute) 460
  - chronic 472.0
- cat-scratch 078.3
- cerebral 323.9
  - late effect — *see* category 326
- cerebrospinal (meningococcal) (*see also* Meningitis, cerebrospinal) 036.0
- Chagres 084.0
- Chandipura 066.8
- changuinola 066.0
- Charcot's (biliary) (hepatic) (intermittent) *see* Choledocholithiasis
- Chikungunya (viral) 066.3
  - hemorrhagic 065.4
- childbed 670
- Chitral 066.0
- Colombo (*see also* Fever, paratyphoid) 002.9
- Colorado tick (virus) 066.1
- congestive
  - malarial (*see also* Malaria) 084.6
  - remittent (*see also* Malaria) 084.6
- Congo virus 065.0
- continued 780.6
  - malarial 084.0
- Corsican (*see also* Malaria) 084.6
- Crimean hemorrhagic 065.0
- Cyprus (*see also* Brucellosis) 023.9
- dandy 061
- deer fly (*see also* Tularemia) 021.9
- dehydration, newborn 778.4
- dengue (virus) 061
  - hemorrhagic 065.4
- desert 114.0
- due to heat 992.0
- Dumdum 085.0
- enteric 002.0
- ephemeral (of unknown origin) (*see also* Pyrexia) 780.6
- epidemic, hemorrhagic of the Far East 065.0
- erysipelatous (*see also* Erysipelas) 035
- estivo-autumnal (malarial) 084.0
- etiocholanolone 277.3

Fever — continued
- famine — *see also* Fever, relapsing
  - meaning typhus — *see* Typhus
- Far Eastern hemorrhagic 065.0
- five day 083.1
- Fort Bragg 100.89
- gastroenteric 002.0
- gastromalarial (*see also* Malaria) 084.6
- Gibraltar (*see also* Brucellosis) 023.9
- glandular 075
- Guama (viral) 066.3
- Haverhill 026.1
- hay (allergic) (with rhinitis) 477.9
  - with
    - asthma (bronchial) (*see also* Asthma) 493.0
  - due to
    - dander 477.8
    - dust 477.8
    - fowl 477.8
    - pollen, any plant or tree 477.0
    - specified allergen other than pollen 477.8
- heat (effects) 992.0
- hematuric, bilious 084.8
- hemoglobinuric (malarial) 084.8
  - bilious 084.8
- hemorrhagic (arthropod-borne) NEC 065.9
  - with renal syndrome 078.6
  - arenaviral 078.7
  - Argentine 078.7
  - Bangkok 065.4
  - Bolivian 078.7
  - Central Asian 065.0
  - chikungunya 065.4
  - Crimean 065.0
  - dengue (virus) 065.4
  - epidemic 078.6
    - of Far East 065.0
  - Far Eastern 065.0
  - Junin virus 078.7
  - Korean 078.6
  - Kyasanur forest 065.2
  - Machupo virus 078.7
  - mite-borne NEC 065.8
  - mosquito-borne 065.4
  - Omsk 065.1
  - Philippine 065.4
  - Russian (Yaroslav) 078.6
  - Singapore 065.4
  - Southeast Asia 065.4
  - Thailand 065.4
  - tick-borne NEC 065.3
- hepatic (*see also* Cholecystitis) 575.8
  - intermittent (Charcot's) — *see* Choledocholithiasis
- herpetic (*see also* Herpes) 054.9
- Hyalomma tick 065.0
- icterohemorrhagic 100.0
- inanition 780.6
  - newborn 778.4
- infective NEC 136.9
- intermittent (bilious) (*see also* Malaria) 084.6
  - hepatic (Charcot) — *see* Choledocholithiasis
  - of unknown origin (*see also* Pyrexia) 780.6
  - pernicious 084.0
- iodide
  - correct substance properly administered 780.6
  - overdose or wrong substance given or taken 975.5
- Japanese river 081.2
- jungle yellow 060.0
- Junin virus 078.7
- Katayama 120.2
- Kedani 081.2
- Kenya 082.1
- Korean hemorrhagic 078.6

Fever — continued
- Lassa 078.89
- Lone Star 082.8
- lung — *see* Pneumonia
- Machupo virus, hemorrhagic 078.7
- malaria, malarial (*see also* Malaria) 084.6
- Malta (*see also* Brucellosis) 023.9
- Marseilles 082.1
- marsh (*see also* Malaria) 084.6
- Mayaro (viral) 066.3
- Mediterranean (*see also* Brucellosis) 023.9
  - familial 277.3
  - tick 082.1
- meningeal — *see* Meningitis
- metal fumes NEC 985.8
- Meuse 083.1
- Mexican — *see* Typhus, Mexican
- Mianeh 087.1
- miasmatic (*see also* Malaria) 084.6
- miliary 078.2
- milk, female 672
- mill 504
- mite-borne hemorrhagic 065.8
- Monday 504
- mosquito-borne NEC 066.3
  - hemorrhagic NEC 065.4
- mountain 066.1
  - meaning
    - Rocky Mountain spotted 082.0
    - undulant fever (*see also* Brucellosis) 023.9
  - tick (American) 066.1
- Mucambo (viral) 066.3
- mud 100.89
- Neapolitan (*see also* Brucellosis) 023.9
- nine-mile 083.0
- nonexanthematous tick 066.1
- North Asian tick-borne typhus 082.2
- Omsk hemorrhagic 065.1
- O'nyong-nyong (viral) 066.3
- Oropouche (viral) 066.3
- Oroya 088.0
- paludal (*see also* Malaria) 084.6
- Panama 084.0
- pappataci 066.0
- paratyphoid 002.9
  - A 002.1
  - B (Schottmüller's) 002.2
  - C (Hirschfeld) 002.3
- parrot 073.9
- periodic 277.3
- pernicious, acute 084.0
- persistent (of unknown origin) (*see also* Pyrexia) 780.6
- petechial 036.0
- pharyngoconjunctival 077.2
  - adenoviral type 3 077.2
- Philippine hemorrhagic 065.4
- phlebotomus 066.0
- Piry 066.8
- Pixuna (viral) 066.3
- Plasmodium ovale 084.3
- pleural (*see also* Pleurisy) 511.0
- pneumonic — *see* Pneumonia
- polymer fume 987.8
- postoperative 998.89 ◆
  - due to infection 998.5
- pretibial 100.89
- puerperal, postpartum 670
- putrid — *see* Septicemia
- pyemic — *see* Septicemia
- Q 083.0
  - with pneumonia 083.0 [484.8]
- quadrilateral 083.0
- quartan (malaria) 084.2
- Queensland (coastal) 083.0
  - seven-day 100.89
- Quintan (A) 083.1
- quotidian 084.0
- rabbit (*see also* Tularemia) 021.9

Fever—continued
- rat-bite 026.9
  - due to
    - Spirillum minor or minus 026.0
    - Spirochaeta morsus muris 026.0
    - Streptobacillus moniliformis 026.1
- recurrent — see Fever, relapsing
- relapsing 087.9
  - Carter's (Asiatic) 087.0
  - Dutton's (West African) 087.1
  - Koch's 087.9
  - louse-borne (epidemic) 087.0
  - Novy's (American) 087.1
  - Obermeyer's (European) 087.0
  - spirillum NEC 087.9
  - tick-borne (endemic) 087.1
- remittent (bilious) (congestive) (gastric) (see also Malaria) 084.6
- rheumatic (active) (acute) (chronic) (subacute) 390
  - with heart involvement 391.9
    - carditis 391.9
    - endocarditis (aortic) (mitral) (pulmonary) (tricuspid) 391.1
    - multiple sites 391.8
    - myocarditis 391.2
    - pancarditis, acute 391.8
    - pericarditis 391.0
    - specified type NEC 391.8
    - valvulitis 391.1
  - inactive or quiescent with cardiac hypertrophy 398.99
    - carditis 398.90
    - endocarditis 397.9
      - aortic (valve) 395.9
        - with mitral (valve) disease 396.9
      - mitral (valve) 394.9
        - with aortic (valve) disease 396.9
      - pulmonary (valve) 397.1
      - tricuspid (valve) 397.0
    - heart conditions (classifiable to 429.3, 429.6, 429.9) 398.99
      - failure (congestive) (conditions classifiable to 428.0, 428.9) 398.91
      - left ventricular failure (conditions classifiable to 428.1) 398.91
    - myocardial degeneration (conditions classifiable to 429.1) 398.0
    - myocarditis (conditions classifiable to 429.0) 398.0
    - pancarditis 398.99
    - pericarditis 393
- Rift Valley (viral) 066.3
- Rocky Mountain spotted 082.0
- rose 477.0
- Ross river (viral) 066.3
- Russian hemorrhagic 078.6
- sandfly 066.0
- San Joaquin (valley) 114.0
- São Paulo 082.0
- scarlet 034.1
- septic — see Septicemia
- seven-day 061
  - Japan 100.89
  - Queensland 100.89
- shin bone 083.1
- Singapore hemorrhagic 065.4
- solar 061
- sore 054.9
- South African tick-bite 087.1

Fever—continued
- Southeast Asia hemorrhagic 065.4
- spinal — see Meningitis
- spirillary 026.0
- splenic (see also Anthrax) 022.9
- spotted (Rocky Mountain) 082.0
  - American 082.0
  - Brazilian 082.0
  - Colombian 082.0
  - meaning
    - cerebrospinal meningitis 036.0
    - typhus 082.9
- spring 309.23
- steroid
  - correct substance properly administered 780.6
  - overdose or wrong substance given or taken 962.0
- streptobacillary 026.1
- subtertian 084.0
- Sumatran mite 081.2
- sun 061
- swamp 100.89
- sweating 078.2
- swine 003.8
- sylvatic yellow 060.0
- Tahyna 062.5
- tertian — see Malaria, tertian
- Thailand hemorrhagic 065.4
- thermic 992.0
- three day 066.0
  - with Coxsackie exanthem 074.8
- tick
  - American mountain 066.1
  - Colorado 066.1
  - Kemerovo 066.1
  - Mediterranean 082.1
  - mountain 066.1
  - nonexanthematous 066.1
  - Quaranfil 066.1
- tick-bite NEC 066.1
- tick-borne NEC 066.1
  - hemorrhagic NEC 065.3
- transitory of newborn 778.4
- trench 083.1
- tsutsugamushi 081.2
- typhogastric 002.0
- typhoid (abortive) (ambulant) (any site) (hemorrhagic) (infection) (intermittent) (malignant) (rheumatic) 002.0
- typhomalarial (see also Malaria) 084.6
- typhus — see Typhus
- undulant (see also Brucellosis) 023.9
- unknown origin (see also Pyrexia) 780.6
- uremic — see Uremia
- uveoparotid 135
- valley (Coccidioidomycosis) 114.0
- Venezuelan equine 066.2
- Volhynian 083.1
- Wesselsbron (viral) 066.3
- West
  - African 084.8
  - Nile (viral) 066.3
- Whitmore's 025
- Wolhynian 083.1
- worm 128.9
- Yaroslav hemorrhagic 078.6
- yellow 060.9
  - jungle 060.0
  - sylvatic 060.0
  - urban 060.1
  - vaccination, prophylactic (against) V04.4
- Zika (viral) 066.3

Fibrillation
- atrial (established) (paroxysmal) 427.31

Fibrillation—continued
- auricular (atrial) (established) 427.31
- cardiac (ventricular) 427.41
- coronary (see also Infarct, myocardium) 410.9
- heart (ventricular) 427.41
- muscular 728.9
- postoperative 997.1
- ventricular 427.41

Fibrin
- ball or bodies, pleural (sac) 511.0
- chamber, anterior (eye) (gelatinous exudate) 364.04

Fibrinogenolysis (hemorrhagic) — see Fibrinolysis

Fibrinogenopenia (congenital) (hereditary) (see also Defect, coagulation) 286.3
- acquired 286.6

Fibrinolysis (acquired) (hemorrhagic) (pathologic) 286.6
- with
  - abortion — see Abortion, by type, with hemorrhage, delayed or excessive
  - ectopic pregnancy (see also categories 633.0-633.9) 639.1
  - molar pregnancy (see also categories 630-632) 639.1
- antepartum or intrapartum 641.3
  - affecting fetus or newborn 762.1
- following
  - abortion 639.1
  - ectopic or molar pregnancy 639.1
- newborn, transient 776.2
- postpartum 666.3

Fibrinopenia (hereditary) (see also Defect, coagulation) 286.3
- acquired 286.6

Fibrinopurulent — see condition

Fibrinous — see condition

Fibroadenoma (M9010/0)
- cellular intracanalicular (M9020/0) 217
- giant (intracanalicular) (M9020/0) 217
- intracanalicular (M9011/0)
  - cellular (M9020/0) 217
  - giant (M9020/0) 217
  - specified site — see Neoplasm, by site, benign
  - unspecified site 217
- juvenile (M9030/0) 217
- pericanicular (M9012/0)
  - specified site — see Neoplasm, by site, benign
  - unspecified site 217
- phyllodes (M9020/0) 217
- prostate 600
- specified site — see Neoplasm, by site, benign
- unspecified site 217

Fibroadenosis, breast (chronic) (cystic) (diffuse) (periodic) (segmental) 610.2

Fibroangioma (M9160/0) — see also Neoplasm, by site, benign
- juvenile (M9160/0)
  - specified site — see Neoplasm, by site, benign
  - unspecified site 210.7

Fibrocellulitis progressiva ossificans 728.11

Fibrochondrosarcoma (M9220/3) — see Neoplasm, cartilage, malignant

Fibrocystic
- disease 277.00
  - bone NEC 733.29
  - breast 610.1
  - jaw 526.2
  - kidney (congenital) 753.19
  - liver 751.62
  - lung 518.89
    - congenital 748.4
  - pancreas 277.00
  - kidney (congenital) 753.19

Fibrodysplasia ossificans multiplex (progressiva) 728.11

Fibroelastosis (cordis) (endocardial) (endomyocardial) 425.3

Fibroid (tumor) (M8890/0) — see also Neoplasm, connective tissue, benign
- disease, lung (chronic) (see also Fibrosis, lung) 515
- heart (disease) (see also Myocarditis) 429.0
- induration, lung (chronic) (see also Fibrosis, lung) 515
- in pregnancy or childbirth 654.1
  - affecting fetus or newborn 763.8
  - causing obstructed labor 660.2
    - affecting fetus or newborn 763.1
- liver — see Cirrhosis, liver
- lung (see also Fibrosis, lung) 515
- pneumonia (chronic) (see also Fibrosis, lung) 515
- uterus (M8890/0) (see also Leiomyoma, uterus) 218.9

Fibrolipoma (M8851/0) (see also Lipoma, by site) 214.9

Fibroliposarcoma (M8850/3) — see Neoplasm, connective tissue, malignant

Fibroma (M8810/0) — see also Neoplasm, connective tissue, benign
- ameloblastic (M9330/0) 213.1
  - upper jaw (bone) 213.0
- bone (nonossifying) 733.99
  - ossifying (M9262/0) — see Neoplasm, bone, benign
- cementifying (M9274/0) — see Neoplasm, bone, benign
- chondromyxoid (M9241/0) — see Neoplasm, bone, benign
- desmoplastic (M8823/1) — see Neoplasm, connective tissue, uncertain behavior
- facial (M8813/0) — see Neoplasm, connective tissue, benign
- invasive (M8821/1) — see Neoplasm, connective tissue, uncertain behavior
- molle (M8851/0) (see also Lipoma, by site) 214.9
- myxoid (M8811/0) — see Neoplasm, connective tissue, benign
- nasopharynx, nasopharyngeal (juvenile) (M9160/0) 210.7
- nonosteogenic (nonossifying) — see Dysplasia, fibrous
- odontogenic (M9321/0) 213.1
  - upper jaw (bone) 213.0
- ossifying (M9262/0) — see Neoplasm, bone, benign
- periosteal (M8812/0) — see Neoplasm, bone, benign
- prostate 600
- soft (M8851/0) (see also Lipoma, by site) 214.9

Fibromatosis
- abdominal (M8822/1) — see Neoplasm, connective tissue, uncertain behavior

Fibromatosis—continued
  aggressive (M8821/1) — see
    Neoplasm, connective
    tissue, uncertain behavior
  Dupuytren's 728.6
  gingival 523.8
  plantar fascia 728.71
  proliferative 728.79
  pseudosarcomatous (proliferative)
    (subcutaneous) 728.79
  subcutaneous pseudosarcomatous
    (proliferative) 728.79
Fibromyalgia 729.1 ◆
Fibromyoma (M8890/0) — see also
    Neoplasm, connective tissue,
    benign
  uterus (corpus) (see also
      Leiomyoma, uterus) 218.9
    in pregnancy or childbirth
      654.1
      affecting fetus or newborn
        763.8
      causing obstructed labor
        660.2
        affecting fetus or
          newborn 763.1
Fibromyositis (see also Myositis)
  729.1
  scapulohumeral 726.2
Fibromyxolipoma (M8852/0) (see
    also Lipoma, by site) 214.9
Fibromyxoma (M8811/0) — see
    Neoplasm, connective tissue,
    benign
Fibromyxosarcoma (M8811/3) — see
    Neoplasm, connective tissue,
    malignant
Fibro-odontoma, ameloblastic
  (M9290/0) 213.1
  upper jaw (bone) 213.0
Fibro-osteoma (M9262/0) — see
    Neoplasm, bone, benign
Fibroplasia, retrolental 362.21
Fibropurulent — see condition
Fibrosarcoma (M8810/3) — see also
    Neoplasm, connective tissue,
    malignant
  ameloblastic (M9330/3) 170.1
    upper jaw (bone) 170.0
  congenital (M8814/3) — see
    Neoplasm, connective
    tissue, malignant
  fascial (M8813/3) — see
    Neoplasm, connective
    tissue, malignant
  infantile (M8814/3) — see
    Neoplasm, connective
    tissue, malignant
  odontogenic (M9330/3) 170.1
    upper jaw (bone) 170.0
  periosteal (M8812/3) — see
    Neoplasm, bone, malignant
Fibrosclerosis
  breast 610.3
  corpora cavernosa (penis) 607.89
  familial multifocal NEC 710.8
  multifocal (idiopathic) NEC 710.8
  penis (corpora cavernosa) 607.89
Fibrosis, fibrotic
  adrenal (gland) 255.8
  alveolar (diffuse) 516.3
  amnion 658.8
  anal papillae 569.49
  anus 569.49
  appendix, appendiceal,
    noninflammatory 543.9
  arteriocapillary — see
    Arteriosclerosis
  bauxite (of lung) 503
  biliary 576.8
    due to Clonorchis sinensis
      121.1

Fibrosis, fibrotic—continued
  bladder 596.8
    interstitial 595.1
    localized submucosal 595.1
    panmural 595.1
  bone, diffuse 756.59
  breast 610.3
  capillary — see also
      Arteriosclerosis
    lung (chronic) (see also
      Fibrosis, lung) 515
  cardiac (see also Myocarditis)
    429.0
  cervix 622.8
  chorion 658.8
  corpus cavernosum 607.89
  cystic (of pancreas) 277.00
  due to (presence of) any device,
    implant, or graft — see
    Complications, due to
    (presence of) any device,
    implant, or graft classified
    to 996.0-996.5 NEC
  ejaculatory duct 608.89
  endocardium (see also
    Endocarditis) 424.90
  endomyocardial (African) 425.0
  epididymis 608.89
  eye muscle 378.62
  graphite (of lung) 503
  heart (see also Myocarditis) 429.0
  hepatic — see also Cirrhosis, liver
    due to Clonorchis sinensis
      121.1
  hepatolienal — see Cirrhosis,
    liver
  hepatosplenic — see Cirrhosis,
    liver
  infrapatellar fat pad 729.31
  interstitial pulmonary, newborn
    770.7
  intrascrotal 608.89
  kidney (see also Sclerosis, renal)
    587
  liver — see Cirrhosis, liver
  lung (atrophic) (capillary)
      (chronic) (confluent)
      (massive) (perialveolar)
      (peribronchial) 515
    with
      anthracosilicosis
        (occupational) 500
      anthracosis (occupational)
        500
      asbestosis (occupational)
        501
      bagassosis (occupational)
        495.1
      bauxite 503
      berylliosis (occupational)
        503
      byssinosis (occupational)
        504
      calcicosis (occupational)
        502
      chalicosis (occupational)
        502
      dust reticulation
        (occupational) 504
      farmers' lung 495.0
      gannister disease
        (occupational) 502
      graphite 503
      pneumoconiosis
        (occupational) 505
      pneumosiderosis
        (occupational) 503
      siderosis (occupational)
        503
      silicosis (occupational) 502
      tuberculosis (see also
        Tuberculosis) 011.4
    diffuse (idiopathic) (interstitial)
      516.3

Fibrosis, fibrotic—continued
  lung—continued
    due to
      bauxite 503
      fumes or vapors (chemical)
        (inhalation) 506.4
      graphite 503
      following radiation 508.1
      postinflammatory 515
      silicotic (massive)
        (occupational) 502
      tuberculous (see also
        Tuberculosis) 011.4
  lymphatic gland 289.3
  median bar 600
  mediastinum (idiopathic) 519.3
  meninges 349.2
  muscle NEC 728.2
    iatrogenic (from injection)
      999.9
  myocardium, myocardial (see
    also Myocarditis) 429.0
  oral submucous 528.8
  ovary 620.8
  oviduct 620.8
  pancreas 577.8
    cystic 277.00
  penis 607.89
  periappendiceal 543.9
  periarticular (see also Ankylosis)
    718.5
  pericardium 423.1
  perineum, in pregnancy or
      childbirth 654.8
    affecting fetus or newborn
      763.8
    causing obstructed labor 660.2
      affecting fetus or newborn
        763.1
  perineural NEC 355.9
    foot 355.6
  periureteral 593.89
  placenta — see Placenta,
    abnormal
  pleura 511.0
  popliteal fat pad 729.31
  preretinal 362.56
  prostate (chronic) 600
  pulmonary (chronic) (see also
      Fibrosis, lung) 515
    alveolar capillary block 516.3
    interstitial
      diffuse (idiopathic) 516.3
      newborn 770.7
  radiation — see Effect, adverse,
    radiation
  rectal sphincter 569.49
  retroperitoneal, idiopathic 593.4
  scrotum 608.89
  seminal vesicle 608.89
  senile 797
  skin NEC 709.2
  spermatic cord 608.89
  spleen 289.59
    bilharzial (see also
      Schistosomiasis) 120.9
  subepidermal nodular (M8832/0)
    — see Neoplasm, skin,
    benign
  submucous NEC 709.2
    oral 528.8
    tongue 528.8
  syncytium — see Placenta,
    abnormal
  testis 608.89
    chronic, due to syphilis 095.8
  thymus (gland) 254.8
  tunica vaginalis 608.89
  ureter 593.89
  urethra 599.84
  uterus (nonneoplastic) 621.8
    bilharzial (see also
      Schistosomiasis) 120.9
    neoplastic (see also
      Leiomyoma, uterus)
      218.9
  vagina 623.8

Fibrosis, fibrotic—continued
  valve, heart (see also
    Endocarditis) 424.90
  vas deferens 608.89
  vein 459.89
    lower extremities 459.89
  vesical 595.1
Fibrositis (periarticular) (rheumatoid)
  729.0
  humeroscapular region 726.2
  nodular, chronic
    Jaccoud's 714.4
    rheumatoid 714.4
  ossificans 728.11
  scapulohumeral 726.2
Fibrothorax 511.0
Fibrotic — see Fibrosis
Fibrous — see condition
Fibroxanthoma (M8831/0) — see
    also Neoplasm, connective
    tissue, benign
  atypical (M8831/1) — see
    Neoplasm, connective
    tissue, uncertain behavior
  malignant (M8831/3) — see
    Neoplasm, connective
    tissue, malignant
Fibroxanthosarcoma (M8831/3) —
    see Neoplasm, connective
    tissue, malignant
Fiedler's
  disease (leptospiral jaundice)
    100.0
  myocarditis or syndrome (acute
    isolated myocarditis)
    422.91
Fiessinger-Leroy (-Reiter) syndrome
  099.3
Fiessinger-Rendu syndrome
  (erythema muliforme
  exudativum) 695.1
Fifth disease (eruptive) 057.0
  venereal 099.1
Filaria, filarial — see Infestation,
  filarial
Filariasis (see also Infestation, filarial)
  125.9
  bancroftian 125.0
  Brug's 125.1
  due to
    bancrofti 125.0
    Brugia (Wuchereria) (malayi)
      125.1
    Loa loa 125.2
    malayi 125.1
    organism NEC 125.6
    Wuchereria (bancrofti) 125.0
      malayi 125.1
  Malayan 125.1
  ozzardi 125.1
  specified type NEC 125.6
Filatoff's, Filatov's, Filatow's disease
  (infectious mononucleosis)
  075
File-cutters' disease 984.9
  specified type of lead — see
    Table of drugs and
    chemicals
Filling defect
  biliary tract 793.3
  bladder 793.5
  duodenum 793.4
  gallbladder 793.3
  gastrointestinal tract 793.4
  intestine 793.4
  kidney 793.5
  stomach 793.4
  ureter 793.5
Filtering bleb, eye (postglaucoma)
  (status) V45.6
  with complication or rupture
    997.9
  postcataract extraction
    (complication) 997.9

Fimbrial cyst / Fissure, fissured

Fimbrial cyst (congenital) 752.11
Fimbriated hymen 752.49
Financial problem affecting care V60.2
Findings, abnormal, without diagnosis (examination) (laboratory test) 796.4
   17-ketosteroids, elevated 791.9
   acetonuria 791.6
   acid phosphatase 790.5
   albumin-globulin ratio 790.99
   albuminuria 791.0
   alcohol in blood 790.3
   alkaline phosphatase 790.5
   amniotic fluid 792.3
   amylase 790.5
   anisocytosis 790.0
   antibody titers, elevated 795.79 ▼
   antigen-antibody reaction 795.79 ▲
   bacteriuria 599.0
   ballistocardiogram 794.39
   bicarbonate 276.9
   bile in urine 791.4
   bilirubin 277.4
   bleeding time (prolonged) 790.92
   blood culture, positive 790.7
   blood gas level 790.91
   blood sugar level 790.2
      high 790.2
      low 251.2
   calcium 275.4
   carbonate 276.9
   casts, urine 791.7
   catecholamines 791.9
   cells, urine 791.7
   cerebrospinal fluid (color) (content) (pressure) 792.0
   chloride 276.9
   cholesterol 272.9
   chromosome analysis 795.2
   chyluria 791.1
   circulation time 794.39
   cloudy urine 791.9
   coagulation study 790.92
   cobalt, blood 790.6
   color of urine (unusual) NEC 791.9
   copper, blood 790.6
   crystals, urine 791.9
   culture, positive NEC 795.3
      blood 790.7
      HIV V08 ▼
      human immunodeficiency virus V08 ▲
      nose 795.3
      skin lesion NEC 795.3
      spinal fluid 792.0
      sputum 795.3
      stool 792.1
      throat 795.3
      urine 599.0
      viral
         human immunodeficiency V08 ◆
      wound 795.3
   echocardiogram 793.2
   echoencephalogram 794.01
   echogram NEC — see Findings, abnormal, structure
   electrocardiogram (ECG) (EKG) 794.31
   electroencephalogram (EEG) 794.02
   electrolyte level, urinary 791.9
   electromyogram (EMG) 794.17
      ocular 794.14
   electro-oculogram (EOG) 794.12
   electroretinogram (ERG) 794.11
   enzymes, serum NEC 790.5
   fibrinogen titer coagulation study 790.92
   filling defect — see Filling defect
   function study NEC 794.9
      auditory 794.15
      bladder 794.9
      brain 794.00

Findings, abnormal, without diagnosis—continued
   function study NEC—continued
      cardiac 794.30
      endocrine NEC 794.6
         thyroid 794.5
      kidney 794.4
      liver 794.8
      nervous system
         central 794.00
         peripheral 794.19
      oculomotor 794.14
      pancreas 794.9
      placenta 794.9
      pulmonary 794.2
      retina 794.11
      special senses 794.19
      spleen 794.9
      vestibular 794.16
   gallbladder, nonvisualization 793.3
   glucose 790.2
      tolerance test 790.2
   glycosuria 791.5
   heart
      shadow 793.2
      sounds 785.3
   hematinuria 791.2
   hematocrit
      elevated 282.7
      low 285.9
   hematologic NEC 790.99
   hematuria 599.7
   hemoglobin
      elevated 282.7
      low 285.9
   hemoglobinuria 791.2
   histological NEC 795.4
   hormones 259.9
   immunoglobulins, elevated 795.79 ◆
   indolacetic acid, elevated 791.9
   iron 790.6
   karyotype 795.2
   ketonuria 791.6
   lactic acid dehydrogenase (LDH) 790.4
   lipase 790.5
   lipids NEC 272.9
   lithium, blood 790.6
   lung field (coin lesion) (shadow) 793.1
   magnesium, blood 790.6
   mammogram 793.8
   mediastinal shift 793.2
   melanin, urine 791.9
   microbiologic NEC 795.3
   mineral, blood NEC 790.6
   myoglobinuria 791.3
   nitrogen derivatives, blood 790.6
   nonvisualization of gallbladder 793.3
   nose culture, positive 795.3
   odor of urine (unusual) NEC 791.9
   oxygen saturation 790.91
   Papanicolaou (smear) 795.1
      cervix (dyskaryotic) 795.0
      other site 795.1
   peritoneal fluid 792.9
   phonocardiogram 794.39
   phosphorus 275.3
   pleural fluid 792.9
   pneumoencephalogram 793.0
   PO_2-oxygen ratio 790.91
   poikilocytosis 790.0
   potassium
      deficiency 276.8
      excess 276.7
   PPD 795.5
   prostate specific antigen (PSA) 790.93
   protein, serum NEC 790.99
   proteinuria 791.0
   prothrombin time (partial) (prolonged) (PT) (PTT) 790.92

Findings, abnormal, without diagnosis—continued
   pyuria 599.0
   radiologic (x-ray) 793.9
      abdomen 793.6
      biliary tract 793.3
      breast 793.8
      gastrointestinal tract 793.4
      genitourinary organs 793.5
      head 793.0
      intrathoracic organs NEC 793.2
      lung 793.1
      musculoskeletal 793.7
      placenta 793.9
      retroperitoneum 793.6
      skin 793.9
      skull 793.0
      subcutaneous tissue 793.9
   red blood cell 790.0
      count 790.0
      morphology 790.0
      sickling 790.0
      volume 790.0
   saliva 792.4
   scan NEC 794.9
      bladder 794.9
      bone 794.9
      brain 794.09
      kidney 794.4
      liver 794.8
      lung 794.2
      pancreas 794.9
      placental 794.9
      spleen 794.9
      thyroid 794.5
   sedimentation rate, elevated 790.1
   semen 792.2
   serological (for)
      human immunodeficiency virus (HIV) ▼
         inconclusive 795.71
         positive V08 ▲
      syphilis — see Findings, serology for syphilis
   serology for syphilis
      false positive 795.6
      positive 097.1
         false 795.6
         follow-up of latent syphilis — see Syphilis, latent
         only finding — see Syphilis, latent
   serum 790.99
      blood NEC 790.99
      enzymes NEC 790.5
      proteins 790.99
   SGOT 790.4
   SGPT 790.4
   sickling of red blood cells 790.0
   skin test, positive 795.79 ◆
      tuberculin (without active tuberculosis) 795.5
   sodium 790.6
      deficiency 276.1
      excess 276.0
   spermatozoa 792.2
   spinal fluid 792.0
      culture, positive 792.0
   sputum culture, positive 795.3
      for acid-fast bacilli 795.3
   stool NEC 792.1
      bloody 578.1
         occult 792.1
      color 792.1
      culture, positive 792.1
      occult blood 792.1
   structure, body (echogram) (thermogram) (ultrasound) (x-ray) NEC 793.9
      abdomen 793.6
      breast 793.8
      gastrointestinal tract 793.4
      genitourinary organs 793.5

Findings, abnormal, without diagnosis—continued
   structure, body—continued
      head 793.0
         echogram (ultrasound) 794.01
      intrathoracic organs NEC 793.2
      lung 793.1
      musculoskeletal 793.7
      placenta 793.9
      retroperitoneum 793.6
      skin 793.9
      subcutaneous tissue NEC 793.9
   synovial fluid 792.9
   thermogram — see Finding, abnormal, structure
   throat culture, positive 795.3
   thyroid (function) 794.5
      metabolism (rate) 794.5
      scan 794.5
      uptake 794.5
   total proteins 790.99
   toxicology (drugs) (heavy metals) 796.0
   transaminase (level) 790.4
   triglycerides 272.9
   tuberculin skin test (without active tuberculosis) 795.5
   ultrasound — see also Finding, abnormal, structure
      cardiogram 793.2
   uric acid, blood 790.6
   urine, urinary constituents 791.9
      acetone 791.6
      albumin 791.0
      bacteria 599.0
      bile 791.4
      blood 599.7
      casts or cells 791.7
      chyle 791.1
      culture, positive 599.0
      glucose 791.5
      hemoglobin 791.2
      ketone 791.6
      protein 791.0
      pus 599.0
      sugar 791.5
   vaginal fluid 792.9
   vanillylmandelic acid, elevated 791.9
   vectorcardiogram (VCG) 793.2
   ventriculogram (cerebral) 793.0
   VMA, elevated 791.9
   Wassermann reaction
      false positive 795.6
      positive 097.1
         follow-up of latent syphilis — see Syphilis, latent
         only finding — see Syphilis, latent
   white blood cell 288.9
      count 288.9
         elevated 288.8
         low 288.0
      differential 288.9
      morphology 288.9
   wound culture 795.3
   xerography 793.8
   zinc, blood 790.6
Finger — see condition
Fire, St. Anthony's (see also Erysipelas) 035
Fish
   hook stomach 537.89
   meal workers' lung 495.8
Fisher's syndrome 357.0
Fissure, fissured
   abdominal wall (congenital) 756.7
   anus, anal 565.0
      congenital 751.5
   buccal cavity 528.9
   clitoris (congenital) 752.49

Fissure, fissured—*continued*
- ear, lobule (congenital) 744.29
- epiglottis (congenital) 748.3
- larynx 478.79
  - congenital 748.3
- lip 528.5
  - congenital (*see also* Cleft, lip) 749.10
- nipple 611.2
  - puerperal, postpartum 676.1
- palate (congenital) (*see also* Cleft, palate) 749.00
- postanal 565.0
- rectum 565.0
- skin 709.8
  - streptococcal 686.9
- spine (congenital) (*see also* Spina bifida) 741.9
- sternum (congenital) 756.3
- tongue (acquired) 529.5
  - congenital 750.13

Fistula (sinus) 686.9
- abdomen (wall) 569.81
  - bladder 596.2
  - intestine 569.81
  - ureter 593.82
  - uterus 619.2
- abdominorectal 569.81
- abdominosigmoidal 569.81
- abdominothoracic 510.0
- abdominouterine 619.2
  - congenital 752.3
- abdominovesical 596.2
- accessory sinuses (*see also* Sinusitis) 473.9
- actinomycotic — *see* Actinomycosis
- alveolar
  - antrum (*see also* Sinusitis, maxillary) 473.0
  - process 522.7
- anorectal 565.1
- antrobuccal (*see also* Sinusitis, maxillary) 473.0
- antrum (*see also* Sinusitis, maxillary) 473.0
- anus, anal (infectional) (recurrent) 565.1
  - congenital 751.5
  - tuberculous (*see also* Tuberculosis) 014.8
- aortic sinus 747.29
- aortoduodenal 447.2
- appendix, appendicular 543.9
- arteriovenous (acquired) 447.0
  - brain 437.3
    - congenital 747.81
      - ruptured (*see also* Hemorrhage, subarachnoid) 430
    - ruptured (*see also* Hemorrhage, subarachnoid) 430
  - cerebral 437.3
    - congenital 747.81
  - congenital (peripheral) 747.60
    - brain — *see* Fistula, arteriovenous, brain, congenital
    - coronary 746.85
    - gastrointestinal 747.61
    - lower limb 747.64
    - pulmonary 747.3
    - renal 747.62
    - specified NEC 747.69
    - upper limb 747.63
  - coronary 414.19
    - congenital 746.85
  - heart 414.19
  - pulmonary (vessels) 417.0
    - congenital 747.3

Fistula—*continued*
- arteriovenous—*continued*
  - surgically created (for dialysis) V45.1
    - complication NEC 996.73
      - atherosclerosis — *see* Arteriosclerosis, extremities ▼
      - embolism 996.74 ▲
      - infection or inflammation 996.62
      - mechanical 996.1
      - occlusion NEC 996.74▼
      - thrombus 996.74 ▲
  - traumatic — *see* Injury, blood vessel, by site
- artery 447.2
- aural 383.81
  - congenital 744.49
- auricle 383.81
  - congenital 744.49
- Bartholin's gland 619.8
- bile duct (*see also* Fistula, biliary) 576.4
- biliary (duct) (tract) 576.4
  - congenital 751.69
- bladder (neck) (sphincter) 596.2
  - into seminal vesicle 596.2
- bone 733.99
- brain 348.8
  - arteriovenous — *see* Fistula, arteriovenous, brain
- branchial (cleft) 744.41
- branchiogenous 744.41
- breast 611.0
  - puerperal, postpartum 675.1
- bronchial 510.0
- bronchocutaneous, bronchomediastinal, bronchopleural, bronchopleuromediastinal (infective) 510.0
  - tuberculous (*see also* Tuberculosis) 011.3
- bronchoesophageal 530.89
  - congenital 750.3
- buccal cavity (infective) 528.3
- canal, ear 380.89
- carotid-cavernous ▼
  - congenital 747.81
    - with hemorrhage 430
  - traumatic 900.82
    - with hemorrhage (*see also* Hemorrhage, brain, traumatic) 853.0
    - late effect 908.3 ▲
- cecosigmoidal 569.81
- cecum 569.81
- cerebrospinal (fluid) 349.81
- cervical, lateral (congenital) 744.41
- cervicoaural (congenital) 744.49
- cervicosigmoidal 619.1
- cervicovesical 619.0
- cervix 619.8
- chest (wall) 510.0
- cholecystocolic (*see also* Fistula, gallbladder) 575.5
- cholecystocolonic (*see also* Fistula, gallbladder) 575.5
- cholecystoduodenal (*see also* Fistula, gallbladder) 575.5
- cholecystoenteric (*see also* Fistula, gallbladder) 575.5
- cholecystogastric (*see also* Fistula, gallbladder) 575.5
- cholecystointestinal (*see also* Fistula, gallbladder) 575.5
- choledochoduodenal 576.4
- cholocolic (*see also* Fistula, gallbladder) 575.5
- coccyx 685.1
  - with abscess 685.0
- colon 569.81
- colostomy 569.6
- colovaginal (acquired) 619.1

Fistula—*continued*
- common duct (bile duct) 576.4
- congenital, NEC — *see* Anomaly, specified type NEC
- cornea, causing hypotony 360.32
- coronary, arteriovenous 414.19
  - congenital 746.85
- costal region 510.0
- cul-de-sac, Douglas' 619.8
- cutaneous 686.9
- cystic duct (*see also* Fistula, gallbladder) 575.5
  - congenital 751.69
- dental 522.7
- diaphragm 510.0
  - bronchovisceral 510.0
  - pleuroperitoneal 510.0
  - pulmonoperitoneal 510.0
- duodenum 537.4
- ear (canal) (external) 380.89
- enterocolic 569.81
- enterocutaneous 569.81
- enteroenteric 569.81
- entero-uterine 619.1
  - congenital 752.3
- enterovaginal 619.1
  - congenital 752.49
- enterovesical 596.1
- epididymis 608.89
  - tuberculous (*see also* Tuberculosis) 016.4
- esophagobronchial 530.89
  - congenital 750.3
- esophagocutaneous 530.89
- esophagopleurocutaneous 530.89
- esophagotracheal 530.84
  - congenital 750.3
- esophagus 530.89
  - congenital 750.4
- ethmoid (*see also* Sinusitis, ethmoidal) 473.2
- eyeball (cornea) (sclera) 360.32
- eyelid 373.11
- fallopian tube (external) 619.2
- fecal 569.81
  - congenital 751.5
- from periapical lesion 522.7
- frontal sinus (*see also* Sinusitis, frontal) 473.1
- gallbladder 575.5
  - with calculus, cholelithiasis, stones (*see also* Cholelithiasis) 574.2
  - congenital 751.69
- gastric 537.4
- gastrocolic 537.4
  - congenital 750.7
  - tuberculous (*see also* Tuberculosis) 014.8
- gastroenterocolic 537.4
- gastroesophageal 537.4
- gastrojejunal 537.4
- gastrojejunocolic 537.4
- genital
  - organs
    - female 619.9
      - specified site NEC 619.8
    - male 608.89
  - tract-skin (female) 619.2
- hepatopleural 510.0
- hepatopulmonary 510.0
- horseshoe 565.1
- ileorectal 569.81
- ileosigmoidal 569.81
- ileostomy 569.6
- ileovesical 596.1
- ileum 569.81
- in ano 565.1
  - tuberculous (*see also* Tuberculosis) 014.8
- inner ear (*see also* Fistula, labyrinth) 386.40
- intestine 569.81
- intestinocolonic (abdominal) 569.81
- intestinoureteral 593.82
- intestinouterine 619.1

Fistula—*continued*
- intestinovaginal 619.1
  - congenital 752.49
- intestinovesical 596.1
- involving female genital tract 619.9
  - digestive-genital 619.1
  - genital tract-skin 619.2
  - specified site NEC 619.8
  - urinary-genital 619.0
- ischiorectal (fossa) 566
- jejunostomy 569.6
- jejunum 569.81
- joint 719.89
  - ankle 719.87
  - elbow 719.82
  - foot 719.87
  - hand 719.84
  - hip 719.85
  - knee 719.86
  - multiple sites 719.89
  - pelvic region 719.85
  - shoulder (region) 719.81
  - specified site NEC 719.88
  - tuberculous — *see* Tuberculosis, joint
  - wrist 719.83
- kidney 593.89
- labium (majus) (minus) 619.8
- labyrinth, labyrinthine NEC 386.40
  - combined sites 386.48
  - multiple sites 386.48
  - oval window 386.42
  - round window 386.41
  - semicircular canal 386.43
- lacrimal, lachrymal (duct) (gland) (sac) 375.61
- lacrimonasal duct 375.61
- laryngotracheal 748.3
- larynx 478.79
- lip 528.5
  - congenital 750.25
- lumbar, tuberculous (*see also* Tuberculosis) 015.0 [730.8]
- lung 510.0
- lymphatic (node) (vessel) 457.8
- mamillary 611.0
- mammary (gland) 611.0
  - puerperal, postpartum 675.1
- mastoid (process) (region) 383.1
- maxillary (*see also* Sinusitis, maxillary) 473.0
- mediastinal 510.0
- mediastinobronchial 510.0
- mediastinocutaneous 510.0
- middle ear 385.89
- mouth 528.3
- nasal 478.1
  - sinus (*see also* Sinusitis) 473.9
- nasopharynx 478.29
- nipple — *see* Fistula, breast
- nose 478.1
- oral (cutaneous) 528.3
  - maxillary (*see also* Sinusitis, maxillary) 473.0
  - nasal (with cleft palate) (*see also* Cleft, palate) 749.00
- orbit, orbital 376.10
- oro-antral (*see also* Sinusitis, maxillary) 473.0
- oval window (internal ear) 386.42
- oviduct (external) 619.2
- palate (hard) 526.89
  - soft 528.9
- pancreatic 577.8
- pancreaticoduodenal 577.8
- parotid (gland) 527.4
  - region 528.3
- pelvoabdominointestinal 569.81
- penis 607.89
- perianal 565.1
- pericardium (pleura) (sac) (*see also* Pericarditis) 423.8
- pericecal 569.81
- perineal — *see* Fistula, perineum

Fistula—*continued*
  perineorectal 569.81
  perineosigmoidal 569.81
  perineo-urethroscrotal 608.89
  perineum, perineal (with urethral involvement) NEC 599.1
    tuberculous (*see also* Tuberculosis) 017.9
    ureter 593.82
  perirectal 565.1
    tuberculous (*see also* Tuberculosis) 014.8
  peritoneum (*see also* Peritonitis) 567.2
  periurethral 599.1
  pharyngo-esophageal 478.29
  pharynx 478.29
    branchial cleft (congenital) 744.41
  pilonidal (infected) (rectum) 685.1
    with abscess 685.0
  pleura, pleural, pleurocutaneous, pleuroperitoneal 510.0
    stomach 510.0
    tuberculous (*see also* Tuberculosis) 012.0
  pleuropericardial 423.8
  postauricular 383.81
  postoperative, persistent 998.6
  preauricular (congenital) 744.46
  prostate 602.8
  pulmonary 510.0
    arteriovenous 417.0
      congenital 747.3
    tuberculous (*see also* Tuberculosis, pulmonary) 011.9
  pulmonoperitoneal 510.0
  rectolabial 619.1
  rectosigmoid (intercommunicating) 569.81
  rectoureteral 593.82
  rectourethral 599.1
    congenital 753.8
  rectouterine 619.1
    congenital 752.3
  rectovaginal 619.1
    congenital 752.49
    old, postpartal 619.1
    tuberculous (*see also* Tuberculosis) 014.8
  rectovesical 596.1
    congenital 753.8
  rectovesicovaginal 619.1
  rectovulvar 619.1
    congenital 752.49
  rectum (to skin) 565.1
    tuberculous (*see also* Tuberculosis) 014.8
  renal 593.89
  retroauricular 383.81
  round window (internal ear) 386.41
  salivary duct or gland 527.4
    congenital 750.24
  sclera 360.32
  scrotum (urinary) 608.89
    tuberculous (*see also* Tuberculosis) 016.5
  semicircular canals (internal ear) 386.43
  sigmoid 569.81
    vesicoabdominal 596.1
  sigmoidovaginal 619.1
    congenital 752.49
  skin 686.9
    ureter 593.82
    vagina 619.2
  sphenoidal sinus (*see also* Sinusitis, sphenoidal) 473.3
  splenocolic 289.59
  stercoral 569.81
  stomach 537.4
  sublingual gland 527.4
    congenital 750.24

Fistula—*continued*
  submaxillary
    gland 527.4
      congenital 750.24
    region 528.3
  thoracic 510.0
    duct 457.8
  thoracicoabdominal 510.0
  thoracicogastric 510.0
  thoracicointestinal 510.0
  thoracoabdominal 510.0
  thoracogastric 510.0
  thorax 510.0
  thyroglossal duct 759.2
  thyroid 246.8
  trachea (congenital) (external) (internal) 748.3
  tracheoesophageal 530.84
    congenital 750.3
    following tracheostomy 519.0
  traumatic
    arteriovenous (*see also* Injury, blood vessel, by site) 904.9
      brain — *see* Injury, intracranial
  tuberculous — *see* Tuberculosis, by site
  typhoid 002.0
  umbilical 759.89
  umbilico-urinary 753.8
  urachal, urachus 753.7
  ureter (persistent) 593.82
  ureteroabdominal 593.82
  ureterocervical 593.82
  ureterorectal 593.82
  ureterosigmoido-abdominal 593.82
  ureterovaginal 619.0
  ureterovesical 596.2
  urethra 599.1
    congenital 753.8
    tuberculous (*see also* Tuberculosis) 016.3
  urethroperineal 599.1
  urethroperineovesical 596.2
  urethrorectal 599.1
    congenital 753.8
  urethroscrotal 608.89
  urethrovaginal 619.0
  urethrovesical 596.2
  urethrovesicovaginal 619.0
  urinary (persistent) (recurrent) 599.1
  uteroabdominal (anterior wall) 619.2
    congenital 752.3
  uteroenteric 619.1
  uterofecal 619.1
  uterointestinal 619.1
    congenital 752.3
  uterorectal 619.1
    congenital 752.3
  uteroureteric 619.0
  uterovaginal 619.8
  uterovesical 619.0
    congenital 752.3
  uterus 619.8
  vagina (wall) 619.8
    postpartal, old 619.8
  vaginocutaneous (postpartal) 619.2
  vaginoileal (acquired) 619.1
  vaginoperineal 619.2
  vesical NEC 596.2
  vesicoabdominal 596.2
  vesicocervicovaginal 619.0
  vesicocolic 596.1
  vesicocutaneous 596.2
  vesicoenteric 596.1
  vesicointestinal 596.1
  vesicometrorectal 619.1
  vesicoperineal 596.2
  vesicorectal 596.1
    congenital 753.8
  vesicosigmoidal 596.1
  vesicosigmoidovaginal 619.1

Fistula—*continued*
  vesicoureteral 596.2
  vesicoureterovaginal 619.0
  vesicourethral 596.2
  vesicourethrorectal 596.1
  vesicouterine 619.0
    congenital 752.3
  vesicovaginal 619.0
  vulvorectal 619.1
    congenital 752.49

Fit 780.3
  apoplectic (*see also* Disease, cerebrovascular, acute) 436
    late effect — *see* category 438
  epileptic (*see also* Epilepsy) 345.9
  fainting 780.2
  hysterical 300.11
  newborn 779.0

Fitting (of)
  artificial
    arm (complete) (partial) V52.0
    breast V52.4
    eye(s) V52.2
    leg(s) (complete) (partial) V52.1
  brain neuropacemaker V53.0
  cardiac pacemaker V53.31 ▼
  carotid sinus pacemaker V53.39 ▲
  colostomy belt V53.5
  contact lenses V53.1
  cystostomy device V53.6
  defibrillator, automatic implantable cardiac V53.32 ◆
  dentures V52.3
  device NEC V53.9
    abdominal V53.5
    cardiac ▼
      defibrillator, automatic implantable V53.32
      pacemaker V53.31
      specified NEC V53.39 ▲
    intrauterine contraceptive V25.1
    nervous system V53.0
    orthodontic V53.4
    orthoptic V53.1
    prosthetic V52.9
      breast V52.4
      dental V52.3
      eye V52.2
      specified type NEC V52.8
    special senses V53.0
    substitution
      auditory V53.0
      nervous system V53.0
      visual V53.0
    urinary V53.6
  diaphragm (contraceptive) V25.02
  glasses (reading) V53.1
  hearing aid V53.2
  ileostomy device V53.5
  intestinal appliance or device NEC V53.5
  intrauterine contraceptive device V25.1
  neuropacemaker (brain) (peripheral nerve) (spinal cord) V53.0
  orthodontic device V53.4
  orthopedic (device) V53.7
    brace V53.7
    cast V53.7
    corset V53.7
    shoes V53.7
  pacemaker (cardiac) V53.31 ◆
    brain V53.0
    carotid sinus V53.39 ◆
    peripheral nerve V53.0
    spinal cord V53.0
  prosthesis V52.9
    arm (complete) (partial) V52.0
    breast V52.4
    dental V52.3
    eye V52.2

Fitting (of)—*continued*
  prosthesis—*continued*
    leg (complete) (partial) V52.1
    specified type NEC V52.8
  spectacles V53.1
  wheelchair V53.8

Fitz's syndrome (acute hemorrhagic pancreatitis) 577.0

Fitz-Hugh and Curtis syndrome (gonococcal peritonitis) 098.86

Fixation
  joint — *see* Ankylosis
  larynx 478.79
  pupil 364.76
  stapes 385.22
    deafness (*see also* Deafness, conductive) 389.04
  uterus (acquired) — *see* Malposition, uterus
  vocal cord 478.5

Flaccid — *see also* condition
  foot 736.79
  forearm 736.09
  palate, congenital 750.26

Flail
  chest 807.4
    newborn 767.3
  joint (paralytic) 718.80
    ankle 718.87
    elbow 718.82
    foot 718.87
    hand 718.84
    hip 718.85
    knee 718.86
    multiple sites 718.89
    pelvic region 718.85
    shoulder (region) 718.81
    specified site NEC 718.88
    wrist 718.83

Flajani (-Basedow) syndrome or disease (exophthalmic goiter) 242.0

Flap, liver 572.8

Flare, anterior chamber (aqueous) (eye) 364.04

Flashback phenomena (drug) (hallucinogenic) 292.89

Flat
  chamber (anterior) (eye) 360.34
  chest, congenital 754.89
  electroencephalogram (EEG) 348.8
  foot (acquired) (fixed type) (painful) (postural) (spastic) 734
    congenital 754.61
      rocker bottom 754.61
      vertical talus 754.61
    rachitic 268.1
    rocker bottom (congenital) 754.61
    vertical talus, congenital 754.61
  organ or site, congenital NEC — *see* Anomaly, specified type NEC
  pelvis 738.6
    with disproportion (fetopelvic) 653.2
      affecting fetus or newborn 763.1
      causing obstructed labor 660.1
        affecting fetus or newborn 763.1
    congenital 755.69

Flatau-Schilder disease 341.1

Flattening
  head, femur 736.39
  hip 736.39
  lip (congenital) 744.89
  nose (congenital) 754.0
    acquired 738.0

Flatulence 787.3

Flatus 787.3
   vaginalis 629.8
Flax dressers' disease 504
Flea bite — *see* Injury, superficial, by site
Fleischer (-Kayser) ring (corneal pigmentation) 275.1 [371.14]
Fleischner's disease 732.3
Fleshy mole 631
Flexibilitas cerea (*see also* Catalepsy) 300.11
Flexion
   cervix (*see also* Malposition, uterus) 621.6
   contracture, joint (*see also* Contraction, joint) 718.4
   deformity, joint (*see also* Contraction, joint) 718.4
   hip, congenital (*see also* Subluxation, congenital, hip) 754.32
   uterus (*see also* Malposition, uterus) 621.6
Flexner's
   bacillus 004.1
   diarrhea (ulcerative) 004.1
   dysentery 004.1
Flexner-Boyd dysentery 004.2
Flexure — *see* condition
Floater, vitreous 379.24
Floating
   cartilage (joint) (*see also* Disorder, cartilage, articular) 718.0
      knee 717.6
   gallbladder (congenital) 751.69
   kidney 593.0
      congenital 753.3
   liver (congenital) 751.69
   rib 756.3
   spleen 289.59
Flooding 626.2
Floor — *see* condition
Floppy
   infant NEC 781.9
   valve syndrome (mitral) 424.0
Flu — *see also* Influenza
   gastric NEC 008.8
Fluctuating blood pressure 796.4
Fluid
   abdomen 789.5
   chest (*see also* Pleurisy, with effusion) 511.9
   heart (*see also* Failure, heart, congestive) 428.0
   joint (*see also* Effusion, joint) 719.0
   loss (acute) 276.5
      with
         hypernatremia 276.0
         hyponatremia 276.1
   lung — *see also* Edema, lung
      encysted 511.8
   peritoneal cavity 789.5
   pleural cavity (*see also* Pleurisy, with effusion) 511.9
   retention 276.6
Flukes NEC (*see also* Infestation, fluke) 121.9
   blood NEC (*see also* Infestation, Schistosoma) 120.9
   liver 121.3
Fluor (albus) (vaginalis) 623.5
   trichomonal (Trichomonas vaginalis) 131.00
Fluorosis (dental) (chronic) 520.3
Flushing 782.62
   menopausal 627.2
Flush syndrome 259.2
Flutter
   atrial or auricular 427.32
   heart (ventricular) 427.42
      atrial 427.32
      impure 427.32

Flutter—*continued*
   postoperative 997.1
   ventricular 427.42
Flux (bloody) (serosanguineous) 009.0
Focal — *see* condition
Fochier's abscess — *see* Abscess, by site
Focus, Assmann's (*see also* Tuberculosis) 011.0
Fogo selvagem 694.4
Foix-Alajouanine syndrome 336.1
Folds, anomalous — *see also* Anomaly, specified type NEC
   Bowman's membrane 371.31
   Descemet's membrane 371.32
   epicanthic 743.63
   heart 746.89
   posterior segment of eye, congenital 743.54
Folie à deux 297.3
Follicle
   cervix (nabothian) (ruptured) 616.0
   graafian, ruptured, with hemorrhage 620.0
   nabothian 616.0
Folliclis (primary) (*see also* Tuberculosis) 017.0
Follicular — *see also* condition
   cyst (atretic) 620.0
Folliculitis 704.8
   abscedens et suffodiens 704.8
   decalvans 704.09
   gonorrheal (acute) 098.0
      chronic or duration of 2 months or more 098.2
   keloid, keloidalis 706.1
   pustular 704.8
   ulerythematosa reticulata 701.8
Folliculosis, conjunctival 372.02
Følling's disease (phenylketonuria) 270.1
Follow-up (examination) (routine) (following) V67.9
   cancer chemotherapy V67.2
   chemotherapy V67.2
   fracture V67.4
   high-risk medication V67.51
   injury NEC V67.59
   postpartum
      immediately after delivery V24.0
      routine V24.2
   psychiatric V67.3
   psychotherapy V67.3
   radiotherapy V67.1
   specified condition NEC V67.59
   surgery V67.0
   treatment V67.9
      combined NEC V67.6
      fracture V67.4
      involving high-risk medication NEC V67.51
      mental disorder V67.3
      specified NEC V67.59
Fong's syndrome (hereditary osteoonychodysplasia) 756.89
Food
   allergy 693.1
   anaphylactic shock — *see* Anaphylactic shock, due to, food
   asphyxia (from aspiration or inhalation) (*see also* Asphyxia, food) 933.1
   choked on (*see also* Asphyxia, food) 933.1
   deprivation 994.2
      specified kind of food NEC 269.8
   intoxication (*see also* Poisoning, food) 005.9
   lack of 994.2

Food—*continued*
   poisoning (*see also* Poisoning, food) 005.9
   refusal or rejection NEC 307.59
   strangulation or suffocation (*see also* Asphyxia, food) 933.1
   toxemia (*see also* Poisoning, food) 005.9
Foot — *see also* condition
   and mouth disease 078.4
   process disease 581.3
Foramen ovale (nonclosure) (patent) (persistent) 745.5
Forbes' (glycogen storage) disease 271.0
Forbes-Albright syndrome (nonpuerperal amenorrhea and lactation associated with pituitary tumor) 253.1
Forced birth or delivery NEC 669.8
   affecting fetus or newborn NEC 763.8
Forceps
   delivery NEC 669.6
      affecting fetus or newborn 763.2
Fordyce's disease (ectopic sebaceous glands) (mouth) 750.26
Fordyce-Fox disease (apocrine miliaria) 705.82
Forearm — *see* condition
Foreign body

Note — For foreign body with open wound or other injury, see Wound, open, or the type of injury specified.

   accidentally left during a procedure 998.4
   anterior chamber (eye) 871.6
      magnetic 871.5
         retained or old 360.51
      retained or old 360.61
   ciliary body (eye) 871.6
      magnetic 871.5
         retained or old 360.52
      retained or old 360.62
   entering through orifice (current) (old)
      accessory sinus 932
      air passage (upper) 933.0
         lower 934.8
      alimentary canal 938
      alveolar process 935.0
      antrum (Highmore) 932
      anus 937
      appendix 936
      asphyxia due to (*see also* Asphyxia, food) 933.1
      auditory canal 931
      auricle 931
      bladder 939.0
      bronchioles 934.8
      bronchus (main) 934.1
      buccal cavity 935.0
      canthus (inner) 930.1
      cecum 936
      cervix (canal) uterine 939.1
      coil, ileocecal 936
      colon 936
      conjunctiva 930.1
      conjunctival sac 930.1
      cornea 930.0
      digestive organ or tract NEC 938
      duodenum 936
      ear (external) 931
      esophagus 935.1
      eye (external) 930.9
         combined sites 930.8
         intraocular — *see* Foreign body, by site
         specified site NEC 930.8

Foreign body—*continued*
   entering through orifice—*continued*
      eyeball 930.8
         intraocular — *see* Foreign body, intraocular
      eyelid 930.1
         retained or old 374.86
      frontal sinus 932
      gastrointestinal tract 938
      genitourinary tract 939.9
      globe 930.8
         penetrating 871.6
            magnetic 871.5
               retained or old 360.50
            retained or old 360.60
      gum 935.0
      Highmore's antrum 932
      hypopharynx 933.0
      ileocecal coil 936
      ileum 936
      inspiration (of) 933.1
      intestine (large) (small) 936
      lacrimal apparatus, duct, gland, or sac 930.2
      larynx 933.1
      lung 934.8
      maxillary sinus 932
      mouth 935.0
      nasal sinus 932
      nasopharynx 933.0
      nose (passage) 932
      nostril 932
      oral cavity 935.0
      palate 935.0
      penis 939.3
      pharynx 933.0
      pyriform sinus 933.0
      rectosigmoid 937
         junction 937
      rectum 937
      respiratory tract 934.9
         specified part NEC 934.8
      sclera 930.1
      sinus 932
         accessory 932
         frontal 932
         maxillary 932
         nasal 932
         pyriform 933.0
      small intestine 936
      stomach (hairball) 935.2
      suffocation by (*see also* Asphyxia, food) 933.1
      swallowed 938
         tongue 933.0
      tear ducts or glands 930.2
      throat 933.0
      tongue 935.0
         swallowed 933.0
      tonsil, tonsillar 933.1
         fossa 933.1
      trachea 934.0
      ureter 939.0
      urethra 939.0
      uterus (any part) 939.1
      vagina 939.2
      vulva 939.2
      wind pipe 934.0
   granuloma (old) 728.82
      bone 733.99
      in operative wound (inadvertently left) 998.4
      due to surgical material intentionally left — *see* Complications, due to (presence of) any device, implant, or graft classified to 996.0-996.5 NEC
      muscle 728.82
      skin 709.4
      soft tissue NEC 728.82
      subcutaneous tissue 709.4

Foreign body—continued

in
- bone (residual) 733.99
- open wound — see Wound, open, by site complicated
- soft tissue (residual) 729.6
- inadvertently left in operation wound (causing adhesions, obstruction, or perforation) 998.4
- ingestion, ingested NEC 938
- inhalation or inspiration (see also Asphyxia, food) 933.1
- internal organ, not entering through an orifice — see Injury, internal, by site, with open wound
- intraocular (nonmagnetic) 871.6
  - combined sites 871.6
    - magnetic 871.5
      - retained or old 360.59
    - retained or old 360.69
  - magnetic 871.5
    - retained or old 360.50
  - retained or old 360.60
  - specified site NEC 871.6
    - magnetic 871.5
      - retained or old 360.59
    - retained or old 360.69
- iris (nonmagnetic) 871.6
  - magnetic 871.5
    - retained or old 360.52
  - retained or old 360.62
- lens (nonmagnetic) 871.6
  - magnetic 871.5
    - retained or old 360.53
  - retained or old 360.63
- lid, eye 930.1
- ocular muscle 870.4
  - retained or old 376.6
- old or residual
  - bone 733.99
  - eyelid 374.86
  - middle ear 385.83
  - muscle 729.6
    - ocular 376.6
  - retrobulbar 376.6
  - skin 709.4
  - soft tissue 729.6
  - subcutaneous tissue 709.4
- operation wound, left accidentally 998.4
- orbit 870.4
  - retained or old 376.6
- posterior wall, eye 871.6
  - magnetic 871.5
    - retained or old 360.55
  - retained or old 360.65
- respiratory tree 934.9
  - specified site NEC 934.8
- retained (old) (nonmagnetic) (in)
  - anterior chamber (eye) 360.61
    - magnetic 360.51
  - ciliary body 360.62
    - magnetic 360.52
  - eyelid 374.86
  - globe 360.60
    - magnetic 360.50
  - intraocular 360.60
    - magnetic 360.50
    - specified site NEC 360.69
      - magnetic 360.59
  - iris 360.62
    - magnetic 360.52
  - lens 360.63
    - magnetic 360.53
  - muscle 729.6
  - orbit 376.6
  - posterior wall of globe 360.65
    - magnetic 360.55
  - retina 360.65
    - magnetic 360.55
  - retrobulbar 376.6
  - soft tissue 729.6
  - vitreous 360.64
    - magnetic 360.54

Foreign body—continued

- retina 871.6
  - magnetic 871.5
    - retained or old 360.55
  - retained or old 360.65
- superficial, without major open wound (see also Injury, superficial, by site) 919.6
- swallowed NEC 938
- vitreous (humor) 871.6
  - magnetic 871.5
    - retained or old 360.54
  - retained or old 360.64

Forking, aqueduct of Sylvius 742.3
- with spina bifida (see also Spina bifida) 741.0

Formation
- bone in scar tissue (skin) 709.3
- connective tissue in vitreous 379.25
- Elschnig pearls (postcataract extraction) 366.51
- hyaline in cornea 371.49
- sequestrum in bone (due to infection) (see also Osteomyelitis) 730.1
- valve
  - colon, congenital 751.5
  - ureter (congenital) 753.2

Formication 782.0
Fort Bragg fever 100.89
Fossa — see also condition
- pyriform — see condition

Foster-Kennedy syndrome 377.04
Fothergill's
- disease, meaning scarlatina anginosa 034.1
- neuralgia (see also Neuralgia, trigeminal) 350.1

Foul breath 784.9
Found dead (cause unknown) 798.9
Foundling V20.0
Fournier's disease (idiopathic gangrene) 608.83
Fourth
- cranial nerve — see condition
- disease 057.8
- molar 520.1

Foville's syndrome 344.89
Fox's
- disease (apocrine miliaria) 705.82
- impetigo (contagiosa) 684

Fox-Fordyce disease (apocrine miliaria) 705.82

Fracture (abduction) (adduction) (avulsion) (compression) (crush) (dislocation) (oblique) (separation) (closed) 829.0

> Note — For fracture of any of the following sites with fracture of other bones — see Fracture, multiple.
> "Closed" includes the following descriptions of fractures, with or without delayed healing, unless they are specified as open or compound:
>   comminuted
>   depressed
>   elevated
>   fissured
>   greenstick
>   impacted
>   linear
>   march
>   simple
>   slipped epiphysis
>   spiral
>   unspecified
> "Open" includes the following descriptions of fractures, with or without delayed healing:
>   compound
>   infected
>   missile
>   puncture
>   with foreign body
> For late effect of fracture, see Late, effect, fracture, by site.

with
- internal injuries in same region (conditions classifiable to 860-869) — see also Injury, internal, by site pelvic region — see Fracture, pelvis
- acetabulum (with visceral injury) (closed) 808.0
  - open 808.1
- acromion (process) (closed) 811.01
  - open 811.11
- alveolus (closed) 802.8
  - open 802.9
- ankle (malleolus) (closed) 824.8
  - bimalleolar (Dupuytren's) (Pott's) 824.4
    - open 824.5
  - bone 825.21
    - open 825.31
  - lateral malleolus only (fibular) 824.2
    - open 824.3
  - medial malleolus only (tibial) 824.0
    - open 824.1
  - open 824.9
  - pathologic 733.16
  - talus 825.21
    - open 825.31
  - trimalleolar 824.6
    - open 824.7
- antrum — see Fracture, skull, base
- arm (closed) 818.0
  - and leg(s) (any bones) 828.0
    - open 828.1
  - both (any bones) (with rib(s)) (with sternum) 819.0
    - open 819.1
  - lower 813.80
    - open 813.90
  - open 818.1
  - upper — see Fracture, humerus

Fracture—continued

- astragalus (closed) 825.21
  - open 825.31
- atlas — see Fracture, vertebra, cervical, first
- axis — see Fracture, vertebra, cervical, second
- back — see Fracture, vertebra, by site
- Barton's — see Fracture, radius, lower end
- basal (skull) — see Fracture, skull, base
- Bennett's (closed) 815.01
  - open 815.11
- bimalleolar (closed) 824.4
  - open 824.5
- bone (closed) NEC 829.0
  - birth injury NEC 767.3
  - open 829.1
  - pathologic NEC (see also Fracture, pathologic) 733.10
- boot top — see Fracture, fibula
- boxers' — see Fracture, metacarpal bone(s)
- breast bone — see Fracture, sternum
- bucket handle (semilunar cartilage) — see Tear, meniscus
- bursting — see Fracture, phalanx, hand, distal
- calcaneus (closed) 825.0
  - open 825.1
- capitate (bone) (closed) 814.07
  - open 814.17
- capitellum (humerus) (closed) 812.49
  - open 812.59
- carpal bone(s) (wrist NEC) (closed) 814.00
  - open 814.10
  - specified site NEC 814.09
    - open 814.19
- cartilage, knee (semilunar) — see Tear, meniscus
- cervical — see Fracture, vertebra, cervical
- chauffeur's — see Fracture, ulna, lower end
- chisel — see Fracture, radius, upper end
- clavicle (interligamentous part) (closed) 810.00
  - acromial end 810.03
    - open 810.13
  - due to birth trauma 767.2
  - open 810.10
  - shaft (middle third) 810.02
    - open 810.12
  - sternal end 810.01
    - open 810.11
- clayshovelers' — see Fracture, vertebra, cervical
- coccyx — see also Fracture, vertebra, coccyx
  - complicating delivery 665.6
- collar bone — see Fracture, clavicle
- Colles' (reversed) (closed) 813.41
  - open 813.51
- comminuted — see Fracture, by site
- compression — see also Fracture, by site
  - nontraumatic — see Fracture, pathologic
- congenital 756.9
- coracoid process (closed) 811.02
  - open 811.12
- coronoid process (ulna) (closed) 813.02
  - mandible (closed) 802.23
    - open 802.33
  - open 813.12

Fracture—continued
  costochondral junction — see Fracture, rib
  costosternal junction — see Fracture, rib
  cranium — see Fracture, skull, by site
  cricoid cartilage (closed) 807.5
    open 807.6
  cuboid (ankle) (closed) 825.23
    open 825.33
  cuneiform
    foot (closed) 825.24
      open 825.34
    wrist (closed) 814.03
      open 814.13
  due to
    birth injury — see Birth injury, fracture
    gunshot — see Fracture, by site, open
    neoplasm — see Fracture, pathologic
    osteoporosis — see Fracture, pathologic
  Dupuytren's (ankle) (fibula) (closed) 824.4
    open 824.5
    radius 813.42
      open 813.52
  Duverney's — see Fracture, ilium
  elbow — see also Fracture, humerus, lower end
    olecranon (process) (closed) 813.01
      open 813.11
    supracondylar (closed) 812.41
      open 812.51
  ethmoid (bone) (sinus) — see Fracture, skull, base
  face bone(s) (closed) NEC 802.8
    with
      other bone(s) — see Fracture, multiple, skull
      skull — see also Fracture, skull
        involving other bones — see Fracture, multiple, skull
    open 802.9
  fatigue — see Fracture, march
  femur, femoral (closed) 821.00
    cervicotrochanteric 820.03
      open 820.13
    condyles, epicondyles 821.21
      open 821.31
    distal end — see Fracture, femur, lower end
    epiphysis (separation)
      capital 820.01
        open 820.11
      head 820.01
        open 820.11
      lower 821.22
        open 821.32
      trochanteric 820.01
        open 820.11
      upper 820.01
        open 820.11
    head 820.09
      open 820.19
    lower end or extremity (distal end) (closed) 821.20
      condyles, epicondyles 821.21
        open 821.31
      epiphysis (separation) 821.22
        open 821.32
      multiple sites 821.29
        open 821.39
      specified site NEC 821.29
        open 821.39
      supracondylar 821.23
        open 821.33

Fracture—continued
  femur, femoral—continued
    lower end or extremity—continued
      T-shaped 821.21
        open 821.31
    neck (closed) 820.8
      base (cervicotrochanteric) 820.03
        open 820.13
      extracapsular 820.20
        open 820.30
      intertrochanteric (section) 820.21
        open 820.31
      intracapsular 820.00
        open 820.10
      intratrochanteric 820.21
        open 820.31
      midcervical 820.02
        open 820.12
      open 820.9
      pathologic 733.14
        specified part NEC 733.15
      specified site NEC 820.09
        open 820.19
      transcervical 820.02
        open 820.12
      transtrochanteric 820.20
        open 820.30
    open 821.10
    pathologic 733.14
      specified part NEC 733.15
    peritrochanteric (section) 820.20
      open 820.30
    shaft (lower third) (middle third) (upper third) 821.01
      open 821.11
    subcapital 820.09
      open 820.19
    subtrochanteric (region) (section) 820.22
      open 820.32
    supracondylar 821.23
      open 821.33
    transepiphyseal 820.01
      open 820.11
    trochanter (greater) (lesser) (see also Fracture, femur, neck, by site) 820.20
      open 820.30
    T-shaped, into knee joint 821.21
      open 821.31
    upper end 820.8
      open 820.9
  fibula (closed) 823.81
    with tibia 823.82
      open 823.92
    distal end 824.8
      open 824.9
    epiphysis
      lower 824.8
        open 824.9
      upper — see Fracture, fibula, upper end
    head — see Fracture, fibula, upper end
    involving ankle 824.2
      open 824.3
    lower end or extremity 824.8
      open 824.9
    malleolus (external) (lateral) 824.2
      open 824.3
    open NEC 823.91
    pathologic 733.16
    proximal end — see Fracture, fibula, upper end
    shaft 823.21
      with tibia 823.22
        open 823.32
      open 823.31

Fracture—continued
  fibula—continued
    upper end or extremity (epiphysis) (head) (proximal end) (styloid) 823.01
      with tibia 823.02
        open 823.12
      open 823.11
    finger(s), of one hand (closed) (see also Fracture, phalanx, hand) 816.00
      with
        metacarpal bone(s), of same hand 817.0
          open 817.1
        thumb of same hand 816.03
          open 816.13
      open 816.10
    foot, except toe(s) alone (closed) 825.20
      open 825.30
    forearm (closed) NEC 813.80
      lower end (distal end) (lower epiphysis) 813.40
        open 813.50
      open 813.90
      shaft 813.20
        open 813.30
      upper end (proximal end) (upper epiphysis) 813.00
        open 813.10
    fossa, anterior, middle, or posterior — see Fracture, skull, base
    frontal (bone) — see also Fracture, skull, vault
      sinus — see Fracture, skull, base
    Galeazzi's — see Fracture, radius, lower end
    glenoid (cavity) (fossa) (scapula) (closed) 811.03
      open 811.13
    Gosselin's — see Fracture, ankle
    greenstick — see Fracture, by site
    grenade-throwers' — see Fracture, humerus, shaft
    gutter — see Fracture, skull, vault
    hamate (closed) 814.08
      open 814.18
    hand, one (closed) 815.00
      carpals 814.00
        open 814.10
        specified site NEC 814.09
          open 814.19
      metacarpals 815.00
        open 815.10
      multiple, bones of one hand 817.0
        open 817.1
      open 815.10
      phalanges (see also Fracture, phalanx, hand) 816.00
        open 816.10
    healing or old
      aftercare or convalescence V54.9
      change of cast V54.8
      complications — see condition
      removal of
        cast V54.8
        fixation device
          external V54.8
          internal V54.0
    heel bone (closed) 825.0
      open 825.1
    hip (closed) (see also Fracture, femur, neck) 820.8
      open 820.9
      pathologic 733.14
    humerus (closed) 812.20
      anatomical neck 812.02
        open 812.12

Fracture—continued
  humerus—continued
    articular process (see also Fracture humerus, condyle(s)) 812.44
      open 812.54
    capitellum 812.49
      open 812.59
    condyle(s) 812.44
      lateral (external) 812.42
        open 812.52
      medial (internal epicondyle) 812.43
        open 812.53
      open 812.54
    distal end — see Fracture, humerus, lower end
    epiphysis
      lower (see also Fracture, humerus, condyle(s)) 812.44
        open 812.54
      upper 812.09
        open 812.19
    external condyle 812.42
      open 812.52
    great tuberosity 812.03
      open 812.13
    head 812.09
      open 812.19
    internal epicondyle 812.43
      open 812.53
    lesser tuberosity 812.09
      open 812.19
    lower end or extremity (distal end) (see also Fracture, humerus, by site) 812.40
      multiple sites NEC 812.49
        open 812.59
      open 812.50
      specified site NEC 812.49
        open 812.59
    neck 812.01
      open 812.11
      open 812.30
    pathologic 733.11
    proximal end — see Fracture, humerus, upper end
    shaft 812.21
      open 812.31
    supracondylar 812.41
      open 812.51
    surgical neck 812.01
      open 812.11
    trochlea 812.49
      open 812.59
    T-shaped 812.44
      open 812.54
    tuberosity — see Fracture, humerus, upper end
    upper end or extremity (proximal end) (see also Fracture, humerus, by site) 812.00
      open 812.10
      specified site NEC 812.09
        open 812.19
  hyoid bone (closed) 807.5
    open 807.6
  hyperextension — see Fracture, radius, lower end
  ilium (with visceral injury) (closed) 808.41
    open 808.51
  impaction, impacted — see Fracture, by site
  incus — see Fracture, skull, base
  innominate bone (with visceral injury) (closed) 808.49
    open 808.59
  instep, of one foot (closed) 825.20
    with toe(s) of same foot 827.0
      open 827.1
    open 825.30

Fracture INDEX TO DISEASES Fracture

Fracture—*continued*
 internal
  ear — *see* Fracture, skull, base
  semilunar cartilage, knee — *see* Tear, meniscus, medial
 intertrochanteric — *see* Fracture, femur, neck, intertrochanteric
 ischium (with visceral injury) (closed) 808.42
  open 808.52
 jaw (bone) (lower) (closed) (*see also* Fracture, mandible) 802.20
  angle 802.25
   open 802.35
  open 802.30
  upper — *see* Fracture, maxilla
 knee
  cap (closed) 822.0
   open 822.1
  cartilage (semilunar) — *see* Tear, meniscus
 labyrinth (osseous) — *see* Fracture, skull, base
 larynx (closed) 807.5
  open 807.6
 late effect — *see* Late, effects (of), fracture
 Le Fort's — *see* Fracture, maxilla
 leg (closed) 827.0
  with rib(s) or sternum 828.0
   open 828.1
  both (any bones) 828.0
   open 828.1
  lower — *see* Fracture, tibia
  open 827.1
  upper — *see* Fracture, femur
 limb
  lower (multiple) (closed) NEC 827.0
   open 827.1
  upper (multiple) (closed) NEC 818.0
   open 818.1
 long bones, due to birth trauma — *see* Birth injury, fracture
 lumbar — *see* Fracture, vertebra, lumbar
 lunate bone (closed) 814.02
  open 814.12
 malar bone (closed) 802.4
  open 802.5
 Malgaigne's (closed) 808.43
  open 808.53
 malleolus (closed) 824.8
  bimalleolar 824.4
   open 824.5
  lateral 824.2
   and medial — *see also* Fracture, malleolus, bimalleolar
    with lip of tibia — *see* Fracture, malleolus, trimalleolar
   open 824.3
  medial (closed) 824.0
   and lateral — *see also* Fracture, malleolus, bimalleolar
    with lip of tibia — *see* Fracture, malleolus, trimalleolar
   open 824.1
  open 824.9
  trimalleolar (closed) 824.6
   open 824.7
 malleus — *see* Fracture, skull, base
 malunion 733.81
 mandible (closed) 802.20
  angle 802.25
   open 802.35

Fracture—*continued*
 mandible—*continued*
  body 802.28
   alveolar border 802.27
    open 802.37
   open 802.38
   symphysis 802.26
    open 802.36
  condylar process 802.21
   open 802.31
  coronoid process 802.23
   open 802.33
  multiple sites 802.29
   open 802.39
  open 802.30
  ramus NEC 802.24
   open 802.34
  subcondylar 802.22
   open 802.32
  manubrium — *see* Fracture, sternum
  march (closed) 825.20
   open 825.30
  maxilla, maxillary (superior) (upper jaw) (closed) 802.4
   inferior — *see* Fracture, mandible
   open 802.5
  meniscus, knee — *see* Tear, meniscus
  metacarpus, metacarpal (bone(s)), of one hand (closed) 815.00
   with phalanx, phalanges, hand (finger(s)) (thumb) of same hand 817.0
    open 817.1
   base 815.02
    first metacarpal 815.01
     open 815.11
    open 815.12
    thumb 815.01
     open 815.11
   multiple sites 815.09
    open 815.19
   neck 815.04
    open 815.14
   open 815.10
   shaft 815.03
    open 815.13
  metatarsus, metatarsal (bone(s)), of one foot (closed) 825.25
   with tarsal bone(s) 825.29
    open 825.39
   open 825.35
  Monteggia's (closed) 813.03
   open 813.13
  Moore's — *see* Fracture, radius, lower end multangular bone (closed)
   larger 814.05
    open 814.15
   smaller 814.06
    open 814.16

Fracture—*continued*
 multiple (closed) 829.0

> Note — Multiple fractures of sites classifiable to the same three- or four-digit category are coded to that category, except for sites classifiable to 810-818 or 820-827 in different limbs.
> Multiple fractures of sites classifiable to different fourth-digit subdivisions within the same three-digit category should be dealt with according to coding rules.
> Multiple fractures of sites classifiable to different three-digit categories (identifiable from the listing under "Fracture"), and of sites classifiable to 810-818 or 820-827 in different limbs should be coded according to the following list, which should be referred to in the following priority order: skull or face bones, pelvis or vertebral column, legs, arms.

  arm (multiple bones in same arm except in hand alone) (sites classifiable to 810-817 with sites classifiable to a different three-digit category in 810-817 in same arm) (closed) 818.0
   open 818.1
  arms, both or arm(s) with rib(s) or sternum (sites classifiable to 810-818 with sites classifiable to same range of categories in other limb or to 807) (closed) 819.0
   open 819.1
  bones of trunk NEC (closed) 809.0
   open 809.1
  hand, metacarpal bone(s) with phalanx or phalanges of same hand (sites classifiable to 815 with sites classifiable to 816 in same hand) (closed) 817.0
   open 817.1
  leg (multiple bones in same leg) (sites classifiable to 820-826 with sites classifiable to a different three-digit category in that range in same leg) (closed) 827.0
   open 827.1
  legs, both or leg(s) with arm(s), rib(s), or sternum (sites classifiable to 820-827 with sites classifiable to same range of categories in other leg or to 807 or 810-819) (closed) 828.0
   open 828.1
  open 829.1
  pelvis with other bones except skull or face bones (sites classifiable to 808 with sites classifiable to 805-807 or 810-829) (closed) 809.0
   open 809.1
  skull, specified or unspecified bones, or face bone(s) with any other bone(s) (sites classifiable to 800-803 with sites classifiable to 805-829) (closed) 804.0

Fracture—*continued*
 multiple—*continued*
  skull—*continued*

> Note — Use the following fifth-digit subclassification with categories 800, 801, 803, and 804:
> 0 unspecified state of consciousness
> 1 with no loss of consciousness
> 2 with brief [less than one hour] loss of consciousness
> 3 with moderate [1-24 hours] loss of consciousness
> 4 with prolonged [more than 24 hours] loss of consciousness and return to pre-existing conscious level
> 5 with prolonged [more than 24 hours] loss of consciousness, without return to pre-existing conscious level
> 6 with loss of consciousness of unspecified duration
> 9 with concussion, unspecified

   with
    contusion, cerebral 804.1
    epidural hemorrhage 804.2
    extradural hemorrhage 804.2
    hemorrhage (intracranial) NEC 804.3
    intracranial injury NEC 804.4
    laceration, cerebral 804.1
    subarachnoid hemorrhage 804.2
    subdural hemorrhage 804.2
   open 804.5
    with
     contusion, cerebral 804.6
     epidural hemorrhage 804.7
     extradural hemorrhage 804.7
     hemorrhage (intracranial) NEC 804.8
     intracranial injury NEC 804.9
     laceration, cerebral 804.6
     subarachnoid hemorrhage 804.7
     subdural hemorrhage 804.7
  vertebral column with other bones, except skull or face bones (sites classifiable to 805 or 806 with sites classifiable to 807-808 or 810-829) (closed) 809.0
   open 809.1
 nasal (bone(s)) (closed) 802.0
  open 802.1
  sinus — *see* Fracture, skull, base

Fracture—*continued*
  navicular
    carpal (wrist) (closed) 814.01
      open 814.11
    tarsal (ankle) (closed) 825.22
      open 825.32
  neck — *see* Fracture, vertebra, cervical
  neural arch — *see* Fracture, vertebra, by site
  nose, nasal, (bone) (septum) (closed) 802.0
    open 802.1
  occiput — *see* Fracture, skull, base
  odontoid process — *see* Fracture, vertebra, cervical
  olecranon (process) (ulna) (closed) 813.01
    open 813.11
  open 829.1
  orbit, orbital (bone) (region) (closed) 802.8
    floor (blow-out) 802.6
      open 802.7
    open 802.9
    roof — *see* Fracture, skull, base
    specified part NEC 802.8
      open 802.9
  os
    calcis (closed) 825.0
      open 825.1
    magnum (closed) 814.07
      open 814.17
    pubis (with visceral injury) (closed) 808.2
      open 808.3
    triquetrum (closed) 814.03
      open 814.13
  osseous
    auditory meatus — *see* Fracture, skull, base
    labyrinth — *see* Fracture, skull, base ossicles, auditory (incus) (malleus) (stapes) — *see* Fracture, skull, base
  osteoporotic — *see* Fracture, pathologic
  palate (closed) 802.8
    open 802.9
  paratrooper — *see* Fracture, tibia, lower end
  parietal bone — *see* Fracture, skull, vault
  parry — *see* Fracture, Monteggia's
  patella (closed) 822.0
    open 822.1
  pathologic (cause unknown) 733.10
    ankle 733.16
    femur (neck) 733.14
      specified NEC 733.15
    fibula 733.16
    hip 733.14
    humerus 733.11
    radius 733.12
    specified site NEC 733.19
    tibia 733.16
    ulna 733.12
    vertebrae (collapse) 733.13
    wrist 733.12
  pedicle (of vertebral arch) — *see* Fracture, vertebra, by site
  pelvis, pelvic (bone(s)) (with visceral injury) (closed) 808.8
    multiple (with disruption of pelvic circle) 808.43
      open 808.53
    open 808.9
    rim (closed) 808.49
      open 808.59
  peritrochanteric (closed) 820.20
    open 820.30

Fracture—*continued*
  phalanx, phalanges, of one
    foot (closed) 826.0
      with bone(s) of same lower limb 827.0
        open 827.1
      open 826.1
    hand (closed) 816.00
      with metacarpal bone(s) of same hand 817.0
        open 817.1
      distal 816.02
        open 816.12
      middle 816.01
        open 816.11
      multiple sites NEC 816.03
        open 816.13
      open 816.10
      proximal 816.01
        open 816.11
  pisiform (closed) 814.04
    open 814.14
  pond — *see* Fracture, skull, vault
  Pott's (closed) 824.4
    open 824.5
  prosthetic device, internal — *see* Complications, mechanical
  pubis (with visceral injury) (closed) 808.2
    open 808.3
  Quervain's (closed) 814.01
    open 814.11
  radius (alone) (closed) 813.81
    with ulna NEC 813.83
      open 813.93
    distal end — *see* Fracture, radius, lower end
    epiphysis
      lower — *see* Fracture, radius, lower end
      upper — *see* Fracture, radius, upper end
    head — *see* Fracture, radius, upper end
    lower end or extremity (distal end) (lower epiphysis) 813.42
      with ulna (lower end) 813.44
        open 813.54
      open 813.52
    neck — *see* Fracture, radius, upper end
    open NEC 813.91
    pathologic 733.12
    proximal end — *see* Fracture, radius, upper end
    shaft (closed) 813.21
      with ulna (shaft) 813.23
        open 813.33
      open 813.31
    upper end 813.07
      with ulna (upper end) 813.08
        open 813.18
      epiphysis 813.05
        open 813.15
      head 813.05
        open 813.15
      multiple sites 813.07
        open 813.17
      neck 813.06
        open 813.16
      open 813.17
      specified site NEC 813.07
        open 813.17
  ramus
    inferior or superior (with visceral injury) (closed) 808.2
      open 808.3
    ischium — *see* Fracture, ischium
    mandible 802.24
      open 802.34

Fracture—*continued*
  rib(s) (closed) 807.0

  Note — Use the following fifth-digit subclassification with categories 807.0-807.1:
0	rib(s), unspecified
1	one rib
2	two ribs
3	three ribs
4	four ribs
5	five ribs
6	six ribs
7	seven ribs
8	eight or more ribs
9	multiple ribs, unspecified

    with flail chest (open) 807.4
    open 807.1
    root, tooth 873.63
      complicated 873.73
  sacrum — *see* Fracture, vertebra, sacrum
  scaphoid
    ankle (closed) 825.22
      open 825.32
    wrist (closed) 814.01
      open 814.11
  scapula (closed) 811.00
    acromial, acromion (process) 811.01
      open 811.11
    body 811.09
      open 811.19
    coracoid process 811.02
      open 811.12
    glenoid (cavity) (fossa) 811.03
      open 811.13
    neck 811.03
      open 811.13
    open 811.10
  semilunar
    bone, wrist (closed) 814.02
      open 814.12
    cartilage (interior) (knee) — *see* Tear, meniscus
  sesamoid bone — *see* Fracture, by site
  Shepherd's (closed) 825.21
    open 825.31
  shoulder — *see also* Fracture, humerus, upper end
    blade — *see* Fracture, scapula
  silverfork — *see* Fracture, radius, lower end
  sinus (ethmoid) (frontal) (maxillary) (nasal) (sphenoidal) — *see* Fracture, skull, base
  Skillern's — *see* Fracture, radius, shaft

Fracture—*continued*
  skull (multiple NEC) (with face bones) (closed) 803.0

  Note — Use the following fifth digit subclassification with categories 800, 801, 803, and 804:
0	unspecified state of consciousness
1	with no loss of consciousness
2	with brief [less than one hour] loss of consciousness
3	with moderate [1-24 hours] loss of consciousness
4	with prolonged [more than 24 hours] loss of consciousness and return to pre-existing conscious level
5	with prolonged [more than 24 hours] loss of consciousness, without return to pre-existing conscious level
6	with loss of consciousness of unspecified duration
9	with concussion, unspecified

    with
      contusion, cerebral 803.1
      epidural hemorrhage 803.2
      extradural hemorrhage 803.2
      hemorrhage (intracranial) NEC 803.3
      intracranial injury NEC 803.4
      laceration, cerebral 803.1
      other bones — *see* Fracture, multiple, skull
      subarachnoid hemorrhage 803.2
      subdural hemorrhage 803.2
    base (antrum) (ethmoid bone) (fossa) (internal ear) (nasal sinus) (occiput) (sphenoid) (temporal bone) (closed) 801.0
      with
        contusion, cerebral 801.1
        epidural hemorrhage 801.2
        extradural hemorrhage 801.2
        hemorrhage (intracranial) NEC 801.3
        intracranial injury NEC 801.4
        laceration, cerebral 801.1
        subarachnoid hemorrhage 801.2
        subdural hemorrhage 801.2
      open 801.5
        with
          contusion, cerebral 801.6
          epidural hemorrhage 801.7
          extradural hemorrhage 801.7
          hemorrhage (intracranial) NEC 801.8

Fracture INDEX TO DISEASES Fracture

Fracture—continued
  skull—continued
    base—continued
      open—continued
        with—continued
          intracranial injury NEC 801.9
          laceration, cerebral 801.6
          subarachnoid hemorrhage 801.7
          subdural hemorrhage 801.7
    birth injury 767.3
    face bones — see Fracture, face bones
    open 803.5
      with
        contusion, cerebral 803.6
        epidural hemorrhage 803.7
        extradural hemorrhage 803.7
        hemorrhage (intracranial) NEC 803.8
        intracranial injury NEC 803.9
        laceration, cerebral 803.6
        subarachnoid hemorrhage 803.7
        subdural hemorrhage 803.7
    vault (frontal bone) (parietal bone) (vertex) (closed) 800.0
      with
        contusion, cerebral 800.1
        epidural hemorrhage 800.2
        extradural hemorrhage 800.2
        hemorrhage (intracranial) NEC 800.3
        intracranial injury NEC 800.4
        laceration, cerebral 800.1
        subarachnoid hemorrhage 800.2
        subdural hemorrhage 800.2
    open 800.5
      with
        contusion, cerebral 800.6
        epidural hemorrhage 800.7
        extradural hemorrhage 800.7
        hemorrhage (intracranial) NEC 800.8
        intracranial injury NEC 800.9
        laceration, cerebral 800.6
        subarachnoid hemorrhage 800.7
        subdural hemorrhage 800.7
  Smith's 813.41
    open 813.51
  sphenoid (bone) (sinus) — see Fracture, skull, base
  spine — see also Fracture, vertebra, by site due to birth trauma 767.4
  spinous process — see Fracture, vertebra, by site

Fracture—continued
  spontaneous — see Fracture, pathologic
  sprinters' — see Fracture, ilium
  stapes — see Fracture, skull, base
  stave — see also Fracture, metacarpus, metacarpal bone(s)
    spine — see Fracture, tibia, upper end
  sternum (closed) 807.2
    with flail chest (open) 807.4
    open 807.3
  Stieda's — see Fracture, femur, lower end
  stress — see Fracture, pathologic
  styloid process
    metacarpal (closed) 815.02
      open 815.12
    radius — see Fracture, radius, lower end
    temporal bone — see Fracture, skull, base
    ulna — see Fracture, ulna, lower end
  supracondylar, elbow 812.41
    open 812.51
  symphysis pubis (with visceral injury) (closed) 808.2
    open 808.3
  talus (ankle bone) (closed) 825.21
    open 825.31
  tarsus, tarsal bone(s) (with metatarsus) of one foot (closed) NEC 825.29
    open 825.39
  temporal bone (styloid) — see Fracture, skull, base
  tendon — see Sprain, by site
  thigh — see Fracture, femur, shaft
  thumb (and finger(s)) of one hand (closed) (see also Fracture, phalanx, hand) 816.00
    with metacarpal bone(s) of same hand 817.0
      open 817.1
    metacarpal(s) — see Fracture, metacarpus
    open 816.10
  thyroid cartilage (closed) 807.5
    open 807.6
  tibia (closed) 823.80
    with fibula 823.82
      open 823.92
    condyles — see Fracture, tibia, upper end
    distal end 824.8
      open 824.9
    epiphysis
      lower 824.8
        open 824.9
      upper — see Fracture, tibia, upper end
    head (involving knee joint) — see Fracture, tibia, upper end
    intercondyloid eminence — see Fracture, tibia, upper end
    involving ankle 824.0
      open 824.9
    malleolus (internal) (medial) 824.0
      open 824.1
    open NEC 823.90
    pathologic 733.16
    proximal end — see Fracture, tibia, upper end
    shaft 823.20
      with fibula 823.22
        open 823.32
      open 823.30
    spine — see Fracture, tibia, upper end
    tuberosity — see Fracture, tibia, upper end

Fracture—continued
  tibia—continued
    upper end or extremity (condyle) (epiphysis) (head) (spine) (proximal end) (tuberosity) 823.00
      with fibula 823.02
        open 823.12
      open 823.10
  toe(s), of one foot (closed) 826.0
    with bone(s) of same lower limb 827.0
      open 827.1
    open 826.1
  tooth (root) 873.63
    complicated 873.73
  trachea (closed) 807.5
    open 807.6
  transverse process — see Fracture, vertebra, by site
  trapezium (closed) 814.05
    open 814.15
  trapezoid bone (closed) 814.06
    open 814.16
  trimalleolar (closed) 824.6
    open 824.7
  triquetral (bone) (closed) 814.03
    open 814.13
  trochanter (greater) (lesser) (closed) (see also Fracture, femur, neck, by site) 820.20
    open 820.30
  trunk (bones) (closed) 809.0
    open 809.1
  tuberosity (external) — see Fracture, by site
  ulna (alone) (closed) 813.82
    with radius NEC 813.83
      open 813.93
    coronoid process (closed) 813.02
      open 813.12
    distal end — see Fracture, ulna, lower end
    epiphysis
      lower — see Fracture, ulna, lower end
      upper — see Fracture, ulna, upper end
    head — see Fracture, ulna, lower end
    lower end (distal end) (head) (lower epiphysis) (styloid process) 813.43
      with radius (lower end) 813.44
        open 813.54
      open 813.53
    olecranon process (closed) 813.01
      open 813.11
    open NEC 813.92
    pathologic 733.12
    proximal end — see Fracture, ulna, upper end
    shaft 813.22
      with radius (shaft) 813.23
        open 813.33
      open 813.32
    styloid process — see Fracture, ulna, lower end
    transverse — see Fracture, ulna, by site
    upper end (epiphysis) 813.04
      with radius (upper end) 813.08
        open 813.18
      multiple sites 813.04
        open 813.14
      specified site NEC 813.04
        open 813.14
  unciform (closed) 814.08
    open 814.18

Fracture—continued
  vertebra, vertebral (back) (body) (column) (neural arch) (pedicle) (spine) (spinous process) (transverse process) (closed) 805.8
    with
      hematomyelia — see Fracture, vertebra, by site, with spinal cord injury
      injury to
        cauda equina — see Fracture, vertebra, sacrum, with spinal cord injury
        nerve — see Fracture, vertebra, by site, with spinal cord injury
      paralysis — see Fracture, vertebra, by site, with spinal cord injury
      paraplegia — see Fracture, vertebra, by site, with spinal cord injury
      quadriplegia — see Fracture, vertebra, by site, with spinal cord injury
      spinal concussion — see Fracture, vertebra, by site, with spinal cord injury
      spinal cord injury (closed) NEC 806.8

> Note — Use the following fifth-digit subclassification with categories 806.0-806.3:
>
> C_1-C_4 or unspecified level and D_1-D_6 (T_1-T_6) or unspecified level with
>
> 0 unspecified spinal cord injury
> 1 complete lesion of cord
> 2 anterior cord syndrome
> 3 central cord syndrome
> 4 specified injury NEC
>
> C_5-C_7 level and D_7-D_{12} level with:
>
> 5 unspecified spinal cord injury
> 6 complete lesion of cord
> 7 anterior cord syndrome
> 8 central cord syndrome
> 9 specified injury NEC

        cervical 806.0
          open 806.1
        dorsal, dorsolumbar 806.2
          open 806.3
        open 806.9
        thoracic, thoracolumbar 806.2
          open 806.3
    atlanto-axial — see Fracture, vertebra, cervical
    cervical (hangman) (teardrop) (closed) 805.00
      with spinal cord injury — see Fracture, vertebra, with spinal cord injury, cervical
      first (atlas) 805.01
        open 805.11
      second (axis) 805.02
        open 805.12
      third 805.03
        open 805.13
      fourth 805.04
        open 805.14

Fracture—*continued*
    vertebra, vertebral—*continued*
        cervical—*continued*
            fifth 805.05
                open 805.15
            sixth 805.06
                open 805.16
            seventh 805.07
                open 805.17
            multiple sites 805.08
                open 805.18
            open 805.10
        coccyx (closed) 805.6
            with spinal cord injury
                (closed) 806.60
                cauda equina injury
                    806.62
                complete lesion
                    806.61
                    open 806.71
                open 806.72
                open 806.70
                specified type NEC
                    806.69
                  open 806.79
            open 805.7
        collapsed 733.13
        compression, not due to
            trauma 733.13
        dorsal (closed) 805.2
            with spinal cord injury —
                see Fracture,
                vertebra, with spinal
                cord injury, dorsal
            open 805.3
        dorsolumbar (closed) 805.2
            with spinal cord injury —
                see Fracture,
                vertebra, with spinal
                cord injury, dorsal
            open 805.3
        due to osteoporosis 733.13
        fetus or newborn 767.4
        lumbar (closed) 805.4
            with spinal cord injury
                (closed) 806.4
                open 806.5
            open 805.5
        nontraumatic 733.13
        open NEC 805.9
        pathologic (any site) 733.13
        sacrum (closed) 805.6
            with spinal cord injury
                806.60
                cauda equina injury
                    806.62
                complete lesion
                    806.61
                  open 806.71
                open 806.72
                open 806.70
                specified type NEC
                    806.69
                  open 806.79
            open 805.7
        site unspecified (closed) 805.8
            with spinal cord injury
                (closed) 806.8
                open 806.9
            open 805.9
        thoracic (closed) 805.2
            with spinal cord injury —
                see Fracture,
                vertebra, with spinal
                cord injury, thoracic
            open 805.3
    vertex — *see* Fracture, skull, vault
    vomer (bone) 802.0
        open 802.1
    Wagstaffe's — *see* Fracture, ankle
    wrist (closed) 814.00
        open 814.10
        pathologic 733.12
    xiphoid (process) — *see* Fracture, sternum

Fracture—*continued*
    zygoma (zygomatic arch) (closed) 802.4
        open 802.5
Fragile X syndrome 759.83 ◆
Fragilitas
    crinium 704.2
    hair 704.2
    ossium 756.51
        with blue sclera 756.51
    unguium 703.8
        congenital 757.5
Fragility
    bone 756.51
        with deafness and blue sclera 756.51
    capillary (hereditary) 287.8
    hair 704.2
    nails 703.8
Fragmentation — *see* Fracture, by site
Frambesia, frambesial (tropica) (*see also* Yaws) 102.9
    initial lesion or ulcer 102.0
    primary 102.0
Frambeside
    gummatous 102.4
    of early yaws 102.2
Frambesioma 102.1
Franceschetti's syndrome (mandibulofacial dysotosis) 756.0
Francis' disease (*see also* Tularemia) 021.9
Frank's essential thrombocytopenia (*see also* Purpura, thrombocytopenic) 287.3
Franklin's disease (heavy chain) 273.2
Fraser's syndrome 759.89
Freckle 709.09 ◆
    malignant melanoma in (M8742/3) — *see* Melanoma
    melanotic (of Hutchinson) (M8742/2) — *see* Neoplasm, skin, in situ
Freeman-Sheldon syndrome 759.89
Freezing 991.9
    specified effect NEC 991.8
Frei's disease (climatic bubo) 099.1
Freiberg's
    disease (osteochondrosis, second metatarsal) 732.5
    infraction of metatarsal head 732.5
    osteochondrosis 732.5
Fremitus, friction, cardiac 785.3
Frenulum linguae 750.0
Frenum
    external os 752.49
    tongue 750.0
Frequency (urinary) NEC 788.41
    micturition 788.41
    nocturnal 788.43
    psychogenic 306.53
Frey's syndrome (auriculotemporal syndrome) 350.8
Friction
    burn (*see also* Injury, superficial, by site) 919.0
    fremitus, cardiac 785.3
    precordial 785.3
    sounds, chest 786.7
Friderichsen-Waterhouse syndrome or disease 036.3
Friedländer's
    B (bacillus) NEC (*see also* condition) 041.3
    sepsis or septicemia 038.49
    disease (endarteritis obliterans) — *see* Arteriosclerosis

Friedreich's
    ataxia 334.0
    combined systemic disease 334.0
    disease 333.2
        combined systemic 334.0
        myoclonia 333.2
        sclerosis (spinal cord) 334.0
Friedrich-Erb-Arnold syndrome (acropachyderma) 757.39
Frigidity 302.72
    psychic or psychogenic 302.72
Fröhlich's disease or syndrome (adiposogenital dystrophy) 253.8
Froin's syndrome 336.8
Frommel's disease 676.6
Frommel-Chiari syndrome 676.6
Frontal — *see also* condition
    lobe syndrome 310.0
Frostbite 991.3
    face 991.0
    foot 991.2
    hand 991.1
    specified site NEC 991.3
Frotteurism 302.89 ◆
Frozen 991.9
    pelvis 620.8
    shoulder 726.0
Fructosemia 271.2
Fructosuria (benign) (essential) 271.2
Fuchs'
    black spot (myopic) 360.21
    corneal dystrophy (endothelial) 371.57
    heterochromic cyclitis 364.21
Fucosidosis 271.8
Fugue 780.9
    hysterical (dissociative) 300.13 ◆
    reaction to exceptional stress (transient) 308.1
Fuller Albright's syndrome (osteitis fibrosa disseminata) 756.59
Fuller's earth disease 502
Fulminant, fulminating — *see* condition
Functional — *see* condition
Fundus — *see also* condition
    flavimaculatus 362.76
Fungemia 117.9
Fungus, fungous
    cerebral 348.8
    disease NEC 117.9
    infection — *see* Infection, fungus
    testis (*see also* Tuberculosis) 016.5 [608.81]
Funiculitis (acute) 608.4
    chronic 608.4
    endemic 608.4
    gonococcal (acute) 098.14
        chronic or duration of 2 months or over 098.34
    tuberculous (*see also* Tuberculosis) 016.5
F.U.O. (*see also* Pyrexia) 780.6
Funnel
    breast (acquired) 738.3
        congenital 754.81
        late effect of rickets 268.1
    chest (acquired) 738.3
        congenital 754.81
        late effect of rickets 268.1
    pelvis (acquired) 738.6
        with disproportion (fetopelvic) 653.3
            affecting fetus or newborn 763.1
            causing obstructed labor 660.1
                affecting fetus or newborn 763.1
        congenital 755.69
        tuberculous (*see also* Tuberculosis) 016.9

Furfur 690
    microsporon 111.0
Furor, paroxysmal (idiopathic) (*see also* Epilepsy) 345.8
Furriers' lung 495.8
Furrowed tongue 529.5
    congenital 750.13
Furrowing nail(s) (transverse) 703.8
    congenital 757.5
Furuncle 680.9
    abdominal wall 680.2
    ankle 680.6
    anus 680.5
    arm (any part, above wrist) 680.3
    auditory canal, external 680.0
    axilla 680.3
    back (any part) 680.2
    breast 680.2
    buttock 680.5
    chest wall 680.2
    corpus cavernosum 607.2
    ear (any part) 680.0
    eyelid 373.13
    face (any part, except eye) 680.0
    finger (any) 680.4
    flank 680.2
    foot (any part) 680.7
    forearm 680.3
    gluteal (region) 680.5
    groin 680.2
    hand (any part) 680.4
    head (any part, except face) 680.8
    heel 680.7
    hip 680.6
    kidney (*see also* Abscess, kidney) 590.2
    knee 680.6
    labium (majus) (minus) 616.4
    lacrimal
        gland (*see also* Dacryoadenitis) 375.00
        passages (duct) (sac) (*see also* Dacryocystitis) 375.30
    leg, any part except foot 680.6
    malignant 022.0
    multiple sites 680.9
    neck 680.1
    nose (external) (septum) 680.0
    orbit 376.01
    partes posteriores 680.5
    pectoral region 680.2
    penis 607.2
    perineum 680.2
    pinna 680.0
    scalp (any part) 680.8
    scrotum 608.4
    seminal vesicle 608.0
    shoulder 680.3
    skin NEC 680.9
    specified site NEC 680.8
    spermatic cord 608.4
    temple (region) 680.0
    testis 604.90
    thigh 680.6
    thumb 680.4
    toe (any) 680.7
    trunk 680.2
    tunica vaginalis 608.4
    umbilicus 680.2
    upper arm 680.3
    vas deferens 608.4
    vulva 616.4
    wrist 680.4
Furunculosis (*see also* Furuncle) 680.9
    external auditory meatus 680.0 [380.13]
Fusarium (infection) 118
Fusion, fused (congenital)
    anal (with urogenital canal) 751.5
    aorta and pulmonary artery 745.0
    astragaloscaphoid 755.67
    atria 745.5
    atrium and ventricle 745.69
    auditory canal 744.02
    auricles, heart 745.5

Fusion, fused—continued
- binocular, with defective stereopsis 368.33
- bone 756.9
- cervical spine — see Fusion, spine
- choanal 748.0
- commissure, mitral valve 746.5
- cranial sutures, premature 756.0
- cusps, heart valve NEC 746.89
    - mitral 746.5
    - tricuspid 746.89
- ear ossicles 744.04
- fingers (see also Syndactylism, fingers) 755.11
- hymen 752.42
- hymeno-urethral 599.89
    - causing obstructed labor 660.1
        - affecting fetus or newborn 763.1
- joint (acquired) — see also Ankylosis
    - congenital 755.8
- kidneys (incomplete) 753.3
- labium (majus) (minus) 752.49
- larynx and trachea 748.3
- limb 755.8
    - lower 755.69
    - upper 755.59
- lobe, lung 748.5
- lumbosacral (acquired) 724.6
    - congenital 756.15
    - surgical V45.4
- nares (anterior) (posterior) 748.0
- nose, nasal 748.0
- nostril(s) 748.0
- organ or site NEC — see Anomaly, specified type NEC
- ossicles 756.9
    - auditory 744.04
- pulmonary valve segment 746.02
- pulmonic cusps 746.02
- ribs 756.3
- sacroiliac (acquired) (joint) 724.6
    - congenital 755.69
    - surgical V45.4
- skull, imperfect 756.0
- spine (acquired) 724.9
    - arthrodesis status V45.4
    - congenital (vertebra) 756.15
    - postoperative status V45.4
- sublingual duct with submaxillary duct at opening in mouth 750.26
- talonavicular (bar) 755.67
- teeth, tooth 520.2
- testes 752.8
- toes (see also Syndactylism, toes) 755.13
- trachea and esophagus 750.3
- twins 759.4
- urethral-hymenal 599.89
- vagina 752.49
- valve cusps — see Fusion, cusps, heart valve
- ventricles, heart 745.4
- vertebra (arch) — see Fusion, spine
- vulva 752.49

Fusospirillosis (mouth) (tongue) (tonsil) 101

Gafsa boil 085.1
Gain, weight (abnormal) (excessive) (see also Weight, gain) 783.1
Gaisböck's disease or syndrome (polycythemia hypertonica) 289.0
Gait
  abnormality 781.2
    hysterical 300.11
  ataxic 781.2
    hysterical 300.11
  disturbance 781.2
    hysterical 300.11
  paralytic 781.2
  scissor 781.2
  spastic 781.2
  staggering 781.2
    hysterical 300.11
Galactocele (breast) (infected) 611.5
  puerperal, postpartum 676.8
Galactophoritis 611.0
  puerperal, postpartum 675.2
Galactorrhea 676.6
  not associated with childbirth 611.6
Galactosemia (classic) (congenital) 271.1
Galactosuria 271.1
Galacturia 791.1
  bilharziasis 120.0
Galen's vein — see condition
Gallbladder — see also condition
  acute (see also Disease, gallbladder) 575.0
Gall duct — see condition
Gallop rhythm 427.89
Gallstone (cholemic) (colic) (impacted) — see also Cholelithiasis
  causing intestinal obstruction 560.31
Gambling, pathological 312.31 ◆
Gammaloidosis 277.3
Gammopathy 273.9
  macroglobulinemia 273.3
  monoclonal (benign) (essential) (idiopathic) (with lymphoplasmacytic dyscrasia) 273.1
Gamna's disease (sideritic splenomegaly) 289.51
Gampsodactylia (congenital) 754.71
Gamstorp's disease (adynamia episodica hereditaria) 359.3
Gandy-Nanta disease (sideritic splenomegaly) 289.51
Gang activity, without manifest psychiatric disorder V71.09
  adolescent V71.02
  adult V71.01
  child V71.02
Gangliocytoma (M9490/0) — see Neoplasm, connective tissue, benign
Ganglioglioma (M9505/1) — see Neoplasm, by site, uncertain behavior
Ganglion 727.43
  joint 727.41
  of yaws (early) (late) 102.6
  periosteal (see also Periostitis) 730.3
  tendon sheath (compound) (diffuse) 727.42
  tuberculous (see also Tuberculosis) 015.9
Ganglioneuroblastoma (M9490/3) — see Neoplasm, connective tissue, malignant

Ganglioneuroma (M9490/0) — see also Neoplasm, connective tissue, benign
  malignant (M9490/3) — see Neoplasm, connective tissue, malignant
Ganglioneuromatosis (M9491/0) — see Neoplasm, connective tissue, benign
Ganglionitis
  fifth nerve (see also Neuralgia, trigeminal) 350.1
  gasserian 350.1
  geniculate 351.1
    herpetic 053.11
    newborn 767.5
  herpes zoster 053.11
  herpetic geniculate (Hunt's syndrome) 053.11
Gangliosidosis 330.1
Gangosa 102.5
Gangrene, gangrenous (anemia) (artery) (cellulitis) (dermatitis) (dry) (infective) (moist) (pemphigus) (septic) (skin) (stasis) (ulcer) 785.4
  with
    arteriosclerosis (native artery) 440.24 ▼
      bypass graft 440.30
        autologous vein 440.31
        nonautologous biological 440.32 ▲
    diabetes (mellitus) 250.7 [785.4]
  abdomen (wall) 785.4
    arteriosclerosis 440.29 [785.4]
  adenitis 683
  alveolar 526.5
  angina 462
    diphtheritic 032.0
  anus 569.49
  appendices epiploicae — see Gangrene, mesentery
  appendix — see Appendicitis, acute ▼
  arteriosclerotic — see Arteriosclerosis, with, gangrene ▲
  auricle 785.4
  Bacillus welchii (see also Gangrene, gas) 040.0
  bile duct (see also Cholangitis) 576.8
  bladder 595.89
  bowel — see Gangrene, intestine
  cecum — see Gangrene, intestine
  Clostridium perfringens or welchii (see also Gangrene, gas) 040.0
  colon — see Gangrene, intestine
  connective tissue 785.4
  cornea 371.40
  corpora cavernosa (infective) 607.2
    noninfective 607.89
  cutaneous, spreading 785.4
  decubital 707.0 [785.4]
  diabetic (any site) 250.7 [785.4]
  dropsical 785.4
  emphysematous (see also Gangrene, gas) 040.0
  epidemic (ergotized grain) 988.2
  epididymis (infectional) (see also Epididymitis) 604.99
  erysipelas (see also Erysipelas) 035
  extremity (lower) (upper) 785.4
  gallbladder or duct (see also Cholecystitis, acute) 575.0

Gangrene, gangrenous—continued
  gas (bacillus) 040.0
    with
      abortion — see Abortion, by type, with sepsis
      ectopic pregnancy (see also categories 633.0-633.9) 639.0
      molar pregnancy (see also categories 630-632) 639.0
    following
      abortion 639.0
      ectopic or molar pregnancy 639.0
    puerperal, postpartum, childbirth 670
  glossitis 529.0
  gum 523.8
  hernia — see Hernia, by site, with gangrene
  hospital noma 528.1
  intestine, intestinal (acute) (hemorrhagic) (massive) 557.0
    with
      hernia — see Hernia, by site, with gangrene
      mesenteric embolism or infarction 557.0
      obstruction (see also Obstruction, intestine) 560.9
  laryngitis 464.0
  liver 573.8
  lung 513.0
    spirochetal 104.8
  lymphangitis 457.2
  Meleney's (cutaneous) 686.0
  mesentery 557.0
    with
      embolism or infarction 557.0
      intestinal obstruction (see also Obstruction, intestine) 560.9
  mouth 528.1
  noma 528.1
  orchitis 604.90
  ovary (see also Salpingo-oophoritis) 614.2
  pancreas 577.0
  penis (infectional) 607.2
    noninfective 607.89
  perineum 785.4
  pharynx 462
    septic 034.0
  pneumonia 513.0
  Pott's 440.24
  presenile 443.1
  pulmonary 513.0
  pulp, tooth 522.1
  quinsy 475
  Raynaud's (symmetric gangrene) 443.0 [785.4]
  rectum 569.49
  retropharyngeal 478.24
  rupture — see Hernia, by site, with gangrene
  scrotum 608.4
    noninfective 608.83
  senile 440.24
  sore throat 462
  spermatic cord 608.4
    noninfective 608.89
  spine 785.4
  spirochetal NEC 104.8
  spreading cutaneous 785.4
  stomach 537.89
  stomatitis 528.1
  symmetrical 443.0 [785.4]
  testis (infectional) (see also Orchitis) 604.99
    noninfective 608.89
  throat 462
    diphtheritic 032.0
  thyroid (gland) 246.8

Gangrene, gangrenous—continued
  tonsillitis (acute) 463
  tooth (pulp) 522.1
  tuberculous NEC (see also Tuberculosis) 011.9
  tunica vaginalis 608.4
    noninfective 608.89
  umbilicus 785.4
  uterus (see also Endometritis) 615.9
  uvulitis 528.3
  vas deferens 608.4
    noninfective 608.89
  vulva (see also Vulvitis) 616.10
Gannister disease (occupational) 502
  with tuberculosis — see Tuberculosis, pulmonary
Ganser's syndrome, hysterical 300.16
Gardner-Diamond syndrome (autoerythrocyte sensitization) 287.2
Gargoylism 277.5
Garré's
  disease (see also Osteomyelitis) 730.1
  osteitis (sclerosing) (see also Osteomyelitis) 730.1
  osteomyelitis (see also Osteomyelitis) 730.1
Garrod's pads, knuckle 728.79
Gartner's duct
  cyst 752.11
  persistent 752.11
Gas
  asphyxia, asphyxiation, inhalation, poisoning, suffocation NEC 987.9
    specified gas — see Table of drugs and chemicals
  bacillus gangrene or infection — see Gas, gangrene
  cyst, mesentery 568.89
  excessive 787.3
  gangrene 040.0
    with
      abortion — see Abortion, by type, with sepsis
      ectopic pregnancy (see also categories 633.0-633.9) 639.0
      molar pregnancy (see also categories 630-632) 639.0
    following
      abortion 639.0
      ectopic or molar pregnancy 639.0
    puerperal, postpartum, childbirth 670
  on stomach 787.3
  pains 787.3
Gastradenitis 535.0
Gastralgia 536.8
  psychogenic 307.89
Gastrectasis, gastrectasia 536.1
  psychogenic 306.4
Gastric — see condition
Gastrinoma (M8153/1)
  malignant (M8153/3)
    pancreas 157.4
    specified site NEC — see Neoplasm, by site, malignant
    unspecified site 157.4
  specified site — see Neoplasm, by site, uncertain behavior
  unspecified site 235.5

Gastritis 535.5

Note — Use the following fifth-digit subclassification for category 535:

    0   without mention of hemorrhage
    1   with hemorrhage

    acute 535.0
    alcoholic 535.3
    allergic 535.4
    antral 535.4
    atrophic 535.1
    atrophic-hyperplastic 535.1
    bile-induced 535.4
    catarrhal 535.0
    chronic (atrophic) 535.1
    cirrhotic 535.4
    corrosive (acute) 535.4
    dietetic 535.4
    due to diet deficiency 269.9 [535.4]
    eosinophilic 535.4
    follicular 535.4
        chronic 535.1
    giant hypertrophic 535.2
    glandular 535.4
        chronic 535.1
    hypertrophic (mucosa) 535.2
        chronic giant 211.1
    irritant 535.4
    nervous 306.4
    phlegmonous 535.0
    psychogenic 306.4
    sclerotic 535.4
    spastic 536.8
    subacute 535.0
    superficial 535.4
    suppurative 535.0
    toxic 535.4
    tuberculous (see also Tuberculosis) 017.9

Gastrocarcinoma (M8010/3) 151.9
Gastrocolic — see condition
Gastrocolitis — see Enteritis
Gastrodisciasis 121.8
Gastroduodenitis (see also Gastritis) 535.5
    catarrhal 535.0
    infectional 535.0
    virus, viral 008.8
        specified type NEC 008.69
Gastrodynia 536.8
Gastroenteritis (acute) (catarrhal) (chronic) (congestive) (hemorrhagic) (noninfectious) (see also Enteritis) 558.9
    aertrycke infection 003.0
    allergic 558.9
    chronic 558.9
        ulcerative (see also Colitis, ulcerative) 556.9
    dietetic 558.9
    due to
        food poisoning (see also Poisoning, food) 005.9
        radiation 558.1
    epidemic 009.0
    functional 558.9
    infectious (see also Enteritis, due to, by organism) 009.0
        presumed 009.1
    salmonella 003.0
    septic (see also Enteritis, due to, by organism) 009.0
    toxic 558.2
    tuberculous (see also Tuberculosis) 014.8
    ulcerative (see also Colitis, ulcerative) 556.9
    viral NEC 008.8
        specified type NEC 008.69
    zymotic 009.0
Gastroenterocolitis — see Enteritis

Gastroenteropathy, protein-losing 579.8
Gastroenteroptosis 569.89
Gastroesophageal laceration-hemorrhage syndrome 530.7
Gastroesophagitis 530.19
Gastrohepatitis (see also Gastritis) 535.5
Gastrointestinal — see condition
Gastrojejunal — see condition
Gastrojejunitis (see also Gastritis) 535.5
Gastrojejunocolic — see condition
Gastroliths 537.89
Gastromalacia 537.89
Gastroparalysis 536.8
    diabetic 250.6 [337.1]
Gastroparesis 536.3
    diabetic 250.6 [337.1]
Gastropathy, exudative 579.8
Gastroptosis 537.5
Gastrorrhagia 578.0
Gastorrhea 536.8
    psychogenic 306.4
Gastroschisis (congenital) 756.7
    acquired 569.89
Gastrospasm (neurogenic) (reflex) 536.8
    neurotic 306.4
    psychogenic 306.4
Gastrostaxis 578.0
Gastrostenosis 537.89
Gastrostomy status V44.1
    with complication 997.4
Gastrosuccorrhea (continous) (intermittent) 536.8
    neurotic 306.4
    psychogenic 306.4
Gaucher's
    disease (adult) (cerebroside lipidosis) (infantile) 272.7
    hepatomegaly 272.7
    splenomegaly (cerebroside lipidosis) 272.7
Gayet's disease (superior hemorrhagic polioencephalitis) 265.1
Gayet-Wernicke's syndrome (superior hemorrhagic polioencephalitis) 265.1
Gee (-Herter) (-Heubner) (-Thaysen) disease or syndrome (nontropical sprue) 579.0
Gélineau's syndrome 347
Gemination, teeth 520.2
Gemistocytoma (M9411/3)
    specified site — see Neoplasm, by site, malignant
    unspecified site 191.9
General, generalized — see condtion
Genital — see condition
Genito-anorectal syndrome 099.1
Genitourinary system — see condition
Genu
    congenital 755.64
    extrorsum (acquired) 736.42
        congenital 755.64
        late effects of rickets 268.1
    introrsum (acquired) 736.41
        congenital 755.64
        late effects of rickets 268.1
    rachitic (old) 268.1
    recurvatum (acquired) 736.5
        congenital 754.40
        with dislocation of knee 754.41
        late effects or rickets 268.1

Genu—continued
    valgum (acquired) (knock-knee) 736.41
        congenital 755.64
        late effects of rickets 268.1
    varum (acquired) (bowleg) 736.42
        congenital 755.64
        late effect of rickets 268.1
Geographic tongue 529.1
Geophagia 307.52
Geotrichosis 117.9
    intestine 117.9
    lung 117.9
    mouth 117.9
Gephyrophobia 300.29
Gerbode defect 745.4
Gerhardt's
    disease (erythromelalgia) 443.89
    syndrome (vocal cord paralysis) 478.30
Gerlier's disease (epidemic vertigo) 078.81
German measles 056.9
    exposure to V01.4
Germinoblastoma (diffuse) (M9614/3) 202.8
    follicular (M9692/3) 202.0
Germinoma (M9064/3) — see Neoplasm, by site, malignant
Gerontoxon 371.41
Gerstmann's syndrome (finger agnosia) 784.69
Gestation (period) — see also Pregnancy
    ectopic NEC (see also Pregnancy, ectopic) 633.9
Gestational proteinuria 646.2
    with hypertension — see Toxemia, of pregnancy
Ghon tubercle primary infection (see also Tuberculosis) 010.0
Ghost
    teeth 520.4
    vessels, cornea 370.64
Ghoul hand 102.3
Giant
    cell
        epulis 523.8
        peripheral (gingiva) 523.8
        tumor, tendon sheath 727.02
    colon (congenital) 751.3
    esophagus (congenital) 750.4
    kidney 753.3
    urticaria 995.1
        hereditary 277.6
Giardia lamblia infestation 007.1
Giardiasis 007.1
Gibert's disease (pityriasis rosea) 696.3
Gibraltar fever — see Brucellosis
Giddiness 780.4
    hysterical 300.11
    psychogenic 306.9
Gierke's disease (glycogenosis I) 271.0
Gigantism (cerebral) (hypophyseal) (pituitary) 253.0
Gilbert's disease or cholemia (familial nonhemolytic jaundice) 277.4
Gilchrist's disease (North American blastomycosis) 116.0
Gilford (-Hutchinson) disease or syndrome (progeria) 259.8
Gilles de la Tourette's disease (motor-verbal tic) 307.23
Gillespie's syndrome (dysplasia oculodentodigitalis) 759.89
Gingivitis 523.1
    acute 523.0
        necrotizing 101
    catarrhal 523.0

Gingivitis—continued
    chronic 523.1
    desquamative 523.1
    expulsiva 523.4
    hyperplastic 523.1
    marginal, simple 523.1
    necrotizing, acute 101
    pellagrous 265.2
    ulcerative 523.1
        acute necrotizing 101
        Vincent's 101
Gingivoglossitis 529.0
Gingivopericementitis 523.4
Gingivosis 523.1
Gingivostomatitis 523.1
    herpetic 054.2
Giovannini's disease 117.9
Gland, glandular — see condition
Glanders 024
Glanzmann (-Naegeli) disease or thrombasthenia 287.1
Glassblowers' disease 527.1
Glaucoma (capsular) (inflammatory) (noninflammatory) (primary) 365.9
    with increased episcleral venous pressure 365.82
    absolute 360.42
    acute 365.22
        narrow angle 365.22
        secondary 365.60
    angle closure 365.20
        acute 365.22
        chronic 365.23
        intermittent 365.21
        interval 365.21
        residual stage 365.24
        subacute 365.21
    borderline 365.00
    chronic 365.11
        noncongestive 365.11
        open angle 365.11
        simple 365.11
    closed angle — see Glaucoma, angle closure
    congenital 743.20
        associated with other eye anomalies 743.22
        simple 743.21
    congestive — see Glaucoma, narrow angle
    corticosteroid-induced (glaucomatous stage) 365.31
        residual stage 365.32
    hemorrhagic 365.60
    hypersecretion 365.81
    in or with
        aniridia 743.45 [365.42]
        Axenfeld's anomaly 743.44 [365.41]
        concussion of globe 921.3 [365.65]
        congenital syndromes NEC 759.89 [365.44]
        dislocation of lens
            anterior 379.33 [365.59]
            posterior 379.34 [365.59]
        disorder of lens NEC 365.59
        epithelial down-growth 364.61 [365.64]
        glaucomatocyclitic crisis 364.22 [365.62]
        hypermature cataract 366.18 [365.51]
        hyphema 364.41 [365.63]
        inflammation, ocular 365.62
        iridocyclitis 364.3 [365.62]
        iris
            anomalies NEC 743.46 [365.42]
            atrophy, essential 364.51 [365.42]
            bombé 364.74 [365.61]
            rubeosis 364.42 [365.63]

Glaucoma—continued
in or with—continued
microcornea 743.41 [365.43]
neurofibromatosis 237.71 [365.44]
ocular
cysts NEC 365.64
disorders NEC 365.60
trauma 365.65
tumors NEC 365.64
postdislocation of lens
anterior 379.33 [365.59]
posterior 379.34 [365.59]
pseudoexfoliation of capsule 366.11 [365.52]
pupillary block or seclusion 364.74 [365.61]
recession of chamber angle 364.77 [365.65]
retinal vein occlusion 362.35 [365.63]
Rieger's anomaly or syndrome 743.44 [365.41]
rubeosis of iris 364.42 [365.63]
seclusion of pupil 364.74 [365.61]
spherophakia 743.36 [365.59]
Sturge-Weber (-Dimitri) syndrome 759.6 [365.44]
systemic syndrome NEC 365.44
tumor of globe 365.64
vascular disorders NEC 365.63
infantile 365.14
congenital 743.20
associated with other eye anomalies 743.22
simple 743.21
juvenile 365.14
low tension 365.12
malignant 365.20
narrow angle (primary) 365.20
acute 365.22
chronic 365.23
intermittent 365.21
interval 365.21
residual stage 365.24
subacute 365.21
newborn 743.20
associated with other eye anomalies 743.22
simple 743.21
noncongestive (chronic) 365.11
nonobstructive (chronic) 365.11
obstructive 365.60
due to lens changes 365.59
open angle 365.10
with
borderline intraocular pressure 365.01
cupping of optic discs 365.01
primary 365.11
residual stage 365.15
phacolytic 365.51
with hypermature cataract 366.18 [365.51]
pigmentary 365.13
postinfectious 365.60
pseudoexfoliation 365.52
with pseudoexfoliation of capsule 366.11 [365.52]
secondary NEC 365.60
simple (chronic) 365.11
simplex 365.11
steroid responders 365.03
suspect 365.00
syphilitic 095.8
traumatic NEC 365.65
newborn 767.8
tuberculous (see also Tuberculosis) 017.3 [365.62]
wide angle (see also Glaucoma, open angle) 365.10

Glaucomatous flecks (subcapsular) 366.31
Glazed tongue 529.4
Gleet 098.2
Glénard's disease or syndrome (enteroptosis) 569.89
Glinski-Simmonds syndrome (pituitary cachexia) 253.2
Glioblastoma (multiforme) (M9440/3)
with sarcomatous component (M9442/3)
specified site — see Neoplasm, by site, malignant
unspecified site 191.9
giant cell (M9441/3)
specified site — see Neoplasm, by site, malignant
unspecified site 191.9
specified site — see Neoplasm, by site, malignant
unspecified site 191.9
Glioma (malignant) (M9380/3)
astrocytic (M9400/3)
specified site — see Neoplasm, by site, malignant
unspecified site 191.9
mixed (M9382/3)
specified site — see Neoplasm, by site, malignant
unspecified site 191.9
nose 748.1
specified site NEC — see Neoplasm, by site, malignant
subependymal (M9383/1) 237.5
unspecified site 191.9
Gliomatosis cerebri (M9381/3) 191.0
Glioneuroma (M9505/1) — see Neoplasm, by site, uncertain behavior
Gliosarcoma (M9380/3)
specified site — see Neoplasm, by site, malignant
unspecified site 191.9
Gliosis (cerebral) 349.89
spinal 336.0
Glisson's
cirrhosis — see Cirrhosis, portal
disease (see also Rickets) 268.0
Glissonitis 573.3
Globinuria 791.2
Globus 306.4
hystericus 300.11
Glomangioma (M8712/0) (see also Hemangioma) 228.00
Glomangiosarcoma (M8710/3) — see Neoplasm, connective tissue, malignant
Glomerular nephritis (see also Nephritis) 583.9
Glomerulitis (see also Nephritis) 583.9
Glomerulonephritis (see also Nephritis) 583.9
with
edema (see also Nephrosis) 581.9
lesion of
exudative nephritis 583.89
interstitial nephritis (diffuse) (focal) 583.89
necrotizing glomerulitis 583.4
acute 580.4
chronic 582.4
renal necrosis 583.9
cortical 583.6
medullary 583.7

Glomerulonephritis—continued
with—continued
lesion of—continued
specified pathology NEC 583.89
acute 580.89
chronic 582.89
necrosis, renal 583.9
cortical 583.6
medullary (papillary) 583.7
specified pathology or lesion NEC 583.89
acute 580.9
with
exudative nephritis 580.89
interstitial nephritis (diffuse) (focal) 580.89
necrotizing glomerulitis 580.4
extracapillary with epithelial crescents 580.4
poststreptococcal 580.0
proliferative (diffuse) 580.0
rapidly progressive 580.4
specified pathology NEC 580.89
arteriolar (see also Hypertension, kidney) 403.90
arteriosclerotic (see also Hypertension, kidney) 403.90
ascending (see also Pyelitis) 590.80
basement membrane NEC 583.89
with
pulmonary hemorrhage (Goodpasture's syndrome) 446.21 [583.81]
chronic 582.9
with
exudative nephritis 582.89
interstitial nephritis (diffuse) (focal) 582.89
necrotizing glomerulitis 582.4
specified pathology or lesion NEC 582.89
endothelial 582.2
extracapillary with epithelial crescents 582.4
hypocomplementemic persistent 582.2
lobular 582.2
membranoproliferative 582.2
membranous 582.1
and proliferative (mixed) 582.2
sclerosing 582.1
mesangiocapillary 582.2
mixed membranous and proliferative 582.2
proliferative (diffuse) 582.0
rapidly progressive 582.4
sclerosing 582.1
cirrhotic — see Sclerosis, renal
desquamative — see Nephrosis
due to or associated with
amyloidosis 277.3 [583.81]
with nephrotic syndrome 277.3 [581.81]
chronic 277.3 [582.81]
diabetes mellitus 250.4 [583.81]
with nephrotic syndrome 250.4 [581.81]
diphtheria 032.89 [580.81]
gonococcal infection (acute) 098.19 [583.81]
chronic or duration of 2 months or over 098.39 [583.81]
infectious hepatitis 070.9 [580.81]
malaria (with nephrotic syndrome) 084.9 [581.81]

Glomerulonephritis—continued
due to or associated with—continued
mumps 072.79 [580.81]
polyarteritis (nodosa) (with nephrotic syndrome) 446.0 [581.81]
specified pathology NEC 583.89
acute 580.89
chronic 582.89
streptotrichosis 039.8 [583.81]
subacute bacterial endocarditis 421.0 [580.81]
syphilis (late) 095.4
congenital 090.5 [583.81]
early 091.69 [583.81]
systemic lupus erythematosus 710.0 [583.81]
with nephrotic syndrome 710.0 [581.81]
chronic 710.0 [582.81]
tuberculosis (see also Tuberculosis) 016.0 [583.81]
typhoid fever 002.0 [580.81]
extracapillary with epithelial crescents 583.4
acute 580.4
chronic 582.4
exudative 583.89
acute 580.89
chronic 582.89
focal (see also Nephritis) 583.9
embolic 580.4
granular 582.89
granulomatous 582.89
hydremic (see also Nephrosis) 581.9
hypocomplementemic persistent 583.2
with nephrotic syndrome 581.2
chronic 582.2
immune complex NEC 583.89
infective (see also Pyelitis) 590.80
interstitial (diffuse) (focal) 583.89
with nephrotic syndrome 581.89
acute 580.89
chronic 582.89
latent or quiescent 582.9
lobular 583.2
with nephrotic syndrome 581.2
chronic 582.2
membranoproliferative 583.2
with nephrotic syndrome 581.2
chronic 582.2
membranous 583.1
with nephrotic syndrome 581.1
and proliferative (mixed) 583.2
with nephrotic syndrome 581.2
chronic 582.2
chronic 582.1
sclerosing 582.1
with nephrotic syndrome 581.1
mesangiocapillary 583.2
with nephrotic syndrome 581.2
chronic 582.2
minimal change 581.3
mixed membranous and proliferative 583.2
with nephrotic syndrome 581.2
chronic 582.2
necrotizing 583.4
acute 580.4
chronic 582.4
nephrotic (see also Nephrosis) 581.9

Glomerulonephritis—continued
  old — see Glomerulonephritis, chronic
  parenchymatous 581.89
  poststreptococcal 580.0
  proliferative (diffuse) 583.0
    with nephrotic syndrome 581.0
    acute 580.0
    chronic 582.0
  purulent (see also Pyelitis) 590.80
  quiescent — see Nephritis, chronic
  rapidly progressive 583.4
    acute 580.4
    chronic 582.4
  sclerosing membranous (chronic) 582.1
    with nephrotic syndrome 581.1
  septic (see also Pyelitis) 590.80
  specified pathology or lesion NEC 583.89
    with nephrotic syndrome 581.89
    acute 580.89
    chronic 582.89
  suppurative (acute) (disseminated) (see also Pyelitis) 590.80
  toxic — see Nephritis, acute
  tubal, tubular — see Nephrosis, tubular
  type II (Ellis) — see Nephrosis
  vascular — see Hypertension, kidney
Glomerulosclerosis (see also Sclerosis, renal) 587
  focal 582.1
    with nephrotic syndrome 581.1
  intercapillary (nodular) (with diabetes) 250.4 [581.81]
Glossagra 529.6
Glossalgia 529.6
Glossitis 529.0
  areata exfoliativa 529.1
  atrophic 529.4
  benign migratory 529.1
  gangrenous 529.0
  Hunter's 529.4
  median rhomboid 529.2
  Moeller's 529.4
  pellagrous 265.2
Glossocele 529.8
Glossodynia 529.6
  exfoliativa 529.4
Glossoncus 529.8
Glossophytia 529.3
Glossoplegia 529.8
Glossoptosis 529.8
Glossopyrosis 529.6
Glossotrichia 529.3
Glossy skin 710.9
Glottis — see condition
Glottitis — see Glossitis
Glucagonoma (M8152/0)
  malignant (M8152/3)
    pancreas 157.4
    specified site NEC — see Neoplasm, by site, malignant
    unspecified site 157.4
  pancreas 211.7
  specified site NEC — see Neoplasm, by site, benign
  unspecified site 211.7
Glucoglycinuria 270.7
Glue ear syndrome 381.20
Glue sniffing (airplane glue) (see also Dependence) 304.6
Glycinemia (with methylmalonic acidemia) 270.7

Glycinuria (renal) (with ketosis) 270.0
Glycogen
  infiltration (see also Disease, glycogen storage) 271.0
  storage disease (see also Disease, glycogen storage) 271.0
Glycogenosis (see also Disease, glycogen storage) 271.0
  cardiac 271.0 [425.7]
  Cori, types I-VII 271.0
  diabetic, secondary 250.8 [259.8]
  diffuse (with hepatic cirrhosis) 271.0
  generalized 271.0
  glucose-6-phosphatase deficiency 271.0
  hepatophosphorylase deficiency 271.0
  hepatorenal 271.0
  myophosphorylase deficiency 271.0
Glycopenia 251.2
Glycoprolinuria 270.8
Glycosuria 791.5
  renal 271.4
Gnathostoma (spinigerum) (infection) (infestation) 128.1
  wandering swellings from 128.1
Gnathostomiasis 128.1
Goiter (adolescent) (colloid) (diffuse) (dipping) (due to iodine deficiency) (endemic) (euthyroid) (heart) (hyperplastic) (internal) (intrathoracic) (juvenile) (mixed type) (nonendemic) (parenchymatous) (plunging) (sporadic) (subclavicular) (substernal) 240.9
  with
    hyperthyroidism (recurrent) (see also Goiter, toxic) 242.0
    thyrotoxicosis (see also Goiter, toxic) 242.0
  adenomatous (see also Goiter, nodular) 241.9
  cancerous (M8000/3) 193
  complicating pregnancy, childbirth, or puerperium 648.1
  congenital 246.1
  cystic (see also Goiter, nodular) 241.9
  due to enzyme defect in synthesis of thyroid hormone (butane-insoluble iodine) (coupling) (deiodinase) (iodide trapping or organificaiton) (iodotyrosine dehalogenase) (peroxidase) 246.1
  dyshormonogenic 246.1
  exophthalmic (see also Goiter, toxic) 242.0
  familial (with deaf-mutism) 243
  fibrous 245.3
  lingual 759.2
  lymphadenoid 245.2
  malignant (M8000/3) 193
  multinodular (nontoxic) 241.1
    toxic or with hyperthyroidism (see also Goiter, toxic) 242.2
  nodular (nontoxic) 241.9
    with
      hyperthyroidism (see also Goiter, toxic) 242.3
      thyrotoxicosis (see also Goiter, toxic) 242.3
    endemic 241.9
    exophthalmic (diffuse) (see also Goiter, toxic) 242.0
    multinodular (nontoxic) 241.1

Goiter—continued
  nodular—continued
    sporadic 241.9
    toxic (see also Goiter, toxic) 242.3
    uninodular (nontoxic) 241.0
  nontoxic (nodular) 241.9
    multinodular 241.1
    uninodular 241.0
  pulsating (see also Goiter, toxic) 242.0
  simple 240.0
  toxic 242.0

> Note — Use the following fifth-digit subclassification with category 242:
>
> 0 without mention of thyrotoxic crisis or storm
>
> 1 with mention of thyrotoxic crisis or storm

    adenomatous 242.3
      multinodular 242.2
      uninodular 242.1
    multinodular 242.2
    nodular 242.3
      multinodular 242.2
      uninodular 242.1
    uninodular 242.1
  uninodular (nontoxic) 241.0
    toxic or with hyperthyroidism (see also Goiter, toxic) 242.1
Goldberg (-Maxwell) (-Morris) syndrome (testicular feminization) 257.8
Goldblatt's
  hypertension 440.1
  kidney 440.1
Goldenhar's syndrome (oculoauriculovertebral dysplasia) 756.0
Goldflam-Erb disease or syndrome 358.0
Goldscheider's disease (epidermolysis bullosa) 757.39
Goldstein's disease (familial hemorrhagic telangiectasia) 448.0
Golfer's elbow 726.32
Goltz-Gorlin syndrome (dermal hypoplasia) 757.39
Gonadoblastoma (M9073/1)
  specified site — see Neoplasm, by site uncertain behavior
  unspecified site
    female 236.2
    male 236.4
Gonecystitis (see also Vesiculitis) 608.0
Gongylonemiasis 125.6
  mouth 125.6
Goniosynechiae 364.73
Gonococcemia 098.89
Gonococcus, gonococcal (disease) (infection) (see also condition) 098.0
  anus 098.7
  bursa 098.52
  chronic NEC 098.2
  complicating pregnancy, childbirth, or puerperium 647.1
  affecting fetus or newborn 760.2
  conjunctiva, conjunctivitis (neonatorum) 098.40
  dermatosis 098.89
  endocardium 098.84

Gonococcus, gonococcal—continued
  epididymo-orchitis 098.13
    chronic or duration of 2 months or over 098.33
  eye (newborn) 098.40
  fallopian tube (chronic) 098.37
    acute 098.17
  genitourinary (acute) (organ) (system) (tract) (see also Gonnorrhea) 098.0
    lower 098.0
      chronic 098.2
    upper 098.10
      chronic 098.30
  heart NEC 098.85
  joint 098.50
  keratoderma 098.81
  keratosis (blennorrhagica) 098.81
  lymphatic (gland) (node) 098.89
  meninges 098.82
  orchitis (acute) 098.13
    chronic or duration of 2 months or over 098.33
  pelvis (acute) 098.19
    chronic or duration of 2 months or over 098.39
  pericarditis 098.83
  peritonitis 098.86
  pharyngitis 098.6
  pharynx 098.6
  proctitis 098.7
  pyosalpinx (chronic) 098.37
    acute 098.17
  rectum 098.7
  septicemia 098.89
  skin 098.89
  specified site NEC 098.89
  synovitis 098.51
  tendon sheath 098.51
  throat 098.6
  urethra (acute) 098.0
    chronic or duration of 2 months or over 098.2
  vulva (acute) 098.0
    chronic or duration of 2 months or over 098.2
Gonocytoma (M9073/1)
  specified site — see Neoplasm, by site, uncertain behavior
  unspecified site
    female 236.2
    male 236.4
Gonorrhea 098.0
  acute 098.0
  Bartholin's gland (acute) 098.0
    chronic or duration of 2 months or over 098.2
  bladder (acute) 098.11
    chronic or duration of 2 months or over 098.31
  carrier (suspected of) V02.7
  cervix (acute) 098.15
    chronic or duration of 2 months or over 098.35
  chronic 098.2
  complicating pregnancy, childbirth, or puerperium 647.1
    affecting fetus or newborn 760.2
  conjunctiva, conjunctivitis (neonatorum) 098.40
  contact V01.6
  Cowper's gland (acute) 098.0
    chronic or duration of 2 months or over 098.2
  duration of two months or over 098.2
  exposure to V01.6
  fallopian tube (chronic) 098.37
    acute 098.17
  genitourinary (acute) (organ) (system) (tract) 098.0
    chronic 098.2
    duration of two months or over 098.2

Gonorrhea—continued
kidney (acute) 098.19
  chronic or duration of 2 months or over 098.39
ovary (acute) 098.19
  chronic or duration of 2 months or over 098.39
pelvis (acute) 098.19
  chronic or duration of 2 months or over 098.39
penis (acute) 098.0
  chronic or duration of 2 months or over 098.2
prostate (acute) 098.12
  chronic or duration of 2 months or over 098.32
seminal vesicle (acute) 098.14
  chronic or duration of 2 months or over 098.34
specified site NEC — see Gonococcus
spermatic cord (acute) 098.14
  chronic or duration of 2 months or over 098.34
urethra (acute) 098.0
  chronic or duration of 2 months or over 098.2
vagina (acute) 098.0
  chronic or duration of 2 months or over 098.2
vas deferens (acute) 098.14
  chronic or duration of 2 months or over 098.34
vulva (acute) 098.0
  chronic or duration of 2 months or over 098.2

Goodpasture's syndrome (pneumorenal) 446.21

Gopalan's syndrome (burning feet) 266.2

Gordon's disease (exudative enteropathy) 579.8

Gorlin-Chaudhry-Moss syndrome 759.89

Gougerot's syndrome (trisymptomatic) 709.1

Gougerot-Blum syndrome (pigmented purpuric lichenoid dermatitis) 709.1

Gougerot-Carteaud disease or syndrome (confluent reticulate papillomatosis) 701.8

Gougerot-Hailey-Hailey disease (benign familial chronic pemphigus) 757.39

Gougerot (-Houwer) - Sjögren syndrome (keratoconjunctivitis sicca) 710.2

Gouley's syndrome (constrictive pericarditis) 423.2

Goundou 102.6

Gout, gouty 274.9
with specified manifestations NEC 274.89
arthritis (acute) 274.0
arthropathy 274.0
degeneration, heart 274.82
diathesis 274.9
eczema 274.89
episcleritis 274.89 [379.09]
external ear (tophus) 274.81
glomerulonephritis 274.10
iritis 274.89 [364.11]
joint 274.0
kidney 274.10
lead 984.9
  specified type of lead — see Table of drugs and chemicals
nephritis 274.10
neuritis 274.89 [357.4]
phlebitis 274.89 [451.9]
rheumatic 714.0

Gout, gouty—continued
saturnine 984.9
  specified type of lead — see Table of drugs and chemicals
spondylitis 274.0
synovitis 274.0
syphilitic 095.8
tophi 274.0
  ear 274.81
  heart 274.82
  specified site NEC 274.82

Gowers'
muscular dystrophy 359.1
syndrome (vasovagal attack) 780.2

Gowers-Paton-Kennedy syndrome 377.04

Gradenigo's syndrome 383.02

Graft-versus-host disease (bone marrow) 996.85
due to organ transplant NEC — see Complications, transplant, organ

Graham Steell's murmur (pulmonic regurgitation) (see also Endocarditis, pulmonary) 424.3

Grain-handlers' disease or lung 495.8

Grain mite (itch) 133.8

Grand
mal (idiopathic) (see also Epilepsy) 345.1
  hysteria of Charcot 300.11
  nonrecurrent or isolated 780.3
multipara
  affecting management of labor and delivery 659.4
  status only (not pregnant) V61.5

Granite workers' lung 502

Granular — see also condition
inflammation, pharynx 472.1
kidney (contracting) (see also Sclerosis, renal) 587
liver — see Cirrhosis, liver
nephritis — see Nephritis

Granulation tissue, abnormal — see also Granuloma
abnormal or excessive 701.5
postmastoidectomy cavity 383.33
postoperative 701.5
skin 701.5

Granulocytopenia, granulocytopenic (primary) 288.0
malignant 288.0

Granuloma NEC 686.1
abdomen (wall) 568.89
  skin (pyogenicum) 686.1
    from residual foreign body 709.4
annulare 695.89
anus 569.49
apical 522.6
appendix 543.9
aural 380.23
beryllium (skin) 709.4
  lung 503
bone (see also Osteomyelitis) 730.1
  eosinophilic 277.8
  from residual foreign body 733.99
canaliculus lacrimalis 375.81
cerebral 348.8
cholesterin, middle ear 385.82
coccidioidal (progressive) 114.3
  lung 114.4
  meninges 114.2
  primary (lung) 114.0
colon 569.89
conjunctiva 372.61
dental 522.6

Granuloma—continued
ear, middle (cholesterin) 385.82
  with otitis media — see Otitis media
eosinophilic 277.8
  bone 277.8
  lung 277.8
  oral mucosa 528.9
exuberant 701.5
eyelid 374.89
facial
  lethal midline 446.3
  malignant 446.3
fissuratum (gum) 523.8
foot NEC 686.1
foreign body (in soft tissue) NEC 728.82
  bone 733.99
  in operative wound 998.4
  muscle 728.82
  skin 709.4
  subcutaneous tissue 709.4
fungoides 202.1
gangraenescens 446.3
giant cell (central) (jaw) (reparative) 526.3
  gingiva 523.8
  peripheral (gingiva) 523.8
gland (lymph) 289.3
Hodgkins (M9661/3) 201.1
ileum 569.89
infectious NEC 136.9
inguinale (Donovan) 099.2
  venereal 099.2
intestine 569.89
iridocyclitis 364.10
jaw (bone) 526.3
  reparative giant cell 526.3
kidney (see also Infection, kidney) 590.9
lacrimal sac 375.81
larynx 478.79
lethal midline 446.3
lipid 999.9
lipoid 277.8
liver 572.8
lung (infectious) (see also Fibrosis, lung) 515
  coccidioidal 114.4
  eosinophilic 277.8
lymph gland 289.3
Majocchi's 110.6
malignant, face 446.3
mandible 526.3
mediastinum 519.3
midline 446.3
monilial 112.3
muscle 728.82
  from residual foreign body 728.82
nasal sinus (see also Sinusitis) 473.9
operation wound 998.5
  foreign body 998.4
  stitch (external) 998.8
    internal wound 996.7
  talc 998.7
oral mucosa, eosinophilic or pyogenic 528.9
orbit, orbital 376.11
paracoccidioidal 116.1
penis, venereal 099.2
periapical 522.6
peritoneum 568.89
  due to ova of helminths NEC (see also Helminthiasis) 128.9
postmastoidectomy cavity 383.33
postoperative — see Granuloma, operation wound
prostate 601.8
pudendi (ulcerating) 099.2
pudendorum (ulcerative) 099.2
pulp, internal (tooth) 521.4
pyogenic, pyogenicum (skin) 686.1
  maxillary alveolar ridge 522.6

Granuloma—continued
pyogenic, pyogenicum—continued
  oral mucosa 528.9
rectum 569.49
reticulohistiocytic 277.8
rubrum nasi 705.89
sarcoid 135
Schistosoma 120.9
septic (skin) 686.1
silica (skin) 709.4
sinus (accessory) (infectional) (nasal) (see also Sinusitis) 473.9
skin (pyogenicum) 686.1
  from foreign body or material 709.4
sperm 608.89
spine
  syphilitic (epidural) 094.89
  tuberculous (see also Tuberculosis) 015.0 [730.88]
stitch (postoperative) 998.8
  internal wound 996.7
suppurative (skin) 686.1
suture (postoperative) 998.8
  internal wound 996.7
swimming pool 031.1
talc 728.82
  in operation wound 998.7
telangiectaticum (skin) 686.1
trichophyticum 110.6
tropicum 102.4
umbilicus 686.1
  newborn 771.4
urethra 599.84
uveitis 364.10
vagina 099.2
venereum 099.2
vocal cords 478.5
Wegener's (necrotizing respiratory granulomatosis) 446.4

Granulomatosis NEC 686.1
disciformis chronica et progressiva 709.3
infantiseptica 771.2
lipoid 277.8
lipohagic, intestinal 040.2
miliary 027.0
necrotizing, respiratory 446.4
progressive, septic 288.1
Wegener's (necrotizing respiratory) 446.4

Granulomatous tissue — see Granuloma

Granulosis rubra nasi 705.89

Graphite fibrosis (of lung) 503

Graphospasm 300.89
organic 333.84

Grating scapula 733.99

Gravel (urinary) (see also Calculus) 592.9

Graves' disease (exophthalmic goiter) (see also Goiter, toxic) 242.0

Gravis — see condition

Grawitz's tumor (hypernephroma) (M8312/3) 189.0

Grayness, hair (premature) 704.3
congenital 757.4

Gray or grey syndrome (chloramphenicol) (newborn) 779.4

Greenfield's disease 330.0

Green sickness 280.9

Greenstick fracture — see Fracture, by site

Greig's syndrome (hypertelorism) 756.0

Griesinger's disease (see also Ancylostomiasis) 126.9

Grinders'
asthma 502
lung 502
phthisis (see also Tuberculosis) 011.4
Grinding, teeth 306.8
Grip
Dabney's 074.1
devil's 074.1
Grippe, grippal — see also Influenza
Balkan 083.0
intestinal 487.8
summer 074.8
Grippy cold 487.1
Grisel's disease 723.5
Groin — see condition
Grooved
nails (transverse) 703.8
tongue 529.5
congenital 750.13
Ground itch 126.9
Growing pains, children 781.9
Growth (fungoid) (neoplastic) (new) (M8000/1) — see also Neoplasm, by site, unspecified nature
adenoid (vegetative) 474.12
benign (M8000/0) — see Neoplasm, by site, benign
fetal, poor 764.9
affecting management of pregnancy 656.5
malignant (M8000/3) — see Neoplasm, by site, malignant
rapid, childhood V21.0
secondary (M8000/6) — see Neoplasm, by site, malignant, secondary
Gruber's hernia — see Hernia, Gruber's
Gruby's disease (tinea tonsurans) 110.0
G-trisomy 758.0
Guama fever 066.3
Gubler (-Millard) **paralysis or syndrome** 344.89
Guérin-Stern syndrome (arthorgryposis multiplex congenita) 754.89
Guertin's disease (electric chorea) 049.8
Guillain-Barré disease or syndrome 357.0
Guinea worms (infection) (infestation) 125.7
Guinon's disease (motor-verbal tic) 307.23
Gull's disease (thyroid atrophy with myxedema) 244.8
Gull and Sutton's disease — see Hypertension, kidney
Gum — see condition
Gumboil 522.7
Gumma (syphilitic) 095.9
artery 093.89
cerebral or spinal 094.89
bone 095.5
of yaws (late) 102.6
brain 094.89
cauda equina 094.89
central nervous system NEC 094.9
ciliary body 095.8 [364.11]
congenital 090.5
testis 090.5
eyelid 095.8 [373.5]
heart 093.89
intracranial 094.89
iris 095.8 [364.11]
kidney 095.4
larynx 095.8
leptomeninges 094.2

Gumma—continued
liver 095.3
meninges 094.2
myocardium 093.82
nasopharynx 095.8
neurosyphilitic 094.9
nose 095.8
orbit 095.8
palate (soft) 095.8
penis 095.8
pericardium 093.81
pharynx 095.8
pituitary 095.8
scrofulous (see also Tuberculosis) 017.0
skin 095.8
specified site NEC 095.8
spinal cord 094.89
tongue 095.8
tonsil 095.8
trachea 095.8
tuberculous (see also Tuberculosis) 017.0
ulcerative due to yaws 102.4
ureter 095.8
yaws 102.4
bone 102.6
Gunn's syndrome (jaw-winking syndrome) 742.8
Gunshot wound — see also Wound, open, by site
fracture — see Fracture, by site, open
internal organs (abdomen, chest, or pelvis) — see Injury, internal, by site, with open wound
intracranial — see Laceration, brain, with open intracranial wound
Günther's disease or syndrome (congenital erythropoietic porphyria) 277.1
Gustatory hallucination 780.1
Gynandrism 752.7
Gynanadroblastoma (M8632/1)
specified site — see Neoplasm, by site, uncertain behavior
unspecified site
female 236.2
male 236.4
Gynandromorphism 752.7
Gynatresia (congenital) 752.49
Gynecoid pelvis, male 738.6
Gynecological examination V72.3
for contraceptive maintenance V25.40
Gynecomastia 611.1
Gynephobia 300.29
Gyrate scalp 757.39

H

Haas' disease (osteochondrosis head of humerus) 732.3
Habermann's disease (acute parapsoriasis varioliformis) 696.2
Habit, habituation
chorea 307.22
disturbance, child 307.9
drug (see also Dependence) 304.9
laxative (see also Abuse, drugs, nondependent) 305.9
spasm 307.20
chronic 307.22
transient of childhood 307.21
tic 307.20
chronic 307.22
transient of childhood 307.21

Habit, habituation—continued
use of
nonprescribed drugs (see also Abuse, drugs, nondependent) 305.9
patent medicines (see also Abuse, drugs, nondependent) 305.9
vomiting 536.2
Hadfield-Clarke syndrome (pancreatic infantilism) 577.8
Haff disease 985.1
Hageman factor defect, deficiency, or disease (see also Defect, coagulation) 286.3
Haglund's disease (osteochondrosis os tibiale externum) 732.5
Haglund-Läwen-Fründ syndrome 717.89
Hagner's disease (hypertrophic pulmonary osteoarthropathy) 731.2
Hag teeth, tooth 524.3
Hailey-Hailey disease (benign familial chronic pemphigus) 757.39
Hair — see also condition
plucking 307.9
Hairball in stomach 935.2
Hairy black tongue 529.3
Half vertebra 756.14
Halitosis 784.9
Hallermann-Streiff syndrome 756.0
Hallervorden-Spatz disease or syndrome 333.0
Hallopeau's
acrodermatitis (continua) 696.1
disease (lichen sclerosis et atrophicus) 701.0
Hallucination (auditory) (gustatory) (olfactory) (tactile) 780.1
alcoholic 291.3
drug-induced 292.12
visual 368.16
Hallucinosis 298.9
alcoholic (acute) 291.3
drug-induced 292.12
Hallus — see Hallux
Hallux 735.9
malleus (acquired) 735.3
rigidus (acquired) 735.2
congenital 755.66
late effects of rickets 268.1
valgus (acquired) 735.0
congenital 755.66
varus (acquired) 735.1
congenital 755.66
Halo, visual 368.15
Hamartoblastoma 759.6
Hamartoma 759.6
epithelial (gingival), odontogenic, central, or peripheral (M9321/0) 213.1
upper jaw (bone) 213.0
vascular 757.32
Hamartosis, hamartoses NEC 759.6
Hamman's disease or syndrome (spontaneous mediastinal emphysema) 518.1
Hamman-Rich syndrome (diffuse interstitial pulmonary fibrosis) 516.3
Hammer toe (acquired) 735.4
congenital 755.66
late effects of rickets 268.1
Hand — see condition
Hand-Schüller-Christian disease or syndrome (chronic histiocytosis x) 277.8
Hand-foot syndrome 282.61
Hanging (asphyxia) (strangulation) (suffocation) 994.7

Hangnail (finger) (with lymphangitis) 681.02
Hangover (alcohol) (see also Abuse, drugs, nondependent) 305.0
Hanot's cirrhosis or disease — see Cirrhosis, biliary
Hanot-Chauffard (-Troisier) **syndrome** (bronze diabetes) 275.0
Hansen's disease (leprosy) 030.9
benign form 030.1
malignant form 030.0
Harada's disease or syndrome 363.22
Hard chancre 091.0
Hardening
artery — see Arteriosclerosis
brain 348.8
liver 571.8
Hare's syndrome (M8010/3) (carcinoma, pulmonary apex) 162.3
Harelip (see also Cleft, lip) 749.10
Harkavy's syndrome 446.0
Harlequin (fetus) 757.1
color change syndrome 779.8
Harley's disease (intermittent hemoglobinuria) 283.2
Harris'
lines 733.91
syndrome (organic hyperinsulinism) 251.1
Hart's disease or syndrome (pellagra-cerebellar ataxia-renal aminoaciduria) 270.0
Hartmann's pouch (abnormal sacculation of gallbladder neck) 575.8
Hartnup disease (pellagra-cerebellar ataxia-renal aminoaciduria) 270.0
Harvester lung 495.0
Hashimoto's disease or struma (struma lymphomatosa) 245.2
Hassell-Henle bodies (corneal warts) 371.41
Haut mal (see also Epilepsy) 345.1
Haverhill fever 026.1
Hawaiian wood rose dependence 304.5
Hawkins' keloid 701.4
Hay
asthma (see also Asthma) 493.0
fever (allergic) (with rhinitis) 477.9
with asthma (bronchial) (see also Asthma) 493.0
allergic, due to grass, pollen, ragweed, or tree 477.0
conjunctivitis 372.05
due to
dander 477.8
dust 477.8
fowl 477.8
pollen 477.0
specified allergen other than pollen 477.8
Hayem-Faber syndrome (achlorhydric anemia) 280.9
Hayem-Widal syndrome (acquired hemolytic jaundice) 283.9
Haygarth's nodosities 715.04
Hazard-Crile tumor (M8350/3) 193
Hb (abnormal)
disease — see Disease, hemoglobin
trait — see Trait
H disease 270.0
Head — see also condition
banging 307.3

Headache / INDEX TO DISEASES / Hematoma

Headache 784.0
  allergic 346.2
  cluster 346.2
  due to
    loss, spinal fluid 349.0
    lumbar puncture 349.0
    saddle block 349.0
  emotional 307.81
  histamine 346.2
  lumbar puncture 349.0
  menopausal 627.2
  migraine 346.9
  nonorganic origin 307.81
  postspinal 349.0
  psychogenic 307.81
  psychophysiologic 307.81
  sick 346.1
  spinal fluid loss 349.0
  tension 307.81
  vascular 784.0
    migraine type 346.9
  vasomotor 346.9
Health
  advice V65.4
  audit V70.0
  checkup V70.0
  education V65.4
  hazard (see also History of) V15.9
    specified cause NEC V15.89
  instruction V65.4
  services provided because (of)
    boarding school residence V60.6
    holiday relief for person providing home care V60.5
    inadequate
      housing V60.1
      resources V60.2
    lack of housing V60.0
    no care available in home V60.4
    person living alone V60.3
    poverty V60.3
    residence in institution V60.6
    specified cause NEC V60.8
    vacation relief for person providing home care V60.5
Healthy
  donor (see also Donor) V59.9
  infant or child
    accompanying sick mother V65.0
    receiving care V20.1
  person
    accompanying sick relative V65.0
    admitted for sterilization V25.2
    receiving prophylactic inoculation or vaccination (see also Vaccination, prophylactic) V05.9
Hearing examination V72.1
Heart — see condition
Heartburn 787.1
  psychogenic 306.4
Heat (effects) 992.9
  apoplexy 992.0
  burn — see also Burn, by site
    from sun 692.71
  collapse 992.1
  cramps 992.2
  dermatitis or eczema 692.89
  edema 992.7
  erythema — see Burn, by site
  excessive 992.9
    specified effect NEC 992.8
  exhaustion 992.5
    anhydrotic 992.3
    due to
      salt (and water) depletion 992.4
      water depletion 992.3

Heat—continued
  fatigue (transient) 992.6
  fever 992.0
  hyperpyrexia 992.0
  prickly 705.1
  prostration — see Heat, exhaustion
  pyrexia 992.0
  rash 705.1
  specified effect NEC 992.8
  stroke 992.0
  sunburn 692.71
  syncope 992.1
Heavy-chain disease 273.2
Heavy-for-dates (fetus or infant) 766.1
  4500 grams or more 766.0
  exceptionally 766.0
Hebephrenia, hebephrenic (acute) (see also Schizophrenia) 295.1
  dementia (praecox) (see also Schizophrenia) 295.1
  schizophrenia (see also Schizophrenia) 295.1
Heberden's
  disease or nodes 715.04
  syndrome (angina pectoris) 413.9
Hebra's disease
  dermatitis exfoliativa 695.89
  erythema multiforme exudativum 695.1
  pityriasis 695.89
    maculata et circinata 696.3
    rubra 695.89
    pilaris 696.4
  prurigo 698.2
Hebra, nose 040.1
Hedinger's syndrome (malignant carcinoid) 259.2
Heel — see condition
Heerfordt's disease or syndrome (uveoparotitis) 135
Hegglin's anomaly or syndrome 288.2
Heidenhain's disease 290.10
  with dementia 290.10
Heilmeyer-Schöner disease (M9842/3) 207.1
Heine-Medin disease (see also Poliomyelitis) 045.9
Heinz-body anemia, congenital 282.7
Heller's disease or syndrome (infantile psychosis) (see also Psychosis, childhood) 299.1
Helminthiasis (see also Infestation, by specific parasite) 128.9
  Ancylostoma (see also Ancylostoma) 126.9
  intestinal 127.9
    mixed types (types classifiable to more than one of the titles 120.0-127.7) 127.8
    specified type 127.7
  mixed types (intestinal) (types classifiable to more than one of the titles 120.0-127.7) 127.8
  Necator americanus 126.1
  specified type NEC 128.8
  Trichinella 124
Heloma 700
Hemangioblastoma (M9161/1) — see also Neoplasm, connective tissue, uncertain behavior
  malignant (M9161/3) — see Neoplasm, connective tissue, malignant
Hemangioblastomatosis, cerebelloretinal 759.6
Hemangioendothelioma (M9130/1) — see also Neoplasm, by site, uncertain behavior
  benign (M9130/0) 228.00

Hemangioendothelioma—continued
  bone (diffuse) (M9130/3) — see Neoplasm, bone, malignant
  malignant (M9130/3) — see Neoplasm, connective tissue, malignant
  nervous system (M9130/0) 228.09
Hemangioendotheliosarcoma (M9130/3) — see Neoplasm, connective tissue, malignant
Hemangiofibroma (M9160/0) — see Neoplasm, by site, benign
Hemangiolipoma (M8861/0) — see Lipoma
Hemangioma (M9120/0) 228.00
  arteriovenous (M9123/0) — see Hemangioma, by site
  brain 228.02
  capillary (M9131/0) — see Hemangioma, by site
  cavernous (M9121/0) — see Hemangioma, by site
  central nervous system NEC 228.09
  choroid 228.09
  heart 228.09
  infantile (M9131/0) — see Hemangioma, by site
  intra-abdominal structures 228.04
  intracranial structures 228.02
  intramuscular (M9132/0) — see Hemangioma, by site
  iris 228.09
  juvenile (M9131/0) — see Hemangioma, by site
  malignant (M9120/3) — see Neoplasm, connective tissue, malignant
  meninges 228.09
    brain 228.02
    spinal cord 228.09
  peritoneum 228.04
  placenta — see Placenta, abnormal
  plexiform (M9131/0) — see Hemangioma, by site
  racemose (M9123/0) — see Hemangioma, by site
  retina 228.03
  retroperitoneal tissue 228.04
  sclerosing (M8832/0) — see Neoplasm, skin, benign
  simplex (M9131/0) — see Hemangioma, by site
  skin and subcutaneous tissue 228.01
  specified site NEC 228.09
  spinal cord 228.09
  venous (M9122/0) — see Hemangioma, by site
  verrucous keratotic (M9142/0) — see Hemangioma, by site
Hemangiomatosis (systemic) 757.32
  involving single site — see Hemangioma
Hemangiopericytoma (M9l50/1) — see also Neoplasm, connective tissue, uncertain behavior
  benign (M9150/0) — see Neoplasm, connective tissue, benign
  malignant (M9150/3) — see Neoplasm, connective tissue, malignant
Hemangiosarcoma (M9120/3) — see Neoplasm, connective tissue, malignant
Hemarthrosis (nontraumatic) 719.10
  ankle 719.17
  elbow 719.12
  foot 719.17
  hand 719.14
  hip 719.15
  knee 719.16
  multiple sites 719.19
  pelvic region 719.15

Hemarthrosis—continued
  shoulder (region) 719.11
  specified site NEC 719.18
  traumatic — see Sprain, by site
  wrist 719.13
Hematemesis 578.0
  with ulcer — see Ulcer, by site, with hemorrhage
  due to S. japonicum 120.2
  Goldstein's (familial hemorrhagic telangiectasia) 448.0
  newborn 772.4
    due to swallowed maternal blood 777.3
Hematidrosis 705.89
Hematinuria (see also Hemoglobinuria) 791.2
  malarial 084.8
  paroxysmal 283.2
Hematite miners' lung 503
Hematobilia 576.8
Hematocele (congenital) (diffuse) (idiopathic) 608.83
  broad ligament 620.7
  canal of Nuck 629.0
  cord male 608.83
  fallopian tube 620.8
  female NEC 629.0
  ischiorectal 569.89
  male NEC 608.83
  ovary 629.0
  pelvis, pelvic
    female 629.0
      with ectopic pregnancy (see also Pregnancy, ectopic) 633.9
    male 608.83
  periuterine 629.0
  retrouterine 629.0
  scrotum 608.83
  spermatic cord (diffuse) 608.83
  testis 608.84
  traumatic — see Injury, internal, pelvis
  tunica vaginalis 608.83
  uterine ligament 629.0
  uterus 621.4
  vagina 623.6
  vulva 624.5
Hematocephalus 742.4
Hematochezia (see also Melena) 578.1
Hematochyluria (see also Infestation, filarial) 125.9
Hematocolpos 626.8
Hematocornea 371.12
Hematogenous — see condition
Hematoma (skin surface intact) (traumatic) — see also Contusion

> Note — Hematomas are coded according to origin and the nature and site of the hematoma or the accompanying injury. Hematomas of unspecified origin are coded as injuries of the sites involved, except:
>
> (a) hematomas of genital organs which are coded as diseases of the organ involved unless they complicate pregnancy or delivery
>
> (b) hematomas of the eye which are coded as diseases of the eye.
>
> For late effect of hematoma classifiable to 920-924 see Late, effect, contusion

Hematoma—*continued*
  with
    crush injury — *see* Crush
    fracture — *see* Fracture, by site
    injury of internal organs — *see also* Injury, internal, by site
    kidney — *see* Hematoma, kidney traumatic
    liver — *see* Hematoma, liver, traumatic
    spleen — *see* Hematoma, spleen
    nerve injury — *see* Injury, nerve
    open wound — *see* Wound, open, by site
    skin surface intact — *see* Contusion
  abdomen (wall) — *see* Contusion, abdomen
  amnion 658.8
  aorta, dissecting 441.00 ▼
    abdominal 441.02
    thoracic 441.01
    thoracoabdominal 441.03 ▲
  arterial (complicating trauma) 904.9
    specified site — *see* Injury, blood vessel, by site
  auricle (ear) 380.31
  birth injury 767.8
    skull 767.1
  brain (traumatic) 853.0

> Note — Use the following fifth-digit subclassification with categories 851-854:
>
> 0   unspecified state of consciousness
> 1   with no loss of consciousness
> 2   with brief [less than one hour] loss of consciousness
> 3   with moderate [1-24 hours] loss of consciousness
> 4   with prolonged [more than 24 hours] loss of consciousness and return to pre-existing conscious level
> 5   with prolonged [more than 24 hours] loss of consciousness, without return to pre-existing conscious level
> 6   with loss of consciousness of unspecified duration
> 9   with concussion, unspecified

    with
      cerebral
        contusion — *see* Contusion, brain
        laceration — *see* Laceration, brain
      open intracranial wound 853.1
      skull fracture — *see* Fracture, skull, by site
    extradural or epidural 852.4
      with open intracranial wound 852.5
      fetus or newborn 767.0
      nontraumatic 432.0
    fetus or newborn NEC 767.0
    nontraumatic (*see also* Hemorrhage, brain) 431

Hematoma—*continued*
  brain—*continued*
    nontraumatic—*continued*
      epidural or extradural 432.0
      newborn NEC 772.8
      subarachnoid, arachnoid, or meningeal (*see also* Hemorrhage, subarachnoid) 430
      subdural (*see also* Hemorrhage, subdural) 432.1
    subarachnoid, arachnoid, or meningeal 852.0
      with open intracranial wound 852.1
      fetus or newborn 772.2
      nontraumatic (*see also* Hemorrhage, subarachnoid) 430
    subdural 852.2
      with open intracranial wound 852.3
      fetus or newborn (localized) 767.0
      nontraumatic (*see also* Hemorrhage, subdural) 432.1
  breast (nontraumatic) 611.8
  broad ligament (nontraumatic) 620.7
    complicating delivery 665.7
    traumatic — *see* Injury, internal, broad ligament
  calcified NEC 959.9
  capitis 920
    due to birth injury 767.1
    newborn 767.1
  cerebral — *see* Hematoma, brain
  cesarean section wound 674.3
  chorion — *see* Placenta, abnormal
  complicating delivery (perineum) (vulva) 664.5
    pelvic 665.7
    vagina 665.7
  corpus
    cavernosum (nontraumatic) 607.82
    luteum (nontraumatic) (ruptured) 620.1
  dura (mater) — *see* Hematoma, brain, subdural
  epididymis (nontraumatic) 608.83
  epidural (traumatic) — *see also* Hematoma, brain, extradural
    spinal — *see* Injury, spinal, by site
  episiotomy 674.3
  external ear 380.31
  extradural — *see also* Hematoma, brain, extradural
    fetus or newborn 767.0
    nontraumatic 432.0
      fetus or newborn 767.0
  fallopian tube 620.8
  genital organ (nontraumatic)
    female NEC 629.8
    male NEC 608.83
    traumatic (external site) 922.4
      internal — *see* Injury, internal, genital organ
  graafian follicle (ruptured) 620.0
  internal organs (abdomen, chest, or pelvis) — *see also* Injury, internal, by site
    kidney — *see* Hematoma, kidney, traumatic
    liver — *see* Hematoma, liver, traumatic
    spleen — *see* Hematoma, brain
  intracrainal — *see* Hematoma, brain

Hematoma—*continued*
  kidney, cystic 593.81
    traumatic 866.01
      with open wound into cavity 866.11
  labia (nontraumatic) 624.5
  lingual (and other parts of neck, scalp, or face, except eye) 920
  liver (subcapsular) 573.8
    birth injury 767.8
    fetus or newborn 767.8
    traumatic NEC 864.01
      with
        laceration — *see* Laceration, liver
        open wound into cavity 864.11
  mediastinum — *see* Injury, internal, mediastinum
  meninges, meningeal (brain) — *see also* Hematoma, brain, subarachnoid
    spinal — *see* Injury, spinal, by site
  mesosalpinx (nontraumatic) 620.8
    traumatic — *see* Injury, internal, pelvis
  muscle (traumatic) — *see* Contusion, by site
  nasal (septum) (and other part(s) of neck, scalp, or face, except eye) 920
  obstetrical surgical wound 674.3
  orbit, orbital (nontraumatic) 376.32
    traumatic 921.2
  ovary (corpus luteum) (nontraumatic) 620.1
    traumatic — *see* Injury, internal, ovary
  pelvis (female) (nontraumatic) 629.8
    complicating delivery 665.7
    male 608.83
    traumatic — *see also* Injury, internal, pelvis
      specified organ NEC (*see also* Injury, internal, pelvis) 867.6
  penis (nontraumatic) 607.82
  pericranial (and neck, or face any part, except eye) 920
    due to injury at birth 767.1
  perineal wound (obstetrical) 674.3
    complicating delivery 664.5
  perirenal, cystic 593.81
  pinna 380.31
  placenta — *see* Placenta, abnormal
  postoperative 998.1
  retroperitoneal (nontraumatic) 568.81
    traumatic — *see* Injury, internal, retroperitoneum
  retropubic, male 568.81
  scalp (and neck, or face any part, except eye) 920
    fetus or newborn 767.1
  scrotum (nontraumatic) 608.83
    traumatic 922.4
  seminal vesicle (nontraumatic) 608.83
    traumatic — *see* Injury, internal, seminal, vesicle
  spermatic cord — *see also* Injury, internal, spermatic cord
    nontraumatic 608.83
  spinal (cord) (meninges) — *see* Injury, spinal, by site
    fetus or newborn 767.4
    nontraumatic 336.1

Hematoma—*continued*
  spleen 865.01
    with
      laceration — *see* Laceration, spleen
      open wound into cavity 865.11
  sternocleidomastoid, birth injury 767.8
  sternomastoid, birth injury 767.8
  subarachnoid — *see also* Hematoma, brain, subarachnoid
    fetus or newborn 772.2
    nontraumatic (*see also* Hemorrhage, subarachnoid) 430
      newborn 772.2
  subdural — *see also* Hematoma, brain, subdural
    fetus or newborn (localized) 767.0
    nontraumatic (*see also* Hemorrhage, subdural) 432.1
  subperiosteal (syndrome) 267
    traumatic — *see* Hematoma, by site
  superficial, fetus or newborn 772.6
  syncytium — *see* Placenta, abnormal
  testis (nontraumatic) 608.83
    birth injury 767.8
    traumatic 922.4
  tunica vaginalis (nontraumatic) 608.83
  umbilical cord 663.6
    affecting fetus or newborn 762.6
  uterine ligament (nontraumatic) 620.7
    traumatic — *see* Injury, internal, pelvis
  uterus 621.4
    traumatic — *see* Injury, internal, pelvis
  vagina (nontraumatic) (ruptured) 623.6
    complicating delivery 665.7
    traumatic 922.4
  vas deferens (nontraumatic) 608.83
    traumatic — *see* Injury, internal, vas deferens
  vitreous 379.23
  vocal cord 920
  vulva (nontraumatic) 624.5
    complicating delivery 664.5
    fetus or newborn 767.8
    traumatic 922.4

Hematometra 621.4

Hematomyelia 336.1
  with fracture of vertebra (*see also* Fracture, vertebra, by site, with spinal cord injury) 806.8
  fetus or newborn 767.4

Hematomyelitis 323.9
  late effect — *see* category 326

Hematoperitoneum (*see also* Hemoperitoneum) 568.81

Hematopneumothorax (*see also* Hemothorax) 511.8

Hematoporphyria (acquired) (congenital) 277.1

Hematoporphyrinuria (acquired) (congenital) 277.1

Hematorachis, hematorrhachis 336.1
  fetus or newborn 767.4

Hematosalpinx 620.8
  with
    ectopic pregnancy (*see also*
        categories 633.0-633.9)
        639.2
    molar pregnancy (*see also*
        categories 630-632)
        639.2
    infectional (*see also* Salpingo-
        oophoritis) 614.2
Hematospermia 608.83
Hematothorax (*see also*
    Hemothorax) 511.8
Hematotympanum 381.03
Hematuria (benign) (essential)
    (idiopathic) 599.7
  due to S. hematobium 120.0
  endemic 120.0
  intermittent 599.7
  malarial 084.8
  paroxysmal 599.7
  sulfonamide
    correct substance properly
        administered 599.7
    overdose or wrong substance
        given or taken 961.0
  tropical (bilharziasis) 120.0
  tuberculous (*see also*
    Tuberculosis) 016.9
Hematuric bilious fever 084.8
Hemeralopia 368.60
  meaning day blindness 368.10
  vitamin A deficiency 264.5
Hemiabiotrophy 799.8
Hemi-akinesia 781.8 ◆
Hemianalgesia (*see also*
    Disturbance, sensation) 782.0
Hemianencephaly 740.0
Hemianesthesia (*see also*
    Disturbance, sensation) 782.0
Hemianopia, hemianopsia
    (altitudinal) (homonymous)
    368.46
  binasal 368.47
  bitemporal 368.47
  heteronymous 368.47
  syphilitic 095.8
Hemiasomatognosia 307.9
Hemiathetosis 781.0
Hemiatrophy 799.8
  cerebellar 334.8
  face 349.89
    progressive 349.89
  fascia 728.9
  leg 728.2
  tongue 529.8
Hemiballism(us) 333.5
Hemiblock (cardiac) (heart) (left)
    426.2
Hemicardia 746.89
Hemicephalus, hemicephaly 740.0
Hemichorea 333.5
Hemicrania 346.9
  congenital malformation 740.0
Hemidystrophy — *see* Hemiatrophy
Hemiectromelia 755.4
Hemihypalgesia (*see also*
    Disturbance, sensation) 782.0
Hemihypertrophy (congenital)
    759.89
  cranial 756.0
Hemihypesthesia (*see also*
    Disturbance, sensation) 782.0
Hemi-inattention 781.8 ◆
Hemimelia 755.4
  lower limb 755.30
    paraxial (complete)
        (incomplete)
        (intercalary) (terminal)
        755.32
      fibula 755.37
      tibia 755.36

Hemimelia—*continued*
  lower limb—*continued*
    transverse (complete) (partial)
        755.31
  upper limb 755.20
    paraxial (complete)
        (incomplete)
        (intercalary) (terminal)
        755.22
      radial 755.26
      ulnar 755.27
    transverse (complete) (partial)
        755.21
Hemiparalysis (*see also* Hemiplegia)
    342.9
Hemiparesis (*see also* Hemiplegia)
    342.9
Hemiparesthesia (*see also*
    Disturbance, sensation) 782.0
Hemiplegia 342.9
  acute (*see also* Disease,
      cerebrovascular, acute) 436
  alternans facialis 344.89
  apoplectic (*see also* Disease,
      cerebrovascular, acute) 436
    late effect or residual — *see*
        category 438
  arteriosclerotic 437.0
    late effect or residual — *see*
        category 438
  ascending (spinal) NEC 344.89
  attack (*see also* Disease,
      cerebrovascular, acute) 436
  brain, cerebral (current episode)
      437.8
    congenital 343.1
  cerebral — *see* Hemiplegia, brain
  congenital (cerebral) (spastic)
      (spinal) 343.1
  conversion neurosis (hysterical)
      300.11
  cortical — *see* Hemiplegia, brain
  due to
    arteriosclerosis 437.0
      late effect or residual — *see*
          category 438
    cerebrovascular lesion (*see
        also* Disease,
        cerebrovascular, acute)
        436
      late effect — *see* category
          438
  embolic (current) (*see also*
      Embolism, brain) 434.1
    late effect — *see* category 438
  flaccid 342.0
  hypertensive (current episode)
      437.8
  infantile (postnatal) 343.4
  late effect
    birth injury, intracranial or
        spinal 343.4
    cerebrovascular lesion — *see*
        category 438
    viral encephalitis 139.0
  middle alternating NEC 344.89
  newborn NEC 767.0
  seizure (current episode) (*see also*
      Disease, cerebrovascular,
      acute) 436
  spastic 342.1
    congenital or infantile 343.1
  specified NEC 342.8 ◆
  thrombotic (current) (*see also*
      Thrombosis, brain) 434.0
    late effect — *see* category 438
Hemisection, spinal cord — *see*
    Fracture, vertebra, by site, with
    spinal cord injury
Hemispasm 781.0
  facial 781.0
Hemispatial neglect 781.8 ◆
Hemisporosis 117.9
Hemitremor 781.0
Hemivertebra 756.14

Hemobilia 576.8
Hemocholecyst 575.8
Hemochromatosis (acquired)
    (diabetic) (hereditary) (liver)
    (myocardium) (primary)
    (idiopathic) (secondary) 275.0
  with refractory anemia 285.0
Hemodialysis V56.0
Hemoglobin — *see also* condition
  abnormal (disease) — *see*
      Disease, hemoglobin
  AS genotype 282.5
  fetal, hereditary persistence 282.7
  high-oxygen-affinity 289.0
  low NEC 285.9
  S (Hb-S), heterozygous 282.5
Hemoglobinemia 283.2
  due to blood transfusion NEC
      999.8
    bone marrow 996.85
  paroxysmal 283.2
Hemoglobinopathy (mixed) (*see also*
    Disease, hemoblobin) 282.7
  with thalassemia 282.4
  sickle-cell 282.60
    with thalassemia 282.4
Hemoglobinuria, hemoglobinuric
    791.2
  with anemia, hemolytic, acquired
      (chronic) NEC 283.2
  cold (agglutinin) (paroxysmal)
      (with Raynaud's syndrome)
      283.2
  due to
    exertion 283.2
    hemolysis (from external
        causes) NEC 283.2
  exercise 283.2
  fever (malaria) 084.8
  infantile 791.2
  intermittent 283.2
  malarial 084.8
  march 283.2
  nocturnal (paroxysmal) 283.2
  paroxysmal (cold) (nocturnal)
      283.2
Hemolymphangioma (M9175/0)
    228.1
Hemolysis
  fetal — *see* Jaundice, fetus or
      newborn
  intravascular (disseminated) NEC
      286.6
    with
      abortion — *see* Abortion,
          by type, with
          hemorrhage, delayed
          or excessive
      ectopic pregnancy (*see also*
          categories 633.0-
          633.9) 639.1
      hemorrhage of pregnancy
          641.3
        affecting fetus or
            newborn 762.1
      molar pregnancy (*see also*
          categories 630-632)
          639.1
    acute 283.2
    following
      abortion 639.1
      ectopic or molar pregnancy
          639.1
  neonatal — *see* Jaundice, fetus or
      newborn
  transfusion NEC 999.8
    bone marrow 996.85
Hemolytic — *see also* condition
  anemia — *see* Anemia, hemolytic
  uremic syndrome 283.11
Hemometra 621.4

Hemopericardium (with effusion)
    423.0
  newborn 772.8
  traumatic (*see also* Hemothorax,
      traumatic) 860.2
    with open wound into thorax
        860.3
Hemoperitoneum 568.81
  infectional (*see also* Peritonitis)
      567.2
  traumatic — *see* Injury, internal,
      peritoneum
Hemophilia (familial) (hereditary)
    286.0
  A 286.0
  B (Leyden) 286.1
  B$_m$ 286.1
  C 286.2
  calcipriva (*see also* Fibrinolysis)
      286.7
  classical 286.0
  nonfamilial 286.7
  vascular 286.4
Hemophilus influenzae NEC 041.5
  arachnoiditis (basic) (brain)
      (spinal) 320.0
    late effect — *see* category 326
  bronchopneumonia 482.2
  cerebral ventriculitis 320.0
    late effect — *see* category 326
  cerebrospinal inflammation 320.0
    late effect — *see* category 326
  infection NEC 041.5
  leptomeningitis 320.0
    late effect — *see* category 326
  meningitis (cerebral)
      (cerebrospinal) (spinal)
      320.0
    late effect — *see* category 326
  meningomyelitis 320.0
    late effect — *see* category 326
  pachymeningitis (adhesive)
      (fibrous) (hemorrhagic)
      (hypertrophic) (spinal)
      320.0
    late effect — *see* category 326
  pneumonia (broncho-) 482.2
Hemophthalmos 360.43
Hemopneumothorax (*see also*
    Hemothorax) 511.8
  traumatic 860.4
    with open wound into thorax
        860.5
Hemoptysis 786.3
  due to Paragonimus (westermani)
      121.2
  newborn 770.3
  tuberculous (*see also*
      Tuberculosis, pulmonary)
      011.9
Hemorrhage, hemorrhagic
    (nontraumatic) 459.0
  abdomen 459.0
  accidental (antepartum) 641.2
    affecting fetus or newborn
        762.1
  adenoid 474.8
  adrenal (capsule) (gland)
      (medulla) 255.4
    newborn 772.5
  after labor — *see* Hemorrhage,
      postpartum
  alveolar
    lung, newborn 770.3
    process 525.8
  alveolus 525.8
  amputation stump (surgical) 998.1
    secondary, delayed 997.69
  anemia (chronic) 280.0
    acute 285.1
  antepartum — *see* Hemorrhage,
      pregnancy
  anus (sphincter) 569.3
  apoplexy (stroke) 432.9
  arachnoid — *see* Hemorrhage,
      subarachnoid

Hemorrhage, hemorrhagic

Hemorrhage, hemorrhagic—*continued*
  artery NEC 459.0
    brain (*see also* Hemorrhage, brain) 431
    middle meningeal — *see* Hemorrhage, subarachnoid
  basilar (ganglion) (*see also* Hemorrhage, brain) 431
  bladder 596.8
  blood dyscrasia 289.9
  bowel 578.9
    newborn 772.4
  brain (miliary) (nontraumatic) 431
    with
      birth injury 767.0
      arachnoid — *see* Hemorrhage, subarachnoid
    due to
      birth injury 767.0
      rupture of aneurysm (congenital) (*see also* Hemorrhage, subarachnoid) 430
        mycotic 431
      syphilis 094.89
    epidural or extradural — *see* Hemorrhage, extradural
    fetus or newborn (anoxic) (hypoxic) (due to birth trauma) (nontraumatic) 767.0
    puerperal, postpartum, childbirth 674.0
    stem 431
    subarachnoid, arachnoid, or meningeal — *see* Hemorrhage, subarachnoid
    subdural — *see* Hemorrhage, subdural
    traumatic NEC 853.0

> Note — Use the following fifth-digit subclassification with categories 851-854:
>
> 0   unspecified state of consciousness
> 1   with no loss of consciousness
> 2   with brief [less than one hour] loss of consciousness
> 3   with moderate [1-24 hours] loss of consciousness
> 4   with prolonged [more than 24 hours] loss of consciousness and return to pre-existing conscious level
> 5   with prolonged [more than 24 hours] loss of consciousness, without return to pre-existing conscious level
> 6   with loss of consciousness of unspecified duration
> 9   with concussion, unspecified

    with
      cerebral
        contusion — *see* Contusion, brain
        laceration — *see* Laceration, brain
      open intracranial wound 853.1

Hemorrhage, hemorrhagic—*continued*
  brain—*continued*
    traumatic—*continued*
      with—*continued*
        skull fracture — *see* Fracture, skull, by site
      extradural or epidural 852.4
        with open intracranial wound 852.5
      subarachnoid 852.0
        with open intracranial wound 852.1
      subdural 852.2
        with open intracranial wound 852.3
  breast 611.79
  bronchial tube — *see* Hemorrhage, lung
  bronchopulmonary — *see* Hemorrhage, lung
  bronchus (cause unknown) (*see also* Hemorrhage, lung) 786.3
  bulbar (*see also* Hemorrhage, brain) 431
  bursa 727.89
  capillary 448.9
    primary 287.8
  capsular — *see* Hemorrhage, brain
  cardiovascular 429.89
  cecum 578.9
  cephalic (*see also* Hemorrhage, brain) 431
  cerebellar (*see also* Hemorrhage, brain) 431
  cerebellum (*see also* Hemorrhage, brain) 431
  cerebral (*see also* Hemorrhage, brain) 431
    fetus or newborn (anoxic) (traumatic) 767.0
  cerebromeningeal (*see also* Hemorrhage, brain) 431
  cerebrospinal (*see also* Hemorrhage, brain) 431
  cerebrum (*see also* Hemorrhage, brain) 431
  cervix (stump) (uteri) 622.8
  cesarean section wound 674.3
  chamber, anterior (eye) 364.41
  childbirth — *see* Hemorrhage, complicating, delivery
  choroid 363.61
    expulsive 363.62
  ciliary body 364.41
  cochlea 386.8
  colon — *see* Hemorrhage, intestine
  complicating
    delivery 641.9
      affecting fetus or newborn 762.1
      associated with
        afibrinogenemia 641.3
          affecting fetus or newborn 763.8
        coagulation defect 641.3
          affecting fetus or newborn 763.8
        hyperfibrinolysis 641.3
          affecting fetus or newborn 763.8
        hypofibrinogenemia 641.3
          affecting fetus or newborn 763.8
      due to
        low-lying placenta 641.1
          affecting fetus or newborn 762.0

Hemorrhage, hemorrhagic—*continued*
  complicating—*continued*
    delivery—*continued*
      due to—*continued*
        placenta previa 641.1
          affecting fetus or newborn 762.0
        premature separation of placenta 641.2
          affecting fetus or newborn 762.1
        retained
          placenta 666.0
          secundines 666.2
        trauma 641.8
          affecting fetus or newborn 763.8
        uterine leiomyoma 641.8
          affecting fetus or newborn 763.8
      surgical procedure 998.1
  concealed NEC 459.0
  congenital 772.9
  conjunctiva 372.72
    newborn 772.8
  cord, newborn 772.0
    slipped ligature 772.3
    stump 772.3
  corpus luteum (ruptured) 620.1
  cortical (*see also* Hemorrhage, brain) 431
  cranial 432.9
  cutaneous 782.7
    newborn 772.6
  cyst, pancreas 577.2
  cystitis — *see* Cystitis
  delayed
    with
      abortion — *see* Abortion, by type, with hemorrhage, delayed or excessive
      ectopic pregnancy (*see also* categories 633.0-633.9) 639.1
      molar pregnancy (*see also* categories 630-632) 639.1
    following
      abortion 639.1
      ectopic or molar pregnancy 639.1
  postpartum 666.2
  diathesis (familial) 287.9
    newborn 776.0
  disease 287.9
    newborn 776.0
    specified type NEC 287.8
  disorder 287.9
    due to circulating anticoagulants 286.5
    specified type NEC 287.8
  due to
    any device, implant or graft (presence of) classifiable to 996.0-996.5 — *see* Complications, due to (presence of) any device, implant, or graft classified to 996.0-996.5 NEC
    circulating anticoagulant 286.5
  duodenum, duodenal 537.89
    ulcer — *see* Ulcer, duodenum, with hemorrhage
  dura mater — *see* Hemorrhage, subdural
  endotracheal — *see* Hemorrhage, lung
  epidural — *see* Hemorrhage, extradural
  episiotomy 674.3

Hemorrhage, hemorrhagic—*continued*
  esophagus 530.82
    varix (*see also* Varix, esophagus, bleeding) 456.0
  excessive
    with
      abortion — *see* Abortion, by type, with hemorrhage, delayed or excessive
      ectopic pregnancy (*see also* categories 633.0-633.9) 639.1
      molar pregnancy (*see also* categories 630-632) 639.1
    following
      abortion 639.1
      ectopic or molar pregnancy 639.1
  external 459.0
  extradural (traumatic) — *see also* Hemorrhage, brain, traumatic, extradural
    birth injury 767.0
    fetus or newborn (anoxic) (traumatic) 767.0
    nontraumatic 432.0
  eye 360.43
    chamber (anterior) (aqueous) 364.41
    fundus 362.81
  eyelid 374.81
  fallopian tube 620.8
  fetomaternal 772.0
    affecting management of pregnancy or puerperium 656.0
  fetus, fetal 772.0
    from
      cut end of co-twin's cord 772.0
      placenta 772.0
      ruptured cord 772.0
      vasa previa 772.0
    into
      co-twin 772.0
      mother's circulation 772.0
        affecting management of pregnancy or puerperium 656.0
  fever (*see also* Fever, hemorrhagic) 065.9
    with renal syndrome 078.6
    arthropod-borne NEC 065.9
    Bangkok 065.4
    Crimean 065.0
    dengue virus 065.4
    epidemic 078.6
    Junin virus 078.7
    Korean 078.6
    Machupo virus 078.7
    mite-borne 065.8
    mosquito-borne 065.4
    Philippine 065.4
    Russian (Yaroslav) 078.6
    Singapore 065.4
    southeast Asia 065.4
    Thailand 065.4
    tick-borne NEC 065.3
  fibrinogenolysis (*see also* Fibrinolysis) 286.6
  fibrinolytic (acquired) (*see also* Fibrinolysis) 286.6
  fontanel 767.1
  from tracheostomy stoma 519.0
  fundus, eye 362.81
  funis
    affecting fetus or newborn 772.0
    complicating delivery 663.8
  gastric (*see also* Hemorrhage, stomach) 578.9
  gastroenteric 578.9
    newborn 772.4

Hemorrhage, hemorrhagic — *continued*
  gastrointestinal (tract) 578.9
    newborn 772.4
  genitourinary (tract) NEC 599.89
  gingiva 523.8
  globe 360.43
  gravidarum — see Hemorrhage, pregnancy
  gum 523.8
  heart 429.89
  hypopharyngeal (throat) 784.8
  intermenstrual 626.8
    irregular 626.6
    regular 626.5
  internal (organs) 459.0
    capsule (see also Hemorrhage, brain) 431
    ear 386.8
    newborn 772.8
  intestine 578.9
    congenital 772.4
    newborn 772.4
  into
    bladder wall 596.7
    bursa 727.89
    corpus luysii (see also Hemorrhage, brain) 431
  intra-abdominal 459.0
    during or following surgery 998.1
  intra-alveolar, newborn (lung) 770.3
  intracerebral (see also Hemorrhage, brain) 431
  intracranial NEC 432.9
    puerperal, postpartum, childbirth 674.0
    traumatic — see Hemorrhage, brain, traumatic
  intramedullary NEC 336.1
  intraocular 360.43
  intraoperative 998.1
  intrapartum — see Hemorrhage, complicating, delivery
  intrapelvic
    female 629.8
    male 459.0
  intraperitoneal 459.0
  intrapontine (see also Hemorrhage, brain) 431
  intrauterine 621.4
    complicating delivery — see Hemorrhage, complicating, delivery
    in pregnancy or childbirth — see Hemorrhage, pregnancy
    postpartum (see also Hemorrhage, postpartum) 666.1
  intraventricular (see also Hemorrhage, brain) 431
    fetus or newborn (anoxic) (traumatic) 772.1
  intravesical 596.7
  iris (postinfectional) (postinflammatory) (toxic) 364.41
  joint (nontraumatic) 719.10
    ankle 719.17
    elbow 719.12
    foot 719.17
    forearm 719.13
    hand 719.14
    hip 719.15
    knee 719.16
    lower leg 719.16
    multiple sites 719.19
    pelvic region 719.15
    shoulder (region) 719.11
    specified site NEC 719.18
    thigh 719.15
    upper arm 719.12
    wrist 719.13
  kidney 593.81
  knee (joint) 719.16

Hemorrhage, hemorrhagic — *continued*
  labyrinth 386.8
  leg NEC 459.0
  lenticular striate artery (see also Hemorrhage, brain) 431
  ligature, vessel 998.1
  liver 573.8
  lower extremity NEC 459.0
  lung 786.3
    newborn 770.3
    tuberculous (see also Tuberculosis, pulmonary) 011.9
  malaria 084.8
  marginal sinus 641.2
  massive subaponeurotic, birth injury 767.1
  maternal, affecting fetus or newborn 762.1
  mediastinum 786.3
  medulla (see also Hemorrhage, brain) 431
  membrane (brain) (see also Hemorrhage, subarachnoid) 430
    spinal cord — see Hemorrhage, spinal cord
  meninges, meningeal (brain) (middle) (see also Hemorrhage, subarachnoid) 430
    spinal cord — see Hemorrhage, spinal cord
  mesentery 568.81
  metritis 626.8
  midbrain (see also Hemorrhage, brain) 431
  mole 631
  mouth 528.9
  mucous membrane NEC 459.0
    newborn 728.8
  muscle 728.89
  nail (subungual) 703.8
  nasal turbinate 784.7
    newborn 772.8
  nasopharynx 478.29
  navel, newborn 772.3
  newborn 772.9
    adrenal 772.5
    alveolar (lung) 770.3
    brain (anoxic) (hypoxic) (due to birth trauma) 767.0
    cerebral (anoxic) (hypoxic) (due to birth trauma) 767.0
    conjunctiva 772.8
    cutaneous 772.6
    diathesis 776.0
    due to vitamin K deficiency 776.0
    gastrointestinal 772.4
    internal (organs) 772.8
    intestines 772.4
    intra-alveolar (lung) 770.3
    intracranial (from any perinatal cause) 767.0
    intraventricular (from any perinatal cause) 772.1
    lung 770.3
    pulmonary (massive) 770.3
    spinal cord, traumatic 767.4
    stomach 772.4
    subaponeurotic (massive) 767.1
    subarachnoid (from any perinatal cause) 772.2
    subconjunctival 772.8
    umbilicus 772.0
      slipped ligature 772.3
      vasa previa 772.0
  nipple 611.79
  nose 784.7
    newborn 772.8
  obstetrical surgical wound 674.3

Hemorrhage, hemorrhagic — *continued*
  omentum 568.89
    newborn 772.4
  optic nerve (sheath) 377.42
  orbit 376.32
  ovary 620.1
  oviduct 620.8
  pancreas 577.8
  parathyroid (gland) (spontaneous) 252.8
  parturition — see Hemorrhage, complicating, delivery
  penis 607.82
  pericardium, paricarditis 423.0
  perineal wound (obstetrical) 674.3
  peritoneum, peritoneal 459.0
  peritonsillar tissue 474.8
    after operation on tonsils 998.1
    due to infection 475
  petechial 782.7
  pituitary (gland) 253.8
  placenta NEC 641.9
    affecting fetus or newborn 762.1
    from surgical or instrumental damage 641.8
      affecting fetus or newborn 762.1
    previa 641.8
      affecting fetus or newborn 762.0
  pleura — see Hemorrhage, lung
  polioencephalitis, superior 265.1
  polymyositis — see Polymyositis
  pons (see also Hemorrhage, brain) 431
  pontine (see also Hemorrhage, brain) 431
  popliteal 459.0
  postcoital 626.7
  postextraction (dental) 998.1
  postmenopausal 627.1
  postnasal 784.7
  postoperative 998.1
  postpartum (atonic) (following delivery of placenta) 666.1
    delayed or secondary (after 24 hours) 666.2
    retained placenta 666.0
    third stage 666.0
  pregnancy (concealed) 641.9
    accidental 641.2
      affecting fetus or newborn 762.1
    affecting fetus or newborn 762.1
    before 22 completed weeks gestation 640.9
      affecting fetus or newborn 762.1
    due to
      abruptio placenta 641.2
        affecting fetus or newborn 762.1
      afibrinogenemia or other coagulation defect (conditions classifiable to 286.0-286.9) 641.3
        affecting fetus or newborn 762.1
      coagulation defect 641.3
        affecting fetus or newborn 762.1
      hyperfibrinolysis 641.3
        affecting fetus or newborn 762.1
      hypofibrinogenemia 641.3
        affecting fetus or newborn 762.1
      leiomyoma, uterus 641.8
        affecting fetus or newborn 762.1

Hemorrhage, hemorrhagic — *continued*
  pregnancy — *continued*
    due to — *continued*
      low-lying placenta 641.1
        affecting fetus or newborn 762.1
      marginal sinus (rupture) 641.2
        affecting fetus or newborn 762.1
      placenta previa 641.1
        affecting fetus or newborn 762.0
      premature separation of placenta (normally implanted) 641.2
        affecting fetus or newborn 762.1
      threatended abortion 640.0
        affecting fetus or newborn 762.1
      trauma 641.8
        affecting fetus or newborn 762.1
    early (before 22 completed weeks gestation) 640.9
      affecting fetus or newborn 762.1
    previous, affecting management of pregnancy or childbirth V23.4
    unavoidable — see Hemorrhage, pregnancy, due to placenta previa
  prepartum (mother) — see Hemorrhage, pregnancy
  preretinal, cause unspecified 362.81
  prostate 602.1
  puerperal (see also Hemorrhage, postpartum) 666.1
  pulmonary — see also Hemorrhage, lung
    newborn (massive) 770.3
    renal syndrome 446.21
  purpura (primary) (see also Purpura, thrombocytopenic) 287.3
  rectum (sphincter) 569.3
  recurring, following initial hemorrhage at time of injury 958.2
  renal 593.81
    pulmonary syndrome 446.21
  respiratory tract (see also Hemorrhage, lung) 786.3
  retina, retinal (deep) (superficial) (vessels) 362.81
    diabetic 250.5 [362.01]
    due to birth injury 772.8
  retrobulbar 376.89
  retroperitoneal 459.0
  retroplacental (see also Placenta, separation) 641.2
  scalp 459.0
    due to injury at birth 767.1
  scrotum 608.83
  secondry (nontraumatic) 459.0
    following initial hemorrhage at time of injury 958.2
  seminal vesicle 608.83
  skin 782.7
    newborn 772.6
  spermatic cord 608.83
  spinal (cord) 336.1
    aneurysm (ruptured) 336.1
    syphilitic 094.89
    due to birth injury 767.4
    fetus or newborn 767.4
  spleen 289.59
  spontaneous NEC 459.0
    petechial 782.7

Hemorrhage, hemorrhagic—
continued
  stomach 578.9
    newborn 772.4
    ulcer — *see* Ulcer, stomach, with hemorrhage
  subaponeurotic, newborn 767.1
    massive (birth injury) 767.1
  subarachnoid (nontraumatic) 430
    fetus or newborn (anoxic) (traumatic) 772.2
    puerperal, postpartum, childbirth 674.0
    traumatic — *see* Hemorrhage, brain, traumatic, subarachnoid
  subconjunctival 372.72
    due to birth injury 772.8
    newborn 772.8
  subcortical (*see also* Hemorrhage, brain) 431
  subcutaneous 782.7
  subdiaphragmatic 459.0
  subdural (nontraumatic) 432.1
    due to birth injury 767.0
    fetus or newborn (anoxic) (hypoxic) (due to birth trauma) 767.0
    puerperal, postpartum, childbirth 674.0
    spinal 336.1
    traumatic — *see* Hemorrhage, brain, traumatic, subdural
  subhyaloid 362.81
  subperiosteal 733.99
  subretinal 362.81
  subtentorial (*see also* Hemorrhage, subdural) 432.1
  subungual 703.8
    due to blood dyscrasia 287.8
  suprarenal (capsule) (gland) 255.4
    fetus or newborn 772.5
  tentorium (traumatic) — *see also* Hemorrhage, brain, traumatic
    fetus or newborn 767.0
    nontraumatic — *see* Hemorrhage, subdural
  testis 608.83
  thigh 459.0
  third stage 666.0
  thorax — *see* Hemorrhage, lung
  throat 784.8
  thrombocythemia 238.7
  thymus (gland) 254.8
  thyroid (gland) 246.3
    cyst 246.3
  tongue 529.8
  tonsil 474.8
    postoperative 998.1
  tooth socket (postextraction) 998.1
  trachea — *see* Hemorrhage, lung
  traumatic — *see also* nature of injury
    brain — *see* Hemorrhage, brain, traumatic
    recurring or secondary (following initial hemorrhage at time of injury) 958.2
  tuberculous NEC (*see also* Tuberculosis, pulmonary) 011.9
  tunica vaginalis 608.83
  ulcer — *see* Ulcer, by site, with hemorrhage
  umbilicus, umbilical cord 772.0
    after birth, newborn 772.3
    complicating delivery 663.8
      affecting fetus or newborn 772.0
    slipped ligature 772.3
    stump 772.3

Hemorrhage, hemorrhagic—
continued
  unavoidable (due to placenta previa) 641.1
    affecting fetus or newborn 762.0
  upper extremity 459.0
  urethra (idiopathic) 599.84
  uterus, uterine (abnormal) 626.9
    climacteric 627.0
    complicating delivery — *see* Hemorrhage, complicating delivery
    due to
      intrauterine contraceptive device 997.76
      perforating uterus 996.32
    functional or dysfunctional 626.8
    in pregnancy — *see* Hemorrhage, pregnancy
    intermenstrual 626.8
      irregular 626.6
      regular 626.5
    postmenopausal 627.1
    postpartum (*see also* Hemorrhage, postpartum) 666.1
    prepubertal 626.8
    pubertal 626.3
    puerperal (immediate) 666.1
  vagina 623.8
  vasa previa 663.5
    affecting fetus or newborn 772.0
  vas deferens 608.83
  ventricular (*see also* Hemorrhage, brain) 431
  vesical 596.8
  viscera 459.0
    newborn 772.8
  vitreous (humor) (intraocular) 379.23
  vocal cord 478.5
  vulva 624.8
Hemorrhoids (anus) (rectum) (without complication) 455.6
  bleeding, prolapsed, strangulated, or ulcerated NEC 455.8
    external 455.5
    internal 455.2
  complicated NEC 455.8
  complicating pregnancy and puerperium 671.8
  external 455.3
    with complication NEC 455.5
      bleeding, prolapsed, strangulated, or ulcerated 455.5
      thrombosed 455.4
  internal 455.0
    with complication NEC 455.2
      bleeding, prolapsed, strangulated, or ulcerated 455.2
      thrombosed 455.1
  residual skin tag 455.9
  sentinel pile 455.9
  thrombosed NEC 455.7
    external 455.4
    internal 455.1
Hemosalpinx 620.8
Hemosiderosis 275.0
  dietary 275.0
  pulmonary (idiopathic) 275.0 [516.1]
  transfusion NEC 999.8
    bone marrow 996.85
Hemospermia 608.83
Hemothorax 511.8
  bacterial, nontuberculous 511.1
  newborn 772.8
  nontuberculous 511.8
    bacterial 511.1
  pneumococcal 511.1

Hemothorax—*continued*
  staphylococcal 511.1
  streptococcal 511.1
  traumatic 860.2
    with
      open wound into thorax 860.3
      pneumothorax 860.4
        with open wound into thorax 860.5
  tuberculous (*see also* Tuberculosis, pleura) 012.0
Hemotympanum 385.89
Hench-Rosenberg syndrome (palindromic arthritis) (*see also* Rheumatism, palindromic) 719.3
Henle's warts 371.41
Henoch (-Schönlein)
  disease or syndrome (allergic purpura) 287.0
  purpura (allergic) 287.0
Henpue, henpuye 102.6
Heparitinuria 277.5
Hepar lobatum 095.3
Hepatalgia 573.8
Hepatic — *see also* condition
  flexure syndrome 569.89
Hepatitis 573.3
  acute (*see also* Necrosis, liver) 570
    alcoholic 571.1
    infective 070.1
      with hepatic coma 070.0
  alcoholic 571.1
  amebic — *see* Abscess, liver, amebic
  anicteric (acute) — *see* Hepatitis, viral
  antigen-associated (HAA) — *see* Hepatitis, viral, type B
  Australian antigen (positive) — *see* Hepatitis, viral, type B
  catarrhal (acute) 070.1
    with hepatic coma 070.0
    chronic 571.40
    newborn 070.1
      with hepatic coma 070.0
  chemical 573.3
  cholangiolitic 573.8
  cholestatic 573.8
  chronic 571.40
    active 571.49
      viral — *see* Hepatitis, viral
    aggressive 571.49
    persistent 571.41
    viral — *see* Hepatitis, viral
  cytomegalic inclusion virus 078.5 [573.1]
  diffuse 573.3
  "dirty needle" — *see* Hepatitis, viral
    with hepatic coma 070.2
  drug-induced 573.3
  due to
    Coxsackie 074.8 [573.1]
    cytomegalic inclusion virus 078.5 [573.1]
    infectious mononucleosis 075 [573.1]
    malaria 084.9 [573.2]
    mumps 072.71
    secondary syphilis 091.62
    toxoplasmosis (acquired) 130.5
      congenital (active) 771.2
  epidemic — *see* Hepatitis, viral, type A
  fetus or newborn 774.4
  fibrous (chronic) 571.49
    acute 570

Hepatitis—*continued*
  from injection, inoculation, or transfusion (blood) (other substance) (plasma) serum) (onset within 8 months after administration) — *see* Hepatitis, viral
  fulminant (viral) (*see also* Hepatitis, viral) 070.9
    with hepatic coma 070.6
    type A 070.1
      with hepatic coma 070.0
    type B — *see* Hepatitis, viral, type B
  giant cell (neonatal) 774.4
  hemorrhagic 573.8
  homologous serum — *see* Hepatitis, viral
  hypertrophic (chronic) 571.49
    acute 570
  infectious, infective (acute) (chronic) (subacute) 070.1
    with hepatic coma 070.0
  inoculation — *see* Hepatitis, viral
  interstitial (chronic) 571.49
    acute 570
  lupoid 571.49
  malarial 084.9 [573.2]
  malignant (*see also* Necrosis, liver) 570
  neonatal (toxic) 774.4
  newborn 774.4
  parenchymatous (acute) (*see also* Necrosis, liver) 570
  peliosis 573.3
  persistent, chronic 571.41
  plasma cell 571.49
  postimmunization — *see* Hepatitis, viral
  postnecrotic 571.49
  posttransfusion — *see* Hepatitis, viral
  recurrent 571.49
  septic 573.3
  serum — *see* Hepatitis, viral
    carrier (suspected) of V02.6
  subacute (*see also* Necrosis, liver) 570
  suppurative (diffuse) 572.0
  syphilitic (late) 095.3
    congenital (early) 090.0 [573.2]
    late 090.5 [573.2]
    secondary 091.62
  toxic (noninfectious) 573.3
    fetus or newborn 774.4
  tuberculous (*see also* Tuberculosis) 017.9
  viral (acute) (anicteric) (cholangiolitic) (cholestatic) (chronic) (subacute) 070.9
    with hepatic coma 070.6
    AU-SH type virus — *see* Hepatitis, viral, type B
    Australian antigen — *see* Hepatitis, viral, type B
    B-antigen — *see* Hepatitis, viral, type B
    Coxsackie 074.8 [573.1]
    cytomegalic inclusion 078.5 [573.1]
    IH (virus) — *see* Hepatitis, viral, type A
    infectious hepatitis, viral, type A
    serum hepatitis virus — *see* Hepatitis, viral, type B
    SH — *see* Hepatitis, viral, type B
    specified type NEC 070.59
      with hepatic coma 070.49
    type A 070.1
      with hepatic coma 070.0

Hepatitis

Hepatitis—*continued*
  viral—*continued*
    type B (acute) 070.30
      with
        hepatic coma 070.20
          with hepatitis delta 070.21
        hepatitis delta 070.31
          with hepatic coma 070.21
      chronic 070.32
        with
          hepatic coma 070.22
            with hepatitis delta 070.23
          hepatitis delta 070.33
            with hepatic coma 070.23
    type C (acute) 070.51
      with hepatic coma 070.41
      chronic 070.54
        with hepatic coma 070.44
    type delta (with hepatitis B carrier state) 070.52
      with
        active hepatitis B disease — *see* Hepatitis, viral, type B
        hepatic coma 070.42
    type E 070.53
      with hepatic coma 070.43
    vaccination and inoculation (prophylactic) V05.3
    Waldenstrom's (lupoid hepatitis) 571.49
Hepatization, lung (acute) — *see also* Pneumonia, lobar
  chronic (*see also* Fibrosis, lung) 515
Hepatoblastoma (M8970/3) 155.0
Hepatocarcinoma (M8170/3) 155.0
Hepatocholangiocarcinoma (M8180/3) 155.0
Hepatocholangioma, benign (M8180/0) 211.5
Hepatocholangitis 573.8
Hepatocystitis (*see also* Cholecystitis) 575.1
Hepatodystrophy 570
Hepatolenticular degeneration 275.1
Hepatolithiasis — *see* Choledocholithiasis
Hepatoma (malignant) (M8170/3) 155.0
  benign (M8170/0) 211.5
  congenital (M8970/3) 155.0
  embryonal (M8970/3) 155.0
Hepatomegalia glycogenica diffusa 271.0
Hepatomegaly (*see also* Hypertrophy, liver) 789.1
  congenital 751.69
    syphilitic 090.0
  due to Clonorchis sinensis 121.1
  Gaucher's 272.7
  syphilitic (congenital) 090.0
Hepatoptosis 573.8
Hepatorrhexis 573.8
Hepatosis, toxic 573.8
Hepatosplenomegaly 571.8
  due to S. japonicum 120.2
  hyperlipemic (Burger-Grutz type) 272.3
Herald patch 696.3
Hereditary — *see* condition
Heredodegeneration 330.9
  macular 362.70

Heredopathia atactica polyneuritiformis 356.3
Heredosyphilis (*see also* Syphilis, congenital) 090.9
Hermaphroditism (true) 752.7
  with specified chromosomal anomaly — *see* Anomaly, chromosomes, sex
Hernia, hernial (acquired) (recurrent) 553.9
  with
    gangrene (obstructed) NEC 551.9
    obstruction NEC 552.9
      and gangrene 551.9
  abdomen (wall) — *see* Hernia, ventral
  abdominal, specified site NEC 553.8
    with
      gangrene (obstructed) 551.8
      obstruction 552.8
        and gangrene 551.8
  appendix 553.8
    with
      gangrene (obstructed) 551.8
      obstruction 552.8
        and gangrene 551.8
  bilateral (inguinal) — *see* Hernia, inguinal
  bladder (sphincter)
    congenital (female) (male) 753.8
    female 618.0
    male 596.8
  brain 348.4
    congenital 742.0
  broad ligament 553.8
  cartilage, vertebral — *see* Displacement, intervertebral disc
  cerebral 348.4
    congenital 742.0
    endaural 742.0
  ciliary body 364.8
    traumatic 871.1
  colic 553.9
    with
      gangrene (obstructed) 551.9
      obstruction 552.9
        and gangrene 551.9
  colon 553.9
    with
      gangrene (obstructed) 551.9
      obstruction 552.9
        and gangrene 551.9
  colostomy (stoma) 569.6
  Cooper's (retroperitoneal) 553.8
    with
      gangrene (obstructed) 551.8
      obstruction 552.8
        and gangrene 551.8
  crural — *see* Hernia, femoral
  diaphragm, diaphragmatic 553.3
    with
      gangrene (obstructed) 551.3
      obstruction 552.3
        and gangrene 551.3
    congenital 756.6
    due to gross defect of diaphragm 756.6
    traumatic 862.0
      with open wound into cavity 862.1
  direct (inguinal) — *see* Hernia, inguinal
  disc, intervertebral — *see* Displacement, intervertebral disc

Hernia, hernial—*continued*
  diverticulum, intestine 553.9
    with
      gangrene (obstructed) 551.9
      obstruction 552.9
        and gangrene 551.9
  double (inguinal) — *see* Hernia, inguinal
  duodenojejunal 553.8
    with
      gangrene (obstructed) 551.8
      obstruction 552.8
        and gangrene 551.8
  en glissade — *see* Hernia, inguinal
  enterostomy (stoma) 569.6
  epigastric 553.29
    with
      gangrene (obstruction) 551.29
      obstruction 552.29
        and gangrene 551.29
    recurrent 553.21
      with
        gangrene (obstructed) 551.21
        obstruction 552.21
          and gangrene 551.21
  esophageal hiatus (sliding) 553.3
    with
      gangrene (obstructed) 551.3
      obstruction 552.3
        and gangrene 551.3
    congenital 750.6
  external (inguinal) — *see* Hernia, inguinal
  fallopian tube 620.4
  fascia 728.89
  fat 729.30
    eyelid 374.34
    orbital 374.34
    pad 729.30
      eye, eyelid 374.34
      knee 729.31
      orbit 374.34
      popliteal (space) 729.31
      specified site NEC 729.39
  femoral (unilateral) 553.00
    with
      gangrene (obstructed) 551.00
      obstruction 552.00
        with gangrene 551.0
    bilateral 553.02
      gangrenous (obstructed) 551.02
      obstructed 552.02
        with gangrene 551.02
      recurrent 553.03
        gangrenous (obstructed) 551.03
        obstructed 552.03
          with gangrene 551.03
    recurrent (unilateral) 553.01
      bilateral 553.03
        gangrenous (obstructed) 551.03
        obstructed 552.03
          with gangrene 551.03
      gangrenous (obstructed) 551.01
      obstructed 552.01
        with gangrene
  foramen
    Bochdalek 553.3
      with
        gangrene (obstructed) 551.3
        obstruction 552.3
          and gangrene 551.3
      congenital 756.6
    magnum 348.4

Hernia, hernial—*continued*
  foramen—*continued*
    Morgagni, morgagnian 553.3
      with
        gangrene 551.3
        obstruction 552.3
          and gangrene 551.3
      congenital 756.6
  funicular (umbilical) 553.1
    with
      gangrene (obstructed) 551.1
      obstruction 552.1
        and gangrene 551.1
    spermatic cord — *see* Hernia, inguinal
  gangrenous — *see* Hernia, by site, with gangrene
  gastrointestinal tract 553.9
    with
      gangrene (obstructed) 551.9
      obstruction 552.9
        and gangrene 551.9
  gluteal — *see* Hernia, femoral
  Gruber's (internal mesogastric) 553.8
    with
      gangrene (obstructed) 551.8
      obstruction 552.8
        and gangrene 551.8
  Hesselbach's 553.8
    with
      gangrene (obstructed) 551.8
      obstruction 552.8
        and gangrene 551.8
  hiatal (esophageal) (sliding) 553.3
    with
      gangrene (obstructed) 551.3
      obstruction 552.3
        and gangrene 551.3
    congenital 750.6
  incarcerated (*see also* Hernia, by site, with obstruction) 529.9
    gangrenous (*see also* Hernia, by site, with gangrene) 551.9
  incisional 553.21
    with
      gangrene (obstructed) 551.21
      obstruction 552.21
        and gangrene 551.21
    lumbar — *see* Hernia, lumbar
    recurrent 553.21
      with
        gangrene (obstructed) 551.21
        obstruction 552.21
          and gangrene 551.21
  indirect (inguinal) — *see* Hernia, inguinal
  infantile — *see* Hernia, inguinal
  infrapatellar fat pad 729.31
  inguinal (direct) (double) (encysted) (external) (funicular) (indirect) (infantile) (internal) (interstitial) (oblique) (scrotal) (sliding) 550.9

Note — Use the following fifth-digit subclassification with category 550:

0	unilateral or unspecified (not specified as recurrent)
1	unilateral or unspecified, recurrent
2	bilateral (not specified as recurrent)
3	bilateral, recurrent

Hernia, hernial—continued
  inguinal—continued
    with
      gangrene (obstructed) 550.0
      obstruction 550.1
        and gangrene 550.0
    internal 553.8
      with
        gangrene (obstructed) 551.8
        obstruction 552.8
          and gangrene 551.8
      inguinal — see Hernia, inguinal
    interstitial 553.9
      with
        gangrene (obstructed) 551.9
        obstruction 552.9
          and gangrene 551.9
      inguinal — see Hernia, inguinal
    intervertebral cartilage or disc — see Displacement, intervertebral disc
    intestine, intestinal 553.9
      with
        gangrene (obstructed) 551.9
        obstruction 552.9
          and gangrene 551.9
    intra-abdominal 553.9
      with
        gangrene (obstructed) 551.9
        obstruction 552.9
          and gangrene 551.9
    intraparietal 553.9
      with
        gangrene (obstructed) 551.9
        obstruction 552.9
          and gangrene 551.9
    iris 364.8
      traumatic 871.1
    irreducible (see also Hernia, by site, with obstruction) 552.9
      gangrenous (with obstruction) (see also Hernia, by site, with gangrene) 551.9
    ischiatic 553.8
      with
        gangrene (obstructed) 551.8
        obstruction 552.8
          and gangrene 551.8
    ischiorectal 553.8
      with
        gangrene (obstructed) 551.8
        obstruction 552.8
          and gangrene 551.8
    lens 379.32
      traumatic 871.1
    linea
      alba — see Hernia, epigastric
      semilunaris — see Hernia, spigelian
    Littre's (diverticular) 553.9
      with
        gangrene (obstructed) 551.9
        obstruction 552.9
          and gangrene 551.9
    lumbar 553.8
      with
        gangrene (obstructed) 551.8
        obstruction 552.8
          and gangrene 551.8
      intervertebral disc 722.10
    lung (subcutaneous) 518.89
      congenital 748.69
    mediastinum 519.3

Hernia, hernial—continued
  mesenteric (internal) 553.8
    with
      gangrene (obstructed) 551.8
      obstruction 552.8
        and gangrene 551.8
  mesocolon 553.8
    with
      gangrene (obstructed) 551.8
      obstruction 552.8
        and gangrene 551.8
  muscle (sheath) 728.89
  nucleus pulposus — see Displacement, intervertebral disc
  oblique (inguinal) — see Hernia, inguinal
  obstructive (see also Hernia, by site, with obstruction) 552.9
    gangrenous (with obstruction) (see also Hernia, by site, with gangrene) 551.9
  obturator 553.8
    with
      gangrene (obstructed) 551.8
      obstruction 552.8
        and gangrene 551.8
  omental 553.8
    with
      gangrene (obstructed) 551.8
      obstruction 552.8
        and gangrene 551.8
  orbital fat (pad) 374.34
  ovary 620.4
  oviduct 620.4
  paracolostomy (stoma) 569.6
  paraduodenal 553.8
    with
      gangrene (obstructed) 551.8
      obstruction 552.8
        and gangrene 551.8
  paraesophageal 553.3
    with
      gangrene (obstructed) 551.3
      obstruction 552.3
        and gangrene 551.3
    congenital 750.6
  parahiatal 553.3
    with
      gangrene (obstructed) 551.3
      obstruction 552.3
        and gangrene 551.3
  paraumbilical 553.1
    with
      gangrene (obstructed) 551.1
      obstruction 552.1
        and gangrene 551.1
  parietal 553.9
    with
      gangrene (obstructed) 551.9
      obstruction 552.9
        and gangrene 551.9
  perineal 553.8
    with
      gangrene (obstructed) 551.8
      obstruction 552.8
        and gangrene 551.8
  peritoneal sac, lesser 553.8
    with
      gangrene (obstructed) 551.8
      obstruction 552.8
        and gangrene 551.8
  popliteal fat pad 729.31

Hernia, hernial—continued
  postoperative 553.21
    with
      gangrene (obstructed) 551.21
      obstruction 552.21
        and gangrene 551.21
  pregnant uterus 654.4
  prevesical 596.8
  properitoneal 553.8
    with
      gangrene (obstructed) 551.8
      obstruction 552.8
        and gangrene 551.8
  pudendal 553.8
    with
      gangrene (obstructed) 551.8
      obstruction 552.8
        and gangrene 551.8
  rectovaginal 618.6
  retroperitoneal 553.8
    with
      gangrene (obstructed) 551.8
      obstruction 552.8
        and gangrene 551.8
  Richter's (parietal) 553.9
    with
      gangrene (obstructed) 551.9
      obstruction 552.9
        and gangrene 551.9
  Rieux's, Riex's (retrocecal) 553.8
    with
      gangrene (obstructed) 551.8
      obstruction 552.8
        and gangrene 551.8
  sciatic 553.8
    with
      gangrene (obstructed) 551.8
      obstruction 552.8
        and gangrene 551.8
  scrotum, scrotal — see Hernia, inguinal
  sliding (inguinal) — see also Hernia, inguinal
    hiatus — see Hernia, hiatal
  spigelian 553.29
    with
      gangrene (obstructed) 551.29
      obstruction 552.29
        and gangrene 551.29
  spinal (see also Spina bifida) 741.9
    with hydrocephalus 741.0
  strangulated (see also Hernia, by site, with obstruction) 552.9
    gangrenous (with obstruction) (see also Hernia, by site, with gangrene) 551.9
  supraumbilicus (linea alba) — see Hernia, epigastric
  tendon 727.9
  testis (nontraumatic) 095.8
  Treitz's (fossa) 553.8
    with
      gangrene (obstructed) 551.8
      obstruction 552.8
        and gangrene 551.8
  tunica
    albuginea 608.89
    vaginalis 752.8
  umbilicus, umbilical 553.1
    with
      gangrene (obstructed) 551.1
      obstruction 552.1
        and gangrene 551.1
  ureter 593.89
    with obstruction 593.4

Hernia, hernial—continued
  uterus 621.8
    pregnant 654.4
  vaginal (posterior) 618.6
  Velpeau's (femoral) (see also Hernia, femoral) 553.00
  ventral 553.20
    with
      gangrene (obstructed) 551.20
      obstruction 552.20
        and gangrene 551.20
    recurrent 553.21
      with
        gangrene (obstructed) 551.21
        obstruction 552.21
          and gangrene 551.21
  vesical
    congenital (female) (male) 753.8
    female 618.0
    male 596.8
  vitreous (into anterior chamber) 379.21
    traumatic 871.1
Herniation — see also Hernia
  brain (stem) 348.4
  cerebral 348.4
  gastric mucosa (into duodenal bulb) 537.89
  mediastinum 519.3
  nucleus pulposus — see Displacement, intervertebral disc
Herpangina 074.0
Herpes, herpetic 054.9
  auricularis (zoster) 053.71
    simplex 054.73
  blepharitis (zoster) 053.20
    simplex 054.41
  circinate 110.5
  circinatus 110.5
    bullous 694.5
  conjunctiva (simplex) 054.43
    zoster 053.21
  cornea (simplex) 054.43
    disciform (simplex) 054.43
    zoster 053.21
  encephalitis 054.3
  eye (zoster) 053.29
    simplex 054.40
  eyelid (zoster) 053.20
    simplex 054.41
  febrilis 054.9
  fever 054.9
  geniculate ganglionitis 053.11
  genital, genitalis 054.10
    specified site NEC 054.19
  gestationis 646.8
  gingivostomatitis 054.2
  iridocyclitis (simplex) 054.44
    zoster 053.22
  iris (any site) 695.1
  iritis (simplex) 054.44
  keratitis (simplex) 054.43
    dendritic 054.42
    disciform 054.43
    interstitial 054.43
    zoster 053.21
  keratoconjunctivitis (simplex) 054.43
    zoster 053.21
  labialis 054.9
    meningococcal 036.89
  lip 054.9
  meningitis (simplex) 054.72
    zoster 053.0
  ophthalmicus (zoster) 053.20
    simplex 054.40
  otitis externa (zoster) 053.71
    simplex 054.73
  penis 054.13
  perianal 054.10
  pharyngitis 054.79
  progenitalis 054.10
  scrotum 054.19

Herpes, herpetic—continued
  septicemia 054.4
  simplex 054.9
    complicated 054.8
      ophthalmic 054.40
        specified NEC 054.49
      specified NEC 054.79
    congenital 771.2
    external ear 054.73
    keratitis 054.43
      dendritic 054.42
    meningitis 054.72
    neuritis 054.79
    specified complication NEC 054.79
    ophthalmic 054.49
    visceral 054.71
  stomatitis 054.2
  tonsurans 110.0
    maculosus (of Hebra) 696.3
  visceral 054.71
  vulva 054.12
  vulvovaginitis 054.11
  whitlow 054.6
  zoster 053.9
    auricularis 053.71
    complicated 053.8
      specified NEC 053.79
    conjunctiva 053.21
    cornea 053.21
    ear 053.71
    eye 053.29
    geniculate 053.11
    keratitis 053.21
      interstitial 053.21
    neuritis 053.10
    ophthalmicus(a) 053.20
    oticus 053.71
    otitis externa 053.71
    specified complication NEC 053.79
    specified site NEC 053.9
  zosteriform, intermediate type 053.9

Herrick's
  anemia (hemoglobin S disease) 282.61
  syndrome (hemoglobin S disease) 282.61

Hers' disease (glycogenosis VI) 271.0
Herter's infantilism (nontropical sprue) 579.0
Herter (-Gee) **disease or syndrome** (nontropical sprue) 579.0
Herxheimer's disease (diffuse idiopathic cutaneous atrophy) 701.8
Herxheimer's reaction 995.0
Hesselbach's hernia — see Hernia, Hesselbach's
Heterochromia (congenital) 743.46
  acquired 364.53
  cataract 366.33
  cyclitis 364.21
  hair 704.3
  iritis 364.21
  retained metallic foreign body 360.62
    magnetic 360.52
  uveitis 364.21
Heterophoria 378.40
  alternating 378.45
  vertical 378.43
Heterophyes, small intestine 121.6
Heterophyiasis 121.6
Heteropsia 368.8
Heterotopia, heterotopic — see also Malposition, congenital
  cerebralis 742.4
  pancreas, pancreatic 751.7
  spinalis 742.59

Heterotropia 378.30
  intermittent 378.20
    vertical 378.31
  vertical (constant) (intermittent) 378.31
Heubner's disease 094.89
Heubner-Herter disease or syndrome (nontropical sprue) 579.0
Hexadactylism 755.0
Heyd's syndrome (hepatorenal) 572.4
Hibernoma (M8880/0) — see Lipoma
Hiccough 786.8
  epidemic 078.89
  psychogenic 306.1
Hiccup (see also Hiccough) 786.8
Hicks (-Braxton) **contractures** 644.1
Hidradenitis (axillaris) (suppurative) 705.83
Hidradenoma (nodular) (M8400/0) — see also Neoplasm, skin, benign
  clear cell (M8402/0) — see Neoplasm, skin, benign
  papillary (M8405/0) — see Neoplasm, skin, benign
Hidrocystoma (M8404/0) — see Neoplasm, skin, benign
High
  A_2 anemia 282.4
  altitude effects 993.2
    anoxia 993.2
    on
      ears 993.0
      sinuses 993.1
    polycythemia 289.0
  arch
    foot 755.67
    palate 750.26
  artery (arterial) tension (see also Hypertension) 401.9
    without diagnosis of hypertension 796.2
  basal metabolic rate (BMR) 794.7
  blood pressure (see also Hypertension) 401.9
    incidental reading (isolated) (nonspecific), no diagnosis of hypertension 796.2
  compliance bladder 596.4
  diaphragm (congenital) 756.6
  frequency deafness (congenital) (regional) 389.8
  head at term 652.5
    affecting fetus or newborn 763.1
    causing obstructed labor 660.0
      affecting fetus or newborn 763.1
  output failure (cardiac) (see also Failure, heart) 428.9
  oxygen-affinity hemoglobin 289.0
  palate 750.26
  risk
    family situation V61.9
      specified circumstance NEC V61.8
    individual NEC V62.89
    infant NEC V20.1
    patient taking drugs
      (prescribed) V67.51
      nonprescribed (see also Abuse, drugs, nondependent) 305.9
    pregnancy V23.9
      inadequate prenatal care V23.7
      specified problem NEC V23.8
  temperature (of unknown origin) (see also Pyrexia) 780.6
  thoracic rib 756.3

Hildenbrand's disease (typhus) 081.9
Hilger's syndrome 337.0
Hill diarrhea 579.1
Hilliard's lupus (see also Tuberculosis) 017.0
Hilum — see condition
Hip — see condition
Hippel's disease (retinocerebral angiomatosis) 759.6
Hippus 379.49
Hirschfeld's disease (acute diabetes mellitus) (see also Diabetes) 250.0
Hirschsprung's disease or megacolon (congenital) 751.3
Hirsuties (see also Hypertrichosis) 704.1
Hirsutism (see also Hypertrichosis) 704.1
Hirudiniasis (external) (internal) 134.2
His-Werner disease (trench fever) 083.1
Hiss-Russell dysentery 004.1
Histamine cephalgia 346.2
Histidinemia 270.5
Histidinuria 270.5
Histiocytoma (M8832/0) — see also Neoplasm, skin, benign
  fibrous (M8830/0) — see also Neoplasm, skin, benign
  atypical (M8830/1) — see Neoplasm, connective tissue, uncertain behavior
  malignant (M8830/3) — see Neoplasm, connective tissue, malignant
Histiocytosis (acute) (chronic) (subacute) 277.8
  acute differentiated progressive (M9722/3) 202.5
  cholesterol 277.8
  essential 277.8
  lipid, lipoid (essential) 272.7
  lipochrome (familial) 288.1
  malignant (M9720/3) 202.3
  X (chronic) 277.8
    acute (progressive) (M9722/3) 202.5
Histoplasmosis 115.90
  with
    endocarditis 115.94
    meningitis 115.91
    pericarditis 115.93
    pneumonia 115.95
    retinitis 115.92
    specified manifestation NEC 115.99
  African (due to Histoplasma duboisii) 115.10
    with
      endocarditis 115.14
      meningitis 115.11
      pericarditis 115.13
      pneumonia 115.15
      retinitis 115.12
      specified manifestation NEC 115.19
  American (due to Histoplasma capsulatum) 115.00
    with
      endocarditis 115.04
      meningitis 115.01
      pericarditis 115.03
      pneumonia 115.05
      retinitis 115.02
      specified manifestation NEC 115.09
  Darling's — see Histoplasmosis, American
  large form (see also Histoplasmosis, African) 115.10

Histoplasmosis—continued
  lung 115.05
  small form (see also Histoplasmosis, American) 115.00
History (personal) of
  affective psychosis V11.1
  alcoholism V11.3
    specified as drinking problem (see also Abuse, drugs, nondependent) 305.0
  allergy to
    analgesic agent NEC V14.6
    anesthetic NEC V14.4
    antibiotic agent NEC V14.1
      penicillin V14.0
    anti-infective agent NEC V14.3
    diathesis V15.0
    drug V14.9
      specified type NEC V14.8
    medicinal agents V14.9
      specified type NEC V14.8
    narcotic agent NEC V14.5
    penicillin V14.0
    radiographic dye V15.0
    serum V14.7
    specified nonmedicinal agents NEC V15.0
    sulfa V14.2
    sulfonamides V14.2
    therapeutic agent NEC V15.0
    vaccine V14.7
  anemia V12.3
  arthritis V13.4
  blood disease V12.3
  calculi, urinary V13.01 ◆
  cardiovascular disease V12.5
    myocardial infarction 412
  child abuse V61.21
  cigarette smoking V15.82 ◆
  circulatory system disease V12.5
    myocardial infarction 412
  congenital malformation V13.6
  contraception V15.7
  diathesis, allergic V15.0
  digestive system disease V12.70 ▼
    peptic ulcer V12.71
    polyps, colonic V12.72
    specified NEC V12.79 ▲
  disease (of) V13.9
    blood V12.3
    blood-forming organs V12.3
    cardiovascular system V12.5
    circulatory system V12.5
    digestive system V12.70 ▼
      peptic ulcer V12.71
      polyps, colonic V12.72
      specified NEC V12.79
    infectious V12.00
      malaria V12.03
      poliomyelitis V12.02
      specified NEC V12.09
      tuberculosis V12.01
    parasitic V12.00
      specified NEC V12.09 ▲
    respiratory system V12.6
    skin V13.3
    specified site NEC V13.8
    subcutaneous tissue V13.3
    trophoblastic V13.1
      affecting management of pregnant V23.1
  disorder (of) V13.9
    endocrine V12.2
    genital system V13.2
    hematological V12.3
    immunity V12.2
    mental V11.9
      affective type V11.1
      manic-depressive V11.1
      neurosis V11.2
      schizophrenia V11.0
      specified type NEC V11.8
    metabolic V12.2
    musculoskeletal NEC V13.5
    nervous system V12.4

History—continued
disorder (of)—continued
  obstetric V13.2
    affecting management of current pregnancy V23.4
  sense organs V12.4
  specified site NEC V13.8
  urinary system V13.00 ▼
    calculi V13.01
    specified NEC V13.09 ▲
drug use
  nonprescribed (see also Abuse, drugs, nondependent) 305.9
  patent (see also Abuse, drugs, nondependent) 305.9
effect NEC of external cause V15.89
endocrine disorder V12.2
family
  allergy V19.6
  anemia V18.2
  arteriosclerosis V17.4
  arthritis V17.7
  asthma V17.5
  blindness V19.0
  blood disorder NEC V18.3
  cardiovascular disease V17.4
  cerebrovascular disease V17.1
  chronic respiratory condition NEC V17.6
  congenital anomalies V19.5
  consanguinity V19.7
  coronary artery disease V17.3
  cystic fibrosis V18.1
  deafness V19.2
  diabetes mellitus V18.0
  digestive disorders V18.5
  disease or disorder (of)
    allergic V19.6
    blood NEC V18.3
    cardiovascular NEC V17.4
    cerebrovascular V17.1
    coronary artery V17.3
    digestive V18.5
    ear NEC V19.3
    endocrine V18.1
    eye NEC V19.1
    genitourinary NEC V18.7
    hypertensive V17.4
    infectious V18.8
    ischemic heart V17.3
    kidney V18.6
    mental V17.0
    metabolic V18.1
    musculoskeletal NEC V17.8
    neurological NEC V17.2
    parasitic V18.8
    psychiatric condition V17.0
    skin condition V19.4
  ear disorder NEC V19.1
  endocrine disease V18.1
  epilepsy V17.2
  eye disorder NEC V19.1
  genitourinary disease NEC V18.7
  glomerulonephritis V18.6
  gout V18.1
  hay fever V17.6
  hearing loss V19.2
  hematopoietic neoplasia V16.7
  Hodgkin's disease V16.7
  Huntington's chorea V17.2
  hydrocephalus V19.5
  hypertension V17.4
  infectious disease V18.8
  ischemic heart disease V17.3
  kidney disease V18.6
  leukemia V16.6
  lymphatic malignant neoplasia NEC V16.7
  malignant neoplasm (of) NEC V16.9
    anorectal V16.0
    anus V16.0

History—continued
family—continued
  malignant neoplasm—continued
    appendix V16.0
    bladder V16.5
    bone V16.8
    brain V16.8
    breast V16.3
      male V16.8
    bronchus V16.1
    cecum V16.0
    cervix V16.4
    colon V16.0
    duodenum V16.0
    esophagus V16.0
    eye V16.8
    gallbladder V16.0
    gastrointestinal tract V16.0
    genital organs V16.4
    hemopoietic NEC V16.7
    ileum V16.0
    ilium V16.8
    intestine V16.0
    intrathoracic organs NEC V16.2
    kidney V16.5
    larynx V16.2
    liver V16.0
    lung V16.1
    lymphatic NEC V16.7
    ovary V16.4
    oviduct V16.4
    pancreas V16.0
    penis V16.4
    prostate V16.4
    rectum V16.0
    respiratory organs NEC V16.2
    skin V16.8
    specified site NEC V16.8
    stomach V16.0
    testis V16.4
    trachea V16.1
    ureter V16.5
    urinary organs V16.5
    uterus V16.4
    vagina V16.4
    vulva 16.4
  mental retardation V18.4
  metabolic disease NEC V18.1
  mongolism V19.5
  multiple myeloma V16.7
  musculoskeletal disease NEC V17.8
  nephritis V18.6
  nephrosis V18.6
  parasitic disease V18.8
  psychiatric disorder V17.0
  psychosis V17.0
  retardation, mental V18.4
  retinitis pigmentosa V19.1
  schizophrenia V17.0
  skin conditions V19.4
  specified condition NEC V19.8
  stroke (cerebrovascular) V17.1
  visual loss V19.0
genital system disorder V13.2
health hazard V15.9
  specified cause NEC V15.89
Hodgkin's disease V10.72
immunity disorder V12.2
infectious disease V12.00 ▼
  malaria V12.03
  poliomyelitis V12.02
  specified NEC V12.09
  tuberculosis V12.01 ▲
injury NEC V15.5
insufficient prenatal care V23.7
irradiation V15.3
leukemia V10.60
  lymphoid V10.61
  monocytic V10.63
  myeloid V10.62
  specified type NEC V10.69
little or no prenatal care V23.7

History—continued
lymphosarcoma V10.71
malaria V12.03 ◆
malignant neoplasm (of) V10.9
  accessory sinus V10.22
  adrenal V10.88
  anus V10.06
  bile duct V10.09
  bladder V10.51
  bone V10.81
  brain V10.85
  breast V10.3
  bronchus V10.11
  cervix uteri V10.41
  colon V10.05
  connective tissue NEC V10.89
  corpus uteri V10.42
  digestive system V10.00
    specified part NEC V10.09
  duodenum V10.09
  endocrine gland NEC V10.88
  esophagus V10.03
  eye V10.84
  fallopian tube V10.44
  female genital organ V10.40
    specified site NEC V10.44
  gallbladder V10.09
  gastrointestinal tract V10.00
  gum V10.02
  hematopoietic NEC V10.79
  hypopharynx V10.02
  ileum V10.09
  intrathoracic organs NEC V10.20
  jejunum V10.09
  kidney V10.52
  large intestine V10.05
  larynx V10.21
  lip V10.02
  liver V10.07
  lung V10.11
  lymphatic NEC V10.79
  lymph glands or nodes NEC V10.79
  male genital organ V10.45
    specified site NEC V10.49
  mediastinum V10.29
  melanoma (of skin) V10.82
  middle ear V10.22
  mouth V10.02
    specified part NEC V10.02
  nasal cavities V10.22
  nasopharynx V10.02
  nervous system NEC V10.86
  nose V10.22
  oropharynx V10.02
  ovary V10.43
  pancreas V10.09
  parathyroid V10.88
  penis V10.49
  pharynx V10.02
  pineal V10.88
  pituitary V10.88
  placenta V10.44
  pleura V10.29
  prostate V10.46
  rectosigmoid junction V10.06
  rectum V10.06
  respiratory organs NEC V10.20
  salivary gland V10.02
  skin V10.83
    melanoma V10.82
  small intestine NEC V10.09
  soft tissue NEC V10.89
  specified site NEC V10.89
  stomach V10.04
  testis V10.47
  thymus V10.29
  thyroid V10.87
  tongue V10.01
  trachea V10.12
  ureter V10.59
  urethra V10.59
  urinary organ V10.50
  uterine adnexa V10.44
  uterus V10.42

History—continued
malignant neoplasm—continued
  vagina V10.44
  vulva V10.44
manic-depressive psychosis V11.1
mental disorder V11.9
  affective type V11.1
  manic-depressive V11.1
  neurosis V11.2
  schizophrenia V11.0
  specified type NEC V11.8
metabolic disorder V12.2
musculoskeletal disorder NEC V13.5
myocardial infarction 412
nervous system disorder V12.4
neurosis V11.2
noncompliance with medical treatment V15.81
nutritional deficiency V12.1
obstetric disorder V13.2
  affecting management of current pregnancy V23.4
parasitic disease V12.00 ▼
  specified NEC V12.09 ▲
perinatal problems V13.7
poisoning V15.6
poliomyelitis V12.02 ▼
polyps, colonic V12.72 ▲
poor obstetric V23.4
psychiatric disorder V11.9
  affective type V11.1
  manic-depressive V11.1
  neurosis V11.2
  schizophrenia V11.0
  specified type NEC V11.8
psychological trauma V15.4
psychoneurosis V11.2
radiation therapy V15.3
respiratory system disease V12.6
reticulosarcoma V10.71
schizophrenia V11.0
skin disease V13.3
smoking (tobacco) V15.82 ◆
subcutaneous tissue disease V13.3
surgery (major) to
  great vessels V15.1
  heart V15.1
  major organs NEC V15.2
tobacco use V15.82 ◆
trophoblastic disease V13.1
  affecting management of pregnancy V23.1
tuberculosis V12.01 ▼
ulcer, peptic V12.71
urinary system disorder V13.00
  calculi V13.01
  specified NEC V13.09 ▲
HIV infection (disease) (illness) — see Human immunodeficiency virus (disease) (illness) (infection)
Hives (bold) (see also Urticaria) 708.9
Hoarseness 784.49
Hobnail liver — see Cirrhosis, portal
Hobo, hoboism V60.0
Hodgkins
  disease (M9650/3) 201.9
    lymphocytic
      depletion (M9653/3) 201.7
        diffuse fibrosis (M9654/3) 201.7
        reticular type (M9655/3) 201.7
      predominance (M9651/3) 201.4
    lymphocytic-histiocytic predominance (M9651/3) 201.4
    mixed cellularity (M9652/3) 201.6

Hodgkins—continued
   disease—continued
      nodular sclerosis (M9656/3) 201.5
         cellular phase (M9657/3) 201.5
      granuloma (M9661/3) 201.1
      lymphogranulomatosis (M9650/3) 201.9
      lymphoma (M9650/3) 201.9
      lymphosarcoma (M9650/3) 201.9
      paragranuloma (M9660/3) 201.0
      sarcoma (M9662/3) 201.2
Hodgson's disease (aneurysmal dilatation of aorta) 441.9
   ruptured 441.5
Hodi-potsy 111.0
Hoffa (-Kastert) disease or syndrome (liposynovitis prepatellaris) 272.8
Hoffman's syndrome 244.9 [359.5]
Hoffmann-Bouveret syndrome (paroxysmal tachycardia) 427.2
Hole
   macula 362.54
   optic disc, crater-like 377.22
   retina (macula) 362.54
      round 361.31
         with detachment 361.01
Holla disease (see also Spherocytosis) 282.0
Holländer-Simons syndrome (progressive lipodystrophy) 272.6
Hollow foot (congenital) 754.71
   acquired 736.73
Holmes' syndrome (visual disorientation) 368.16
Holoprosencephaly 742.2
   due to
      trisomy 13 758.1
      trisomy 18 758.2
Holthouse's hernia — see Hernia, inguinal
Homesickness 309.89
Homocystinemia 270.4
Homocystinuria 270.4
Homologous serum jaundice (prophylactic) (therapeutic) — see Hepatitis, viral
Homosexuality — omit code
   ego-dystonic 302.0
   pedophilic 302.2
   problems with 302.0
Homozygous Hb-S disease 282.61
Honeycomb lung 518.89
   congenital 748.4
Hong Kong ear 117.3
HOOD (hereditary osteo-onychodyplasia) 756.89
Hooded
   clitoris 752.49
   penis 752.8
Hookworm (anemia) (disease) (infestation) — see Ancylostomiasis
Hoppe-Goldflam syndrome 358.0
Hordeolum (external) (eyelid) 373.11
   internal 373.12
Horn
   cutaneous 702.8
      cheek 702.8
      eyelid 702.8
      penis 702.8
   iliac 756.89
   nail 703.8
      congenital 757.5
   papillary 700

Horner's
   syndrome (see also Neuropathy, peripheral, autonomic) 337.9
      traumatic 954.0
   teeth 520.4
Horseshoe kidney (congenital) 753.3
Horton's
   disease (temporal arteritis) 446.5
   headache or neuralgia 346.2
Hospitalism (in children) NEC 309.83
Hourglass contraction, contracture
   bladder 596.8
   gallbladder 575.2
      congenital 751.69
   stomach 536.8
      congenital 750.7
      psychogenic 306.4
   uterus 661.4
      affecting fetus or newborn 763.7
Household circumstance affecting care V60.9
   specified type NEC V60.8
Housemaid's knee 727.2
Housing circumstance affecting care V60.9
   specified type NEC V60.8
Huchard's disease (continued arterial hypertension) 401.9
Hudson-Stähli lines 371.11
Huguier's disease (uterine fibroma) 218.9
Hum, venous — omit code
Human bite (open wound) — see also Wound, open, by site
   intact skin surface — see Contusion
Human immunodeficiency virus (disease) (illness) 042 ▼
   infection V08
      with symptoms, symptomatic 042 ▲
Human immunodeficiency virus-2 infection 079.53
Human immunovirus (disease) (illness) (infection) — see Human immunodeficiency virus (disease) (illness) (infection)
Human T-cell lymphotrophic virus-I infection 079.51
Human T-cell lymphotrophic virus-II infection 079.52
Human T-cell lymphotrophic virus-III (disease) (illness) (infection) — see Human immunodeficiency virus (disease) (illness) (infection)
HTLV-I infection 079.51
HTLV-II infection 079.52
HTLV-III (disease) (illness) (infection) — see Human immunodeficiency virus (disease) (illness) (infection)
HTLV-III/LAV (disease) (illness) (infection) — see Human immunodeficiency virus (disease) (illness) (infection)
Humpback (acquired) 737.9
   congenital 756.19
Hunchback (acquired) 737.9
   congenital 756.19
Hunger 994.2
   air, psychogenic 306.1
   disease 251.1
Hunner's ulcer (see also Cystitis) 595.1

Hunt's
   neuralgia 053.11
   syndrome (herpetic geniculate ganglionitis) 053.11
   dyssynergia cerebellaris myoclonica 334.2
Hunter's glossitis 529.4
Hunter (-Hurler) syndrome (mucopolysaccharidosis II) 277.5
Hunterian chancre 091.0
Huntington's
   chorea 333.4
   disease 333.4
Huppert's disease (multiple myeloma) (M9730/3) 203.0
Hurler (-Hunter) disease or syndrome (mucopolysaccharidosis II) 277.5
Hürthle cell
   adenocarcinoma (M8290/3) 193
   adenoma (M8290/0) 226
   carcinoma (M8290/3) 193
   tumor (M8290/0) 226
Hutchinson's
   disease meaning
      angioma serpiginosum 709.1
      cheiropompholyx 705.81
      prurigo estivalis 692.72
      summer eruption, or summer prurigo 692.72
   incisors 090.5
   melanotic freckle (M8742/2) — see also Neoplasm, skin, in situ
      malignant melanoma in (M8742/3) — see Melanoma
   teeth or incisors (congenital syphilis) 090.5
Hutchinson-Boeck disease or syndrome (sarcoidosis) 135
Hutchinson-Gilford disease or syndrome (progeria) 259.8
Hyaline
   degeneration (diffuse) (generalized) 728.9
      localized — see Degeneration, by site
   membrane (disease) (lung) (newborn) 769
Hyalinosis cutis et mucosae 272.8
Hyalin plaque, sclera, senile 379.16
Hyalitis (asteroid) 379.22
   syphilitic 095.8
Hydatid
   cyst or tumor — see also Echinococcus
      fallopian tube 752.11
   mole — see Hydatidiform mole
   Morgagni (congenital) 752.8
      fallopian tube 752.11
Hydatidiform mole (benign) (complicating pregnancy) (delivered) (undelivered) 630
   invasive (M9100/1) 236.1
   malignant (M9100/1) 236.1
   previous, affecting management of pregnancy V23.1
Hydatidosis — see Echinococcus
Hyde's disease (prurigo nodularis) 698.3
Hydradenitis 705.83
Hydradenoma (M8400/0) — see Hidradenoma
Hydralazine lupus or syndrome
   correct substance properly administered 695.4
   overdose or wrong substance given or taken 972.6

Hydramnios 657
   affecting fetus or newborn 761.3
Hydrancephaly 742.3
   with spina bifida (see also Spina bifida) 741.0
Hydranencephaly 742.3
   with spina bifida (see also Spina bifida) 741.0
Hydrargyrism NEC 985.0
Hydrarthrosis (see also Effusion, joint) 719.0
   gonococcal 098.50
   intermittent (see also Rheumatism, palindromic) 719.3
   of yaws (early) (late) 102.6
   syphilitic 095.8
      congenital 090.5
Hydremia 285.9
Hydrencephalocele (congenital) 742.0
Hydrencephalomeningocele (congenital) 742.0
Hydroa 694.0
   aestivale 692.72
   gestationis 646.8
   herpetiformis 694.0
   pruriginosa 694.0
   vacciniforme 692.72
Hydroadenitis 705.83
Hydrocalycosis (see also Hydronephrosis) 591
   congenital 753.2
Hydrocalyx (see also Hydronephrosis) 591
Hydrocele (calcified) (chylous) (idiopathic) (infantile) (inguinal canal) (recurrent) (senile) (spermatic cord) (testis) (tunica vaginalis) 603.9
   canal of Nuck (female) 629.1
      male 603.9
   congenital 778.6
   encysted 603.0
      congenital 778.6
   female NEC 629.8
   infected 603.1
   round ligament 629.8
   specified type NEC 603.8
      congenital 778.6
   spinalis (see also Spina bifida) 741.9
   vulva 624.8
Hydrocephalic fetus
   affecting management or pregnancy 655.0
   causing disproportion 653.6
      with obstructed labor 660.1
         affecting fetus or newborn 763.1
Hydrocephalus (acquired) (external) (internal) (malignant) (noncommunicating) (obstructive) (recurrent) 331.4
   aqueduct of Sylvius structure 742.3
      with spina bifida (see also Spina bifida) 741.0
   chronic 742.3
      with spina bifida (see also Spina bifida) 741.0
   communicating 331.3
   congenital (external) (internal) 742.3
      with spina bifida (see also Spina bifida) 741.0
   due to
      structure of aqueduct of Sylvius 742.3
         with spina bifida (see also Spina bifida) 741.0
      toxoplasmosis (congenital) 771.2
   fetal affecting management of pregnancy 655.0

Hydrocephalus—continued
  foramen Magendie block
      (acquired) 331.3
  congenital 742.3
    with spina bifida (see also
        Spina bifida) 741.0
  newborn 742.3
    with spina bifida (see also
        Spina bifida) 741.0
  otitic 331.4
  syphilitic, congenital 090.49
  tuberculous (see also
      Tuberculosis) 013.8
Hydrocolpos (congenital) 623.8
Hydrocystoma (M8404/0) — see
    Neoplasm, skin, benign
Hydroencephalocele (congenital)
    742.0
Hydroencephalomeningocele
    (congenital) 742.0
Hydrohematopneumothorax (see
    also Hemothorax) 511.8
Hydromeningitis — see Meningitis
Hydromeningocele (spinal) (see also
    Spina bifida) 741.9
  cranial 742.0
Hydrometra 621.8
Hydrometrocolpos 623.8
Hydromicrocephaly 742.1
Hydromphalus (congenital) (since
    birth) 757.39
Hydromyelia 742.53
Hydromyelocele (see also Spina
    bifida) 741.9
Hydronephrosis 591
  atrophic 591
  congenital 753.2
  due to S. hematobium 120.0
  early 591
  functionless (infected) 591
  infected 591
  intermittent 591
  primary 591
  secondary 591
  tuberculous (see also
      Tuberculosis) 016.0
Hydropericarditis (see also
    Pericarditis) 423.9
Hydropericardium (see also
    Pericarditis) 423.9
Hydroperitoneum 789.5
Hydrophobia 071
Hydrophthalmos (see also
    Buphthalmia) 743.20
Hydropneumohemothorax (see also
    Hemothorax) 511.8
Hydropneumopericarditis (see also
    Pericarditis) 423.9
Hydropneumopericardium (see also
    Pericarditis) 423.9
Hydropneumothorax 511.8
  nontuberculous 511.8
    bacterial 511.1
    pneumococcal 511.1
    staphylococcal 511.1
    streptococcal 511.1
  traumatic 860.0
    with open wound into thorax
        860.1
  tuberculous (see also
      Tuberculosis, pleura) 012.0
Hydrops 782.3
  abdominis 789.5
  amnii (complicating pregnancy)
      (see also Hydramnios) 657
  articulorum intermittens (see also
      Rheumatism, palindromic)
      719.3
  cardiac (see also Failure, heart,
      congestive) 428.0
  congenital — see Hydrops, fetalis
  endolymphatic (see also Disease,
      Ménière's) 386.00

Hydrops—continued
  fetal(is) or newborn 778.0
    due to isoimmunization 773.3
    not due to isoimmunization
        778.0
  gallbladder 575.3
  idiopathic (fetus or newborn)
      778.0
  joint (see also Effusion, joint)
      719.0
  labyrinth (see also Disease,
      Ménière's) 386.00
  meningeal NEC 331.4
  nutritional 262
  pericardium — see Pericarditis
  pleura (see also Hydrothorax)
      511.8
  renal (see also Nephrosis) 581.9
  spermatic cord (see also
      Hydrocele) 603.9
Hydropyonephrosis (see also
    Pyelitis) 590.80
  chronic 590.00
Hydrorachis 742.53
Hydrorrhea (nasal) 478.1
  gravidarum 658.1
  pregnancy 658.1
Hydrosadenitis 705.83
Hydrosalpinx (fallopian tube)
    (follicularis) 614.1
Hydrothorax (double) (pleural) 511.8
  chylous (nonfilarial) 457.8
    filaria (see also Infestation,
        filarial) 125.9
  nontuberculous 511.8
    bacterial 511.1
    pneumococcal 511.1
    staphylococcal 511.1
    streptococcal 511.1
  traumatic 862.29
    with open wound into thorax
        862.39
  tuberculous (see also
      Tuberculosis, pleura) 012.0
Hydroureter 593.5
  congenital 753.2
Hydroureteronephrosis (see also
    Hydronephrosis) 591
Hydrourethra 599.84
Hydroxykynureninuria 270.2
Hydroxyprolinemia 270.8
Hydroxyprolinuria 270.8
Hygroma (congenital) (cystic)
    (M9173/0) 228.1
  prepatellar 727.3
  subdural — see Hematoma,
      subdural
Hymen — see condition
Hymenolepiasis (diminuta)
    (infection) (infestation) (nana)
    123.6
Hymenolepis (diminuta) (infection)
    (infestation) (nana) 123.6
Hypalgesia (see also Disturbance,
    sensation) 782.0
Hyperabduction syndrome 447.8
Hyperacidity, gastric 536.8
  psychogenic 306.4
Hyperactive, hyperactivity
  basal cell, uterine cervix 622.1
  bladder 596.51
  bowel (syndrome) 564.1
    sounds 787.5
  cervix epithelial (basal) 622.1
  child 314.01
  colon 564.1
  gastrointestinal 536.8
    psychogenic 306.4
  intestine 564.1
  labyrinth (unilateral) 386.51
    with loss of labyrinthine
        reactivity 386.58
    bilateral 386.52
  nasal mucous membrane 478.1

Hyperactive, hyperactivity—
    continued
  stomach 536.8
  thyroid (gland) (see also
      Thyrotoxicosis) 242.9
Hyperacusis 388.42
Hyperadrenalism (cortical) 255.3
  medullary 255.6
Hyperadrenocorticism 255.3
  congenital 255.2
  iatrogenic
    correct substance properly
        administered 255.3
    overdose or wrong substance
        given or taken 962.0
Hyperaffectivity 301.11
Hyperaldosteronism (atypical)
    (hyperplastic)
    (normoaldosteronal)
    (normotensive) (primary)
    (secondary) 255.1
Hyperalgesia (see also Disturbance,
    sensation) 782.0
Hyperalimentation 783.6
  carotene 278.3
  specified NEC 278.8
  vitamin A 278.2
  vitamin D 278.4
Hyperaminoaciduria 270.9
  arginine 270.6
  citrulline 270.6
  cystine 270.0
  glycine 270.0
  lysine 270.7
  ornithine 270.6
  renal (types I, II, III) 270.0
Hyperammonemia (congenital)
    270.6
Hyperamnesia 780.9
Hyperamylasemia 790.5
Hyperaphia 782.0
Hyperazotemia 791.9
Hyperbetalipoproteinemia
    (acquired) (essential) (familial)
    (hereditary) (primary)
    (secondary) 272.0
  with prebetalipoproteinemia
      272.2
Hyperbilirubinemia 782.4
  congenital 277.4
  constitutional 277.4
  neonatal (transient) (see also
      Jaundice, fetus or newborn)
      774.6
  of prematurity 774.2
Hyperbilirubinemica
    encephalopathia, newborn
    774.7
  due to isoimmunization 773.4
Hypercalcemia, hypercalcemic
    (idiopathic) 275.4
  nephropathy 588.8
Hypercalcinuria 275.4
Hypercapnia 786.09
  with mixed acid-base disorder
      276.4
Hypercarotinemia 278.3
Hypercementosis 521.5
Hyperchloremia 276.9
Hyperchlorhydria 536.8
  neurotic 306.4
  psychogenic 306.4
Hypercholesterinemia — see
    Hypercholesterolemia
Hypercholesterolemia 272.0
  with hyperglyceridemia,
      endogenous 272.2
  essential 272.0
  familial 272.0
  hereditary 272.0
  primary 272.0
  pure 272.0

Hypercholesterolosis 272.0
Hyperchylia gastrica 536.8
  psychogenic 306.4
Hyperchylomicronemia (familial)
    (with
    hyperbetalipoproteinemia)
    272.3
Hypercoagulation syndrome 289.8
Hypercorticosteronism
  correct substance properly
      administered 255.3
  overdose or wrong substance
      given or taken 962.0
Hypercortisonism
  correct substance properly
      administered 255.3
  overdose or wrong substance
      given or taken 962.0
**Hyperdynamic beta-adrenergic state
    or syndrome** (circulatory)
    429.82
Hyperelectrolytemia 276.9
Hyperemesis 536.2
  arising during pregnancy — see
      Hyperemesis, gravidarum
  gravidarum (mild) (before 22
      completed weeks gestation)
      643.0
    with
      carbohydrate depletion
          643.1
      dehydration 643.1
      electrolyte imbalance
          643.1
      metabolic disturbance
          643.1
    affecting fetus or newborn
        761.8
    severe (with metabolic
        disturbance) 643.1
  psychogenic 306.4
Hyperemia (acute) 780.9
  anal mucosa 569.49
  bladder 596.7
  cerebral 437.8
  conjunctiva 372.71
  ear, internal, acute 386.30
  enteric 564.8
  eye 372.71
  eyelid (active) (passive) 374.82
  intestine 564.8
  iris 364.41
  kidney 593.81
  labyrinth 386.30
  liver (active) (passive) 573.8
  lung 514
  ovary 620.8
  passive 780.9
  pulmonary 514
  renal 593.81
  retina 362.89
  spleen 289.59
  stomach 537.89
Hyperesthesia (body surface) (see
    also Disturbance, sensation)
    782.0
  larynx (reflex) 478.79
    hysterical 300.11
  pharynx (reflex) 478.29
Hyperestrinism 256.0
Hyperestrogenism 256.0
Hyperestrogenosis 256.0
Hyperextension, joint 718.80
  ankle 718.87
  elbow 718.82
  foot 718.87
  hand 718.84
  hip 718.85
  knee 718.86
  multiple sites 718.89
  pelvic region 718.85
  shoulder (region) 718.81
  specified site NEC 718.88
  wrist 718.83

Hyperfibrinolysis — INDEX TO DISEASES — Hyperplasia, hyperplastic

Hyperfibrinolysis — *see* Fibrinolysis
Hyperfolliculinism 256.0
Hyperfructosemia 271.2
Hyperfunction
   adrenal (cortex) 255.3
      androgenic, acquired benign 255.3
      medulla 255.6
      virilism 255.2
   corticoadrenal NEC 255.3
   labyrinth — *see* Hyperactive, labyrinth
   medulloadrenal 255.6
   ovary 256.1
      estrogen 256.0
   pancreas 577.8
   parathyroid (gland) 252.0
   pituitary (anterior) (gland) (lobe) 253.1
   testicular 257.0
Hypergammaglobulinemia 289.8
   monoclonal, benign (BMH) 273.1
   polyclonal 273.0
   Waldenström's 273.0
Hyperglobulinemia 273.8
Hyperglycemia 790.6
   maternal
      affecting fetus or newborn 775.0
      manifest diabetes in infant 775.1
   postpancreatectomy (complete) (partial) 251.3
Hyperglyceridemia 272.1
   endogenous 272.1
   essential 272.1
   familial 272.1
   hereditary 272.1
   mixed 272.3
   pure 272.1
Hyperglycinemia 270.7
Hypergonadism
   ovarian 256.1
   testicular (infantile) (primary) 257.0
Hyperheparinemia (*see also* Circulating anticoagulants) 286.5
Hyperhidrosis, hyperidrosis 780.8
   psychogenic 306.3
Hyperhistidinemia 270.5
Hyperinsulinism (ectopic) (functional) (organic) NEC 251.1
   iatrogenic 251.0
   reactive 251.2
   spontaneous 251.2
   therapeutic misadventure (from administration of insulin) 962.3
Hyperiodemia 276.9
Hyperirritability (cerebral), in newborn 779.1
Hyperkalemia 276.7
Hyperkeratosis (*see also* Keratosis) 701.1
   cervix 622.1
   congenital 757.39
   cornea 371.89
   due to yaws (early) (late) (palmar or plantar) 102.3
   eccentrica 757.39
   figurata centrifuga atrophica 757.39
   follicularis 757.39
      in cutem penetrans 701.1
   limbic (cornea) 371.89
   palmoplantaris climacterica 701.1
   pinta (carate) 103.1
   senile (with pruritus) 702.0
   tongue 528.7
   universalis congenita 757.1
   vagina 623.1

Hyperkeratosis—*continued*
   vocal cord 478.5
   vulva 624.0
Hyperkinesia, hyperkinetic (disease) (reaction) (syndrome) 314.9
   with
      attention deficit — *see* Disorder, attention deficit
      conduct disorder 314.2
      developmental delay 314.1
      simple disturbance of activity and attention 314.01
      specified manifestation NEC 314.8
   heart (disease) 429.82
   of childhood or adolescence NEC 314.9
Hyperlacrimation (*see also* Epiphora) 375.20
Hyperlipemia (*see also* Hyperlipidemia) 272.4
Hyperlipidemia 272.4
   carbohydrate-induced 272.1
   combined 272.4
   endogenous 272.1
   exogenous 272.3
   fat-induced 272.3
   group
      A 272.0
      B 272.1
      C 272.2
      D 272.3
   mixed 272.2
   specified type NEC 272.4
Hyperlipidosis 272.7
   hereditary 272.7
Hyperlipoproteinemia (acquired) (essential) (familial) (hereditary) (primary) (secondary) 272.4
   Fredrickson type
      I 272.3
      IIa 272.0
      IIb 272.2
      III 272.2
      IV 272.1
      V 272.3
   low-density-lipoid-type (LDL) 272.0
   very-low-density-lipoid-type (VLDL) 272.1
Hyperlucent lung, unilateral 492.8
Hyperluteinization 256.1
Hyperlysinemia 270.7
Hypermagnesemia 275.2
   neonatal 775.5
Hypermaturity (fetus or newborn) 766.2
Hypermenorrhea 626.2
Hypermetabolism 794.7
Hypermethioninemia 270.4
Hypermetropia (congenital) 367.0
Hypermobility
   cecum 564.1
   coccyx 724.71
   colon 564.1
      psychogenic 306.4
   ileum 564.8
   joint (acquired) 718.80
      ankle 718.87
      elbow 718.82
      foot 718.87
      hand 718.84
      hip 718.85
      knee 718.86
      multiple sites 718.89
      pelvic region 718.85
      shoulder (region) 718.81
      specified site NEC 718.88
      wrist 718.83
   kidney, congenital 753.3
   meniscus (knee) 717.5
   scapula 718.81

Hypermobility—*continued*
   stomach 536.8
      psychogenic 306.4
   syndrome 728.5
   testis, congenital 752.5
   urethral 599.81
Hypermotility
   gastrointestinal 536.8
   intestine 564.1
      psychogenic 306.4
   stomach 536.8
Hypernasality 784.49
Hypernatremia 276.0
   with water depletion 276.0
Hypernephroma (M8312/3) 189.0
Hyperopia 367.0
Hyperorexia 783.6
Hyperornithinemia 270.6
Hyperosmia (*see also* Disturbance, sensation) 781.1
Hyperosmolality 276.0
Hyperosteogenesis 733.99
Hyperostosis 733.99
   calvarial 733.3
   cortical 733.3
      infantile 756.59
   frontal, internal of skull 733.3
   interna frontalis 733.3
   monomelic 733.99
   skull 733.3
      congenital 756.0
   vertebral 721.8
      with spondylosis — *see* Spondylosis
      ankylosing 721.6
Hyperovarianism 256.1
Hyperovarism, hyperovaria 256.1
Hyperoxaluria (primary) 271.8
Hyperoxia 987.8
Hyperparathyroidism 252.0
   ectopic 259.3
   secondary, of renal origin 588.8
Hyperpathia (*see also* Disturbance, sensation) 782.0
   psychogenic 307.80
Hyperperistalsis 787.4
   psychogenic 306.4
Hyperpermeability, capillary 448.9
Hyperphagia 783.6
Hyperphenylalaninemia 270.1
Hyperphoria 378.40
   alternating 378.45
Hyperphosphatemia 275.3
Hyperpiesia (*see also* Hypertension) 401.9
Hyperpiesis (*see also* Hypertension) 401.9
Hyperpigmentation — *see* Pigmentation
Hyperpinealism 259.8
Hyperpipecolatemia 270.7
Hyperpituitarism 253.1
Hyperplasia, hyperplastic
   adenoids (lymphoid tissue) 474.12
      and tonsils 474.10
   adrenal (capsule) (cortex) (gland) 255.8
      with
         sexual precocity (male) 255.2
         virilism, adrenal 255.2
         virilization (female) 255.2
      congenital 255.2
      due to excess ACTH (ectopic) (pituitary) 255.0
      medulla 255.8
   alpha cells (pancreatic)
      with
         gastrin excess 251.5
         glucagon excess 251.4
   appendix (lymphoid) 543.0

Hyperplasia, hyperplastic—*continued*
   artery, fibromuscular NEC 447.8
      carotid 447.8
      renal 447.3
   bone 733.99
      marrow 289.9
   breast (*see also* Hypertrophy, breast) 611.1
   carotid artery 447.8
   cementation, cementum (teeth) (tooth) 521.5
   cervical gland 785.6
   cervix (uteri) 622.1
      basal cell 622.1
      congenital 752.49
      endometrium 622.1
      polypoid 622.1
   chin 524.05
   clitoris, congenital 752.49
   dentin 521.5
   endocervicitis 616.0
   endometrium, endometrial (adenomatous) (atypical) (cystic) (glandular) (polypoid) (uterus) 621.3
      cervix 622.1
   epithelial 709.8
      focal, oral, including tongue 528.7
      mouth (focal) 528.7
      nipple 611.8
      skin 709.8
      tongue (focal) 528.7
      vaginal wall 623.0
   erythroid 289.9
   fascialis ossificans (progressiva) 728.11
   fibromuscular, artery NEC 447.8
      carotid 447.8
      renal 447.3
   genital
      female 629.8
      male 608.89
   gingiva 523.8
   glandularis
      cystica uteri 621.3
      endometrium (uterus) 621.3
      interstitialis uteri 621.3
   granulocytic 288.8
   gum 523.8
   hymen, congenital 752.49
   islands of Langerhans 251.1
   islet cell (pancreatic) 251.9
      alpha cells
         with excess
            gastrin 251.5
            glucagon 251.4
      beta cells 251.1
   juxtaglomerular (complex) (kidney) 593.89
   kidney (congenital) 753.3
   liver (congenital) 751.69
   lymph node (gland) 785.6
   lymphoid (diffuse) (nodular) 785.6
      appendix 543.0
      intestine 569.89
   mandibular 524.02
      alveolar 524.72
      unilateral condylar 526.89
   Marchand multiple nodular (liver) — *see* Cirrhosis, postnecrotic
   maxillary 524.01
      alveolar 524.71
   medulla, adrenal 255.8
   myometrium, myometrial 621.2
   nose (lymphoid) (polypoid) 478.1
   oral soft tissue (inflammatory) (irritative) (mucosa) NEC 528.9
      gingiva 523.8
      tongue 529.8
   organ or site, congenital NEC — *see* Anomaly, specified type NEC
   ovary 620.8

Hyperplasia, hyperplastic—
continued
  palate, papillary 528.9
  pancreatic islet cells 251.9
    alpha
      with excess
        gastrin 251.5
        glucagon 251.4
    beta 251.1
  parathyroid (gland) 252.0
  persistent, vitreous (primary) 743.51
  pharynx (lymphoid) 478.29
  prostate (adenofibromatous) (nodular) 600
  renal artery (fibromuscular) 447.3
  reticuloendothelial (cell) 289.9
  salivary gland (any) 527.1
  Schimmelbusch's 610.1
  suprarenal (capsule) (gland) 255.8
  thymus (gland) (persistent) 254.0
  thyroid (*see also* Goiter) 240.9
    primary 242.0
    secondary 242.2
  tonsil (lymphoid tissue) 474.11
    and adenoids 474.10
  urethrovaginal 599.89
  uterus, uterine (myometrium) 621.2
    endometrium 621.3
  vitreous (humor), primary persistent 743.51
  vulva 624.3
  zygoma 738.11

Hyperpnea (*see also* Hyperventilation) 786.01

Hyperpotassemia 276.7

Hyperprebetalipoproteinemia 272.1
  with chylomicronemia 272.3
  familial 272.1

Hyperprolinemia 270.8

Hyperproteinemia 273.8

Hyperprothrombinemia 289.8

Hyperpselaphesia 782.0

Hyperpyrexia 780.6
  heat (effects of) 992.0
  malarial (*see also* Malaria) 084.6
  malignant, due to anesthetic 995.89
  rheumatic — *see* Fever, rheumatic
  unknown origin (*see also* Pyrexia) 780.6

Hyperreactor, vascular 780.2

Hyperreflexia 796.1
  bladder, autonomic 596.54
    with cauda equina 344.61
  detrusor 344.61

Hypersalivation (*see also* Ptyalism) 527.7

Hypersarcosinemia 270.8

Hypersecretion
  ACTH 255.3
  androgens (ovarian) 256.1
  calcitonin 246.0
  corticoadrenal 255.3
  cortisol 255.0
  estrogen 256.0
  gastric 536.8
    psychogenic 306.4
  gastrin 251.5
  glucagon 251.4
  hormone
    ACTH 255.3
    anterior pituitary 253.1
    growth NEC 253.0
    ovarian androgen 256.1
    testicular 257.0
    thyroid stimulating 242.8
  insulin — *see* Hyperinsulinism
  lacrimal glands (*see also* Epiphora) 375.20
  medulloadrenal 255.6
  milk 676.6
  ovarian androgens 256.1

Hypersecretion—*continued*
  pituitary (anterior) 253.1
  salivary gland (any) 527.7
  testicular hormones 257.0
  thyrocalcitonin 246.0
  upper respiratory 478.9

Hypersegmentation, hereditary 288.2
  eosinophils 288.2
  neutrophil nuclei 288.2

Hypersensitive, hypersensitiveness, hypersensitivity — *see also* Allergy
  angiitis 446.20
    specified NEC 446.29
  carotid sinus 337.0
  colon 564.1
    psychogenic 306.4
  DNA (deoxyribonucleic acid) NEC 287.2
  drug (*see also* Allergy, drug) 995.2
  esophagus 530.89
  insect bites — *see* Injury, superficial, by site
  labyrinth 386.58
  pain (*see also* Disturbance, sensation) 782.0
  pneumonitis NEC 495.9
  reaction (*see also* Allergy) 995.3
    upper respiratory tract NEC 478.8
  stomach (allergic) (nonallergic) 536.8
    psychogenic 306.4

Hypersomatotropism (classic) 253.0

Hypersomnia 780.54
  with sleep apnea 780.53
  nonorganic origin 307.43
    persistent (primary) 307.44 ◆
    transient 307.43

Hypersplenia 289.4

Hypersplenism 289.4

Hypersteatosis 706.3

Hypersuprarenalism 255.3

Hypersusceptibility — *see* Allergy

Hyper-TBG-nemia 246.8

Hypertelorism 756.0
  orbit, orbital 376.41

	Malignant	Benign	Unspecified
Hypertension, hypertensive (arterial) (arteriolar) (crisis) (degeneration) (disease) (essential) (fluctuating) (idiopathic) (intermittent) (labile) (low renin) (orthostatic) (paroxysmal) (primary) (systemic) (uncontrolled) (vascular)	401.0	401.1	401.9
with			
heart involvement (conditions classifiable to 425.8, 428, 429.0-429.3, 429.8, 429.9 due to hypertension) (*see also* Hypertension, heart)	402.00	402.10	402.90 ◆
with kidney involvement — *see* Hypertension, cardiorenal			
renal involvement (*only* conditions classifiable to 585, 586, 587) (*excludes conditions classifiable to 584*)			
(*see also* Hypertension, kidney)	403.00	403.10	403.90
renal sclerosis or failure	403.00	403.10	403.90
with heart involvement — *see* Hypertension, cardiorenal			
failure (and sclerosis) (*see also* Hypertension, kidney)	403.01	403.11	403.91
sclerosis without failure (*see also* Hypertension, kidney)	403.00	403.10	403.90
accelerated — (*see also* Hypertension, by type, malignant)	401.0	—	—
antepartum — *see* Hypertension, complicating pregnancy, childbirth, or the puerperium			
cardiorenal (disease)	404.00	404.10	404.90
with			
heart failure (congestive)	404.01	404.11	404.91
and renal failure	404.03	404.13	404.93
renal failure	404.02	404.12	404.92
and heart failure (congestive)	404.03	404.13	404.93
cardiovascular disease (arteriosclerotic) (sclerotic)	402.00	402.10	402.90
with			
heart failure (congestive)	402.01	402.11	402.91
renal involvement (conditions classifiable to 403) (*see also* Hypertension, cardiorenal)	404.00	404.10	404.90
cardiovascular renal (disease) (sclerosis) (*see also* Hypertension, cardiorenal)	404.00	404.10	404.90
cerebrovascular disease NEC	437.2	437.2	437.2
complicating pregnancy, childbirth, or the puerperium	642.2	642.0	642.9
with			
albuminuria (and edema) (mild)	—	—	642.4
severe	—	—	642.5
edema (mild)	—	—	642.4
severe	—	—	642.5
heart disease	642.2	642.2	642.2
and renal disease	642.2	642.2	642.2
renal disease	642.2	642.2	642.2
and heart disease	642.2	642.2	642.2
chronic	642.2	642.0	642.0
with pre-eclampsia or eclampsia	642.7	642.7	642.7
fetus or newborn	760.0	760.0	760.0
essential	—	642.0	642.0
with pre-eclampsia or eclampsia	—	642.7	642.7
fetus or newborn	760.0	760.0	760.0
fetus or newborn	760.0	760.0	760.0
gestational	—	—	642.3
pre-existing	642.2	642.0	642.0
with pre-eclampsia or eclampsia	642.7	642.7	642.7
fetus or newborn	760.0	760.0	760.0
secondary to renal disease	642.1	642.1	642.1
with pre-eclampsia or eclampsia	642.7	642.7	642.7
fetus or newborn	760.0	760.0	760.0
transient	—	—	642.3
due to			
aldosteronism, primary	405.09	405.19	405.99
brain tumor	405.09	405.19	405.99
bulbar poliomyelitis	405.09	405.19	405.99
calculus			
kidney	405.09	405.19	405.99
ureter	405.09	405.19	405.99
coarctation, aorta	405.09	405.19	405.99
Cushing's disease	405.09	405.19	405.99
glomerulosclerosis (*see also* Hypertension, kidney)	403.00	403.10	403.90
periarteritis nodosa	405.09	405.19	405.99
pheochromocytoma	405.09	405.19	405.99
polycystic kidney(s)	405.09	405.19	405.99
polycythemia	405.09	405.19	405.99
porphyria	405.09	405.19	405.99
pyelonephritis	405.09	405.19	405.99
renal (artery)			
aneurysm	405.01	405.11	405.91
anomaly	405.01	405.11	405.91
embolism	405.01	405.11	405.91
fibromuscular hyperplasia	405.01	405.11	405.91
occlusion	405.01	405.11	405.91
stenosis	405.01	405.11	405.91
thrombosis	405.01	405.11	405.91
encephalopathy	437.2	437.2	437.2
gestational (transient) NEC	—	—	642.3
Goldblatt's	440.1	440.1	440.1
heart (disease) (conditions classifiable to 425.8, 428, 429.0-429.3, 429.8, 429.9 due to hypertension)	402.00	402.10	402.90 ◆
with heart failure	402.01	402.11	402.91 ◆
congestive	402.01	402.11	402.91
hypertensive kidney disease (conditions classifiable to 403) (*see also* Hypertension, cardiorenal)	404.00	404.10	404.90
renal sclerosis (*see also* Hypertension, cardiorenal)	404.00	404.10	404.90
intracranial, benign	—	348.2	—

Hypertension — INDEX TO DISEASES

	Malignant	Benign	Unspecified
intraocular	—	—	365.04
kidney	403.00	403.10	403.90
with			
heart involvement (conditions classifiable to 425.8, 428, 429.0-429.3, 429.8, 429.9 due to hypertension) (*see also* Hypertension, cardiorenal)	404.00	404.10	404.90 ◆
hypertensive heart (disease) (conditions classifiable to 402) (*see also* Hypertension, cardiorenal)	404.00	404.10	404.90
lesser circulation	—	—	416.0
necrotizing	401.0	—	—
ocular	—	—	365.04
portal (due to chronic liver disease)	—	—	572.3
postoperative	—	—	997.9 ◆
psychogenic	—	—	306.2
puerperal, postpartum — *see* Hypertension, complicating pregnancy, childbirth, or the puerperium			
pulmonary (artery) (idiopathic) (primary) (solitary)	—	—	416.0
with cor pulmonale (chronic)	—	—	416.8
acute	—	—	415.0
secondary	—	—	416.8
renal (disease) (*see also* Hypertension, kidney)	403.00	403.10	403.90
renovascular NEC	405.01	405.11	405.91
secondary NEC	405.09	405.19	405.99
due to			
aldosteronism, primary	405.09	405.19	405.99
brain tumor	405.09	405.19	405.99
bulbar poliomyelitis	405.09	405.19	405.99
calculus			
kidney	405.09	405.19	405.99
ureter	405.09	405.19	405.99
coarctation, aorta	405.09	405.19	405.99
Cushing's disease	405.09	405.19	405.99
glomerulosclerosis (*see also* Hypertension, kidney)	403.00	403.10	403.90
periarteritis nodosa	405.09	405.19	405.99
pheochromocytoma	405.09	405.19	405.99
polycystic kidney(s)	405.09	405.19	405.99
polycythemia	405.09	405.19	405.99
porphyria	405.09	405.19	405.99
pyelonephritis	405.09	405.19	405.99
renal (artery)			
aneurysm	405.01	405.11	405.91
anomaly	405.01	405.11	405.91
embolism	405.01	405.11	405.91
fibromuscular hyperplasia	405.01	405.11	405.91
occlusion	405.01	405.11	405.91
stenosis	405.01	405.11	405.91
thrombosis	405.01	405.11	405.91
transient	—	—	796.2
of pregnancy	—	—	642.3

Hyperthecosis, ovary 256.8
Hyperthermia (of unknown origin)
  (see also Pyrexia) 780.6
  malignant (due to anesthesia)
    995.89
  newborn 778.4
Hyperthymergasia (see also
    Psychosis, affective) 296.0
  reactive (from emotional stress,
    psychological trauma)
    298.1
  recurrent episode 296.1
  single episode 296.0
Hyperthymism 254.8
Hyperthyroid (recurrent) — see
    Hyperthyroidism
Hyperthyroidism (latent) (preadult)
  (recurrent) (without goiter)
  242.9

Note — Use the following fifth-
digit subclassification with
category 242:

0 without mention of
   thyrotoxic crisis or
   storm
1 with mention of
   thyrotoxic crisis or
   storm

  with
    goiter (diffuse) 242.0
      adenomatous 242.3
        multinodular 242.2
        uninodular 242.1
      nodular 242.3
        multinodular 242.2
        uninodular 242.1
      thyroid nodule 242.1
  complicating pregnancy,
    childbirth, or puerperium
    648.1
  neonatal (transient) 775.3
Hypertonia — see Hypertonicity
Hypertonicity
  bladder 596.51
  fetus or newborn 779.8
  gastrointestinal (tract) 536.8
  infancy 779.8
    due to electrolyte imbalance
      779.8
  muscle 728.85
  stomach 536.8
    psychogenic 306.4
  uterus, uterine (contractions)
    661.4
    affecting fetus or newborn
      763.7
Hypertony — see Hypertonicity
Hypertransaminemia 790.4
Hypertrichosis 704.1
  congenital 757.4
  eyelid 374.54
  lanuginosa 757.4
    acquired 704.1
Hypertriglyceridemia, essential
  272.1
Hypertrophy, hypertrophic
  adenoids (infectional) 474.12
    and tonsils (faucial) (infective)
      (lingual) (lymphoid)
      474.10
  adrenal 255.8
  alveolar process or ridge 525.8
  anal papillae 569.49
  apocrine gland 705.82
  artery NEC 447.8
    carotid 447.8
    congenital (peripheral) NEC
      747.60
      gastrointestinal 747.61
      lower limb 747.64
      renal 747.62
      specified NEC 747.69

Hypertrophy, hypertrophic—
  continued
  artery NEC—continued
    congenital—continued
      spinal 747.82
      upper limb 747.63
  arthritis (chronic) (see also
    Osteoarthrosis) 715.9
    spine (see also Spondylosis)
      721.90
  arytenoid 478.79
  asymmetrical (heart) 429.9
  auricular — see Hypertrophy,
    cardiac
  Bartholin's gland 624.8
  bile duct 576.8
  bladder (sphincter) (trigone) 596.8
  blind spot, visual field 368.42
  bone 733.99
  brain 348.8
  breast 611.1
    cystic 610.1
    fetus or newborn 778.7
    fibrocystic 610.1
    massive pubertal 611.1
    puerperal, postpartum 676.3
    senile (parenchymatous) 611.1
  cardiac (chronic) (idiopathic)
    429.3
    with
      rheumatic fever (conditions
        classifiable to 390)
        active 391.8
          with chorea 392.0
        inactive or quiescent
          (with chorea)
          398.99
    congenital NEC 746.89
    fatty (see also Degeneration,
      myocardial) 429.1
    hypertensive (see also
      Hypertension, heart)
      402.90
    rheumatic (with chorea)
      398.99
      active or acute 391.8
        with chorea 392.0
    valve (see also Endocarditis)
      424.90
      congenital NEC 746.89
  cartilage 733.99
  cecum 569.89
  cervix (uteri) 622.6
    congenital 752.49
    elongation 622.6
  clitoris (cirrhotic) 624.2
    congenital 752.49
  colon 569.89
    congenital 751.3
  conjunctiva, lymphoid 372.73
  cornea 371.89
  corpora cavernosa 607.89
  duodenum 537.89
  endometrium (uterus) 621.3
    cervix 622.6
  epididymis 608.89
  esophageal hiatus (congenital)
    756.6
    with hernia — see Hernia,
      diaphragm
  eyelid 374.30
  falx, skull 733.99
  fat pad 729.30
    infrapatellar 729.31
    knee 729.31
    orbital 374.34
    popliteal 729.31
    prepatellar 729.31
    retropatellar 729.31
    specified site NEC 729.39
  foot (congenital) 755.67
  frenum, frenulum (tongue) 529.8
    linguae 529.8
    lip 528.5
  gallbladder or cystic duct 575.8
  gastric mucosa 535.2
  gingiva 523.8

Hypertrophy, hypertrophic—
  continued
  gland, glandular (general) NEC
    785.6
  gum (mucous membrane) 523.8
  heart (idiopathic) — see also
    Hypertrophy, cardiac
    valve — see also Endocarditis
      congenital NEC 746.89
  hemifacial 754.0
  hepatic — see Hypertrophy, liver
  hiatus (esophageal) 756.6
  hilus gland 785.6
  hymen, congenital 752.49
  ileum 569.89
  infrapatellar fat pad 729.31
  intestine 569.89
  jejunum 569.89
  kidney (compensatory) 593.1
    congenital 753.3
  labial frenulum 528.5
  labium (majus) (minus) 624.3
  lacrimal gland, chronic 375.03
  ligament 728.9
    spinal 724.8
  linguae frenulum 529.8
  lingual tonsil (infectional) 474.11
  lip (frenum) 528.5
    congenital 744.81
  liver 789.1
    acute 573.8
    cirrhotic — see Cirrhosis, liver
    congenital 751.69
    fatty — see Fatty, liver
  lymph gland 785.6
    tuberculous — see
      Tuberculosis, lymph
      gland
  mammary gland — see
    Hypertrophy, breast
  maxillary frenulum 528.5
  Meckel's diverticulum
    (congenital) 751.0
  medial meniscus, acquired 717.3
  median bar 600
  mediastinum 519.3
  meibomian gland 373.2
  meniscus, knee, congenital
    755.64
  metatarsal head 733.99
  metatarsus 733.99
  mouth 528.9
  mucous membrane
    alveolar process 523.8
    nose 478.1
    turbinate (nasal) 478.0
  muscle 728.9
  muscular coat, artery NEC 447.8
    carotid 447.8
    renal 447.3
  myocardium (see also
    Hypertrophy, cardiac)
    429.3
    idiopathic 425.4
  myometrium 621.2
  nail 703.8
    congenital 757.5
  nasal 478.1
    alae 478.1
    bone 738.0
    cartilage 478.1
    mucous membrane (septum)
      478.1
    sinus (see also Sinusitis) 473.9
    turbinate 478.0
  nasopharynx, lymphoid
    (infectional) (tissue) (wall)
    478.29
  neck, uterus 622.6
  nipple 611.1
  normal aperture diaphragm
    (congenital) 756.6
  nose (see also Hypertrophy, nasal)
    478.1
  orbit 376.46

Hypertrophy, hypertrophic—
  continued
  organ or site, congenital NEC —
    see Anomaly, specified type
    NEC
  osteoarthropathy (pulmonary)
    731.2
  ovary 620.8
  palate (hard) 526.89
    soft 528.9
  pancreas (congenital) 751.7
  papillae
    anal 569.49
    tongue 529.3
  parathyroid (gland) 252.0
  parotid gland 527.1
  penis 607.89
  phallus 607.89
    female (clitoris) 624.2
  pharyngeal tonsil 474.12
  pharyngitis 472.1
  pharynx 478.29
    lymphoid (infectional) (tissue)
      (wall) 478.29
  pituitary (fossa) (gland) 253.8
  popliteal fat pad 729.31
  preauricular (lymph) gland
    (Hampstead) 785.6
  prepuce (congenital) 605
    female 624.2
  prostate (adenofibromatous)
    (asymptomatic) (benign)
    (early) (recurrent) 600
    congenital 752.8
  pseudoedematous hypodermal
    757.0
  pseudomuscular 359.1
  pylorus (muscle) (sphincter) 537.0
    congenital 750.5
    infantile 750.5
  rectal sphincter 569.49
  rectum 569.49
  renal 593.1
  rhinitis (turbinate) 472.0
  salivary duct or gland 527.1
    congenital 750.26
  scaphoid (tarsal) 733.99
  scar 701.4
  scrotum 608.89
  sella turcica 253.8
  seminal vesicle 608.89
  sigmoid 569.89
  skin condition NEC 701.9
  spermatic cord 608.89
  spinal ligament 728.9
  spleen — see Splenomegaly
  spondylitis (spine) (see also
    Spondylosis) 721.90
  stomach 537.89
  subaortic stenosis (idiopathic)
    425.1
  sublingual gland 527.1
    congenital 750.26
  submaxillary gland 527.1
  suprarenal (gland) 255.8
  tendon 727.9
  testis 608.89
    congenital 752.8
  thymic, thymus (congenital)
    (gland) 254.0
  thyroid (gland) (see also Goiter)
    240.9
    primary 242.0
    secondary 242.2
  toe (congenital) 755.65
    acquired 735.8
  tongue 529.8
    congenital 750.15
    frenum 529.8
    papillae (foliate) 529.3
  tonsil (faucial) (infective) (lingual)
    (lymphoid) 474.11
    with tonsillitis 474.0
      and adenoids 474.10
  tunica vaginalis 608.89
  turbinate (mucous membrane)
    478.0

Hypertrophy, hypertrophic—
continued
- ureter 593.89
- urethra 599.84
- uterus 621.2
  - puerperal, postpartum 674.8
- uvula 528.9
- vagina 623.8
- vas deferens 608.89
- vein 459.89
- ventricle, ventricular (heart) (left) (right) — *see also* Hypertrophy, cardiac
  - congenital 746.89
  - due to hypertension (left) (right) (*see also* Hypertension, heart) 402.90
    - benign 402.10
    - malignant 402.00
  - right with ventricular septal defect, pulmonary stenosis or atresia, and dextraposition of aorta 745.2
- verumontanum 599.89
- vesical 596.8
- vocal cord 478.5
- vulva 624.3
  - stasis (nonfilarial) 624.3

Hypertropia (intermittent) (periodic) 378.31
Hypertyrosinemia 270.2
Hyperuricemia 790.6
Hypervalinemia 270.3
Hyperventilation (tetany) 786.01
- hysterical 300.11
- psychogenic 306.1
- syndrome 306.1

Hyperviscidosis 277.00
Hyperviscosity (of serum) (syndrome) NEC 273.3
- polycythemic 289.0
- sclerocythemic 282.8

Hypervitaminosis (dietary) NEC 278.8
- A (dietary) 278.2
- D (dietary) 278.4
- from excessive administration or use of vitamin preparations (chronic) 278.8
  - reaction to sudden overdose 963.5
- vitamin A 278.2
  - reaction to sudden overdose 963.5
- vitamin D 278.4
  - reaction to sudden overdose 963.5
- vitamin K
  - correct substance properly administered 278.8
  - overdose or wrong substance given or taken 964.3

Hypervolemia 276.6
Hypesthesia (*see also* Disturbance, sensation) 782.0
- cornea 371.81

Hyphema (anterior chamber) (ciliary body) (iris) 364.41
- traumatic 921.3

Hyphemia — *see* Hyphema
Hypoacidity, gastric 536.8
- psychogenic 306.4

Hypoactive labyrinth (function) — *see* Hypofunction, labyrinth
Hypoadrenalism 255.4
- tuberculous (*see also* Tuberculosis) 017.6

Hypoadrenocorticism 255.4
- pituitary 253.4

Hypoalbuminemia 273.8
Hypoalphalipoproteinemia 272.5

Hypobarism 993.2
Hypobaropathy 993.2
Hypobetalipoproteinemia (familial) 272.5
Hypocalcemia 275.4
- cow's milk 775.4
- dietary 269.3
- neonatal 775.4
- phosphate-loading 775.4

Hypocalcification, teeth 520.4
Hypochloremia 276.9
Hypochlorhydria 536.8
- neurotic 306.4
- psychogenic 306.4

Hypocholesteremia 272.5
Hypochondria (reaction) 300.7
Hypochondriac 300.7
Hyponchondriasis 300.7
Hypochromasia blood cells 280.9
Hypochromic anemia 280.9
- due to blood loss (chronic) 280.0
  - acute 285.1
- microcytic 280.9

Hypocoagulability (*see also* Defect, coagulation) 286.9
Hypocomplementemia 279.8
Hypocythemia (progressive) 284.9
Hypodontia (*see also* Anodontia) 520.0
Hypoeosinophilia 288.8
Hypoesthesia (*see also* Disturbance, sensation) 782.0
- cornea 371.81
- tactile 782.0

Hypoestrinism 256.3
Hypoestrogenism 256.3
Hypoferremia 280.9
- due to blood loss (chronic) 280.0

Hypofertility
- female 628.9
- male 606.1

Hypofibrinogenemia 286.3
- acquired 286.6
- congenital 286.3

Hypofunction
- adrenal (gland) 255.4
  - cortex 255.4
  - medulla 255.5
  - specified NEC 255.5
- cerebral 331.9
- corticoadrenal NEC 255.4
- intestinal 564.8
- labyrinth (unilateral) 386.53
  - with loss of labyrinthine reactivity 386.55
  - bilateral 386.54
    - with loss of labyrinthine reactivity 386.56
- Leydig cell 257.2
- ovary 256.3
  - postablative 256.2
- pituitary (anterior) (gland) (lobe) 253.2
  - posterior 253.5
- testicular 257.2
  - iatrogenic 257.1
  - postablative 257.1
  - postirradiation 257.1
  - postsurgical 257.1

Hypogammaglobulinemia 279.00
- acquired primary 279.06
- non-sex-linked, congenital 279.06
- sporadic 279.06
- transient of infancy 279.09

Hypogenitalism (congenital) (female) (male) 752.8
Hypoglycemia (spontaneous) 251.2
- coma 251.0
  - diabetic 250.3
- diabetic 250.8

Hypoglycemia—*continued*
- due to insulin 251.0
  - therapeutic misadventure 962.3
- familial (idiopathic) 251.2
- following gastrointestinal surgery 579.3
- infantile (idiopathic) 251.2
- in infant of diabetic mother 775.0
- leucine-induced 270.3
- neonatal 775.6
- reactive 251.2
- specified NEC 251.1

Hypoglycemic shock 251.0
- diabetic 250.8
- due to insulin 251.0
- functional (syndrome) 251.1

Hypogonadism
- female 256.3
- gonadotrophic (isolated) 253.4
- hypogonadotropic (isolated) (with anosmia) 253.4
- isolated 253.4
- male 257.2
- ovarian (primary) 256.3
- pituitary (secondary) 253.4
- testicular (primary) (secondary) 257.2

Hypohidrosis 705.0
Hypohidrotic ectodermal dysplasia 757.31
Hypoidrosis 705.0
Hypoinsulinemia, postsurgical 251.3
- postpancreatectomy (complete) (partial) 251.3

Hypokalemia 276.8
Hypokinesia 780.9
Hypoleukia splenica 289.4
Hypoleukocytosis 288.8
Hypolipidemia 272.5
Hypolipoproteinemia 272.5
Hypomagnesemia 275.2
- neonatal 775.4

Hypomania, hypomanic reaction (*see also* Psychosis, affective) 296.0
- recurrent episode 296.1
- single episode 296.0

Hypomastia (congenital) 757.6
Hypomenorrhea 626.1
Hypometabolism 783.9
Hypomotility
- gastrointestinal tract 536.8
  - psychogenic 306.4
- intestine 564.8
  - psychogenic 306.4
- stomach 536.8
  - psychogenic 306.4

Hyponasality 784.49
Hyponatremia 276.1
- with water depletion 276.1

Hypo-ovarianism 256.3
Hypo-ovarism 256.3
Hypoparathyroidism (idiopathic) (surgically induced) 252.1
- neonatal 775.4

Hypopharyngitis 462
Hypophoria 378.40
Hypophosphatasia 275.3
Hypophosphatemia (acquired) (congenital) (familial) 275.3
- renal 275.3

Hypophyseal, hypophysis — *see also* condition
- dwarfism 253.3
- gigantism 253.0
- syndrome 253.8

Hypophyseothalamic syndrome 253.8
Hypopiesis — *see* Hypotension
Hypopigmentation 709.00 ◆
- eyelid 374.53

Hypopinealism 259.8
Hypopituitarism (juvenile) (syndrome) 253.2
- due to
  - hormone therapy 253.7
  - hypophysectomy 253.7
  - radiotherapy 253.7
- postablative 253.7
- postpartum hemorrhage 253.2

Hypoplasia, hypoplasis 759.89
- adrenal (gland) 759.1
- alimentary tract 751.8
  - lower 751.2
  - upper 750.8
- anus, anal (canal) 751.2
- aorta 747.22
- aortic
  - arch (tubular) 747.10
  - orifice or valve with hypoplasia of ascending aorta and defective development of left ventricle (with mitral valve atresia) 746.7
- appendix 751.2
- areola 757.6
- arm (*see also* Absence, arm, congenital) 755.20
- artery (congenital) (peripheral) NEC 747.60
  - brain 747.81
  - cerebral 747.81
  - coronary 746.85
  - gastrointestinal 747.61
  - lower limb 747.64
  - pulmonary 747.3
  - renal 747.62
  - retinal 743.58
  - specified NEC 747.69
  - spinal 747.82
  - umbilical 747.5
  - upper limb 747.63
- auditory canal 744.29
  - causing impairment of hearing 744.02
- biliary duct (common) or passage 751.61
- bladder 753.8
- bone NEC 756.9
  - face 756.0
  - malar 756.0
  - mandible 524.04
    - alveolar 524.74
  - marrow 284.9
    - acquired (secondary) 284.8
    - congenital 284.0
    - idiopathic 284.9
  - maxilla 524.03
    - alveolar 524.73
  - skull (*see also* Hypoplasia, skull) 756.0
- brain 742.1
  - gyri 742.2
  - specified part 742.2
- breast (areola) 757.6
- bronchus (tree) 748.3
- cardiac 746.89
  - valve — *see* Hypoplasia, heart, valve
  - vein 746.89
- carpus (*see also* Absence, carpal, congenital) 755.28
- cartilaginous 756.9
- cecum 751.2
- cementum 520.4
  - hereditary 520.5
- cephalic 742.1
- cerebellum 742.2
- cervix (uteri) 752.49
- chin 524.06
- clavicle 755.51
- coccyx 756.19
- colon 751.2
- corpus callosum 742.2
- cricoid cartilage 748.3
- dermal, focal (Goltz) 757.39

Hypoplasia, hypoplasis—continued
 digestive organ(s) or tract NEC 751.8
  lower 751.2
  upper 750.8
 ear 744.29
  auricle 744.23
  lobe 744.29
  middle, except ossicles 744.03
   ossicles 744.04
  ossicles 744.04
 enamel of teeth (neonatal) (postnatal) (prenatal) 520.4
  hereditary 520.5
 endocrine (gland) NEC 759.2
 endometrium 621.8
 epididymis 752.8
 epiglottis 748.3
 erythroid, congenital 284.0
 erythropoietic, chronic acquired 284.8
 esophagus 750.3
 Eustachian tube 744.24
 eye (see also Microphthalmos) 743.10
  lid 743.62
 face 744.89
  bone(s) 756.0
 fallopian tube 752.19
 femur (see also Absence, femur, congenital) 755.34
 fibula (see also Absence, fibula, congenital) 755.37
 finger (see also Absence, finger, congenital) 755.29
 focal dermal 757.39
 foot 755.31
 gallbladder 751.69
 genitalia, genital organ(s)
  female 752.8
   external 752.49
   internal NEC 752.8
   in adiposogenital dystrophy 253.8
  male 752.8
 glottis 748.3
 hair 757.4
 hand 755.21
 heart 746.89
  left (complex) (syndrome) 746.7
  valve NEC 746.89
   pulmonary 746.01
 humerus (see also Absence, humerus, congenital) 755.24
 hymen 752.49
 intestine (small) 751.1
  large 751.2
 iris 743.46
 jaw 524.09
 kidney(s) 753.0
 labium (majus) (minus) 752.49
 labyrinth, membranous 744.05
 lacrimal duct (apparatus) 743.65
 larynx 748.3
 leg (see also Absence, limb, congenital, lower) 755.30
 limb 755.4
  lower (see also Absence, limb, congenital, lower) 755.30
  upper (see also Absence, limb, congenital, upper) 755.20
 liver 751.69
 lung (lobe) 748.5
 mammary (areolar) 757.6
 mandibular 524.04
  alveolar 524.74
  unilateral condylar 526.89
 maxillary 524.03
  alveolar 524.73
 medullary 248.9
 megakaryocytic 287.3

Hypoplasia, hypoplasis—continued
 metacarpus (see also Absence, metacarpal, congenital) 755.28
 metatarsus (see also Absence, metatarsal, congenital) 755.38
 muscle 756.89
  eye 743.69
 myocardium (congenital) (Uhl's anomaly) 746.84
 nail(s) 757.5
 nasolacrimal duct 743.65
 nervous system NEC 742.8
 neural 742.8
 nose, nasal 748.1
 ophthalmic (see also Microphthalmos) 743.10
 organ
  of Corti 744.05
  or site NEC — see Anomaly, by site
 osseous meatus (ear) 744.03
 ovary 752.0
 oviduct 752.19
 pancreas 751.7
 parathyroid (gland) 759.2
 parotid gland 750.26
 patella 755.64
 pelvis, pelvic girdle 755.69
 penis 752.8
 peripheral vascular system (congenital) NEC 747.60
  gastrointestinal 747.61
  lower limb 747.64
  renal 747.62
  specified NEC 747.69
  spinal 747.82
  upper limb 747.63
 pituitary (gland) 759.2
 pulmonary 748.5
  arteriovenous 747.3
  artery 747.3
  valve 746.01
 punctum lacrimale 743.65
 radioulnar (see also Absence, radius, congenital, with ulna) 755.25
 radius (see also Absence, radius, congenital) 755.26
 rectum 751.2
 respiratory system NEC 748.9
 rib 756.3
 sacrum 756.19
 scapula 755.59
 shoulder girdle 755.59
 skin 757.39
 skull (bone) 756.0
  with
   anencephalus 740.0
   encephalocele 742.0
   hydrocephalus 742.3
    with spina bifida (see also Spina bifida) 741.0
   microcephalus 742.1
 spinal (cord) (ventral horn cell) 742.59
  vessel 747.82
 spine 756.19
 spleen 759.0
 sternum 756.3
 tarsus (see also Absence, tarsal, congenital) 755.38
 testis, testicle 752.8
 thymus (gland) 279.11
 thyroid (gland) 243
  cartilage 748.3
 tibiofibular (see also Absence, tibia, congenital, with fibula) 755.35
 toe (see also Absence, toe, congenital) 755.39
 tongue 750.16
 trachea (cartilage) (rings) 748.3
 Turner's (tooth) 520.4

Hypoplasia, hypoplasis—continued
 ulna (see also Absence, ulna, congenital) 755.27
 umbilical artery 747.5
 ureter 753.2
 uterus 752.3
 vagina 752.49
 vascular (peripheral) NEC (see also Hypoplasia, peripheral vascular system) 747.60
  brain 747.81
 vein(s) (peripheral) NEC (see also Hypoplasia, peripheral vascular system) 747.60
  brain 747.81
  cardiac 746.89
  great 747.49
  portal 747.49
  pulmonary 747.49
  vena cava (inferior) (superior) 747.49
 vertebra 756.19
 vulva 752.49
 zonule (ciliary) 743.39
 zygoma 738.12
Hypopotassemia 276.8
Hypoproaccelerinemia (see also Defect, coagulation) 286.3
Hypoproconvertinemia (congenital) (see also Defect, coagulation) 286.3
Hypoproteinemia (essential) (hypermetabolic) (idiopathic) 273.8
Hypoproteinosis 260
Hypoprothrombinemia (congenital) (hereditary) (idiopathic) (see also Defect, coagulation) 286.3
 acquired 286.7
 newborn 776.3
Hypopselaphesia 782.0
Hypopyon (anterior chamber) (eye) 364.05
 iritis 364.05
 ulcer (cornea) 370.04
Hypopyrexia 780.9
Hyporeflex 796.1
Hyporeninemia, extreme 790.99
 in primary aldosteronism 255.1
Hyposecretion
 ACTH 253.4
 ovary 256.3
  postblative 256.2
 salivary gland (any) 527.7
Hyposegmentation of neutrophils, hereditary 288.2
Hyposiderinemia 280.9
Hyposmolality 276.1
 syndrome 276.1
Hyposomatotropism 253.3
Hyposomnia (see also Insomnia) 780.52
Hypospadias (male) 752.6
 female 753.8
Hypospermatogenesis 606.1
Hyposphagma 372.72
Hyposplenism 289.59
Hypostasis, pulmonary 514
Hypostatic — see condition
Hyposthenuria 593.89
Hyposuprarenalism 255.4
Hypo-TBG-nemia 246.8
Hypotension (arterial) (constitutional) 458.9
 chronic 458.1
 maternal, syndrome (following labor and delivery) 669.2
 orthostatic (chronic) 458.0
  dysautonomic-dyskinetic syndrome 333.0
 permanent idiopathic 458.1

Hypotension—continued
 postural 458.0
 transient 796.3
Hypothermia (accidental) 991.6
 anesthetic 995.89
 newborn NEC 778.3
 not associated with low environmental temperature 780.9
Hypothymergasia (see also Psychosis, affective) 296.2
 recurrent episode 296.3
 single episode 296.2
Hypothyroidism (acquired) 244.9
 complicating pregnancy, childbirth, or puerperium 648.1
 congenital 243
 due to
  ablation 244.1
   radioactive iodine 244.1
   surgical 244.0
  iodine (administration) (ingestion) 244.2
   radioactive 244.1
  irradiation therapy 244.1
  p-aminosalicylic acid (PAS) 244.3
  phenylbutazone 244.3
  resorcinol 244.3
  specified cause NEC 244.8
  surgery 244.0
 goitrous (sporadic) 246.1
 iatrogenic NEC 244.3
 iodine 244.2
 pituitary 244.8
 postablative NEC 244.1
 postsurgical 244.0
 primary 244.9
 secondary NEC 244.8
 specified cause NEC 244.8
 sporadic goitrous 246.1
Hypotonia, hypotonicity, hypotony 781.3
 benign congenital 358.8
 bladder 596.4
 congenital 779.8
  benign 358.8
 eye 360.30
  due to
   fistula 360.32
   ocular disorder NEC 360.33
   following loss of aqueous or vitreous 360.33
  primary 360.31
 infantile muscular (benign) 359.0
 muscle 728.9
 uterus, uterine (contractions) — see Inertia, uterus
Hypotrichosis 704.09
 congenital 757.4
 lid (congenital) 757.4
  acquired 374.55
 postinfectional NEC 704.09
Hypotropia 378.32
Hypoventilation 786.09
Hypovitaminosis (see also Deficiency, vitamin) 269.2
Hypovolemia 276.5
 surgical shock 998.0
 traumatic (shock) 958.4
Hypoxemia (see also Anoxia) 799.0
Hypoxia (see also Anoxia) 799.0
 cerebral 348.1
  during or resulting from a procedure 997.0
 newborn 768.9
  mild or moderate 768.6
  severe 768.5
 fetal — see Distress, fetal
 intrauterine — see Distress, fetal

Hypoxia

Hypoxia—continued
  myocardial (see also
      Insufficiency, coronary)
      411.89
    arteriosclerotic — see
      Arteriosclerosis,
      coronary
    newborn — see Asphyxia,
      newborn
Hypsarrhythmia (see also Epilepsy)
    345.6
Hysteralgia, pregnant uterus 646.8
Hysteria, hysterical 300.10
  anxiety 300.20
  Charcot's gland 300.11
  conversion (any manifestation)
      300.11
  dissociative type NEC 300.15
  psychosis, acute 298.1
Hysteroepilepsy 300.11
**Hysterotomy, affecting fetus or
    newborn** 763.8

I

**Iatrogenic syndrome of excess
    cortisol** 255.0
Iceland disease (epidemic
    neuromyasthenia) 049.8
Ichthyosis (congenita) 757.1
  acquired 701.1
  fetalis gravior 757.1
  follicularis 757.1
  hystrix 757.39
  lamellar 757.1
  lingual 528.6
  palmaris and plantaris 757.39
  simplex 757.1
  vera 757.1
  vulgaris 757.1
Ichthyotoxism 988.0
  bacterial (see also Poisoning,
      food) 005.9
Icteroanemia, hemolytic (acquired)
    283.9
  congenital (see also
      Spherocytosis) 282.0
Icterus (see also Jaundice) 782.4
  catarrhal — see Icterus, infectious
  conjunctiva 782.4
    newborn 774.6
  epidemic — see Icterus,
      infectious
  febrilis — see Icterus, infectious
  fetus or newborn — see Jaundice,
      fetus or newborn
  gravis (see also Necrosis, liver)
      570
    complicating pregnancy 646.7
      affecting fetus or newborn
        760.8
    fetus or newborn NEC 773.0
    obstetrical 646.7
      affecting fetus or newborn
        760.8
  hematogenous (acquired) 283.9
  hemolytic (acquired) 283.9
    congenital (see also
        Spherocytosis) 282.0
  hemorrhagic (acute) 100.0
    leptospiral 100.0
    newborn 776.0
    spirochetal 100.0
  infectious 070.1
    with hepatic coma 070.0
    leptospiral 100.0
    spirochetal 100.0
  intermittens juvenilis 277.4
  malignant (see also Necrosis,
      liver) 570
  neonatorum (see also Jaundice,
      fetus or newborn) 774.6

INDEX TO DISEASES

Icterus—continued
  pernicious (see also Necrosis,
      liver) 570
  spirochetal 100.0
Ictus solaris, solis 992.0
Identity disorder 313.82
  dissociative 300.14
  gender role (child) 302.6
    adult 302.85
  psychosexual (child) 302.6
    adult 302.85
Idioglossia 307.9
Idiopathic — see condition
Idiosyncrasy (see also Allergy) 995.3
  drug, medicinal substance, and
      biological — see Allergy,
      drug
Idiot, idiocy (congenital) 318.2
  amaurotic (Bielschowsky) (-
      Jansky) (family) (infantile
      (late)) (juvenile (late)) (Vogt-
      Spielmeyer) 330.1
  microcephalic 742.1
  Mongolian 758.0
  oxycephalic 756.0
Id reaction (due to bacteria) 692.89
IgE asthma 493.0
Ileitis (chronic) (see also Enteritis)
    558.9
  infectious 009.0
  noninfectious 558.9
  regional (ulcerative) 555.0
    with large intestine 555.2
  segmental 555.0
    with large intestine 555.2
  terminal (ulcerative) 555.0
    with large intestine 555.2
Ileocolitis (see also Enteritis) 558.9
  infectious 009.0
  regional 555.2
  ulcerative 556.1
Ileostomy status V44.2
  with complication 569.6
Ileotyphus 002.0
Ileum — see condition
Ileus (adynamic) (bowel) (colon)
    (inhibitory) (intestine)
    (neurogenic) (paralytic) 560.1
  arteriomesenteric duodenal 537.2
  due to gallstone (in intestine)
      560.31
  duodenal, chronic 537.2
  following gastrointestinal surgery
      997.4
  gallstone 560.31
  mechanical (see also Obstruction,
      intestine) 560.9
  meconium 777.1
    due to cystic fibrosis 277.01
  myxedema 564.8
  postoperative 997.4
  transitory, newborn 777.4
Iliac — see condition
Ill, louping 063.1
Illegitimacy V61.6
Illness — see also Disease
  factitious (with physical
      symptoms) 300.19
    with psychological symptoms
        300.16
    chronic (with physical
        symptoms) 301.51
  heart — see Disease, heart
  manic-depressive (see also
      Psychosis, affective) 296.80
  mental (see also Disorder, mental)
      300.9

Imbalance 781.2
  autonomic (see also Neuropathy,
      peripheral, autonomic)
      337.9
  electrolyte 276.9
    with
      abortion — see Abortion,
          by type, with
          metabolic disorder
      ectopic pregnancy (see also
          categories 633.0-
          633.9) 639.4
      hyperemesis gravidarum
          (before 22 completed
          weeks gestation)
          643.1
      molar pregnancy (see also
          categories 630-632)
          639.4
    following
      abortion 639.4
      ectopic or molar pregnancy
          639.4
    neonatal, transitory NEC 775.5
  endocrine 259.9
  eye muscle NEC 378.9
    heterophoria — see
        Heterophoria
  glomerulotubular NEC 593.89
  hormone 259.9
  hysterical (see also Hysteria)
      300.10
  labyrinth NEC 386.50
  posture 729.9
  sympathetic (see also
      Neuropathy, peripheral,
      autonomic) 337.9
Imbecile, imbecility 318.0
  moral 301.7
  old age 290.9
  senile 290.9
  specified IQ — see IQ
  unspecified IQ 318.0
Imbedding, intrauterine device
    996.32
Imbibition, cholesterol (gallbladder)
    575.6
Imerslund (-Gräsbeck) syndrome
    (anemia due to familial
    selective vitamin B_{12}
    malabsorption) 281.1
Iminoacidopathy 270.8
Iminoglycinuria, familial 270.8
Immature — see also Immaturity
  personality 301.89
Immaturity 765.1
  extreme 765.0
  fetus or infant light-for-dates —
      see Light-for-dates
  lung, fetus or newborn 770.4
  organ or site NEC — see
      Hypoplasia
  pulmonary, fetus or newborn
      770.4
  reaction 301.89
  sexual (female) (male) 259.0
Immersion 994.1
  foot 991.4
  hand 991.4
Immobile, immobility
  intestine 564.8
  joint — see Ankylosis
  syndrome (paraplegic) 728.2
Immunization
  ABO
    affecting management of
        pregnancy 656.2
    fetus or newborn 773.1
    complication — see
        Complications, vaccination
  Rh factor
    affecting management of
        pregnancy 656.1
    fetus or newborn 773.0
    from transfusion 999.7

Impaired, impairment

Immunodeficiency 279.3
  with
    adenosine-deaminase
        deficiency 279.2
    defect, predominant
      B-cell 279.00
      T-cell 279.10
    hyperimmunoglobulinemia
        279.2
    lymphopenia, hereditary 279.2
    thrombocytopenia and
        eczema 279.12
    thymic
      aplasia 279.2
      dysplasia 279.2
    autosomal recessive, Swiss-type
        279.2
    common variable 279.06
    severe combined (SCID) 279.2
  to Rh factor
    affecting management of
        pregnancy 656.1
    fetus or newborn 773.0
  X-linked, with increased IgM
      279.05
Immunotherapy, prophylactic V07.2
Impaction, impacted
  bowel, colon, rectum 560.30
    with hernia — see also
        Hernia, by site, with
        obstruction
      gangrenous — see Hernia,
          by site, with
          gangrene
    by
      calculus 560.39
      gallstone 560.31
      fecal 560.39
      specified type NEC 560.39
  calculus — see Calculus
  cerumen (ear) (external) 380.4
  cuspid 520.6
    with abnormal position (same
        or adjacent tooth) 524.3
  dental 520.6
    with abnormal position (same
        or adjacent tooth) 524.3
  fecal, feces 560.39
    with hernia — see also
        Hernia, by site, with
        obstruction
      gangrenous — see Hernia,
          by site, with
          gangrene
  fracture — see Fracture, by site
  gallbladder — see Cholelithiasis
  gallstone(s) — see Cholelithiasis
    in intestine (any part) 560.31
  intestine(s) 560.30
    with hernia — see also
        Hernia, by site, with
        obstruction
      grangrenous — see Hernia,
          by site, with
          gangrene
    by
      calculus 560.39
      gallstone 560.31
      fecal 560.39
      specified type NEC 560.39
  intrauterine device (IUD) 996.32
  molar 520.6
    with abnormal position (same
        or adjacent tooth) 524.3
  shoulder 660.4
    affecting fetus or newborn
        763.1
  tooth, teeth 520.6
    with abnormal position (same
        or adjacent tooth) 524.3
  turbinate 733.99
Impaired, impairment (function)
  arm V49.1
    movement, involving
        musculoskeletal system
        V49.1
    nervous system V49.2

Impaired, impairment—*continued*
  auditory discrimination 388.43
  back V48.3
  body (entire) V49.8
  hearing (*see also* Deafness) 389.9
  heart — *see* Disease, heart
  kidney (*see also* Disease, renal) 593.9
    disorder resulting from 588.9
    specified NEC 588.8
  leg V49.1
    movement, involving
      musculoskeletal system V49.1
      nervous system V49.2
  limb V49.1
    movement, involving
      musculoskeletal system V49.1
      nervous system V49.2
  liver 573.8
  mastication 524.9
  mobility
    ear ossicles NEC 385.22
    incostapedial joint 385.22
    malleus 385.21
  myocardium, myocardial (*see also* Insufficiency, myocardial) 428.0
  neuromusculoskeletal NEC V49.8
    back V48.3
    head V48.2
    limb V49.2
    neck V48.3
    spine V48.3
    trunk V48.3
  rectal sphincter 787.9
  renal (*see also* Disease, renal) 593.9
    disorder resulting from 588.9
    specified NEC 588.8
  spine V48.3
  vision NEC 369.9
    both eyes NEC 369.3
    moderate 369.74
      both eyes 369.25
        with impairment of lesser eye (specified as)
          blind, not further specified 369.15
          low vision, not further specified 369.23
          near-total 369.17
          profound 369.18
          severe 369.24
          total 369.16
      one eye 369.74
        with vision of other eye (specified as)
          near-normal 369.75
          normal 369.76
    near-total 369.64
      both eyes 369.04
        with impairment of lesser eye (specified as)
          blind, not further specified 369.02
          total 369.03
      one eye 369.64
        with vision of other eye (specified as)
          near normal 369.65
          normal 369.66
    one eye 369.60
      with low vision of other eye 369.10

Impaired, impairment—*continued*
  vision NEC—*continued*
    profound 369.67
      both eyes 369.08
        with impairment of lesser eye (specified as)
          blind, not further specified 369.05
          near-total 369.07
          total 369.06
      one eye 369.67
        with vision of other eye (specified as)
          near-normal 369.68
          normal 369.69
    severe 369.71
      both eyes 369.22
        with impairment of lesser eye (specified as)
          blind, not further specified 369.11
          low vision, not further specified 369.21
          near-total 369.13
          profound 369.14
          total 369.12
      one eye 369.71
        with vision of other eye (specified as)
          near-normal 369.72
          normal 369.73
    total
      both eyes 369.01
      one eye 369.61
        with vision of other eye (specified as)
          near-normal 369.62
          normal 369.63

Impaludism — *see* Malaria
Impediment, speech NEC 784.5
  psychogenic 307.9
  secondary to organic lesion 784.5
Impending
  cerebrovascular accident or attack 435.9
  coronary syndrome 411.1
  delirium tremens 291.0
  myocardial infarction 411.1
Imperception, auditory (acquired) (congenital) 389.9
Imperfect
  aeration, lung (newborn) 770.5
  closure (congenital)
    alimentary tract NEC 751.8
      lower 751.5
      upper 750.8
    atrioventricular ostium 745.69
    atrium (secundum) 745.5
      primum 745.61
    branchial cleft or sinus 744.41
    choroid 743.59
    cricoid cartilage 748.3
    cusps, heart valve NEC 746.89
      pulmonary 746.09
    ductus
      arteriosus 747.0
      Botalli 747.0
    ear drum 744.29
      causing impairment of hearing 744.03
    endocardial cushion 745.60
    epiglottis 748.3
    esophagus with communication to bronchus or trachea 750.3
    Eustachian valve 746.89
    eyelid 743.62
    face, facial (*see also* Cleft, lip) 749.10

Imperfect—*continued*
  closure—*continued*
    foramen
      Botalli 745.5
      ovale 745.5
    genitalia, genital organ(s) or system
      female 752.8
        external 752.49
        internal NEC 752.8
        uterus 752.3
      male 752.8
    glottis 748.3
    heart valve (cusps) NEC 746.89
    interatrial ostium or septum 745.5
    interauricular ostium or septum 745.5
    interventricular ostium or septum 745.4
    iris 743.46
    kidney 753.3
    larynx 748.3
    lens 743.36
    lip (*see also* Cleft, lip) 749.10
    nasal septum or sinus 748.1
    nose 748.1
    omphalomesenteric duct 751.0
    optic nerve entry 743.57
    organ or site NEC — *see* Anomaly, specified type, by site
    ostium
      interatrial 745.5
      interauricular 745.5
      interventricular 745.4
    palate (*see also* Cleft, palate) 749.00
    preauricular sinus 744.46
    retina 743.56
    roof of orbit 742.0
    sclera 743.47
    septum
      aortic 745.0
      aorticopulmonary 745.0
      atrial (secundum) 745.5
        primum 745.61
      between aorta and pulmonary artery 745.0
      heart 745.9
      interatrial (secundum) 745.5
        primum 745.61
      interauricular (secundum) 745.5
        primum 745.61
      interventricular 745.4
        with pulmonary stenosis or atresia, dextraposition of aorta, and hypertrophy of right ventricle 745.2
          in tetralogy of Fallot 745.2
      nasal 748.1
      ventricular 745.4
        with pulmonary stenosis or atresia, dextraposition of aorta, and hypertrophy of right ventricle 745.2
          in tetralogy of Fallot 745.2
    skull 756.0
      with
        anencephalus 740.0
        encephalocele 742.0

Imperfect—*continued*
  closure—*continued*
    skull—*continued*
      with—*continued*
        hydrocephalus 742.3
          with spina bifida (*see also* Spina bifida) 741.0
        microcephalus 742.1
    spine (with meningocele) (*see also* Spina bifida) 741.90
    thyroid cartilage 748.3
    trachea 748.3
    tympanic membrane 744.29
      causing impairment of hearing 744.03
    uterus (with communication to bladder, intestine, or rectum) 752.3
    uvula 749.02
      with cleft lip (*see also* Cleft, palate, with cleft lip) 749.20
    vitelline duct 751.0
  development — *see* Anomaly, by site
  erection 607.84
  fusion — *see* Imperfect, closure
  inflation lung (newborn) 770.5
  intestinal canal 751.5
  poise 729.9
  rotation — *see* Malrotation
  septum, ventricular 745.4
Imperfectly descended testis 752.5
Imperforate (congenital) — *see also* Atresia
  anus 751.2
  bile duct 751.61
  cervix (uteri) 752.49
  esophagus 750.3
  hymen 752.42
  intestine (small) 751.1
    large 751.2
  jejunum 751.1
  pharynx 750.29
  rectum 751.2
  salivary duct 750.23
  ureter 753.2
  urethra 753.6
  urinary meatus 753.6
  vagina 752.49
Impervious (congenital) — *see also* Atresia
  anus 751.2
  bile duct 751.61
  esophagus 750.3
  intestine (small) 751.1
    large 751.5
  rectum 751.2
  ureter 753.2
  urethra 753.6
Impetiginization of other dermatoses 684
Impetigo (any organism) (any site) (bullous) (circinate) (contagiosa) (neonatorum) (simplex) 684
  Bockhart's (superficial folliculitis) 704.8
  external ear 684 [380.13]
  eyelid 684 [373.5]
  Fox's (contagiosa) 684
  furfuracea 696.5
  herpetiformis 694.3
    nonobstetrical 694.3
  staphylococcal infection 684
  ulcerative 686.8
  vulgaris 684
Impingement, soft tissue between teeth 524.2
Implant, endometrial 617.9

Implantation
- anomalous — see also Anomaly, specified type, by site
    - ureter 753.4
- cyst
    - external area or site (skin) NEC 709.8
    - iris 364.61
    - vagina 623.8
    - vulva 624.8
- dermoid (cyst)
    - external area or site (skin) NEC 709.8
    - iris 364.61
    - vagina 623.8
    - vulva 624.8
- placenta, low or marginal — see Placenta previa

Impotence (sexual) (psychogenic) 302.72
- organic origin NEC 607.84

Impoverished blood 285.9

Impression, basilar 756.0

Imprisonment V62.5

Improper
- care (child) (newborn) 995.5
    - affecting parent or family V61.21
    - as reason for family seeking advice V61.21
    - specified person other than child 995.81
- development, infant 764.9

Improperly tied umbilical cord (causing hemorrhage) 772.3

Impulses, obsessional 300.3

Impulsive neurosis 300.3

Inaction, kidney (see also Disease, renal) 593.9

Inactive — see condition

Inadequate, inadequacy
- biologic 301.6
- cardiac and renal — see Hypertension, cardiorenal
- constitutional 301.6
- development
    - child 783.4
    - fetus 764.9
        - affecting management of pregnancy 656.5
    - genitalia
        - after puberty NEC 259.0
        - congenital — see Hypoplasia, genitalia
    - lungs 748.5
    - organ or site NEC — see Hypoplasia, by site
- dietary 269.9
- education V62.3
- environment
    - economic problem V60.2
    - household condition NEC V60.1
    - poverty V60.2
    - unemployment V62.0
- functional 301.6
- household care, due to family member
    - handicapped or ill V60.4
    - temporarily away from home V60.4
    - on vacation V60.5
    - technical defects in home V60.1
    - temporary absence from home of person rendering care V60.4
- housing (heating) (space) V60.1
- material resources V60.2
- mental (see also Retardation, mental) 319
- nervous system 799.2
- personality 301.6
- prenatal care in current pregnancy V23.7

Inadequate, inadequacy—continued
- pulmonary
    - function 786.09
        - newborn 770.8
    - ventilation, newborn 770.8
    - respiration 786.09
        - newborn 770.8
- social 301.6

Inanition 263.9
- with edema 262
- due to
    - deprivation of food 994.2
    - malnutrition 263.9
- fever 780.6

Inappropriate secretion
- ACTH 255.0
- antidiuretic hormone (ADH) (excessive) 253.6
    - deficiency 253.5
- ectopic hormone NEC 259.3
- pituitary (posterior) 253.6

Inattention after or at birth 995.5
- affecting parent or family V61.21

Inborn errors of metabolism — see Disorder, metabolism

Incarceration, incarcerated
- bubonocele — see also Hernia, inguinal, with obstruction
    - gangrenous — see Hernia, inguinal, with gangrene
- colon (by hernia) — see also Hernia, by site with obstruction
    - gangrenous — see Hernia, by site, with gangrene
- enterocele 552.9
    - gangrenous 551.9
- epigastrocele 552.29
    - gangrenous 551.29
- epiplocele 552.9
    - gangrenous 551.9
- exomphalos 552.1
    - gangrenous 551.1
- fallopian tube 620.8
- hernia — see also Hernia, by site, with obstruction
    - gangrenous — see Hernia, by site, with gangrene
- iris, in wound 871.1
- lens, in wound 871.1
- merocele (see also Hernia, femoral, with obstruction) 552.00
- omentum (by hernia) — see also Hernia, by site, with obstruction
    - gangrenous — see Hernia, by site, with gangrene
- omphalocele 756.7
- rupture (meaning hernia) (see also Hernia, by site, with obstruction) 552.9
    - gangrenous (see also Hernia, by site, with gangrene) 551.9
- sarcoepiplocele 552.9
    - gangrenous 551.9
- sarcoepiplomphalocele 552.1
    - with gangrene 551.1
- uterus 621.8
    - gravid 654.3
        - causing obstructed labor 660.2
        - affecting fetus or newborn 763.1

Incident, cerebrovascular (see also Disease, cerebrovascular, acute) 436

Incineration (entire body) (from fire, conflagration, electricity, or lightning) — see Burn, multiple, specified sites

Incised wound
- external — see Wound, open, by site
- internal organs (abdomen, chest, or pelvis) — see Injury, internal, by site, with open wound

Incision, incisional
- hernia — see Hernia, incisional
- surgical, complication — see Complications, surgical procedures
- traumatic
    - external — see Wound, open, by site
    - internal organs (abdomen, chest, or pelvis) — see Injury, internal, by site, with open wound

Inclusion
- azurophilic leukocytic 288.2
- blennorrhea (neonatal) (newborn) 771.6
- cyst — see Cyst, skin
- gallbladder in liver (congenital) 751.69

Incompatibility
- ABO
    - affecting management of pregnancy 656.2
    - fetus or newborn 773.1
    - infusion or transfusion reaction 999.6
- blood (group) (Duffy) (E) (K(ell)) (Kidd) (Lewis) (M) (N) (P) (S) NEC
    - affecting management of pregnancy 656.2
    - fetus or newborn 773.2
    - infusion or transfusion reaction 999.6
- marital V61.1
    - involving divorce or estrangement V61.0
- Rh (blood group) (factor)
    - affecting management of pregnancy 656.1
    - fetus or newborn 773.0
    - infusion or transfusion reaction 999.7
- Rhesus — see Incompatibility, Rh

Incompetency, incompetence, incompetent
- annular
- aortic (valve) (see also Insufficiency, aortic) 424.1
- mitral (valve) — (see also Insufficiency, mitral) 424.0
- pulmonary valve (heart) (see also Endocarditis, pulmonary) 424.3
- aortic (valve) (see also Insufficiency, aortic) 424.1
    - syphilitic 093.22
- cardiac (orifice) 530.0
- valve — see Endocarditis
- cervix, cervical (os) 622.5
    - in pregnancy 654.5
        - affecting fetus or newborn 761.0
- esophagogastric (junction) (sphincter) 530.0
- heart valve, congenital 746.89
- mitral (valve) — see Insufficiency, mitral
- papillary muscle (heart) 429.81
- pelvic fundus 618.8
- pulmonary valve (heart) (see also Endocarditis, pulmonary) 424.3
    - congenital 746.09

Incompetency, incompetence, incompetent—continued
- tricuspid (annular) (rheumatic) (valve) (see also Endocarditis, tricuspid) 397.0
- valvular — see Endocarditis
- vein, venous (saphenous) (varicose) (see also Varicose, vein) 454.9
- velopharyngeal (closure)
    - acquired 528.9
    - congenital 750.29

Incomplete — see also condition
- bladder emptying 788.21
- expansion lungs (newborn) 770.5
- gestation (liveborn) — see Immaturity
- rotation — see Malrotation

Incontinence 788.30
- without sensory awareness 788.34
- anal sphincter 787.6
- continuous leakage 788.37
- feces 787.6
    - due to hysteria 300.11
    - nonorganic origin 307.7
- hysterical 300.11
- mixed (male) (female) (urge and stress) 788.33
- overflow 788.39
- paradoxical 788.39
- rectal 787.6
- specified NEC 788.39
- stress (female) 625.6
    - male NEC 788.32
- urethral sphincter 599.84
- urge 788.31
    - and stress (male) (female) 788.33
- urine 788.30
    - active 788.30
    - male 788.30
        - stress 788.32
            - and urge 788.33
    - neurogenic 788.39
    - nonorganic origin 307.6
    - stress (female) 625.6
        - male NEC 788.32
    - urge 788.31
        - and stress 788.33

Incontinentia pigmenti 757.33

Incoordinate
- uterus (action) (contractions) 661.4
    - affecting fetus or newborn 763.7

Incoordination
- esophageal-pharyngeal (newborn) 787.2
- muscular 781.3
- papillary muscle 429.81

Increase, increased
- abnormal, in development 783.9
- androgens (ovarian) 256.1
- anticoagulants (antithrombin) (anti-VIIIa) (anti-IXa) (anti-Xa) (anti-XIa) 286.5
    - postpartum 666.3
- cold sense (see also Disturbance, sensation) 782.0
- estrogen 256.0
- function
    - adrenal (cortex) 255.3
        - medulla 255.6
    - pituitary (anterior) (gland) (lobe) 253.1
        - posterior 253.6
- heat sense (see also Disturbance, sensation) 782.0
- intracranial pressure 348.2
    - injury at birth 767.8
- light reflex of retina 362.13
- permeability, capillary 448.9

Increase, increased—continued
  pressure
    intracranial 348.2
      injury at birth 767.8
    intraocular 365.00
  pulsations 785.9
  pulse pressure 785.9
  sphericity, lens 743.36
  splenic activity 289.4
  venous pressure 459.89
    portal 572.3
Incrustation, cornea, lead or zinc 930.0
Incyclophoria 378.44
Incyclotropia 378.33
Indeterminate sex 752.7
India rubber skin 756.83
Indicanuria 270.2
Indigestion (bilious) (functional) 536.8
  acid 536.8
  catarrhal 536.8
  due to decomposed food NEC 005.9
  fat 579.8
  nervous 306.4
  psychogenic 306.4
Indirect — see condition
Indolent bubo NEC 099.8
Induced
  abortion — see Abortion, induced
  birth, affecting fetus or newborn 763.8
  delivery — see Delivery
  labor — see Delivery
Induration, indurated
  brain 348.8
  breast (fibrous) 611.79
    puerperal, postpartum 676.3
  broad ligament 620.8
  chancre 091.0
    anus 091.1
    congenital 090.0
    extragenital NEC 091.2
  corpora cavernosa (penis) (plastic) 607.89
  liver (chronic) 573.8
    acute 573.8
  lung (black) (brown) (chronic) (fibroid) (see also Fibrosis, lung) 515
    essential brown 275.0 [516.1]
  penile 607.89
  phlebitic — see Phlebitis
  skin 782.8
  stomach 537.89
Induratio penis plastica 607.89
Industrial — see condition
Inebriety (see also Abuse, drugs, nondependent) 305.0
Inefficiency
  kidney (see also Disease, renal) 593.9
  thyroid (acquired) (gland) 244.9
Inelasticity, skin 782.8
Inequality, leg (acquired) (length) 736.81
  congenital 755.30
Inertia
  bladder 596.4
    neurogenic 596.54
      with cauda equina syndrome 344.61
  stomach 536.8
    psychogenic 306.4
  uterus, uterine 661.2
    affecting fetus or newborn 763.7
    primary 661.0
    secondary 661.1
  vesical 596.4
    neurogenic 596.54
      with cauda equina 344.61

Infant — see also condition
  held for adoption V68.89
  newborn — see Newborn
  syndrome of diabetic mother 775.0
"Infant Hercules" syndrome 255.2
Infantile — see also condition
  genitalia, genitals 259.0
    in pregnancy or childbirth NEC 654.4
      affecting fetus or newborn 763.8
      causing obstructed labor 660.2
        affecting fetus or newborn 763.1
  heart 746.9
  kidney 753.3
  lack of care 995.5
    affecting parent or family V61.21
  macula degeneration 362.75
  melanodontia 521.0
  os, uterus (see also Infantile, genitalia) 259.0
  pelvis 738.6
    with disproportion (fetopelvic) 653.1
      affecting fetus or newborn 763.1
      causing obstructed labor 660.1
        affecting fetus or newborn 763.1
  penis 259.0
  testis 257.2
  uterus (see also Infantile, genitalia) 259.0
  vulva 752.49
Infantilism 259.9
  with dwarfism (hypophyseal) 253.3
  Brissaud's (infantile myxedema) 244.9
  celiac 579.0
  Herter's (nontropical sprue) 579.0
  hypophyseal 253.3
  hypothalamic (with obesity) 253.8
  idiopathic 259.9
  intestinal 579.0
  pancreatic 577.8
  pituitary 253.3
  renal 588.0
  sexual (with obesity) 259.0
Infants, healthy liveborn — see Newborn
Infarct, infarction
  adrenal (capsule) (gland) 255.4
  amnion 658.8
  anterior (with contiguous portion of intraventricular septum) NEC (see also Infarct, myocardium) 410.1
  appendices epiploicae 557.0
  bowel 557.0
  brain (stem) 434.91
    embolic (see also Embolism, brain) 434.11
    healed or old — see also category 438
      without residuals V12.5
    late effect — see category 438
    puerperal, postpartum, childbirth 674.0
    thrombotic (see also Thrombosis, brain) 434.01
  breast 611.8
  Brewer's (kidney) 593.81
  cardiac (see also Infarct, myocardium) 410.9
  cerebellar (see also Infarct, brain) 434.91
    embolic (see also Embolism, brain) 434.11

Infarct, infarction—continued
  cerebral (see also Infarct, brain) 434.91
    embolic (see also Embolism, brain) 434.11
  chorion 658.8
  colon (acute) (agnogenic) (embolic) (hemorrhagic) (nonocclusive) (nonthrombotic) (occlusive) (segmental) (thrombotic) (with gangrene) 557.0
  coronary artery (see also Infarct, myocardium) 410.9
  embolic (see also Embolism) 444.9
  fallopian tube 620.8
  gallbladder 575.8
  heart (see also Infarct, myocardium) 410.9
  hepatic 573.4
  hypophysis (anterior lobe) 253.8
  impending (myocardium) 411.1
  intestine (acute) (agnogenic) (embolic) (hemorrhagic) (nonocclusive) (nonthrombotic) (occlusive) (thrombotic) (with gangrene) 557.0
  kidney 593.81
  liver 573.4
  lung (embolic) (thrombotic) 415.1
    with
      abortion — see Abortion, by type, with embolism
      ectopic pregnancy (see also categories 633.0-633.9) 639.6
      molar pregnancy (see also categories 630-632) 639.6
    following
      abortion 639.6
      ectopic or molar pregnancy 639.6
    in pregnancy, childbirth, or puerperium — see Embolism, obstetrical
  lymph node or vessel 457.8
  medullary (brain) — see Infarct, brain
  meibomian gland (eyelid) 374.85
  mesentary, mesenteric (embolic) (thrombotic) (with gangrene) 557.0
  midbrain — see Infarct, brain
  myocardium, myocardial (acute or with a stated duration of 8 weeks or less) (with hypertension) 410.9

Note — Use the following fifth-digit subclassification with category 410:
  0 episode unspecified
  1 initial episode
  2 subsequent episode without recurrence

  with symptoms after 8 weeks from date of infarction 414.8
  anterior (wall) (with contiguous portion of intraventricular septum) NEC 410.1
  anteroapical (with contiguous portion of intraventricular septum) 410.1
  anterolateral (wall) 410.0
  anteroseptal (with contiguous portion of intraventricular septum) 410.1
  apical-lateral 410.5

Infarct, infarction—continued
  myocardium, myocardial—continued
    atrial 410.8
    basal-lateral 410.5
    chronic (with symptoms after 8 weeks from date of infarction) 414.8
    diagnosed on ECG, but presenting no symptoms 412
    diaphragmatic wall (with contiguous portion of intraventricular septum) 410.4
    healed or old, currently presenting no symptoms 412
    high lateral 410.5
    impending 411.1
    inferior (wall) (with contiguous portion of intraventricular septum) 410.4
    inferolateral (wall) 410.2
    inferoposterior wall 410.3
    lateral wall 410.5
    nontransmural 410.7
    papillary muscle 410.8
    past (diagnosed on ECG or other special investigation, but currently presenting no symptoms) 412
      with symptoms NEC 414.8
    posterior (strictly) (true) (wall) 410.6
    posterobasal 410.6
    posteroinferior 410.3
    posterolateral 410.5
    previous, currently presenting no symptoms 412
    septal 410.8
    specified site NEC 410.8
    subendocardial 410.7
    syphilitic 093.82
  nontransmural 410.7
  omentum 557.0
  ovary 620.8
  pancreas 577.8
  papillary muscle (see also Infarct, myocardium) 410.8
  parathyroid gland 252.8
  pituitary (gland) 253.8
  placenta (complicating pregnancy) 656.7
    affecting fetus or newborn 762.2
  pontine — see Infarct, brain
  posterior NEC (see also Infarct, myocardium) 410.6
  prostate 602.8
  pulmonary (artery) (hemorrhagic) (vein) 415.1
    with
      abortion — see Abortion, by type, with embolism
      ectopic pregnancy (see also categories 633.0-633.9) 639.6
      molar pregnancy (see also categories 630-632) 639.6
    following
      abortion 639.6
      ectopic or molar pregnancy 639.6
    in pregnancy, childbirth, or puerperium — see Embolism, obstetrical
  renal 593.81
    embolic or thrombotic 593.81
  retina, retinal 362.84
    with occlusion — see Occlusion, retina

Infarct, infarction—continued
    spinal (acute) (cord) (embolic) (nonembolic) 336.1
    spleen 289.59
        embolic or thrombotic 444.89
    subchorionic — *see* Infarct, placenta
    subendocardial (*see also* Infarct, myocardium) 410.7
    suprarenal (capsule) (gland) 255.4
    syncytium — *see* Infarct, placenta
    testis 608.83
    thrombotic (*see also* Thrombosis) 453.9
        artery, arterial — *see* Embolism
    thyroid (gland) 246.3
    ventricle (heart) (*see also* Infarct, myocardium) 410.9

Infecting — *see* condition

Infection, infected, infective
    (opportunistic) 136.9
    with lymphangitis — *see* Lymphangitis
    abortion — *see* Abortion, by type, with sepsis
    abscess (skin) — *see* Abscess, by site
    Absidia 117.7
    Acanthocheilonema (perstans) 125.4
        streptocerca 125.6
    accessory sinus (chronic) (*see also* Sinusitis) 473.9
    Achorion — *see* Dermatophytosis
    Acremonium falciforme 117.4
    acromioclavicular (joint) 711.91
    actinobacillus
        lignieresii 027.8
        mallei 024
        muris 026.1
    actinomadura — *see* Actinomycosis
    Actinomyces (israelii) — *see also* Actinomycosis
        muris-ratti 026.1
    Actinomycetales (actinomadura) (Actinomyces) (Nocardia) (Streptomyces) — *see* Actinomycosis
    actinomycotic NEC (*see also* Actinomycosis) 039.9
    adenoid (chronic) 474.0
        acute 463
        and tonsil (chronic) 474.0
            acute or subacute 463
    adenovirus NEC 079.0
        in diseases classified elsewhere — *see* category 079
        unspecified nature or site 079.0
    Aerobacter aerogenes NEC 041.85
        enteritis 008.2
    aerogenes capsulatus (*see also* Gangrene, gas) 040.0
    aertrycke (*see also* Infection, Salmonella) 003.9
    ajellomyces dermatitidis 116.0
    alimentary canal NEC (*see also* Enteritis, due to, by organism) 009.0
    Allescheria boydii 117.6
    Alternaria 118
    alveolus, alveolar (process) (pulpal origin) 522.4
    ameba, amebic (histolytica) (*see also* Amebiasis) 006.9
        acute 006.0
        chronic 006.1
        free-living 136.2
        hartmanni 007.8
        specified
            site NEC 006.8
            type NEC 007.8

Infection, infected, infective—continued
    amniotic fluid or cavity 658.4
        affecting fetus or newborn 762.7
    anaerobes (cocci) (gram-negative) (gram-positive) (mixed) NEC 041.84
    anal canal 569.49
    Ancylostoma braziliense 126.2
    Angiostrongylus cantonensis 128.8
    anisakiasis 127.1
    Anisakis larva 127.1
    anthrax (*see also* Anthrax) 022.9
    antrum (chronic) (*see also* Sinusitis, maxillary) 473.0
    anus (papillae) (sphincter) 569.49
    arbor virus NEC 066.9
    arbovirus NEC 066.9
    argentophil-rod 027.0
    Ascaris lumbricoides 127.0
    ascomycetes 117.4
    Aspergillus (flavus) (fumigatus) (terreus) 117.3
    atypical
        acid-fast (bacilli) (*see also* Mycobacterium, atypical) 031.9
        mycobacteria (*see also* Mycobacterium, atypical) 031.9
    auditory meatus (circumscribed) (diffuse) (external) (*see also* Otitis, externa) 380.10
    auricle (ear) (*see also* Otitis, externa) 380.10
    axillary gland 683
    Babesiasis 088.82
    Babesiosis 088.82
    Bacillus NEC 041.89
        abortus 023.1
        anthracis (*see also* Anthrax) 022.9
        cereus (food poisoning) 005.8
        coli — *see* Infection, Escherichia coli
        coliform NEC 041.85
        Ducrey's (any location) 099.0
        Flexner's 004.1
        fragilis NEC 041.82
        Friedländer's NEC 041.3
        fusiformis 101
        gas (gangrene) (*see also* Gangrene, gas) 040.0
        mallei 024
        melitensis 023.0
        paratyphoid, paratyphosus 002.9
            A 002.1
            B 002.2
            C 002.3
        Schmorl's 040.3
        Shiga 004.0
        suipestifer (*see also* Infection, Salmonella) 003.9
        swimming pool 031.1
        typhosa 002.0
        welchii (*see also* Gangrene, gas) 040.0
        Whitmore's 025
    bacterial NEC 041.9
        specified NEC 041.89
            anaerobic NEC 041.84
            gram-negative NEC 041.85
                anaerobic NEC 041.84
    Bacterium
        paratyphosum 002.9
            A 002.1
            B 002.2
            C 002.3
        typhosum 002.0
    Bacteroides (fragilis) (melaninogenicus) (oralis) NEC 041.84
    balantidium coli 007.0
    Bartholin's gland 616.8

Infection, infected, infective—continued
    Basidiobolus 117.7
    Bedsonia 079.98
        specified NEC 079.88
    bile duct 576.1
    bladder (*see also* Cystitis) 595.9
    Blastomyces, blastomycotic 116.0
        brasiliensis 116.1
        dermatitidis 116.0
        European 117.5
        Loboi 116.2
        North American 116.0
        South American 116.1
    blood stream — *see* Septicemia
    bone 730.9
        specified — *see* Osteomyelitis
    Bordetella 033.9
        bronchiseptica 033.8
        parapertussis 033.1
        pertussis 033.0
    Borrelia
        bergdorfi 088.81
        vincentii (mouth) (pharynx) (tonsil) 101
    brain (*see also* Encephalitis) 323.9
        late effect — *see* category 326
        membranes — (*see also* Meningitis) 322.9
        septic 324.0
            late effect — *see* category 326
        meninges (*see also* Meningitis) 320.9
    branchial cyst 744.42
    breast 611.0
        puerperal, postpartum 675.2
            with nipple 675.9
                specified type NEC 675.8
            nonpurulent 675.2
            purulent 675.1
    bronchus (*see also* Bronchitis) 490
        fungus NEC 117.9
    Brucella 023.9
        abortus 023.1
        canis 023.3
        melitensis 023.0
        mixed 023.8
        suis 023.2
    Brugia (Wuchereria) malayi 125.1
    bursa — *see* Bursitis
    buttocks (skin) 686.9
    Candida (albicans) (tropicalis) (*see also* Candidiasis) 112.9
        congenital 771.7
    Candiru 136.8
    Capillaria
        hepatica 128.8
        philippinensis 127.5
    cartilage 733.99
    cat liver fluke 121.0
    cellulitis — *see* Cellulitis, by site
    Cephalosporum falciforme 117.4
    Cercomonas hominis (intestinal) 007.3
    cerebrospinal (*see also* Meningitis) 322.9
        late effect — *see* category 326
    cervical gland 683
    cervix (*see also* Cervicitis) 616.0
    cesarean section wound 674.3
    Chilomastix (intestinal) 007.8
    Chlamydia 079.98
        specified NEC 079.88
    cholera (*see also* Cholera) 001.9
    chorionic plate 658.8
    Cladosporium
        bantianum 117.8
        carrionii 117.2
        mansoni 111.1
        trichoides 117.8
        wernecki 111.1
    Clonorchis (sinensis) (liver) 121.1

Infection, infected, infective—continued
    Clostridium (haemolyticum) (novyi) NEC 041.84
        botulinum 005.1
        congenital 771.8
        histolyticum (*see also* Gangrene, gas) 040.0
        oedematiens (*see also* Gangrene, gas) 040.0
        perfringens 041.83
            due to food 005.2
        septicum (*see also* Gangrene, gas) 040.0
        sordellii (*see also* Gangrene, gas) 040.0
        welchii (*see also* Gangrene, gas) 040.0
            due to food 005.2
    Coccidioides (immitis) (*see also* Coccidioidomycosis) 114.9
    coccus NEC 041.89
    colon (*see also* Enteritis, due to, by organism) 009.0
        bacillus — *see* Infection, Escherichia coli
    common duct 576.1
    complicating pregnancy, childbirth, or puerperium NEC 647.9
        affecting fetus or newborn 760.2
    Condiobolus 117.7
    congenital NEC 771.8
        Candida albicans 771.7
        chronic 771.2
        clostridial 771.8
        cytomegalovirus 771.1
        Escherichia coli 771.8
        hepatitis, viral 771.2
        herpes simplex 771.2
        listeriosis 771.2
        malaria 771.2
        poliomyelitis 771.2
        rubella 771.0
        Salmonella 771.8
        streptococcal 771.8
        toxoplasmosis 771.2
        tuberculosis 771.2
        urinary (tract) 771.8
        vaccinia 771.2
    corpus luteum (*see also* Salpingo-oophoritis) 614.2
    Corynebacterium diphtheriae — *see* Diphtheria
    Coxsackie (*see also* Coxsackie) 079.2
        endocardium 074.22
        heart NEC 074.20
        in diseases classified elsewhere — *see* category 079
        meninges 047.0
        myocardium 074.23
        pericardium 074.21
        pharynx 074.0
        specified disease NEC 074.8
        unspecified nature or site 079.2
    Cryptococcus neoformans 117.5
    Cunninghamella 117.7
    cyst — *see* Cyst
    Cysticercus cellulosae 123.1
    cytomegalovirus 078.5
        congenital 771.1
    dental (pulpal origin) 522.4
    deuteromycetes 117.4
    Dicrocoelium dendriticum 121.8
    Dipetalonema (perstans) 125.4
        streptocerca 125.6
    diphtherial — *see* Diphtheria
    Diphyllobothrium (adult) (latum) (pacificum) 123.4
        larval 123.5
    Diplogonoporus (grandis) 123.8
    Dipylidium (caninum) 123.8
    Dirofilaria 125.6

Infection, infected, infective—
continued
- dog tapeworm 123.8
- Dracunculus medinensis 125.7
- Dreschlera 118
  - hawaiiensis 117.8
- Ducrey's bacillus (any site) 099.0
- due to or resulting from
  - device, implant, or graft (any) (presence of) — *see* Complications, infection and inflammation, due to (presence of) any device, implant, or graft classified to 996.0-996.5 NEC
  - injection, inoculation, infusion, transfusion, or vaccination (prophylactic) (therapeutic) 999.3
  - injury NEC — *see* Wound, open, by site, complicated
  - surgery 998.5
- duodenum 535.6
- ear — *see also* Otitis
  - external (*see also* Otitis, externa) 380.10
  - inner (*see also* Labyrinthitis) 386.30
  - middle — *see* Otitis, media
- Eaton's agent NEC 041.81
- Eberthella typhosa 002.0
- echinococcosis 122.9
- Echinococcus (*see also* Echinococcus) 122.9
- Echinostoma 121.8
- ECHO virus 079.1
  - in diseases classified elsewhere — *see* category 079
  - unspecified nature or site 079.1
- Endamoeba — *see* Infection, ameba
- endocardium (*see also* Endocarditis) 421.0
- endocervix (*see also* Cervicitis) 616.0
- Entamoeba — *see* Infection, ameba
- enteric (*see also* Enteritis, due to, by organism) 009.0
- Enterobacter aerogenes NEC 041.85
- Enterobius vermicularis 127.4
- enterococcus NEC 041.00 ◆
- enterovirus NEC 079.89
  - central nervous system NEC 048
  - enteritis 008.67
  - meningitis 047.9
- Entomophthora 117.7
- Epidermophyton — *see* Dermatophytosis
- epidermophytosis — *see* Dermatophytosis
- episiotomy 674.3
- Epstein-Barr virus 075
- erysipeloid 027.1
- Erysipelothrix (insidiosa) (rhusiopathiae) 027.1
- erythema infectiosum 057.0
- Escherichia coli NEC 041.4
  - congenital 771.8
  - enteritis — *see* Enteritis, E. coli
  - generalized 038.42
  - intestinal — *see* Enteritis, E. coli
- ethmoidal (chronic) (sinus) (*see also* Sinusitis, ethmoidal) 473.2
- Eubacterium 041.84
- Eustachian tube (ear) 381.50
  - acute 381.51
  - chronic 381.52

Infection, infected, infective—
continued
- exanthema subitum 057.8
- external auditory canal (meatus) (*see also* Otitis, externa) 380.10
- eye NEC 360.00
- eyelid 373.9
  - specified NEC 373.8
- fallopian tube (*see also* Salpingo-oophoritis) 614.2
- fascia 728.89
- Fasciola
  - gigantica 121.3
  - hepatica 121.3
- Fasciolopsis (buski) 121.4
- fetus (intra-amniotic) — *see* Infection, congenital
- filarial — *see* Infestation, filarial
- finger (skin) 686.9
  - abscess (with lymphangitis) 681.00
    - pulp 681.01
  - cellulitis (with lymphangitis) 681.00
  - distal closed space (with lymphangitis) 681.00
  - nail 681.02
    - fungus 110.1
- fish tapeworm 123.4
  - larval 123.5
- flagellate, intestinal 007.9
- fluke — *see* Infestation, fluke
- focal
  - teeth (pulpal origin) 522.4
  - tonsils 474.0
- Fonsecaea
  - compactum 117.2
  - pedrosoi 117.2
- food (*see also* Poisoning, food) 005.9
- foot (skin) 686.9
  - fungus 110.4
- Francisella tularensis (*see also* Tularemia) 021.9
- frontal sinus (chronic) (*see also* Sinusitis, frontal) 473.1
- fungus NEC 117.9
  - beard 110.0
  - body 110.5
  - dermatiacious NEC 117.8
  - foot 110.4
  - groin 110.3
  - hand 110.2
  - nail 110.1
  - pathogenic to compromised host only 118
  - perianal (area) 110.3
  - scalp 110.0
  - scrotum 110.8
  - skin 111.9
    - foot 110.4
    - hand 110.2
  - toenails 110.1
  - trachea 117.9
- Fusarium 118
- Fusobacterium 041.84
- gallbladder (*see also* Cholecystitis, acute) 575.0
- gas bacillus (*see also* Gas, gangrene) 040.0
- gastric (*see also* Gastritis) 535.5
- Gastrodiscoides hominis 121.8
- gastroenteric (*see also* Enteritis, due to, by organism) 009.0
- gastrointestinal (*see also* Enteritis, due to, by organism) 009.0
- generalized NEC (*see also* Septicemia) 038.9
- genital organ or tract NEC female 614.9
  - with
    - abortion — *see* Abortion, by type, with sepsis

Infection, infected, infective—
continued
- genital organ or tract NEC—
  continued
  - female—*continued*
    - with—*continued*
      - ectopic pregnancy (*see also* categories 633.0-633.9) 639.0
      - molar pregnancy (*see also* categories 630-632) 639.0
      - complicating pregnancy 646.6
        - affecting fetus or newborn 760.8
      - following
        - abortion 639.0
        - ectopic or molar pregnancy 639.0
      - puerperal, postpartum, childbirth 670
      - minor or localized 646.6
        - affecting fetus or newborn 760.8
  - male 608.4
- genitourinary tract NEC 599.0
- Ghon tubercle, primary (*see also* Tuberculosis) 010.0
- Giardia lamblia 007.1
- gingival (chronic) 523.1
  - acute 523.0
  - Vincent's 101
- glanders 024
- Glenosporopsis amazonica 116.2
- Gnathostoma spinigerum 128.1
- Gongylonema 125.6
- gonococcal NEC (*see also* Gonococcus) 098.0
- gram-negative bacilli NEC 041.85
  - anaerobic 041.84
- guinea worm 125.7
- gum (*see also* Infection, gingival) 523.1
- heart 429.89
- helminths NEC 128.9
  - intestinal 127.9
    - mixed (types classifiable to more than one category in 120.0-127.7) 127.8
    - specified type NEC 127.7
  - specified type NEC 128.8
- Hemophilus influenzae NEC 041.5
  - generalized 038.41
- herpes (simplex) (*see also* Herpes, simplex) 054.9
  - congenital 771.2
  - zoster (*see also* Herpes, zoster) 053.9
  - eye NEC 053.29
- Heterophyes heterophyes 121.6
- Histoplasma (*see also* Histoplasmosis) 115.90
  - capsulatum (*see also* Histoplasmosis, American) 115.00
  - duboisii (*see also* Histoplasmosis, African) 115.10
- HIV V08 ▼
  - with symptoms, symptomatic 042 ▲
- hookworm (*see also* Ancylostomiasis) 126.9
- human immunodeficiency virus V08 ▼
  - with symptoms, symptomatic 042 ▲
- human papilloma virus 079.4
- hydrocele 603.1
- hydronephrosis 591
- Hymenolepis 123.6
- hypopharynx 478.29

Infection, infected, infective—
continued
- inguinal glands 683
  - due to soft chancre 099.0
- intestine, intestinal (*see also* Enteritis, due to, by organism) 009.0
- intrauterine (*see also* Endometritis) 615.9
  - complicating delivery 646.6
  - specified infection NEC in fetus or newborn 771.8
- isospora belli or hominis 007.2
- Japanese B encephalitis 062.0
- jaw (bone) (acute) (chronic) (lower) (subacute) (upper) 526.4
- joint — *see* Arthritis, infectious or infective
- kidney (cortex) (hematogenous) 590.9
  - with
    - abortion — *see* Abortion, by type, with urinary tract infection
    - calculus 592.0
    - ectopic pregnancy (*see also* categories 633.0-633.9) 639.8
    - molar pregnancy (*see also* categories 630-632) 639.8
    - complicating pregnancy or puerperium 646.6
      - affecting fetus or newborn 760.1
    - following
      - abortion 639.8
      - ectopic or molar pregnancy 639.8
  - pelvis and ureter 590.3
- Klebsiella pneumoniae NEC 041.3
- knee (skin) NEC 686.9
  - joint — *see* Arthritis, infectious
- Koch's (*see also* Tuberculosis, pulmonary) 011.9
- labia (majora) (minora) (*see also* Vulvitis) 616.10
- lacrimal
  - gland (*see also* Dacryoadenitis) 375.00
  - passages (duct) (sac) (*see also* Dacryocystitis) 375.30
- larynx NEC 478.79
- leg (skin) NEC 686.9
- Leishmania (*see also* Leishmaniasis) 085.9
  - aethiopica 085.3
  - braziliensis 085.5
  - donovani 085.0
  - furunculosa 085.1
  - infantum 085.0
  - mexicana 085.4
  - tropica (minor) 085.1
    - major 085.2
- Leptosphaeria senegalensis 117.4
- leptospira (*see also* Leptospirosis) 100.9
  - Australis 100.89
  - Bataviae 100.89
  - pyrogenes 100.89
  - specified type NEC 100.89
- leptospirochetal NEC (*see also* Leptospirosis) 100.9
- Leptothrix — *see* Actinomycosis
- Listeria monocytogenes (listeriosis) 027.0
  - congenital 771.2
- liver fluke — *see* Infestation, fluke, liver
- Loa loa 125.2
  - eyelid 125.2 [373.6]
- Loboa loboi 116.2

Infection, infected, infective— continued
local, skin (staphylococcal) (streptococcal) NEC 686.9
  abscess — see Abscess, by site
  cellulitis — see Cellulitis, by site
  ulcer (see also Ulcer, skin) 707.9
Loefflerella
  mallei 024
  whitmori 025
lung 518.89
  atypical Mycobacterium 031.0
  tuberculous (see also Tuberculosis, pulmonary) 011.9
  basilar 518.89
  chronic 518.89
  fungus NEC 117.9
  spirochetal 104.8
  virus — see Pneumonia, virus
lymph gland (axillary) (cervical) (inguinal) 683
  mesenteric 289.2
lymphoid tissue, base of tongue or posterior pharynx, NEC 474.0
madurella
  grisea 117.4
  mycetomii 117.4
major
  with
    abortion — see Abortion, by type, with sepsis
    ectopic pregnancy (see also categories 633.0-633.9) 639.0
    molar pregnancy (see also categories 630-632) 639.0
  following
    abortion 639.0
    ectopic or molar pregnancy 639.0
  puerperal, postpartum, childbirth 670
malarial — see Malaria
Malassezia furfur 111.0
Malleomyces
  mallei 024
  pseudomallei 025
mammary gland 611.0
  puerperal, postpartum 675.2
Mansonella (ozzardi) 125.5
mastoid (suppurative) — see Mastoiditis
maxilla, maxillary 526.4
  sinus (chronic) (see also Sinusitis, maxillary) 473.0
mediastinum 519.2
medina 125.7
meibomian
  cyst 373.12
  gland 373.12
melioidosis 025
meninges (see also Meningitis) 320.9
meningococcal (see also condition) 036.9
  brain 036.1
  cerebrospinal 036.0
  endocardium 036.42
  generalized 036.2
  meninges 036.0
  meningococcemia 036.2
  specified site NEC 036.89
mesenteric lymph nodes or glands NEC 289.2
Metagonimus 121.5
metatarsophalangeal 711.97
microorganism resistant to drugs — see Resistance (to), drugs by microorganisms
microsporum, microsporic — see Dermatophytosis

Infection, infected, infective— continued
Mima polymorpha NEC 041.85
mixed flora NEC 041.89
Monilia (see also Candidiasis) 112.9
  neonatal 771.7
Microsporidia 136.8
Monosporium apiospermum 117.6
mouth (focus) NEC 528.9
  parasitic 112.0
Mucor 117.7
muscle NEC 728.89
mycelium NEC 117.9
mycetoma
  actinomycotic NEC (see also Actinomycosis) 039.9
  mycotic NEC 117.4
Mycobacterium, mycobacterial (see also Mycobacterium) 031.9
mycoplasma NEC 041.81
mycotic NEC 117.9
  pathogenic to compromised host only 118
  skin NEC 111.9
  systemic 117.9
myocardium NEC 422.90
nail (chronic) (with lymphangitis) 681.9
  finger 681.02
  fungus 110.1
  ingrowing 703.0
  toe 681.11
  fungus 110.1
nasal sinus (chronic) (see also Sinusitis) 473.9
nasopharynx (chronic) 478.29
  acute 460
navel 686.9
  newborn 771.4
Neisserian — see Gonococcus
Neotestudina rosatii 117.4
newborn, generalized 771.8
nipple 611.0
  puerperal, postpartum 675.0
    with breast 675.9
    specified type NEC 675.8
Nocardia — see Actinomycosis
nose 478.1
nostril 478.1
obstetrical surgical wound 674.3
Oesophagostomum (apiostomum) 127.7
Oestrus ovis 134.0
Oidium albicans (see also Candidiasis) 112.9
Onchocerca (volvulus) 125.3
  eye 125.3 [360.13]
  eyelid 125.3 [373.6]
operation wound 998.5
Opisthorchis (felineus) (tenuicollis) (viverrini) 121.0
orbit 376.00
  chronic 376.10
ovary (see also Salpingo-oophoritis) 614.2
Oxyuris vermicularis 127.4
pancreas 577.0
Paracoccidioides brasiliensis 116.1
Paragonimus (westermani) 121.2
parainfluenza virus 079.89
parameningococcus NEC 036.9
  with meningitis 036.0
parasitic NEC 136.9 ◆
paratyphoid 002.9
  Type A 002.1
  Type B 002.2
  Type C 002.3
paraurethral ducts 597.89
parotid gland 527.2

Infection, infected, infective— continued
Pasteurella NEC 027.2
  multocida (cat-bite) (dog-bite) 027.2
  pestis (see also Plague) 020.9
  pseudotuberculosis 027.2
  septica (cat-bite) (dog-bite) 027.2
  tularensis (see also Tularemia) 021.9
pelvic, female (see also Disease, pelvis, inflammatory) 614.9
penis (glans) (retention) NEC 607.2
  herpetic 054.13
Peptococcus 041.84
Peptostreptococcus 041.84
periapical (pulpal origin) 522.4
peridental 523.3
perineal wound (obstetrical) 674.3
periodontal 523.3
periorbital 376.00
  chronic 376.10
perirectal 569.49
perirenal (see also Infection, kidney) 590.9
peritoneal (see also Peritonitis) 567.9
periureteral 593.89
periurethral 597.89
Petriellidium boydii 117.6
pharynx 478.29
  Coxsackievirus 074.0
  phlegmonous 462
  posterior, lymphoid 474.0
Phialophora
  gougerotii 117.8
  jeanselmei 117.8
  verrucosa 117.2
Piedraia hortai 111.3
pinna, acute 380.11
pinta 103.9
  intermediate 103.1
  late 103.2
  mixed 103.3
  primary 103.0
pinworm 127.4
pityrosporum furfur 111.0
pleuropneumonia-like organisms NEC (PPLO) 041.81
pneumococcal NEC 041.2
  generalized (purulent) 038.2
Pneumococcus NEC 041.2
postoperative wound 998.5
posttraumatic NEC 958.3
postvaccinal 999.3
prepuce NEC 607.1
Proprionibacterium 041.84
prostate (capsule) (see also Prostatitis) 601.9
Proteus (mirabilis) (morganii) (vulgaris) NEC 041.6
  enteritis 008.3
protozoal NEC 136.8
  intestinal NEC 007.9
Pseudomonas NEC 041.7
  mallei 024
  pneumonia 482.1
  pseudomallei 025
psittacosis 073.9
puerperal, postpartum (major) 670
  minor 646.6
pulmonary — see Infection, lung
purulent — see Abscess
putrid, generalized — see Septicemia
pyemic — see Septicemia
Pyrenochaeta romeroi 117.4
Q fever 083.0
rabies 071
rectum (sphincter) 569.49
renal (see also Infection, kidney) 590.9
  pelvis and ureter 590.3

Infection, infected, infective— continued
resistant to drugs — see Resistance (to), drugs by microorganisms
respiratory 519.8
  chronic 519.8
  influenzal (acute) (upper) 487.1
  lung 518.89
  rhinovirus 460
  upper (acute) (infectious) NEC 465.9
    with flu, grippe, or influenza 487.1
    influenzal 487.1
    multiple sites NEC 465.8
    streptococcal 034.0
    viral NEC 465.9
resulting from presence of shunt or other internal prosthetic device — see Complications, infection and inflammation, due to (presence of) any device, implant, or graft classified to 996.0-996.5 NEC
retrovirus 079.50
  human immunodeficiency virus type 2 [HIV 2] 079.53
  human T-cell lymphotrophic virus type I [HTLV-I] 079.51
  human T-cell lymphotrophic virus type II [HTLV-II] 079.52
  specified NEC 079.59
Rhinocladium 117.1
Rhinosporidium (seeberi) 117.0
rhinovirus
  in diseases classified elsewhere — see category 079
  unspecified nature or site 079.3
Rhizopus 117.7
rickettsial 083.9
rickettsialpox 083.2
rubella (see also Rubella) 056.9
  congenital 771.0
Saccharomyces (see also Candidiasis) 112.9
Saksenaea 117.7
salivary duct or gland (any) 527.2
Salmonella (aertrycke) (callinarum) (choleraesuis) (enteritidis) (suipestifer) (typhimurium) 003.9
  with
    arthritis 003.23
    gastroenteritis 003.0
    localized infection 003.20
      specified type NEC 003.29
    meningitis 003.21
    osteomyelitis 003.24
    pneumonia 003.22
    septicemia 003.1
    specified manifestation NEC 003.8
  congenital 771.8
  due to food (poisoning) (any serotype) (see also Poisoning, food, due to, Salmonella)
  hirschfeldii 002.3
  localized 003.20
    specified type NEC 003.29
  paratyphi 002.9
    A 002.1
    B 002.2
    C 002.3
  schottmuelleri 002.2
  specified type NEC 003.8
  typhi 002.0
  typhosa 002.0

Infection, infected, infective—
continued
saprophytic 136.8
Sarcocystis, lindemanni 136.5
scabies 133.0
Schistosoma — *see* Infestation, Schistosoma
Schmorl's bacillus 040.3
scratch or other superficial injury — *see* Injury, superficial, by site
scrotum (acute) NEC 608.4
secondary, burn or open wound (dislocation) (fracture) 958.3
seminal vesicle (*see also* Vesiculitis) 608.0
septic
 generalized — *see* Septicemia
 localized, skin (*see also* Abscess) 682.9
septicemic — *see* Septicemia
Serratia (marcescens) 041.85
 generalized 038.44
sheep liver fluke 121.3
Shigella 004.9
 boydii 004.2
 dysenteriae 004.0
 flexneri 004.1
 group
  A 004.0
  B 004.1
  C 004.2
  D 004.3
 Schmitz (-Stutzer) 004.0
 schmitzii 004.0
 shiga 004.0
 sonnei 004.3
 specified type NEC 004.8
sinus (*see also* Sinusitis) 473.9
 pilonidal 685.1
  with abscess 685.0
 skin NEC 686.9
Skene's duct or gland (*see also* Urethritis) 597.89
skin (local) (staphylococcal) (streptococcal) NEC 686.9
 abscess — *see* Abscess, by site
 cellulitis — *see* Cellulitis, by site
 due to fungus 111.9
  specified type NEC 111.8
 mycotic 111.9
  specified type NEC 111.8
 ulcer (*see also* Ulcer, skin) 707.9
slow virus 046.9
 specified condition NEC 046.8
Sparganum (mansoni) (proliferum) 123.5
specific (*see also* Syphilis) 097.9
 to perinatal period NEC 771.8
spermatic cord NEC 608.4
sphenoidal (chronic) (sinus) (*see also* Sinusitis,
Spherophorus necrophorus 040.3
spinal cord NEC (*see also* Encephalitis) 323.9
 abscess 324.1
  late effect — *see* category 326
 late effect — *see* category 326
 meninges — *see* Meningitis
 streptococcal 320.2
Spirillum
 minus or minor 026.0
 morsus muris 026.0
 obermeieri 087.0
spirochetal NEC 104.9
 lung 104.8
 specified nature or site NEC 104.8
spleen 289.59
Sporothrix schenckii 117.1
Sporotrichum (schenckii) 117.1
Sporozoa 136.8

Infection, infected, infective—
continued
staphylococcal NEC 041.10
 aureus 041.11
 food poisoning 005.0
 generalized (purulent) 038.1
 pneumonia 482.4
 septicemia 038.1
 specified NEC 041.19
steatoma 706.2
Stellantchasmus falcatus 121.6
Streptobacillus moniliformis 026.1
streptococcal NEC 041.00
 congenital 771.8
 generalized (purulent) 038.0
 Group
  A 041.01
  B 041.02
  C 041.03
  D 041.04
  G 041.05
 pneumonia — *see* Pneumonia, streptococcal 482.3
 septicemia 038.0
 sore throat 034.0
 specified NEC 041.09
Streptomyces — *see* Actinomycosis
streptotrichosis — *see* Actinomycosis
Strongyloides (stercoralis) 127.2
stump (amputation) (surgical) 997.62
 traumatic — *see* Amputation, traumatic, by site, complicated
subcutaneous tissue, local NEC 686.9
submaxillary region 528.9
suipestifer (*see also* Infection, Salmonella) 003.9
swimming pool bacillus 031.1
syphilitic — *see* Syphilis
systemic — *see* Septicemia
Taenia — *see* Infestation, Taenia
Taeniarhynchus saginatus 123.2
tapeworm — *see* Infestation, tapeworm
tendon (sheath) 727.89
Ternidens diminutus 127.7
testis (*see also* Orchitis) 604.90
thigh (skin) 686.9
threadworm 127.4
throat 478.29
 pneumococcal 462
 staphylococcal 462
 streptococcal 034.0
 viral NEC (*see also* Pharyngitis) 462
thumb (skin) 686.9
 abscess (with lymphangitis) 681.00
 pulp 681.01
 cellulitis (with lymphangitis) 681.00
 nail 681.02
thyroglossal duct 529.8
toe (skin) 686.9
 abscess (with lymphangitis) 681.10
 cellulitis (with lymphangitis) 681.10
 nail 681.11
 fungus 110.1
tongue NEC 529.0
 parasitic 112.0
tonsil (and adenoid) (faucial) (lingual) (pharyngeal) 474.0
 acute or subacute 463
 tag 474.0
tooth, teeth 522.4
 periapical (pulpal origin) 522.4
 peridental 523.3
 periodontal 523.3
 pulp 522.0

Infection, infected, infective—
continued
tooth, teeth—*continued*
 socket 526.5
Torula histolytica 117.5
Toxocara (cani) (cati) (felis) 128.0
Toxoplasma gondii (*see also* Toxoplasmosis) 130.9
trachea, chronic 491.8
 fungus 117.9
traumatic NEC 958.3
trematode NEC 121.9
trench fever 083.1
Treponema
 denticola 041.84
 macrodenticum 041.84
 pallidum (*see also* Syphillis) 097.9
Trichinella (spiralis) 124
Trichomonas 131.9
 bladder 131.09
 cervix 131.09
 hominis 007.3
 intestine 007.3
 prostate 131.03
 specified site NEC 131.8
 urethra 131.02
 urogenitalis 131.00
 vagina 131.01
 vulva 131.01
Trichophyton, trichophytid — *see* Dermatophytosis
Trichosporon (beigelii) cutaneum 111.2
Trichostrongylus 127.6
Trichuris (trichiuria) 127.3
Trombicula (irritans) 133.8
Trypanosoma (*see also* Trypanosomiasis) 086.9
 cruzi 086.2
tubal (*see also* Salpingo-oophoritis) 614.2
tuberculous NEC (*see also* Tuberculosis) 011.9
tubo-ovarian (*see also* Salpingo-oophoritis) 614.2
tunica vaginalis 608.4
tympanic membrane — *see* Myringitis
typhoid (abortive) (ambulant) (bacillus) 002.0
typhus 081.9
 flea-borne (endemic) 081.0
 louse-borne (epidemic) 080
 mite-borne 081.2
 recrudescent 081.1
 tick-borne 082.9
  African 082.1
  North Asian 082.2
umbilicus (septic) 686.9
 newborn NEC 771.4
ureter 593.89
urethra (*see also* Urethritis) 597.80
urinary (tract) NEC 599.0
 with
  abortion — *see* Abortion, by type, with urinary tract infection
  ectopic pregnancy (*see also* categories 633.0-633.9) 639.8
  molar pregnancy (*see also* categories 630-632) 639.8
 complicating pregnancy, childbirth, or puerperium 646.6
  affecting fetus or newborn 760.1
  asymptomatic 646.5
   affecting fetus or newborn 760.1
 diplococcal (acute) 098.0
  chronic 098.2

Infection, infected, infective—
continued
urinary (tract) NEC—*continued*
 due to Trichomonas (vaginalis) 131.00
 following
  abortion 639.8
  ectopic or molar pregnancy 639.8
 gonococcal (acute) 098.0
  chronic or duration of 2 months or over 098.2
 newborn 771.8
 trichomonal 131.00
 tuberculous (*see also* Tuberculosis) 016.3
uterus, uterine (*see also* Endometritis) 615.9
utriculus masculinus NEC 597.89
vaccination 999.3
vagina (granulation tissue) (wall) (*see also* Vaginitis) 616.10
varicella 052.9
varicose veins — *see* Varicose, veins
variola 050.9
 major 050.0
 minor 050.1
vas deferens NEC 608.4
Veillonella 041.84
verumontanum 597.89
vesical (*see also* Cystitis) 595.9
Vibrio
 cholerae 001.0
  El Tor 001.1
 parahaemolyticus (food poisoning) 005.4
 vulnificus 041.85
Vincent's (gums) (mouth) (tonsil) 101
virus, viral 079.99
 adenovirus
  in diseases classified elsewhere — *see* category 079
  unspecified nature or site 079.0
 central nervous system NEC 049.9
  enterovirus 048
  meningitis 047.9
   specified type NEC 047.8
  slow virus 046.9
   specified condition NEC 046.8
 chest 519.8
 conjunctivitis 077.99
  specified type NEC 077.8
 Coxsackie (*see also* Infection, Coxsackie) 079.2
 ECHO
  in diseases classified elsewhere — *see* category 079
  unspecified nature or site 079.1
 encephalitis 049.9
  arthropod-borne NEC 064
  tick-borne 063.9
   specified type NEC 063.8
 enteritis NEC (*see also* Enteritis, viral) 008.8
 exanthem NEC 057.9
 human papilloma 079.4
 in diseases classified elsewhere — *see* category 079
 intestine (*see also* Enteritis, viral) 008.8
 lung — *see* Pneumonia, viral

Infection, infected, infective—
  continued
  virus, viral—*continued*
    rhinovirus
      in diseases classified
          elsewhere — *see*
          category 079
      unspecified nature or site
          079.3
    salivary gland disease 078.5
    slow 046.9
      specified condition NEC
          046.8
    specified type NEC 079.89
      in diseases classified
          elsewhere — *see*
          category 079
      unspecified nature or site
          079.99
    warts NEC 078.10
  vulva (*see also* Vulvitis) 616.10
  whipworm 127.3
  Whitmore's bacillus 025
  wound (local) (posttraumatic)
      NEC 958.3
    with
      dislocation — *see*
          Dislocation, by site,
          open
      fracture — *see* Fracture, by
          site, open
      open wound — *see*
          Wound, open, by
          site, complicated
    postoperative 998.5
    surgical 998.5
  Wuchereria 125.0
    bancrofti 125.0
    malayi 125.1
  yaws — *see* Yaws
  yeast (*see also* Candidiasis) 112.9
  yellow fever (*see also* Fever,
      yellow) 060.9
  Yersinia pestis (*see also* Plague)
      020.9
  Zeis' gland 373.12
  zoonotic bacterial NEC 027.9
  Zopfia senegalensis 117.4
Infective, infectious — *see* condition
Inferiority complex 301.9
  constitutional psychopathic 301.9
Infertility
  female 628.9
    associated with
      adhesions, peritubal 614.6
          [628.2]
      anomaly
        cervical mucus 628.4
        congenital
          cervix 628.4
          fallopian tube 628.2
          uterus 628.3
          vagina 628.4
      anovulation 628.0
      dysmucorrhea 628.4
      endometritis, tuberculous
          (*see also*
          Tuberculosis) 016.7
          [628.3]
      Stein-Leventhal syndrome
          256.4 [628.0]
    due to
      adiposogenital dystrophy
          253.8 [628.1]
      anterior pituitary disorder
          NEC 253.4 [628.1]
        hyperfunction 253.1
          [628.1]
      cervical anomaly 628.4
      fallopian tube anomaly
          628.2
      ovarian failure 256.3
          [628.0]
      Stein-Leventhal syndrome
          256.4 [628.0]
      uterine anomaly 628.3
      vaginal anomaly 628.4

Infertility—*continued*
  female—*continued*
    nonimplantation 628.3
    origin
      cervical 628.4
      pituitary-hypothalamus
          NEC 253.8 [628.1]
        anterior pituitary NEC
            253.4 [628.1]
          hyperfunction NEC
              253.1 [628.1]
          dwarfism 253.3 [628.1]
          panhypopituitarism
              253.2 [628.1]
        specified NEC 628.8
      tubal (block) (occlusion)
          (stenosis) 628.2
        adhesions 614.6 [628.2]
      uterine 628.3
      vaginal 628.4
    previous, requiring supervision
        of pregnancy V23.0
  male 606.9
    absolute 606.0
    due to
      azoospermia 606.0
      drug therapy 606.8
      extratesticular cause NEC
          606.8
      germinal cell
        aplasia 606.0
        desquamation 606.1
      hypospermatogenesis 606.1
      infection 606.8
      obstruction, afferent ducts
          606.8
      oligospermia 606.1
      radiation 606.8
      spermatogenic arrest
          (complete) 606.0
        incomplete 606.1
      systemic disease 606.8
Infestation 134.9
  Acanthocheilonema (perstans)
      125.4
    streptocerca 125.6
  Acariasis 133.9
    demodex folliculorum 133.8
    Sarcoptes scabiei 133.0
    trombiculae 133.8
  Agamofilaria streptocerca 125.6
  Ancylostoma, Ankylostoma 126.9
    americanum 126.1
    braziliense 126.2
    canium 126.8
    ceylanicum 126.3
    duodenale 126.0
    new world 126.1
    old world 126.0
  Angiostrongylus cantonensis
      128.8
  anisakiasis 127.1
  Anisakis larva 127.1
  arthropod NEC 134.1
  Ascaris lumbricoides 127.0
  Bacillus fusiformis 101
  Balantidium coli 007.0
  beef tapeworm 123.2
  Bothriocephalus (latus) 123.4
    larval 123.5
  broad tapeworm 123.4
    larval 123.5
  Brugia malayi 125.1
  Candiru 136.8
  Capillaria
    hepatica 128.8
    philippinensis 127.5
  cat liver fluke 121.0
  Cercomonas hominis (intestinal)
      007.3
  cestodes 123.9
    specified type NEC 123.8
  chigger 133.8
  chigoe 134.1
  Chilomastix 007.8
  Clonorchis (sinensis) (liver) 121.1
  coccidia 007.2

Infestation—*continued*
  complicating pregnancy,
      childbirth, or puerperium
      647.9
    affecting fetus or newborn
        760.8
  Cysticercus cellulosae 123.1
  Demodex folliculorum 133.8
  Dermatobia (hominis) 134.0
  Dibothriocephalus (latus) 123.4
    larval 123.5
  Dicrocoelium dendriticum 121.8
  Diphyllobothrium (adult)
      (intestinal) (latum)
      (pacificum) 123.4
    larval 123.5
  Diplogonoporus (grandis) 123.8
  Dipylidium (caninum) 123.8
  Distoma hepaticum 121.3
  dog tapeworm 123.8
  Dracunculus medinensis 125.7
  dragon worm 125.7
  dwarf tapeworm 123.6
  Echinococcus (*see also*
      Echinococcus) 122.9
  Echinostoma ilocanum 121.8
  Embadomonas 007.8
  Endamoeba (histolytica) — *see*
      Infection, ameba
  Entamoeba (histolytica) — *see*
      Infection, ameba
  Enterobius vermicularis 127.4
  Epidermophyton — *see*
      Dermatophytosis
  eyeworm 125.2
  Fasciola
    gigantica 121.3
    hepatica 121.3
  Fasciolopsis (buski) (small
      intestine) 121.4
  filarial 125.9
    due to
      Acanthocheilonema
          (perstans) 125.4
        streptocerca 125.6
      Brugia (Wuchereria)
          malayi 125.1
      Dracunculus medinensis
          125.7
      guinea worms 125.7
      Mansonella (ozzardi)
          125.5
      Onchocerca volvulus
          125.3
        eye 125.3 [360.13]
        eyelid 125.3 [373.6]
      Wuchereria (bancrofti)
          125.0
        malayi 125.1
    specified type NEC 125.6
  fish tapeworm 123.4
    larval 123.5
  fluke 121.9
  blood NEC (*see also*
      Schistosomiasis) 120.9
  cat liver 121.0
  intestinal (giant) 121.4
  liver (sheep) 121.3
    cat 121.0
    Chinese 121.1
    clonorchiasis 121.1
    fascioliasis 121.3
    Oriental 121.1
  lung (oriental) 121.2
  sheep liver 121.3
  fly larva 134.0
  Gasterophilus (intestinalis) 134.0
  Gastrodiscoides hominis 121.8
  Giardia lamblia 007.1
  Gnathostoma (spinigerum) 128.1
  Gongylonema 125.6
  guinea worm 125.7

Infestation—*continued*
  helminth NEC 128.9
    intestinal 127.9
      mixed (types classifiable to
          more than one
          category in 120.0-
          127.7) 127.8
      specified type NEC 127.7
    specified type NEC 128.8
  Heterophyes heterophyes (small
      intestine) 121.6
  hookworm (*see also* Infestation,
      ancylostoma) 126.9
  Hymenolepis (diminuta) (nana)
      123.6
  intestinal NEC 129
  leeches (aquatic) (land) 134.2
  Leishmania — *see* Leishmaniasis
  lice (*see also* Infestation,
      pediculus) 132.9
  Linguatulidae, linguatula
      (pentastoma) (serrata) 134.1
  Loa loa 125.2
    eyelid 125.2 [373.6]
  louse (*see also* Infestation,
      pediculus) 132.9
    body 132.1
    head 132.0
    pubic 132.2
  maggots 134.0
  Mansonella (ozzardi) 125.5
  medina 125.7
  Metagonimus yokogawai (small
      intestine) 121.5
  Microfilaria streptocerca 125.3
    eye 125.3 [360.13]
    eyelid 125.3 [373.6]
  Microsporon furfur 111.0
  microsporum — *see*
      Dermatophytosis
  mites 133.9
    scabic 133.0
    specified type NEC 133.8
  Monilia (albicans) (*see also*
      Candidiasis) 112.9
    vagina 112.1
    vulva 112.1
  mouth 112.0
  Necator americanus 126.1
  nematode (intestinal) 127.9
    Ancylostoma (*see also*
        Ancylostoma) 126.9
    Ascaris lumbricoides 127.0
    conjunctiva NEC 128.9
    Dioctophyma 128.8
    Enterobius vermicularis 127.4
    Gnathostoma spinigerum
        128.1
    Oesophagostomum
        (apiostomum) 127.7
    Physaloptera 127.4
    specified type NEC 127.7
    Strongyloides stercoralis 127.2
    Ternidens diminutus 127.7
    Trichinella spiralis 124
    Trichostrongylus 127.6
    Trichuris (trichiuria) 127.3
  Oesophagostomum (apiostomum)
      127.7
  Oestrus ovis 134.0
  Onchocerca (volvulus) 125.3
    eye 125.3 [360.13]
    eyelid 125.3 [373.6]
  Opisthorchis (felineus)
      (tenuicollis) (viverrini)
      121.0
  Oxyuris vermicularis 127.4
  Paragonimus (westermani) 121.2
  parasite, parasitic NEC 136.9
    eyelid 134.9 [373.6]
    intestinal 129
    mouth 112.0
    orbit 376.13
    skin 134.9
    tongue 112.0

Infestation—continued
pediculus 132.9
　capitis (humanus) (any site) 132.0
　corporis (humanus) (any site) 132.1
　eyelid 132.0 [373.6]
　mixed (classifiable to more than one category in 132.0-132.2) 132.3
　pubis (any site) 132.2
phthirus (pubis) (any site) 132.2
　with any infestation classifiable to 132.0, 132.1 and 132.3
pinworm 127.4
pork tapeworm (adult) 123.0
protozoal NEC 136.8
pubic louse 132.2
rat tapeworm 123.6
red bug 133.8
roundworm (large) NEC 127.0
sand flea 134.1
saprophytic NEC 136.8
Sarcoptes scabiei 133.0
scabies 133.0
Schistosoma 120.9
　bovis 120.8
　cercariae 120.3
　hematobium 120.0
　intercalatum 120.8
　japonicum 120.2
　mansoni 120.1
　mattheii 120.8
　specified
　　site — see Schistosomiasis
　　type NEC 120.8
　spindale 120.8
screw worms 134.0
skin NEC 134.9
Sparganum (mansoni) (proliferum) 123.5
　larval 123.5
specified type NEC 134.8
Spirometra larvae 123.5
Sporozoa NEC 136.8
Stellantchasmus falcatus 121.6
Strongyloides 127.2
Strongylus (gibsoni) 127.7
Taenia 123.3
　diminuta 123.6
　Echinococcus (see also Echinococcus) 122.9
　mediocanellata 123.2
　nana 123.6
　saginata (mediocanellata) 123.2
　solium (intestinal form) 123.0
　　larval form 123.1
Taeniarhynchus saginatus 123.2
tapeworm 123.9
　beef 123.2
　broad 123.4
　　larval 123.5
　dog 123.8
　dwarf 123.6
　fish 123.4
　　larval 123.5
　pork 123.0
　rat 123.6
Ternidens diminutus 127.7
Tetranychus molestissimus 133.8
threadworm 127.4
tongue 112.0
Toxocara (cani) (cati) (felis) 128.0
trematode(s) NEC 121.9
Trichina spiralis 124
Trichinella spiralis 124
Trichocephalus 127.3
Trichomonas 131.9
　bladder 131.09
　cervix 131.09
　intestine 007.3
　prostate 131.03
　specified site NEC 131.8
　urethra (female) (male) 131.02
　urogenital 131.00

Infestation—continued
Trichomonas—continued
　vagina 131.01
　vulva 131.01
Trichophyton — see Dermatophytosis
Trichostrongylus instabilis 127.6
Trichuris (trichiuria) 127.3
Trombicula (irritans) 133.8
Trypanosoma — see Trypanosomiasis
Tunga penetrans 134.1
Uncinaria americana 126.1
whipworm 127.3
worms NEC 128.9
　intestinal 127.9
Wuchereria 125.0
　bancrofti 125.0
　malayi 125.1

Infiltrate, infiltration
with an iron compound 275.0
amyloid (any site) (generalized) 277.3
calcareous (muscle) NEC 275.4
　localized — see Degeneration, by site
calcium salt (muscle) 275.4
corneal (see also Edema, cornea) 371.20
eyelid 373.9
fatty (diffuse) (generalized) 272.8
　localized — see Degeneration, by site, fatty
glycogen, glycogenic (see also Disease, glycogen storage) 271.0
heart, cardiac
　fatty (see also Degeneration, myocardial) 429.1
　glycogenic 271.0 [425.7]
inflammatory in vitreous 379.29
kidney (see also Disease, renal) 593.9
leukemic (M9800/3) — see Leukemia
liver 573.8
　fatty — see Fatty, liver
　glycogen (see also Disease, glycogen storage) 271.0
lung (see also Infiltrate, pulmonary) 518.3
　eosinophilic 518.3
　x-ray finding only 793.1
lymphatic (see also Leukemia, lymphatic) 204.9
　gland, pigmentary 289.3
muscle, fatty 728.9
myelogenous (see also Leukemia, myeloid) 205.9
myocardium, myocardial
　fatty (see also Degeneration, myocardial) 429.1
　glycogenic 271.0 [425.7]
pulmonary 518.3
　with
　　eosinophilia 518.3
　　pneumonia — see Pneumonia, by type
　x-ray finding only 793.1
Ranke's primary (see also Tuberculosis) 010.0
skin, lymphocytic (benign) 709.8
thymus (gland) (fatty) 254.8
urine 788.8
vitreous humor 379.29

Infirmity 799.8
senile 797

Inflammation, inflamed, inflammatory (with exudation)
abducens (nerve) 378.54
accessory sinus (chronic) (see also Sinusitis) 473.9
adrenal (gland) 255.8
alimentary canal — see Enteritis
alveoli (teeth) 526.5
　scorbutic 267
amnion — see Amnionitis

Inflammation, inflamed, inflammatory—continued
anal canal 569.49
antrum (chronic) (see also Sinusitis, maxillary) 473.0
anus 569.49
appendix (see also Appendicitis) 541
arachnoid — see Meningitis
areola 611.0
　puerperal, postpartum 675.0
areolar tissue NEC 686.9
artery — see Arteritis
auditory meatus (external) (see also Otitis, externa) 380.10
Bartholin's gland 616.8
bile duct or passage 576.1
bladder (see also Cystitis) 595.9
bone — see Osteomyelitis
bowel (see also Enteritis) 558.9
brain (see also Encephalitis) 323.9
　late effect — see category 326
　membrane — see Meningitis
breast 611.0
　puerperal, postpartum 675.2
broad ligament (see also Disease, pelvis, inflammatory) 614.4
　acute 614.3
bronchus — see Bronchitis
bursa — see Bursitis
capsule
　liver 573.3
　spleen 289.59
catarrhal (see also Catarrh) 460
　vagina 616.10
cecum (see also Appendicitis) 541
cerebral (see also Encephalitis) 323.9
　late effect — see category 326
　membrane — see Meningitis
cerebrospinal (see also Meningitis) 322.9
　late effect — see category 326
　meningococcal 036.0
　tuberculous (see also Tuberculosis) 013.6
cervix (uteri) (see also Cervicitis) 616.0
chest 519.9
choroid NEC (see also Choroiditis) 363.20
cicatrix (tissue) — see Cicatrix
colon (see also Enteritis) 558.9
　granulomatous 555.1
　newborn 558.9
connective tissue (diffuse) NEC 728.9
cornea (see also Keratitis) 370.9
　with ulcer (see also Ulcer, cornea) 370.00
corpora cavernosa (penis) 607.2
cranial nerve — see Disorder, nerve, cranial
diarrhea — see Diarrhea
disc (intervertebral) (space) 722.90
　cervical, cervicothoracic 722.91
　lumbar, lumbosacral 722.93
　thoracic, thoracolumbar 722.92
Douglas' cul-de-sac or pouch (chronic) (see also Disease, pelvis, inflammatory) 614.4
　acute 614.3
due to (presence of) any device, implant, or graft classifiable to 996.0-996.5 — see Complications, infection and inflammation, due to (presence of) any device, implant, or graft classified to 996.0-996.5 NEC
duodenum 535.6
dura mater — see Meningitis

Inflammation, inflamed, inflammatory—continued
ear — see also Otitis
　external (see also Otitis, externa) 380.10
　inner (see also Labyrinthitis) 386.30
　middle — see Otitis media
esophagus 530.10
ethmoidal (chronic) (sinus) (see also Sinusitis, ethmoidal) 473.2
Eustachian tube (catarrhal) 381.50
　acute 381.51
　chronic 381.52
extrarectal 569.49
eye 379.99
eyelid 373.9
　specified NEC 373.8
fallopian tube (see also Salpingo-oophoritis) 614.2
fascia 728.9
fetal membranes (acute) 658.4
　affecting fetus or newborn 762.7
follicular, pharynx 472.1
frontal (chronic) (sinus) (see also Sinusitis, frontal) 473.1
gallbladder (see also Cholecystitis, acute) 575.0
gall duct (see also Cholecystitis) 575.1
gastrointestinal (see also Enteritis) 558.9
genital organ (diffuse) (internal)
　female 614.9
　　with
　　　abortion — see Abortion, by type, with sepsis
　　　ectopic pregnancy (see also categories 633.0-633.9) 639.0
　　　molar pregnancy (see also categories 630-632) 639.0
　　　complicating pregnancy, childbirth, or puerperium 646.6
　　　　affecting fetus or newborn 760.8
　　following
　　　abortion 639.0
　　　ectopic or molar pregnancy 639.0
　male 608.4
gland (lymph) (see also Lymphadenitis) 289.3
glottis (see also Laryngitis) 464.0
granular, pharynx 472.1
gum 523.1
heart (see also Carditis) 429.89
hepatic duct 576.8
hernial sac — see Hernia, by site
ileum (see also Enteritis) 558.9
　terminal or regional 555.0
　with large intestine 555.2
intervertebral disc 722.90
　cervical, cervicothoracic 722.91
　lumbar, lumbosacral 722.93
　thoracic, thoracolumbar 722.92
intestine (see also Enteritis) 558.9
jaw (acute) (bone) (chronic) (lower) (suppurative) (upper) 526.4
jejunum — see Enteritis
joint NEC (see also Arthritis) 716.9
　sacroiliac 720.2
kidney (see also Nephritis) 583.9
knee (joint) 716.66
　tuberculous (active) (see also Tuberculosis) 015.2

Inflammation, inflamed, inflammatory—continued

labium (majus) (minus) (see also Vulvitis) 616.10
lacrimal
  gland (see also Dacryoadenitis) 375.00
  passages (duct) (sac) (see also Dacryocystitis) 375.30
larynx (see also Laryngitis) 464.0
  diphtheritic 032.3
leg NEC 686.9
lip 528.5
liver (capsule) (see also Hepatitis) 573.3
  acute 570
  chronic 571.40
  suppurative 572.0
lung (acute) (see also Pneumonia) 486
  chronic (interstitial) 518.89
lymphatic vessel (see also Lymphangitis) 457.2
lymph node or gland (see also Lymphadenitis) 289.3
mammary gland 611.0
  puerperal, postpartum 675.2
maxilla, maxillary 526.4
  sinus (chronic) (see also Sinusitis, maxillary) 473.0
membranes of brain or spinal cord — see Meningitis
meninges — see Meningitis
mouth 528.0
muscle 728.9
myocardium (see also Myocarditis) 429.0
nasal sinus (chronic) (see also Sinusitis) 473.9
nasopharynx — see Nasopharyngitis
navel 686.9
  newborn NEC 771.4
nerve NEC 729.2
nipple 611.0
  puerperal, postpartum 675.0
nose 478.1
  suppurative 472.0
oculomotor nerve 378.51
optic nerve 377.30
orbit (chronic) 376.10
  acute 376.00
  chronic 376.10
ovary (see also Salpingo-oophoritis) 614.2
oviduct (see also Salpingo-oophoritis) 614.2
pancreas — see Pancreatitis
parametrium (chronic) (see also Disease, pelvis, inflammatory) 614.4
  acute 614.3
parotid region 686.9
  gland 527.2
pelvis, female (see also Disease, pelvis, inflammatory) 614.9
penis (corpora cavernosa) 607.2
perianal 569.49
pericardium (see also Pericarditis) 423.9
perineum (female) (male) 686.9
perirectal 569.49
peritoneum (see also Peritonitis) 567.9
periuterine (see also Disease, pelvis, inflammatory) 614.9
perivesical (see also Cystitis) 595.9
petrous bone (see also Petrositis) 383.20
pharynx (see also Pharyngitis) 462
  follicular 472.1
  granular 472.1
pia mater — see Meningitis
pleura — see Pleurisy

Inflammation, inflamed, inflammatory—continued

postmastoidectomy cavity 383.30
  chronic 383.33
prostate (see also Prostatitis) 601.9
rectosigmoid — see Rectosigmoiditis
rectum (see also Proctitis) 569.49
respiratory, upper (see also Infection, respiratory, upper) 465.9
  chronic, due to external agent — see Condition, respiratory, chronic, due to, external agent
  due to
    fumes or vapors (chemical) (inhalation) 506.2
    radiation 508.1
retina (see also Retinitis) 363.20
retrocecal (see also Appendicitis) 541
retroperitoneal (see also Peritonitis) 567.9
salivary duct or gland (any) (suppurative) 527.2
scorbutic, alveoli, teeth 267
scrotum 608.4
sigmoid — see Enteritis
sinus (see also Sinusitis) 473.9
Skene's duct or gland (see also Urethritis) 597.89
skin 686.9
spermatic cord 608.4
sphenoidal (sinus) (see also Sinusitis, sphenoidal) 473.3
spinal
  cord (see also Encephalitis) 323.9
  late effect — see category 326
  membrane — see Meningitis
  nerve — see Disorder, nerve
spine (see also Spondylitis) 720.9
spleen (capsule) 289.59
stomach — see Gastritis
stricture, rectum 569.49
subcutaneous tissue NEC 686.9
suprarenal (gland) 255.8
synovial (fringe) (membrane) — see Bursitis
tendon (sheath) NEC 727.9
testis (see also Orchitis) 604.90
thigh 686.9
throat (see also Sore throat) 462
thymus (gland) 254.8
thyroid (gland) (see also Thyroiditis) 245.9
tongue 529.0
tonsil — see Tonsillitis
trachea — see Tracheitis
trochlear nerve 378.53
tubal (see also Salpingo-oophoritis) 614.2
tuberculous NEC (see also Tuberculosis) 011.9
tubo-ovarian (see also Salpingo-oophoritis) 614.2
tunica vaginalis 608.4
tympanic membrane — see Myringitis
umbilicus, umbilical 686.9
  newborn NEC 771.4
uterine ligament (see also Disease, pelvis, inflammatory) 614.4
  acute 614.3
uterus (catarrhal) (see also Endometritis) 615.9
uveal tract (anterior) (see also Iridocyclitis) 364.3
  posterior — see Chorioretinitis
  sympathetic 360.11
vagina (see also Vaginitis) 616.10
vas deferens 608.4

Inflammation, inflamed, inflammatory—continued

vein (see also Phlebitis) 451.9
  thrombotic 451.9
  cerebral (see also Thrombosis, brain) 434.0
  leg 451.2
    deep (vessels) NEC 451.19
    superficial (vessels) 451.0
  lower extremity 451.2
    deep (vessels) NEC 451.19
    superficial (vessels) 451.0
vocal cord 478.5
vulva (see also Vulvitis) 616.10

Inflation, lung imperfect (newborn) 770.5

Influenza, influenzal 487.1
  with
    bronchitis 487.1
    bronchopneumonia 487.0
    cold (any type) 487.1
    digestive manifestations 487.8
    hemoptysis 487.1
    involvement of
      gastrointestinal tract 487.8
      nervous system 487.8
    laryngitis 487.1
    manifestations NEC 487.8
      respiratory 487.1
        pneumonia 487.0
    pharyngitis 487.1
    pneumonia (any form classifiable to 480-483, 485-486) 487.0
    respiratory manifestations NEC 487.1
    sinusitis 487.1 ◆
    sore throat 487.1
    tonsillitis 487.1
    tracheitis 487.1
    upper respiratory infection (acute) 487.1
  abdominal 487.8
  Asian 487.1
  bronchial 487.1
  bronchopneumonia 487.0
  catarrhal 487.1
  epidemic 487.1
  gastric 487.8
  intestinal 487.8
  laryngitis 487.1
  maternal affecting fetus or newborn 760.2
    manifest influenza in infant 771.2
  pharyngitis 487.1
  pneumonia (any form) 487.0
  respiratory (upper) 487.1
  stomach 487.8
  vaccination, prophylactic (against) V04.8

Influenza-like disease 487.1

Infraction, Freiberg's (metatarsal head) 732.5

Infusion complication, misadventure, or reaction — see Complication, infusion

Ingestion
  chemical — see Table of drugs and chemicals
  drug or medicinal substance
    correct substance properly administered 995.2
    overdose or wrong substance given or taken 977.9
    specified drug — see Table of drugs and chemicals
  foreign body NEC (see also Foreign body) 938

Ingrowing
  hair 704.8
  nail (finger) (toe) (infected) 703.0

Inguinal — see also condition
  testis 752.5

Inhalation
  carbon monoxide 986
  flame (asphyxia) (see also Burn, by site) 949.0
  food or foreign body (see also Asphyxia, food or foreign body) 933.1
  gas, fumes, or vapor (noxious) 987.9
    specified agent — see Table of drugs and chemicals
  liquid or vomitus (see also Asphyxia, food or foreign body) 933.1
  lower respiratory tract NEC 934.9
  meconium (fetus or newborn) 770.1
  mucus (see also Asphyxia, mucus) 933.1
  oil (causing suffocation) (see also Asphyxia, food or foreign body) 933.1
  pneumonia — see Pneumonia, aspiration
  smoke 987.9
  steam 987.9
  stomach contents or secretions (see also Asphyxia, food or foreign body) 933.1
    in labor and delivery 668.0

Inhibition, inhibited
  academic as adjustment reaction 309.23
  orgasm
    female 302.73
    male 302.74
  sexual
    desire 302.71
    excitement 302.72
  work as adjustment reaction 309.23

Inhibitor, systemic lupus erythematosus (presence of) 286.5

Iniencephalus, iniencephaly 740.2

Injected eye 372.74

Injury 959.9

> Note — For abrasion, insect bite (nonvenomous), blister, or scratch, see Injury, superficial.
>
> For laceration, traumatic rupture, tear, or penetrating wound of internal organs, such as heart, lung, liver, kidney, pelvic organs, whether or not accompanied by open wound in the same region, see Injury, internal.
>
> For nerve injury, see Injury, nerve.
>
> For late effect of injuries classifiable to 850-854, 860-869, 900-919, 950-959, see Late, effect, injury, by type.

abdomen, abdominal (viscera) — see also Injury, internal, abdomen
  muscle or wall 959.1
acoustic, resulting in deafness 951.5
adenoid 959.0
adrenal (gland) — see Injury, internal, adrenal
alveolar (process) 959.0
ankle (and foot) (and knee) (and leg, except thigh) 959.7
anterior chamber, eye 921.3
anus 959.1

Injury—continued
  aorta (thoracic) 901.0
    abdominal 902.0
  appendix — see Injury, internal, appendix
  arm, upper (and shoulder) 959.2
  artery (complicating trauma) (see also Injury, blood vessel, by site) 904.9
    cerebral or meningeal (see also Hemorrhage, brain, traumatic, subarachnoid) 852.0
  auditory canal (external) (meatus) 959.0
  auricle, auris, ear 959.0
  axilla 959.2
  back 959.1
  bile duct — see Injury, internal, bile duct
  birth — see also Birth, injury
    canal NEC, complicating delivery 665.9
  bladder (sphincter) — see Injury, internal, bladder
  blast (air) (hydraulic) (immersion) (underwater) NEC 869.0
    with open wound into cavity NEC 869.1
    abdomen or thorax — see Injury, internal, by site
    brain — see Concussion, brain
    ear (acoustic nerve trauma) 951.5
      with perforation of tympanic membrane — see Wound, open, ear, drum
  blood vessel NEC 904.9
    abdomen 902.9
      multiple 902.87
      specified NEC 902.89
    aorta (thoracic) 901.0
      abdominal 902.0
    arm NEC 903.9
    axillary 903.00
      artery 903.01
      vein 903.02
    azygos vein 901.89
    basilic vein 903.1
    brachial (artery) (vein) 903.1
    bronchial 901.89
    carotid artery 900.00
      common 900.01
      external 900.02
      internal 900.03
    celiac artery 902.20
      specified branch NEC 902.24
    cephalic vein (arm) 903.1
    colica dextra 902.26
    cystic
      artery 902.24
      vein 902.39
    deep plantar 904.6
    digital (artery) (vein) 903.5
    due to accidental puncture or laceration during procedure 998.2
    extremity
      lower 904.8
        multiple 904.7
        specified NEC 904.7
      upper 903.9
        multiple 903.8
        specified NEC 903.8
    femoral
      artery (superficial) 904.1
        above profunda origin 904.0
        common 904.0
      vein 904.2
    gastric
      artery 902.21
      vein 902.39

Injury—continued
  blood vessel NEC—continued
    head 900.9
      intracranial — see Injury, intracranial
      multiple 900.82
      specified NEC 900.89
    hemiazygos vein 901.89
    hepatic
      artery 902.22
      vein 902.11
    hypogastric 902.59
      artery 902.51
      vein 902.52
    ileocolic
      artery 902.26
      vein 902.31
    iliac 902.50
      artery 902.53
      specified branch NEC 902.59
      vein 902.54
    innominate
      artery 901.1
      vein 901.3
    intercostal (artery) (vein) 901.81
    jugular vein (external) 900.81
      internal 900.1
    leg NEC 904.8
    mammary (artery) (vein) 901.82
    mesenteric
      artery 902.20
        inferior 902.27
        specified branch NEC 902.29
        superior (trunk) 902.25
          branches, primary 902.26
      vein 902.39
        inferior 902.32
        superior (and primary subdivisions) 902.31
    neck 900.9
      multiple 900.82
      specified NEC 900.89
    ovarian 902.89
      artery 902.81
      vein 902.82
    palmar artery 903.4
    pelvis 902.9
      multiple 902.87
      specified NEC 902.89
    plantar (deep) (artery) (vein) 904.6
    popliteal 904.40
      artery 904.41
      vein 904.42
    portal 902.33
    pulmonary 901.40
      artery 901.41
      vein 901.42
    radial (artery) (vein) 903.2
    renal 902.40
      artery 902.41
      specified NEC 902.49
      vein 902.42
    saphenous
      artery 904.7
      vein (greater) (lesser) 904.3
    splenic
      artery 902.23
      vein 902.34
    subclavian
      artery 901.1
      vein 901.3
    suprarenal 902.49
    thoracic 901.9
      multiple 901.83
      specified NEC 901.89
    tibial 904.50
      artery 904.50
        anterior 904.51
        posterior 904.53

Injury—continued
  blood vessel NEC—continued
    tibial—continued
      vein 904.50
        anterior 904.52
        posterior 904.54
    ulnar (artery) (vein) 903.3
    uterine 902.59
      artery 902.55
      vein 902.56
    vena cava
      inferior 902.10
        specified branches NEC 902.19
      superior 901.2
  brachial plexus 953.4
    newborn 767.6
  brain NEC (see also Injury, intracranial) 854.0
  breast 959.1
  broad ligament — see Injury, internal, broad ligament
  bronchus, bronchi — see Injury, internal, bronchus
  brow 959.0
  buttock 959.1
  canthus, eye 921.1
  cathode ray 990
  cauda equina 952.4
    with fracture, vertebra — see Fracture, vertebra, sacrum
  cavernous sinus (see also Injury, intracranial) 854.0
  cecum — see Injury, internal, cecum
  celiac ganglion or plexus 954.1
  cerebellum (see also Injury, intracranial) 854.0
  cervix (uteri) — see Injury, internal, cervix
  cheek 959.0
  chest — see also Injury, internal, chest
    wall 959.1
  childbirth — see also Birth, injury
    maternal NEC 665.9
  chin 959.0
  choroid (eye) 921.3
  clitoris 959.1
  coccyx 959.1
    complicating delivery 665.6
  colon — see Injury, internal, colon
  common duct — see Injury, internal, common duct
  conjunctiva 921.1
    superficial 918.2
  cord
    spermatic — see Injury, internal, spermatic cord
    spinal — see Injury, spinal, by site
  cornea 921.3
    abrasion 918.1
    due to contact lens 371.82
    penetrating — see Injury, eyeball, penetrating
    superficial 918.1
      due to contact lens 371.82 ◆
  cortex (cerebral) (see also Injury, intracranial) 854.0
    visual 950.3
  costal region 959.1
  costochondral 959.1
  cranial
    bones — see Fracture, skull, by site
    cavity (see also Injury, intracranial) 854.0
    nerve — see Injury, nerve, cranial
  crushing — see Crush
  cutaneous sensory nerve
    lower limb 956.4
    upper limb 955.5

Injury—continued
  delivery — see also Birth, injury
    maternal NEC 665.9
  Descemet's membrane — see Injury, eyeball, penetrating
  diaphragm — see Injury, internal, diaphragm
  duodenum — see Injury, internal, duodenum
  ear (auricle) (canal) (drum) (external) 959.0
  elbow (and forearm) (and wrist) 959.3
  epididymis 959.1
  epigastric region 959.1
  epiglottis 959.1
  epiphyseal, current — see Fracture, by site
  esophagus — see Injury, internal, esophagus
  Eustachian tube 959.0
  extremity (lower) (upper) NEC 959.8
  eye 921.9
    penetrating eyeball — see Injury, eyeball, penetrating
    superficial 918.9
  eyeball 921.3
    penetrating 871.7
      with
        partial loss (of intraocular tissue) 871.2
        prolapse or exposure (of intraocular tissue) 871.1
        without prolapse 871.0
      foreign body (nonmagnetic) 871.6
        magnetic 871.5
    superficial 918.9
  eyebrow 959.0
  eyelid(s) 921.1
    laceration — see Laceration, eyelid
    superficial 918.0
  face (and neck) 959.0
  fallopian tube — see Injury, internal, fallopian tube
  finger(s) (nail) 959.5
  flank 959.1
  foot (and ankle) (and knee) (and leg except thigh) 959.7
  forceps NEC 767.9
    scalp 767.1
  forearm (and elbow) (and wrist) 959.3
  forehead 959.0
  gallbladder — see Injury, internal, gallbladder
  gasserian ganglion 951.2
  gastrointestinal tract — see Injury, internal, gastrointestinal tract
  genital organ(s)
    with
      abortion — see Abortion, by type, with, damage to pelvic organs
      ectopic pregnancy (see also categories 633.0-633.9) 639.2
      molar pregnancy (see also categories 630-632) 639.2
    external 959.1
    following
      abortion 639.2
      ectopic or molar pregnancy 639.2
    internal — see Injury, internal, genital organs
    obstetrical trauma NEC 665.9
      affecting fetus or newborn 763.8

Injury—continued
  gland
    lacrimal 921.1
      laceration 870.8
    parathyroid 959.0
    salivary 959.0
    thyroid 959.0
  globe (eye) (see also Injury, eyeball) 921.3
  grease gun — see Wound, open, by site, complicated
  groin 959.1
  gum 959.0
  hand(s) (except fingers) 959.4
  head NEC (see also Injury, intracranial) 854.0
    with
      skull fracture — see Fracture, skull, by site
  heart — see Injury, internal, heart
  heel 959.7
  hip (and thigh) 959.6
  hymen 959.1
  hyperextension (cervical) (vertebra) 847.0
  ileum — see Injury, internal, ileum
  iliac region 959.1
  infrared rays NEC 990
  instrumental (during surgery) 998.2
    birth injury — see Birth, injury
    nonsurgical (see also Injury, by site) 959.9
    obstetrical 665.9
      affecting fetus or newborn 763.8
      bladder 665.5
      cervix 665.3
      high vaginal 665.4
      perineal NEC 664.9
      urethra 665.5
      uterus 665.5
  internal 869.0

> Note — For injury of internal organ(s) by foreign body entering through a natural orifice (e.g., inhaled, ingested, or swallowed) — see Foreign body, entering through orifice.
>
> For internal injury of any of the following sites with internal injury of any other of the sites — see Injury, internal, multiple.

    with
      fracture
        pelvis — see Fracture, pelvis
        specified site, except pelvis — see Injury, internal, by site
      open wound into cavity 869.1
    abdomen, abdominal (viscera) NEC 868.00
      with
        fracture, pelvis — see Fracture, pelvis
        open wound into cavity 868.10
      specified site NEC 868.09
        with open wound into cavity 868.19
    adrenal (gland) 868.01
      with open wound into cavity 868.11
    aorta (thoracic) 901.0
      abdominal 902.0

Injury—continued
  internal—continued
    with—continued
      appendix 863.85
        with open wound into cavity 863.95
      bile duct 868.02
        with open wound into cavity 868.12
      bladder (sphincter) 867.0
        with
          abortion — see Abortion, by type, with damage to pelvic organs
          ectopic pregnancy (see also categories 633.0-633.9) 639.2
          molar pregnancy (see also categories 630-632) 639.2
          open wound into cavity 867.1
        following
          abortion 639.2
          ectopic or molar pregnancy 639.2
        obstetrical trauma 665.5
          affecting fetus or newborn 763.8
      blood vessel — see Injury, blood vessel, by site
      broad ligament 867.6
        with open wound into cavity 867.7
      bronchus, bronchi 862.21
        with open wound into cavity 862.31
      cecum 863.89
        with open wound into cavity 863.99
      cervix (uteri) 867.4
        with
          abortion — see Abortion, by type, with damage to pelvic organs
          ectopic pregnancy (see also categories 633.0-633.9) 639.2
          molar pregnancy (see also categories 630-632) 639.2
          open wound into cavity 867.5
        following
          abortion 639.2
          ectopic or molar pregnancy 639.2
        obstetrical trauma 665.3
          affecting fetus or newborn 763.8
      chest (see also Injury, internal, intrathoracic organs) 862.8
        with open wound into cavity 862.9
      colon 863.40
        with
          open wound into cavity 863.50
          rectum 863.46
            with open wound into cavity 863.56
        ascending (right) 863.41
          with open wound into cavity 863.51
        descending (left) 863.43
          with open wound into cavity 863.53

Injury—continued
  internal—continued
    colon—continued
      multiple sites 863.46
        with open wound into cavity 863.56
      sigmoid 863.44
        with open wound into cavity 863.54
      specified site NEC 863.49
        with open wound into cavity 863.59
      transverse 863.42
        with open wound into cavity 863.52
    common duct 868.02
      with open wound into cavity 868.12
    complicating delivery 665.9
      affecting fetus or newborn 763.8
    diaphragm 862.0
      with open wound into cavity 862.1
    duodenum 863.21
      with open wound into cavity 863.31
    esophagus (intrathoracic) 862.22
      with open wound into cavity 862.32
      cervical region 874.4
        complicated 874.5
    fallopian tube 867.6
      with open wound into cavity 867.7
    gallbladder 868.02
      with open wound into cavity 868.12
    gastrointestinal tract NEC 863.80
      with open wound into cavity 863.90
    genital organ NEC 867.6
      with open wound into cavity 867.7
    heart 861.00
      with open wound into thorax 861.10
    ileum 863.29
      with open wound into cavity 863.39
    intestine NEC 863.89
      with open wound into cavity 863.99
      large NEC 863.40
        with open wound into cavity 863.50
      small NEC 863.20
        with open wound into cavity 863.30
    intra-abdominal (organ) 868.00
      with open wound into cavity 868.10
      multiple sites 868.09
        with open wound into cavity 868.19
      specified site NEC 868.09
        with open wound into cavity 868.19
    intrathoracic organs (multiple) 862.8
      with open wound into cavity 862.9
      diaphragm (only) — see Injury, internal, diaphragm
      heart (only) — see Injury, internal, heart
      lung (only) — see Injury, internal, lung
      specified site NEC 862.29
        with open wound into cavity 862.39

Injury—continued
  internal—continued
    intrauterine (see also Injury, internal, uterus) 867.4
      with open wound into cavity 867.5
    jejunum 863.29
      with open wound into cavity 863.39
    kidney (subcapsular) 866.00
      with
        disruption of parenchyma (complete) 866.03
          with open wound into cavity 866.13
        hematoma (without rupture of capsule) 866.01
          with open wound into cavity 866.11
        laceration 866.02
          with open wound into cavity 866.12
        open wound into cavity 866.10
    liver 864.00
      with
        contusion 864.01
          with open wound into cavity 864.11
        hematoma 864.01
          with open wound into cavity 864.11
        laceration 864.09
          with open wound into cavity 864.19
        major (disruption of hepatic parenchyma) 864.04
          with open wound into cavity 864.14
        minor (capsule only) 864.02
          with open wound into cavity 864.12
        moderate (involving parenchyma) 864.03
          with open wound into cavity 864.13
        multiple 864.04
        stellate 864.04
          with open wound into cavity 864.14
      open wound into cavity 864.10
    lung 861.20
      with open wound into thorax 861.30
      hemopneumothorax — see Hemopneumothorax, traumatic
      hemothorax — see Hemothorax, traumatic
      pneumohemothorax — see Pneumohemothorax, traumatic
      pneumothorax — see Pneumothorax, traumatic
    mediastinum 862.29
      with open wound into cavity 862.39

Injury—continued
    internal—continued
        mesentery 863.89
            with open wound into cavity 863.99
        mesosalpinx 867.6
            with open wound into cavity 867.7
        multiple 869.0

> Note — Multiple internal injuries of sites classifiable to the same three- or four-digit category should be classified to that category.
>
> Multiple injuries classifiable to different fourth-digit subdivisions of 861 (heart and lung injuries) should be dealt with according to coding rules.

            with open wound into cavity 869.1
        intra-abdominal organ (sites classifiable to 863-868)
            with
                intrathoracic organ(s) (sites classifiable to 861-862) 869.0
                    with open wound into cavity 869.1
                other intra-abdominal organ(s) (sites classifiable to 863-868, except where classifiable to the same three-digit category) 868.09
                    with open wound into cavity 868.19
        intrathoracic organ (sites classifiable to 861-862)
            with
                intra-abdominal organ(s) (sites classifiable to 863-868) 869.0
                    with open wound into cavity 869.1
                other intrathoracic organ(s) (sites classifiable to 861-862, except where classifiable to the same three-digit category) 862.8
                    with open wound into cavity 862.9
        myocardium — see Injury, internal, heart
        ovary 867.6
            with open wound into cavity 867.7
        pancreas (multiple sites) 863.84
            with open wound into cavity 863.94
            body 863.82
                with open wound into cavity 863.92

Injury—continued
    internal—continued
        pancreas—continued
            head 863.81
                with open wound into cavity 863.91
            tail 863.83
                with open wound into cavity 863.93
        pelvis, pelvic (organs) (viscera) 867.8
            with
                fracture, pelvis — see Fracture, pelvis
                open wound into cavity 867.9
            specified site NEC 867.6
                with open wound into cavity 867.7
        peritoneum 868.03
            with open wound into cavity 868.13
        pleura 862.29
            with open wound into cavity 862.39
        prostate 867.6
            with open wound into cavity 867.7
        rectum 863.45
            with
                colon 863.46
                    with open wound into cavity 863.56
                open wound into cavity 863.55
        retroperitoneum 868.04
            with open wound into cavity 868.14
        round ligament 867.6
            with open wound into cavity 867.7
        seminal vesicle 867.6
            with open wound into cavity 867.7
        spermatic cord 867.6
            with open wound into cavity 867.7
        scrotal — see Wound, open, spermatic cord
        spleen 865.00
            with
                disruption of parenchyma (massive) 865.04
                    with open wound into cavity 865.14
                hematoma (without rupture of capsule) 865.01
                    with open wound into cavity 865.11
                open wound into cavity 865.10
                tear, capsular 865.02
                    with open wound into cavity 865.12
                extending into parenchyma 865.03
                    with open wound into cavity 865.13
        stomach 863.0
            with open wound into cavity 863.1
        suprarenal gland (multiple) 868.01
            with open wound into cavity 868.11

Injury—continued
    internal—continued
        thorax, thoracic (cavity) (organs) (multiple) (see also Injury, internal, intrathoracic organs) 862.8
            with open wound into cavity 862.9
        thymus (gland) 862.29
            with open wound into cavity 862.39
        trachea (intrathoracic) 862.29
            with open wound into cavity 862.39
            cervical region (see also Wound, open, trachea) 874.02
        ureter 867.2
            with open wound into cavity 867.3
        urethra (sphincter) 867.0
            with
                abortion — see Abortion, by type, with damage to pelvic organs
                ectopic pregnancy (see also categories 633.0-633.9) 639.2
                molar pregnancy (see also categories 630-632) 639.2
                open wound into cavity 867.1
            following
                abortion 639.2
                ectopic or molar pregnancy 639.2
            obstetrical trauma 665.5
            affecting fetus or newborn 763.8
        uterus 867.4
            with
                abortion — see Abortion, by type, with damage to pelvic organs
                ectopic pregnancy (see also categories 633.0-633.9) 639.2
                molar pregnancy (see also categories 630-632) 639.2
                open wound into cavity 867.5
            following
                abortion 639.2
                ectopic or molar pregnancy 639.2
            obstetrical trauma NEC 665.5
            affecting fetus or newborn 763.8
        vas deferens 867.6
            with open wound into cavity 867.7
        vesical (sphincter) 867.0
            with open wound into cavity 867.1
        viscera (abdominal) (see also Injury, internal, multiple) 868.00
            with
                fracture, pelvis — see Fracture, pelvis
                open wound into cavity 868.10
        thoracic NEC (see also Injury, internal, intrathoracic organs) 862.8
            with open wound into cavity 862.9
    interscapular region 959.1

Injury—continued
    intervertebral disc 959.1
    intestine — see Injury, internal, intestine
    intra-abdominal (organs) NEC — see Injury, internal, intra-abdominal
    intracranial 854.0

> Note — Use the following fifth-digit subclassification with categories 851-854:
>
> 0   unspecified state of consciousness
> 1   with no loss of consciousness
> 2   with brief [less than one hour] loss of consciousness
> 3   with moderate [1-24 hours] loss of consciousness
> 4   with prolonged [more than 24 hours] loss of consciousness and return to pre-existing conscious level
> 5   with prolonged [more than 24 hours] loss of consciousness, without return to pre-existing conscious level
> 6   with loss of consciousness of unspecified duration
> 9   with concussion, unspecified

        with
            open intracranial wound 854.1
            skull fracture — see Fracture, skull, by site
        contusion 851.8
            with open intracranial wound 851.9
            brain stem 851.4
                with open intracranial wound 851.5
            cerebellum 851.4
                with open intracranial wound 851.5
            cortex (cerebral) 851.0
                with open intracranial wound 851.2
        hematoma — see Injury, intracranial, hemorrhage
        hemorrhage 853.0
            with
                laceration — see Injury, intracranial, laceration
                open intracranial wound 853.1
            extradural 852.4
                with open intracranial wound 852.5
            subarachnoid 852.0
                with open intracranial wound 852.1
            subdural 852.2
                with open intracranial wound 852.3
        laceration 851.8
            with open intracranial wound 851.9
            brain stem 851.6
                with open intracranial wound 851.7
            cerebellum 851.6
                with open intracranial wound 851.7

Injury—continued
  intracranial—continued
    laceration—continued
      cortex (cerebral) 851.2
        with open intracranial
          wound 851.3
  intraocular — see Injury, eyeball,
    penetrating
  intrathoracic organs (multiple) —
    see Injury, internal,
    intrathoracic organs
  intrauterine — see Injury,
    internal, intrauterine
  iris 921.3
    penetrating — see Injury,
      eyeball, penetrating
  jaw 959.0
  jejunum — see Injury, internal,
    jejunum
  joint NEC 959.9
    old or residual 718.80
      ankle 718.87
      elbow 718.82
      foot 718.87
      hand 718.84
      hip 718.85
      knee 718.86
      multiple sites 718.89
      pelvic region 718.85
      shoulder (region) 718.81
      specified site NEC 718.88
      wrist 718.83
  kidney — see Injury, internal,
    kidney
  knee (and ankle) (and foot) (and
    leg, except thigh) 959.7
  labium (majus) (minus) 959.1
  labyrinth, ear 959.0
  lacrimal apparatus, gland, or sac
    921.1
    laceration 870.8
  larynx 959.0
  late effect — see Late, effects (of),
    injury
  leg except thigh (and ankle) (and
    foot) (and knee) 959.7
    upper or thigh 959.6
  lens, eye 921.3
    penetrating — see Injury,
      eyeball, penetrating
  lid, eye — see Injury, eyelid
  lip 959.0
  liver — see Injury, internal, liver
  lobe, parietal — see Injury,
    intracranial
  lumbar (region) 959.1
    plexus 953.5
  lumbosacral (region) 959.1
    plexus 953.5
  lung — see Injury, internal, lung
  malar region 959.0
  mastoid region 959.0
  maternal, during pregnancy,
    affecting fetus or newborn
    760.5
  maxilla 959.0
  mediastinum — see Injury,
    internal, mediastinum
  membrane
    brain (see also Injury,
      intracranial) 854.0
    tympanic 959.0
  meningeal artery — see
    Hemorrhage, brain,
    traumatic, subarachnoid
  meninges (cerebral) — see Injury,
    intracranial
  mesenteric
    artery — see Injury, blood
      vessel, mesenteric,
      artery
    plexus, inferior 954.1
    vein — see Injury, blood
      vessel, mesenteric, vein
  mesentery — see Injury, internal,
    mesentery

Injury—continued
  mesosalpinx — see Injury,
    internal, mesosalpinx
  middle ear 959.0
  midthoracic region 959.1
  mouth 959.0
  multiple (sites not classifiable to
    the same four-digit category
    in 959.0-959.7) 959.8
    internal 869.0 ▼
      with open wound into
        cavity 869.1 ▲
  musculocutaneous nerve 955.4
  nail
    finger 959.5
    toe 959.7
  nasal (septum) (sinus) 959.0
  nasopharynx 959.0
  neck (and face) 959.0
  nerve 957.9
    abducens 951.3
    abducent 951.3
    accessory 951.6
    acoustic 951.5
    ankle and foot 956.9
    anterior crural, femoral 956.1
    arm (see also Injury, nerve,
      upper limb) 955.9
    auditory 951.5
    axillary 955.0
    brachial plexus 953.4
    cervical sympathetic 954.0
    cranial 951.9
      first or olfactory 951.8
      second or optic 950.0
      third or oculomotor 951.0
      fourth or trochlear 951.1
      fifth or trigeminal 951.2
      sixth or abducens 951.3
      seventh or facial 951.4
      eighth, acoustic, or
        auditory 951.5
      ninth or glossopharyngeal
        951.8
      tenth, pneumogastric, or
        vagus 951.8
      eleventh or accessory
        951.6
      twelfth or hypoglossal
        951.7
      newborn 767.7
    cutaneous sensory
      lower limb 956.4
      upper limb 955.5
    digital (finger) 955.6
      toe 956.5
    facial 951.4
      newborn 767.5
    femoral 956.1
    finger 955.9
    foot and ankle 956.9
    forearm 955.9
    glossopharyngeal 951.8
    hand and wrist 955.9
    head and neck, superficial
      957.0
    hypoglossal 951.7
    involving several parts of body
      957.8
    leg (see also Injury, nerve,
      lower limb) 956.9
    lower limb 956.9
      multiple 956.8
      specified site NEC 956.5
    lumbar plexus 953.5
    lumbosacral plexus 953.5
    median 955.1
      forearm 955.1
      wrist and hand 955.1
    multiple (in several parts of
      body) (sites not
      classifiable to the same
      three-digit category)
      957.8
    musculocutaneous 955.4
    musculospiral 955.3
      upper arm 955.3

Injury—continued
  nerve—continued
    oculomotor 951.0
    olfactory 951.8
    optic 950.0
    pelvic girdle 956.9
      multiple sites 956.8
      specified site NEC 956.5
    peripheral 957.9
      multiple (in several regions)
        (sites not classifiable
        to the same three-
        digit category) 957.8
      specified site NEC 957.1
    peroneal 956.3
      ankle and foot 956.3
      lower leg 956.3
    plantar 956.5
    plexus 957.9
      celiac 954.1
      mesenteric, inferior 954.1
      spinal 953.9
        brachial 953.4
        lumbosacral 953.5
        multiple sites 953.8
      sympathetic NEC 954.1
    pneumogastric 951.8
    radial 955.3
      wrist and hand 955.3
    sacral plexus 953.5
    sciatic 956.0
      thigh 956.0
    shoulder girdle 955.9
      multiple 955.8
      specified site NEC 955.7
    specified site NEC 957.1
    spinal 953.9
      plexus — see Injury, nerve,
        plexus, spinal
      root 953.9
        cervical 953.0
        dorsal 953.1
        lumbar 953.2
        multiple sites 953.8
        sacral 953.3
    splanchnic 954.1
    sympathetic NEC 954.1
      cervical 954.0
    thigh 956.9
    tibial 956.5
      ankle and foot 956.2
      lower leg 956.5
      posterior 956.2
    toe 956.9
    trigeminal 951.2
    trochlear 951.1
    trunk, excluding shoulder and
      pelvic girdles 954.9
      specified site NEC 954.8
      sympathetic NEC 954.1
    ulnar 955.2
      forearm 955.2
      wrist (and hand) 955.2
    upper limb 955.9
      multiple 955.8
      specified site NEC 955.7
    vagus 951.8
    wrist and hand 955.9
  nervous system, diffuse 957.8
  nose (septum) 959.0
  obstetrical NEC 665.9
    affecting fetus or newborn
      763.8
  occipital (region) (scalp) 959.0
    lobe (see also Injury,
      intracranial) 854.0
  optic 950.9
    chiasm 950.1
    cortex 950.3
    nerve 950.0
    pathways 950.2
  orbit, orbital (region) 921.2
    penetrating 870.3
      with foreign body 870.4
  ovary — see Injury, internal,
    ovary

Injury—continued
  paint-gun — see Wound, open,
    by site, complicated
  palate (soft) 959.0
  pancreas — see Injury, internal,
    pancreas
  parathyroid (gland) 959.0
  parietal (region) (scalp) 959.0
    lobe — see Injury, intracranial
  pelvic
    floor 959.1
      complicating delivery
        664.1
        affecting fetus or
          newborn 763.8
      joint or ligament, complicating
        delivery 665.6
        affecting fetus or newborn
          763.8
    organs — see also Injury,
      internal, pelvis
      with
        abortion — see
          Abortion, by type,
          with damage to
          pelvic organs
        ectopic pregnancy (see
          also categories
          633.0-633.9)
          639.2
        molar pregnancy (see
          also categories
          633.0-633.9)
          639.2
      following
        abortion 639.2
        ectopic or molar
          pregnancy 639.2
      obstetrical trauma 665.5
        affecting fetus or
          newborn 763.8
  pelvis 959.1
  penis 959.1
  perineum 959.1
  peritoneum — see Injury,
    internal, peritoneum
  periurethral tissue
    with
      abortion — see Abortion,
        by type, with
        damage to pelvic
        organs
      ectopic pregnancy (see also
        categories 633.0-
        633.9) 639.2
      molar pregnancy (see also
        categories 630-632)
        639.2
    complicating delivery 665.5
      affecting fetus or newborn
        763.8
    following
      abortion 639.2
      ectopic or molar pregnancy
        639.2
  phalanges
    foot 959.7
    hand 959.5
  pharynx 959.0
  pleura — see Injury, internal,
    pleura
  popliteal space 959.7
  prepuce 959.1
  prostate — see Injury, internal,
    prostate
  pubic region 959.1
  pudenda 959.1
  radiation NEC 990
  radioactive substance or radium
    NEC 990
  rectovaginal septum 959.1
  rectum — see Injury, internal,
    rectum
  retina 921.3
    penetrating — see Injury,
      eyeball, penetrating

Injury—continued
- retroperitoneal — *see* Injury, internal, retroperitoneum
- roentgen rays NEC 990
- round ligament — *see* Injury, internal, round ligament
- sacral (region) 959.1
  - plexus 953.5
- sacroiliac ligament NEC 959.1
- sacrum 959.1
- salivary ducts or glands 959.0
- scalp 959.0
  - due to birth trauma 767.1
  - fetus or newborn 767.1
- scapular region 959.2
- sclera 921.3
  - penetrating — *see* Injury, eyeball, penetrating
  - superficial 918.2
- scrotum 959.1
- seminal vesicle — *see* Injury, internal, seminal vesicle
- shoulder (and upper arm) 959.2
- sinus
  - cavernous (*see also* Injury, intracranial) 854.0
  - nasal 959.0
- skeleton NEC, birth injury 767.3
- skin NEC 959.9
- skull — *see* Fracture, skull, by site
- soft tissue (of external sites) (severe) — *see* Wound, open, by site
- specified site NEC 959.8
- spermatic cord — *see* Injury, internal, spermatic cord
- spinal (cord) 952.9
  - with fracture, vertebra — *see* Fracture, vertebra, by site, with spinal cord injury
  - cervical (C_1-C_4) 952.00
    - with
      - anterior cord syndrome 952.02
      - central cord syndrome 952.03
      - complete lesion of cord 952.01
      - incomplete lesion NEC 952.04
      - posterior cord syndrome 952.04
    - C_5-C_7 level 952.05
      - with
        - anterior cord syndrome 952.07
        - central cord syndrome 952.08
        - complete lesion of cord 952.06
        - incomplete lesion NEC 952.09
        - posterior cord syndrome 952.09
        - specified type NEC 952.09
    - specified type NEC 952.04
  - dorsal (D_1-D_6) (T_1-T_6) (thoracic) 952.10
    - with
      - anterior cord syndrome 952.12
      - central cord syndrome 952.13
      - complete lesion of cord 952.11
      - incomplete lesion NEC 952.14
      - posterior cord syndrome 952.14

Injury—continued
- spinal (cord)—continued
  - dorsal—continued
    - D_7-D_{12} level (T_7-T_{12}) 952.15
      - with
        - anterior cord syndrome 952.17
        - central cord syndrome 952.18
        - complete lesion of cord 952.16
        - incomplete lesion NEC 952.19
        - posterior cord syndrome 952.19
        - specified type NEC 952.19
    - specified type NEC 952.14
  - lumbar 952.2
  - multiple sites 952.8
  - nerve (root) NEC — *see* Injury, nerve, spinal, root
  - plexus 953.9
    - brachial 953.4
    - lumbosacral 953.5
    - multiple sites 953.8
  - sacral 952.3
  - thoracic (*see also* Injury, spinal, dorsal) 952.10
- spleen — *see* Injury, internal, spleen
- stellate ganglion 954.1
- sternal region 959.1
- stomach — *see* Injury, internal, stomach
- subconjunctival 921.1
- subcutaneous 959.9
- subdural — *see* Injury, intracranial
- submaxillary region 959.0
- submental region 959.0
- subungual
  - fingers 959.5
  - toes 959.7
- superficial 919

> Note — Use the following fourth-digit subdivisions with categories 910-919:
>
> 0 Abrasion or friction burn without mention of infection
> 1 Abrasion or friction burn, infected
> 2 Blister without mention of infection
> 3 Blister, infected
> 4 Insect bite, nonvenomous, without mention of infection
> 5 Insect bite, nonvenomous, infected
> 6 Superficial foreign body (splinter) without major open wound and without mention of infection
> 7 Superficial foreign body (splinter) without major open wound, infected
> 8 Other and unspecified superficial injury without mention of infection
> 9 Other and unspecified superficial injury, infected
>
> *For late effects of superficial injury, see category 906.2.*

Injury—continued
- superficial—continued
  - abdomen, abdominal (muscle) (wall) (and other part(s) of trunk) 911
  - ankle (and hip, knee, leg, or thigh) 916
  - anus (and other part(s) of trunk) 911
  - arm 913
    - upper (and shoulder) 912
  - auditory canal (external) (meatus) (and other part(s) of face, neck, or scalp, except eye) 910
  - axilla (and upper arm) 912
  - back (and other part(s) of trunk) 911
  - breast (and other part(s) of trunk) 911
  - brow (and other part(s) of face, neck, or scalp, except eye) 910
  - buttock (and other part(s) of trunk) 911
  - canthus, eye 918.0
  - cheek(s) (and other part(s) of face, neck, or scalp, except eye) 910
  - chest wall (and other part(s) of trunk) 911
  - chin (and other part(s) of face, neck, or scalp, except eye) 910
  - clitoris (and other part(s) of trunk) 911
  - conjunctiva 918.2
  - cornea 918.1
    - due to contact lens 371.82 ◆
  - costal region (and other part(s) of trunk) 911
  - ear(s) (auricle) (canal) (drum) (external) (and other part(s) of face, neck, or scalp, except eye) 910
  - elbow (and forearm) (and wrist) 913
  - epididymis (and other part(s) of trunk) 911
  - epigastric region (and other part(s) of trunk) 911
  - epiglottis (and other part(s) of face, neck, or scalp, except eye) 910
  - eye(s) (and adnexa) NEC 918.9
  - eyelid(s) (and periocular area) 918.0
  - face (any part(s), except eye) (and neck or scalp) 910
  - finger(s) (nail) (any) 915
  - flank (and other part(s) of trunk) 911
  - foot (phalanges) (and toe(s)) 917
  - forearm (and elbow) (and wrist) 913
  - forehead (and other part(s) of face, neck, or scalp, except eye) 910
  - globe (eye) 918.9
  - groin (and other part(s) of trunk) 911
  - gum(s) (and other part(s) of face, neck, or scalp, except eye) 910
  - hand(s) (except fingers alone) 914
  - head (and other part(s) of face, neck, or scalp, except eye) 910
  - heel (and foot or toe) 917
  - hip (and ankle, knee, leg, or thigh) 916
  - iliac region (and other part(s) of trunk) 911

Injury—continued
- superficial—continued
  - interscapular region (and other part(s) of trunk) 911
  - iris 918.9
  - knee (and ankle, hip, leg, or thigh) 916
  - labium (majus) (minus) (and other part(s) of trunk) 911
  - lacrimal (apparatus) (gland) (sac) 918.0
  - leg (lower) (upper) (and ankle, hip, knee, or thigh) 916
  - lip(s) (and other part(s) of face, neck, or scalp, except eye) 910
  - lower extremity (except foot) 916
  - lumbar region (and other part(s) of trunk) 911
  - malar region (and other part(s) of face, neck, or scalp, except eye) 910
  - mastoid region (and other part(s) of face, neck, or scalp, except eye) 910
  - midthoracic region (and other part(s) of trunk) 911
  - mouth (and other part(s) of face, neck, or scalp, except eye) 910
  - multiple sites (not classifiable to the same three-digit category) 919
  - nasal (septum) (and other part(s) of face, neck, or scalp, except eye) 910
  - neck (and face or scalp, any part(s), except eye) 910
  - nose (septum) (and other part(s) of face, neck, or scalp, except eye) 910
  - occipital region (and other part(s) of face, neck, or scalp, except eye) 910
  - orbital region 918.0
  - palate (soft) (and other part(s) of face, neck, or scalp, except eye) 910
  - parietal region (and other part(s) of face, neck, or scalp, except eye) 910
  - penis (and other part(s) of trunk) 911
  - perineum (and other part(s) of trunk) 911
  - periocular area 918.0
  - pharynx (and other part(s) of face, neck, or scalp, except eye) 910
  - popliteal space (and ankle, hip, leg, or thigh) 916
  - prepuce (and other part(s) of trunk) 911
  - pubic region (and other part(s) of trunk) 911
  - pudenda (and other part(s) of trunk) 911
  - sacral region (and other part(s) of trunk) 911
  - salivary (ducts) (glands) (and other part(s) of face, neck, or scalp, except eye) 910
  - scalp (and other part(s) of face or neck, except eye) 910
  - scapular region (and upper arm) 912
  - sclera 918.2
  - scrotum (and other part(s) of trunk) 911
  - shoulder (and upper arm) 912
  - skin NEC 919
  - specified site(s) NEC 919
  - sternal region (and other part(s) of trunk) 911

Injury—continued
  superficial—continued
    subconjunctival 918.2
    subcutaneous NEC 919
    submaxillary region (and other part(s) of face, neck, or scalp, except eye) 910
    submental region (and other part(s) of face, neck, or scalp, except eye) 910
    supraclavicular fossa (and other part(s) of face, neck or scalp, except eye) 910
    supraorbital 918.0
    temple (and other part(s) of face, neck, or scalp, except eye) 910
    temporal region (and other part(s) of face, neck, or scalp, except eye) 910
    testis (and other part(s) of trunk) 911
    thigh (and ankle, hip, knee, or leg) 916
    thorax, thoracic (external) (and other part(s) of trunk) 911
    throat (and other part(s) of face, neck, or scalp, except eye) 910
    thumb(s) (nail) 915
    toe(s) (nail) (subungual) (and foot) 917
    tongue (and other part(s) of face, neck, or scalp, except eye) 910
    tooth, teeth 521.2
    trunk (any part(s)) 911
    tunica vaginalis (and other part(s) of trunk) 911
    tympanum, tympanic membrane (and other part(s) of face, neck, or scalp, except eye) 910
    upper extremity NEC 913
    uvula (and other part(s) of face, neck, or scalp, except eye) 910
    vagina (and other part(s) of trunk) 911
    vulva (and other part(s) of trunk) 911
    wrist (and elbow) (and forearm) 913
  supraclavicular fossa 959.1
  supraorbital 959.0
  surgical complication (external or internal site) 998.2
  symphysis pubis 959.1
    complicating delivery 665.6
      affecting fetus or newborn 763.8
  temple 959.0
  temporal region 959.0
  testis 959.1
  thigh (and hip) 959.6
  thorax, thoracic (external) 959.1
    cavity — see Injury, internal, thorax
    internal — see Injury, internal, intrathoracic organs
  throat 959.0
  thumb(s) (nail) 959.5
  thymus — see Injury, internal, thymus
  thyroid (gland) 959.0
  toe (nail) (any) 959.7
  tongue 959.0
  tonsil 959.0
  tooth NEC 873.63
    complicated 873.73
  trachea — see Injury, internal, trachea
  trunk 959.1
  tunica vaginalis 959.1

Injury—continued
  tympanum, tympanic membrane 959.0
  ultraviolet rays NEC 990
  ureter — see Injury, internal, ureter
  urethra (sphincter) — see Injury, internal, urethra
  uterus — see Injury, internal, uterus
  uvula 959.0
  vagina 959.1
  vascular — see Injury, blood vessel
  vas deferens — see Injury, internal, vas deferens
  vein (see also Injury, blood vessel, by site) 904.9
  vena cava
    inferior 902.10
    superior 901.2
  vesical (sphincter) — see Injury, internal, vesical
  viscera (abdominal) — see also Injury, internal, viscera
    with fracture, pelvis — see Fracture, pelvis
  visual 950.9
    cortex 950.3
  vitreous (humor) 871.2
  vulva 959.1
  whiplash (cervical spine) 847.0
  wringer — see Crush, by site
  wrist (and elbow) (and forearm) 959.3
  x-ray NEC 990
Inoculation — see also Vaccination
  complication or reaction — see Complication, vaccination
Insanity, insane (see also Psychosis) 298.9
  adolescent (see also Schizophrenia) 295.9
  alternating (see also Psychosis, affective, circular) 296.7
  confusional 298.9
    acute 293.0
    subacute 293.1
  delusional 298.9
  paralysis, general 094.1
    progressive 094.1
  paresis, general 094.1
  senile 290.20
Insect
  bite — see Injury, superficial, by site
  venomous, poisoning by 989.5
Insemination, artificial V26.1
Insertion
  cord (umbilical) lateral or velamentous 663.5
    affecting fetus or newborn 762.6
  intrauterine contraceptive device V25.1
  placenta, vicious — see Placenta, previa
  subdermal implantable contraceptive V25.5
  velamentous, umbilical cord 663.5
    affecting fetus or newborn 762.6
Insolation 992.0
  meaning sunstroke 992.0
Insomnia 780.52
  with sleep apnea 780.51
  nonorganic origin 307.41
    persistent 307.42
    transient 307.41
  subjective complaint 307.49
Inspiration
  food or foreign body (see also Asphyxia, food or foreign body) 933.1

Inspiration—continued
  mucus (see also Asphyxia, mucus) 933.1
Inspissated bile syndrome, newborn 774.4
Instability
  detrusor 596.59
  emotional (excessive) 301.3
  joint (posttraumatic) 718.80
    ankle 718.87
    elbow 718.82
    foot 718.87
    hand 718.84
    hip 718.85
    knee 718.86
    lumbosacral 724.6
    multiple sites 718.89
    pelvic region 718.85
    sacroiliac 724.6
    shoulder (region) 718.81
    specified site NEC 718.88
    wrist 718.83
  lumbosacral 724.6
  nervous 301.89
  personality (emotional) 301.59
  thyroid, paroxysmal 242.9
  urethral 599.83
  vasomotor 780.2
Insufficiency, insufficient
  accommodation 367.4
  adrenal (gland) (acute) (chronic) 255.4
    medulla 255.5
    primary 255.4
    specified NEC 255.5
  adrenocortical 255.4
  anus 569.49
  aortic (valve) 424.1
    with
      mitral (valve) disease 396.1
        insufficiency, incompetence, or regurgitation 396.3
        stenosis or obstruction 396.1
      stenosis or obstruction 424.1
        with mitral (valve) disease 396.8
    congenital 746.4
    rheumatic 395.1
      with
        mitral (valve) disease 396.1
          insufficiency, incompetence, or regurgitation 396.3
          stenosis or obstruction 396.1
        stenosis or obstruction 395.2
          with mitral (valve) disease 396.8
    specified cause NEC 424.1
    syphilitic 093.22
  arterial 447.1
    basilar artery 435.0
    carotid artery 435.8
    cerebral 437.1
    coronary (acute or subacute) 411.89
    mesenteric 557.1
    peripheral 443.9
    precerebral 435.9
    vertebral artery 435.1
  arteriovenous 459.9
  basilar artery 435.0
  biliary 575.8
  cardiac (see also Insufficiency, myocardial) 428.0
    complicating surgery 997.1
    due to presence of (cardiac) prosthesis 429.4

Insufficiency, insufficient—continued
  cardiac—continued
    postoperative 997.1
      long-term effect of cardiac surgery 429.4
    specified during or due to a procedure 997.1
      long-term effect of cardiac surgery 429.4
  cardiorenal (see also Hypertension, cardiorenal) 404.90
  cardiovascular (see also Disease, cardiovascular) 429.2
    renal (see also Hypertension, cardiorenal) 404.90
  carotid artery 435.8
  cerebral (vascular) 437.9
  cerebrovascular 437.9
    with transient focal neurological signs and symptoms 435.9
    acute 437.1
      with transient focal neurological signs and symptoms 435.9
  circulatory NEC 459.9
    fetus or newborn 779.8
  convergence 378.83
  coronary (acute or subacute) 411.89
    chronic or with a stated duration of over 8 weeks 414.8
  corticoadrenal 255.4
  dietary 269.9
  divergence 378.85
  food 994.2
  gastroesophageal 530.89
  gonadal
    ovary 256.3
    testis 257.2
  gonadotropic hormone secretion 253.4
  heart — see also Insufficiency, myocardial
    fetus or newborn 779.8
    valve (see also Endocarditis) 424.90
      congenital NEC 746.89
  hepatic 573.8
  idiopathic autonomic 333.0
  kidney (see also Disease, renal) 593.9
  labyrinth, labyrinthine (function) 386.53
    bilateral 386.54
    unilateral 386.53
  lacrimal 375.15
  liver 573.8
  lung (acute) (see also Insufficiency, pulmonary) 518.82
    following trauma, surgery, or shock 518.5
    newborn 770.8
  mental (congenital) (see also Retardation, mental) 319
  mesenteric 557.1
  mitral (valve) 424.0
    with
      aortic (valve) disease 396.3
        insufficiency, incompetence, or regurgitation 396.3
        stenosis or obstruction 396.2
      obstruction or stenosis 394.2
        with aortic valve disease 396.8
    congenital 746.6

Insufficiency, insufficient—
continued
  mitral—*continued*
    rheumatic 394.1
      with
        aortic (valve) disease
          396.3
          insufficiency,
            incompetence,
            or regurgitation
            396.3
          stenosis or
            obstruction
            396.2
        obstruction or stenosis
          394.2
          with aortic valve
            disease 396.8
        active or acute 391.1
          with chorea, rheumatic
            (Sydenham's)
            392.0
        congenital 243
        specified cause, except
          rheumatic 424.0
  muscle
    heart — *see* Insufficiency,
      myocardial
    ocular (*see also* Strabismus)
      378.9
  myocardial, myocardium (with
    arteriosclerosis) 428.0
    with rheumatic fever
      (conditions classifiable
      to 390)
      active, acute, or subacute
        391.2
        with chorea 392.0
      inactive or quiescent (with
        chorea) 398.0
    congenital 746.89
    due to presence of (cardiac)
      prosthesis 429.4
    fetus or newborn 779.8
    following cardiac surgery
      429.4
    hypertensive (*see also*
      Hypertension, heart)
      402.91
      benign 402.11
      malignant 402.01
    postoperative 997.1
      long-term effect of cardiac
        surgery 429.4
    rheumatic 398.0
      active, acute, or subacute
        391.2
        with chorea
          (Sydenham's)
          392.0
    syphilitic 093.82
  nourishment 994.2
  organic 799.8
  ovary 256.3
    postablative 256.2
  pancreatic 577.8
  parathyroid (gland) 252.1
  peripheral vascular (arterial)
    443.9
  pituitary (anterior) 253.2
    posterior 253.5
  placental — *see* Placenta,
    insufficiency
  platelets 287.5
  prenatal care in current
    pregnancy V23.7
  progressive pluriglandular 258.9
  pseudocholinesterase 289.8
  pulmonary (acute) 518.82
    following
      shock 518.5
      surgery 518.5
      trauma 518.5
    newborn 770.8
    valve (*see also* Endocarditis,
      pulmonary) 424.3
      congenital 746.09
  pyloric 537.0

Insufficiency, insufficient—
continued
  renal (acute) (chronic) (*see also*
    Disease, renal) 593.9 ◆
    due to a procedure 997.5
  respiratory 786.09
    acute 518.82
      following shock, surgery, or
        trauma 518.5
    newborn 770.8
  rotation — *see* Malrotation
  suprarenal 255.4
    medulla 255.5
  tarso-orbital fascia, congenital
    743.66
  tear film 375.15
  testis 257.2
  thyroid (gland) (acquired) — *see
    also* Hypothyroidism
    congenital 243
  tricuspid (*see also* Endocarditis,
    tricuspid) 397.0
    congenital 746.89
    syphilitic 093.23
  urethral sphincter 599.84
  valve, valvular (heart) (*see also*
    Endocarditis) 424.90
  vascular 459.9
    intestine NEC 557.9
    mesenteric 557.1
    peripheral 443.9
    renal (*see also* Hypertension,
      kidney) 403.90
  velopharyngeal
    acquired 528.9
    congenital 750.29
  venous (peripheral) 459.81
  ventricular — *see* Insufficiency,
    myocardial
  vertebral artery 435.1
  weight gain during pregnancy
    646.8
  zinc 269.3
Insufflation
  fallopian V26.2
  meconium 770.1
Insular — *see* condition
Insulinoma (M8151/0)
  malignant (M8151/3)
    pancreas 157.4
    specified site — *see*
      Neoplasm, by site,
      malignant
    unspecified site 157.4
  pancreas 211.7
  specified site — *see* Neoplasm,
    by site, benign
  unspecified site 211.7
Insuloma — *see* Insulinoma
Insult
  brain 437.9
    acute 436
  cerebral 437.9
    acute 436
  cerebrovascular 437.9
    acute 436
  vascular NEC 437.9
    acute 436
Insurance examination (certification)
  V70.3
Intemperance (*see also* Alcoholism)
  303.9
Interception of pregnancy
  (menstrual extraction) V25.3
Intermenstrual
  bleeding 626.4
    irregular 626.6
    regular 626.5
  hemorrhage 626.4
    irregular 626.6
    regular 626.5
  pain(s) 625.2
Intermittent — *see* condition
Internal — *see* condition
Interproximal wear 521.1

Interruption
  aortic arch 747.11
  bundle of His 426.50
  fallopian tube (for sterilization)
    V25.2
  phase-shift, sleep cycle 307.45
  repeated REM-sleep 307.48
  sleep
    due to perceived
      environmental
      disturbances 307.48
    phase-shift, of 24-hour sleep-
      wake cycle 307.45
    repeated REM-sleep type
      307.48
  vas deferens (for sterilization)
    V25.2
Intersexuality 752.7
Interstitial — *see* condition
Intertrigo 695.89
  labialis 528.5
Intervertebral disc — *see* condition
Intestine, intestinal — *see also*
  condition
  flu 487.8
Intolerance
  carbohydrate NEC 579.8
  cardiovascular exercise, with pain
    (at rest) (with less than
    ordinary activity) (with
    ordinary activity) V47.2
  dissaccharide (hereditary) 271.3
  drug
    correct substance properly
      administered 995.2
    wrong substance given or
      taken in error 977.9
    specified drug — *see* Table
      of drugs and
      chemicals
  effort 306.2
  fat NEC 579.8
  foods NEC 579.8
  fructose (hereditary) 271.2
  glucose (-galactose) (congenital)
    271.3
  gluten 579.0
  lactose (hereditary) (infantile)
    271.3
  lysine (congenital) 270.7
  milk NEC 579.8
  protein (familial) 270.7
  starch NEC 579.8
  sucrose (-isomaltose) (congenital)
    271.3
Intoxicated NEC (*see also*
  Alcoholism) 305.0
Intoxication
  acid 276.2
  acute
    alcoholic 305.0
      with alcoholism 303.0
      hangover effects 305.0
    caffeine 305.9 ◆
    hallucinogenic (*see also*
      Abuse, drugs,
      nondependent) 305.3
  alcohol (acute) 305.0
    with alcoholism 303.0
    hangover effects 305.0
    idiosyncratic 291.4
    pathological 291.4
  alimentary canal 558.2
  ammonia (hepatic) 572.2
  chemical — *see also* Table of
    drugs and chemicals
    via placenta or breast milk
      760.70
      alcohol 760.71
      anti-infective agents 760.74
      cocaine 760.75
      "crack" 760.75
      hallucinogenic agents NEC
        760.73
      medicinal agents NEC
        760.79

Intoxication—*continued*
  chemical—*continued*
    via placenta or breast milk—
      continued
      narcotics 760.72
      obstetric anesthetic or
        analgesic drug 763.5
      specified agent NEC 760.79
      suspected, affecting
        management of
        pregnancy 655.5
    cocaine, through placenta or
      breast milk 760.75
  drug
    correct substance properly
      administered (*see also*
      Allergy, drug) 995.2
    newborn 779.4
    obstetric anesthetic or sedation
      668.9
    affecting fetus or newborn
      763.5
    overdose or wrong substance
      given or taken — *see*
      Table of drugs and
      chemicals
    pathologic 292.2
    specific to newborn 779.4
    via placenta or breast milk
      760.70
      alcohol 760.71
      anti-infective agents 760.74
      cocaine 760.75
      "crack" 760.75
      hallucinogenic agents
        760.73
      medicinal agents NEC
        760.79
      narcotics 760.72
      obstetric anesthetic or
        analgesic drug 763.5
      specified agent NEC 760.79
      suspected, affecting
        management of
        pregnancy 655.5
  enteric — *see* Intoxication,
    intestinal
  fetus or newborn, via placenta or
    breast milk 760.70
    alcohol 760.71
    anti-infective agents 760.74
    cocaine 760.75
    "crack" 760.75
    hallucinogenic agents 760.73
    medicinal agents NEC 760.79
    narcotics 760.72
    obstetric anesthetic or
      analgesic drug 763.5
    specified agent NEC 760.79
    suspected, affecting
      management of
      pregnancy 655.5
  food — *see* Poisoning, food
  gastrointestinal 558.2
  hallucinogenic (acute) 305.3
  hepatocerebral 572.2
  idiosyncratic alcohol 291.4
  intestinal 569.89
    due to putrefaction of food
      005.9
  methyl alcohol (*see also*
    Alcoholism) 305.0
    with alcoholism 303.0
  pathologic 291.4
    drug 292.2
  potassium (K) 276.7
  septic
    with
      abortion — *see* Abortion,
        by type, with sepsis
      ectopic pregnancy (*see also*
        categories 633.0-
        633.9) 639.0
      molar pregnancy (*see also*
        categories 630-632)
        639.0
    during labor 659.3

Intoxication—continued
septic—continued
following
abortion 639.0
ectopic or molar pregnancy 639.0
generalized — see Septicemia
puerperal, postpartum, childbirth 670
serum (prophylactic) (therapeutic) 999.5
uremic — see Uremia
water 276.6

Intracranial — see condition

Intrahepatic gallbladder 751.69

Intraligamentous — see also condition
pregnancy — see Pregnancy, cornual

Intraocular — see also condition
sepsis 360.00

Intrathoracic — see also condition
kidney 753.3
stomach — see Hernia, diaphragm

Intrauterine contraceptive device
checking V25.42
insertion V25.1
in situ V45.51
management V25.42
prescription V25.02
repeat V25.42
reinsertion V25.42
removal V25.42

Intraventricular — see condition

Intrinsic deformity — see Deformity

Intrusion, repetitive, of sleep (due to environmental disturbances) (with atypical polysomnographic features) 307.48

Intumescent, lens (eye) NEC 366.9
senile 366.12

Intussusception (colon) (enteric) (intestine) (rectum) 560.0
appendix 543.9
congenital 751.5
fallopian tube 620.8
ileocecal 560.0
ileocolic 560.0
ureter (with obstruction) 593.4

Invagination
basilar 756.0
colon or intestine 560.0

Invalid (since birth) 799.8

Invalidism (chronic) 799.8

Inversion
albumin-globulin (A-G) ratio 273.8
bladder 596.8
cecum (see also Intussusception) 560.0
cervix 622.8
nipple 611.79
congenital 757.6
puerperal, postpartum 676.3
optic papilla 743.57
organ or site, congenital NEC — see Anomaly, specified type NEC
sleep rhythm 780.55
nonorganic origin 307.45
testis (congenital) 752.5
uterus (postinfectional) (postpartal, old) 621.7
chronic 621.7
complicating delivery 665.2
affecting fetus or newborn 763.8
vagina — see Prolapse, vagina

Investigation
allergens V72.7
clinical research V70.7

Inviability — see Immaturity

Involuntary movement, abnormal 781.0

Involution, involutional — see also condition
breast, cystic or fibrocystic 610.1
depression (see also Psychosis, affective) 296.2
recurrent episode 296.3
single episode 296.2
melancholia (see also Psychosis, affective) 296.2
recurrent episode 296.3
single episode 296.2
ovary, senile 620.3
paranoid state (reaction) 297.2
paraphrenia (climacteric) (menopause) 297.2
psychosis 298.8
thymus failure 254.8

IQ
under 20 318.2
20-34 318.1
35-49 318.0
50-70 317

IRDS 769

Irideremia 743.45

Iridis rubeosis 364.42
diabetic 250.5 [364.42]

Iridochoroiditis (panuveitis) 360.12

Iridocyclitis NEC 364.3
acute 364.00
primary 364.01
recurrent 364.02
chronic 364.10
in
lepromatous leprosy 030.0 [364.11]
sarcoidosis 135 [364.11]
tuberculosis (see also Tuberculosis) 017.3 [364.11]
due to allergy 364.04
endogenous 364.01
gonococcal 098.41
granulomatous 364.10
herpetic (simplex) 054.44
zoster 053.22
hypopyon 364.05
lens induced 364.23
nongranulomatous 364.00
primary 364.01
recurrent 364.02
rheumatic 364.10
secondary 364.04
infectious 364.03
noninfectious 364.04
subacute 364.00
primary 364.01
recurrent 364.02
sympathetic 360.11
syphilitic (secondary) 091.52
tuberculous (chronic) (see also Tuberculosis) 017.3 [364.11]

Iridocyclochoroiditis (panuveitis) 360.12

Iridodialysis 364.76

Iridodonesis 364.8

Iridoplegia (complete) (partial) (reflex) 379.49

Iridoschisis 364.52

Iris — see condition

Iritis 364.3
acute 364.00
primary 364.01
recurrent 364.02
chronic 364.10
in
sarcoidosis 135 [364.11]
tuberculosis (see also Tuberculosis) 017.3 [364.11]
diabetic 250.5 [364.42]

Iritis—continued
due to
allergy 364.04
herpes simplex 054.44
leprosy 030.0 [364.11]
endogenous 364.01
gonococcal 098.41
gouty 274.89 [364.11]
granulomatous 364.10
hypopyon 364.05
lens induced 364.23
nongranulomatous 364.00
papulosa 095.8 [364.11]
primary 364.01
recurrent 364.02
rheumatic 364.10
secondary 364.04
infectious 364.03
noninfectious 364.04
subacute 364.00
primary 364.01
recurrent 364.02
sympathetic 360.11
syphilitic (secondary) 091.52
congenital 090.0 [364.11]
late 095.8 [364.11]
tuberculous (see also Tuberculosis) 017.3 [364.11]
uratic 274.89 [364.11]

Iron
deficiency anemia 280.9
metabolism disease 275.0
storage disease 275.0

Iron-miners' lung 503

Irradiated enamel (tooth, teeth) 521.8

Irradiation
burn — see Burn, by site
effects, adverse 990

Irreducible, irreducibility — see condition

Irregular, irregularity
action, heart 427.9
alveolar process 525.8
bleeding NEC 626.4
breathing 786.09
colon 569.89
contour of cornea 743.41
acquired 371.70
dentin in pulp 522.3
eye movements NEC 379.59
menstruation (cause unknown) 626.4
periods 626.4
prostate 602.9
pupil 364.75
respiratory 786.09
septum (nasal) 470
shape, organ or site, congenital NEC — see Distortion
sleep-wake rhythm (non-24-hour) 780.55
nonorganic origin 307.45
vertebra 733.99

Irritability (nervous) 799.2
bladder 596.8
neurogenic 596.54
with cauda equina syndrome 344.61
bowel (syndrome) 564.1
bronchial (see also Bronchitis) 490
cerebral, newborn 779.1
colon 564.1
psychogenic 306.4
duodenum 564.8
heart (psychogenic) 306.2
ileum 564.8
jejunum 564.8
myocardium 306.2
rectum 564.8
stomach 536.9
psychogenic 306.4

Irritability—continued
sympathetic (nervous system) (see also Neuropathy, peripheral, autonomic) 337.9
urethra 599.84
ventricular (heart) (psychogenic) 306.2

Irritable — see Irritability

Irritation
anus 569.49
axillary nerve 353.0
bladder 596.8
brachial plexus 353.0
brain (traumatic) (see also Injury, intracranial) 854.0
nontraumatic — see Encephalitis
bronchial (see also Bronchitis) 490
cerebral (traumatic) (see also Injury, intracranial) 854.0
nontraumatic — see Encephalitis
cervical plexus 353.2
cervix (see also Cervicitis) 616.0
choroid, sympathetic 360.11
cranial nerve — see Disorder, nerve, cranial
digestive tract 536.9
psychogenic 306.4
gastric 536.9
psychogenic 306.4
gastrointestinal (tract) 536.9
functional 536.9
psychogenic 306.4
globe, sympathetic 360.11
intestinal (bowel) 564.1
labyrinth 386.50
lumbosacral plexus 353.1
meninges (traumatic) (see also Injury, intracranial) 854.0
nontraumatic — see Meningitis
myocardium 306.2
nerve — see Disorder, nerve
nervous 799.2
nose 478.1
penis 607.89
perineum 709.9
peripheral
autonomic nervous system (see also Neuropathy, peripheral, autonomic) 337.9
nerve — see Disorder, nerve
peritoneum (see also Peritonitis) 567.9
pharynx 478.29
plantar nerve 355.6
spinal (cord) (traumatic) — see also Injury, spinal, by site
nerve — see also Disorder, nerve
root NEC 724.9
traumatic — see Injury, nerve, spinal
nontraumatic — see Myelitis
stomach 536.9
psychogenic 306.4
sympathetic nerve NEC (see also Neuropathy, peripheral, autonomic) 337.9
ulnar nerve 354.2
vagina 623.9

Isambert's disease 012.3

Ischemia, ischemic 459.9
basilar artery (with transient neurologic deficit) 435.0
bone NEC 733.40
bowel (transient) 557.9
acute 557.0
chronic 557.1
due to mesenteric artery insufficiency 557.1

Ischemia, ischemic—continued
  brain — see also Ischemia, cerebral
    recurrent focal 435.9
  cardiac (see also Ischemia, heart) 414.9
  cardiomyopathy 414.8
  carotid artery (with transient neurologic deficit) 435.8
  cerebral (chronic) (generalized) 437.1
    arteriosclerotic 437.0
    intermittent (with transient neurologic deficit) 435.9
    puerperal, postpartum, childbirth 674.0
    recurrent focal (with transient neurologic deficit) 435.9
    transient (with transient neurologic deficit) 435.9
  colon 557.9
    acute 557.0
    chronic 557.1
    due to mesenteric artery insufficiency 557.1
  coronary (chronic) (see also Ischemia, heart) 414.9
  heart (chronic or with a stated duration of over 8 weeks) 414.9
    acute or with a stated duration of 8 weeks or less (see also Infarct, myocardium) 410.9
      without myocardial infarction 411.89
        with coronary (artery) occlusion 411.81
    subacute 411.89
  intestine (transient) 557.9
    acute 557.0
    chronic 557.1
    due to mesenteric artery insufficiency 557.1
  kidney 593.81
  labyrinth 386.50
  muscles, leg 728.89
  myocardium, myocardial (chronic or with a stated duration of over 8 weeks) 414.8
    acute (see also Infarct, myocardium) 410.9
      without myocardial infarction 411.89
        with coronary (artery) occlusion 411.81
  renal 593.81
  retina, retinal 362.84
  small bowel 557.9
    acute 557.0
    chronic 557.1
    due to mesenteric artery insufficiency 557.1
  spinal cord 336.1
  subendocardial (see also Insufficiency, coronary) 411.89
  vertebral artery (with transient neurologic deficit) 435.1
Ischialgia (see also Sciatica) 724.3
Ischiopagus 759.4
Ischium, ischial — see condition
Ischomenia 626.8
Ischuria 788.5
Iselin's disease or osteochondrosis 732.5
Islands of
  parotid tissue in
    lymph nodes 750.26
    neck structures 750.26
  submaxillary glands in
    fascia 750.26
    lymph nodes 750.26
    neck muscles 750.26
Islet cell tumor, pancreas (M8150/0) 211.7

Isoimmunization NEC (see also Incompatibility) 656.2
  fetus or newborn 773.2
    ABO blood groups 773.1
    Rhesus (Rh) factor 773.0
Isolation V07.0
  social V62.4
Isosporosis 007.2
Issue
  medical certificate NEC V68.0
    cause of death V68.0
    fitness V68.0
    incapacity V68.0
  repeat prescription NEC V68.1
    appliance V68.1
    contraceptive V25.40
      device NEC V25.49
        intrauterine V25.42
        specified type NEC V25.49
      pill V25.41
    glasses V68.1
    medicinal substance V68.1
Itch (see also Pruritus) 698.9
  bakers' 692.89
  barbers' 110.0
  bricklayers' 692.89
  cheese 133.8
  clam diggers' 120.3
  coolie 126.9
  copra 133.8
  Cuban 050.1
  dew 126.9
  dhobie 110.3
  eye 379.99
  filarial (see also Infestation, filarial) 125.9
  grain 133.8
  grocers' 133.8
  ground 126.9
  harvest 133.8
  jock 110.3
  Malabar 110.9
    beard 110.0
    foot 110.4
    scalp 110.0
  meaning scabies 133.0
  Norwegian 133.0
  perianal 698.0
  poultrymen's 133.8
  sarcoptic 133.0
  scrub 134.1
  seven year V61.1
    meaning scabies 133.0
  straw 133.8
  swimmers' 120.3
  washerwoman's 692.4
  water 120.3
  winter 698.8
Itsenko-Cushing syndrome (pituitary basophilism) 255.0
Ivemark's syndrome (asplenia with congenital heart disease) 759.0
Ivory bones 756.52
Ixodes 134.8
Ixodiasis 134.8

Jacoud's nodular fibrositis, chronic
(Jaccoud's syndrome) 714.4
Jackson's
membrane 751.4
paralysis or syndrome 344.89
veil 751.4
Jacksonian
epilepsy (see also Epilepsy) 345.5
seizures (focal) (see also Epilepsy) 345.5
Jacob's ulcer (M8090/3) — see Neoplasm, skin, malignant, by site
Jacquet's dermatitis (diaper dermatitis) 691.0
Jadassohn's
blue nevus (M8780/0) — see Neoplasm, skin, benign
disease (maculopapular erythroderma) 696.2
intraepidermal epithelioma (M8096/0) — see Neoplasm, skin, benign
Jadassohn-Lewandowski syndrome (pachyonychia congenita) 757.5
Jadassohn-Pellizari's disease (anetoderma) 701.3
Jadassohn-Tièche nevus (M8780/0) — see Neoplasm, skin, benign
Jaffe-Lichtenstein (-Uehlinger) syndrome 252.0
Jahnke's syndrome (encephalocutaneous angiomatosis) 759.6
Jakob-Creutzfeldt disease or syndrome 046.1
with dementia 290.10
Jaksch (-Luzet) disease or syndrome (pseudoleukemia infantum) 285.8
Jamaican
neuropathy 349.82
paraplegic tropical ataxic-spastic syndrome 349.82
Janet's disease (psychasthenia) 300.89
Janiceps 759.4
Jansky-Bielschowsky amaurotic familial idiocy 330.1
Japanese
B type encephalitis 062.0
river fever 081.2
seven-day fever 100.89
Jaundice (yellow) 782.4
acholuric (familial) (splenomegalic) (see also Spherocytosis) 282.0
acquired 283.9
breast milk 774.39
catarrhal (acute) 070.1
with hepatic coma 070.0
chronic 571.9
epidemic — see Jaundice, epidemic
cholestatic (benign) 782.4
chronic idiopathic 277.4
epidemic (catarrhal) 070.1
with hepatic coma 070.0
leptospiral 100.0
spirochetal 100.0
febrile (acute) 070.1
with hepatic coma 070.0
leptospiral 100.0
spirochetal 100.0
fetus or newborn 774.6
due to or associated with ABO
antibodies 773.1
incompatibility, maternal/fetal 773.1
isoimmunization 773.1

Jaundice—continued
fetus or newborn—continued
due to or associated with—continued
absence or deficiency of enzyme system for bilirubin conjugation (congenital) 774.39
blood group incompatibility NEC 773.2
breast milk inhibitors to conjugation 774.39
associated with preterm delivery 774.2
bruising 774.1
Crigler-Najjar syndrome 277.4 [774.31]
delayed conjugation 774.30
associated with preterm delivery 774.2
development 774.39
drugs or toxins transmitted from mother 774.1
G-6-PD deficiency 282.2 [774.0]
galactosemia 271.1 [774.5]
Gilbert's syndrome 277.4 [774.31]
hepatocellular damage 774.4
hereditary hemolytic anemia (see also Anemia, hemolytic) 282.9 [774.0]
hypothyroidism, congenital 243 [774.31]
incompatibility, maternal/fetal NEC 773.2
infection 774.1
inspissated bile syndrome 774.4
isoimmunization NEC 773.2
mucoviscidosis 277.01 [774.5]
obliteration of bile duct, congenital 751.61 [774.5]
polycythemia 774.1
preterm delivery 774.2
red cell defect 282.9 [774.0]
Rh
antibodies 773.0
incompatibility, maternal/fetal 773.0
isoimmunization 773.0
spherocytosis (congenital) 282.0 [774.0]
swallowed maternal blood 774.1
physiological NEC 774.6
from injection, inoculation, infusion, or transfusion (blood) (plasma) (serum) (other substance) (onset within 8 months after administration) — see Hepatitis, viral
Gilbert's (familial nonhemolytic) 277.4
hematogenous 283.9
hemolytic (acquired) 283.9
congenital (see also Spherocytosis) 282.0
hemorrhagic (acute) 100.0
leptospiral 100.0
newborn 776.0
spirochetal 100.0
hepatocellular 573.8

Jaundice—continued
homologous (serum) — see Hepatitis, viral
idiopathic, chronic 277.4
infectious (acute) (subacute) 070.1
with hepatic coma 070.0
leptospiral 100.0
spirochetal 100.0
leptospiral 100.0
malignant (see also Necrosis, liver) 570
newborn (physiological) (see also Jaundice, fetus or newborn) 774.6
nonhemolytic, congenital familial (Gilbert's) 277.4
nuclear, newborn (see also Kernicterus of newborn) 774.7
obstructive NEC (see also Obstruction, biliary) 576.8
postimmunization — see Hepatitis, viral
posttransfusion — see Hepatitis, viral
regurgitation (see also Obstruction, biliary) 576.8
serum (homologous) (prophylactic) (therapeutic) — see Hepatitis, viral
spirochetal (hemorrhagic) 100.0
symptomatic 782.4
newborn 774.6
Jaw — see condition
Jaw-blinking 374.43
congenital 742.8
Jaw-winking phenomenon or syndrome 742.8
Jealousy
alcoholic 291.5
childhood 313.3
sibling 313.3
Jejunitis (see also Enteritis) 558.9
Jejunostomy status V44.4
Jejunum, jejunal — see condition
Jensen's disease 363.05
Jericho boil 085.1
Jerks, myoclonic 333.2
Jeune's disease or syndrome (asphyxiating thoracic dystrophy) 756.4
Jigger disease 134.1
Job's syndrome (chronic granulomatous disease) 288.1
Jod-Basedow phenomenon 242.8
Johnson-Stevens disease (erythema multiforme exudativum) 695.1
Joint — see also condition
Charcot's 094.0 [713.5]
false 733.82
flail — see Flail, joint
mice — see also Loose, body, joint
knee 717.6
sinus to bone 730.9
von Gies' 095.8
Jordan's anomaly or syndrome 288.2
Josephs-Diamond-Blackfan anemia (congenital hypoplastic) 284.0
Jumpers' knee 727.2
Jungle yellow fever 060.0
Jüngling's disease (sarcoidosis) 135
Junin virus hemorrhagic fever 078.7
Juvenile — see also condition
delinquent 312.9
group (see also Disturbance, conduct) 312.2
neurotic 312.4

K

Kahler (-Bozzolo) disease (multiple myeloma) (M9730/3) 203.0
Kakergasia 300.9
Kakke 265.0
Kala-azar (Indian) (infantile) (Mediterranean) (Sudanese) 085.0
Kalischer's syndrome (encephalocutaneous angiomatosis) 759.6
Kallmann's syndrome (hypogonadotropic hypogonadism with anosmia) 253.4
Kanner's syndrome (autism) (see also Psychosis, childhood) 299.0
Kaolinosis 502
Kaposi's
disease 757.33
lichen ruber 696.4
acuminatus 696.4
moniliformis 697.8
xeroderma pigmentosum 757.33
sarcoma (M9140/3) 176.9
adipose tissue 176.1
aponeurosis 176.1
artery 176.1
blood vessel 176.1
bursa 176.1
connective tissue 176.1
external genitalia 176.8
fascia 176.1
fatty tissue 176.1
fibrous tissue 176.1
gastrointestinal tract NEC 176.3
ligament 176.1
lung 176.4
lymph
gland(s) 176.5
node(s) 176.5
lymphatic(s) NEC 176.1
muscle (skeletal) 176.1
oral cavity NEC 176.8
palate 176.2
scrotum 176.8
skin 176.0
soft tissue 176.1
specified site NEC 176.8
subcutaneous tissue 176.1
synovia 176.1
tendon (sheath) 176.1
vein 176.1
vessel 176.1
viscera NEC 176.9
vulva 176.8
varicelliform eruption 054.0
vaccinia 999.0
Kartagener's syndrome or triad (sinusitis, bronchiectasis, situs inversus) 759.3
Kasabach-Merritt syndrome (capillary hemangioma associated with thrombocytopenic purpura) 287.3
Kaschin-Beck disease (endemic polyarthritis) — see Disease, Kaschin-Beck
Kast's syndrome (dyschondroplasia with hemangiomas) 756.4
Katatonia (see also Schizophrenia) 295.2
Katayama disease or fever 120.2
Kathisophobia 781.0
Kawasaki disease 446.1
Kayser-Fleischer ring (cornea) (pseudosclerosis) 275.1 [371.14]
Kaznelson's syndrome (congenital hypoplastic anemia) 284.0

Kedani fever 081.2
Kelis 701.4
Kelly (-Patterson) syndrome
	(sideropenic dysphagia) 280.8
Keloid, cheloid 701.4
	Addison's (morphea) 701.0
	cornea 371.00
	Hawkins' 701.4
	scar 701.4
Keloma 701.4
Kenya fever 082.1
Keratectasia 371.71
	congenital 743.41
Keratitis (nodular) (nonulcerative)
		(simple) (zonular) NEC 370.9
	with ulceration (see also Ulcer,
		cornea) 370.00
	actinic 370.24
	arborescens 054.42
	areolar 370.22
	bullosa 370.8
	deep — see Keratitis, interstitial
	dendritic(a) 054.42
	desiccation 370.34
	diffuse interstitial 370.52
	disciform(is) 054.43
		varicella 052.7 [370.44]
	epithelialis vernalis 372.13
		[370.32]
	exposure 370.34

	oyster-shuckers 370.8
	parenchymatous — see Keratitis,
		interstitial
	petrificans 370.8
	phlyctenular 370.31
	postmeasles 055.71
	punctata, punctate 370.21
		leprosa 030.0 [370.21]
		profunda 090.3
		superficial (Thygeson's) 370.21
	purulent 370.8
	pustuliformis profunda 090.3
	rosacea 695.3 [370.49]
	sclerosing 370.54
	specified type NEC 370.8
	stellate 370.22
	striate 370.22

Keratitis—continued
	superficial 370.20
		with conjunctivitis (see also
			Keratoconjunctivitis)
			370.40
		punctate (Thygeson's) 370.21
	suppurative 370.8
	syphilitic (congenital) (prenatal)
		090.3
	trachomatous 076.1
		late effect 139.1
	tuberculous (phlyctenular) (see
		also Tuberculosis) 017.3
		[370.31]
	ulcerated (see also Ulcer, cornea)
		370.00
	vesicular 370.8
	welders' 370.24
	xerotic (see also Keratomalacia)
		371.45
	vitamin A deficiency 264.4
Keratoacanthoma 238.2 ◆
Keratocele 371.72
Keratoconjunctivitis (see also
		Keratitis) 370.40
	adenovirus type 8 077.1
	epidemic 077.1
	exposure 370.34
	gonococcal 098.43
	herpetic (simplex) 054.43

	gonorrheal 098.81
	punctata 701.1
	tylodes, progressive 701.1
Keratodermatocele 371.72
Keratoglobus 371.70
	congenital 743.41
		associated with buphthalmos
			743.22
Keratohemia 371.12
Keratoiritis (see also Iridocyclitis)
	364.3
	syphilitic 090.3
	tuberculous (see also
		Tuberculosis) 017.3
		[364.11]
Keratolysis exfoliativa (congenital)
	757.39
	acquired 695.89
	neonatorum 757.39

Keratoma 701.1
	congenital 757.39
	malignum congenitale 757.1
	palmaris et plantaris hereditarium
		757.39
	senile 702.0
Keratomalacia 371.45
	vitamin A deficiency 264.4
Keratomegaly 743.41
Keratomycosis 111.1
	nigricans (palmaris) 111.1
Keratopathy 371.40
	band (see also Keratitis) 371.43
	bullous (see also Keratitis) 371.23
	degenerative (see also
		Degeneration, cornea)
		371.40
		hereditary (see also Dystrophy,
			cornea) 371.50
	discrete colliquative 371.49
Keratoscleritis, tuberculous (see also
	Tuberculosis) 017.3 [370.31]
Keratosis 701.1
	actinic 702.0
	arsenical 692.4
	blennorrhagica 701.1
		gonococcal 098.81
	congenital (any type) 757.39
	ear (middle) (see also
		Cholesteatoma) 385.30
	female genital (external) 629.8
	follicular, vitamin A deficiency
		264.8
	follicularis 757.39
		acquired 701.1
		congenital (acneiformis)
			(Siemens) 757.39
		spinulosa (decalvans) 757.39
		vitamin A deficiency 264.8
	gonococcal 098.81
	larynx, laryngeal 478.79
	male genital (external) 608.89
	middle ear (see also
		Cholesteatoma) 385.30
	nigricans 701.2
		congenital 757.39
	obturans 380.21
	palmaris et plantaris (symmetrical)
		757.39
	penile 607.89
	pharyngeus 478.29
	pilaris 757.39
		acquired 701.1
	punctata (palmaris et plantaris)
		701.1
	scrotal 608.89
	seborrheic 702.19 ▼
		inflamed 702.11 ▲
	senilis 702.0
	solar 702.0
	suprafollicularis 757.39
	tonsillaris 478.29
	vagina 623.1
	vegetans 757.39
	vitamin A deficiency 264.8
Kerato-uveitis (see also Iridocyclitis)
	364.3
Keraunoparalysis 994.0
Kerion (celsi) 110.0
Kernicterus of newborn (not due to
	isoimmunization) 774.7
	due to isoimmunization
		(conditions classifiable to
		773.0-773.2) 773.4
Ketoacidosis 276.2
	diabetic 250.1
Ketonuria 791.6
	branched-chain, intermittent
		270.3
Ketosis 276.2
	diabetic 250.1
Kidney — see condition

Kienböck's
	disease 732.3
		adult 732.8
	osteochondrosis 732.3
Kimmelstiel (-Wilson) disease or
	syndrome (intercapillary
	glomerulosclerosis) 250.4
	[581.81]
Kink, kinking
	appendix 543.9
	artery 447.1
	cystic duct, congenital 751.61
	hair (acquired) 704.2
	ileum or intestine (see also
		Obstruction, intestine)
		560.9
	Lane's (see also Obstruction,
		intestine) 560.9
	organ or site, congenital NEC —
		see Anomaly, specified type
		NEC, by site
	ureter (pelvic junction) 593.3
		congenital 753.2
	vein(s) 459.2
		caval 459.2
		peripheral 459.2
Kinnier Wilson's disease
	(hepatolenticular
	degeneration) 275.1
Kissing
	osteophytes 721.5
	spine 721.5
	vertebra 721.5
Klauder's syndrome (erythema
	multiforme, exudativum) 695.1
Klebs' disease (see also Nephritis)
	583.9
Klein-Waardenburg syndrome
	(ptosis-epicanthus) 270.2
Kleine-Levin syndrome 349.89
Kleptomania 312.32
Klinefelter's syndrome 758.7
Klinger's disease 446.4
Klippel's disease 723.8
Klippel-Feil disease or syndrome
	(brevicollis) 756.16
Klippel-Trenaunay syndrome 759.89
Klumpke (-Déjérine) palsy, paralysis
	(birth) (newborn) 767.6
Klüver-Bucy (-Terzian) syndrome
	310.0
Knee — see condition
Knifegrinders' rot (see also
	Tuberculosis) 011.4
Knock-knee (acquired) 736.41
	congenital 755.64
Knot
	intestinal, syndrome (volvulus)
		560.2
	umbilical cord (true) 663.2
		affecting fetus or newborn
		762.5
Knots, surfer 919.8
	infected 919.9
Knotting (of)
	hair 704.2
	intestine 560.2
Knuckle pads (Garrod's) 728.79
Köbner's disease (epidermolysis
	bullosa) 757.39
Koch's
	infection (see also Tuberculosis,
		pulmonary) 011.9
	relapsing fever 087.9
Koch-Weeks conjunctivitis 372.03
Koenig-Wichman disease
	(pemphigus) 694.4
Köhler's disease (osteochondrosis)
	732.5
	first (osteochondrosis juvenilis)
		732.5

Köhler's disease—continued
  second (Freiburg's infarction, metatarsal head) 732.5
  patellar 732.4
  tarsal navicular (bone) (osteoarthrosis juvenilis) 732.5
Köhler-Mouchet disease (osteoarthrosis juvenilis) 732.5
Köhler-Pellegrini-Stieda disease or syndrome (calcification, knee joint) 726.62
Koilonychia 703.8
  congenital 757.5
Kojevnikov's, Kojewnikoff's epilepsy (see also Epilepsy) 345.7
König's
  disease (osteochondritis dissecans) 732.7
  syndrome 564.8
Koniophthisis (see also Tuberculosis) 011.4
Koplik's spots 055.9
Kopp's asthma 254.8
Korean hemorrhagic fever 078.6
Korsakoff (-Wernicke) disease, psychosis, or syndrome (nonalcoholic) 294.0
  alcoholic 291.1
Korsakov's disease — see Korsakoff's disease
Korsakow's disease — see Korsakoff's disease
Kostmann's disease or syndrome (infantile genetic agranulocytosis) 288.0
Krabbe's
  disease (leukodystrophy) 330.0
  syndrome
    congenital muscle hypoplasia 756.89
    cutaneocerebral angioma 759.6
Kraepelin-Morel disease (see also Schizophrenia) 295.9
Kraft-Weber-Dimitri disease 759.6
Kraurosis
  ani 569.49
  penis 607.0
  vagina 623.8
  vulva 624.0
Kreotoxism 005.9
Krukenberg's
  spindle 371.13
  tumor (M8490/6) 198.6
Kufs' disease 330.1
Kugelberg-Welander disease 335.11
Kuhnt-Junius degeneration or disease 362.52
Kulchitsky's cell carcinoma (carcinoid tumor of intestine) 259.2
Kümmell's disease or spondylitis 721.7
Kundrat's disease (lymphosarcoma) 200.1
Kunekune — see Dermatophytosis
Kunkel syndrome (lupoid hepatitis) 571.49
Kupffer cell sarcoma (M9124/3) 155.0
Kuru 046.0
Kussmaul's
  coma (diabetic) 250.3
  disease (polyarteritis nodosa) 446.0
  respiration (air hunger) 786.09
Kwashiorkor (marasmus type) 260
Kyasanur Forest disease 065.2

Kyphoscoliosis, kyphoscoliotic (acquired) (see also Scoliosis) 737.30
  congenital 756.19
  due to radiation 737.33
  heart (disease) 416.1
  idiopathic 737.30
  infantile
    progressive 737.32
    resolving 737.31
  late effect of rickets 268.1 [737.43]
  specified NEC 737.39
  thoracogenic 737.34
  tuberculous (see also Tuberculosis) 015.0 [737.43]
Kyphosis, kyphotic (acquired) (postural) 737.10
  adolescent postural 737.0
  congenital 756.19
  dorsalis juvenilis 732.0
  due to or associated with
    Charcot-Marie-Tooth disease 356.1 [737.41]
    mucopolysaccharidosis 277.5 [737.41]
    neurofibromatosis 237.71 [737.41]
    osteitis
      deformans 731.0 [737.41]
      fibrosa cystica 252.0 [737.41]
    osteoporosis (see also Osteoporosis) 733.0 [737.41]
    poliomyelitis (see also Poliomyelitis) 138 [737.41]
    radiation 737.11
    tuberculosis (see also Tuberculosis) 015.0 [737.41]
  Kümmell's 721.7
  late effect of rickets 268.1 [737.41]
  Morquio-Brailsford type (spinal) 277.5 [737.41]
  pelvis 738.6
  postlaminectomy 737.12
  specified cause NEC 737.19
  syphilitic, congenital 090.5 [737.41]
  tuberculous (see also Tuberculosis) 015.0 [737.41]
Kyrle's disease (hyperkeratosis follicularis in cutem penetrans) 701.1

L

Labia, labium — see condition
Labiated hymen 752.49
Labile
  blood pressure 796.4
  emotions, emotionality 301.3
  vasomotor system 443.9
Labioglossal paralysis 335.22
Labium leporinum (see also Cleft, lip) 749.10
Labor (see also Delivery)
  with complications — see Delivery, complicated
  abnormal NEC 661.9
    affecting fetus or newborn 763.7
  arrested active phase 661.1
    affecting fetus or newborn 763.7
  desultory 661.2
    affecting fetus or newborn 763.7

Labor—continued
  dyscoordinate 661.4
    affecting fetus or newborn 763.7
  early onset (22-36 weeks gestation) 644.2
  failed
    induction 659.1
      mechanical 659.0
      medical 659.1
      surgical 659.0
    trial (vaginal delivery) 660.6
  false 644.1
  forced or induced, affecting fetus or newborn 763.8
  hypertonic 661.4
    affecting fetus or newborn 763.7
  hypotonic 661.2
    affecting fetus or newborn 763.7
    primary 661.0
      affecting fetus or newborn 763.7
    secondary 661.1
      affecting fetus or newborn 763.7
  incoordinate 661.4
    affecting fetus or newborn 763.7
  irregular 661.2
    affecting fetus or newborn 763.7
  long — see Labor, prolonged
  missed (at or near term) 656.4
  obstructed NEC 660.9
    affecting fetus or newborn 763.1
    specified cause NEC 660.8
      affecting fetus or newborn 763.1
  pains, spurious 644.1
  precipitate 661.3
    affecting fetus or newborn 763.6
  premature 644.2
    threatened 644.0
  prolonged or protracted 662.1
    first stage 662.0
      affecting fetus or newborn 763.8
    second stage 662.2
      affecting fetus or newborn 763.8
      affecting fetus or newborn 763.8
  threatened NEC 644.1
  undelivered 644.1
Labored breathing (see also Hyperventilation) 786.09
Labyrinthitis (inner ear) (destructive) (latent) 386.30
  circumscribed 386.32
  diffuse 386.31
  focal 386.32
  purulent 386.33
  serous 386.31
  suppurative 386.33
  syphilitic 095.8
  toxic 386.34
  viral 386.35
Laceration — see also Wound, open, by site, accidental,
  complicating surgery 998.2
  Achilles tendon 845.09
    with open wound 892.2
  anus (sphincter) 863.89
    with
      abortion — see Abortion, by type, with damage to pelvic organs
      ectopic pregnancy (see also categories 633.0-633.9) 639.2
      molar pregnancy (see also categories 630-632) 639.2

Laceration—continued
  anus—continued
    complicating delivery 664.2
      with laceration of anal or rectal mucosa 664.3
    following
      abortion 639.2
      ectopic or molar pregnancy 639.2
    nontraumatic, nonpuerperal 565.0
  bladder (urinary)
    with
      abortion — see Abortion, by type, with damage to pelvic organs
      ectopic pregnancy (see also categories 633.0-633.9) 639.2
      molar pregnancy (see also categories 630-632) 639.2
    following
      abortion 639.2
      ectopic or molar pregnancy 639.2
    obstetrical trauma 665.5
  blood vessel — see Injury, blood vessel, by site
  bowel
    with
      abortion — see Abortion, by type, with damage to pelvic organs
      ectopic pregnancy (see also categories 633.0-633.9) 639.2
      molar pregnancy (see also categories 630-632) 639.2
    following
      abortion 639.2
      ectopic or molar pregnancy 639.2
    obstetrical trauma 665.5
  brain (with hemorrhage) (cerebral) (membrane) 851.8
  brain (cerebral) (membrane) 851.8

Note — Use the following fifth-digit subclassification with categories 851–854:

0	unspecified state of consciousness
1	with no loss of consciousness
2	with brief [less than one hour] loss of consciousness
3	with moderate [1-24 hours] loss of consciousness
4	with prolonged [more than 24 hours] loss of consciousness and return to pre-existing conscious level
5	with prolonged [more than 24 hours] loss of consciousness, without return to pre-existing conscious level
6	with loss of consciousness of unspecified duration
9	with concussion, unspecified

  with
    open intracranial wound 851.9
    skull fracture — see Fracture, skull, by site

Laceration—continued
- brain—continued
  - cerebellum 851.6
    - with open intracranial wound 851.7
  - cortex 851.2
    - with open intracranial wound 851.3
  - during birth 767.0
  - stem 851.6
    - with open intracranial wound 851.7
- broad ligament
  - with
    - abortion — see Abortion, by type, with damage to pelvic organs
    - ectopic pregnancy (see also categories 633.0-633.9) 639.2
    - molar pregnancy (see also categories 630-632) 639.2
  - following
    - abortion 639.2
    - ectopic or molar pregnancy 639.2
  - nontraumatic 620.6
  - obstetrical trauma 665.6
  - syndrome (nontraumatic) 620.6
- capsule, joint — see Sprain, by site
- cardiac — see Laceration, heart
- causing eversion of cervix uteri (old) 622.0
- central, complicating delivery 664.4
- cerebellum — see Laceration, brain, cerebellum
- cerebral — see also Laceration, brain during birth 767.0
- cervix (uteri)
  - with
    - abortion — see Abortion, by type, with damage to pelvic organs
    - ectopic pregnancy (see also categories 633.0-633.9) 639.2
    - molar pregnancy (see also categories 630-632) 639.2
  - following
    - abortion 639.2
    - ectopic or molar pregnancy 639.2
  - nonpuerperal, nontraumatic 622.3
  - obstetrical trauma (current) 665.3
  - old (postpartal) 622.3
  - traumatic — see Injury, internal, cervix
- chordae heart 429.5
- complicated 879.9
- cornea — see Laceration, eyeball
- cortex (cerebral) — see Laceration, brain, cortex
- esophagus 530.89
- eye(s) — see Laceration, ocular
- eyeball NEC 871.4
  - with prolapse or exposure of intraocular tissue 871.1
  - penetrating — see Penetrating wound, eyeball
  - specified as without prolapse of intraocular tissue 871.0
- eyelid NEC 870.8
  - full thickness 870.1
    - involving lacrimal passages 870.2
  - skin (and periocular area) 870.0

Laceration—continued
- eyelid NEC—continued
  - skin—continued
    - penetrating — see Penetrating wound, orbit
- fourchette
  - with
    - abortion — see Abortion, by type, with damage to pelvic organs
    - ectopic pregnancy (see also categories 633.0-633.9) 639.2
    - molar pregnancy (see also categories 630-632) 639.2
  - complicating delivery 664.0
  - following
    - abortion 639.2
    - ectopic or molar pregnancy 639.2
- heart (without penetration of heart chambers) 861.02
  - with
    - open wound into thorax 861.12
    - penetration of heart chambers 861.03
      - with open wound into thorax 861.13
- hernial sac — see Hernia, by site
- internal organ (abdomen) (chest) (pelvis)
  - NEC — see Injury, internal, by site
- kidney (parenchyma) 866.02
  - with
    - complete disruption of parenchyma (rupture) 866.03
      - with open wound into cavity 866.13
    - open wound into cavity 866.12
- labia
  - complicating delivery 664.0
- ligament — see also Sprain, by site
  - with open wound — see Wound, open, by site
- liver 864.09
  - with open wound into cavity 864.19
  - major (disruption of hepatic parenchyma) 864.04
    - with open wound into cavity 864.14
  - minor (capsule only) 864.02
    - with open wound into cavity 864.12
  - moderate (involving parenchyma without major disruption) 864.03
    - with open wound into cavity 864.13
  - multiple 864.04
    - with open wound into cavity 864.14
  - stellate 864.04
    - with open wound into cavity 864.14
- lung 861.22
  - with open wound into thorax 861.32
- meninges — see Laceration, brain
- meniscus (knee) (see also Tear, meniscus) 836.2
  - old 717.5
  - site other than knee — see also Sprain, by site
  - old NEC (see also Disorder, cartilage, articular) 718.0

Laceration—continued
- muscle — see also Sprain, by site
  - with open wound — see Wound, open, by site
- myocardium — see Laceration, heart
- nerve — see Injury, nerve, by site
- ocular NEC (see also Laceration, eyeball) 871.4
  - adnexa NEC 870.8
    - penetrating 870.3
      - with foreign body 870.4
- orbit (eye) 870.8
  - penetrating 870.3
    - with foreign body 870.4
- pelvic
  - floor (muscles)
    - with
      - abortion — see Abortion, by type, with damage to pelvic organs
      - ectopic pregnancy (see also categories 633.0-633.9) 639.2
      - molar pregnancy (see also categories 630-632) 639.2
    - complicating delivery 664.1
    - following
      - abortion 639.2
      - ectopic or molar pregnancy 639.2
    - nonpuerperal 618.7
    - old (postpartal) 618.7
  - organ NEC
    - with
      - abortion — see Abortion, by type, with damage to pelvic organs
      - ectopic pregnancy (see also categories 633.0-633.9) 639.2
      - molar pregnancy (see also categories 630-632) 639.2
    - complicating delivery 665.5
      - affecting fetus or newborn 763.8
    - following
      - abortion 639.2
      - ectopic or molar pregnancy 639.2
    - obstetrical trauma 665.5
- perineum, perineal (old) (postpartal) 618.7
  - with
    - abortion — see Abortion, by type, with damage to pelvic floor
    - ectopic pregnancy (see also categories 633.0-633.9) 639.2
    - molar pregnancy (see also categories 630-632) 639.2
  - complicating delivery 664.4
    - first degree 664.0
    - second degree 664.1
    - third degree 664.2
    - fourth degree 664.3
    - central 664.4
    - involving
      - anal sphincter 664.2
      - fourchette 664.0
      - hymen 664.0
      - labia 664.0
      - pelvic floor 664.1
      - perineal muscles 664.1

Laceration—continued
- perineum, perineal—continued
  - complicating delivery—continued
    - involving—continued
      - rectovaginal septum 664.2
        - with anal mucosa 664.3
      - skin 664.0
      - sphincter (anal) 664.2
        - with anal mucosa 664.3
      - vagina 664.0
      - vaginal muscles 664.1
      - vulva 664.0
    - secondary 674.2
  - following
    - abortion 639.2
    - ectopic or molar pregnancy 639.2
  - male 879.6
    - complicated 879.7
  - muscles, complicating delivery 664.1
  - nonpuerperal, current injury 879.6
    - complicated 879.7
  - secondary (postpartal) 674.2
- peritoneum
  - with
    - abortion — see Abortion, by type, with damage to pelvic organs
    - ectopic pregnancy (see also categories 633.0-633.9) 639.2
    - molar pregnancy (see also categories 630-632) 639.2
  - following
    - abortion 639.2
    - ectopic or molar pregnancy 639.2
  - obstetrical trauma 665.5
- periurethral tissue
  - with
    - abortion — see Abortion, by type, with damage to pelvic organs
    - ectopic pregnancy (see also categories 633.0-633.9) 639.2
    - molar pregnancy (see also categories 630-632) 639.2
  - following
    - abortion 639.2
    - ectopic or molar pregnancy 639.2
  - obstetrical trauma 665.5
- rectovaginal (septum)
  - with
    - abortion — see Abortion, by type, with damage to pelvic organs
    - ectopic pregnancy (see also categories 633.0-633.9) 639.2
    - molar pregnancy (see also categories 630-632) 639.2
  - complicating delivery 665.4
    - with perineum 664.2
      - involving anal or rectal mucosa 664.3
  - following
    - abortion 639.2
    - ectopic or molar pregnancy 639.2
  - nonpuerperal 623.4
  - old (postpartal) 623.4

Laceration—continued
  spinal cord (meninges) — see also
    Injury, spinal, by site
    due to injury at birth 767.4
    fetus or newborn 767.4
  spleen 865.09
    with
      disruption of parenchyma
        (massive) 865.04
        with open wound into
          cavity 865.14
      open wound into cavity
        865.19
      capsule (without disruption of
        parenchyma) 865.02
        with open wound into
          cavity 865.12
      parenchyma 865.03
        with open wound into
          cavity 865.13
        massive disruption (rupture)
          865.04
          with open wound into
            cavity 865.14
  tendon 848.9
    with open wound — see
      Wound, open, by site
    Achilles 845.09
      with open wound 892.2
    lower limb NEC 844.9
      with open wound NEC
        894.2
    upper limb NEC 840.9
      with open wound NEC
        884.2
  tentorium cerebelli — see
    Laceration, brain,
    cerebellum
  urethra
    with
      abortion — see Abortion,
        by type, with damage
        to pelvic organs
      ectopic pregnancy (see also
        categories 633.0-
        633.9) 639.2
      molar pregnancy (see also
        categories 630-632)
        639.2
    following
      abortion 639.2
      ectopic or molar pregnancy
        639.2
    nonpuerperal, nontraumatic
      599.84
    obstetrical trauma 665.5
  uterus
    with
      abortion — see Abortion,
        by type, with damage
        to pelvic organs
      ectopic pregnancy (see also
        categories 633.0-
        633.9) 639.2
      molar pregnancy (see also
        categories 630-632)
        639.2
    following
      abortion 639.2
      ectopic or molar pregnancy
        639.2
    nonpuerperal, nontraumatic
      621.8
    obstetrical trauma NEC 665.1
    old (postpartal) 621.8
  vagina
    with
      abortion — see Abortion,
        by type, with damage
        to pelvic organs
      ectopic pregnancy (see also
        categories 633.0-
        633.9) 639.2
      molar pregnancy (see also
        categories 630-632)
        639.2

Laceration—continued
  vagina—continued
    with—continued
      perineal involvement,
        complicating delivery
        664.0
    complicating delivery 665.4
      first degree 664.0
      second degree 664.1
      third degree 664.2
      fourth degree 664.3
      high 665.4
      muscles 664.1
      sulcus 665.4
      wall 665.4
    following
      abortion 639.2
      ectopic or molar pregnancy
        639.2
    nonpuerperal, nontraumatic
      623.4
    old (postpartal) 623.4
  valve, heart — see Endocarditis
  vulva
    with
      abortion — see Abortion,
        by type, with damage
        to pelvic organs,
      ectopic pregnancy (see also
        categories 633.0-
        633.9) 639.2
      molar pregnancy (see also
        categories 630-632)
        639.2
    complicating delivery 664.0
    following
      abortion 639.2
      ectopic or molar pregnancy
        639.2
    nonpuerperal, nontraumatic
      624.4
    old (postpartal) 624.4
Lachrymal — see condition
Lachrymonasal duct — see
  condition
Lack of
  appetite (see also Anorexia) 783.0
  care
    in home V60.4
    of infant (at or after birth)
      995.5
      affecting parent or family
        V61.21
    specified person NEC 995.81
  coordination 781.3
  development — see also
    Hypoplasia
    physiological 783.4
  education V62.3
  energy 780.7
  financial resources V60.2
  food 994.2
    in environment V60.8
  growth 783.4
  heating V60.1
  housing (permanent) (temporary)
    V60.0
    adequate V60.1
  material resources V60.2
  medical attention 799.8
  memory (see also Amnesia) 780.9
    mild, following organic brain
      damage 310.1
  ovulation 628.0
  person able to render necessary
    care V60.4
  physical exercise V69.0 ◆
  physiologic development 783.4
  prenatal care in current
    pregnancy V23.7
  shelter V60.0
  water 994.3
Lacrimal — see condition
Lacrimation, abnormal (see also
  Epiphora) 375.20
Lacrimonasal duct — see condition

Lactation, lactating (breast)
  (puerperal) (postpartum)
  defective 676.4
  disorder 676.9
    specified type NEC 676.8
  excessive 676.6
  failed 676.4
  mastitis NEC 675.2
  mother (care and/or examination)
    V24.1
  nonpuerperal 611.6
  suppressed 676.5
Lacticemia 271.3
  excessive 276.2
Lactosuria 271.3
Lacunar skull 756.0
Laennec's cirrhosis (alcoholic) 571.2
  nonalcoholic 571.5
Lafora's disease 333.2
Lag, lid (nervous) 374.41
Lagleyze-von Hippel disease
  (retinocerebral angiomatosis)
  759.6
Lagophthalmos (eyelid) (nervous)
  374.20
  cicatricial 374.23
  keratitis (see also Keratitis) 370.34
  mechanical 374.22
  paralytic 374.21
La grippe — see Influenza
Lahore sore 085.1
Lakes, venous (cerebral) 437.8
Laki-Lorand factor deficiency (see
  also Defect, coagulation)
  286.3
Lalling 307.9
Lambliasis 007.1
Lame back 724.5
Lancereaux's diabetes (diabetes
  mellitus with marked
  emaciation) 250.8 [261]
Landouzy-Déjérine dystrophy
  (fascioscapulohumeral
  atrophy) 359.1
Landry's disease or paralysis 357.0
Landry-Guillain-Barré syndrome
  357.0
Lane's
  band 751.4
  disease 569.89
  kink (see also Obstruction,
    intestine) 560.9
Langdon Down's syndrome
  (mongolism) 758.0
Language abolition 784.69
Lanugo (persistent) 757.4
Lardaceous
  degeneration (any site) 277.3
  disease 277.3
  kidney 277.3 [583.81]
  liver 277.3
Large
  baby (regardless of gestational
    age) 766.1
    exceptionally (weight of 4500
      grams or more) 766.0
    of diabetic mother 775.0
  ear 744.22
  fetus — see also Oversize, fetus
    causing disproportion 653.5
      with obstructed labor 660.1
    for dates
      fetus or newborn (regardless of
        gestational age) 766.1
        affecting management of
          pregnancy 656.6
        exceptionally (weight of
          4500 grams or more)
          766.0
  physiological cup 743.57
  waxy liver 277.3
  white kidney — see Nephrosis

Larsen's syndrome (flattened facies
  and multiple congenital
  dislocations) 755.8
Larsen-Johansson disease (juvenile
  osteopathia patellae) 732.4
Larva migrans
  cutaneous NEC 126.9
    ancylostoma 126.9
  of Diptera in vitreous 128.0
  visceral NEC 128.0
Laryngeal — see also condition
  syncope 786.2
Laryngismus (acute) (infectious)
  (stridulous) 478.75
  congenital 748.3
  diphtheritic 032.3
Laryngitis (acute) (edematous)
  (fibrinous) (gangrenous)
  (infective) (infiltrative)
  (malignant) (membranous)
  (phlegmonous)
  (pneumococcal)
  (pseudomembranous) (septic)
  (subglottic) (suppurative)
  (ulcerative) (viral) 464.0
  with
    influenza, flu, or grippe 487.1
    tracheitis (see also
      Laryngotracheitis)
      464.20
      with obstruction 464.21
      acute 464.20
        with obstruction 464.21
      chronic 476.1
  atrophic 476.0
  Borrelia vincentii 101
  catarrhal 476.0
  chronic 476.0
    with tracheitis (chronic) 476.1
    due to external agent — see
      Condition, respiratory,
      chronic, due to
  diphtheritic (membranous) 032.3
  due to external agent — see
    Inflammation, respiratory,
    upper, due to
  H. influenzae 464.0
  Hemophilus influenzae 464.0
  hypertrophic 476.0
  influenzal 487.1
  pachydermic 478.79
  sicca 476.0
  spasmodic 478.75
    acute 464.0
  streptococcal 034.0
  stridulous 478.75
  syphilitic 095.8
    congenital 090.5
  tuberculous (see also
    Tuberculosis, larynx) 012.3
  Vincent's 101
Laryngocele (congenital) (ventricular)
  748.3
Laryngofissure 478.79
  congenital 748.3
Laryngomalacia (congenital) 748.3
Laryngopharyngitis (acute) 465.0
  chronic 478.9
    due to external agent — see
      Condition, respiratory,
      chronic, due to
  due to external agent — see
    Inflammation, respiratory,
    upper, due to
  septic 034.0
Laryngoplegia (see also Paralysis,
  vocal cord) 478.30
Laryngoptosis 478.79
Laryngospasm 478.75
  due to external agent — see
    Condition, respiratory,
    acute, due to

Laryngostenosis / INDEX TO DISEASES / Lateroflexion

Laryngostenosis 478.74
  congenital 748.3
Laryngotracheitis (acute)
  (infectional) (viral) (see also
  Laryngitis) 464.20
  with obstruction 464.21
  atrophic 476.1
  Borrelia vincenti 101
  catarrhal 476.1
  chronic 476.1
    due to external agent — see
      Condition, respiratory,
      chronic, due to
  diphtheritic (membranous) 032.3
  due to external agent — see
    Inflammation, respiratory,
    upper, due to
  H. influenzae 464.20
    with obstruction 464.21
  hypertrophic 476.1
  influenzal 487.1
  pachydermic 478.75
  sicca 476.1
  spasmodic 478.75
    acute 464.20
      with obstruction 464.21
  streptococcal 034.0
  stridulous 478.75
  syphilitic 095.8
    congenital 090.5
  tuberculous (see also
    Tuberculosis, larynx) 012.3
  Vincent's 101
Laryngotracheobronchitis (see also
  Bronchitis) 490
  acute 466.0
  chronic 491.8
  viral 466.0
Laryngotracheobronchopneumonitis
  — see Pneumonia, broncho-
Larynx, laryngeal — see condition
Lasegue's disease (persecution
  mania) 297.9
Lassa fever 078.89
Lassitude (see also Weakness) 780.7
Late — see also condition —
  Allergic Reaction 909.9
  effect(s) (of) — see also condition
    abscess
      intracranial or intraspinal
        (conditions
        classifiable to 324)
        — see category 326
    adverse effect of drug,
      medicinal or biological
      substance 909.5 ◆
    amputation
      postoperative (late) 997.60
      traumatic (injury
        classifiable to 885-
        887 and 895-897)
        905.9
    burn (injury classifiable to
      948-949) 906.9
    extremities NEC (injury
      classifiable to 943 or
      945) 906.7
    hand or wrist (injury
      classifiable to
      944) 906.6
    eye (injury classifiable to
      940) 906.5
    face, head, and neck
      (injury classifiable to
      941) 906.5
    specified site NEC (injury
      classifiable to 942
      and 946-947) 906.8
    cerebrovascular disease
      (conditions classifiable
      to 430-437) — see
      category 438
    childbirth complication(s)
      677 ◆

Late—continued
  effect(s) (of)—continued
    complication(s) of
      childbirth 677 ▼
      delivery 677
      pregnancy 677
      puerperium 677 ▲
      surgical and medical care
        (conditions
        classifiable to 996-
        999) 909.3
      trauma (conditions
        classifiable to 958)
        908.6
    contusion (injury classifiable
      to 920-924) 906.3
    crushing (injury classifiable to
      925-929) 906.4
    delivery complication(s) 677 ◆
    dislocation (injury classifiable
      to 830-839) 905.6
    encephalitis or
      encephalomyelitis
      (conditions classifiable
      to 323) — see category
      326
      in infectious diseases 139.8
      viral (conditions
        classifiable to
        049.8, 049.9,
        062-064) 139.0
    external cause NEC
      (conditions classifiable
      to 995) 909.9
      certain conditions
        classifiable to
        categories 991-994
        909.4
    foreign body in orifice (injury
      classifiable to 930-939)
      908.5
    fracture (multiple) (injury
      classifiable to 828-829)
      905.5
      extremity
        lower (injury classifiable
          to 821-827) 905.4
        neck of femur (injury
          classifiable to
          820) 905.3
        upper (injury classifiable
          to 810-819) 905.2
      face and skull (injury
        classifiable to 800-
        804) 905.0
      skull and face (injury
        classifiable to 800-
        804) 905.0
      spine and trunk (injury
        classifiable to 805
        and 807-809) 905.1
        with spinal cord lesion
          (injury classifiable
          to 806) 907.2
    infection
      pyogenic, intracranial —
        see category 326
    infectious diseases (conditions
      classifiable to 001-136)
      NEC 139.8
    injury (injury classifiable to
      959) 908.9
      blood vessel 908.3
        abdomen and pelvis
          (injury classifiable
          to 902) 908.4
        extremity (injury
          classifiable to
          903-904) 908.3
        head and neck (injury
          classifiable to
          900) 908.3
        intracranial (injury
          classifiable to
          850-854)
          907.0

Late—continued
  effect(s) (of)—continued
    injury—continued
      blood vessel—continued
        head and neck—
          continued
          intracranial—
            continued
            with skull fracture
              905.0
        thorax (injury
          classifiable to
          901) 908.4
        internal organ NEC (injury
          classifiable to 867
          and 869) 908.2
        abdomen (injury
          classifiable to
          863-866 and 868)
          908.1
        thorax (injury
          classifiable to
          860-862) 908.0
      intracranial (injury
        classifiable to 850-
        854) 907.0
        with skull fracture
          (injury classifiable
          to 800-801 and
          803-804) 905.0
      nerve NEC (injury
        classifiable to 957)
        907.9
        cranial (injury
          classifiable to
          950-951) 907.1
        peripheral NEC (injury
          classifiable to
          957) 907.9
        lower limb and
          pelvic girdle
          (injury
          classifiable to
          956) 907.5
        upper limb and
          shoulder girdle
          (injury
          classifiable to
          955) 907.4
        roots and plexus(es),
          spinal (injury
          classifiable to
          953) 907.3
      trunk (injury classifiable
        to 954) 907.3
      spinal
        cord (injury classifiable
          to 806 and 952)
          907.2
        nerve root(s) and
          plexus(es) (injury
          classifiable to
          953) 907.3
      superficial (injury
        classifiable to 910-
        919) 906.2
      tendon (tendon injury
        classifiable to 840-
        848, 880-884 with
        .2, and 890-894 with
        .2) 905.8
    meningitis
      bacterial (conditions
        classifiable to 320)
        — see category 326
      unspecified cause
        (conditions
        classifiable to 322)
        — see category 326
    myelitis (see also Late, effect(s)
      (of), encephalitis) — see
      category 326
    parasitic diseases (conditions
      classifiable to 001-136
      NEC) 139.8

Late—continued
  effect(s) (of)—continued
    phlebitis or thrombophlebitis
      of intracranial venous
      sinuses (conditions
      classifiable to 325) —
      see category 326
    poisoning due to drug,
      medicinal or biological
      substance (conditions
      classifiable to 960-979)
      909.0
    poliomyelitis, acute
      (conditions classifiable
      to 045) 138
    pregnancy complication(s)
      677 ▼
    puerperal complication(s)
      677 ▲
    radiation (conditions
      classifiable to 990)
      909.2
    rickets 268.1
    sprain and strain without
      mention of tendon
      injury (injury classifiable
      to 840-848, except
      tendon injury) 905.7
    tendon involvement 905.8
    toxic effect of
      drug, medicinal or
        biological substance
        (conditions
        classifiable to 960-
        979) 909.0
      nonmedical substance
        (conditions
        classifiable to 980-
        989) 909.1
    trachoma (conditions
      classifiable to 076)
      139.1
    tuberculosis 137.0
      bones and joints
        (conditions
        classifiable to 015)
        137.3
      central nervous system
        (conditions
        classifiable to 013)
        137.1
      genitourinary (conditions
        classifiable to 016)
        137.2
      pulmonary (conditions
        classifiable to 010-
        012) 137.0
      specified organs NEC
        (conditions
        classifiable to 014,
        017-018) 137.4
    viral encephalitis (conditions
      classifiable to 049.8,
      049.9, 062-064) 139.0
    wound, open
      extremity (injury
        classifiable to 880-
        884 and 890-894,
        except .2) 906.1
      tendon (injury
        classifiable to
        880-884 with .2
        and 890-894
        with.2) 905.8
      head, neck, and trunk
        (injury classifiable to
        870-879) 906.0
Latent — see condition
Lateral — see condition
Laterocession — see Lateroversion
Lateroflexion — see Lateroversion

Lateroversion

Lateroversion
  cervix — *see* Lateroversion, uterus
  uterus, uterine (cervix) (postinfectional) (postpartal, old) 621.6
    congenital 752.3
    in pregnancy or childbirth 654.4
      affecting fetus or newborn 763.8
Lathyrism 988.2
Launois' syndrome (pituitary gigantism) 253.0
Launois-Bensaude's lipomatosis 272.8
Launois-Cléret syndrome (adiposogenital dystrophy) 253.8
Laurence-Moon-Biedl syndrome (obesity, polydactyly, and mental retardation) 759.89
LAV (disease) (illness) (infection) — *see* Human immunodeficiency virus (disease) (illness) (infection)
LAV/HTLV-III (disease) (illness) (infection) — *see* Human immunodeficiency virus (disease) (illness) (infection)
Lawford's syndrome (encephalocutaneous angiomatosis) 759.6
Lax, laxity — *see also* Relaxation
  ligament 728.4
  skin (acquired) 701.8
    congenital 756.83
Laxative habit (*see also* Abuse, drugs, nondependent) 305.9
Lazy leukocyte syndrome 288.0
Lead — *see also* condition
  incrustation of cornea 371.15
  poisoning 984.9
    specified type of lead — *see* Table of drugs and chemicals
Lead miners' lung 503
Leakage
  amniotic fluid 658.1
    with delayed delivery 658.2
    affecting fetus or newborn 761.1
  bile from drainage tube (T tube) 997.4
  blood (microscopic), fetal, into maternal circulation 656.0
    affecting management of pregnancy or puerperium 656.0
  device, implant, or graft — *see* Complications, mechanical
  spinal fluid at lumbar puncture site 997.0
  urine, continuous 788.37
Leaky heart — *see* Endocarditis
Learning defect, specific NEC (strephosymbolia) 315.2
Leather bottle stomach (M8142/3) 151.9
Leber's
  congenital amaurosis 362.76
  optic atrophy (hereditary) 377.16
Lederer's anemia or disease (acquired infectious hemolytic anemia) 283.19
Lederer-Brill syndrome (acquired infectious hemolytic anemia) 283.19
Leeches (aquatic) (land) 134.2
Left-sided neglect 781.8 ◆
Leg — *see* condition
Legal investigation V62.5

Legg (-Calvé) — Perthes disease or syndrome (osteochondrosis, femoral capital) 732.1
Legionnaires' disease 482.83
Leigh's disease 330.8
Leiner's disease (exfoliative dermatitis) 695.89
Leiofibromyoma (M8890/0) — *see also* Leiomyoma
  uterus (cervix) (corpus) (*see also* Leiomyoma, uterus) 218.9
Leiomyoblastoma (M8891/1) — *see* Neoplasm, connective tissue, uncertain behavior
Leiomyofibroma (M8890/0) — *see also* Neoplasm, connective tissue, benign
  uterus (cervix) (corpus) (*see also* Leiomyoma, uterus) 218.9
Leiomyoma (M8890/0) — *see also* Neoplasm, connective tissue, benign
  bizarre (M8893/0) — *see* Neoplasm, connective tissue, benign
  cellular (M8892/1) — *see* Neoplasm, connective tissue, uncertain behavior
  epithelioid (M8891/1) — *see* Neoplasm, connective tissue, uncertain behavior
  prostate (polypoid) 600
  uterus (cervix) (corpus) 218.9
    interstitial 218.1
    intramural 218.1
    submucous 218.0
    subperitoneal 218.2
    subserous 218.2
  vascular (M8894/0) — *see* Neoplasm, connective tissue, benign
Leiomyomatosis (intravascular) (M8890/1) — *see* Neoplasm, connective tissue, uncertain behavior
Leiomyosarcoma (M8890/3) — *see also* Neoplasm, connective tissue, malignant
  epithelioid (M8891/3) — *see* Neoplasm, connective tissue, malignant
Leishmaniasis 085.9
  American 085.5
    cutaneous 085.4
    mucocutaneous 085.5
  Asian desert 085.2
  Brazilian 085.5
  cutaneous 085.9
    acute necrotizing 085.2
    American 085.4
    Asian desert 085.2
    diffuse 085.3
    dry form 085.1
    Ethiopian 085.3
    eyelid 085.5 [373.6]
    late 085.1
    lepromatous 085.3
    recurrent 085.1
    rural 085.2
    ulcerating 085.1
    urban 085.1
    wet form 085.2
    zoonotic form 085.2
  dermal — *see also* Leishmaniasis, cutaneous
    post kala-azar 085.0
  eyelid 085.5 [373.6]
  infantile 085.0
  Mediterranean 085.0
  mucocutaneous (American) 085.5
  naso-oral 085.5
  nasopharyngeal 085.5
  Old World 085.1
  tegumentaria diffusa 085.4

INDEX TO DISEASES

Leishmaniasis—*continued*
  vaccination, prophylactic (against) V05.2
  visceral (Indian) 085.0
Leishmanoid, dermal — *see also* Leishmaniasis, cutaneous
  post kala-azar 085.0
Leloir's disease 695.4
Lenegre's disease 426.0
Lengthening, leg 736.81
Lennox's syndrome (*see also* Epilepsy) 345.0
Lens — *see* condition
Lenticonus (anterior) (posterior) (congenital) 743.36
Lenticular degeneration, progressive 275.1
Lentiglobus (posterior) (congenital) 743.36
Lentigo (congenital) 709.09 ▼
  juvenile 709.09 ▲
  Maligna (M8742/2) — *see also* Neoplasm, skin, in situ
    melanoma (M8742/3) — *see* Melanoma
  senile 709.09 ◆
Leonine leprosy 030.0
Leontiasis
  ossium 733.3
  syphilitic 095.8
    congenital 090.5
Léopold-Lévi's syndrome (paroxysmal thyroid instability) 242.9
Lepore hemoglobin syndrome 282.4
Lepothrix 039.0
Lepra 030.9
  Willan's 696.1
Leprechaunism 259.8
Lepromatous leprosy 030.0
Leprosy 030.9
  anesthetic 030.1
  beriberi 030.1
  borderline (group B) (infiltrated) (neuritic) 030.3
  cornea (*see also* Leprosy, by type) 030.9 [371.89]
  dimorphous (group B) (infiltrated) (lepromatous) (neuritic) (tuberculoid) 030.3
  eyelid 030.0 [373.4]
  indeterminate (group I) (macular) (neuritic) (uncharacteristic) 030.2
  leonine 030.0
  lepromatous (diffuse) (infiltrated) (macular) (neuritic) (nodular) (type L) 030.0
  macular (early) (neuritic) (simple) 030.2
  maculoanesthetic 030.1
  mixed 030.0
  neuro 030.1
  nodular 030.0
  primary neuritic 030.3
  specified type or group NEC 030.8
  tubercular 030.1
  tuberculoid (macular) (maculoanesthetic) (major) (minor) (neuritic) (type T) 030.1
Leptocytosis, hereditary 282.4
Leptomeningitis (chronic) (circumscribed) (hemorrhagic) (nonsuppurative) (*see also* Meningitis) 322.9
  aseptic 047.9
    adenovirus 049.1
    Coxsackie virus 047.0
    ECHO virus 047.1
    enterovirus 047.9

Lesion

Leptomeningitis—*continued*
  aseptic—*continued*
    lymphocytic choriomeningitis 049.0
  epidemic 036.0
  late effect — *see* category 326
  meningococcal 036.0
  pneumococcal 320.1
  syphilitic 094.2
  tuberculous (*see also* Tuberculosis, meninges) 013.0
Leptomeningopathy (*see also* Meningitis) 322.9
Leptospiral — *see* condition
Leptospirochetal — *see* condition
Leptospirosis 100.9
  autumnalis 100.89
  canicula 100.89
  grippotyphosa 100.89
  hebdomidis 100.89
  icterohemorrhagica 100.0
  nanukayami 100.89
  pomona 100.89
  Weil's disease 100.0
Leptothricosis — *see* Actinomycosis
Leptothrix infestation — *see* Actinomycosis
Leptotricosis — *see* Actinomycosis
Leptus dermatitis 133.8
Léris pleonosteosis 756.89
Léri-Weill syndrome 756.59
Leriche's syndrome (aortic bifurcation occlusion) 444.0
Lermoyez's syndrome (*see also* Disease, Ménière's) 386.00
Lesbianism — *omit code*
  ego-dystonic 302.0
  problems with 302.0
Lesch-Nyhan syndrome (hypoxanthineguanine-phosphoribosyltransferase deficiency) 277.2
Lesion
  abducens nerve 378.54
  alveolar process 525.8
  anorectal 569.49
  aortic (valve) — *see* Endocarditis, aortic
  auditory nerve 388.5
  basal ganglion 333.90
  bile duct (*see also* Disease, biliary) 576.8
  bladder 596.9
  bone 733.90
  brachial plexus 353.0
  brain 348.8
    congenital 742.9
    vascular (*see also* Lesion, cerebrovascular) 437.9
      degenerative 437.1
      healed or old — *see also* category 438
        without residuals V12.5
      hypertensive 437.2
      late effect — *see* category 438
  buccal 528.9
  calcified — *see* Calcification
  canthus 373.9
  carate — *see* Pinta, lesions
  cardia 537.89
  cardiac — *see also* Disease, heart
    congenital 746.9
    valvular — *see* Endocarditis
  cauda equina 344.60
    with neurogenic bladder 344.61
  cecum 569.89
  cerebral — *see* Lesion, brain
  cerebrovascular (*see also* Disease, cerebrovascular NEC) 437.9
    degenerative 437.1

Lesion—continued

cerebrovascular—continued
  healed or old — see also
      category 438
    without residuals V12.5
  hypertensive 437.2
  late effect — see category 438
  specified type NEC 437.8
cervical root (nerve) NEC 353.2
chiasmal 377.54
  associated with
      inflammatory disorders
      377.54
    neoplasm NEC 377.52
      pituitary 377.51
    pituitary disorders 377.51
    vascular disorders 377.53
chorda tympani 351.8
coin, lung 793.1
colon 569.89
congenital — see Anomaly
conjunctiva 372.9
coronary artery (see also
    Ischemia, heart) 414.9
cranial nerve 352.9
  first 352.0
  second 377.49
  third
    partial 378.51
    total 378.52
  fourth 378.53
  fifth 350.9
  sixth 378.54
  seventh 351.9
  eighth 388.5
  ninth 352.2
  tenth 352.3
  eleventh 352.4
  twelfth 352.5
cystic — see Cyst
degenerative — see Degeneration
dermal (skin) 709.9
duodenum 537.89
  with obstruction 537.3
eyelid 373.9
gasserian ganglion 350.8
gastric 537.89
gastroduodenal 537.89
gastrointestinal 569.89
glossopharyngeal nerve 352.2
heart (organic) — see also
    Disease, heart
  vascular — see Disease,
    cardiovascular
helix (ear) 709.9
hyperchromic, due to pinta
    (carate) 103.1
hyperkeratotic (see also
    Hyperkeratosis) 701.1
hypoglossal nerve 352.5
hypopharynx 478.29
hypothalamic 253.9
ileocecal coil 569.89
ileum 569.89
iliohypogastric nerve 355.79
ilioinguinal nerve 355.79
in continuity — see Injury, nerve,
    by site
inflammatory — see Inflammation
intestine 569.89
intracerebral — see Lesion, brain
intrachiasmal (optic) (see also
    Lesion, chiasmal) 377.54
intracranial, space-occupying
    NEC 784.2
joint 719.90
  ankle 719.97
  elbow 719.92
  foot 719.97
  hand 719.94
  hip 719.95
  knee 719.96
  multiple sites 719.99
  pelvic region 719.95
  sacroiliac (old) 724.6
  shoulder (region) 719.91
  specified site NEC 719.98

Lesion—continued

joint—continued
  wrist 719.93
keratotic (see also Keratosis)
    701.1
kidney (see also Disease, renal)
    593.9
laryngeal nerve (recurrent) 352.3
leonine 030.0
lip 528.5
liver 573.8
lumbosacral
  plexus 353.1
  root (nerve) NEC 353.4
lung 518.89
  coin 793.1
maxillary sinus 473.0
mitral — see Endocarditis, mitral
motor cortex 348.8
nerve (see also Disorder, nerve)
    355.9
nervous system 349.9
  congenital 742.9
nonallopathic NEC 739.9
  in region (of)
    abdomen 739.9
    acromioclavicular 739.7
    cervical, cervicothoracic
        739.1
    costochondral 739.8
    costovertebral 739.8
    extremity
      lower 739.6
      upper 739.7
    head 739.0
    hip 739.5
    lower extremity 739.6
    lumbar, lumbosacral 739.3
    occipitocervical 739.0
    pelvic 739.5
    pubic 739.5
    rib cage 739.8
    sacral, sacrococcygeal,
        sacroiliac 739.4
    sternochondral 739.8
    sternoclavicular 739.7
    thoracic, thoracolumbar
        739.2
    upper extremity 739.7
nose (internal) 478.1
obstructive — see Obstruction
obturator nerve 355.79
occlusive
  artery — see Embolism, artery
organ or site NEC — see Disease,
    by site
osteolytic 733.90
paramacular, of retina 363.32
peptic 537.89
periodontal, due to traumatic
    occlusion 523.8
perirectal 569.49
peritoneum (granulomatous)
    568.89
pigmented (skin) 709.00 ◆
pinta — see Pinta, lesions
polypoid — see Polyp
prechiasmal (optic) (see also
    Lesion, chiasmal) 377.54
primary — see also Syphilis,
    primary
  carate 103.0
  pinta 103.0
  yaws 102.0
pulmonary 518.89
  valve (see also Endocarditis,
      pulmonary) 424.3
pylorus 537.89
radiation NEC 990
radium NEC 990
rectosigmoid 569.89
retina, retinal — see also
    Retinopathy
  vascular 362.17
retroperitoneal 568.89
romanus 720.1
sacroiliac (joint) 724.6

Lesion—continued

salivary gland 527.8
  benign lymphoepithelial 527.8
saphenous nerve 355.79
secondary — see Syphilis,
    secondary
sigmoid 569.89
sinus (accessory) (nasal) (see also
    Sinusitis) 473.9
skin 709.9
  suppurative 686.0
space-occupying, intracranial
    NEC 784.2
spinal cord 336.9
  congenital 742.9
  traumatic (complete)
      (incomplete) (transverse)
      — see also Injury,
      spinal, by site
    with
      broken
        back — see Fracture,
            vertebra, by
            site, with
            spinal cord
            injury
        neck — see Fracture,
            vertebra,
            cervical, with
            spinal cord
            injury
      fracture, vertebra — see
          Fracture, vertebra,
          by site, with
          spinal cord injury
spleen 289.50
stomach 537.89
syphilitic — see Syphilis
tertiary — see Syphilis, tertiary
thoracic root (nerve) 353.3
tonsillar fossa 474.9
tooth, teeth 525.8
  white spot 521.0
traumatic NEC (see also nature
    and site of injury) 959.9
tricuspid (valve) — see
    Endocarditis, tricuspid
trigeminal nerve 350.9
ulcerated or ulcerative — see
    Ulcer
uterus NEC 621.9
vagus nerve 352.3
valvular — see Endocarditis
vascular 459.9
  affecting central nervous
      system (see also Lesion,
      cerebrovascular) 437.9
  following trauma (see also
      Injury, blood vessel, by
      site) 904.9
  retina 362.17
  traumatic — see Injury, blood
      vessel, by site
  umbilical cord 663.6
    affecting fetus or newborn
        762.6
visual
  cortex NEC (see also Disorder,
      visual, cortex) 377.73
  pathway NEC (see also
      Disorder, visual,
      pathway) 377.63
warty — see Verruca
white spot, on teeth 521.0
x-ray NEC 990

Lethargic — see condition
Lethargy 780.7
Letterer-Siwe disease (acute
    histiocytosis X) (M9722/3)
    202.5
Leucinosis 270.3
Leucocoria 360.44
Leucosarcoma (M9850/3) 207.8
Leukasmus 270.2

Leukemia, leukemic (congenital) (M9800/3) 208.9

Note — Use the following fifth-digit subclassification for categories 203–208:
  0 without mention of remission
  1 with remission

acute NEC (M9801/3) 208.0
aleukemic NEC (M9804/3) 208.8
  granulocytic (M9864/3) 205.8
basophilic (M9870/3) 205.1
blast (cell) (M9801/3) 208.0
blastic (M9801/3) 208.0
  granulocytic (M9861/3) 205.0
chronic NEC (M9803/3) 208.1
compound (M9810/3) 207.8
eosinophilic (M9880/3) 205.1
giant cell (M9910/3) 207.2
granulocytic (M9860/3) 205.9
  acute (M9861/3) 205.0
  aleukemic (M9864/3) 205.8
  blastic (M9861/3) 205.0
  chronic (M9863/3) 205.1
  subacute (M9862/3) 205.2
  subleukemic (M9864/3) 205.8
hairy cell (M9940/3) 202.4
hemoblastic (M9801/3) 208.0
histiocytic (M9890/3) 206.9
lymphatic (M9820/3) 204.9
  acute (M9821/3) 204.0
  aleukemic (M9824/3) 204.8
  chronic (M9823/3) 204.1
  subacute (M9822/3) 204.2
  subleukemic (M9824/3) 204.8
lymphoblastic (M9821/3) 204.0
lymphocytic (M9820/3) 204.9
  acute (M9821/3) 204.0
  aleukemic (M9824/3) 204.8
  chronic (M9823/3) 204.1
  subacute (M9822/3) 204.2
  subleukemic (M9824/3) 204.8
lymphogenous (M9820/3) — see
    Leukemia, lymphoid
lymphoid (M9820/3) 204.9
  acute (M9821/3) 204.0
  aleukemic (M9824/3) 204.8
  blastic (M9821/3) 204.0
  chronic (M9823/3) 204.1
  subacute (M9822/3) 204.2
  subleukemic (M9824/3) 204.8
lymphosarcoma cell (M9850/3)
    207.8
mast cell (M9900/3) 207.8
megakaryocytic (M9910/3) 207.2
megakaryocytoid (M9910/3)
    207.2
mixed (cell) (M9810/3) 207.8
monoblastic (M9891/3) 206.0
monocytic (Schilling-type)
    (M9890/3) 206.9
  acute (M9891/3) 206.0
  aleukemic (M9894/3) 206.8
  chronic (M9893/3) 206.1
  Naegeli-type (M9863/3) 205.1
  subacute (M9892/3) 206.2
  subleukemic (M9894/3) 206.8
monocytoid (M9890/3) 206.9
  acute (M9891/3) 206.0
  aleukemic (M9894/3) 206.8
  chronic (M9893/3) 206.1
  myelogenous (M9863/3) 205.1
  subacute (M9892/3) 206.2
  subleukemic (M9894/3) 206.8
monomyelocytic (M9860/3) —
    see Leukemia,
    myelomonocytic
myeloblastic (M9861/3) 205.0
myelocytic (M9863/3) 205.1
  acute (M9861/3) 205.0
myelogenous (M9860/3) 205.9
  acute (M9861/3) 205.0
  aleukemic (M9864/3) 205.8
  chronic (M9863/3) 205.1
  monocytoid (M9863/3) 205.1

Leukemia, leukemic—*continued*
  myelogenous—*continued*
    subacute (M9862/3) 205.2
    subleukemic (M9864) 205.8
  myeloid (M9860/3) 205.9
    acute (M9861/3) 205.0
    aleukemic (M9864/3) 205.8
    chronic (M9863/3) 205.1
    subacute (M9862/3) 205.2
    subleukemic (M9864/3) 205.8
  myelomonocytic (M9860/3) 205.9
    acute (M9861/3) 205.0
    chronic (M9863/3) 205.1
  Naegeli-type monocytic (M9863/3) 205.1
  neutrophilic (M9865/3) 205.1
  plasma cell (M9830/3) 203.1
  plasmacytic (M9830/3) 203.1
  prolymphocytic (M9825/3) — see Leukemia, lymphoid
  promyelocytic, acute (M9866/3) 205.0
  Schilling-type monocytic (M9890/3) — see Leukemia, monocytic
  stem cell (M9801/3) 208.0
  subacute NEC (M9802/3) 208.2
  subleukemic NEC (M9804/3) 208.8
  thrombocytic (M9910/3) 207.2
  undifferentiated (M9801/3) 208.0
Leukemoid reaction (lymphocytic) (monocytic) (myelocytic) 288.8
Leukocoria 360.44
Leukocythemia — see Leukemia
Leukocytosis 288.8
  basophilic 288.8
  eosinophilic 288.3
  lymphocytic 288.8
  monocytic 288.8
  neutrophilic 288.8
Leukoderma 709.09 ◆
  syphilitic 091.3
    late 095.8
Leukodermia (see also Leukoderma) 709.09 ◆
Leukodystrophy (cerebral) (globoid cell) (metachromatic) (progressive) (sudanophilic) 330.0
Leukoedema, mouth or tongue 528.7
Leukoencephalitis
  acute hemorrhagic (postinfectious) NEC 136.9 [323.6]
    postimmunization or postvaccinal 323.5
  subacute sclerosing 046.2
  van Bogaert's 046.2
  van Bogaert's (sclerosing) 046.2
Leukoencephalopathy (see also Encephalitis) 323.9
  acute necrotizing hemorrhagic (postinfectious) 136.9 [323.6]
    postimmunization or postvaccinal 323.5
  metachromatic 330.0
  multifocal (progressive) 046.3
  progressive multifocal 046.3
Leukoerythroblastosis 289.0
Leukoerythrosis 289.0
Leukokeratosis (see also Leukoplakia) 702.8
  mouth 528.6
  nicotina palati 528.7
  tongue 528.6
Leukokoria 360.44
Leukokraurosis vulva, vulvae 624.0
Leukolymphosarcoma (M9850/3) 207.8

Leukoma (cornea) (interfering with central vision) 371.03
  adherent 371.04
Leukomelanopathy, hereditary 288.2
Leukonychia (punctata) (striata) 703.8
  congenital 757.5
Leukopathia
  unguium 703.8
    congenital 757.5
Leukopenia 288.0
  cyclic 288.0
  familial 288.0
  malignant 288.0
  periodic 288.0
  transitory neonatal 776.7
Leukopenic — see condition
Leukoplakia 702.8
  anus 569.49
  bladder (postinfectional) 596.8
  buccal 528.6
  cervix (uteri) 622.2
  esophagus 530.83
  gingiva 528.6
  kidney (pelvis) 593.89
  larynx 478.79
  lip 528.6
  mouth 528.6
  oral soft tissue (including tongue) (mucosa) 528.6
  palate 528.6
  pelvis (kidney) 593.89
  penis (infectional) 607.0
  rectum 569.49
  syphilitic 095.8
  tongue 528.6
  tonsil 478.29
  ureter (postinfectional) 593.89
  urethra (postinfectional) 599.84
  uterus 621.8
  vagina 623.1
  vesical 596.8
  vocal cords 478.5
  vulva 624.0
Leukopolioencephalopathy 330.0
Leukorrhea (vagina) 623.5
  due to trichomonas (vaginalis) 131.00
  trichomonal (Trichomonas vaginalis) 131.00
Leukosarcoma (M9850/3) 207.8
Leukosis (M9800/3) — see Leukemia
Lev's disease or syndrome (acquired complete heart block) 426.0
Levi's syndrome (pituitary dwarfism) 253.3
Levocardia (isolated) 746.87
  with situs inversus 759.3
Levulosuria 271.2
Lewandowski's disease (primary) (see also Tuberculosis) 017.0
Lewandowski-Lutz disease (epidermodysplasia verruciformis) 078.19
Leyden's disease (periodic vomiting) 536.2
Leyden-Möbius dystrophy 359.1
Leydig cell
  carcinoma (M8650/3)
    specified site — see Neoplasm, by site, malignant
    unspecified site
      female 183.0
      male 186.9
  tumor (M8650/1)
    benign (M8650/0)
      specified site — see Neoplasm, by site, benign
      unspecified site
        female 220
        male 222.0

Leydig cell—*continued*
  tumor—*continued*
    malignant (M8650/3)
      specified site — see Neoplasm, by site, malignant
      unspecified site
        female 183.0
        male 186.9
    specified site — see Neoplasm, by site, uncertain behavior
    unspecified site
      female 236.2
      male 236.4
Leydig-Sertoli cell tumor (M8631/0)
  specified site — see Neoplasm, by site, benign
  unspecified site
    female 220
    male 222.0
Liar, pathologic 301.7
Libman-Sacks disease or syndrome 710.0 [424.91]
Lice (infestation) 132.9
  body (pediculus corporis) 132.1
  crab 132.2
  head (pediculus capitis) 132.0
  mixed (classifiable to more than one of the categories 132.0-132.2) 132.3
  pubic (pediculus pubis) 132.2
Lichen 697.9
  albus 701.0
  annularis 695.89
  atrophicus 701.0
  corneus obtusus 698.3
  myxedematous 701.8
  nitidus 697.1
  pilaris 757.39
    acquired 701.1
  planopilaris 697.0
  planus (acute) (chronicus) (hypertrophic) (verrucous) 697.0
    morphoeicus 701.0
    sclerosus (et atrophicus) 701.0
  ruber 696.4
    acuminatus 696.4
    moniliformis 697.8
    obtusus corneus 698.3
    of Wilson 697.0
    planus 697.0
  sclerosus (et atrophicus) 701.0
  scrofulosus (primary) (see also Tuberculosis) 017.0
  simplex (Vidal's) 698.3
    chronicus 698.3
    circumscriptus 698.3
  spinulosus 757.39
    mycotic 117.9
  striata 697.8
  urticatus 698.2
Lichenification 698.3
  nodular 698.3
Lichenoides tuberculosis (primary) (see also Tuberculosis) 017.0
Lichtheim's disease or syndrome (subacute combined sclerosis with pernicious anemia) 281.0 [336.2]
Lien migrans 289.59
Lientery (see also Diarrhea) 558.9
  infectious 009.2
Life circumstance problem NEC V62.89
Ligament — see condition
Light-for-dates (infant) 764.0
  with signs of fetal malnutrition 764.1
  affecting management of pregnancy 656.5
Light-headedness 780.4

Lightning (effects) (shock) (stroke) (struck by) 994.0
  burn — see Burn, by site
  foot 266.2
Lightwood's disease or syndrome (renal tubular acidosis) 588.8
Lignac's disease (cystinosis) 270.0
Lignac (-de Toni) (-Fanconi) (-Debré) syndrome (cystinosis) 270.0
Lignac (-Fanconi) syndrome (cystinosis) 270.0
Ligneous thyroiditis 245.3
Likoff's syndrome (angina in menopausal women) 413.9
Limb — see condition
Limitation of joint motion (see also Stiffness, joint) 719.5
  sacroiliac 724.6
Limit dextrinosis 271.0
Limited
  cardiac reserve — see Disease, heart
  duction, eye NEC 378.63
Lindau's disease (retinocerebral angiomatosis) 759.6
Lindau (-von Hippel) disease (angiomatosis retinocerebellosa) 759.6
Linea corneae senilis 371.41
Lines
  Beau's (transverse furrows on fingernails) 703.8
  Harris' 733.91
  Hudson-Stähli 371.11
  Stähli's 371.11
Lingua
  geographical 529.1
  nigra (villosa) 529.3
  plicata 529.5
    congenital 750.13
  tylosis 528.6
Lingual (tongue) — see also condition
  thyroid 759.2
Linitis (gastric) 535.4
  plastica (M8142/3) 151.9
Lioderma essentialis (cum melanosis et telangiectasia) 757.33
Lip — see also condition
  biting 528.9
Lipalgia 272.8
Lipedema — see Edema
Lipemia (see also Hyperlipidemia) 272.4
  retina, retinalis 272.3
Lipidosis 272.7
  cephalin 272.7
  cerebral (infantile) (juvenile) (late) 330.1
  cerebroretinal 330.1 [362.71]
  cerebroside 272.7
  cerebrospinal 272.7
  chemically-induced 272.7
  cholesterol 272.7
  diabetic 250.8 [272.7]
  dystopic (hereditary) 272.7
  glycolipid 272.7
  hepatosplenomegalic 272.3
  hereditary, dystopic 272.7
  sulfatide 330.0
Lipoadenoma (M8324/0) — see Neoplasm, by site, benign
Lipoblastoma (M8881/0) — see Lipoma, by site
Lipoblastomatosis (M8881/0) — see Lipoma, by site
Lipochondrodystrophy 277.5
Lipochrome histiocytosis (familial) 288.1
Lipodystrophia progressiva 272.6

Lipodystrophy (progressive) 272.6
  insulin 272.6
  intestinal 040.2
Lipofibroma (M8851/0) — see Lipoma, by site
Lipoglycoproteinosis 272.8
Lipogranuloma, sclerosing 709.8
Lipogranulomatosis (disseminated) 272.8
  kidney 272.8
Lipoid — see also condition
  histiocytosis 272.7
    essential 272.7
  nephrosis (see also Nephrosis) 581.3
  proteinosis of Urbach 272.8
Lipoidemia (see also Hyperlipidemia) 272.4
Lipoidosis (see also Lipidosis) 272.7
Lipoma (M8850/0) 214.9
  breast (skin) 214.1
  face 214.0
  fetal (M8881/0) — see also Lipoma, by site
  fat cell (M8880/0) — see Lipoma, by site
  infiltrating (M8856/0) — see Lipoma, by site
  intra-abdominal 214.3
  intramuscular (M8856/0) — see Lipoma, by site
  intrathoracic 214.2
  kidney 214.3
  mediastinum 214.2
  muscle 214.8
  peritoneum 214.3
  retroperitoneum 214.3
  skin 214.1
    face 214.0
  spermatic cord 214.4
  spindle cell (M8857/0) — see Lipoma, by site
  stomach 214.3
  subcutaneous tissue 214.1
    face 214.0
  thymus 214.2
  thyroid gland 214.2
Lipomatosis (dolorosa) 272.8
  fetal (M8881/0) — see Lipoma, by site
  Launois-Bensaude's 272.8
Lipomyohemangioma (M8860/0)
  specified site — see Neoplasm, connective tissue, benign
  unspecified site 223.0
Lipomyoma (M8860/0)
  specified site — see Neoplasm, connective tissue, benign
  unspecified site 223.0
Lipomyxoma (M8852/0) — see Lipoma, by site
Lipomyxosarcoma (M8852/3) — see Neoplasm, connective tissue, malignant
Lipophagocytosis 289.8
Lipoproteinemia (alpha) 272.4
  broad-beta 272.2
  floating-beta 272.2
  hyper-pre-beta 272.1
Lipoproteinosis (Rössle-Urbach-Wiethe) 272.8
Liposarcoma (M8850/3) — see also Neoplasm, connective tissue, malignant
  differentiated type (M8851/3) — see Neoplasm, connective tissue, malignant
  embryonal (M8852/3) — see Neoplasm, connective tissue, malignant
  mixed type (M8855/3) — see Neoplasm, connective tissue, malignant

Liposarcoma—continued
  myxoid (M8852/3) — see Neoplasm, connective tissue, malignant
  pleomorphic (M8854/3) — see Neoplasm, connective tissue, malignant
  round cell (M8853/3) — see Neoplasm, connective tissue, malignant
  well differentiated type (M8851/3) — see Neoplasm, connective tissue, malignant
Lipsynovitis prepatellaris 272.8
Lipping
  cervix 622.0
  spine (see also Spondylosis) 721.90
  vertebra (see also Spondylosis) 721.90
Lip pits (mucus), congenital 750.25
Lipschütz disease or ulcer 616.50
Lipuria 791.1
  bilharziasis 120.0
Liquefaction, vitreous humor 379.21
Lisping 307.9
Lissauer's paralysis 094.1
Lissencephalia, lissencephaly 742.2
Listerellose 027.0
Listeriose 027.0
Listeriosis 027.0
  congenital 771.2
  fetal 771.2
  suspected fetal damage affecting management of pregnancy 655.4
Listlessness 780.7
Lithemia 790.6
Lithiasis — see also Calculus
  hepatic (duct) — see Choledocholithiasis
  urinary 592.9
Lithopedion 779.9
  affecting management of pregnancy 656.8
Lithosis (occupational) 502
  with tuberculosis — see Tuberculosis, pulmonary
Lithuria 791.9
Litigation V62.5
Little
  league elbow 718.82
  stroke syndrome 435.9
Little's disease — see Palsy, cerebral
Littre's
  gland — see condition
  hernia — see Hernia, Littre's
Littritis (see also Urethritis) 597.89
Livedo 782.61
  annularis 782.61
  racemose 782.61
  reticularis 782.61
Live flesh 781.0
Liver — see also condition
  donor V59.8
Livida, asphyxia
  newborn 768.6
Living
  alone V60.3
    with handicapped person V60.4
Lloyd's syndrome 258.1
Loa loa 125.2
Loasis 125.2
Lobe, lobar — see condition
Lobo's disease or blastomycosis 116.2
Lobomycosis 116.2
Lobotomy syndrome 310.0

Lobstein's disease (brittle bones and blue sclera) 756.51
Lobster-claw hand 755.58
Lobulation (congenital) — see also Anomaly, specified type NEC, by site
  kidney, fetal 753.3
  liver, abnormal 751.69
  spleen 759.0
Lobule, lobular — see condition
Local, localized — see condition
Locked bowel or intestine (see also Obstruction, intestine) 560.9
Locked-in state 344.81
Locked twins 660.5
  affecting fetus or newborn 763.1
Locking
  joint (see also Derangement, joint) 718.90
  knee 717.9
Lockjaw (see also Tetanus) 037
Locomotor ataxia (progressive) 094.0
Löffler's
  endocarditis 421.0
  eosinophilia or syndrome 518.3
  pneumonia 518.3
  syndrome (eosinophilic pneumonitis) 518.3
Löfgren's syndrome (sarcoidosis) 135
Loiasis 125.2
  eyelid 125.2 [373.6]
Loneliness V62.89
Lone star fever 082.8
Long labor 662.1
  affecting fetus or newborn 763.8
  first stage 662.0
  second stage 662.2
Longitudinal stripes or grooves, nails 703.8
  congenital 757.5
Loop
  intestine (see also Volvulus) 560.2
  intrascleral nerve 379.29
  vascular on papilla (optic) 743.57
Loose — see also condition
  body
    in tendon sheath 727.82
    joint 718.10
      ankle 718.17
      elbow 718.12
      foot 718.17
      hand 718.14
      hip 718.15
      knee 717.6
      multiple sites 718.19
      pelvic region 718.15
      prosthetic implant — see Complications, mechanical
      shoulder (region) 718.11
      specified site NEC 718.18
      wrist 718.13
    cartilage (joint) (see also Loose, body, joint) 718.1
      knee 717.6
    facet (vertebral) 724.9
    prosthetic implant — see Complications, mechanical
    sesamoid, joint (see also Loose, body, joint) 718.1
  tooth, teeth 525.8
Loosening epiphysis 732.9
Looser (-Debray) — Milkman syndrome (osteomalacia with pseudofractures) 268.2
Lop ear (deformity) 744.29
Lorain's disease or syndrome (pituitary dwarfism) 253.3
Lorain-Levi syndrome (pituitary dwarfism) 253.3

Lordosis (acquired) (postural) 737.20
  congenital 754.2
  due to or associated with
    Charcot-Marie-Tooth disease 356.1 [737.42]
    mucopolysaccharidosis 277.5 [737.42]
    neurofibromatosis 237.71 [737.42]
    osteitis
      deformans 731.0 [737.42]
      fibrosa cystica 252.0 [737.42]
    osteoporosis (see also Osteoporosis) 733.00 [737.42]
    poliomyelitis (see also Poliomyelitis) 138 [737.42]
    tuberculosis (see also Tuberculosis) 015.0 [737.42]
  late effect of rickets 268.1 [737.42]
  postlaminectomy 737.21
  postsurgical NEC 737.22
  rachitic 268.1 [737.42]
  specified NEC 737.29
  tuberculous (see also Tuberculosis) 015.0 [737.42]
Loss
  appetite 783.0
    hysterical 300.11
    nonorganic origin 307.59
    psychogenic 307.59
  blood — see Hemorrhage
  central vision 368.41
  consciousness 780.09
    transient 780.2
  control, sphincter, rectum 787.6
    nonorganic origin 307.7
  ear ossicle, partial 385.24
  elasticity, skin 782.8
  extremity or member, traumatic, current — see Amputation, traumatic
  fluid (acute) 276.5
    with
      hypernatremia 276.0
      hyponatremia 276.1
    fetus or newborn 775.5
  hair 704.00
  hearing — see also Deafness
    central 389.14
    conductive (air) 389.00
      with sensorineural hearing loss 389.2
      combined types 389.08
      external ear 389.01
      inner ear 389.04
      middle ear 389.03
      multiple types 389.08
      tympanic membrane 389.02
    mixed type 389.2
    nerve 389.12
    neural 389.12
    noise-induced 388.12
    perceptive NEC (see also Loss, hearing, sensorineural) 389.10
    sensorineural 389.10
      with conductive hearing loss 389.2
      central 389.14
      combined types 389.18
      multiple types 389.18
      neural 389.12
      sensory 389.11
    sensory 389.11
    specified type NEC 389.8
    sudden NEC 388.2
  labyrinthine reactivity (unilateral) 386.55
    bilateral 386.56

Loss—continued
memory (see also Amnesia) 780.9
   mild, following organic brain damage 310.1
mind (see also Psychosis) 298.9
organ or part — see Absence, by site, acquired
sensation 782.0
sense of
   smell (see also Disturbance, sensation) 781.1
   taste (see also Disturbance, sensation) 781.1
   touch (see also Disturbance, sensation) 781.1
sight (acquired) (complete) (congenital) see Blindness
spinal fluid
   headache 349.0
substance of
   bone (see also Osteoporosis) 733.00
   cartilage 733.99
   ear 380.32
   vitreous (humor) 379.26
tooth, teeth, due to accident, extraction, or local periodontal disease 525.1
vision, visual (see also Blindness) 369.9
   both eyes (see also Blindness, both eyes) 369.3
   complete (see also Blindness, both eyes) 369.00
   one eye 369.8
   sudden 368.11
   transient 368.12
vitreous 379.26
voice (see also Aphonia) 784.41
weight (cause unknown) 783.2
Louis-Bar syndrome (ataxia-telangiectasia) 334.8
Louping ill 063.1
Lousiness — see Lice
Low
back syndrome 724.2
basal metabolic rate (BMR) 794.7
birthweight 765.1
   extreme (less than 1000 grams) 765.0
   for gestational age 764.0
bladder compliance 596.52
blood pressure (see also Hypotension) 458.9
   reading (incidental) (isolated) (nonspecific) 796.3
cardiac reserve — see Disease, heart
compliance bladder 596.52
frequency deafness — see Disorder, hearing
function — see also Hypofunction
   kidney (see also Disease, renal) 593.9
   liver 573.9
hemoglobin 285.9
implantation, placenta — see Placenta, previa
insertion, placenta — see placenta, previa
lying
   kidney 593.0
   organ or site, congenital — see Malposition, congenital
   placenta — see Placenta, previa
output syndrome (cardiac) (see also Failure, heart) 428.9
platelets (blood) (see also Thrombocytopenia) 287.5
reserve, kidney (see also Disease, renal) 593.9
salt syndrome 593.9
tension glaucoma 365.12

Low—continued
vision 369.9
   both eyes 369.20
   one eye 369.70
Lowe (-Terrey-MacLachlan) syndrome (oculocerebrorenal dystrophy) 270.8
Lower extremity — see condition
Lown (-Ganong) — Levine syndrome (short P-R interval, normal QRS complex, and paroxysmal supraventricular tachycardia) 426.81
LSD reaction (see also Abuse, drugs, nondependent) 305.3
L-shaped kidney 753.3
Lucas-Championnière disease (fibrinous bronchitis) 466.0
Lucey-Driscoll syndrome (jaundice due to delayed conjugation) 774.30
Ludwig's
angina 528.3
disease (submaxillary cellulitis) 528.3
Lues (venerea), luetic — see Syphilis
Luetscher's syndrome (dehydration) 276.5
Lumbago 724.2
due to displacement, intervertebral disc 722.10
Lumbalgia 724.2
due to displacement, intervertebral disc 722.10
Lumbar — see condition
Lumbarization, vertebra 756.15
Lumbermen's itch 133.8
Lump — see also Mass
abdominal 789.3
breast 611.72
chest 786.6
epigastric 789.3
head 784.2
kidney 753.3
liver 789.1
lung 786.6
mediastinal 786.6
neck 784.2
nose or sinus 784.2
pelvic 789.3
skin 782.2
substernal 786.6
throat 784.2
umbilicus 789.3
Lunacy (see also Psychosis) 298.9
Lunatomalacia 732.3
Lung — see also condition
donor V59.8
drug addict's 417.8
mainliners' 417.8
vanishing 492.0
Lupoid (miliary) of Boeck 135
Lupus 710.0
Cazenave's (erythematosus) 695.4
discoid (local) 695.4
disseminated 710.0
erythematodes (discoid) (local) 695.4
erythematosus (discoid) (local) 695.4
   disseminated 710.0
   eyelid 373.34
   systemic 710.0
      with lung involvement 710.0 [517.8]
      inhibitor (presence of) 286.5
exedens 017.0
eyelid (see also Tuberculosis) 017.0 [373.4]
Hilliard's 017.0

Lupus—continued
hydralazine
   correct substance properly administered 695.4
   overdose or wrong substance given or taken 972.6
miliaris disseminatus faciei 017.0
nephritis 710.0 [583.81]
   acute 710.0 [580.81]   ◆
   chronic 710.0 [582.81]
nontuberculous, not disseminated 695.4
pernio (Besnier) 135
tuberculous (see also Tuberculosis) 017.0
   eyelid (see also Tuberculosis) 017.0 [373.4]
vulgaris 017.0
Luschka's joint disease 721.90
Luteinoma (M8610/0) 220
Lutembacher's disease or syndrome (atrial septal defect with mitral stenosis) 745.5
Luteoma (M8610/0) 220
Lutz-Miescher disease (elastosis perforans serpiginosa) 701.1
Lutz-Splendore-de Almeida disease (Brazilian blastomycosis) 116.1
Luxatio
bulbi due to birth injury 767.8
coxae congenita (see also Dislocation, hip, congenital) 754.30
erecta — see Dislocation, shoulder
imperfecta — see Sprain, by site
perinealis — see Dislocation, hip
Luxation — see also Dislocation, by site
eyeball 360.81
   due to birth injury 767.8
   lateral 376.36
genital organs (external) NEC — see Wound, open, genital organs
globe (eye) 360.81
   lateral 376.36
lacrimal gland (postinfectional) 375.16
lens (old) (partial) 379.32
   congenital 743.37
   syphilitic 090.49 [379.32]
   Marfan's disease 090.49
   spontaneous 379.32
penis — see Wound, open, penis
scrotum — see Wound, open, scrotum
testis — see Wound, open, testis
L-xyloketosuria 271.8
Lycanthropy (see also Psychosis) 298.9
Lyell's disease or syndrome (toxic epidermal necrolysis) 695.1
due to drug
   correct substance properly administered 695.1
   overdose or wrong substance given or taken 977.9
   specified drug — see Table of drugs and chemicals
Lyme disease 088.81
Lymph
gland or node — see condition
scrotum (see also Infestation, filarial) 125.9
Lymphadenitis 289.3
with
   abortion — see Abortion, by type, with sepsis
   ectopic pregnancy (see also categories 633.0-633.9) 639.0

Lymphadenitis—continued
with—continued
   molar pregnancy (see also categories 630-632) 639.0
acute 683
   mesenteric 289.2
any site, except mesenteric 289.3
   acute 683
   chronic 289.1
   mesenteric (acute) (chronic) (nonspecific) (subacute) 289.2
   subacute 289.1
      mesenteric 289.2
breast, puerperal, postpartum 675.2
chancroidal (congenital) 099.0
chronic 289.1
   mesenteric 289.2
dermatopathic 695.89
due to
   anthracosis (occupational) 500
   Brugia (Wuchereria) malayi 125.1
   diphtheria (toxin) 032.89
   lymphogranuloma venereum 099.1
   Wuchereria bancrofti 125.0
following
   abortion 639.0
   ectopic or molar pregnancy 639.0
generalized 289.3
gonorrheal 098.89
granulomatous 289.1
infectional 683
mesenteric (acute) (chronic) (nonspecific) (subacute) 289.2
   due to Bacillus typhi 002.0
   tuberculous (see also Tuberculosis) 014.8
mycobacterial 031.8
purulent 683
pyogenic 683
regional 078.3
septic 683
streptococcal 683
subacute, unspecified site 289.1
suppurative 683
syphilitic (early) (secondary) 091.4
   late 095.8
tuberculous — see Tuberculosis, lymph gland
venereal 099.1
Lymphadenoid goiter 245.2
Lymphadenopathy (general) 785.6
due to toxoplasmosis (acquired) 130.7
congenital (active) 771.2
Lymphadenopathy-associated virus (disease) (illness) (infection) — see Human immunodeficiency virus (disease) (illness) (infection)
Lymphadenosis 785.6
acute 075
Lymphangiectasis 457.1
conjunctiva 372.8
postinfectional 457.1
scrotum 457.1
Lymphangiectatic elephantiasis, nonfilarial 457.1
Lymphangioendothelioma (M9170/0) 228.1
malignant (M9170/3) — see Neoplasm, connective tissue, malignant
Lymphangioma (M9170/0) 228.1
capillary (M9171/0) 228.1
cavernous (M9172/0) 228.1
cystic (M9173/0) 228.1

Lymphangioma—continued
   malignant (M9170/3) — see
     Neoplasm, connective
     tissue, malignant
Lymphangiomyoma (M9174/0) 228.1
Lymphangiomyomatosis (M9174/1)
   — see Neoplasm, connective
   tissue, uncertain behavior
Lymphangiosarcoma (M9170/3) —
   see Neoplasm, connective
   tissue, malignant
Lymphangitis 457.2
   with
     abortion — see Abortion, by
       type, with sepsis
     abscess — see Abscess, by site
     cellulitis — see Abscess, by
       site
     ectopic pregnancy (see also
       categories 633.0-633.9)
       639.0
     molar pregnancy (see also
       categories 630-632)
       639.0
   acute (with abscess or cellulitis)
     682.9
     specified site — see Abscess,
       by site
   breast, puerperal, postpartum
     675.2
   chancroidal 099.0
   chronic (any site) 457.2
   due to
     Brugia (Wuchereria) malayi
       125.1
     Wuchereria bancrofti 125.0
   following
     abortion 639.0
     ectopic or molar pregnancy
       639.0
   gangrenous 457.2
   penis
     acute 607.2
     gonococcal (acute) 098.0
       chronic or duration of 2
         months or more
         098.2
   puerperal, postpartum, childbirth
     670
   strumous, tuberculous (see also
     Tuberculosis) 017.2
   subacute (any site) 457.2
   tuberculous — see Tuberculosis,
     lymph gland
Lymphatic (vessel) — see condition
Lymphatism 254.8
   scrofulous (see also Tuberculosis)
     017.2
Lymphectasia 457.1
Lymphedema (see also Elephantiasis)
   457.1
   acquired (chronic) 457.1
   chronic hereditary 757.0
   congenital 757.0
   idiopathic hereditary 757.0
   praecox 457.1
   secondary 457.1
   surgical NEC 997.9
     postmastectomy (syndrome)
       457.0
Lymph-hemangioma (M9120/0) —
   see Hemangioma, by site
Lymphoblastic — see condition
Lymphoblastoma (diffuse) (M9630/3)
   200.1
   giant follicular (M9690/3) 202.0
   macrofollicular (M9690/3) 202.0
Lymphoblastosis, acute benign 075
Lymphocele 457.8
Lymphocythemia 288.8

Lymphocytic — see also condition
   chorioencephalitis (acute) (serous)
     049.0
   choriomeningitis (acute) (serous)
     049.0
Lymphocytoma (diffuse) (malignant)
   (M9620/3) 200.1
Lymphocytomatosis (M9620/3)
   200.1
Lymphocytopenia 288.8
Lymphocytosis (symptomatic) 288.8
   infectious (acute) 078.89
Lymphoepithelioma (M8082/3) —
   see Neoplasm, by site,
   malignant
Lymphogranuloma (malignant)
   (M9650/3) 201.9
   inguinale 099.1
   venereal (any site) 099.1
     with stricture of rectum 099.1
   venereum 099.1
Lymphogranulomatosis (malignant)
   (M9650/3) 201.9
   benign (Boeck's sarcoid)
     (Schaumann's) 135
   Hodgkin's (M9650/3) 201.9
Lymphoid — see condition
Lympholeukoblastoma (M9850/3)
   207.8
Lympholeukosarcoma (M9850/3)
   207.8
Lymphoma (malignant) (M9590/3)
   202.8

> Note — Use the following fifth-
> digit subclassification with
> categories 200–202:
>
> 0   unspecified site
> 1   lymph nodes of head,
>   face, and neck
> 2   intrathoracic lymph
>   nodes
> 3   intra-abdominal lymph
>   nodes
> 4   lymph nodes of axilla
>   and upper limb
> 5   lymph nodes of inguinal
>   region and lower limb
> 6   intrapelvic lymph nodes
> 7   spleen
> 8   lymph nodes of multiple
>   sites

   benign (M9590/0) — see
     Neoplasm, by site, benign
   Burkitt's type (lymphoblastic)
     (undifferentiated)
     (M9750/3) 200.2
   Castleman's (mediastinal lymph
     node hyperplasia) 785.6
   centroblastic-centrocytic
     diffuse (M9614/3) 202.8
     follicular (M9692/3) 202.0
   centroblastic type (diffuse)
     (M9632/3) 202.8
     follicular (M9697/3) 202.0
   centrocytic (M9622/3) 202.8
   compound (M9613/3) 200.8
   convoluted cell type
     (lymphoblastic) (M9602/3)
     202.8
   diffuse NEC (M9590/3) 202.8
   follicular (giant) (M9690/3) 202.0
     center cell (diffuse) (M9615/3)
       202.8
     cleaved (diffuse) (M9623/3)
       202.8
       follicular (M9695/3)
         202.0
     non-cleaved (diffuse)
       (M9633/3) 202.8
       follicular (M9698/3)
         202.0

Lymphoma—continued
   follicular—continued
     centroblastic-centrocytic
       (M9692/3) 202.0
     centroblastic type (M9697/3)
       202.0
     lymphocytic
       intermediate differentiation
         (M9694/3) 202.0
       poorly differentiated
         (M9696/3) 202.0
     mixed (cell type)
       (lymphocytic-histiocytic)
       (small cell and large
       cell) (M9691/3) 202.0
   germinocytic (M9622/3) 202.8
   giant, follicular or follicle
     (M9690/3) 202.0
   histiocytic (diffuse) (M9640/3)
     200.0
     nodular (M9642/3) 200.0
     pleomorphic cell type
       (M9641/3) 200.0
   Hodgkin's (M9650/3) (see also
     Disease, Hodgkin's) 201.9
   immunoblastic (type) (M9612/3)
     200.8
   large cell (M9640/3) 200.0
     nodular (M9642/3) 200.0
     pleomorphic cell type
       (M9641/3) 200.0
   lymphoblastic (diffuse) (M9630/3)
     200.1
     Burkitt's type (M9750/3) 200.2
     convoluted cell type
       (M9602/3) 202.8
   lymphocytic (cell type) (diffuse)
     (M9620/3) 200.1
     with plasmacytoid
       differentiation, diffuse
       (M9611/3) 200.8
     intermediate differentiation
       (diffuse) (M9621/3)
       200.1
       follicular (M9694/3) 202.0
       nodular (M9694/3) 202.0
     nodular (M9690/3) 202.0
     poorly differentiated (diffuse)
       (M9630/3) 200.1
       follicular (M9696/3) 202.0
       nodular (M9696/3) 202.0
     well differentiated (diffuse)
       (M9620/3) 200.1
       follicular (M9693/3) 202.0
       nodular (M9693/3) 202.0
   lymphocytic-histiocytic, mixed
     (diffuse) (M9613/3) 200.8
     follicular (M9691/3) 202.0
     nodular (M9691/3) 202.0
   lymphoplasmacytoid type
     (M9611/3) 200.8
   lymphosarcoma type (M9610/3)
     200.1
   macrofollicular (M9690/3) 202.0
   mixed cell type (diffuse)
     (M9613/3) 200.8
     follicular (M9691/3) 202.0
     nodular (M9691/3) 202.0
   nodular (M9690/3) 202.0
     histiocytic (M9642/3) 200.0
     lymphocytic (M9690/3) 202.0
       intermediate differentiation
         (M9694/3) 202.0
       poorly differentiated
         (M9696/3) 202.0
     mixed (cell type)
       (lymphocytic-histiocytic)
       (small cell and large
       cell) (M9691/3) 202.0
   non-Hodgkin's type NEC
     (M9591/3) 202.8
   reticulum cell (type) (M9640/3)
     200.0
   small cell and large cell, mixed
     (diffuse) (M9613/3) 200.8
     follicular (M9691/3) 202.0
     nodular (9691/3) 202.0

Lymphoma—continued
   stem cell (type) (M9601/3) 202.8
   undifferentiated (cell type) (non-
     Burkitt's) (M9600/3) 202.8
     Burkitt's type (M9750/3) 200.2
Lymphomatosis (M9590/3) — see
   also Lymphoma
   granulomatous 099.1
Lymphopathia
   venereum 099.1
   veneris 099.1
Lymphopenia 288.8
   familial 279.2
Lymphoreticulosis, benign (of
   inoculation) 078.3
Lymphorrhea 457.8
Lymphosarcoma (M9610/3) 200.1
   diffuse (M9610/3) 200.1
     with plasmacytoid
       differentiation (M9611/3)
       200.8
     lymphoplasmacytic (M9611/3)
       200.8
   follicular (giant) (M9690/3) 202.0
     lymphoblastic (M9696/3)
       202.0
     lymphocytic, intermediate
       differentiation
       (M9694/3) 202.0
     mixed cell type (M9691/3)
       202.0
   giant follicular (M9690/3) 202.0
   Hodgkin's (M9650/3) 201.9
   immunoblastic (M9612/3) 200.8
   lymphoblastic (diffuse) (M9630/3)
     200.1
     follicular (M9696/3) 202.0
     nodular (M9696/3) 202.0
   lymphocytic (diffuse) (M9620/3)
     200.1
     intermediate differentiation
       (diffuse) (M9621/3)
       200.1
       follicular (M9694/3) 202.0
       nodular (M9694/3) 202.0
   mixed cell type (diffuse)
     (M9613/3) 200.8
     follicular (M9691/3) 202.0
     nodular (M9691/3) 202.0
   nodular (M9690/3) 202.0
     lymphoblastic (M9696/3)
       202.0
     lymphocytic, intermediate
       differentiation
       (M9694/3) 202.0
     mixed cell type (M9691/3)
       202.0
   prolymphocytic (M9631/3) 200.1
   reticulum cell (M9640/3) 200.0
Lymphostasis 457.8
Lypemania (see also Melancholia)
   296.2
Lyssa 071

M

Macacus ear 744.29
Maceration
   fetus (cause not stated) 779.9
   wet feet, tropical (syndrome)
     991.4
Machupo virus hemorrhagic fever
   078.7
Macleod's syndrome (abnormal
   transradiancy, one lung) 492.8
Macrocephalia, macrocephaly 756.0
Macrocheilia (congenital) 744.81
Macrochilia (congenital) 744.81
Macrocolon (congenital) 751.3
Macrocornea 743.41
   associated with buphthalmos
     743.22
Macrocytic — see condition

Macrocytosis — Malfunction

Macrocytosis 289.8
Macrodactylia, macrodactylism
  (fingers) (thumbs) 755.57
  toes 755.65
Macrodontia 520.2
Macroencephaly 742.4
Macrogenia 524.05
Macrogenitosomia (female) (male)
  (praecox) 255.2
Macrogingivae 523.8
Macroglobulinemia (essential)
  (idiopathic) (monoclonal)
  (primary) (syndrome)
  (Waldenström's) 273.3
Macroglossia (congenital) 750.15
  acquired 529.8
Macrognathia, macrognathism
  (congenital) 524.00
  mandibular 524.02
    alveolar 524.72
  maxillary 524.01
    alveolar 524.71
Macrogyria (congenital) 742.4
Macrohydrocephalus (see also
  Hydrocephalus) 331.4
Macromastia (see also Hypertrophy,
  breast) 611.1
Macropsia 368.14
Macrosigmoid 564.7
  congenital 751.3
Macrospondylitis, acromegalic
  253.0
Macrostomia (congenital) 744.83
Macrotia (external ear) (congenital)
  744.22
Macula
  cornea, corneal
    congenital 743.43
      interfering with vision
        743.42
    interfering with central vision
      371.03
    not interfering with central
      vision 371.02
  degeneration (see also
    Degeneration, macula)
    362.50
  hereditary (see also Dystrophy,
    retina) 362.70
Maculae ceruleae 132.1
Macules and papules 709.8
Maculopathy, toxic 362.55
Madarosis 374.55
Madelung's
  deformity (radius) 755.54
  disease (lipomatosis) 272.8
  lipomatosis 272.8
Madness (see also Psychosis) 298.9
  myxedema (acute) 293.0
    subacute 293.1
Madura
  disease (actinomycotic) 039.9
    mycotic 117.4
  foot (actinomycotic) 039.9
    mycotic 117.4
Maduromycosis (actinomycotic)
  039.9
  mycotic 117.4
Maffucci's syndrome
  (dyschondroplasia with
  hemangiomas) 756.4
Magenblase syndrome 306.4
Main en griffe (acquired) 736.06
  congenital 755.59
Maintenance
  chemotherapy regimen or
    treatment V58.1
  dialysis regimen or treatment
    extracorporeal (renal) V56.0
    peritoneal V56.8
    renal V56.0
  drug therapy or regimen V58.1

Maintenance—continued
  external fixation NEC V54.8
  radiotherapy V58.0
  traction NEC V54.8
Majocchi's
  disease (purpura annularis
    telangiectodes) 709.1
  granuloma 110.6
Major — see condition
Mal
  cerebral (idiopathic) (see also
    Epilepsy) 345.9
  comital (see also Epilepsy) 345.9
  de los pintos (see also Pinta)
    103.9
  de Meleda 757.39
  de mer 994.6
  lie — see Presentation, fetal
  perforant (see also Ulcer, lower
    extremity) 707.1
Malabar itch 110.9
  beard 110.0
  foot 110.4
  scalp 110.0
Malabsorption 579.9
  calcium 579.8
  carbohydrate 579.8
  disaccharide 271.3
  drug-induced 579.8
  due to bacterial overgrowth 579.8
  fat 579.8
  folate, congenital 281.2
  galactose 271.1
  glucose-galactose (congenital)
    271.3
  intestinal 579.9
  isomaltose 271.3
  lactose (hereditary) 271.3
  methionine 270.4
  monosaccharide 271.8
  postgastrectomy 579.3
  postsurgical 579.3
  protein 579.8
  sucrose (-isomaltose) (congenital)
    271.3
  syndrome 579.9
    postgastrectomy 579.3
    postsurgical 579.3
Malacia, bone 268.2
  juvenile (see also Rickets) 268.0
  Kienböck's (juvenile) (lunate)
    (wrist) 732.3
  adult 732.8
Malacoplakia
  bladder 596.8
  colon 569.89
  pelvis (kidney) 593.89
  ureter 593.89
  urethra 599.84
Malacosteon 268.2
  juvenile (see also Rickets) 268.0
Maladaptation — see Maladjustment
Maladie de Roger 745.4
Maladjustment
  conjugal V61.1
    involving divorce or
      estrangement V61.0
  educational V62.3
  family V61.9
    specified circumstance NEC
      V61.8
  marital V61.1
    involving divorce or
      estrangement V61.0
  occupational V62.2
  simple, adult (see also Reaction,
    adjustment) 309.9
  situational acute (see also
    Reaction, adjustment)
    309.9
  social V62.4
Malaise 780.7
Malakoplakia — see Malacoplakia

Malaria, malarial (fever) 084.6
  algid 084.9
  any type, with
    algid malaria 084.9
    blackwater fever 084.8
    fever
      blackwater 084.8
      hemoglobinuric (bilious)
        084.8
    hemoglobinuria, malarial
      084.8
    hepatitis 084.9 [573.2]
    nephrosis 084.9 [581.81]
    pernicious complication NEC
      084.9
      cardiac 084.9
      cerebral 084.9
  cardiac 084.9
  carrier (suspected) of V02.9
  cerebral 084.9
  complicating pregnancy,
    childbirth, or puerperium
    647.4
  congenital 771.2
  congestion, congestive 084.6
    brain 084.9
  continued 084.0
  estivo-autumnal 084.0
  falciparum (malignant tertian)
    084.0
  hematinuria 084.8
  hematuria 084.8
  hemoglobinuria 084.8
  hemorrhagic 084.6
  induced (therapeutically) 084.7
    accidental — see Malaria, by
      type
  liver 084.9 [573.2]
  malariae (quartan) 084.2
  malignant (tertian) 084.0
  mixed infections 084.5
  monkey 084.4
  ovale 084.3
  pernicious, acute 084.0
  Plasmodium, P.
    falciparum 084.0
    malariae 084.2
    ovale 084.3
    vivax 084.1
  quartan 084.2
  quotidian 084.0
  recurrent 084.6
    induced (therapeutically)
      084.7
      accidental — see Malaria,
        by type
  remittent 084.6
  specified types NEC 084.4
  spleen 084.6
  subtertian 084.0
  tertian (benign) 084.1
    malignant 084.0
  tropical 084.0
  typhoid 084.6
  vivax (benign tertian) 084.1
Malassez's disease (testicular cyst)
  608.89
Malassimilation 579.9
Maldescent, testis 752.5
Maldevelopment — see also
  Anomaly, by site
  brain 742.9
  colon 751.5
  hip (joint) 755.63
    congenital dislocation (see
      also Dislocation, hip,
      congenital) 754.30
  mastoid process 756.0
  middle ear, except ossicles
    744.03
    ossicles 744.04
  newborn (not malformation)
    764.9
  ossicles, ear 744.04
  spine 756.10
  toe 755.66

Male type pelvis 755.69
  with disproportion (fetopelvic)
    653.2
    affecting fetus or newborn
      763.1
    causing obstructed labor 660.1
      affecting fetus or newborn
        763.1
Malformation (congenital) — see
  also Anomaly
  bone 756.9
  bursa 756.9
  circulatory system NEC 747.9
    specified type NEC 747.89
  Chiari
    type I 348.4
    type II (see also Spina bifida)
      741.0
    type III 742.0
    type IV 742.2
  cochlea 744.05
  digestive system NEC 751.9
    lower 751.5
    specified type NEC 751.8
    upper 750.9
  eye 743.9
  gum 750.9
  heart NEC 746.9
    specified type NEC 746.89
    valve 746.9
  internal ear 744.05
  joint NEC 755.9
    specified type NEC 755.8
  Mondini's (congenital)
    (malformation, cochlea)
    744.05
  muscle 756.9
  nervous system (central) 742.9
  pelvic organs or tissues
    in pregnancy or childbirth
      654.9
      affecting fetus or newborn
        763.8
      causing obstructed labor
        660.2
      affecting fetus or
        newborn 763.1
  placenta (see also Placenta,
    abnormal) 656.7
  respiratory organs 748.9
    specified type NEC 748.8
  Rieger's 743.44
  sense organs NEC 742.9
    specified type NEC 742.8
  skin 757.9
    specified type NEC 757.8
  spinal cord 742.9
  teeth, tooth NEC 520.9
  tendon 756.9
  throat 750.9
  umbilical cord (complicating
    delivery) 663.9
    affecting fetus or newborn
      762.6
  umbilicus 759.9
  urinary system NEC 753.9
    specified type NEC 753.8
Malfunction — see also Dysfunction
  arterial graft 996.1
  cardiac pacemaker 996.01
  catheter device — see
    Complications, mechanical,
    catheter
  colostomy 569.6
  cystostomy 997.5
  device, implant, or graft NEC —
    see Complications,
    mechanical
  enteric stoma 569.6
  enterostomy 569.6
  gastroenteric 536.8
  nephrostomy 997.5
  pacemaker — see Complications,
    mechanical, pacemaker
  prosthetic device, internal —
    see Complications, mechanical
  tracheostomy 519.0

Malfunction

Malfunction—continued
  vascular graft or shunt 996.1
Malgaigne's fracture (closed) 808.43
  open 808.53
Malherbe's
  calcifying epithelioma (M8110/0) — see Neoplasm, skin, benign
  tumor (M8110/0) — see Neoplasm, skin, benign
Malibu disease 919.8
  infected 919.9
Malignancy (M8000/3) — see Neoplasm, by site, malignant
Malignant — see condition
Malingerer, malingering V65.2
Mallet, finger (acquired) 736.1
  congenital 755.59
  late effect of rickets 268.1
Malleus 024
Mallory's bodies 034.1
Mallory-Weiss syndrome 530.7
Malnutrition (calorie) 263.9
  complicating pregnancy 648.9
  degree
    first 263.1
    second 263.0
    third 262
    mild 263.1
    moderate 263.0
    severe 261
      protein-calorie 262
  fetus 764.2
  "light-for-dates" 764.1
  following gastrointestinal surgery 579.3
  intrauterine or fetal 764.2
    fetus or infant "light-for-dates" 764.1
  lack of care, or neglect (child) (infant) 995.5
    affecting parent or family V61.21
    specified person NEC 995.81
  malignant 260
  mild 263.1
  moderate 263.0
  protein 260
  protein-calorie 263.9
    severe 262
    specified type NEC 263.8
  severe 261
    protein-calorie NEC 262
Malocclusion (teeth) 524.4
  due to
    abnormal swallowing 524.5
    accessory teeth (causing crowding) 524.3
    dentofacial abnormality NEC 524.8
    impacted teeth (causing crowding) 524.3
    missing teeth 524.3
    mouth breathing 524.5
    supernumerary teeth (causing crowding) 524.3
    thumb sucking 524.5
    tongue, lip, or finger habits 524.5
  temporomandibular (joint) 524.69
Malposition
  cardiac apex (congenital) 746.87
  cervix — see Malposition, uterus
  congenital
    adrenal (gland) 759.1
    alimentary tract 751.8
      lower 751.5
      upper 750.8
    aorta 747.21
    appendix 751.5
    arterial trunk 747.29

Malposition—continued
  congenital—continued
    artery (peripheral) NEC (see also Malposition, congenital, peripheral vascular system) 747.60
      coronary 746.85
      pulmonary 747.3
    auditory canal 744.29
      causing impairment of hearing 744.02
    auricle (ear) 744.29
      causing impairment of hearing 744.02
      cervical 744.43
    biliary duct or passage 751.69
    bladder (mucosa) 753.8
      exteriorized or extroverted 753.5
    brachial plexus 742.8
    brain tissue 742.4
    breast 757.6
    bronchus 748.3
    cardiac apex 746.87
    cecum 751.5
    clavicle 755.51
    colon 751.5
    digestive organ or tract NEC 751.8
      lower 751.5
      upper 750.8
    ear (auricle) (external) 744.29
      ossicles 744.04
    endocrine (gland) NEC 759.2
    epiglottis 748.3
    Eustachian tube 744.24
    eye 743.8
    facial features 744.89
    fallopian tube 752.19
    finger(s) 755.59
      supernumerary 755.01
    foot 755.67
    gallbladder 751.69
    gastrointestinal tract 751.8
    genitalia, genital organ(s) or tract
      female 752.8
        external 752.49
        internal NEC 752.8
      male 752.8
    glottis 748.3
    hand 755.59
    heart 746.87
      dextrocardia 746.87
        with complete transposition of viscera 759.3
    hepatic duct 751.69
    hip (joint) (see also Dislocation, hip, congenital) 754.30
    intestine (large) (small) 751.5
      with anomalous adhesions, fixation, or malrotation 751.4
    joint NEC 755.8
    kidney 753.3
    larynx 748.3
    limb 755.8
      lower 755.69
      upper 755.59
    liver 751.69
    lung (lobe) 748.69
    nail(s) 757.5
    nerve 742.8
    nervous system NEC 742.8
    nose, nasal (septum) 748.1
    organ or site NEC — see Anomaly, specified type NEC, by site
    ovary 752.0
    pancreas 751.7
    parathyroid (gland) 759.2
    patella 755.64
    peripheral vascular system 747.60
      gastrointestinal 747.61

Malposition—continued
  congenital—continued
    peripheral vascular system—continued
      lower limb 747.64
      renal 747.62
      specified NEC 747.69
      spinal 747.82
      upper limb 747.63
    pituitary (gland) 759.2
    respiratory organ or system NEC 748.9
    rib (cage) 756.3
      supernumerary in cervical region 756.2
    scapula 755.59
    shoulder 755.59
    spinal cord 742.59
    spine 756.19
    spleen 759.0
    sternum 756.3
    stomach 750.7
    symphysis pubis 755.69
    testis (undescended) 752.5
    thymus (gland) 759.2
    thyroid (gland) (tissue) 759.2
      cartilage 748.3
    toe(s) 755.66
      supernumerary 755.02
    tongue 750.19
    trachea 748.3
    uterus 752.3
    vein(s) (peripheral) NEC (see also Malposition, congenital, peripheral vascular system) 747.60
      great 747.49
      portal 747.49
      pulmonary 747.49
      vena cava (inferior) (superior) 747.49
  device, implant, or graft — see Complications, mechanical
  fetus NEC — (see also Presentation, fetal) 652.9
    with successful version 652.1
    affecting fetus or newborn 763.1
    before labor, affecting fetus or newborn 761.7
    causing obstructed labor 660.0
    in multiple gestation (one fetus or more) 652.6
      with locking 660.5
      causing obstructed labor 660.0
  gallbladder — (see also Disease, gallbladder) 575.8
  gastrointestinal tract 569.89
    congenital 751.8
  heart (see also Malposition, congenital, heart) 746.87
  intestine 569.89
    congenital 751.5
  pelvic organs or tissues
    in pregnancy or childbirth 654.4
    affecting fetus or newborn 763.8
    causing obstructed labor 660.2
    affecting fetus or newborn 763.1
  placenta — see Placenta, previa
  stomach 537.89
    congenital 750.7
  tooth, teeth (with impaction) 524.3
  uterus or cervix (acquired) (acute) (adherent) (any degree) (asymptomatic) (postinfectional) (postpartal, old) 621.6
    anteflexion or anteversion (see also Anteversion, uterus) 621.6
    congenital 752.3

Malposition—continued
  uterus or cervix—continued
    flexion 621.6
      lateral (see also Lateroversion, uterus) 621.6
      in pregnancy or childbirth 654.4
        affecting fetus or newborn 763.8
        causing obstructed labor 660.2
          affecting fetus or newborn 763.1
    inversion 621.6
    lateral (flexion) (version) (see also Lateroversion, uterus) 621.6
    lateroflexion (see also Lateroversion, uterus) 621.6
    lateroversion (see also Lateroversion, uterus) 621.6
    retroflexion or retroversion (see also Retroversion, uterus) 621.6
Malposture 729.9
Malpresentation, fetus — (see also Presentation, fetal) 652.9
Malrotation
  cecum 751.4
  colon 751.4
  intestine 751.4
  kidney 753.3
Malta fever (see also Brucellosis) 023.9
Maltosuria 271.3
Maltreatment (of)
  adult (emotional) 995.81
  child (emotional) (nutritional) 995.5
    affecting parent or family V61.21
  specified person NEC 995.81
  spouse (emotional) 995.81
Malt workers' lung 495.4
Malum coxae senilis 715.25
Malunion, fracture 733.81
Mammillitis (see also Mastitis) 611.0
  puerperal, postpartum 675.2
Mammitis (see also Mastitis) 611.0
  puerperal, postpartum 675.2
Mammoplasia 611.1
Management
  contraceptive V25.9
    specified type NEC V25.8
  procreative V26.9
    specified type NEC V26.8
Mangled NEC (see also nature and site of injury) 959.9
Mania (monopolar) — (see also Psychosis, affective) 296.0
  alcoholic (acute) (chronic) 291.9
  Bell's — see Mania, chronic
  chronic 296.0
    recurrent episode 296.1
    single episode 296.0
  compulsive 300.3
  delirious (acute) 296.0
    recurrent episode 296.1
    single episode 296.0
  epileptic (see also Epilepsy) 345.4
  hysterical 300.10
  inhibited 296.89
  puerperal (after delivery) 296.0
    recurrent episode 296.1
    single episode 296.0
  recurrent episode 296.1
  senile 290.8
  single episode 296.0
  stupor 296.89
  stuporous 296.89
  unproductive 296.89

Manic-depressive insanity, psychosis, reaction, or syndrome (see also Psychosis, affective) 296.80
 circular (alternating) 296.7
  currently
   depressed 296.5
    episode unspecified 296.7
    hypomanic, previously depressed 296.4
    manic 296.4
   mixed 296.6
  depressed (type), depressive 296.2
   atypical 296.82
   recurrent episode 296.3
   single episode 296.2
  hypomanic 296.0
   recurrent episode 296.1
   single episode 296.0
  manic 296.0
   atypical 296.81
   recurrent episode 296.1
   single episode 296.0
  mixed NEC 296.89
  perplexed 296.89
  stuporous 296.89
Manifestations, rheumatoid
 lungs 714.81
 pannus — see Arthritis, rheumatoid
 subcutaneous nodules — see Arthritis, rheumatoid
Mankowsky's syndrome (familial dysplastic osteopathy) 731.2
Mannoheptulosuria 271.8
Mannosidosis 271.8
Manson's
 disease (schistosomiasis) 120.1
 pyosis (pemphigus contagiosus) 684
 schistosomiasis 120.1
Mansonellosis 125.5
Manual — see condition
Maple bark disease 495.6
Maple bark-strippers' lung 495.6
Maple syrup (urine) disease or syndrome 270.3
Marable's syndrome (celiac artery compression) 447.4
Marasmus 261
 brain 331.9
 due to malnutrition 261
 intestinal 569.89
 nutritional 261
 senile 797
 tuberculous NEC (see also Tuberculosis) 011.9
Marble
 bones 756.52
 skin 782.61
Marburg disease (virus) 078.89
March
 foot (closed) 825.20
  open 825.30
 hemoglobinuria 283.2
Marchand multiple nodular hyperplasia (liver) 571.5
Marchesani (-Weill) syndrome (brachymorphism and ectopia lentis) 759.89
Marchiafava (-Bignami) disease or syndrome 341.8
Marchiafava-Micheli syndrome (paroxysmal nocturnal hemoglobinuria) 283.2
Marcus Gunn's syndrome (jaw-winking syndrome) 742.8

Marfan's
 congenital syphilis 090.49
 disease 090.49
 syndrome (arachnodactyly) 759.82
  meaning congenital syphilis 090.49
  with luxation of lens 090.49 [379.32]
Marginal
 implantation, placenta — see Placenta, previa
 placenta — see Placenta, previa
 sinus (hemorrhage) (rupture) 641.2
  affecting fetus or newborn 762.1
Marie's
 cerebellar ataxia 334.2
 syndrome (acromegaly) 253.0
Marie-Bamberger disease or syndrome (hypertrophic) (pulmonary) (secondary) 731.2
 idiopathic (acropachyderma) 757.39
 primary (acropachyderma) 757.39
Marie-Charcot-Tooth neuropathic atrophy, muscle 356.1
Marie-Strümpell arthritis or disease (ankylosing spondylitis) 720.0
Marihuana, marijuana
 abuse (see also Abuse, drugs, nondependent) 305.2
 dependence (see also Dependence) 304.3
Marion's disease (bladder neck obstruction) 596.0
Marital conflict V61.1
Mark
 port wine 757.32
 raspberry 757.32
 strawberry 757.32
 stretch 701.3
 tattoo 709.09
Maroteaux-Lamy syndrome (mucopolysaccharidosis VI) 277.5
Marriage license examination V70.3
Marrow (bone)
 arrest 284.9
 megakaryocytic 287.3
 poor function 289.9
Marseilles fever 082.1
Marsh's disease (exophthalmic goiter) 242.0
Marshall's (hidrotic) ectodermal dysplasia 757.31
Marsh fever (see also Malaria) 084.6
Martin's disease 715.27
Martin-Albright syndrome (pseudohypoparathyroidism) 275.4
Martorell-Fabre syndrome (pulseless disease) 446.7
Masculinization, female, with adrenal hyperplasia 255.2
Masculinovoblastoma (M8670/0) 220
Masochism 302.83
Masons' lung 502
Mass
 abdominal 789.3
 anus 787.9
 bone 733.90
 breast 611.72
 cheek 784.2
 chest 786.6
 cystic — see Cyst
 ear 388.8
 epigastric 789.3
 eye 379.92
 female genital organ 625.8
 gum 784.2

Mass—continued
 head 784.2
 intracranial 784.2
 joint 719.60
  ankle 719.67
  elbow 719.62
  foot 719.67
  hand 719.64
  hip 719.65
  knee 719.66
  multiple sites 719.69
  pelvic region 719.65
  shoulder (region) 719.61
  specified site NEC 719.68
  wrist 719.63
 kidney (see also Disease, kidney) 593.9
 lung 786.6
 lymph node 785.6
 malignant (M8000/3) — see Neoplasm, by site, malignant
 mediastinal 786.6
 mouth 784.2
 muscle (limb) 729.89
 neck 784.2
 nose or sinus 784.2
 palate 784.2
 pelvis, pelvic 789.3
 penis 607.89
 perineum 625.8
 rectum 787.9
 scrotum 608.89
 skin 782.2
 specified organ NEC — see Disease of specified organ or site
 splenic 789.2
 substernal 786.6
  thyroid (see also Goiter) 240.9
 superficial (localized) 782.2
 testes 608.89
 throat 784.2
 tongue 784.2
 umbilicus 789.3
 uterus 625.8
 vagina 625.8
 vulva 625.8
Massive — see condition
Mastalgia 611.71
 psychogenic 307.89
Mast cell
 disease 757.33
  systemic (M9741/3) 202.6
 leukemia (M9900/3) 207.8
 sarcoma (M9742/3) 202.6
 tumor (M9740/1) 238.5
  malignant (M9740/3) 202.6
Masters-Allen syndrome 620.6
Mastitis (acute) (adolescent) (diffuse) (interstitial) (lobular) (nonpuerperal) (nonsuppurative) (parenchymatous) (phlegmonous) (simple) (subacute) (suppurative) 611.0
 chronic (cystic) (fibrocystic) 610.1
 cystic 610.1
  Schimmelbusch's type 610.1
 fibrocystic 610.1
 infective 611.0
 lactational 675.2
 lymphangitis 611.0
 neonatal (noninfective) 778.7
  infective 771.5
 periductal 610.4
 plasma cell 610.4
 puerperal, postpartum, (interstitial) (nonpurulent) (parenchymatous) 675.2
  purulent 675.1
  stagnation 676.2
 puerperalis 675.2
 retromammary 611.0
  puerperal, postpartum 675.1

Mastitis —continued
 submammary 611.0
  puerperal, postpartum 675.1
Mastocytoma (M9740/1) 238.5
 malignant (M9740/3) 202.6
Mastocytosis 757.33
 malignant (M9741/3) 202.6
 systemic (M9741/3) 202.6
Mastodynia 611.71
 psychogenic 307.89
Mastoid — see condition
Mastoidalgia (see also Otalgia) 388.70
Mastoiditis (coalescent) (hemorrhagic) (pneumococcal) (streptococcal) (suppurative) 383.9
 acute or subacute 383.00
  with
   Gradenigo's syndrome 383.02
   petrositis 383.02
   specified complication NEC 383.02
   subperiosteal abscess 383.01
 chronic (necrotic) (recurrent) 383.1
 tuberculous (see also Tuberculosis) 015.6
Mastopathy, mastopathia 611.9
 chronica cystica 610.1
 diffuse cystic 610.1
 estrogenic 611.8
 ovarian origin 611.8
Mastoplasia 611.1
Masturbation 307.9
Maternal condition, affecting fetus or newborn
 acute yellow atrophy of liver 760.8
 albuminuria 760.1
 anesthesia or analgesia 763.5
 blood loss 762.1
 chorioamnionitis 762.7
 circulatory disease, chronic (conditions classifiable to 390-459, 745-747) 760.3
 congenital heart disease (conditions classifiable to 745-746) 760.3
 cortical necrosis of kidney 760.1
 death 761.6
 diabetes mellitus 775.0
  manifest diabetes in the infant 775.1
 disease NEC 760.9
  circulatory system, chronic (conditions classifiable to 390-459, 745-747) 760.3
  genitourinary system (conditions classifiable to 580-599) 760.1
  respiratory (conditions classifiable to 490-519, 748) 760.3
 eclampsia 760.0
 hemorrhage NEC 762.1
 hepatitis acute, malignant, or subacute 760.8
 hyperemesis (gravidarum) 761.8
 hypertension (arising during pregnancy) (conditions classifiable to 642) 760.0
 infection
  disease classifiable to 001-136 760.2
  genital tract NEC 760.8
  urinary tract 760.1
 influenza 760.2
  manifest influenza in the infant 771.2
 injury (conditions classifiable to 800-996) 760.5

Maternal condition, affecting fetus or newborn—continued
  malaria 760.2
    manifest malaria in infant or fetus 771.2
  malnutrition 760.4
  necrosis of liver 760.8
  nephritis (conditions classifiable to 580-583) 760.1
  nephrosis (conditions classifiable to 581) 760.1
  noxious substance transmitted via breast milk or placenta 760.70
    alcohol 760.71
    anti-infective agents 760.74
    cocaine 760.75
    "crack" 760.75
    diethylstilbestrol [DES] 760.76
    hallucinogenic agents 760.73
    medicinal agents NEC 760.79
    narcotics 760.72
    obstetric anesthetic or analgesic drug 760.72
    specified agent NEC 760.79
  nutritional disorder (conditions classifiable to 260-269) 760.4
  operation unrelated to current delivery 760.6
  preeclampsia 760.0
  pyelitis or pyelonephritis, arising during pregnancy (conditions classifiable to 590) 760.1
  renal disease or failure 760.1
  respiratory disease, chronic (conditions classifiable to 490-519, 748) 760.3
  rheumatic heart disease (chronic) (conditions classifiable to 393-398) 760.3
  rubella (conditions classifiable to 056) 760.2
    manifest rubella in the infant or fetus 771.0
  surgery unrelated to current delivery 760.6
    to uterus or pelvic organs 763.8
  syphilis (conditions classifiable to 090-097) 760.2
    manifest syphilis in the infant or fetus 090.0
  thrombophlebitis 760.3
  toxemia (of pregnancy) 760.0
    preeclampsia 760.0
  toxoplasmosis (conditions classifiable to 130) 760.2
    manifest toxoplasmosis in the infant or fetus 771.2
  transmission of chemical substance through the placenta 760.70
    alcohol 760.71
    anti-infective 760.74
    cocaine 760.75
    "crack" 760.75
    diethylstilbestrol [DES] 760.76
    hallucinogenic agents 760.73
    narcotics 760.72
    specified substance NEC 760.79
  uremia 760.1
  urinary tract conditions (conditions classifiable to 580-599) 760.1
  vomiting (pernicious) (persistent) (vicious) 761.8

Maternity — *see* Delivery
Matheiu's disease (leptospiral jaundice) 100.0
Mauclaire's disease or osteochondrosis 732.3
Maxcy's disease 081.0
Maxilla, maxillary — *see* condition
May (-Hegglin) anomaly or syndrome 288.2
Mayaro fever 066.3
Mazoplasia 610.8
MBD (minimal brain dysfunction), child (*see also* Hyperkinesia) 314.9
McArdle (-Schmid-Pearson) disease or syndrome (glycogenosis V) 271.0
McCune-Albright syndrome (osteitis fibrosa disseminata) 756.59
MCLS (mucocutaneous lymph node syndrome) 446.1
McQuarrie's syndrome (idiopathic familial hypoglycemia) 251.2
Measles (black) (hemorrhagic) (suppressed) 055.9
  with
    encephalitis 055.0
    keratitis 055.71
    keratoconjunctivitis 055.71
    otitis media 055.2
    pneumonia 055.1
    complication 055.8
      specified type NEC 055.79
  encephalitis 055.0
  French 056.9
  German 056.9
  keratitis 055.71
  keratoconjunctivitis 055.71
  liberty 056.9
  otitis media 055.2
  pneumonia 055.1
  specified complications NEC 055.79
  vaccination, prophylactic (against) V04.2
Meatitis, urethral (*see also* Urethritis) 597.89
Meat poisoning — *see* Poisoning, food
Meatus, meatal — *see* condition
Meat-wrappers' asthma 506.9
Meckel's
  diverticulitis 751.0
  diverticulum (displaced) (hypertrophic) 751.0
Meconium
  aspiration 770.1
  delayed passage in newborn 777.1
  ileus 777.1
    due to cystic fibrosis 277.01
  in liquor 792.3
    noted during delivery — omit code
  insufflation 770.1
  obstruction
    fetus or newborn 777.1
      in mucoviscidosis 277.01
    passage of 792.3
      noted during delivery — omit code
  peritonitis 777.6
  plug syndrome (newborn) NEC 777.1
Median — *see also* condition
  arcuate ligament syndrome 447.4
  bar (prostate) 600
    vesical orifice 600
  rhomboid glossitis 529.2
Mediastinal shift 793.2
Mediastinitis (acute) (chronic) 519.2
  actinomycotic 039.8
  syphilitic 095.8
  tuberculous (*see also* Tuberculosis) 012.8

Mediastinopericarditis (*see also* Pericarditis) 423.9
  acute 420.90
  chronic 423.8
    rheumatic 393
  rheumatic, chronic 393
Mediastinum, mediastinal — *see* condition
Medical services provided for — *see* Health, services provided because (of)
Medicine poisoning (by overdose) (wrong substance given or taken in error) 977.9
  specified drug or substance — *see* Table of drugs and chemicals
Medin's disease (poliomyelitis) 045.9
Mediterranean
  anemia (with other hemoglobinopathy) 282.4
  disease or syndrome (hemipathic) 282.4
  fever (*see also* Brucellosis) 023.9
    familial 277.3
    kala-azar 085.0
    leishmaniasis 085.0
    tick fever 082.1
Medulla — *see* condition
Medullary
  cystic kidney 753.16
  sponge kidney 753.17
Medullated fibers
  optic (nerve) 743.57
  retina 362.85
Medulloblastoma (M9470/3)
  desmoplastic (M9471/3) 191.6
  specified site — *see* Neoplasm, by site, malignant
  unspecified site 191.6
Medulloepithelioma (M9501/3) — *see also* Neoplasm, by site, malignant
  teratoid (M9502/3) — *see* Neoplasm, by site, malignant
Medullomyoblastoma (M9472/3)
  specified site — *see* Neoplasm, by site, malignant
  unspecified site 191.6
Meekeren-Ehlers-Danlos syndrome 756.83
Megacaryocytic — *see* condition
Megacolon (acquired) (functional) (not Hirschsprung's disease) 564.7
  aganglionic 751.3
  congenital, congenitum 751.3
  Hirschsprung's (disease) 751.3
  psychogenic 306.4
  toxic (*see also* Colitis, ulcerative) 556.9
Megaduodenum 537.3
Megaesophagus (functional) 530.0
  congenital 750.4
Megakaryocytic — *see* condition
Megalencephaly 742.4
Megalerythema (epidermicum) (infectiosum) 057.0
Megalia, cutis et ossium 757.39
Megaloappendix 751.5
Megalocephalus, megalocephaly NEC 756.0
Megalocornea 743.41
  associated with buphthalmos 743.22
Megalocytic anemia 281.9
Megalodactylia (fingers) (thumbs) 755.57
  toes 755.65
Megaloduodenum 751.5

Megaloesophagus (functional) 530.0
  congenital 750.4
Megalogastria (congenital) 750.7
Megalomania 307.9
Megalophthalmos 743.8
Megalopsia 368.14
Megalosplenia (*see also* Splenomegaly) 789.2
Megaloureter 593.89
  congenital 753.2
Megarectum 569.49
Megasigmoid 564.7
  congenital 751.3
Megaureter 593.89
  congenital 753.2
Megrim 346.9
Meibomian
  cyst 373.2
    infected 373.12
  gland — *see* condition
  infarct (eyelid) 374.85
  stye 373.11
Meibomitis 373.12
Meige
  -Milroy disease (chronic hereditary edema) 757.0
  syndrome (blepharospasm-oromandibular dystonia) 333.82
Melalgia, nutritional 266.2
Melancholia (*see also* Psychosis, affective) 296.90
  climacteric 296.2
    recurrent episode 296.3
    single episode 296.2
  hypochondriac 300.7
  intermittent 296.2
    recurrent episode 296.3
    single episode 296.2
  involutional 296.2
    recurrent episode 296.3
    single episode 296.2
  menopausal 296.2
    recurrent episode 296.3
    single episode 296.2
  puerperal 296.2
  reactive (from emotional stress, psychological trauma) 298.0
  recurrent 296.3
  senile 290.21
  stuporous 296.2
    recurrent episode 296.3
    single episode 296.2
Melanemia 275.0
Melanoameloblastoma (M9363/0) — *see* Neoplasm, bone, benign
Melanoblastoma (M8720/3) — *see* Melanoma
Melanoblastosis
  Block-Sulzberger 757.33
  cutis linearis sive systematisata 757.33
Melanocarcinoma (M8720/3) — *see* Melanoma
Melanocytoma, eyeball (M8726/0) 224.0
Melanoderma, melanodermia 709.09
  Addison's (primary adrenal insufficiency) 255.4
Melanodontia, infantile 521.0
Melanoepithelioma (M8720/3) — *see* Melanoma

Melanoma — INDEX TO DISEASES — Meningitis

Melanoma (malignant) (M8720/3) 172.9

> Note — Except where otherwise indicated, the morphological varieties of melanoma in the list below should be coded by site as for "Melanoma (malignant)". Internal sites should be coded to malignant neoplasm of those sites.

abdominal wall 172.5
ala nasi 172.3
amelanotic (M8730/3) — see Melanoma, by site
ankle 172.7
anus, anal 154.3
   canal 154.2
arm 172.6
auditory canal (external) 172.2
auricle (ear) 172.2
auricular canal (external) 172.2
axilla 172.5
axillary fold 172.5
back 172.5
balloon cell (M8722/3) — see Melanoma, by site
benign (M8720/0) — see Neoplasm, skin, benign
breast (female) (male) 172.5
brow 172.3
buttock 172.5
canthus (eye) 172.1
cheek (external) 172.3
chest wall 172.5
chin 172.3
choroid 190.6
conjunctiva 190.3
ear (external) 172.2
epithelioid cell (M8771/3) — see also Melanoma, by site
   and spindle cell, mixed (M8775/3) — see Melanoma, by site
external meatus (ear) 172.2
eye 190.9
eyebrow 172.3
eyelid (lower) (upper) 172.1
face NEC 172.3
female genital organ (external) NEC 184.4
finger 172.6
flank 172.5
foot 172.7
forearm 172.6
forehead 172.3
foreskin 187.1
gluteal region 172.5
groin 172.5
hand 172.6
heel 172.7
helix 172.2
hip 172.7
in
   giant pigmented nevus (M8761/3) — see Melanoma, by site
   Hutchinson's melanotic freckle (M8742/3) — see Melanoma, by site
   junctional nevus (M8740/3) — see Melanoma, by site
   precancerous melanosis (M8741/3) — see Melanoma, by site
interscapular region 172.5
iris 190.0
jaw 172.3
juvenile (M8770/0) — see Neoplasm, skin, benign
knee 172.7
labium
   majus 184.1
   minus 184.2
lacrimal gland 190.2
leg 172.7

Melanoma—continued
lip (lower) (upper) 172.0
liver 197.7
lower limb NEC 172.7
male genital organ (external) NEC 187.9
meatus, acoustic (external) 172.2
meibomian gland 172.1
metastatic
   of or from specified site — see Melanoma, by site
   site not of skin — see Neoplasm, by site, malignant, secondary
   to specified site — see Neoplasm, by site, malignant, secondary
   unspecified site 172.9
nail 172.9
   finger 172.6
   toe 172.7
neck 172.4
nodular (M8721/3) — see Melanoma, by site
nose, external 172.3
orbit 190.1
penis 187.4
perianal skin 172.5
perineum 172.5
pinna 172.2
popliteal (fossa) (space) 172.7
prepuce 187.1
pubes 172.5
pudendum 184.4
retina 190.5
scalp 172.4
scrotum 187.7
septum nasal (skin) 172.3
shoulder 172.6
skin NEC 172.8
spindle cell (M8772/3) — see also Melanoma, by site
   type A (M8773/3) 190.0
   type B (M8774/3) 190.0
submammary fold 172.5
superficial spreading (M8743/3) — see Melanoma, by site
temple 172.3
thigh 172.7
toe 172.7
trunk NEC 172.5
umbilicus 172.5
upper limb NEC 172.6
vagina vault 184.0
vulva 184.4

Melanoplakia 528.9

Melanosarcoma (M8720/3) — see also Melanoma, by site
epithelioid cell (M8771/3) — see Melanoma

Melanosis 709.09 ◆
addisonian (primary adrenal insufficiency) 255.4
   tuberculous (see also Tuberculosis) 017.6
adrenal 255.4
colon 569.89
conjunctiva 372.55
   congenital 743.49
corii degenerativa 757.33
cornea (presenile) (senile) 371.12
   congenital 743.43
      interfering with vision 743.42
   prenatal 743.43
      interfering with vision 743.42
eye 372.55
   congenital 743.49
jute spinners' 709.09 ◆
lenticularis progressiva 757.33
liver 573.8
precancerous (M8741/2) — see also Neoplasm, skin, in situ
   malignant melanoma in (M8741/3) — see Melanoma

Melanosis—continued
Riehl's 709.09 ◆
sclera 379.19
   congenital 743.47
suprarenal 255.4
tar 709.09 ▼
toxic 709.09 ▲

Melanuria 791.9

Melasma 709.09 ◆
adrenal (gland) 255.4
suprarenal (gland) 255.4

Melena 578.1
due to
   swallowed maternal blood 777.3
   ulcer — see Ulcer, by site, with hemorrhage
newborn 772.4
   due to swallowed maternal blood 777.3

Meleney's
gangrene (cutaneous) 686.0
ulcer (chronic undermining) 686.0

Melioidosis 025

Melitensis, febris 023.0

Melitococcosis 023.0

Melkersson (-Rosenthal) syndrome 351.8

Mellitus, diabetes — see Diabetes

Melorheostosis (bone) (leri) 733.99

Meloschisis 744.83

Melotia 744.29

Membrana
capsularis lentis posterior 743.39
epipapillaris 743.57

Membranacea placenta — see Placenta, abnormal

Membranaceous uterus 621.8

Membrane, membranous — see also condition
folds, congenital — see Web
Jackson's 751.4
over face (causing asphyxia), fetus or newborn 768.9
premature rupture — see Rupture, membranes, premature
pupillary 364.74
   persistent 743.46
retained (complicating delivery)
   (with hemorrhage) 666.2
   without hemorrhage 667.1
secondary (eye) 366.50
unruptured (causing asphyxia) 768.9
vitreous humor 379.25

Membranitis, fetal 658.4
affecting fetus or newborn 762.7

Memory disturbance, loss or lack
(see also Amnesia) 780.9
mild, following organic brain damage 310.1

Menadione (vitamin K) deficiency 269.0

Menarche, precocious 259.1

Mendacity, pathologic 301.7

Mende's syndrome (ptosis-epicanthus) 270.2

Mendelson's syndrome (resulting from a procedure) 997.3
obstetric 668.0

Ménétrier's disease or syndrome (hypertrophic gastritis) 535.2

Ménière's disease, syndrome, or vertigo 386.00
cochlear 386.02
cochleovestibular 386.01
inactive 386.04
in remission 386.04
vestibular 386.03

Meninges, meningeal — see condition

Meningioma (M9530/0) — see also Neoplasm, meninges, benign
angioblastic (M9535/0) — see Neoplasm, meninges, benign
angiomatous (M9534/0) — see Neoplasm, meninges, benign
endotheliomatous (M9531/0) — see Neoplasm, meninges, benign
fibroblastic (M9532/0) — see Neoplasm, meninges, benign
fibrous (M9532/0) — see Neoplasm, meninges, benign
hemangioblastic (M9535/0) — see Neoplasm, meninges, benign
hemangiopericytic (M9536/0) — see Neoplasm, meninges, benign
malignant (M9530/3) — see Neoplasm, meninges, malignant
meningiothelial (M9531/0) — see Neoplasm, meninges, benign
meningotheliomatous (M9531/0) — see Neoplasm, meninges, benign
mixed (M9537/0) — see Neoplasm, meninges, benign
multiple (M9530/1) 237.6
papillary (M9538/1) 237.6
psammomatous (M9533/0) — see Neoplasm, meninges, benign
syncytial (M9531/0) — see Neoplasm, meninges, benign
transitional (M9537/0) — see Neoplasm, meninges, benign

Meningiomatosis (diffuse) (M9530/1) 237.6

Meningism (see also Meningismus) 781.6

Meningismus (infectional) (pneumococcal) 781.6
due to serum or vaccine 997.0 [321.8]
influenzal NEC 487.8

Meningitis (basal) (basic) (basilar) (brain) (cerebral) (cervical) (congestive) (diffuse) (hemorrhagic) (infantile) (membranous) (metastatic) (nonspecific) (pontine) (progressive) (simple) (spinal) (subacute) (sympathetica) (toxic) 322.9
abacterial NEC (see also Meningitis, aseptic) 047.9
actinomycotic 039.8 [320.7]
adenoviral 049.1
Aerobacter acrogenes 320.82
anaerobes (cocci) (gram-negative) (gram-positive) (mixed) (NEC) 320.81
arbovirus NEC 066.9 [321.2]
   specified type NEC 066.8 [321.2]
aseptic (acute) NEC 047.9
adenovirus 049.1
Coxsackievirus 047.0
due to
   adenovirus 049.1
   Coxsackievirus 047.0
   ECHO virus 047.1
   enterovirus 047.9
   mumps 072.1

Meningitis—*continued*
  aseptic—*continued*
    due to—*continued*
      poliovirus (*see also*
        Poliomyelitis) 045.2
        [321.2]
      ECHO virus 047.1
      herpes (simplex) virus 054.72
        zoster 053.0
      leptospiral 100.81
      lymphocytic choriomeningitis
        049.0
      noninfective 322.0
  Bacillus pyocyaneus 320.89
  bacterial NEC 320.9
    anaerobic 320.81
    gram-negative 320.82
      anaerobic 320.81
  Bacteroides (fragilis) (oralis)
    (melaninogenicus) 320.81
  cancerous (M8000/6) 198.4
  candidal 112.83
  carcinomatous (M8010/6) 198.4
  caseous (*see also* Tuberculosis,
    meninges) 013.0
  cerebrospinal (acute) (chronic)
    (diplococcal) (endemic)
    (epidemic) (fulminant)
    (infectious) (malignant)
    (meningococcal) (sporadic)
    036.0
    carrier (suspected) of V02.5
  chronic NEC 322.2
  clear cerebrospinal fluid NEC
    322.0
  Clostridium (haemolyticum)
    (novyi) NEC 320.81
  coccidioidomycosis 114.2
  Coxsackievirus 047.0
  cryptococcal 117.5 *[321.0]*
  diplococcal 036.0
    gram-negative 036.0
    gram-positive 320.1
  Diplococcus pneumoniae 320.1
  due to
    actinomycosis 039.8 *[320.7]*
    adenovirus 049.1
    coccidiomycosis 114.2
    enterovirus 047.9
      specified NEC 047.8
    histoplasmosis (*see also*
      Histoplasmosis) 115.91
    Listerosis 027.0 *[320.7]*
    Lyme disease 088.81 *[320.7]*
    moniliasis 112.83
    mumps 072.1
    neurosyphilis 094.2
    nonbacterial organisms NEC
      321.8
    oidiomycosis 112.83
    poliovirus (*see also*
      Poliomyelitis) 045.9
      [321.2]
    preventive immunization,
      inoculation, or
      vaccination 997.0
      [321.8]
    sarcoidosis 135 *[321.4]*
    sporotrichosis 117.1 *[321.1]*
    syphilis 094.2
      acute 091.81
      congenital 090.42
      secondary 091.81
    trypanosomiasis (*see also*
      Trypanosomiasis) 086.9
      [321.3]
    whooping cough 033.9
      [320.7]
  E. coli 320.82
  ECHO virus 047.1
  endothelial-leukocytic, benign,
    recurrent 047.9
  Enterobacter aerogenes 320.82
  enteroviral 047.9
    specified type NEC 047.8
  enterovirus 047.9
    specified NEC 047.8

Meningitis—*continued*
  eosinophilic 322.1
  epidemic NEC 036.0
  Escherichia coli (E. coli) 320.82
  Eubacterium 320.81
  fibrinopurulent NEC 320.9
    specified type NEC 320.89
  Friedländer (bacillus) 320.82
  fungal NEC 117.9 *[321.1]*
  Fusobacterium 320.81
  gonococcal 098.82
  gram-negative bacteria NEC
    320.82
    anaerobic 320.81
    cocci 036.0
      specified NEC 320.82
  gram-negative cocci NEC 036.0
    specified NEC 320.82
  gram-positive cocci NEC 320.9
  H. influenzae 320.0
  herpes (simplex) virus 054.72
    zoster 053.0
  infectious NEC 320.9
  influenzal 320.0
  Klebsiella pneumoniae 320.82
  late effect — *see* Late, effect,
    meningitis
  leptospiral (aseptic) 100.81
  Listerella (monocytogenes) 027.0
    [320.7]
  Listeria monocytogenes 027.0
    [320.7]
  lymphocytic (acute) (benign)
    (serous) 049.0
    choriomeningitis virus 049.0
  meningococcal (chronic) 036.0
  Mima polymorpha 320.82
  Mollaret's 047.9
  monilial 112.83
  mumps (virus) 072.1
  mycotic NEC 117.9 *[321.1]*
  Neisseria 036.0
  neurosyphilis 094.2
  nonbacterial NEC (*see also*
    Meningitis, aseptic) 047.9
  nonpyogenic NEC 322.0
  oidiomycosis 112.83
  ossificans 349.2
  Peptococcus 320.81
  Peptostreptococcus 320.81
  pneumococcal 320.1
  poliovirus (*see also* Poliomyelitis)
    045.2 *[321.2]*
  Proprionibacterium 320.81
  Proteus morganii 320.82
  Pseudomonas (aeruginosa)
    (pyocyaneus) 320.82
  purulent NEC 320.9
    specified organism NEC
      320.89
  pyogenic NEC 320.9
    specified organism NEC
      320.89
  Salmonella 003.21
  septic NEC 320.9
    specified organism NEC
      320.89
  serosa circumscripta NEC 322.0
  serous NEC (*see also* Meningitis,
    aseptic) 047.9
    lymphocytic 049.0
    syndrome 348.2
  Serratia (marcescens) 320.82
  specified organism NEC 320.89
  sporadic cerebrospinal 036.0
  sporotrichosis 117.1 *[321.1]*
  staphylococcal 320.3
  sterile 997.0
  streptococcal (acute) 320.2
  suppurative 320.9
    specified organism NEC
      320.89
  syphilitic 094.2
    acute 091.81
    congenital 090.42
    secondary 091.81
  torula 117.5 *[321.0]*

Meningitis—*continued*
  traumatic (complication of injury)
    958.8
  Treponema (denticola)
    (Macrodenticum) 320.81
  trypanosomiasis 086.1 *[321.3]*
  tuberculous (*see also*
    Tuberculosis, meninges)
    013.0
  typhoid 002.0 *[320.7]*
  Veillonella 320.81
  Vibrio vulnificus 320.82
  viral, virus NEC (*see also*
    Meningitis, aseptic) 047.9
  Wallgren's (*see also* Meningitis,
    aseptic) 047.9
Meningocele (congenital) (spinal)
  (*see also* Spina bifida) 741.9▼
  acquired (traumatic) 349.2 ▲
  cerebral 742.0
  cranial 742.0
Meningocerebritis — *see*
  Meningoencephalitis
Meningococcemia (acute) (chronic)
  036.2
Meningococcus, meningococcal (*see*
  also condition) 036.9
  adrenalitis, hemorrhagic 036.3
  carditis 036.40
  carrier (suspected) of V02.5
  cerebrospinal fever 036.0
  encephalitis 036.1
  endocarditis 036.42
  infection NEC 036.9
  meningitis (cerebrospinal) 036.0
  myocarditis 036.43
  optic neuritis 036.81
  pericarditis 036.41
  septicemia (chronic) 036.2
Meningoencephalitis (*see also*
  Encephalitis) 323.9
  acute NEC 048
  bacterial, purulent, pyogenic, or
    septic — *see* Meningitis
  chronic NEC 094.1
  diffuse NEC 094.1
  diphasic 063.2
  due to
    actinomycosis 039.8 *[320.7]*
    blastomycosis NEC (*see also*
      Blastomycosis) 116.0
      [323.4]
    free-living amebae 136.2
    Listeria monocytogenes 027.0
      [320.7]
    Lyme disease 088.81 *[320.7]*
    mumps 072.2
    Naegleria (amebae) (gruberi)
      (organisms) 136.2
    rubella 056.01
    sporotrichosis 117.1 *[321.1]*
    toxoplasmosis (acquired)
      130.0
      congenital (active) 771.2
      [323.4]
    Trypanosoma 086.1 *[323.2]*
  epidemic 036.0
  herpes 054.3
  herpetic 054.3
  H. influenzae 320.0
  infectious (acute) 048
  influenzal 320.0
  late effect — *see* category 326
  Listeria monocytogenes 027.0
    [320.7]
  lymphocytic (serous) 049.0
  mumps 072.2
  parasitic NEC 123.9 *[323.4]*
  pneumococcal 320.1
  primary amebic 136.2
  rubella 056.01
  serous 048
    lymphocytic 049.0
  specific 094.2
  staphylococcal 320.3
  streptococcal 320.2

Meningoencephalitis—*continued*
  syphilitic 094.2
  toxic NEC 989.9 *[323.7]*
    due to
      carbon tetrachloride 987.8
        [323.7]
      hydroxyquinoline
        derivatives poisoning
        961.3 *[323.7]*
      lead 984.9 *[323.7]*
      mercury 985.0 *[323.7]*
      thallium 985.8 *[323.7]*
  toxoplasmosis (acquired) 130.0
  trypanosomic 086.1 *[323.2]*
  tuberculous (*see also*
    Tuberculosis, meninges)
    013.0
  virus NEC 048
Meningoencephalocele 742.0
  syphilitic 094.89
  congenital 090.49
Meningoencephalomyelitis (*see also*
  Meningoencephalitis) 323.9
  acute NEC 048
    disseminated (postinfectious)
      136.9 *[323.6]*
      postimmunization or
        postvaccination
        323.5
  due to
    actinomycosis 039.8 *[320.7]*
    torula 117.5 *[323.4]*
    toxoplasma or toxoplasmosis
      (acquired) 130.0
      congenital (active) 771.2
        [323.4]
  late effect — *see* category 326
Meningoencephalomyelopathy (*see*
  also Meningoencephalomyelitis) 349.9
Meningoencephalopathy (*see also*
  Meningoencephalitis) 348.3
Meningoencephalopoliomyelitis (*see*
  also Poliomyelitis, bulbar)
  045.0
  late effect 138
Meningomyelitis (*see also*
  Meningoencephalitis) 323.9
  blastomycotic NEC (*see also*
    Blastomycosis) 116.0
    [323.4]
  due to
    actinomycosis 039.8 *[320.7]*
    blastomycosis (*see also*
      Blastomycosis) 116.0
      [323.4]
    Meningococcus 036.0
    sporotrichosis 117.1 *[323.4]*
    torula 117.5 *[323.4]*
  late effect — *see* category 326
  lethargic 049.8
  meningococcal 036.0
  syphilitic 094.2
  tuberculous (*see also*
    Tuberculosis, meninges)
    013.0
Meningomyelocele (*see also* Spina
  bifida) 741.9
  syphilitic 094.89
Meningomyeloneuritis — *see*
  Meningoencephalitis
Meningoradiculitis — *see* Meningitis
Meningovascular — *see* condition
Meniscocytosis 282.60
Menkes' syndrome — *see* Syndrome,
  Menkes'
Menolipsis 626.0
Menometrorrhagia 626.2
Menopause, menopausal (symptoms)
  (syndrome) 627.2
  arthritis (any site) NEC 716.3
  artificial 627.4
  bleeding 627.0

Menopause, menopausal—continued
crisis 627.2
depression (see also Psychosis, affective) 296.2
  agitated 296.2
    recurrent episode 296.3
    single episode 296.2
  psychotic 296.2
    recurrent episode 296.3
    single episode 296.2
  recurrent episode 296.3
  single episode 296.2
melancholia (see also Psychosis, affective) 296.2
  recurrent episode 296.3
  single episode 296.2
paranoid state 297.2
paraphrenia 297.2
postsurgical 627.4
premature 256.3
  postirradiation 256.2
  postsurgical 256.2
psychoneurosis 627.2
psychosis NEC 298.8
surgical 627.4
toxic polyarthritis NEC 716.39

Menorrhagia (primary) 626.2
climacteric 627.0
menopausal 627.0
postclimacteric 627.1
postmenopausal 627.1
preclimacteric 627.0
premenopausal 627.0
puberty (menses retained) 626.3

Menorrhalgia 625.3
Menoschesis 626.8
Menostaxis 626.2
Menses, retention 626.8
Menstrual — see also Menstruation
cycle, irregular 626.4
disorders NEC 626.9
extraction V25.3
fluid, retained 626.8
molimen 625.4
period, normal V65.5
regulation V25.3

Menstruation
absent 626.0
anovulatory 628.0
delayed 626.8
difficult 625.3
disorder 626.9
  psychogenic 306.52
  specified NEC 626.8
during pregnancy 640.8
excessive 626.2
frequent 626.2
infrequent 626.1
irregular 626.4
latent 626.8
membranous 626.8
painful (primary) (secondary) 625.3
  psychogenic 306.52
passage of clots 626.2
precocious 626.8
protracted 626.8
retained 626.8
retrograde 626.8
scanty 626.1
suppression 626.8
vicarious (nasal) 625.8

Mentagra (see also Sycosis) 704.8
Mental — see also condition
deficiency (see also Retardation, mental) 319
deterioration (see also Psychosis) 298.9
disorder (see also Disorder, mental) 300.9
exhaustion 300.5
insufficiency (congenital) (see also Retardation, mental) 319

Mental—continued
observation without need for further medical care NEC V71.09
retardation (see also Retardation, mental) 319
subnormality (see also Retardation, mental) 319
  mild 317
  moderate 318.0
  profound 318.2
  severe 318.1
upset (see also Disorder, mental) 300.9

Meralgia paresthetica 355.1
Mercurial — see condition
Mercurialism NEC 985.0
Merergasia 300.9
Merocele (see also Hernia, femoral) 553.00
Meromelia 755.4
lower limb 755.30
  intercalary 755.32
    femur 755.34
    tibiofibular (complete) (incomplete) 755.33
    fibula 755.37
    metatarsal(s) 755.38
    tarsal(s) 755.38
    tibia 755.36
    tibiofibular 755.35
  terminal (complete) (partial) (transverse) 755.31
    longitudinal 755.32
      metatarsal(s) 755.38
      phalange(s) 755.39
      tarsal(s) 755.38
  transverse 755.31
upper limb 755.20
  intercalary 755.22
    carpal(s) 755.28
    humeral 755.24
    radioulnar (complete) (incomplete) 755.23
    metacarpal(s) 755.28
    phalange(s) 755.29
    radial 755.26
    radioulnar 755.25
    ulnar 755.27
  terminal (complete) (partial) (transverse) 755.21
    longitudinal 755.22
      carpal(s) 755.28
      metacarpal(s) 755.28
      phalange(s) 755.29
  transverse 755.21

Merosmia 781.1
Merycism — see also Vomiting
psychogenic 307.53
Merzbacher-Pelizaeus disease 330.0
Mesaortitis — see Aortitis
Mesarteritis — see Arteritis
Mesencephalitis (see also Encephalitis) 323.9
late effect — see category 326
Mesenchymoma (M8990/1) — see also Neoplasm, connective tissue, uncertain behavior
benign (M8990/0) — see Neoplasm, connective tissue, benign
malignant (M8990/3) — see Neoplasm, connective tissue, malignant
Mesentery, mesenteric — see condition
Mesiodens, mesiodentes 520.1
causing crowding 524.3
Mesio-occlusion 524.2
Mesocardia (with asplenia) 746.87
Mesocolon — see condition

Mesonephroma (malignant) (M9110/3) — see also Neoplasm, by site, malignant
benign (M9110/0) — see Neoplasm, by site, benign
Mesophlebitis — see Phlebitis
Mesostromal dysgenesis 743.51
Mesothelioma (malignant) (M9050/3) — see also Neoplasm, by site, malignant
benign (M9050/0) — see Neoplasm, by site, benign
biphasic type (M9053/3) — see also Neoplasm, by site, malignant
  benign (M9053/0) — see Neoplasm, by site, benign
epithelioid (M9052/3) — see also Neoplasm, by site, malignant
  benign (M9052/0) — see Neoplasm, by site, benign
fibrous (M9051/3) — see also Neoplasm, by site, malignant
  benign (M9051/0) — see Neoplasm, by site, benign

Metabolism disorder 277.9
specified type NEC 277.8
Metagonimiasis 121.5
Metagonimus infestation (small intestine) 121.5
Metal
pigmentation (skin) 709.00 ◆
polishers' disease 502
Metalliferous miners' lung 503
Metamorphopsia 368.14
Metaplasia
bone, in skin 709.3
breast 611.8
cervix — omit code
endometrium (squamous) 621.8
intestinal, of gastric mucosa 537.89
kidney (pelvis) (squamous) (see also Disease, renal) 593.89
myelogenous 289.8
myeloid (agnogenic) (megakaryocytic) 289.8
spleen 289.59
squamous cell
  amnion 658.8
  bladder 596.8
  cervix — see condition
  trachea 519.1
  tracheobronchial tree 519.1
  uterus 621.8
    cervix — see condition
Metastasis, metastatic
abscess — see Abscess
calcification 275.4
cancer, neoplasm, or disease from specified site (M8000/3) — see Neoplasm, by site, malignant
  to specified site (M8000/6) — see Neoplasm, by site, secondary
deposits (in) (M8000/6) — see Neoplasm, by site, secondary
pneumonia 038.8 [484.8]
spread (to) (M8000/6) — see Neoplasm, by site, secondary
Metatarsalgia 726.70
anterior 355.6
due to Freiberg's disease 732.5
Morton's 355.6

Metatarsus, metatarsal — see also condition
adductus (congenital)
  valgus 754.60
  varus 754.53
primus varus 754.52
valgus (adductus) (congenital) 754.60
varus (adductus) (congenital) 754.53
primus 754.52
Methemoglobinemia 289.7
acquired (with sulfhemoglobinemia) 289.7
congenital 289.7
enzymatic 289.7
Hb-M disease 289.7
hereditary 289.7
toxic 289.7
Methemoglobinuria (see also Hemoglobinuria) 791.2
Methioninemia 270.4
Metritis (catarrhal) (septic) (suppurative) (see also Endometritis) 615.9
blennorrhagic 098.16
  chronic or duration of 2 months or over 098.36
cervical (see also Cervicitis) 616.0
gonococcal 098.16
  chronic or duration of 2 months or over 098.36
hemorrhagic 626.8
puerperal, postpartum, childbirth 670
tuberculous (see also Tuberculosis) 016.7
Metropathia hemorrhagica 626.8
Metroperitonitis (see also Peritonitis, pelvic, female) 614.5
Metrorrhagia 626.6
arising during pregnancy — see Hemorrhage, pregnancy
postpartum NEC 666.2
primary 626.6
psychogenic 306.59
puerperal 666.2
Metrorrhexis — see Rupture, uterus
Metrosalpingitis (see also Salpingo-oophoritis) 614.2
Metrostaxis 626.6
Metrovaginitis (see also Endometritis) 615.9
gonococcal (acute) 098.16
  chronic or duration of 2 months or over 098.36
Mexican fever — see Typhus, Mexican
Meyenburg-Altherr-Uehlinger syndrome 733.99
Meyer-Schwickerath and Weyers syndrome (dysplasia oculodentodigitalis) 759.89
Meynert's amentia (nonalcoholic) 294.0
alcoholic 291.1
Mibelli's disease 757.39
Mice, joint (see also Loose, body, joint) 718.1
knee 717.6
Micheli-Rietti syndrome (thalassemia minor) 282.4
Michotte's syndrome 721.5
Micrencephalon, micrencephaly 742.1
Microaneurysm, retina 362.14
diabetic 250.5 [362.01]
Microangiopathy 443.9
diabetic (peripheral) 250.7 [443.81]
  retinal 250.5 [362.01]
peripheral 443.9
  diabetic 250.7 [443.81]

Microangiopathy—continued
  retinal 362.18
    diabetic 250.5 [362.01]
  thrombotic 446.6
    Moschcowitz's (thrombotic thrombocytopenic purpura) 446.6
Microcephalus, microcephalic, microcephaly 742.1
  due to toxoplasmosis (congenital) 771.2
Microcheilia 744.82
Microcolon (congenital) 751.5
Microcornea (congenital) 743.41
Microcytic — see condition
Microdontia 520.2
Microdrepanocytosis (thalassemia-Hb-S disease) 282.4
Microembolism, retina 362.33
Microencephalon 742.1
Microfilaria streptocerca infestation 125.3
Microgastria (congenital) 750.7
Microgenia 524.0
Microgenitalia (congenital) 752.8
Microglioma (M9710/3)
  specified site — see Neoplasm, by site, malignant
  unspecified site 191.9
Microglossia (congenital) 750.16
Micrognathia, micrognathism (congenital) 524.00
  mandibular 524.04
    alveolar 524.74
  maxillary 524.03
    alveolar 524.73
Microgyria (congenital) 742.2
Microinfarct, heart (see also Insufficiency, coronary) 411.89
Microlithiasis, alveolar, pulmonary 516.2
Micromyelia (congenital) 742.59
Microphakia (congenital) 743.36
Microphthalmia (congenital) (see also Microphthalmos) 743.10
Microphthalmos (congenital) 743.10
  associated with eye and adnexal anomalies NEC 743.12
  due to toxoplasmosis (congenital) 771.2
  isolated 743.11
  simple 743.11
  syndrome 759.89
Micropsia 368.14
Microsporidiosis 136.8
Microsporon furfur infestation 111.0
Microsporosis (see also Dermatophytosis) 110.9
  nigra 111.1
Microstomia (congenital) 744.84
Microthelia 757.6
Microthromboembolism — see Embolism
Microtia (congenital) (external ear) 744.23
Microtropia 378.34
Micturition
  disorder NEC 788.69
    psychogenic 306.53
  frequency 788.41
    psychogenic 306.53
  nocturnal 788.43
  painful 788.1
    psychogenic 306.53
Middle
  ear — see condition
  lobe (right) syndrome 518.0
Midplane — see condition
Miescher's disease 709.3
  cheilitis 351.8
  granulomatosis disciformis 709.3

Miescher-Leder syndrome or granulomatosis 709.3
Mieten's syndrome 759.89
Migraine (idiopathic) 346.9
  with aura 346.0
  abdominal (syndrome) 346.2
  allergic (histamine) 346.2
  atypical 346.1
  basilar 346.2
  classical 346.0
  common 346.1
  hemiplegic 346.8
  lower-half 346.2
  menstrual 625.4
  ophthalmic 346.8
  ophthalmoplegic 346.8
  retinal 346.8
  variant 346.2
Migrant, social V60.0
Migratory, migrating — see also condition
  person V60.0
  testis, congenital 752.5
Mikulicz's disease or syndrome (dryness of mouth, absent or decreased lacrimation) 527.1
Milian atrophia blanche 701.3
Miliaria (crystallina) (rubra) (tropicalis) 705.1
  apocrine 705.82
Miliary — see condition
Milium (see also Cyst, sebaceous) 706.2
  colloid 709.3
  eyelid 374.84
Milk
  crust 691.8
  excess secretion 676.6
  fever, female 672
  poisoning 988.8
  retention 676.2
  sickness 988.8
  spots 423.1
Milkers' nodes 051.1
Milk-leg (deep vessels) 671.4
  complicating pregnancy 671.3
  nonpuerperal 451.19
  puerperal, postpartum, childbirth 671.4
Milkman (-Looser) disease or syndrome (osteomalacia with pseudofractures) 268.2
Milky urine (see also Chyluria) 791.1
Millar's asthma (laryngismus stridulus) 478.75
Millard-Gubler paralysis or syndrome 344.89
Millard-Gubler-Foville paralysis 344.89
Miller's disease (osteomalacia) 268.2
Miller Fisher's syndrome 357.0
Milles' syndrome (encephalocutaneous angiomatosis) 759.6
Mills' disease 335.29
Millstone makers' asthma or lung 502
Milroy's disease (chronic hereditary edema) 757.0
Miners' — see also condition
  asthma 500
  elbow 727.2
  knee 727.2
  lung 500
  nystagmus 300.89
  phthisis (see also Tuberculosis) 011.4
  tuberculosis (see also Tuberculosis) 011.4
Minkowski-Chauffard syndrome (see also Spherocytosis) 282.0
Minor — see condition

Minor's disease 336.1
Minot's disease (hemorrhagic disease, newborn) 776.0
Minot-von Willebrand (-Jürgens) disease or syndrome (angiohemophilia) 286.4
Minus (and plus) hand (intrinsic) 736.09
Miosis (persistent) (pupil) 379.42
Mirizzi's syndrome (hepatic duct stenosis) (see also Obstruction, biliary) 576.2
  with calculus, cholelithiasis, or stones — see Choledocholithiasis
Mirror writing 315.09
  secondary to organic lesion 784.69
Misadventure (prophylactic) (therapeutic) (see also Complications) 999.9
  administration of insulin 962.3
  infusion — see Complications, infusion
  local applications (of fomentations, plasters, etc.) 999.9
    burn or scald — see Burn, by site
  medical care (early) (late) NEC 999.9
    adverse effect of drugs or chemicals — see Table of drugs and chemicals
    burn or scald — see Burn, by site
  radiation NEC 990
  radiotherapy NEC 990
  surgical procedure (early) (late) — see Complications, surgical procedure
  transfusion — see Complications, transfusion
  vaccination or other immunological procedure — see Complications, vaccination
Misanthropy 301.7
Miscarriage — see Abortion, spontaneous
Mischief, malicious, child (see also Disturbance, conduct) 312.0
Mismanagement, feeding 783.3
Misplaced, misplacement
  kidney (see also Disease, renal) 593.0
    congenital 753.3
  organ or site, congenital NEC — see Malposition, congenital
Missed
  abortion 632
  delivery (at or near term) 656.4
  labor (at or near term) 656.4
Missing — see also Absence
  teeth (acquired) 525.1
    congenital (see also Anodontia) 520.0
  vertebrae (congenital) 756.13
Misuse of drugs NEC (see also Abuse, drug, nondependent) 305.9
Mitchell's disease (erythromelalgia) 443.89
Mite(s)
  diarrhea 133.8
  grain (itch) 133.8
  hair follicle (itch) 133.8
  in sputum 133.8
Mitral — see condition
Mittelschmerz 625.2
Mixed — see condition
Mljet disease (mal de Meleda) 757.39

Mobile, mobility
  cecum 751.4
  coccyx 733.99
  excessive — see Hypermobility
  gallbladder 751.69
  kidney 593.0
    congenital 753.3
  organ or site, congenital NEC — see Malposition, congenital
  spleen 289.59
Mobitz heart block (atrioventricular) 426.10
  type I (Wenckebach's) 426.13
  type II 426.12
Möbius'
  disease 346.8
  syndrome
    congenital oculofacial paralysis 352.6
    ophthalmoplegic migraine 346.8
Moeller (-Barlow) disease (infantile scurvy) 267
  glossitis 529.4
Mohr's syndrome (types I and II) 759.89
Mola destruens (M9100/1) 236.1
Molarization, premolars 520.2
Molar pregnancy 631
  hydatidiform (delivered) (undelivered) 630
Mold(s) in vitreous 117.9
Molding, head (during birth) 767.3
Mole (pigmented) (M8720/0) — see also Neoplasm, skin, benign
  blood 631
  Breus' 631
  cancerous (M8720/3) — see Melanoma
  carneous 631
  destructive (M9100/1) 236.1
  ectopic — see Pregnancy, ectopic
  fleshy 631
  hemorrhagic 631
  hydatid, hydatidiform (benign) (complicating pregnancy) (delivered) (undelivered) (see also Hydatidiform mole) 630
    invasive (M9100/1) 236.1
    malignant (M9100/1) 236.1
  previous, affecting management of pregnancy V23.1
  invasive (hydatidiform) (M9100/1) 236.1
  malignant
    meaning
      malignant hydatidiform mole (9100/1) 236.1
      melanoma (M8720/3) — see Melanoma
  nonpigmented (M8730/0) — see Neoplasm, skin, benign
  pregnancy NEC 631
  skin (M8720/0) — see Neoplasm, skin, benign
  tubal — see Pregnancy, tubal
  vesicular (see also Hydatidiform mole) 630
Molimen, molimina (menstrual) 625.4
Mollaret's meningitis 047.9
Mollities (cerebellar) (cerebral) 437.8
  ossium 268.2
Molluscum
  contagiosum 078.0
  epitheliale 078.0
  fibrosum (M8851/0) — see Lipoma, by site
  pendulum (M8851/0) — see Lipoma, by site

Mönckeberg's arteriosclerosis, degeneration, disease, or sclerosis (see also Arteriosclerosis, extremities) 440.20
Monday fever 504
Monday morning dyspnea or asthma 504
Mondini's malformation (cochlea) 744.05
Mondor's disease (thrombophlebitis of breast) 451.89
Mongolian, mongolianism, mongolism, mongoloid 758.0
  spot 757.33
Monilethrix (congenital) 757.4
Monilia infestation — see Candidiasis
Moniliasis — see also Candidiasis
  neonatal 771.7
  vulvovaginitis 112.1
Monoarthritis 716.60
  ankle 716.67
  arm 716.62
    lower (and wrist) 716.63
    upper (and elbow) 716.62
  foot (and ankle) 716.67
  forearm (and wrist) 716.63
  hand 716.64
  leg 716.66
    lower 716.66
    upper 716.65
  pelvic region (hip) (thigh) 716.65
  shoulder (region) 716.61
  specified site NEC 716.68
Monoblastic — see condition
Monochromatism (cone) (rod) 368.54
Monocytic — see condition
Monocytosis (symptomatic) 288.8
Monofixation syndrome 378.34
Monomania (see also Psychosis) 298.9
Mononeuritis 355.9
  cranial nerve — see Disorder, nerve, cranial
  femoral nerve 355.2
  lateral
    cutaneous nerve of thigh 355.1
    popliteal nerve 355.3
  lower limb 355.8
    specified nerve NEC 355.79
  medial popliteal nerve 355.4
  median nerve 354.1
  multiplex 354.5
  plantar nerve 355.6
  posterior tibial nerve 355.5
  radial nerve 354.3
  sciatic nerve 355.0
  ulnar nerve 354.2
  upper limb 354.9
    specified nerve NEC 354.8
  vestibular 388.5
Mononeuropathy (see also Mononeuritis) 355.9
  diabetic NEC 250.6 [355.9]
    lower limb 250.6 [355.8]
    upper limb 250.6 [354.9]
  iliohypogastric 355.79
  ilioinguinal 355.79
  obturator 355.79
  saphenous 355.79
Mononucleosis, infectious 075
  with hepatitis 075 [573.1]
Monoplegia 344.5
  brain (current episode) (see also Paralysis, brain) 437.8
  fetus or newborn 767.8
  cerebral (current episode) (see also Paralysis, brain) 437.8
  congenital or infantile (cerebral) (spastic) (spinal) 343.3

Monoplegia—continued
  embolic (current) (see also Embolism, brain) 434.1
    late effect — see category 438
  infantile (cerebral) (spastic) (spinal) 343.3
  lower limb 344.30
    affecting
      dominant side 344.31
      nondominant side 344.32▲
  newborn 767.8
  psychogenic 306.0
    specified as conversion reaction 300.11
  thrombotic (current) (see also Thrombosis, brain) 434.0
    late effect — see category 438
  transient 781.4
  upper limb 344.40
    affecting
      dominant side 344.41
      nondominant side 344.42▲
Monorchism, monorchidism 752.8
Monster, monstrosity — see Anomaly ◆
Monteggia's fracture (closed) 813.03
  open 813.13
Mood swings
  brief compensatory 296.99
  rebound 296.99
Moore's syndrome (see also Epilepsy) 345.5
Mooren's ulcer (cornea) 370.07
Mooser-Neill reaction 081.0
Mooser bodies 081.0
Moral
  deficiency 301.7
  imbecility 301.7
Morax-Axenfeld conjunctivitis 372.03
Morbilli (see also Measles) 055.9
Morbus
  anglicus, anglorum 268.0
  Beigel 111.2
  caducus (see also Epilepsy) 345.9
  caeruleus 746.89
  celiacus 579.0
  comitialis (see also Epilepsy) 345.9
  cordis — see also Disease, heart
    valvulorum — see Endocarditis
  coxae 719.95
    tuberculous (see also Tuberculosis) 015.1
  hemorrhagicus neonatorum 776.0
  maculosus neonatorum 772.6
  renum 593.0
  senilis (see also Osteoarthrosis) 715.9
Morel-Kraepelin disease (see also Schizophrenia) 295.9
Morel-Moore syndrome (hyperostosis frontalis interna) 733.3
Morel-Morgagni syndrome (hyperostosis frontalis interna) 733.3
Morgagni
  cyst, organ, hydatid, or appendage 752.8
  fallopian tube 752.11
  disease or syndrome (hyperostosis frontalis interna) 733.3
Morgagni-Adams-Stokes syndrome (syncope with heart block) 426.9
Morgagni-Stewart-Morel syndrome (hyperostosis frontalis interna) 733.3
Moria (see also Psychosis) 298.9
Morning sickness 643.0
Moron 317

Morphea (guttate) (linear) 701.0
Morphine dependence (see also Dependence) 304.0
Morphinism (see also Dependence) 304.0
Morphinomania (see also Dependence) 304.0
Morphoea 701.0
Morquio (-Brailsford) (-Ullrich) disease or syndrome (mucopolysaccharidosis IV) 277.5
  kyphosis 277.5
Morris syndrome (testicular feminization) 257.8
Morsus humanus (open wound) — see also Wound, open, by site
  skin surface intact — see Contusion
Mortification (dry) (moist) (see also Gangrene) 785.4
Morton's
  disease 355.6
  foot 355.6
  metatarsalgia (syndrome) 355.6
  neuralgia 355.6
  neuroma 355.6
  syndrome (metatarsalgia) (neuralgia) 355.6
  toe 355.6
Morvan's disease 336.0
Mosaicism, mosaic (chromosomal) 758.9
  autosomal 758.5
  sex 758.8
Moschcowitz's syndrome (thrombotic thrombocytopenic purpura) 446.6
Mother yaw 102.0
Motion sickness (from travel, any vehicle) (from roundabouts or swings) 994.6
Mottled teeth (enamel) (endemic) (nonendemic) 520.3
Mottling enamel (endemic) (nonendemic) (teeth) 520.3
Mouchet's disease 732.5
Mould(s) (in vitreous) 117.9
Moulders'
  bronchitis 502
  tuberculosis (see also Tuberculosis) 011.4
Mounier-Kuhn syndrome 494
Mountain
  fever — see Fever, mountain
  sickness 993.2
    with polycythemia, acquired 289.0
    acute 289.0
  tick fever 066.1
Mouse, joint (see also Loose, body, joint) 718.1
  knee 717.6
Mouth — see condition
Movable
  coccyx 724.71
  kidney (see also Disease, renal) 593.0
    congenital 753.3
  organ or site, congenital NEC — see Malposition, congenital
  spleen 289.59
Movement, abnormal (dystonic) (involuntary) 781.0
  paradoxical facial 374.43
Moya Moya disease 437.5
Mozart's ear 744.29
Mucha's disease (acute parapsoriasis varioliformis) 696.2
Mucha-Haberman syndrome (acute parapsoriasis varioliformis) 696.2

Mu-chain disease 273.2
Mucinosis (cutaneous) (papular) 701.8
Mucocele
  appendix 543.9
  buccal cavity 528.9
  gallbladder (see also Disease, gallbladder) 575.3
  lacrimal sac 375.43
  orbit (eye) 376.81
  salivary gland (any) 527.6
  sinus (accessory) (nasal) 478.1
  turbinate (bone) (middle) (nasal) 478.1
  uterus 621.8
Mucocutaneous lymph node syndrome (acute) (febrile) (infantile) 446.1
Mucoenteritis 564.1
Mucolipidosis I, II, III 272.7
Mucopolysaccharidosis (types 1-6) 277.5
  cardiopathy 277.5 [425.7]
Mucormycosis (lung) 117.7
Mucositis — see also Inflammation by site
  necroticans agranulocytica 288.0
Mucous — see also condition
  patches (syphilitic) 091.3
    congenital 090.0
Mucoviscidosis 277.00
  with meconium obstruction 277.01
Mucus
  asphyxia or suffocation (see also Asphyxia, mucus) 933.1
    newborn 770.1
  in stool 792.1
  plug (see also Asphyxia, mucus) 933.1
    aspiration, of newborn 770.1
    tracheobronchial 934.8
    newborn 770.1
Muguet 112.0
Mulberry molars 090.5
Mullerian mixed tumor (M8950/3) — see Neoplasm, by site, malignant
Multicystic kidney 753.19
Multilobed placenta — see Placenta, abnormal
Multiparity V61.5
  affecting
    fetus or newborn 763.8
    management of
      labor and delivery 659.4
      pregnancy V23.3
    requiring contraceptive management (see also Contraception) V25.9
Multipartita placenta — see Placenta, abnormal
Multiple, multiplex — see also condition
  birth
    affecting fetus or newborn 761.5
    healthy liveborn — see Newborn, multiple
  digits (congenital) 755.00
    fingers 755.01
    toes 755.02
  organ or site NEC — see Accessory
  personality 300.14
  renal arteries 747.62
Mumps 072.9
  with complication 072.8
    specified type NEC 072.79
  encephalitis 072.2
  hepatitis 072.71
  meningitis (aseptic) 072.1
  meningoencephalitis 072.2
  oophoritis 072.79

Mumps—continued
  orchitis 072.0
  pancreatitis 072.3
  polyneuropathy 072.72
  vaccination, prophylactic
    (against) V04.6
Mumu (see also Infestation, filarial)
  125.9
Münchausen syndrome 301.51
Münchmeyer's disease or syndrome
  (exostosis luxurians) 728.11
Mural — see condition
Murmur (cardiac) (heart)
    (nonorganic) (organic) 785.2
  abdominal 787.5
  aortic (valve) (see also
    Endocarditis, aortic) 424.1
  benign — omit code
  cardiorespiratory 785.2
  diastolic — see condition
  Flint (see also Endocarditis, aortic)
    424.1
  functional — omit code
  Graham Steell (pulmonic
    regurgitation) (see also
    Endocarditis, pulmonary)
    424.3
  innocent — omit code
  insignificant — omit code
  midsystolic 785.2
  mitral (valve) — see Stenosis,
    mitral
  physiologic — see condition
  presystolic, mitral — see
    Insufficiency, mitral
  pulmonic (valve) (see also
    Endocarditis, pulmonary)
    424.3
  Still's (vibratory) — omit code
  systolic (valvular) — see
    condition
  tricuspid (valve) — see
    Endocarditis, tricuspid
  valvular — see condition
  vibratory — omit code
  undiagnosed 785.2
Murri's disease (intermittent
  hemoglobinuria) 283.2
Muscae volitantes 379.24
Muscle, muscular — see condition
Musculoneuralgia 729.1
Mushrooming hip 718.95
Mushroom workers' (pickers') lung
  495.5
Mutism (see also Aphasia) 784.3
  akinetic 784.3
  deaf (acquired) (congenital) 389.7
  elective (selective) 313.23 ▼
    adjustment reaction 309.83 ▲
  hysterical 300.11
Myà's disease (congenital dilation,
  colon) 751.3
Myalgia (intercostal) 729.1
  eosinophilia syndrome 710.5
  epidemic 074.1
    cervical 078.89
  psychogenic 307.89
  traumatic NEC 959.9
Myasthenia, myasthenic 358.0
  cordis — see Failure, heart
  gravis 358.0
    neonatal 775.2
    pseudoparalytica 358.0
  stomach 536.8
  psychogenic 306.4
  syndrome
    in
      botulism 005.1 [358.1]
      diabetes mellitus 250.6
        [358.1]
      hypothyroidism (see also
        Hypothyroidism)
        244.9 [358.1]

Myasthenia, myasthenic—continued
  syndrome—continued
    in—continued
      malignant neoplasm NEC
        199.1 [358.1]
      pernicious anemia 281.0
        [358.1]
      thyrotoxicosis (see also
        Thyrotoxicosis) 242.9
        [358.1]
Mycelium infection NEC 117.9
Mycetismus 988.1
Mycetoma (actinomycotic) 039.9
  bone 039.8
    mycotic 117.4
  foot 039.4
    mycotic 117.4
  madurae 039.9
    mycotic 117.4
  maduromycotic 039.9
    mycotic 117.4
  mycotic 117.4
  nocardial 039.9
Mycobacteriosis — see
  Mycobacterium
Mycobacterium, mycobacterial
    (infection) 031.9
  acid-fast (bacilli) 031.9
  anonymous (see also
    Mycobacterium, atypical)
    031.9
  atypical (acid-fast bacilli) 031.9
    cutaneous 031.1
    pulmonary 031.0
      tuberculous (see also
        Tuberculosis,
        pulmonary) 011.9
    specified site NEC 031.8
  avium 031.0
  balnei 031.1
  Battey 031.0
  cutaneous 031.1
  fortuitum 031.0
  intracellulare (battey bacillus)
    031.0
  kakerifu 031.8
  kansasii 031.0
  kasongo 031.8
  leprae — see Leprosy
  luciflavum 031.0
  marinum 031.1
  pulmonary 031.0
    tuberculous (see also
      Tuberculosis,
      pulmonary) 011.9
  scrofulaceum 031.1
  tuberculosis (human, bovine) —
    see also Tuberculosis
    avian type 031.0
  ulcerans 031.1
  xenopi 031.0
Mycosis, mycotic 117.9
  cutaneous NEC 111.9
  ear 111.8 [380.15]
  fungoides (M9700/3) 202.1
  mouth 112.0
  pharynx 117.9
  skin NEC 111.9
  stomatitis 112.0
  systemic NEC 117.9
  tonsil 117.9
  vagina, vaginitis 112.1
Mydriasis (persistent) (pupil) 379.43
Myelatelia 742.59
Myelinoclasis, perivascular, acute
  (postinfectious) NEC 136.9
    [323.6]
  postimmunization or postvaccinal
    323.5
Myelinosis, central pontine 341.8

Myelitis (acute) (ascending)
    (cerebellar) (childhood)
    (chronic) (descending) (diffuse)
    (disseminated) (pressure)
    (progressive) (spinal cord)
    (subacute) (transverse) (see
    also Encephalitis) 323.9
  late effect — see category 326
  optic neuritis in 341.0
  postchickenpox 052.7
  postvaccinal 323.5
  syphilitic (transverse) 094.89
  tuberculous (see also
    Tuberculosis) 013.6
  virus 049.9
Myeloblastic — see condition
Myelocele (see also Spina bifida)
  741.9
  with hydrocephalus 741.0
Myelocystocele (see also Spina
  bifida) 741.9
Myelocytic — see condition
Myelocytoma 205.1
Myelodysplasia (spinal cord) 742.59
  meaning myelodysplastic
    syndrome — see
    Syndrome, myelodysplastic
Myeloencephalitis — see
  Encephalitis
Myelofibrosis (osteosclerosis) 289.8
Myelogenous — see condition
Myeloid — see condition
Myelokathexis 288.0
Myeloleukodystrophy 330.0
Myelolipoma (M8870/0) — see
  Neoplasm, by site, benign
Myeloma (multiple) (plasma cell)
    (plasmacytic) (M9730/3) 203.0
  monostotic (M9731/1) 238.6
  solitary (M9731/1) 238.6
Myelomalacia 336.8
Myelomata, multiple (M9730/3)
  203.0
Myelomatosis (M9730/3) 203.0
Myelomeningitis — see
  Meningoencephalitis
Myelomeningocele (spinal cord) (see
  also Spina bifida) 741.9
  fetal, causing fetopelvic
    disproportion 653.7
Myelo-osteo-musculodysplasia
  hereditaria 756.89
Myelopathic — see condition
Myelopathy (spinal cord) 336.9
  cervical 721.1
  diabetic 250.6 [336.3]
  drug-induced 336.8
  due to or with
    carbon tetrachloride 987.8
      [323.7]
    degeneration or displacement,
      intervertebral disc
      722.70
      cervical, cervicothoracic
        722.71
      lumbar, lumbosacral
        722.73
      thoracic, thoracolumbar
        722.72
    hydroxyquinoline derivatives
      961.3 [323.7]
    infection — see Encephalitis
    intervertebral disc disorder
      722.70
      cervical, cervicothoracic
        722.71
      lumbar, lumbosacral
        722.73
      thoracic, thoracolumbar
        722.72
    lead 984.9 [323.7]
    mercury 985.0 [323.7]

Myelopathy—continued
  due to or with—continued
    neoplastic disease (see also
      Neoplasm, by site)
      239.9 [336.3]
    pernicious anemia 281.0
      [336.3]
  spondylosis 721.91
    cervical 721.1
    lumbar, lumbosacral
      721.42
    thoracic 721.41
  thallium 985.8 [323.7]
  lumbar, lumbosacral 721.42
  necrotic (subacute) 336.1
  radiation-induced 336.8
  spondylogenic NEC 721.91
    cervical 721.1
    lumbar, lumbosacral 721.42
    thoracic 721.41
  thoracic 721.41
  toxic NEC 989.9 [323.7]
  transverse (see also Encephalitis)
    323.9
  vascular 336.1
Myeloproliferative disease
  (M9960/1) 238.7
Myeloradiculitis (see also
  Polyneuropathy) 357.0
Myeloradiculodysplasia (spinal)
  742.59
Myelosarcoma (M9930/3) 205.3
Myelosclerosis 289.8
  with myeloid metaplasia
    (M9961/1) 238.7
  disseminated, of nervous system
    340
  megakaryocytic (M9961/1) 238.7
Myelosis (M9860/3) (see also
    Leukemia, myeloid) 205.9
  acute (M9861/3) 205.0
  aleukemic (M9864/3) 205.8
  chronic (M9863/3) 205.1
  erythremic (M9840/3) 207.0
    acute (M9841/3) 207.0
  megakaryocytic (M9920/3) 207.2
  nonleukemic (chronic) 288.8
  subacute (M9862/3) 205.2
Myesthenia — see Myasthenia
Myiasis (cavernous) 134.0
  orbit 134.0 [376.13]
Myoadenoma, prostate 600
Myoblastoma
  granular cell (M9580/0) —
    also see Neoplasm, connective
    tissue, benign
    malignant (M9580/3) — see
      Neoplasm, connective
      tissue, malignant
  tongue (M9580/0) 210.1
Myocardial — see condition
Myocardiopathy (congestive)
    (constrictive) (familial)
    (hypertrophic nonobstructive)
    (idiopathic) (infiltrative)
    (obstructive) (primary)
    (restrictive) (sporadic) 425.4
  alcoholic 425.5
  amyloid 277.3 [425.7]
  beriberi 265.0 [425.7]
  cobalt-beer 425.5
  due to
    amyloidosis 277.3 [425.7]
    beriberi 265.0 [425.7]
    cardiac glycogenosis 271.0
      [425.7]
    Chagas' disease 086.0
    Friedreich's ataxia 334.0
      [425.8]
    influenza 487.8 [425.8]
    mucopolysaccharidosis 277.5
      [425.7]
    myotonia atrophica 359.2
      [425.8]

Myocardiopathy—continued
  due to—continued
    progressive muscular
      dystrophy 359.1 *[425.8]*
    sarcoidosis 135 *[425.8]*
    glycogen storage 271.0 *[425.7]*
    hypertrophic obstructive 425.1
    metabolic NEC 277.9 *[425.7]*
    nutritional 269.9 *[425.7]*
    obscure (African) 425.2
    postpartum 674.8
    secondary 425.9
    thyrotoxic (see also
      Thyrotoxicosis) 242.9
      [425.7]
    toxic NEC 425.9
Myocarditis (fibroid) (interstitial)
  (old) (progressive) (senile)
  (with arteriosclerosis) 429.0
  with
    rheumatic fever (conditions
      classifiable to 390)
      398.0
      active (see also
        Myocarditis, acute,
        rheumatic) 391.2
      inactive or quiescent (with
        chorea) 398.0
  active (nonrheumatic) 422.90
    rheumatic 391.2
      with chorea (acute)
        (rheumatic)
        (Sydenham's) 392.0
  acute or subacute (interstitial)
    422.90
    due to Streptococcus (beta-
      hemolytic) 391.2
    idiopathic 422.91
    rheumatic 391.2
      with chorea (acute)
        (rheumatic)
        (Sydenham's) 392.0
    specified type NEC 422.99
  aseptic of newborn 074.23
  bacterial (acute) 422.92
  chagasic 086.0
  chronic (interstitial) 429.0
  congenital 746.89
  constrictive 425.4
  Coxsackie (virus) 074.23
  diphtheritic 032.82
  due to or in
    Coxsackie (virus) 074.23
    diphtheria 032.82
    epidemic louse-borne typhus
      080 *[422.0]*
    influenza 487.8 *[422.0]*
    Lyme disease 088.81 *[422.0]*
    scarlet fever 034.1 *[422.0]*
    toxoplasmosis (acquired)
      130.3
    tuberculosis (see also
      Tuberculosis) 017.9
      [422.0]
    typhoid 002.0 *[422.0]*
    typhus NEC 081.9 *[422.0]*
  eosinophilic 422.91
  epidemic of newborn 074.23
  Fiedler's (acute) (isolated)
    (subacute) 422.91
  giant cell (acute) (subacute)
    422.91
  gonococcal 098.85
  granulomatous (idiopathic)
    (isolated) (nonspecific)
    422.91
  hypertensive (see also
    Hypertension, heart)
    402.90
  idiopathic 422.91
    granulomatous 422.91
  infective 422.92
  influenzal 487.8 *[422.0]*
  isolated (diffuse) (granulomatous)
    422.91
  malignant 422.99
  meningococcal 036.43

Myocardiopathy—continued
  nonrheumatic, active 422.90
  parenchymatous 422.90
  pneumococcal (acute) (subacute)
    422.92
  rheumatic (chronic) (inactive)
    (with chorea) 398.0
    active or acute 391.2
      with chorea (acute)
        (rheumatic)
        (Sydenham's) 392.0
  septic 422.92
  specific (giant cell) (productive)
    422.91
  staphylococcal (acute) (subacute)
    422.92
  suppurative 422.92
  syphilitic (chronic) 093.82
  toxic 422.93
    rheumatic (see also
      Myocarditis, acute
      rheumatic) 391.2
  tuberculous (see also
    Tuberculosis) 017.9 *[422.0]*
  typhoid 002.0 *[422.0]*
  valvular — see Endocarditis
  viral, except Coxsackie 422.91
    Coxsackie 074.23
    of newborn (Coxsackie)
      074.23
Myocardium, myocardial — see
  condition
Myocardosis (see also
  Cardiomyopathy) 425.4
Myoclonia (essential) 333.2
  epileptica 333.2
  Friedrich's 333.2
  massive 333.2
Myoclonic
  epilepsy, familial (progressive)
    333.2
  jerks 333.2
Myoclonus (familial essential)
  (multifocal) (simplex) 333.2
  facial 351.8
  massive (infantile) 333.2
  pharyngeal 478.29
Myodiastasis 728.84
Myoendocarditis — see also
  Endocarditis
  acute or subacute 421.9
Myoepithelioma (M8982/0) — see
  Neoplasm, by site, benign
Myofascitis (acute) 729.1
  low back 724.2
Myofibroma (M8890/0) — see also
  Neoplasm, connective tissue,
  benign
  uterus (cervix) (corpus) (see also
    Leiomyoma) 218.9
Myofibrosis 728.2
  heart (see also Myocarditis) 429.0
  humeroscapular region 726.2
  scapulohumeral 726.2
Myofibrositis (see also Myositis)
  729.1
  scapulohumeral 726.2
Myogelosis (occupational) 728.89
Myoglobinuria 791.3
Myoglobulinuria, primary 791.3
Myokymia — see also Myoclonus
  facial 351.8
Myolipoma (M8860/0)
  specified site — see Neoplasm,
    connective tissue, benign
  unspecified site 223.0
Myoma (M8895/0) — see also
  Neoplasm, connective tissue,
  benign
  cervix (stump) (uterus) (see also
    Leiomyoma) 218.9
  malignant (M8895/3) — see
    Neoplasm, connective
    tissue, malignant

Myoma—continued
  prostate 600
  uterus (cervix) (corpus) (see also
    Leiomyoma) 218.9
    in pregnancy or childbirth
      654.1
      affecting fetus or newborn
        763.8
      causing obstructed labor
        660.2
        affecting fetus or
          newborn 763.1
Myomalacia 728.9
  cordis, heart (see also
    Degeneration, myocardial)
    429.1
Myometritis (see also Endometritis)
  615.9
Myometrium — see condition
Myonecrosis, clostridial 040.0
Myopathy 359.9
  alcoholic 359.4
  amyloid 277.3 *[359.6]*
  benign congenital 359.0
  central core 359.0
  centronuclear 359.0
  congenital (benign) 359.0
  distal 359.1
  due to drugs 359.4
  endocrine 259.9 *[359.5]*
    specified type NEC 259.8
      [359.5]
  extraocular muscles 376.82
  facioscapulohumeral 359.1
  in
    Addison's disease 255.4
      [359.5]
    amyloidosis 277.3 *[359.6]*
    cretinism 243 *[359.5]*
    Cushing's syndrome 255.0
      [359.5]
    disseminated lupus
      erythematosus 710.0
      [359.6]
    giant cell arteritis 446.5
      [359.6]
    hyperadrenocorticism NEC
      255.3 *[359.5]*
    hyperparathyroidism 252.0
      [359.5]
    hypopituitarism 253.2 *[359.5]*
    hypothyroidism (see also
      Hypothyroidism) 244.9
      [359.5]
    malignant neoplasm NEC
      (M8000/3) 199.1
      [359.6]
    myxedema (see also
      Myxedema) 244.9
      [359.5]
    polyarteritis nodosa 446.0
      [359.6]
    rheumatoid arthritis 714.0
      [359.6]
    sarcoidosis 135 *[359.6]*
    scleroderma 710.1 *[359.6]*
    Sjögren's disease 710.2
      [359.6]
    thyrotoxicosis (see also
      Thyrotoxicosis) 242.9
      [359.5]
  inflammatory 359.8
  limb-girdle 359.1
  myotubular 359.0
  nemaline 359.0
  ocular 359.1
  oculopharyngeal 359.1
  primary 359.8
  progressive NEC 359.8
  rod body 359.0
  scapulohumeral 359.1
  specified type NEC 359.8
  toxic 359.4
Myopericarditis (see also
  Pericarditis) 423.9

Myopia (axial) (congenital)
  (increased curvature or
  refraction, nucleus of lens)
  367.1
  degenerative, malignant 360.21
  malignant 360.21
  progressive high (degenerative)
    360.21
Myosarcoma (M8895/3) — see
  Neoplasm, connective tissue,
  malignant
Myosis (persistent) 379.42
  stromal (endolymphatic)
    (M8931/1) 236.0
Myositis 729.1
  clostridial 040.0
  due to posture 729.1
  epidemic 074.1
  fibrosa or fibrous (chronic) 728.2
    Volkmann's (complicating
      trauma) 958.6
  infective 728.1
  interstitial 728.81
  multiple — see Polymyositis
  occupational 729.1
  orbital, chronic 376.12
  ossificans 728.12
    circumscribed 728.12
    progressive 728.11
    traumatic 728.12
  progressive fibrosing 728.11
  purulent 728.0
  rheumatic 729.1
  rheumatoid 729.1
  suppurative 728.0
  syphilitic 095.6
  traumatic (old) 729.1
Myospasia impulsiva 307.23
Myotonia (acquisita) (intermittens)
  728.85
  atrophica 359.2
  congenita 359.2
  dystrophica 359.2
Myotonic pupil 379.46
Myriapodiasis 134.1
Myringitis
  with otitis media — see Otitis
    media
  acute 384.00
    specified type NEC 384.09
  bullosa hemorrhagica 384.01
  bullous 384.01
  chronic 384.1
Mysophobia 300.29
Mytilotoxism 988.0
Myxadenitis labialis 528.5
Myxedema (adult) (idiocy) (infantile)
  (juvenile) (thyroid gland) (see
  also Hypothyroidism) 244.9
  circumscribed 242.9
  congenital 243
  cutis 701.8
  localized (pretibial) 242.9
  madness (acute) 293.0
    subacute 293.1
  papular 701.8
  pituitary 244.8
  postpartum 674.8
  pretibial 242.9
  primary 244.9
Myxochondrosarcoma (M9220/3) —
  see Neoplasm, cartilage,
  malignant
Myxofibroma (M8811/0) — see also
  Neoplasm, connective tissue,
  benign
  odontogenic (M9320/0) 213.1
    upper jaw (bone) 213.0
Myxofibrosarcoma (M8811/3) — see
  Neoplasm, connective tissue,
  malignant
Myxolipoma (M8852/0) (see also
  Lipoma, by site) 214.9

Myxoliposarcoma (M8852/3) — see
Neoplasm, connective tissue,
malignant
Myxoma (M8840/0) — see also
Neoplasm, connective tissue,
benign
odontogenic (M9320/0) 213.1
upper jaw (bone) 213.0
Myxosarcoma (M8840/3) — see
Neoplasm, connective tissue,
malignant

N

Naegeli's
disease (hereditary hemorrhagic
thrombasthenia) 287.1
leukemia, monocytic (M9863/3)
205.1
syndrome (incontinentia
pigmenti) 757.33
Naffziger's syndrome 353.0
Naga sore (see also Ulcer, skin)
707.9
Nägele's pelvis 738.6
with disproportion (fetopelvic)
653.0
affecting fetus or newborn
763.1
causing obstructed labor 660.1
affecting fetus or newborn
763.1
Nager-de Reynier syndrome
(dysostosis mandibularis)
756.0
Nail — see also condition
biting 307.9
patella syndrome (hereditary
osteoonychodysplasia)
756.89
Nanism, nonosomia (see also
Dwarfism) 259.4
hypophyseal 253.3
pituitary 253.3
renis, renalis 588.0
Nanukayami 100.89
Napkin rash 691.0
Narcissism 301.81
Narcolepsy 347
Narcosis
carbon dioxide (respiratory)
786.09
due to drug
correct substance properly
administered 780.09
overdose or wrong substance
given or taken 977.9
specified drug — see Table
of drugs and
chemicals
Narcotism (chronic) (see also listing
under Dependence) 304.9
acute
correct substance properly
administered 349.82
overdose or wrong substance
given or taken 967.8
specified drug — see Table
of drugs and
chemicals
Narrow
anterior chamber angle 365.02
pelvis (inlet) (outlet) — see
Contraction, pelvis
Narrowing
artery NEC 447.1
auditory, internal 433.8
basilar 433.0
with other precerebral
artery 433.3
bilateral 433.3
carotid 433.1

Narrowing—continued
artery—continued
carotid—continued
with other precerebral
artery 433.3
bilateral 433.3
cerebellar 433.8
choroidal 433.8
communicating posterior
433.8
coronary — see also
Arteriosclerosis,
coronary
congenital 746.85
due to syphilis 090.5
hypophyseal 433.8
pontine 433.8
precerebral NEC 433.9
multiple or bilateral 433.3
specified NEC 433.8
vertebral 433.2
with other precerebral
artery 433.3
bilateral 433.3
auditory canal (external) (see also
Stricture, ear canal,
acquired) 380.50
cerebral arteries 437.0
cicatricial — see Cicatrix
congenital — see Anomaly,
congenital
coronary artery — see Narrowing,
artery, coronary
ear, middle 385.22
Eustachian tube (see also
Obstruction, Eustachian
tube) 381.60
eyelid 374.46
congenital 743.62
intervertebral disc or space NEC
— see Degeneration,
intervertebral disc
joint space, hip 719.85
larynx 478.74
lids 374.46
congenital 743.62
mesenteric artery (with gangrene)
557.0
palate 524.8
palpebral fissure 374.46
retinal artery 362.13
ureter 593.3
urethra (see also Stricture,
urethra) 598.9
Narrowness, abnormal, eyelid
743.62
Nasal — see condition
Nasolacrimal — see condition
Nasopharyngeal — see also
condition
bursa 478.29
pituitary gland 759.2
torticollis 723.5
Nasopharyngitis (acute) (infective)
(subacute) 460
chronic 472.2
due to external agent — see
Condition, respiratory,
chronic, due to
due to external agent — see
Condition, respiratory, due
to
septic 034.0
streptococcal 034.0
suppurative (chronic) 472.2
ulcerative (chronic) 472.2
Nasopharynx, nasopharyngeal —
see condition
Natal tooth, teeth 520.6
Nausea (see also Vomiting) 787.02
with vomiting 787.01
epidemic 078.82
gravidarum — see Hyperemesis,
gravidarum
marina 994.6

Navel — see condition
Neapolitan fever (see also
Brucellosis) 023.9
Nearsightedness 367.1
Near-syncope 780.2
Nebécourt's syndrome 253.3
Nebula, cornea (eye) 371.01
congenital 743.43
interfering with vision 743.42
Necator americanus infestation
126.1
Necatoriasis 126.1
Neck — see condition
Necrencephalus (see also Softening,
brain) 437.8
Necrobacillosis 040.3
Necrobiosis 799.8
brain or cerebral (see also
Softening, brain) 437.8
lipoidica 709.3
diabeticorum 250.8 [709.3]
Necrodermolysis 695.1
Necrolysis, toxic epidermal 695.1
due to drug
correct substance properly
administered 695.1
overdose or wrong substance
given or taken 977.9
specified drug — see Table
of drugs and
chemicals
Necrophilia 302.89
Necrosis, necrotic (ischemic) (see
also Gangrene) 785.4
adrenal (capsule) (gland) 255.8
antrum, nasal sinus 478.1
aorta (hyaline) (see also
Aneurysm, aorta) 441.9
cystic medial 441.00
abdominal 441.02
thoracic 441.01
thoracoabdominal
441.03
ruptured 441.5
arteritis 446.0
artery 447.5
aseptic, bone 733.40
femur (head) (neck) 733.42
medial condyle 733.43
humoral head 733.41
medial femoral condyle
733.43
specific site NEC 733.49
talus 733.44
avascular, bone NEC (see also
Necrosis, aseptic, bone)
733.40
bladder (aseptic) (sphincter) 596.8
bone (see also Osteomyelitis)
730.1
acute 730.0
aseptic or avascular 733.40
femur (head) (neck) 733.42
medial condyle 733.43
humoral head 733.41
medial femoral condyle
733.43
specified site NEC 733.49
talus 733.44
ethmoid 478.1
ischemic 733.40
jaw 526.4
marrow 289.8
Paget's (osteitis deformans)
731.0
tuberculous — see
Tuberculosis, bone
brain (softening) (see also
Softening, brain) 437.8
breast (aseptic) (fat) (segmental)
611.3
bronchus, bronchi 519.1
central nervous system NEC (see
also Softening, brain) 437.8

Necrosis, necrotic—continued
cerebellar (see also Softening,
brain) 437.8
cerebral (softening) (see also
Softening, brain) 437.8
cerebrospinal (softening) (see also
Softening, brain) 437.8
cornea (see also Keratitis) 371.40
cortical, kidney 583.6
cystic medial (aorta) 441.00
abdominal 441.02
thoracic 441.01
thoracoabdominal 441.03
dental 521.0
pulp 522.1
due to swallowing corrosive
substance — see Burn, by
site
ear (ossicle) 385.24
esophagus 530.89
ethmoid (bone) 478.1
eyelid 374.50
fat, fatty (generalized) (see also
Degeneration, fatty) 272.8
breast (aseptic) (segmental)
611.3
intestine 569.89
localized — see Degeneration,
by site, fatty
mesentery 567.8
omentum 567.8
pancreas 577.8
peritoneum 567.8
skin (subcutaneous) 709.3
newborn 778.1
femur (aseptic) (avascular) 733.42
head 733.42
medial condyle 733.43
neck 733.42
gallbladder (see also
Cholecystitis, acute) 575.0
gastric 537.89
glottis 478.79
heart (myocardium) — see Infarct,
myocardium
hepatic (see also Necrosis, liver)
570
hip (aseptic) (avascular) 733.42
intestine (acute) (hemorrhagic)
(massive) 557.0
jaw 526.4
kidney (bilateral) 583.9
acute 584.9
cortical 583.6
acute 584.6
with
abortion — see
Abortion, by
type, with
renal failure
ectopic pregnancy
(see also
categories
633.0-633.9)
639.3
molar pregnancy (see
also categories
630-632)
639.3
complicating pregnancy
646.2
affecting fetus or
newborn 760.1
following labor and
delivery 669.3
medullary (papillary) (see also
Pyelitis) 590.80
in
acute renal failure 584.7
nephritis, nephropathy
583.7

Necrosis, necrotic—continued
  kidney—continued
    papillary (see also Pyelitis) 590.80
      in
        acute renal failure 584.7
        nephritis, nephropathy 583.7
    tubular 584.5
      with
        abortion — see Abortion, by type, with renal failure
        ectopic pregnancy (see also categories 633.0-633.9) 639.3
        molar pregnancy (see also categories 630-632) 639.3
      complicating
        abortion 639.3
        ectopic or molar pregnancy 639.3
        pregnancy 646.2
          affecting fetus or newborn 760.1
      following labor and delivery 669.3
      traumatic 958.5
  larynx 478.79
  liver (acute) (congenital) (diffuse) (massive) (subacute) 570
    with
      abortion — see Abortion, by type, with specified complication NEC
      ectopic pregnancy (see also categories 633.0-633.9) 639.8
      molar pregnancy (see also categories 630-632) 639.8
    complicating pregnancy 646.7
      affecting fetus or newborn 760.8
    following
      abortion 639.8
      ectopic or molar pregnancy 639.8
    obstetrical 646.7
    postabortal 639.8
    puerperal, postpartum 674.8
    toxic 573.3
  lung 513.0
  lymphatic gland 683
  mammary gland 611.3
  mastoid (chronic) 383.1
  mesentery 557.0
    fat 567.8
  mitral valve — see Insufficiency, mitral
  myocardium, myocardial — see Infarct, myocardium
  nose (septum) 478.1
  omentum 557.0
    with mesenteric infarction 557.0
    fat 567.8
  orbit, orbital 376.10
  ossicles, ear (aseptic) 385.24
  ovary (see also Salpingo-oophoritis) 614.2
  pancreas (aseptic) (duct) (fat) 577.8
    acute 577.0
    infective 577.0
  papillary, kidney (see also Pyelitis) 590.80
  peritoneum 557.0
    with mesenteric infarction 557.0
    fat 567.8
  pharynx 462
    in granulocytopenia 288.0
  phosphorus 983.9

Necrosis, necrotic—continued
  pituitary (gland) (postpartum) (Sheehan) 253.2
  placenta (see also Placenta, abnormal) 656.7
  pneumonia 513.0
  pulmonary 513.0
  pulp (dental) 522.1
  pylorus 537.89
  radiation — see Necrosis, by site
  radium — see Necrosis, by site
  renal — see Necrosis, kidney
  sclera 379.19
  scrotum 608.89
  skin or subcutaneous tissue NEC 785.4
  spine, spinal (column) 730.18
    acute 730.18
    cord 336.1
  spleen 289.59
  stomach 537.89
  stomatitis 528.1
  subcutaneous fat 709.3
    fetus or newborn 778.1
  subendocardial — see Infarct, myocardium
  suprarenal (capsule) (gland) 255.8
  teeth, tooth 521.0
  testis 608.89
  thymus (gland) 254.8
  tonsil 474.8
  trachea 519.1
  tuberculous NEC — see Tuberculosis
  tubular (acute) (anoxic) (toxic) 584.5
    due to a procedure 997.5
  umbilical cord, affecting fetus or newborn 762.6
  vagina 623.8
  vertebra (lumbar) 730.18
    acute 730.18
    tuberculous (see also Tuberculosis) 015.0 [730.8]
  vesical (aseptic) (bladder) 596.8
  x-ray — see Necrosis, by site

Necrospermia 606.0

Necrotizing angiitis 446.0

Negativism 301.7

Neglect (child) (newborn) NEC 995.5
  affecting parent or family V61.21
  after or at birth 995.5
    affecting parent or family V61.21
  hemispatial 781.8 ▼
  left-sided 781.8
  sensory 781.8 ▲
  specified person other than child 995.81
  visuospatial 781.8 ◆

Negri bodies 071

Neill-Dingwall syndrome (microcephaly and dwarfism) 759.89

Neisserian infection NEC — see Gonococcus

Nematodiasis NEC (see also Infestation, Nematode) 127.9
  ancylostoma (see also Ancylostomiasis) 126.9

Neoformans cryptococcus infection 117.5

Neonatal — see also condition
  teeth, tooth 520.6

Neonatorum — see condition

	Malignant					
	Primary	Secondary	Ca in situ	Benign	Uncertain Behavior	Unspecified
Neoplasm, neoplastic	199.1	199.1	234.9	229.9	238.9	239.9

Notes — 1. The list below gives the code numbers for neoplasms by anatomical site. For each site there are six possible code numbers according to whether the neoplasm in question is malignant, benign, in situ, of uncertain behavior, or of unspecified nature. The description of the neoplasm will often indicate which of the six columns is appropriate; e.g., malignant melanoma of skin, benign fibroadenoma of breast, carcinoma in situ of cervix uteri.

Where such descriptors are not present, the remainder of the Index should be consulted where guidance is given to the appropriate column for each morphological (histological) variety listed; e.g., Mesonephroma — see Neoplasm, malignant; Embryoma — see also Neoplasm, uncertain behavior; Disease, Bowen's — see Neoplasm, skin, in situ. However, the guidance in the Index can be overridden if one of the descriptors mentioned above is present; e.g., malignant adenoma of colon is coded to 153.9 and not to 211.3 as the adjective "malignant" overrides the Index entry "Adenoma — see also Neoplasm, benign."

2. Sites marked with the sign * (e.g., face NEC*) should be classified to malignant neoplasm of skin of these sites if the variety of neoplasm is a squamous cell carcinoma or an epidermoid carcinoma, and to benign neoplasm of skin of these sites if the variety of neoplasm is a papilloma (any type).

	Primary	Secondary	Ca in situ	Benign	Uncertain Behavior	Unspecified
abdomen, abdominal	195.2	198.89	234.8	229.8	238.8	239.8
cavity 195.2	198.89	234.8	229.8	238.8	239.8	
organ 195.2	198.89	234.8	229.8	238.8	239.8	
viscera	195.2	198.89	234.8	229.8	238.8	239.8
wall 173.5	198.2	232.5	216.5	238.2	239.2	
connective tissue	171.5	198.89	—	215.5	238.1	239.2
abdominopelvic	195.8	198.89	234.8	229.8	238.8	239.8
accessory sinus — see Neoplasm, sinus						
acoustic nerve	192.0	198.4	—	225.1	237.9	239.7
acromion (process)	170.4	198.5	—	213.4	238.0	239.2
adenoid (pharynx) (tissue)	147.1	198.89	230.0	210.7	235.1	239.0
adipose tissue (see also Neoplasm, connective tissue)	171.9	198.89	—	215.9	238.1	239.2
adnexa (uterine)	183.9	198.82	233.3	221.8	236.3	239.5
adrenal (cortex) (gland) (medulla)	194.0	198.7	234.8	227.0	237.2	239.7
ala nasi (external)	173.3	198.2	232.3	216.3	238.2	239.2
alimentary canal or tract NEC	159.9	197.8	230.9	211.9	235.5	239.0
alveolar	143.9	198.89	230.0	210.4	235.1	239.0
mucosa	143.9	198.89	230.0	210.4	235.1	239.0
lower 143.1	198.89	230.0	210.4	235.1	239.0	
upper 143.0	198.89	230.0	210.4	235.1	239.0	
ridge or process	170.1	198.5	—	213.1	238.0	239.2
carcinoma	143.9	—	—	—	—	
lower 143.1	—	—	—	—	—	
upper 143.0	—	—	—	—	—	
lower 170.1	198.5	—	213.1	238.0	239.2	
mucosa	143.9	198.89	230.0	210.4	235.1	239.0
lower 143.1	198.89	230.0	210.4	235.1	239.0	
upper 143.0	198.89	230.0	210.4	235.1	239.0	
upper 170.0	198.5	—	213.0	238.0	239.2	
sulcus 145.1	198.89	230.0	210.4	235.1	239.0	
alveolus	143.9	198.89	230.0	210.4	235.1	239.0
lower 143.1	198.89	230.0	210.4	235.1	239.0	
upper 143.0	198.89	230.0	210.4	235.1	239.0	
ampulla of Vater	156.2	197.8	230.8	211.5	235.3	239.0
ankle NEC*	195.5	198.89	232.7	229.8	238.8	239.8
anorectum, anorectal (junction)	154.8	197.5	230.7	211.4	235.2	239.0
antecubital fossa or space*	195.4	198.89	232.6	229.8	238.8	239.8
antrum (Highmore) (maxillary)	160.2	197.3	231.8	212.0	235.9	239.1
pyloric	151.2	197.8	230.2	211.1	235.2	239.0
tympanicum	160.1	197.3	231.8	212.0	235.9	239.1
anus, anal	154.3	197.5	230.6	211.4	235.5	239.0
canal 154.2	197.5	230.5	211.4	233.5	239.0	
contiguous sites with rectosigmoid junction or rectum	154.8	—	—	—	—	—
margin	173.5	198.2	232.5	216.5	238.2	239.2
skin 173.5	198.2	232.5	216.5	238.2	239.2	
sphincter	154.2	197.5	230.5	211.4	235.5	239.0
aorta (thoracic)	171.4	198.89	—	215.4	238.1	239.2
abdominal	171.5	198.89	—	215.5	238.1	239.2
aortic body	194.6	198.89	—	227.6	237.3	239.7
aponeurosis	171.9	198.89	—	215.9	238.1	239.2
palmar	171.2	198.89	—	215.2	238.1	239.2
plantar	171.3	198.89	—	215.3	238.1	239.2
appendix	153.5	197.5	230.3	211.3	235.2	239.0
arachnoid (cerebral)	192.1	198.4	—	225.2	237.6	239.7
spinal 192.3	198.4	—	225.4	237.6	239.7	
areola (female)	174.0	198.81	233.0	217	238.3	239.3
male 175.0	198.81	233.0	217	238.3	239.3	
arm NEC*	195.4	198.89	232.6	229.8	238.8	239.8
artery — see Neoplasm, connective tissue						

	Malignant			Benign	Uncertain Behavior	Unspecified
	Primary	Seconday	Ca in situ			
Neoplasm, neoplastic—*continued*						
aryepiglottic fold	148.2	198.89	230.0	210.8	235.1	239.0
hypopharyngeal aspect	148.2	198.89	230.0	210.8	235.1	239.0
laryngeal aspect	161.1	197.3	231.0	212.1	235.6	239.1
marginal zone	148.2	198.89	230.0	210.8	235.1	239.0
arytenoid (cartilage)	161.3	197.3	231.0	212.1	235.6	239.1
fold — see Neoplasm, aryepiglottic						
atlas	170.2	198.5	—	213.2	238.0	239.2
atrium, cardiac	164.1	198.89	—	212.7	238.8	239.8
auditory						
canal (external) (skin)	173.2	198.2	232.2	216.2	238.2	239.2
internal	160.1	197.3	231.8	212.0	235.9	239.1
nerve	192.0	198.4	—	225.1	237.9	239.7
tube	160.1	197.3	231.8	212.0	235.9	239.1
opening	147.2	198.89	230.0	210.7	235.1	239.0
auricle, ear	173.2	198.2	232.2	216.2	238.2	239.2
cartilage	171.0	198.89	—	215.0	238.1	239.2
auricular canal (external)	173.2	198.2	232.2	216.2	238.2	239.2
internal	160.1	197.3	231.8	212.0	235.9	239.1
autonomic nerve or nervous system NEC	171.9	198.89	—	215.9	238.1	239.2
axilla, axillary	195.1	198.89	234.8	229.8	238.8	239.8
fold	173.5	198.2	232.5	216.5	238.2	239.2
back NEC*	195.8	198.89	232.5	229.8	238.8	239.8
Bartholin's gland	184.1	198.82	233.3	221.2	236.3	239.5
basal ganglia	191.0	198.3	—	225.0	237.5	239.6
basis pedunculi	191.7	198.3	—	225.0	237.5	239.6
bile or biliary (tract)	156.9	197.8	230.8	211.5	235.3	239.0
canaliculi (biliferi) (intrahepatic)	155.1	197.8	230.8	211.5	235.3	239.0
canals, interlobular	155.1	197.8	230.8	211.5	235.3	239.0
contiguous sites	156.8	—	—	—	—	—
duct or passage (common) (cystic) (extrahepatic)	156.1	197.8	230.8	211.5	235.3	239.0
contiguous sites with gallbladder	156.8	—	—	—	—	—
interlobular	155.1	197.8	230.8	211.5	235.3	239.0
intrahepatic	155.1	197.8	230.8	211.5	235.3	239.0
and extrahepatic	156.9	197.8	230.8	211.5	235.3	239.0
bladder (urinary)	188.9	198.1	233.7	223.3	236.7	239.4
contiguous sites	188.8	—	—	—	—	—
dome	188.1	198.1	233.7	223.3	236.7	239.4
neck	188.5	198.1	233.7	223.3	236.7	239.4
orifice	188.9	198.1	233.7	223.3	236.7	239.4
ureteric	188.6	198.1	233.7	223.3	236.7	239.4
urethral	188.5	198.1	233.7	223.3	236.7	239.4
sphincter	188.8	198.1	233.7	223.3	236.7	239.4
trigone	188.0	198.1	233.7	223.3	236.7	239.4
urachus	188.7	—	233.7	223.3	236.7	239.4
wall	188.9	198.1	233.7	223.3	236.7	239.4
anterior	188.3	198.1	233.7	223.3	236.7	239.4
lateral	188.2	198.1	233.7	223.3	236.7	239.4
posterior	188.4	198.1	233.7	223.3	236.7	239.4
blood vessel — see Neoplasm, connective tissue						
bone (periosteum)	170.9	198.5	—	213.9	238.0	239.2

Note — Carcinomas and adenocarcinomas, of any type other than intraosseous or odontogenic, of the sites listed under "Neoplasm, bone" should be considered as constituting metastatic spread from an unspecified primary site and coded to 198.5 for morbidity coding and to 199.1 for underlying cause of death coding.

acetabulum	170.6	198.5	—	213.6	238.0	239.2
acromion (process)	170.4	198.5	—	213.4	238.0	239.2
ankle	170.8	198.5	—	213.8	238.0	239.2
arm NEC	170.4	198.5	—	213.4	238.0	239.2
astragalus	170.8	198.5	—	213.8	238.0	239.2
atlas	170.2	198.5	—	213.2	238.0	239.2
axis	170.2	198.5	—	213.2	238.0	239.2
back NEC	170.2	198.5	—	213.2	238.0	239.2
calcaneus	170.8	198.5	—	213.8	238.0	239.2
calvarium	170.0	198.5	—	213.0	238.0	239.2
carpus (any)	170.5	198.5	—	213.5	238.0	239.2
cartilage NEC	170.9	198.5	—	213.9	238.0	239.2
clavicle	170.3	198.5	—	213.3	238.0	239.2
clivus	170.0	198.5	—	213.0	238.0	239.2
coccygeal vertebra	170.6	198.5	—	213.6	238.0	239.2
coccyx	170.6	198.5	—	213.6	238.0	239.2
costal cartilage	170.3	198.5	—	213.3	238.0	239.2
costovertebral joint	170.3	198.5	—	213.3	238.0	239.2
cranial	170.0	198.5	—	213.0	238.0	239.2

	Malignant			Benign	Uncertain Behavior	Unspecified
	Primary	Secondary	Ca in situ			
Neoplasm, neoplastic—*continued*						
bone (periosteum)—*continued*						
cuboid	170.8	198.5	—	213.8	238.0	239.2
cuneiform	170.9	198.5	—	213.9	238.0	239.2
ankle	170.8	198.5	—	213.8	238.0	239.2
wrist	170.5	198.5	—	213.5	238.0	239.2
digital	170.9	198.5	—	213.9	238.0	239.2
finger	170.5	198.5	—	213.5	238.0	239.2
toe	170.8	198.5	—	213.8	238.0	239.2
elbow	170.4	198.5	—	213.4	238.0	239.2
ethmoid (labyrinth)	170.0	198.5	—	213.0	238.0	239.2
face	170.0	198.5	—	213.0	238.0	239.2
lower jaw	170.1	198.5	—	213.1	238.0	239.2
femur (any part)	170.7	198.5	—	213.7	238.0	239.2
fibula (any part)	170.7	198.5	—	213.7	238.0	239.2
finger (any)	170.5	198.5	—	213.5	238.0	239.2
foot	170.8	198.5	—	213.8	238.0	239.2
forearm	170.4	198.5	—	213.4	238.0	239.2
frontal	170.0	198.5	—	213.0	238.0	239.2
hand	170.5	198.5	—	213.5	238.0	239.2
heel	170.8	198.5	—	213.8	238.0	239.2
hip	170.6	198.5	—	213.6	238.0	239.2
humerus (any part)	170.4	198.5	—	213.4	238.0	239.2
hyoid	170.0	198.5	—	213.0	238.0	239.2
ilium	170.6	198.5	—	213.6	238.0	239.2
innominate	170.6	198.5	—	213.6	238.0	239.2
intervertebral cartilage or disc	170.2	198.5	—	213.2	238.0	239.2
ischium	170.6	198.5	—	213.6	238.0	239.2
jaw (lower)	170.1	198.5	—	213.1	238.0	239.2
upper	170.0	198.5	—	213.0	238.0	239.2
knee	170.7	198.5	—	213.7	238.0	239.2
leg NEC	170.7	198.5	—	213.7	238.0	239.2
limb NEC	170.9	198.5	—	213.9	238.0	239.2
lower (long bones)	170.7	198.5	—	213.7	238.0	239.2
short bones	170.8	198.5	—	213.8	238.0	239.2
upper (long bones)	170.4	198.5	—	213.4	238.0	239.2
short bones	170.5	198.5	—	213.5	238.0	239.2
long	170.9	198.5	—	213.9	238.0	239.2
lower limbs NEC	170.7	198.5	—	213.7	238.0	239.2
upper limbs NEC	170.4	198.5	—	213.4	238.0	239.2
malar	170.0	198.5	—	213.0	238.0	239.2
mandible	170.1	198.5	—	213.1	238.0	239.2
marrow NEC	202.9	198.5	—	—	—	238.7
mastoid	170.0	198.5	—	213.0	238.0	239.2
maxilla, maxillary (superior)	170.0	198.5	—	213.0	238.0	239.2
inferior	170.1	198.5	—	213.1	238.0	239.2
metacarpus (any)	170.5	198.5	—	213.5	238.0	239.2
metatarsus (any)	170.8	198.5	—	213.8	238.0	239.2
navicular (ankle)	170.8	198.5	—	213.8	238.0	239.2
hand	170.5	198.5	—	213.5	238.0	239.2
nose, nasal	170.0	198.5	—	213.0	238.0	239.2
occipital	170.0	198.5	—	213.0	238.0	239.2
orbit	170.0	198.5	—	213.0	238.0	239.2
parietal	170.0	198.5	—	213.0	238.0	239.2
patella	170.8	198.5	—	213.8	238.0	239.2
pelvic	170.6	198.5	—	213.6	238.0	239.2
phalanges	170.9	198.5	—	213.9	238.0	239.2
foot	170.8	198.5	—	213.8	238.0	239.2
hand	170.5	198.5	—	213.5	238.0	239.2
pubic	170.6	198.5	—	213.6	238.0	239.2
radius (any part)	170.4	198.5	—	213.4	238.0	239.2
rib	170.3	198.5	—	213.3	238.0	239.2
sacral vertebra	170.6	198.5	—	213.6	238.0	239.2
sacrum	170.6	198.5	—	213.6	238.0	239.2
scaphoid (of hand)	170.5	198.5	—	213.5	238.0	239.2
of ankle	170.8	198.5	—	213.8	238.0	239.2
scapula (any part)	170.4	198.5	—	213.4	238.0	239.2
sella turcica	170.0	198.5	—	213.0	238.0	239.2
short	170.9	198.5	—	213.9	238.0	239.2
lower limb	170.8	198.5	—	213.8	238.0	239.2
upper limb	170.5	198.5	—	213.5	238.0	239.2
shoulder	170.4	198.5	—	213.4	238.0	239.2
skeleton, skeletal NEC	170.9	198.5	—	213.9	238.0	239.2
skull	170.0	198.5	—	213.0	238.0	239.2

	Malignant			Benign	Uncertain Behavior	Unspecified
	Primary	Secondary	Ca in situ			
Neoplasm, neoplastic—*continued*						
bone (periosteum)—*continued*						
sphenoid	170.0	198.5	—	213.0	238.0	239.2
spine, spinal (column)	170.2	198.5	—	213.2	238.0	239.2
coccyx	170.6	198.5	—	213.6	238.0	239.2
sacrum	170.6	198.5	—	213.6	238.0	239.2
sternum	170.3	198.5	—	213.3	238.0	239.2
tarsus (any)	170.8	198.5	—	213.8	238.0	239.2
temporal	170.0	198.5	—	213.0	238.0	239.2
thumb	170.5	198.5	—	213.5	238.0	239.2
tibia (any part)	170.7	198.5	—	213.7	238.0	239.2
toe (any)	170.8	198.5	—	213.8	238.0	239.2
trapezium	170.5	198.5	—	213.5	238.0	239.2
trapezoid	170.5	198.5	—	213.5	238.0	239.2
turbinate	170.0	198.5	—	213.0	238.0	239.2
ulna (any part)	170.4	198.5	—	213.4	238.0	239.2
unciform	170.5	198.5	—	213.5	238.0	239.2
vertebra (column)	170.2	198.5	—	213.2	238.0	239.2
coccyx	170.6	198.5	—	213.6	238.0	239.2
sacrum	170.6	198.5	—	213.6	238.0	239.2
vomer	170.0	198.5	—	213.0	238.0	239.2
wrist	170.5	198.5	—	213.5	238.0	239.2
xiphoid process	170.3	198.5	—	213.3	238.0	239.2
zygomatic	170.0	198.5	—	213.0	238.0	239.2
book-leaf (mouth)	145.8	198.89	230.0	210.4	235.1	239.0
bowel — *see* Neoplasm, intestine						
brachial plexus	171.2	198.89	—	215.2	238.1	239.2
brain NEC	191.9	198.3	—	225.0	237.5	239.6
basal ganglia	191.0	198.3	—	225.0	237.5	239.6
cerebellopontine angle	191.6	198.3	—	225.0	237.5	239.6
cerebellum NOS	191.6	198.3	—	225.0	237.5	239.6
cerebrum	191.0	198.3	—	225.0	237.5	239.6
choroid plexus	191.5	198.3	—	225.0	237.5	239.6
contiguous sites	191.8	—	—	—	—	—
corpus callosum	191.8	198.3	—	225.0	237.5	239.6
corpus striatum	191.0	198.3	—	225.0	237.5	239.6
cortex (cerebral)	191.0	198.3	—	225.0	237.5	239.6
frontal lobe	191.1	198.3	—	225.0	237.5	239.6
globus pallidus	191.0	198.3	—	225.0	237.5	239.6
hippocampus	191.2	198.3	—	225.0	237.5	239.6
hypothalamus	191.0	198.3	—	225.0	237.5	239.6
internal capsule	191.0	198.3	—	225.0	237.5	239.6
medulla oblongata	191.7	198.3	—	225.0	237.5	239.6
meninges	192.1	198.4	—	225.2	237.6	239.7
midbrain	191.7	198.3	—	225.0	237.5	239.6
occipital lobe	191.4	198.3	—	225.0	237.5	239.6
parietal lobe	191.3	198.3	—	225.0	237.5	239.6
peduncle	191.7	198.3	—	225.0	237.5	239.6
pons	191.7	198.3	—	225.0	237.5	239.6
stem	191.7	198.3	—	225.0	237.5	239.6
tapetum	191.8	198.3	—	225.0	237.5	239.6
temporal lobe	191.2	198.3	—	225.0	237.5	239.6
thalamus	191.0	198.3	—	225.0	237.5	239.6
uncus	191.2	198.3	—	225.0	237.5	239.6
ventricle (floor)	191.5	198.3	—	225.0	237.5	239.6
branchial (cleft) (vestiges)	146.8	198.89	230.0	210.6	235.1	239.0
breast (connective tissue) (female) (glandular tissue) (soft parts)	174.9	198.81	233.0	217	238.3	239.3
areola	174.0	198.81	233.0	217	238.3	239.3
male	175.0	198.81	233.0	217	238.3	239.3
axillary tail	174.6	198.81	233.0	217	238.3	239.3
central portion	174.1	198.81	233.0	217	238.3	239.3
contiguous sites	174.8	—	—	—	—	—
ectopic sites	174.8	198.81	233.0	217	238.3	239.3
inner	174.8	198.81	233.0	217	238.3	239.3
lower	174.8	198.81	233.0	217	238.3	239.3
lower-inner quadrant	174.3	198.81	233.0	217	238.3	239.3
lower-outer quadrant	174.5	198.81	233.0	217	238.3	239.3
male	175.9	198.81	233.0	217	238.3	239.3
areola	175.0	198.81	233.0	217	238.3	239.3
ectopic tissue	175.9	198.81	233.0	217	238.3	239.3
nipple	175.0	198.81	233.0	217	238.3	239.3
mastectomy site (skin)	173.5	198.2	—	—	—	—
specified as breast tissue	174.8	198.81	—	—	—	—
midline	174.8	198.81	233.0	217	238.3	239.3

	Malignant			Benign	Uncertain Behavior	Unspecified
	Primary	Seconday	Ca in situ			

	Primary	Seconday	Ca in situ	Benign	Uncertain Behavior	Unspecified
Neoplasm, neoplastic—*continued*						
breast (connective tissue) (female) (glandular tissue) (soft parts)—*continued*						
nipple	174.0	198.81	233.0	217	238.3	239.3
male	175.0	198.81	233.0	217	238.3	239.3
outer	174.8	198.81	233.0	217	238.3	239.3
skin	173.5	198.2	232.5	216.5	238.2	239.2
tail (axillary)	174.6	198.81	233.0	217	238.3	239.3
upper	174.8	198.81	233.0	217	238.3	239.3
upper-inner quadrant	174.2	198.81	233.0	217	238.3	239.3
upper-outer quadrant	174.4	198.81	233.0	217	238.3	239.3
broad ligament	183.3	198.82	233.3	221.0	236.3	239.5
bronchiogenic, bronchogenic (lung)	162.9	197.0	231.2	212.3	235.7	239.1
bronchiole	162.9	197.0	231.2	212.3	235.7	239.1
bronchus	162.9	197.0	231.2	212.3	235.7	239.1
carina	162.2	197.0	231.2	212.3	235.7	239.1
contiguous sites with lung or trachea	162.8	—	—	—	—	—
lower lobe of lung	162.5	197.0	231.2	212.3	235.7	239.1
main	162.2	197.0	231.2	212.3	235.7	239.1
middle lobe of lung	162.4	197.0	231.2	212.3	235.7	239.1
upper lobe of lung	162.3	197.0	231.2	212.3	235.7	239.1
brow	173.3	198.2	232.3	216.3	238.2	239.2
buccal (cavity)	145.9	198.89	230.0	210.4	235.1	239.0
commissure	145.0	198.89	230.0	210.4	235.1	239.0
groove (lower) (upper)	145.1	198.89	230.0	210.4	235.1	239.0
mucosa	145.0	198.89	230.0	210.4	235.1	239.0
sulcus (lower) (upper)	145.1	198.89	230.0	210.4	235.1	239.0
bulbourethral gland	189.3	198.1	233.9	223.81	236.99	239.5
bursa — *see* Neoplasm, connective tissue						
buttock NEC*	195.3	198.89	232.5	229.8	238.8	239.8
calf*	195.5	198.89	232.7	229.8	238.8	239.8
calvarium	170.0	198.5	—	213.0	238.0	239.2
calyx, renal	189.1	198.0	233.9	223.1	236.91	239.5
canal						
anal	154.2	197.5	230.5	211.4	235.5	239.0
auditory (external)	173.2	198.2	232.2	216.2	238.2	239.2
auricular (external)	173.2	198.2	232.2	216.2	238.2	239.2
canaliculi, biliary (biliferi) (intrahepatic)	155.1	197.8	230.8	211.5	235.3	239.0
canthus (eye) (inner) (outer)	173.1	198.2	232.1	216.1	238.2	239.2
capillary — *see* Neoplasm, connective tissue						
caput coli	153.4	197.5	230.3	211.3	235.2	239.0
cardia (gastric)	151.0	197.8	230.2	211.1	235.2	239.0
cardiac orifice (stomach)	151.0	197.8	230.2	211.1	235.2	239.0
cardio-esophageal junction	151.0	197.8	230.2	211.1	235.2	239.0
cardio-esophagus	151.0	197.8	230.2	211.1	235.2	239.0
carina (trachea) (bronchus)	162.2	197.0	231.2	212.3	235.7	239.1 ◆
carotid (artery)	171.0	198.89	—	215.0	238.1	239.2
body	194.5	198.89	—	227.5	237.3	239.7
carpus (any bone)	170.5	198.5	—	213.5	238.0	239.2
cartilage (articular) (joint) NEC — *see also* Neoplasm, bone	170.9	198.5	—	213.9	238.0	239.2
arytenoid	161.3	197.3	231.0	212.1	235.6	239.1
auricular	171.0	198.89	—	215.0	238.1	239.2
bronchi	162.2	197.3	—	212.3	235.7	239.1
connective tissue — *see* Neoplasm, connective tissue						
costal	170.3	198.5	—	213.3	238.0	239.2
cricoid	161.3	197.3	231.0	212.1	235.6	239.1
cuneiform	161.3	197.3	231.0	212.1	235.6	239.1
ear (external)	171.0	198.89	—	215.0	238.1	239.2
ensiform	170.3	198.5	—	213.3	238.0	239.2
epiglottis	161.1	197.3	231.0	212.1	235.6	239.1
anterior surface	146.4	198.89	230.0	210.6	235.1	239.0
eyelid	171.0	198.89	—	215.0	238.1	239.2
intervertebral	170.2	198.5	—	213.2	238.0	239.2
larynx, laryngeal	161.3	197.3	231.0	212.1	235.6	239.1
nose, nasal	160.0	197.3	231.8	212.0	235.9	239.1
pinna	171.0	198.89	—	215.0	238.1	239.2
rib	170.3	198.5	—	213.3	238.0	239.2
semilunar (knee)	170.7	198.5	—	213.7	238.0	239.2
thyroid	161.3	197.3	231.0	212.1	235.6	239.1
trachea	162.0	197.3	231.1	212.2	235.7	239.1
cauda equina	192.2	198.3	—	225.3	237.5	239.7
cavity						
buccal	145.9	198.89	230.0	210.4	235.1	239.0
nasal	160.0	197.3	231.8	212.0	235.9	239.1
oral	145.9	198.89	230.0	210.4	235.1	239.0

	Malignant			Benign	Uncertain Behavior	Unspecified
	Primary	Secondary	Ca in situ			
Neoplasm, neoplastic—continued						
cavity—continued						
peritoneal	158.9	197.6	—	211.8	235.4	239.0
tympanic	160.1	197.3	231.8	212.0	235.9	239.1
cecum	153.4	197.5	230.3	211.3	235.2	239.0
central						
nervous system — see Neoplasm, nervous system						
white matter	191.0	198.3	—	225.0	237.5	239.6
cerebellopontine (angle)	191.6	198.3	—	225.0	237.5	239.6
cerebellum, cerebellar	191.6	198.3	—	225.0	237.5	239.6
cerebrum, cerebral (cortex) (hemisphere) (white matter)	191.0	198.3	—	225.0	237.5	239.6
meninges	192.1	198.4	—	225.2	237.6	239.7
peduncle	191.7	198.3	—	225.0	237.5	239.6
ventricle (any)	191.5	198.3	—	225.0	237.5	239.6
cervical region	195.0	198.89	234.8	229.8	238.8	239.8
cervix (cervical) (uteri) (uterus)	180.9	198.82	233.1	219.0	236.0	239.5
canal	180.0	198.82	233.1	219.0	236.0	239.5
contiguous sites	180.8	—	—	—	—	—
endocervix (canal) (gland)	180.0	198.82	233.1	219.0	236.0	239.5
exocervix	180.1	198.82	233.1	219.0	236.0	239.5
external os	180.1	198.82	233.1	219.0	236.0	239.5
internal os	180.0	198.82	233.1	219.0	236.0	239.5
nabothian gland	180.0	198.82	233.1	219.0	236.0	239.5
squamocolumnar junction	180.8	198.82	233.1	219.0	236.0	239.5
stump	180.8	198.82	233.1	219.0	236.0	239.5
cheek	195.0	198.89	234.8	229.8	238.8	239.8
external	173.3	198.2	232.3	216.3	238.2	239.2
inner aspect	145.0	198.89	230.0	210.4	235.1	239.0
internal	145.0	198.89	230.0	210.4	235.1	239.0
mucosa	145.0	198.89	230.0	210.4	235.1	239.0
chest (wall) NEC	195.1	198.89	234.8	229.8	238.8	239.8
chiasma opticum	192.0	198.4	—	225.1	237.9	239.7
chin	173.3	198.2	232.3	216.3	238.2	239.2
choana	147.3	198.89	230.0	210.7	235.1	239.0
cholangiole	155.1	197.8	230.8	211.5	235.3	239.0
choledochal duct	156.1	197.8	230.8	211.5	235.3	239.0
choroid	190.6	198.4	234.0	224.6	238.8	239.8
plexus	191.5	198.3	—	225.0	237.5	239.6
ciliary body	190.0	198.4	234.0	224.0	238.8	239.8
clavicle	170.3	198.5	—	213.3	238.0	239.2
clitoris	184.3	198.82	233.3	221.2	236.3	239.5
clivus	170.0	198.5	—	213.0	238.0	239.2
cloacogenic zone	154.8	197.5	230.7	211.4	235.5	239.0
coccygeal						
body or glomus	194.6	198.89	—	227.6	237.3	239.7
vertebra	170.6	198.5	—	213.6	238.0	239.2
coccyx	170.6	198.5	—	213.6	238.0	239.2
colon — see also Neoplasm, intestine, large						
and rectum	154.0	197.5	230.4	211.4	235.2	239.0
column, spinal — see Neoplasm, spine						
columnella	173.3	198.2	232.3	216.3	238.2	239.2
commissure						
labial, lip	140.6	198.89	230.0	210.4	235.1	239.0
laryngeal	161.0	197.3	231.0	212.1	235.6	239.1
common (bile) duct	156.1	197.8	230.8	211.5	235.3	239.0
concha	173.2	198.2	232.2	216.2	238.2	239.2
nose	160.0	197.3	231.8	212.0	235.9	239.1
conjunctiva	190.3	198.4	234.0	224.3	238.8	239.8
connective tissue NEC	171.9	198.89	—	215.9	238.1	239.2

Note — For neoplasms of connective tissue (blood vessel, bursa, fascia, ligament, muscle, peripheral nerves, sympathetic and parasympathetic nerves and ganglia, synovia, tendon, etc.) or of morphological types that indicate connective tissue, code according to the list under "Neoplasm, connective tissue"; for sites that do not appear in this list, code to neoplasm of that site; e.g.,

> liposarcoma, shoulder 171.2
> leiomyosarcoma, stomach 151.9
> neurofibroma, chest wall 215.4

Morphological types that indicate connective tissue appear in the proper place in the alphabetic index with the instruction "see Neoplasm, connective tissue..."

abdomen	171.5	198.89	—	215.5	238.1	239.2
abdominal wall	171.5	198.89	—	215.5	238.1	239.2
ankle	171.3	198.89	—	215.3	238.1	239.2
antecubital fossa or space	171.2	198.89	—	215.2	238.1	239.2
arm	171.2	198.89	—	215.2	238.1	239.2
auricle (ear)	171.0	198.89	—	215.0	238.1	239.2

	Malignant			Benign	Uncertain Behavior	Unspecified
	Primary	Secondary	Ca in situ			

Neoplasm, neoplastic—*continued*						
connective tissue NEC—*continued*						
axilla	171.4	198.89	—	215.4	238.1	239.2
back	171.7	198.89	—	215.7	238.1	239.2
breast (female) (see also Neoplasm, breast)	174.9	198.81	233.0	217	238.3	239.3
male	175.9	198.81	233.0	217	238.3	239.3
buttock	171.6	198.89	—	215.6	238.1	239.2
calf	171.3	198.89	—	215.3	238.1	239.2
cervical region	171.0	198.89	—	215.0	238.1	239.2
cheek	171.0	198.89	—	215.0	238.1	239.2
chest (wall)	171.4	198.89	—	215.4	238.1	239.2
chin	171.0	198.89	—	215.0	238.1	239.2
contiguous sites	171.8	—	—	—	—	—
diaphragm	171.4	198.89	—	215.4	238.1	239.2
ear (external)	171.0	198.89	—	215.0	238.1	239.2
elbow	171.2	198.89	—	215.2	238.1	239.2
extrarectal	171.6	198.89	—	215.6	238.1	239.2
extremity	171.8	198.89	—	215.8	238.1	239.2
lower	171.3	198.89	—	215.3	238.1	239.2
upper	171.2	198.89	—	215.2	238.1	239.2
eyelid	171.0	198.89	—	215.0	238.1	239.2
face	171.0	198.89	—	215.0	238.1	239.2
finger	171.2	198.89	—	215.2	238.1	239.2
flank	171.7	198.89	—	215.7	238.1	239.2
foot	171.3	198.89	—	215.3	238.1	239.2
forearm	171.2	198.89	—	215.2	238.1	239.2
forehead	171.0	198.89	—	215.0	238.1	239.2
gluteal region	171.6	198.89	—	215.6	238.1	239.2
great vessels NEC	171.4	198.89	—	215.4	238.1	239.2
groin	171.6	198.89	—	215.6	238.1	239.2
hand	171.2	198.89	—	215.2	238.1	239.2
head	171.0	198.89	—	215.0	238.1	239.2
heel	171.3	198.89	—	215.3	238.1	239.2
hip	171.3	198.89	—	215.3	238.1	239.2
hypochondrium	171.5	198.89	—	215.5	238.1	239.2
iliopsoas muscle	171.6	198.89	—	215.5	238.1	239.2
infraclavicular region	171.4	198.89	—	215.4	238.1	239.2
inguinal (canal) (region)	171.6	198.89	—	215.6	238.1	239.2
intrathoracic	171.4	198.89	—	215.4	238.1	239.2
ischorectal fossa	171.6	198.89	—	215.6	238.1	239.2
jaw	143.9	198.89	230.0	210.4	235.1	239.0
knee	171.3	198.89	—	215.3	238.1	239.2
leg	171.3	198.89	—	215.3	238.1	239.2
limb NEC	171.9	198.89	—	215.8	238.1	239.2
lower	171.3	198.89	—	215.3	238.1	239.2
upper	171.2	198.89	—	215.2	238.1	239.2
nates	171.6	198.89	—	215.6	238.1	239.2
neck	171.0	198.89	—	215.0	238.1	239.2
orbit	190.1	198.4	234.0	224.1	238.8	239.8
pararectal	171.6	198.89	—	215.6	238.1	239.2
para-urethral	171.6	198.89	—	215.6	238.1	239.2
paravaginal	171.6	198.89	—	215.6	238.1	239.2
pelvis (floor)	171.6	198.89	—	215.6	238.1	239.2
pelvo-abdominal	171.8	198.89	—	215.8	238.1	239.2
perineum	171.6	198.89	—	215.6	238.1	239.2
perirectal (tissue)	171.6	198.89	—	215.6	238.1	239.2
periurethral (tissue)	171.6	198.89	—	215.6	238.1	239.2
popliteal fossa or space	171.3	198.89	—	215.3	238.1	239.2
presacral	171.6	198.89	—	215.6	238.1	239.2
psoas muscle	171.5	198.89	—	215.5	238.1	239.2
pterygoid fossa	171.0	198.89	—	215.0	238.1	239.2
rectovaginal septum or wall	171.6	198.89	—	215.6	238.1	239.2
rectovesical	171.6	198.89	—	215.6	238.1	239.2
retroperitoneum	158.0	197.6	—	211.8	235.4	239.0
sacrococcygeal region	171.6	198.89	—	215.6	238.1	239.2
scalp	171.0	198.89	—	215.0	238.1	239.2
scapular region	171.4	198.89	—	215.4	238.1	239.2
shoulder	171.2	198.89	—	215.2	238.1	239.2
skin (dermis) NEC	173.9	198.2	232.9	216.9	238.2	239.2
submental	171.0	198.89	—	215.0	238.1	239.2
supraclavicular region	171.0	198.89	—	215.0	238.1	239.2
temple	171.0	198.89	—	215.0	238.1	239.2
temporal region	171.0	198.89	—	215.0	238.1	239.2
thigh	171.3	198.89	—	215.3	238.1	239.2

	Malignant			Benign	Uncertain Behavior	Unspecified
	Primary	Seconday	Ca in situ			
Neoplasm, neoplastic—*continued*						
connective tissue NEC—*continued*						
thoracic (duct) (wall)	171.4	198.89	—	215.4	238.1	239.2
thorax	171.4	198.89	—	215.4	238.1	239.2
thumb	171.2	198.89	—	215.2	238.1	239.2
toe	171.3	198.89	—	215.3	238.1	239.2
trunk	171.7	198.89	—	215.7	238.1	239.2
umbilicus	171.5	198.89	—	215.5	238.1	239.2
vesicorectal	171.6	198.89	—	215.6	238.1	239.2
wrist	171.2	198.89	—	215.2	238.1	239.2
conus medullaris	192.2	198.3	—	225.3	237.5	239.7
cord (true) (vocal)	161.0	197.3	231.0	212.1	235.6	239.1
false	161.1	197.3	231.0	212.1	235.6	239.1
spermatic	187.6	198.82	233.6	222.8	236.6	239.5
spinal (cervical) (lumbar) (thoracic)	192.2	198.3	—	225.3	237.5	239.7
cornea (limbus)	190.4	198.4	234.0	224.4	238.8	239.8
corpus						
albicans	183.0	198.6	233.3	220	236.2	239.5
callosum, brain	191.8	198.3	—	225.0	237.5	239.6
cavernosum	187.3	198.82	233.5	222.1	236.6	239.5
gastric	151.4	197.8	230.2	211.1	235.2	239.0
penis	187.3	198.82	233.5	222.1	236.6	239.5
striatum, cerebrum	191.0	198.3	—	225.0	237.5	239.6
uteri	182.0	198.82	233.2	219.1	236.0	239.5
isthmus	182.1	198.82	233.2	219.1	236.0	239.5
cortex						
adrenal	194.0	198.7	234.8	227.0	237.2	239.7
cerebral	191.0	198.3	—	225.0	237.5	239.6
costal cartilage	170.3	198.5	—	213.3	238.0	239.2
costovertebral joint	170.3	198.5	—	213.3	238.0	239.2
Cowper's gland	189.3	198.1	233.9	223.81	236.99	239.5
cranial (fossa, any)	191.9	198.3	—	225.0	237.5	239.6
meninges	192.1	198.4	—	225.2	237.6	239.7
nerve (any)	192.0	198.4	—	225.1	237.9	239.7
craniobuccal pouch	194.3	198.89	234.8	227.3	237.0	239.7
craniopharyngeal (duct) (pouch)	194.3	198.89	234.8	227.3	237.0	239.7
cricoid	148.0	198.89	230.0	210.8	235.1	239.0
cartilage	161.3	197.3	231.0	212.1	235.6	239.1
cricopharynx	148.0	198.89	230.0	210.8	235.1	239.0
crypt of Morgagni	154.8	197.5	230.7	211.4	235.2	239.0
crystalline lens	190.0	198.4	234.0	224.0	238.8	239.8
cul-de-sac (Douglas')	158.8	197.6	—	211.8	235.4	239.0
cuneiform cartilage	161.3	197.3	231.0	212.1	235.6	239.1
cutaneous — *see* Neoplasm, skin						
cutis — *see* Neoplasm, skin						
cystic (bile) duct (common)	156.1	197.8	230.8	211.5	235.3	239.0
dermis — *see* Neoplasm, skin						
diaphragm	171.4	198.89	—	215.4	238.1	239.2
digestive organs, system, tube, or tract NEC	159.9	197.8	230.9	211.9	235.5	239.0
contiguous sites with peritoneum	159.8	—	—	—	—	—
disc, intervertebral	170.2	198.5	—	213.2	238.0	239.2
disease, generalized	199.0	199.0	234.9	229.9	238.9	199.0
disseminated	199.0	199.0	234.9	229.9	238.9	199.0
Douglas' cul-de-sac or pouch	158.8	197.6	—	211.8	235.4	239.0
duodenojejunal junction	152.8	197.4	230.7	211.2	235.2	239.0
duodenum	152.0	197.4	230.7	211.2	235.2	239.0
dura (cranial) (mater)	192.1	198.4	—	225.2	237.6	239.7
cerebral	192.1	198.4	—	225.2	237.6	239.7
spinal	192.3	198.4	—	225.4	237.6	239.7
ear (external)	173.2	198.2	232.2	216.2	238.2	239.2
auricle or auris	173.2	198.2	232.2	216.2	238.2	239.2
canal, external	173.2	198.2	232.2	216.2	238.2	239.2
cartilage	171.0	198.89	—	215.0	238.1	239.2
external meatus	173.2	198.2	232.2	216.2	238.2	239.2
inner	160.1	197.3	231.8	212.0	235.9	239.1
lobule	173.2	198.2	232.2	216.2	238.2	239.2
middle	160.1	197.3	231.8	212.0	235.9	239.1
contiguous sites with accessory sinuses or nasal cavities	160.8	—	—	—	—	—
skin	173.2	198.2	232.2	216.2	238.2	239.2
earlobe	173.2	198.2	232.2	216.2	238.2	239.2
ejaculatory duct	187.8	198.82	233.6	222.8	236.6	239.5
elbow NEC*	195.4	198.89	232.6	229.8	238.8	239.8
endocardium	164.1	198.89	—	212.7	238.8	239.8
endocervix (canal) (gland)	180.0	198.82	233.1	219.0	236.0	239.5

	Malignant			Benign	Uncertain Behavior	Unspecified
	Primary	Secondary	Ca in situ			
Neoplasm, neoplastic—*continued*						
endocrine gland NEC	194.9	198.89	—	227.9	237.4	239.7
pluriglandular NEC	194.8	198.89	234.8	227.8	237.4	239.7
endometrium (gland) (stroma)	182.0	198.82	233.2	219.1	236.0	239.5
ensiform cartilage	170.3	198.5	—	213.3	238.0	239.2
enteric — *see* Neoplasm, intestine						
ependyma (brain)	191.5	198.3	—	225.0	237.5	239.6
epicardium	164.1	198.89	—	212.7	238.8	239.8
epididymis	187.5	198.82	233.6	222.3	236.6	239.5
epidural	192.9	198.4	—	225.9	237.9	239.7
epiglottis	161.1	197.3	231.0	212.1	235.6	239.1
anterior aspect or surface	146.4	198.89	230.0	210.6	235.1	239.0
cartilage	161.3	197.3	231.0	212.1	235.6	239.1
free border (margin)	146.4	198.89	230.0	210.6	235.1	239.0
junctional region	146.5	198.89	230.0	210.6	235.1	239.0
posterior (laryngeal) surface	161.1	197.3	231.0	212.1	235.6	239.1
suprahyoid portion	161.1	197.3	231.0	212.1	235.6	239.1
esophagogastric junction	151.0	197.8	230.2	211.1	235.2	239.0
esophagus	150.9	197.8	230.1	211.0	235.5	239.0
abdominal	150.2	197.8	230.1	211.0	235.5	239.0
cervical	150.0	197.8	230.1	211.0	235.5	239.0
contiguous sites	150.8	—	—	—	—	—
distal (third)	150.5	197.8	230.1	211.0	235.5	239.0
lower (third)	150.5	197.8	230.1	211.0	235.5	239.0
middle (third)	150.4	197.8	230.1	211.0	235.5	239.0
proximal (third)	150.3	197.8	230.1	211.0	235.5	239.0
specified part NEC	150.8	197.8	230.1	211.0	235.5	239.0
thoracic	150.1	197.8	230.1	211.0	235.5	239.0
upper (third)	150.3	197.8	230.1	211.0	235.5	239.0
ethmoid (sinus)	160.3	197.3	231.8	212.0	235.9	239.1
bone or labyrinth	170.0	198.5	—	213.0	238.0	239.2
Eustachian tube	160.1	197.3	231.8	212.0	235.9	239.1
exocervix	180.1	198.82	233.1	219.0	236.0	239.5
external						
meatus (ear)	173.2	198.2	232.2	216.2	238.2	239.2
os, cervix uteri	180.1	198.82	233.1	219.0	236.0	239.5
extradural	192.9	198.4	—	225.9	237.9	239.7
extrahepatic (bile) duct	156.1	197.8	230.8	211.5	235.3	239.0
contiguous sites with gallbladder	156.8	—	—	—	—	—
extraocular muscle	190.1	198.4	234.0	224.1	238.8	239.8
extrarectal	195.3	198.89	234.8	229.8	238.8	239.8
extremity*	195.8	198.89	232.8	229.8	238.8	239.8
lower*	195.5	198.89	232.7	229.8	238.8	239.8
upper*	195.4	198.89	232.6	229.8	238.8	239.8
eye NEC	190.9	198.4	234.0	224.9	238.8	239.8
contiguous sites	190.8	—	—	—	—	—
specified sites NEC	190.8	198.4	234.0	224.8	238.8	239.8
eyeball	190.0	198.4	234.0	224.0	238.8	239.8
eyebrow	173.3	198.2	232.3	216.3	238.2	239.2
eyelid (lower) (skin) (upper)	173.1	198.2	232.1	216.1	238.2	239.2
cartilage	171.0	198.89	—	215.0	238.1	239.2
face NEC*	195.0	198.89	232.3	229.8	238.8	239.8
fallopian tube (accessory)	183.2	198.82	233.3	221.0	236.3	239.5
falx (cerebelli) (cerebri)	192.1	198.4	—	225.2	237.6	239.7
fascia — *see also* Neoplasm, connective tissue						
palmar	171.2	198.89	—	215.2	238.1	239.2
plantar	171.3	198.89	—	215.3	238.1	239.2
fatty tissue — *see* Neoplasm, connective tissue						
fauces, faucial NEC	146.9	198.89	230.0	210.6	235.1	239.0
pillars	146.2	198.89	230.0	210.6	235.1	239.0
tonsil	146.0	198.89	230.0	210.5	235.1	239.0
femur (any part)	170.7	198.5	—	213.7	238.0	239.2
fetal membrane	181	198.82	233.2	219.8	236.1	239.5
fibrous tissue — *see* Neoplasm, connective tissue						
fibula (any part)	170.7	198.5	—	213.7	238.0	239.2
filum terminale	192.2	198.3	—	225.3	237.5	239.7
finger NEC*	195.4	198.89	232.6	229.8	238.8	239.8
flank NEC*	195.8	198.89	232.5	229.8	238.8	239.8
follicle, nabothian	180.0	198.82	233.1	219.0	236.0	239.5
foot NEC*	195.5	198.89	232.7	229.8	238.8	239.8
forearm NEC*	195.4	198.89	232.6	229.8	238.8	239.8
forehead (skin)	173.3	198.2	232.3	216.3	238.2	239.2
foreskin	187.1	198.82	233.5	222.1	236.6	239.5

	Malignant			Benign	Uncertain Behavior	Unspecified
	Primary	Secondary	Ca in situ			
Neoplasm, neoplastic—*continued*						
fornix						
pharyngeal	147.3	198.89	230.0	210.7	235.1	239.0
vagina	184.0	198.82	233.3	221.1	236.3	239.5
fossa (of)						
anterior (cranial)	191.9	198.3	—	225.0	237.5	239.6
cranial	191.9	198.3	—	225.0	237.5	239.6
ischiorectal	195.3	198.89	234.8	229.8	238.8	239.8
middle (cranial)	191.9	198.3	—	225.0	237.5	239.6
pituitary	194.3	198.89	234.8	227.3	237.0	239.7
posterior (cranial)	191.9	198.3	—	225.0	237.5	239.6
pterygoid	171.0	198.89	—	215.0	238.1	239.2
pyriform	148.1	198.89	230.0	210.8	235.1	239.0
Rosenmüller	147.2	198.89	230.0	210.7	235.1	239.0
tonsillar	146.1	198.89	230.0	210.6	235.1	239.0
fourchette	184.4	198.82	233.3	221.2	236.3	239.5
frenulum						
labii — *see* Neoplasm, lip, internal						
linguae	141.3	198.89	230.0	210.1	235.1	239.0
frontal						
bone	170.0	198.5	—	213.0	238.0	239.2
lobe, brain	191.1	198.3	—	225.0	237.5	239.6
meninges	192.1	198.4	—	225.2	237.6	239.7
pole	191.1	198.3	—	225.0	237.5	239.6
sinus	160.4	197.3	231.8	212.0	235.9	239.1
fundus						
stomach	151.3	197.8	230.2	211.1	235.2	239.0
uterus	182.0	198.82	233.2	219.1	236.0	239.5
gall duct (extrahepatic)	156.1	197.8	230.8	211.5	235.3	239.0
intrahepatic	155.1	197.8	230.8	211.5	235.3	239.0
gallbladder	156.0	197.8	230.8	211.5	235.3	239.0
contiguous sites with extrahepatic bile ducts	156.8	—	—	—	—	—
ganglia (*see also* Neoplasm, connective tissue)	171.9	198.89	—	215.9	238.1	239.2
basal	191.0	198.3	—	225.0	237.5	239.6
ganglion (*see also* Neoplasm, connective tissue)	171.9	198.89	—	215.9	238.1	239.2
cranial nerve	192.0	198.4	—	225.1	237.9	239.7
Gartner's duct	184.0	198.82	233.3	221.1	236.3	239.5
gastric — *see* Neoplasm, stomach						
gastrocolic	159.8	197.8	230.9	211.9	235.5	239.0
gastroesophageal junction	151.0	197.8	230.2	211.1	235.2	239.0
gastrointestinal (tract) NEC	159.9	197.8	230.9	211.9	235.5	239.0
generalized	199.0	199.0	234.9	229.9	238.9	199.0
genital organ or tract						
female NEC	184.9	198.82	233.3	221.9	236.3	239.5
contiguous sites	184.8	—	—	—	—	—
specified site NEC	184.8	198.82	233.3	221.8	236.3	239.5
male NEC	187.9	198.82	233.6	222.9	236.6	239.5
contiguous sites	187.8	—	—	—	—	—
specified site NEC	187.8	198.82	233.6	222.8	236.6	239.5
genitourinary tract						
female	184.9	198.82	233.3	221.9	236.3	239.5
male	187.9	198.82	233.6	222.9	236.6	239.5
gingiva (alveolar) (marginal)	143.9	198.89	230.0	210.4	235.1	239.0
lower	143.1	198.89	230.0	210.4	235.1	239.0
mandibular	143.1	198.89	230.0	210.4	235.1	239.0
maxillary	143.0	198.89	230.0	210.4	235.1	239.0
upper	143.0	198.89	230.0	210.4	235.1	239.0
gland, glandular (lymphatic) (system) — *see also* Neoplasm, lymph gland						
endocrine NEC	194.9	198.89	—	227.9	237.4	239.7
salivary — *see* Neoplasm, salivary, gland						
glans penis	187.2	198.82	233.5	222.1	236.6	239.5
globus pallidus	191.0	198.3	—	225.0	237.5	239.6
glomus						
coccygeal	194.6	198.89	—	227.6	237.3	239.7
jugularis	194.6	198.89	—	227.6	237.3	239.7
glosso-epiglottic fold(s)	146.4	198.89	230.0	210.6	235.1	239.0
glossopalatine fold	146.2	198.89	230.0	210.6	235.1	239.0
glossopharyngeal sulcus	146.1	198.89	230.0	210.6	235.1	239.0
glottis	161.0	197.3	231.0	212.1	235.6	239.1
gluteal region*	195.3	198.89	232.5	229.8	238.8	239.8
great vessels NEC	171.4	198.89	—	215.4	238.1	239.2
groin NEC*	195.3	198.89	232.5	229.8	238.8	239.8

	Malignant			Benign	Uncertain Behavior	Unspecified
	Primary	Secondary	Ca in situ			

	Primary	Secondary	Ca in situ	Benign	Uncertain Behavior	Unspecified
Neoplasm, neoplastic—*continued*						
gum	143.9	198.89	230.0	210.4	235.1	239.0
contiguous sites	143.8	—	—	—	—	—
lower	143.1	198.89	230.0	210.4	235.1	239.0
upper	143.0	198.89	230.0	210.4	235.1	239.0
hand NEC*	195.4	198.89	232.6	229.8	238.8	239.8
head NEC*	195.0	198.89	232.4	229.8	238.8	239.8
heart	164.1	198.89	—	212.7	238.8	239.8
contiguous sites with mediastinum or thymus	164.8	—	—	—	—	—
heel NEC*	195.5	198.89	232.7	229.8	238.8	239.8
helix	173.2	198.2	232.2	216.2	238.2	239.2
hematopoietic, hemopoietic tissue NEC	202.8	198.89	—	—	—	238.7
hemisphere, cerebral	191.0	198.3	—	225.0	237.5	239.6
hemorrhoidal zone	154.2	197.5	230.5	211.4	235.5	239.0
hepatic	155.2	197.7	230.8	211.5	235.3	239.0
duct (bile)	156.1	197.8	230.8	211.5	235.3	239.0
flexure (colon)	153.0	197.5	230.3	211.3	235.2	239.0
primary	155.0	—	—	—	—	—
hilus of lung	162.2	197.0	231.2	212.3	235.7	239.1
hip NEC*	195.5	198.89	232.7	229.8	238.8	239.8
hippocampus, brain	191.2	198.3	—	225.0	237.5	239.6
humerus (any part)	170.4	198.5	—	213.4	238.0	239.2
hymen	184.0	198.82	233.3	221.1	236.3	239.5
hypopharynx, hypopharyngeal NEC	148.9	198.89	230.0	210.8	235.1	239.0
contiguous sites	148.8	—	—	—	—	—
postcricoid region	148.0	198.89	230.0	210.8	235.1	239.0
posterior wall	148.3	198.89	230.0	210.8	235.1	239.0
pyriform fossa (sinus)	148.1	198.89	230.0	210.8	235.1	239.0
specified site NEC	148.8	198.89	230.0	210.8	235.1	239.0
wall	148.9	198.89	230.0	210.8	235.1	239.0
posterior	148.3	198.89	230.0	210.8	235.1	239.0
hypophysis	194.3	198.89	234.8	227.3	237.0	239.7
hypothalamus	191.0	198.3	—	225.0	237.5	239.6
ileocecum, ileocecal (coil) (junction) (valve)	153.4	197.5	230.3	211.3	235.2	239.0
ileum	152.2	197.4	230.7	211.2	235.2	239.0
ilium	170.6	198.5	—	213.6	238.0	239.2
immunoproliferative NEC	203.8	—	—	—	—	—
infraclavicular (region)*	195.1	198.89	232.5	229.8	238.8	239.8
inguinal (region)*	195.3	198.89	232.5	229.8	238.8	239.8
insula	191.0	198.3	—	225.0	237.5	239.6
insular tissue (pancreas)	157.4	197.8	230.9	211.7	235.5	239.0
brain	191.0	198.3	—	225.0	237.5	239.6
interarytenoid fold	148.2	198.89	230.0	210.8	235.1	239.0
hypopharyngeal aspect	148.2	198.89	230.0	210.8	235.1	239.0
laryngeal aspect	161.1	197.3	231.0	212.1	235.6	239.1
marginal zone	148.2	198.89	230.0	210.8	235.1	239.0
interdental papillae	143.9	198.89	230.0	210.4	235.1	239.0
lower	143.1	198.89	230.0	210.4	235.1	239.0
upper	143.0	198.89	230.0	210.4	235.1	239.0
internal						
capsule	191.0	198.3	—	225.0	237.5	239.6
os (cervix)	180.0	198.82	233.1	219.0	236.0	239.5
intervertebral cartilage or disc	170.2	198.5	—	213.2	238.0	239.2
intestine, intestinal	159.0	197.8	230.7	211.9	235.2	239.0
large	153.9	197.5	230.3	211.3	235.2	239.0
appendix	153.5	197.5	230.3	211.3	235.2	239.0
caput coli	153.4	197.5	230.3	211.3	235.2	239.0
cecum	153.4	197.5	230.3	211.3	235.2	239.0
colon	153.9	197.5	230.3	211.3	235.2	239.0
and rectum	154.0	197.5	230.4	211.4	235.2	239.0
ascending	153.6	197.5	230.3	211.3	235.2	239.0
caput	153.4	197.5	230.3	211.3	235.2	239.0
contiguous sites	153.8	—	—	—	—	—
descending	153.2	197.5	230.3	211.3	235.2	239.0
distal	153.2	197.5	230.3	211.3	235.2	239.0
left	153.2	197.5	230.3	211.3	235.2	239.0
pelvic	153.3	197.5	230.3	211.3	235.2	239.0
right	153.6	197.5	230.3	211.3	235.2	239.0
sigmoid (flexure)	153.3	197.5	230.3	211.3	235.2	239.0
transverse	153.1	197.5	230.3	211.3	235.2	239.0
contiguous sites	153.8	—	—	—	—	—
hepatic flexure	153.0	197.5	230.3	211.3	235.2	239.0
ileocecum, ileocecal (coil) (valve)	153.4	197.5	230.3	211.3	235.2	239.0
sigmoid flexure (lower) (upper)	153.3	197.5	230.3	211.3	235.2	239.0

	Malignant			Benign	Uncertain Behavior	Unspecified
	Primary	Secondary	Ca in situ			
Neoplasm, neoplastic—*continued*						
intestine, intestinal—*continued*						
large—*continued*						
splenic flexure	153.7	197.5	230.3	211.3	235.2	239.0
small	152.9	197.4	230.7	211.2	235.2	239.0
contiguous sites	152.8	—	—	—	—	—
duodenum	152.0	197.4	230.7	211.2	235.2	239.0
ileum	152.2	197.4	230.7	211.2	235.2	239.0
jejunum	152.1	197.4	230.7	211.2	235.2	239.0
tract NEC	159.0	197.8	230.7	211.9	235.2	239.0
intra-abdominal	195.2	198.89	234.8	229.8	238.8	239.8
intracranial NEC	191.9	198.3	—	225.0	237.5	239.6
intrahepatic (bile) duct	155.1	197.8	230.8	211.5	235.3	239.0
intraocular	190.0	198.4	234.0	224.0	238.8	239.8
intraorbital	190.1	198.4	234.0	224.1	238.8	239.8
intrasellar	194.3	198.89	234.8	227.3	237.0	239.7
intrathoracic (cavity) (organs NEC)	195.1	198.89	234.8	229.8	238.8	239.8
contiguous sites with respiratory organs	165.8	—	—	—	—	—
iris	190.0	198.4	234.0	224.0	238.8	239.8
ischiorectal (fossa)	195.3	198.89	234.8	229.8	238.8	239.8
ischium	170.6	198.5	—	213.6	238.0	239.2
island of Reil	191.0	198.3	—	225.0	237.5	239.6
islands or islets of Langerhans	157.4	197.8	230.9	211.7	235.5	239.0
isthmus uteri	182.1	198.82	233.2	219.1	236.0	239.5
jaw	195.0	198.89	234.8	229.8	238.8	239.8
bone	170.1	198.5	—	213.1	238.0	239.2
carcinoma	143.9	—	—	—	—	—
lower	143.1	—	—	—	—	—
upper	143.0	—	—	—	—	—
lower	170.1	198.5	—	213.1	238.0	239.2
upper	170.0	198.5	—	213.0	238.0	239.2
carcinoma (any type) (lower) (upper)	195.0	—	—	—	—	—
skin	173.3	198.2	232.3	216.3	238.2	239.2
soft tissues	143.9	198.89	230.0	210.4	235.1	239.0
lower	143.1	198.89	230.0	210.4	235.1	239.0
upper	143.0	198.89	230.0	210.4	235.1	239.0
jejunum	152.1	197.4	230.7	211.2	235.2	239.0
joint NEC (*see also* Neoplasm, bone)	170.9	198.5	—	213.9	238.0	239.2
acromioclavicular	170.4	198.5	—	213.4	238.0	239.2
bursa or synovial membrane — *see* Neoplasm, connective tissue						
costovertebral	170.3	198.5	—	213.3	238.0	239.2
sternocostal	170.3	198.5	—	213.3	238.0	239.2
temporomandibular	170.1	198.5	—	213.1	238.0	239.2
junction						
anorectal	154.8	197.5	230.7	211.4	235.5	239.0
cardioesophageal	151.0	197.8	230.2	211.1	235.2	239.0
esophagogastric	151.0	197.8	230.2	211.1	235.2	239.0
gastroesophageal	151.0	197.8	230.2	211.1	235.2	239.0
hard and soft palate	145.5	198.89	230.0	210.4	235.1	239.0
ileocecal	153.4	197.5	230.3	211.3	235.2	239.0
pelvirectal	154.0	197.5	230.4	211.4	235.2	239.0
pelviureteric	189.1	198.0	233.9	223.1	236.91	239.5
rectosigmoid	154.0	197.5	230.4	211.4	235.2	239.0
squamocolumnar, of cervix	180.8	198.82	233.1	219.0	236.0	239.5
kidney (parenchyma)	189.0	198.0	233.9	223.0	236.91	239.5
calyx	189.1	198.0	233.9	223.1	236.91	239.5
hilus	189.1	198.0	233.9	223.1	236.91	239.5
pelvis	189.1	198.0	233.9	223.1	236.91	239.5
knee NEC*	195.5	198.89	232.7	229.8	238.8	239.8
labia (skin)	184.4	198.82	233.3	221.2	236.3	239.5
majora	184.1	198.82	233.3	221.2	236.3	239.5
minora	184.2	198.82	233.3	221.2	236.3	239.5
labial — *see also* Neoplasm, lip						
sulcus (lower) (upper)	145.1	198.89	230.0	210.4	235.1	239.0
labium (skin)	184.4	198.82	233.3	221.2	236.3	239.5
majus	184.1	198.82	233.3	221.2	236.3	239.5
minus	184.2	198.82	233.3	221.2	236.3	239.5
lacrimal						
canaliculi	190.7	198.4	234.0	224.7	238.8	239.8
duct (nasal)	190.7	198.4	234.0	224.7	238.8	239.8
gland	190.2	198.4	234.0	224.2	238.8	239.8
punctum	190.7	198.4	234.0	224.7	238.8	239.8
sac	190.7	198.4	234.0	224.7	238.8	239.8
Langerhans, islands or islets	157.4	197.8	230.9	211.7	235.5	239.0

	Malignant			Benign	Uncertain Behavior	Unspecified
	Primary	Secondary	Ca in situ			
Neoplasm, neoplastic—*continued*						
laryngopharynx	148.9	198.89	230.0	210.8	235.1	239.0
larynx, laryngeal NEC	161.9	197.3	231.0	212.1	235.6	239.1
aryepiglottic fold	161.1	197.3	231.0	212.1	235.6	239.1
cartilage (arytenoid) (cricoid) (cuneiform) (thyroid)	161.3	197.3	231.0	212.1	235.6	239.1
commissure (anterior) (posterior)	161.0	197.3	231.0	212.1	235.6	239.1
contiguous sites	161.8	—	—	—	—	—
extrinsic NEC	161.1	197.3	231.0	212.1	235.6	239.1
meaning hypopharynx	148.9	198.89	230.0	210.8	235.1	239.0
interarytenoid fold	161.1	197.3	231.0	212.1	235.6	239.1
intrinsic	161.0	197.3	231.0	212.1	235.6	239.1
ventricular band	161.1	197.3	231.0	212.1	235.6	239.1
leg NEC*	195.5	198.89	232.7	229.8	238.8	239.8
lens, crystalline	190.0	198.4	234.0	224.0	238.8	239.8
lid (lower) (upper)	173.1	198.2	232.1	216.1	238.2	239.2
ligament — *see also* Neoplasm, connective tissue						
broad	183.3	198.82	233.3	221.0	236.3	239.5
Mackenrodt's	183.8	198.82	233.3	221.8	236.3	239.5
non-uterine — *see* Neoplasm, connective tissue						
round	183.5	198.82	—	221.0	236.3	239.5
sacro-uterine	183.4	198.82	—	221.0	236.3	239.5
uterine	183.4	198.82	—	221.0	236.3	239.5
utero-ovarian	183.8	198.82	233.3	221.8	236.3	239.5
uterosacral	183.4	198.82	—	221.0	236.3	239.5
limb*	195.8	198.89	232.8	229.8	238.8	239.8
lower*	195.5	198.89	232.7	229.8	238.8	239.8
upper*	195.4	198.89	232.6	229.8	238.8	239.8
limbus of cornea	190.4	198.4	234.0	224.4	238.8	239.8
lingual NEC (*see also* Neoplasm, tongue)	141.9	198.89	230.0	210.1	235.1	239.0
lingula, lung	162.3	197.0	231.2	212.3	235.7	239.1
lip (external) (lipstick area) (vermillion border)	140.9	198.89	230.0	210.0	235.1	239.0
buccal aspect — *see* Neoplasm, lip, internal						
commissure	140.6	198.89	230.0	210.4	235.1	239.0
contiguous sites	140.8	—	—	—	—	—
with oral cavity or pharynx	149.8	—	—	—	—	—
frenulum — *see* Neoplasm, lip, internal						
inner aspect — *see* Neoplasm, lip, internal						
internal (buccal) (frenulum) (mucosa) (oral)	140.5	198.89	230.0	210.0	235.1	239.0
lower	140.4	198.89	230.0	210.0	235.1	239.0
upper	140.3	198.89	230.0	210.0	235.1	239.0
lower	140.1	198.89	230.0	210.0	235.1	239.0
internal (buccal) (frenulum) (mucosa) (oral)	140.4	198.89	230.0	210.0	235.1	239.0
mucosa — *see* Neoplasm, lip, internal						
oral aspect — *see* Neoplasm, lip, internal						
skin (commissure) (lower) (upper)	173.0	198.2	232.0	216.0	238.2	239.2
upper	140.0	198.89	230.0	210.0	235.1	239.0
internal (buccal) (frenulum) (mucosa) (oral)	140.3	198.89	230.0	210.0	235.1	239.0
liver	155.2	197.7	230.8	211.5	235.3	239.0
primary	155.0	—	—	—	—	—
lobe						
azygos	162.3	197.0	231.2	212.3	235.7	239.1
frontal	191.1	198.3	—	225.0	237.5	239.6
lower	162.5	197.0	231.2	212.3	235.7	239.1
middle	162.4	197.0	231.2	212.3	235.7	239.1
occipital	191.4	198.3	—	225.0	237.5	239.6
parietal	191.3	198.3	—	225.0	237.5	239.6
temporal	191.2	198.3	—	225.0	237.5	239.6
upper	162.3	197.0	231.2	212.3	235.7	239.1
lumbosacral plexus	171.6	198.4	—	215.6	238.1	239.2
lung	162.9	197.0	231.2	212.3	235.7	239.1
azgos lobe	162.3	197.0	231.2	212.3	235.7	239.1
carina	162.2	197.0	231.2	212.3	235.7	239.1
contiguous sites with bronchus or trachea	162.8	—	—	—	—	—
hilus	162.2	197.0	231.2	212.3	235.7	239.1
lingula	162.3	197.0	231.2	212.3	235.7	239.1
lobe NEC	162.9	197.0	231.2	212.3	235.7	239.1
lower lobe	162.5	197.0	231.2	212.3	235.7	239.1
main bronchus	162.2	197.0	231.2	212.3	235.7	239.1
middle lobe	162.4	197.0	231.2	212.3	235.7	239.1
upper lobe	162.3	197.0	231.2	212.3	235.7	239.1

	Malignant			Benign	Uncertain Behavior	Unspecified
	Primary	Seconday	Ca in situ			
Neoplasm, neoplastic—*continued*						
lymph, lymphatic						
channel NEC (*see also* Neoplasm, connective tissue)	171.9	198.89	—	215.9	238.1	239.2
gland (secondary)	—	196.9	—	229.0	238.8	239.8
abdominal	—	196.2	—	229.0	238.8	239.
aortic	—	196.2	—	229.0	238.8	239.8
arm	—	196.3	—	229.0	238.8	239.8
auricular (anterior) (posterior)	—	196.0	—	229.0	238.8	239.8
axilla, axillary	—	196.3	—	229.0	238.8	239.8
brachial	—	196.3	—	229.0	238.8	239.8
bronchial	—	196.1	—	229.0	238.8	239.8
bronchopulmonary	—	196.1	—	229.0	238.8	239.8
celiac	—	196.2	—	229.0	238.8	239.8
cervical	—	196.0	—	229.0	238.8	239.8
cervicofacial	—	196.0	—	229.0	238.8	239.8
Cloquet	—	196.5	—	229.0	238.8	239.8
colic	—	196.2	—	229.0	238.8	239.8
common duct	—	196.2	—	229.0	238.8	239.8
cubital	—	196.3	—	229.0	238.8	239.8
diaphragmatic	—	196.1	—	229.0	238.8	239.8
epigastric, inferior	—	196.6	—	229.0	238.8	239.8
epitrochlear	—	196.3	—	229.0	238.8	239.8
esophageal	—	196.1	—	229.0	238.8	239.8
face	—	196.0	—	229.0	238.8	239.8
femoral	—	196.5	—	229.0	238.8	239.8
gastric	—	196.2	—	229.0	238.8	239.8
groin	—	196.5	—	229.0	238.8	239.8
head	—	196.0	—	229.0	238.8	239.8
hepatic	—	196.2	—	229.0	238.8	239.8
hilar (pulmonary)	—	196.1	—	229.0	238.8	239.8
splenic	—	196.2	—	229.0	238.8	239.8
hypogastric	—	196.6	—	229.0	238.8	239.8
ileocolic	—	196.2	—	229.0	238.8	239.8
iliac	—	196.6	—	229.0	238.8	239.8
infraclavicular	—	196.3	—	229.0	238.8	239.8
inguina, inguinal	—	196.5	—	229.0	238.8	239.8
innominate	—	196.1	—	229.0	238.8	239.8
intercostal	—	196.1	—	229.0	238.8	239.8
intestinal	—	196.2	—	229.0	238.8	239.8
intra-abdominal	—	196.2	—	229.0	238.8	239.8
intrapelvic	—	196.6	—	229.0	238.8	239.8
intrathoracic	—	196.1	—	229.0	238.8	239.9
jugular	—	196.0	—	229.0	238.8	239.8
leg	—	196.5	—	229.0	238.8	239.8
limb						
lower	—	196.5	—	229.0	238.8	239.8
upper	—	196.3	—	229.0	238.8	239.8
lower limb	—	196.5	—	229.0	238.8	238.9
lumbar	—	196.2	—	229.0	238.8	239.8
mandibular	—	196.0	—	229.0	238.8	239.8
mediastinal	—	196.1	—	229.0	238.8	239.8
mesenteric (inferior) (superior)	—	196.2	—	229.0	238.8	239.8
midcolic	—	196.2	—	229.0	238.8	239.8
multiple sites in categories 196.0-196.6	—	196.8	—	229.0	238.8	239.8
neck	—	196.0	—	229.0	238.8	239.8
obturator	—	196.6	—	229.0	238.8	239.8
occipital	—	196.0	—	229.0	238.8	239.8
pancreatic	—	196.2	—	229.0	238.8	239.8
para-aortic	—	196.2	—	229.0	238.8	239.8
paracervical	—	196.6	—	229.0	238.8	239.8
parametrial	—	196.6	—	229.0	238.8	239.8
parasternal	—	196.1	—	229.0	238.8	239.8
parotid	—	196.0	—	229.0	238.8	239.8
pectoral	—	196.3	—	229.0	238.8	239.8
pelvic	—	196.6	—	229.0	238.8	239.8
peri-aortic	—	196.2	—	229.0	238.8	239.8
peripancreatic	—	196.2	—	229.0	238.8	239.8
popliteal	—	196.5	—	229.0	238.8	239.8
porta hepatis	—	196.2	—	229.0	238.8	239.8
portal	—	196.2	—	229.0	238.8	239.8
preauricular	—	196.0	—	229.0	238.8	239.8
prelaryngeal	—	196.0	—	229.0	238.8	239.8
presymphysial	—	196.6	—	229.0	238.8	239.8
pretracheal	—	196.0	—	229.0	238.8	239.8

	Malignant			Benign	Uncertain Behavior	Unspecified
	Primary	Secondary	Ca in situ			
Neoplasm, neoplastic—continued						
lymph, lymphatic—continued						
gland (secondary)—continued						
primary (any site) NEC	202.9	—	—	—	—	—
pulmonary (hiler)	—	196.1	—	229.0	238.8	239.8
pyloric	—	196.2	—	229.0	238.8	239.8
retroperitoneal	—	196.2	—	229.0	238.8	239.8
retropharyngeal	—	196.0	—	229.0	238.8	239.8
Rosenmüller's	—	196.5	—	229.0	238.8	239.8
sacral —	196.6	—	229.0	238.8	239.8	
scalene	—	196.0	—	229.0	238.8	239.8
site NEC	—	196.9	—	229.0	238.8	239.8
splenic (hilar)	—	196.2	—	229.0	238.8	239.8
subclavicular	—	196.3	—	229.0	238.8	239.8
subinguinal	—	196.5	—	229.0	238.8	239.8
sublingual	—	196.0	—	229.0	238.8	239.8
submandibular	—	196.0	—	229.0	238.8	239.8
submaxillary	—	196.0	—	229.0	238.8	239.8
submental	—	196.0	—	229.0	238.8	239.8
subscapular	—	196.3	—	229.0	238.8	239.8
supraclavicular	—	196.0	—	229.0	238.8	239.8
thoracic	—	196.1	—	229.0	238.8	239.8
tibial —	196.5	—	229.0	238.8	239.8	
tracheal	—	196.1	—	229.0	238.8	239.8
tracheobronchial	—	196.1	—	229.0	238.8	239.8
upper limb	—	196.3	—	229.0	238.8	239.8
Virchow's	—	196.0	—	229.0	238.8	239.8
node — see also Neoplasm, lymph gland						
primary NEC	202.9	—	—	—	—	—
vessel (see also Neoplasm, connective tissue)	171.9	198.89	—	215.9	238.1	239.2
Nackenrodt's ligament	183.8	198.82	233.3	221.8	236.3	239.5
malar	170.0	198.5	—	213.0	238.0	239.2
region — see Neoplasm, cheek						
mammary gland — see Neoplasm, breast						
mandible	170.1	198.5	—	213.1	238.0	239.2
alveolar						
mucose	143.1	198.89	230.0	210.4	235.1	239.0
ridge or process	170.1	198.5	—	213.1	238.0	239.2
carcinoma	143.1	—	—	—	—	—
carcinoma	143.1	—	—	—	—	—
marrow (bone) NEC	202.9	198.5	—	—	—	238.7
mastectomy site (skin)	173.5	198.2	—	—	—	—
specified as breast tissue	174.8	198.81	—	—	—	—
mastoid (air cells) (antrum) (cavity)	160.1	197.3	231.8	212.0	235.9	239.1
bone or process	170.0	198.5	—	213.0	238.0	239.2
maxilla, maxillary (superior)	170.0	198.5	—	213.0	238.0	239.2
alveolar						
mucosa	143.0	198.89	230.0	210.4	235.1	239.0
ridge or process	170.0	198.5	—	213.0	238.0	239.2
carcinoma	143.0	—	—	—	—	—
antrum	160.2	197.3	231.8	212.0	235.9	239.1
carcinoma	143.0	—	—	—	—	—
inferior — see Neoplasm, mandible						
sinus	160.2	197.3	231.8	212.0	235.9	239.1
meatus						
external (ear)	173.2	198.2	232.2	216.2	238.2	239.2
Meckel's diverticulum	152.3	197.4	230.7	211.2	235.2	239.0
mediastinum, mediastinal	164.9	197.1	—	212.5	235.8	239.8
anterior	164.2	197.1	—	212.5	235.8	239.8
contiguous sites with heart and thymus	164.8	—	—	—	—	—
posterior	164.3	197.1	—	212.5	235.8	239.8
medulla						
adrenal	194.0	198.7	234.8	227.0	237.2	239.7
oblongata	191.7	198.3	—	225.0	237.5	239.6
meibomian gland	173.1	198.2	232.1	216.1	238.2	239.2
melanoma — see Melanoma						◆
meninges (brain) (cerebral) (cranial) (intracranial)	192.1	198.4	—	225.2	237.6	239.7
spinal (cord)	192.3	198.4	—	225.4	237.6	239.7
meniscus, knee joint (lateral) (medial)	170.7	198.5	—	213.7	238.0	239.2
mesentery, mesenteric	158.8	197.6	—	211.8	235.4	239.0
mesoappendix	158.8	197.6	—	211.8	235.4	239.0
mesocolon	158.8	197.6	—	211.8	235.4	239.0
mesopharynx — see Neoplasm, oropharynx						
mesosalpinx	183.3	198.82	233.3	221.0	236.3	239.5

	Malignant			Benign	Uncertain Behavior	Unspecified
	Primary	Seconday	Ca in situ			
Neoplasm, neoplastic—*continued*						
mesovarium	183.3	198.82	233.3	221.0	236.3	239.5
metacarpus (any bone)	170.5	198.5	—	213.5	238.0	239.2
metastatic NEC — *see also* Neoplasm, by site, secondary	—	199.1	—	—	—	—
metatarsus (any bone)	170.8	198.5	—	213.8	238.0	239.2
midbrain	191.7	198.3	—	225.0	237.5	239.6
milk duct — *see* Neoplasm, breast						
mons						
pubis	184.4	198.82	233.3	221.2	236.3	239.5
veneris	184.4	198.82	233.3	221.2	236.3	239.5
motor tract	192.9	198.4	—	225.9	237.9	239.7
brain	191.9	198.3	—	225.0	237.5	239.6
spinal	192.2	198.3	—	225.3	237.5	239.7
mouth	145.9	198.89	230.0	210.4	235.1	239.0
contiguous sites	145.8	—	—	—	—	—
floor	144.9	198.89	230.0	210.3	235.1	239.0
anterior portion	144.0	198.89	230.0	210.3	235.1	239.0
contiguous sites	144.8	—	—	—	—	—
lateral portion	144.1	198.89	230.0	210.3	235.1	239.0
roof	145.5	198.89	230.0	210.4	235.1	239.0
specified part NEC	145.8	198.89	230.0	210.4	235.1	239.0
vestibule	145.1	198.89	230.0	210.4	235.1	239.0
mucosa						
alveolar (ridge or process)	143.9	198.89	230.0	210.4	235.1	239.0
lower	143.1	198.89	230.0	210.4	235.1	239.0
upper	143.0	198.89	230.0	210.4	235.1	239.0
buccal	145.0	198.89	230.0	210.4	235.1	239.0
cheek	145.0	198.89	230.0	210.4	235.1	239.0
lip — *see* Neoplasm, lip, internal						
nasal	160.0	197.3	231.8	212.0	235.9	239.1
oral	145.0	198.89	230.0	210.4	235.1	239.0
Müllerian duct						
female	184.8	198.82	233.3	221.8	236.3	239.5
male	187.8	198.82	233.6	222.8	236.6	239.5
multiple sites NEC	199.0	199.0	234.9	229.9	238.9	199.0
muscle — *see also* Neoplasm, connective tissue						
extraocular	190.1	198.4	234.0	224.1	238.8	239.8
myocardium	164.1	198.89	—	212.7	238.8	239.8
myometrium	182.0	198.82	233.2	219.1	236.0	239.5
myopericardium	164.1	198.89	—	212.7	238.8	239.8
nabothian gland (follicle)	180.0	198.82	233.1	219.0	236.0	239.5
nail	173.9	198.2	232.9	216.9	238.2	239.2
finger	173.6	198.2	232.6	216.6	238.2	239.2
toe	173.7	198.2	232.7	216.7	238.2	239.2
nares, naris (anterior) (posterior)	160.0	197.3	231.8	212.0	235.9	239.1
nasal — *see* Neoplasm, nose						
nasolabial groove	173.3	198.2	232.3	216.3	238.2	239.2
nasolacrimal duct	190.7	198.4	234.0	224.7	238.8	239.8
nasopharynx, nasopharyngeal	147.9	198.89	230.0	210.7	235.1	239.0
contiguous sites	147.8	—	—	—	—	—
floor	147.3	198.89	230.0	210.7	235.1	239.0
roof	147.0	198.89	230.0	210.7	235.1	239.0
specified site NEC	147.8	198.89	230.0	210.7	235.1	239.0
wall	147.9	198.89	230.0	210.7	235.1	239.0
anterior	147.3	198.89	230.0	210.7	235.1	239.0
lateral	147.2	198.89	230.0	210.7	235.1	239.0
posterior	147.1	198.89	230.0	210.7	235.1	239.0
superior	147.0	198.89	230.0	210.7	235.1	239.0
nates	173.5	198.2	232.5	216.5	238.2	239.2
neck NEC*	195.0	198.89	234.8	229.8	238.8	239.8
nerve (autonomic) (ganglion) (parasympathetic) (peripheral) (sympathetic) — *see also* Neoplasm, connective tissue						
abducens	192.0	198.4	—	225.1	237.9	239.7
accessory (spinal)	192.0	198.4	—	225.1	237.9	239.7
acoustic	192.0	198.4	—	225.1	237.9	239.7
auditory	192.0	198.4	—	225.1	237.9	239.7
brachial	171.2	198.89	—	215.2	238.1	239.2
cranial (any)	192.0	198.4	—	225.1	237.9	239.7
facial	192.0	198.4	—	225.1	237.9	239.7
femoral	171.3	198.89	—	215.3	238.1	239.2
glossopharyngeal	192.0	198.4	—	225.1	237.9	239.7
hypoglossal	192.0	198.4	—	225.1	237.9	239.7
intercostal	171.4	198.89	—	215.4	238.1	239.2
lumbar	171.7	198.89	—	215.7	238.1	239.2

	Malignant			Benign	Uncertain Behavior	Unspecified
	Primary	Secondary	Ca in situ			
Neoplasm, neoplastic—*continued*						
nerve—*continued*						
median	171.2	198.89	—	215.2	238.1	239.2
obturator	171.3	198.89	—	215.3	238.1	239.2
oculomotor	192.0	198.4	—	225.1	237.9	239.7
olfactory	192.0	198.4	—	225.1	237.9	239.7
optic	192.0	198.4	—	225.1	237.9	239.7
peripheral NEC	171.9	198.89	—	215.9	238.1	239.2
radial	171.2	198.89	—	215.2	238.1	239.2
sacral	171.6	198.89	—	215.6	238.1	239.2
sciatic	171.3	198.89	—	215.3	238.1	239.2
spinal NEC	171.9	198.89	—	215.9	238.1	239.2
trigeminal	192.0	198.4	—	225.1	237.9	239.7
trochlear	192.0	198.4	—	225.1	237.9	239.7
ulnar	171.2	198.89	—	215.2	238.1	239.2
vagus	192.0	198.4	—	225.1	237.9	239.7
nervous system (central) NEC	192.9	198.4	—	225.9	237.9	239.7
autonomic NEC	171.9	198.89	—	215.9	238.1	239.2
brain — *see also* Neoplasm, brain						
membrane or meninges	192.1	198.4	—	225.2	237.6	239.7
contiguous sites	192.8	—	—	—	—	—
parasympathetic NEC	171.9	198.89	—	215.9	238.1	239.2
sympathetic NEC	171.9	198.89	—	215.9	238.1	239.2
nipple (female)	174.0	198.81	233.0	217	238.3	239.3
male	175.0	198.81	233.0	217	238.3	239.3
nose, nasal	195.0	198.89	234.8	229.8	238.8	239.8
ala (external)	173.3	198.2	232.3	216.3	238.2	239.2
bone	170.0	198.5	—	213.0	238.0	239.2
cartilage	160.0	197.3	231.8	212.0	235.9	239.1
cavity	160.0	197.3	231.8	212.0	235.9	239.1
contiguous sites with accessory sinuses or middle ear	160.8	—	—	—	—	—
choana	147.3	198.89	230.0	210.7	235.1	239.0
external (skin)	173.3	198.2	232.3	216.3	238.2	239.2
fossa	160.0	197.3	231.8	212.0	235.9	239.1
internal	160.0	197.3	231.8	212.0	235.9	239.1
mucosa	160.0	197.3	231.8	212.0	235.9	239.1
septum	160.0	197.3	231.8	212.0	235.9	239.1
posterior margin	147.3	198.89	230.0	210.7	235.1	239.0
sinus — *see* Neoplasm, sinus						
skin	173.3	198.2	232.3	216.3	238.2	239.2
turbinate (mucosa)	160.0	197.3	231.8	212.0	235.9	239.1
bone	170.0	198.5	—	213.0	238.0	239.2
vestibule	160.0	197.3	231.8	212.0	235.9	239.1
nostril	160.0	197.3	231.8	212.0	235.9	239.1
nucleus pulposus	170.2	198.5	—	213.2	238.0	239.2
occipital						
bone	170.0	198.5	—	213.0	238.0	239.2
lobe or pole, brain	191.4	198.3	—	225.0	237.5	239.6
odontogenic — *see* Neoplasm, jaw bone						
oesophagus — *see* Neoplasm, esophagus						
olfactory nerve or bulb	192.0	198.4	—	225.1	237.9	239.7
olive (brain)	191.7	198.3	—	225.0	237.5	239.6
omentum	158.8	197.6	—	211.8	235.4	239.0
operculum (brain)	191.0	198.3	—	225.0	237.5	239.6
optic nerve, chiasm, or tract	192.0	198.4	—	225.1	237.9	239.7
oral (cavity)	145.9	198.89	230.0	210.4	235.1	239.0
contiguous sites with lip or pharynx	149.8	—	—	—	—	—
ill-defined	149.9	198.89	230.0	210.4	235.1	239.0
mucosa	145.9	198.89	230.0	210.4	235.1	239.0
orbit	190.1	198.4	234.0	224.1	238.8	239.8
bone	170.0	198.5	—	213.0	238.0	239.2
eye	190.1	198.4	234.0	224.1	238.8	239.8
soft parts	190.1	198.4	234.0	224.1	238.8	239.8
organ of Zuckerkandl	194.6	198.89	—	227.6	237.3	239.7
oropharynx	146.9	198.89	230.0	210.6	235.1	239.0
branchial cleft (vestige)	146.8	198.89	230.0	210.6	235.1	239.0
contiguous sites	146.8	—	—	—	—	—
junctional region	146.5	198.89	230.0	210.6	235.1	239.0
lateral wall	146.6	198.89	230.0	210.6	235.1	239.0
pillars of fauces	146.2	198.89	230.0	210.6	235.1	239.0
posterior wall	146.7	198.89	230.0	210.6	235.1	239.0
specified part NEC	146.8	198.89	230.0	210.6	235.1	239.0
vallecula	146.3	198.89	230.0	210.6	235.1	239.0

	Malignant			Benign	Uncertain Behavior	Unspecified
	Primary	Secondary	Ca in situ			

	Primary	Secondary	Ca in situ	Benign	Uncertain Behavior	Unspecified
Neoplasm, neoplastic—*continued*						
os						
external	180.1	198.82	233.1	219.0	236.0	239.5
internal	180.0	198.82	233.1	219.0	236.0	239.5
ovary	183.0	198.6	233.3	220	236.2	239.5
oviduct	183.2	198.82	233.3	221.0	236.3	239.5
palate	145.5	198.89	230.0	210.4	235.1	239.0
hard	145.2	198.89	230.0	210.4	235.1	239.0
junction of hard and soft palate	145.5	198.89	230.0	210.4	235.1	239.0
soft	145.3	198.89	230.0	210.4	235.1	239.0
nasopharyngeal surface	147.3	198.89	230.0	210.7	235.1	239.0
posterior surface	147.3	198.89	230.0	210.7	235.1	239.0
superior surface	147.3	198.89	230.0	210.7	235.1	239.0
palatoglossal arch	146.2	198.89	230.0	210.6	235.1	239.0
palatopharyngeal arch	146.2	198.89	230.0	210.6	235.1	239.0
pallium	191.0	198.3	—	225.0	237.5	239.6
palpebra	173.1	198.2	232.1	216.1	238.2	239.2
pancreas	157.9	197.8	230.9	211.6	235.5	239.0
body	157.1	197.8	230.9	211.6	235.5	239.0
contiguous sites	157.8	—	—	—	—	—
duct (of Santorini) (of Wirsung)	157.3	197.8	230.9	211.6	235.5	239.0
ectopic tissue	157.8	197.8	230.9	211.6	235.5	239.0
head	157.0	197.8	230.9	211.6	235.5	239.0
islet cells	157.4	197.8	230.9	211.7	235.5	239.0
neck	157.8	197.8	230.9	211.6	235.5	239.0
tail	157.2	197.8	230.9	211.6	235.5	239.0
para-aortic body	194.6	198.89	—	227.6	237.3	239.7
paraganglion NEC	194.6	198.89	—	227.6	237.3	239.7
parametrium	183.4	198.82	—	221.0	236.3	239.5
paranephric	158.0	197.6	—	211.8	235.4	239.0
pararectal	195.3	198.89	—	229.8	238.8	239.8
parasagittal (region)	195.0	198.89	234.8	229.8	238.8	239.8
parasellar	192.9	198.4	—	225.9	237.9	239.7
parathyroid (gland)	194.1	198.89	234.8	227.1	237.4	239.7
paraurethral	195.3	198.89	—	229.8	238.8	239.8
gland	189.4	198.1	233.9	223.89	236.99	239.5
paravaginal	195.3	198.89	—	229.8	238.8	239.8
parenchyma, kidney	189.0	198.0	233.9	223.0	236.91	239.5
parietal						
bone	170.0	198.5	—	213.0	238.0	239.2
lobe, brain	191.3	198.3	—	225.0	237.5	239.6
paroophoron	183.3	198.82	233.3	221.0	236.3	239.5
parotid (duct) (gland)	142.0	198.89	230.0	210.2	235.0	239.0
parovarium	183.3	198.82	233.3	221.0	236.3	239.5
patella	170.8	198.5	—	213.8	238.0	239.2
peduncle, cerebral	191.7	198.3	—	225.0	237.5	239.6
pelvirectal junction	154.0	197.5	230.4	211.4	235.2	239.0
pelvis, pelvic	195.3	198.89	234.8	229.8	238.8	239.8
bone	170.6	198.5	—	213.6	238.0	239.2
floor	195.3	198.89	234.8	229.8	238.8	239.8
renal	189.1	198.0	233.9	223.1	236.91	239.5
viscera	195.3	198.89	234.8	229.8	238.8	239.8
wall	195.3	198.89	234.8	229.8	238.8	239.8
pelvo-abdominal	195.8	198.89	234.8	229.8	238.8	239.8
penis	187.4	198.82	233.5	222.1	236.6	239.5
body	187.3	198.82	233.5	222.1	236.6	239.5
corpus (cavernosum)	187.3	198.82	233.5	222.1	236.6	239.5
glans	187.2	198.82	233.5	222.1	236.6	239.5
skin NEC	187.4	198.82	233.5	222.1	236.6	239.5
periadrenal (tissue)	158.0	197.6	—	211.8	235.4	239.0
perianal (skin)	173.5	198.2	232.5	216.5	238.2	239.2
pericardium	164.1	198.89	—	212.7	238.8	239.8
perinephric	158.0	197.6	—	211.8	235.4	239.0
perineum	195.3	198.89	234.8	229.8	238.8	239.8
periodontal tissue NEC	143.9	198.89	230.0	210.4	235.1	239.0
periosteum — *see* Neoplasm, bone						
peripancreatic	158.0	197.6	—	211.8	235.4	239.0
peripheral nerve NEC	171.9	198.89	—	215.9	238.1	239.2
perirectal (tissue)	195.3	198.89	—	229.8	238.8	239.8
perirenal (tissue)	158.0	197.6	—	211.8	235.4	239.0
peritoneum, peritoneal (cavity)	158.9	197.6	—	211.8	235.4	239.0
contiguous sites	158.8	—	—	—	—	—
with digestive organs	159.8	—	—	—	—	—
parietal	158.8	197.6	—	211.8	235.4	239.0

	Malignant			Benign	Uncertain Behavior	Unspecified
	Primary	Secondary	Ca in situ			
Neoplasm, neoplastic—*continued*						
peritoneum, peritoneal (cavity)—*continued*						
pelvic	158.8	197.6	—	211.8	235.4	239.0
specified part NEC	158.8	197.6	—	211.8	235.4	239.0
peritonsillar (tissue)	195.0	198.89	234.8	229.8	238.8	239.8
periurethral tissue	195.3	198.89	—	229.8	238.8	239.8
phalanges	170.9	198.5	—	213.9	238.0	239.2
foot	170.8	198.5	—	213.8	238.0	239.2
hand	170.5	198.5	—	213.5	238.0	239.2
pharynx, pharyngeal	149.0	198.89	230.0	210.9	235.1	239.0
bursa	147.1	198.89	230.0	210.7	235.1	239.0
fornix	147.3	198.89	230.0	210.7	235.1	239.0
recess	147.2	198.89	230.0	210.7	235.1	239.0
region	149.0	198.89	230.0	210.9	235.1	239.0
tonsil	147.1	198.89	230.0	210.7	235.1	239.0
wall (lateral) (posterior)	149.0	198.89	230.0	210.9	235.1	239.0
pia mater (cerebral) (cranial)	192.1	198.4	—	225.2	237.6	239.7
spinal	192.3	198.4	—	225.4	237.6	239.7
pillars of fauces	146.2	198.89	230.0	210.6	235.1	239.0
pineal (body) (gland)	194.4	198.89	234.8	227.4	237.1	239.7
pinna (ear) NEC	173.2	198.2	232.2	216.2	238.2	239.2
cartilage	171.0	198.89	—	215.0	238.1	239.2
piriform fossa or sinus	148.1	198.89	230.0	210.8	235.1	239.0
pituitary (body) (fossa) (gland) (lobe)	194.3	198.89	234.8	227.3	237.0	239.7
placenta	181	198.82	233.2	219.8	236.1	239.5
pleura, pleural (cavity)	163.9	197.2	—	212.4	235.8	239.1
contiguous sites	163.8	—	—	—	—	—
parietal	163.0	197.2	—	212.4	235.8	239.1
visceral	163.1	197.2	—	212.4	235.8	239.1
plexus						
brachial	171.2	198.89	—	215.2	238.1	239.2
cervical	171.0	198.89	—	215.0	238.1	239.2
choroid	191.5	198.3	—	225.0	237.5	239.6
lumbosacral	171.6	198.89	—	215.6	238.1	239.2
sacral	171.6	198.89	—	215.6	238.1	239.2
pluri-endocrine	194.8	198.89	234.8	227.8	237.4	239.7
pole						
frontal	191.1	198.3	—	225.0	237.5	239.6
occipital	191.4	198.3	—	225.0	237.5	239.6
pons (varolii)	191.7	198.3	—	225.0	237.5	239.6
popliteal fossa or space*	195.5	198.89	234.8	229.8	238.8	239.8
postcricoid (region)	148.0	198.89	230.0	210.8	235.1	239.0
posterior fossa (cranial)	191.6	198.3	—	225.0	237.5	239.6
postnasal space	147.9	198.89	230.0	210.7	235.1	239.0
prepuce	187.1	198.82	233.5	222.1	236.6	239.5
prepylorus	151.1	197.8	230.2	211.1	235.2	239.0
presacral (region)	195.3	198.89	—	229.8	238.8	239.8
prostate (gland)	185	198.82	233.4	222.2	236.5	239.5
utricle	189.3	198.1	233.9	223.81	236.99	239.5
pterygoid fossa	171.0	198.89	—	215.0	238.1	239.2
pubic bone	170.6	198.5	—	213.6	238.0	239.2
pudenda, pudendum (female)	184.4	198.82	233.3	221.2	236.3	239.5
pulmonary	162.9	197.0	231.2	212.3	235.7	239.1
putamen	191.0	198.3	—	225.0	237.5	239.6
pyloric						
antrum	151.2	197.8	230.2	211.1	235.2	239.0
canal	151.1	197.8	230.2	211.1	235.2	239.0
pylorus	151.1	197.8	230.2	211.1	235.2	239.0
pyramid (brain)	191.7	198.3	—	225.0	237.5	239.6
pyriform fossa or sinus	148.1	198.89	230.0	210.8	235.1	239.0
radius (any part)	170.4	198.5	—	213.4	238.0	239.2
Rathke's pouch	194.3	198.89	234.8	227.3	237.0	239.7
rectosigmoid (colon) (junction)	154.0	197.5	230.4	211.4	235.2	239.0
contiguous sites with anus or rectum	154.8	—	—	—	—	—
rectouterine pouch	158.8	197.6	—	211.8	235.4	239.0
rectovaginal septum or wall	195.3	198.89	234.8	229.8	238.8	239.8
rectovesical septum	195.3	198.89	234.8	229.8	238.8	239.8
rectum (ampulla)	154.1	197.5	230.4	211.4	235.2	239.0
and colon	154.0	197.5	230.4	211.4	235.2	239.0
contiguous sites with anus or rectosigmoid junction	154.8	—	—	—	—	—
renal	189.0	198.0	233.9	223.0	236.91	239.5
calyx	189.1	198.0	233.9	223.1	236.91	239.5
hilus	189.1	198.0	233.9	223.1	236.91	239.5

	Malignant Primary	Secondary	Ca in situ	Benign	Uncertain Behavior	Unspecified
Neoplasm, neoplastic—*continued*						
renal—*continued*						
parenchyma	189.0	198.0	233.9	223.0	236.91	239.5
pelvis	189.1	198.0	233.9	223.1	236.91	239.5
respiratory						
organs or system NEC	165.9	197.3	231.9	212.9	235.9	239.1
contiguous sites with intrathoracic organs	165.8	—	—	—	—	—
specified sites NEC	165.8	197.3	231.8	212.8	235.9	239.1
tract NEC	165.9	197.3	231.9	212.9	235.9	239.1
upper	165.0	197.3	231.9	212.9	235.9	239.1
retina	190.5	198.4	234.0	224.5	238.8	239.8
retrobulbar	190.1	198.4	—	224.1	238.8	239.8
retrocecal	158.0	197.6	—	211.8	235.4	239.0
retromolar (area) (triangle) (trigone)	145.6	198.89	230.0	210.4	235.1	239.0
retro-orbital	195.0	198.89	234.8	229.8	238.8	239.8
retroperitoneal (space) (tissue)	158.0	197.6	—	211.8	235.4	239.0
contiguous sites	158.8	—	—	—	—	—
retroperitoneum	158.0	197.6	—	211.8	235.4	239.0
contiguous sites	158.8	—	—	—	—	—
retropharyngeal	149.0	198.89	230.0	210.9	235.1	239.0
retrovesical (septum)	195.3	198.89	234.8	229.8	238.8	239.8
rhinencephalon	191.0	198.3	—	225.0	237.5	239.6
rib	170.3	198.5	—	213.3	238.0	239.2
Rosenmüller's fossa	147.2	198.89	230.0	210.7	235.1	239.0
round ligament	183.5	198.82	—	221.0	236.3	239.5
sacrococcyx, sacrococcygeal	170.6	198.5	—	213.6	238.0	239.2
region	195.3	198.89	234.8	229.8	238.8	239.8
sacrouterine ligament	183.4	198.82	—	221.0	236.3	239.5
sacrum, sacral (vertebra)	170.6	198.5	—	213.6	238.0	239.2
salivary gland or duct (major)	142.9	198.89	230.0	210.2	235.0	239.0
contiguous sites	142.8	—	—	—	—	—
minor NEC	145.9	198.89	230.0	210.4	235.1	239.0
parotid	142.0	198.89	230.0	210.2	235.0	239.0
pluriglandular	142.8	198.89	230.0	210.2	235.0	239.0
sublingual	142.2	198.89	230.0	210.2	235.0	239.0
submandibular	142.1	198.89	230.0	210.2	235.0	239.0
submaxillary	142.1	198.89	230.0	210.2	235.0	239.0
salpinx (uterine)	183.2	198.82	233.3	221.0	236.3	239.5
Santorini's duct	157.3	197.8	230.9	211.6	235.5	239.0
scalp	173.4	198.2	232.4	216.4	238.2	239.2
scapula (any part)	170.4	198.5	—	213.4	238.0	239.2
scapular region	195.1	198.89	234.8	229.8	238.8	239.8
scar NEC (*see also* Neoplasm, skin)	173.9	198.2	232.9	216.9	238.2	239.2
sciatic nerve	171.3	198.89	—	215.3	238.1	239.2
sclera	190.0	198.4	234.0	224.0	238.8	239.8
scrotum (skin)	187.7	198.82	233.6	222.4	236.6	239.5
sebaceous gland — *see* Neoplasm, skin						
sella turcica	194.3	198.89	234.8	227.3	237.0	239.7
bone	170.0	198.5	—	213.0	238.0	239.2
semilunar cartilage (knee)	170.7	198.5	—	213.7	238.0	239.2
seminal vesicle	187.8	198.82	233.6	222.8	236.6	239.5
septum						
nasal	160.0	197.3	231.8	212.0	235.9	239.1
posterior margin	147.3	198.89	230.0	210.7	235.1	239.0
rectovaginal	195.3	198.89	234.8	229.8	238.8	239.8
rectovesical	195.3	198.89	234.8	229.8	238.8	239.8
urethrovaginal	184.9	198.82	233.3	221.9	236.3	239.5
vesicovaginal	184.9	198.82	233.3	221.9	236.3	239.5
shoulder NEC*	195.4	198.89	232.6	229.8	238.8	239.8
sigmoid flexure (lower) (upper)	153.3	197.5	230.3	211.3	235.2	239.0
sinus (accessory)	160.9	197.3	231.8	212.0	235.9	239.1
bone (any)	170.0	198.5	—	213.0	238.0	239.2
contiguous sites with middle ear or nasal cavities	160.8	—	—	—	—	—
ethmoidal	160.3	197.3	231.8	212.0	235.9	239.1
frontal	160.4	197.3	231.8	212.0	235.9	239.1
maxillary	160.2	197.3	231.8	212.0	235.9	239.1
nasal, paranasal NEC	160.9	197.3	231.8	212.0	235.9	239.1
pyriform	148.1	198.89	230.0	210.8	235.1	239.0
sphenoidal	160.5	197.3	231.8	212.0	235.9	239.1
skeleton, skeletal NEC	170.9	198.5	—	213.9	238.0	239.2
Skene's gland	189.4	198.1	233.9	223.89	236.99	239.5

Neoplasm, skin

	Malignant			Benign	Uncertain Behavior	Unspecified
	Primary	Secondary	Ca in situ			

	Primary	Secondary	Ca in situ	Benign	Uncertain Behavior	Unspecified
Neoplasm, neoplastic—*continued*						
skin NEC	173.9	198.2	232.9	216.9	238.2	239.2
abdominal wall	173.5	198.2	232.5	216.5	238.2	239.2
ala nasi	173.3	198.2	232.3	216.3	238.2	239.2
ankle	173.7	198.2	232.7	216.7	238.2	239.2
antecubital space	173.6	198.2	232.6	216.6	238.2	239.2
anus	173.5	198.2	232.5	216.5	238.2	239.2
arm	173.6	198.2	232.6	216.6	238.2	239.2
auditory canal (external)	173.2	198.2	232.2	216.2	238.2	239.2
auricle (ear)	173.2	198.2	232.2	216.2	238.2	239.2
auricular canal (external)	173.2	193.2	232.2	216.2	238.2	239.2
axilla, axillary fold	173.5	198.2	232.5	216.5	238.2	239.2
back	173.5	198.2	232.5	216.5	238.2	239.2
breast	173.5	198.2	232.5	216.5	238.2	239.2
brow	173.3	198.2	232.3	216.3	238.2	239.2
buttock	173.5	198.2	232.5	216.5	238.2	239.2
calf	173.7	198.2	232.7	216.7	238.2	239.2
canthus (eye) (inner) (outer)	173.1	198.2	232.1	216.1	238.2	239.2
cervical region	173.4	198.2	232.4	216.4	238.2	239.2
cheek (external)	173.3	198.2	232.3	216.3	238.2	239.2
chest (wall)	173.5	198.2	232.5	216.5	238.2	239.2
chin	173.3	198.2	232.3	216.3	238.2	239.2
clavicular area	173.5	198.2	232.5	216.5	238.2	239.2
clitoris	184.3	198.82	233.3	221.2	236.3	239.5
columnella	173.3	198.2	232.3	216.3	238.2	239.2
concha	173.2	198.2	232.2	216.2	238.2	239.2
contiguous sites	173.8	—	—	—	—	—
ear (external)	173.2	198.2	232.2	216.2	238.2	239.2
elbow	173.6	198.2	232.6	216.6	238.2	239.2
eyebrow	173.3	198.2	232.3	216.3	238.2	239.2
eyelid	173.1	198.2	232.1	216.1	238.2	239.2
face NEC	173.3	198.2	232.3	216.3	238.2	239.2
female genital organs (external)	184.4	198.82	233.3	221.2	236.3	239.5
clitoris	184.3	198.82	233.3	221.2	236.3	239.5
labium NEC	184.4	198.82	233.3	221.2	236.3	239.5
majus	184.1	198.82	233.3	221.2	236.3	239.5
minus	184.2	198.82	233.3	221.2	236.3	239.5
pudendum	184.4	198.82	233.3	221.2	236.3	239.5
vulva	184.4	198.82	233.3	221.2	236.3	239.5
finger	173.6	198.2	232.6	216.6	238.2	239.2
flank	173.5	198.2	232.5	216.5	238.2	239.2
foot	173.7	198.2	232.7	216.7	238.2	239.2
forearm	173.6	198.2	232.6	216.6	238.2	239.2
forehead	173.3	198.2	232.3	216.3	238.2	239.2
glabella	173.3	198.2	232.3	216.3	238.2	239.2
gluteal region	173.5	198.2	232.5	216.5	238.2	239.2
groin	173.5	198.2	232.5	216.5	238.2	239.2
hand	173.6	198.2	232.6	216.6	238.2	239.2
head NEC	173.4	198.2	232.4	216.4	238.2	239.2
heel	173.7	198.2	232.7	216.7	238.2	239.2
helix	173.2	198.2	232.2	216.2	238.2	239.2
hip	173.7	198.2	232.7	216.7	238.2	239.2
infraclavicular region	173.5	198.2	232.5	216.5	238.2	239.2
inguinal region	173.5	198.2	232.5	216.5	238.2	239.2
jaw	173.3	198.2	232.3	216.3	238.2	239.2
knee	173.7	198.2	232.7	216.7	238.2	239.2
labia						
majora	184.1	198.82	233.3	221.2	236.3	239.5
minora	184.2	198.82	233.3	221.2	236.3	239.5
leg	173.7	198.2	232.7	216.7	238.2	239.2
lid (lower) (upper)	173.1	198.2	232.1	216.1	238.2	239.2
limb NEC	173.9	198.2	232.9	216.9	238.2	239.5
lower	173.7	198.2	232.7	216.7	238.2	239.2
upper	173.6	198.2	232.6	216.6	238.2	239.2
lip (lower) (upper)	173.0	198.2	232.0	216.0	238.2	239.2
male genital organs	187.9	198.82	233.6	222.9	236.6	239.5
penis	187.4	198.82	233.5	222.1	236.6	239.5
prepuce	187.1	198.82	233.5	222.1	236.6	239.5
scrotum	187.7	198.82	233.6	222.4	236.6	239.5
mastectomy site	173.5	198.2	—	—	—	—
specified as breast tissue	174.8	198.81	—	—	—	—
meatus, acoustic (external)	173.2	198.2	232.2	216.2	238.2	239.2
melanoma — *see* Melanoma						
nates	173.5	198.2	232.5	216.5	238.2	239.0

	Malignant			Benign	Uncertain Behavior	Unspecified
	Primary	Secondary	Ca in situ			

	Primary	Secondary	Ca in situ	Benign	Uncertain Behavior	Unspecified
Neoplasm, neoplastic—*continued*						
skin NEC—*continued*						
neck	173.4	198.2	232.4	216.4	238.2	239.2
nose (external)	173.3	198.2	232.3	216.3	238.2	239.2
palm	173.6	198.2	232.6	216.6	238.2	239.2
palpebra	173.1	198.2	232.1	216.1	238.2	239.2
penis NEC	187.4	198.82	233.5	222.1	236.6	239.5
perianal	173.5	198.2	232.5	216.5	238.2	239.2
perineum	173.5	198.2	232.5	216.5	238.2	239.2
pinna	173.2	198.2	232.2	216.2	238.2	239.2
plantar	173.7	198.2	232.7	216.7	238.2	239.2
popliteal fossa or space	173.7	198.2	232.7	216.7	238.2	239.2
prepuce	187.1	198.82	233.5	222.1	236.6	239.5
pubes	173.5	198.2	232.5	216.5	238.2	239.2
sacrococcygeal region	173.5	198.2	232.5	216.5	238.2	239.2
scalp	173.4	198.2	232.4	216.4	238.2	239.2
scapular region	173.5	198.2	232.5	216.5	238.2	239.2
scrotum	187.7	198.82	233.6	222.4	236.6	239.5
shoulder	173.6	198.2	232.6	216.6	238.2	239.2
sole (foot)	173.7	198.2	232.7	216.7	238.2	239.2
specified sites NEC	173.8	198.2	232.8	216.8	232.8	239.2
submammary fold	173.5	198.2	232.5	216.5	238.2	239.2
supraclavicular region	173.4	198.2	232.4	216.4	238.2	239.2
temple	173.3	198.2	232.3	216.3	238.2	239.2
thigh	173.7	198.2	232.7	216.7	238.2	239.2
thoracic wall	173.5	198.2	232.5	216.5	238.2	239.2
thumb	173.6	198.2	232.6	216.6	238.2	239.2
toe	173.7	198.2	232.7	216.7	238.2	239.2
tragus	173.2	198.2	232.2	216.2	238.2	239.2
trunk	173.5	198.2	232.5	216.5	238.2	239.2
umbilicus	173.5	198.2	232.5	216.5	238.2	239.2
vulva	184.4	198.82	233.3	221.2	236.3	239.5
wrist	173.6	198.2	232.6	216.6	238.2	239.2
skull	170.0	198.5	—	213.0	238.0	239.2
soft parts or tissues — *see* Neoplasm, connective tissue						
specified site NEC	195.8	198.89	234.8	229.8	238.8	239.8
spermatic cord	187.6	198.82	233.6	222.8	236.6	239.5
sphenoid	160.5	197.3	231.8	212.0	235.9	239.1
bone	170.0	198.5	—	213.0	238.0	239.2
sinus	160.5	197.3	231.8	212.0	235.9	239.1
sphincter						
anal	154.2	197.5	230.5	211.4	235.5	239.0
of Oddi	156.1	197.8	230.8	211.5	235.3	239.0
spine, spinal (column)	170.2	198.5	—	213.2	238.0	239.2
bulb	191.7	198.3	—	225.0	237.5	239.6
coccyx	170.6	198.5	—	213.6	238.0	239.2
cord (cervical) (lumbar) (sacral) (thoracic)	192.2	198.3	—	225.3	237.5	239.7
dura mater	192.3	198.4	—	225.4	237.6	239.7
lumbosacral	170.2	198.5	—	213.2	238.0	239.2
membrane	192.3	198.4	—	225.4	237.6	239.7
meninges	192.3	198.4	—	225.4	237.6	239.7
nerve (root)	171.9	198.89	—	215.9	238.1	239.2
pia mater	192.3	198.4	—	225.4	237.6	239.7
root	171.9	198.89	—	215.9	238.1	239.2
sacrum	170.6	198.5	—	213.6	238.0	239.2
spleen, splenic NEC	159.1	197.8	230.9	211.9	235.5	239.0
flexure (colon)	153.7	197.5	230.3	211.3	235.2	239.0
stem, brain	191.7	198.3	—	225.0	237.5	239.6
Stensen's duct	142.0	198.89	230.0	210.2	235.0	239.0
sternum	170.3	198.5	—	213.3	238.0	239.2
stomach	151.9	197.8	230.2	211.1	235.2	239.0
antrum (pyloric)	151.2	197.8	230.2	211.1	235.2	239.0
body	151.4	197.8	230.2	211.1	235.2	239.0
cardia	151.0	197.8	230.2	211.1	235.2	239.0
cardiac orifice	151.0	197.8	230.2	211.1	235.2	239.0
contiguous sites	151.8	—	—	—	—	—
corpus	151.4	197.8	230.2	211.1	235.2	239.0
fundus	151.3	197.8	230.2	211.1	235.2	239.0
greater curvature NEC	151.6	197.8	230.2	211.1	235.2	239.0
lesser curvature NEC	151.5	197.8	230.2	211.1	235.2	239.0
prepylorus	151.1	197.8	230.2	211.1	235.2	239.0
pylorus	151.1	197.8	230.2	211.1	235.2	239.0

	Malignant			Benign	Uncertain Behavior	Unspecified
	Primary	Seconday	Ca in situ			
Neoplasm, neoplastic—*continued*						
stomach—*continued*						
wall NEC	151.9	197.8	230.2	211.1	235.2	239.0
anterior NEC	151.8	197.8	230.2	211.1	235.2	239.0
posterior NEC	151.8	197.8	230.2	211.1	235.2	239.0
stroma, endometrial	182.0	198.82	233.2	219.1	236.0	239.5
stump, cervical	180.8	198.82	233.1	219.0	236.0	239.5
subcutaneous (nodule) (tissue) NEC — *see* Neoplasm, connective tissue						
subdural	192.1	198.4	—	225.2	237.6	239.7
subglottis, subglottic	161.2	197.3	231.0	212.1	235.6	239.1
sublingual	144.9	198.89	230.0	210.3	235.1	239.0
gland or duct	142.2	198.89	230.0	210.2	235.0	239.0
submandibular gland	142.1	198.89	230.0	210.2	235.0	239.0
submaxillary gland or duct	142.1	198.89	230.0	210.2	235.0	239.0
submental	195.0	198.89	234.8	229.8	238.8	239.8
subpleural	162.9	197.0	—	212.3	235.7	239.1
substernal	164.2	197.1	—	212.5	235.8	239.8
sudoriferous, sudoriparous gland, site unspecified	173.9	198.2	232.9	216.9	238.2	239.2
specified site — *see* Neoplasm, skin						
supraclavicular region	195.0	198.89	234.8	229.8	238.8	239.8
supraglottis	161.1	197.3	231.0	212.1	235.6	239.1
suprarenal (capsule) (cortex) (gland) (medulla)	194.0	198.7	234.8	227.0	237.2	239.7
suprasellar (region)	191.9	198.3	—	225.0	237.5	239.6
sweat gland (apocrine) (eccrine), site unspecified	173.9	198.2	232.9	216.9	238.2	239.2
specified site — *see* Neoplasm, skin						
sympathetic nerve or nervous system NEC	171.9	198.89	—	215.9	238.1	239.2
symphysis pubis	170.6	198.5	—	213.6	238.0	239.2
synovial membrane — *see* Neoplasm, connective tissue						
tapetum, brain	191.8	198.3	—	225.0	237.5	239.6
tarsus (any bone)	170.8	198.5	—	213.8	238.0	239.2
temple (skin)	173.3	198.2	232.3	216.3	238.2	239.2
temporal						
bone	170.0	198.5	—	213.0	238.0	239.2
lobe or pole	191.2	198.3	—	225.0	237.5	239.6
region	195.0	198.89	234.8	229.8	238.8	239.8
skin	173.3	198.2	232.3	216.3	238.2	239.2
tendon (sheath) — *see* Neoplasm, connective tissue						
tentorium (cerebelli)	192.1	198.4	—	225.2	237.6	239.7
testis, testes (descended) (scrotal)	186.9	198.82	233.6	222.0	236.4	239.5
ectopic	186.0	198.82	233.6	222.0	236.4	239.5
retained	186.0	198.82	233.6	222.0	236.4	239.5
undescended	186.0	198.82	233.6	222.0	236.4	239.5
thalamus	191.0	198.3	—	225.0	237.5	239.6
thigh NEC*	195.5	198.89	234.8	229.8	238.8	239.8
thorax, thoracic (cavity) (organs NEC)	195.1	198.89	234.8	229.8	238.8	239.8
duct	171.4	198.89	—	215.4	238.1	239.2
wall NEC	195.1	198.89	234.8	229.8	238.8	239.8
throat	149.0	198.89	230.0	210.9	235.1	239.0
thumb NEC*	195.4	198.89	232.6	229.8	238.8	239.8
thymus (gland)	164.0	198.89	—	212.6	235.8	239.8
contiguous sites with heart and mediastinum	164.8	—	—	—	—	—
thyroglossal duct	193	198.89	234.8	226	237.4	239.7
thyroid (gland)	193	198.89	234.8	226	237.4	239.7
cartilage	161.3	197.3	231.0	212.1	235.6	239.1
tibia (any part)	170.7	198.5	—	213.7	238.0	239.2
toe NEC*	195.5	198.89	232.7	229.8	238.8	239.8
tongue	141.9	198.89	230.0	210.1	235.1	239.0
anterior (two-thirds) NEC	141.4	198.89	230.0	210.1	235.1	239.0
dorsal surface	141.1	198.89	230.0	210.1	235.1	239.0
ventral surface	141.3	198.89	230.0	210.1	235.1	239.0
base (dorsal surface)	141.0	198.89	230.0	210.1	235.1	239.0
border (lateral)	141.2	198.89	230.0	210.1	235.1	239.0
contiguous sites	141.8	—	—	—	—	—
dorsal surface NEC	141.1	198.89	230.0	210.1	235.1	239.0
fixed part NEC	141.0	198.89	230.0	210.1	235.1	239.0
foreamen cecum	141.1	198.89	230.0	210.1	235.1	239.0
frenulum linguae	141.3	198.89	230.0	210.1	235.1	239.0
junctional zone	141.5	198.89	230.0	210.1	235.1	239.0
margin (lateral)	141.2	198.89	230.0	210.1	235.1	239.0
midline NEC	141.1	198.89	230.0	210.1	235.1	239.0
mobile part NEC	141.4	198.89	230.0	210.1	235.1	239.0
posterior (third)	141.0	198.89	230.0	210.1	235.1	239.0
root	141.0	198.89	230.0	210.1	235.1	239.0

	Malignant			Benign	Uncertain Behavior	Unspecified
	Primary	Seconday	Ca in situ			
Neoplasm, neoplastic—*continued*						
tongue—*continued*						
surface (dorsal)	141.1	198.89	230.0	210.1	235.1	239.0
base	141.0	198.89	230.0	210.1	235.1	239.0
ventral	141.3	198.89	230.0	210.1	235.1	239.0
tip	141.2	198.89	230.0	210.1	235.1	239.0
tonsil	141.6	198.89	230.0	210.1	235.1	239.0
tonsil	146.0	198.89	230.0	210.5	235.1	239.0
fauces, faucial	146.0	198.89	230.0	210.5	235.1	239.0
lingual	141.6	198.89	230.0	210.1	235.1	239.0
palatine	146.0	198.89	230.0	210.5	235.1	239.0
pharyngeal	147.1	198.89	230.0	210.7	235.1	239.0
pillar (anterior) (posterior)	146.2	198.89	230.0	210.6	235.1	239.0
tonsillar fossa	146.1	198.89	230.0	210.6	235.1	239.0
tooth socket NEC	143.9	198.89	230.0	210.4	235.1	239.0
trachea (cartilage) (mucosa)	162.0	197.3	231.1	212.2	235.7	239.1
contiguous sites with bronchus or lung	162.8	—	—	—	—	—
tracheobronchial	162.8	197.3	231.1	212.2	235.7	239.1
contiguous sites with lung	162.8	—	—	—	—	—
tragus	173.2	198.2	232.2	216.2	238.2	239.2
trunk NEC*	195.8	198.89	232.5	229.8	238.8	239.8
tubo-ovarian	183.8	198.82	233.3	221.8	236.3	239.5
tunica vaginalis	187.8	198.82	233.6	222.8	236.6	239.5
turbinate (bone)	170.0	198.5	—	213.0	238.0	239.2
nasal	160.0	197.3	231.8	212.0	235.9	239.1
tympanic cavity	160.1	197.3	231.8	212.0	235.9	239.1
ulna (any part)	170.4	198.5	—	213.4	238.0	239.2
umbilicus, umbilical	173.5	198.2	232.5	216.5	238.2	239.2
uncus, brain	191.2	198.3	—	225.0	237.5	239.6
unknown site or unspecified	199.1	199.1	234.9	229.9	238.9	239.9
urachus	188.7	198.1	233.7	223.3	236.7	239.4
ureter, ureteral	189.2	198.1	233.9	223.2	236.91	239.5
orifice (bladder)	188.6	198.1	233.7	223.3	236.7	239.4
ureter-bladder junction)	188.6	198.1	233.7	223.3	236.7	239.4
urethra, urethral (gland)	189.3	198.1	233.9	223.81	236.99	239.5
orifice, internal	188.5	198.1	233.7	223.3	236.7	239.4
urethrovaginal (septum)	184.9	198.82	233.3	221.9	236.3	239.5
urinary organ or system NEC	189.9	198.1	233.9	223.9	236.99	239.5
bladder — *see* Neoplasm, bladder						
contiguous sites	189.8	—	—	—	—	—
specified sites NEC	189.8	198.1	233.9	223.89	236.99	239.5
utero-ovarian	183.8	198.82	233.3	221.8	236.3	239.5
ligament	183.3	198.82	—	221.0	236.3	239.5
uterosacral ligament	183.4	198.82	—	221.0	236.3	239.5
uterus, uteri, uterine	179	198.82	233.2	219.9	236.0	239.5
adnexa NEC	183.9	198.82	233.3	221.8	236.3	239.5
contiguous sites	183.8	—	—	—	—	—
body	182.0	198.82	233.2	219.1	236.0	239.5
contiguous sites	182.8	—	—	—	—	—
cervix	180.9	198.82	233.1	219.0	236.0	239.5
tornu	182.0	198.82	233.2	219.1	236.0	239.5
corpus	182.0	198.82	233.2	219.1	236.0	239.5
endocervix (canal) (gland)	180.0	198.82	233.1	219.0	236.0	239.5
endometrium	182.0	198.82	233.2	219.1	236.0	239.5
exocervix	180.1	198.82	233.1	219.0	236.0	239.5
external os	180.1	198.82	233.1	219.0	236.0	239.5
fundus	182.0	198.82	233.2	219.1	236.0	239.5
internal os	180.0	198.82	233.1	219.0	236.0	239.5
isthmus	182.1	198.82	233.2	219.1	236.0	239.5
ligament	183.4	198.82	—	221.0	236.3	239.5
broad	183.3	198.82	233.3	221.0	236.3	239.5
round	183.5	198.82	—	221.0	236.3	239.5
lower segment	182.1	198.82	233.2	219.1	236.0	239.5
myometrium	182.0	198.82	233.2	219.1	236.0	239.5
squamocolumnar junction	180.8	198.82	233.1	219.0	236.0	239.5
tube	183.2	198.82	233.3	221.0	236.3	239.5
utricle, prostatic	189.3	198.1	233.9	223.81	236.99	239.5
uveal tract	190.0	198.4	234.0	224.0	238.8	239.8
uvula	145.4	198.89	230.0	210.4	235.1	239.0
vagina, vaginal (fornix) (vault) (wall)	184.0	198.82	233.3	221.1	236.3	239.5
vaginovesical	184.9	198.82	233.3	221.9	236.3	239.5
septum	194.9	198.82	233.3	221.9	236.3	239.5
vallecula (epiglottis)	146.3	198.89	230.0	210.6	235.1	239.0
vascular — *see* Neoplasm, connective tissue						

	Malignant			Benign	Uncertain Behavior	Unspecified
	Primary	Secondary	Ca in situ			
Neoplasm, neoplastic—*continued*						
vas deferens	187.6	198.82	233.6	222.8	236.6	239.5
Vater's ampulla	156.2	197.8	230.8	211.5	235.3	239.0
vein, venous — *see* Neoplasm, connective tissue						
vena cava (abdominal) (inferior)	171.5	198.89	—	215.5	238.1	239.2
superior	171.4	198.89	—	215.4	238.1	239.2
ventricle (cerebral) (floor) (fourth) (lateral) (third)	191.5	198.3	—	225.0	237.5	239.6
cardiac (left) (right)	164.1	198.89	—	212.7	238.8	239.8
ventricular band of larynx	161.1	197.3	231.0	212.1	235.6	239.1
ventriculus — *see* Neoplasm, stomach						
vermillion border — *see* Neoplasm, lip						
vermis, cerebellum	191.6	198.3	—	225.0	237.5	239.6
vertebra (column)	170.2	198.5	—	213.2	238.0	239.2
coccyx	170.6	198.5	—	213.6	238.0	239.2
sacrum	170.6	198.5	—	213.6	238.0	239.2
vesical — *see* Neoplasm, bladder						
vesicle, seminal	187.8	198.82	233.6	222.8	236.6	239.5
vesicocervical tissue	184.9	198.82	233.3	221.9	236.3	239.5
vesicorectal	195.3	198.89	234.8	229.8	238.8	239.8
vesicovaginal	184.9	198.82	233.3	221.9	236.3	239.5
septum	184.9	198.82	233.3	221.9	236.3	239.5
vessel (blood) — *see* Neoplasm, connective tissue						
vestibular gland, greater	184.1	198.82	233.3	221.2	236.3	239.5
vestibule						
mouth	145.1	198.89	230.0	210.4	235.1	239.0
nose	160.0	197.3	231.8	212.0	235.9	239.1
Virchow's gland	—	196.0	—	229.0	238.8	239.8
viscera NEC	195.8	198.89	234.8	229.8	238.8	239.8
vocal cords (true)	161.0	197.3	231.0	212.1	235.6	239.1
false	161.1	197.3	231.0	212.1	235.6	239.1
vomer	170.0	198.5	—	213.0	238.0	239.2
vulva	184.4	198.82	233.3	221.2	236.3	239.5
vulvovaginal gland	184.4	198.82	233.3	221.2	236.3	239.5
Waldeyer's ring	149.1	198.89	230.0	210.9	235.1	239.0
Wharton's duct	142.1	198.89	230.0	210.2	235.0	239.0
white matter (central) (cerebral)	191.0	198.3	—	225.0	237.5	239.6
windpipe	162.0	197.3	231.1	212.2	235.7	239.1
Wirsung's duct	157.3	197.8	230.9	211.6	235.5	239.0
wolffian (body) (duct)						
female	184.8	198.82	233.3	221.8	236.3	239.5
male	187.8	198.82	233.6	222.8	236.6	239.5
womb — *see* Neoplasm, uterus						
wrist NEC*	195.4	198.89	232.6	229.8	238.8	239.8
xiphoid process	170.3	198.5	—	213.3	238.0	239.2
Zuckerkandl's organ	194.6	198.89	—	227.6	237.3	239.7

Neovascularization
    choroid 362.16
    ciliary body 364.42
    cornea 370.60
        deep 370.63
        localized 370.61
    iris 364.42
    retina 362.16
    subretinal 362.16
Nephralgia 788.0
Nephritis, nephritic (albuminuric)
    (azotemic) (congenital)
    (degenerative) (diffuse)
    (disseminated) (epithelial)
    (familial) (focal)
    (granulomatous) (hemorrhagic)
    (infantile) (nonsuppurative,
    excretory) (uremic) 583.9
    with
        edema — see Nephrosis
        lesion of
            glomerulonephritis
                hypocomplementemic
                      persistent 583.2
                      with nephrotic
                          syndrome
                          581.2
                      chronic 582.2
                lobular 583.2
                    with nephrotic
                        syndrome
                        581.2
                    chronic 582.2
                membranoproliferative
                    583.2
                    with nephrotic
                        syndrome
                        581.2
                    chronic 582.2
                membranous 583.1
                    with nephrotic
                        syndrome
                        581.1
                    chronic 582.1
                mesangiocapillary 583.2
                    with nephrotic
                        syndrome
                        581.2
                    chronic 582.2
                mixed membranous and
                    proliferative 583.2
                    with nephrotic
                        syndrome
                        581.2
                    chronic 582.2
                proliferative (diffuse)
                    583.0
                    with nephrotic
                        syndrome
                        581.0
                    acute 580.0
                    chronic 582.0
                    rapidly progressive
                      583.4
                    acute 580.4
                    chronic 582.4
                interstitial nephritis (diffuse)
                    (focal) 583.89
                    with nephrotic
                        syndrome 581.89
                    acute 580.89
                    chronic 582.89
                necrotizing glomerulitis
                    583.4
                    acute 580.4
                    chronic 582.4
                renal necrosis 583.9
                    cortical 583.6
                    medullary 583.7
                specified pathology NEC
                    583.89
                    with nephrotic
                        syndrome 581.89
                    acute 580.89
                    chronic 582.89

Nephritis, nephritic—continued
    with—continued
        necrosis, renal 583.9
            cortical 583.6
            medullary (papillary) 583.7
        nephrotic syndrome (see also
            Nephrosis) 581.9
        papillary necrosis 583.7
        specified pathology NEC
            583.89
    acute 580.9
        extracapillary with epithelial
            crescents 580.4
        hypertensive (see also
            Hypertension, kidney)
            403.90
        necrotizing 580.4
        poststreptococcal 580.0
        proliferative (diffuse) 580.0
        rapidly progressive 580.4
        specified pathology NEC
            580.89
    amyloid 277.3 [583.81]
        chronic 277.3 [582.81]
    arteriolar (see also Hypertension,
        kidney) 403.90
    arteriosclerotic (see also
        Hypertension, kidney)
        403.90
    ascending (see also Pyelitis)
        590.80
    atrophic 582.9
    basement membrane NEC 583.89
        with
            pulmonary hemorrhage
                (Goodpasture's
                syndrome) 446.21
                [583.81]
    calculous, calculus 592.0
    cardiac (see also Hypertension,
        kidney) 403.90
    cardiovascular (see also
        Hypertension, kidney)
        403.90
    chronic 582.9
        arteriosclerotic (see also
            Hypertension, kidney)
            403.90
        hypertensive (see also
            Hypertension, kidney)
            403.90
    cirrhotic (see also Sclerosis, renal)
        587
    complicating pregnancy,
        childbirth, or puerperium
        646.2
        with hypertension 642.1
            affecting fetus or newborn
                760.0
        affecting fetus or newborn
            760.1
    croupous 580.9
    desquamative — see Nephrosis
    due to
        amyloidosis 277.3 [583.81]
            chronic 277.3 [582.81]
        arteriosclerosis (see also
            Hypertension, kidney)
            403.90
        diabetes mellitus 250.4
            [583.81]
            with nephrotic syndrome
                250.4 [581.81]
        diphtheria 032.89 [580.81]
        gonococcal infection (acute)
            098.19 [583.81]
            chronic or duration of 2
                months or over
                098.39 [583.81]
        gout 274.10
        infectious hepatitis 070.9
            [580.81]
        mumps 072.79 [580.81]
        specified kidney pathology
            NEC 583.89
            acute 580.89
            chronic 582.89

Nephritis, nephritic—continued
    due to—continued
        streptotrichosis 039.8 [583.81]
        subacute bacterial endocarditis
            421.0
        systemic lupus erythematosus
            710.0 [583.81]
            chronic 710.0 [582.81]
        typhoid fever 002.0 [580.81]
    endothelial 582.2
    end stage (chronic) (terminal)
        NEC 585
    epimembranous 581.1
    exudative 583.89
        with nephrotic syndrome
            581.89
        acute 580.89
        chronic 582.89
    gonococcal (acute) 098.19
        [583.81]
        chronic or duration of 2
            months or over 098.39
            [583.81]
    gouty 274.10
    hereditary (Alport's syndrome)
        759.89
    hydremic — see Nephrosis
    hypertensive (see also
        Hypertension, kidney)
        403.90
    hypocomplementemic persistent
        583.2
        with nephrotic syndrome
            581.2
        chronic 582.2
    immune complex NEC 583.89
    infective (see also Pyelitis) 590.80
    interstitial (diffuse) (focal) 583.89
        with nephrotic syndrome
            581.89
        acute 580.89
        chronic 582.89
    latent or quiescent — see
        Nephritis, chronic
    lead 984.9
        specified type of lead — see
            Table of drugs and
            chemicals
    lobular 583.2
        with nephrotic syndrome
            581.2
        chronic 582.2
    lupus 710.0 [583.81]
        acute 710.0 [580.81]   ◆
        chronic 710.0 [582.81]
    membranoproliferative 583.2
        with nephrotic syndrome
            581.2
        chronic 582.2
    membranous 583.1
        with nephrotic syndrome
            581.1
        chronic 582.1
    mesangiocapillary 583.2
        with nephrotic syndrome
            581.2
        chronic 582.2
    minimal change 581.3
    mixed membranous and
        proliferative 583.2
        with nephrotic syndrome
            581.2
        chronic 582.2
    necrotic, necrotizing 583.4
        acute 580.4
        chronic 582.4
    nephrotic — see Nephrosis
    old — see Nephritis, chronic
    parenchymatous 581.89
    polycystic 753.12
        adult type (APKD) 753.13
        autosomal dominant 753.13
        autosomal recessive 753.14
        childhood type (CPKD) 753.14
        infantile type 753.14
    poststreptococcal 580.0

Nephritis, nephritic—continued
    pregnancy — see Nephritis,
        complicating pregnancy
    proliferative 583.0
        with nephrotic syndrome
            581.0
        acute 580.0
        chronic 582.0
    purulent (see also Pyelitis) 590.80
    rapidly progressive 583.4
        acute 580.4
        chronic 582.4
    salt-losing or salt-wasting (see
        also Disease, renal) 593.9
    saturnine 984.9
        specified type of lead — see
            Table of drugs and
            chemicals
    septic (see also Pyelitis) 590.80
    specified pathology NEC 583.89
        acute 580.89
        chronic 582.89
    staphylococcal (see also Pyelitis)
        590.80
    streptotrichosis 039.8 [583.81]
    subacute (see also Nephrosis)
        581.9
    suppurative (see also Pyelitis)
        590.80
    syphilitic (late) 095.4
        congenital 090.5 [583.81]
        early 091.69 [583.81]
    terminal (chronic) (end-stage)
        NEC 585
    toxic — see Nephritis, acute
    tubal, tubular — see Nephrosis,
        tubular
    tuberculous (see also
        Tuberculosis) 016.0
        [583.81]
    type II (Ellis) — see Nephrosis
    vascular — see Hypertension,
        kidney
    war 580.9
Nephroblastoma (M8960/3) 189.0
    epithelial (M8961/3) 189.0
    mesenchymal (M8962/3) 189.0
Nephrocalcinosis 275.4
Nephrocystitis, pustular (see also
    Pyelitis) 590.80
Nephrolithiasis (congenital) (pelvis)
    (recurrent) 592.0
    uric acid 274.11
Nephroma (M8960/3) 189.0
    mesoblastic (M8960/1) 236.9
Nephronephritis (see also Nephrosis)
    581.9
Nephronopthisis 753.16
Nephropathy (see also Nephritis)
    583.9
    with
        exudative nephritis 583.89
        interstitial nephritis (diffuse)
            (focal) 583.89
        medullary necrosis 583.7
        necrosis 583.9
            cortical 583.6
            medullary or papillary
                583.7
        papillary necrosis 583.7
        specified lesion or cause NEC
            583.89
    analgesic 583.89
        with medullary necrosis, acute
            584.7
    arteriolar (see also Hypertension,
        kidney) 403.90
    arteriosclerotic (see also
        Hypertension, kidney)
        403.90
    complicating pregnancy 646.2
    diabetic 250.4 [583.81]
    gouty 274.10
        specified type NEC 274.19
    hypercalcemic 588.8

Nephropathy—continued
  hypertensive (see also
      Hypertension, kidney)
      403.90
  hypokalemic (vacuolar) 588.8
  obstructive 593.89
    congenital 753.2
  phenacetin 584.7
  phosphate-losing 588.0
  potassium depletion 588.8
  proliferative (see also Nephritis,
      proliferative) 583.0
  protein-losing 588.8
  salt-losing or salt-wasting (see
      also Disease, renal) 593.9
  sickle-cell (see also Disease,
      sickle-cell) 282.60 [583.81]
  toxic 584.5
  vasomotor 584.5
  water-losing 588.8
Nephroptosis (see also Disease,
    renal) 593.0
  congenital (displaced) 753.3
Nephropyosis (see also Abscess,
    kidney) 590.2
Nephrorrhagia 593.81
Nephrosclerosis (arteriolar)
    (arteriosclerotic) (chronic)
    (hyaline) (see also
    Hypertension, kidney) 403.90
  gouty 274.10
  hyperplastic (arteriolar) (see also
      Hypertension, kidney)
      403.90
  senile (see also Sclerosis, renal)
      587
Nephrosis, nephrotic (Epstein's)
    (syndrome) 581.9
  with
    lesion of
      focal glomerulosclerosis
        581.1
      glomerulonephritis
        endothelial 581.2
          hypocomplementemic
            persistent 581.2
        lobular 581.2
        membranoproliferative
          581.2
        membranous 581.1
        mesangiocapillary 581.2
        minimal change 581.3
        mixed membranous and
          proliferative 581.2
        proliferative 581.0
      segmental hyalinosis 581.1
      specified pathology NEC
        581.89
  acute — see Nephrosis, tubular
  anoxic — see Nephrosis, tubular
  arteriosclerotic (see also
      Hypertension, kidney)
      403.90
  chemical — see Nephrosis,
      tubular
  cholemic 572.4
  complicating pregnancy,
      childbirth, or puerperium
      — see Nephritis,
      complicating pregnancy
  diabetic 250.4 [581.81]
  hemoglobinuric — see Nephrosis,
      tubular
  in
    amyloidosis 277.3 [581.81]
    diabetes mellitus 250.4
      [581.81]
    epidemic hemorrhagic fever
      078.6
    malaria 084.9 [581.81]
    polyarteritis 446.0 [581.81]
    systemic lupus erythematosus
      710.0 [581.81]
  ischemic — see Nephrosis,
      tubular
  lipoid 581.3

Nephrosis, nephrotic—continued
  lower nephron — see Nephrosis,
      tubular
  lupoid 710.0 [581.81]
  lupus 710.0 [581.81]
  malarial 084.9 [581.81]
  minimal change 581.3
  necrotizing — see Nephrosis,
      tubular
  osmotic (sucrose) 588.8
  polyarteritic 446.0 [581.81]
  radiation 581.9
  specified lesion or cause NEC
    581.89
  syphilitic 095.4
  toxic — see Nephrosis, tubular
  tubular (acute) 584.5
    due to a procedure 997.5
    radiation 581.9
Nephrosonephritis hemorrhagic
    (endemic) 078.6
Nephrostomy status V44.6
  with complication 997.5
Nerve — see condition
Nerves 799.2
Nervous (see also condition) 799.2
  breakdown 300.9
  heart 306.2
  stomach 306.4
  tension 799.2
Nervousness 799.2
Nesidioblastoma (M8150/0)
  pancreas 211.7
  specified site NEC — see
      Neoplasm, by site, benign
  unspecified site 211.7
Netherton's syndrome
    (ichthyosiform erythroderma)
    757.1
Nettle rash 708.8
Nettleship's disease (urticaria
    pigmentosa) 757.33
Neumann's disease (pemphigus
    vegetans) 694.4
Neuralgia, neuralgic (acute) (see also
    Neuritis) 729.2
  accessory (nerve) 352.4
  acoustic (nerve) 388.5
  ankle 355.8
  anterior crural 355.8
  anus 787.9
  arm 723.4
  auditory (nerve) 388.5
  axilia 353.0
  bladder 788.1
  brachial 723.4
  brain — see Disorder, nerve,
      cranial
  broad ligament 625.9
  cerebral — see Disorder, nerve,
      cranial
  ciliary 346.2
  cranial nerve — see also
      Disorder, nerve, cranial
    fifth or trigeminal (see also
        Neuralgia, trigeminal)
        350.1
  ear 388.71
    middle 352.1
  facial 351.8
  finger 354.9
  flank 355.8
  foot 355.8
  forearm 354.9
  Fothergill's (see also Neuralgia,
      trigeminal) 350.1
    postherpetic 053.12
  glossopharyngeal (nerve) 352.1
  groin 355.8
  hand 354.9
  heel 355.8
  Horton's 346.2
  Hunt's 053.11
  hypoglossal (nerve) 352.5
  iliac region 355.8

Neuralgia, neuralgic—continued
  infraorbital (see also Neuralgia,
      trigeminal) 350.1
  inguinal 355.8
  intercostal (nerve) 353.8
    postherpetic 053.19
  jaw 352.1
  kidney 788.0
  knee 355.8
  loin 355.8
  malarial (see also Malaria) 084.6
  mastoid 385.89
  maxilla 352.1
  median thenar 354.1
  metatarsal 355.6
  middle ear 352.1
  migrainous 346.2
  Morton's 355.6
  nerve, cranial — see Disorder,
      nerve, cranial
  nose 352.0
  olfactory (nerve) 352.0
  ophthalmic 377.30
    postherpetic 053.19
  optic (nerve) 377.30
  penis 607.9
  perineum 355.8
  pleura 511.0
  postherpetic NEC 053.19
    geniculate ganglion 053.11
    ophthalmic 053.19
    trifacial 053.12
    trigeminal 053.12
  pubic region 355.8
  radial (nerve) 723.4
  rectum 787.9
  sacroiliac joint 724.3
  sciatic (nerve) 724.3
  scrotum 608.9
  seminal vesicle 608.9
  shoulder 354.9
  Sluder's 337.0
  specified nerve NEC — see
      Disorder, nerve
  spermatic cord 608.9
  sphenopalatine (ganglion) 337.0
  subscapular (nerve) 723.4
  suprascapular (nerve) 723.4
  testis 608.89
  thenar (median) 354.1
  thigh 355.8
  tongue 352.5
  trifacial (nerve) (see also
      Neuralgia, trigeminal)
      350.1
  trigeminal (nerve) 350.1
    postherpetic 053.12
  tympanic plexus 388.71
  ulnar (nerve) 723.4
  vagus (nerve) 352.3
  wrist 354.9
  writers' 300.89
    organic 333.84
Neurapraxia — see Injury, nerve, by
    site
Neurasthenia 300.5
  cardiac 306.2
  gastric 306.4
  heart 306.2
  postfebrile 780.7
  postviral 780.7
Neurilemmoma (M9560/0) — see
    also Neoplasm, connective
    tissue, benign
  acoustic (nerve) 225.1
  malignant (M9560/3) — see also
      Neoplasm, connective
      tissue, malignant
    acoustic (nerve) 192.0
Neurilemmosarcoma (M9560/3) —
    see Neoplasm, connective
    tissue, malignant
Neurilemoma — see Neurilemmoma
Neurinoma (M9560/0) — see
    Neurilemmoma

Neurinomatosis (M9560/1) — see
    also Neoplasm, connective
    tissue, uncertain behavior
  centralis 759.5
Neuritis (see also Neuralgia) 729.2
  abducens (nerve) 378.54
  accessory (nerve) 352.4
  acoustic (nerve) 388.5
    syphilitic 094.86
  alcoholic 357.5
    with psychosis 291.1
  amyloid, any site 277.3 [357.4]
  anterior crural 355.8
  arising during pregnancy 646.4
  arm 723.4
  ascending 355.2
  auditory (nerve) 388.5
  brachial (nerve) NEC 723.4
    due to displacement,
        intervertebral disc 722.0
  cervical 723.4
  chest (wall) 353.8
  costal region 353.8
  cranial nerve — see also
      Disorder, nerve, cranial
    first or olfactory 352.0
    second or optic 377.30
    third or oculomotor 378.52
    fourth or trochlear 378.53
    fifth or trigeminal (see also
        Neuralgia, trigeminal)
        350.1
    sixth or abducens 378.54
    seventh or facial 351.8
      newborn 767.5
    eighth or acoustic 388.5
    ninth or glossopharyngeal
        352.1
    tenth or vagus 352.3
    eleventh or accessory 352.4
    twelfth or hypoglossal 352.5
  Déjérine-Sottas 356.0
  diabetic 250.6 [357.2]
  diphtheritic 032.89 [357.4]
  due to
    beriberi 265.0 [357.4]
    displacement, prolapse,
        protrusion, or rupture of
        intervertebral disc 722.2
      cervical 722.0
      lumbar, lumbosacral
        722.10
      thoracic, thoracolumbar
        722.11
    herniation, nucleus pulposus
        722.2
      cervical 722.0
      lumbar, lumbosacral
        722.10
      thoracic, thoracolumbar
        722.11
  endemic 265.0 [357.4]
  facial (nerve) 351.8
    newborn 767.5
  general — see Polyneuropathy
  geniculate ganglion 351.1
    due to herpes 053.11
  glossopharyngeal (nerve) 352.1
  gouty 274.89 [357.4]
  hypoglossal (nerve) 352.5
  ilioinguinal (nerve) 355.8
  in diseases classified elsewhere
      — see Polyneuropathy, in
  infectious (multiple) 357.0
  intercostal (nerve) 353.8
  interstitial hypertrophic
      progressive NEC 356.9
  leg 355.8
  lumbosacral NEC 724.4
  median (nerve) 354.1
    thenar 354.1
  multiple (acute) (infective) 356.9
    endemic 265.0 [357.4]
    multiplex endemica 265.0
      [357.4]
  nerve root (see also Radiculitis)
      729.2

Neuritis—continued
- oculomotor (nerve) 378.52
- olfactory (nerve) 352.0
- optic (nerve) 377.30
  - in myelitis 341.0
  - meningococcal 036.81
- pelvic 355.8
- peripheral (nerve) — see also Neuropathy, peripheral
  - complicating pregnancy or puerperium 646.4
  - specified nerve NEC — see Mononeuritis
- pneumogastric (nerve) 352.3
- postchickenpox 052.7
- postherpetic 053.19
- progressive hypertrophic interstitial NEC 356.9
- puerperal, postpartum 646.4
- radial (nerve) 723.4
- retrobulbar 377.32
  - syphilitic 094.85
- rheumatic (chronic) 729.2
- sacral region 355.8
- sciatic (nerve) 724.3
  - due to displacement of intervertebral disc 722.10
- serum 999.5
- specified nerve NEC — see Disorder, nerve
- spinal (nerve) 355.9
  - root (see also Radiculitis) 729.2
- subscapular (nerve) 723.4
- suprascapular (nerve) 723.4
- syphilitic 095.8
- thenar (median) 354.1
- thoracic NEC 724.4
- toxic NEC 357.7
- trochlear (nerve) 378.53
- ulnar (nerve) 723.4
- vagus (nerve) 352.3

Neuroangiomatosis, encephalofacial 759.6

Neuroastrocytoma (M9505/1) — see Neoplasm, by site, uncertain behavior

Neuro-avitaminosis 269.2

Neuroblastoma (M9500/3)
- olfactory (M9522/3) 160.0
- specified site — see Neoplasm, by site, malignant
- unspecified site 194.0

Neurochorioretinitis (see also Chorioretinitis) 363.20

Neurocirculatory asthenia 306.2

Neurocytoma (M9506/0) — see Neoplasm, by site, benign

Neurodermatitis (circumscribed) (circumscripta) (local) 698.3
- atopic 691.8
- diffuse (Brocq) 691.8
- disseminated 691.8
- nodulosa 698.3

Neuroencephalomyelopathy, optic 341.0

Neuroepithelioma (M9503/3) — see also Neoplasm, by site, malignant
- olfactory (M9521/3) 160.0

Neurofibroma (M9540/0) — see also Neoplasm, connective tissue, benign
- melanotic (M9541/0) — see Neoplasm, connective tissue, benign
- multiple (M9540/1) 237.70
  - Type 1 237.71
  - Type 2 237.72
- plexiform (M9550/0) — see Neoplasm, connective tissue, benign

Neurofibromatosis (multiple) (M9540/1) 237.70
- acoustic 237.72
- malignant (M9540/3) — see Neoplasm, connective tissue, malignant
  - Type 1 237.71
  - Type 2 237.72
- von Recklinghausen's 237.71

Neurofibrosarcoma (M9540/3) — see Neoplasm, connective tissue, malignant

Neurogenic — see also condition
- bladder (atonic) (automatic) (autonomic) (flaccid) (hypertonic) (hypotonic) (inertia) (infranuclear) (irritable) (motor) (nonreflex) (nuclear) (paralysis) (reflex) (sensory) (spastic) (supranuclear) (uninhibited) 596.54
  - with cauda equina syndrome 344.61
- heart 306.2

Neuroglioma (M9505/1) — see Neoplasm, by site, uncertain behavior

Neurolabyrinthitis (of Dix and Hallpike) 386.12

Neurolathyrism 988.2

Neuroleprosy 030.1

Neuroleptic malignant syndrome 333.92 ◆

Neurolipomatosis 272.8

Neuroma (M9570/0) — see also Neoplasm, connective tissue, benign
- acoustic (nerve) (M9560/0) 225.1
- amputation (traumatic) — see also Injury, nerve, by site
  - surgical complication (late) 997.61
- appendix 211.3
- auditory nerve 225.1
- digital 355.6
  - toe 355.6
- interdigital (toe) 355.6
- intermetatarsal 355.6
- Morton's 355.6
- multiple 237.70
  - Type 1 237.71
  - Type 2 237.72
- nonneoplastic 355.9
  - arm NEC 354.9
  - leg NEC 355.8
  - lower extremity NEC 355.8
  - specified site NEC — see Mononeuritis, by site
  - upper extremity NEC 354.9
- optic (nerve) 225.1
- plantar 355.6
- plexiform (M9550/0) — see Neoplasm, connective tissue, benign
- surgical (nonneoplastic) 355.9
  - arm NEC 354.9
  - leg NEC 355.8
  - lower extremity NEC 355.8
  - upper extremity NEC 354.9
- traumatic — see also Injury, nerve, by site
  - old — see Neuroma, nonneoplastic

Neuromyalgia 729.1

Neuromyasthenia (epidemic) 049.8

Neuromyelitis 341.8
- ascending 357.0
- optica 341.0

Neuromyopathy NEC 358.9

Neuromyositis 729.1

Neuronevus (M8725/0) — see Neoplasm, skin, benign

Neuronitis 357.0
- ascending (acute) 355.2
- vestibular 386.12

Neuroparalytic — see condition

Neuropathy, neuropathic (see also Disorder, nerve) 355.9
- alcoholic 357.5
  - with psychosis 291.1
- arm NEC 354.9
- autonomic (peripheral) — see Neuropathy, peripheral, autonomic
- axillary nerve 353.0
- brachial plexus 353.0
- cervical plexus 353.2
- chronic
  - progressive segmentally demyelinating 357.8
  - relapsing demyelinating 357.8
- congenital sensory 356.2
- Déjérine-Sottas 356.0
- diabetic 250.6 [357.2]
- entrapment 355.9
  - iliohypogastric nerve 355.79
  - ilioinguinal nerve 355.79
  - lateral cutaneous nerve of thigh 355.1
  - median nerve 354.0
  - obturator nerve 355.79
  - peroneal nerve 355.3
  - posterior tibial nerve 355.5
  - saphenous nerve 355.79
  - ulnar nerve 354.2
- facial nerve 351.9
- hereditary 356.9
  - peripheral 356.0
  - sensory (radicular) 356.2
- hypertrophic
  - Charcot-Marie-Tooth 356.1
  - Déjérine-Sottas 356.0
  - interstitial 356.9
  - Refsum 356.3
- intercostal nerve 354.8
- ischemic — see Disorder, nerve
- Jamaican (ginger) 357.7
- leg NEC 355.8
- lower extremity NEC 355.8
- lumbar plexus 353.1
- median nerve 354.1
- multiple (acute) (chronic) (see also Polyneuropathy) 356.9
- optic 377.39
  - ischemic 377.41
  - nutritional 377.33
  - toxic 377.34
- peripheral (nerve) (see also Polyneuropathy) 356.9
  - arm NEC 354.9
  - autonomic 337.9
    - amyloid 277.3 [337.1]
    - idiopathic 337.0
    - in
      - amyloidosis 277.3 [337.1]
      - diabetes (mellitus) 250.6 [337.1]
      - diseases classified elsewhere 337.1
      - gout 274.89 [337.1]
      - hyperthyroidism 242.9 [337.1]
    - due to
      - antitetanus serum 357.6
      - arsenic 357.7
      - drugs 357.6
      - lead 357.7
      - organophosphate compounds 357.7
      - toxic agent NEC 357.7
  - hereditary 356.0
  - idiopathic 356.9
    - progressive 356.4
    - specified type NEC 356.8
  - in diseases classified elsewhere — see Polyneuropathy, in
  - leg NEC 355.8

Neuropathy, neuropathic—continued
- peripheral—continued
  - lower extremity NEC 355.8
  - upper extremity NEC 354.9
  - plantar nerves 355.6
  - progressive hypertrophic interstitial 356.9
  - radicular NEC 729.2
    - brachial 723.4
    - cervical NEC 723.4
    - hereditary sensory 356.2
    - lumbar 724.4
    - lumbosacral 724.4
    - thoracic NEC 724.4
  - sacral plexus 353.1
  - sciatic 355.0
  - spinal nerve NEC 355.9
    - root (see also Radiculitis) 729.2
  - toxic 357.7
  - trigeminal sensory 350.8
  - ulnar nerve 354.2
  - upper extremity NEC 354.9
  - uremic 585 [357.4]
  - vitamin B_{12} 266.2 [357.4]
    - with anemia (pernicious) 281.0 [357.4]
    - due to dietary deficiency 281.1 [357.4]

Neurophthisis — (see also Disorder, nerve peripheral) 356.9
- diabetic 250.6 [357.2]

Neuroretinitis 363.05
- syphilitic 094.85

Neurosarcoma (M9540/3) — see Neoplasm, connective tissue, malignant

Neurosclerosis — see Disorder, nerve

Neurosis, neurotic 300.9
- accident 300.16
- anancastic, anankastic 300.3
- anxiety (state) 300.00
  - generalized 300.02
  - panic type 300.01
- asthenic 300.5
- bladder 306.53
- cardiac (reflex) 306.2
- cardiovascular 306.2
- climacteric, unspecified type 627.2
- colon 306.4
- compensation 300.16
- compulsive, compulsion 300.3
- conversion 300.11
- craft 300.89
- cutaneous 306.3
- depersonalization 300.6
- depressive (reaction) (type) 300.4
- endocrine 306.6
- environmental 300.89
- fatigue 300.5
- functional (see also Disorder, psychosomatic) 306.9
- gastric 306.4
- gastrointestinal 306.4
- genitourinary 306.50
- heart 306.2
- hypochondriacal 300.7
- hysterical 300.10
  - conversion type 300.11
  - dissociative type 300.15
- impulsive 300.3
- incoordination 306.0
  - larynx 306.1
  - vocal cord 306.1
- intestine 306.4
- larynx 306.1
  - hysterical 300.11
  - sensory 306.1
- menopause, unspecified type 627.2
- mixed NEC 300.89
- musculoskeletal 306.0

Neurosis, neurotic—continued
obsessional 300.3
phobia 300.3
obsessive-compulsive 300.3
occupational 300.89
ocular 306.7
oral 307.0
organ (see also Disorder,
psychosomatic) 306.9
pharynx 306.1
phobic 300.20
posttraumatic (acute) (situational) 308.3
chronic 309.81
psychasthenic (type) 300.89
railroad 300.16
rectum 306.4
respiratory 306.1
rumination 306.4
senile 300.89
sexual 302.70
situational 300.89
specified type NEC 300.89
state 300.9
with depersonalization episode 300.6
stomach 306.4
vasomotor 306.2
visceral 306.4
war 300.16
Neurospongioblastosis diffusa 759.5
Neurosyphilis (arrested) (early)
(inactive) (late) (latent)
(recurrent) 094.9
with ataxia (cerebellar)
(locomotor) (spastic)
(spinal) 094.0
acute meningitis 094.2
aneurysm 094.89
arachnoid (adhesive) 094.2
arteritis (any artery) 094.89
asymptomatic 094.3
congenital 090.40
dura (mater) 094.89
general paresis 094.1
gumma 094.9
hemorrhagic 094.9
juvenile (asymptomatic)
(meningeal) 090.40
leptomeninges (aseptic) 094.2
meningeal 094.2
meninges (adhesive) 094.2
meningovascular (diffuse) 094.2
optic atrophy 094.84
parenchymatous (degenerative) 094.1
paresis (see also Paresis, general) 094.1
paretic (see also Paresis, general) 094.1
relapse 094.9
remission in (sustained) 094.9
serological 094.3
specified nature or site NEC 094.89
tabes (dorsalis) 094.0
juvenile 090.40
tabetic 094.0
juvenile 090.40
taboparesis 094.1
juvenile 090.40
thrombosis 094.89
vascular 094.89
Neurotic (see also Neurosis) 300.9
excoriation 698.4
psychogenic 306.3
Neurotmesis — see Injury, nerve, by site
Neurotoxemia — see Toxemia
Neutroclusion 524.2

Neutropenia, neutropenic (chronic)
(cyclic) (drug-induced)
(genetic) (idiopathic) (immune)
(infantile) (malignant)
(periodic) (pernicious)
(primary) (splenic)
(splenomegaly) (toxic) 288.0
chronic hypoplastic 288.0
congenital (nontransient) 288.0
neonatal, transitory (isoimmune)
(maternal transfer) 776.7
Neutrophilia, hereditary giant 288.2
Nevocarcinoma (M8720/3) — see Melanoma
Nevus (M8720/0) — see also Neoplasm, skin, benign

Note — Except where otherwise indicated, varieties of nevus in the list below that are followed by a morphology code number (M----/0) should be coded by site as for "Neoplasm, skin, benign."

acanthotic 702.8
achromic (M8730/0)
amelanotic (M8730/0)
anemic, anemicus 709.09 ◆
angiomatous (M9120/0) (see also Hemangioma) 228.00
araneus 448.1
avasculosus 709.09 ◆
balloon cell (M8722/0)
bathing trunk (M8761/1) 238.2
blue (M8780/0)
cellular (M8790/0)
giant (M8790/0)
Jadassohn's (M8780/0)
malignant (M8780/3) — see Melanoma
capillary (M9131/0) (see also Hemangioma) 228.00
cavernous (M9121/0) (see also Hemangioma) 228.00
cellular (M8720/0)
blue (M8790/0)
comedonicus 757.33
compound (M8760/0)
conjunctiva (M8720/0) 224.3
dermal (M8750/0)
and epidermal (M8760/0)
epithelioid cell (and spindle cell) (M8770/0)
flammeus 757.32
osteohypertrophic 759.89
hairy (M8720/0)
halo (M8723/0)
hemangiomatous (M9120/0) (see also Hemangioma) 228.00
intradermal (M8750/0)
intraepidermal (M8740/0)
involuting (M8724/0
Jadassohn's (blue) (M8780/0)
junction, junctional (M8740/0)
malignant melanoma in (M8740/3) — see Melanoma
juvenile (M8770/0)
lymphatic (M9170/0) 228.1
magnocellular (M8726/0)
specified site — see Neoplasm, by site, benign
unspecified site 224.0
malignant (M8720/3) — see Melanoma
meaning hemangioma (M9120/0) (see also Hemangioma) 228.00
melanotic (pigmented) (M8720/0)
multiplex 759.5
nonneoplastic 448.1
nonpigmented (M8730/0)
nonvascular (M8720/0)
oral mucosa, white sponge 750.26

Nevus—continued
osteohypertrophic, flammeus 759.89
papillaris (M8720/0)
papillomatosus (M8720/0)
pigmented (M8720/0)
giant (M8761/1) — see also Neoplasm, skin, uncertain behavior
malignant melanoma in (M8761/3) — see Melanoma
systematicus 757.33
pilosus (M8720/0)
port wine 757.32
sanguineous 757.32
sebaceous (senile) 702.8
senile 448.1
spider 448.1
spindle cell (and epithelioid cell) (M8770/0)
stellar 448.1
strawberry 757.32
syringocystadenomatous papilliferous (M8406/0)
unius lateris 757.33
Unna's 757.32
vascular 757.32
verrucous 757.33
white sponge (oral mucosa) 750.26
Newborn (infant) (liveborn)
multiple NEC
born in hospital (without mention of cesarean delivery or section) V37.00
with cesarean delivery or section V37.01
born outside hospital
hospitalized V37.1
not hospitalized V37.2
mates all liveborn
born in hospital (without mention of cesarean delivery or section) V34.00
with cesarean delivery or section V34.01
born outside hospital
hospitalized V34.1
not hospitalized V34.2
mates all stillborn
born in hospital (without mention of cesarean delivery or section) V35.00
with cesarean delivery or section V35.01
born outside hospital
hospitalized V35.1
not hospitalized V35.2
mates liveborn and stillborn
born in hospital (without mention of cesarean delivery or section) V36.00
with cesarean delivery or section V36.01
born outside hospital
hospitalized V36.1
not hospitalized V36.2
single
born in hospital (without mention of cesarean delivery or section) V30.00
with cesarean delivery or section V30.01
born outside hospital
hospitalized V30.1
not hospitalized V30.2

Newborn—continued
twin NEC
born in hospital (without mention of cesarean delivery or section) V33.00
with cesarean delivery or section V33.01
born outside hospital
hospitalized V33.1
not hospitalized V33.2
mate liveborn
born in hospital V31.0
born outside hospital
hospitalized V31.1
not hospitalized V31.2
mate stillborn
born in hospital V32.0
born outside hospital
hospitalized V32.1
not hospitalized V32.2
unspecified as to single or multiple birth
born in hospital (without mention of cesarean delivery or section) V39.00
with cesarean delivery or section V39.01
born outside hospital
hospitalized V39.1
not hospitalized V39.2
Newcastle's conjunctivitis or disease 077.8
Nezelof's syndrome (pure alymphocytosis) 279.13
Niacin (amide) deficiency 265.2
Nicolas-Durand-Favre disease (climatic bubo) 099.1
Nicolas-Favre disease (climatic bubo) 099.1
Nicotinic acid (amide) deficiency 265.2
Niemann-Pick disease (lipid histiocytosis) (splenomegaly) 272.7
Night
blindness (see also Blindness, night) 368.60
congenital 368.61
vitamin A deficiency 264.5
cramps 729.82
sweats 780.8
terrors, child 307.46
Nightmare 307.47
REM-sleep type 307.47
Nipple — see condition
Nisbet's chancre 099.0
Nishimoto (-Takeuchi) disease 437.5
Nitritoid crisis or reaction — see Crisis, nitritoid
Nitrogen retention, extrarenal 788.9
Nitrosohemoglobinemia 289.8
Njovera 104.0
No
diagnosis 799.9
disease (found) V71.9
room at the inn V65.0
Nocardiasis — see Nocardiosis
Nocardiosis 039.9
with pneumonia 039.1
lung 039.1
specified type NEC 039.8
Nocturia 788.43
psychogenic 306.53
Nocturnal — see also condition
dyspnea (paroxysmal) 786.09
emissions 608.89
enuresis 788.36
psychogenic 307.6
frequency (micturition) 788.43
psychogenic 306.53
Nodal rhythm disorder 427.89

Nodding of head 781.0
Node(s) — see also Nodule
　Heberden's 715.04
　larynx 478.79
　lymph — see condition
　milkers' 051.1
　Osler's 421.0
　rheumatic 729.89
　Schmorl's 722.30
　　lumbar, lumbosacral 722.32
　　specified region NEC 722.39
　　thoracic, thoracolumbar 722.31
　singers' 478.5
　skin NEC 782.2
　tuberculous — see Tuberculosis, lymph gland
　vocal cords 478.5
Nodosities, Haygarth's 715.04
Nodule(s), nodular
　actinomycotic (see also Actinomycosis) 039.9
　arthritic — see Arthritis, nodosa
　cutaneous 782.2
　Haygarth's 715.04
　inflammatory — see Inflammation
　juxta-articular 102.7
　　syphilitic 095.7
　　yaws 102.7
　larynx 478.79
　lung, solitary 518.89
　　emphysematous 492.8
　milkers' 051.1
　prostate 600
　rheumatic 729.89
　rheumatoid — see Arthritis, rheumatoid
　scrotum (inflammatory) 608.4
　singers' 478.5
　skin NEC 782.2
　solitary, lung 518.89
　　emphysematous 492.8
　subcutaneous 782.2
　thyroid (gland) (nontoxic) (uninodular) 241.0
　　with
　　　hyperthyroidism 242.1
　　　thyrotoxicosis 242.1
　　toxic or with hyperthyroidism 242.1
　vocal cords 478.5
Noma (gangrenous) (hospital) (infective) 528.1
　auricle (see also Gangrene) 785.4
　mouth 528.1
　pudendi (see also Vulvitis) 616.10
　vulvae (see also Vulvitis) 616.10
Nomadism V60.0
Non-autoimmune hemolytic anemia NEC 283.10
Nonclosure — see also Imperfect, closure
　ductus
　　arteriosus 747.0
　　Botalli 747.0
　Eustachian valve 746.89
　foramen
　　Botalli 745.5
　　ovale 745.5
Nondescent (congenital) — see also Malposition, congenital
　cecum 751.4
　colon 751.4
　testis 752.5
Nondevelopment
　brain 742.1
　　specified part 742.2
　heart 746.89
　organ or site, congenital NEC — see Hypoplasia
Nonengagement
　head NEC 652.5
　　in labor 660.1
　　　affecting fetus or newborn 763.1

Nonexanthematous tick fever 066.1
Nonexpansion, lung (newborn) NEC 770.4
Nonfunctioning
　cystic duct (see also Disease, gallbladder) 575.8
　gallbladder (see also Disease, gallbladder) 575.8
　kidney (see also Disease, renal) 593.9
　labyrinth 386.58
Nonhealing stump (surgical) 997.60
Nonimplantation of ovum, causing infertility 628.3
Noninsufflation, fallopian tube 628.2
Nonne-Milroy-Meige syndrome (chronic hereditary edema) 757.0
Nonovulation 628.0
Nonpatent fallopian tube 628.2
Nonpneumatization, lung NEC 770.4
Nonreflex bladder 596.54
　with cauda equina 344.61
Nonretention of food — see Vomiting
Nonrotation — see Malrotation
Nonsecretion, urine (see also Anuria) 788.5
　newborn 753.3
Nonunion
　fracture 733.82
　organ or site, congenital NEC — see Imperfect, closure
　symphysis pubis, congenital 755.69
　top sacrum, congenital 756.19
Nonviability 765.0
Nonvisualization, gallbladder 793.3
Nonvitalized tooth 522.9
Normal
　delivery — see category 650
　menses V65.5
　state (feared complaint unfounded) V65.5
Normoblastosis 289.8
Normocytic anemia (infectional) 285.9
　due to blood loss (chronic) 280.0
　　acute 285.1
Norrie's disease (congenital) (progressive oculoacousticocerebral degeneration) 743.8
North American blastomycosis 116.0
Norwegian itch 133.0
Nose, nasal — see condition
Nosebleed 784.7
Nosomania 298.9
Nosophobia 300.29
Nostalgia 309.89
Notch of iris 743.46
Notched lip, congenital (see also Cleft, lip) 749.10
Notching nose, congenital (tip) 748.1
Nothnagel's
　syndrome 378.52
　vasomotor acroparesthesia 443.89
Novy's relapsing fever (American) 087.1
Noxious
　foodstuffs, poisoning by
　　fish 988.0
　　fungi 988.1
　　mushrooms 988.1
　　plants (food) 988.2

Noxious—continued
　foodstuffs, poisoning by—continued
　　shellfish 988.0
　　specified type NEC 988.8
　　toadstool 988.1
　substances transmitted through placenta or breast milk 760.70
　　alcohol 760.71
　　anti-infective agents 760.74
　　cocaine 760.75
　　"crack" 760.75
　　hallucinogenic agents NEC 760.73
　　medicinal agents NEC 760.79
　　narcotics 760.72
　　obstetric anesthetic or analgesic 763.5
　　specified agent NEC 760.79
　　suspected, affecting management of pregnancy 655.5
Nuchal hitch (arm) 652.8
Nucleus pulposus — see condition
Numbness 782.0
Nuns' knee 727.2
Nutmeg liver 573.8
Nutrition, deficient or insufficient (particular kind of food) 269.9
　due to
　　insufficient food 994.2
　　lack of
　　　care 995.5
　　　food 994.2
Nyctalopia (see also Blindness, night) 368.60
　vitamin A deficiency 264.5
Nycturia 788.43
　psychogenic 306.53
Nymphomania 302.89
Nystagmus 379.50
　associated with vestibular system disorders 379.54
　benign paroxysmal positional 386.11
　central positional 386.2
　congenital 379.51
　deprivation 379.53
　dissociated 379.55
　latent 379.52
　miners' 300.89
　positional
　　benign paroxysmal 386.11
　　central 386.2
　specified NEC 379.56
　vestibular 379.54
　visual deprivation 379.53

Oasthouse urine disease 270.2
Obermeyer's relapsing fever
  (European) 087.0
Obesity (constitutional) (exogenous)
  (familial) (nutritional) (simple)
  278.0
  adrenal 255.8
  due to hyperalimentation 278.0
  endocrine NEC 259.9
  endogenous 259.9
  Fröhlich's (adiposogenital
    dystrophy) 253.8
  glandular NEC 259.9
  hypothyroid (see also
    Hypothyroidism) 244.9
  of pregnancy 646.1
  pituitary 253.8
  thyroid (see also Hypothyroidism)
    244.9
Oblique — see also condition
  lie before labor, affecting fetus or
    newborn 761.7
Obliquity, pelvis 738.6
Obliteration
  abdominal aorta 446.7
  appendix (lumen) 543.9
  artery 447.1
  ascending aorta 446.7
  bile ducts 576.8
    with calculus,
      choledocholithiasis, or
      stones — see
      Choledocholithiasis
    congenital 751.61
      jaundice from 751.61
        [774.5]
  common duct 576.8
    with calculus,
      choledocholithiasis, or
      stones — see
      Choledocholithiasis
    congenital 751.61
  cystic duct 575.8
    with calculus,
      choledocholithiasis, or
      stones — see
      Choledocholithiasis
  disease, arteriolar 447.1
  endometrium 621.8
  eye, anterior chamber 360.34
  fallopian tube 628.2
  lymphatic vessel 457.1
    postmastectomy 457.0
  organ or site, congenital NEC —
    see Atresia
  placental blood vessels — see
    Placenta, abnormal
  supra-aortic branches 446.7
  ureter 593.89
  urethra 599.84
  vein 459.9
  vestibule (oral) 525.8
Observation (for) V71.9
  without need for further medical
    care V71.9
  accident NEC V71.4
    at work V71.3
  criminal assault V71.6
  deleterious agent ingestion V71.8
  disease V71.9
    cardiovascular V71.7
    heart V71.7
    mental V71.09
    specified condition NEC V71.8
  foreign body ingestion V71.8
  growth and development
    variations V21.8
  injuries (accidental) V71.4
    inflicted NEC V71.6
      during alleged rape or
        seduction V71.5
  malignant neoplasm, suspected
    V71.1

Observation—continued
  postpartum
    immediately after delivery
      V24.0
    routine follow-up V24.2
  pregnancy
    high-risk V23.9
      specified problem NEC
        V23.8
    normal (without complication)
      V22.1
      with nonobstetric
        complication V22.2
      first V22.0
  rape or seduction, alleged V71.5
    injury during V71.5
  suicide attempt, alleged V71.8
  suspected (undiagnosed)
    (unproven)
    cardiovascular disease V71.7
    child or wife battering victim
      V71.6
    concussion (cerebral) V71.6
    condition NEC V71.8
      infant — see Observation,
        suspected, condition,
        newborn
      newborn V29.9
        cardiovascular disease
          V29.8
        congenital anomaly
          V29.8
        infectious V29.0
        ingestion foreign object
          V29.8
        injury V29.8
        neoplasm V29.8
        neurological V29.1
        poison, poisoning V29.8
        respiratory V29.2 ◆
        specified NEC V29.8
    infectious disease not
      requiring isolation
      V71.8
    malignant neoplasm V71.l
    mental disorder V71.09
    neoplasm
      benign V71.8
      malignant V71.1
    specified condition NEC V71.8
    tuberculosis V71.2
  tuberculosis, suspected V71.2
Obsession, obsessional 300.3
  ideas and mental images 300.3
  impulses 300.3
  neurosis 300.3
  phobia 300.3
  psychasthenia 300.3
  ruminations 300.3
  state 300.3
  syndrome 300.3
Obsessive-compulsive 300.3
  neurosis 300.3
  reaction 300.3
Obstetrical trauma NEC
  (complicating delivery) 665.9
  with
    abortion — see Abortion, by
      type, with damage to
      pelvic organs
    ectopic pregnancy (see also
      categories 633.0-633.9)
      639.2
    molar pregnancy (see also
      categories 630-632)
      639.2
  affecting fetus or newborn 763.8
  following
    abortion 639.2
    ectopic or molar pregnancy
      639.2
Obstipation (see also Constipation)
  564.0
  psychogenic 306.4

Obstruction, obstructed, obstructive
  airway NEC 519.8
    with
      allergic alveolitis NEC
        495.9
      asthma NEC (see also
        Asthma) 493.9
      bronchiectasis 494
      bronchitis (chronic) (see
        also Bronchitis,
        with, obstruction)
        491.20 ◆
      emphysema NEC 492.8
    chronic 496
      with
        allergic alveolitis NEC
          495.5
        asthma NEC (see also
          Asthma) 493.9
        bronchiectasis 494
        bronchitis (chronic) (see
          also Bronchitis,
          with, obstruction)
          491.20 ◆
        emphysema NEC 492.8
    due to
      bronchospasm 519.1
      foreign body 934.9
      inhalation of fumes or
        vapors 506.9
      laryngospasm 478.75
  alimentary canal (see also
    Obstruction, intestine)
    560.9
  ampulla of Vater 576.2
    with calculus, cholelithiasis, or
      stones — see
      Choledocholithiasis
  aortic (heart) (valve) (see also
    Stenosis, aortic) 424.1
    rheumatic (see also Stenosis,
      aortic, rheumatic) 395.0
  aortoiliac 444.0
  aqueduct of Sylvius 331.4
    congenital 742.3
      with spina bifida (see also
        Spina bifida) 741.0
    Arnold-Chiari (see also Spina
      bifida) 741.0
  artery (see also Embolism, artery)
    444.9
    basilar (complete) (partial) (see
      also Occlusion, artery,
      basilar) 433.0
    carotid (complete) (partial) (see
      also Occlusion, artery,
      carotid) 433.1
    precerebral — see Occlusion,
      artery, precerebral NEC
    retinal (central) (see also
      Occlusion, retina)
      362.30
    vertebral (complete) (partial)
      (see also Occlusion,
      artery, vertebral) 433.2
  asthma (chronic) (with obstructive
    pulmonary disease) 493.2
  band (intestinal) 560.81
  bile duct or passage (see also
    Obstruction, biliary) 576.2
    congenital 751.61
      jaundice from 751.61
        [774.5]
  biliary (duct) (tract) 576.2
    with calculus 574.51
      with cholecystitis (chronic)
        574.41
        acute 574.31
    congenital 751.61
      jaundice from 751.61
        [774.5]
    gallbladder 575.2
      with calculus 574.21
        with cholecystitis
          (chronic) 574.11
          acute 574.01

**Obstruction, obstructed,
  obstructive**—continued
  bladder neck (acquired) 596.0
    congenital 753.6
  bowel (see also Obstruction,
    intestine) 560.9
  bronchus 519.1
  canal, ear (see also Stricture, ear
    canal, acquired) 380.50
  cardia 537.89
  caval veins (inferior) (superior)
    459.2
  cecum (see also Obstruction,
    intestine) 560.9
  circulatory 459.9
  colon (see also Obstruction,
    intestine) 560.9
    sympathicotonic 560.89
  common duct (see also
    Obstruction, biliary) 576.2
    congenital 751.61
  coronary (artery) (heart) —see
    Arteriosclerosis, coronary ◆
  cystic duct (see also Obstruction,
    gallbladder) 575.2
    congenital 751.61
  device, implant, or graft — see
    Complications, due to
    (presence of) any device,
    implant, or graft classified
    to 996.0-996.5 NEC
  due to foreign body accidentally
    left in operation wound
    998.4
  duodenum 537.3
    congenital 751.1
    due to
      compression NEC 537.3
      cyst 537.3
      intrinsic lesion or disease
        NEC 537.3
      scarring 537.3
      torsion 537.3
      ulcer 532.91
      volvulus 537.3
  ejaculatory duct 608.89
  endocardium 424.90
    arteriosclerotic 424.99
    specified cause, except
      rheumatic 424.99
  esophagus 530.3
  eustachian tube (complete)
    (partial) 381.60
    cartilaginous
      extrinsic 381.63
      intrinsic 381.62
    due to
      cholesteatoma 381.61
      osseous lesion NEC 381.61
      polyp 381.61
    osseous 381.61
  fallopian tube (bilateral) 628.2
  fecal 560.39
    with hernia — see also
      Hernia, by site, with
      obstruction
    gangrenous — see Hernia,
      by site, with
      gangrene
  foramen of Monro (congenital)
    742.3
    with spina bifida (see also
      Spina bifida) 741.0
  foreign body — see Foreign body
  gallbladder 575.2
    with calculus, cholelithiasis, or
      stones 574.21
      with cholecystitis (chronic)
        574.11
        acute 574.01
    congenital 751.69
      jaundice from 751.69
        [774.5]
  gastric outlet 537.0
  gastrointestinal (see also
    Obstruction, intestine)
    560.9

Obstruction, obstructed, obstructive—continued
glottis 478.79
hepatic 573.8
  duct (see also Obstruction, biliary) 576.2
    congenital 751.61
  icterus (see also Obstruction, biliary) 576.8
    congenital 751.61
ileocecal coil (see also Obstruction, intestine) 560.9
ileum (see also Obstruction, intestine) 560.9
iliofemoral (artery) 444.81
internal anastomosis — see Complications, mechanical, graft
intestine (mechanical) (neurogenic) (paroxysmal) (postinfectional) (reflex) 560.9
  with
    adhesions (intestinal) (peritoneal) 560.81
    hernia — see also Hernia, by site, with obstruction
      gangrenous — see Hernia, by site, with gangrene
  adynamic (see also Ileus) 560.1
  by gallstone 560.31
  congenital or infantile (small) 751.1
    large 751.2
  due to
    Ascaris lumbricoides 127.0
    mural thickening 560.89
    procedure 997.4
      involving urinary tract 997.5
  impaction 560.39
  infantile — see Obstruction, intestine, congenital
  newborn
    due to
      fecaliths 777.1
      inspissated milk 777.2
      meconium (plug) 777.1
        in mucoviscidosis 277.01
      transitory 777.4
    specified cause NEC 560.89
    transitory, newborn 777.4
    volvulus 560.2
intracardiac ball valve prosthesis 996.02
jaundice (see also Obstruction, biliary) 576.8
  congenital 751.61
jejunum (see also Obstruction, intestine) 560.9
kidney 593.89
labor 660.9
  affecting fetus or newborn 763.1
  by
    bony pelvis (conditions classifiable to 653.0-653.9) 660.1
    deep transverse arrest 660.3
    impacted shoulder 660.4
    locked twins 660.5
    malposition (fetus) (conditions classifiable to 652.0-652.9) 660.0
      head during labor 660.3
    persistent occipitoposterior position 660.3

Obstruction, obstructed, obstructive—continued
labor—continued
  by—continued
    soft tissue, pelvic (conditions classifiable to 654.0-654.9) 660.2
lacrimal
  canaliculi 375.53
    congenital 743.65
  punctum 375.52
  sac 375.54
lacrimonasal duct 375.56
  congenital 743.65
  neonatal 375.55
lacteal, with steatorrhea 579.2
laryngitis (see also Laryngitis) 464.0
larynx 478.79
  congenital 748.3
liver 573.8
  cirrhotic (see also Cirrhosis, liver) 571.5
lung 518.89
  with
    asthma — see Asthma
    bronchitis (chronic) 491.2
    emphysema NEC 492.8
  airway, chronic 496
  chronic NEC 496
    with
      asthma (chronic) (obstructive) 493.2
  disease, chronic 496
    with
      asthma (chronic) (obstructive) 493.2
  emphysematous 492.8
lymphatic 457.1
meconium
  fetus or newborn 777.1
    in mucoviscidosis 277.01
  newborn due to fecaliths 777.1
mediastinum 519.3
mitral (rheumatic) — see Stenosis, mitral
nasal 478.1
  duct 375.56
    neonatal 375.55
  sinus — see Sinusitis
nasolacrimal duct 375.56
  congenital 743.65
  neonatal 375.55
nasopharynx 478.29
nose 478.1
organ or site, congenital NEC — see Atresia
pancreatic duct 577.8
parotid gland 527.8
pelviureteral junction (see also Obstruction, ureter) 593.4
pharynx 478.29
portal (circulation) (vein) 452
prostate 600
  valve (urinary) 596.0
pulmonary
  valve (heart) (see also Endocarditis, pulmonary) 424.3
  vein, isolated 747.49
pyemic — see Septicemia
pylorus (acquired) 537.0
  congenital 750.5
  infantile 750.5
rectosigmoid (see also Obstruction, intestine) 560.9
rectum 569.49
renal 593.89
respiratory 519.8
  chronic 496

Obstruction, obstructed, obstructive—continued
retinal (artery) (vein) (central) (see also Occlusion, retina) 362.30
salivary duct (any) 527.8
  with calculus 527.5
sigmoid (see also Obstruction, intestine) 560.9
sinus (accessory) (nasal) (see also Sinusitis) 473.9
Stensen's duct 527.8
stomach 537.89
  acute 536.1
  congenital 750.7
submaxillary gland 527.8
  with calculus 527.5
thoracic duct 457.1
thrombotic — see Thrombosis
tooth eruption 520.6
trachea 519.1
tracheostomy airway 519.0
tricuspid — see Endocarditis, tricuspid
upper respiratory, congenital 748.8
ureter (pelvic juncture) (functional) 593.4
  congenital 753.2
  due to calculus 592.1
urethra 599.6
  congenital 753.6
urinary (moderate) 599.6
  organ or tract (lower) 599.6
  prostatic valve 596.0
uropathy 599.6
uterus 621.8
vagina 623.2
valvular — see Endocarditis
vascular graft or shunt 996.1
  atherosclerosis — see Arteriosclerosis, coronary ▼
  embolism 996.74
  occlusion NEC 996.74
  thrombus 996.74 ▲
vein, venous 459.2
  caval (inferior) (superior) 459.2
  thrombotic — see Thrombosis
  vena cava (inferior) (superior) 459.2
ventricular shunt 996.2
vesical 596.0
vesicourethral orifice 596.0
vessel NEC 459.9

Obturator — see condition
Occlusal wear, teeth 521.1
Occlusion
anus 569.49
  congenital 751.2
  infantile 751.2
aortoiliac (chronic) 444.0
aqueduct of Sylvius 331.4
  congenital 742.3
    with spina bifida (see also Spina bifida) 741.0
arteries of extremities, lower 444.22
  without thrombus or embolus (see also Arteriosclerosis, extremities) 440.20
  due to stricture or stenosis 447.1
  upper 444.21
    without thrombus or embolus (see also Arteriosclerosis, extremities) 440.20
    due to stricture or stenosis 447.1
artery NEC (see also Embolism, artery) 444.9
  auditory, internal 433.8

Occlusion—continued
artery NEC—continued
  basilar 433.0
    with other precerebral artery 433.3
    bilateral 433.3
  brain or cerebral (see also Infarct, brain) 434.9
  carotid 433.1
    with other precerebral artery 433.3
    bilateral 433.3
  cerebellar (anterior inferior) (posterior inferior) (superior) 433.8
  cerebral (see also Infarct, brain) 434.9
  choroidal (anterior) 433.8
  communicating posterior 433.8
  coronary (acute) (thrombotic) (see also Infarct, myocardium) 410.9
    healed or old 412
    without myocardial infarction 411.81
  hypophyseal 433.8
  iliac (see also Arteriosclerosis, extremities) 440.20
  mesenteric (embolic) (thrombotic) (with gangrene) 557.0
  pontine 433.8
  precerebral NEC 433.9
    late effect — see category 438
    multiple or bilateral 433.3
    puerperal, postpartum, childbirth 674.0
    specified NEC 433.8
  renal 593.81
  retinal — see Occlusion, retina, artery
  spinal 433.8
  vertebral 433.2
    with other precerebral artery 433.3
    bilateral 433.3
basilar (artery) — see Occlusion, artery, basilar
bile duct (any) (see also Obstruction, biliary) 576.2
bowel (see also Obstruction, intestine) 560.9
brain (artery) (vascular) (see also Infarct, brain) 434.9
breast (duct) 611.8
carotid (artery) (common) (internal) — see Occlusion, artery, carotid
cerebellar (anterior inferior) (artery) (posterior inferior) (superior) 433.8
cerebral (artery) (see also Infarct, brain) 434.9
cerebrovascular (see also Infarct, brain) 434.9
  diffuse 437.0
cervical canal (see also Stricture, cervix) 622.4
  by falciparum malaria 084.0
cervix (uteri) (see also Stricture, cervix) 622.4
choanal 748.0
choroidal (artery) 433.8
colon (see also Obstruction, intestine) 560.9
communicating posterior artery 433.8
coronary (acute) (artery) (thrombotic) (see also Infarct, myocardium) 410.9
  healed or old 412
  without myocardial infarction 411.81

Occlusion—*continued*
  cystic duct (*see also* Obstruction, gallbladder) 575.2
    congenital 751.69
  embolic — *see* Embolism
  fallopian tube 628.2
    congenital 752.19
  gallbladder (*see also* Obstruction, gallbladder) 575.2
    congenital 751.69
      jaundice from 751.69
        [774.5]
  gingiva, traumatic 523.8
  hymen 623.3
    congenital 752.41
  hypophyseal (artery) 433.8
  iliac artery 444.81
  intestine (*see also* Obstruction, intestine) 560.9
  kidney 593.89
  lacrimal apparatus — *see* Stenosis, lacrimal
  lung 518.89
  lymph or lymphatic channel 457.1
  mammary duct 611.8
  mesenteric artery (embolic) (thrombotic) (with gangrene) 557.0
  nose 478.1
    congenital 748.0
  organ or site, congenital NEC — *see* Atresia
  oviduct 628.2
    congenital 752.19
  periodontal, traumatic 523.8
  peripheral arteries (lower extremity) 444.22
    without thrombus or embolus (*see also* Arteriosclerosis, extremities) 440.20
    due to stricture or stenosis 447.1
    upper extremity 444.21
      without thrombus or embolus (*see also* Arteriosclerosis, extremities 440.20
      due to stricture or stenosis 447.1
  pontine (artery) 433.8
  posterior lingual, of mandibular teeth 524.2
  precerebral artery — *see* Occlusion, artery, precerebral NEC
  puncta lacrimalia 375.52
  pupil 364.74
  pylorus (*see also* Stricture, pylorus) 537.0
  renal artery 593.81
  retina, retinal (vascular) 362.30
    artery, arterial 362.30
      branch 362.32
      central (total) 362.31
      partial 362.33
      transient 362.34
      tributary 362.32
    vein 362.30
      branch 362.36
      central (total) 362.35
      incipient 362.37
      partial 362.37
      tributary 362.36
  spinal artery 433.8
  teeth (mandibular) (posterior lingual) 524.2
  thoracic duct 457.1
  tubal 628.2
  ureter (complete) (partial) 593.4
    congenital 753.2
  urethra (*see also* Stricture, urethra) 598.9
    congenital 753.6
  uterus 621.8

Occlusion—*continued*
  vagina 623.2
  vascular NEC 459.9
  vein — *see* Thrombosis
  vena cava (inferior) (superior) 453.2
  ventricle (brain) NEC 331.4
  vertebral (artery) — *see* Occlusion, artery, vertebral
  vessel (blood) NEC 459.9
  vulva 624.8
Occlusio pupillae 364.74
Occupational
  problems NEC V62.2
  therapy V57.21 ◆
Ochlophobia 300.29
Ochronosis (alkaptonuric) (congenital) (endogenous) 270.2
  with chloasma of eyelid 270.2
Ocular muscle — *see also* condition
  myopathy 359.1
Oculoauriculovertebral dysplasia 756.0
Oculogyric
  crisis or disturbance 378.87
    psychogenic 306.7
Oculomotor syndrome 378.81
Oddi's sphincter spasm 576.5
Odelberg's disease (juvenile osteochondrosis) 732.1
Odontalgia 525.9
Odontoameloblastoma (M9311/0) 213.1
  upper jaw (bone) 213.0
Odontoclasia 521.0
Odontoclasis 873.63
  complicated 873.73
Odontodysplasia, regional 520.4
Odontogenesis imperfecta 520.5
Odontoma (M9280/0) 213.1
  ameloblastic (M9311/0) 213.1
    upper jaw (bone) 213.0
  calcified (M9280/0) 213.1
    upper jaw (bone) 213.0
  complex (M9282/0) 213.1
    upper jaw (bone) 213.0
  compound (M9281/0) 213.1
    upper jaw (bone) 213.0
  fibroameloblastic (M9290/0) 213.1
    upper jaw (bone) 213.0
  follicular 526.0
    upper jaw (bone) 213.0
Odontomyelitis (closed) (open) 522.0
Odontonecrosis 521.0
Odontorrhagia 525.8
Odontosarcoma, ameloblastic (M9290/3) 170.1
  upper jaw (bone) 170.0
Oesophagostomiasis 127.7
Oesophagostomum infestation 127.7
Oestriasis 134.0
Ogilvie's syndrome (sympathicotonic colon obstruction) 560.89
Oguchi's disease (retina) 368.61
Ohara's disease (*see also* Tularemia) 021.9
Oidiomycosis (*see also* Candidiasis) 112.9
Oidiomycotic meningitis 112.83
Oidium albicans infection (*see also* Candidiasis) 112.9
Old age 797
  dementia (of) 290.0
Olfactory — *see* condition
Oligemia 285.9
Oligergasia (*see also* Retardation, mental) 319

Oligoamnios 658.0
  affecting fetus or newborn 761.2
Oligoastrocytoma, mixed (M9382/3)
  specified site — *see* Neoplasm, by site, malignant
  unspecified site 191.9
Oligocythemia 285.9
Oligodendroblastoma (M9460/3)
  specified site — *see* Neoplasm, by site, malignant
  unspecified site 191.9
Oligodendroglioma (M9450/3)
  anaplastic type (M9451/3)
    specified site — *see* Neoplasm, by site, malignant
    unspecified site 191.9
  specified site — *see* Neoplasm, by site, malignant
  unspecified site 191.9
Oligodendroma — *see* Oligodendroglioma
Oligodontia (*see also* Anodontia) 520.0
Oligoencephalon 742.1
Oligohydramnios 658.0
  affecting fetus or newborn 761.2
  due to premature rupture of membranes 658.1
    affecting fetus or newborn 761.2
Oligohydrosis 705.0
Oligomenorrhea 626.1
Oligophrenia (*see also* Retardation, mental) 319
  phenylpyruvic 270.1
Oligospermia 606.1
Oligotrichia 704.09
  congenita 757.4
Oliguria 788.5
  with
    abortion — *see* Abortion, by type, with renal failure
    ectopic pregnancy (*see also* categories 633.0-633.9) 639.3
    molar pregnancy (*see also* categories 630-632) 639.3
  complicating
    abortion 639.3
    ectopic or molar pregnancy 639.3
    pregnancy 646.2
      with hypertension — *see* Toxemia, of pregnancy
  due to a procedure 997.5
  following labor and delivery 669.3
  heart or cardiac — *see* Failure, heart, congestive
  puerperal, postpartum 669.3
  specified due to a procedure 997.5
Ollier's disease (chondrodysplasia) 756.4
Omentitis (*see also* Peritonitis) 567.9
Omentocele (*see also* Hernia, omental) 553.8
Omentum, omental — *see* condition
Omphalitis (congenital) (newborn) 771.4
  not of newborn 686.9
  tetanus 771.3
Omphalocele 756.7
Omphalomesenteric duct, persistent 751.0
Omphalorrhagia, newborn 772.3
Omsk hemorrhagic fever 065.1
Onanism 307.9
Onchocerciasis 125.3
  eye 125.3 [360.13]

Onchocercosis 125.3
Oncocytoma (M8290/0) — *see* Neoplasm, by site, benign
Ondine's curse 348.8
Oneirophrenia (*see also* Schizophrenia) 295.4
Onychauxis 703.8
  congenital 757.5
Onychia (with lymphangitis) 681.9
  dermatophytic 110.1
  finger 681.02
  toe 681.11
Onychitis (with lymphangitis) 681.9
  finger 681.02
  toe 681.11
Onychocryptosis 703.0
Onychodystrophy 703.8
  congenital 757.5
Onychogryphosis 703.8
Onychogryposis 703.8
Onycholysis 703.8
Onychomadesis 703.8
Onychomalacia 703.8
Onychomycosis 110.1
  finger 110.1
  toe 110.1
Onycho-osteodysplasia 756.89
Onychophagy 307.9
Onychoptosis 703.8
Onychorrhexis 703.8
  congenital 757.5
Onychoschizia 703.8
Onychotrophia (*see also* Atrophy, nail) 703.8
O'nyong-nyong fever 066.3
Onyxis (finger) (toe) 703.0
Onyxitis (with lymphangitis) 681.9
  finger 681.02
  toe 681.11
Oophoritis (cystic) (infectional) (interstitial) (*see also* Salpingo-oophoritis) 614.2
  complicating pregnancy 646.6
  fetal (acute) 752.0
  gonococcal (acute) 098.19
    chronic or duration of 2 months or over 098.39
  tuberculous (*see also* Tuberculosis) 016.6
Opacity, opacities
  cornea 371.00
    central 371.03
    congenital 743.43
      interfering with vision 743.42
    degenerative (*see also* Degeneration, cornea) 371.40
    hereditary (*see also* Dystrophy, cornea) 371.50
    inflammatory (*see also* Keratitis) 370.9
    late effect of trachoma (healed) 139.1
    minor 371.01
    peripheral 371.02
  enamel (fluoride) (nonfluoride) (teeth) 520.3
  lens (*see also* Cataract) 366.9
  snowball 379.22
  vitreous (humor) 379.24
    congenital 743.51
Opalescent dentin (hereditary) 520.5
Open, opening
  abnormal, organ or site, congenital — *see* Imperfect, closure
  angle with
    borderline intraocular pressure 365.01
    cupping of discs 365.01
  bite (anterior) (posterior) 524.2

Open, opening

Open, opening—continued
  false — see Imperfect, closure
  wound — see Wound, open, by site
Operation
  causing mutilation of fetus 763.8
  destructive, on live fetus, to facilitate birth 763.8
  for delivery, fetus or newborn 763.8
  maternal, unrelated to current delivery, affecting fetus or newborn 760.6
Operational fatigue 300.89
Operative — see condition
Operculitis (chronic) 523.4
  acute 523.3
Operculum, retina 361.32
  with detachment 361.01
Ophiasis 704.01
Ophthalmia (see also Conjunctivitis) 372.30
  actinic rays 370.24
  allergic (acute) 372.05
    chronic 372.14
  blennorrhagic (neonatorum) 098.40
  catarrhal 372.03
  diphtheritic 032.81
  Egyptian 076.1
  electric, electrica 370.24
  gonococcal (neonatorum) 098.40
  metastatic 360.11
  migraine 346.8
  neonatorum, newborn 771.6
    gonococcal 098.40
  nodosa 360.14
  phlyctenular 370.31
    with ulcer (see also Ulcer, cornea) 370.00
  sympathetic 360.11
Ophthalmitis — see Ophthalmia
Ophthalmocele (congenital) 743.66
Ophthalmoneuromyelitis 341.0
Ophthalmopathy, infiltrative with thyrotoxicosis 242.0
Ophthalmoplegia (see also Strabismus) 378.9
  anterior internuclear 378.86
  ataxia-areflexia syndrome 357.0
  bilateral 378.9
  diabetic 250.5 [378.86]
  exophthalmic 242.0 [376.22]
  external 378.55
    progressive 378.72
    total 378.56
  interna(l) (complete) (total) 367.52
  internuclear 378.86
  migraine 346.8
  painful 378.55
  Parinaud's 378.81
  progressive external 378.72
  supranuclear, progressive 333.0
  total (external) 378.56
    internal 367.52
  unilateral 378.9
Opisthognathism 524.00
Opisthorchiasis (felineus) (tenuicollis) (viverrini) 121.0
Opisthotonos, opisthotonus 781.0
Opitz's disease (congestive splenomegaly) 289.51
Opiumism (see also Dependence) 304.0
Oppenheim's disease 358.8
Oppenheim-Urbach disease or syndrome (necrobiosis lipoidica diabeticorum) 250.8 [709.3]
Opsoclonia 379.59
Optic nerve — see condition
Orbit — see condition

Orchioblastoma (M9071/3) 186.9
Orchitis (nonspecific) (septic) 604.90
  with abscess 604.0
  blennorrhagic (acute) 098.13
    chronic or duration of 2 months or over 098.33
  diphtheritic 032.89 [604.91]
  filarial 125.9 [604.91]
  gangrenous 604.99
  gonococcal (acute) 098.13
    chronic or duration of 2 months or over 098.33
  mumps 072.0
  parotidea 072.0
  suppurative 604.99
  syphilitic 095.8 [604.91]
  tuberculous (see also Tuberculosis) 016.5 [608.81]
Orf 051.2
Organic — see also condition
  heart — see Disease, heart
  insufficiency 799.8
Oriental
  bilharziasis 120.2
  schistosomiasis 120.2
  sore 085.1
Orifice — see condition
Origin, both great vessels from right ventricle 745.11
Ormond's disease or syndrome 593.4
Ornithosis 073.9
  with
    complication 073.8
      specified NEC 073.7
    pneumonia 073.0
    pneumonitis (lobular) 073.0
Orodigitofacial dysostosis 759.89
Oropouche fever 066.3
Orotaciduria, oroticaciduria (congenital) (hereditary) (pyrimidine deficiency) 281.4
Oroya fever 088.0
Orthodontics V58.5
  adjustment V53.4
  aftercare V58.5
  fitting V53.4
Orthopnea 786.02
Orthoptic training V57.4
Os, uterus — see condition
Osgood-Schlatter
  disease 732.4
  osteochondrosis 732.4
Osler's
  disease (M9950/1) (polycythemia vera) 238.4
  nodes 421.0
Osler-Rendu disease (familial hemorrhagic telangiectasia) 448.0
Osler-Vaquez disease (M9950/1) (polycythemia vera) 238.4
Osler-Weber-Rendu syndrome (familial hemorrhagic telangiectasia) 448.0
Osmidrosis 705.89
Osseous — see condition
Ossification
  artery — see Arteriosclerosis
  auricle (ear) 380.39
  bronchus 519.1
  cardiac (see also Degeneration, myocardial) 429.1
  cartilage (senile) 733.99
  coronary (artery) — see Arteriosclerosis, coronary◆
  diaphragm 728.10
  ear 380.39
    middle (see also Otosclerosis) 387.9
  falx cerebri 349.2
  fascia 728.10

INDEX TO DISEASES

Ossification—continued
  fontanel
    defective or delayed 756.0
    premature 756.0
  heart (see also Degeneration, myocardial) 429.1
    valve — see Endocarditis
  larynx 478.79
  ligament
    posterior longitudinal 724.8
      cervical 723.7
  meninges (cerebral) 349.2
    spinal 336.8
  multiple, eccentric centers 733.99
  muscle 728.10
    heterotopic, postoperative 728.13
  myocardium, myocardial (see also Degeneration, myocardial) 429.1
  penis 607.81
  periarticular 728.89
  sclera 379.16
  tendon 727.82
  trachea 519.1
  tympanic membrane (see also Tympanosclerosis) 385.00
  vitreous (humor) 360.44
Osteitis (see also Osteomyelitis) 730.2
  acute 730.0
  alveolar 526.5
  chronic 730.1
  condensans (ilii) 733.5
  deformans (Paget's) 731.0
    due to or associated with malignant neoplasm (see also Neoplasm, bone, malignant) 170.9 [731.1]
  due to yaws 102.6
  fibrosa NEC 733.29
    cystica (generalisata) 252.0
    disseminata 756.59
    osteoplastica 252.0
  fragilitans 756.51
  Garré's (sclerosing) 730.1
  infectious (acute) (subacute) 730.0
    chronic or old 730.1
  jaw (acute) (chronic) (lower) (neonatal) (suppurative) (upper) 526.4
  parathyroid 252.0
  petrous bone (see also Petrositis) 383.20
  pubis 733.5
  sclerotic, nonsuppurative 730.1
  syphilitic 095.5
  tuberculosa
    cystica (of Jüngling) 135
    multiplex cystoides 135
Osteoarthritica spondylitis (spine) (see also Spondylosis) 721.90
Osteoarthritis (see also Osteoarthrosis) 715.9
  distal interphalangeal 715.9
  hyperplastic 731.2
  interspinalis (see also Spondylosis) 721.90
  spine, spinal NEC (see also Spondylosis) 721.90
Osteoarthropathy (see also Osteoarthrosis) 715.9
  chronic idiopathic hypertrophic 757.39
  familial idiopathic 757.39
  hypertrophic pulmonary 731.2
    secondary 731.2
  idiopathic hypertrophic 757.39
  primary hypertrophic 731.2
  pulmonary hypertrophic 731.2
  secondary hypertrophic 731.2

Osteochondrosis

Osteoarthrosis (degenerative) (hypertrophic) (rheumatoid) 715.9

> Note — Use the following fifth-digit subclassification with category 715:
> 0 site unspecified
> 1 shoulder region
> 2 upper arm
> 3 forearm
> 4 hand
> 5 pelvic region and thigh
> 6 lower leg
> 7 ankle and foot
> 8 other specified sites except spine
> 9 multiple sites

  deformans alkaptonurica 270.2
  generalized 715.09
  juvenilis (Köhler's) 732.5
  localized 715.3
    idiopathic 715.1
    primary 715.1
    secondary 715.2
  multiple sites, not specified as generalized 715.89
  polyarticular 715.09
  spine (see also Spondylosis) 721.90
Osteoblastoma (M9200/0) — see Neoplasm, bone, benign
Osteochondritis (see also Osteochondrosis) 732.9
  dissecans 732.7
    hip 732.7
  ischiopubica 732.1
  multiple 756.59
  syphilitic (congenital) 090.0
Osteochondrodermodysplasia 756.59
Osteochondrodystrophy 277.5
  deformans 277.5
  familial 277.5
  fetalis 756.4
Osteochondrolysis 732.7
Osteochondroma (M9210/0) — see also Neoplasm, bone, benign
  multiple, congenital 756.4
Osteochondromatosis (M9210/1) 238.0
  synovial 727.82
Osteochondromyxosarcoma (M9180/3) — see Neoplasm, bone, malignant
Osteochondropathy NEC 732.9
Osteochondrosarcoma (M9180/3) — see Neoplasm, bone, malignant
Osteochondrosis 732.9
  acetabulum 732.1
  adult spine 732.8
  astragalus 732.5
  Blount's 732.4
  Buchanan's (juvenile osteochondrosis of iliac crest) 732.1
  Buchman's (juvenile osteochondrosis) 732.1
  Burns' 732.3
  calcaneus 732.5
  capitular epiphysis (femur) 732.1
  carpal
    lunate (wrist) 732.3
    scaphoid 732.3
  coxae juvenilis 732.1
  deformans juvenilis (coxae) (hip) 732.1
    Scheuermann's 732.0
    spine 732.0
    tibia 732.4
    vertebra 732.0

Osteochondrosis—continued
  Diaz's (astragalus) 732.5
  dissecans (knee) (shoulder) 732.7
  femoral capital epiphysis 732.1
  femur (head) (juvenile) 732.1
  foot (juvenile) 732.5
  Freiberg's (disease) (second metatarsal) 732.5
  Haas' 732.3
  Haglund's (os tibiale externum) 732.5
  hand (juvenile) 732.3
  head of
    femur 732.1
    humerus (juvenile) 732.3
  hip (juvenile) 732.1
  humerus (juvenile) 732.3
  iliac crest (juvenile) 732.1
  ilium (juvenile) 732.1
  ischiopubic synchondrosis 732.1
  Iselin's (osteochondrosis fifth metatarsal) 732.5
  juvenile, juvenilis 732.6
    arm 732.3
    capital femoral epiphysis 732.1
    capitellum humeri 732.3
    capitular epiphysis 732.1
    carpal scaphoid 732.3
    clavicle, sternal epiphysis 732.6
    coxae 732.1
    deformans 732.1
    foot 732.5
    hand 732.3
    hip and pelvis 732.1
    lower extremity, except foot 732.4
    lunate, wrist 732.3
    medial cuneiform bone 732.5
    metatarsal (head) 732.5
    metatarsophalangeal 732.5
    navicular, ankle 732.5
    patella 732.4
    primary patellar center (of Köhler) 732.4
    specified site NEC 732.6
    spine 732.0
    tarsal scaphoid 732.5
    tibia (epiphysis) (tuberosity) 732.4
    upper extremity 732.3
    vertebra (body) (Calvé) 732.0
      epiphyseal plates (of Scheuermann) 732.0
  Kienböck's (disease) 732.3
  Köhler's (disease) (navicular, ankle) 732.5
  patellar 732.4
  tarsal navicular 732.5
  Legg-Calvé-Perthes (disease) 732.1
  lower extremity (juvenile) 732.4
  lunate bone 732.3
  Mauclaire's 732.3
  metacarpal heads (of Mauclaire) 732.3
  metatarsal (fifth) (head) (second) 732.5
  navicular, ankle 732.5
  os calcis 732.5
  Osgood-Schlatter 732.4
  os tibiale externum 732.5
  Panner's 732.3
  patella (juvenile) 732.4
  patellar center
    primary (of Köhler) 732.4
    secondary (of Sinding-Larsen) 732.4
  pelvis (juvenile) 732.1
  Pierson's 732.1
  radial head (juvenile) 732.3
  Scheuermann's 732.0
  Sever's (calcaneum) 732.5
  Sinding-Larsen (secondary patellar center) 732.4

Osteochondrosis—continued
  spine (juvenile) 732.0
    adult 732.8
  symphysis pubis (of Pierson) (juvenile) 732.1
  syphilitic (congenital) 090.0
  tarsal (navicular) (scaphoid) 732.5
  tibia (proximal) (tubercle) 732.4
  tuberculous — see Tuberculosis, bone
  ulna 732.3
  upper extremity (juvenile) 732.3
  van Neck's (juvenile osteochondrosis) 732.1
  vertebral (juvenile) 732.0
    adult 732.8
Osteoclastoma (M9250/1) 238.0
  malignant (M9250/3) — see Neoplasm, bone, malignant
Osteocopic pain 733.90
Osteodynia 733.90
Osteodystrophy
  azotemic 588.0
  chronica deformans hypertrophica 731.0
  congenital 756.50
    specified type NEC 756.59
  deformans 731.0
  fibrosa localisata 731.0
  parathyroid 252.0
  renal 588.0
Osteofibroma (M9262/0) — see Neoplasm, bone, benign
Osteofibrosarcoma (M9182/3) — see Neoplasm, bone, malignant
Osteogenesis imperfecta 756.51
Osteogenic — see condition
Osteoma (M9180/0) — see also Neoplasm, bone, benign
  osteoid (M9191/0) — see also Neoplasm, bone, benign
    giant (M9200/0) — see Neoplasm, bone, benign
Osteomalacia 268.2
  chronica deformans hypertrophica 731.0
  due to vitamin D deficiency 268.2
  infantile (see also Rickets) 268.0
  juvenile (see also Rickets) 268.0
  pelvis 268.2
  vitamin D-resistant 275.3
Osteomalacic bone 268.2
Osteomalacosis 268.2
Osteomyelitis (general) (infective) (localized) (neonatal) (purulent) (pyogenic) (septic) (staphylococcal) (streptococcal) (suppurative) (with periostitis) 730.2

> Note — Use the following fifth-digit subclassification with category 730:
>
> 0 site unspecified
> 1 shoulder region
> 2 upper arm
> 3 forearm
> 4 hand
> 5 pelvic region and thigh
> 6 lower leg
> 7 ankle and foot
> 8 other specified sites
> 9 multiple sites

  acute or subacute 730.0
  chronic or old 730.1

Osteomyelitis—continued
  due to, associated with
    tuberculosis (see also Tuberculosis, bone) 015.9 [730.8]
      limb bones 015.5 [730.8]
      specified bones NEC 015.7 [730.8]
      spine 015.0 [730.8]
    typhoid 002.0 [730.8]
  Garré's 730.1
  jaw (acute) (chronic) (lower) (neonatal) (suppurative) (upper) 526.4
  nonsuppurating 730.1
  orbital 376.03
  petrous bone (see also Petrositis) 383.20
  Salmonella 003.24
  sclerosing, nonsuppurative 730.1
  sicca 730.1
  syphilitic 095.5
    congenital 090.0 [730.8]
  tuberculous — see Tuberculosis, bone
  typhoid 002.0 [730.8]
Osteomyelofibrosis 289.8
Osteomyelosclerosis 289.8
Osteonecrosis (see also Osteomyelitis) 730.1
Osteo-onycho-arthro dysplasia 756.89
Osteo-onychodysplasia, hereditary 756.89
Osteopathia
  condensans disseminata 756.53
  hyperostotica multiplex infantilis 756.59
  hypertrophica toxica 731.2
  striata 756.4
Osteopathy resulting from poliomyelitis (see also Poliomyelitis) 045.9 [730.7]
  familial dysplastic 731.2
Osteopecilia 756.53
Osteopenia 733.90
Osteoperiostitis (see also Osteomyelitis) 730.2
  ossificans toxica 731.2
  toxica ossificans 731.2
Osteopetrosis (familial) 756.52
Osteophyte — see Exostosis
Osteophytosis — see Exostosis
Osteopoikilosis 756.53
Osteoporosis (generalized) 733.00
  circumscripta 731.0
  disuse 733.03
  drug-induced 733.09
  idiopathic 733.02
  postmenopausal 733.01
  posttraumatic 733.7
  senile 733.01
  specified type NEC 733.09
Osteoporosis-osteomalacia syndrome 268.2
Osteopsathyrosis 756.51
Osteoradionecrosis, jaw 526.89
Osteosarcoma (M9180/3) — see also Neoplasm, bone, malignant
  chondroblastic (M9181/3) — see Neoplasm, bone, malignant
  fibroblastic (M9182/3) — see Neoplasm, bone, malignant
  in Paget's disease of bone (M9184/3) — see Neoplasm, bone, malignant
  juxtacortical (M9190/3) — see Neoplasm, bone, malignant
  parosteal (M9190/3) — see Neoplasm, bone, malignant
  telangiectatic (M9183/3) — see Neoplasm, bone, malignant

Osteosclerosis 756.52
  fragilis (generalisata) 756.52
  myelofibrosis 289.8
Osteosclerotic anemia 289.8
Osteosis
  acromegaloid 757.39
  cutis 709.3
  parathyroid 252.0
  renal fibrocystic 588.0
Österreicher-Turner syndrome 756.89
Ostium
  atrioventriculare commune 745.69
  primum (arteriosum) (defect) (persistent) 745.61
  secundum (arteriosum) (defect) (patent) (persistent) 745.5
Ostrum-Furst syndrome 756.59
Otalgia 388.70
  otogenic 388.71
  referred 388.72
Othematoma 380.31
Otitic hydrocephalus 348.2
Otitis 382.9
  with effusion 381.4
    purulent 382.4
    secretory 381.4
    serous 381.4
    suppurative 382.4
  acute 382.9
  adhesive (see also Adhesions, middle ear) 385.10
  chronic 382.9
    with effusion 381.3
    mucoid, mucous (simple) 381.20
    purulent 382.3
    secretory 381.3
    serous 381.10
    suppurative 382.3
  diffuse parasitic 136.8
  externa (acute) (diffuse) (hemorrhagica) 380.10
    actinic 380.22
    candidal 112.82
    chemical 380.22
    chronic 380.23
      mycotic — see Otitis, externa, mycotic
      specified type NEC 380.23
    circumscribed 380.10
    contact 380.22
    due to
      erysipelas 035 [380.13]
      impetigo 684 [380.13]
      seborrheic dermatitis 690 [380.13]
    eczematoid 380.22
    furuncular 680.0 [380.13]
    infective 380.10
      chronic 380.16
    malignant 380.14
    mycotic (chronic) 380.15
      due to
        aspergillosis 117.3 [380.15]
        moniliasis 112.82
        otomycosis 111.8 [380.15]
    reactive 380.22
    specified type NEC 380.22
    tropical 111.8 [380.15]
  insidiosa (see also Otosclerosis) 387.9
  interna (see also Labyrinthitis) 386.30
  media (hemorrhagic) (staphylococcal) (streptococcal) 382.9
    acute 382.9
      with effusion 381.00
      allergic 381.04
        mucoid 381.05
        sanguineous 381.06

Otitis—continued
  media—continued
    acute—continued
      allergic—continued
        serous 381.04
      catarrhal 381.00
      exudative 381.00
      mucoid 381.02
        allergic 381.05
      necrotizing 382.00
        with spontaneous
          rupture of ear
          drum 382.01
        in
          influenza 487.8
            [382.02]
          measles 055.2
          scarlet fever 034.1
            [382.02]
      nonsuppurative 381.00
      purulent 382.00
        with spontaneous
          rupture of ear
          drum 382.01
      sanguineous 381.03
        allergic 381.06
      secretory 381.01
      seromucinous 381.02
      serous 381.01
        allergic 381.04
      suppurative 382.00
        with spontaneous
          rupture of ear
          drum 382.01
        due to
          influenza 487.8
            [382.02]
          scarlet fever 034.1
            [382.02]
      transudative 381.00
    adhesive (see also Adhesions, middle ear) 385.10
    allergic 381.4
      acute 381.04
        mucoid 381.05
        sanguineous 381.06
        serous 381.04
      chronic 381.3
    catarrhal 381.4
      acute 381.00
      chronic (simple) 381.10
    chronic 382.9
      with effusion 381.3
      adhesive (see also
        Adhesions, middle
        ear) 385.10
      allergic 381.3
      atticoantral, suppurative
        (with posterior or
        superior marginal
        perforation of ear
        drum) 382.2
      benign suppurative (with
        anterior perforation
        of ear drum) 382.1
      catarrhal 381.10
      exudative 381.3
      mucinous 381.20
      mucoid, mucous (simple) 381.20
      mucosanguineous 381.29
      nonsuppurative 381.3
      purulent 382.3
      secretory 381.3
      seromucinous 381.3
      serosanguineous 381.19
      serous (simple) 381.10
      suppurative 382.3
        atticoantral (with
          posterior or
          superior marginal
          perforation of ear
          drum) 382.2
        benign (with anterior
          perforation of ear
          drum) 382.1

Otitis—continued
  media—continued
    chronic—continued
      suppurative—continued
        tuberculous (see also
          Tuberculosis)
          017.4
        tubotympanic 382.1
      transudative 381.3
    exudative 381.4
      acute 381.00
      chronic 381.3
    fibrotic (see also Adhesions, middle ear) 385.10
    mucoid, mucous 381.4
      acute 381.02
      chronic (simple) 381.20
    mucosanguineous, chronic 381.29
    nonsuppurative 381.4
      acute 381.00
      chronic 381.3
    postmeasles 055.2
    purulent 382.4
      acute 382.00
        with spontaneous
          rupture of ear
          drum 382.01
      chronic 382.3
    sanguineous, acute 381.03
      allergic 381.06
    secretory 381.4
      acute or subacute 381.01
      chronic 381.3
    seromucinous 381.4
      acute or subacute 381.02
      chronic 381.3
    serosanguineous, chronic 381.19
    serous 381.4
      acute or subacute 381.01
      chronic (simple) 381.10
    subacute — see Otitis, media, acute
    suppurative 382.4
      acute 382.00
        with spontaneous
          rupture of ear
          drum 382.01
      chronic 382.3
        atticoantral 382.2
        benign 382.1
        tuberculous (see also
          Tuberculosis)
          017.4
        tubotympanic 382.1
    transudative 381.4
      acute 381.00
      chronic 381.3
    tuberculous (see also Tuberculosis) 017.4
  postmeasles 055.2
Otoconia 386.8
Otolith syndrome 386.19
Otomycosis 111.8 [380.15]
  in
    aspergillosis 117.3 [380.15]
    moniliasis 112.82
Otopathy 388.9
Otoporosis (see also Otosclerosis) 387.9
Otorrhagia 388.69
  traumatic — see nature of injury
Otorrhea 388.60
  blood 388.69
  cerebrospinal (fluid) 388.61
Otosclerosis (general) 387.9
  cochlear (endosteal) 387.2
  involving
    otic capsule 387.2
    oval window
      nonobliterative 387.0
      obliterative 387.1
    round window 387.2
  nonobliterative 387.0

Otosclerosis—continued
  obliterative 387.1
  specified type NEC 387.8
Otospongiosis (see also Otosclerosis) 387.9
Otto's disease or pelvis 715.35
Outburst, aggressive (see also Disturbance, conduct) 312.0
  in children and adolescents 313.9
Outcome of delivery
  multiple birth NEC V27.9
    all liveborn V27.5
    all stillborn V27.7
    some liveborn V27.6
    unspecified V27.9
  single V27.9
    liveborn V27.0
    stillborn V27.1
  twins V27.9
    both liveborn V27.2
    both stillborn V27.4
    one liveborn, one stillborn V27.3
Outlet — see also condition
  syndrome (thoracic) 353.0
Outstanding ears (bilateral) 744.29
Ovalocytosis (congenital) (hereditary) (see also Elliptocytosis) 282.1
Ovarian — see also condition
  pregnancy — see Pregnancy, ovarian
  vein syndrome 593.4
Ovaritis (cystic) (see also Salpingo-oophoritis) 614.2
Ovary, ovarian — see condition
Overactive — see also Hyperfunction
  eye muscle (see also Strabismus) 378.9
  hypothalamus 253.8
  thyroid (see also Thyrotoxicosis) 242.9
Overactivity, child 314.01
Overbite (deep) (excessive) (horizontal) (vertical) 524.2
Overbreathing (see also Hyperventilation) 786.01
Overconscientious personality 301.4
Overdevelopment — see also Hypertrophy
  breast (female) (male) 611.1
  nasal bones 738.0
  prostate, congenital 752.8
Overdistention — see Distention
Overdose, overdosage (drug) 977.9
  specified drug or substance — see Table of drugs and chemicals
Overeating 783.6
  with obesity 278.0
  nonorganic origin 307.51
Overexertion (effects) (exhaustion) 994.5
Overexposure (effects) 994.9
  exhaustion 994.4
Overfeeding (see also Overeating) 783.6
Overgrowth, bone NEC 733.99
Overheated (effects) (places) — see Heat
Overinhibited child 313.0
Overjet 524.2
Overlaid, overlying (suffocation) 994.7
Overlapping toe (acquired) 735.8
  congenital (fifth toe) 755.66
Overload
  fluid 276.6
  potassium (K) 276.7
  sodium (Na) 276.0

Overnutrition (see also Hyperalimentation) 783.6
Overproduction — see also Hypersecretion
  ACTH 255.3
  cortisol 255.0
  growth hormone 253.0
  thyroid-stimulating hormone (TSH) 242.8
Overriding
  aorta 747.21
  finger (acquired) 736.29
    congenital 755.59
  toe (acquired) 735.8
    congenital 755.66
Oversize
  fetus (weight of 4500 grams or more) 766.0
    affecting management of pregnancy 656.6
    causing disproportion 653.5
      with obstructed labor 660.1
    affecting fetus or newborn 763.1
Overstrained 780.7
  heart — see Hypertrophy, cardiac
Overweight (see also Obesity) 278.0
Overwork 780.7
Oviduct — see condition
Ovotestis 752.7
Ovulation (cycle)
  failure or lack of 628.0
  pain 625.2
Ovum
  blighted 631
  dropsical 631
  pathologic 631
Owren's disease or syndrome (parahemophilia) (see also Defect, coagulation) 286.3
Oxalosis 271.8
Oxaluria 271.8
Ox heart — see Hypertrophy, cardiac
OX syndrome 758.6
Oxycephaly, oxycephalic 756.0
  syphilitic, congenital 090.0
Oxyuriasis 127.4
Oxyuris vermicularis (infestation) 127.4
Ozena 472.0

P

Pacemaker syndrome 429.4 ◆
Pachyderma, pachydermia 701.8
  laryngis 478.5
  laryngitis 478.79
  larynx (verrucosa) 478.79
Pachydermatitis 701.8
Pachydermatocele (congenital) 757.39
  acquired 701.8
Pachydermatosis 701.8
Pachydermoperiostitis
  secondary 731.2
Pachydermoperiostosis
  primary idiopathic 757.39
  secondary 731.2
Pachymeningitis (adhesive) (basal) (brain) (cerebral) (cervical) (chronic) (circumscribed) (external) (fibrous) (hemorrhagic) (hypertrophic) (internal) (purulent) (spinal) (suppurative) (see also Meningitis) 322.9
  gonococcal 098.82
Pachyonychia (congenital) 757.5
  acquired 703.8

Pachyperiosteodermia
  primary or idiopathic 757.39
  secondary 731.2
Pachyperiostosis
  primary or idiopathic 757.39
  secondary 731.2
Pacinian tumor (M9507/0) — *see* Neoplasm, skin, benign
Pads, knuckle or Garrod's 728.79
Paget's disease (osteitis deformans) 731.0
  with infiltrating duct carcinoma of the breast (M8541/3) — *see* Neoplasm, breast, malignant
  bone 731.0
    osteosarcoma in (M9184/3) — *see* Neoplasm, bone, malignant
  breast (M8540/3) 174.0
  extramammary (M8542/3) — *see also* Neoplasm, skin, malignant
    anus 154.3
    skin 173.5
  malignant (M8540/3)
    breast 174.0
    specified site NEC (M8542/3) — *see* Neoplasm, skin, malignant
    unspecified site 174.0
  mammary (M8540/3) 174.0
  necrosis of bone 731.0
  nipple (M8540/3) 174.0
  osteitis deformans 731.0
Paget-Schroetter syndrome (intermittent venous claudication) 453.8
Pain(s)
  abdominal 789.0
  adnexa (uteri) 625.9
  alimentary, due to vascular insufficiency 557.9
  anginoid (*see also* Pain, precordial) 786.51
  anus 569.42
  arch 729.5
  arm 729.5
  back (postural) 724.5
    low 724.2
      psychogenic 307.89
  bile duct 576.9
  bladder 788.9
  bone 733.90
  breast 611.71
    psychogenic 307.89
  broad ligament 625.9
  cartilage NEC 733.90
  cecum 789.0
  cervicobrachial 723.3
  chest (central) 786.50
    wall (anterior) 786.52
  coccyx 724.79
  colon 789.0
  common duct 576.9
  coronary — *see* Angina
  costochondral 786.52
  diaphragm 786.52
  due to (presence of) any device, implant, or graft classifiable to 996.0-996.5 — *see* Complications, due to (presence of) any device, implant, or graft classified to 996.0-996.5 NEC
  ear (*see also* Otalgia) 388.70
  epigastric, epigastrium 789.0
  extremity (lower) (upper) 729.5
  eye 379.91
  face, facial 784.0
    atypical 350.2
    nerve 351.8
  false (labor) 644.1
  female genital organ NEC 625.9
    psychogenic 307.89
  finger 729.5

Pain(s)—*continued*
  flank 789.0
  foot 729.5
  gallbladder 575.9
  gas (intestinal) 787.3
  gastric 536.8
  generalized 780.9
  genital organ
    female 625.9
    male 608.9
    psychogenic 307.89
  groin 789.0
  growing 781.9
  hand 729.5
  head (*see also* Headache) 784.0
  heart (*see also* Pain, precordial) 786.51
  infraorbital (*see also* Neuralgia, trigeminal) 350.1
  intermenstrual 625.2
  jaw 526.9
  joint 719.40
    ankle 719.47
    elbow 719.42
    foot 719.47
    hand 719.44
    hip 719.45
    knee 719.46
    multiple sites 719.49
    pelvic region 719.45
    psychogenic 307.89
    shoulder (region) 719.41
    specified site NEC 719.48
    wrist 719.43
  kidney 788.0
  labor, false or spurious 644.1
  laryngeal 784.1
  leg 729.5
  limb 729.5
  low back 724.2
  lumbar region 724.2
  mastoid (*see also* Otalgia) 388.70
  maxilla 526.9
  metacarpophalangeal (joint) 719.44
  metatarsophalangeal (joint) 719.47
  mouth 528.9
  muscle 729.1
    intercostal 786.52
  nasal 478.1
  nasopharynx 478.29
  neck NEC 723.1
    psychogenic 307.89
  nerve NEC 729.2
  neuromuscular 729.1
  nose 478.1
  ocular 379.91
  ophthalmic 379.91
  orbital region 379.91
  osteocopic 733.90
  ovary 625.9
    psychogenic 307.89
  over heart (*see also* Pain, precordial) 786.51
  ovulation 625.2
  pelvic (female) 625.9
    male NEC 789.0
      psychogenic 307.89
    psychogenic 307.89
  penis 607.9
    psychogenic 307.89
  pericardial (*see also* Pain, precordial) 786.51
  perineum
    female 625.9
    male 608.9
  pharynx 478.29
  pleura, pleural, pleuritic 786.52
  post-operative — *see* Pain, by site
  preauricular 388.70
  precordial (region) 786.51
    psychogenic 307.89
  psychogenic 307.80
    cardiovascular system 307.89
    gastrointestinal system 307.89
    genitourinary system 307.89

Pain(s)—*continued*
  psychogenic—*continued*
    heart 307.89
    musculoskeletal system 307.89
    respiratory system 307.89
    skin 306.3
  radicular (spinal) (*see also* Radiculitis) 729.2
  rectum 569.42
  respiration 786.52
  retrosternal 786.51
  rheumatic NEC 729.0
    muscular 729.1
  rib 786.50
  root (spinal) (*see also* Radiculitis) 729.2
  round ligament (stretch) 625.9
  sacroiliac 724.6
  sciatic 724.3
  scrotum 608.9
    psychogenic 307.89
  seminal vesicle 608.9
  sinus 478.1
  skin 782.0
  spermatic cord 608.9
  spinal root (*see also* Radiculitis) 729.2
  stomach 536.8
    psychogenic 307.89
  substernal 786.51
  temporomandibular (joint) 524.62
  temporomaxillary joint 524.62
  testis 608.9
    psychogenic 307.89
  thoracic spine 724.1
    with radicular and visceral pain 724.4
  throat 784.1
  tibia 733.90
  toe 729.5
  tongue 529.6
  tooth 525.9
  trigeminal (*see also* Neuralgia, trigeminal) 350.1
  umbilicus 789.0
  ureter 788.0
  urinary (organ) (system) 788.0
  uterus 625.9
    psychogenic 307.89
  vagina 625.9
  vertebrogenic (syndrome) 724.5
  vesical 788.9
  vulva 625.9
  xiphoid 733.90
Painful — *see also* Pain
  arc syndrome 726.19
  coitus
    female 625.0
    male 608.89
    psychogenic 302.76
  ejaculation (semen) 608.89
    psychogenic 302.79
  erection 607.3
  feet syndrome 266.2
  menstruation 625.3
    psychogenic 306.52
  micturition 788.1
  ophthalmoplegia 378.55
  respiration 786.52
  scar NEC 709.2
  urination 788.1
  wire sutures 998.89 ◆
Painters' colic 984.9
  specified type of lead — *see* Table of drugs and chemicals
Palate — *see* condition
Palatoplegia 528.9
Palatoschisis (*see also* Cleft, palate) 749.00
Palilalia 784.69
Palindromic arthritis (*see also* Rheumatism, palindromic) 719.3
Pallor 782.61
  temporal, optic disc 377.15

Palmar — *see also* condition
  fascia — *see* condition
Palpable
  cecum 569.89
  kidney 593.89
  liver 573.9
  lymph nodes 785.6
  ovary 620.8
  prostate 602.9
  spleen (*see also* Splenomegaly) 789.2
  uterus 625.8
Palpitation (heart) 785.1
  psychogenic 306.2
Palsy (*see also* Paralysis) 344.9
  atrophic diffuse 335.20
  Bell's 351.0
    newborn 767.5
  birth 767.7
  brachial plexus 353.0
    fetus or newborn 767.6
  brain — *see also* Palsy, cerebral
    noncongenital or noninfantile 344.8
    due to vascular lesion — *see* category 438
  syphilitic 094.89
    congenital 090.49
  bulbar (chronic) (progressive) 335.22
    pseudo NEC 335.23
    supranuclear NEC 344.8
  cerebral (congenital) (infantile) (spastic) 343.9
    athetoid 333.7
    diplegic 343.0
    due to previous vascular lesion — *see* category 438
    hemiplegic 343.1
    monoplegic 343.3
    noncongenital or noninfantile 437.8
    due to previous vascular lesion — *see* category 438
    paraplegic 343.0
    quadriplegic 343.2
    spastic, not congenital or infantile 344.8
    syphilitic 094.89
      congenital 090.49
    tetraplegic 343.2
  cranial nerve — *see also* Disorder, nerve, cranial
    multiple 352.6
  creeping 335.21
  divers' 993.3
  Erb's (birth injury) 767.6
  facial 351.0
    newborn 767.5
  glossopharyngeal 352.2
  Klumpke (-Déjérine) 767.6
  lead 984.9
    specified type of lead — *see* Table of drugs and chemicals
  median nerve (tardy) 354.0
  peroneal nerve (acute) (tardy) 355.3
  pseudobulbar NEC 335.23
  radial nerve (acute) 354.3
  seventh nerve 351.0
    newborn 767.5
  shaking (*see also* Parkinsonism) 332.0
  spastic (cerebral) (spinal) 343.9
    hemiplegic 343.1
  specified nerve NEC — *see* Disorder, nerve
  supranuclear NEC 356.8
  ulnar nerve (tardy) 354.2
  wasting 335.21
Paltauf-Sternberg disease 201.9
Paludism — *see* Malaria
Panama fever 084.0

Panaris (with lymphangitis) 681.9
  finger 681.02
  toe 681.11
Panaritium (with lymphangitis) 681.9
  finger 681.02
  toe 681.11
Panarteritis (nodosa) 446.0
  brain or cerebral 437.4
Pancake heart 793.2
  with cor pulmonale (chronic) 416.9
Pancarditis (acute) (chronic) 429.89
  with
    rheumatic
      fever (active) (acute) (chronic) (subacute) 391.8
        inactive or quiescent 398.99
    rheumatic, acute 391.8
      chronic or inactive 398.99
Pancoast's syndrome or tumor (carcinoma, pulmonary apex) (M8010/3) 162.3
Pancoast-Tobias syndrome (M8010/3) (carcinoma, pulmonary apex) 162.3
Pancolitis 556.6 ◆
Pancreas, pancreatic — *see* condition
Pancreatitis 577.0
  acute (edematous) (hemorrhagic) (recurrent) 577.0
  annular 577.0
  apoplectic 577.0
  calcerous 577.0
  chronic (infectious) 577.1
    recurrent 577.1
  cystic 577.2
  fibrous 577.8
  gangrenous 577.0
  hemorrhagic (acute) 577.0
  interstitial (chronic) 577.1
    acute 577.0
  malignant 577.0
  mumps 072.3
  painless 577.1
  recurrent 577.1
  relapsing 577.1
  subacute 577.0
  suppurative 577.0
  syphilitic 095.8
Pancreatolithiasis 577.8
Pancytolysis 289.9
Pancytopenia (acquired) 284.8
  with malformations 284.0
  congenital 284.0
Panencephalitis — *see also* Encephalitis
  subacute, sclerosing 046.2
Panhematopenia 284.8
  congenital 284.0
  constitutional 284.0
  splenic, primary 289.4
Panhemocytopenia 284.8
  congenital 284.0
  constitutional 284.0
Panhypogonadism 257.2
Panhypopituitarism 253.2
  prepubertal 253.3
Panic (attack) (state) 300.01
  reaction to exceptional stress (transient) 308.0
Panmyelopathy, familial constitutional 284.0
Panmyelophthisis 284.9
  acquired (secondary) 284.8
  congenital 284.0
  idiopathic 284.9
Panmyelosis (acute) (M9951/1) 238.7

Panner's disease 732.3
  capitellum humeri 732.3
  head of humerus 732.3
  tarsal navicular (bone) (osteochondrosis) 732.5
Panneuritis endemica 265.0 *[357.4]*
Panniculitis 729.30
  back 724.8
  knee 729.31
  neck 723.6
  nodular, nonsuppurative 729.30
  sacral 724.8
  specified site NEC 729.39
Panniculus adiposus (abdominal) 278.1
Pannus 370.62
  allergic eczematous 370.62
  degenerativus 370.62
  keratic 370.62
  rheumatoid — *see* Arthritis, rheumatoid
  trachomatosus, trachomatous (active) 076.1 *[370.62]*
    late effect 139.1
Panophthalmitis 360.02
Panotitis — *see* Otitis media
Pansinusitis (chronic) (hyperplastic) (nonpurulent) (purulent) 473.8
  acute 461.8
  due to fungus NEC 117.9
  tuberculous (*see also* Tuberculosis) 012.8
Panuveitis 360.12
  sympathetic 360.11
Panvalvular disease — *see* Endocarditis, mitral
Papageienkrankheit 073.9
Papanicolaou smear
  cervix (screening test) V76.2
    as part of gynecological examination V72.3
    for suspected malignant neoplasm V76.2
    no disease found V71.1
    nonspecific abnormal finding 795.0
  specified site, except cervix — *see also* Screening, malignant neoplasm
    for suspected malignant neoplasm — *see also* Screening, malignant neoplasm
    no disease found V71.1
    nonspecific abnormal finding 795.1
Papilledema 377.00
  associated with
    decreased ocular pressure 377.02
    increased intracranial pressure 377.01
    retinal disorder 377.03
  choked disc 377.00
  infectional 377.00
Papillitis 377.31
  anus 569.49
  chronic lingual 529.4
  necrotizing, kidney 584.7
  optic 377.31
  rectum 569.49
  renal, necrotizing 584.7
  tongue 529.0
Papilloma (M8050/0) — *see also* Neoplasm, by site, benign

Note — Except where otherwise indicated, the morphological varieties of papilloma in the list below should be coded by site as for "Neoplasm, benign."

  acuminatum (female) (male) 078.1

Papilloma—*continued*
  bladder (urinary) (transitional cell) (M8120/1) 236.7
    benign (M8120/0) 223.3
  choroid plexus (M9390/0) 225.0
    anaplastic type (M9390/3) 191.5
    malignant (M9390/3) 191.5
  ductal (M8503/0)
  dyskeratotic (M8052/0)
  epidermoid (M8052/0)
  hyperkeratotic (M8052/0)
  intracystic (M8504/0)
  intraductal (M8503/0)
  inverted (M8053/0)
  keratotic (M8052/0)
  parakeratotic (M8052/0)
  pinta (primary) 103.0
  renal pelvis (transitional cell) (M8120/1) 236.99
    benign (M8120/0) 223.1
  Schneiderian (M8121/0)
    specified site — *see* Neoplasm, by site, benign
    unspecified site 212.0
  serous surface (M8461/0)
    borderline malignancy (M8461/1)
      specified site — *see* Neoplasm, by site, uncertain behavior
      unspecified site 236.2
    specified site — *see* Neoplasm, by site, benign
    unspecified site 220
  squamous (cell) (M8052/0)
  transitional (cell) (M8120/0)
    bladder (urinary) (M8120/1) 236.7
    inverted type (M8121/1) — *see* Neoplasm, by site, uncertain behavior
    renal pelvis (M8120/1) 236.91
    ureter (M8120/1) 236.91
  ureter (transitional cell) (M8120/1) 236.91
    benign (M8120/0) 223.2
  urothelial (M8120/1) — *see* Neoplasm, by site, uncertain behavior
  verrucous (M8051/0)
  villous (M8261/1) — *see* Neoplasm, by site, uncertain behavior
  yaws, plantar or palmar 102.1
Papillomata, multiple, of yaws 102.1
Papillomatosis (M8060/0) — *see also* Neoplasm, by site, benign
  confluent and reticulate 701.8
  cutaneous 701.8
  ductal, breast 610.1
  Gougerot-Carteaud (confluent reticulate) 701.8
  intraductal (diffuse) (M8505/0) — *see* Neoplasm, by site, benign
  subareolar duct (M8506/0) 217
Papillon-Léage and Psaume syndrome (orodigitofacial dysostosis) 759.89
Papule 709.8
  carate (primary) 103.0
  fibrous, of nose (M8724/0) 216.3
  pinta (primary) 103.0
Papulosis, malignant 447.8
Papyraceous fetus 779.8
  complicating pregnancy 646.0
Paracephalus 759.7
Parachute mitral valve 746.5
Paracoccidioidomycosis 116.1
  mucocutaneous-lymphangitic 116.1
  pulmonary 116.1
  visceral 116.1

Paracoccidiomycosis — *see* Paracoccidioidomycosis
Paracusis 388.40
Paradentosis 523.5
Paradoxical facial movements 374.43
Paraffinoma 999.9
Paraganglioma (M8680/1)
  adrenal (M8700/0) 227.0
    malignant (M8700/3) 194.0
  aortic body (M8691/1) 237.3
    malignant (M8691/3) 194.6
  carotid body (M8692/1) 237.3
    malignant (M8692/3) 194.5
  chromaffin (M8700/0) — *see also* Neoplasm, by site, benign
    malignant (M8700/3) — *see* Neoplasm, by site, malignant
  extra-adrenal (M8693/1)
    malignant (M8693/3)
      specified site — *see* Neoplasm, by site, malignant
      unspecified site 194.6
    specified site — *see* Neoplasm, by site, uncertain behavior
    unspecified site 237.3
  glomus jugulare (M8690/1) 237.3
    malignant (M8690/3) 194.6
  jugular (M8690/1) 237.3
    malignant (M8680/3)
      specified site — *see* Neoplasm, by site, malignant
      unspecified site 194.6
  nonchromaffin (M8693/1)
    malignant (M8693/3)
      specified site — *see* Neoplasm, by site, malignant
      unspecified site 194.6
    specified site — *see* Neoplasm, by site, uncertain behavior
    unspecified site 237.3
  parasympathetic (M8682/1)
    specified site — *see* Neoplasm, by site, uncertain behavior
    unspecified site 237.3
  specified site — *see* Neoplasm, by site, uncertain behavior
  sympathetic (M8681/1)
    specified site — *see* Neoplasm, by site, uncertain behavior
    unspecified site 237.3
  unspecified site 237.3
Parageusia 781.1
  psychogenic 306.7
Paragonimiasis 121.2
Paragranuloma, Hodgkin's (M9660/3) 201.0
Parahemophilia (*see also* Defect, coagulation) 286.3
Parakeratosis 690
  psoriasiformis 696.2
  variegata 696.2
Paralysis, paralytic (complete) (incomplete) 344.9
  with
    broken
      back — *see* Fracture, vertebra, by site, with spinal cord injury
      neck — *see* Fracture, vertebra, cervical, with spinal cord injury

Paralysis, paralytic—continued
- with—continued
  - fracture, vertebra — see Fracture, vertebra, by site, with spinal cord injury
  - syphilis 094.89
- abdomen and back muscles 355.9
- abdominal muscles 355.9
- abducens (nerve) 378.54
- abductor 355.9
  - lower extremity 355.8
  - upper extremity 354.9
- accessory nerve 352.4
- accommodation 367.51
  - hysterical 300.11
- acoustic nerve 388.5
- agitans 332.0
  - arteriosclerotic 332.0
- alternating 344.8
  - oculomotor 344.8
- amyotrophic 335.20
- ankle 355.8
- anterior serratus 355.9
- anus (sphincter) 569.49
- apoplectic (current episode) (see also Disease, cerebrovascular, acute) 436
  - late effect — see category 438
- arm 344.40
  - affecting
    - dominant side 344.41
    - nondominant side 344.42 ▲
  - both 344.2
  - due to old CVA — see category 438
  - hysterical 300.11
  - psychogenic 306.0
  - transient 781.4
  - traumatic NEC (see also Injury, nerve, upper limb) 955.9
- arteriosclerotic (current episode) 437.0
  - late effect — see category 438
- ascending (spinal), acute 357.0
- associated, nuclear 344.8
- asthenic bulbar 358.0
- ataxic NEC 334.9
  - general 094.1
- athetoid 333.7
- atrophic 356.9
  - infantile, acute (see also Poliomyelitis, with paralysis) 045.1
  - muscle NEC 355.9
  - progressive 335.21
  - spinal (acute) (see also Poliomyelitis, with paralysis) 045.1
- attack (see also Disease, cerebrovascular, acute) 436
- axillary 353.0
- Babinski-Nageotte's 344.8
- Bell's 351.0
  - newborn 767.5
- Benedikt's 344.8
- birth (injury) 767.7
  - brain 767.0
  - intracranial 767.0
  - spinal cord 767.4
- bladder (sphincter) 596.53
  - neurogenic 596.54
    - with cauda equina syndrome 344.61
  - puerperal, postpartum, childbirth 665.5
  - sensory 344.61
    - with cauda equina 344.61
  - spastic 344.61
    - with cauda equina 344.61
- bowel, colon, or intestine (see also Ileus) 560.1
- brachial plexus 353.0
  - due to birth injury 767.6
  - newborn 767.6

Paralysis, paralytic—continued
- brain
  - congenital — see Palsy, cerebral
  - current episode 437.8
  - diplegia 344.2
  - due to previous vascular lesion — see category 438
  - hemiplegia 342.9
    - due to previous vascular lesion — see category 438
  - infantile — see Palsy, cerebral
  - monoplegia — see also Monoplegia
    - due to previous vascular lesion — see category 438
  - paraplegia 344.1
  - quadriplegia — see Quadriplegia
  - syphilitic, congenital 090.49
  - triplegia 344.8
- bronchi 519.1
- Brown-Séquard's 344.8
- bulbar (chronic) (progessive) 335.22
  - infantile (see also Poliomyelitis, bulbar) 045.0
  - poliomyelitic (see also Poliomyelitis, bulbar) 045.0
  - pseudo 335.23
  - supranuclear 344.8
- bulbospinal 358.0
- cardiac (see also Failure, heart) 428.9
- cerebral
  - current episode 437.8
  - spastic, infantile — see Palsy, cerebral
- cerebrocerebellar 437.8
  - diplegic infantile 343.0
- cervical
  - plexus 353.2
  - sympathetic NEC 337.0
- Céstan-Chenais 344.8
- Charcot-Marie-Tooth type 356.1
- childhood — see Palsy, cerebral
- Clark's 343.9
- colon (see also Ileus) 560.1
- compressed air 993.3
- compression
  - arm NEC 354.9
  - cerebral — see Paralysis, brain
  - leg NEC 355.8
  - lower extremity NEC 355.8
  - upper extremity NEC 354.9
- congenital (cerebral) (spastic) (spinal) — see Palsy, cerebral
- conjugate movement (of eye) 378.81
  - cortical (nuclear) (supranuclear) 378.81
- convergence 378.83
- cordis (see also Failure, heart) 428.9
- cortical (see also Paralysis, brain) 437.8
- cranial or cerebral nerve (see also Disorder, nerve, cranial) 352.9
- creeping 335.21
- crossed leg 344.8
- crutch 953.4
- deglutition 784.9
  - hysterical 300.11
- dementia 094.1
- descending (spinal) NEC 335.9
- diaphragm (flaccid) 519.4
  - due to accidental section of phrenic nerve during procedure 998.2
- digestive organs NEC 564.8
- diplegic — see Diplegia

Paralysis, paralytic—continued
- divergence (nuclear) 378.85
- divers' 993.3
- Duchenne's 335.22
- due to intracranial or spinal birth injury — see Palsy, cerebral
- embolic (current episode) (see also Embolism, brain) 434.1
  - late effect or old — see category 438
- enteric (see also Ileus) 560.1
  - with hernia — see Hernia, by site, with obstruction
- Erb's syphilitic spastic spinal 094.89
- Erb (-Duchenne) (birth) (newborn) 767.6
- esophagus 530.8
- essential, infancy (see also Poliomyelitis) 045.9
- extremity
  - lower — see Paralysis, leg
  - spastic (hereditary) 343.3
    - noncongenital or noninfantile 344.1
  - transient (cause unknown) 781.4
  - upper — see Paralysis, arm
- eye muscle (extrinsic) 378.55
  - intrinsic 367.51
- facial (nerve) 351.0
  - birth injury 767.5
  - congenital 767.5
  - following operation NEC 998.2
  - newborn 767.5
- familial 359.3
  - periodic 359.3
  - spastic 334.1
- fauces 478.29
- finger NEC 354.9
- foot NEC 355.8
- gait 781.2
- gastric nerve 352.3
- gaze 378.81
- general 094.1
  - ataxic 094.1
  - insane 094.1
  - juvenile 090.40
  - progressive 094.1
  - tabetic 094.1
- glossopharyngeal (nerve) 352.2
- glottis (see also Paralysis, vocal cord) 478.30
- gluteal 353.4
- Gubler (-Millard) 344.8
- hand 354.9
  - hysterical 300.11
  - psychogenic 306.0
- heart (see also Failure, heart) 428.9
- hemifacial, progressive 349.89
- hemiplegic — see Hemiplegia
- hyperkalemic periodic (familial) 359.3
- hypertensive (current episode) 437.8
- hypoglossal (nerve) 352.5
- hypokalemic periodic 359.3
- Hyrtl's sphincter (rectum) 569.49
- hysterical 300.11
- ileus (see also Ileus) 560.1
- infantile (see also Poliomyelitis) 045.9
  - atrophic acute 045.1
  - bulbar 045.0
  - cerebral — see Palsy, cerebral
  - paralytic 045.1
  - progressive acute 045.9
  - spastic — see Palsy, cerebral
  - spinal 045.9
- infective (see also Poliomyelitis) 045.9
- inferior nuclear 344.9
- insane, general or progressive 094.1

Paralysis, paralytic—continued
- internuclear 378.86
- interosseous 355.9
- intestine (see also Ileus) 560.1
- intracranial (current episode) (see also Paralysis, brain) 437.8
  - due to birth injury 767.0
- iris 379.49
  - due to diphtheria (toxin) 032.81 [379.49]
- ischemic, Volkmann's (complicating trauma) 958.6
- Jackson's 344.8
- jake 357.7
- Jamaica ginger (jake) 357.7
- juvenile general 090.40
- Klumpke (-Déjérine) (birth) (newborn) 767.6
- labioglossal (laryngeal) (pharyngeal) 335.22
- Landry's 357.0
- laryngeal nerve (recurrent) (superior) (see also Paralysis, vocal cord) 478.30
- larynx (see also Paralysis, vocal cord) 478.30
  - due to diphtheria (toxin) 032.3
- late effect
  - due to
    - birth injury, brain or spinal (cord) — see Palsy, cerebral
    - edema, brain or cerebral — see Paralysis, brain
  - lesion
    - cerebrovascular — see category 438
    - spinal (cord) — see Paralysis, spinal
- lateral 335.24
- lead 984.9
  - specified type of lead — see Table of drugs and chemicals
- left side — see Hemiplegia
- leg 344.30
  - affecting
    - dominant side 344.31
    - nondominant side 344.32 ▲
  - both (see also Paraplegia) 344.1
  - crossed 344.8
  - hysterical 300.11
  - psychogenic 306.0
  - transient or transitory 781.4
  - traumatic NEC (see also Injury, nerve, lower limb) 956.9
- levator palpebrae superioris 374.31
- limb NEC 344.5
  - all four — see Quadriplegia
  - quadriplegia — see Quadriplegia
- lip 528.5
- Lissauer's 094.1
- local 355.9
- lower limb — see also Paralysis, leg
  - both (see also Paraplegia) 344.1
- lung 518.89
  - newborn 770.8
- median nerve 354.1
- medullary (tegmental) 344.8
- mesencephalic NEC 344.8
  - tegmental 344.8
- middle alternating 344.8
- Millard-Gubler-Foville 344.8
- monoplegic — see Monoplegia
- motor NEC 344.9
  - cerebral — see Paralysis, brain
  - spinal — see Paralysis, spinal

Paralysis, paralytic—continued
multiple
  cerebral — see Paralysis, brain
  spinal — see Paralysis, spinal
muscle (flaccid) 359.9
  due to nerve lesion NEC 355.9
  eye (extrinsic) 378.55
    intrinsic 367.51
    oblique 378.51
    iris sphincter 364.8
  ischemic (complicating
    trauma) (Volkmann's)
    958.6
  pseudohypertrophic 359.1
muscular (atrophic) 359.9
  progressive 335.21
musculocutaneous nerve 354.9
musculospiral 354.9
nerve — see also Disorder, nerve
  third or oculomotor (partial)
    378.51
    total 378.52
  fourth or trochlear 378.53
  sixth or abducens 378.54
  seventh or facial 351.0
    birth injury 767.5
    due to
      injection NEC 999.9
      operation NEC 997.0
    newborn 767.5
  accessory 352.4
  auditory 388.5
  birth injury 767.7
  cranial or cerebral (see also
    Disorder, nerve, cranial)
    352.9
  facial 351.0
    birth injury 767.5
    newborn 767.5
  laryngeal (see also Paralysis,
    vocal cord) 478.30
  newborn 767.7
  phrenic 354.8
    newborn 767.7
  radial 354.3
    birth injury 767.6
    newborn 767.6
  syphilitic 094.89
  traumatic NEC (see also Injury,
    nerve, by site) 957.9
  trigeminal 350.9
  ulnar 354.2
newborn NEC 767.0
normokalemic periodic 359.3
obstetrical, newborn 767.7
ocular 378.9
oculofacial, congenital 352.6
oculomotor (nerve) (partial)
  378.51
  alternating 344.8
  external bilateral 378.55
  total 378.52
olfactory nerve 352.0
palate 528.9
palatopharyngolaryngeal 352.6
paratrigeminal 350.9
periodic (familial) (hyperkalemic)
  (hypokalemic)
  (normokalemic) (secondary)
  359.3
peripheral
  autonomic nervous system —
    see Neuropathy,
    peripheral, autonomic
  nerve NEC 355.9
peroneal (nerve) 355.3
pharynx 478.29
phrenic nerve 354.8
plantar nerves 355.6
pneumogastric nerve 352.3
poliomyelitis (current) (see also
  Poliomyelitis, with
  paralysis) 045.1
  bulbar 045.0
popliteal nerve 355.3
pressure (see also Neuropathy,
  entrapment) 355.9

Paralysis, paralytic—continued
progressive 335.21
  atrophic 335.21
  bulbar 335.22
  general 094.1
  hemifacial 349.89
  infantile, acute (see also
    Poliomyelitis) 045.9
  multiple 335.20
pseudobulbar 335.23
pseudohypertrophic 359.1
  muscle 359.1
psychogenic 306.0
pupil, pupillary 379.49
quadriceps 355.8
quadriplegic (see also
  Quadriplegia) 344.0
radial nerve 354.3
  birth injury 767.6
rectum (sphincter) 569.49
rectus muscle (eye) 378.55
recurrent laryngeal nerve (see
  also Paralysis, vocal cord)
  478.30
respiratory (muscle) (system)
  (tract) 786.09
  center NEC 344.8
    fetus or newborn 770.8
  congenital 768.9
  newborn 768.9
right side — see Hemiplegia
Saturday night 354.3
saturnine 984.9
  specified type of lead — see
    Table of drugs and
    chemicals
sciatic nerve 355.0
secondary — see Paralysis, late
  effect
seizure (cerebral) (current
  episode) (see also Disease,
  cerebrovascular, acute) 436
  late effect — see category 438
senile NEC 344.9
serratus magnus 355.9
shaking (see also Parkinsonism)
  332.0
shock (see also Disease,
  cerebrovascular, acute) 436
  late effect — see category 438
shoulder 354.9
soft palate 528.9
spasmodic — see Paralysis,
  spastic
spastic 344.9
  cerebral infantile — see Palsy,
    cerebral
  congenital (cerebral) — see
    Palsy, cerebral
  familial 334.1
  hereditary 334.1
  infantile 343.9
  noncongenital or noninfantile,
    cerebral 344.9
  syphilitic 094.0
    spinal 094.89
sphincter, bladder (see also
  Paralysis, bladder) 596.53
spinal (cord) NEC 344.1
  accessory nerve 352.4
  acute (see also Poliomyelitis)
    045.9
  ascending acute 357.0
  atrophic (acute) (see also
    Poliomyelitis, with
    paralysis) 045.1
    spastic, syphilitic 094.89
  congenital NEC 343.9
  hemiplegic — see
    Hemiplegia
  hereditary 336.8
  infantile (see also
    Poliomyelitis) 045.9
  late effect NEC 344.8
  monoplegic — see
    Monoplegia
  nerve 355.9

Paralysis, paralytic—continued
spinal (cord)—continued
  progressive 335.10
  quadriplegic — see
    Quadriplegia
  spastic NEC 343.9
  traumatic — see Injury, spinal,
    by site
sternomastoid 352.4
stomach 536.3
  nerve 352.3
stroke (current episode) (see also
  Disease, cerebrovascular,
  acute) 436
  late effect — see category 438
subscapularis 354.8
superior nuclear NEC 334.9
supranuclear 356.8
sympathetic
  cervical NEC 337.0
  nerve NEC (see also
    Neuropathy, peripheral,
    autonomic) 337.9
  nervous system — see
    Neuropathy, peripheral,
    autonomic
syndrome 344.9
  specified NEC 344.8
syphilitic spastic spinal (Erb's)
  094.89
tabetic general 094.1
thigh 355.8
throat 478.29
  diphtheritic 032.0
  muscle 478.29
thrombotic (current episode) (see
  also Thrombosis, brain)
  434.0
  old — see category 438
thumb NEC 354.9
tick (-bite) 989.5
Todd's (postepileptic transitory
  paralysis) 344.8
toe 355.6
tongue 529.8
transient
  arm or leg NEC 781.4
  traumatic NEC (see also Injury,
    nerve, by site) 957.9
trapezius 352.4
traumatic, transient NEC (see also
  Injury, nerve, by site) 957.9
trembling (see also Parkinsonism)
  332.0
triceps brachii 354.9
trigeminal nerve 350.9
trochlear nerve 378.53
ulnar nerve 354.2
upper limb — see also Paralysis,
  arm
  both (see also Diplegia) 344.2
uremic — see Uremia
uveoparotitic 135
uvula 528.9
  hysterical 300.11
  postdiphtheritic 032.0
vagus nerve 352.3
vasomotor NEC 337.9
velum palati 528.9
vesical (see also Paralysis,
  bladder) 596.53
vestibular nerve 388.5
visual field, psychic 368.16
vocal cord 478.30
  bilateral (partial) 478.33
    complete 478.34
  complete (bilateral) 478.34
  unilateral (partial) 478.31
    complete 478.32
Volkmann's (complicating trauma)
  958.6
wasting 335.21
Weber's 344.8
wrist NEC 354.9

Paramedial orifice, urethrovesical
  753.8
Paramenia 626.9

Parametritis (chronic) (see also
  Disease, pelvis, inflammatory)
  614.4
  acute 614.3
  puerperal, postpartum, childbirth
    670
Parametrium, parametric — see
  condition
Paramnesia (see also Amnesia) 780.9
Paramolar 520.1
  causing crowding 524.3
Paramyloidosis 277.3
Paramyoclonus multiplex 333.2
Paramyotonia 359.2
  congenita 359.2
Parangi (see also Yaws) 102.9
Paranoia 297.1
  alcoholic 291.5
  querulans 297.8
  senile 290.20
Paranoid
  dementia (see also Schizophrenia)
    295.3
    praecox (acute) 295.3
    senile 290.20
  personality 301.0
  psychosis 297.9
    alcoholic 291.5
    climacteric 297.2
    drug-induced 292.11
    involutional 297.2
    menopausal 297.2
    protracted reactive 298.4
    psychogenic 298.4
      acute 298.3
    senile 290.20
  reaction (chronic) 297.9
    acute 298.3
  schizophrenia (acute) (see also
    Schizophrenia) 295.3
  state 297.9
    alcohol-induced 291.5
    climacteric 297.2
    drug-induced 292.11
    due to or associated with
      arteriosclerosis
      (cerebrovascular)
      290.42
      presenile brain disease
        290.12
      senile brain disease 290.20
    involutional 297.2
    menopausal 297.2
    senile 290.20
    simple 297.0
    specified type NEC 297.8
  tendencies 301.0
  traits 301.0
  trends 301.0
  type, psychopathic personality
    301.0
Paraparesis (see also Paralysis) 344.9
Paraphasia 784.3
Paraphilia (see also Deviation,
  sexual) 302.9
Paraphimosis (congenital) 605
  chancroidal 099.0
Paraphrenia, paraphrenic (late)
  297.2
  climacteric 297.2
  dementia (see also Schizophrenia)
    295.3
  involutional 297.2
  menopausal 297.2
  schizophrenia (acute) (see also
    Schizophrenia) 295.3
Paraplegia 344.1
  with
    broken back — see Fracture,
      vertebra, by site, with
      spinal cord injury

Paraplegia—continued
  with—continued
    fracture, vertebra — see Fracture, vertebra, by site, with spinal cord injury
    ataxic — see Degeneration, combined, spinal cord
    brain (current episode) (see also Paralysis, brain) 437.8
    cerebral (current episode) (see also Paralysis, brain) 437.8
    congenital or infantile (cerebral) (spastic) (spinal) 343.0
    cortical — see Paralysis, brain
    familial spastic 334.1
    functional (hysterical) 300.11
    hysterical 300.11
    infantile 343.0
    late effect 344.1
    Pott's (see also Tuberculosis) 015.0 [730.88]
    psychogenic 306.0
    spastic
      Erb's spinal 094.89
      hereditary 334.1
      not infantile or congenital 344.1
    spinal (cord)
      traumatic NEC — see Injury, spinal, by site
    syphilitic (spastic) 094.89
    traumatic NEC — see Injury, spinal, by site
Paraproteinemia 273.2
  benign (familial) 273.1
  monoclonal 273.1
  secondary to malignant or inflammatory disease 273.1
Parapsoriasis 696.2
  en plaques 696.2
  guttata 696.2
  lichenoides chronica 696.2
  retiformis 696.2
  varioliformis (acuta) 696.2
Parascarlatina 057.8
Parasitic — see also condition
  disease NEC (see also Infestation, parasitic) 136.9
    contact V01.8
    exposure to V01.8
    intestinal NEC 129
    skin NEC 134.9
  stomatitis 112.0
  sycosis 110.0
    beard 110.0
    scalp 110.0
  twin 759.4
Parasitism NEC 136.9
  intestinal NEC 129
  skin NEC 134.9
  specified — see Infestation
Parasitophobia 300.29
Parasomnia 780.59
  nonorganic origin 307.47
Paraspadias 752.8
Paraspasm facialis 351.8
Parathyroid gland — see condition
Parathyroiditis (autoimmune) 252.1
Parathyroprival tetany 252.1
Paratrachoma 077.0
Paratyphilitis (see also Appendicitis) 541
Paratyphoid (fever) — see Fever, paratyphoid
Paratyphus — see Fever, paratyphoid
Paraurethral duct 753.8
Para-urethritis 597.89
  gonococcal (acute) 098.0
  chronic or duration of 2 months or over 098.2
Paravaccinia NEC 051.9
  milkers' node 051.1

Paravaginitis (see also Vaginitis) 616.10
Parencephalitis (see also Encephalitis) 323.9
  late effect — see category 326
Parergasia 298.9
Paresis (see also Paralysis) 344.9
  accommodation 367.51
  bladder (spastic) (sphincter) (see also Paralysis, bladder) 596.53
    tabetic 094.0
  bowel, colon, or intestine (see also Ileus) 560.1
  brain or cerebral — see Paralysis, brain
  extrinsic muscle, eye 378.55
  general 094.1
    arrested 094.1
    brain 094.1
    cerebral 094.1
    insane 094.1
    juvenile 090.40
      remission 090.49
    progressive 094.1
    remission (sustained) 094.1
    tabetic 094.1
  heart (see also Failure, heart) 428.9
  infantile (see also Poliomyelitis) 045.9
  insane 094.1
  juvenile 090.40
  late effect — see Paralysis, late effect
  luetic (general) 094.1
  peripheral progressive 356.9
  pseudohypertrophic 359.1
  senile NEC 344.9
  stomach 536.3
  syphilitic (general) 094.1
    congenital 090.40
  transient, limb 781.4
  vesical (sphincter) NEC 596.53
Paresthesia (see also Disturbance, sensation) 782.0
  Berger's (paresthesia of lower limb) 782.0
  Bernhardt 355.1
  Magnan's 782.0
Paretic — see condition
Parinaud's
  conjunctivitis 372.02
  oculoglandular syndrome 372.02
  ophthalmoplegia 378.81
  syndrome (paralysis of conjugate upward gaze) 378.81
Parkes Weber and Dimitri syndrome (encephalocutaneous angiomatosis) 759.6
Parkinson's disease, syndrome, or tremor — see Parkinsonism
Parkinsonism (arteriosclerotic) (idiopathic) (primary) 332.0
  associated with orthostatic hypotension (idiopathic) (symptomatic) 333.0
  due to drugs 332.1
  secondary 332.1
  syphilitic 094.82
Parodontitis 523.4
Parodontosis 523.5
Paronychia (with lymphangitis) 681.9
  candidal (chronic) 112.3
  chronic 681.9
    candidal 112.3
    finger 681.02
    toe 681.11
  finger 681.02
  toe 681.11
  tuberculous (primary) (see also Tuberculosis) 017.0
Parorexia NEC 307.52
  hysterical 300.11

Parosmia 781.1
  psychogenic 306.7
Parotid gland — see condition
Parotiditis (see also Parotitis) 527.2
  epidemic 072.9
  infectious 072.9
Parotitis 527.2
  allergic 527.2
  chronic 527.2
  epidemic (see also Mumps) 072.9
  infectious (see also Mumps) 072.9
  noninfectious 527.2
  nonspecific toxic 527.2
  not mumps 527.2
  postoperative 527.2
  purulent 527.2
  septic 527.2
  suppurative (acute) 527.2
  surgical 527.2
  toxic 527.2
Paroxysmal — see also condition
  dyspnea (nocturnal) 786.09
Parrot's disease (syphilitic osteochondritis) 090.0
Parrot fever 073.9
Parry's disease or syndrome (exophthalmic goiter) 242.0
Parry-Romberg syndrome 349.89
Parson's disease (exophthalmic goiter) 242.0
Parsonage-Aldren-Turner syndrome 353.5
Parsonage-Turner syndrome 353.5
Pars planitis 363.21
Particolored infant 757.39
Parturition — see Delivery
Passage
  false, urethra 599.4
  of sounds or bougies (see also Attention to artificial opening) V55.9
Passive — see condition
Pasteurella septica 027.2
Pasteurellosis (see also Infection, Pasteurella) 027.2
PAT (paroxysmal atrial tachycardia) 427.0
Patau's syndrome (trisomy D) 758.1
Patch
  herald 696.3
Patches
  mucous (syphilitic) 091.3
    congenital 090.0
  smokers' (mouth) 528.6
Patellar — see condition
Patent — see also Imperfect closure
  atrioventricular ostium 745.69
  canal of Nuck 752.41
  cervix 622.5
    complicating pregnancy 654.5
    affecting fetus or newborn 761.0
  ductus arteriosus or Botalli 747.0
  eustachian
    tube 381.7
    valve 746.89
  foramen
    Botalli 745.5
    ovale 745.5
  interauricular septum 745.5
  interventricular septum 745.4
  omphalomesenteric duct 751.0
  os (uteri) — see Patent, cervix
  ostium secundum 745.5
  urachus 753.7
  vitelline duct 751.0
Paterson's syndrome (sideropenic dysphagia) 280.8
Paterson (-Brown) (-Kelly) syndrome (sideropenic dysphagia) 280.8
Paterson-Kelly syndrome or web (sideropenic dysphagia) 280.8

Pathologic, pathological — see also condition
  asphyxia 799.0
  drunkenness 291.4
  emotionality 301.3
  liar 301.7
  personality 301.9
  resorption, tooth 521.4
  sexuality (see also Deviation, sexual) 302.9
Pathology (of) — see Disease
Patterned motor discharge, idiopathic (see also Epilepsy) 345.5
Patulous — see also Patent
  anus 569.49
  Eustachian tube 381.7
Pause, sinoatrial 427.81
Pavor nocturnus 307.46
Pavy's disease 593.6
Paxton's disease (white piedra) 111.2
Payr's disease or syndrome (splenic flexure syndrome) 569.89
Pearls
  Elschnig 366.51
  enamel 520.2
Pearl-workers' disease (chronic osteomyelitis) (see also Osteomyelitis) 730.1
Pectenitis 569.49
Pectenosis 569.49
Pectoral — see condition
Pectus
  carinatum (congenital) 754.82
    acquired 738.3
    rachitic (see also Rickets) 268.0
  excavatum (congenital) 754.81
    acquired 738.3
    rachitic (see also Rickets) 268.0
  recurvatum (congenital) 754.81
    acquired 738.3
Pedatrophia 261
Pederosis 302.2
Pediculosis (infestation) 132.9
  capitis (head louse) (any site) 132.0
  corporis (body louse) (any site) 132.1
  eyelid 132.0 [373.6]
  mixed (classifiable to more than one category in 132.0-132.2) 132.3
  pubis (pubic louse) (any site) 132.2
  vestimenti 132.1
  vulvae 132.2
Pediculus (infestation) — see Pediculosis
Pedophilia 302.2
Peg-shaped teeth 520.2
Pel's crisis 094.0
Pel-Ebstein disease — see Disease, Hodgkin's
Pelade 704.01
Pelger-Huët anomaly or syndrome (hereditary hyposegmentation) 288.2
Peliosis (rheumatica) 287.0
Pelizaeus-Merzbacher
  disease 330.0
  sclerosis, diffuse cerebral 330.0
Pellagra (alcoholic or with alcoholism) 265.2
  with polyneuropathy 265.2 [357.4]
Pellagra-cerebellar-ataxia-renal aminoaciduria syndrome 270.0
Pellegrini's disease (calcification, knee joint) 726.62

Pellegrini (-Stieda) disease or syndrome (calcification, knee joint) 726.62
Pellizzi's syndrome (pineal) 259.8
Pelvic — see also condition
 congestion-fibrosis syndrome 625.5
 kidney 753.3
Pelvioectasis 591
Pelviolithiasis 592.0
Pelviperitonitis
 female (see also Peritonitis, pelvic, female) 614.5
 male (see also Peritonitis) 567.2
Pelvis, pelvic — see also condition or type
 infantile 738.6
 Nägele's 738.6
 obliquity 738.6
 Robert's 755.69
Pemphigoid 694.5
 benign, mucous membrane 694.60
  with ocular involvement 694.61
 bullous 694.5
 cicatricial 694.60
  with ocular involvement 694.61
 juvenile 694.2
Pemphigus 694.4
 benign 694.5
  chronic familial 757.39
 Brazilian 694.4
 circinatus 694.0
 congenital, traumatic 757.39
 conjunctiva 694.61
 contagiosus 684
 erythematodes 694.4
 erythematosus 694.4
 foliaceus 694.4
 frambesiodes 694.4
 gangrenous (see also Gangrene) 785.4
 malignant 694.4
 neonatorum, newborn 684
 ocular 694.61
 papillaris 694.4
 seborrheic 694.4
 South American 694.4
 syphilitic (congenital) 090.0
 vegetans 694.4
 vulgaris 694.4
 wildfire 694.4
Pendred's syndrome (familial goiter with deaf-mutism) 243
Pendulous
 abdomen 701.9
  in pregnancy or childbirth 654.4
   affecting fetus or newborn 763.8
 breast 611.8
Penetrating wound — see also Wound, open, by site
 with internal injury — see Injury, internal, by site, with open wound
 eyeball 871.7
  with foreign body (nonmagnetic) 871.6
   magnetic 871.5
 ocular (see also Penetrating wound, eyeball) 871.7
  adnexa 870.3
   with foreign body 870.4
  orbit 870.3
   with foreign body 870.4
Penetration, pregnant uterus by instrument
 with
  abortion — see Abortion, by type, with damage to pelvic organs
  ectopic pregnancy (see also categories 633.0-633.9) 639.2
  molar pregnancy (see also categories 630-632) 639.2
  complication of delivery 665.1
   affecting fetus or newborn 763.8
  following
   abortion 639.2
   ectopic or molar pregnancy 639.2
Penfield's syndrome (see also Epilepsy) 345.5
Penicilliosis of lung 117.3
Penis — see condition
Penitis 607.2
Penta X syndrome 758.8
Pentalogy (of Fallot) 745.2
Pentosuria (benign) (essential) 271.8
Peptic acid disease 536.8
Peregrinating patient V65.2
Perforated — see Perforation
Perforation, perforative (nontraumatic)
 antrum (see also Sinusitis, maxillary) 473.0
 appendix 540.0
  with peritoneal abcess 540.1◆
 atrial septum, multiple 745.5
 attic, ear 384.22
  healed 384.81
 bile duct, except cystic (see also Disease, biliary) 576.3
  cystic 575.4
 bladder (urinary) — see also Injury, internal, bladder
  with
   abortion — see Abortion, by type, with damage to pelvic organs
   ectopic pregnancy (see also categories 633.0-633.9) 639.2
   molar pregnancy (see also categories 630-632) 639.2
  following
   abortion 639.2
   ectopic or molar pregnancy 639.2
  obstetrical trauma 665.5
 bowel 569.83
  with
   abortion — see Abortion, by type, with damage to pelvic organs
   ectopic pregnancy (see also categories 633.0-633.9) 639.2
   molar pregnancy (see also categories 630-632) 639.2
  fetus or newborn 777.6
  following
   abortion 639.2
   ectopic or molar pregnancy 639.2
  obstetrical trauma 665.5
 broad ligament
  with
   abortion — see Abortion, by type, with damage to pelvic organs
   ectopic pregnancy (see also categories 633.0-633.9) 639.2
   molar pregnancy (see also categories 630-632) 639.2
  following
   abortion 639.2
   ectopic or molar pregnancy 639.2
  obstetrical trauma 665.6
  by
   device, implant, or graft — see Complications, mechanical
   foreign body left accidentally in operation wound 998.4
   instrument (any) during a procedure, accidental 998.2
 cecum 540.0
  with peritoneal abcess 540.1◆
 cervix (uteri) — see also Injury, internal, cervix
  with
   abortion — see Abortion, by type, with damage to pelvic organs
   ectopic pregnancy (see also categories 633.0-633.9) 639.2
   molar pregnancy (see also categories 630-632) 639.2
  following
   abortion 639.2
   ectopic or molar pregnancy 639.2
  obstetrical trauma 665.3
 colon 569.83
 common duct (bile) 576.3
 cornea (see also Ulcer, cornea) 370.00
  due to ulceration 370.06
 cystic duct 575.4
 diverticulum (see also Diverticula) 562.10
  small intestine 562.00
 duodenum, duodenal (ulcer) — see Ulcer, duodenum, with perforation
 ear drum — see Perforation, tympanum
 enteritis — see Enteritis
 esophagus 530.4
 ethmoidal sinus (see also Sinusitis, ethmoidal) 473.2
 foreign body (external site) — see also Wound, open, by site, complicated
  internal site, by ingested object — see Foreign body
 frontal sinus (see also Sinusitis, frontal) 473.1
 gallbladder or duct (see also Disease, gallbladder) 575.4
 gastric (ulcer) — see Ulcer, stomach, with perforation
 heart valve — see Endocarditis
 ileum 569.83
 instrumental
  external — see Wound, open, by site
  pregnant uterus, complicating delivery 665.9
  surgical (accidental) (blood vessel) (nerve) (organ) 998.2
 intestine 569.83
  with
   abortion — see Abortion, by type, with damage to pelvic organs
   ectopic pregnancy (see also categories 633.0-633.9) 639.2
   molar pregnancy (see also categories 630-632) 639.2
  fetus or newborn 777.6
  obstetrical trauma 665.5
  ulcerative NEC 569.83
 jejunum, jejunal 569.83
  ulcer — see Ulcer, gastrojejunal, with perforation
 mastoid (antrum) (cell) 383.89
 maxillary sinus (see also Sinusitis, maxillary) 473.0
 membrana tympani — see Perforation, tympanum
 nasal
  septum 478.1
   congenital 748.1
   syphilitic 095.8
  sinus (see also Sinusitis) 473.9
   congenital 748.1
 palate (hard) 526.89
  soft 528.9
   syphilitic 095.8
  syphilitic 095.8
 palatine vault 526.89
  syphilitic 095.8
   congenital 090.5
 pelvic
  floor
   with
    abortion — see Abortion, by type, with damage to pelvic organs
    ectopic pregnancy (see also categories 633.0-633.9) 639.2
    molar pregnancy (see also categories 630-632) 639.2
   obstetrical trauma 664.1
  organ
   with
    abortion — see Abortion, by type, with damage to pelvic organs
    ectopic pregnancy (see also categories 633.0-633.9) 639.2
    molar pregnancy (see also categories 630-632) 639.2
   following
    abortion 639.2
    ectopic or molar pregnancy 639.2
   obstetrical trauma 665.5
 perineum — see Laceration, perineum
 periurethral tissue
  with
   abortion — see Abortion, by type, with damage to pelvic organs
   ectopic pregnancy (see also categories 630-632) 639.2
   molar pregnancy (see also categories 630-632) 639.2
 pharynx 478.29
 pylorus, pyloric (ulcer) — see Ulcer, stomach, with perforation
 rectum 569.49
 sigmoid 569.83
 sinus (accessory) (chronic) (nasal) (see also Sinusitis) 473.9

Perforation, perforative—continued
  sphenoidal sinus (see also
      Sinusitis, sphenoidal) 473.3
  stomach (due to ulcer) — see
      Ulcer, stomach, with
      perforation
  surgical (accidental) (by
      instrument) (blood vessel)
      (nerve) (organ) 998.2
  traumatic
    external — see Wound, open,
      by site
    eye (see also Penetrating
      wound, ocular) 871.7
    internal organ — see Injury,
      internal, by site
  tympanum (membrane) (persistent
      posttraumatic)
      (postinflammatory) 384.20
    attic 384.22
    central 384.21
    healed 384.81
    marginal NEC 384.23
    multiple 384.24
    pars flaccida 384.22
    total 384.25
    traumatic — see Wound,
      open, ear, drum
  typhoid, gastrointestinal 002.0
  ulcer — see Ulcer, by site, with
      perforation
  ureter 593.89
  urethra
    with
      abortion — see Abortion,
        by type, with damage
        to pelvic organs
      ectopic pregnancy (see also
        categories 633.0-
        633.9) 639.2
      molar pregnancy (see also
        categories 630-632)
        639.2
    following
      abortion 639.2
      ectopic or molar pregnancy
        639.2
    obstetrical trauma 665.5
  uterus — see also Injury, internal,
      uterus
    with
      abortion — see Abortion,
        by type, with
        damage to pelvic
        organs
      ectopic pregnancy (see also
        categories 633.0-
        633.9) 639.2
      molar pregnancy (see also
        categories 630-632)
        639.2
    by intrauterine contraceptive
      device 996.32
    following
      abortion 639.2
      ectopic or molar pregnancy
        639.2
    obstetrical trauma — see
      Injury, internal, uterus,
      obstetrical trauma
  uvula 528.9
    syphilitic 095.8
  vagina — see Laceration, vagina
  viscus NEC 799.8
    traumatic 868.00
      with open wound into
        cavity 868.10

Periadenitis mucosa necrotica recurrens 528.2

Periangiitis 446.0

Periantritis 535.4

Periappendicitis (acute) (see also Appendicitis) 541

Periarteritis (disseminated) (infectious) (necrotizing) (nodosa) 446.0

Periarthritis (joint) 726.90
  Duplay's 726.2
  gonococcal 098.50
  humeroscapularis 726.2
  scapulohumeral 726.2
  shoulder 726.2
  wrist 726.4

Periarthrosis (angioneural) — see Periarthritis

Peribronchitis 491.9
  tuberculous (see also Tuberculosis) 011.3

Pericapsulitis, adhesive (shoulder) 726.0

Pericarditis (granular) (with decompensation) (with effusion) 423.9
  with
    rheumatic fever (conditions
      classifiable to 390)
      active (see also Pericarditis,
        rheumatic) 391.0
      inactive or quiescent 393
  actinomycotic 039.8 [420.0]
  acute (nonrheumatic) 420.90
    with chorea (acute)
      (rheumatic)
      (Sydenham's) 392.0
    bacterial 420.99
    benign 420.91
    hemorrhagic 420.90
    idiopathic 420.91
    infective 420.90
    nonspecific 420.91
    rheumatic 391.0
      with chorea (acute)
        (rheumatic)
        (Sydenham's) 392.0
    sicca 420.90
    viral 420.91
  adhesive or adherent (external)
      (internal) 423.1
    acute — see Pericarditis, acute
    rheumatic (external) (internal)
      393
  amebic 006.8 [420.0]
  bacterial (acute) (subacute) (with
      serous or seropurulent
      effusion) 420.99
  calcareous 423.2
  cholesterol (chronic) 423.8
    acute 420.90
  chronic (nonrheumatic) 423.8
    rheumatic 393
  constrictive 423.2
  Coxsackie 074.21
  due to
    actinomycosis 039.8 [420.0]
    amebiasis 006.8 [420.0]
    Coxsackie (virus) 074.21
    histoplasmosis (see also
      Histoplasmosis) 115.93
    nocardiosis 039.8 [420.0]
    tuberculosis (see also
      Tuberculosis) 017.9
      [420.0]
  fibrinocaseous (see also
      Tuberculosis) 017.9 [420.0]
  fibrinopurulent 420.99
  fibrinous — see Pericarditis,
      rheumatic
  fibropurulent 420.99
  fibrous 423.1
  gonococcal 098.83
  hemorrhagic 423.0
  idiopathic (acute) 420.91
  infective (acute) 420.90
  meningococcal 036.41
  neoplastic (chronic) 423.8
    acute 420.90
  nonspecific 420.91
  obliterans, obliterating 423.1
  plastic 423.1
  pneumococcal (acute) 420.99
  postinfarction 411.0
  purulent (acute) 420.99

Pericarditis—continued
  rheumatic (active) (acute) (with
      effusion) (with pneumonia)
      391.0
    with chorea (acute)
      (rheumatic)
      (Sydenham's) 392.0
    chronic or inactive (with
      chorea) 393
  septic (acute) 420.99
  serofibrinous — see Pericarditis,
      rheumatic
  staphylococcal (acute) 420.99
  streptococcal (acute) 420.99
  suppurative (acute) 420.99
  syphilitic 093.81
  tuberculous (acute) (chronic) (see
      also Tuberculosis) 017.9
      [420.0]
  uremic 585 [420.0]
  viral (acute) 420.91

Pericardium, pericardial — see condition

Pericellulitis (see also Cellulitis) 682.9

Pericementitis 523.4
  acute 523.3
  chronic (suppurative) 523.4

Pericholecystitis (see also Cholecystitis) 575.1

Perichondritis
  auricle 380.00
    acute 380.01
    chronic 380.02
  bronchus 491.9
  ear (external) 380.00
    acute 380.01
    chronic 380.02
  larynx 478.71
    syphilitic 095.8
    typhoid 002.0 [478.71]
  nose 478.1
  pinna 380.00
    acute 380.01
    chronic 380.02
  trachea 478.9

Periclasia 523.5

Pericolitis 569.89

Pericoronitis (chronic) 523.4
  acute 523.3

Pericystitis (see also Cystitis) 595.9

Pericytoma (M9150/1) — see also
  Neoplasm, connective tissue,
  uncertain behavior
  benign (M9150/0) — see
    Neoplasm, connective
    tissue, benign
  malignant (M9150/3) — see
    Neoplasm, connective
    tissue, malignant

Peridacryocystitis, acute 375.32

Peridiverticulitis (see also Diverticulitis) 562.11

Periduodenitis 535.6

Periendocarditis (see also Endocarditis) 424.90
  acute or subacute 421.9

Periepididymitis (see also Epididymitis) 604.90

Perifolliculitis (abscedens) 704.8
  capitis, abscedens et suffodiens
      704.8
  dissecting, scalp 704.8
  scalp 704.8
  superficial pustular 704.8

Perigastritis (acute) 535.0

Perigastrojejunitis (acute) 535.0

Perihepatitis (acute) 573.3
  chlamydial 099.56
  gonococcal 098.86

Peri-ileitis (subacute) 569.89

Perilabyrinthitis (acute) — see Labyrinthitis

Perimeningitis — see Meningitis

Perimetritis (see also Endometritis) 615.9

Perimetrosalpingitis (see also Salpingo-oophoritis) 614.2

Perinephric — see condition

Perinephritic — see condition

Perinephritis (see also Infection, kidney) 590.9
  purulent (see also Abscess, kidney) 590.2

Perineum, perineal — see condition

Perineuritis NEC 729.2

Periodic — see also condition
  disease (familial) 277.3
  edema 995.1
    hereditary 277.6
  fever 277.3
  paralysis (familial) 359.3
  peritonitis 277.3
  polyserositis 277.3
  somnolence 347

Periodontal
  cyst 522.8
  pocket 523.8

Periodontitis (chronic) (complex) (compound) (local) (simplex) 523.4
  acute 523.3
  apical 522.6
    acute (pulpal origin) 522.4

Periodontoclasia 523.5

Periodontosis 523.5

Periods — see also Menstruation
  heavy 626.2
  irregular 626.4

Perionychia (with lymphangitis) 681.9
  finger 681.02
  toe 681.11

Perioophoritis (see also Salpingo-oophoritis) 614.2

Periorchitis (see also Orchitis) 604.90

Periosteum, periosteal — see condition

Periostitis (circumscribed) (diffuse) (infective) 730.3

> Note — Use the following fifth-digit subclassification with category 730:
>
> 0   site unspecified
> 1   shoulder region
> 2   upper arm
> 3   forearm
> 4   hand
> 5   pelvic region and thigh
> 6   lower leg
> 7   ankle and foot
> 8   other specified sites
> 9   multiple sites

  with osteomyelitis (see also Osteomyelitis) 730.2
  acute or subacute 730.0
  chronic or old 730.1
  albuminosa, albuminosus 730.3
  alveolar 526.5
  alveolodental 526.5
  dental 526.5
  gonorrheal 098.89
  hyperplastica, generalized 731.2
  jaw (lower) (upper) 526.4
  monomelic 733.99
  orbital 376.02
  syphilitic 095.5
    congenital 090.0 [730.8]
    secondary 091.61

Periostitis

Periostitis—continued
  tuberculous (see also
      Tuberculosis, bone) 015.9
      [730.8]
  yaws (early) (hypertrophic) (late)
      102.6
Periostosis (see also Periostitis) 730.3
  with osteomyelitis (see also
      Osteomyelitis) 730.2
  acute or subacute 730.0
  chronic or old 730.1
  hyperplastic 756.59
Periphlebitis (see also Phlebitis)
    451.9
  lower extremity 451.2
    deep (vessels) 451.19
    superficial (vessels) 451.0
  portal 572.1
  retina 362.18
  superficial (vessels) 451.0
  tuberculous (see also
      Tuberculosis) 017.9
    retina 017.3 [362.18]
Peripneumonia — see Pneumonia
Periproctitis 569.49
Periprostatitis (see also Prostatitis)
    601.9
Perirectal — see condition
Perirenal — see condition
Perisalpingitis (see also Salpingo-
    oophoritis) 614.2
Perisigmoiditis 569.89
Perisplenitis (infectional) 289.59
Perispondylitis — see Spondylitis
Peristalsis reversed or visible 787.4
Peritendinitis (see also
    Tenosynovitis) 726.90
  adhesive (shoulder) 726.0
Perithelioma (M9150/1) — see
    Pericytoma
Peritoneum, peritoneal — see
    condition
Peritonitis (acute) (adhesive)
    (fibrinous) (hemorrhagic)
    (idiopathic) (localized)
    (perforative) (primary) (with
    adhesions) (with effusion)
    567.9
  with or following
    abortion — see Abortion, by
        type, with sepsis
    abscess 567.2
    appendicitis 540.0
      with peritoneal abcess
          540.1 ◆
    ectopic pregnancy (see also
        categories 633.0-633.9)
        639.0
    molar pregnancy (see also
        categories 630-632)
        639.0
  aseptic 998.7
  bacterial 567.2
  bile, biliary 567.8
  chemical 998.7
  chlamydial 099.56
  chronic proliferative 567.8
  congenital NEC 777.6
  diaphragmatic 567.2
  diffuse NEC 567.2
  diphtheritic 032.83
  disseminated NEC 567.2
  due to
    bile 567.8
    foreign
      body or object accidentally
          left during a
          procedure
          (instrument) (sponge)
          (swab) 998.4
      substance accidentally left
          during a procedure
          (chemical) (powder)
          (talc) 998.7

INDEX TO DISEASES

Peritonitis—continued
  due to—continued
    talc 998.7
    urine 567.8
  fibrinopurulent 567.2
  fibrinous 567.2
  fibrocaseous (see also
      Tuberculosis) 014.0
  fibropurulent 567.2
  general, generalized (acute) 567.2
  gonococcal 098.86
  in infective disease NEC 136.9
      [567.0]
  meconium (newborn) 777.6
  pancreatic 577.8
  paroxysmal, benign 277.3
  pelvic
    female (acute) 614.5
      chronic NEC 614.7
        with adhesions 614.6
      puerperal, postpartum,
          childbirth 670
    male (acute) 567.2
  periodic (familial) 277.3
  phlegmonous 567.2
  pneumococcal 567.1
  postabortal 639.0
  proliferative, chronic 567.8
  puerperal, postpartum, childbirth
      670
  purulent 567.2
  septic 567.2
  staphylococcal 567.2
  streptococcal 567.2
  subdiaphragmatic 567.2
  subphrenic 567.2
  suppurative 567.2
  syphilitic 095.2
    congenital 090.0 [567.0]
  talc 998.7
  tuberculous (see also
      Tuberculosis) 014.0
  urine 567.8
Peritonsillar — see condition
Peritonsillitis 475
Perityphlitis (see also Appendicitis)
    541
Periureteritis 593.89
Periurethral — see condition
Periurethritis (gangrenous) 597.89
Periuterine — see condition
Perivaginitis (see also Vaginitis)
    616.10
Perivasculitis, retinal 362.18
Perivasitis (chronic) 608.4
Perivesiculitis (seminal) (see also
    Vesiculitis) 608.0
Perlèche 686.8
  due to
    moniliasis 112.0
    riboflavin deficiency 266.0
Pernicious — see condition
Pernio, perniosis 991.5
Persecution
  delusion 297.9
  social V62.4
Perseveration (tonic) 784.69
Persistence, persistent (congenital)
    759.89
  anal membrane 751.2
  arteria stapedia 744.04
  atrioventricular canal 745.69
  bloody ejaculate 792.2
  branchial cleft 744.41
  bulbus cordis in left ventricle
      745.8
  canal of Cloquet 743.51
  capsule (opaque) 743.51
  cilioretinal artery or vein 743.51
  cloaca 751.5
  communication — see Fistula,
      congenital

Persistence, persistent—continued
  convolutions
    aortic arch 747.21
    fallopian tube 752.19
    oviduct 752.19
    uterine tube 752.19
  double aortic arch 747.21
  ductus
    arteriosus 747.0
    Botalli 747.0
  fetal
    circulation 747.9
    form of cervix (uteri) 752.49
    hemoglobin (hereditary)
        ("Swiss variety") 282.7
  foramen
    Botalli 745.5
    ovale 745.5
  Gartner's duct 752.11
  hemoglobin, fetal (hereditary)
      (HPFH) 282.7
  hyaloid
    artery (generally incomplete)
        743.51
    system 743.51
  hymen (tag)
    in pregnancy or childbirth
        654.8
      causing obstructed labor
          660.2
  lanugo 757.4
  left
    posterior cardinal vein 747.49
    root with right arch of aorta
        747.21
    superior vena cava 747.49
  Meckel's diverticulum 751.0
  mesonephric duct 752.8
    fallopian tube 752.11
  mucosal disease (middle ear)
      (with posterior or superior
      marginal perforation of ear
      drum) 382.2
  nail(s), anomalous 757.5
  occiput, anterior or posterior
      660.3
    fetus or newborn 763.1
  omphalomesenteric duct 751.0
  organ or site NEC — see
      Anomaly, specified type
      NEC
  ostium
    atrioventriculare commune
        745.69
    primum 745.61
    secundum 745.5
  ovarian rests in fallopian tube
      752.19
  pancreatic tissue in intestinal tract
      751.5
  primary (deciduous)
    teeth 520.6
    vitreous hyperplasia 743.51
  pupillary membrane 743.46
    iris 743.46
  Rhesus (Rh) titer 999.7
  right aortic arch 747.21
  sinus
    urogenitalis 752.8
    venosus with imperfect
        incorporation in right
        auricle 747.49
  thymus (gland) 254.8
    hyperplasia 254.0
  thyroglossal duct 759.2
  thyrolingual duct 759.2
  truncus arteriosus or communis
      745.0
  tunica vasculosa lentis 743.39
  umbilical sinus 753.7
  urachus 753.7
  vegetative state 780.03
  vitelline duct 751.0
  wolffian duct 752.8

Personality

Person (with)
  admitted for clinical research, as
      control subject V70.7
  awaiting admission to adequate
      facility elsewhere V63.2
    undergoing social agency
        investigation V63.8
  concern (normal) about sick
      person in family V61.49
  consulting on behalf of another
      V65.1
  feared
    complaint in whom no
        diagnosis was made
        V65.5
    condition not demonstrated
        V65.5
  feigning illness V65.2
  healthy, accompanying sick
      person V65.0
  living (in)
    alone V60.3
    boarding school V60.6
    residence remote from hospital
        or medical care facility
        V63.0
    residential institution V60.6
    without
      adequate
        financial resources
            V60.2
        housing (heating)
            (space) V60.1
        housing (permanent)
            (temporary) V60.0
        material resources V60.2
        person able to render
            necessary care V60.4
        shelter V60.0
      medical services in home not
          available V63.1
  on waiting list V63.2
    undergoing social agency
        investigation V63.8
  sick or handicapped in family
      V61.49
  "worried well" V65.5
Personality
  affective 301.10
  aggressive 301.3
  amoral 301.7
  anancastic, anankastic 301.4
  antisocial 301.7
  asocial 301.7
  asthenic 301.6
  avoidant 301.82
  borderline 301.83
  change 310.1 ◆
  compulsive 301.4
  cycloid 301.13
  cyclothymic 301.13
  dependent 301.6
  depressive (chronic) 301.12
  disorder, disturbance NEC
      301.9 ▼
    with
      antisocial disturbance
          301.7
      pattern disturbance NEC
          301.9
      sociopathic disturbance
          301.7
      trait disturbance 301.9 ▲
  dual 300.14
  dyssocial 301.7
  eccentric 301.89
    "haltlose" type 301.89
  emotionally unstable 301.59
  epileptoid 301.3
  explosive 301.3
  fanatic 301.0
  histrionic 301.50
  hyperthymic 301.11
  hypomanic 301.11
  hypothymic 301.12
  hysterical 301.50
  immature 301.89

Personality — INDEX TO DISEASES — Phlebitis

Personality—continued
  inadequate 301.6
  labile 301.59
  masochistic 301.89
  morally defective 301.7
  multiple 300.14
  narcissistic 301.81
  obsessional 301.4
  obsessive (-compulsive) 301.4
  overconscientious 301.4
  paranoid 301.0
  passive (-dependent) 301.6
  passive-aggressive 301.84
  pathologic NEC 301.9
  pattern defect or disturbance 301.9
  pseudosocial 301.7
  psychoinfantile 301.59
  psychoneurotic NEC 301.89
  psychopathic 301.9
   with
     amoral trend 301.7
     antisocial trend 301.7
     asocial trend 301.7
     pathologic sexuality (see also Deviation, sexual) 302.9
  mixed types 301.9
  schizoid 301.20
     introverted 301.21
     schizotypal 301.22
     with sexual deviation (see also Deviation, sexual) 302.9
     antisocial 301.7
     dyssocial 301.7
  type A 301.4
  unstable (emotional) 301.59
Perthes' disease (capital femoral osteochondrosis) 732.1
Pertussis (see also Whooping cough) 033.9
  vaccination, prophylactic (against) V03.6
Peruvian wart 088.0
Perversion, perverted
  appetite 307.52
     hysterical 300.11
  function
     pineal gland 259.8
     pituitary gland 253.9
        anterior lobe
           deficient 253.2
           excessive 253.1
        posterior lobe 253.6
     placenta — see Placenta, abnormal
  sense of smell or taste 781.1
     psychogenic 306.7
  sexual (see also Deviation, sexual) 302.9
Pervious, congenital — see also Imperfect, closure
  ductus arteriosus 747.0
Pes (congenital) (see also Talipes) 754.70
  abductus (congenital) 754.60
     acquired 736.79
  acquired NEC 736.79
     planus 734
  adductus (congenital) 754.79
     acquired 736.79
  cavus 754.71
     acquired 736.73
  planovalgus (congenital) 754.69
     acquired 736.79
  planus (acquired) (any degree) 734
     congenital 754.61
     rachitic 268.1
  valgus (congenital) 754.61
     acquired 736.79
  varus (congenital) 754.50
     acquired 736.79
Pest (see also Plague) 020.9

Pestis (see also Plague) 020.9
  bubonica 020.0
  fulminans 020.0
  minor 020.8
  pneumonica — see Plague, pneumonic
Petechia, petechiae 782.7
  fetus or newborn 772.6
Petechial
  fever 036.0
  typhus 081.9
Petges-Cléjat or Petges-Clégat syndrome (poikilodermatomyositis) 710.3
Petit's
  disease (see also Hernia, lumbar) 553.8
Petit mal (idiopathic) (see also Epilepsy) 345.0
  status 345.2
Petrellidosis 117.6
Petrositis 383.20
  acute 383.21
  chronic 383.22
Peutz-Jeghers disease or syndrome 759.6
Peyronie's disease 607.89
Pfeiffer's disease 075
Phacentocele 379.32
  traumatic 921.3
Phacoanaphylaxis 360.19
Phacocele (old) 379.32
  traumatic 921.3
Phaehyphomycosis 117.8
Phagedena (dry) (moist) (see also Gangrene) 785.4
  arteriosclerotic 440.2 [785.4]
  geometric 686.0
  penis 607.89
  senile 440.2 [785.4]
  sloughing 785.4
  tropical (see also Ulcer, skin) 707.9
  vulva 616.50
Phagedenic — see also condition
  abscess — see also Abscess
     chancroid 099.0
  bubo NEC 099.8
  chancre 099.0
  ulcer (tropical) (see also Ulcer, skin) 707.9
Phagomania 307.52
Phakoma 362.89
Phantom limb (syndrome) 353.6
Pharyngeal — see also condition
  arch remnant 744.41
  pouch syndrome 279.11
Pharyngitis (acute) (catarrhal) (gangrenous) (infective) (malignant) (membranous) (phlegmonous) (pneumococcal) (pseudomembranous) (simple) (staphylococcal) (subacute) (suppurative) (ulcerative) (viral) 462
  with influenza, flu, or grippe 487.1
  aphthous 074.0
  atrophic 472.1
  chronic 472.1
  chlamydial 099.51
  coxsackievirus 074.0
  diphtheritic (membranous) 032.0
  follicular 472.1
  fusospirochetal 101
  gonococcal 098.6
  granular (chronic) 472.1
  herpetic 054.79
  hypertrophic 472.1
  infectional, chronic 472.1
  influenzal 487.1
  lymphonodular, acute 074.8

Pharyngitis—continued
  septic 034.0
  streptococcal 034.0
  tuberculous (see also Tuberculosis) 012.8
  vesicular 074.0
Pharyngoconjunctival fever 077.2
Pharyngoconjunctivitis, viral 077.2
Pharyngolaryngitis (acute) 465.0
  chronic 478.9
  septic 034.0
Pharyngoplegia 478.29
Pharyngotonsillitis 465.8
  tuberculous 012.8
Pharyngotracheitis (acute) 465.8
  chronic 478.9
Pharynx, pharyngeal — see condition
Phase of life problem NEC V62.89
Phenomenon
  Arthus' — see Arthus' phenomenon
  flashback (drug) 292.89
  jaw-winking 742.8
  Jod-Basedow 242.8
  L. E. cell 710.0
  lupus erythematosus cell 710.0
  Pelger-Huët (hereditary hyposegmentation) 288.2
  Raynaud's (paroxysmal digital cyanosis) (secondary) 443.0
  Reilly's (see also Neuropathy, peripheral, autonomic) 337.9
  vasomotor 780.2
  vasospastic 443.9
  vasovagal 780.2
  Wenckebach's, heart block (second degree) 426.13
Phenylketonuria (PKU) 270.1
Phenylpyruvicaciduria 270.1
Pheochromoblastoma (M8700/3)
  specified site — see Neoplasm, by site, malignant
  unspecified site 194.0
Pheochromocytoma (M8700/0)
  malignant (M8700/3)
     specified site — see Neoplasm, by site, malignant
     unspecified site 194.0
  specified site — see Neoplasm, by site, benign
  unspecified site 227.0
Phimosis (congenital) 605
  chancroidal 099.0
  due to infection 605
Phlebectasia (see also Varicose, vein) 454.9
  congenital 747.6
  esophagus (see also Varix, esophagus) 456.1
     with hemorrhage (see also Varix, esophagus, bleeding) 456.0
Phlebitis (infective) (pyemic) (septic) (suppurative) 451.9
  antecubital vein 451.82
  arm NEC 451.84
     axillary vein 451.89
     basilic vey 451.82
     deep 451.83
     superficial 451.82
  basilic vein 451.82
  blue 451.19
  brachial vein 451.83
  breast, superficial 451.89
  cavernous (venous) sinus — see Phlebitis, intracranial sinus
  cephalic vein 451.82
  cerebral (venous) sinus — see Phlebitis, intracranial sinus
  chest wall, superficial 451.89

Phlebitis—continued
  complicating pregnancy or puerperium 671.9
     affecting fetus or newborn 760.3
  cranial (venous) sinus — see Phlebitis, intracranial sinus
  deep (vessels) 451.19
     femoral vein 451.11
     specified vessel NEC 451.19
  due to implanted device — see Complications, due to (presence of) any device, implant or graft classified to 996.0-996.5 NEC
  during or resulting from a procedure 997.2
  femoral vein (deep) 451.11
  femoropopliteal 451.0
  following infusion, perfusion, or transfusion 999.2
  gouty 274.89 [451.9]
  hepatic veins 451.89
  iliac vein 451.81
  iliofemoral 451.11
  intracranial sinus (any) (venous) 325
     late effect — see category 326
     nonpyogenic 437.6
        in pregnancy or puerperium 671.5
  jugular vein 451.89
  lateral (venous) sinus — see Phlebitis, intracranial sinus
  leg 451.2
     deep (vessels) 451.19
        femoral vein 451.11
        specified vessel NEC 451.19
     superficial (vessels) 451.0
        femoral vein 451.11
  longitudinal sinus — see Phlebitis, intracranial sinus
  lower extremity 451.2
     deep (vessels) 451.19
        femoral vein 451.11
        specified vessel NEC 451.19
     superficial (vessels) 451.0
        femoral vein 451.11
  migrans, migrating (superficial) 453.1
  pelvic
     with
        abortion — see Abortion, by type, with sepsis
        ectopic pregnancy (see also categories 633.0-633.9) 639.0
        molar pregnancy (see also categories 630-632) 639.0
     following
        abortion 639.0
        ectopic or molar pregnancy 639.0
     puerperal, postpartum 671.4
  popliteal vein 451.19
  portal (vein) 572.1
  postoperative 997.2
  pregnancy 671.9
     deep 671.3
     specified type NEC 671.5
     superficial 671.2
  puerperal, postpartum, childbirth 671.9
     deep 671.4
     lower extremities 671.2
     pelvis 671.4
     specified site NEC 671.5
     superficial 671.2
  radial vein 451.83
  retina 362.18
  saphenous (great) (long) 451.0
     accessory or small 451.0
  sinus (meninges) — see Phlebitis, intracranial sinus

Phlebitis—continued
specified site NEC 451.89
subclavian vein 451.89
syphilitic 093.89
tibial vein 451.19
ulcer, ulcerative 451.9
    leg 451.2
        deep (vessels) 451.19
            femoral vein 451.11
            specified vessel NEC 451.19
        superficial (vessels) 451.0
            femoral vein 451.11
    lower extremity 451.2
        deep (vessels) 451.19
            femoral vein 451.11
            specified vessel NEC 451.19
        superficial (vessels) 451.0
ulnar vein 451.83
upper extremity — see Phlebitis, arm
umbilicus 451.89
uterus (septic) (see also Endometritis) 615.9
varicose (leg) (lower extremity) (see also Varicose, vein) 454.1

Phlebofibrosis 459.89
Phleboliths 459.89
Phlebosclerosis 459.89
Phlebothrombosis — see Thrombosis
Phlebotomus fever 066.0
Phlegm, choked on 933.1
Phlegmasia
alba dolens (deep vessels) 451.19
    complicating pregnancy 671.3
    nonpuerperal 451.19
    puerperal, postpartum, childbirth 671.4
cerulea dolens 451.19

Phlegmon (see also Abscess) 682.9
erysipelatous (see also Erysipelas) 035
iliac 682.2
    fossa 540.1
throat 478.29

Phlegmonous — see condition
Phlyctenulosis (allergic) (keratoconjuctivitis) (nontuberculous) 370.31
cornea 370.31
    with ulcer (see also Ulcer, cornea) 370.00
tuberculous (see also Tuberculosis) 017.3 [370.31]

Phobia, phobic (reaction) 300.20
animal 300.29
isolated NEC 300.29
obsessional 300.3
simple NEC 300.29
social 300.23
specified NEC 300.29 ◆
state 300.20

Phocas' disease 610.1
Phocomelia 755.4
lower limb 755.32
    complete 755.33
    distal 755.35
    proximal 755.34
upper limb 755.22
    complete 755.23
    distal 755.25
    proximal 755.24

Phoria (see also Heterophoria) 378.40
Phosphate-losing tubular disorder 588.0
Phosphatemia 275.3
Phosphaturia 275.3
Photoallergic response 692.72
Photocoproporphyria 277.1

Photodermatitis (sun) 692.72
light other than sun 692.82
Photokeratitis 370.24
Photo-ophthalmia 370.24
Photophobia 368.13
Photopsia 368.15
Photoretinitis 363.31
Photoretinopathy 363.31
Photosensitiveness (sun) 692.72
light other than sun 692.82
Photosensitization (sun) skin 692.72
light other than sun 692.82
Phototoxic response 692.72
Phrenitis 323.9
Phrynoderma 264.8
Phthiriasis (pubis) (any site) 132.2
with any infestation classifiable to 132.0, 132.1 and 132.3
Phthirus infestation — see Phthiriasis
Phthisis (see also Tuberculosis) 011.9
bulbi (infectional) 360.41
colliers' 011.4
cornea 371.05
eyeball (due to infection) 360.41
millstone makers' 011.4
miners' 011.4
potters' 011.4
sandblasters' 011.4
stonemasons' 011.4

Phycomycosis 117.7
Physalopteriasis 127.7
Physical therapy NEC V57.1
breathing exercises V57.0
Physiological cup, optic papilla
borderline, glaucoma suspect 365.00
enlarged 377.14
glaucomatous 377.14
Phytobezoar 938
intestine 936
stomach 935.2
Pian (see also Yaws) 102.9
Pianoma 102.1
Piarhemia, piarrhemia (see also Hyperlipemia) 272.4
bilharziasis 120.9
Pica 307.52
hysterical 300.11
Pick's
cerebral atrophy 331.1
    with dementia 290.10
disease
    brain 331.1
        dementia in 290.10
    lipid histiocytosis 272.7
    liver (pericardial pseudocirrhosis of liver) 423.2
    pericardium (pericardial pseudocirrhosis of liver) 423.2
    polyserositis (pericardial pseudocirrhosis of liver) 423.2
syndrome
    heart (pericardial pseudocirrhosis of liver) 423.2
    liver (pericardial pseudocirrhosis of liver) 423.2
tubular adenoma (M8640/0)
    specified site — see Neoplasm, by site, benign
    unspecified site
        female 220
        male 222.0

Pick-Herxheimer syndrome (diffuse idiopathic cutaneous atrophy) 701.8

Pick-Niemann disease (lipid histiocytosis) 272.7
Pickwickian syndrome (cardiopulmonary obesity) 278.8
Piebaldism, classic 709.09 ◆
Piedra 111.2
beard 111.2
    black 111.3
    white 111.2
black 111.3
scalp 111.3
    black 111.3
    white 111.2
white 111.2
Pierre Marie's syndrome (pulmonary hypertrophic osteoarthropathy) 731.2
Pierre Marie-Bamberger syndrome (hypertrophic pulmonary osteoarthropathy) 731.2
Pierre Mauriac's syndrome (diabetes-dwarfism-obesity) 258.1
Pierre Robin deformity or syndrome (congenital) 756.0
Pierson's disease or osteochondrosis 732.1
Pigeon
breast or chest (acquired) 738.3
    congenital 754.82
    rachitic (see also Rickets) 268.0
breeders' disease or lung 495.2
fanciers' disease or lung 495.2
toe 735.8
Pigmentation (abnormal) 709.00 ▼
anomaly 709.00 ▲
    congenital 757.33
    specified NEC 709.09 ◆
conjunctiva 372.55
cornea 371.10
    anterior 371.11
    posterior 371.13
    stromal 371.12
lids (congenital) 757.33
    acquired 374.52
limbus corneae 371.10
metals 709.00 ◆
optic papilla, congenital 743.57
retina (congenital) (grouped) (nevoid) 743.53
    acquired 362.74
scrotum, congenital 757.33
Piles — see Hemorrhoids
Pili
annulati or torti (congenital) 757.4
incarnati 704.8
Pill roller hand (intrinsic) 736.09
Pilomatrixoma (M8110/0) — see Neoplasm, skin, benign
Pilonidal — see condition
Pimple 709.8
Pinched nerve — see Neuropathy, entrapment
Pineal body or gland — see condition
Pineaoblastoma (M9362/3) 194.4
Pinealoma (M9360/1) 237.1
malignant (M9360/3) 194.4
Pineoblastoma (M9362/3) 194.4
Pineocytoma (M9361/1) 237.1
Pinguecula 372.51
Pinhole meatus (see also Stricture, urethra) 598.9
Pink
disease 985.0
eye 372.03
puffer 492.8
Pinkus' disease (lichen nitidus) 697.1

Pinpoint
meatus (see also Stricture, urethra) 598.9
os uteri) (see also Stricture, cervix) 622.4
Pinselhaare (congenital) 757.4
Pinta 103.9
cardiovascular lesions 103.2
chancre (primary) 103.0
erythematous plaques 103.1
hyperchromic lesions 103.1
hyperkeratosis 103.1
lesions 103.9
    cardiovascular 103.2
    hyperchromic 103.1
    intermediate 103.1
    late 103.2
    mixed 103.3
    primary 103.0
    skin (achromic) (cicatricial) (dyschromic) 103.2
        hyperchromic 103.1
        mixed (achromic and hyperchromic) 103.3
papule (primary) 103.0
skin lesions (achromic) (cicatricial) (dyschromic) 103.2
    hyperchromic 103.1
    mixed (achromic and hyperchromic) 103.3
vitiligo 103.2
Pintid 103.0
Pinworms (disease) (infection) (infestation) 127.4
Piry fever 066.8
Pistol wound — see Gunshot wound
Pit, lip (mucus), congenital 750.25
Pitchers' elbow 718.82
Pithecoid pelvis 755.69
with disproportion (fetopelvic) 653.2
    affecting fetus or newborn 763.1
    causing obstructed labor 660.1
Pithiatism 300.11
Pitted — see also Pitting
teeth 520.4
Pitting (edema) (see also Edema) 782.3
lip 782.3
nail 703.8
    congenital 757.5
Pituitary gland — see condition
Pituitary snuff-takers' disease 495.8
Pityriasis 696.5
alba 696.5
capitis 690
circinata (et maculata) 696.3
Hebra's (exfoliative dermatitis) 695.89
lichenoides et varioliformis 696.2
maculata (et circinata) 696.3
nigra 111.1
pilaris 757.39
    acquired 701.1
    Hebra's 696.4
rosea 696.3
rotunda 696.3
rubra (Hebra) 695.89
    pilaris 696.4
sicca 690
simplex 690
specified type NEC 696.5
streptogenes 696.5
versicolor 111.0
    scrotal 111.0

Placenta, placental
- ablatio 641.2
  - affecting fetus or newborn 762.1
- abnormal, abnormality 656.7
  - with hemorrhage 641.8
    - affecting fetus or newborn 762.1
  - affecting fetus or newborn 762.2
- abruptio 641.2
  - affecting fetus or newborn 762.1
- accessory lobe — see Placenta, abnormal
- accreta (without hemorrhage) 667.0
  - with hemorrhage 666.0
- adherent (without hemorrhage) 667.0
  - with hemorrhage 666.0
- apoplexy — see Placenta, separation
- battledore — see Placenta, abnormal
- bilobate — see Placenta, abnormal
- bipartita — see Placenta, abnormal
- carneous mole 631
- centralis — see Placenta, previa
- circumvallata — see Placenta, abnormal
- cyst (amniotic) — see Placenta, abnormal
- deficiency — see Placenta, insufficiency
- degeneration — see Placenta, insufficiency
- detachment (partial) (premature) (with hemorrhage) 641.2
  - affecting fetus or newborn 762.1
- dimidiata — see Placenta, abnormal
- disease 656.7
  - affecting fetus or newborn 762.2
- duplex — see Placenta, abnormal
- dysfunction — see Placenta, insufficiency
- fenestrata — see Placenta, abnormal
- fibrosis — see Placenta, abnormal
- fleshy mole 631
- hematoma — see Placenta, abnormal
- hemorrhage NEC — see Placenta, separation
- hormone disturbance or malfunction — see Placenta, abnormal
- hyperplasia — see Placenta, abnormal
- increta (without hemorrhage) 667.0
  - with hemorrhage 666.0
- infarction 656.7
  - affecting fetus or newborn 762.2
- insertion, vicious — see Placenta, previa
- insufficiency
  - affecting
    - fetus or newborn 762.2
    - management of pregnancy 656.5
- lateral — see Placenta, previa
- low implantation or insertion — see Placenta, previa
- low-lying — see Placenta, previa
- malformation — see Placenta, abnormal
- malposition — see Placenta, previa
- marginalis, marginata — see Placenta, previa

Placenta, placental—continued
- marginal sinus (hemorrhage) (rupture) 641.2
  - affecting fetus or newborn 762.1
- membranacea — see Placenta, abnormal
- multilobed — see Placenta, abnormal
- multipartita — see Placenta, abnormal
- necrosis — see Placenta, abnormal
- percreta (without hemorrhage) 667.0
  - with hemorrhage 666.0
- polyp 674.4
- previa (central) (centralis) (complete) (lateral) (marginal) (marginalis) (partial) (partialis) (total) (with hemorrhage) 641.1
  - affecting fetus or newborn 762.0
  - noted
    - before labor, without hemorrhage (with cesarean delivery) 641.1
    - during pregnancy (without hemorrhage) 641.0
  - without hemorrhage (before labor and delivery) (during pregnancy) 641.0
- retention (with hemorrhage) 666.0
  - fragments, complicating puerperium (delayed hemorrhage) 666.2
    - without hemorrhage 667.1
  - postpartum, puerperal 666.2
  - without hemorrhage 667.0
- separation (normally implanted) (partial) (premature) (with hemorrhage) 641.2
  - affecting fetus or newborn 762.1
- septuplex — see Placenta, abnormal
- small — see Placenta, insufficiency
- softening (premature) — see Placenta, abnormal
- spuria — see Placenta, abnormal
- succenturiata — see Placenta, abnormal
- syphilitic 095.8
- transfusion syndromes 762.3
- transmission of chemical substance — see Absorption, chemical, through placenta
- trapped (with hemorrhage) 666.0
  - without hemorrhage 667.0
- trilobate — see Placenta, abnormal
- tripartita — see Placenta, abnormal
- triplex — see Placenta, abnormal
- varicose vessel — see Placenta, abnormal
- vicious insertion — see Placenta, previa

Placentitis
- affecting fetus or newborn 762.7
- complicating pregnancy 658.4

Plagiocephaly (skull) 754.0

Plague 020.9
- abortive 020.8
- ambulatory 020.8
- bubonic 020.0
- cellulocutaneous 020.1
- lymphatic gland 020.0
- pneumonic 020.5
  - primary 020.3
  - secondary 020.4

Plague—continued
- pulmonary — see Plague, pneumonic
- pulmonic — see Plague, pneumonic
- septicemic 020.2
- tonsillar 020.9
  - septicemic 020.2
- vaccination, prophylactic (against) V03.3

Planning, family V25.09
- contraception V25.9
- procreation V26.4

Plaque
- artery, arterial — see Arteriosclerosis
- calcareous — see Calcification
- Hollenhorst's (retinal) 362.33
- tongue 528.6

Plasma cell myeloma 203.0

Plasmacytoma, plasmocytoma (solitary) (M9731/1) 238.6
- benign (M9731/0) — see Neoplasm, by site, benign
- malignant (M9731/3) 203.8

Plasmacytosis 288.8

Plaster ulcer (see also Decubitus) 707.0

Platybasia 756.0

Platyonychia (congenital) 757.5
- acquired 703.8

Platypelloid pelvis 738.6
- with disproportion (fetopelvic) 653.2
  - affecting fetus or newborn 763.1
- causing obstructed labor 660.1
  - affecting fetus or newborn 763.1
- congenital 755.69

Platyspondylia 756.19

Plethora 782.62
- newborn 776.4

Pleura, pleural — see condition

Pleuralgia 786.52

Pleurisy (acute) (adhesive) (chronic) (costal) (diaphragmatic) (double) (dry) (fetid) (fibrinous) (fibrous) (interlobar) (latent) (lung) (old) (plastic) (primary) (residual) (sicca) (sterile) (subacute) (unresolved) (with adherent pleura) 511.0
- with
  - effusion (without mention of cause) 511.9
    - bacterial, nontuberculous 511.1
    - nontuberculous NEC 511.9
      - bacterial 511.1
    - pneumococcal 511.1
    - specified type NEC 511.8
    - staphylococcal 511.1
    - streptococcal 511.1
    - tuberculous (see also Tuberculosis, pleura) 012.0
      - primary, progressive 010.1
  - influenza, flu, or grippe 487.1
  - tuberculosis — see Pleurisy, tuberculous
- encysted 511.8
- exudative (see also Pleurisy, with effusion) 511.9
  - bacterial, nontuberculous 511.1
- fibrinopurulent 510.9
  - with fistula 510.0
- fibropurulent 510.9
  - with fistula 510.0
- hemorrhagic 511.8
- influenzal 487.1
- pneumococcal 511.0
  - with effusion 511.1

Pleurisy—continued
- purulent 510.9
  - with fistula 510.0
- septic 510.9
  - with fistula 510.0
- serofibrinous (see also Pleurisy, with effusion) 511.9
  - bacterial, nontuberculous 511.1
- seropurulent 510.9
  - with fistula 510.0
- serous (see also Pleurisy, with effusion) 511.9
  - bacterial, nontuberculous 511.1
- staphylococcal 511.0
  - with effusion 511.1
- streptococcal 511.0
  - with effusion 511.1
- suppurative 510.9
  - with fistula 510.0
- traumatic (post) (current) 862.29
  - with open wound into cavity 862.39
- tuberculous (with effusion) (see also Tuberculosis, pleura) 012.0
  - primary, progressive 010.1

Pleuritis sicca — see Pleurisy

Pleurobronchopneumonia (see also Pneumonia, broncho-) 485

Pleurodynia 786.52
- epidemic 074.1
- viral 074.1

Pleurohepatitis 573.8

Pleuropericarditis (see also Pericarditis) 423.9
- acute 420.90

Pleuropneumonia (acute) (bilateral) (double) (septic) (see also Pneumonia) 486
- chronic (see also Fibrosis, lung) 515

Pleurorrhea (see also Hydrothorax) 511.8

Plexitis, brachial 353.0

Plica
- polonica 132.0
- tonsil 474.8

Plicae dysphonia ventricularis 784.49

Plicated tongue 529.5
- congenital 750.13

Plug
- bronchus NEC 519.1
- meconium (newborn) NEC 777.1
- mucus — see Mucus, plug

Plumbism 984.9
- specified type of lead — see Table of drugs and chemicals

Plummer's disease (toxic nodular goiter) 242.3

Plummer-Vinson syndrome (sideropenic dysphagia) 280.8

Pluricarential syndrome of infancy 260

Plurideficiency syndrome of infancy 260

Plus (and minus) hand (intrinsic) 736.09

Pneumathemia — see Air, embolism, by type

Pneumatic drill or hammer disease 994.9

Pneumatocele (lung) 518.89
- intracranial 348.8
- tension 492.0

Pneumatosis
- cystoides intestinalis 569.89
- peritonei 568.89
- pulmonum 492.8

Pneumaturia 599.84

Pneumoblastoma (M8981/3) — see
    Neoplasm, lung, malignant
Pneumocephalus 348.8
Pneumococcemia 038.2
Pneumococcus, pneumococcal —
    see condition
Pneumoconiosis (due to) (inhalation
    of) 505
    aluminum 503
    asbestos 501
    bagasse 495.1
    bauxite 503
    beryllium 503
    carbon electrode makers' 503
    coal
        miners' (simple) 500
        workers' (simple) 500
    cotton dust 504
    diatomite fibrosis 502
    dust NEC 504
        inorganic 503
        lime 502
        marble 502
        organic NEC 504
    fumes or vapors (from silo) 506.9
    graphite 503
    hard metal 503
    mica 502
    moldy hay 495.0
    rheumatoid 714.81
    silica NEC 502
        and carbon 500
    silicate NEC 502
    talc 502
Pneumocystis carinii pneumonia
    136.3
Pneumocystosis 136.3
    with pneumonia 136.3
Pneumoenteritis 025
Pneumohemopericardium (see also
    Pericarditis) 423.9
Pneumohemothorax (see also
    Hemothorax) 511.8
    traumatic 860.4
        with open wound into thorax
            860.5
Pneumohydropericardium (see also
    Pericarditis) 423.9
Pneumohydrothorax (see also
    Hydrothorax) 511.8
Pneumomediastinum 518.1
    congenital 770.2
    fetus or newborn 770.2
Pneumomycosis 117.9
Pneumonia (acute) (Alpenstich)
    (benign) (bilateral) (brain)
    (cerebral) (circumscribed)
    (congestive) (creeping)
    (delayed resolution) (double)
    (epidemic) (fever) (flash)
    (fulminant) (fungoid)
    (granulomatous) (hemorrhagic)
    (incipient) (infantile)
    (infectious) (infiltration)
    (insular) (intermittent) (latent)
    (lobe) (migratory) (newborn)
    (organized) (overwhelming)
    (primary) (progressive)
    (pseudolobar) (purulent)
    (resolved) (secondary) (senile)
    (septic) (suppurative) (terminal)
    (true) (unresolved) (vesicular)
    486
    with influenza, flu, or grippe
        487.0
    adenoviral 480.0
    adynamic 514
    alba 090.0
    allergic 518.3
    alveolar — see Pneumonia, lobar
    anthrax 022.1 [484.5]
    apex, apical — see Pneumonia,
        lobar
    ascaris 127.0 [484.8]

Pneumonia—continued
    aspiration 507.0
        due to
            aspiration of
                microorganisms
                    bacterial 482.9
                        specified type NEC
                            482.89
                        specified organism NEC
                            483.8
                            bacterial NEC 482.89
                        viral 480.9
                            specified type NEC
                                480.8
            food (regurgitated) 507.0
            gastric secretions 507.0
            milk 507.0
            oils, essences 507.1
            solids, liquids NEC 507.8
            vomitus 507.0
        newborn 770.1
    asthenic 514
    atypical (disseminated, focal)
        (primary) 486
        with influenza 487.0
    bacillus 482.9
        specified type NEC 482.89
    bacterial 482.9
        specified type NEC 482.89
    Bacteroides (fragilis) (oralis)
        (melaninogenicus) 482.81
    basal, basic, basilar — see
        Pneumonia, lobar
    broncho-, bronchial (confluent)
        (croupous) (diffuse)
        (disseminated)
        (hemorrhagic) (involving
        lobes) (lobar) (terminal) 485
        with influenza 487.0
        allergic 518.3
        aspiration (see also
            Pneumonia, aspiration)
            507.0
        bacterial 482.9
            specified type NEC 482.89
        capillary 466.1
            with bronchospasm or
                obstruction 466.1
        chronic (see also Fibrosis,
            lung) 515
        congenital (infective) 770.0
        diplococcal 481
        Eaton's agent 483.0
        Escherichia coli (E. coli)
            482.82
        Friedländer's bacillus 482.0
        Hemophilus influenzae 482.2
        hiberno-vernal 083.0 [484.8]
        hypostatic 514
        influenzal 487.0
        inhalation (see also
            Pneumonia, aspiration)
            507.0
            due to fumes or vapors
                (chemical) 506.0
        Klebsiella 482.0
        lipid 507.1
            endogenous 516.8
        Mycoplasma (pneumoniae)
            483.0
        ornithosis 073.0
        pleuropneumonia-like
            organisms (PPLO) 483.0
        pneumococcal 481
        Proteus 482.83
        pseudomonas 482.1
        specified organism NEC 483.8
            bacterial NEC 482.89
        staphylococcal 482.4
        streptococcal — see
            Pneumonia,
            streptococcal
        typhoid 002.0 [484.8]
        viral, virus (see also
            Pneumonia, viral) 480.9
    Butyrivibrio (fibriosolvens) 482.81
    Candida 112.4

Pneumonia—continued
    capillary 466.1
        with bronchospasm or
            obstruction 466.1
    caseous (see also Tuberculosis)
        011.6
    catarrhal — see Pneumonia,
        broncho-central — see
        Pneumonia, lobar
    Chlamydia, chlamydial 078.89
        [484.8]
        pneumoniae 078.89 [484.8]
        psittaci 073.0
        specified type NEC 078.89
            [484.8]
        trachomatis 078.89 [484.8]
    cholesterol 516.8
    Clostridium (haemolyticum)
        (novyi) NEC 482.81
    confluent — see Pneumonia,
        broncho-
    congenital (infective) 770.0
        aspiration 770.1
    croupous — see Pneumonia,
        lobar
    cytomegalic inclusion 078.5
        [484.1]
    deglutition (see also Pneumonia,
        aspiration) 507.0
    desquamative interstitial 516.8
    diffuse — see Pneumonia,
        broncho-
    diplococcal, diplococcus
        (broncho-) (lobar) 481
    disseminated (focal) — see
        Pneumonia, broncho-
    due to
        adenovirus 480.0
        Bacterium anitratum 482.83
        Chlamydia, chlamydial 078.89
            [484.8]
            pneumoniae 078.89
                [484.8]
            psittaci 073.0
            specified type NEC 078.89
                [484.8]
            trachomatis 078.89 [484.8]
        coccidioidomycosis 114.0
        Diplococcus (pneumoniae)
            481
        Eaton's agent 483.0
        Escherichia coli (E. coli)
            482.82
        Friedländer's bacillus 482.0
        fumes or vapors (chemical)
            (inhalation) 506.0
        fungus NEC 117.9 [484.7]
            coccidioidomycosis 114.0
        Hemophilus influenzae (H.
            influenzae) 482.2
        Herellea 482.83
        influenza 487.0
        Klebsiella pneumoniae 482.0
        Mycoplasma (pneumoniae)
            483.0
        parainfluenza virus 480.2
        pleuropneumonia-like
            organism (PPLO) 483.0
        Pneumococcus 481
        Pneumocystis carinii 136.3
        Proteus 482.83
        pseudomonas 482.1
        respiratory syncytial virus
            480.1
        rickettsia 083.9 [484.8]
        specified
            bacteria NEC 482.89
            organism NEC 483.8
            virus NEC 480.8
        Staphylococcus 482.4

Pneumonia—continued
    due to—continued
        Streptococcus — see also
            Pneumonia,
            streptococcal
            pneumoniae 481
        virus (see also Pneumonia,
            viral) 480.9
    Eaton's agent 483.0
    embolic, embolism (see also
        Embolism, pulmonary)
        415.1
    eosinophilic 518.3
    Escherichia coli (E. coli) 482.82
    Eubacterium 482.81
    fibrinous — see Pneumonia,
        lobar
    fibroid (chronic)(see also Fibrosis,
        lung) 515
    fibrous (see also Fibrosis, lung)
        515
    Friedländer's bacillus 482.0
    Fusobacterium (nucleatum)
        482.81
    gangrenous 513.0
    giant cell (see also Pneumonia,
        viral) 480.9
    gram-negative bacteria NEC
        482.83
        anaerobic 482.81
    grippal 487.0
    Hemophilus influenzae
        (bronchial) (lobar) 482.2
    hypostatic (broncho-) (lobar) 514
    in
        actinomycosis 039.1
        anthrax 022.1 [484.5]
        aspergillosis 117.3 [484.6]
        candidiasis 112.4
        coccidioidomycosis 114.0
        cytomegalic inclusion disease
            078.5 [484.1]
        histoplasmosis (see also
            Histoplasmosis) 115.95
        infectious disease NEC 136.9
            [484.8]
        measles 055.1
        mycosis, systemic NEC 117.9
            [484.7]
        nocardiasis, nocardiosis 039.1
        ornithosis 073.0
        pneumocystosis 136.3
        psittacosis 073.0
        Q fever 083.0 [484.8]
        salmonellosis 003.22
        toxoplasmosis 130.4
        tularemia 021.2
        typhoid (fever) 002.0 [484.8]
        varicella 052.1
        whooping cough (see also
            Whooping cough) 033.9
            [484.3]
    infective, acquired prenatally
        770.0
    influenzal (broncho) (lobar) (virus)
        487.0
    inhalation (see also Pneumonia,
        aspiration) 507.0
        fumes or vapors (chemical)
            506.0
    interstitial 516.8
        with influenzal 487.0
        acute 136.3
        chronic (see also Fibrosis,
            lung) 515
        desquamative 516.8
        hypostatic 514
        lipid 507.1
        lymphoid 516.8
        plasma cell 136.3
        pseudomonas 482.1
    intrauterine (infective) 770.0
        aspiration 770.1
    Klebsiella pneumoniae 482.0
    lipid, lipoid (exogenous)
        (interstitial) 507.1
        endogenous 516.8

Pneumonia—continued
  lobar (diplococcal) (disseminated) (double) (interstitial) (pneumococcal, any type) 481
    with influenza 487.0
    bacterial 482.9
      specified type NEC 482.89
    chronic (see also Fibrosis, lung) 515
    Escherichia coli (E. coli) 482.82
    Friedländer's bacillus 482.0
    Hemophilus influenzae (H. influenzae) 482.2
    hypostatic 514
    influenzal 487.0
    Klebsiella 482.0
    ornithosis 073.0
    Proteus 482.83
    pseudomonas 482.1
    psittacosis 073.0
    specified organism NEC 483.8
      bacterial NEC 482.89
    staphylococcal 482.4
    streptococcal — see Pneumonia, streptococcal
    viral, virus (see also Pneumonia, viral) 480.9
  lobular (confluent) — see Pneumonia, broncho-
  Löffler's 518.3
  massive — see Pneumonia, lobar
  meconium 770.1
  metastatic NEC 038.8 [484.8]
  Mycoplasma (pneumoniae) 483.0
  necrotic 513.0
  nitrogen dioxide 506.9
  orthostatic 514
  parainfluenza virus 480.2
  parenchymatous (see also Fibrosis, lung) 515
  passive 514
  patchy — see Pneumonia, broncho-
  Peptococcus 482.81
  Peptostreptococcus 482.81
  plasma cell 136.3
  pleurolobar — see Pneumonia, lobar
  pleuropneumonia-like organism (PPLO) 483.0
  pneumococcal (broncho) (lobar) 481
  Pneumocystis (carinii) 136.3
  postinfectional NEC 136.9 [484.8]
  postmeasles 055.1
  postoperative 997.3
  primary atypical 486
  Proprionibacterium 482.81
  Proteus 482.83
  pseudomonas 482.1
  psittacosis 073.0
  radiation 508.0
  respiratory syncytial virus 480.1
  resulting from a procedure 997.3
  rheumatic 390 [517.1]
  Salmonella 003.22
  segmented, segmental — see Pneumonia, broncho-
  Serratia (marcescens) 482.83
  specified
    bacteria NEC 482.89
    organism NEC 483.8
    virus NEC 480.8
  spirochetal 104.8 [484.8]
  staphylococcal (broncho) (lobar) 482.4
  static, stasis 514
  streptococcal (broncho) (lobar) NEC 482.30
    Group
      A 482.31
      B 482.32
      specified NEC 482.39

Pneumonia—continued
  streptococcal—continued
    pneumoniae 481
    specified type NEC 482.39
  Streptococcus pneumoniae 481
  traumatic (complication) (early) (secondary) 958.8
  tuberculous (any) (see also Tuberculosis) 011.6
  tularemic 021.2
  TWAR agent 078.89 [484.8]
  varicella 052.1
  Veillonella 482.81
  viral, virus (broncho) (interstitial) (lobar) 480.9
    with influenza, flu, or grippe 487.0
    adenoviral 480.0
    parainfluenza 480.2
    respiratory syncytial 480.1
    specified type NEC 480.8
  white (congenital) 090.0
Pneumonic — see condition
Pneumonitis (acute) (primary) (see also Pneumonia) 486
  allergic 495.9
    specified type NEC 495.8
  aspiration 507.0
    due to fumes or gases 506.0
    newborn 770.1
    obstetric 668.0
  chemical 506.0
    due to fumes or gases 506.0
  cholesterol 516.8
  chronic (see also Fibrosis, lung) 515
  congenital rubella 771.0
  due to
    fumes or vapors 506.0
    inhalation
      food (regurgitated), milk, vomitus 507.0
      oils, essences 507.1
      saliva 507.0
      solids, liquids NEC 507.8
    toxoplasmosis (acquired) 130.4
      congenital (active) 771.2 [484.8]
  eosinophilic 518.3
  fetal aspiration 770.1
  hypersensitivity 495.9
  interstitial (chronic) (see also Fibrosis, lung) 515
    lymphoid 516.8
  lymphoid, interstitial 516.8
  meconium 770.1
  postanesthetic
    correct substance properly administered 507.0
    obstetric 668.0
    overdose or wrong substance given 968.4
    specified anesthetic — see Table of drugs and chemicals
  postoperative 997.3
    obstetric 668.0
  radiation 508.0
  rubella, congenital 771.0
  "ventilation" 495.7
  wood-dust 495.8
Pneumonoconiosis — see Pneumoconiosis
Pneumoparotid 527.8
Pneumopathy NEC 518.89
  alveolar 516.9
    specified NEC 516.8
  due to dust NEC 504
  parietoalveolar 516.9
    specified condition NEC 516.8
Pneumopericarditis (see also Pericarditis) 423.9
  acute 420.90

Pneumopericardium — see also Pericarditis
  congenital 770.2
  fetus or newborn 770.2
  traumatic (post) (see also Pneumothorax, traumatic) 860.0
    with open wound into thorax 860.1
Pneumoperitoneum 568.89
  fetus or newborn 770.2
Pneumophagia (psychogenic) 306.4
Pneumopleurisy, pneumopleuritis (see also Pneumonia) 486
Pneumopyopericardium 420.99
Pneumopyothorax (see also Pyopneumothorax) 510.9
  with fistula 510.0
Pneumorrhagia 786.3
  newborn 770.3
  tuberculous (see also Tuberculosis, pulmonary) 011.9
Pneumosiderosis (occupational) 503
Pneumothorax (acute) (chronic) 512.8
  congenital 770.2
  due to operative injury of chest wall or lung 512.1 ▼
    accidental puncture or laceration 512.1 ▲
  fetus or newborn 770.2
  iatrogenic 512.1 ▼
  postoperative 512.1 ▲
  spontaneous 512.8
    fetus or newborn 770.2
    tension 512.0
  sucking 512.8
    iatrogenic 512.1 ▼
    postoperative 512.1 ▲
  tense valvular, infectional 512.0
  tension 512.0
    iatrogenic 512.1 ▼
    postoperative 512.1 ▲
    spontaneous 512.0 ▲
  traumatic 860.0
    with
      hemothorax 860.4
        with open wound into thorax 860.5
      open wound into thorax 860.1
  tuberculous (see also Tuberculosis) 011.7
Pocket(s)
  endocardial (see also Endocarditis) 424.90
  periodontal 523.8
Podagra 274.9
Podencephalus 759.89
Poikilocytosis 790.0
Poikiloderma 709.09 ▼
  Civatte's 709.09 ▲
  congenital 757.33
  vasculare atrophicans 696.2
Poikilodermatomyositis 710.3
Pointed ear 744.29
Poise imperfect 729.9
Poisoned — see Poisoning
Poisoning (acute) — see also Table of drugs and chemicals
  Bacillus, B.
    aertrycke (see also Infection, Salmonella) 003.9
    botulinus 005.1
    cholerae (suis) (see also Infection, Salmonella) 003.9
    paratyphosus (see also Infection, Salmonella) 003.9
    suipestifer (see also Infection, Salmonella) 003.9
  bacterial toxins NEC 005.9

Poisoning—continued
  berries, noxious 988.2
  blood (general) — see Septicemia
  botulism 005.1
  bread, moldy, mouldy — see Poisoning, food
  damaged meat — see Poisoning, food
  death-cap (Amanita phalloides) (Amanita verna) 988.1
  decomposed food — see Poisoning, food
  diseased food — see Poisoning, food
  drug — see Table of drugs and chemicals
  epidemic, fish, meat, or other food — see Poisoning, food
  fava bean 282.2
  fish (bacterial) — see also Poisoning, food
    noxious 988.0
  food (acute) (bacterial) (diseased) (infected) NEC 005.9
    due to
      Bacillus
        aertrycke (see also Poisoning, food, due to Salmonella) 003.9
        botulinus 005.1
        cereus 005.8
        choleraesuis (see also Poisoning, food, due to Salmonella) 003.9
        paratyphosus (see also Poisoning, food, due to Salmonella) 003.9
        suipestifer (see also Poisoning, food, due to Salmonella) 003.9
      Clostridium 005.3
        botulinum 005.1
        perfringens 005.2
        welchii 005.2
      Salmonella (aertrycke) (callinarum) (choleraesuis) (enteritidis) (paratyphi) (suipestifer) 003.9
        with
          gastroenteritis 003.0
          localized infection(s) (see also Infection, Salmonella) 003.20
          septicemia 003.1
          specified manifestation NEC 003.8
      specified bacterium NEC 005.8
      Staphylococcus 005.0
      Streptococcus 005.8
      Vibrio parahaemolyticus 005.4
    noxious or naturally toxic 988.0
      berries 988.2
      fish 988.0
      mushroom 988.1
      plants NEC 988.2
  ice cream — see Poisoning, food
  ichthyotoxism (bacterial) 005.9
  kreotoxism, food 005.9
  malarial — see Malaria
  meat — see Poisoning, food
  mushroom (noxious) 988.1

Poisoning

Poisoning—*continued*
    mussel — *see also* Poisoning, food
      noxious 988.0
    noxious foodstuffs (*see also* Poisoning, food, noxious) 988.9
      specified type NEC 988.8
    plants, noxious 988.2
    pork — *see also* Poisoning, food
      specified NEC 988.8
      Trichinosis 124
    ptomaine — *see* Poisoning, food
    putrefaction, food — *see* Poisoning, food
    radiation 508.0
    Salmonella (*see also* Infection, Salmonella) 003.9
    sausage — *see also* Poisoning, food
      Trichinosis 124
    saxitoxin 988.0
    shellfish — *see also* Poisoning, food
      noxious 988.0
    Staphylococcus, food 005.0
    toxic, from disease NEC 799.8
    truffles — *see* Poisoning, food
    uremic — *see* Uremia
    uric acid 274.9

Poison ivy, oak, sumac or other plant dermatitis 692.6
Poker spine 720.0
Policeman's disease 729.2
Polioencephalitis (acute) (bulbar) (*see also* Poliomyelitis, bulbar) 045.0
    inferior 335.22
    influenzal 487.8
    superior hemorrhagic (acute) (Wernicke's) 265.1
    Wernicke's (superior hemorrhagic) 265.1
Polioencephalomyelitis (acute) (anterior) (bulbar) (*see also* Polioencephalitis) 045.0
Polioencephalopathy, superior hemorrhagic 265.1
    with
      beriberi 265.0
      pellagra 265.2
Poliomeningoencephalitis — *see* Meningoencephalitis
Poliomyelitis (acute) (anterior) (epidemic) 045.9

Note — Use the following fifth-digit subclassification with category 045:

    0   poliovirus, unspecified type
    1   poliovirus, type I
    2   poliovirus, type II
    3   poliovirus, type III

    with
      paralysis 045.1
        bulbar 045.0
    abortive 045.2
    ascending 045.9
      progressive 045.9
    bulbar 045.0
    cerebral 045.0
    chronic 335.21
    congenital 771.2
    contact V01.2
    deformities 138
    exposure to V01.2
    late effect 138
    nonepidemic 045.9
    nonparalytic 045.2
    old with deformity 138
    posterior, acute 053.19
    residual 138
    sequelae 138

Poliomyelitis—*continued*
    spinal, acute 045.9
    syphilitic (chronic) 094.89
    vaccination, prophylactic (against) V04.0
Poliosis (eyebrow) (eyelashes) 704.3
    circumscripta (congenital) 757.4
      acquired 704.3
    congenital 757.4
Pollakiuria 788.4
    psychogenic 306.53
Pollinosis 477.0
Pollitzer's disease (hidradenitis suppurativa) 705.83
Polyadenitis (*see also* Adenitis) 289.3
    malignant 020.0
Polyalgia 729.9
Polyangiitis (essential) 446.0
Polyarteritis (nodosa) (renal) 446.0
Polyarthralgia 719.49
    psychogenic 306.0
Polyarthritis, polyarthropathy NEC 716.59
    due to or associated with other specified conditions — *see* Arthritis, due to or associated with
    endemic (*see also* Disease, Kaschin-Beck) 716.0
    inflammatory 714.9
      specified type NEC 714.89
    juvenile (chronic) 714.30
      acute 714.31
    migratory — *see* Fever, rheumatic
    rheumatic 714.0
      fever (acute) — *see* Fever, rheumatic
Polycarential syndrome of infancy 260
Polychondritis (atrophic) (chronic) (relapsing) 733.99
Polycoria 743.46
Polycystic (congenital) (disease) 759.89
    degeneration, kidney — *see* Polycystic, kidney
    kidney (congenital) 753.12
      adult type (APKD) 753.13
      autosomal dominant 753.13
      autosomal recessive 753.14
      childhood type (CPKD) 753.14
      infantile type 753.14
    liver 751.62
    lung 518.89
      congenital 748.4
    ovary, ovaries 256.4
    spleen 759.0
Polycythemia (primary) (rubra) (vera) (M9950/1) 238.4
    acquired 289.0
    benign 289.0
      familial 289.6
    due to
      donor twin 776.4
      fall in plasma volume 289.0
      high altitude 289.0
      maternal-fetal transfusion 776.4
      stress 289.0
    emotional 289.0
    erythropoietin 289.0
    familial (benign) 289.6
    Gaisböck's (hypertonica) 289.0
    high altitude 289.0
    hypertonica 289.0
    hypoxemic 289.0
    neonatorum 776.4
    nephrogenous 289.0
    relative 289.0
    secondary 289.0
    spurious 289.0
    stress 289.0
Polycytosis cryptogenica 289.0

Polydactylism, polydactyly 755.00
    fingers 755.01
    toes 755.02
Polydipsia 783.5
Polydystrophic oligophrenia 277.5
Polyembryoma (M9072/3) — *see* Neoplasm, by site, malignant
Polygalactia 676.6
Polyglandular
    deficiency 258.9
    dyscrasia 258.9
    dysfunction 258.9
    syndrome 258.8
Polyhydramnios (*see also* Hydramnios) 657
Polymastia 757.6
Polymenorrhea 626.2
Polymicrogyria 742.2
Polymyalgia 725
    arteritica 446.5
    rheumatica 725
Polymyositis (acute) (chronic) (hemorrhagic) 710.4
    with involvement of
      lung 710.4 [517.8]
      skin 710.3
    ossificans (generalisata) (progressiva) 728.19
    Wagner's (dermatomyositis) 710.3
Polyneuritis, polyneuritic (*see also* Polyneuropathy) 356.9
    alcoholic 357.5
      with psychosis 291.1
    cranialis 352.6
    diabetic 250.6 [357.2]
    due to lack of vitamin NEC 269.2 [357.4]
    endemic 265.0 [357.4]
    erythredema 985.0
    febrile 357.0
    hereditary ataxic 356.3
    idiopathic, acute 357.0
    infective (acute) 357.0
    nutritional 269.9 [357.4]
    postinfectious 357.0
Polyneuropathy (peripheral) 356.9
    alcoholic 357.5
    amyloid 277.3 [357.4]
    arsenical 357.7
    diabetic 250.6 [357.2]
    due to
      antitetanus serum 357.6
      arsenic 357.7
      drug or medicinal substance 357.6
        correct substance properly administered 357.6
        overdose or wrong substance given or taken 977.9
        specified drug — *see* Table of drugs and chemicals
      lack of vitamin NEC 269.2 [357.4]
      lead 357.7
      organophosphate compounds 357.7
      pellagra 265.2 [357.4]
      porphyria 277.1 [357.4]
      serum 357.6
      toxic agent NEC 357.7
    hereditary 356.0
    idiopathic 356.9
      progressive 356.4
    in
      amyloidosis 277.3 [357.4]
      avitaminosis 269.2 [357.4]
        specified NEC 269.1 [357.4]
      beriberi 265.0 [357.4]
      collagen vascular disease NEC 710.9 [357.1]
      deficiency

Polyneuropathy—*continued*
    in—*continued*
      B-complex NEC 266.2 [357.4]
        vitamin B 266.9 [357.4]
        vitamin B 266.1 [357.4]
      diabetes 250.6 [357.2]
      diphtheria (*see also* Diphtheria) 032.89 [357.4]
      disseminated lupus erythematosus 710.0 [357.1]
      herpes zoster 053.13
      hypoglycemia 251.2 [357.4]
      malignant neoplasm (M8000/3) NEC 199.1 [357.3]
      mumps 072.72
      pellagra 265.2 [357.4]
      polyarteritis nodosa 446.0 [357.1]
      porphyria 277.1 [357.4]
      rheumatoid arthritis 714.0 [357.1]
      sarcoidosis 135 [357.4]
      uremia 585 [357.4]
    lead 357.7
    nutritional 269.9 [357.4]
      specified NEC 269.8 [357.4]
    postherpetic 053.13
    progressive 356.4
    sensory (hereditary) 356.2
Polyonychia 757.5
Polyopia 368.2
    refractive 368.15
Polyorchism, polyorchidism (three testes) 752.8
Polyorrhymenitis (peritoneal) (*see also* Polyserositis) 568.82
    pericardial 423.2
Polyostotic fibrous dysplasia 756.54
Polyotia 744.1
Polyp, polypus

Note — Polyps of organs or sites that do not appear in the list below should be coded to the residual category for diseases of the organ or site concerned.

    accessory sinus 471.8
    adenoid tissue 471.0
    adenomatous (M8210/0) — *see also* Neoplasm, by site, benign
      adenocarcinoma in (M8210/3) — *see* Neoplasm, by site, malignant
      carcinoma in (M8210/3) — *see* Neoplasm, by site, malignant
      multiple (M8221/0) — *see* Neoplasm, by site, benign
    antrum 471.8
    anus, anal (canal) 569.0
    Bartholin's gland 624.6
    bladder (M8120/1) 236.7
    broad ligament 620.8
    cervix (uteri) 622.7
      adenomatous 219.0
      in pregnancy or childbirth 654.6
        affecting fetus or newborn 763.8
        causing obstructed labor 660.2
      mucous 622.7
      nonneoplastic 622.7
    choanal 471.0
    cholesterol 575.6
    clitoris 624.6
    colon (M8210/0) (*see also* Polyp, adenomatous) 211.3
    corpus uteri 621.0
    dental 522.0

Polyp, polypus—continued
  ear (middle) 385.30
  endometrium 621.0
  ethmoidal (sinus) 471.8
  fallopian tube 620.8
  female genital organs NEC 624.8
  frontal (sinus) 471.8
  gallbladder 575.6
  gingiva 523.8
  gum 523.8
  labia 624.6
  larynx (mucous) 478.4
  malignant (M8000/3) — see Neoplasm, by site, malignant
  maxillary (sinus) 471.8
  middle ear 385.30
  myometrium 621.0
  nares
    anterior 471.9
    posterior 471.0
  nasal (mucous) 471.9
    cavity 471.0
    septum 471.9
  nasopharyngeal 471.0
  neoplastic (M8210/0) — see Neoplasm, by site, benign
  nose (mucous) 471.9
  oviduct 620.8
  paratubal 620.8
  pharynx 478.29
    congenital 750.29
  placenta, placental 674.4
  prostate 600
  pudenda 624.6
  pulp (dental) 522.0
  rectum 569.0
  septum (nasal) 471.9
  sinus (accessory) (ethmoidal) (frontal) (maxillary) (sphenoidal) 471.8
  sphenoidal (sinus) 471.8
  stomach (M8210/0) 211.1
  tube, fallopian 620.8
  turbinate, mucous membrane 471.8
  ureter 593.89
  urethra 599.3
  uterine
    ligament 620.8
    tube 620.8
  uterus (body) (corpus) (mucous) 621.0
    in pregnancy or childbirth 654.1
      affecting fetus or newborn 763.8
      causing obstructed labor 660.2
  vagina 623.7
  vocal cord (mucous) 478.4
  vulva 624.6
Polyphagia 783.6
Polypoid — see condition
Polyposis — see also Polyp
  coli (adenomatous) (M8220/0) 211.3
    adenocarcinoma in (M8220/3) 153.9
    carcinoma in (M8220/3) 153.9
  familial (M8220/0) 211.3
  intestinal (adenomatous) (M8220/0) 211.3
  multiple (M8221/0) — see Neoplasm, by site, benign
Polyradiculitis (acute) 357.0
Polyradiculoneuropathy (acute) (segmentally demyelinating) 357.0
Polysarcia 278.0
Polyserositis (peritoneal) 568.82
  due to pericarditis 423.2
  paroxysmal (familial) 277.3
  pericardial 423.2
  periodic 277.3
  pleural — see Pleurisy

Polyserositis—continued
  recurrent 277.3
  tuberculous (see also Tuberculosis, polyserositis) 018.9
Polysialia 527.7
Polysplenia syndrome 759.0
Polythelia 757.6
Polytrichia (see also Hypertrichosis) 704.1
Polyunguia (congenital) 757.5
  acquired 703.8
Polyuria 788.42
Pompe's disease (glycogenosis II) 271.0
Pompholyx 705.81
Poncet's disease (tuberculous rheumatism) (see also Tuberculosis) 015.9
Pond fracture — see Fracture, skull, vault
Ponos 085.0
Pons, pontine — see condition
Poor
  contractions, labor 661.2
    affecting fetus or newborn 763.7
  fetal growth NEC 764.9
    affecting management of pregnancy 656.5
  obstetrical history V23.4
  sucking reflex (newborn) 796.1
  vision NEC 369.9
Poradenitis, nostras 099.1
Porencephaly (congenital) (developmental) (true) 742.4
  acquired 348.0
  nondevelopmental 348.0
  traumatic (post) 310.2
Porocephaliasis 134.1
Porokeratosis 757.39
Poroma, eccrine (M8402/0) — see Neoplasm, skin, benign
Porphyria (acute) (congenital) (constitutional) (erythropoietic) (familial) (hepatica) (idiopathic) (idiosyncratic) (intermittent) (latent) (mixed hepatic) (photosensitive) (South African genetic) (Swedish) 277.1
  acquired 277.1
  cutaneatarda
    hereditaria 277.1
    symptomatica 277.1
  due to drugs
    correct substance properly administered 277.1
    overdose or wrong substance given or taken 977.9
    specified drug — see Table of drugs and chemicals
  secondary 277.1
  toxic NEC 277.1
  variegata 277.1
Porphyrinuria (acquired) (congenital) (secondary) 277.1
Porphyruria (acquired) (congenital) 277.1
Portal — see condition
Port wine nevus or mark 757.32
Posadas-Wernicke disease 114.9
Position
  fetus, abnormal (see also Presentation, fetal) 652.9
  teeth, faulty 524.3
Positive
  culture (nonspecific) 795.3
    AIDS virus V08
    blood 790.7
    HIV V08

Positive—continued
  culture—continued
    human immunodeficiency virus V08
    nose 795.3
    skin lesion NEC 795.3
    spinal fluid 792.0
    sputum 795.3
    stool 792.1
    throat 795.3
    urine 599.0
    wound 795.3
  HIV V08
  human immunodeficiency virus (HIV) V08
  PPD 795.5
  serology
    AIDS virus V08
      inconclusive 795.71
    HIV V08
      inconclusive 795.71
    human immunodeficiency virus (HIV) V08
      inconclusive 795.71
    syphilis 097.1
      with signs or symptoms — see Syphilis, by site and stage
      false 795.6
  skin test 795.7
    tuberculin (without active tuberculosis) 795.5
  VDRL 097.1
    with signs or symptoms — see Syphilis, by site and stage
    false 795.6
  Wassermann reaction 097.1
    false 795.6
Postcardiotomy syndrome 429.4
Postcaval ureter 753.4
Postcholecystectomy syndrome 576.0
Postclimacteric bleeding 627.1
Postcommissurotomy syndrome 429.4
Postconcussional syndrome 310.2
Postcontusional syndrome 310.2
Postcricoid region — see condition
Post-dates (pregnancy) 645
Postencephalitic — see also condition
  syndrome 310.8
Posterior — see condition
Posterolateral sclerosis (spinal cord) — see Degeneration, combined
Postexanthematous — see condition
Postfebrile — see condition
Postgastrectomy dumping syndrome 564.2
Posthemiplegic chorea 344.89
Posthemorrhagic anemia (chronic) 280.0
  acute 285.1
  newborn 776.5
Posthepatitis syndrome 780.7
Postherpetic neuralgia (intercostal) (syndrome) (zoster) 053.19
  geniculate ganglion 053.11
  ophthalmica 053.19
  trigeminal 053.12
Posthitis 607.1
Postimmunization complication or reaction — see Complications, vaccination
Postinfectious — see condition
Postinfluenzal syndrome 780.7
Postlaminectomy syndrome 722.80
  cervical, cervicothoracic 722.81
  kyphosis 737.12
  lumbar, lumbosacral 722.83
  thoracic, thoracolumbar 722.82

Postleukotomy syndrome 310.0
Postlobectomy syndrome 310.0
Postmastectomy lymphedema (syndrome) 457.0
Postmaturity, postmature (fetus or newborn) 766.2
  affecting management of pregnancy 645
  syndrome 766.2
Postmeasles — see also condition
  complication 055.8
  specified NEC 055.79
Postmenopausal endometrium (atrophic) 627.8
  suppurative (see also Endometritis) 615.9
Postnasal drip — see Sinusitis
Postnatal — see condition
Postoperative — see also condition
  confusion state 293.9
  psychosis 293.9
  status NEC (see also Status (post)) V45.89
Postpancreatectomy hyperglycemia 251.3
Postpartum — see also condition
  observation
    immediately after delivery V24.0
    routine follow-up V24.2
Postperfusion syndrome NEC 999.8
  bone marrow 996.85
Postpoliomyelitic — see condition
Postsurgery status NEC (see also Status (post)) V45.89
Post-term (pregnancy) 645
  infant (294 days or more gestation) 766.2
Posttraumatic — see condition
Posttraumatic brain syndrome, nonpsychotic 310.2
Post-typhoid abscess 002.0
Postures, hysterical 300.11
Postvaccinal reaction or complication — see Complications, vaccination
Postvagotomy syndrome 564.2
Postvalvulotomy syndrome 429.4
Postvasectomy sperm count V25.8
Potain's disease (pulmonary edema) 514
Potain's syndrome (gastrectasis with dyspepsia) 536.1
Pott's
  curvature (spinal) (see also Tuberculosis) 015.0 [737.43]
  disease or paraplegia (see also Tuberculosis) 015.0 [730.88]
  fracture (closed) 824.4
    open 824.5
  gangrene 440.24
  osteomyelitis (see also Tuberculosis) 015.0 [730.88]
  spinal curvature (see also Tuberculosis) 015.0 [737.43]
  tumor, puffy (see also Osteomyelitis) 730.2
Potter's
  asthma 502
  disease 753.0
  facies 754.0
  lung 502
  syndrome (with renal agenesis) 753.0
Pouch
  bronchus 748.3
  Douglas' — see condition

Pouch—continued
esophagus, esophageal (congenital) 750.4
  acquired 530.6
gastric 537.1
Hartmann's (abnormal sacculation of gallbladder neck) 575.8
pharynx, pharyngeal (congenital) 750.27

Poulet's disease 714.2
Poultrymen's itch 133.8
Poverty V60.2
Prader-Labhart-Willi-Fanconi syndrome (hypogenital dystrophy with diabetic tendency) 759.81
Prader-Willi syndrome (hypogenital dystrophy with diabetic tendency) 759.81
Preachers' voice 784.49
Pre-AIDS — see Human immunodeficiency virus (disease) (illness) (infection)
Preauricular appendage 744.1
Prebetalipoproteinemia (acquired) (essential) (familial) (hereditary) (primary) (secondary) 272.1
  with chylomicronemia 272.3
Precipitate labor 661.3
  affecting fetus or newborn 763.6
Preclimacteric bleeding 627.0
  menorrhagia 627.0
Precocious
  adrenarche 259.1
  menarche 259.1
  menstruation 626.8
  pubarche 259.1
  puberty NEC 259.1
  sexual development NEC 259.1
  thelarche 259.1
Precocity, sexual (constitutional) (cryptogenic) (female) (idiopathic) (male) NEC 259.1
  with adrenal hyperplasia 255.2
Precordial pain 786.51
  psychogenic 307.89
Predeciduous teeth 520.2
Prediabetes, prediabetic 790.2
  complicating pregnancy, childbirth, or puerperium 648.8
  fetus or newborn 775.8
Predislocation status of hip, at birth (see also Subluxation, congenital, hip) 754.32
Preeclampsia (mild) 642.4
  with pre-existing hypertension 642.7
  affecting fetus or newborn 760.0
  severe 642.5
  superimposed on pre-existing hypertensive disease 642.7
Preeruptive color change, teeth, tooth 520.8
Preexcitation 426.7
  atrioventricular conduction 426.7
  ventricular 426.7
Preglaucoma 365.00

Pregnancy (single) (uterine) (without sickness) V22.2

> Note — Use the following fifth-digit subclassification with categories 640-648, 651-676:
>
> 0 unspecified as to episode of care
> 1 delivered, with or without mention of antepartum condition
> 2 delivered, with mention of postpartum complication
> 3 antepartum condition or complication
> 4 postpartum condition or complication

abdominal (ectopic) 633.0
  affecting fetus or newborn 761.4
abnormal NEC 646.9
ampullar — see Pregnancy, tubal
broad ligament — see Pregnancy, cornual
cervical — see Pregnancy, cornual
combined (extrauterine and intrauterine) — see Pregnancy, cornual
complicated (by) 646.9
  abnormal, abnormality NEC 646.9
    cervix 654.6
    cord (umbilical) 663.9
    glucose tolerance (conditions classifiable to 790.2) 648.8
    injury 648.9
      obstetrical NEC 665.9 ▼
    obstetrical trauma NEC 665.9 ▲
    pelvic organs or tissues NEC 654.9
    pelvis (bony) 653.0
    perineum or vulva 654.8
    placenta, placental (vessel) 656.7
    position
      cervix 654.4
      placenta 641.1
        without hemorrhage 641.0
      uterus 654.4
    size, fetus 653.5
    trauma 648.9
      obstetrical NEC 665.9 ▲
    uterus (congenital) 654.0
  abscess or cellulitis
    bladder 646.6
    genitourinary tract (conditions classifiable to 590, 595, 597, 599.0, 614-616) 646.6
    kidney 646.6
    urinary tract NEC 646.6
  air embolism 673.0
  albuminuria 646.2
    with hypertension — see Toxemia, of pregnancy
  amnionitis 658.4
  amniotic fluid embolism 673.1
  anemia (conditions classifiable to 280-285) 648.2
  atrophy, yellow (acute) (liver) (subacute) 646.7
  bacilluria, asymptomatic 646.5
  bacteriuria, asymptomatic 646.5
  bicornis or bicornuate uterus 654.0

Pregnancy—continued
complicated (by)—continued
  bone and joint disorders (conditions classifiable to 720-724 or conditions affecting lower limbs classifiable to 711-719, 725-738) 648.7
  breech presentation 652.2
    with successful version 652.1
  cardiovascular disease (conditions classifiable to 390-398, 410-429, 435, 440-459) 648.6
    congenital (conditions classifiable to 745-747) 648.5
  cerebrovascular disorders (conditions classifiable to 430-434, 436-437) 674.0
  cervicitis (conditions classifiable to 616.0) 646.6
  chloasma (gravidarum) 646.8
  chorea (gravidarum) — see Eclampsia, pregnancy
  contraction, pelvis (general) 653.1
    inlet 653.2
    outlet 653.3
  convulsions (eclamptic) (uremic) 642.6
    with pre-existing hypertension 642.7
  current disease or condition (nonobstetric)
    abnormal glucose tolerance 648.8
    anemia 648.2
    bone and joint (lower limb) 648.7
    cardiovascular 648.6
    congenital 648.5
    cerebrovascular 674.0
    diabetic 648.0
    drug dependence 648.3
    genital organ or tract 646.6
    gonorrheal 647.1
    hypertensive 642.2
      renal 642.1
    infectious 647.9
      specified type NEC 647.8
    liver 646.7
    malarial 647.4
    nutritional deficiency 648.9
    parasitic NEC 647.8
    renal 646.2
      hypertensive 642.1
    rubella 647.5
    specified condition NEC 648.9
    syphilitic 647.0
    thyroid 648.1
    tuberculous 647.3
    urinary 646.6
    venereal 647.2
    viral NEC 647.6
  cystitis 646.6
  cystocele 654.4
  death of fetus (near term) 656.4
    early pregnancy (before 22 completed weeks gestation) 632
  deciduitis 646.6
  diabetes (mellitus) (conditions classifiable to 250) 648.0
  disorders of liver 646.7
  displacement, uterus NEC 654.4
  disproportion — see Disproportion

Pregnancy—continued
complicated (by)—continued
  double uterus 654.0
  drug dependence (conditions classifiable to 304) 648.3
  dysplasia, cervix 654.6
  early onset of delivery (spontaneous) 644.2
  eclampsia, eclamptic (coma) (convulsions) (delirium) (nephritis) (uremia) 642.6
    with pre-existing hypertension 642.7
  edema 646.1
    with hypertension — see Toxemia, of pregnancy
  effusion, amniotic fluid 658.1
    delayed delivery following 658.2
  embolism
    air 673.0
    amniotic fluid 673.1
    blood-clot 673.2
    cerebral 674.0
    pulmonary NEC 673.2
    pyemic 673.3
    septic 673.3
  emesis (gravidarum) — see Pregnancy, complicated, vomiting
  endometritis (conditions classifiable to 615.0-615.9) 646.6
  decidual 646.6
  excessive weight gain NEC 646.1
  face presentation 652.4
  failure, fetal head to enter pelvic brim 652.5
  false labor (pains) 644.1
  fatigue 646.8
  fatty metamorphosis of liver 646.7
  fetal
    death (near term) 656.4
      early (before 22 completed weeks gestation) 632
    deformity 653.7
    distress 656.3
  fibroid (tumor) (uterus) 654.1
  goiter 648.1
  gonococcal infection (conditions classifiable to 098) 647.1
  gonorrhea (conditions classifiable to 098) 647.1
  hemorrhage 641.9
    accidental 641.2
    before 22 completed weeks gestation NEC 640.9
    cerebrovascular 674.0
    due to
      afibrinogenemia or other coagulation defect (conditions classifiable to 286.0-286.9) 641.3
    leiomyoma, uterine 641.8
    marginal sinus (rupture) 641.2
    premature separation, placenta 641.2
    trauma 641.8
    early (before 22 completed weeks gestation) 640.9
    threatened abortion 640.0
    unavoidable 641.1
  hepatitis (acute) (malignant) (subacute) 646.7

Pregnancy—continued
    complicated (by)—continued
        herniation of uterus 654.4
        high head at term 652.5
        hydatidiform mole (delivered) (undelivered) 630
        hydramnios 657
        hydrocephalic fetus 653.6
        hydrops amnii 657
        hydrorrhea 658.1
        hyperemesis (gravidarum) — see Hyperemesis, gravidarum
        hypertension — see Hypertension, complicating pregnancy
        hypertensive
            heart and renal disease 642.2
            heart disease 642.2
            renal disease 642.2
        hyperthyroidism 648.1
        hypothyroidism 648.1
        hysteralgia 646.8
        icterus gravis 646.7
        incarceration, uterus 654.3
        incompetent cervix (os) 654.5
        infection 647.9
            amniotic fluid 658.4
            bladder 646.6
            genital organ (conditions classifiable to 614-616) 646.6
            kidney (conditions classifiable to 590.0-590.9) 646.6
            urinary (tract) 646.6
                asymptomatic 646.5
        infective and parasitic diseases NEC 647.8
        inflammation
            bladder 646.6
            genital organ (conditions classifiable to 614-616) 646.6
            urinary tract NEC 646.6
        insufficient weight gain 646.8
        intrauterine fetal death (near term) NEC 656.4
            early (before 22 completed weeks' gestation) 632
        malaria (conditions classifiable to 084) 647.4
        malformation, uterus (congenital) 654.0
        malnutrition (conditions classifiable to 260-269) 648.9
        malposition
            fetus — see Pregnancy, complicated, malpresentation
            uterus or cervix 654.4
        malpresentation 652.9
            with successful version 652.1
            in multiple gestation 652.6
            specified type NEC 652.8
        marginal sinus hemorrhage or rupture 641.2
        maternal obesity syndrome 646.1
        menstruation 640.8
        mental disorders (conditions classifiable to 290-303, 305-316, 317-319) 648.4
        mentum presentation 652.4
        missed
            abortion 632
            delivery (at or near term) 656.4
            labor (at or near term) 656.4

Pregnancy—continued
    complicated (by)—continued
        necrosis
            genital organ or tract (conditions classifiable to 614-616) 646.6
            liver (conditions classifiable to 570) 646.7
            renal, cortical 646.2
        nephritis or nephrosis (conditions classifiable to 580-589) 646.2
            with hypertension 642.1
        nephropathy NEC 646.2
        neuritis (peripheral) 646.4
        nutritional deficiency (conditions classifiable to 260-269) 648.9
        oblique lie or presentation 652.3
            with successful version 652.1
        oligohydramnios NEC 658.0
        onset of contractions before 37 weeks 644.0
        oversize fetus 653.5
        papyraceous fetus 646.0
        patent cervix 654.5
        pelvic inflammatory disease (conditions classifiable to 614-616) 646.6
        placenta, placental
            abnormality 656.7
            abruptio or ablatio 641.2
            detachment 641.2
            disease 656.7
            infarct 656.7
            low implantation 641.1
                without hemorrhage 641.0
            malformation 656.7
            malposition 641.1
                without hemorrhage 641.0
            marginal sinus hemorrhage 641.2
            previa 641.1
                without hemorrhage 641.0
            separation (premature) (undelivered) 641.2
        placentitis 658.4
        polyhydramnios 657
        postmaturity 645
        prediabetes 648.8
        pre-eclampsia (mild) 642.4
            severe 642.5
            superimposed on pre-existing hypertensive disease 642.7
        premature rupture of membranes 658.1
            with delayed delivery 658.2
        previous
            infertility V23.0
            nonobstetric condition V23.8
            poor obstetrical history V23.4
            premature delivery V23.4
            trophoblastic disease (conditions classifiable to 630) V23.1
        prolapse, uterus 654.4
        proteinuria (gestational) 646.2
            with hypertension — see Toxemia, of pregnancy
        pruritus (neurogenic) 646.8
        psychosis or psychoneurosis 648.4
        ptyalism 646.8
        pyelitis (conditions classifiable to 590.0-590.9) 646.6

Pregnancy—continued
    complicated (by)—continued
        renal disease or failure NEC 646.2
            with secondary hypertension 642.1
            hypertensive 642.2
        retention, retained dead ovum 631
        retroversion, uterus 654.3
        Rh immunization, incompatibility, or sensitization 656.1
        rubella (conditions classifiable to 056) 647.5
        rupture
            amnion (premature) 658.1
                with delayed delivery 658.2
            marginal sinus (hemorrhage) 641.2
            membranes (premature) 658.1
                with delayed delivery 658.2
            uterus (before onset of labor) 665.0
        salivation (excessive) 646.8
        salpingo-oophoritis (conditions classifiable to 614.0-614.2) 646.6
        septicemia (conditions classifiable to 038.0-038.9) 647.8
        spasms, uterus (abnormal) 646.8
        specified condition NEC 646.8
        spurious labor pains 644.1
        superfecundation 651.9
        superfetation 651.9
        syphilis (conditions classifiable to 090-097) 647.0
        threatened
            abortion 640.0
            premature delivery 644.2
            premature labor 644.0
        thrombophlebitis (superficial) 671.2
            deep 671.3
        thrombosis 671.9
            venous (superficial) 671.2
            deep 671.3
        thyroid dysfunction (conditions classifiable to 240-246) 648.1
        thyroiditis 648.1
        thyrotoxicosis 648.1
        torsion of uterus 654.4
        toxemia — see Toxemia, of pregnancy
        transverse lie or presentation 652.3
            with successful version 652.1
        tuberculosis (conditions classifiable to 010-018) 647.3
        tumor
            cervix 654.6
            ovary 654.4
            pelvic organs or tissue NEC 654.4
            uterus (body) 654.1
                cervix 654.6
            vagina 654.7
            vulva 654.8
        unstable lie 652.0
        uremia — see also Pregnancy, complicated, renal disease
        urethritis 646.6
        vaginitis or vulvitis (conditions classifiable to 616.1) 646.6

Pregnancy—continued
    complicated (by)—continued
        varicose
            placental vessels 656.7
            veins (legs) 671.0
                perineum 671.1
                vulva 671.1
        varicosity, labia or vulva 671.1
        venereal disease NEC (conditions classifiable to 099) 647.2
        viral disease NEC (conditions classifiable to 050-055, 057-079) 647.6
        vomiting (incoercible) (pernicious) (persistent) (uncontrollable) (vicious) 643.9
            due to organic disease or other cause 643.8
            early — see Hyperemesis, gravidarum
            late (after 22 completed weeks gestation) 643.2
    complications NEC 646.9
    cornual 633.8
        affecting fetus or newborn 761.4
    death, maternal NEC 646.9
    delivered — see Delivery
    ectopic (ruptured) NEC 633.9
        abdominal — see Pregnancy, abdominal
        affecting fetus or newborn 761.4
        combined (extrauterine and intrauterine) — see Pregnancy, cornual
        ovarian — see Pregnancy, ovarian
        specified type NEC 633.8
            affecting fetus or newborn 761.4
        tubal — see Pregnancy, tubal
    examination, pregnancy not confirmed V72.4
    extrauterine — see Pregnancy, ectopic
    fallopian — see Pregnancy, tubal
    false 300.11
        labor (pains) 644.1
    fatigue 646.8
    illegitimate V61.6
    incidental finding V22.2
    in double uterus 654.0
    interstitial — see Pregnancy, cornual
    intraligamentous — see Pregnancy, cornual
    intramural — see Pregnancy, cornual
    intraperitoneal — see Pregnancy, abdominal
    isthmian — see Pregnancy, tubal
    management affected by
        abnormal, abnormality
            fetus (suspected) 655.9
                specified NEC 655.8
            placenta 656.7
        advanced maternal age NEC 659.6
            primigravida 659.5
        antibodies (maternal)
            anti-c 656.1
            anti-d 656.1
            anti-e 656.1
            blood group (ABO) 656.2
                Rh(esus) 656.1
        elderly primigravida 659.5
        fetal (suspected)
            abnormality 655.9
                acid-base balance 656.3
                heart rate or rhythm 656.3
                specified NEC 655.8
            acidemia 656.3

Pregnancy—continued
   complicated (by)—continued
     fetal—continued
      anencephaly 655.0
      bradycardia 656.3
      central nervous system malformation 655.0
      chromosomal abnormalities (conditions classifiable to 758.0-758.9) 655.1
      damage from
       drugs 655.5
        obstetric, anesthetic, or sedative 655.5
       environmental toxins 655.8
       intrauterine contraceptive device 655.8
       maternal
        alcohol addiction 655.4
        disease NEC 655.4
        drug use 655.5
        listeriosis 655.4
        rubella 655.3
        toxoplasmosis 655.4
        viral infection 655.3
       radiation 655.6
     death (near term) 656.4
      early (before 22 completed weeks' gestation) 632
     distress 656.3
     excessive growth 656.6
     growth retardation 656.5
     hereditary disease 655.2
     hydrocephalus 655.0
     intrauterine death 656.4
     poor growth 656.5
     spina bifida (with myelomeningocele) 655.0
    fetal-maternal hemorrhage 656.0
    hereditary disease in family (possibly) affecting fetus 655.2
    hydrocephalus 655.0
    incompatibility, blood groups (ABO) 656.2
     rh(esus) 656.1
    insufficient prenatal care V23.7
    intrauterine death 656.4
    isoimmunization (ABO) 656.2
     rh(esus) 656.1
    large-for-dates fetus 656.6
    light-for-dates fetus 656.5
    meconium in liquor 656.3
    mental disorder (conditions classifiable to 290-303, 305-316, 317-319) 648.4
    multiparity (grand) 659.4
    poor obstetric history V23.4
    postmaturity 645
    previous
     abortion V23.2
      habitual 646.3
     cesarean delivery 654.2
     difficult delivery V23.4
     forceps delivery V23.4
     habitual abortions 646.3
     hemorrhage, antepartum or postpartum V23.4
     hydatidiform mole V23.1
     infertility V23.0
     malignancy NEC V23.8
     nonobstetrical conditions V23.8
     premature delivery V23.4
     trophoblastic disease (conditions in 630) V23.1
     vesicular mole V23.1

Pregnancy—continued
   complicated (by)—continued
    prolonged pregnancy 645
    small-for-dates fetus 656.5
    maternal death NEC 646.9
    mesometric (mural) — see Pregnancy, cornual
    molar 631
     hydatidiform (see also Hydatidiform mole) 630
      previous, affecting management of pregnancy V23.1
     previous, affecting management of pregnancy V23.4
    multiple NEC 651.9
     with fetal loss and retention of one or more fetus(es) 651.6
     affecting fetus or newborn 761.5
     specified type NEC 651.8
      with fetal loss and retention of one or more fetus(es) 651.6
    mural — see Pregnancy, cornual
    observation NEC V22.1
     first pregnancy V22.0
     high-risk V23.9
      specified problem NEC V23.8
    ovarian 633.2
     affecting fetus or newborn 761.4
    postmature 645
    post-term 645
    prenatal care only V22.1
     first pregnancy V22.0
     high-risk V23.9
      specified problem NEC V23.8
    prolonged 645
    quadruplet NEC 651.2
     with fetal loss and retention of one or more fetus(es) 651.5
     affecting fetus or newborn 761.5
    quintuplet NEC 651.8
     with fetal loss and retention of one or more fetus(es) 651.6
     affecting fetus or newborn 761.5
    sextuplet NEC 651.8
     with fetal loss and retention of one or more fetus(es) 651.6
     affecting fetus or newborn 761.5
    spurious 300.11
    superfecundation NEC 651.9
     with fetal loss and retention of one or more fetus(es) 651.6
    superfetation NEC 651.9
     with fetal loss and retention of one or more fetus(es) 651.6
    supervision (of) (for) — see also Pregnancy, management affected by
     high-risk V23.9
      insufficient prenatal care V23.7
      specified problem NEC V23.8
     multiparity V23.3
     normal NEC V22.1
      first V22.0
     poor
      obstetric history V23.4
      reproductive history V23.5

Pregnancy—continued
   complicated (by)—continued
    previous
     abortion V23.2
     hydatidiform mole V23.1
     infertility V23.0
     neonatal death V23.5
     stillbirth V23.5
     trophoblastic disease V23.1
     vesicular mole V23.1
     specified problem NEC V23.8
    triplet NEC 651.1
     with fetal loss and retention of one or more fetus(es) 651.4
     affecting fetus or newborn 761.5
    tubal (with rupture) 633.1
     affecting fetus or newborn 761.4
    twin NEC 651.0
     with fetal loss and retention of one fetus 651.3
     affecting fetus or newborn 761.5
    unconfirmed V72.4
    undelivered (no other diagnosis) V22.2
     with false labor 644.1
     high-risk V23.9
      specified problem NEC V23.8
    unwanted NEC V61.7
Pregnant uterus — see condition
Preiser's disease (osteoporosis) 733.09
Prekwashiorkor 260
Preleukemia 238.7
Preluxation of hip, congenital (see also Subluxation, congenital, hip) 754.32
Premature — see also condition
   beats (nodal) 427.60
    atrial 427.61
    auricular 427.61
    postoperative 997.1
    specified type NEC 427.69
    supraventricular 427.61
    ventricular 427.69
   birth NEC 765.1
   closure
    cranial suture 756.0
    fontanel 756.0
    foramen ovale 745.8
   contractions 427.60
    atrial 427.61
    auricular 427.61
    auriculoventricular 427.61
    heart (extrasystole) 427.60
    junctional 427.60
    nodal 427.60
    postoperative 997.1
    ventricular 427.69
   ejaculation 302.75
   infant NEC 765.1
    excessive 765.0
    light-for-dates — see Light-for-dates
   labor 644.2
    threatened 644.0
   lungs 770.4
   menopause 256.3
   puberty 259.1
   rupture of membranes or amnion 658.1
    affecting fetus or newborn 761.1
    delayed delivery following 658.2
   senility (syndrome) 259.8
   separation, placenta (partial) — see Placenta, separation
   ventricular systole 427.69
Prematurity NEC 765.1
   extreme 765.0
Premenstrual tension 625.4

Premolarization, cuspids 520.2
Premyeloma 273.1
Prenatal
   care, normal pregnancy V22.1
    first V22.0
   death, cause unknown — see Death, fetus
   screening — see Antenatal, screening
Prepartum — see condition
Preponderance, left or right ventricular 429.3
Prepuce — see condition
Presbycardia 797
   hypertensive (see also Hypertension, heart) 402.90
Presbycusis 388.01
Presbyesophagus 530.89
Presbyophrenia 310.1
Presbyopia 367.4
Prescription of contraceptives NEC V25.02
   diaphragm V25.02
   oral (pill) V25.01
    repeat V25.41
   repeat V25.40
    oral (pill) V25.41
Presenile — see also condition
   aging 259.8
   dementia (see also Dementia, presenile) 290.10
Presenility 259.8
Presentation, fetal
   abnormal 652.9
    with successful version 652.1
    before labor, affecting fetus or newborn 761.7
    causing obstructed labor 660.0
     affecting fetus or newborn, any, except breech 763.1
    in multiple gestation (one or more) 652.6
    specified NEC 652.8
   arm 652.7
    causing obstructed labor 660.0
   breech 652.2
    with successful version 652.1
    before labor, affecting fetus or newborn 761.7
    before labor, affecting fetus or newborn 761.7
    causing obstructed labor 660.0
     affecting fetus or newborn 763.0
   brow 652.4
    causing obstructed labor 660.0
   chin 652.4
    causing obstructed labor 660.0
   compound 652.8
    causing obstructed labor 660.0
   cord 663.0
   extended head 652.4
    causing obstructed labor 660.0
   face 652.4
    causing obstructed labor 660.0
    to pubes 652.8
     causing obstructed labor 660.3
   hand, leg, or foot NEC 652.8
    causing obstructed labor 660.0
   mentum 652.4
    causing obstructed labor 660.0
   multiple gestation (one fetus or more) 652.6
   oblique 652.3
    with successful version 652.1
    causing obstructed labor 660.0
   shoulder 652.8
    affecting fetus or newborn 763.1
    causing obstructed labor 660.0

Presentation, fetal—continued
  transverse 652.3
    with successful version 652.1
    causing obstructed labor 660.0
  umbilical cord 663.0
  unstable 652.0
Prespondylolisthesis (congenital) (lumbosacral) 756.11
Pressure
  area, skin ulcer (see also Decubitus) 707.0
  atrophy, spine 733.99
  birth, fetus or newborn NEC 767.9
  brachial plexus 353.0
  brain 348.4
    injury at birth 767.0
  cerebral — see Pressure, brain
  chest 786.59
  cone, tentorial 348.4
    injury at birth 767.0
  funis — see Compression, umbilical cord
  hyposystolic (see also Hypotension) 458.9
  increased
    intracranial 348.2
      injury at birth 767.8
    intraocular 365.00
  lumbosacral plexus 353.1
  mediastinum 519.3
  necrosis (chronic) (skin) (see also Decubitus) 707.0
  nerve — see Compression, nerve
  paralysis (see also Neuropathy, entrapment) 355.9
  sore (chronic) (see also Decubitus) 707.0
  spinal cord 336.9
  ulcer (chronic) (see also Decubitus) 707.0
  umbilical cord — see Compression, umbilical cord
  venous, increased 459.89
Pre-syncope 780.2
Preterm infant NEC 765.1
  extreme 765.0
Priapism (penis) 607.3
Prickling sensation (see also Disturbance, sensation) 782.0
Prickly heat 705.1
Primary — see condition
Primigravida, elderly
  affecting
    fetus or newborn 763.8
    management of pregnancy, labor, and delivery 659.5
Primipara, old
  affecting
    fetus or newborn 763.8
    management of pregnancy, labor, and delivery 659.5
Primula dermatitis 692.6
Primus varus (bilateral) (metatarsus) 754.52
P.R.I.N.D. 436
Pringle's disease (tuberous sclerosis) 759.5
Prinzmetal's angina 413.1
Prinzmetal-Massumi syndrome (anterior chest wall) 786.52
Prizefighter ear 738.7
Problem (with) V49.9
  academic V62.3
  acculturation V62.4
  adopted child V61.29
  aged
    in-law V61.3
    parent V61.3
    person NEC V61.8
  alcoholism in family V61.41

Problem (with)—continued
  anger reaction (see also Disturbance, conduct) 312.0
  behavior, child 312.9
  behavioral V40.9
    specified NEC V40.3
  betting V69.3
  cardiorespiratory NEC V47.2
  care of sick or handicapped person in family or household V61.49
  career choice V62.2
  child abuse, maltreatment or neglect V61.21
    affecting the child 995.5
  communication V40.1
  conscience regarding medical care V62.6
  delinquency (juvenile) 312.9
  diet, inappropriate V69.1
  digestive NEC V47.3
  ear NEC V41.3
  eating habits, inappropriate V69.1
  economic V60.2
    affecting care V60.9
      specified type NEC V60.8
  educational V62.3
  enuresis, child 307.6
  exercise, lack of V69.0
  eye NEC V41.1
  family V61.9
    specified circumstance NEC V61.8
  fear reaction, child 313.0
  feeding (elderly) (infant) 783.3
    newborn 779.3
    nonorganic 307.50
  fetal, affecting management of pregnancy 656.9
    specified type NEC 656.8
  financial V60.2
  foster child V61.29
    specified NEC V41.8
  functional V41.9
    specified type NEC V41.8
  gambling V69.3
  genital NEC V47.5
  head V48.9
    deficiency V48.0
    disfigurement V48.6
    mechanical V48.2
    motor V48.2
    movement of V48.2
    sensory V48.4
    specified condition NEC V48.8
  hearing V41.2
  high-risk sexual behavior V69.2
  influencing health status NEC V49.8
  internal organ NEC V47.9
    deficiency V47.0
    mechanical or motor V47.1
  interpersonal NEC V62.81
  jealousy, child 313.3
  learning V40.0
  legal V62.5
  life circumstance NEC V62.89
  lifestyle V69.9
    specified NEC V69.8
  limb V49.9
    deficiency V49.0
    disfigurement V49.4
    mechanical V49.1
    motor V49.2
    movement, involving musculoskeletal system V49.1
    nervous system V49.2
    sensory V49.3
    specified condition NEC V49.5
  litigation V62.5
  living alone V60.3
  loneliness NEC V62.89

Problem (with)—continued
  marital V61.1
    involving
      divorce V61.0
      estrangement V61.0
      psychosexual disorder 302.9
      sexual function V41.7
  mastication V41.6
  medical care, within family V61.49
  mental V40.9
    specified NEC V40.2
  mental hygiene, adult V40.9
  multiparity V61.5
  nail biting, child 307.9
  neck V48.9
    deficiency V48.1
    disfigurement V48.7
    mechanical V48.3
    motor V48.3
    movement V48.3
    sensory V48.5
    specified condition NEC V48.8
  neurological NEC 781.9
  none (feared complaint unfounded) V65.5
  occupational V62.2
  parent-child V61.20
  partner V61.1
  personal NEC V62.89
    interpersonal conflict NEC V62.81
  personality (see also Disorder, personality) 301.9
  phase of life V62.89
  placenta, affecting managment of pregnancy 656.9
    specified type NEC 656.8
  poverty V60.2
  presence of sick or handicapped person in family or household V61.49
  psychiatric 300.9
  psychosocial V62.9
    specified type NEC V62.89
  relational NEC V62.81
  relationship, childhood 313.3
  religious or spiritual belief other than medical care V62.89
    regarding medical care V62.6
  self-damaging behavior V69.8
  sexual
    behavior, high-risk V69.2
    function NEC V41.7
  sibling relational V61.8
  sight V41.0
  sleep disorder, child 307.40
  smell V41.5
  speech V40.1
  spite reaction, child (see also Disturbance, conduct) 312.0
  spoiled child reaction (see also Disturbance, conduct) 312.1
  swallowing V41.6
  tantrum, child (see also Disturbance, conduct) 312.1
  taste V41.5
  thumb sucking, child 307.9
  tic, child 307.21
  trunk V48.9
    deficiency V48.1
    disfigurement V48.7
    mechanical V48.3
    motor V48.3
    movement V48.3
    sensory V48.5
    specified condition NEC V48.8
  unemployment V62.0
  urinary NEC V47.4
  voice production V41.4

Procedure (surgical) not done NEC V64.3
  because of
    contraindication V64.1
    patient's decision V64.2
      for reasons of conscience or religion V62.6
    specified reason NEC V64.3
Procidentia
  anus (sphincter) 569.1
  rectum (sphincter) 569.1
  stomach 537.89
  uteri 618.1
Proctalgia 569.42
  fugax 564.6
  spasmodic 564.6
    psychogenic 307.89
Proctitis 569.49
  amebic 006.8
  chlamydial 099.52
  gonococcal 098.7
  granulomatous 555.1
  idiopathic 556.2
    with ulcerative sigmoiditis 556.3
  tuberculous (see also Tuberculosis) 014.8
  ulcerative (chronic) (nonspecific) 556.2
    with ulcerative sigmoiditis 556.3
Proctocele
  female (without uterine prolapse) 618.0
    with uterine prolapse 618.4
      complete 618.3
      incomplete 618.2
  male 569.49
Proctocolitis, idiopathic 556.2
  with ulcerative sigmoiditis 556.3
Proctoptosis 569.1
Proctosigmoiditis 569.89
  ulcerative (chronic) 556.3
Proctospasm 564.6
  psychogenic 306.4
Prodromal-AIDS — see Human immunodeficiency virus (disease) (illness) (infection)
Profichet's disease or syndrome 729.9
Progeria (adultorum) (syndrome) 259.8
Prognathism (mandibular) (maxillary) 524.00
Progonoma (melanotic) (M9363/0) — see Neoplasm, by site, benign
Progressive — see condition
Prolapse, prolapsed
  anus, anal (canal) (sphincter) 569.1
  arm or hand, complicating delivery 652.7
    causing obstructed labor 660.0
      affecting fetus or newborn 763.1
    fetus or newborn 763.1
  bladder (acquired) (mucosa) (sphincter)
    congenital (female) (male) 753.8
    female 618.0
    male 596.8
  breast implant (prosthetic) 996.54
  cecostomy 569.6
  cecum 569.89
  cervix, cervical (stump) (hypertrophied) 618.1
    anterior lip, obstructing labor 660.2
      affecting fetus or newborn 763.1
    congenital 752.49

Prolapse, prolapsed—continued
   cervix, cervical—continued
      postpartal (old) 618.1
   ciliary body 871.1
   colon (pedunculated) 569.89
   colostomy 569.6
   conjunctiva 372.73
   cord — see Prolapse, umbilical cord
   disc (intervertebral) — see Displacement, intervertebral disc
   duodenum 537.89
   eye implant (orbital) 996.59
      lens (ocular) 996.53
   fallopian tube 620.4
   fetal extremity, complicating delivery 652.8
      causing obstructed labor 660.0
      fetus or newborn 763.1
   funis — see Prolapse, umbilical cord
   gastric (mucosa) 537.89
   genital, female 618.9
      specified NEC 618.8
   globe 360.81
   ileostomy bud 569.6
   intervertebral disc — see Displacement, intervertebral disc
   intestine (small) 569.89
   iris 364.8
      traumatic 871.1
   kidney (see also Disease, renal) 593.0
      congenital 753.3
   laryngeal muscles or ventricle 478.79
   leg, complicating delivery 652.8
      causing obstructed labor 660.0
      fetus or newborn 763.1
   liver 573.8
   meatus urinarius 599.5
   mitral valve 424.0
   ocular lens implant 996.53
   organ or site, congenital NEC — see Malposition, congenital
   ovary 620.4
   pelvic (floor), female 618.8
   perineum, female 618.8
   pregnant uterus 654.4
   rectum (mucosa) (sphincter) 569.1
      due to Trichuris trichiuria 127.3
   spleen 289.59
   stomach 537.89
   umbilical cord
      affecting fetus or newborn 762.4
      complicating delivery 663.0
   ureter 593.89
      with obstruction 593.4
   ureterovesical orifice 593.89
   urethra (acquired) (infected) (mucosa) 599.5
      congenital 753.8
   uterovaginal 618.4
      complete 618.3
      incomplete 618.2
      specified NEC 618.8
   uterus (first degree) (second degree) (third degree) (complete) (without vaginal wall prolapse) 618.1
      with mention of vaginal wall prolapse — see Prolapse, uterovaginal
      congenital 752.3
      in pregnancy or childbirth 654.4
         affecting fetus or newborn 763.1
         causing obstructed labor 660.2
            affecting fetus or newborn 763.1

Prolapse, prolapsed—continued
   uterus—continued
      postpartal (old) 618.1
   uveal 871.1
   vagina (anterior) (posterior) (vault) (wall) (without uterine prolapse) 618.0
      with uterine prolapse 618.4
         complete 618.3
         incomplete 618.2
      posthysterectomy 618.5
   vitreous (humor) 379.26
      traumatic 871.1
   womb — see Prolapse, uterus
Prolapsus, female 618.9
Proliferative — see condition
Prolinemia 270.8
Prolinuria 270.8
Prolonged, prolongation
   bleeding time (see also Defect, coagulation) 790.92
      "idiopathic" (in von Willebrand's disease) 286.4
   coagulation time (see also Defect, coagulation) 790.92
   gestation syndrome 766.2
   labor 662.1
      first stage 662.0
      second stage 662.2
      affecting fetus or newborn 763.8
   PR interval 426.11
   prothrombin time (see also Defect, coagulation) 790.92
   rupture of membranes (24 hours or more prior to onset of labor) 658.2
   uterine contractions in labor 661.4
      affecting fetus or newborn 763.7
Prominauris 744.29
Prominence
   auricle (ear) (congenital) 744.29
      acquired 380.32
   ischial spine or sacral promontory with disproportion (fetopelvic) 653.3
      affecting fetus or newborn 763.1
      causing obstructed labor 660.1
         affecting fetus or newborn 763.1
   nose (congenital) 748.1
      acquired 738.0
Pronation
   ankle 736.79
   foot 736.79
      congenital 755.67
Prophylactic
   administration of
      antibiotics V07.39 ◆
      antitoxin, any V07.2
      antivenin V07.2
      chemotherapeutic agent NEC V07.39 ▼
         fluoride V07.31 ▲
      diphtheria antitoxin V07.2
      gamma globulin V07.2
      immune sera (gamma globulin) V07.2
      RhoGAM V07.2
      tetanus antitoxin V07.2
   chemotherapy NEC V07.39 ▼
      fluoride V07.31 ▲
   immunotherapy V07.2
   measure V07.9
      specified type NEC V07.8
   sterilization V25.2
Proptosis (ocular) (see also Exophthalmos) 376.30
   thyroid 242.0

Propulsion
   eyeball 360.81
Prosecution, anxiety concerning V62.5
Prostate, prostatic — see condition
Prostatism 600
Prostatitis (congestive) (suppurative) 601.9
   acute 601.0
   cavitary 601.8
   chlamydial 099.54
   chronic 601.1
   diverticular 601.8
   due to Trichomonas (vaginalis) 131.03
   fibrous 600
   gonococcal (acute) 098.12
      chronic or duration of 2 months or over 098.32
   granulomatous 601.8
   hypertrophic 600
   specified type NEC 601.8
   subacute 601.1
   trichomonal 131.03
   tuberculous (see also Tuberculosis) 016.5 [601.4]
Prostatocystitis 601.3
Prostatorrhea 602.8
Prostatoseminovesiculitis, trichomonal 131.03
Prostration 780.7
   heat 992.5
      anhydrotic 992.3
      due to
         salt (and water) depletion 992.4
         water depletion 992.3
   nervous 300.5
   newborn 779.8
   senile 797
Protanomaly 368.51
Protanopia (anomalous trichromat) (complete) (incomplete) 368.51
Protein
   deficiency 260
   malnutrition 260
   sickness (prophylactic) (therapeutic) 999.5
Proteinemia 790.99
Proteinosis
   alveolar, lung or pulmonary 516.0
   lipid 272.8
   lipoid (of Urbach) 272.8
Proteinuria (see also Albuminuria) 791.0
   Bence-Jones NEC 791.0
   gestational 646.2
      with hypertension — see Toxemia, of pregnancy
   orthostatic 593.6
   postural 593.6
Proteolysis, pathologic 286.6
Protocoproporphyria 277.1
Protoporphyria (erythrohepatic) (erythropoietic) 277.1
Protrusio acetabuli 718.65
Protrusion
   acetabulum (into pelvis) 718.65
   device, implant, or graft — see Complications, mechanical
   ear, congenital 744.29
   intervertebral disc — see Displacement, intervertebral disc
   nucleus pulposus — see Displacement, intervertebral disc
Proud flesh 701.5
Prune belly (syndrome) 756.7

Prurigo (ferox) (gravis) (Hebra's) (hebrae) (mitis) (simplex) 698.2
   agria 698.3
   asthma syndrome 691.8
   Besnier's (atopic dermatitis) (infantile eczema) 691.8
   eczematodes allergicum 691.8
   estivalis (Hutchinson's) 692.72
   Hutchinson's 692.72
   nodularis 698.3
   psychogenic 306.3
Pruritus, pruritic 698.9
   ani 698.0
      psychogenic 306.3
   conditions NEC 698.9
      psychogenic 306.3
   due to Onchocerca volvulus 125.3
   ear 698.9
   essential 698.9
   genital organ(s) 698.1
      psychogenic 306.3
   gravidarum 646.8
   hiemalis 698.8
   neurogenic (any site) 306.3
   perianal 698.0
   psychogenic (any site) 306.3
   scrotum 698.1
      psychogenic 306.3
   senile, senilis 698.8
   Trichomonas 131.9
   vulva, vulvae 698.1
      psychogenic 306.3
Psammocarcinoma (M8140/3) — see Neoplasm, by site, malignant
Pseudarthrosis, pseudoarthrosis (bone) 733.82
   joint following fusion V45.4
Pseudoacanthosis
   nigricans 701.8
Pseudoaneurysm — see Aneurysm
Pseudoangina (pectoris) — see Angina
Pseudoangioma 452
Pseudo-Argyll-Robertson pupil 379.45
Pseudoarteriosus 747.89
Pseudoarthrosis — see Pseudarthrosis
Pseudoataxia 799.8
Pseudobursa 727.89
Pseudocholera 025
Pseudochromidrosis 705.89
Pseudocirrhosis, liver, pericardial 423.2
Pseudocoarctation 747.21
Pseudocowpox 051.1
Pseudocoxalgia 732.1
Pseudocroup 478.75
Pseudocyesis 300.11
Pseudocyst
   lung 518.89
   pancreas 577.2
   retina 361.19
Pseudodementia 300.16
Pseudoelephantiasis neuroarthritica 757.0
Pseudoemphysema 518.89
Pseudoencephalitis
   superior (acute) hemorrhagic 265.1
Pseudoerosion cervix, congenital 752.49
Pseudoexfoliation, lens capsule 366.11
Pseudofracture (idiopathic) (multiple) (spontaneous) (symmetrical) 268.2
Pseudoglanders 025
Pseudoglioma 360.44
Pseudogout — see Chondrocalcinosis

Pseudohallucination 780.1
Pseudohemianesthesia 782.0
Pseudohemophilia (Bernuth's) (hereditary) (type B) 286.4
 type A 287.8
 vascular 287.8
Pseudohermaphroditism 752.7
 with chromosomal anomaly —
  see Anomaly, chromosomal
 adrenal 255.2
 female (without adrenocortical disorder) 752.7
  with adrenocortical disorder 255.2
   adrenal 255.2
 male (without gonadal disorder) 752.7
  with
   adrenocortical disorder 255.2
    cleft scrotum 752.7
   feminizing testis 257.8
   gonadal disorder 257.9
    adrenal 255.2
Pseudohole, macula 362.54
Pseudo-Hurler's disease (mucolipidosis III) 272.7
Pseudohydrocephalus 348.2
Pseudohypertrophic muscular dystrophy (Erb's) 359.1
Pseudohypertrophy, muscle 359.1
Pseudohypoparathyroidism 275.4
Pseudoinfluenza 487.1
Pseudoinsomnia 307.49
Pseudoleukemia 288.8
 infantile 285.8
Pseudomembranous — see condition
Pseudomeningocele (cerebral) (infective) (surgical) 349.81
 spinal 349.81
Pseudomenstruation 626.8
Pseudomucinous
 cyst (ovary) (M8470/0) 220
 peritoneum 568.89
Pseudomyeloma 273.1
Pseudomyxoma peritonei (M8480/6) 197.6
Pseudoneuritis optic (nerve) 377.24
 papilla 377.24
  congenital 743.57
Pseudoneuroma — see Injury, nerve, by site
Pseudo-obstruction
 intestine 564.8
Pseudopapilledema 377.24.
Pseudoparalysis
 arm or leg 781.4
 atonic, congenital 358.8
Pseudopelade 704.09
Pseudophakia V43.1
Pseudopolycythemia 289.0
Pseudopolyposis, colon 556.4 ◆
Pseudoporencephaly 348.0
Pseudopseudohypoparathyroidism 275.4
Pseudopsychosis 300.16
Pseudopterygium 372.52
Pseudoptosis (eyelid) 374.34
Pseudorabies 078.89
Pseudoretinitis, pigmentosa 362.65
Pseudorickets 588.0
 senile (Pozzi's) 731.0
Pseudorubella 057.8
Pseudoscarlatina 057.8
Pseudoscleroma 778.1

Pseudosclerosis (brain)
 Jakob's 046.1
 of Westphal (-Strümpell) (hepatolenticular degeneration) 275.1
 spastic 046.1
 with dementia (see also Dementia, presenile) 290.10
Pseudotabes 799.8
 diabetic 250.6 [337.1]
Pseudotetanus (see also Convulsions) 780.3
Pseudotetany 781.7
 hysterical 300.11
Pseudothalassemia 285.0
Pseudotrichinosis 710.3
Pseudotruncus arteriosus 747.29
Pseudotuberculosis, pasteurella (infection) 027.2
Pseudotumor
 cerebri 348.2
 orbit (inflammatory) 376.11
Pseudo-Turner's syndrome 759.89
Pseudoxanthoma elasticum 757.39
Psilosis (sprue) (tropical) 579.1
 Monilia 112.89
 nontropical 579.0
 not sprue 704.00
Psittacosis 073.9
Psoitis 728.89
Psora NEC 696.1
Psoriasis 696.1
 any type, except arthropathic 696.1
 arthritic, arthropathic 696.0
 buccal 528.6
 flexural 696.1
 follicularis 696.1
 guttate 696.1
 inverse 696.1
 mouth 528.6
 nummularis 696.1
 psychogenic 316 [696.1]
 punctata 696.1
 pustular 696.1
 rupioides 696.1
 vulgaris 696.1
Psorospermiasis 136.4
Psorospermosis 136.4
 follicularis (vegetans) 757.39
Psychalgia 307.80
Psychasthenia 300.89
 compulsive 300.3
 mixed compulsive states 300.3
 obsession 300.3
Psychiatric disorder or problem NEC 300.9
Psychogenic — see also condition
 factors associated with physical conditions 316
Psychoneurosis, psychoneurotic (see also Neurosis) 300.9
 anxiety (state) 300.00
 climacteric 627.2
 compensation 300.16
 compulsion 300.3
 conversion hysteria 300.11
 depersonalization 300.6
 depressive type 300.4
 dissociative hysteria 300.15
 hypochondriacal 300.7
 hysteria 300.10
  conversion type 300.11
  dissociative type 300.15
 mixed NEC 300.89
 neurasthenic 300.5
 obsessional 300.3
 obsessive-compulsive 300.3
 occupational 300.89
 personality NEC 301.89
 phobia 300.20
 senile NEC 300.89

Psychopathic — see also condition
 constitution, posttraumatic 310.2
  with psychosis 293.9
 personality 301.9
  amoral trends 301.7
  antisocial trends 301.7
  asocial trends 301.7
  mixed types 301.7
 state 301.9
Psychopathy, sexual (see also Deviation, sexual) 302.9
Psychophysiologic, psychophysiological condition — see Reaction, psychophysiologic
Psychose passionelle 297.8
Psychosexual identity disorder 302.6
 adult-life 302.85
 childhood 302.6
Psychosis 298.9
 acute hysterical 298.1
 affecting management of pregnancy, childbirth, or puerperium 648.4
 affective NEC 296.90

Note — Use the following fifth-digit subclassification with categories 296.0-296.6:

 0 unspecified
 1 mild
 2 moderate
 3 severe, without mention of psychotic behavior
 4 severe, specified as with psychotic behavior
 5 in partial or unspecified remission
 6 in full remission

 involutional 296.2
  recurrent episode 296.3
  single episode 296.2
 manic-depressive 296.80
  circular (alternating) 296.7
   currently depressed 296.5
   currently manic 296.4
  depressed type 296.2
   atypical 296.82
   recurrent episode 296.3
   single episode 296.2
  manic 296.0
   atypical 296.81
   recurrent episode 296.1
   single episode 296.0
  mixed type NEC 296.89
  specified type NEC 296.89
 senile 290.21
 specified type NEC 296.99
 alcoholic 291.9
  with
   anxiety 291.8 ◆
   delirium tremens 291.0
   delusions 291.5 ◆
   dementia 291.2
   hallucinosis 291.3
   mood disturbance 291.8 ◆
   jealousy 291.5
   paranoia 291.5
   persisting amnesia 291.1 ▼
   sexual dysfunction 292.8
   sleep disturbance 291.8 ▲
  amnestic confabulatory 291.1
  delirium tremens 291.0
  hallucinosis 291.3
  Korsakoff's, Korsakov's, Korsakow's 291.1
  paranoid type 291.5
  pathological intoxication 291.4
  polyneuritic 291.1
  specified type NEC 291.8

Psychosis—continued
 alternating (see also Psychosis, manic-depressive, circular) 296.7
 anergastic (see also Psychosis, organic) 294.9
 arteriosclerotic 290.40
  with
   acute confusional state 290.41
   delirium 290.41
   delusional features 290.42
   depressive features 290.43
  depressed type 290.43
  paranoid type 290.42
  simple type 290.40
  uncomplicated 290.40
 atypical 298.9
  depressive 296.82
  manic 296.81
 borderline (schizophrenia) (see also Schizophrenia) 295.5
  of childhood (see also Psychosis, childhood) 299.8
  prepubertal 299.8
 brief reactive 298.8
 childhood, with origin specific to 299.9

Note — Use the following fifth-digit subclassification with category 299:

 0 current or active state
 1 residual state

 atypical 299.8
 specified type NEC 299.8
 circular (see also Psychosis, manic-depressive, circular) 296.7
 climacteric (see also Psychosis, involutional) 298.8
 confusional 298.9
  acute 293.0
  reactive 298.2
  subacute 293.1
 depressive (see also Psychosis, affective) 296.2
  atypical 296.82
  involutional 296.2
   recurrent episode 296.3
   single episode 296.2
  psychogenic 298.0
  reactive (emotional stress) (psychological trauma) 298.0
   recurrent episode 296.3
   with hypomania (bipolar II) 296.89 ◆
   single episode 296.2
 disintegrative (childhood) (see also Psychosis, childhood) 299.1
 drug 292.9
  with
   affective syndrome 292.84
   amnestic syndrome 292.83
   anxiety 292.89 ◆
   delirium 292.81
    withdrawal 292.0
   delusional syndrome 292.11
   dementia 292.82
   depressive state 292.84
   hallucinosis 292.12
   mood disturbance 292.84 ◆
   organic personality syndrome NEC 292.89
   sexual dysfunction 292.89 ▼
   sleep disturbance 292.89 ▲
   withdrawal syndrome (and delirium) 292.0
  affective syndrome 292.84
  delusional state 292.11
  hallucinatory state 292.12

Psychosis—continued
  drug—continued
    hallucinosis 292.12
    paranoid state 292.11
    specified type NEC 292.89
    withdrawal syndrome (and delirium) 292.0
  due to or associated with physical condition (see also Psychosis, organic) 294.9
  epileptic NEC 294.8
  excitation (psychogenic) (reactive) 298.1
  exhaustive (see also Reaction, stress, acute) 308.9
  hypomanic (see also Psychosis, affective) 296.0
    recurrent episode 296.1
    single episode 296.0
  hysterical 298.8
    acute 298.1
  incipient 298.8
    schizophrenic (see also Schizophrenia) 295.5
  induced 297.3
  infantile (see also Psychosis, childhood) 299.0
  infective 293.9
    acute 293.0
    subacute 293.1
  in pregnancy, childbirth, or puerperium 648.4
  interactional (childhood) (see also Psychosis, childhood) 299.1
  involutional 298.8
    depressive (see also Psychosis, affective) 296.2
      recurrent episode 296.3
      single episode 296.2
    melancholic 296.2
      recurrent episode 296.3
      single episode 296.2
    paranoid state 297.2
    paraphrenia 297.2
  Korsakoff's, Korakov's, Korsakow's (nonalcoholic) 294.0
    alcoholic 291.1
  mania (phase) (see also Psychosis, affective) 296.0
    recurrent episode 296.1
    single episode 296.0
  manic (see also Psychosis, affective) 296.0
    atypical 296.81
    recurrent episode 296.1
    single episode 296.0
  manic-depressive 296.80
    circular 296.7
      currently
        depressed 296.5
        manic 296.4
        mixed 296.6
    depressive 296.2
      recurrent episode 296.3
        with hypomania (bipolar II) 296.89 ◆
      single episode 296.2
    hypomanic 296.0
      recurrent episode 296.1
      single episode 296.0
    manic 296.0
      atypical 296.81
      recurrent episode 296.1
      single episode 296.0
    mixed NEC 296.89
    perplexed 296.89
    stuporous 296.89
  menopausal (see also Psychosis, involutional) 298.8
  mixed schizophrenic and affective (see also Schizophrenia) 295.7
  multi-infarct (cerebrovascular) (see also Psychosis, arteriosclerotic) 290.40

Psychosis—continued
  organic NEC 294.9
    due to or associated with addiction
      alcohol (see also Psychosis, alcoholic) 291.9
      drug (see also Psychosis, drug) 292.9
    alcohol intoxication, acute (see also Psychosis, alcoholic) 291.9
    alcoholism (see also Psychosis, alcoholic) 291.9
    arteriosclerosis (cerebral) (see also Psychosis, arteriosclerotic) 290.40
    cerebrovascular disease
      acute (psychosis) 293.0
      arteriosclerotic (see also Psychosis, arteriosclerotic) 290.40
    childbirth — see Psychosis, puerperal
    conditions classified elsewhere 294.1
    dependence
      alcohol (see also Psychosis, alcoholic) 291.9
      drug 292.9
    disease
      alcoholic liver (see also Psychosis, alcoholic) 291.9
      brain
        arteriosclerotic (see also Psychosis, arteriosclerotic) 290.40
        cerebrovascular
          acute (psychosis) 293.0
          arteriosclerotic (see also Psychosis, arteriosclerotic) 290.40
        endocrine or metabolic 293.9
          acute (psychosis) 293.0
          subacute (psychosis) 293.1
        Jakob-Creutzfeldt 290.10
        liver, alcoholic (see also Psychosis, alcoholic) 291.9
    disorder
      cerebrovascular
        acute (psychosis) 293.0
      endocrine or metabolic 293.9
        acute (psychosis) 293.0
        subacute (psychosis) 293.1
      epilepsy 294.1
        transient (acute) 293.0
      Huntington's chorea 294.1
      infection
        brain 293.9
          acute (psychosis) 293.0
          chronic 294.8
          subacute (psychosis) 293.1
        intracranial NEC 293.9

Psychosis—continued
  organic—continued
    due to or associated with—continued
      disorder—continued
        infection—continued
          intracranial NEC—continued
            acute (psychosis) 293.0
            chronic 294.8
            subacute (psychosis) 293.1
        intoxication
          alcoholic (acute) (see also Psychosis, alcoholic) 291.9
          pathological 291.4
          drug (see also Psychosis, drug) 292.2
        ischemia
          cerebrovascular (generalized) (see also Psychosis, arteriosclerotic) 290.40
        Jakob-Creutzfeldt disease or syndrome 290.10
        multiple sclerosis 294.1
        physical condition NEC 294.9
        presenility 290.10
        puerperium — see Psychosis, puerperal
        sclerosis, multiple 294.1
        senility 290.20
        status epilepticus 294.1
        trauma
          brain (birth) (from electrical current) (surgical) 293.9
            acute (psychosis) 293.0
            chronic 294.8
            subacute (psychosis) 293.1
        unspecified physical condition 294.9
    infective 293.9
      acute (psychosis) 293.0
      subacute 293.1
    posttraumatic 293.9
      acute 293.0
      subacute 293.1
    specified type NEC 294.8
    transient 293.9
      with
        delusions 293.81
        depression 293.83
        hallucinations 293.82
      depressive type 293.83
      hallucinatory type 293.82
      paranoid type 293.81
      specified type NEC 293.89
  paranoic 297.1
  paranoid (chronic) 297.9
    alcoholic 291.5
    chronic 297.1
    climacteric 297.2
    involutional 297.2
    menopausal 297.2
    protracted reactive 298.4
    psychogenic 298.4
      acute 298.3

Psychosis—continued
  paranoid—continued
    schizophrenic (see also Schizophrenia) 295.3
    senile 290.20
  paroxysmal 298.9
    senile 290.20
  polyneuritic, alcoholic 291.1
  postoperative 293.9
  postpartum — see Psychosis, puerperal
  prepsychotic (see also Schizophrenia) 295.5
  presbyophrenic (type) 290.8
  presenile (see also Dementia, presenile) 290.10
  prison 300.16
  psychogenic 298.8
    depressive 298.0
    paranoid 298.4
      acute 298.3
  puerperal
    specified type — see categories 295-298
    unspecified type 293.89
      acute 293.0
      chronic 293.89
      subacute 293.1
  reactive (emotional stress) (psychological trauma) 298.8
    brief 298.8
    confusion 298.2
    depressive 298.0
    excitation 298.1
  schizo-affective (depressed) (excited) (see also Schizophrenia) 295.7
  schizophrenia, schizophrenic (see also Schizophrenia) 295.9
    borderline type 295.5
    of childhood (see also Psychosis, childhood) 299.8
    catatonic (excited) (withdrawn) 295.2
    childhood type (see also Psychosis, childhood) 299.9
    hebephrenic 295.1
    incipient 295.5
    latent 295.5
    paranoid 295.3
    prepsychotic 295.5
    prodromal 295.5
    pseudoneurotic 295.5
    pseudopsychopathic 295.5
    schizophreniform 295.4 ◆
    simple 295.0
  schizophreniform 295.4 ◆
  senile NEC 290.20
    with
      delusional features 290.20
      depressive features 290.21
    depressed type 290.21
    paranoid type 290.20
    simple deterioration 290.20
    specified type — see categories 295-298
  shared 297.3
  situational (reactive) 298.8
  symbiotic (childhood) (see also Psychosis, childhood) 299.1
  toxic (acute) 293.9
Psychotic (see also condition) 298.9
  episode 298.9
    due to or associated with physical conditions (see also Psychosis, organic) 294.9
Pterygium (eye) 372.40
  central 372.43
  colli 744.5
  double 372.44
  peripheral (stationary) 372.41
    progressive 372.42

Pterygium—continued
  recurrent 372.45
Ptilosis 374.55
Ptomaine (poisoning) (see also
      Poisoning, food) 005.9
Ptosis (adiposa) 374.30
  breast 611.8
  cecum 569.89
  colon 569.89
  congenital (eyelid) 743.61
    specified site NEC — see
        Anomaly, specified type
        NEC
  epicanthus syndrome 270.2
  eyelid 374.30
    congenital 743.61
    mechanical 374.33
    myogenic 374.32
    paralytic 374.31
  gastric 537.5
  intestine 569.89
  kidney (see also Disease, renal)
        593.0
    congenital 753.3
  liver 573.8
  renal (see also Disease, renal)
        593.0
    congenital 753.3
  splanchnic 569.89
  spleen 289.59
  stomach 537.5
  viscera 569.89
Ptyalism 527.7
  hysterical 300.11
  periodic 527.2
  pregnancy 646.8
  psychogenic 306.4
Ptyalolithiasis 527.5
Pubarche, precocious 259.1
Pubertas praecox 259.1
Puberty V21.1
  abnormal 259.9
  bleeding 626.3
  delayed 259.0
  precocious (constitutional)
        (cryptogenic) (idiopathic)
        NEC 259.1
    due to
      adrenal
        cortical hyperfunction
            255.2
          hyperplasia 255.2
      cortical hyperfunction
            255.2
      ovarian hyperfunction
            256.1
        estrogen 256.0
      pineal tumor 259.8
      testicular hyperfunction
            257.0
  premature 259.1
    due to
      adrenal cortical
            hyperfunction 255.2
      pineal tumor 259.8
      pituitary (anterior)
            hyperfunction 253.1
Puckering, macula 362.56
Pudenda, pudendum — see
      condition
Puente's disease (simple glandular
      cheilitis) 528.5
Puerperal
  abscess
    areola 675.1
    Bartholin's gland 646.6
    breast 675.1
    cervix (uteri) 670
    fallopian tube 670
    genital organ 670
    kidney 646.6
    mammary 675.1
    mesosalpinx 670
    nabothian 646.6
    nipple 675.0

Puerperal—continued
  abscess—continued
    ovary, ovarian 670
    oviduct 670
    parametric 670
    para-uterine 670
    pelvic 670
    perimetric 670
    periuterine 670
    retro-uterine 670
    subareolar 675.1
    suprapelvic 670
    tubal (ruptured) 670
    tubo-ovarian 670
    urinary tract NEC 646.6
    uterine, uterus 670
    vagina (wall) 646.6
    vaginorectal 646.6
    vulvovaginal gland 646.6
  accident 674.9
  adnexitis 670
  afibrinogenemia, or other
        coagulation defect 666.3
  albuminuria (acute) (subacute)
        646.2
    pre-eclamptic 642.4
  anemia (conditions classifiable to
        280-285) 648.2
  anuria 669.3
  apoplexy 674.0
  asymptomatic bacteriuria 646.5
  atrophy, breast 676.3
  bacteremia 670
  blood dyscrasia 666.3
  caked breast 676.2
  cardiomyopathy 674.8
  cellulitis — see Puerperal,
        abscess
  cerebrovascular disorder
        (conditions classifiable to
        430-434, 436-437) 674.0
  cervicitis (conditions classifiable
        to 616.0) 646.6
  coagulopathy (any) 666.3
  complications 674.9
    specified type NEC 674.8
  convulsions (eclamptic) (uremic)
        642.6
    with pre-existing hypertension
        642.7
  cracked nipple 676.1
  cystitis 646.6
  cystopyelitis 646.6
  deciduitis (acute) 670
  delirium NEC 293.9
  diabetes (mellitus) (conditions
        classifiable to 250) 648.0
  disease 674.9
    breast NEC 676.3
    cerebrovascular (acute) 674.0
    nonobstetric NEC (see also
        Pregnancy, complicated,
        current disease or
        condition) 648.9
    pelvis inflammatory 670
    renal NEC 646.2
    tubo-ovarian 670
    Valsuani's (progressive
        pernicious anemia)
        648.2
  disorder
    lactation 676.9
      specified type NEC 676.8
    nonobstetric NEC (see also
        Pregnancy, complicated,
        current disease or
        condition) 648.9
  disruption
    cesarean wound 674.1
    episiotomy wound 674.2
    perineal laceration wound
        674.2
  drug dependence (conditions
        classifiable to 304) 648.3
  eclampsia 642.6
    with pre-existing hypertension
        642.7

Puerperal—continued
  embolism (pulmonary) 673.2
    air 673.0
    amniotic fluid 673.1
    blood-clot 673.2
    brain or cerebral 674.0
    cardiac 674.8
    fat 673.8
    intracranial sinus (venous)
        671.5
    pyemic 673.3
    septic 673.3
    spinal cord 671.5
  endometritis (conditions
        classifiable to 615.0-615.9)
        670
  endophlebitis — see Puerperal,
        phlebitis
  endotrachelitis 646.6
  engorgement, breasts 676.2
  erysipelas 670
  failure
    lactation 676.4
    renal, acute 669.3
  fever (meaning sepsis) 670
    meaning pyrexia (of unknown
        origin) 672
  fissure, nipple 676.1
  fistula
    breast 675.1
    mammary gland 675.1
    nipple 675.0
  galactophoritis 675.2
  galactorrhea 676.6
  gangrene
    gas 670
    uterus 670
  gonorrhea (conditions classifiable
        to 098) 647.1
  hematoma, subdural 674.0
  hematosalpinx, infectional 670
  hemiplegia, cerebral 674.0
  hemorrhage 666.1
    brain 674.0
    bulbar 674.0
    cerebellar 674.0
    cerebral 674.0
    cortical 674.0
    delayed (after 24 hours)
        (uterine) 666.2
    extradural 674.0
    internal capsule 674.0
    intracranial 674.0
    intrapontine 674.0
    meningeal 674.0
    pontine 674.0
    subarachnoid 674.0
    subcortical 674.0
    subdural 674.0
    uterine, delayed 666.2
    ventricular 674.0
  hemorrhoids 671.8
  hepatorenal syndrome 674.8
  hypertrophy
    breast 676.3
    mammary gland 676.3
  induration breast (fibrous) 676.3
  infarction
    lung — see Puerperal,
        embolism
    pulmonary — see Puerperal,
        embolism
  infection
    Bartholin's gland 646.6
    breast 675.2
      with nipple 675.9
        specified type NEC
            675.8
    cervix 646.6
    endocervix 646.6
    fallopian tube 670
    generalized 670
    genital tract (major) 670
      minor or localized 646.6
    kidney (bacillus coli) 646.6

Puerperal—continued
  infection—continued
    mammary gland 675.2
      with nipple 675.9
        specified type NEC
            675.8
    nipple 675.0
      with breast 675.9
        specified type NEC
            675.8
    ovary 670
    pelvic 670
    peritoneum 670
    renal 646.6
    tubo-ovarian 670
    urinary (tract) NEC 646.6
      asymptomatic 646.5
    uterus, uterine 670
    vagina 646.6
  inflammation — see also
        Puerperal, infection
    areola 675.1
    Bartholin's gland 646.6
    breast 675.2
    broad ligament 670
    cervix (uteri) 646.6
    fallopian tube 670
    genital organs 670
      localized 646.6
      mammary gland 675.2
      nipple 675.0
      ovary 670
      oviduct 670
      pelvis 670
      periuterine 670
      tubal 670
      vagina 646.6
      vein — see Puerperal,
          phlebitis
  inversion, nipple 676.3
  ischemia, cerebral 674.0
  lymphangitis 670
    breast 675.2
  malaria (conditions classifiable to
        084) 647.4
  malnutrition 648.9
  mammillitis 675.0
  mammitis 675.2
  mania 296.0
    recurrent episode 296.1
    single episode 296.0
  mastitis 675.2
    purulent 675.1
    retromammary 675.1
    submammary 675.1
  melancholia 296.2
    recurrent episode 296.3
    single episode 296.2
  mental disorder (conditions
        classifiable to 290-303,
        305-316, 317-319) 648.4
  metritis (septic) (suppurative) 670
  metroperitonitis 670
  metrorrhagia 666.2
  metrosalpingitis 670
  metrovaginitis 670
  milk leg 671.4
  monoplegia, cerebral 674.0
  necrosis
    kidney, tubular 669.3
    liver (acute) (subacute)
        (conditions classifiable
        to 570) 674.8
    ovary 670
    renal cortex 669.3
  nephritis or nephrosis (conditions
        classifiable to 580-589)
        646.2
    with hypertension 642.1
  nutritional deficiency (conditions
        classifiable to 260-269)
        648.9
  occlusion, precerebral artery
        674.0
  oliguria 669.3
  oophoritis 670
  ovaritis 670

Puerperal—continued
  paralysis
    bladder (sphincter) 665.5
      cerebral 674.0
  paralytic stroke 674.0
  parametritis 670
  paravaginitis 646.6
  pelviperitonitis 670
  perimetritis 670
  perimetrosalpingitis 670
  perinephritis 646.6
  perioophoritis 670
  periphlebitis — see Puerperal, phlebitis
  perisalpingitis 670
  peritoneal infection 670
  peritonitis (pelvic) 670
  perivaginitis 646.6
  phlebitis 671.9
    deep 671.4
      intracranial sinus (venous) 671.5
    pelvic 671.4
    specified site NEC 671.5
    superficial 671.2
  phlegmasia alba dolens 671.4
  placental polyp 674.4
  pneumonia, embolic — see Puerperal, embolism
  prediabetes 648.8
  pre-eclampsia (mild) 642.4
    with pre-existing hypertension 642.7
    severe 642.5
  psychosis, unspecified (see also Psychosis, puerperal) 293.89
  pyelitis 646.6
  pyelocystitis 646.6
  pyelohydronephrosis 646.6
  pyelonephritis 646.6
  pyelonephrosis 646.6
  pyemia 670
  pyocystitis 646.6
  pyohemia 670
  pyometra 670
  pyonephritis 646.6
  pyonephrosis 646.6
  pyo-oophoritis 670
  pyosalpingitis 670
  pyosalpinx 670
  pyrexia (of unknown origin) 672
  renal
    disease NEC 646.2
    failure, acute 669.3
  retention
    decidua (fragments) (with delayed hemorrhage) 666.2
      without hemorrhage 667.1
    placenta (fragments) (with delayed hemorrhage) 666.2
      without hemorrhage 667.1
    secundines (fragments) (with delayed hemorrhage) 666.2
      without hemorrhage 667.1
  retracted nipple 676.0
  rubella (conditions classifiable to 056) 647.5
  salpingitis 670
  salpingo-oophoritis 670
  salpingo-ovaritis 670
  salpingoperitonitis 670
  sapremia 670
  secondary perineal tear 674.2
  sepsis (pelvic) 670
  septicemia 670
  subinvolution (uterus) 674.8
  sudden death (cause unknown) 674.9
  suppuration — see Puerperal, abscess
  syphilis (conditions classifiable to 090-097) 647.0
  tetanus 670

Puerperal—continued
  thelitis 675.0
  thrombocytopenia 666.3
  thrombophlebitis (superficial) 671.2
    deep 671.4
    pelvic 671.4
    specified site NEC 671.5
  thrombosis (venous) — see Thrombosis, puerperal
  thyroid dysfunction (conditions classifiable to 240-246) 648.1
  toxemia (see also Toxemia, of pregnancy) 642.4
    eclamptic 642.6
      with pre-existing hypertension 642.7
    pre-eclamptic (mild) 642.4
      with
        convulsions 642.6
        pre-existing hypertension 642.7
      severe 642.5
  tuberculosis (conditions classifiable to 010-018) 647.3
  uremia 669.3
  vaginitis (conditions classifiable to 616.1) 646.6
  varicose veins (legs) 671.0
    vulva or perineum 671.1
  vulvitis (conditions classifiable to 616.1) 646.6
  vulvovaginitis (conditions classifiable to 616.1) 646.6
  white leg 671.4
Pulled muscle — see Sprain, by site
Pulmolithiasis 518.89
Pulmonary — see condition
Pulmonitis (unknown etiology) 486
Pulpitis (acute) (anachoretic) (chronic) (hyperplastic) (putrescent) (suppurative) (ulcerative) 522.0
Pulpless tooth 522.9
Pulse
  alternating 427.89
    psychogenic 306.2
  bigeminal 427.89
  fast 785.0
  feeble, rapid, due to shock following injury 958.4
  rapid 785.0
  slow 427.89
  strong 785.9
  trigeminal 427.89
  water-hammer (see also Insufficiency, aortic) 424.1
  weak 785.9
Pulseless disease 446.7
Pulsus
  alternans or trigeminy 427.89
    psychogenic 306.2
Punch drunk 310.2
Puncta lacrimalia occlusion 375.52
Punctiform hymen 752.49
Puncture (traumatic) — see also Wound, open, by site
  accidental, complicating surgery 998.2
  bladder, nontraumatic 596.6
  by
    device, implant, or graft — see Complications, mechanical
    foreign body
      internal organs — see also Injury, internal, by site
      by ingested object — see Foreign body

Puncture—continued
  by—continued
    foreign body—continued
      left accidentally in operation wound 998.4
      instrument (any) during a procedure, accidental 998.2
    internal organs, abdomen, chest, or pelvis — see Injury, internal, by site
    kidney, nontraumatic 593.89
Pupil — see condition
Pupillary membrane 364.74
  persistent 743.46
Pupillotonia 379.46
  pseudotabetic 379.46
Purpura 287.2
  abdominal 287.0
  allergic 287.0
  anaphylactoid 287.0
  annularis telangiectodes 709.1
  arthritic 287.0
  autoerythrocyte sensitization 287.2
  autoimmune 287.0
  bacterial 287.0
  Bateman's (senile) 287.2
  capillary fragility (hereditary) (idiopathic) 287.8
  cryoglobulinemic 273.2
  devil's pinches 287.2
  fibrinolytic (see also Fibrinolysis) 286.6
  fulminans, fulminous 286.6
  gangrenous 287.0
  hemorrhagic (see also Purpura, thrombocytopenic) 287.3
    nodular 272.7
    nonthrombocytopenic 287.0
    thrombocytopenic 287.3
  Henoch's (purpura nervosa) 287.0
  Henoch-Schönlein (allergic) 287.0
  hypergammaglobulinemic (benign primary) (Waldenström's) 273.0
  idiopathic 287.3
    nonthrombocytopenic 287.0
    thrombocytopenic 287.3
  infectious 287.0
  malignant 287.0
  neonatorum 772.6
  nervosa 287.0
  newborn NEC 772.6
  nonthrombocytopenic 287.2
    hemorrhagic 287.0
    idiopathic 287.0
  nonthrombopenic 287.2
  peliosis rheumatica 287.0
  pigmentaria, progressiva 709.09◆
  posttransfusion 287.4
  primary 287.0
  primitive 287.0
  red cell membrane sensitivity 287.2
  rheumatica 287.0
  Schönlein (-Henoch) (allergic) 287.0
  scorbutic 267
  senile 287.2
  simplex 287.2
  symptomatica 287.0
  telangiectasia annularis 709.1
  thrombocytopenic (congenital) (essential) (hereditary) (idiopathic) (primary) (see also Thrombocytopenia) 287.3
  neonatal, transitory (see also Thrombocytopenia, neonatal transitory) 776.1
  puerperal, postpartum 666.3
  thrombotic 446.6

Purpura—continued
  thrombohemolytic (see also Fibrinolysis) 286.6
  thrombopenic (congenital) (essential) (see also Thrombocytopenia) 287.3
  thrombotic 446.6
    thrombocytic 446.6
    thrombocytopenic 446.6
  toxic 287.0
  variolosa 050.0
  vascular 287.0
  visceral symptoms 287.0
  Werlhof's (see also Purpura, thrombocytopenic) 287.3
Purpuric spots 782.7
Purulent — see condition
Pus
  absorption, general — see Septicemia
  in
    stool 792.1
    urine 599.0
  tube (rupture) (see also Salpingo-oophoritis) 614.2
Pustular rash 782.1
Pustule 686.9
  malignant 022.0
  nonmalignant 686.9
Putnam's disease (subacute combined sclerosis with pernicious anemia) 281.0 [336.2]
Putnam-Dana syndrome (subacute combined sclerosis with pernicious anemia) 281.0 [336.2]
Putrefaction, intestinal 569.89
Putrescent pulp (dental) 522.1
Pyarthritis — see Pyarthrosis
Pyarthrosis (see also Arthritis, pyogenic) 711.0
  tuberculous — see Tuberculosis, joint
Pycnoepilepsy, pycnolepsy (idiopathic) (see also Epilepsy) 345.0
Pyelectasia 593.89
Pyelectasis 593.89
Pyelitis (congenital) (uremic) 590.80
  with
    abortion — see Abortion, by type, with specified complication NEC
    calculus or stones 592.9
    contracted kidney 590.00
    ectopic pregnancy (see also categories 633.0-633.9) 639.8
    molar pregnancy (see also categories 630-632) 639.8
  acute 590.10
    with renal medullary necrosis 590.11
  chronic 590.00
    with
      calculus 592.9
      renal medullary necrosis 590.01
  complicating pregnancy, childbirth, or puerperium 646.6
  affecting fetus or newborn 760.1
  cystica 590.3
  following
    abortion 639.8
    ectopic or molar pregnancy 639.8
  gonococcal 098.19
    chronic or duration of 2 months or over 098.39

Pyelitis—continued
  tuberculous (see also
    Tuberculosis) 016.0
    [590.81]
Pyelocaliectasis 593.89
Pyelocystitis (see also Pyelitis)
  590.80
Pyelohydronephrosis 591
Pyelonephritis (see also Pyelitis)
  590.80
  acute 590.10
    with renal medullary necrosis
      590.11
  calculus 592.9
  chronic 590.00
  syphilitic (late) 095.4
  tuberculous (see also
    Tuberculosis) 016.0
    [590.81]
Pyelonephrosis (see also Pyelitis)
  590.80
  chronic 590.00
Pyelophlebitis 451.89
Pyelo-ureteritis cystica 590.3
Pyemia, pyemic (purulent) (see also
    Septicemia) 038.9
  abscess — see Abscess
  arthritis (see also Arthritis,
    pyogenic) 711.0
  Bacillus coli 038.42
  embolism — see Embolism,
    pyemic
  fever 038.9
  infection 038.9
  joint (see also Arthritis, pyogenic)
    711.0
  liver 572.1
  meningococcal 036.2
  newborn 771.8
  phlebitis — see Phlebitis
  pneumococcal 038.2
  portal 572.1
  postvaccinal 999.3
  specified organism NEC 038.8
  staphylococcal 038.1
  streptococcal 038.0
  tuberculous — see Tuberculosis,
    miliary
Pygopagus 759.4
Pykno-epilepsy, pyknolepsy
  (idiopathic) (see also Epilepsy)
  345.0
Pyle (-Cohn) disease
  (craniometaphyseal dysplasia)
  756.89
Pylephlebitis (suppurative) 572.1
Pylethrombophlebitis 572.1
Pylethrombosis 572.1
Pyloritis (see also Gastritis) 535.5
Pylorospasm (reflex) 537.81
  congenital or infantile 750.5
  neurotic 306.4
  newborn 750.5
  psychogenic 306.4
Pylorus, pyloric — see condition
Pyoarthrosis — see Pyarthrosis
Pyocele
  mastoid 383.00
  sinus (accessory) (nasal) (see also
    Sinusitis) 473.9
  turbinate (bone) 473.9
  urethra (see also Urethritis) 597.0
Pyococcal dermatitis 686.0
Pyococcide, skin 686.0
Pyocolpos (see also Vaginitis) 616.10
Pyocyaneus dermatitis 686.0
Pyocystitis (see also Cystitis) 595.9
Pyoderma, pyodermia NEC 686.0
  gangrenosum 686.0
  vegetans 686.8
Pyodermatitis 686.0
  vegetans 686.8

Pyogenic — see condition
Pyohemia — see Septicemia
Pyohydronephrosis (see also Pyelitis)
  590.80
Pyometra 615.9
Pyometritis (see also Endometritis)
  615.9
Pyometrium (see also Endometritis)
  615.9
Pyomyositis 728.0
  ossificans 728.19
  tropical (bungpagga) 040.81
Pyonephritis (see also Pyelitis)
  590.80
  chronic 590.00
Pyonephrosis (congenital) (see also
  Pyelitis) 590.80
  acute 590.10
Pyo-oophoritis (see also Salpingo-
  oophoritis) 614.2
Pyo-ovarium (see also Salpingo-
  oophoritis) 614.2
Pyopericarditis 420.99
Pyopericardium 420.99
Pyophlebitis — see Phlebitis
Pyopneumopericardium 420.99
Pyopneumothorax (infectional)
  510.9
  with fistula 510.0
  subdiaphragmatic (see also
    Peritonitis) 567.2
  subphrenic (see also Peritonitis)
    567.2
  tuberculous (see also
    Tuberculosis, pleura) 012.0
Pyorrhea (alveolar) (alveolaris) 523.4
  degenerative 523.5
Pyosalpingitis (see also Salpingo-
  oophoritis) 614.2
Pyosalpinx (see also Salpingo-
  oophoritis) 614.2
Pyosepticemia — see Septicemia
Pyosis
  Corlett's (impetigo) 684
  Manson's (pemphigus
    contagiosus) 684
Pyothorax 510.9
  with fistula 510.0
  tuberculous (see also
    Tuberculosis, pleura) 012.0
Pyoureter 593.89
  tuberculous (see also
    Tuberculosis) 016.2
Pyramidopallidonigral syndrome
  332.0
Pyrexia (of unknown origin) (P.U.O.)
  780.6
  atmospheric 992.0
  during labor 659.2
  environmentally-induced
    newborn 778.4
  heat 992.0
  newborn, environmentally-
    induced 778.4
  puerperal 672
Pyroglobulinemia 273.8
Pyromania 312.33
Pyrosis 787.1
Pyrroloporphyria 277.1
Pyuria (bacterial) 599.0

Q

Q fever 083.0
  with pneumonia 083.0 [484.8]
Quadricuspid aortic valve 746.89
Quadrilateral fever 083.0
Quadriparesis — see Quadriplegia ◆

Quadriplegia 344.00 ◆
  with fracture, vertebra (process)
    — see Fracture, vertebra,
    cervical, with spinal cord
    injury
  brain (current episode) 437.8
  C1-C4 ▼
    complete 344.01
    incomplete 344.02
  C5-C7
    complete 344.03
    incomplete 344.04 ▲
  cerebral (current episode) 437.8
  congenital or infantile (cerebral)
    (spastic) (spinal) 343.2
  cortical 437.8
  embolic (current episode) (see
    also Embolism, brain)
    434.1
  infantile (cerebral) (spastic)
    (spinal) 343.2
  newborn NEC 767.0
  spinal 344.0
  specified NEC 344.09 ◆
  thrombotic (current episode) (see
    also Thrombosis, brain)
    434.0
  traumatic — see Injury, spinal,
    cervical
Quadruplet
  affected by maternal
    complications of pregnancy
    761.5
  healthy liveborn — see Newborn,
    multiple
  pregnancy (complicating delivery)
    NEC 651.8
    with fetal loss and retention of
      one or more fetus(es)
      651.5
Quarrelsomeness 301.3
Quartan
  fever 084.2
  malaria (fever) 084.2
Queensland fever 083.0
  coastal 083.0
  seven-day 100.89
Quervain's disease 727.04
  thyroid (subacute granulomatous
    thyroiditis) 245.1
Queyrat's erythroplasia (M8080/2)
  specified site — see Neoplasm,
    skin, in situ
  unspecified site 233.5
Quincke's disease or edema — see
  Edema, angioneurotic
Quinquaud's disease (acne
  decalvans) 704.09
Quinsy (gangrenous) 475
Quintan fever 083.1
Quintuplet
  affected by maternal
    complications of pregnancy
    761.5
  healthy liveborn — see Newborn,
    multiple
  pregnancy (complicating delivery)
    NEC 651.2
    with fetal loss and retention of
      one or more fetus(es)
      651.6
Quotidian
  fever 084.0
  malaria (fever) 084.0

R

Rabbia 071
Rabbit fever (see also Tularemia)
  021.9
Rabies 071
  contact V01.5
  exposure to V01.5

Rabies—continued
  inoculation V04.5
    reaction — see Complications,
      vaccination
  vaccination, prophylactic
    (against) V04.5
Rachischisis (see also Spina bifida)
  741.9
Rachitic — see also condition
  deformities of spine 268.1
  pelvis 268.1
    with disproportion (fetopelvic)
      653.2
      affecting fetus or newborn
        763.1
      causing obstructed labor
        660.1
        affecting fetus or
          newborn 763.1
Rachitis, rachitism — see also
    Rickets
  acute 268.0
  fetalis 756.4
  renalis 588.0
  tarda 268.0
Racket nail 757.5
Radial nerve — see condition
Radiation effects or sickness — see
    also Effect, adverse, radiation
  cataract 366.46
  dermatitis 692.82
  sunburn 692.71
Radiculitis (pressure) (vertebrogenic)
  729.2
  accessory nerve 723.4
  anterior crural 724.4
  arm 723.4
  brachial 723.4
  cervical NEC 723.4
  due to displacement of
    intervertebral disc — see
    Neuritis, due to,
    displacement intervertebral
    disc
  leg 724.4
  lumbar NEC 724.4
  lumbosacral 724.4
  rheumatic 729.2
  syphilitic 094.89
  thoracic (with visceral pain)
    724.4
Radiculomyelitis 357.0
  toxic, due to
    Clostridium tetani 037
    Corynebacterium diphtheriae
      032.89
Radiculopathy (see also Radiculitis)
  729.2
**Radioactive substances, adverse
  effect** — see Effect, adverse,
    radioactive substance
Radiodermal burns (acute) (chronic)
    (occupational) — see Burn, by
    site
Radiodermatitis 692.82
Radionecrosis — see Effect, adverse,
    radiation
Radiotherapy session V58.0
Radium, adverse effect — see Effect,
    adverse, radioactive substance
Raeder-Harbitz syndrome (pulseless
    disease) 446.7
Rage (see also Disturbance, conduct)
  312.0
  meaning rabies 071
Rag sorters' disease 022.1
Raillietiniasis 123.8
Railroad neurosis 300.16
Railway spine 300.16
Raised — see Elevation
Raiva 071
Rake teeth, tooth 524.3
Rales 786.7

Ramifying renal pelvis 753.3
Ramsay Hunt syndrome (herpetic geniculate ganglionitis) 053.11
  meaning dyssynergia cerebellaris myoclonica 334.2
Ranke's primary infiltration (see also Tuberculosis) 010.0
Ranula 527.6
  congenital 750.26
Rape (see also nature and site of injury) 959.9
  alleged, observation or examination V71.5
Rapid
  feeble pulse, due to shock, following injury 958.4
  heart (beat) 785.0
    psychogenic 306.2
  respiration 786.09
    psychogenic 306.1
  second stage (delivery) 661.3
    affecting fetus or newborn 763.6
  time-zone change syndrome 307.45
Rarefaction, bone 733.99
Rash 782.1
  canker 034.1
  diaper 691.0
  drug (internal use) 693.0
    contact 692.3
  ECHO 9 virus 078.89
  enema 692.89
  food (see also Allergy, food) 693.1
  heat 705.1
  napkin 691.0
  nettle 708.8
  pustular 782.1
  rose 782.1
    epidemic 056.9
    of infants 057.8
  scarlet 034.1
  serum (prophylactic) (therapeutic) 999.5
  toxic 782.1
  wandering tongue 529.1
Rasmussen's aneurysm (see also Tuberculosis) 011.2
Rat-bite fever 026.9
  due to Streptobacillus moniliformis 026.1
  spirochetal (morsus muris) 026.0
Rathke's pouch tumor (M9350/1) 237.0
Raymond (-Céstan) syndrome 433.8
Raynaud's
  disease or syndrome (paroxysmal digital cyanosis) 443.0
  gangrene (symmetric) 443.0 [785.4]
  phenomenon (paroxysmal digital cyanosis) (secondary) 443.0
RDS 769
Reaction
  acute situational maladjustment (see also Reaction, adjustment) 309.9
  adaptation (see also Reaction, adjustment) 309.9
  adjustment 309.9
    with
      anxious mood 309.24
        with depressed mood 309.28
      conduct disturbance 309.3
        combined with disturbance of emotions 309.4
      depressed mood 309.0
        brief 309.0
          with anxious mood 309.28
        prolonged 309.1
      elective mutism 309.83

Reaction—continued
  adjustment—continued
    with—continued
      mixed emotions and conduct 309.4
      mutism, elective 309.83
      physical symptoms 309.82
      predominant disturbance (of)
        conduct 309.3
        emotions NEC 309.29
          mixed 309.28
        mixed, emotions and conduct 309.4
      specified type NEC 309.89
      specific academic or work inhibition 309.23
      withdrawal 309.83
    depressive 309.0
      with conduct disturbance 309.4
      brief 309.0
      prolonged 309.1
      specified type NEC 309.89
    affective (see also Psychosis, affective) 296.90
    specified type NEC 296.99
  aggressive 301.3
    unsocialized (see also Disturbance, conduct) 312.0
  allergic (see also Allergy) 995.3
    drug, medicinal substance, and biological — see Allergy, drug
    food — see Allergy, food
    serum 999.5
  anaphylactic — see Shock, anaphylactic
  anesthesia — see Anesthesia, complication
  anger 312.0
  antisocial 301.7
  antitoxin (prophylactic) (therapeutic) — see Complications, vaccination
  anxiety 300.00
  asthenic 300.5
  compulsive 300.3
  conversion (anesthetic) (autonomic) (hyperkinetic) (mixed paralytic) (paresthetic) 300.11
  deoxyribonuclease (DNA) (DNase) hypersensitivity NEC 287.2
  depressive 300.4
    acute 309.0
    affective (see also Psychosis, affective) 296.2
      recurrent episode 296.3
      single episode 296.2
    brief 309.0
    manic (see also Psychosis, affective) 296.80
    neurotic 300.4
    psychoneurotic 300.4
    psychotic 298.0
  dissociative 300.15
  drug NEC (see also Table of drugs and chemicals) 995.2
    allergic — see Allergy, drug
    correct substance properly administered 995.2
    obstetric anesthetic or analgesic NEC 668.9
      affecting fetus or newborn 763.5
    specified drug — see Table of drugs and chemicals
    overdose or poisoning 977.9
    specified drug — see Table of drugs and chemicals
    specific to newborn 779.4

Reaction—continued
  drug NEC—continued
    transmitted via placenta or breast milk — see Absorption, drug, through placenta
    withdrawal NEC 292.0
      infant of dependent mother 779.5
    wrong substance given or taken in error 977.9
    specified drug — see Table of drugs and chemicals
  dyssocial 301.7
  erysipeloid 027.1
  fear 300.20
    child 313.0
  fluid loss, cerebrospinal 349.0
  food — see also Allergy, food
    anaphylactic shock — see Anaphylactic shock, due to, food
  foreign
    body NEC 728.82
      in operative wound (inadvertently left) 998.4
      due to surgical material intentionally left — see Complications, due to (presence of) any device, implant, or graft classified to 996.0-996.5 NEC
    substance accidentally left during a procedure (chemical) (powder) (talc) 998.7
      body or object (instrument) (sponge) (swab) 998.4
  graft-versus-host (GVH) 996.85
  grief (acute) (brief) 309.0
    prolonged 309.1
  gross stress (see also Reaction, stress, acute) 308.9
  group delinquent (see also Disturbance, conduct) 312.2
  Herxheimer's 995.0
  hyperkinetic (see also Hyperkinesia) 314.9
  hypochondriacal 300.7
  hypoglycemic, due to insulin 251.2
    therapeutic misadventure 962.3
  hypomanic (see also Psychosis, affective) 296.0
    recurrent episode 296.1
    single episode 296.0
  hysterical 300.10
    conversion type 300.11
    dissociative 300.15
  id (bacterial cause) 692.89
  immaturity NEC 301.89
    aggressive 301.3
    emotional instability 301.59
  immunization — see Complications, vaccination
  incompatibility
    blood group (ABO) (infusion) (transfusion) 999.6
    Rh (factor) (infusion) (transfusion) 999.7
  inflammatory — see Infection
  infusion — see Complications, infusion
  inoculation (immune serum) — see Complications, vaccination
  insulin 995.2

Reaction—continued
  involutional
    paranoid 297.2
    psychotic (see also Psychosis, affective, depressive) 296.2
  leukemoid (lymphocytic) (monocytic) (myelocytic) 288.8
  LSD (see also Abuse, drugs, nondependent) 305.3
  lumbar puncture 349.0
  manic-depressive (see also Psychosis, affective) 296.80
    depressed 296.2
      recurrent episode 296.3
      single episode 296.2
    hypomanic 296.0
  neurasthenic 300.5
  neurogenic (see also Neurosis) 300.9
  neurotic NEC 300.9
  neurotic-depressive 300.4
  nitritoid — see Crisis, nitritoid
  obsessive (-compulsive) 300.3
  organic 293.9
    acute 293.0
    subacute 293.1
  overanxious, child or adolescent 313.0
  paranoid (chronic) 297.9
    acute 298.3
    climacteric 297.2
    involutional 297.2
    menopausal 297.2
    senile 290.20
    simple 297.0
  passive
    aggressive 301.84
    dependency 301.6
  personality (see also Disorder, personality) 301.9
  phobic 300.20
  postradiation — see Effect, adverse, radiation
  psychogenic NEC 300.9
  psychoneurotic (see also Neurosis) 300.9
    anxiety 300.00
    compulsive 300.3
    conversion 300.11
    depersonalization 300.6
    depressive 300.4
    dissociative 300.15
    hypochondriacal 300.7
    hysterical 300.10
      conversion type 300.11
      dissociative type 300.15
    neurasthenic 300.5
    obsessive 300.3
    obsessive-compulsive 300.3
    phobic 300.20
    tension state 300.9
  psychophysiologic NEC (see also Disorder, psychosomatic) 306.9
    cardiovascular 306.2
    digestive 306.4
    endocrine 306.6
    gastrointestinal 306.4
    genitourinary 306.50
    heart 306.2
    hemic 306.8
    intestinal (large) (small) 306.4
    laryngeal 306.1
    lymphatic 306.8
    musculoskeletal 306.0
    pharyngeal 306.1
    respiratory 306.1
    skin 306.3
    special sense organs 306.7
  psychosomatic (see also Disorder, psychosomatic) 306.9

Reaction—continued
  psychotic (see also Psychosis) 298.9
    depressive 298.0
    due to or associated with physical condition (see also Psychosis, organic) 294.9
    involutional (see also Psychosis, affective) 296.2
      recurrent episode 296.3
      single episode 296.2
    pupillary (myotonic) (tonic) 379.46
  radiation — see Effect, adverse, radiation
  runaway — see also Disturbance, conduct
    socialized 312.2
    undersocialized, unsocialized 312.1
  scarlet fever toxin — see Complications, vaccination
  schizophrenic (see also Schizophrenia) 295.9
    latent 295.5
  serological for syphilis — see Serology for syphilis
  serum (prophylactic) (therapeutic) 999.5
    immediate 999.4
  situational (see also Reaction, adjustment) 309.9
    acute, to stress 308.3
  adjustment (see also Reaction, adjustment) 309.9
  somatization (see also Disorder, psychosomatic) 306.9
  spinal puncture 349.0
  spite, child (see also Disturbance, conduct) 312.0
  stress, acute 308.9
    with predominant disturbance (of)
      consciousness 308.1
      emotions 308.0
      mixed 308.4
      psychomotor 308.2
      specified type NEC 308.3
  surgical procedure — see Complications, surgical procedure
  tetanus antitoxin — see Complications, vaccination
  toxin-antitoxin — see Complications, vaccination
  transfusion (blood) (bone marrow) (lymphocytes) (allergic) — see Complications, transfusion
  tuberculin skin test, nonspecific (without active tuberculosis) 795.5
    positive (without active tuberculosis) 795.5
  ultraviolet — see Effect, adverse, ultraviolet
  undersocialized, unsocialized — see also Disturbance, conduct
    aggressive (type) 312.0
    unaggressive (type) 312.1
  vaccination (any) — see Complications, vaccination
  white graft (skin) 996.52
  withdrawing, child or adolescent 313.22
  x-ray — see Effect, adverse, x-rays

Reactive depression (see also Reaction, depressive) 300.4
  neurotic 300.4
  psychoneurotic 300.4
  psychotic 298.0

Rebound tenderness 789.6 ◆

Recalcitrant patient V15.81

Recanalization, thrombus — see Thrombosis

Recession, receding
  chamber angle (eye) 364.77
  chin 524.06
  gingival (generalized) (localized) (postinfective) (postoperative) 523.2

Recklinghausen's disease (M9540/1) 237.71
  bones (osteitis fibrosa cystica) 252.0

Recklinghausen-Applebaum disease (hemochromatosis) 275.0

Reclus' disease (cystic) 610.1

Recrudescent typhus (fever) 081.1

Recruitment, auditory 388.44

Rectalgia 569.42

Rectitis 569.49

Rectocele
  female (without uterine prolapse) 618.0
    with uterine prolapse 618.4
      complete 618.3
      incomplete 618.2
    in pregnancy or childbirth 654.4
      causing obstructed labor 660.2
        affecting fetus or newborn 763.1
  male 569.49
  vagina, vaginal (outlet) 618.0

Rectosigmoiditis 569.89
  ulcerative (chronic) 556.3 ◆

Rectosigmoid junction — see condition

Rectourethral — see condition

Rectovaginal — see condition

Rectovesical — see condition

Rectum, rectal — see condition

Recurrent — see condition

Red bugs 133.8

Red cedar asthma 495.8

Redness
  conjunctiva 379.93
  eye 379.93
  nose 478.1

Reduced ventilatory or vital capacity 794.2

Reduction
  function
    kidney (see also Disease, renal) 593.9
    liver 573.8
  ventilatory capacity 794.2
  vital capacity 794.2

Redundant, redundancy
  abdomen 701.9
  anus 751.5
  cardia 537.89
  clitoris 624.2
  colon (congenital) 751.5
  foreskin (congenital) 605
  intestine 751.5
  labia 624.3
  organ or site, congenital NEC — see Accessory
  panniculus (abdominal) 278.1
  prepuce (congenital) 605
  pylorus 537.89
  rectum 751.5
  scrotum 608.89
  sigmoid 751.5
  skin (of face) 701.9
    eyelids 374.30
  stomach 537.89
  uvula 528.9
  vagina 623.8

Reduplication — see Duplication

Referral
  adoption (agency) V68.89
  nursing care V63.8
  patient without examination or treatment V68.81

Referral—continued
  social services V63.8

Reflex — see also condition
  blink, deficient 374.45
  hyperactive gag 478.29
  neurogenic bladder NEC 596.54
    atonic 596.54
    with cauda equina syndrome 344.61
  vasoconstriction 443.9
  vasovagal 780.2

Reflux
  esophageal 530.81
  esophagitis 530.11
  gastroesophageal 530.81
  mitral — see Insufficiency, mitral
  ureteral — see Reflux, vesicoureteral
  vesicoureteral 593.70
    with
      reflux nephropathy 593.73
        bilateral 593.72
        unilateral 593.71 ▲

Reformed gallbladder 576.0

Reforming, artificial openings (see also Attention to, artificial, opening) V55.9

Refractive error (see also Error, refractive) 367.9

Refsum's disease or syndrome (heredopathia atactica polyneuritiformis) 356.3

Refusal of
  food 307.59
    hysterical 300.11
  treatment because of, due to patient's decision NEC V64.2
    reason of conscience or religion V62.6

Regaud
  tumor (M8082/3) — see Neoplasm, nasopharynx, malignant
  type carcinoma (M8082/3) — see Neoplasm, nasopharynx, malignant

Regional — see condition

Regulation feeding (elderly) (infant) 783.3
  newborn 779.3

Regurgitated
  food, choked on 933.1
  stomach contents, choked on 933.1

Regurgitation
  aortic (valve) (see also Insufficiency, aortic) 424.1
    congenital 746.4
    syphilitic 093.22
  food — see also Vomiting ◆
    with reswallowing — see Rumination
    newborn 779.3
  gastric contents — see Vomiting ◆
  heart — see Endocarditis
  mitral (valve) — see also Insufficiency, mitral
    congenital 746.6
  myocardial — see Endocarditis
  pulmonary (heart) (valve) (see also Endocarditis, pulmonary) 424.3
  stomach — see Vomiting ◆
  tricuspid — see Endocarditis, tricuspid
  valve, valvular — see Endocarditis
  vesicoureteral — see Reflux, vesicoureteral ◆

Rehabilitation V57.9
  multiple types V57.89 ▼
  occupational V57.21 ▲
  specified type NEC V57.89
  speech V57.3
  vocational V57.22 ◆

Reichmann's disease or syndrome (gastrosuccorrhea) 536.8

Reifenstein's syndrome (hereditary familial hypogonadism, male) 257.2

Reilly's syndrome or phenomenon (see also Neuropathy, peripheral, autonomic) 337.9

Reimann's periodic disease 277.3

Reinsertion, contraceptive device V25.42

Reiter's disease, syndrome, or urethritis 099.3

Rejection
  food, hysterical 300.11
  transplant 996.80
    bone marrow 996.85
    corneal 996.51
    organ (immune or nonimmune cause) 996.80
      bone marrow 996.85
      heart 996.83
      intestines 996.89
      kidney 996.81
      liver 996.82
      lung 996.84
      pancreas 996.86
      specified NEC 996.89
    skin 996.52

Relapsing fever 087.9
  Carter's (Asiatic) 087.0
  Dutton's (West African) 087.1
  Koch's 087.9
  louse-borne (epidemic) 087.0
  Novy's (American) 087.1
  Obermeyer's (European) 087.0
  Spirillum 087.9
  tick-borne (endemic) 087.1

Relaxation
  anus (sphincter) 569.49
    due to hysteria 300.11
  arch (foot) 734
    congenital 754.61
  back ligaments 728.4
  bladder (sphincter) 596.59
  cardio-esophageal 530.89
  cervix (see also Incompetency, cervix) 622.5
  diaphragm 519.4
  inguinal rings — see Hernia, inguinal
  joint (capsule) (ligament) (paralytic) (see also Derangement, joint) 718.90
    congenital 755.8
  lumbosacral joint 724.6
  pelvic floor 618.8
  pelvis 618.8
  perineum 618.8
  posture 729.9
  rectum (sphincter) 569.49
  sacroiliac (joint) 724.6
  scrotum 680.89
  urethra (sphincter) 599.84
  uterus (outlet) 618.8
  vagina (outlet) 618.8
  vesical 596.59

Remains
  canal of Cloquet 743.51
  capsule (opaque) 743.51

Remittent fever (malarial) 084.6

Remnant
  canal of Cloquet 743.51
  capsule (opaque) 743.51
  cervix, cervical stump (acquired) (postoperative) 622.8
  cystic duct, postcholecystectomy 576.0
  fingernail 703.8
    congenital 757.5
  meniscus, knee 717.5
  thyroglossal duct 759.2
  tonsil 474.8
    infected 474.0
  urachus 753.7

Removal

Removal (of)
- catheter (urinary) (indwelling) V53.6
  - from artificial opening — see Attention to, artificial, opening
  - vascular V58.81
- device — see also Fitting (of)
  - contraceptive V25.42
  - fixation
    - external V54.8
    - internal V54.0
  - traction V54.8
- dressing V58.3
- ileostomy V55.2
- Kirschner wire V54.8
- pin V54.0
- plaster cast V54.8
- plate (fracture) V54.0
- rod V54.0
- screw V54.0
- splint, external V54.8
- subdermal implantable contraceptive V25.43
- suture V58.3
- traction device, external V54.8
- vascular catheter V58.81

Ren
- arcuatus 753.3
- mobile, mobilis (see also Disease, renal) 593.0
  - congenital 753.3
- unguliformis 753.3

Renal — see also condition
- glomerulohyalinosis-diabetic syndrome 250.4 [581.81]

Rendu-Osler-Weber disease or syndrome (familial hemorrhagic telangiectasia) 448.0

Reninoma (M8361/1) 236.91

Rénon-Delille syndrome 253.8

Repair
- pelvic floor, previous, in pregnancy or childbirth 654.4
  - affecting fetus or newborn 763.8
- scarred tissue V51

Replacement by artificial or mechanical device or prosthesis of (see also Fitting (of))
- bladder V43.5
- blood vessel V43.4
- eye globe V43.0
- heart V43.2
  - valve V43.3
- intestine V43.8
- joint V43.60
  - ankle V43.66
  - elbow V43.62
  - finger V43.69
  - hip (partial) (total) V43.64
  - knee V43.65
  - shoulder V43.61
  - specified NEC V43.69
  - wrist V43.63
- kidney V43.8
- larynx V43.8
- lens V43.1
- limb(s) V43.7
- liver V43.8
- lung V43.8
- organ NEC V43.8
- pancreas V43.8
- tissue NEC V43.8

Reprogramming
- cardiac pacemaker V53.31

Request for expert evidence V68.2

Reserve, decreased or low
- cardiac — see Disease, heart
- kidney (see also Disease, renal) 593.9

Residual — see also condition
- bladder 596.8
- foreign body — see Retention, foreign body
- state, schizophrenic (see also Schizophrenia) 295.6
- urine 788.69

Resistance, resistant (to)

Note — use the following subclassification for categories V09.5, V09.7, V09.8, V09.9:	
0	without mention of resistance to multiple drugs
1	with resistance to multiple drugs
V09.5	quinolones and fluoroquinolones
V09.7	antimycobacterial agents
V09.8	specified drugs NEC
V09.9	unspecified drugs 9

- drugs by microorganisms V09.9
  - amikacin V09.4
  - aminoglycosides V09.4
  - amodiaquine V09.5
  - amoxicillin V09.0
  - ampicillin V09.0
  - antimycobacterial agents V09.7
  - azithromycin V09.2
  - azlocillin V09.0
  - Aztreonam V09.1
  - B-lactam antibiotics V09.1
  - bacampicillin V09.0
  - bacitracin V09.8
  - Benznidazole V09.8
  - capreomycin V09.7
  - carbenicillin V09.0
  - cefaclor V09.1
  - cefadroxil V09.1
  - cefamandole V09.1
  - Cefatetan V09.1
  - cefazolin V09.1
  - Cefixime V09.1
  - Cefonicid V09.1
  - Cefoperazone V09.1
  - ceforanide V09.1
  - cefotaxime V09.1
  - cefoxitin V09.1
  - ceftazidine V09.1
  - ceftizoxime V09.1
  - ceftriaxone V09.1
  - Cefuroxime V09.1
  - cephalexin V09.1
  - cephaloglycin V09.1
  - cephaloridine V09.1
  - cephalosporins V09.1
  - cephalothin V09.1
  - cephapirin V09.1
  - cephradine V09.1
  - chloramphenicol V09.8
  - Chloraquine V09.5
  - chlorguanide V09.8
  - Chlorproguanil V09.8
  - chlortetracyline V09.3
  - cinoxacin V09.5
  - Ciprofloxacin V09.5
  - Clarithromycin V09.2
  - clindamycin V09.8
  - clioquinol V09.5
  - clofazimine V09.7
  - cloxacillin V09.0
  - cyclacillin V09.0
  - cycloserine V09.7
  - dapsone [DZ] V09.7
  - demeclocycline V09.3
  - dicloxacillin V09.0
  - doxycycline V09.3
  - enoxacin V09.5
  - erythromycin V09.2
  - ethambutol [EMB] V09.7
  - ethionamide [ETA] V09.7
  - fluoroquinolones V09.5

Resistance, resistant (to)—continued
- drugs by microorganisms—continued
  - Gentamicin V09.4
  - Halofantrine V09.8
  - Imipenem V09.1
  - iodoquinol V09.5
  - isoniazid [INH] V09.7
  - kanamycin V09.4
  - macrolides V09.2
  - mafenide V09.6
  - Mefloquine V09.8
  - Melassoprol V09.8
  - Methacillin V09.0
  - methacycline V09.3
  - Methenamine V09.8
  - metronidazole V09.8
  - mezlocillin V09.0
  - minocycline V09.3
  - nafcillin V09.0
  - nalidixic acid V09.5
  - natamycin V09.2
  - neomycin V09.4
  - netilmicin V09.4
  - Nimorazole V09.8
  - nitrofurantoin V09.8
  - Nitrofurtimox V09.8
  - norfloxacin V09.5
  - nystatin V09.2
  - Ofloxacin V09.5
  - oleandomycin V09.2
  - oxacillin V09.0
  - Oxytetracycline V09.3
  - para-amino salicylic acid [PAS] V09.7
  - paromomycin V09.4
  - penicillin (G) (V) (VK) V09.0
  - penicillins V09.0
  - pentamidine V09.8
  - piperacillin V09.0
  - primaquine V09.5
  - proguanil V09.8
  - pyrazinamide [PZA] V09.7
  - pyrimethamine/sulfalene V09.8
  - pyrimethamine/sulfodoxine V09.8
  - quinacrine V09.5
  - quinidine V09.8
  - quinine V09.8
  - quinolones V09.5
  - Rifabutin V09.7
  - rifampin [RIF] V09.7
  - rifamycin V09.7
  - rolitetracycline V09.3
  - specified drugs NEC V09.8
  - spectinomycin V09.8
  - spiramycin V09.2
  - streptomycin [SM] V09.4
  - sulfacetamide V09.6
  - sulfacytine V09.6
  - sulfadiazine V09.6
  - sulfadoxine V09.6
  - sulfamethoxazole V09.6
  - sulfapyridine V09.6
  - sulfasalizine V09.6
  - Sulfasoxazone V09.6
  - sulfonamides V09.6
  - sulfoxone V09.7
  - tetracycline V09.3
  - tetracyclines V09.3
  - thiamphenicol V09.8
  - ticarcillin V09.0
  - tinidazole V09.8
  - tobramycin V09.4
  - Triamphenicol V09.8
  - trimethoprim V09.8
  - vancomycin V09.8

Resorption
- biliary 576.8
  - purulent or putrid (see also Cholecystitis) 576.8
- dental (roots) 521.4
  - alveoli 525.8
- septic — see Septicemia
- teeth (external) (internal) (pathological) (roots) 521.4

Respiration
- asymmetrical 786.09
- bronchial 786.09
- Cheyne-Stokes (periodic respiration) 786.09
- decreased, due to shock following injury 958.4
- disorder of 786.00
  - psychogenic 306.1
  - specified NEC 786.09
- failure 518.81
  - newborn 770.8
- insufficiency 786.09
  - acute 518.82
  - newborn NEC 770.8
- Kussmaul (air hunger) 786.09
- painful 786.52
- periodic 786.09
- poor 786.09
  - newborn NEC 770.8
- sighing 786.7
  - psychogenic 306.1
- wheezing 786.09

Respiratory — see also condition
- distress 786.09
  - acute 518.82
  - fetus or newborn NEC 770.8
  - syndrome (newborn) 769
    - adult (following shock, surgery, or trauma) 518.5
    - specified NEC 518.82
- failure (acute) (chronic) 518.81

Response
- photoallergic 692.72
- phototoxic 692.72

Rest, rests
- mesonephric duct 752.8
  - fallopian tube 752.11
- ovarian, in fallopian tubes 752.19
- wolffian duct 752.8

Restless leg (syndrome) 333.99

Restlessness 799.2

Restoration of organ continuity from previous sterilization (tuboplasty) (vasoplasty) V26.0

Restriction of housing space V60.1

Restzustand, schizophrenic (see also Schizophrenia) 295.6

Retained — see Retention

Retardation
- development, developmental, specific (see also Disorder, development, specific) 315.9
  - learning, specific 315.2
    - arithmetical 315.1
    - language (skills) 315.31
      - expressive 315.31
      - mixed receptive-expressive 315.31
    - mathematics 315.1
    - reading 315.00
      - phonological 315.39
      - written expression 315.2
  - motor 315.4
- endochondral bone growth 733.91
- growth (physical) 783.4
  - due to malnutrition 263.2
  - fetal (intrauterine) 764.9
    - affecting management of pregnancy 656.5
- intrauterine growth 764.9
  - affecting management of pregnancy 656.5
- mental 319
  - borderline V62.89
  - mild, IQ 50-70 317
  - moderate, IQ 35-49 318.0
  - profound, IQ under 20 318.2
  - severe, IQ 20-34 318.1
- motor, specific 315.4

Retardation—continued
　physical 783.4
　　child 783.4
　　due to malnutrition 263.2
　　fetus (intrauterine) 764.9
　　　affecting management of
　　　　pregnancy 656.5
　psychomotor NEC 307.9
　reading 315.00
Retching — see Vomiting
Retention, retained
　bladder NEC (see also Retention,
　　urine) 788.20
　　psychogenic 306.53
　carbon dioxide 276.2
　cyst — see Cyst
　dead
　　fetus (after 22 completed
　　　weeks gestation) 656.4
　　　early fetal death (before 22
　　　　completed weeks
　　　　gestation) 632
　　ovum 631
　decidua (following delivery)
　　(fragments) (with
　　hemorrhage) 666.2
　　without hemorrhage 667.1
　deciduous tooth 520.6
　dental root 525.3
　fecal (see also Constipation)
　　564.0
　fluid 276.6
　foreign body — see also Foreign
　　body, retained
　　bone 733.99
　　current trauma — see Foreign
　　　body, by site or type
　　middle ear 385.83
　　muscle 729.6
　　soft tissue NEC 729.6
　gastric 536.8
　membranes (following delivery)
　　(with hemorrhage) 666.2
　　with abortion — see Abortion,
　　　by type
　　without hemorrhage 667.1
　menses 626.8
　milk (puerperal) 676.2
　nitrogen, extrarenal 788.9
　placenta (total) (with hemorrhage)
　　666.0
　　with abortion — see Abortion,
　　　by type
　　portions or fragments 666.2
　　　without hemorrhage 667.1
　　without hemorrhage 667.0
　products of conception
　　early pregnancy (fetal death
　　　before 22 completed
　　　weeks gestation) 632
　　following
　　　abortion — see Abortion,
　　　　by type
　　　delivery 666.2
　　　　with hemorrhage 666.2
　　　　without hemorrhage
　　　　　667.1
　secundines (following delivery)
　　(with hemorrhage) 666.2
　　with abortion — see Abortion,
　　　by type
　　complicating puerperium
　　　(delayed hemorrhage)
　　　666.2
　　without hemorrhage 667.1
　smegma, clitoris 624.8
　urine NEC 788.20
　　bladder, incomplete emptying
　　　788.21
　　psychogenic 306.53
　　specified NEC 788.29
　water (in tissue) (see also Edema)
　　782.3
Reticulation, dust (occupational) 504
Reticulocytosis NEC 790.99

Reticuloendotheliosis
　acute infantile (M9722/3) 202.5
　leukemic (M9940/3) 202.4
　malignant (M9720/3) 202.3
　nonlipid (M9722/3) 202.5
Reticulohistiocytoma (giant cell)
　277.8
Reticulohistiocytosis, multicentric
　272.8
Reticulolymphosarcoma (diffuse)
　(M9613/3) 200.8
　follicular (M9691/3) 202.0
　nodular (M9691/3) 202.0
Reticulosarcoma (M9640/3) 200.0
　nodular (M9642/3) 200.0
　pleomorphic cell type (M9641/3)
　　200.0
Reticulosis (skin)
　acute of infancy (M9722/3) 202.5
　histiocytic medullary (M9721/3)
　　202.3
　lipomelanotic 695.89
　malignant (M9720/3) 202.3
　Sézary's (M9701/3) 202.2
Retina, retinal — see condition
Retinitis (see also Chorioretinitis)
　363.20
　albuminurica 585 [363.10]
　arteriosclerotic 440.8 [362.13]
　central angiospastic 362.41
　Coat's 362.12
　diabetic 250.5 [362.01]
　disciformis 362.52
　disseminated 363.10
　　metastatic 363.14
　　neurosyphilitic 094.83
　　pigment epitheliopathy 363.15
　exudative 362.12
　focal 363.00
　　in histoplasmosis 115.92
　　　capsulatum 115.02
　　　duboisii 115.12
　　juxtapapillary 363.05
　　macular 363.06
　　paramacular 363.06
　　peripheral 363.08
　　posterior pole NEC 363.07
　gravidarum 646.8
　hemorrhagica externa 362.12
　juxtapapillary (Jensen's) 363.05
　luetic — see Retinitis, syphilitic
　metastatic 363.14
　pigmentosa 362.74
　proliferans 362.29
　proliferating 362.29
　punctata albescens 362.76
　renal 585 [363.13]
　syphilitic (secondary) 091.51
　　congenital 090.0 [363.13]
　　early 091.51
　　late 095.8 [363.13]
　syphilitica, central, recurrent
　　095.8 [363.13]
　tuberculous (see also
　　Tuberculous) 017.3
　　[363.13]
Retinoblastoma (M9510/3) 190.5
　differentiated type (M9511/3)
　　190.5
　undifferentiated type (M9512/3)
　　190.5
Retinochoroiditis (see also
　Chorioretinitis) 363.20
　central angiospastic 362.41
　disseminated 363.10
　　metastatic 363.14
　　neurosyphilitic 094.83
　　pigment epitheliopathy 363.15
　　syphilitic 094.83
　due to toxoplasmosis (acquired)
　　(focal) 130.2
　focal 363.00
　　in histoplasmosis 115.92
　　　capsulatum 115.02
　　　duboisii 115.12

Retinochoroiditis—continued
　focal—continued
　　juxtapapillary (Jensen's)
　　　363.05
　　macular 363.06
　　paramacular 363.06
　　peripheral 363.08
　　posterior pole NEC 363.07
　juxtapapillaris 363.05
　syphilitic (disseminated) 094.83
Retinopathy (background) 362.10
　arteriosclerotic 440.8 [362.13]
　atherosclerotic 440.8 [362.13]
　central serous 362.41
　circinate 362.10
　Coat's 362.12
　diabetic 250.5 [362.01]
　　proliferative 250.5 [362.02]
　exudative 362.12
　hypertensive 362.11
　of prematurity 362.21
　pigmentary, congenital 362.74
　proliferative 362.29
　　diabetic 250.5 [362.021]
　　sickle-cell 282.60 [362.29]
　solar 363.31
Retinoschisis 361.10
　bullous 361.12
　congenital 743.56
　flat 361.11
　juvenile 362.73
Retraction
　cervix (see also Retroversion,
　　uterus) 621.6
　drum (membrane) 384.82
　eyelid 374.41
　finger 736.29
　head 781.0
　lid 374.41
　lung 518.89
　mediastinum 519.3
　nipple 611.79
　　congenital 757.6
　　puerperal, postpartum 676.0
　palmar fascia 728.6
　pleura (see also Pleurisy) 511.0
　ring, uterus (Bandl's)
　　(pathological) 661.4
　　affecting fetus or newborn
　　　763.7
　sternum (congenital) 756.3
　　acquired 738.3
　　during respiration 786.9
　substernal 738.3
　supraclavicular 738.8
　syndrome (Duane's) 378.71
　uterus (see also Retroversion,
　　uterus) 621.6
　valve (heart) — see Endocarditis
Retrobulbar — see condition
Retrocaval ureter 753.4
Retrocecal — see also condition
　appendix (congenital) 751.5
Retrocession — see Retroversion
Retrodisplacement — see
　Retroversion
Retroflection, retroflexion — see
　Retroversion
Retrognathia, retrognathism
　(mandibular) (maxillary)
　524.06
Retrograde menstruation 626.8
Retroiliac ureter 753.4
Retroperineal — see condition
Retroperitoneal — see condition
Retroperitonitis (see also Peritonitis)
　567.9
Retropharyngeal — see condition
Retroplacental — see condition
Retroposition — see Retroversion
Retrosternal thyroid (congenital)
　759.2

Retroversion, retroverted
　cervix (see also Retroversion,
　　uterus) 621.6
　female NEC (see also
　　Retroversion, uterus) 621.6
　iris 364.70
　testis (congenital) 752.5
　uterus, uterine (acquired) (acute)
　　(adherent) (any degree)
　　(asymptomatic) (cervix)
　　(postinfectional) (postpartal,
　　old) 621.6
　　congenital 752.3
　　in pregnancy or childbirth
　　　654.3
　　　affecting fetus or newborn
　　　　763.8
　　　causing obstructed labor
　　　　660.2
　　　　affecting fetus or
　　　　　newborn 763.1
Retrusion, premaxilla
　(developmental) 524.04
Rett's syndrome 330.8
Reverse, reversed
　peristalsis 787.4
Reye's syndrome 331.81
Reye-Sheehan syndrome (postpartum
　pituitary necrosis) 253.2
Rh (factor)
　hemolytic disease 773.0
　incompatibility, immunization, or
　　sensitization
　　affecting management of
　　　pregnancy 656.1
　　fetus or newborn 773.0
　　transfusion reaction 999.7
　negative mother, affecting fetus or
　　newborn 773.0
　titer elevated 999.7
　transfusion reaction 999.7
Rhabdomyolysis (idiopathic) 728.89
Rhabdomyoma (M8900/0) — see
　also Neoplasm, connective
　tissue, benign
　adult (M8904/0) — see
　　Neoplasm, connective
　　tissue, benign
　fetal (M8903/0) — see Neoplasm,
　　connective tissue, benign
　glycogenic (M8904/0) — see
　　Neoplasm, connective
　　tissue, benign
Rhabdomyosarcoma (M8900/3) —
　see also Neoplasm, connective
　tissue, malignant
　alveolar (M8920/3) — see
　　Neoplasm, connective
　　tissue, malignant
　embryonal (M8910/3) — see
　　Neoplasm, connective
　　tissue, malignant
　mixed type (M8902/3) — see
　　Neoplasm, connective
　　tissue, malignant
　pleomorphic (M8901/3) — see
　　Neoplasm, connective
　　tissue, malignant
Rhabdosarcoma (M8900/3) — see
　Rhabdomyosarcoma
Rhesus (factor) (Rh) incompatibility
　— see Rh, incompatibility
Rheumaticosis — see Rheumatism
Rheumatism, rheumatic (acute NEC)
　729.0
　adherent pericardium 393
　arthritis
　　acute or subacute — see
　　　Fever, rheumatic
　　chronic 714.0
　　　spine 720.0
　articular (chronic) NEC (see also
　　Arthritis) 716.9
　　acute or subacute — see
　　　Fever, rheumatic

Rheumatism, rheumatic—continued
back 724.9
blennorrhagic 098.59
carditis — see Disease, heart, rheumatic
cerebral — see Fever, rheumatic
chorea (acute) — see Chorea, rheumatic
chronic NEC 729.0
coronary arteritis 391.9
    chronic 398.99
degeneration, myocardium (see also Degeneration, myocardium, with rheumatic fever) 398.0
desert 114.0
febrile — see Fever, rheumatic
fever — see Fever, rheumatic
gonococcal 098.59
gout 274.0
heart
    disease (see also Disease, heart, rheumatic) 398.90
    failure (chronic) (congestive) (inactive) 398.91
hemopericardium — see Rheumatic, pericarditis
hydropericardium — see Rheumatic, pericarditis
inflammatory (acute) (chronic) (subacute) — see Fever, rheumatic
intercostal 729.0
    meaning Tietze's disease 733.6
joint (chronic) NEC (see also Arthritis) 716.9
    acute — see Fever, rheumatic
mediastinopericarditis — see Rheumatic, pericarditis
muscular 729.0
myocardial degeneration (see also Degeneration, myocardium, with rheumatic fever) 398.0
myocarditis (chronic) (inactive) (with chorea) 398.0
    active or acute 391.2
        with chorea (acute) (rheumatic) (Sydenham's) 392.0
myositis 729.1
neck 724.9
neuralgic 729.0
neuritis (acute) (chronic) 729.2
neuromuscular 729.0
nodose — see Arthritis, nodosa
nonarticular 729.0
palindromic 719.30
    ankle 719.37
    elbow 719.32
    foot 719.37
    hand 719.34
    hip 719.35
    knee 719.36
    multiple sites 719.39
    pelvic region 719.35
    shoulder (region) 719.31
    specified site NEC 719.38
    wrist 719.33
pancarditis, acute 391.8
    with chorea (acute) (rheumatic) (Sydenham's) 392.0
    chronic or inactive 398.99
pericarditis (active) (acute) (with effusion) (with pneumonia) 391.0
    with chorea (acute) (rheumatic) (Sydenham's) 392.0
    chronic or inactive 393
pericardium — see Rheumatic, pericarditis
pleuropericarditis — see Rheumatic, pericarditis
pneumonia 390 [517.1]

Rheumatism, rheumatic—continued
pneumonitis 390 [517.1]
pneumopericarditis — see Rheumatic, pericarditis
polyarthritis
    acute or subacute — see Fever, rheumatic
    chronic 714.0
polyarticular NEC (see also Arthritis) 716.9
psychogenic 306.0
radiculitis 729.2
sciatic 724.3
septic — see Fever, rheumatic
spine 724.9
subacute NEC 729.0
torticollis 723.5
tuberculous NEC (see also Tuberculosis) 015.9
typhoid fever 002.0

Rheumatoid — see also condition
lungs 714.81

Rhinitis (atrophic) (catarrhal) (chronic) (croupous) (fibrinous) (hyperplastic) (hypertrophic) (membranous) (purulent) (suppurative) (ulcerative) 472.0
with
    hay fever (see also Fever, hay) 477.9
        with asthma (bronchial) 493.0
    sore throat — see Nasopharyngitis
acute 460
allergic (nonseasonal) (seasonal) (see also Fever, hay) 477.9
    with asthma (see also Asthma) 493.0
granulomatous 472.0
infective 460
obstructive 472.0
pneumococcal 460
syphilitic 095.8
    congenital 090.0
tuberculous (see also Tuberculosis) 012.8
vasomotor (see also Fever, hay) 477.9

Rhinoantritis (chronic) 473.0
    acute 461.0
Rhinodacryolith 375.57
Rhinolalia (aperta) (clausa) (open) 784.49
Rhinolith 478.1
    nasal sinus (see also Sinusitis) 473.9
Rhinomegaly 478.1
Rhinopharyngitis (acute) (subacute) (see also Nasopharyngitis) 460
    chronic 472.2
    destructive ulcerating 102.5
    mutilans 102.5
Rhinophyma 695.3
Rhinorrhea 478.1
    cerebrospinal (fluid) 349.81
    paroxysmal (see also Fever, hay) 477.9
    spasmodic (see also Fever, hay) 477.9
Rhinosalpingitis 381.50
    acute 381.51
    chronic 381.52
Rhinoscleroma 040.1
Rhinosporidiosis 117.0
Rhinovirus infection 079.3
Rhizomelique, pseudopolyarthritic 446.5
Rhoads and Bomford anemia (refractory) 284.9

Rhus
diversiloba dermatitis 692.6
radicans dermatitis 692.6
toxicodendron dermatitis 692.6
venenata dermatitis 692.6
verniciflua dermatitis 692.6

Rhythm
atrioventricular nodal 427.89
disorder 427.9
    coronary sinus 427.89
    ectopic 427.89
    nodal 427.89
escape 427.89
heart, abnormal 427.9
idioventricular 426.89
    accelerated 427.89
nodal 427.89
sleep, inversion 780.55
    nonorganic origin 307.45

Rhytidosis facialis 701.8
Rib — see also condition
cervical 756.2
Riboflavin deficiency 266.0
Rice bodies (see also Loose, body, joint) 718.1
    knee 717.6
Richter's hernia — see Hernia, Richter's
Ricinism 988.2
Rickets (active) (acute) (adolescent) (adult) (chest wall) (congenital) (current) (infantile) (intestinal) 268.0
celiac 579.0
fetal 756.4
hemorrhagic 267
hypophosphatemic with nephroticglycosuric dwarfism 270.0
kidney 588.0
late effect 268.1
renal 588.0
scurvy 267
vitamin D-resistant 275.3

Rickettsial disease 083.9
    specified type NEC 083.8
Rickettsialpox 083.2
Rickettsiosis NEC 083.9
    specified type NEC 083.8
    tick-borne 082.9
        specified type NEC 082.8
    vesicular 083.2
Ricord's chancre 091.0
Riddoch's syndrome (visual disorientation) 368.16
Rider's
bone 733.99
chancre 091.0
Ridge, alveolus — see also condition
flabby 525.2
Ridged ear 744.29
Riedel's
disease (ligneous thyroiditis) 245.3
lobe, liver 751.69
struma (ligneous thyroiditis) 245.3
thyroiditis (ligneous) 245.3
Rieger's anomaly or syndrome (mesodermal dysgenesis, anterior ocular segment) 743.44
Riehl's melanosis 709.09 ◆
Rietti-Greppi-Micheli anemia or syndrome 282.4
Rieux's hernia — see Hernia, Rieux's
Rift Valley fever 066.3
Riga's disease (cachectic aphthae) 529.0
Riga-Fede disease (cachectic aphthae) 529.0
Riggs' disease (compound periodontitis) 523.4

Right middle lobe syndrome 518.0
Rigid, rigidity — see also condition
abdominal 789.4
articular, multiple congenital 754.89
back 724.8
cervix uteri
    in pregnancy or childbirth 654.6
        affecting fetus or newborn 763.8
        causing obstructed labor 660.2
            affecting fetus or newborn 763.1
hymen (acquired) (congenital) 623.3
nuchal 781.6
pelvic floor
    in pregnancy or childbirth 654.4
        affecting fetus or newborn 763.8
        causing obstructed labor 660.2
            affecting fetus or newborn 763.1
perineum or vulva
    in pregnancy or childbirth 654.8
        affecting fetus or newborn 763.8
        causing obstructed labor 660.2
            affecting fetus or newborn 763.1
spine 724.8
vagina
    in pregnancy or childbirth 654.7
        affecting fetus or newborn 763.8
        causing obstructed labor 660.2
            affecting fetus or newborn 763.1

Rigors 780.9
Riley-Day syndrome (familial dysautonomia) 742.8
Ring(s)
aorta 747.21
Bandl's, complicating delivery 661.4
    affecting fetus or newborn 763.7
contraction, complicating delivery 661.4
    affecting fetus or newborn 763.7
esophageal (congenital) 750.3
Fleischer (-Kayser) (cornea) 275.1 [371.14]
hymenal, tight (acquired) (congenital) 623.3
Kayser-Fleischer (cornea) 275.1 [371.14]
retraction, uterus, pathological 661.4
    affecting fetus or newborn 763.7
Schatzki's (esophagus) (congenital) (lower) 750.3
    acquired 530.3
Soemmering's 366.51
trachea, abnormal 748.3
vascular (congenital) 747.21
Vossius' 921.3
late effect 366.21
Ringed hair (congenital) 757.4
Ringing in the ear (see also Tinnitus) 388.30
Ringworm 110.9
beard 110.0
body 110.5
Burmese 110.9
corporeal 110.5

Ringworm / INDEX TO DISEASES / Rupture, ruptured

Ringworm—*continued*
 foot 110.4
 groin 110.3
 hand 110.2
 honeycomb 110.0
 nails 110.1
 perianal (area) 110.3
 scalp 110.0
 specified site NEC 110.8
 Tokelau 110.5
Rise, venous pressure 459.89
Risk, suicidal 300.9
Ritter's disease (dermatitis exfoliativa neonatorum) 695.81
Rivalry, sibling 313.3
Rivalta's disease (cervicofacial actinomycosis) 039.3
River blindness 125.3 [360.13]
Robert's pelvis 755.69
 with disproportion (fetopelvic) 653.0
  affecting fetus or newborn 763.1
  causing obstructed labor 660.1
   affecting fetus or newborn 763.1
Robin's syndrome 756.0
Robinson's (hidrotic) ectodermal dysplasia 757.31
Robles' disease (onchocerciasis) 125.3 [360.13]
Rocky Mountain fever (spotted) 082.0
Rodent ulcer (M8090/3) — *see also* Neoplasm, skin, malignant
 cornea 370.07
Roentgen ray, adverse effect — *see* Effect, adverse, x-ray
Roetheln 056.9
Roger's disease (congenital interventricular septal defect) 745.4
Rokitansky's
 disease (*see also* Necrosis, liver) 570
 tumor 620.2
Rokitansky-Aschoff sinuses (mucosal outpouching of gallbladder) (*see also* Disease, gallbladder) 575.8
Rokitansky-Kuster-Hauser syndrome (congenital absence vagina) 752.49
Rollet's chancre (syphilitic) 091.0
Rolling of head 781.0
Romano-Ward syndrome (prolonged Q-T interval) 794.31
Romanus lesion 720.1
Romberg's disease or syndrome 349.89
Roof, mouth — *see* condition
Rosacea 695.3
 acne 695.3
 keratitis 695.3 [370.49]
Rosary, rachitic 268.0
Rose
 cold 477.0
 fever 477.0
 rash 782.1
  epidemic 056.9
  of infants 057.8
Rosen-Castleman-Liebow syndrome (pulmonary proteinosis) 516.0
Rosenbach's erysipelatoid or erysipeloid 027.1
Rosenthal's disease (factor XI deficiency) 286.2
Roseola 056.9
 complicated 056.8
 congenital 771.0
 infantum, infantilis 057.8

Rossbach's disease (hyperchlorhydria) 536.8
 psychogenic 306.4
Rössle-Urbach-Wiethe lipoproteinosis 272.8
Ross river fever 066.3
Rostan's asthma (cardiac) (*see also* Failure, ventricular, left) 428.1
Rot
 Barcoo (*see also* Ulcer, skin) 707.9
 knife-grinders' (*see also* Tuberculosis) 011.4
Rot-Bernhardt disease 355.1
Rotation
 anomalous, incomplete or insufficient — *see* Malrotation
 cecum (congenital) 751.4
 colon (congenital) 751.4
 manual, affecting fetus or newborn 763.8
 spine, incomplete or insufficient 737.8
 tooth, teeth 524.3
 vertebra, incomplete or insufficient 737.8
Röteln 056.9
Roth's disease or meralgia 355.1
Roth-Bernhardt disease or syndrome 355.1
Rothmund (-Thomson) **syndrome** 757.33
Rotor's disease or syndrome (idiopathic hyperbilirubinemia) 277.4
Rotundum ulcus — *see* Ulcer, stomach
Round
 back (with wedging of vertebrae) 737.10
  late effect of rickets 268.1
 hole, retina 361.31
  with detachment 361.01
 ulcer (stomach) — *see* Ulcer, stomach
 worms (infestation) (large) NEC 127.0
Roussy-Lévy syndrome 334.3
Routine postpartum follow-up V24.2
Roy (-Jutras) **syndrome** (acropachyderma) 757.39
Rubella (German measles) 056.9
 complicating pregnancy, childbirth, or puerperium 647.5
 complication 056.8
  neurological 056.00
   encephalomyelitis 056.01
   specified type NEC 056.09
  specified type NEC 056.79
 congenital 771.0
 contact V01.4
 exposure to V01.4
 maternal
  with suspected fetal damage affecting management of pregnancy 655.3
  affecting fetus or newborn 760.2
   manifest rubella in infant 771.0
 specified complications NEC 056.79
 vaccination, prophylactic (against) V04.3
Rubeola (measles) (*see also* Measles) 055.9
 complicated 055.8
 meaning rubella (*see also* Rubella) 056.9
 scarlatinosis 057.8
Rubeosis iridis 364.42
 diabetica 250.5 [364.42]

Rubinstein-Taybi's syndrome (brachydactylia, short stature, and mental retardation) 759.89
Rud's syndrome (mental deficiency, epilepsy, and infantilism) 759.89
Rudimentary (congenital) — *see also* Agenesis
 arm 755.22
 bone 756.9
 cervix uteri 752.49
 eye (*see also* Microphthalmos) 743.10
 fallopian tube 752.19
 leg 755.32
 lobule of ear 744.21
 patella 755.64
 respiratory organs in thoracopagus 759.4
 tracheal bronchus 748.3
 uterine horn 752.3
 uterus 752.3
  in male 752.7
  solid or with cavity 752.3
 vagina 752.49
Ruiter-Pompen (-Wyers) **syndrome** (angiokeratoma corporis diffusum) 272.7
Ruled out condition (*see also* Observation, suspected) V71.9
Rumination — *see* Vomiting ◆
 neurotic 300.3
 obsessional 300.3
 psychogenic 307.53
Runaway reaction — *see also* Disturbance, conduct
 socialized 312.2
 undersocialized, unsocialized 312.1
Runeberg's disease (progressive pernicious anemia) 281.0
Runge's syndrome (postmaturity) 766.2
Rupia 091.3
 congenital 090.0
 tertiary 095.9
Rupture, ruptured 553.9
 abdominal viscera NEC 799.8
  obstetrical trauma 665.5
 abscess (spontaneous) — *see* Abscess, by site
 amnion — *see* Rupture, membranes
 aneurysm — *see* Aneurysm
 anus (sphincter) — *see* Laceration, anus
 aorta, aortic 441.5
  abdominal 441.3
  arch 441.1
  ascending 441.1
  descending 441.5
   abdominal 441.3
   thoracic 441.1
  syphilitic 093.0
  thoracoabdominal 441.6
  thorax, thoracic 441.1
  transverse 441.1
  traumatic (thoracic) 901.0
   abdominal 902.0
  valve or cusp (*see also* Endocarditis, aortic) 424.1
 appendix (with peritonitis) 540.0
  with peritoneal abscess 540.1 ◆
  traumatic — *see* Injury, internal, gastrointestinal tract
 arteriovenous fistula, brain (congenital) 430
 artery 447.2
  brain (*see also* Hemorrhage, brain) 431

Rupture, ruptured—*continued*
 artery—*continued*
  coronary (*see also* Infarct, myocardium) 410.9
  heart (*see also* Infarct, myocardium) 410.9
  pulmonary 417.8
  traumatic (complication) (*see also* Injury, blood vessel, by site) 904.9
 bile duct, except cystic (*see also* Disease, biliary) 576.3
  cystic 575.4
  traumatic — *see* Injury, internal, intra-abdominal
 bladder (sphincter) 596.6
  with
   abortion — *see* Abortion, by type, with damage to pelvic organs
   ectopic pregnancy (*see also* categories 633.0-633.9) 639.2
   molar pregnancy (*see also* categories 630-632) 639.2
  following
   abortion 639.2
   ectopic or molar pregnancy 639.2
  nontraumatic 596.6
  obstetrical trauma 665.5
  spontaneous 596.6
  traumatic — *see* Injury, internal, bladder
 blood vessel (*see also* Hemorrhage) 459.0
  brain (*see also* Hemorrhage, brain) 431
  heart (*see also* Infarct, myocardium) 410.9
  traumatic (complication) (*see also* Injury, blood vessel, by site) 904.9
 bone — *see* Fracture, by site
 bowel 569.89
  traumatic — *see* Injury, internal, intestine
 Bowman's membrane 371.31
 brain
  aneurysm (congenital) (*see also* Hemorrhage, subarachnoid) 430
   late effect — *see* category 438
  syphilitic 094.87
  hemorrhagic (*see also* Hemorrhage, brain) 431
  injury at birth 767.0
  syphilitic 094.89
 capillaries 448.9
 cardiac (*see also* Infarct, myocardium) 410.9
 cartilage (articular) (current) — *see also* Sprain, by site
  knee — *see* Tear, meniscus
  semilunar — *see* Tear, meniscus
 cecum (with peritonitis) 540.0
  with peritoneal abscess 540.1 ◆
  traumatic 863.89
   with open wound into cavity 863.99
 cerebral aneurysm (congenital) (*see also* Hemorrhage, subarachnoid) 430
  late effect — *see* category 438
 cervix (uteri)
  with
   abortion — *see* Abortion, by type, with damage to pelvic organs
   ectopic pregnancy (*see also* categories 633.0-633.9) 639.2

Rupture, ruptured—continued
   cervix (uteri)—continued
      with—continued
         molar pregnancy (see also categories 630-632) 639.2
      following
         abortion 639.2
         ectopic or molar pregnancy 639.2
      obstetrical trauma 665.3
      traumatic — see Injury, internal, cervix
   chordae tendineae 429.5
   choroid (direct) (indirect) (traumatic) 363.63
   circle of Willis (see also Hemorrhage, subarachnoid) 430
      late effect — see category 438
   colon 569.89
      traumatic — see Injury, internal, colon
   cornea (traumatic) — see also Rupture, eye
      due to ulcer 370.00
   coronary (artery) (thrombotic) (see also Infarct, myocardium) 410.9
   corpus luteum (infected) (ovary) 620.1
   cyst — see Cyst
   cystic duct (see also Disease, gallbladder) 575.4
   Descemet's membrane 371.33
      traumatic — see Rupture, eye
   diaphragm (see also Hernia, diaphragm)
      traumatic — see Injury, internal, diaphragm
   diverticulum
      bladder 596.3
      intestine (large) (see also Diverticula) 562.10
         small 562.00
   duodenal stump 537.89
   duodenum (ulcer) — see Ulcer, duodenum, with perforation
   ear drum (see also Perforation, tympanum) 384.20
      with otitis media — see Otitis media
      traumatic — see Wound, open, ear
   esophagus 530.4
      traumatic 862.22
         with open wound into cavity 862.32
         cervical region — see Wound, open, esophagus
   eye (without prolapse of intraocular tissue) 871.0
      with
         exposure of intraocular tissue 871.1
         partial loss of intraocular tissue 871.2
         prolapse of intraocular tissue 871.1
      due to burn 940.5
   fallopian tube 620.8
      due to pregnancy — see Pregnancy, tubal
      traumatic — see Injury, internal, fallopian tube
   fontanel 767.3
   free wall (ventricle) (see also Infarct, myocardium) 410.9
   gallbladder or duct (see also Disease, gallbladder) 575.4
      traumatic — see Injury, internal, gallbladder
   gastric (see also Rupture, stomach) 537.89
      vessel 459.0

Rupture, ruptured—continued
   globe (eye) (traumatic) — see Rupture, eye
   graafian follicle (hematoma) 620.0
   heart (auricle) (ventricle) (see also Infarct, myocardium) 410.9
      infectional 422.90
      traumatic — see Rupture, myocardium, traumatic
   hymen 623.8
   internal
      organ, traumatic — see also Injury, internal, by site
         heart — see Rupture, myocardium, traumatic
         kidney — see Rupture, kidney
         liver — see Rupture, liver
         spleen — see Rupture, spleen, traumatic
      semilunar cartilage — see Tear, meniscus
   intervertebral disc — see Displacement, intervertebral disc
      traumatic (current) — see Dislocation, vertebra
   intestine 569.89
      traumatic — see Injury, internal, intestine
   intracranial, birth injury 767.0
   iris 364.76
      traumatic — see Rupture, eye
   joint capsule — see Sprain, by site
   kidney (traumatic) 866.03
      with open wound into cavity 866.13
      due to birth injury 767.8
      nontraumatic 593.89
   lacrimal apparatus (traumatic) 870.2
   lens (traumatic) 366.20
   ligament — see also Sprain, by site
      with open wound — see Wound, open, by site
      old (see also Disorder, cartilage, articular) 718.0
   liver (traumatic) 864.04
      with open wound into cavity 864.14
      due to birth injury 767.8
      nontraumatic 573.8
   lymphatic (node) (vessel) 457.8
   marginal sinus (placental) (with hemorrhage) 641.2
      affecting fetus or newborn 762.1
   meaning hernia — see Hernia
   membrana tympani (see also Perforation, tympanum) 384.20
      with otitis media — see Otitis media
      traumatic — see Wound, open, ear
   membranes (spontaneous)
      artificial
         delayed delivery following 658.3
         affecting fetus or newborn 761.1
         fetus or newborn 761.1
      delayed delivery following 658.2
         affecting fetus or newborn 761.1
      premature (less than 24 hours prior to onset of labor) 658.1
         affecting fetus or newborn 761.1

Rupture, ruptured—continued
   membranes—continued
      premature—continued
         delayed delivery following 658.2
         affecting fetus or newborn 761.1
   meningeal artery (see also Hemorrhage, subarachnoid) 430
      late effect — see category 438
   meniscus (knee) — see also Tear, meniscus
      old (see also Derangement, meniscus) 717.5
      site other than knee — see Disorder, cartilage, articular
      site other than knee — see Sprain, by site
   mesentery 568.89
      traumatic — see Injury, internal, mesentery
   mitral — see Insufficiency, mitral
   muscle (traumatic) NEC — see also Sprain, by site
      with open wound — see Wound, open, by site
      nontraumatic 728.83
   musculotendinous cuff (nontraumatic) (shoulder) 840.4
   mycotic aneurysm, causing cerebral hemorrhage (see also Hemorrhage, subarachnoid) 430
      late effect — see category 438
   myocardium, myocardial (see also Infarct, myocardium) 410.9
      traumatic 861.03
         with open wound into thorax 861.13
   nontraumatic (meaning hernia) (see also Hernia, by site) 553.9
      obstructed (see also Hernia, by site, with obstruction) 552.9
      gangrenous (see also Hernia, by site, with gangrene) 551.9
   operation wound 998.3
   ovary, ovarian 620.8
      corpus luteum 620.1
      follicle (graafian) 620.0
   oviduct 620.8
      due to pregnancy — see Pregnancy, tubal
   pancreas 577.8
      traumatic — see Injury, internal, pancreas
   papillary muscle (ventricular) 429.6
   pelvic
      floor, complicating delivery 664.1
      organ NEC — see Injury, pelvic, organs
   penis (traumatic) — see Wound, open, penis
   perineum 624.8
      during delivery (see also Laceration, perineum, complicating delivery) 664.4
   pharynx (nontraumatic) (spontaneous) 478.29
   postoperative 998.3
   pregnant uterus (before onset of labor) 665.0
   prostate (traumatic) — see Injury, internal, prostate

Rupture, ruptured—continued
   pulmonary
      artery 417.8
      valve (heart) (see also Endocarditis, pulmonary) 424.3
      vein 417.8
      vessel 417.8
   pupil, sphincter 364.75
   pus tube (see also Salpingo-oophoritis) 614.2
   pyosalpinx (see also Salpingo-oophoritis) 614.2
   rectum 569.49
      traumatic — see Injury, internal, rectum
   retina, retinal (traumatic) (without detachment) 361.30
      with detachment (see also Detachment, retina, with retinal defect) 361.00
   rotator cuff (capsule) (traumatic) 840.4
      nontraumatic, complete 727.61
   sclera 871.0
   semilunar cartilage, knee (see also Tear, meniscus) 836.2
      old (see also Derangement, meniscus) 717.5
   septum (cardiac) 410.8
   sigmoid 569.89
      traumatic — see Injury, internal, colon, sigmoid
   sinus of Valsalva 747.29
   spinal cord — see also Injury, spinal, by site
      due to injury at birth 767.4
      fetus or newborn 767.4
      syphilitic 094.89
      traumatic — see also Injury, spinal, by site
         with fracture — see Fracture, vertebra, by site, with spinal cord injury
   spleen 289.59
      congenital 767.8
      due to injury at birth 767.8
      malarial 084.9
      nontraumatic 289.59
      spontaneous 289.59
      traumatic 865.04
         with open wound into cavity 865.14
   splenic vein 459.0
   stomach 537.89
      due to injury at birth 767.8
      traumatic — see Injury, internal, stomach
      ulcer — see Ulcer, stomach, with perforation
   synovium 727.50
      specified site NEC 727.59
   tendon (traumatic) — see also Sprain, by site
      with open wound — see Wound, open, by site
      Achilles 845.09
         nontraumatic 727.67
      ankle 845.09
         nontraumatic 727.68
      biceps (long bead) 840.8
         nontraumatic 727.62
      foot 845.10
         interphalangeal (joint) 845.13
         metatarsophalangeal (joint) 845.12
         nontraumatic 727.68
         specified site NEC 845.19
         tarsometatarsal (joint) 845.11

Rupture, ruptured—continued
  tendon—continued
    hand 842.10
      carpometacarpal (joint) 842.11
      interphalangeal (joint) 842.13
      metacarpophalangeal (joint) 842.12
      nontraumatic 727.63
        extensors 727.63
        flexors 727.64
      specified site NEC 842.19
    nontraumatic 727.60
      specified site NEC 727.69
    patellar 844.8
      nontraumatic 727.66
    quadriceps 844.8 ◆
      nontraumatic 727.65
    rotator cuff (capsule) 840.4
      nontraumatic, complete 727.61
    wrist 842.00
      carpal (joint) 842.01
      nontraumatic 727.63
        extensors 727.63
        flexors 727.64
      radiocarpal (joint) (ligament) 842.02
      radioulnar (joint), distal 842.09
      specified site NEC 842.09
  testis (traumatic) 878.2
    complicated 878.3
    due to syphilis 095.8
  thoracic duct 457.8
  tonsil 474.8
  traumatic
    with open wound — *see* Wound, open, by site
    aorta — *see* Rupture, aorta, traumatic
    ear drum — *see* Wound, open, ear, drum
    external site — *see* Wound, open, by site
    eye 871.2
    globe (eye) — *see* Wound, open, eyeball
    internal organ (abdomen, chest, or pelvis) — *see also* Injury, internal, by site
    heart — *see* Rupture, myocardium, traumatic
    kidney — *see* Rupture, kidney
    liver — *see* Rupture, liver
    spleen — *see* Rupture, spleen, traumatic
    ligament, muscle, or tendon — *see also* Sprain, by site
      with open wound — *see* Wound, open, by site
    meaning hernia — *see* Hernia
  tricuspid (heart) (valve) — *see* Endocarditis, tricuspid
  tube, tubal 620.8
    abscess (*see also* Salpingo-oophoritis) 614.2
    due to pregnancy — *see* Pregnancy, tubal
  tympanum, tympanic (membrane) (*see also* Perforation, tympanum) 384.20
    with otitis media — *see* Otitis media
    traumatic — *see* Wound, open, ear, drum
  umbilical cord 663.8
    fetus or newborn 772.0
  ureter (traumatic) (*see also* Injury, internal, ureter) 867.2
    nontraumatic 593.89

Rupture, ruptured—continued
  urethra 599.84
    with
      abortion — *see* Abortion, by type, with damage to pelvic organs
      ectopic pregnancy (*see also* categories 633.0-633.9) 639.2
      molar pregnancy (*see also* categories 630-632) 639.2
    following
      abortion 639.2
      ectopic or molar pregnancy 639.2
    obstetrical trauma 665.5
    traumatic — *see* Injury, internal urethra
  uterosacral ligament 620.8
  uterus (traumatic) — *see also* Injury, internal uterus
    affecting fetus or newborn 763.8
    during labor 665.1
    nonpuerperal, nontraumatic 621.8
    nontraumatic 621.8
    pregnant (during labor) 665.1
      before labor 665.0
  vagina 878.6
    complicated 878.7
    complicating delivery — *see* Laceration, vagina, complicating delivery
  valve, valvular (heart) — *see* Endocarditis
  varicose vein — *see* Varicose, vein
  varix — *see* Varix
  vena cava 459.0
  ventricle (free wall) (left) (*see also* Infarct, myocardium) 410.9
  vesical (urinary) 596.6
    traumatic — *see* Injury, internal, bladder
  vessel (blood) 459.0
    pulmonary 417.8
  viscus 799.8
  vulva 878.4
    complicated 878.5
    complicating delivery 664.0

Russell's dwarf (uterine dwarfism and craniofacial dysostosis) 759.89

Russell's dysentery 004.8

Russell (-Silver) syndrome (congenital hemihypertrophy and short stature) 759.89

Russian spring-summer type encephalitis 063.0

Rust's disease (tuberculous spondylitis) 015.0 *[720.81]*

Rustitskii's disease (multiple myeloma) (M9730/3) 203.0

Ruysch's disease (Hirschsprung's disease) 751.3

Rytand-Lipsitch syndrome (complete atrioventricular block) 426.0

Saber
- shin 090.5
- tibia 090.5

Sac, lacrimal — see condition

Saccharomyces infection (see also Candidiasis) 112.9

Saccharopinuria 270.7

Saccular — see condition

Sacculation
- aorta (nonsyphilitic) (see also Aneurysm, aorta) 441.9
  - ruptured 441.5
  - syphilitic 093.0
- bladder 596.3
- colon 569.89
- intralaryngeal (congenital) (ventricular) 748.3
- larynx (congenital) (ventricular) 748.3
- organ or site, congenital — see Distortion
- pregnant uterus, complicating delivery 654.4
  - affecting fetus or newborn 763.1
  - causing obstructed labor 660.2
    - affecting fetus or newborn 763.1
- rectosigmoid 569.89
- sigmoid 569.89
- ureter 593.89
- urethra 599.2
- vesical 596.3

Sachs (-Tay) disease (amaurotic familial idiocy) 330.1

Sacks-Libman disease 710.0 [424.91]

Sacralgia 724.6

Sacralization
- fifth lumbar vertebra 756.15
- incomplete (vertebra) 756.15

Sacrodynia 724.6

Sacroiliac joint — see condition

Sacroiliitis NEC 720.2

Sacrum — see condition

Saddle
- back 737.8
- embolus, aorta 444.0
- nose 738.0
  - congenital 754.0
  - due to syphilis 090.5

Sadism (sexual) 302.84

Seamisch's ulcer 370.04

Saenger's syndrome 379.46

Sago spleen 277.3

Sailors' skin 692.74

Saint
- Anthony's fire (see also Erysipelas) 035
- Guy's dance — see Chorea
- Louis-type encephalitis 062.3
- triad (see also Hernia, diaphragm) 553.3
- Vitus' dance — see Chorea

Salicylism
- correct substance properly administered 535.4
- overdose or wrong substance given or taken 965.1

Salivary duct or gland — see also condition
- virus disease 078.5

Salivation (excessive) (see also Ptyalism) 527.7

Salmonella (aertrycke) (choleraesuis) (enteritidis) (gallinarum) (suipestifer) (typhimurium) (see also Infection, Salmonella) 003.9
- arthritis 003.23
- carrier (suspected) of V02.3
- meningitis 003.21

Salmonella—continued
- osteomyelitis 003.24
- pneumonia 003.22
- septicemia 003.1
- typhosa 002.0
  - carrier (suspected) of V02.1

Salmonellosis 003.0
- with pneumonia 003.22

Salpingitis (catarrhal) (fallopian tube) (nodular) (pseudofollicular) (purulent) (septic) (see also Salpingo-oophoritis) 614.2
- ear 381.50
  - acute 381.51
  - chronic 381.52
- Eustachian (tube) 381.50
  - acute 381.51
  - chronic 381.52
- follicularis 614.1
- gonococcal (chronic) 098.37
  - acute 098.17
- interstitial, chronic 614.1
- isthmica nodosa 614.1
- old — see Salpingo-oophoritis, chronic
- puerperal, postpartum, childbirth 670
- specific (chronic) 098.37
  - acute 098.17
- tuberculous (acute) (chronic) (see also Tuberculosis) 016.6
- venereal (chronic) 098.37
  - acute 098.17

Salpingocele 620.4

Salpingo-oophoritis (catarrhal) (purulent) (ruptured) (septic) (suppurative) 614.2
- acute 614.0
  - with
    - abortion — see Abortion, by type, with sepsis
    - ectopic pregnancy (see also categories 633.0-633.9) 639.0
    - molar pregnancy (see also categories 630-632) 639.0
  - following
    - abortion 639.0
    - ectopic or molar pregnancy 639.0
  - gonococcal 098.17
  - puerperal, postpartum, childbirth 670
  - tuberculous (see also Tuberculosis) 016.6
- chronic 614.1
  - gonococcal 098.37
  - tuberculous (see also Tuberculosis) 016.6
- complicating pregnancy 646.6
  - affecting fetus or newborn 760.8
- gonococcal (chronic) 098.37
  - acute 098.17
- old — see Salpingo-oophoritis, chronic
- puerperal 670
- specific — see Salpingo-oophoritis, gonococcal
- subacute (see also Salpingo-oophoritis, acute) 614.0
- tuberculous (acute) (chronic) (see also Tuberculosis) 016.6
- venereal — see Salpingo-oophoritis, gonococcal

Salpingo-ovaritis (see also Salpingoophoritis) 614.2

Salpingoperitonitis (see also Salpingo-oophoritis) 614.2

Salt-losing
- nephritis (see also Disease, renal) 593.9
- syndrome (see also Disease, renal) 593.9

Salt-rheum (see also Eczema) 692.9

Salzmann's nodular dystrophy 371.46

Sampson's cyst or tumor 617.1

Sandblasters'
- asthma 502
- lung 502

Sander's disease (paranoia) 297.1

Sandfly fever 066.0

Sandhoff's disease 330.1

Sanfilippo's syndrome (mucopolysaccharidosis III) 277.5

Sanger-Brown's ataxia 334.2

San Joaquin Valley fever 114.0

Sao Paulo fever or typhus 082.0

Saponification, mesenteric 567.8

Sapremia — see Septicemia

Sarcocele (benign)
- syphilitic 095.8
- congenital 090.5

Sarcoepiplocele (see also Hernia) 553.9

Sarcoepiplomphalocele (see also Hernia, umbilicus) 553.1

Sarcoid (any site) 135
- with lung involvement 135 [517.8]
- Boeck's 135
- Darier-Roussy 135
- Spiegler-Fendt 686.8

Sarcoidosis 135
- cardiac 135 [425.8]
- lung 135 [517.8]

Sarcoma (M8800/3) — see also Neoplasm, connective tissue, malignant
- alveolar soft part (M9581/3) — see Neoplasm, connective tissue, malignant
- ameloblastic (M9330/3) 170.1
  - upper jaw (bone) 170.0
- botryoid (M8910/3) — see Neoplasm, connective tissue, malignant
- botryoides (M8910/3) — see Neoplasm, connective tissue, malignant
- cerebellar (M9480/3) 191.6
  - circumscribed (arachnoidal) (M9471/3) 191.6
- circumscribed (arachnoidal) cerebellar (M9471/3) 191.6
- clear cell, of tendons and aponeuroses (M9044/3) — see Neoplasm, connective tissue, malignant
- embryonal (M8991/3) — see Neoplasm, connective tissue, malignant
- endometrial (stromal) (M8930/3) 182.0
  - isthmus 182.1
- endothelial (M9130/3) — see also Neoplasm, connective tissue, malignant
  - bone (M9260/3) — see Neoplasm, bone, malignant
- epithelioid cell (M8804/3) — see Neoplasm, connective tissue, malignant
- Ewing's (M9260/3) — see Neoplasm, bone, malignant
- germinoblastic (diffuse) (M9632/3) 202.8
  - follicular (M9697/3) 202.0
- giant cell (M8802/3) — see also Neoplasm, connective tissue, malignant
  - bone (M9250/3) — see Neoplasm, bone, malignant

Sarcoma—continued
- glomoid (M8710/3) — see Neoplasm, connective tissue, malignant
- granulocytic (M9930/3) 205.3
- hemangioendothelial (M9130/3) — see Neoplasm, connective tissue, malignant
- hemorrhagic, multiple (M9140/3) — see Kaposi's, sarcoma
- Hodgkin's (M9662/3) 201.2
- immunoblastic (M9612/3) 200.8
- Kaposi's (M9140/3) — see Kaposi's, sarcoma
- Kupffer cell (M9124/3) 155.0
- leptomeningeal (M9530/3) — see Neoplasm, meninges, malignant
- lymphangioendothelial (M9170/3) — see Neoplasm, connective tissue, malignant
- lymphoblastic (M9630/3) 200.1
- lymphocytic (M9620/3) 200.1
- mast cell (M9740/3) 202.6
- melanotic (M8720/3) — see Melanoma
- meningeal (M9530/3) — see Neoplasm, meninges, malignant
- meningothelial (M9530/3) — see Neoplasm, meninges, malignant
- mesenchymal (M8800/3) — see also Neoplasm, connective tissue, malignant
  - mixed (M8990/3) — see Neoplasm, connective tissue, malignant
- mesothelial (M9050/3) — see Neoplasm, by site, malignant
- monstrocellular (M9481/3)
  - specified site — see Neoplasm, by site, malignant
  - unspecified site 191.9
- myeloid (M9930/3) 205.3
- neurogenic (M9540/3) — see Neoplasm, connective tissue, malignant
- odontogenic (M9270/3) 170.1
  - upper jaw (bone) 170.0
- osteoblastic (M9180/3) — see Neoplasm, bone, malignant
- osteogenic (M9180/3) — see also Neoplasm, bone, malignant
  - juxtacortical (M9190/3) — see Neoplasm, bone, malignant
  - periosteal (M9190/3) — see Neoplasm, bone, malignant
- periosteal (M8812/3) — see also Neoplasm, bone, malignant
  - osteogenic (M9190/3) — see Neoplasm, bone, malignant
- plasma cell (M9731/3) 203.8
- pleomorphic cell (M8802/3) — see Neoplasm, connective tissue, malignant
- reticuloendothelial (M9720/3) 202.3
- reticulum cell (M9640/3) 200.0
  - nodular (M9642/3) 200.0
  - pleomorphic cell type (M9641/3) 200.0
- round cell (M8803/3) — see Neoplasm, connective tissue, malignant
- small cell (M8803/3) — see Neoplasm, connective tissue, malignant

Sarcoma—continued
- spindle cell (M8801/3) — see Neoplasm, connective tissue, malignant
- stromal (endometrial) (M8930/3) 182.0
  - isthmus 182.1
- synovial (M9040/3) — see also Neoplasm, connective tissue, malignant
  - biphasic type (M9043/3) — see Neoplasm, connective tissue, malignant
  - epithelioid cell type (M9042/3) — see Neoplasm, connective tissue, malignant
  - spindle cell type (M9041/3) — see Neoplasm, connective tissue, malignant

Sarcomatosis
- meningeal (M9539/3) — see Neoplasm, meninges, malignant
- specified site NEC (M8800/3) — see Neoplasm, connective tissue, malignant
- unspecified site (M8800/6) 171.9

Sarcosinemia 270.8
Sarcosporidiosis 136.5
Saturnine — see condition
Saturnism 984.9
- specified type of lead — see Table of drugs and chemicals

Satyriasis 302.89
Sauriasis — see Ichthyosis
Sauriderma 757.39
Sauriosis — see Ichthyosis
Savill's disease (epidemic exfoliative dermatitis) 695.89
SBE (subacute bacterial endocarditis) 421.0
Scabies (any site) 133.0
Scabs 782.8
Scaglietti-Dagnini syndrome (acromegalic macrospondylitis) 253.0
Scald, scalded — see also Burn, by site
- skin syndrome 695.1

Scalenus anticus (anterior) syndrome 353.0
Scales 782.8
Scalp — see condition
Scaphocephaly 756.0
Scaphoiditis, tarsal 732.5
Scapulalgia 733.90
Scapulohumeral myopathy 359.1
Scar, scarring (see also Cicatrix) 709.2
- adherent 709.2
- atrophic 709.2
- cervix
  - in pregnancy or childbirth 654.6
    - affecting fetus or newborn 763.8
    - causing obstructed labor 660.2
      - affecting fetus or newborn 763.1
- cheloid 701.4
- chorioretinal 363.30
  - disseminated 363.35
  - macular 363.32
  - peripheral 363.34
  - posterior pole NEC 363.33
- choroid (see also Scar, chorioretinal) 363.30
- compression, pericardial 423.9

Scar, scarring—continued
- congenital 757.39
- conjunctiva 372.64
- cornea 371.00
  - xerophthalmic 264.6
- due to previous cesarean delivery, complicating pregnancy or childbirth 654.2
  - affecting fetus or newborn 763.8
- duodenal (bulb) (cap) 537.3
- hypertrophic 701.4
- keloid 701.4
- labia 624.4
- lung (base) 518.89
- macula 363.32
  - disseminated 363.35
  - peripheral 363.34
- muscle 728.89
- myocardium, myocardial 412
- painful 709.2
- papillary muscle 429.81
- posterior pole NEC 363.33
  - macular — see Scar, macula
- postnecrotic (hepatic) (liver) 571.9
- psychic V15.4
- retina (see also Scar, chorioretinal) 363.30
- trachea 478.9
- uterus 621.8
  - in pregnancy or childbirth NEC 654.9
    - affecting fetus or newborn 763.8
    - due to previous cesarean delivery 654.2
- vulva 624.4

Scarabiasis 134.1
Scarlatina 034.1
- anginosa 034.1
- maligna 034.1
- myocarditis, acute 034.1 [422.01]
- old (see also Myocarditis) 429.0
- otitis media 034.1 [382.02]
- ulcerosa 034.1

Scarlatinella 057.8
Scarlet fever (albuminuria) (angina) (convulsions) (lesions of lid) (rash) 034.1
Schamberg's disease, dermatitis, or dermatosis (progressive pigmentary dermatosis) 709.09 ◆
Schatzki's ring (esophagus) (lower) (congenital) 750.3
- acquired 530.3

Schaufenster krankheit 413.9
Schaumann's
- benign lymphogranulomatosis 135
- disease (sarcoidosis) 135
- syndrome (sarcoidosis) 135

Scheie's syndrome (mucopolysaccharidosis IS) 277.5
Schenck's disease (sporotrichosis) 117.1
Scheuermann's disease or osteochondrosis 732.0
Scheuthauer-Marie-Sainton syndrome (cleidocranialis dysostosis) 755.59
Schilder (-Flatau) disease 341.1
Schilling-type monocytic leukemia (M9890/3) 206.9
Schimmelbusch's disease, cystic mastitis, or hyperplasia 610.1
Schirmer's syndrome (encephalocutaneous angiomatosis) 759.6
Schistocelia 756.7
Schistoglossia 750.13

Schistosoma infestation — see Infestation, Schistosoma
Schistosomiasis 120.9
- Asiatic 120.2
- bladder 120.0
- chestermani 120.8
- colon 120.1
- cutaneous 120.3
- due to
  - S. hematobium 120.0
  - S. japonicum 120.2
  - S. mansoni 120.1
  - S. mattheii 120.8
- eastern 120.2
- genitourinary tract 120.0
- intestinal 120.1
- lung 120.2
- Manson's (intestinal) 120.1
- Oriental 120.2
- pulmonary 120.2
- specified type NEC 120.8
- vesical 120.0

Schizencephaly 742.4
Schizo-affective psychosis (see also Schizophrenia) 295.7
Schizodontia 520.2
Schizoid personality 301.20
- introverted 301.21
- schizotypal 301.22

Schizophrenia, schizophrenic (reaction) 295.9

Note — Use the following fifth-digit subclassification with category 295

0	unspecified
1	subchronic
2	chronic
3	subchronic with acute exacerbation
4	chronic with acute exacerbation
5	in remission

- acute (attack) NEC 295.8
  - episode 295.4
- atypical form 295.8
- borderline 295.5
- catalepsy 295.2
- catatonic (type) (acute) (excited) (withdrawn) 295.2
- childhood (type) (see also Psychosis, childhood) 299.9
- chronic NEC 295.6
- coenesthesiopathic 295.8
- cyclic (type) 295.7
- disorganized (type) 295.1
- flexibilitas cerea 295.2
- hebephrenic (type) (acute) 295.1
- incipient 295.5
- latent 295.5
- paranoid (type) (acute) 295.3
- paraphrenic (acute) 295.3
- prepsychotic 295.5
- primary (acute) 295.0
- prodromal 295.5
- pseudoneurotic 295.5
- pseudopsychopathic 295.5
- reaction 295.9
- residual (state) (type) 295.6
- restzustand 295.6
- schizo-affective (type) (depressed) (excited) 295.7
- schizophreniform type 295.4 ◆
- simple (type) (acute) 295.0
- simplex (acute) 295.0
- specified type NEC 295.8
- syndrome of childhood NEC (see also Psychosis, childhood) 299.9
- undifferentiated 295.9
  - acute 295.8
  - chronic 295.6

Schizothymia 301.20
- introverted 301.21
- schizotypal 301.22

Schlafkrankheit 086.5
Schlatter's tibia (osteochondrosis) 732.4
Schlatter-Osgood disease (osteochondrosis, tibial tubercle) 732.4
Schloffer's tumor (see also Peritonitis) 567.2
Schmidt's syndrome
- sphallo-pharyngo-laryngeal hemiplegia 352.6
- thyroid-adrenocortical insufficiency 258.1
- vagoaccessory 352.6

Schmincke
- carcinoma (M8082/3) — see Neoplasm, nasopharynx, malignant
- tumor (M8082/3) — see Neoplasm, nasopharynx, malignant

Schmitz (-Stutzer) dysentery 004.0
Schmorl's disease or nodes 722.30
- lumbar, lumbosacral 722.32
- specified region NEC 722.39
- thoracic, thoracolumbar 722.31

Schneider's syndrome 047.9
Schneiderian
- carcinoma (M8121/3)
  - specified site — see Neoplasm, by site, malignant
  - unspecified site 160.0
- papilloma (M8121/0)
  - specified site — see Neoplasm, by site, benign
  - unspecified site 212.0

Schoffer's tumor (see also Peritonitis) 567.2
Scholte's syndrome (malignant carcinoid) 259.2
Scholz's disease 330.0
Scholz (-Bielschowsky-Henneberg) syndrome 330.0
Schönlein (-Henoch) disease (primary) (purpura) (rheumatic) 287.0
School examination V70.3
Schottmüller's disease (see also Fever, paratyphoid) 002.9
Schroeder's syndrome (endocrine-hypertensive) 255.3
Schüller-Christian disease or syndrome (chronic histiocytosis X) 277.8
Schultz's disease or syndrome (agranulocytosis) 288.0
Schultze's acroparesthesia, simple 443.89
Schwalbe-Ziehen-Oppenheimer disease 333.6
Schwannoma (M9560/0) — see also Neoplasm, connective tissue, benign
- malignant (M9560/3) — see Neoplasm, connective tissue, malignant

Schwartz (-Jampel) syndrome 756.89
Schwartz-Bartter syndrome (inappropriate secretion of antidiuretic hormone) 253.6
Schweninger-Buzzi disease (macular atrophy) 701.3
Sciatic — see condition
Sciatica (infectional) 724.3
- due to
  - displacement of intervertebral disc 722.10

Sciatica—continued
   due to—continued
      herniation, nucleus pulposus 722.10
Scimitar syndrome (anomalous venous drainage, right lung to inferior vena cava) 747.49
Sclera — see condition
Sclerectasia 379.11
Scleredema
   adultorum 710.1
   Buschke's 710.1
   newborn 778.1
Sclerema
   adiposum (newborn) 778.1
   adultorum 710.1
   edematosum (newborn) 778.1
   neonatorum 778.1
   newborn 778.1
Scleriasis — see Scleroderma
Scleritis 379.00
   with corneal involvement 379.05
   anterior (annular) (localized) 379.03
   brawny 379.06
   granulomatous 379.09
   posterior 379.07
   specified NEC 379.09
   suppurative 379.09
   syphilitic 095.0
   tuberculous (nodular) (see also Tuberculosis) 017.3 [379.09]
Sclerochoroiditis (see also Scleritis) 379.00
Scleroconjunctivitis (see also Scleritis) 379.00
Sclerocystic ovary (syndrome) 256.4
Sclerodactylia 701.0
Scleroderma, sclerodermia (acrosclerotic) (diffuse) (generalized) (progressive) (pulmonary) 710.1
   circumscribed 701.0
   linear 701.0
   localized (linear) 701.0
   newborn 778.1
Sclerokeratitis 379.05
   meaning sclerosing keratitis 370.54
   tuberculous (see also Tuberculosis) 017.3 [379.09]
Scleroma, trachea 040.1
Scleromalacia
   multiple 731.0
   perforans 379.04
Scleromyxedema 701.8
Scleroperikeratitis 379.05
Sclerose en plaques 340
Sclerosis, sclerotic
   adrenal (gland) 255.8
   Alzheimer's 331.0
      with dementia — see Alzheimer's, dementia
   amyotrophic (lateral) 335.20
   annularis fibrosi
      aortic 424.1
      mitral 424.0
   aorta, aortic 440.0
      valve (see also Endocarditis, aortic) 424.1
   artery, arterial, arteriolar, arteriovascular — see Arteriosclerosis
   ascending multiple 340
   Baló's (concentric) 341.1
   basilar — see Sclerosis, brain
   bone (localized) NEC 733.99
   brain (general) (lobular) 341.9
      Alzheimer's — see Alzheimer's, dementia
      artery, arterial 437.0

Sclerosis, sclerotic—continued
   brain—continued
      atrophic lobar 331.0
         with dementia 290.10
      diffuse 341.1
         familial (chronic) (infantile) 330.0
         infantile (chronic) (familial) 330.0
         Pelizaeus-Merzbacher type 330.0
      disseminated 340
      hereditary 334.2
      infantile, (degenerative) (diffuse) 330.0
      insular 340
      Krabbe's 330.0
      miliary 340
      multiple 340
      Pelizaeus-Merzbacher 330.0
      presenile (Alzheimer's) 331.0
         with dementia 290.10
      progressive familial 330.0
      senile 437.0
      tuberous 759.5
   bulbar, progressive 340
   bundle of His 426.50
      left 426.3
      right 426.4
   cardiac — see Arteriosclerosis, coronary ◆
   cardiorenal (see also Hypertension, cardiorenal) 404.90
   cardiovascular (see also Disease, cardiovascular) 429.2
      renal (see also Hypertension, cardiorenal) 404.90
   centrolobar, familial 330.0
   cerebellar — see Sclerosis, brain
   cerebral — see Sclerosis, brain
   cerebrospinal 340
      disseminated 340
      multiple 340
   cerebrovascular 437.0
   choroid 363.40
      diffuse 363.56
   combined (spinal cord) — see also Degeneration, combined
      multiple 340
   concentric, Baló's 341.1
   cornea 370.54
   coronary (artery) — see Arteriosclerosis, coronary ◆
   corpus cavernosum
      female 624.8
      male 607.89
   Dewitzky's
      aortic 424.1
      mitral 424.0
   diffuse NEC 341.1
   disease, heart — see Arteriosclerosis, coronary ◆
   disseminated 340
   dorsal 340
   dorsolateral (spinal cord) — see Degeneration, combined
   endometrium 621.8
   extrapyramidal 333.90
   eye, nuclear (senile) 366.16
   Friedreich's (spinal cord) 334.0
   funicular (spermatic cord) 608.89
   gastritis 535.4
   general (vascular) — see Arteriosclerosis
   gland (lymphatic) 457.8
   hepatic 571.9
   hereditary
      cerebellar 334.2
      spinal 334.0
   idiopathic cortical (Garré's) (see also Osteomyelitis) 730.1
   ilium, piriform 733.5
   insular 340
      pancreas 251.8
   Islands of Langerhans 251.8

Sclerosis, sclerotic—continued
   kidney — see Sclerosis, renal
   larynx 478.79
   lateral 335.24
      amyotrophic 335.20
      descending 335.24
      primary 335.24
      spinal 335.24
   liver 571.9
   lobar, atrophic (of brain) 331.0
      with dementia 290.10
   lung (see also Fibrosis, lung) 515
   mastoid 383.1
   mitral — see Endocarditis, mitral
   Mönckeberg's (medial) (see also Arteriosclerosis, extremities) 440.20
   multiple (brain stem) (cerebral) (generalized) (spinal cord) 340
   myocardium, myocardial — see Arteriosclerosis, coronary ◆
   nuclear (senile), eye 366.16
   ovary 620.8
   pancreas 577.8
   penis 607.89
   peripheral arteries NEC (see also Arteriosclerosis, extremities) 440.20
   plaques 340
   pluriglandular 258.8
   polyglandular 258.8
   posterior (spinal cord) (syphilitic) 094.0
   posterolateral (spinal cord) — see Degeneration, combined
   prepuce 607.89
   presenile (Alzheimer's) 331.0
      with dementia 290.10
   primary lateral 335.24
   progressive systemic 710.1
   pulmonary (see also Fibrosis, lung) 515
      artery 416.0
      valve (heart) (see also Endocarditis, pulmonary) 424.3
   renal 587
      with
         cystine storage disease 270.0
         hypertension (see also Hypertension, kidney) 403.90
         hypertensive heart disease (conditions classifiable to 402) (see also Hypertension, cardiorenal) 404.90
         arteriolar (hyaline) (see also Hypertension, kidney) 403.90
         hyperplastic (see also Hypertension, kidney) 403.90
   retina (senile) (vascular) 362.17
   rheumatic
      aortic valve 395.9
      mitral valve 394.9
   Schilder's 341.1
   senile — see Arteriosclerosis
   spinal (cord) (general) (progressive) (transverse) 336.8
      ascending 357.0
      combined — see also Degeneration, combined
         multiple 340
         syphilitic 094.89
      disseminated 340
      dorsolateral — see Degeneration, combined
      hereditary (Friedreich's) (mixed form) 334.0
      lateral (amyotrophic) 335.24
      multiple 340

Sclerosis, sclerotic—continued
   spinal—continued
      posterior (syphilitic) 094.0
   stomach 537.89
   subendocardial, congenital 425.3
   systemic (progressive) 710.1
      with lung involvement 710.1 [517.2]
   tricuspid (heart) (valve) — see Endocarditis, tricuspid
   tuberous (brain) 759.5
   tympanic membrane (see also Tympanosclerosis) 385.00
   valve, valvular (heart) — see Endocarditis
   vascular — see Arteriosclerosis
   vein 459.89
Sclerotenonitis 379.07
Sclerotitis (see also Scleritis) 379.00
   syphilitic 095.0
   tuberculous (see also Tuberculosis) 017.3 [379.09]
Scoliosis (acquired) (postural) 737.30
   congenital 754.2
   due to or associated with
      Charcot-Marie-Tooth disease 356.1 [737.43]
      mucopolysaccharidosis 277.5 [737.43]
      neurofibromatosis 237.71 [737.43]
      osteitis
         deformans 731.0 [737.43]
         fibrosa cystica 252.0 [737.43]
      osteoporosis (see also Osteoporosis) 733.00 [737.43]
      poliomyelitis 138 [737.43]
      radiation 737.33
      tuberculosis (see also Tuberculosis) 015.0 [737.43]
   idiopathic 737.30
   infantile
      progressive 737.32
      resolving 737.31
   paralytic 737.39
   rachitic 268.1
   sciatic 724.3
   specified NEC 737.39
   thoracogenic 737.34
   tuberculous (see also Tuberculosis) 015.0 [737.43]
Scoliotic pelvis 738.6
   with disproportion (fetopelvic) 653.0
      affecting fetus or newborn 763.1
      causing obstructed labor 660.1
         affecting fetus or newborn 763.1
Scorbutus, scorbutic 267
   anemia 281.8
Scotoma (ring) 368.44
   arcuate 368.43
   Bjerrum 368.43
   blind spot area 368.42
   central 368.41
   centrocecal 368.41
   paracecal 368.42
   paracentral 368.41
   scintillating 368.12
   Seidel 368.43
Scratch — see Injury, superficial, by site
Screening (for) V82.9
   alcoholism V79.1
   anemia, deficiency NEC V78.1
      iron V78.0
   anomaly, congenital V82.8
   antenatal V28.9
      alphafetoprotein levels, raised V28.1

Screening—continued
    antenatal—continued
        based on amniocentesis V28.2
            chromosomal anomalies V28.0
            raised alpha-fetoprotein levels V28.1
        fetal growth retardation using ultrasonics V28.4
        isoimmunization V28.5
        malformations using ultrasonics V28.3
        raised alphafetoprotein levels V28.1
        specified condition NEC V28.8
    arterial hypertension V81.1
    arthropod-borne viral disease NEC V73.5
    asymptomatic bacteriuria V81.5
    bacterial
        conjunctivitis V74.4
        disease V74.9
            specified condition NEC V74.8
    bacteriuria, asymptomatic V81.5
    blood disorder NEC V78.9
        specified type NEC V78.8
    bronchitis, chronic V81.3
    brucellosis V74.8
    cancer — see Screening, malignant neoplasm
    cardiovascular disease NEC V81.2
    cataract V80.2
    Chagas' disease V75.3
    chemical poisoning V82.5
    cholera V74.0
    chromosomal
        anomalies
            by amniocentesis, antenatal V28.0
            postnatal V82.4
        athletes V70.3
    condition
        cardiovascular NEC V81.2
        eye NEC V80.2
        genitourinary NEC V81.6
        neurological V80.0
        respiratory NEC V81.4
        skin V82.0
        specified NEC V82.8
    congenital
        anomaly V82.8
            eye V80.2
        dislocation of hip V82.3
        eye condition or disease V80.2
    conjunctivitis, bacterial V74.4
    contamination NEC (see also Poisoning) V82.5
    coronary artery disease V81.0
    cystic fibrosis V77.6
    deficiency anemia NEC V78.1
        iron V78.0
    dengue fever V73.5
    depression V79.0
    developmental handicap V79.9
        in early childhood V79.3
        specified type NEC V79.8
    diabetes mellitus V77.1
    diphtheria V74.3
    disease or disorder V82.9
        bacterial V74.9
            specified NEC V74.8
        blood V78.9
            specified type NEC V78.8
        blood-forming organ V78.9
            specified type NEC 78.8
        cardiovascular NEC V81.2
            hypertensive V81.1
            ischemic V81.0
        Chagas' V75.3
        chlamydial V73.98
            specified NEC V73.88
        ear NEC V80.3
        endocrine NEC V77.9
        eye NEC V80.2

Screening—continued
    disease or disorder—continued
        genitourinary NEC V81.6
        heart NEC V81.2
            hypertensive V81.1
            ischemic V81.0
        immunity NEC V77.9
        infectious NEC V75.9
        mental V79.9
            specified type NEC V79.8
        metabolic NEC V77.9
            inborn NEC V77.7
        neurological V80.0
        nutritional NEC V77.9
        rheumatic NEC V82.2
        rickettsial V75.0
        sickle-cell V78.2
            trait V78.2
        specified type NEC V82.8
        thyroid V77.0
        vascular NEC V81.2
            ischemic V81.0
        venereal V74.5
        viral V73.99
            arthropod-borne NEC V73.5
            specified type NEC V73.89
    dislocation of hip, congenital V82.3
    drugs in athletes V70.3
    emphysema (chronic) V81.3
    encephalitis, viral (mosquito or tick borne) V73.5
    endocrine disorder NEC V77.9
    eye disorder NEC V80.2
        congenital V80.2
    fever
        dengue V73.5
        hemorrhagic V73.5
        yellow V73.4
    filariasis V75.6
    galactosemia V77.4
    genitourinary condition NEC V81.6
    glaucoma V80.1
    gonorrhea V74.5
    gout V77.5
    Hansen's disease V74.2
    heart disease NEC V81.2
        hypertensive V81.1
        ischemic V81.0
    heavy metal poisoning V82.5
    helminthiasis, intestinal V75.7
    hematopoietic malignancy V76.8
    hemoglobinopathies NEC V78.3
    hemorrhagic fever V73.5
    Hodgkin's disease V76.8
    hormones in athletes V70.3
    hypertension V81.1
    immunity disorder NEC V77.9
    inborn errors of metabolism NEC V77.7
    infection
        bacterial V74.9
            specified type NEC V74.8
        mycotic V75.4
        parasitic NEC V75.8
    infectious disease V75.9
        specified type NEC V75.8
    ingestion of radioactive substance V82.5
    intestinal helminthiasis V75.7
    iron deficiency anemia V78.0
    ischemic heart disease V81.0
    lead poisoning V82.5
    leishmaniasis V75.2
    leprosy V74.2
    leptospirosis V74.8
    leukemia V76.8
    lymphoma V76.8
    malaria V75.1
    malignant neoplasm (of) V76.9
        bladder V76.3
        blood V76.8
        breast V76.1
        cervix V76.2
        hematopoietic system V76.8

Screening—continued
    malignant neoplasm—continued
        lung V76.0
        lymph (glands) V76.8
        oral cavity V76.42
        rectum V76.41
        respiratory organs V76.0
        skin V76.43
        specified sites NEC V76.49
    malnutrition V77.2
    measles V73.2
    mental
        disorder V79.9
            specified type NEC V79.8
        retardation V79.2
    metabolic errors, inborn V77.7
    mucoviscidosis V77.6
    multiphasic V82.6
    mycosis V75.4
    mycotic infection V75.4
    nephropathy V81.5
    neurological condition V80.0
    nutritional disorder V77.9
    obesity V77.8
    parasitic infection NEC V75.8
    phenylketonuria V77.3
    plague V74.8
    poisoning
        chemical NEC V82.5
        contaminated water supply V82.5
        heavy metal V82.5
    poliomyelitis V73.0
    postnatal chromosomal anomalies V82.4
    prenatal — see Screening, antenatal
    pulmonary tuberculosis V74.1
    radiation exposure 82.5
    renal disease V81.5
    respiratory condition NEC V81.4
    rheumatic disorder NEC V82.2
    rheumatoid arthritis V82.1
    rickettsial disease V75.0
    rubella V73.3
    schistosomiasis V75.5
    senile macular lesions of eye V80.2
    sickle-cell anemia, disease, or trait V78.2
    skin condition V82.0
    sleeping sickness V75.3
    smallpox V73.1
    special V82.9
        specified condition NEC V82.8
    specified type NEC V82.8
    spirochetal disease V74.9
        specified type NEC V74.8
    stimulants in athletes V70.3
    syphilis V74.5
    tetanus V74.8
    thyroid disorder V77.0
    trachoma V73.6
    trypanosomiasis V75.3
    tuberculosis, pulmonary V74.1
    venereal disease V74.5
    viral encephalitis
        mosquito-borne V73.5
        tick-borne V73.5
    whooping cough V74.8
    worms, intestinal V75.7
    yaws V74.6
    yellow fever V73.4

Scrofula (see also Tuberculosis) 017.2

Scrofulide (primary) (see also Tuberculosis) 017.0

Scrofuloderma, scrofulodermia (any site) (primary) (see also Tuberculosis) 017.0

Scrofulosis (universal) (see also Tuberculosis) 017.2

Scrofulosis lichen (primary) (see also Tuberculosis) 017.0

Scrofulous — see condition

Scrotal tongue 529.5
    congenital 750.13

Scrotum — see condition

Scurvy (gum) (infantile) (rickets) (scorbutic) 267

Sea-blue histiocyte syndrome 272.7

Seabright-Bantam syndrome (pseudohypoparathyroidism) 275.4

Seasickness 994.6

Seatworm 127.4

Sebaceous
    cyst (see also Cyst, sebaceous) 706.2
    gland disease NEC 706.9

Sebocystomatosis 706.2

Seborrhea, seborrheic 706.3
    adiposa 706.3
    capitis 704.8
    congestiva 695.4
    corporis 706.3
    dermatitis 690
        infantile 691.8
    diathesis in infants 695.89
    eczema 690
        infantile 691.8
    keratosis 702.19 ▼
        inflamed 702.11 ▲
    nigricans 705.89
    sicca 690
    wart 702.19 ▼
        inflamed 702.11 ▲

Seckel's syndrome 759.89

Seclusion pupil 364.74

Seclusiveness, child 313.22

Secondary — see also condition
    neoplasm — see Neoplasm, by site, malignant, secondary

Secretan's disease or syndrome (posttraumatic edema) 782.3

Secretion
    antidiuretic hormone, inappropriate (syndrome) 253.6
    catecholamine, by pheochromocytoma 255.6
    hormone
        antidiuretic, inappropriate (syndrome) 253.6
        by
            carcinoid tumor 259.2
            pheochromocytoma 255.6
        ectopic NEC 259.3
    urinary
        excessive 788.42
        suppression 788.5

Section
    cesarean
        affecting fetus or newborn 763.4
        post mortem, affecting fetus or newborn 761.6
        previous, in pregnancy or childbirth 654.2
            affecting fetus or newborn 763.8
    nerve, traumatic — see Injury, nerve, by site

Seeligmann's syndrome (ichthyosis congenita) 757.1

Segmentation, incomplete (congenital) — see also Fusion
    bone NEC 756.9
    lumbosacral (joint) 756.15
    vertebra 756.15
        lumbosacral 756.15

Seizure 780.3
    akinetic (idiopathic) (see also Epilepsy) 345.0
        psychomotor 345.4
    apoplexy, apoplectic (see also Disease, cerebrovascular, acute) 436

Seizure—continued
  atonic (see also Epilepsy) 345.0
  autonomic 300.11
  brain or cerebral (see also
      Disease, cerebrovascular,
      acute) 436
  convulsive (see also Convulsions)
      780.3
  cortical (focal) (motor) (see also
      Epilepsy) 345.5
  epilepsy, epileptic (cryptogenic)
      (see also Epilepsy) 345.9
  epileptiform, epileptoid 780.3
    focal (see also Epilepsy) 345.5
  febrile 780.3
  heart — see Disease, heart
  hysterical 300.11
  Jacksonian (focal) (see also
      Epilepsy) 345.5
    motor type 345.5
    sensory type 345.5
  newborn 779.0
  paralysis (see also Disease,
      cerebrovascular, acute) 436
  recurrent 780.3
    epileptic — see Epilepsy
  repetitive 780.3
    epileptic — see Epilepsy
  salaam (see also Epilepsy) 345.6
  uncinate (see also Epilepsy) 345.4
Self-mutilation 300.9
Semicoma 780.09
Semiconsciousness 780.09
Seminal
  vesicle — see condition
  vesiculitis (see also Vesiculitis)
      608.0
Seminoma (M9061/3)
  anaplastic type (M9062/3)
    specified site — see
        Neoplasm, by site,
        malignant
    unspecified site 186.9
  specified site — see Neoplasm,
      by site, malignant
  spermatocytic (M9063/3)
    specified site — see
        Neoplasm, by site,
        malignant
    unspecified site 186.9
  unspecified site 186.9
Semliki Forest encephalitis 062.8
Senear-Usher disease or syndrome
  (pemphigus erythematosus)
  694.4
Senecio jacobae dermatitis 692.6
Senectus 797
Senescence 797
Senile (see also condition) 797
  cervix (atrophic) 622.8
  degenerative atrophy, skin 701.3
  endometrium (atrophic) 621.8
  fallopian tube (atrophic) 620.3
  heart (failure) 797
  lung 492.8
  ovary (atrophic) 620.3
  syndrome 259.8
  vagina, vaginitis (atrophic) 627.3
  wart 702.0
Senility 797
  with
    acute confusional state 290.3
    delirium 290.3
    mental changes 290.9
    psychosis NEC (see also
        Psychosis, senile)
        290.20
  premature (syndrome) 259.8
Sensation
  burning (see also Disturbance,
      sensation) 782.0
  tongue 529.6
  choking 784.9
  loss of (see also Disturbance,
      sensation) 782.0

Sensation—continued
  prickling (see also Disturbance,
      sensation) 782.0
  tingling (see also Disturbance,
      sensation) 782.0
Sense loss (touch) (see also
    Disturbance, sensation) 782.0
  smell 781.1
  taste 781.1
Sensibility disturbance NEC
    (cortical) (deep) (vibratory) (see
    also Disturbance, sensation)
    782.0
Sensitive dentine 521.8
Sensitiver Beziehungswahn 297.8
Sensitivity, sensitization — see also
    Allergy
  autoerythrocyte 287.2
  carotid sinus 337.0
  child (excessive) 313.21
  cold, autoimmune 283.0
  methemoglobin 289.7
  suxamethonium 289.8
  tuberculin, without clinical or
      radiological symptoms
      795.5
Sensory ▼
  extinction 781.8
  neglect 781.8 ▲
Separation
  acromioclavicular — see
      Dislocation,
      acromioclavicular
  anxiety, abnormal 309.21
  apophysis, traumatic — see
      Fracture, by site
  choroid 363.70
    hemorrhagic 363.72
    serous 363.71
  costochondral (simple) (traumatic)
      — see Dislocation,
      costochondral
  epiphysis, epiphyseal
    nontraumatic 732.9
    upper femoral 732.2
    traumatic — see Fracture, by
        site
  fracture — see Fracture, by site
  infundibulum cardiac from right
      ventricle by a partition
      746.83
  joint (current) (traumatic) — see
      Dislocation, by site
  placenta (normally implanted) —
      see Placenta, separation
  pubic bone, obstetrical trauma
      665.6
  retina, retinal (see also
      Detachment, retina) 361.9
    layers 362.40
      sensory (see also
          Retinoschisis) 361.10
    pigment epithelium
        (exudative) 362.42
      hemorrhagic 362.43
  sternoclavicular (traumatic) — see
      Dislocation,
      sternoclavicular
  symphysis pubis, obstetrical
      trauma 665.6
  tracheal ring, incomplete
      (congenital) 748.3
Sepsis (generalized) (see also
    Septicemia) 038.9
  with
    abortion — see Abortion, by
        type, with sepsis
    ectopic pregnancy (see also
        categories 633.0-633.9)
        639.0
    molar pregnancy (see also
        categories 630-632)
        639.0
  buccal 528.3
  complicating labor 659.3
  dental (pulpal origin) 522.4

Sepsis—continued
  female genital organ NEC 614.9
  fetus (intrauterine) 771.8
  following
    abortion 639.0
    ectopic or molar pregnancy
        639.0
    infusion, perfusion, or
        transfusion 999.3
  Friedländer's 038.49
  intraocular 360.00
  localized
    in operation wound 998.5
    skin (see also Abscess) 682.9
  malleus 024
  newborn (umbilical) (organism
      unspecified) NEC 771.8
  of tracheostomy stoma 519.0
  oral 528.3
  puerperal, postpartum, childbirth
      (pelvic) 670
  resulting from infusion, injection,
      transfusion, or vaccination
      999.3
  skin, localized (see also Abscess)
      682.9
  umbilical (newborn) (organism
      unspecified) 771.8
  tetanus 771.3
  urinary 599.0
Septate — see also Septum
Septic — see also condition
  arm (with lymphangitis) 682.3
  embolus — see Embolism
  finger (with lymphangitis) 681.00
  foot (with lymphangitis) 682.7
  gallbladder (see also
      Cholecystitis) 575.8
  hand (with lymphangitis) 682.4
  joint (see also Arthritis, septic)
      711.0
  kidney (see also Infection, kidney)
      590.9
  leg (with lymphangitis) 682.6
  mouth 528.3
  nail 681.9
    finger 681.02
    toe 681.11
  shock (endotoxic) 785.59
  sore (see also Abscess) 682.9
    throat 034.0
      milk-borne 034.0
      streptococcal 034.0
  spleen (acute) 289.59
  teeth (pulpal origin) 522.4
  throat 034.0
  thrombus — see Thrombosis
  toe (with lymphangitis) 681.0
  tonsils 474.0
  umbilical cord (newborn)
      (organism unspecified)
      771.8
  uterus (see also Endometritis)
      615.9
Septicemia, septicemic (generalized)
    (suppurative) 038.9
  with
    abortion — see Abortion, by
        type, with sepsis
    ectopic pregnancy (see also
        categories 633.0-633.9)
        639.0
    molar pregnancy (see also
        categories 630-632)
        639.0
  Aerobacter aerogenes 038.49
  anaerobic 038.3
  anthrax 022.3
  Bacillus coli 038.42
  Bacteroides 038.3
  Clostridium 038.3
  complicating labor 659.3
  cryptogenic 038.9
  enteric gram-negative bacilli
      038.40
  Enterobacter aerogenes 038.49

Septicemia, septicemic—continued
  Erysipelothrix (insidiosa)
      (rhusiopathiae) 027.1
  Escherichia coli 038.42
  following
    abortion 639.0
    ectopic or molar pregnancy
        639.0
    infusion, injection, transfusion,
        or vaccination 999.3
  Friedländer's (bacillus) 038.49
  gangrenous 038.9
  gonococcal 098.89
  gram-negative (organism) 038.40
    anaerobic 038.3
  Hemophilus influenzae 038.41
  herpes (simplex) 054.5
  herpetic 054.5
  Listeria monocytogenes 027.0
  meningeal — see Meningitis
  meningococcal (chronic)
      (fulminating) 036.2
  navel, newborn (organism
      unspecified) 771.8
  newborn (umbilical) (organism
      unspecified) 771.8
  plague 020.2
  pneumococcal 038.2
  postabortal 639.0
  postoperative 998.5
  Proteus vulgaris 038.49
  Pseudomonas (aeruginosa)
      038.43
  puerperal, postpartum 670
  Salmonella (aertrycke)
      (callinarum) (choleraesuis)
      (enteritidis) (suipestifer)
      003.1
  Serratia 038.44
  Shigella (see also Dysentery,
      bacillary) 004.9
  specified organism NEC 038.8
  staphylococcal 038.1
  streptococcal (anaerobic) 038.0
  suipestifer 003.1
  umbilicus, newborn (organism
      unspecified) 771.8
  viral 079.99
  Yersinia enterocolitica 038.49
Septum, septate (congenital) — see
    also Anomaly, specified type
    NEC
  anal 751.2
  aqueduct of Sylvius 742.3
    with spina bifida (see also
        Spina bifida) 741.0
  hymen 752.49
  uterus (see also Double, uterus)
      752.2
  vagina 752.49
    in pregnancy or childbirth
        654.7
      affecting fetus or newborn
          763.8
      causing obstructed labor
          660.2
        affecting fetus or
            newborn 763.1
Sequestration
  lung (congenital) (extralobar)
      (intralobar) 748.5
  orbit 376.10
  pulmonary artery (congenital)
      747.3
Sequestrum
  bone (see also Osteomyelitis)
      730.1
  jaw 526.4
  dental 525.8
  jaw bone 526.4
  sinus (accessory) (nasal) (see also
      Sinusitis) 473.9
    maxillary 473.0
Sequoiosis asthma 495.8

Serology for syphilis
- doubtful
  - with signs or symptoms — *see* Syphilis, by site and stage
  - follow-up of latent syphilis — *see* Syphilis, latent
- false positive 795.6
- negative, with signs or symptoms — *see* Syphilis, by site and stage
- positive 097.1
  - with signs or symptoms — *see* Syphilis, by site and stage
  - false 795.6
  - follow-up of latent syphilis — *see* Syphilis, latent
  - only finding — *see* Syphilis, latent
- reactivated 097.1

Seroma — *see* Hematoma
Seropurulent — *see* condition
Serositis, multiple 569.89
- pericardial 423.2
- peritoneal 568.82
- pleural — *see* Pleurisy

Serous — *see* condition
Sertoli cell
- adenoma (M8640/0)
  - specified site — *see* Neoplasm, by site, benign
  - unspecified site
    - female 220
    - male 222.0
- carcinoma (M8640/3)
  - specified site — *see* Neoplasm, by site, malignant
  - unspecified site 186.9
- syndrome (germinal aplasia) 606.0
- tumor (M8640/0)
  - with lipid storage (M8641/0)
    - specified site — *see* Neoplasm, by site, benign
    - unspecified site
      - female 220
      - male 222.0
  - specified site — *see* Neoplasm, by site, benign
  - unspecified site
    - female 220
    - male 222.0

Sertoli-Leydig cell tumor (M8631/0)
- specified site — *see* Neoplasm, by site, benign
- unspecified site
  - female 220
  - male 222.0

Serum
- allergy, allergic reaction 999.5
  - shock 999.4
- arthritis 999.5 [713.6]
- complication or reaction NEC 999.5
- disease NEC 999.5
- hepatitis — *see* Hepatitis, viral
- carrier (suspected) of V02.6
- intoxication 999.5
- jaundice (homologous) — *see* Hepatitis, viral
- neuritis 999.5
- poisoning NEC 999.5
- rash NEC 999.5
- reaction NEC 999.5
- sickness NEC 999.5

Sesamoiditis 733.99
Seven-day fever 061
- of
  - Japan 100.89
  - Queensland 100.89

Sever's disease or osteochondrosis (calcaneum) 732.5
Sex chromosome mosaics 758.8
Sextuplet
- affected by maternal complications of pregnancy 761.5
- healthy liveborn — *see* Newborn, multiple
- pregnancy (complicating delivery) NEC 651.8
  - with fetal loss and retention of one or more fetus(es) 651.6

Sexual
- anesthesia 302.72
- deviation (*see also* Deviation, sexual) 302.9
- disorder (*see also* Deviation, sexual) 302.9
- frigidity (female) 302.72
- function, disorder of (psychogenic) 302.70
  - specified type NEC 302.79
- immaturity (female) (male) 259.0
- impotence (psychogenic) 302.72
  - organic origin NEC 607.84
- precocity (constitutional) (cryptogenic) (female) (idiopathic) (male) NEC 259.1
  - with adrenal hyperplasia 255.2
- sadism 302.84

Sexuality, pathological (*see also* Deviation, sexual) 302.9
Sézary's disease, reticulosis, or syndrome (M9701/3) 202.2
Shadow, lung 793.1
Shaking
- head (tremor) 781.0
- palsy or paralysis (*see also* Parkinsonism) 332.0

Shallowness, acetabulum 736.39
Shaver's disease or syndrome (bauxite pneumoconiosis) 503
Sheath (tendon) — *see* condition
Shedding
- nail 703.8
- teeth, premature, primary (deciduous) 520.6

Sheehan's disease or syndrome (postpartum pituitary necrosis) 253.2
Shelf, rectal 569.49
Shell
- shock (current) (*see also* Reaction, stress, acute) 308.9
  - lasting state 300.16
- teeth 520.5

Shield kidney 753.3
Shift, mediastinal 793.2
Shifting
- pacemaker 427.89
- sleep-work schedule (affecting sleep) 307.45

Shiga's
- bacillus 004.0
- dysentery 004.0

Shigella (dysentery) (*see also* Dysentery, bacillary) 004.9
- carrier (suspected) of V02.3

Shigellosis (*see also* Dysentery, bacillary) 004.9
Shingles (*see also* Herpes, zoster) 053.9
- eye NEC 053.29

Shin splints 844.9
Shipyard eye or disease 077.1
Shirodkar suture, in pregnancy 654.5

Shock 785.50
- with
  - abortion — *see* Abortion, by type, with shock
  - ectopic pregnancy (*see also* categories 633.0-633.9) 639.5
  - molar pregnancy (*see also* categories 630-632) 639.5
- allergic — *see* Shock, anaphylactic
- anaclitic 309.21
- anaphylactic 995.0
  - chemical — *see* Table of drugs and chemicals
  - correct medicinal substance properly administered 995.0
  - drug or medicinal substance
    - correct substance properly administered 995.0
    - overdose or wrong substance given or taken 977.9
    - specified drug — *see* Table of drugs and chemicals
  - following sting(s) 989.5
  - food — *see* Anaphylactic shock, due to, food
  - immunization 999.4
  - serum 999.4
- anaphylactoid — *see* Shock, anaphylactic
- anesthetic
  - correct substance properly administered 995.4
  - overdose or wrong substance given 968.4
  - specified anesthetic — *see* Table of drugs and chemicals
- birth, fetus or newborn NEC 779.8
- cardiogenic 785.51
- chemical substance — *see* Table of drugs and chemicals
- circulatory 785.59
- complicating
  - abortion — *see* Abortion, by type, with shock
  - ectopic pregnancy (*see also* categories 633.0-633.9) 639.5
  - labor and delivery 669.1
  - molar pregnancy (*see also* categories 630-632) 639.5
- culture 309.29
- due to
  - drug 995.0
    - correct substance properly administered 995.0
    - overdose or wrong substance given or taken 977.9
    - specified drug — *see* Table of drugs and chemicals
  - food — *see* Anaphylactic shock, due to, food
- during labor and delivery 669.1
- electric 994.8
- endotoxic 785.59
  - due to surgical procedure 998.0
- following
  - abortion 639.5
  - ectopic or molar pregnancy 639.5
  - injury (immediate) (delayed) 958.4
  - labor and delivery 669.1
- gram-negative 785.59
- hematogenic 785.59

Shock—*continued*
- hemorrhagic
  - due to
    - disease 785.59
    - surgery (intraoperative) (postoperative) 998.0
    - trauma 958.4
- hypovolemic NEC 785.59
  - surgical 998.0
  - traumatic 958.4
- insulin 251.0
  - therapeutic misadventure 962.3
- kidney 584.5
  - traumatic (following crushing) 958.5
- lightning 994.0
- lung 518.5
- nervous (*see also* Reaction, stress, acute) 308.9
- obstetric 669.1
  - with
    - abortion — *see* Abortion, by type, with shock
    - ectopic pregnancy (*see also* categories 633.0-633.9) 639.5
    - molar pregnancy (*see also* categories 630-632) 639.5
  - following
    - abortion 639.5
    - ectopic or molar pregnancy 639.5
- paralysis, paralytic (*see also* Disease, cerebrovascular, acute) 436
  - late effect — *see* category 438
- pleural (surgical) 998.0
  - due to trauma 958.4
- postoperative 998.0
  - with
    - abortion — *see* Abortion, by type, with shock
    - ectopic pregnancy (*see also* categories 633.0-633.9) 639.5
    - molar pregnancy (*see also* categories 630-632) 639.5
  - following
    - abortion 639.5
    - ectopic or molar pregnancy 639.5
- psychic (*see also* Reaction, stress, acute) 308.9
  - past history (of) V15.4
- psychogenic (*see also* Reaction, stress, acute) 308.9
- septic 785.59
  - with
    - abortion — *see* Abortion, by type, with shock
    - ectopic pregnancy (categories 633.0-633.9) 639.5
    - molar pregnancy (*see also* categories 630-632) 639.5
  - due to
    - surgical procedure 998.0
    - transfusion NEC 999.8
      - bone marrow 996.85
  - following
    - abortion 639.5
    - ectopic or molar pregnancy 639.5
    - surgical procedure 998.0
    - transfusion NEC 999.8
      - bone marrow 996.85
- spinal — *see also* Injury, spinal, by site
  - with spinal bone injury — *see* Fracture, vertebra, by site, with spinal cord injury
- surgical 998.0

Shock—continued
therapeutic misadventure NEC
(see also Complications)
998.89 ◆
thyroxin 962.7
toxic 040.89 ◆
transfusion — see Complications,
transfusion
traumatic (immediate) (delayed)
958.4
Shoemakers' chest 738.3
Short, shortening, shortness
Achilles tendon (acquired) 727.81
arm 736.89
congenital 755.20
back 737.9
bowel syndrome 579.3
breath 786.09
common bile duct, congenital
751.69
cord (umbilical) 663.4
affecting fetus or newborn
762.6
cystic duct, congenital 751.69
esophagus (congenital) 750.4
femur (acquired) 736.81
congenital 755.34
frenulum linguae 750.0
frenum, lingual 750.0
hamstrings 727.81
hip (acquired) 736.39
congenital 755.63
leg (acquired) 736.81
congenital 755.30
metatarsus (congenital) 754.79
acquired 736.79
organ or site, congenital NEC —
see Distortion
palate (congenital) 750.26
P-R interval syndrome 426.81
radius (acquired) 736.09
congenital 755.26
round ligament 629.8
sleeper 307.49
stature, constitutional (hereditary)
783.4
tendon 727.81
Achilles (acquired) 727.81
congenital 754.79
congenital 756.89
thigh (acquired) 736.81
congenital 755.34
tibialis anticus 727.81
umbilical cord 663.4
affecting fetus or newborn
762.6
urethra 599.84
uvula (congenital) 750.26
vagina 623.8
Shortsightedness 367.1
Shoshin (acute fulminating beriberi) 265.0
Shoulder — see condition
Shovel-shaped incisors 520.2
Shower, thromboembolic — see Embolism
Shunt (status)
aortocoronary bypass V45.81
arterial-venous (dialysis) V45.1
arteriovenous, pulmonary
(acquired) 417.0
congenital 747.3
traumatic (complication)
901.40
cerebral ventricle
(communicating) in situ
V45.2
coronary artery bypass V45.81
surgical, prosthetic, with
complications — see
Complications, shunt
vascular NEC V45.89

Shutdown
renal 586
with
abortion — see Abortion,
by type, with renal
failure
ectopic pregnancy (see also
categories 633.0-
633.9) 639.3
molar pregnancy (see also
categories 630-632)
639.3
complicating
abortion 639.3
ectopic or molar pregnancy
639.3
following labor and delivery
669.3
Shwachman's syndrome 288.0
Shy-Drager syndrome (orthostatic hypotension with multisystem degeneration) 333.0
Sialadenitis (any gland) (chronic) (suppurative) 527.2
epidemic — see Mumps
Sialadenosis, periodic 527.2
Sialaporia 527.7
Sialectasia 527.8
Sialitis 527.2
Sialoadenitis (see also Sialadenitis) 527.2
Sioloangitis 527.2
Sialodochitis (fibrinosa) 527.2
Sialodocholithiasis 527.5
Sialolithiasis 527.5
Sialorrhea (see also Ptyalism) 527.7
periodic 527.2
Sialosis 527.8
rheumatic 710.2
Siamese twin 759.4
Sicard's syndrome 352.6
Sicca syndrome (keratoconjunctivitis) 710.2
Sick 799.9
or handicapped person in family
V61.49
Sickle-cell
anemia (see also Disease, sickle-cell) 282.60
disease (see also Disease, sickle-cell) 282.60
hemoglobin
C disease 282.63
D disease 282.69
E disease 282.69
thalassemia 282.4
trait 282.5
Sicklemia (see also Disease, sickle-cell) 282.60
trait 282.5
Sickness
air (travel) 994.6
airplane 994.6
alpine 993.2
altitude 993.2
Andes 993.2
aviators' 993.2
balloon 993.2
car 994.6
compressed air 993.3
decompression 993.3
green 280.9
harvest 100.89
milk 988.8
morning 643.0
motion 994.6
mountain 993.2
acute 289.0
protein (see also Complications, vaccination) 999.5
radiation NEC 990
roundabout (motion) 994.6
sea 994.6

Sickness—continued
serum NEC 999.5
sleeping (African) 086.5
by Trypanosoma 086.5
gambiense 086.3
rhodesiense 086.4
Gambian 086.3
late effect 139.8
Rhodesian 086.4
sweating 078.2
swing (motion) 994.6
train (railway) (travel) 994.6
travel (any vehicle) 994.6
Sick sinus syndrome 427.81
Sideropenia (see also Anemia, iron deficiency) 280.9
Siderosis (lung) (occupational) 503
cornea 371.15
eye (bulbi) (vitreous) 360.23
lens 360.23
Siegal-Cattan-Mamou disease (periodic) 277.3
Siemens' syndrome
ectodermal dysplasia 757.31
keratosis follicularis spinulosa
(decalvans) 757.39
Sighing respiration 786.7
Sigmoid
flexure — see condition
kidney 753.3
Sigmoiditis — see Enteritis
Silfverskiöld's syndrome 756.5
Silicosis, silicotic (complicated) (occupational) (simple) 502
fibrosis, lung (confluent) (massive) (occupational) 502
non-nodular 503
pulmonum 502
Silicotuberculosis (see also Tuberculosis) 011.4
Silo fillers' disease 506.9
Silver's syndrome (congenital hemihypertrophy and short stature) 759.89
Silver wire arteries, retina 362.13
Silvestroni-Bianco syndrome (thalassemia minima) 282.4
Simian crease 757.2
Simmonds' cachexia or disease (pituitary cachexia) 253.2
Simons' disease or syndrome (progressive lipodystrophy) 272.6
Simple, simplex — see condition
Sinding-Larsen disease (juvenile osteopathia patellae) 732.4
Singapore hemorrhagic fever 065.4
Singers' node or nodule 478.5
Single
atrium 745.69
coronary artery 746.85
umbilical artery 747.5
ventricle 745.3
Singultus 786.8
epidemicus 078.89
Sinus — see also Fistula
abdominal 569.81
arrest 426.6
arrhythmia 427.89
bradycardia 427.89
chronic 427.81
branchial cleft (external) (internal)
744.41
coccygeal (infected) 685.1
with abscess 685.0
dental 522.7
dermal (congenital) 685.1
with abscess 685.00
draining — see Fistula
infected, skin NEC 686.9

Sinus—continued
marginal, ruptured or bleeding
641.2
affecting fetus or newborn
762.1
pause 426.6
pericranii 742.0
pilonidal (infected) (rectum)
685.1
with abscess 685.0
preauricular 744.46
rectovaginal 619.1
sacrococcygeal (dermoid)
(infected) 685.1
with abscess 685.0
tachycardia 427.89
tarsi syndrome 355.5
testis 608.89
tract (postinfectional) — see
Fistula
urachus 753.7
Sinuses, Rokitansky-Aschoff (see also Disease, gallbladder) 575.8
Sinusitis (accessory) (nasal) (hyperplastic) (nonpurulent) (purulent) (chronic) 473.9
with influenza, flu, or grippe
487.1
acute 461.9
ethmoidal 461.2
frontal 461.1
maxillary 461.0
specified type NEC 461.8
sphenoidal 461.3
allergic (see also Fever, hay)
477.9
antrum — see Sinusitis, maxillary
due to
fungus, any sinus 117.9
high altitude 993.1
ethmoidal 473.2
acute 461.2
frontal 473.1
acute 461.1
influenzal 478.1
maxillary 473.0
acute 461.0
specified site NEC 473.8
sphenoidal 473.3
acute 461.3
syphilitic, any sinus 095.8
tuberculous, any sinus (see also
Tuberculosis) 012.8
Sinusitis-bronchiectasis-situs inversus (syndrome) (triad) 759.3
Sipple's syndrome (medullary thyroid carcinoma-pheochromocytoma) 193
Sirenomelia 759.89
Siriasis 992.0
Sirkari's disease 085.0
Siti 104.0
Sitophobia 300.29
Situation, psychiatric 300.9
Situational
disturbance (transient) (see also
Reaction, adjustment)
309.9
acute 308.3
maladjustment, acute (see also
Reaction, adjustment)
309.9
reaction (see also Reaction,
adjustment) 309.9
acute 308.3
Situs inversus or transversus 759.3
abdominalis 759.3
thoracis 759.3
Sixth disease 057.8
Sjögren (-Gougerot) syndrome or disease (keratoconjunctivitis sicca) 710.2
with lung involvement 710.2
[517.8]

Sjögren-Larsson syndrome
(ichthyosis congenita) 757.1
Skeletal — see condition
Skene's gland — see condition
Skenitis (see also Urethritis) 597.89
gonorrheal (acute) 098.0
chronic or duration of 2
months or over 098.2
Skerljevo 104.0
Skevas-Zerfus disease 989.5
Skin — see also condition
donor V59.1
hidebound 710.9
Slate-dressers' lung 502
Slate-miners' lung 502
Sleep
disorder 780.50
with apnea — see Apnea,
sleep
child 307.40
nonorganic origin 307.40
specified type NEC 307.49
disturbance 780.50
with apnea — see Apnea,
sleep
nonorganic origin 307.40
specified type NEC 307.49
drunkenness 307.47
paroxysmal 347
rhythm inversion 780.55
nonorganic origin 307.45
walking 307.46
hysterical 300.13
Sleeping sickness 086.5
late effect 139.8
Sleeplessness (see also Insomnia)
780.52
menopausal 627.2
nonorganic origin 307.41
Slipped, slipping
epiphysis (postinfectional) 732.9
traumatic (old) 732.9
current — see Fracture, by
site
upper femoral (nontraumatic)
732.2
intervertebral disc — see
Displacement,
intervertebral disc
ligature, umbilical 772.3
patella 717.89
rib 733.99
sacroiliac joint 724.6
tendon 727.9
ulnar nerve, nontraumatic 354.2
vertebra NEC (see also
Spondylolisthesis) 756.12
Slocumb's syndrome 255.3
Sloughing (multiple) (skin) 686.9
abscess — see Abscess, by site
appendix 543.9
bladder 596.8
fascia 728.9
graft — see Complications, graft
phagedena (see also Gangrene)
785.4
reattached extremity (see also
Complications, reattached
extremity) 996.90
rectum 569.49
scrotum 608.89
tendon 727.9
transplanted organ (see also
Rejection, transplant,
organ, by site) 996.80
ulcer (see also Ulcer, skin) 707.9
Slow
feeding newborn 779.3
fetal, growth NEC 764.9
affecting management of
pregnancy 656.5
Slowing
heart 427.89
urinary stream 788.62

Sluder's neuralgia or syndrome
337.0
Slurred, slurring, speech 784.5
Small, smallness
cardiac reserve — see Disease,
heart
for dates
fetus or newborn 764.0
with malnutrition 764.1
affecting management of
pregnancy 656.5
infant, term 764.0
with malnutrition 764.1
affecting management of
pregnancy 656.5
introitus, vagina 623.3
kidney, unknown cause 589.9
bilateral 589.1
unilateral 589.0
ovary 620.8
pelvis
with disproportion (fetopelvic)
653.1
affecting fetus or newborn
763.1
causing obstructed labor 660.1
affecting fetus or newborn
763.1
placenta — see Placenta,
insufficiency
uterus 621.8
white kidney 582.9
Small-for-dates (see also Light-for-
dates) 764.0
affecting management of
pregnancy 656.5
Smallpox 050.9
contact V01.3
exposure to V01.3
hemorrhagic (pustular) 050.0
malignant 050.0
modified 050.2
vaccination
complications — see
Complications,
vaccination
prophylactic (against) V04.1
Smith's fracture (separation) (closed)
813.41
open 813.51
Smith-Lemli Opitz syndrome
(cerebrohepatorenal
syndrome) 759.89
Smith-Strang disease (oasthouse
urine) 270.2
Smokers'
bronchitis 491.0
cough 491.0
syndrome (see also Abuse, drugs,
nondependent) 305.1
throat 472.1
tongue 528.6
Smothering spells 786.09
Snaggle teeth, tooth 524.3
Snapping
finger 727.05
hip 719.65
jaw 524.69
knee 717.9
thumb 727.05
**Sneddon-Wilkinson disease or
syndrome** (subcorneal pustular
dermatosis) 694.1
Sneezing 784.9
intractable 478.1
Sniffing
cocaine (see also Dependence)
304.2
ether (see also Dependence)
304.6
glue (airplane) (see also
Dependence) 304.6
Snoring 786.09
Snow blindness 370.24

Snuffles (nonsyphilitic) 460
syphilitic (infant) 090.0
Social migrant V60.0
Sodoku 026.0
Soemmering's ring 366.51
Soft — see also condition
nails 703.8
Softening
bone 268.2
brain (necrotic) (progressive)
434.9
arteriosclerotic 437.0
congenital 742.4
embolic (see also Embolism,
brain) 434.1
hemorrhagic (see also
Hemorrhage, brain) 431
occlusive 434.9
thrombotic (see also
Thrombosis, brain)
434.0
cartilage 733.92
cerebellar — see Softening, brain
cerebral — see Softening, brain
cerebrospinal — see Softening,
brain
myocardial, heart (see also
Degeneration, myocardial)
429.1
nails 703.8
spinal cord 336.8
stomach 537.89
Solar fever 061
Soldier's
heart 306.2
patches 423.1
Solitary
cyst
bone 733.21
kidney 593.2
kidney (congenital) 753.0
tubercle, brain (see also
Tuberculosis, brain) 013.2
ulcer, bladder 596.8
**Somatization reaction, somatic
reaction** (see also Disorder,
psychosomatic) 306.9
Somnambulism 307.46
hysterical 300.13
Somnolence 780.09
nonorganic origin 307.43
periodic 349.89
Sonne dysentery 004.3
Soor 112.0
Sore
Delhi 085.1
desert (see also Ulcer, skin) 707.9
eye 379.99
Lahore 085.1
mouth 528.9
canker 528.2
due to dentures 528.9
muscle 729.1
Naga (see also Ulcer, skin) 707.9
oriental 085.1
pressure 707.0
with gangrene 707.0 [785.4]
skin NEC 709.9
soft 099.0
throat 462
with influenza, flu, or grippe
487.1
acute 462
chronic 472.1
clergyman's 784.49
coxsackie (virus) 074.0
diphtheritic 032.0
epidemic 034.0
gangrenous 462
herpetic 054.79
influenzal 487.1
malignant 462
purulent 462
putrid 462
septic 034.0

Sore—continued
throat—continued
streptococcal (ulcerative)
034.0
ulcerated 462
viral NEC 462
Coxsackie 074.0
tropical (see also Ulcer, skin)
707.9
veldt (see also Ulcer, skin) 707.9
Sotos' syndrome (cerebral gigantism)
253.0
Sounds
friction, pleural 786.7
succussion, chest 786.7
**South African cardiomyopathy
syndrome** 425.2
South American
blastomycosis 116.1
trypanosomiasis — see
Trypanosomiasis
Southeast Asian hemorrhagic fever
065.4
Spacing, teeth, abnormal 524.3
Spade-like hand (congenital) 754.89
Spading nail 703.8
congenital 757.5
Spanemia 285.9
Spanish collar 605
Sparganosis 123.5
Spasm, spastic, spasticity (see also
condition) 781.0
accommodation 367.53
ampulla of Vater (see also
Disease, gallbladder) 576.8
anus, ani (sphincter) (reflex) 564.6
psychogenic 306.4
artery NEC 443.9
basilar 435.0
carotid 435.8
cerebral 435.9
specified artery NEC 435.8
retinal (see also Occlusion,
retinal, artery) 362.30
vertebral 435.1
Bell's 351.0
bladder (sphincter, external or
internal) 596.8
bowel 564.1
psychogenic 306.4
bronchus, bronchiole 519.1
cardia 530.0
cardiac — see Angina
carpopedal (see also Tetany)
781.7
cecum 564.1
psychogenic 306.4
cerebral (arteries) (vascular) 435.9
specified artery NEC 435.8
cerebrovascular 435.9
cervix, complicating delivery
661.4
affecting fetus or newborn
763.7
ciliary body (of accommodation)
367.53
colon 564.1
psychogenic 306.4
common duct (see also Disease,
biliary) 576.8
compulsive 307.22
conjugate 378.82
convergence 378.84
coronary (artery) — see Angina
diaphragm (reflex) 786.8
psychogenic 306.1
duodenum, duodenal (bulb)
564.8
esophagus (diffuse) 530.5
psychogenic 306.4
facial 351.8
fallopian tube 620.8
gait 781.2

Spasm, spastic, spasticity—continued
- gastrointestinal (tract) 536.8
  - psychogenic 306.4
- glottis 478.75
  - hysterical 300.11
  - psychogenic 306.1
    - specified as conversion reaction 300.11
  - reflex through recurrent laryngeal nerve 478.75
- habit 307.20
  - chronic 307.22
  - transient of childhood 307.21
- heart — see Angina
- hourglass — see Contraction, hourglass
- hysterical 300.11
- infantile (see also Epilepsy) 345.6
- internal oblique, eye 378.51
- intestinal 564.1
  - psychogenic 306.4
- larynx, laryngeal 478.75
  - hysterical 300.11
  - psychogenic 306.1
    - specified as conversion reaction 300.11
- levator palpebrae superioris 333.81
- lightning (see also Epilepsy) 345.6
- mobile 781.0
- muscle 728.85
  - back 724.8
  - psychogenic 306.0
- nerve, trigeminal 350.1
- nervous 306.0
- nodding 307.3
  - infantile (see also Epilepsy) 345.6
- occupational 300.89
- oculogyric 378.87
- ophthalmic artery 362.30
- orbicularis 781.0
- perineal 625.8
- peroneo-extensor (see also Flat, foot) 734
- pharynx (reflex) 478.29
  - hysterical 300.11
  - psychogenic 306.1
    - specified as conversion reaction 300.11
- pregnant uterus, complicating delivery 661.4
- psychogenic 306.0
- pylorus 537.81
  - adult hypertrophic 537.0
  - congenital or infantile 750.5
  - psychogenic 306.4
- rectum (sphincter) 564.6
  - psychogenic 306.4
- retinal artery NEC (see also Occlusion, retina, artery) 362.30
- sacroiliac 724.6
- salaam (infantile) (see also Epilepsy) 345.6
- saltatory 781.0
- sigmoid 564.1
  - psychogenic 306.4
- sphincter of Oddi (see also Disease, gallbladder) 576.5
- stomach 536.8
  - neurotic 306.4
- throat 478.29
  - hysterical 300.11
  - psychogenic 306.1
    - specified as conversion reaction 300.11
- tic 307.20
  - chronic 307.22
  - transient of childhood 307.21
- tongue 529.8
- torsion 333.6
- trigeminal nerve 350.1
  - postherpetic 053.12
- ureter 593.89
- urethra (sphincter) 599.84

Spasm, spastic, spasticity—continued
- uterus 625.8
  - complicating labor 661.4
    - affecting fetus or newborn 763.7
- vagina 625.1
  - psychogenic 306.51
- vascular NEC 443.9
- vasomotor NEC 443.9
- vein NEC 459.89
- vesical (sphincter, external or internal) 596.8
- viscera 789.0

Spasmodic — see condition
Spasmophilia (see also Tetany) 781.7
Spasmus nutans 307.3
Spastic — see also Spasm
- child 343.9

Spasticity — see also Spasm
- cerebral, child 343.9

Speakers' throat 784.49
Specific, specified — see condition
Speech
- defect, disorder, disturbance, impediment NEC 784.5
  - psychogenic 307.9
- therapy V57.3

Spells 780.3
- breath-holding 786.9

Spencer's disease (epidemic vomiting) 078.82
Spens' syndrome (syncope with heart block) 426.9
Spermatic cord — see condition
Spermatocele 608.1
- congenital 752.8

Spermatocystitis 608.4
Spermatocytoma (M9063/3)
- specified site — see Neoplasm, by site, malignant
- unspecified site 186.9

Spermatorrhea 608.89
Sperm counts V26.2
- postvasectomy V25.8

Sphacelus (see also Gangrene) 785.4
Sphenoidal — see condition
Sphenoiditis (chronic) (see also Sinusitis, sphenoidal) 473.3
Sphenopalatine ganglion neuralgia 337.0
Sphericity, increased, lens 743.36
Spherocytosis (congenital) (familial) (hereditary) 282.0
- hemoglobin disease 282.7
- sickle-cell (disease) 282.60

Spherophakia 743.36
Sphincter — see condition
Sphincteritis, sphincter of Oddi (see also Cholecystitis) 576.8
Sphingolipidosis 272.7
Sphingolipodystrophy 272.7
Sphingomyelinosis 272.7
Spicule tooth 520.2
Spider
- finger 755.59
- nevus 448.1
- vascular 448.1

Spiegler-Fendt sarcoid 686.8
Spielmeyer-Stock disease 330.1
Spielmeyer-Vogt disease 330.1
Spina bifida (aperta) 741.9

> Note — Use the following fifth-digit subclassification with category 741:
>
> 0   unspecified region
> 1   cervical region
> 2   dorsal [thoracic] region
> 3   lumbar region

Spina bifida—continued
- with hydrocephalus 741.0
- fetal (suspected), affecting management of pregnancy 655.0
- occulta 756.17

Spindle, Krukenberg's 371.13
Spine, spinal — see condition
Spiradenoma (eccrine) (M8403/0) — see Neoplasm, skin, benign
Spirillosis NEC (see also Fever, relapsing) 087.9
Spirillum minus 026.0
Spirillum obermeieri infection 087.0
Spirochetal — see condition
Spirochetosis 104.9
- arthritic, arthritica 104.9 [711.8]
- bronchopulmonary 104.8
- icterohemorrhagica 100.0
- lung 104.8

Spitting blood (see also Hemoptysis) 786.3
Splanchnomegaly 569.89
Splanchnoptosis 569.89
Spleen, splenic — see also condition
- agenesis 759.0
- flexure syndrome 569.89
- neutropenia syndrome 288.0
- sequestration syndrome 282.60

Splenectasis (see also Splenomegaly) 789.2
Splenitis (interstitial) (malignant) (nonspecific) 289.59
- malarial (see also Malaria) 084.6
- tuberculous (see also Tuberculosis) 017.7

Splenocele 289.59
Splenomegalia — see Splenomegaly
Splenomegalic — see condition
Splenomegaly 789.2
- Bengal 789.2
- cirrhotic 289.51
- congenital 759.0
- congestive, chronic 289.51
- cryptogenic 789.2
- Egyptian 120.1
- Gaucher's (cerebroside lipidosis) 272.7
- idiopathic 789.2
- malarial (see also Malaria) 084.6
- neutropenic 288.0
- Niemann-Pick (lipid histiocytosis) 272.7
- siderotic 289.51
- syphilitic 095.8
  - congenital 090.0
- tropical (Bengal) (idiopathic) 789.2

Splenopathy 289.50
Splenopneumonia — see Pneumonia
Splenoptosis 289.59
Splinter — see Injury, superficial, by site
Split, splitting
- heart sounds 427.89
- lip, congenital (see also Cleft, lip) 749.10
- nails 703.8
- urinary stream 788.61

Spoiled child reaction (see also Disturbance, conduct) 312.1
Spondylarthritis (see also Spondylosis) 721.90
Spondylarthrosis (see also Spondylosis) 721.90
Spondylitis 720.9
- ankylopoietica 720.0
- ankylosing (chronic) 720.0
- atrophic 720.9
  - ligamentous 720.9
- chronic (traumatic) (see also Spondylosis) 721.90

Spondylitis—continued
- deformans (chronic) (see also Spondylosis) 721.90
- gonococcal 098.53
- gouty 274.0
- hypertrophic (see also Spondylosis) 721.90
- infectious NEC 720.9
- juvenile (adolescent) 720.0
- Kümmell's 721.7
- Marie-Strümpell (ankylosing) 720.0
- muscularis 720.9
- ossificans ligamentosa 721.6
- osteoarthritica (see also Spondylosis) 721.90
- posttraumatic 721.7
- proliferative 720.0
- rheumatoid 720.0
- rhizomelica 720.0
- sacroiliac NEC 720.2
- senescent (see also Spondylosis) 721.90
- senile (see also Spondylosis) 721.90
- static (see also Spondylosis) 721.90
- traumatic (chronic) (see also Spondylosis) 721.90
- tuberculous (see also Tuberculosis) 015.0 [720.81]
- typhosa 002.0 [720.81]

Spondyloarthrosis (see also Spondylosis) 721.90
Spondylolisthesis (congenital) (lumbosacral) 756.12
- with disproportion (fetopelvic) 653.3
  - affecting fetus or newborn 763.1
- causing obstructed labor 660.1
  - affecting fetus or newborn 763.1
- acquired 738.4
- degenerative 738.4
- traumatic 756.12
  - acute (lumbar) — see Fracture, vertebra, lumbar
  - site other than lumbosacral — see Fracture, vertebra, by site

Spondylolysis (congenital) 756.11
- acquired 738.4
- cervical 756.19
- lumbosacral region 756.11
  - with disproportion (fetopelvic) 653.3
    - affecting fetus or newborn 763.1
  - causing obstructed labor 660.1
    - affecting fetus or newborn 763.1

Spondylopathy
- inflammatory 720.9
  - specified type NEC 720.89
- traumatic 721.7

Spondylose rhizomelique 720.0
Spondylosis 721.90
- with
  - disproportion 653.3
    - affecting fetus or newborn 763.1
  - causing obstructed labor 660.1
    - affecting fetus or newborn 763.1
  - myelopathy NEC 721.91
- cervical, cervicodorsal 721.0
  - with myelopathy 721.1
- inflammatory 720.9
- lumbar, lumbosacral 721.3
  - with myelopathy 721.42
- sacral 721.3
  - with myelopathy 721.42

Spondylosis—continued
thoracic 721.2
  with myelopathy 721.41
  traumatic 721.7

Sponge
divers' disease 989.5
inadvertently left in operation wound 998.4
kidney (medullary) 753.17

Spongioblastoma (M9422/3)
multiforme (M9440/3)
  specified site — see Neoplasm, by site, malignant
  unspecified site 191.9
polare (M9423/3)
  specified site — see Neoplasm, by site, malignant
  unspecified site 191.9
primitive polar (M9443/3)
  specified site — see Neoplasm, by site, malignant
  unspecified site 191.9
specified site — see Neoplasm, by site, malignant
unspecified site 191.9

Spongiocytoma (M9400/3)
specified site — see Neoplasm, by site, malignant
unspecified site 191.9

Spongioneuroblastoma (M9504/3) —
see Neoplasm, by site, malignant

Spontaneous — see also condition
fracture — see Fracture, pathologic

Spoon nail 703.8
congenital 757.5

Sporadic — see condition

Sporotrichosis (bones) (cutaneous) (disseminated) (epidermal) (lymphatic) (lymphocutaneous) (mucous membranes) (pulmonary) (skeletal) (visceral) 117.1

Sporotrichum schenckii infection 117.1

Spots, spotting
atrophic (skin) 701.3
Bitôt's (in the young child) 264.1
café au lait 709.09
cayenne pepper 448.1
cotton wool (retina) 362.83
de Morgan's (senile angiomas) 448.1
Fúchs' black (myopic) 360.21
intermenstrual
  irregular 626.6
  regular 626.5
interpalpebral 372.53
Koplik's 055.9
liver 709.09
Mongolian (pigmented) 757.33
of pregnancy 641.9
purpuric 782.7
ruby 448.1

Spotted fever — see Fever, spotted

Sprain, strain (joint) (ligament) (muscle) (tendon) 848.9
abdominal wall (muscle) 848.8
Achilles tendon 845.09
acromioclavicular 840.0
ankle 845.00
  and foot 845.00
anterior longitudinal, cervical 847.0
arm 840.9
  upper 840.9
    and shoulder 840.9
astragalus 845.00
atlanto-axial 847.0
atlanto-occipital 847.0
atlas 847.0

Sprain, strain—continued
axis 847.0
back (see also Sprain, spine) 847.9
breast bone 848.40
broad ligament — see Injury, internal, broad ligament
calcaneofibular 845.02
carpal 842.01
carpometacarpal 842.11
cartilage
  costal, without mention of injury to sternum 848.3
    involving sternum 848.42
  ear 848.8
  knee 844.9
    with current tear (see also Tear, meniscus) 836.2
  semilunar (knee) 844.8
    with current tear (see also Tear, meniscus) 836.2
  septal, nose 848.0
  thyroid region 848.2
  xiphoid 848.49
cervical, cervicodorsal, cervicothoracic 847.0
chondrocostal, without mention of injury to sternum 848.3
  involving sternum 848.42
chondrosternal 848.42
chronic (joint) — see Derangement, joint
clavicle 840.9
coccyx 847.4
collar bone 840.9
collateral, knee (medial) (tibial) 844.1
  lateral (fibular) 844.0
  recurrent or old 717.89
    lateral 717.81
    medial 717.82
coracoacromial 840.8
coracoclavicular 840.1
coracohumeral 840.2
coracoid (process) 840.9
coronary, knee 844.8
costal cartilage, without mention of injury to sternum 848.3
  involving sternum 848.42
cricoarytenoid articulation 848.2
cricothyroid articulation 848.2
cruciate
  knee 844.2
  old 717.89
    anterior 717.83
    posterior 717.84
deltoid
  ankle 845.01
  shoulder 840.8
    dorsal (spine) 847.1
    ear cartilage 848.8
    elbow 841.9
    and forearm 841.9
    specified site NEC 841.8
    femur (proximal end) 843.9
    distal end 844.9
    fibula (proximal end) 844.9
    distal end 845.00
fibulocalcaneal 845.02
finger(s) 842.10
foot 845.10
  and ankle 845.00
forearm 841.9
  and elbow 841.9
  specified site NEC 841.8
glenoid (shoulder) 840.8
hand 842.10
hip 843.9
  and thigh 843.9
humerus (proximal end) 840.9
  distal end 841.9
iliofemoral 843.0
infraspinatus 840.3
innominate
  acetabulum 843.9

Sprain, strain—continued
innominate—continued
  pubic junction 848.5
  sacral junction 846.1
internal
  collateral, ankle 845.01
  semilunar cartilage 844.8
    with current tear (see also Tear, meniscus) 836.2
    old 717.5
interphalangeal
  finger 842.13
  toe 845.13
ischiocapsular 843.1
jaw (cartilage) (meniscus) 848.1
  old 524.69
knee 844.9
  and leg 844.9
  old 717.5
    collateral
      lateral 717.81
      medial 717.82
    cruciate
      anterior 717.83
      posterior 717.84
late effect — see Late, effects (of), sprain
lateral collateral, knee 844.0
  old 717.81
leg 844.9
  and knee 844.9
ligamentum teres femoris 843.8
low back 846.9
lumbar (spine) 847.2
lumbosacral 846.0
  chronic or old 724.6
mandible 848.1
  old 524.69
maxilla 848.1
medial collateral, knee 844.1
  old 717.82
meniscus
  jaw 848.1
    old 524.69
  knee 844.8
    with current tear (see also Tear, meniscus) 836.2
    old 717.5
  mandible 848.1
    old 524.69
  specified site NEC 848.8
metacarpal 842.10
  distal 842.12
  proximal 842.11
metacarpophalangeal 842.12
metatarsal 845.10
metatarsophalangeal 845.12
midcarpal 842.19
midtarsal 845.19
multiple sites, except fingers alone or toes alone 848.8
neck 847.0
nose (septal cartilage) 848.0
occiput from atlas 847.0
old — see Derangement, joint
orbicular, hip 843.8
patella(r) 844.8
  old 717.89
pelvis 848.5
phalanx
  finger 842.10
  toe 845.10
radiocarpal 842.02
radiohumeral 841.2
radioulnar 841.9
  distal 842.09
radius, radial (proximal end) 841.9
  and ulna 841.9
    distal 842.09
    collateral 841.0
    distal end 842.00
recurrent — see Sprain, by site

Sprain, strain—continued
rib (cage), without mention of injury to sternum 848.3
  involving sternum 848.42
rotator cuff (capsule) 840.4
round ligament — see also Injury, internal, round ligament
  femur 843.8
sacral (spine) 847.3
sacrococcygeal 847.3
sacroiliac (region) 846.9
  chronic or old 724.6
  ligament 846.1
  specified site NEC 846.8
sacrospinatus 846.2
sacrospinous 846.2
sacrotuberous 846.3
scaphoid bone, ankle 845.00
scapula(r) 840.9
semilunar cartilage (knee) 844.8
  with current tear (see also Tear, meniscus) 836.2
  old 717.5
septal cartilage (nose) 848.0
shoulder 840.9
  and arm, upper 840.9
  blade 840.9
  specified site NEC 848.8
spine 847.9
  cervical 847.0
  coccyx 847.4
  dorsal 847.1
  lumbar 847.2
  lumbosacral 846.0
    chronic or old 724.6
  sacral 847.3
  sacroiliac (see also Sprain, sacroiliac) 846.9
    chronic or old 724.6
  thoracic 847.1
sternoclavicular 848.41
sternum 848.40
subglenoid 840.8
subscapularis 840.5
supraspinatus 840.6
symphysis
  jaw 848.1
    old 524.69
  mandibular 848.1
    old 524.69
  pubis 848.5
talofibular 845.09
tarsal 845.10
tarsometatarsal 845.11
temporomandibular 848.1
  old 524.69
teres
  ligamentum femoris 843.8
  major or minor 840.8
thigh (proximal end) 843.9
  and hip 843.9
  distal end 844.9
thoracic (spine) 847.1
thorax 848.8
thumb 842.10
thyroid cartilage or region 848.2
tibia (proximal end) 844.9
  distal end 845.00
tibiofibular
  distal 845.03
  superior 844.3
toe(s) 845.10
trachea 848.8
trapezoid 840.8
ulna, ulnar (proximal end) 841.9
  collateral 841.1
  distal end 842.00
ulnohumeral 841.3
vertebrae (see also Sprain, spine) 847.9
  cervical, cervicodorsal, cervicothoracic 847.0
wrist (cuneiform) (scaphoid) (semilunar) 842.00
xiphoid cartilage 848.49

Sprengel's deformity (congenital) 755.52

Spring fever 309.23
Sprue 579.1
  celiac 579.0
  idiopathic 579.0
  meaning thrush 112.0
  nontropical 579.0
  tropical 579.1
Spur — *see also* Exostosis
  bone 726.91
    calcaneal 726.73
  calcaneal 726.73
  iliac crest 726.5
  nose (septum) 478.1
    bone 726.91
  septal 478.1
Spuria placenta — *see* Placenta, abnormal
Spurway's syndrome (brittle bones and blue sclera) 756.51
Sputum, abnormal (amount) (color) (excessive) (odor) (purulent) 786.4
  bloody 786.3
Squamous — *see also* condition
  cell metaplasia
    bladder 596.8
    cervix — *see* condition
  epithelium in
    cervical canal (congenital) 752.49
    uterine mucosa (congenital) 752.3
  metaplasia
    bladder 596.8
    cervix — *see* condition
Squashed nose 738.0
  congenital 754.0
Squeeze, divers' 993.3
Squint (*see also* Strabismus) 378.9
  accommodative (*see also* Esotropia) 378.00
  concomitant (*see also* Heterotropia) 378.30
Stab — *see also* Wound, open, by site
  internal organs — *see* Injury, internal, by site, with open wound
Staggering gait 781.2
  hysterical 300.11
Staghorn calculus 592.0
Stähl's
  ear 744.29
  pigment line (cornea) 371.11
Stähli's pigment lines (cornea) 371.11
Stain
  port wine 757.32
  tooth, teeth (hard tissues) 521.7
    due to
      accretions 523.6
      deposits (betel) (black) (green) (materia alba) (orange) (tobacco) 523.6
      metals (copper) (silver) 521.7
      nicotine 523.6
      pulpal bleeding 521.7
      tobacco 523.6
Stammering 307.0
Standstill
  atrial 426.6
  auricular 426.6
  cardiac (*see also* Arrest, cardiac) 427.5
  sinoatrial 429.6
  sinus 426.6
  ventricular (*see also* Arrest, cardiac) 427.5
Stannosis 503
Stanton's disease (melioidosis) 025

Staphylitis (acute) (catarrhal) (chronic) (gangrenous) (membranous) (suppurative) (ulcerative) 528.3
Staphylococcemia 038.1
Staphylococcus, staphylococcal — *see* condition
Staphyloderma (skin) 686.0
Staphyloma 379.11
  anterior, localized 379.14
  ciliary 379.11
  cornea 371.73
  equatorial 379.13
  posterior 379.12
  posticum 379.12
  ring 379.15
  sclera NEC 379.11
Starch eating 307.52
Stargardt's disease 362.75
Starvation (inanition) (due to lack of food) 994.2
  edema 262
  voluntary NEC 307.1
Stasis
  bile (duct) (*see also* Disease, biliary) 576.8
  bronchus (*see also* Bronchitis) 490
  cardiac (*see also* Failure, heart, congestive) 428.0
  cecum 564.8
  colon 564.8
  dermatitis (*see also* Varix, with stasis dermatitis) 454.1
  duodenal 536.8
  eczema (*see also* Varix, with stasis dermatitis) 454.1
  foot 991.4
  gastric 536.3
  ileocecal coil 564.8
  ileum 564.8
  intestinal 564.8
  jejunum 564.8
  kidney 586
  liver 571.9
    cirrhotic — *see* Cirrhosis, liver
  lymphatic 457.8
  pneumonia 514
  portal 571.9
  pulmonary 514
  rectal 564.8
  renal 586
    tubular 584.5
  stomach 536.3
  ulcer 454.0
  urine NEC (*see also* Retention, urine) 788.20
  venous 459.81
State
  affective and paranoid, mixed, organic psychotic 294.8
  agitated 307.9
    acute reaction to stress 308.2
  anxiety (neurotic) (*see also* Anxiety) 300.00
    specified type NEC 300.09
  apprehension (*see also* Anxiety) 300.00
    specified type NEC 300.09
  climacteric, female 627.2
    following induced menopause 627.4
  clouded
    epileptic (*see also* Epilepsy) 345.9
    paroxysmal (idiopathic) (*see also* Epilepsy) 345.9
  compulsive (mixed) (with obsession) 300.3

State—*continued*
  confusional 298.9
    acute 293.0
      with
        arteriosclerotic dementia 290.41
        presenile brain disease 290.11
        senility 290.3
      alcoholic 291.0
      drug-induced 292.81
      epileptic 293.0
      postoperative 293.9
      reactive (emotional stress) (psychological trauma) 298.2
    subacute 293.1
  constitutional psychopathic 301.9
  convulsive (*see also* Convulsions) 780.3
  depressive NEC 311
    induced by drug 292.84
    neurotic 300.4
  dissociative 300.15
  hallucinatory 780.1
    induced by drug 292.12
  hyperdynamic beta-adrenergic circulatory 429.82
  locked-in 344.81
  menopausal 627.2
    artificial 627.4
    following induced menopause 627.4
  neurotic NEC 300.9
    with depersonalization episode 300.6
  obsessional 300.3
  oneiroid (*see also* Schizophrenia) 295.4
  panic 300.01
  paranoid 297.9
    alcohol-induced 291.5
    arteriosclerotic 290.42
    climacteric 297.2
    drug-induced 292.11
    in
      presenile brain disease 290.12
      senile brain disease 290.20
    involutional 297.2
    menopausal 297.2
    senile 290.20
    simple 297.0
  postleukotomy 310.0
  pregnant (*see also* Pregnancy) V22.2
  psychogenic, twilight 298.2
  psychotic, organic (*see also* Psychosis, organic) 294.9
    mixed paranoid and affective 294.8
    senile or presenile NEC 290.9
    transient NEC 293.9
      with
        delusions 293.81
        depression 293.83
        hallucinations 293.82
  residual schizophrenic (*see also* Schizophrenia) 295.6
  tension (*see also* Anxiety) 300.9
  transient organic psychotic 293.9
    depressive type 293.83
    hallucinatory type 293.83
    paranoid type 293.81
    specified type NEC 293.89
  twilight
    epileptic 293.0
    psychogenic 298.2
  vegetative (persistent) 780.03
Status (post)
  absence
    epileptic (*see also* Epilepsy) 345.2
    of organ, acquired (postsurgical) — *see* Absence, by site, acquired

Status—*continued*
  anastomosis of intestine (for bypass) V45.3
  angioplasty, percutaneous transluminal coronary V45.82
  anginosus 413.9
  ankle prosthesis V43.66
  aortocoronary bypass or shunt V45.81
  arthrodesis V45.4
  artificially induced condition NEC V45.89
  artificial opening (of) V44.9
    gastrointestinal tract NEC V44.4
    specified site NEC V44.8
    urinary tract NEC V44.6
    vagina V44.7
  asthmaticus (*see also* Asthma) 493.9
  cardiac
    device (in situ) V45.00
      carotid sinus V45.09
        fitting or adjustment V53.39
      defibrillator, automatic implantable V45.02
      pacemaker V45.01
        fitting or adjustmanet V53.31
  carotid sinus stimulator V45.09
  cataract extraction V45.6
  chemotherapy V66.2
  colostomy V44.3
  contraceptive device V45.59
    intrauterine V45.51
    subdermal V45.52
  convulsivus idiopathicus (*see also* Epilepsy) 345.3
  coronary artery bypass or shunt V45.81
  cystostomy V44.5
  defibrillator, automatic implantable cardiac V45.02
  dialysis V45.1
  donor V59.9
  drug therapy or regimen V67.59
    high-risk medication NEC V67.51
  elbow prosthesis V43.62
  enterostomy V44.4
  epileptic, epilepticus (absence) (grand mal) (*see also* Epilepsy) 345.3
    focal motor 345.7
    partial 345.7
    petit mal 345.2
    psychomotor 345.7
    temporal lobe 345.7
  eye (adnexa) surgery V45.6
  filtering bleb (eye) (postglaucoma) V45.6
    with rupture or complication 997.9
    pastcataract extraction (complication) 997.9
  finger joint prosthesis V43.69
  gastrostomy V44.1
  grand mal 345.3
  heart valve prosthesis V43.3
  hip prosthesis (joint) (partial) (total) V43.64
  ileostomy V44.2
  intestinal bypass V45.3
  intrauterine contraceptive device V45.51
  jejunostomy V44.4
  knee joint prosthesis V43.65
  lacunaris 437.8
  lacunosis 437.8
  lymphaticus 254.8
  malignant neoplasm, ablated or excised — *see* History, malignant neoplasm
  marmoratus 333.7

Status—continued
  nephrostomy V44.6
  neuropacemaker NEC V45.89
    brain V45.89
    carotid sinus V45.09
    neurologic NEC V45.89
  organ replacement
    by artificial or mechanical
        device or prosthesis of
      artery V43.4
      bladder V43.5
      blood vessel V43.4
      eye globe V43.0
      heart V43.2
        valve V43.3
      intestine V43.8
      joint V43.60
        ankle V43.66
        elbow V43.62
        finger V43.69
        hip (partial) (total)
            V43.64
        knee V43.65
        shoulder V43.61
        specified NEC V43.69
          wrist V43.63
      kidney V43.8
      larynx V43.8
      lens V43.1
      limb(s) V43.7
      liver V43.8
      lung V43.8
      organ NEC V43.8
      pancreas V43.8
      tissue NEC V43.8
      vein V43.4
    by organ transplant
        (heterologous)
        (homologous) — see
        Status, transplant
  pacemaker
    brain V45.89
    cardiac V45.01
    carotid sinus V45.09
    neurologic NEC V45.89
    specified site NEC V45.89
  percutaneous transluminal
      coronary angioplasty
      V45.82
  petit mal 345.2
  postcommotio cerebri 310.2
  postoperative NEC V45.89
  postpartum NEC V24.2
    care immediately following
        delivery V24.0
    routine follow-up V24.2
  postsurgical NEC V45.89
  renal dialysis V45.1
  reversed jejunal transposition (for
      bypass) V45.3
  shoulder prosthesis V43.61
  shunt
    aortocoronary bypass V45.81
    arteriovenous (for dialysis)
        V45.1
    cerebrospinal fluid V45.2
    vascular NEC V45.89
      aortocoronary (bypass)
          V45.81
    ventricular (communicating)
        (for drainage) V45.2
  subdermal contraceptive device
      V45.52
  thymicolymphaticus 254.8
  thymicus 254.8
  thymolymphaticus 254.8
  tracheostomy V44.0
  transplant
    blood vessel V42.8
    bone V42.4
      marrow V42.8
    cornea V42.5
    heart V42.1
      valve V42.2
    intestine V42.8
    kidney V42.0
    liver V42.7

Status—continued
  transplant—continued
    lung V42.6
    organ V42.9
      specified site NEC V42.8
    pancreas V42.8
    skin V42.3
    tissue V42.9
      specified type NEC V42.8
    vessel, blood V42.8
  ureterostomy V44.6
  urethrostomy V44.6
  vagina, artificial V44.7
  vascular shunt NEC V45.89
    aortocoronary (bypass) V45.81
  wrist prosthesis V43.63
Stave fracture — see Fracture,
    metacarpus, metacarpal
    bone(s)
Steal
  subclavian artery 435.2
  vertebral artery 435.1
Stealing, solitary, child problem (see
    also Disturbance, conduct)
    312.1
Steam burn — see Burn, by site
Steatocystoma multiplex 706.2
Steatoma (infected) 706.2
  eyelid (cystic) 374.84
    infected 373.13
Steatorrhea (chronic) 579.8
  with lacteal obstruction 579.2
  idiopathic 579.0
    adult 579.0
    infantile 579.0
  pancreatic 579.4
  primary 579.0
  secondary 579.8
  specified cause NEC 579.8
  tropical 579.1
Steatosis 272.8
  heart (see also Degeneration,
      myocardial) 429.1
  kidney 593.89
  liver 571.8
Stein's syndrome (polycystic ovary)
    256.4
Stein-Leventhal syndrome
    (polycystic ovary) 256.4
Steinbrocker's syndrome (see also
    Neuropathy, peripheral,
    autonomic) 337.9
Steinert's disease 359.2
Stenocardia (see also Angina) 413.9
Stenocephaly 756.0
Stenosis (cicatricial) — see also
    Stricture
  ampulla of Vater 576.2
    with calculus, cholelithiasis, or
        stones — see
        Choledocholithiasis
  anus, anal (canal) (sphincter)
      569.2
    congenital 751.2
  aorta (ascending) 747.22
    arch 747.10
    arteriosclerotic 440.0
    calcified 440.0
  aortic (valve) 424.1
    with
      mitral (valve)
        insufficiency or
            incompetence
            396.2
        stenosis or obstruction
            396.0
    atypical 396.0
    congenital 746.3

Stenosis—continued
  aortic—continued
    rheumatic 395.0
      with
        insufficiency,
            incompetency or
            regurgitation
            395.2
          with mitral (valve)
              disease 396.8
        mitral (valve)
          disease (stenosis)
              396.0
          insufficiency or
              incompetence
              396.2
          stenosis or
              obstruction
              396.0
    specified cause, except
        rheumatic 424.1
    syphilitic 093.22
  aqueduct of Sylvius (congenital)
      742.3
    with spina bifida (see also
        Spina bifida) 741.0
    acquired 331.4
  artery NEC 447.1
    basilar — see Narrowing,
        artery, basilar
    carotid (common) (internal) —
        see Narrowing, artery,
        carotid
    celiac 447.4
    cerebral 437.0
      due to
        embolism (see also
            Embolism, brain)
            434.1
        thrombus (see also
            Thrombosis,
            brain) 434.0
    precerebral — see Narrowing,
        artery, precerebral
    pulmonary (congenital) 747.3
      acquired 417.8
    renal 440.1
    vertebral — see Narrowing,
        artery, vertebral
  bile duct or biliary passage (see
      also Obstruction, biliary)
      576.2
    congenital 751.61
  bladder neck (acquired) 596.0
    congenital 753.6
  brain 348.8
  bronchus 519.1
    syphilitic 095.8
  cardia (stomach) 537.89
    congenital 750.7
  cardiovascular (see also Disease,
      cardiovascular) 429.2
  carotid artery — see Narrowing,
      artery, carotid
  cervix, cervical (canal) 622.4
    congenital 752.49
    in pregnancy or childbirth
        654.6
      affecting fetus or newborn
          763.8
      causing obstructed labor
          660.2
        affecting fetus or
            newborn 763.1
  colon (see also Obstruction,
      intestine) 560.9
    congenital 751.2
  colostomy 569.6
  common bile duct (see also
      Obstruction, biliary) 576.2
    congenital 751.61
  coronary (artery) —see
      Arteriosclerosis, coronary
  cystic duct (see also Obstruction,
      gallbladder) 575.2
    congenital 751.61

Stenosis—continued
  due to (presence of) any device,
      implant, or graft classifiable
      to 996.0-996.5 — see
      Complications, due to
      (presence of) any device,
      implant, or graft classified
      to 996.0-996.5 NEC
  duodenum 537.3
    congenital 751.1
  ejaculatory duct NEC 608.89
  endocervical os — see Stenosis,
      cervix
  enterostomy 569.6
  esophagus 530.3
    congenital 750.3
    syphilitic 095.8
      congenital 090.5
  external ear canal 380.50
    secondary to
      inflammation 380.53
      surgery 380.52
      trauma 380.51
  gallbladder (see also Obstruction,
      gallbladder) 575.2
  glottis 478.74
  heart valve (acquired) — see also
      Endocarditis
    congenital NEC 746.89
      aortic 746.3
      mitral 746.5
      pulmonary 746.02
      tricuspid 746.1
  hepatic duct (see also
      Obstruction, biliary) 576.2
  hymen 623.3
  hypertrophic subaortic
      (idiopathic) 425.1
  infundibulum cardiac 746.83
  intestine (see also Obstruction,
      intestine) 560.9
    congenital (small) 751.1
      large 751.2
  lacrimal
    canaliculi 375.53
    duct 375.56
      congenital 743.65
    punctum 375.52
      congenital 743.65
    sac 375.54
      congenital 743.65
  lacrimonasal duct 375.56
    congenital 743.65
    neonatal 375.55
  larynx 478.74
    congenital 748.3
    syphilitic 095.8
      congenital 090.5
  mitral (valve) (chronic) (inactive)
      394.0
    with
      aortic (valve)
        disease (insufficiency)
            396.1
        insufficiency or
            incompetence
            396.1
        stenosis or obstruction
            396.0
      incompetency, insufficiency
          or regurgitation
          394.2
        with aortic valve disease
            396.8
    active or acute 391.1
      with chorea (acute)
          (rheumatic)
          (Sydenham's) 392.0
    congenital 746.5
    specified cause, except
        rheumatic 424.0
    syphilitic 093.21
  myocardium, myocardial (see
      also Degeneration,
      myocardial) 429.1
    hypertrophic subaortic
        (idiopathic) 425.1

Stenosis—continued
- nares (anterior) (posterior) 478.1
  - congenital 748.0
- nasal duct 375.56
  - congenital 743.65
- nasolacrimal duct 375.56
  - congenital 743.65
  - neonatal 375.55
- organ or site, congenital NEC — see Atresia
- papilla of Vater 576.2
  - with calculus, cholelithiasis, or stones — see Choledocholithiasis
- pulmonary (artery) (congenital) 747.3
  - with ventricular septal defect, dextraposition of aorta and hypertrophy of right ventricle 745.2
  - acquired 417.8
  - infundibular 746.83
  - in tetralogy of Fallot 745.2
  - subvalvular 746.83
  - valve (see also Endocarditis, pulmonary) 424.3
    - congenital 746.02
  - vein 747.49
    - acquired 417.8
  - vessel NEC 417.8
- pulmonic (congenital) 746.02
  - infundibular 746.83
  - subvalvular 746.83
- pylorus (hypertrophic) 537.0
  - adult 537.0
  - congenital 750.5
  - infantile 750.5
- rectum (sphincter) (see also Stricture, rectum) 569.2
- renal artery 440.1
- salivary duct (any) 527.8
- sphincter of Oddi (see also Obstruction, biliary) 576.2
- spinal 724.00
  - cervical 723.0
  - lumbar, lumbosacral 724.02
  - nerve (root) NEC 724.9
    - specified region NEC 724.09
  - thoracic, thoracolumbar 724.01
- stomach, hourglass 537.6
- subaortic 746.81
  - hypertrophic (idiopathic) 425.1
- supra (valvular)-aortic 747.22
- trachea 519.1
  - congenital 748.3
  - syphilitic 095.8
  - tuberculous (see also Tuberculosis) 012.8
- tracheostomy 519.0
- tricuspid (valve) (see also Endocarditis, tricuspid) 397.0
  - congenital 746.1
  - nonrheumatic 424.2
- tubal 628.2
- ureter (see also Stricture, ureter) 593.3
  - congenital 753.2
- urethra (see also Stricture, urethra) 598.9
- vagina 623.2
  - congenital 752.49
  - in pregnancy or childbirth 654.7
    - affecting fetus or newborn 763.8
    - causing obstructed labor 660.2
      - affecting fetus or newborn 763.1
- valve (cardiac) (heart) (see also Endocarditis) 424.90
  - congenital NEC 746.89
    - aortic 746.3
    - mitral 746.5

Stenosis—continued
- valve—continued
  - congenital NEC—continued
    - pulmonary 746.02
    - tricuspid 746.1
    - urethra 753.6
  - valvular (see also Endocarditis) 424.90
    - congenital NEC 746.89
      - urethra 753.6
  - vascular graft or shunt 996.1
    - atherosclerosis — see Arteriosclerosis, extremitites
    - embolism 996.74
    - occlusion NEC 996.74
    - thrombus 996.74
  - vena cava (inferior) (superior) 459.2
    - congenital 747.49
  - ventricular shunt 996.2
  - vulva 624.8
- **Stercolith** (see also Fecalith) 560.39
  - appendix 543.9
- **Stercoraceous, stercoral ulcer** 569.82
  - anus or rectum 569.41
- **Stereopsis, defective**
  - with fusion 368.33
  - without fusion 368.32
- **Stereotypies** NEC 307.3
- **Sterility**
  - female — see Infertility, female
  - male (see also Infertility, male) 606.9
- **Sterilization, admission for** V25.2
- **Sternalgia** (see also Angina) 413.9
- **Sternopagus** 759.4
- **Sternum bifidum** 756.3
- **Sternutation** 784.9
- **Steroid**
  - effects (adverse) (iatrogenic)
    - cushingoid
      - correct substance properly administered 255.0
      - overdose or wrong substance given or taken 962.0
    - diabetes
      - correct substance properly administered 251.8
      - overdose or wrong substance given or taken 962.0
    - due to
      - correct substance properly administered 255.8
      - overdose or wrong substance given or taken 962.0
    - fever
      - correct substance properly administered 780.6
      - overdose or wrong substance given or taken 962.0
    - withdrawal
      - correct substance properly administered 255.4
      - overdose or wrong substance given or taken 962.0
  - responder 365.03
- **Stevens-Johnson disease or syndrome** (erythema multiforme exudativum) 695.1
- **Stewart-Morel syndrome** (hyperostosis frontalis interna) 733.3
- **Sticker's disease** (erythema infectiosum) 057.0
- **Sticky eye** 372.03
- **Stieda's disease** (calcification, knee joint) 726.62

Stiff
- back 724.8
- neck (see also Torticollis) 723.5

Stiff-man syndrome 333.91

Stiffness, joint NEC 719.50
- ankle 719.57
- back 724.8
- elbow 719.52
- finger 719.54
- hip 719.55
- knee 719.56
- multiple sites 719.59
- sacroiliac 724.6
- shoulder 719.51
- specified site NEC 719.58
- spine 724.9
- surgical fusion V45.4
- wrist 719.53

Stigmata, congenital syphilis 090.5

Still's disease or syndrome 714.30

Still-Felty syndrome (rheumatoid arthritis with splenomegaly and leukopenia) 714.1

Stillbirth, stillborn NEC 779.9

Stiller's disease (asthenia) 780.7

Stilling-Türk-Duane syndrome (ocular retraction syndrome) 378.71

Stimulation, ovary 256.1

Sting (animal) (bee) (fish) (insect) (jellyfish) (Portuguese man-o-war) (wasp) (venomous) 989.5
- anaphylactic shock or reaction 989.5
- plant 692.6

Stippled epiphyses 756.59

Stitch
- abscess 998.5
- burst (in operation wound) 998.3
- in back 724.5

Stojano's (subcostal) syndrome 098.86

Stokes' disease (exophthalmic goiter) 242.0

Stokes-Adams syndrome (syncope with heart block) 426.9

Stokvis' (-Talma) disease (enterogenous cyanosis) 289.7

Stomach — see condition

Stoma malfunction
- colostomy 569.6
- cystostomy 997.5
- enterostomy 569.6
- gastrostomy 997.4
- ileostomy 569.6
- nephrostomy 997.5
- tracheostomy 519.0
- ureterostomy 997.5

Stomatitis 528.0
- angular 528.5
  - due to dietary or vitamin deficiency 266.0
- aphthous 528.2
- candidal 112.0
- catarrhal 528.0
- denture 528.9
- diphtheritic (membranous) 032.0
- due to
  - dietary deficiency 266.0
  - thrush 112.0
  - vitamin deficiency 266.0
- epidemic 078.4
- epizootic 078.4
- follicular 528.0
- gangrenous 528.1
- herpetic 054.2
- herpetiformis 528.2
- malignant 528.0
- membranous acute 528.0
- monilial 112.0
- mycotic 112.0
- necrotic 528.1
  - ulcerative 101
- necrotizing ulcerative 101

Stomatitis—continued
- parasitic 112.0
- septic 528.0
- spirochetal 101
- suppurative (acute) 528.0
- ulcerative 528.0
  - necrotizing 101
- ulceromembranous 101
- vesicular 528.0
  - with exanthem 074.3
- Vincent's 101

Stomatocytosis 282.8

Stomatomycosis 112.0

Stomatorrhagia 528.9

Stone(s) — see also Calculus
- bladder 594.1
  - diverticulum 594.0
- cystine 270.0
- heart syndrome (see also Failure, ventricular, left) 428.1
- kidney 592.0
- prostate 602.0
- pulp (dental) 522.2
- renal 592.0
- salivary duct or gland (any) 527.5
- ureter 592.1
- urethra (impacted) 594.2
- urinary (duct) (impacted) (passage) 592.9
  - bladder 594.1
    - diverticulum 594.0
  - lower tract NEC 594.9
  - specified site 594.8
- xanthine 277.2

Stonecutters' lung 502
- tuberculous (see also Tuberculosis) 011.4

Stonemasons'
- asthma, disease, or lung 502
  - tuberculous (see also Tuberculosis) 011.4
- phthisis (see also Tuberculosis) 011.4

Stoppage
- bowel (see also Obstruction, intestine) 560.9
- heart (see also Arrest, cardiac) 427.5
- intestine (see also Obstruction, intestine) 560.9
- urine NEC (see also Retention, urine) 788.20

Storm, thyroid (apathetic) (see also Thyrotoxicosis) 242.9

Strabismus (alternating) (congenital) (nonparalytic) 378.9
- concomitant (see also Heterotropia) 378.30
  - convergent (see also Esotropia) 378.00
  - divergent (see also Exotropia) 378.10
- convergent (see also Esotropia) 378.00
- divergent (see also Exotropia) 378.10
- due to adhesions, scars — see Strabismus, mechanical
- in neuromuscular disorder NEC 378.73
- intermittent 378.20
  - vertical 378.31
- latent 378.40
  - convergent (esophoria) 378.41
  - divergent (exophoria) 378.42
  - vertical 378.43
- mechanical 378.60
  - due to
    - Brown's tendon sheath syndrome 378.61
    - specified musculofascial disorder NEC 378.62

Strabismus — continued
- paralytic 378.50
  - third or oculomotor nerve (partial) 378.51
    - total 378.52
  - fourth or trochlear nerve 378.53
  - sixth or abducens nerve 378.54
- specified type NEC 378.73
- vertical (hypertropia) 378.31

Strain — *see also* Sprain, by site
- eye NEC 368.13
- heart — *see* Disease, heart
- meaning gonorrhea — *see* Gonorrhea
- physical NEC V62.89
- postural 729.9
- psychological NEC V62.89

Strands
- conjunctiva 372.62
- vitreous humor 379.25

Strangulation, strangulated 994.7
- appendix 543.9
- asphyxiation or suffocation by 994.7
- bladder neck 596.0
- bowel — *see* Strangulation, intestine
- colon — *see* Strangulation, intestine
- cord (umbilical) — *see* Compression, umbilical cord
- due to birth injury 767.8
- food or foreign body (*see also* Asphyxia, food) 933.1
- hemorrhoids 455.8
  - external 455.5
  - internal 455.2
- hernia — *see also* Hernia, by site, with obstruction
  - gangrenous — *see* Hernia, by site, with gangrene
- intestine (large) (small) 560.2
  - with hernia — *see also* Hernia, by site, with obstruction
    - gangrenous — *see* Hernia, by site, with gangrene
  - congenital (small) 751.1
    - large 751.2
- mesentery 560.2
- mucus (*see also* Asphyxia, mucus) 933.1
  - newborn 770.1
- omentum 560.2
- organ or site, congenital NEC — *see* Atresia
- ovary 620.8
  - due to hernia 620.4
- penis 607.89
  - foreign body 939.3
- rupture (*see also* Hernia, by site, with obstruction) 552.9
  - gangrenous (*see also* Hernia, by site, with gangrene) 551.9
- stomach, due to hernia (*see also* Hernia, by site, with obstruction) 552.9
  - with gangrene (*see also* Hernia, by site, with gangrene) 551.9
- umbilical cord — *see* Compression, umbilical cord
- vesicourethral orifice 596.0

Strangury 788.1

Strawberry
- gallbladder (*see also* Disease, gallbladder) 575.6
- mark 757.32
- tongue (red) (white) 529.3

Straw itch 133.8

Streak, ovarian 752.0

Strephosymbolia 315.01
- secondary to organic lesion 784.69

Streptobacillary fever 026.1

Streptobacillus moniliformis 026.1

Streptococcemia 038.0

Streptococcicosis — *see* Infection, streptococcal

Streptococcus, streptococcal — *see* condition

Streptoderma 686.0

Streptomycosis — *see* Actinomycosis

Streptothricosis — *see* Actinomycosis

Streptothrix — *see* Actinomycosis

Streptotrichosis — *see* Actinomycosis

Stress
- fracture — *see* Fracture, pathologic
- polycythemia 289.0
- reaction (gross) (*see also* Reaction, stress, acute) 308.9

Stretching, nerve — *see* Injury, nerve, by site

Striae (albicantes) (atrophicae) (cutis distensae) (distensae) 701.3

Striations of nails 703.8

Stricture (*see also* Stenosis) 799.8
- ampulla of Vater 576.2
  - with calculus, cholelithiasis, or stones — *see* Choledocholithiasis
- anus (sphincter) 569.2
  - congenital 751.2
  - infantile 751.2
- aorta (ascending) 747.22
  - arch 747.10
  - arteriosclerotic 440.0
  - calcified 440.0
- aortic (valve) (*see also* Stenosis, aortic) 424.1
  - congenital 746.3
- aqueduct of Sylvius (congenital) 742.3
  - with spina bifida (*see also* Spina bifida) 741.0
  - acquired 331.4
- artery 447.1
  - basilar — *see* Narrowing, artery, basilar
  - carotid (common) (internal) — *see* Narrowing, artery, carotid
  - celiac 447.4
  - cerebral 437.0
    - congenital 747.81
    - due to
      - embolism (*see also* Embolism, brain) 434.1
      - thrombus (*see also* Thrombosis, brain) 434.0
  - congenital (peripheral) 747.60
    - cerebral 747.81
    - coronary 746.85
    - gastrointestinal 747.61
    - lower limb 747.64
    - renal 747.62
    - retinal 743.58
    - specified NEC 747.69
    - spinal 747.82
    - umbilical 747.5
    - upper limb 747.63
  - coronary — *see* Arteriosclerosis, coronary ◆
    - congenital 746.85
  - precerebral — *see* Narrowing, artery, precerebral NEC

Stricture — continued
- artery — *continued*
  - pulmonary (congenital) 747.3
    - acquired 417.8
  - renal 440.1
  - vertebral — *see* Narrowing, artery, vertebral
- auditory canal (congenital) (external) 744.02
  - acquired (*see also* Stricture, ear canal, acquired) 380.50
- bile duct or passage (any) (postoperative) (*see also* Obstruction, biliary) 576.2
  - congenital 751.61
- bladder 596.8
  - congenital 753.6
  - neck 596.0
    - congenital 753.6
- bowel (*see also* Obstruction, intestine) 560.9
- brain 348.8
- bronchus 519.1
  - syphilitic 095.8
- cardia (stomach) 537.89
  - congenital 750.7
- cardiac — *see* Disease, heart
  - orifice (stomach) 537.89
- cardiovascular (*see also* Disease, cardiovascular) 429.2
- carotid artery — *see* Narrowing, artery, carotid
- cecum (*see also* Obstruction, intestine) 560.9
- cervix, cervical (canal) 622.4
  - congenital 752.49
  - in pregnancy or childbirth 654.6
    - affecting fetus or newborn 763.8
    - causing obstructed labor 660.2
      - affecting fetus or newborn 763.1
- colon (*see also* Obstruction, intestine) 560.9
  - congenital 751.2
- colostomy 569.6
- common bile duct (*see also* Obstruction, biliary) 576.2
  - congenital 751.61
- coronary (artery) — *see* Arteriosclerosis, coronary ◆
  - congenital 746.85
- cystic duct (*see also* Obstruction, gallbladder) 575.2
  - congenital 751.61
- cystostomy 997.5
- digestive organs NEC, congenital 751.8
- duodenum 537.3
  - congenital 751.1
- ear canal (external) (congenital) 744.02
  - acquired 380.50
    - secondary to
      - inflammation 380.53
      - surgery 380.52
      - trauma 380.51
- ejaculatory duct 608.85
- enterostomy 569.6
- esophagus (corrosive) (peptic) 530.3
  - congenital 750.3
  - syphilitic 095.8
    - congenital 090.5
- eustachian tube (*see also* Obstruction, Eustachian tube) 381.60
  - congenital 744.24
- fallopian tube 628.2
  - gonococcal (chronic) 098.37
    - acute 098.17
  - tuberculous (*see also* Tuberculosis) 016.6

Stricture — continued
- gallbladder (*see also* Obstruction, gallbladder) 575.2
  - congenital 751.69
- glottis 478.74
- heart — *see also* Disease, heart
  - congenital NEC 746.89
  - valve — *see also* Endocarditis
    - congenital NEC 746.89
      - aortic 746.3
      - mitral 746.5
      - pulmonary 746.02
      - tricuspid 746.1
- hepatic duct (*see also* Obstruction, biliary) 576.2
- hourglass, of stomach 537.6
- hymen 623.3
- hypopharynx 478.29
- intestine (*see also* Obstruction, intestine) 560.9
  - congenital (small) 751.1
    - large 751.2
  - ischemic 557.1
- lacrimal
  - canaliculi 375.53
    - congenital 743.65
  - punctum 375.52
    - congenital 743.65
  - sac 375.54
    - congenital 743.65
- lacrimonasal duct 375.56
  - congenital 743.65
  - neonatal 375.55
- larynx 478.79
  - congenital 748.3
  - syphilitic 095.8
    - congenital 090.5
- lung 518.89
- meatus
  - ear (congenital) 744.02
    - acquired (*see also* Stricture, ear canal, acquired) 380.50
  - osseous (congenital) (ear) 744.03
    - acquired (*see also* Stricture, ear canal, acquired) 380.50
  - urinarius (*see also* Stricture, urethra) 598.9
    - congenital 753.6
- mitral (valve) (*see also* Stenosis, mitral) 394.0
  - congenital 746.5
  - specified cause, except rheumatic 424.0
- myocardium, myocardial (*see also* Degeneration, myocardial) 429.1
  - hypertrophic subaortic (idiopathic) 425.1
- nares (anterior) (posterior) 478.1
  - congenital 748.0
- nasal duct 375.56
  - congenital 743.65
  - neonatal 375.55
- nasolacrimal duct 375.56
  - congenital 743.65
  - neonatal 375.55
- nasopharynx 478.29
  - syphilitic 095.8
- nephrostomy 997.5
- nose 478.1
  - congenital 748.0
- nostril (anterior) (posterior) 478.1
  - congenital 748.0
- organ or site, congenital NEC — *see* Atresia
- osseous meatus (congenital) (ear) 744.03
  - acquired (*see also* Stricture, ear canal, acquired) 380.50
- os uteri (*see also* Stricture, cervix) 622.4
- oviduct — *see* Stricture, fallopian tube

Stricture—continued
  pelviureteric junction 593.3
  pharynx (dilation) 478.29
  prostate 602.8
  pulmonary, pulmonic
    artery (congenital) 747.3
      acquired 417.8
      noncongenital 417.8
    infundibulum (congenital) 746.83
    valve (see also Endocarditis, pulmonary) 424.3
      congenital 746.02
    vein (congenital) 747.49
      acquired 417.8
    vessel NEC 417.8
  punctum lacrimale 375.52
    congenital 743.65
  pylorus (hypertrophic) 537.0
    adult 537.0
    congenital 750.5
    infantile 750.5
  rectosigmoid 569.89
  rectum (sphincter) 569.2
    congenital 751.2
    due to
      chemical burn 947.3
      irradiation 569.2
      lymphogranuloma venereum 099.1
    gonococcal 098.7
    inflammatory 099.1
    syphilitic 095.8
    tuberculous (see also Tuberculosis) 014.8
  renal artery 440.1
  salivary duct or gland (any) 527.8
  sigmoid (flexure) (see also Obstruction, intestine) 560.9
  spermatic cord 608.85
  stoma (following) (of)
    colostomy 569.6
    cystostomy 997.5
    enterostomy 569.6
    gastrostomy 997.4
    ileostomy 569.6
    nephrostomy 997.5
    tracheostomy 519.0
    ureterostomy 997.5
  stomach 537.89
    congenital 750.7
    hourglass 537.6
  subaortic 746.81
    hypertrophic (acquired) (idiopathic) 425.1
  subglottic 478.74
  syphilitic NEC 095.8
  tendon (sheath) 727.81
  trachea 519.1
    congenital 748.3
    syphilitic 095.8
    tuberculous (see also Tuberculosis) 012.8
  tracheostome 519.0
  tricuspid (valve) (see also Endocarditis, tricuspid) 397.0
    congenital 746.1
    nonrheumatic 424.2
  tunica vaginalis 608.85
  ureter (postoperative) 593.3
    congenital 753.2
    tuberculous (see also Tuberculosis) 016.2
  ureteropelvic junction 593.3
    congenital 753.2
  ureterovesical orifice 593.3
    congenital 753.2
  urethra (anterior) (meatal) (organic) (posterior) (spasmodic) 598.9
    associated with schistosomiasis (see also Schistosomiasis) 120.9 [598.01]
    congenital (valvular) 753.6

Stricture—continued
  urethra—continued
    due to
      infection 598.00
        syphilis 095.8 [598.01]
      trauma 598.1
    gonococcal 098.2 [598.01]
    gonorrheal 098.2 [598.01]
    infective 598.00
    late effect of injury 598.1
    postcatheterization 598.2
    postobstetric 598.1
    postoperative 598.2
    specified cause NEC 598.8
    syphilitic 095.8 [598.01]
    traumatic 598.1
    valvular, congenital 753.6
  urinary meatus (see also Stricture, urethra) 598.9
    congenital 753.6
  uterus, uterine 621.5
    os (external) (internal) — see Stricture, cervix
  vagina (outlet) 623.2
    congenital 752.49
  valve (cardiac) (heart) (see also Endocarditis) 424.90
    congenital (cardiac) (heart) NEC 746.89
      aortic 746.3
      mitral 746.5
      pulmonary 746.02
      tricuspid 746.1
      urethra 753.6
  valvular (see also Endocarditis) 424.90
  vascular graft or shunt 996.1
    atherosclerosis — see Arteriosclersis, extremities
    embolism 996.74
    occlusion NEC 996.74
    thrombus 996.74
  vas deferens 608.85
    congenital 752.8
  vein 459.2
  vena cava (inferior) (superior) NEC 459.2
    congenital 747.49
  ventricular shunt 996.2
  vesicourethral orifice 596.0
    congenital 753.6
  vulva (acquired) 624.8
Stridor 786.1
  congenital (larynx) 748.3
Stridulous — see condition
Strippling of nails 703.8
Stroke (see also Disease, cerebrovascular, acute) 436
  apoplectic (see also Disease, cerebrovascular, acute) 436
  brain (see also Disease, cerebrovascular, acute) 436
  epileptic — see Epilepsy
  healed or old — see also category 438
    without residuals V12.5
  heart — see Disease, heart
  heat 992.0
  in evolution 435.9
  late effect — see category 438
  lightning 994.0
  paralytic (see also Disease, cerebrovascular, acute) 436
  progressive 435.9
Stromatosis, endometrial (M8931/1) 236.0
Strong pulse 785.9
Strongyloides stercoralis infestation 127.2
Strongyloidiasis 127.2
Strongyloidosis 127.2
Strongylus (gibsoni) infestation 127.7
Strophulus (newborn) 779.8
  pruriginosus 698.2

Struck by lightning 994.0
Struma (see also Goiter) 240.9
  fibrosa 245.3
  Hashimoto (struma lymphomatosa) 245.2
  lymphomatosa 245.2
  nodosa (simplex) 241.9
    endemic 241.9
    multinodular 241.1
    sporadic 241.9
    toxic or with hyperthyroidism 242.3
      multinodular 242.2
      uninodular 242.1
    toxicosa 242.3
      multinodular 242.2
      uninodular 242.1
    uninodular 241.0
  ovarii (M9090/0) 220
    and carcinoid (M9091/1) 236.2
    malignant (M9090/3) 183.0
  Riedel's (ligneous thyroiditis) 245.3
  scrofulous (see also Tuberculosis) 017.2
  tuberculous (see also Tuberculosis) 017.2
    abscess 017.2
    adenitis 017.2
    lymphangitis 017.2
    ulcer 017.2
Strumipriva cachexia (see also Hypothyroidism) 244.9
Strümpell-Marie disease or spine (ankylosing spondylitis) 720.0
Strümpell-Westphal pseudosclerosis (hepatolenticular degeneration) 275.1
Stuart's disease (congenital factor X deficiency) (see also Defect, coagulation) 286.3
Stuart-Prower factor deficiency (congenital factor X deficiency) (see also Defect, coagulation) 286.3
Students' elbow 727.2
Stuffy nose 478.1
Stump — see also Amputation
  cervix, cervical (healed) 622.8
Stupor 780.09
  catatonic (see also Schizophrenia) 295.2
  circular (see also Psychosis, manic-depressive, circular) 296.7
  manic 296.89
  manic-depressive (see also Psychosis, affective) 296.89
  mental (anergic) (delusional) 298.9
  psychogenic 298.8
  reaction to exceptional stress (transient) 308.2
  traumatic NEC — see also Injury, intracranial
    with spinal (cord)
      lesion — see Injury, spinal, by site
      shock — see Injury, spinal, by site
Sturge (-Weber) (-Dimitri) disease or syndrome (encephalocutaneous angiomatosis) 759.6
Sturge-Kalischer-Weber syndrome (encephalocutaneous angiomatosis) 759.6
Stuttering 307.0
Sty, stye 373.11
  external 373.11
  internal 373.12
  meibomian 373.12

Subacidity, gastric 536.8
  psychogenic 306.4
Subacute — see condition
Subarachnoid — see condition
Subclavian steal syndrome 435.2
Subcortical — see condition
Subcostal syndrome 098.86
  nerve compression 354.8
Subcutaneous, subcuticular — see condition
Subdelirium 293.1
Subdural — see condition
Subendocardium — see condition
Subependymoma (M9383/1) 237.5
Suberosis 495.3
Subglossitis — see Glossitis
Subhemophilia 286.0
Subinvolution (uterus) 621.1
  breast (postlactational) (postpartum) 611.8
  chronic 621.1
  puerperal, postpartum 674.8
Sublingual — see condition
Sublinguitis 527.2
Subluxation — see also Dislocation, by site
  congenital NEC — see also Malposition, congenital
  hip (unilateral) 754.32
    with dislocation of other hip 754.35
    bilateral 754.33
  joint
    lower limb 755.69
    shoulder 755.59
    upper limb 755.59
  lower limb (joint) 755.69
  shoulder (joint) 755.59
  upper limb (joint) 755.59
  lens 379.32
    anterior 379.33
    posterior 379.34
  rotary, cervical region of spine — see Fracture, vertebra, cervical
Submaxillary — see condition
Submersion (fatal) (nonfatal) 994.1
Submissiveness (undue), in child 313.0
Submucous — see condition
Subnormal, subnormality
  accommodation (see also Disorder, accommodation) 367.9
  mental (see also Retardation, mental) 319
    mild 317
    moderate 318.0
    profound 318.2
    severe 318.1
  temperature (accidental) 991.6
    not associated with low environmental temperature 780.9
Subphrenic — see condition
Subscapular nerve — see condition
Subseptus uterus 752.3
Subsiding appendicitis 542
Substernal thyroid (see also Goiter) 240.9
  congenital 759.2
Substitution disorder 300.11
Subtentorial — see condition
Subtertian
  fever 084.0
  malaria (fever) 084.0
Subthyroidism (acquired) (see also Hypothyroidism) 244.9
  congenital 243
Succenturiata placenta — see Placenta, abnormal

Succession sounds, chest 786.7
Sucking thumb, child 307.9
Sudamen 705.1
Sudamina 705.1
Sudanese kala-azar 085.0
Sudden
  death, cause unknown (less than 24 hours) 798.1
    during childbirth 669.9
    infant 798.0
    puerperal, postpartum 674.9
  hearing loss NEC 388.2
  heart failure (*see also* Failure, heart) 428.9
  infant death syndrome 798.0
Sudeck's atrophy, disease, or syndrome 733.7
SUDS (Sudden unexplained death) 798.2
Suffocation (*see also* Asphyxia) 799.0
  by
    bed clothes 994.7
    bunny bag 994.7
    cave-in 994.7
    constriction 994.7
    drowning 994.1
    inhalation
      food or foreign body (*see also* Asphyxia, food or foreign body) 933.1
      oil or gasoline (*see also* Asphyxia, food or foreign body) 933.1
    overlying 994.7
    plastic bag 994.7
    pressure 994.7
    strangulation 994.7
  during birth 768.1
  mechanical 994.7
Sugar
  blood
    high 790.6
    low 251.2
  in urine 791.5
Suicide, suicidal (attempted)
  by poisoning — *see* Table of drugs and chemicals
  risk 300.9
  tendencies 300.9
  trauma NEC (*see also* nature and site of injury) 959.9
Suipestifer infection (*see also* Infection, Salmonella) 003.9
Sulfatidosis 330.0
Sulfhemoglobinemia, sulphemoglobinemia
  (acquired) (congenital) 289.7
Sumatran mite fever 081.2
Summer — *see* condition
Sunburn 692.71
  dermatitis 692.71
Sunken
  acetabulum 718.85
  fontanels 756.0
Sunstroke 992.0
Superfecundation 651.9
  with fetal loss and retention of one or more fetus(es) 651.6
Superfetation 651.9
  with fetal loss and retention of one or more fetus(es) 651.6
Superinvolution uterus 621.8
Supernumerary (congenital)
  aortic cusps 746.89
  auditory ossicles 744.04
  bone 756.9
  breast 757.6
  carpal bones 755.56
  cusps, heart valve NEC 746.89
    mitral 746.5
    pulmonary 746.09

Supernumerary—*continued*
  digit(s) 755.00
    finger 755.01
    toe 755.02
  ear (lobule) 744.1
  fallopian tube 752.19
  finger 755.01
  hymen 752.49
  kidney 753.3
  lacrimal glands 743.64
  lacrimonasal duct 743.65
  lobule (ear) 744.1
  mitral cusps 746.5
  muscle 756.82
  nipples 757.6
  organ or site NEC — *see* Accessory
  ossicles, auditory 744.04
  ovary 752.0
  oviduct 752.19
  pulmonic cusps 746.09
  rib 756.3
    cervical or first 756.2
      syndrome 756.2
  roots (of teeth) 520.2
  spinal vertebra 756.19
  spleen 759.0
  tarsal bones 755.67
  teeth 520.1
    causing crowding 524.3
  testis 752.8
  thumb 755.01
  toe 755.02
  uterus 752.2
  vagina 752.49
  vertebra 756.19
Supervision (of)
  contraceptive method previously prescribed V25.40
    intrauterine device V25.42
    oral contraceptive (pill) V25.41
    specified type NEC V25.49
    subdermal implantable contraceptive V25.43
  dietary (for) V65.3
    allergy (food) V65.3
    colitis V65.3
    diabetes mellitus V65.3
    food allergy intolerance V65.3
    gastritis V65.3
    hypercholesterolemia V65.3
    hypoglycemia V65.3
    intolerance (food) V65.3
    obesity V65.3
    specified NEC V65.3
  lactation V24.1
  pregnancy — *see* Pregnancy, supervision of
Supplemental teeth 520.1
  causing crowding 524.3
Suppression
  binocular vision 368.31
  lactation 676.5
  menstruation 626.8
  ovarian secretion 256.3
  renal 586
  urinary secretion 788.5
  urine 788.5
Suppuration, suppurative — *see also* condition
  accessory sinus (chronic) (*see also* Sinusitis) 473.9
  adrenal gland 255.8
  antrum (chronic) (*see also* Sinusitis, maxillary) 473.0
  bladder (*see also* Cystitis) 595.89
  bowel 569.89
  brain 324.0
    late effect 326
  breast 611.0
    puerperal, postpartum 675.1
  dental periosteum 526.5
  diffuse (skin) 686.0

Suppuration, suppurative—*continued*
  ear (middle) (*see also* Otitis media) 382.4
    external (*see also* Otitis, externa) 380.10
    internal 386.33
  ethmoidal (sinus) (chronic) (*see also* Sinusitis, ethmoidal) 473.2
  fallopian tube (*see also* Salpingo-oophoritis) 614.2
  frontal (sinus) (chronic) (*see also* Sinusitis, frontal) 473.1
  gallbladder (*see also* Cholecystitis, acute) 575.0
  gum 523.3
  hernial sac — *see* Hernia, by site
  intestine 569.89
  joint (*see also* Arthritis, suppurative) 711.0
  labyrinthine 386.33
  lung 513.0
  mammary gland 611.0
    puerperal, postpartum 675.1
  maxilla, maxillary 526.4
    sinus (chronic) (*see also* Sinusitis, maxillary) 473.0
  muscle 728.0
  nasal sinus (chronic) (*see also* Sinusitis) 473.9
  pancreas 577.0
  parotid gland 527.2
  pelvis, pelvic
    female (*see also* Disease, pelvis, inflammatory) 614.4
      acute 614.3
    male (*see also* Peritonitis) 567.2
  pericranial (*see also* Osteomyelitis) 730.2
  salivary duct or gland (any) 527.2
  sinus (nasal) (*see also* Sinusitis) 473.9
  sphenoidal (sinus) (chronic) (*see also* Sinusitis, sphenoidal) 473.3
  thymus (gland) 254.1
  thyroid (gland) 245.0
  tonsil 474.8
  uterus (*see also* Endometritis) 615.9
  vagina 616.10
  wound — *see also* Wound, open, by site, complicated
    dislocation — *see* Dislocation, by site, compound
    fracture — *see* Fracture, by site, open
    scratch or other superficial injury — *see* Injury, superficial, by site
Suprapubic drainage 596.8
Suprarenal (gland) — *see* condition
Suprascapular nerve — *see* condition
Suprasellar — *see* condition
Supraspinatus syndrome 726.10
Surfer knots 919.8
  infected 919.9
Surgery
  cosmetic NEC V50.1
    following healed injury or operation V51
    hair transplant V50.0
  elective V50.9
    breast augmentation or reduction V50.1
    circumcision, ritual or routine (in absence of medical indication) V50.2
    cosmetic NEC V50.1
    ear piercing V50.3
    face-lift V50.1

Surgery—*continued*
  elective—*continued*
    following healed injury or operation V51
    hair transplant V50.0
  not done because of
    contraindication V64.1
    patient's decision V64.2
    specified reason NEC V64.3
  plastic
    breast augmentation or reduction V50.1
    cosmetic V50.1
    face-lift V50.1
    following healed injury or operation V51
    repair of scarred tissue (following healed injury or operation) V51
    specified type NEC V50.8
  previous, in pregnancy or childbirth
    cervix 654.6
      affecting fetus or newborn 763.8
      causing obstructed labor 660.2
        affecting fetus or newborn 763.1
    pelvic soft tissues NEC 654.9
      affecting fetus or newborn 763.8
      causing obstructed labor 660.2
        affecting fetus or newborn 763.1
    perineum or vulva 654.8
    uterus NEC 654.9
      affecting fetus or newborn 763.8
      causing obstructed labor 660.2
        affecting fetus or newborn 763.1
      due to previous cesarean delivery 654.2
    vagina 654.7
Surgical
  abortion — *see* Abortion, legal
  emphysema 998.81
  kidney (*see also* Pyelitis) 590.80
  operation NEC 799.9
  procedures, complication or misadventure — *see* Complications, surgical procedure
  shock 998.0
Suspected condition, ruled out (*see also* Observation, suspected) V71.9
  specified condition NEC V71.8
Suspended uterus, in pregnancy or childbirth 654.4
  affecting fetus or newborn 763.8
  causing obstructed labor 660.2
    affecting fetus or newborn 763.1
Sutton's disease 709.09
Sutton and Gull's disease (arteriolar nephrosclerosis) (*see also* Hypertension, kidney) 403.90
Suture
  burst (in operation wound) 998.3
  inadvertently left in operation wound 998.4
  removal V58.3
  Shirodkar, in pregnancy (with or without cervical incompetence) 654.5
Swab inadvertently left in operation wound 998.4
Swallowed, swallowing
  difficulty (*see also* Dysphagia) 787.2
  foreign body NEC (*see also* Foreign body) 938

Swamp fever 100.89
Swan neck hand (intrinsic) 736.09
Sweat(s), sweating
 disease or sickness 078.2
  excessive 780.8
  fetid 705.89
  fever 078.2
  gland disease 705.9
   specified type NEC 705.89
  miliary 078.2
  night 780.8
Sweeley-Klionsky disease (angiokeratoma corporis diffusum) 272.7
Sweet's syndrome (acute febrile neutrophilic dermatosis) 695.89
Swelling
 abdominal (not referable to specific organ) 789.3
 adrenal gland, cloudy 255.8
 ankle 719.07
 anus 787.9
 arm 729.81
 breast 611.72
 Calabar 125.2
 cervical gland 785.6
 cheek 784.2
 chest 786.6
 ear 388.8
 epigastric 789.3
 extremity (lower) (upper) 729.81
 eye 379.92
 female genital organ 625.8
 finger 729.81
 foot 729.81
 glands 785.6
 gum 784.2
 hand 729.81
 head 784.2
 inflammatory — see Inflammation
 joint (see also Effusion, joint) 719.0
  tuberculous — see Tuberculosis, joint
 kidney, cloudy 593.89
 leg 729.81
 limb 729.81
 liver 573.8
 lung 786.6
 lymph nodes 785.6
 mediastinal 786.6
 mouth 784.2
 muscle (limb) 729.81
 neck 784.2
 nose or sinus 784.2
 palate 784.2
 pelvis 789.3
 penis 607.83
 perineum 625.8
 rectum 787.9
 scrotum 608.86
 skin 782.2
 splenic (see also Splenomegaly) 789.2
 substernal 786.6
 superficial, localized (skin) 782.2
 testicle 608.86
 throat 784.2
 toe 729.81
 tongue 784.2
 tubular (see also Disease, renal) 593.9
 umbilicus 789.3
 uterus 625.8
 vagina 625.8
 vulva 625.8
 wandering, due to Gnathostoma (spinigerum) 128.1
 white — see Tuberculosis, arthritis
Swift's disease 985.0
Swimmers'
 ear (acute) 380.12
 itch 120.3
Swimming in the head 780.4

Swollen — see also Swelling
 glands 785.6
Swyer-James syndrome (unilateral hyperlucent lung) 492.8
Swyer's syndrome (XY pure gonadal dysgenesis) 752.7
Sycosis 704.8
 barbae (not parasitic) 704.8
 contagiosa 110.0
 lupoid 704.8
 mycotic 110.0
 parasitic 110.0
 vulgaris 704.8
Sydenham's chorea — see Chorea, Sydenham's
Sylvatic yellow fever 060.0
Sylvest's disease (epidemic pleurodynia) 074.1
Symblepharon 372.63
 congenital 743.62
Symonds' syndrome 348.2
Sympathetic — see condition
Sympatheticotonia (see also Neuropathy, peripheral, autonomic) 337.9
Sympathicoblastoma (M9500/3)
 specified site — see Neoplasm, by site, malignant
 unspecified site 194.0
Sympathicogonioma (M9500/3) — see Sympathicoblastoma
Sympathoblastoma (M9500/3) — see Sympathicoblastoma
Sympathogonioma (M9500/3) — see Sympathicoblastoma
Symphalangy (see also Syndactylism) 755.10
Symptoms, specified (general) NEC 780.9
 abdomen NEC 789.9
 bone NEC 733.90
 breast NEC 611.79
 cardiac NEC 785.9
 cardiovascular NEC 785.9
 chest NEC 786.9
 development NEC 783.9
 digestive system NEC 787.9
 eye NEC 379.99
 gastrointestinal tract NEC 787.9
 genital organs NEC
  female 625.9
  male 608.9
 head and neck NEC 784.9
 heart NEC 785.9
 joint NEC 719.60
  ankle 719.67
  elbow 719.62
  foot 719.67
  hand 719.64
  hip 719.65
  knee 719.66
  multiple sites 719.69
  pelvic region 719.65
  shoulder (region) 719.61
  specified site NEC 719.68
  wrist 719.63
 larynx NEC 784.9
 limbs NEC 729.89
 lymphatic system NEC 785.9
 menopausal 627.2
 metabolism NEC 783.9
 mouth NEC 528.9
 muscle NEC 728.9
 musculoskeletal NEC 781.9
  limbs NEC 729.89
 nervous system NEC 781.9
 neurotic NEC 300.9
 nutrition, metabolism, and development NEC 783.9
 pelvis NEC 789.9
  female 625.9
 peritoneum NEC 789.9
 respiratory system NEC 786.9
 skin and integument NEC 782.9

Symptoms, specified—continued
 subcutaneous tissue NEC 782.9
 throat NEC 784.9
 tonsil NEC 784.9
 urinary system NEC 788.9
 vascular NEC 785.9
Sympus 759.89
Synarthrosis 719.80
 ankle 719.87
 elbow 719.82
 foot 719.87
 hand 719.84
 hip 719.85
 knee 719.86
 multiple sites 719.89
 pelvic region 719.85
 shoulder (region) 719.81
 specified site NEC 719.88
 wrist 719.83
Syncephalus 759.4
Synchondrosis 756.9
 abnormal (congenital) 756.9
 ischiopubic (van Neck's) 732.1
Synchysis (senile) (vitreous humor) 379.21
 scintillans 379.22
Syncope (near) (pre-) 780.2 ◆
 anginosa 413.9
 bradycardia 427.89
 cardiac 780.2
 carotid sinus 337.0
 complicating delivery 669.2
 due to lumbar puncture 349.0
 fatal 798.1
 heart 780.2
 heat 992.1
 laryngeal 786.2
 tussive 786.2
 vasoconstriction 780.2
 vasodepressor 780.2
 vasomotor 780.2
 vasovagal 780.2
Syncytial infarct — see Placenta, abnormal
Syndactylism, syndactyly (multiple sites) 755.10
 fingers (without fusion of bone) 755.11
  with fusion of bone 755.12
 toes (without fusion of bone) 755.13
  with fusion of bone 755.14
Syndrome — see also Disease
 abdominal
  acute 789.0
  migraine 346.2
  muscle deficiency 756.7
 Abercrombie's (amyloid degeneration) 277.3
 abnormal innervation 374.43
 abstinence
  alcohol 291.8
  drug 292.0
 Abt-Letterer-Siwe (acute histiocytosis X) (M9722/3) 202.5
 Achard-Thiers (adrenogenital) 255.2
 acid pulmonary aspiration 997.3
  obstetric (Mendelson's) 668.0
 acquired immune deficiency 042 ▼
 acquired immunodeficiency 042 ▲
 acrocephalosyndactylism 755.55
 acute abdominal 789.0
 Adair-Dighton (brittle bones and blue sclera, deafness) 756.51
 Adams-Stokes (-Morgagni) (syncope with heart block) 426.9
 addisonian 255.4
 Adie (-Holmes) (pupil) 379.46
 adiposogenital 253.8

Syndrome—continued
 adrenal
  hemorrhage 036.3
  meningococcic 036.3
 adrenocortical 255.3
 adrenogenital (acquired) (congenital) 255.2
  feminizing 255.2
  iatrogenic 760.79
  virilism (acquired) (congenital) 255.2
 adult maltreatment (emotional) 995.81
 affective organic NEC 293.89
  drug-induced 292.84
 afferent loop NEC 537.89
 African macroglobulinemia 273.3
 Ahumada-Del Castillo (nonpuerperal galactorrhea and amenorrhea) 253.1
 air blast concussion — see Injury, internal, by site
 Albright (-Martin) (pseudohypoparathyroidism) 275.4
 Albright-McCune-Sternberg (osteitis fibrosa disseminata) 756.59
 alcohol withdrawal 291.8
 Alder's (leukocyte granulation anomaly) 288.2
 Aldrich (-Wiskott) (eczema-thrombocytopenia) 279.12
 Alibert-Bazin (mycosis fungoides) (M9700/3) 202.1
 Alice in Wonderland 293.89
 Allen-Masters 620.6
 Alligator baby (ichthyosis congenita) 757.1
 Alport's (hereditary hematuria-nephropathy-deafness) 759.89
 Alvarez (transient cerebral ischemia) 435.9
 alveolar capillary block 516.3
 Alzheimer's 331.0
  with dementia — see Alzheimer's, dementia
 amnestic (confabulatory) 294.0
  alcoholic 291.1
  drug-induced 292.83
  posttraumatic 294.0
 amotivational 292.89
 amyostatic 275.1
 amyotrophic lateral sclerosis 335.20
 angina (see also Angina) 413.9
 ankyloglossia superior 750.0
 anterior
  chest wall 786.52
  compartment (tibial) 958.8
  spinal artery 433.8
   compression 721.1
  tibial (compartment) 958.8
 antibody deficiency 279.00
  agammaglobulinemic 279.00
  congenital 279.04
  hypogammaglobulinemic 279.00
 antimongolism 758.3
 Anton (-Babinski) (hemiasomatognosia) 307.9
 anxiety (see also Anxiety) 300.00
 aortic
  arch 446.7
  bifurcation (occlusion) 444.0
  ring 747.21
 Apert's (acrocephalosyndactyly) 755.55
 Apert-Gallais (adrenogenital) 255.2
 aphasia-apraxia-alexia 784.69
 "approximate answers" 300.16
 arcuate ligament (-celiac axis) 447.4
 arcus aortae 446.7
 arc-welders' 370.24

Syndrome—continued

argentaffin, argintaffinoma 259.2
Argonz-Del Castillo (nonpuerperal galactorrhea and amenorrhea) 253.1
Argyll Robertson's (syphilitic) 094.89
  nonsyphilitic 379.45
arm-shoulder (see also Neuropathy, peripheral, autonomic) 337.9
Arnold-Chiari (see also Spina bifida) 741.0
  type I 348.4
  type II 741.0
  type III 742.0
  type IV 742.2
Arrillaga-Ayerza (pulmonary artery sclerosis with pulmonary hypertension) 416.0
arteriomesenteric duodenum occlusion 537.89
arteriovenous steal 996.73
arteritis, young female (obliterative brachiocephalic) 446.7
aseptic meningitis — see Meningitis, aseptic
Asherman's 621.5
asphyctic (see also Anxiety) 300.00
aspiration, of newborn, massive or meconium 770.1
ataxia-telangiectasia 334.8
Audry's (acropachyderma) 757.39
auriculotemporal 350.8
autosomal — see also Abnormal, autosomes NEC
  deletion 758.3
Avellis' 344.89
Axenfeld's 743.44
Ayerza (-Arrillaga) (pulmonary artery sclerosis with pulmonary hypertension) 416.0
Baader's (erythema multiforme exudativum) 695.1
Baastrup's 721.5
Babinski (-Vaquez) (cardiovascular syphilis) 093.89
Babinski-Fröhlich (adiposogenital dystrophy) 253.8
Babinski-Nageotte 344.89
Bagratuni's (temporal arteritis) 446.5
Bakwin-Krida (craniometaphyseal dysplasia) 756.89
Balint's (psychic paralysis of visual disorientation) 368.16
Ballantyne (-Runge) (postmaturity) 766.2
ballooning posterior leaflet 424.0
Banti's — see Cirrhosis, liver
Bard-Pic's (carcinoma, head of pancreas) 157.0
Bardet-Biedl (obesity, polydactyly, and mental retardation) 759.89
Barlow's (mitral valve prolapse) 424.0
Barlow (-Möller) (infantile scurvy) 267
Baron Munchausen's 301.51
Barré-Guillain 357.0
Barré-Liéou (posterior cervical sympathetic) 723.2
Barrett's (chronic peptic ulcer of esophagus) 530.2
Bársony-Polgár (corkscrew esophagus) 530.5
Bársony-Teschendorf (corkscrew esophagus) 530.5

Syndrome—continued

Bartter's (secondary hyperaldosteronism with juxtaglomerular hyperplasia) 255.1
Basedow's (exophthalmic goiter) 242.0
basilar artery 435.0
basofrontal 377.04
Bassen-Kornzweig (abetalipoproteinemia) 272.5
Batten-Steinert 359.2
battered
  adult 995.81
  baby or child 995.5
    affecting parent or family V61.21
    as reason for family seeking advice V61.21
    history V61.21
  specified person NEC 995.81
  spouse 995.81
Baumgarten-Cruveilhier (cirrhosis of liver) 571.5
Bearn-Kunkel (-Slater) (lupoid hepatitis) 571.49
Beau's (see also Degeneration, myocardial) 429.1
Bechterew-Strümpell-Marie (ankylosing spondylitis) 720.0
Beck's (anterior spinal artery occlusion) 433.8
Beckwith (-Wiedemann) 759.89
Behçet's 136.1
Bekhterev-Strümpell-Marie (ankylosing spondylitis) 720.0
Benedikt's 344.89
Béquez César (-Steinbrinck-Chédiak- Higashi) (congenital gigantism of peroxidase granules) 288.2
Bernard-Horner (see also Neuropathy, peripheral, autonomic) 337.9
Bernard-Sergent (acute adrenocortical insufficiency) 255.4
Bernhardt-Roth 355.1
Bernheim's (see also Failure, heart, congestive) 428.1
Bertolotti's (sacralization of fifth lumbar vertebra) 756.15
Besnier-Boeck-Schaumann (sarcoidosis) 135
Bianchi's (aphasia-apraxia-alexia syndrome) 784.69
Biedl-Bardet (obesity, polydactyly, and mental retardation) 759.89
Biemond's (obesity, polydactyly, and mental retardation) 759.89
big spleen 289.4
bilateral polycystic ovarian 256.4
Bing-Horton's 346.2
Biörck (-Thorson) (malignant carcinoid) 259.2
Blackfan-Diamond (congenital hypoplastic anemia) 284.0
black lung 500
black widow spider bite 989.5
bladder neck (see also Incontinence, urine) 788.30
blast (concussion) — see Blast, injury
blind loop (postoperative) 579.2
Bloch-Siemens (incontinentia pigmenti) 757.33
Bloch-Sulzberger (incontinentia pigmenti) 757.33
Bloom (-Machacek) (-Torre) 757.39
Blount-Barber (tibia vara) 732.4

Syndrome—continued

blue
  bloater 491.2
  diaper 270.0
  drum 381.02
  sclera 756.51
  toe — see Atherosclerosis
Boder-Sedgwick (ataxia-telangiectasia) 334.8
Boerhaave's (spontaneous esophageal rupture) 530.4
Bonnevie-Ullrich 758.6
Bonnier's 386.19
Bouillaud's (rheumatic heart disease) 391.9
Bourneville (-Pringle) (tuberous sclerosis) 759.5
Bouveret (-Hoffmann) (paroxysmal tachycardia) 427.2
brachial plexus 353.0
Brachman-de Lange (Amsterdam dwarf, mental retardation, and brachycephaly) 759.89
bradycardia-tachycardia 427.81
Brailsford-Morquio (dystrophy) (mucopolysaccharidosis IV) 277.5
brain (acute) (chronic) (nonpsychotic) (organic) (with behavioral reaction) (with neurotic reaction) 310.9
  with
    presenile brain disease (see also Dementia, presenile) 290.10
    psychosis, psychotic reaction (see also Psychosis, organic) 294.9
  chronic alcoholic 291.2
  congenital (see also Retardation, mental) 319
  postcontusional 310.2
  posttraumatic
    nonpsychotic 310.2
    psychotic 293.9
      acute 293.0
      chronic (see also Psychosis, organic) 294.8
      subacute 293.1
  psycho-organic (see also Syndrome, psycho-organic) 310.9
  psychotic (see also Psychosis, organic) 294.9
  senile (see also Dementia, senile) 290.0
branchial arch 744.41
Brandt's (acrodermatitis enteropathica) 686.8
Brennemann's 289.2
Briquet's 300.81
Brissaud-Meige (infantile myxedema) 244.9
broad ligament laceration 620.6
Brock's (atelectasis due to enlarged lymph nodes) 518.0
Brown's tendon sheath 378.61
Brown-Séquard 344.89
brown spot 756.59
Brugsch's (acropachyderma) 757.39
bubbly lung 770.7
Buchem's (hyperostosis corticalis) 733.3
Budd-Chiari (hepatic vein thrombosis) 453.0
Büdinger-Ludloff-Läwen 717.89
bulbar 335.22
  lateral (see also Disease, cerebrovascular, acute) 436

Syndrome—continued

Bullis fever 082.8
bundle of Kent (anomalous atrioventricular excitation) 426.7
Bürger-Grütz (essential familial hyperlipemia) 272.3
Burke's (pancreatic insufficiency and chronic neutropenia) 577.8
Burnett's (milk-alkali) 999.9
Burnier's (hypophyseal dwarfism) 253.3
burning feet 266.2
Bywaters' 958.5
Caffey's (infantile cortical hyperostosis) 756.59
Calvé-Legg-Perthes (osteochondrosis, femoral capital) 732.1
Caplan (-Colinet) syndrome 714.81
capsular thrombosis (see also Thrombosis, brain) 434.0
carcinogenic thrombophlebitis 453.1
carcinoid 259.2
cardiac asthma (see also Failure, ventricular, left) 428.1
cardiacos negros 416.0
cardiopulmonary obesity 278.8
cardiorenal (see also Hypertension, cardiorenal) 404.90
cardiorespiratory distress (idiopathic), newborn 769
cardiovascular renal (see also Hypertension, cardiorenal) 404.90
cardiovasorenal 272.7
Carini's (ichthyosis congenita) 757.1
carotid
  artery (internal) 435.8
  body or sinus 337.0
carpal tunnel 354.0
Carpenter's 759.89
Cassidy (-Scholte) (malignant carcinoid) 259.2
cat-cry 758.3
cauda equina 344.60
causalgia 355.9
  lower limb 355.71
  upper limb 354.4
cavernous sinus 437.6
celiac 579.0
  artery compression 447.4
  axis 447.4
cerebellomedullary malformation (see also Spina bifida) 741.0
cerebral gigantism 253.0
cerebrohepatorenal 759.89
cervical (root) (spine) NEC 723.8
  disc 722.71
  posterior, sympathetic 723.2
  rib 353.0
  sympathetic paralysis 337.0
  traumatic (acute) NEC 847.0
cervicobrachial (diffuse) 723.3
cervicocranial 723.2
cervicodorsal outlet 353.2
Céstan's 344.89
Céstan (-Raymond) 433.8
Céstan-Chenais 344.89
chancriform 114.1
Charcot's (intermittent claudication) 443.9
  angina cruris 443.9
  due to atherosclerosis 440.21
Charcot-Marie-Tooth 356.1
Charcot-Weiss-Baker 337.0
Cheadle (-Möller) (-Barlow) (infantile scurvy) 267
Chédiak-Higashi (-Steinbrinck) (congenital gigantism of peroxidase granules) 288.2

Syndrome—continued

chest wall 786.52
Chiari's (hepatic vein thrombosis) 453.0
Chiari-Frommel 676.6
chiasmatic 368.41
Chilaiditi's (subphrenic displacement, colon) 751.4
child maltreatment (emotional) (nutritional) 995.5
  affecting parent or family V61.21
  history V61.21
chondroectodermal dysplasia 756.55
chorea-athetosis-agitans 275.1
Christian's (chronic histiocytosis X) 277.8
chromosome 4 short arm deletion 758.3
Clarke-Hadfield (pancreatic infantilism) 577.8
Claude's 352.6
Claude Bernard-Horner (see also Neuropathy, peripheral, autonomic) 337.9
Clérambault's
  automatism 348.8
  erotomania 297.8
Clifford's (postmaturity) 766.2
climacteric 627.2
Clouston's (hidrotic ectodermal dysplasia) 757.31
clumsiness 315.4
Cockayne's (microencephaly and dwarfism) 759.89
Cockayne-Weber (epidermolysis bullosa) 757.39
Cogan's (nonsyphilitic interstitial keratitis) 370.52
cold injury (newborn) 778.2
Collet (-Sicard) 352.6
combined immunity deficiency 279.2
compartment(al) (anterior) (deep) (posterior) (tibial) 958.8
compression 958.5
  cauda equina 344.60
    with neurogenic bladder 344.61
concussion 310.2
congenital
  affecting more than one system 759.7
  specified type NEC 759.89
  facial diplegia 352.6
  muscular hypertrophy-cerebral 759.89
congestion-fibrosis (pelvic) 625.5
conjunctivourethrosynovial 099.3
Conn (-Louis) (primary aldosteronism) 255.1
Conradi (-Hünermann) (chondrodysplasia calcificans congenita) 756.59
conus medullaris 336.8
Cooke-Apert-Gallais (adrenogenital) 255.2
Cornelia de Lange's (Amsterdam dwarf, mental retardation, and brachycephaly) 759.8
coronary insufficiency or intermediate 411.1
cor pulmonale 416.9
corticosexual 255.2
Costen's (complex) 524.60
costochondral junction 733.6
costoclavicular 353.0
costovertebral 253.0
Cotard's (paranoia) 297.1
craniovertebral 723.2
Creutzfeldt-Jakob 046.1
  with dementia 290.10
crib death 798.0
cricopharyngeal 787.2
cri-du-chat 758.3

Syndrome—continued

Crigler-Najjar (congenital hyperbilirubinemia) 277.4
crocodile tears 351.8
Cronkhite-Canada 211.3
croup 464.4
CRST (cutaneous systemic sclerosis) 710.1
crush 958.5
crushed lung (see also Injury, internal, lung) 861.20
Cruveilhier-Baumgarten (cirrhosis of liver) 571.5
cubital tunnel 354.2
Cuiffini-Pancoast (M8010/3) (carcinoma, pulmonary apex) 162.3
Curschmann (-Batten) (-Steinert) 359.2
Cushing's (iatrogenic) (idiopathic) (pituitary basophilism) (pituitary-dependent) 255.0
  overdose or wrong substance given or taken 962.0
Cyriax's (slipping rib) 733.99
cystic duct stump 576.0
Da Costa's (neurocirculatory asthenia) 306.2
Dameshek's (erythroblastic anemia) 282.4
Dana-Putnam (subacute combined sclerosis with pernicious anemia) 281.0 [336.2]
Danbolt (-Closs) (acrodermatitis enteropathica) 686.8
Dandy-Walker (atresia, foramen of Magendie) 742.3
  with spina bifida (see also Spina bifida) 741.0
Danlos' 756.83
Davies-Colley (slipping rib) 733.99
dead fetus 641.3
defeminization 255.2
defibrination (see also Fibrinolysis) 286.6
Degos' 447.8
Deiters' nucleus 386.19
Déjérine-Roussy 348.8
Déjérine-Thomas 333.0
de Lange's (Amsterdam dwarf, mental retardation, and brachycephaly) (Cornelia) 759.89
Del Castillo's (germinal aplasia) 606.0
deletion chromosomes 758.3
delusional
  induced by drug 292.11
dementia-aphonia, of childhood (see also Psychosis, childhood) 299.1
demyelinating NEC 341.9
denial visual hallucination 307.9
depersonalization 300.6
Dercum's (adiposis dolorosa) 272.8
de Toni-Fanconi (-Debré) (cystinosis) 270.0
diabetes-dwarfism-obesity (juvenile) 258.1
diabetes mellitus-hypertension-nephrosis 250.4 [581.81]
diabetes mellitus in newborn infant 775.1
diabetes-nephrosis 250.4 [581.81]
diabetic amyotrophy 250.6 [358.1]
Diamond-Blackfan (congenital hypoplastic anemia) 284.0
Diamond-Gardener (autoerythrocyte sensitization) 287.2

Syndrome—continued

DIC (diffuse or disseminated intravascular coagulopathy) (see also Fibrinolysis) 286.6
diencephalohypophyseal NEC 253.8
diffuse cervicobrachial 723.3
diffuse obstructive pulmonary 496
DiGeorge's (thymic hypoplasia) 279.11
Dighton's 756.51
Di Guglielmo's (erythremic myelosis) (M9841/3) 207.0
disc — see Displacement, intervertebral disc
discogenic — see Displacement, intervertebral disc
disequilibrium 276.9
disseminated platelet thrombosis 446.6
Ditthomska 307.81
Doan-Wiseman (primary splenic neutropenia) 288.0
Döhle body-panmyelopathic 288.2
Donohue's (leprechaunism) 259.8
dorsolateral medullary (see also Disease, cerebrovascular, acute) 436
double whammy 360.81
Down's (mongolism) 758.0
Dresbach's (elliptocytosis) 282.1
Dressler's (postmyocardial infarction) 411.0
  hemoglobinuria 283.2
drug withdrawal, infant, of dependent mother 779.5
dry skin 701.1
  eye 375.15
Duane's (retraction) 378.71
Duane-Stilling-Türk (ocular retraction syndrome) 378.71
Dubin-Johnson (constitutional hyperbilirubinemia) 277.4
Dubin-Sprinz (constitutional hyperbilirubinemia) 277.4
Duchenne's 335.22
due to abnormality
  autosomal NEC (see also Abnormal, autosomes NEC) 758.5
  13 758.1
  18 758.2
  21 or 22 758.0
  D 758.1
  E 758.2
  G 758.0
  chromosomal 758.9
  sex 758.8
dumping 564.2
  nonsurgical 536.8
Duplay's 726.2
Dupré's (meningism) 781.6
Dyke-Young (acquired macrocytic hemolytic anemia) 283.9
dyspraxia 315.4
dystocia, dystrophia 654.9
Eales' 362.18
Eaton-Lambert (see also Neoplasm, by site, malignant) 199.1 [358.1]
Ebstein's (downward displacement, tricuspid valve into right ventricle) 746.2
ectopic ACTH secretion 255.0
eczema-thrombocytopenia 279.12
Eddowes' (brittle bones and blue sclera) 756.51
Edwards' 758.2
efferent loop 537.89
effort (aviators') (psychogenic) 306.2
Ehlers-Danlos 756.83

Syndrome—continued

Eisenmenger's (ventricular septal defect) 745.4
Ekbom's (restless legs) 333.99
Ekman's (brittle bones and blue sclera) 756.51
electric feet 266.2
Ellison-Zollinger (gastric hypersecretion with pancreatic islet cell tumor) 251.5
Ellis-van Creveld (chondroectodermal dysplasia) 756.55
embryonic fixation 270.2
empty sella (turcica) 253.8
endocrine-hypertensive 255.3
Engel-von Recklinghausen (osteitis fibrosa cystica) 252.0
enteroarticular 099.3
entrapment — see Neuropathy, entrapment
eosinophilia myalgia 710.5
epidemic vomiting 078.82
Epstein's — see Nephrosis
Erb (-Oppenheim) — Goldflam 358.0
Erdheim's (acromegalic macrospondylitis) 253.0
Erlacher-Blount (tibia vara) 732.4
erythrocyte fragmentation 283.19
Evans' (thrombocytopenic purpura) 287.3
excess cortisol, iatrogenic 255.0
exhaustion 300.5
extrapyramidal 333.90
eyelid-malar-mandible 756.0
eye retraction 378.71
Faber's (achlorhydric anemia) 280.9
Fabry (-Anderson) (angiokeratoma corporis diffusum) 272.7
facet 724.8
Fallot's 745.2
falx (see also Hemorrhage, brain) 431
familial eczema-thrombocytopenia 279.12
Fanconi's (anemia) (congenital pancytopenia) 284.0
Fanconi (-de Toni) (-Debré) (cystinosis) 270.0
Farber (-Uzman) (disseminated lipogranulomatosis) 272.8
fatigue NEC 300.5
  chronic 780.7
faulty bowel habit (idiopathic megacolon) 564.7
FDH (focal dermal hypoplasia) 757.39
fecal reservoir 560.39
Feil-Klippel (brevicollis) 756.16
Felty's (rheumatoid arthritis with splenomegaly and leukopenia) 714.1
fertile eunuch 257.2
fetal alcohol 760.71
  late effect 760.71
fibrillation-flutter 427.32
fibrositis (periarticular) 729.0
Fiedler's (acute isolated myocarditis) 422.91
Fiessinger-Leroy (-Reiter) 099.3
Fiessinger-Rendu (erythema multiforme exudativum) 695.1
first arch 756.0
Fisher's 357.0
Fitz's (acute hemorrhagic pancreatitis) 577.0
Fitz-Hugh and Curtis (gonococcal peritonitis) 098.86
Flajani (-Basedow) (exophthalmic goiter) 242.0

Syndrome—*continued*
  floppy
    infant 781.9
    valve (mitral) 424.0
  flush 259.2
  Foix-Alajouanine 336.1
  Fong's (hereditary osteo-onychodysplasia) 756.89
  foramen magnum 348.4
  Forbes-Albright (nonpuerperal amenorrhea and lactation associated with pituitary tumor) 253.1
  Foster-Kennedy 377.04
  Foville's (peduncular) 344.89
  fragile X 759.83
  Franceschetti's (mandibulofacial dysostosis) 756.0
  Fraser's 759.89
  Freeman-Sheldon 759.89
  Frey's (auriculotemporal) 350.8
  Friderichsen-Waterhouse 036.3
  Friedrich-Erb-Arnold (acropachyderma) 757.39
  Fröhlich's (adiposogenital dystrophy) 253.8
  Froin's 336.8
  Frommel-Chiari 676.6
  frontal lobe 310.0
  Fuller Albright's (osteitis fibrosa disseminata) 756.59
  functional
    bowel 564.9
    prepubertal castrate 752.8
  Gaisböck's (polycythemia hypertonica) 289.0
  ganglion (basal, brain) 333.90
    geniculi 351.1
  Ganser's, hysterical 300.16
  Gardner-Diamond (autoerythrocyte sensitization) 287.2
  gastroesophageal junction 530.0
  gastroesophageal laceration-hemorrhage 530.7
  gastrojejunal loop obstruction 537.89
  Gayet-Wernicke's (superior hemorrhagic polioencephalitis) 265.1
  Gee-Herter-Heubner (nontropical sprue) 579.0
  Gélineau's 347
  genito-anorectal 099.1
  Gerhardt's (vocal cord paralysis) 478.30
  Gerstmann's (finger agnosia) 784.69
  Gilbert's 277.4
  Gilford (-Hutchinson) (progeria) 259.8
  Gilles de la Tourette's 307.23
  Gillespie's (dysplasia oculodentodigitalis) 759.89
  Glénard's (enteroptosis) 569.89
  Glinski-Simmonds (pituitary cachexia) 253.2
  glucuronyl transferase 277.4
  glue ear 381.20
  Goldberg (-Maxwell) (-Morris) (testicular feminization) 257.8
  Goldenhar's (oculoauriculovertebral dysplasia) 756.0
  Goldflam-Erb 358.0
  Goltz-Gorlin (dermal hypoplasia) 757.39
  Goodpasture's (pneumorenal) 446.21
  Gopalan's (burning feet) 266.2
  Gorlin-Chaudhry-Moss 759.89
  Gougerot (-Houwer) — Sjögren (keratoconjunctivitis sicca) 710.2

Syndrome—*continued*
  Gougerot-Blum (pigmented purpuric lichenoid dermatitis) 709.1
  Gougerot-Carteaud (confluent reticulate papillomatosis) 701.8
  Gouley's (constrictive pericarditis) 423.2
  Gowers' (vasovagal attack) 780.2
  Gowers-Paton-Kennedy 377.04
  Gradenigo's 383.02
  Gray or grey (chloramphenicol) (newborn) 779.4
  Greig's (hypertelorism) 756.0
  Gubler-Millard 344.89
  Guérin-Stern (arthrogryposis multiplex congenita) 754.89
  Guillain-Barré (-Strohl) 357.0
  Gunn's (jaw-winking syndrome) 742.8
  Günther's (congenital erythropoietic porphyria) 277.1
  gustatory sweating 350.8
  H_3O 759.81
  Hadfield-Clarke (pancreatic infantilism) 577.8
  Haglund-Läwen-Fründ 717.89
  hairless women 257.8
  Hallermann-Streiff 756.0
  Hallervorden-Spatz 333.0
  Hamman's (spontaneous mediastinal emphysema) 518.1
  Hamman-Rich (diffuse interstitial pulmonary fibrosis) 516.3
  Hand-Schüller-Christian (chronic histiocytosis X) 277.8
  hand-foot 282.61
  Hanot-Chauffard (-Troisier) (bronze diabetes) 275.0
  Harada's 363.22
  Hare's (M8010/3) (carcinoma, pulmonary apex) 162.3
  Harkavy's 446.0
  harlequin color change 779.8
  Harris' (organic hyperinsulinism) 251.1
  Hart's (pellagra-cerebellar ataxia-renal aminoaciduria) 270.0
  Hayem-Faber (achlorhydric anemia) 280.9
  Hayem-Widal (acquired hemolytic jaundice) 283.9
  Heberden's (angina pectoris) 413.9
  Hedinger's (malignant carcinoid) 259.2
  Hegglin's 288.2
  Heller's (infantile psychosis) (see also Psychosis, childhood) 299.1
  hemolytic-uremic (adult) (child) 283.11
  Hench-Rosenberg (palindromic arthritis) (see also Rheumatism, palindromic) 719.3
  Henoch-Schönlein (allergic purpura) 287.0
  hepatic flexure 569.89
  hepatorenal 572.4
    due to a procedure 997.4
    following delivery 674.8
  hepatourologic 572.4
  Herrick's (hemoglobin S disease) 282.61
  Herter (-Gee) (nontropical sprue) 579.0
  Heubner-Herter (nontropical sprue) 579.0
  Heyd's (hepatorenal) 572.4
  HHHO 759.81
  Hilger's 337.0

Syndrome—*continued*
  Hoffa (-Kastert) (liposynovitis prepatellaris) 272.8
  Hoffmann's 244.9 [359.5]
  Hoffmann-Bouveret (paroxysmal tachycardia) 427.2
  Hoffmann-Werdnig 335.0
  Holländer-Simons (progressive lipodystrophy) 272.6
  Holmes' (visual disorientation) 368.16
  Holmes-Adie 379.46
  Hoppe-Goldflam 358.0
  Horner's (see also Neuropathy, peripheral, autonomic) 337.9
    traumatic — see Injury, nerve, cervical sympathetic
  hospital addiction 301.51
  Hunt's (herpetic geniculate ganglionitis) 053.11
    dyssynergia cerebellaris myoclonica 334.2
  Hunter (-Hurler) (mucopolysaccharidosis II) 277.5
  hunterian glossitis 529.4
  Hurler (-Hunter) (mucopolysaccharidosis II) 277.5
  Hutchinson's incisors or teeth 090.5
  Hutchinson-Boeck (sarcoidosis) 135
  Hutchinson-Gilford (progeria) 259.8
  hydralazine
    correct substance properly administered 695.4
    overdose or wrong substance given or taken 972.6
  hydraulic concussion (abdomen) (see also Injury, internal, abdomen) 868.00
  hyperabduction 447.8
  hyperactive bowel 564.1
  hyperaldosteronism with hypokalemic alkalosis (Bartter's) 255.1
  hypercalcemic 275.4
  hypercoagulation NEC 289.8
  hypereosinophilic (idiopathic) 288.3
  hyperkalemic 276.7
  hyperkinetic — see also Hyperkinesia
    heart 429.82
  hyperlipemia-hemolytic anemia-icterus 571.1
  hypermobility 728.5
  hypernatremia 276.0
  hyperosmolarity 276.0
  hypersomnia-bulimia 349.89
  hypersplenic 289.4
  hypersympathetic (see also Neuropathy, peripheral, autonomic) 337.9
  hypertransfusion, newborn 776.4
  hyperventilation, psychogenic 306.1
  hyperviscosity (of serum) NEC 273.3
    polycythemic 289.0
    sclerothymic 282.8
  hypoglycemic (familial) (neonatal) 251.2
    functional 251.1
  hypokalemic 276.8
  hypophyseal 253.8
  hypophyseothalamic 253.8
  hypopituitarism 253.2
  hypoplastic left heart 746.7
  hypopotassemia 276.8
  hyposmolality 276.1
  hypotension, maternal 669.2

Syndrome—*continued*
  hypotonia-hypomentia-hypogonadism-obesity 759.81
  ICF (intravascular coagulation-fibrinolysis) (see also Fibrinolysis) 286.6
  idiopathic cardiorespiratory distress, newborn 769
  idiopathic nephrotic (infantile) 581.9
  Imerslund (-Gräsbeck) (anemia due to familial selective vitamin B_{12} malabsorption) 281.1
  immobility (paraplegic) 728.3
  immunity deficiency, combined 279.2
  impending coronary 411.1
  impingement
    shoulder 726.2
    vertebral bodies 724.4
  inappropriate secretion of antidiuretic hormone (ADH) 253.6
  incomplete
    mandibulofacial 756.0
  infant
    death, sudden (SIDS) 798.0
    Hercules 255.2
    of diabetic mother 775.0
  infantilism 253.3
  inferior vena cava 459.2
  influenza-like 487.1
  inspissated bile, newborn 774.4
  intermediate coronary (artery) 411.1
  internal carotid artery (see also Occlusion, artery, carotid) 433.1
  interspinous ligament 724.8
  intestinal
    carcinoid 259.2
    gas 787.3
    knot 560.2
  intravascular
    coagulation-fibrinolysis (ICF) (see also Fibrinolysis) 286.6
    coagulopathy (see also Fibrinolysis) 286.6
  inverted Marfan's 759.89
  IRDS (idiopathic respiratory distress, newborn) 769
  irritable
    bowel 564.1
    heart 306.2
    weakness 300.5
  ischemic bowel (transient) 557.9
    chronic 557.1
    due to mesenteric artery insufficiency 557.1
  Itsenko-Cushing (pituitary basophilism) 255.0
  IVC (intravascular coagulopathy) (see also Fibrinolysis) 286.6
  Ivemark's (asplenia with congenital heart disease) 759.0
  Jaccoud's 714.4
  Jackson's 344.89
  Jadassohn-Lewandowski (pachyonchia congenita) 757.5
  Jaffe-Lichtenstein (-Uehlinger) 252.0
  Jahnke's (encephalocutaneous angiomatosis) 759.6
  Jakob-Creutzfeldt 046.1
    with dementia 290.10
  Jaksch's (pseudoleukemia infantum) 285.8
  Jaksch-Hayem (-Luzet) (pseudoleukemia infantum) 285.8
  jaw-winking 742.8
  jejunal 564.2

Syndrome—continued

jet lag 307.45
Jeune's (asphyxiating thoracic dystrophy of newborn) 756.4
Job's (chronic granulomatous disease) 288.1
Jordan's 288.2
Joseph-Diamond-Blackfan (congenital hypoplastic anemia) 284.0
jugular foramen 352.6
Kahler's (multiple myeloma) (M9730/3) 203.0
Kalischer's (encephalocutaneous angiomatosis) 759.6
Kallmann's (hypogonadotropic hypogonadism with anosmia) 253.4
Kanner's (autism) (see also Psychosis, childhood) 299.0
Kartagener's (sinusitis, bronchiectasis, situs inversus) 759.3
Kasabach-Merritt (capillary hemangioma associated with thrombocytopenic purpura) 287.3
Kast's (dyschondroplasia with hemangiomas) 756.4
Kaznelson's (congenital hypoplastic anemia) 284.0
Kelly's (sideropenic dysphagia) 280.8
Kimmelstiel-Wilson (intercapillary glomerulosclerosis) 250.4 [581.81]
Klauder's (erythema multiforme exudativum) 695.1
Klein-Waardenburg (ptosis-epicanthus) 270.2
Kleine-Levin 349.89
Klinefelter's 758.7
Klippel-Feil (brevicollis) 756.16
Klippel-Trenaunay 759.89
Klumpke (-Déjérine) (injury to brachial plexus at birth) 767.6
Klüver-Bucy (-Terzian) 310.0
Köhler-Pellegrini-Stieda (calcification, knee joint) 726.62
König's 564.8
Korsakoff's (nonalcoholic) 294.0
  alcoholic 291.1
Korsakoff (-Wernicke) (nonalcoholic) 294.0
  alcoholic 291.1
Kostmann's (infantile genetic agranulocytosis) 288.0
Krabbe's
  congenital muscle hypoplasia 756.89
  cutaneocerebral angioma 759.6
Kunkel (lupoid hepatitis) 571.49
labyrinthine 386.50
laceration, broad ligament 620.6
Langdon Down (mongolism) 758.0
Larsen's (flattened facies and multiple congenital dislocations) 755.8
lateral
  cutaneous nerve of thigh 355.1
  medullary (see also Disease, cerebrovascular acute) 436
Launois' (pituitary gigantism) 253.0
Launois-Cléret (adiposogenital dystrophy) 253.8
Laurence-Moon (-Bardet) — Biedl (obesity, polydactyly, and mental retardation) 759.89

Syndrome—continued

Lawford's (encephalocutaneous angiomatosis) 759.6
lazy
  leukocyte 288.0
  posture 728.3
Lederer-Brill (acquired infectious hemolytic anemia) 283.19
Legg-Calvé-Perthes (osteochondrosis capital femoral) 732.1
Lennox's (see also Epilepsy) 345.0
lenticular 275.1
Léopold-Lévi's (paroxysmal thyroid instability) 242.9
Lepore hemoglobin 282.4
Léri-Weill 756.59
Leriche's (aortic bifurcation occlusion) 444.0
Lermoyez's (see also Disease, Ménière's) 386.00
Lesch-Nyhan (hypoxanthine-guanine-phosphoribosyltransferase deficiency) 277.2
Lev's (acquired complete heart block) 426.0
Levi's (pituitary dwarfism) 253.3
Lévy-Roussy 334.3
Lichtheim's (subacute combined sclerosis with pernicious anemia) 281.0 [336.2]
Lightwood's (renal tubular acidosis) 588.8
Lignac (-de Toni) (-Fanconi) (-Debré) (cystinosis) 270.0
Likoff's (angina in menopausal women) 413.9
liver-kidney 572.4
Lloyd's 258.1
lobotomy 310.0
Löffler's (eosinophilic pneumonitis) 518.3
Löfgren's (sarcoidosis) 135
long arm 18 or 21 deletion 758.3
Looser (-Debray) — Milkman (osteomalacia with pseudofractures) 268.2
Lorain-Levi (pituitary dwarfism) 253.3
Louis-Bar (ataxia-telangiectasia) 334.8
low
  atmospheric pressure 993.2
  back 724.2
    psychogenic 306.0
  output (cardiac) (see also Failure, heart) 428.9
Lowe's (oculocerebrorenal dystrophy) 270.8
Lowe-Terrey-MacLachlan (oculocerebrorenal dystrophy) 270.8
lower radicular, newborn 767.4
Lown (-Ganong)-Levine (short P-R interval, normal QRS complex, and supraventricular tachycardia) 426.81
Lucey-Driscoll (jaundice due to delayed conjugation) 774.30
Luetscher's (dehydration) 276.5
lumbar vertebral 724.4
Lutembacher's (atrial septal defect with mitral stenosis) 745.5
Lyell's (toxic epidermal necrolysis) 695.1
  due to drug
    correct substance properly administered 695.1
    overdose or wrong substance given or taken 977.9
    specified drug — see Table of drugs and chemicals

Syndrome—continued

MacLeod's 492.8
macrogenitosomia praecox 259.8
macroglobulinemia 273.3
Maffucci's (dyschondroplasia with hemangiomas) 756.4
Magenblase 306.4
magnesium-deficiency 781.7
malabsorption 579.9
  postsurgical 579.3
  spinal fluid 331.3
malignant carcinoid 259.2
Mallory-Weiss 530.7
mandibulofacial dysostosis 756.0
manic-depressive (see also Psychosis, affective) 296.80
Mankowsky's (familial dysplastic osteopathy) 731.2
maple syrup (urine) 270.3
Marable's (celiac artery compression) 447.4
Marchesani (-Weill) (brachymorphism and ectopia lentis) 759.89
Marchiafava-Bignami 341.8
Marchiafava-Micheli (paroxysmal nocturnal hemoglobinuria) 283.2
Marcus Gunn's (jaw-winking syndrome) 742.8
Marfan's (arachnodactyly) 759.82
  meaning congenital syphilis 090.49
  with luxation of lens 090.49 [379.32]
Marie's (acromegaly) 253.0
  primary or idiopathic (acropachyderma) 757.39
  secondary (hypertrophic pulmonary osteoarthropathy) 731.2
Markus-Adie 379.46
Maroteaux-Lamy (mucopolysaccharidosis VI) 277.5
Martin's 715.27
Martin-Albright (pseudohypoparathyroidism) 275.4
Martorell-Fabré (pulseless disease) 446.7
massive aspiration of newborn 770.1
Masters-Allen 620.6
mastocytosis 757.33
maternal hypotension 669.2
maternal obesity 646.1
May (-Hegglin) 288.2
McArdle (-Schmid) (-Pearson) (glycogenosis V) 271.0
McCune-Albright (osteitis fibrosa disseminata) 756.59
McQuarrie's (idiopathic familial hypoglycemia) 251.2
meconium
  aspiration 770.1
  plug (newborn) NEC 777.1
median arcuate ligament 447.4
mediastinal fibrosis 519.3
Meekeren-Ehlers-Danlos 756.83
Meige (blepharospasm-oromandibular dystonia) 333.82
-Milroy (chronic hereditary edema) 757.0
Melkersson (-Rosenthal) 351.8
Mende's (ptosis-epicanthus) 270.2
Mendelson's (resulting from a procedure) 997.3
  during labor 668.0
  obstetric 668.0
Ménétrier's (hypertrophic gastritis) 535.2
Ménière's (see also Disease, Ménière's) 386.00
meningo-eruptive 047.1

Syndrome—continued

Menkes' 759.89
  glutamic acid 759.89
  maple syrup (urine) disease 270.3
menopause 627.2
  postartificial 627.4
menstruation 625.4
mesenteric
  artery, superior 557.1
  vascular insufficiency (with gangrene) 557.1
metastatic carcinoid 259.2
Meyenburg-Altherr-Uehlinger 733.99
Meyer-Schwickerath and Weyers (dysplasia oculodentodigitalis) 759.89
Micheli-Rietti (thalassemia minor) 282.4
Michotte's 721.5
micrognathia-glossoptosis 756.0
microphthalmos (congenital) 759.89
midbrain 348.8
middle
  lobe (lung) (right) 518.0
  radicular 353.0
Miescher's
  familial acanthosis nigricans 701.2
  granulomatosis disciformis 709.3
Mieten's 759.89
migraine 346.0
Mikity-Wilson (pulmonary dysmaturity) 770.7
Mikulicz's (dryness of mouth, absent or decreased lacrimation) 527.1
milk alkali (milk drinkers') 999.9
Milkman (-Looser) (osteomalacia with pseudofractures) 268.2
Millard-Gubler 344.89
Miller Fisher's 357.0
Milles' (encephalocutaneous angiomatosis) 759.6
Minkowski-Chauffard (see also Spherocytosis) 282.0
Mirizzi's (hepatic duct stenosis) 576.2
  with calculus, cholelithiasis, or stones — see Choledocholithiasis
mitral
  click (-murmur) 785.2
  valve prolapse 424.0
Möbius'
  congenital oculofacial paralysis 352.6
  ophthalmoplegic migraine 346.8
Mohr's (types I and II) 759.89
monofixation 378.34
Moore's (see also Epilepsy) 345.5
Morel-Moore (hyperostosis frontalis interna) 733.3
Morel-Morgagni (hyperostosis frontalis interna) 733.3
Morgagni (-Stewart-Morel) (hyperostosis frontalis interna) 733.3
Morgagni-Adams-Stokes (syncope with heart block) 426.9
Morquio (-Brailsford) (-Ullrich) (mucopolysaccharidosis IV) 277.5
Morris (testicular feminization) 257.8
Morton's (foot) (metatarsalgia) (metatarsal neuralgia) (neuralgia) (neuroma) (toe) 355.6
Moschcowitz (-Singer-Symmers) (thrombotic thrombocytopenic purpura) 446.6

Syndrome — INDEX TO DISEASES — Syndrome

Syndrome—continued
- Mounier-Kuhn 494
- Mucha-Haberman (acute parapsoriasis varioliformis) 696.2
- mucocutaneous lymph node (acute) (febrile) (infantile) (MCLS) 446.1
- multiple
  - deficiency 260
  - operations 301.51
- Munchausen's 301.51
- Münchmeyer's (exostosis luxurians) 728.11
- Murchison-Sanderson — see Disease, Hodgkin's
- myasthenic — see Myasthenia, syndrome
- myelodysplastic 238.7
- myeloproliferative (chronic) (M9960/1) 238.7
- myofascial pain NEC 729.1
- Naffziger's 353.0
- Nager-de Reynier (dysostosis mandibularis) 756.0
- nail-patella (hereditary osteo-onychodysplasia) 756.89
- Nebécourt's 253.3
- Neill-Dingwall (microencephaly and dwarfism) 759.89
- nephrotic (see also Nephrosis) 581.9
  - diabetic 250.4 [581.81]
- Netherton's (ichthyosiform erythroderma) 757.1
- neurocutaneous 759.6
- neuroleptic malignant 333.92 ◆
- Nezelof's (pure alymphocytosis) 279.13
- Niemann-Pick (lipid histiocytosis) 272.7
- Nonne-Milroy-Meige (chronic hereditary edema) 757.0
- nonsense 300.16
- Noonan's 759.89 ◆
- Nothnagel's
  - ophthalmoplegia-cerebellar ataxia 378.52
  - vasomotor acroparesthesia 443.89
- nucleus ambiguous-hypoglossal 352.6
- OAV (oculoauriculovertebral dysplasia) 756.0
- obsessional 300.3
- oculocutaneous 364.24
- oculomotor 378.81
- oculourethroarticular 099.3
- Ogilvie's (sympathicotonic colon obstruction) 560.89
- ophthalmoplegia-cerebellar ataxia 378.52
- Oppenheim-Urbach (necrobiosis lipoidica diabeticorum) 250.8 [709.3]
- oral-facial-digital 759.89
- organic
  - affective NEC 293.83
    - drug-induced 292.84
  - delusional 293.81
    - alcohol-induced 291.5
    - drug-induced 292.11
    - due to or associated with
      - arteriosclerosis 290.42
      - presenile brain disease 290.12
      - senility 290.20
  - depressive 293.83
    - drug-induced 292.84
    - due to or associated with
      - arteriosclerosis 290.43
      - presenile brain disease 290.13
      - senile brain disease 290.21
  - hallucinosis 293.82
    - drug-induced 292.84

Syndrome—continued
- organic affective 293.83
  - induced by drug 292.84
- organic personality 310.1
  - induced by drug 292.89
- Ormond's 593.4
- orodigitofacial 759.89
- orthostatic hypotensive-dysautonomic dyskinetic 333.0
- Osler-Weber-Rendu (familial hemorrhagic telangiectasia) 448.0
- osteodermopathic hyperostosis 757.39
- osteoporosis-osteomalacia 268.2
- Österreicher-Turner (hereditary osteo-onychodysplasia) 756.89
- Ostrum-Furst 756.59
- otolith 386.19
- otopalatodigital 759.89
- outlet (thoracic) 353.0
- ovarian vein 593.4
- Owren's (see also Defect, coagulation) 286.3
- OX 758.6
- pacemaker 429.4 ◆
- Paget-Schroetter (intermittent venous claudication) 453.8
- pain — see Pain
- painful
  - apicocostal vertebral (M8010/3) 162.3
  - arc 726.19
  - bruising 287.2
  - feet 266.2
- Pancoast's (carcinoma, pulmonary apex) (M8010/3) 162.3
- panhypopituitary (postpartum) 253.2
- papillary muscle 429.81
  - with myocardial infarction 410.8
- Papillon-Léage and Psaume (orodigitofacial dysostosis) 759.89
- parabiotic (transfusion)
  - donor (twin) 772.0
  - recipient (twin) 776.4
- paralysis agitans 332.0
- paralytic 344.9
  - specified type NEC 344.89
- Parinaud's (paralysis of conjugate upward gaze) 378.81
  - oculoglandular 372.02
- Parkes Weber and Dimitri (encephalocutaneous angiomatosis) 759.6
- Parkinson's (see also Parkinsonism) 332.0
- parkinsonian (see also Parkinsonism) 332.0
- Parry's (exophthalmic goiter) 242.0
- Parry-Romberg 349.89
- Parsonage-Aldren-Turner 353.5
- Parsonage-Turner 353.5
- Patau's (trisomy D) 758.1
- Paterson (-Brown) (-Kelly) (sideropenic dysphagia) 280.8
- Payr's (splenic flexure syndrome) 569.89
- pectoral girdle 447.8
- pectoralis minor 447.8
- Pelger-Huët (hereditary hyposegmentation) 288.2
- pellagra-cerebellar ataxia-renal aminoaciduria 270.0
- Pellegrini-Stieda 726.62
- pellagroid 265.2
- Pellizzi's (pineal) 259.8
- pelvic congestion (-fibrosis) 625.5
- Pendred's (familial goiter with deaf-mutism) 243

Syndrome—continued
- Penfield's (see also Epilepsy) 345.5
- Penta X 758.8
- peptic ulcer — see Ulcer, peptic 533.9
- perabduction 447.8
- periodic 277.3
- periurethral fibrosis 593.4
- persistent fetal circulation 747.9
- Petges-Cléjat (poikilodermatomyositis) 710.3
- Peutz-Jeghers 759.6
- phantom limb 353.6
- pharyngeal pouch 279.11
- Pick's (pericardial pseudocirrhosis of liver) 423.2
  - heart 423.2
  - liver 423.2
- Pick-Herxheimer (diffuse idiopathic cutaneous atrophy) 701.8
- Pickwickian (cardiopulmonary obesity) 278.8
- PIE (pulmonary infiltration with eosinophilia) 518.3
- Pierre Marie-Bamberger (hypertrophic pulmonary osteoarthropathy) 731.2
- Pierre Mauriac's (diabetes-dwarfism-obesity) 258.1
- Pierre Robin 756.0
- pigment dispersion, iris 364.53
- pineal 259.8
- pink puffer 492.8
- pituitary 253.0
- placental
  - dysfunction 762.2
  - insufficiency 762.2
  - transfusion 762.3
- plantar fascia 728.71
- Plummer-Vinson (sideropenic dysphagia) 280.8
- pluricarential of infancy 260
- plurideficiency of infancy 260
- pluriglandular (compensatory) 258.8
- polycarential of infancy 260
- polyglandular 258.8
- polysplenia 759.0
- pontine 433.8
- popliteal
  - artery entrapment 447.8
  - web 756.89
- postartificial menopause 627.4
- postcardiotomy 429.4
- postcholecystectomy 576.0
- postcommissurotomy 429.4
- postconcussional 310.2
- postcontusional 310.2
- postencephalitic 310.8
- posterior
  - cervical sympathetic 723.2
  - fossa compression 348.4
  - inferior cerebellar artery (see also Disease, cerebrovascular, acute) 436
- postgastrectomy (dumping) 564.2
- post-gastric surgery 564.2
- posthepatitis 780.7
- postherpetic (neuralgia) (zoster) 053.19
  - geniculate ganglion 053.11
  - ophthalmica 053.19
- postimmunization — see Complications, vaccination
- postinfarction 411.0
- postinfluenza (asthenia) 780.7
- postirradiation 990
- postlaminectomy 722.80
  - cervical, cervicothoracic 722.1
  - lumbar, lumbosacral 722.83
  - thoracic, thoracolumbar 722.82

Syndrome—continued
- postleukotomy 310.0
- postlobotomy 310.0
- postmastectomy lymphedema 457.0
- postmature (of newborn) 766.2
- postmyocardial infarction 411.0
- postoperative NEC 998.9
  - blind loop 579.2
- postpartum panhypopituitary 253.2
- postperfusion NEC 999.8
  - bone marrow 996.85
- postpericardiotomy 429.4
- postphlebitic 459.1
- postpolio (myelitis) 138
- postvagotomy 564.2
- postvalvulotomy 429.4
- postviral (asthenia) NEC 780.7
- Potain's (gastrectasis with dyspepsia) 536.1
- potassium intoxication 276.7
- Potter's 753.0
- Prader (-Labhart) — Willi (-Fanconi) 759.81
- preinfarction 411.1
- preleukemic 288.8
- premature senility 259.8
- premenstrual tension 625.4
- pre ulcer 536.9
- Prinzmetal-Massumi (anterior chest wall syndrome) 786.52
- Profichet's 729.9
- progeria 259.8
- progressive pallidal degeneration 333.0
- prolonged gestation 766.2
- prune belly 756.7
- prurigo-asthma 691.8
- pseudocarpal tunnel (sublimis) 354.0
- pseudohermaphroditism-virilism-hirsutism 255.2
- pseudoparalytica 358.0
- pseudo-Turner's 759.89
- psycho-organic 293.9
  - acute 293.0
  - depressive type 293.83
  - hallucinatory type 293.82
  - nonpsychotic severity 310.1
    - specified focal (partial) NEC 310.8
  - paranoid type 293.81
  - specified type NEC 293.89
  - subacute 293.1
- pterygolymphangiectasia 758.6
- ptosis-epicanthus 270.2
- pulmonary
  - arteriosclerosis 416.0
  - hypoperfusion (idiopathic) 769
  - renal (hemorrhagic) 446.21
- pulseless 446.7
- Putnam-Dana (subacute combined sclerosis with pernicious anemia) 281.0 [336.2]
- pyloroduodenal 537.89
- pyramidopallidonigral 332.0
- pyriformis 355.0
- Q-T interval prolongation 794.31
- radicular NEC 729.2
  - lower limbs 724.4
  - upper limbs 723.4
  - newborn 767.4
- Raeder-Harbitz (pulseless disease) 446.7
- Ramsay Hunt's
  - dyssynergia cerebellaris myoclonica 334.2
  - herpetic geniculate ganglionitis 053.11
- rapid time-zone change 307.45
- Raymond (-Céstan) 433.8
- Raynaud's (paroxysmal digital cyanosis) 443.0

Syndrome—*continued*
- RDS (respiratory distress syndrome, newborn) 769
- Refsum's (heredopathia atactica polyneuritiformis) 356.3
- Reichmann's (gastrosuccorrhea) 536.8
- Reifenstein's (hereditary familial hypogonadism, male) 257.2
- Reilly's (*see also* Neuropathy, peripheral, autonomic) 337.9
- Reiter's 099.3
- renal glomerulohyalinosis-diabetic 250.4 [581.81]
- Rendu-Osler-Weber (familial hemorrhagic telangiectasia) 448.0
- renofacial (congenital biliary fibroangiomatosis) 753.0
- Rénon-Delille 253.8
- respiratory distress (idiopathic) (newborn) 769
  - adult (following shock, surgery, or trauma) 518.5
  - specified NEC 518.82
- restless leg 333.99
- retraction (Duane's) 378.71
- retroperitoneal fibrosis 593.4
- Rett's 330.8
- Reye's 331.81
- Reye-Sheehan (postpartum pituitary necrosis) 253.2
- Riddoch's (visual disorientation) 368.16
- Ridley's (*see also* Failure, ventricular, left) 428.1
- Rieger's (mesodermal dysgenesis, anterior ocular segment) 743.44
- Rietti-Greppi-Micheli (thalassemia minor) 282.4
- right ventricular obstruction — *see* Failure heart, congestive
- Riley-Day (familial dysautonomia) 742.8
- Robin's 756.0
- Rokitansky-Kuster-Hauser (congenital absence, vagina) 752.49
- Romano-Ward (prolonged Q-T interval) 794.31
- Romberg's 349.89
- Rosen-Castleman-Liebow (pulmonary proteinosis) 516.0
- rotator cuff, shoulder 726.10
- Roth's 355.1
- Rothmund's (congenital poikiloderma) 757.33
- Rotor's (idiopathic hyperbilirubinemia) 277.4
- Roussy-Lévy 334.3
- Roy (-Jutras) (acropachyderma) 757.39
- rubella (congenital) 771.0
- Rubinstein-Taybi's (brachydactylia, short stature, and mental retardation) 759.89
- Rud's (mental deficiency, epilepsy, and infantilism) 759.89
- Ruiter-Pompen (-Wyers) (angiokeratoma corporis diffusum) 272.7
- Runge's (postmaturity) 766.2
- Russell (-Silver) (congenital hemihypertrophy and short stature) 759.89
- Rytand-Lipsitch (complete atrioventricular block) 426.0

Syndrome—*continued*
- sacralization-scoliosis-sciatica 756.15
- sacroiliac 724.6
- Saenger's 379.46
- salt
  - depletion (*see also* Disease, renal) 593.9
    - due to heat NEC 992.8
      - causing heat exhaustion or prostration 992.4
  - low (*see also* Disease, renal) 593.9
  - salt-losing (*see also* Disease, renal) 593.9
- Sanfilippo's (mucopolysaccharidosis III) 277.5
- Scaglietti-Dagnini (acromegalic macrospondylitis) 253.0
- scalded skin 695.1
- scalenus anticus (anterior) 353.0
- scapulocostal 354.8
- scapuloperoneal 359.1
- scapulovertebral 723.4
- Schaumann's (sarcoidosis) 135
- Scheie's (mucopolysaccharidosis IS) 277.5
- Scheuthauer-Marie-Sainton (cleidocranialis dysostosis) 755.59
- Schirmer's (encephalocutaneous angiomatosis) 759.6
- schizophrenic, of childhood NEC (*see also* Psychosis, childhood) 299.9
- Schmidt's
  - sphallo-pharyngo-laryngeal hemiplegia 352.6
  - thyroid-adrenocortical insufficiency 258.1
  - vagoaccessory 352.6
- Schneider's 047.9
- Scholte's (malignant carcinoid) 259.2
- Scholz (-Bielschowsky-Henneberg) 330.0
- Schroeder's (endocrine-hypertensive) 255.3
- Schüller-Christian (chronic histiocytosis X) 277.8
- Schultz's (agranulocytosis) 288.0
- Schwartz (-Jampel) 756.89
- Schwartz-Bartter (inappropriate secretion of antidiuretic hormone) 253.6
- Scimitar (anomalous venous drainage, right lung to inferior vena cava) 747.49
- sclerocystic ovary 256.4
- sea-blue histiocyte 272.7
- Seabright-Bantam (pseudohypoparathyroidism) 275.4
- Seckel's 759.89
- Secretan's (posttraumatic edema) 782.3
- secretoinhibitor (keratoconjunctivitis sicca) 710.2
- Seeligmann's (ichthyosis congenita) 757.1
- Senear-Usher (pemphigus erythematosus) 694.4
- senilism 259.8
- serous meningitis 348.2
- Sertoli cell (germinal aplasia) 606.0
- sex chromosome mosaic 758.8
- Sézary's (reticulosis) (M9701/3) 202.2
- Shaver's (bauxite pneumoconiosis) 503
- Sheehan's (postpartum pituitary necrosis) 253.2

Syndrome—*continued*
- shock (traumatic) 958.4
  - kidney 584.5
    - following crush injury 958.5
  - lung 518.5
  - neurogenic 308.9
  - psychic 308.9
- short
  - bowel 579.3
  - P-R interval 426.81
- shoulder-arm (*see also* Neuropathy, peripheral, autonomic) 337.9
- shoulder-girdle 723.4
- shoulder-hand (*see also* Neuropathy, peripheral, autonomic) 337.9
- Shwachman's 288.0
- Shy-Drager (orthostatic hypotension with multisystem degeneration) 333.0
- Sicard's 352.6
- sicca (keratoconjunctivitis) 710.2
- sick
  - cell 276.1
  - sinus 427.81
- sideropenic 280.8
- Siemens'
  - ectodermal dysplasia 757.31
  - keratosis follicularis spinulosa (decalvans) 757.39
- Silfverskiöld's (osteochondrodystrophy, extremities) 756.50
- Silver's (congenital hemihypertrophy and short stature) 759.89
- Silvestroni-Bianco (thalassemia minima) 282.4
- Simons' (progressive lipodystrophy) 272.6
- sinus tarsi 355.5
- sinusitis-bronchiectasis-situs inversus 759.3
- Sipple's (medullary thyroid carcinoma-pheochromocytoma) 193
- Sjögren (-Gougerot) (keratoconjunctivitis sicca) 710.2
  - with lung involvement 710.2 [517.8]
- Sjögren-Larsson (ichthyosis congenita) 757.1
- Slocumb's 255.3
- Sluder's 337.0
- Smith-Lemli-Opitz (cerebrohepatorenal syndrome) 759.89
- smokers' 305.1
- Sneddon-Wilkinson (subcorneal pustular dermatosis) 694.1
- Sotos' (cerebral gigantism) 253.0
- South African cardiomyopathy 425.2
- spasmodic
  - upward movement, eye(s) 378.82
  - winking 307.20
- Spens' (syncope with heart block) 426.9
- spherophakia-brachymorphia 759.89
- spinal cord injury — *see also* Injury, spinal, by site
  - with fracture, vertebra — *see* Fracture, vertebra, by site, with spinal cord injury
  - cervical — *see* Injury, spinal, cervical
  - fluid malabsorption (acquired) 331.3

Syndrome—*continued*
- splenic
  - agenesis 759.0
  - flexure 569.89
  - neutropenia 288.0
  - sequestration 282.60
- Spurway's (brittle bones and blue sclera) 756.51
- staphylococcal scalded skin 695.1
- Stein's (polycystic ovary) 256.4
- Stein-Leventhal (polycystic ovary) 256.4
- Steinbrocker's (*see also* Neuropathy, peripheral, autonomic) 337.9
- Stevens-Johnson (erythema multiforme exudativum) 695.1
- Stewart-Morel (hyperostosis frontalis interna) 733.3
- stiff-man 333.91
- Still's (juvenile rheumatoid arthritis) 714.30
- Still-Felty (rheumatoid arthritis with splenomegaly and leukopenia) 714.1
- Stilling-Türk-Duane (ocular retraction syndrome) 378.71
- Stojano's (subcostal) 098.86
- Stokes (-Adams) (syncope with heart block) 426.9
- Stokvis-Talma (enterogenous cyanosis) 289.7
- stone heart (*see also* Failure, ventricular, left) 428.1
- straight-back 756.19
- stroke (*see also* Disease, cerebrovascular, acute) 436
  - little 435.9
- Sturge-Kalischer-Weber (encephalotrigeminal angiomatosis) 759.6
- Sturge-Weber (-Dimitri) (encephalocutaneous angiomatosis) 759.6
- subclavian-carotid obstruction (chronic) 446.7
- subclavian steal 435.2
- subcoracoid-pectoralis minor 447.8
- subcostal 098.86
  - nerve compression 354.8
- subperiosteal hematoma 267
- subphrenic interposition 751.4
- sudden infant death (SIDS) 798.0
- Sudeck's 733.7
- Sudeck-Leriche 733.7
- superior
  - cerebellar artery (*see also* Disease, cerebrovascular, acute) 436
  - mesenteric artery 557.1
  - pulmonary sulcus (tumor) (M8010/3) 162.3
  - vena cava 459.2
- suprarenal cortical 255.3
- supraspinatus 726.10
- swallowed blood 777.3
- sweat retention 705.1
- Sweet's (acute febrile neutrophilic dermatosis) 695.89
- Swyer-James (unilateral hyperlucent lung) 492.8
- Swyer's (XY pure gonadal dysgenesis) 752.7
- Symonds' 348.2
- sympathetic
  - cervical paralysis 337.0
  - pelvic 625.5
- syndactylic oxycephaly 755.55
- syphilitic-cardiovascular 093.89
- systemic fibrosclerosing 710.8
- systolic click (-murmur) 785.2
- Tabagism 305.1

Syndrome—continued
  tachycardia-bradycardia 427.81
  Takayasu (-Onishi) (pulseless disease) 446.7
  Tapia's 352.6
  tarsal tunnel 355.5
  Taussig-Bing (transposition, aorta and overriding pulmonary artery) 745.11
  Taybi's (otopalatodigital) 759.89
  Taylor's 625.5
  teething 520.7
  tegmental 344.89
  telangiectasis-pigmentation-cataract 757.33
  temporal 383.02
    lobectomy behavior 310.0
  temporomandibular joint-pain-dysfunction [TMJ] NEC 524.60
    specified NEC 524.69
  Terry's 362.21
  testicular feminization 257.8
  testis, nonvirilizing 257.8
  tethered (spinal) cord 742.59
  thalamic 348.8
  Thibierge-Weissenbach (cutaneous systemic sclerosis) 710.1
  Thiele 724.6
  thoracic outlet (compression) 353.0
  thoracogenous rheumatic (hypertrophic pulmonary osteoarthropathy) 731.2
  Thorn's (see also Disease, renal) 593.9
  Thorson-Biörck (malignant carcinoid) 259.2
  thrombopenia-hemangioma 287.3
  thyroid-adrenocortical insufficiency 258.1
  Tietze's 733.6
  time-zone (rapid) 307.45
  Tobias' (carcinoma, pulmonary apex) (M8010/3) 162.3
  toilet seat 926.0
  Tolosa-Hunt 378.55
  Toni-Fanconi (cystinosis) 270.0
  Touraine's (hereditary osteo-onychodysplasia) 756.89
  Touraine-Solente-Golé (acropachyderma) 757.39
  toxic
    oil 710.5
    shock 040.89
  transfusion
    fetal-maternal 772.0
    twin
      donor (infant) 772.0
      recipient (infant) 776.4
  Treacher Collins' (incomplete mandibulofacial dysostosis) 756.0
  trigeminal plate 259.8
  triplex X female 758.8
  trisomy NEC 758.5
    13 or D_1 758.1
    16-18 or E 758.2
    18 or E_3 758.2
    20 758.5
    21 or G (mongolism) 758.0
    22 or G (mongolism) 758.0
    G 758.0
  Troisier-Hanot-Chauffard (bronze diabetes) 275.0
  tropical wet feet 991.4
  Trousseau's (thrombophlebitis migrans visceral cancer) 453.1
  Türk's (ocular retraction syndrome) 378.71
  Turner's 758.6
  Turner-Varny 758.6
  twin-to-twin transfusion 762.3
    recipient twin 776.4

Syndrome—continued
  Uehlinger's (acropachyderma) 757.39
  Ullrich (-Bonnevie) (-Turner) 758.6
  Ullrich-Feichtiger 759.89
  underwater blast injury (abdominal) (see also Injury, internal, abdomen) 868.00
  universal joint, cervix 620.6
  Unverricht (-Lundborg) 333.2
  Unverricht-Wagner (dermatomyositis) 710.3
  upward gaze 378.81
  Urbach-Oppenheim (necrobiosis lipoidica diabeticorum) 250.8 [709.3]
  Urbach-Wiethe (lipoid proteinosis) 272.8
  uremia, chronic 585
  urethral 597.81
  urethro-oculoarticular 099.3
  urethro-oculosynovial 099.3
  urohepatic 572.4
  uveocutaneous 364.24
  uveomeningeal, uveomeningitis 363.22
  vagohypoglossal 352.6
  vagovagal 780.2
  van Buchem's (hyperostosis corticalis) 733.3
  van der Hoeve's (brittle bones and blue sclera, deafness) 756.51
  van der Hoeve-Halbertsma-Waardenburg (ptosis-epicanthus) 270.2
  van der Hoeve-Waardenburg-Gualdi (ptosis-epicanthus) 270.2
  van Neck-Odelberg (juvenile osteochondrosis) 732.1
  vascular splanchnic 557.0
  vasomotor 443.9
  vasovagal 780.2
  VATER 759.89
  vena cava (inferior) (superior) (obstruction) 459.2
  Verbiest's (claudicatio intermittens spinalis) 435.1
  Vernet's 352.6
  vertebral
    artery 435.1
      compression 721.1
    lumbar 724.4
    steal 435.1
  vertebrogenic (pain) 724.5
  vertiginous NEC 386.9
  video display tube 723.8
  Villaret's 352.6
  Vinson-Plummer (sideropenic dysphagia) 280.8
  virilizing adrenocortical hyperplasia, congenital 255.2
  virus, viral 079.99
  visceral larval migrans 128.0
  visual disorientation 368.16
  vitamin B_6 deficiency 266.1
  vitreous touch 997.9
  Vogt's (corpus striatum) 333.7
  Vogt-Koyanagi 364.24
  Volkmann's 958.6
  von Bechterew-Strümpell (ankylosing spondylitis) 720.0
  von Graefe's 378.72
  von Hippel-Lindau (angiomatosis retinocerebellosa) 759.6
  von Schroetter's (intermittent venous claudication) 453.8
  von Willebrand (-Jürgens) (angiohemophilia) 286.4
  Waardenburg-Klein (ptosis epicanthus) 270.2

Syndrome—continued
  Wagner (-Unverricht) (dermatomyositis) 710.3
  Waldenström's (macroglobulinemia) 273.3
  Waldenström-Kjellberg (sideropenic dysphagia) 280.8
  Wallenberg's (posterior inferior cerebellar artery) (see also Disease, cerebrovascular, acute) 436
  Waterhouse (-Friderichsen) 036.3
  water retention 276.6
  Weber's 344.89
  Weber-Christian (nodular nonsuppurative panniculitis) 729.30
  Weber-Cockayne (epidermolysis bullosa) 757.39
  Weber-Dimitri (encephalocutaneous angiomatosis) 759.6
  Weber-Gubler 344.89
  Weber-Leyden 344.89
  Weber-Osler (familial hemorrhagic telangiectasia) 448.0
  Wegener's (necrotizing respiratory granulomatosis) 446.4
  Weill-Marchesani (brachymorphism and ectopia lentis) 759.89
  Weingarten's (tropical eosinophilia) 518.3
  Weiss-Baker (carotid sinus syncope) 337.0
  Weissenbach-Thibierge (cutaneous systemic sclerosis) 710.1
  Werdnig-Hoffmann 335.0
  Werlhof-Wichmann (see also Purpura, thrombocytopenic) 287.3
  Wermer's (polyendocrine adenomatosis) 258.0
  Werner's (progeria adultorum) 259.8
  Wernicke's (nonalcoholic) (superior hemorrhagic polioencephalitis) 265.1
  Wernicke-Korsakoff (nonalcoholic) 294.0
    alcoholic 291.1
  Westphal-Strümpell (hepatolenticular degeneration) 275.1
  wet
    brain (alcoholic) 303.9
    feet (maceration) (tropical) 991.4
    lung
      adult 518.5
      newborn 770.6
  whiplash 847.0
  Whipple's (intestinal lipodystrophy) 040.2
  "whistling face" (craniocarpotarsal dystrophy) 759.89
  Widal (-Abrami) (acquired hemolytic jaundice) 283.9
  Wilkie's 557.1
  Wilkinson-Sneddon (subcorneal pustular dermatosis) 694.1
  Willan-Plumbe (psoriasis) 696.1
  Willebrand (-Jürgens) (angiohemophilia) 286.4
  Willi-Prader (hypogenital dystrophy with diabetic tendency) 759.81
  Wilson's (hepatolenticular degeneration) 275.1
  Wilson-Mikity 770.7
  Wiskott-Aldrich (eczema-thrombocytopenia) 279.12

Syndrome—continued
  withdrawal
    alcohol 291.8
    drug 292.0
      infant of dependent mother 779.5
  Woakes' (ethmoiditis) 471.1
  Wolff-Parkinson-White (anomalous atrioventricular excitation) 426.7
  Wright's (hyperabduction) 447.8
  X 413.9
  xiphoidalgia 733.99
  XO 758.6
  XXX 758.8
  XXXXY 758.8
  XXY 758.7
  yellow vernix (placental dysfunction) 762.2
  Zahorsky's 074.0
  Zieve's (jaundice, hyperlipemia and hemolytic anemia) 571.1
  Zollinger-Ellison (gastric hypersecretion with pancreatic islet cell tumor) 251.5
  Zuelzer-Ogden (nutritional megaloblastic anemia) 281.2

Synechia (iris) (pupil) 364.70
  anterior 364.72
  peripheral 364.73
  intrauterine (traumatic) 621.5
  posterior 364.71
  vulvae, congenital 752.49

Synesthesia (see also Disturbance, sensation) 782.0

Synodontia 520.2

Synophthalmus 759.89

Synorchidism 752.8

Synorchism 752.8

Synostosis (congenital) 756.59
  astragaloscaphoid 755.67
  radioulnar 755.53
  talonavicular (bar) 755.67
  tarsal 755.67

Synovial — see condition

Synovioma (M9040/3) — see also Neoplasm, connective tissue, malignant
  benign (M9040/0) — see Neoplasm, connective tissue, benign

Synoviosarcoma (M9040/3) — see Neoplasm, connective tissue, malignant

Synovitis 727.00
  chronic crepitant, wrist 727.2
  due to crystals — see Arthritis, due to crystals
  gonococcal 098.51
  gouty 274.0
  syphilitic 095.7
    congenital 090.0
  traumatic, current — see Sprain, by site
  tuberculous — see Tuberculosis, synovitis
  villonodular 719.20
    ankle 719.27
    elbow 719.22
    foot 719.27
    hand 719.24
    hip 719.25
    knee 719.26
    multiple sites 719.29
    pelvic region 719.25
    shoulder (region) 719.21
    specified site NEC 719.28
    wrist 719.23

Syphilide 091.3
  congenital 090.0
  newborn 090.0

Syphilide—continued
- tubercular 095.8
  - congenital 090.0

Syphilis, syphilitic (acquired) 097.9
- with lung involvement 095.1
- abdomen (late) 095.2
- acoustic nerve 094.86
- adenopathy (secondary) 091.4
- adrenal (gland) 095.8
  - with cortical hypofunction 095.8
- age under 2 years NEC (see also Syphilis, congenital) 090.9
  - acquired 097.9
- alopecia (secondary) 091.82
- anemia 095.8
- aneurysm (artery) (ruptured) 093.89
  - aorta 093.0
  - central nervous system 094.89
  - congenital 090.5
- anus 095.8
  - primary 091.1
  - secondary 091.3
- aorta, aortic (arch) (abdominal) (insufficiency) (pulmonary) (regurgitation) (stenosis) (thoracic) 093.89
  - aneurysm 093.0
- arachnoid (adhesive) 094.2
- artery 093.89
  - cerebral 094.89
  - spinal 094.89
- arthropathy (neurogenic) (tabetic) 094.0 [713.5]
- asymptomatic — see Syphilis, latent
- ataxia, locomotor (progressive) 094.0
- atrophoderma maculatum 091.3
- auricular fibrillation 093.89
- Bell's palsy 094.89
- bladder 095.8
- bone 095.5
  - secondary 091.61
- brain 094.89
- breast 095.8
- bronchus 095.8
- bubo 091.0
- bulbar palsy 094.89
- bursa (late) 095.7
- cardiac decompensation 093.89
- cardiovascular (early) (late) (primary) (secondary) (tertiary) 093.9
  - specified type and site NEC 093.89
- causing death under 2 years of age (see also Syphilis, congenital) 090.9
  - stated to be acquired NEC 097.9
- central nervous system (any site) (early) (late) (latent) (primary) (recurrent) (relapse) (secondary) (tertiary) 094.9
  - with
    - ataxia 094.0
    - paralysis, general 094.1
      - juvenile 090.40
    - paresis (general) 094.1
      - juvenile 090.40
    - tabes (dorsalis) 094.0
      - juvenile 090.40
    - taboparesis 094.1
      - juvenile 090.40
  - aneurysm (ruptured) 094.87
  - congenital 090.40
  - juvenile 090.40
  - remission in (sustained) 094.9
  - serology doubtful, negative, or positive 094.9
  - specified nature or site NEC 094.89
  - vascular 094.89

Syphilis, syphilitic—continued
- cerebral 094.89
  - meningovascular 094.2
  - nerves 094.89
  - sclerosis 094.89
  - thrombosis 094.89
- cerebrospinal 094.89
  - tabetic 094.0
- cerebrovascular 094.89
- cervix 095.8
- chancre (multiple) 091.0
  - extragenital 091.2
  - Rollet's 091.0
- Charcot's joint 094.0 [713.5]
- choked disc 094.89 [377.00]
- chorioretinitis 091.51
  - congenital 090.0 [363.13]
  - late 094.83
- choroiditis 091.51
  - congenital 090.0 [363.13]
  - late 094.83
  - prenatal 090.0 [363.13]
- choroidoretinitis (secondary) 091.51
  - congenital 090.0 [363.13]
  - late 094.83
- ciliary body (secondary) 091.52
  - late 095.8 [364.11]
- colon (late) 095.8
- combined sclerosis 094.89
- complicating pregnancy, childbirth or puerperium 647.0
- affecting fetus or newborn 760.2
- condyloma (latum) 091.3
- congenital 090.9
  - with
    - encephalitis 090.41
    - paresis (general) 090.40
    - tabes (dorsalis) 090.40
    - taboparesis 090.40
  - chorioretinitis, choroiditis 090.0 [363.13]
  - early or less than 2 years after birth NEC 090.2
    - with manifestations 090.0
    - latent (without manifestations) 090.1
      - negative spinal fluid test 090.1
      - serology, positive 090.1
    - symptomatic 090.0
  - interstitial keratitis 090.3
  - juvenile neurosyphilis 090.40
  - late or 2 years or more after birth NEC 090.7
    - chorioretinitis, choroiditis 090.5 [363.13]
    - interstitial keratitis 090.3
    - juvenile neurosyphilis NEC 090.40
    - latent (without manifestations) 090.6
      - negative spinal fluid test 090.6
      - serology, positive 090.6
    - symptomatic or with manifestations NEC 090.5
    - interstitial keratitis 090.3
- conjugal 097.9
  - tabes 094.0
- conjunctiva 095.8 [372.10]
- contact V01.6
- cord, bladder 094.0
- cornea, late 095.8 [370.59]
- coronary (artery) 093.89
  - sclerosis 093.89
- coryza 095.8
  - congenital 090.0
- cranial nerve 094.89
- cutaneous — see Syphilis, skin
- dacryocystitis 095.8
- degeneration, spinal cord 094.89
- d'emblée 095.8

Syphilis, syphilitic—continued
- dementia 094.89
  - paralytica 094.1
    - juvenilis 090.40
- destruction of bone 095.5
- dilatation, aorta 093.0
- due to blood transfusion 097.9
- dura mater 094.89
- ear 095.8
  - inner 095.8
    - nerve (eighth) 094.86
    - neurorecurrence 094.86
- early NEC 091.0
  - cardiovascular 093.9
  - central nervous system 094.9
    - paresis 094.1
    - tabes 094.0
  - latent (without manifestations) (less than 2 years after infection) 092.9
    - negative spinal fluid test 092.9
    - serological relapse following treatment 092.0
    - serology positive 092.9
  - paresis 094.1
  - relapse (treated, untreated) 091.7
  - skin 091.3
  - symptomatic NEC 091.89
    - extragenital chancre 091.2
    - primary, except extragenital chancre 091.0
    - secondary (see also Syphilis, secondary) 091.3
      - relapse (treated, untreated) 091.7
  - tabes 094.0
  - ulcer 091.3
- eighth nerve 094.86
- endemic, nonvenereal 104.0
- endocarditis 093.20
  - aortic 093.22
  - mitral 093.21
  - pulmonary 093.24
  - tricuspid 093.23
- epididymis (late) 095.8
- epiglottis 095.8
- epiphysitis (congenital) 090.0
- esophagus 095.8
- Eustachian tube 095.8
- exposure to V01.6
- eye 095.8 [363.13]
  - neuromuscular mechanism 094.85
- eyelid 095.8 [373.5]
  - with gumma 095.8 [373.5]
  - ptosis 094.89
- fallopian tube 095.8
- fracture 095.5
- gallbladder (late) 095.8
- gastric 095.8
  - crisis 094.0
  - polyposis 095.8
- general 097.9
  - paralysis 094.1
    - juvenile 090.40
- genital (primary) 091.0
- glaucoma 095.8
- gumma (late) NEC 095.9
  - cardiovascular system 093.9
  - central nervous system 094.9
  - congenital 090.5
  - heart or artery 093.89
- heart 093.89
  - block 093.89
  - decompensation 093.89
  - disease 093.89
  - failure 093.89
  - valve (see also Syphilis, endocarditis) 093.20
- hemianesthesia 094.89
- hemianopsia 095.8
- hemiparesis 094.89
- hemiplegia 094.89

Syphilis, syphilitic—continued
- hepatic artery 093.89
- hepatitis 095.3
- hepatomegaly 095.3
  - congenital 090.0
- hereditaria tarda (see also Syphilis, congenital, late) 090.7
- hereditary (see also Syphilis, congenital) 090.9
- interstitial keratitis 090.3
- Hutchinson's teeth 090.5
- hyalitis 095.8
- inactive — see Syphilis, latent
- infantum NEC (see also Syphilis, congenital) 090.9
- inherited — see Syphilis, congenital
- internal ear 095.8
- intestine (late) 095.8
- iris, iritis (secondary) 091.52
  - late 095.8 [364.11]
- joint (late) 095.8
- keratitis (congenital) (early) (interstitial) (late) (parenchymatous) (punctata profunda) 090.3
- kidney 095.4
- lacrimal apparatus 095.8
- laryngeal paralysis 095.8
- larynx 095.8
- late 097.0
  - cardiovascular 093.9
  - central nervous system 094.9
  - latent or 2 years or more after infection (without manifestations) 096
    - negative spinal fluid test 096
    - serology positive 096
  - paresis 094.1
  - specified site NEC 095.8
  - symptomatic or with symptoms 095.9
  - tabes 094.0
- latent 097.1
  - central nervous system 094.9
  - date of infection unspecified 097.1
  - early or less than 2 years after infection 092.9
  - late or 2 years or more after infection 096
  - serology
    - doubtful
      - follow-up of latent syphilis 097.1
      - central nervous system 094
      - date of infection unspecified 097.1
      - early or less than 2 years after infection 092
      - late or 2 years or more after infection 096
    - positive, only finding 097.1
      - date of infection unspecified 097.1
      - early or less than 2 years after infection 097.1
      - late or 2 years or more after infection 097.1
- lens 095.8
- leukoderma 091.3
  - late 095.8
- lienis 095.8
- lip 091.3
  - chancre 091.2
  - late 095.8
  - primary 091.2

Syphilis, syphilitic—continued
  Lissauer's paralysis 094.1
  liver 095.3
    secondary 091.62
  locomotor ataxia 094.0
  lung 095.1
  lymphadenitis (secondary) 091.4
  lymph gland (early) (secondary) 091.4
    late 095.8
  macular atrophy of skin 091.3
    striated 095.8
  maternal, affecting fetus or newborn 760.2
    manifest syphilis in newborn — see Syphilis, congenital
  mediastinum (late) 095.8
  meninges (adhesive) (basilar) (brain) (spinal cord) 094.2
  meningitis 094.2
    acute 091.81
    congenital 090.42
  meningoencephalitis 094.2
  meningovascular 094.2
    congenital 090.49
  mesarteritis 093.89
    brain 094.89
    spine 094.89
  middle ear 095.8
  mitral stenosis 093.21
  monoplegia 094.89
  mouth (secondary) 091.3
    late 095.8
  mucocutaneous 091.3
    late 095.8
  mucous
    membrane 091.3
      late 095.8
    patches 091.3
      congenital 090.0
  mulberry molars 090.5
  muscle 095.6
  myocardium 093.82
  myositis 095.6
  nasal sinus 095.8
  neonatorum NEC (see also Syphilis, congenital) 090.9
  nerve palsy (any cranial nerve) 094.89
  nervous system, central 094.9
  neuritis 095.8
    acoustic nerve 094.86
  neurorecidive of retina 094.83
  neuroretinitis 094.85
  newborn (see also Syphilis, congenital) 090.9
  nodular superficial 095.8
  nonvenereal, endemic 104.0
  nose 095.8
    saddle back deformity 090.5
    septum 095.8
      perforated 095.8
  occlusive arterial disease 093.89
  ophthalmic 095.8 [363.13]
  ophthalmoplegia 094.89
  optic nerve (atrophy) (neuritis) (papilla) 094.84
  orbit (late) 095.8
  orchitis 095.8
  organic 097.9
  osseous (late) 095.5
  osteochondritis (congenital) 090.0
  osteoporosis 095.5
  ovary 095.8
  oviduct 095.8
  palate 095.8
    gumma 095.8
    perforated 090.5
  pancreas (late) 095.8
  pancreatitis 095.8
  paralysis 094.89
    general 094.1
    juvenile 090.40
  paraplegia 094.89
  paresis (general) 094.1
    juvenile 090.40

Syphilis, syphilitic—continued
  paresthesia 094.89
  Parkinson's disease or syndrome 094.82
  paroxysmal tachycardia 093.89
  pemphigus (congenital) 090.0
  penis 091.0
    chancre 091.0
    late 095.8
  pericardium 093.81
  perichondritis, larynx 095.8
  periosteum 095.5
    congenital 090.0
    early 091.61
    secondary 091.61
  peripheral nerve 095.8
  petrous bone (late) 095.5
  pharynx 095.8
    secondary 091.3
  pituitary (gland) 095.8
  placenta 095.8
  pleura (late) 095.8
  pneumonia, white 090.0
  pontine (lesion) 094.89
  portal vein 093.89
  primary NEC 091.2
    anal 091.1
    and secondary (see also Syphilis, secondary) 091.9
    cardiovascular 093.9
    central nervous system 094.9
    extragenital chancre NEC 091.2
    fingers 091.2
    genital 091.0
    lip 091.2
    specified site NEC 091.2
    tonsils 091.2
  prostate 095.8
  psychosis (intracranial gumma) 094.89
  ptosis (eyelid) 094.89
  pulmonary (late) 095.1
    artery 093.89
  pulmonum 095.1
  pyelonephritis 095.4
  recently acquired, symptomatic NEC 091.89
  rectum 095.8
  respiratory tract 095.8
  retina
    late 094.83
    neurorecidive 094.83
  retrobulbar neuritis 094.85
  salpingitis 095.8
  sclera (late) 095.0
  sclerosis
    cerebral 094.89
    coronary 093.89
    multiple 094.89
    subacute 094.89
  scotoma (central) 095.8
  scrotum 095.8
  secondary (and primary) 091.9
    adenopathy 091.4
    anus 091.3
    bone 091.61
    cardiovascular 093.9
    central nervous system 094.9
    chorioretinitis, choroiditis 091.51
    hepatitis 091.62
    liver 091.62
    lymphadenitis 091.4
    meningitis, acute 091.81
    mouth 091.3
    mucous membranes 091.3
    periosteum 091.61
    periostitis 091.61
    pharynx 091.3
    relapse (treated) (untreated) 091.7
    skin 091.3
    specified form NEC 091.89
    tonsil 091.3
    ulcer 091.3

Syphilis, syphilitic—continued
  secondary—continued
    viscera 091.69
    vulva 091.3
  seminal vesicle (late) 095.8
  seronegative
    with signs or symptoms — see Syphilis, by site and stage
  seropositive
    with signs or symptoms — see Syphilis, by site and stage
    follow-up of latent syphilis — see Syphilis, latent
    only finding — see Syphilis, latent
  seventh nerve (paralysis) 094.89
  sinus 095.8
  sinusitis 095.8
  skeletal system 095.5
  skin (early) (secondary) (with ulceration) 091.3
    late or tertiary 095.8
  small intestine 095.8
  spastic spinal paralysis 094.0
  spermatic cord (late) 095.8
  spinal (cord) 094.89
    with
      paresis 094.1
      tabes 094.0
  spleen 095.8
  splenomegaly 095.8
  spondylitis 095.5
  staphyloma 095.8
  stigmata (congenital) 090.5
  stomach 095.8
  synovium (late) 095.7
  tabes dorsalis (early) (late) 094.0
    juvenile 090.40
  tabetic type 094.0
    juvenile 090.40
  taboparesis 094.1
    juvenile 090.40
  tachycardia 093.89
  tendon (late) 095.7
  tertiary 097.0
    with symptoms 095.8
    cardiovascular 093.9
    central nervous system 094.9
    multiple NEC 095.8
    specified site NEC 095.8
  testis 095.8
  thorax 095.8
  throat 095.8
  thymus (gland) 095.8
  thyroid (late) 095.8
  tongue 095.8
  tonsil (lingual) 095.8
    primary 091.2
    secondary 091.3
  trachea 095.8
  tricuspid valve 093.23
  tumor, brain 094.89
  tunica vaginalis (late) 095.8
  ulcer (any site) (early) (secondary) 091.3
    late 095.9
    perforating 095.9
      foot 094.0
  urethra (stricture) 095.8
  urogenital 095.8
  uterus 095.8
  uveal tract (secondary) 091.50
    late 095.8 [363.13]
  uveitis (secondary) 091.50
    late 095.8 [363.13]
  uvula (late) 095.8
    perforated 095.8
  vagina 091.0
    late 095.8
  valvulitis NEC 093.20
  vascular 093.89
    brain or cerebral 094.89
  vein 093.89
    cerebral 094.89
  ventriculi 095.8

Syphilis, syphilitic—continued
  vesicae urinariae 095.8
  viscera (abdominal) 095.2
    secondary 091.69
  vitreous (hemorrhage) (opacities) 095.8
  vulva 091.0
    late 095.8
    secondary 091.3
Syphiloma 095.9
  cardiovascular system 093.9
  central nervous system 094.9
  circulatory system 093.9
  congenital 090.5
Syphilophobia 300.29
Syringadenoma (M8400/0) — see also Neoplasm, skin, benign
  papillary (M8406/0) — see Neoplasm, skin, benign
Syringobulbia 336.0
Syringocarcinoma (M8400/3) — see Neoplasm, skin, malignant
Syringocystadenoma (M8400/0) — see also Neoplasm, skin, benign
  papillary (M8406/0) — see Neoplasm, skin, benign
Syringocystoma (M8407/0) — see Neoplasm, skin, benign
Syringoma (M8407/0) — see also Neoplasm, skin, benign
  chondroid (M8940/0) — see Neoplasm, by site, benign
Syringomyelia 336.0
Syringomyelitis 323.9
  late effect — see category 326
Syringomyelocele (see also Spina bifida) 741.9
Syringopontia 336.0
System, systemic — see also condition
  disease, combined — see Degeneration, combined
  fibrosclerosing syndrome 710.8
  lupus erythematosus 710.0
    inhibitor 286.5

T

Tab — see Tag
Tabacism 989.8
Tabacosis 989.8
Tabardillo 080
  flea-borne 081.0
  louse-borne 080
Tabes, tabetic
  with
    central nervous system syphilis 094.0
    Charcot's joint 094.0 [713.5]
    cord bladder 094.0
    crisis, viscera (any) 094.0
    paralysis, general 094.1
    paresis (general) 094.1
    perforating ulcer 094.0
  arthropathy 094.0 [713.5]
  bladder 094.0
  bone 094.0
  cerebrospinal 094.0
  congenital 090.40
  conjugal 094.0
  dorsalis 094.0
    neurosyphilis 094.0
  early 094.0
  juvenile 090.40
  latent 094.0
  mesenterica (see also Tuberculosis) 014.8
  paralysis insane, general 094.1
  peripheral (nonsyphilitic) 799.8
  spasmodic 094.0
    not dorsal or dorsalis 343.9
  syphilis (cerebrospinal) 094.0

Taboparalysis — INDEX TO DISEASES — Tear, torn

Taboparalysis 094.1
Taboparesis (remission) 094.1
  with
    Charcot's joint 094.1 *[713.5]*
    cord bladder 094.1
    perforating ulcer 094.1
  juvenile 090.40
Tachyalimentation 579.3
Tachyarrhythmia, tachyrhythmia — *see also* Tachycardia
  paroxysmal with sinus bradycardia 427.81
Tachycardia 785.0
  atrial 427.89
  auricular 427.89
  nodal 427.89
    nonparoxysmal atrioventricular 426.89
  nonparoxysmal atrioventricular (nodal) 426.89
  paroxysmal 427.2
    with sinus bradycardia 427.81
    atrial (PAT) 427.0
      psychogenic 316 *[427.0]*
    atrioventricular (AV) 427.0
      psychogenic 316 *[427.0]*
    essential 427.2
    junctional 427.0
    nodal 427.0
    psychogenic 316 *[427.2]*
      atrial 316 *[427.0]*
      supraventricular 316 *[427.0]*
      ventricular 316 *[427.1]*
    supraventricular 427.0
      psychogenic 316 *[427.0]*
    ventricular 427.1
      psychogenic 316 *[427.1]*
  postoperative 997.1
  psychogenic 306.2
  sick sinus 427.81
  sinoauricular 427.89
  sinus 427.89
  supraventricular 427.89
  ventricular (paroxysmal) 427.1
    psychogenic 316 *[427.1]*
Tachypnea 786.09
  hysterical 300.11
  newborn (idiopathic) (transitory) 770.6
  psychogenic 306.1
  transitory, of newborn 770.6
Taenia (infection) (infestation) (*see also* Infestation, taenia) 123.3
  diminuta 123.6
  echinococcal infestation (*see also* Echinococcus) 122.9
  nana 123.6
  saginata infestation 123.2
  solium (intestinal form) 123.0
    larval form 123.1
Taeniasis (intestine) (*see also* Infestation, Taenia) 123.3
  saginata 123.2
  solium 123.0
Taenzer's disease 757.4
Tag (hypertrophied skin) (infected) 701.9
  adenoid 474.8
  anus 455.9
  endocardial (*see also* Endocarditis) 424.90
  hemorrhoidal 455.9
  hymen 623.8
  perineal 624.8
  preauricular 744.1
  rectum 455.9
  sentinel 455.9
  skin 701.9
    accessory 757.39
    anus 455.9
    congenital 757.39
    preauricular 744.1
    rectum 455.9
  tonsil 474.8

Tag—*continued*
  urethra, urethral 599.84
  vulva 624.8
Tahyna fever 062.5
Takayasu (-Onishi) **disease or syndrome** (pulseless disease) 446.7
Talc granuloma 728.82
Talcosis 502
Talipes (congenital) 754.70
  acquired NEC 736.79
    planus 734
  asymmetric 754.79
    acquired 736.79
  calcaneovalgus 754.62
    acquired 736.76
  calcaneovarus 754.59
    acquired 736.76
  calcaneus 754.79
    acquired 736.76
  cavovarus 754.59
    acquired 736.75
  cavus 754.71
    acquired 736.73
  equinovalgus 754.69
    acquired 736.72
  equinovarus 754.51
    acquired 736.71
  equinus 754.79
    acquired, NEC 736.72
  percavus 754.71
    acquired 736.73
  planovalgus 754.69
    acquired 736.79
  planus (acquired) (any degree) 734
    congenital 754.61
    due to rickets 268.1
  valgus 754.60
    acquired 736.79
  varus 754.50
    acquired 736.79
Talma's disease 728.85
Tamponade heart (Rose's) (*see also* Pericarditis) 423.9
Tanapox 078.89
Tangier disease (familial high-density lipoprotein deficiency) 272.5
Tank ear 380.12
Tantrum (childhood) (*see also* Disturbance, conduct) 312.1
Tapeworm (infection) (infestation) (*see also* Infestation, tapeworm) 123.9
Tapia's syndrome 352.6
Tarantism 297.8
Target-oval cell anemia 282.4
Tarlov's cyst 355.9
Tarral-Besnier disease (pityriasis rubra pilaris) 696.4
Tarsalgia 729.2
Tarsal tunnel syndrome 355.5
Tarsitis (eyelid) 373.00
  syphilitic 095.8 *[373.00]*
  tuberculous (*see also* Tuberculosis) 017.0 *[373.4]*
Tartar (teeth) 523.6
Tattoo (mark) 709.09 ◆
Taurodontism 520.2
Taussig-Bing defect, heart, or syndrome (transposition, aorta and overriding pulmonary artery) 745.11
Tay's choroiditis 363.41
Tay-Sachs
  amaurotic familial idiocy 330.1
  disease 330.1
Taybi's syndrome (otopalatodigital) 759.89

Taylor's
  disease (diffuse idiopathic cutaneous atrophy) 701.8
  syndrome 625.5
Tear, torn (traumatic) — *see also* Wound, open, by site
  anus, anal (sphincter) 863.89
    with open wound in cavity 863.99
    complicating delivery 664.2
      with mucosa 664.3
    nontraumatic, nonpuerperal 565.0
  articular cartilage, old (*see also* Disorder, cartilage, articular) 718.0
  bladder
    with
      abortion — *see* Abortion, by type, with damage to pelvic organs
      ectopic pregnancy (*see also* categories 633.0-633.9) 639.2
      molar pregnancy (*see also* categories 630-632) 639.2
    following
      abortion 639.2
      ectopic or molar pregnancy 639.2
    obstetrical trauma 665.5
  bowel
    with
      abortion — *see* Abortion, by type, with damage to pelvic organs
      ectopic pregnancy (*see also* categories 633.0-633.9) 639.2
      molar pregnancy (*see also* categories 630-632) 639.2
    following
      abortion 639.2
      ectopic or molar pregnancy 639.2
    obstetrical trauma 665.5
  broad ligament
    with
      abortion — *see* Abortion, by type, with damage to pelvic organs
      ectopic pregnancy (*see also* categories 633.0-633.9) 639.2
      molar pregnancy (*see also* categories 630-632) 639.2
    following
      abortion 639.2
      ectopic or molar pregnancy 639.2
    obstetrical trauma 665.6
  bucket handle (knee) (meniscus) — *see* Tear, meniscus
  capsule
    joint — *see* Sprain, by site
    spleen — *see* Laceration, spleen, capsule
  cartilage — *see also* Sprain, by site
    articular, old (*see also* Disorder, cartilage, articular) 718.0
    knee — *see* Tear, meniscus
    semilunar (knee) (current injury) — *see* Tear, meniscus
  cervix
    with
      abortion — *see* Abortion, by type, with damage to pelvic organs
      ectopic pregnancy (*see also* categories 633.0-633.9) 639.2

Tear, torn—*continued*
  cervix—*continued*
    with—*continued*
      molar pregnancy (*see also* categories 630-632) 639.2
    following
      abortion 639.2
      ectopic or molar pregnancy 639.2
    obstetrical trauma (current) 665.3
    old 622.3
  internal organ (abdomen, chest, or pelvis) — *see* Injury, internal, by site
  ligament — *see also* Sprain, by site
    with open wound — *see* Wound, open by site
  meniscus (knee) (current injury) 836.2
    bucket handle 836.0
      old 717.0
    lateral 836.1
      anterior horn 836.1
        old 717.42
      bucket handle 836.1
        old 717.41
      old 717.40
      posterior horn 836.1
        old 717.43
      specified site NEC 836.1
        old 717.49
    medial 836.0
      anterior horn 836.0
        old 717.1
      bucket handle 836.0
        old 717.0
      old 717.3
      posterior horn 836.0
        old 717.2
    old NEC 717.5
    site other than knee — *see* Sprain, by site
  muscle — *see also* Sprain, by site
    with open wound — *see* Wound, open by site
  pelvic
    floor, complicating delivery 664.1
    organ NEC
      with
        abortion — *see* Abortion, by type, with damage to pelvic organs
        ectopic pregnancy (*see also* categories 633.0-633.9) 639.2
        molar pregnancy (*see also* categories 630-632) 639.2
      following
        abortion 639.2
        ectopic or molar pregnancy 639.2
      obstetrical trauma 665.5
  perineum — *see also* Laceration, perineum
    obstetrical trauma 665.5
  periurethral tissue
    with
      abortion — *see* Abortion, by type, with damage to pelvic organs
      ectopic pregnancy (*see also* categories 633.0-633.9) 639.2
      molar pregnancy (*see also* categories 630-632) 639.2
    following
      abortion 639.2
      ectopic or molar pregnancy 639.2

Tear, torn—continued
  periurethral tissue—continued
    obstetrical trauma 665.5
  rectovaginal septum — see
      Laceration, rectovaginal
      septum
  retina, retinal (recent) (with
      detachment) 361.00
    without detachment 361.30
    dialysis (juvenile) (with
        detachment) 361.04
    giant (with detachment)
        361.03
    horseshoe (without
        detachment) 361.32
    multiple (with detachment)
        361.02
      without detachment 361.33
    old
      delimited (partial) 361.06
      partial 361.06
      total or subtotal 361.07
    partial (without detachment)
      giant 361.03
      multiple defects 361.02
      old (delimited) 361.06
      single defect 361.01
    round hole (without
        detachment) 361.31
      single defect (with
          detachment) 361.01
    total or subtotal (recent)
        361.05
      old 361.07
  rotator cuff 840.4
    current injury 840.4
  semilunar cartilage, knee (see
      also Tear, meniscus) 836.2
    old 717.5
  tendon — see also Sprain, by site
    with open wound — see
        Wound, open by site
  tentorial, at birth 767.0
  umbilical cord
    affecting fetus or newborn
        772.0
    complicating delivery 663.8
  urethra
    with
      abortion — see Abortion,
          by type, with damage
          to pelvic organs
      ectopic pregnancy (see also
          categories 633.0-
          633.9) 639.2
      molar pregnancy (see also
          categories 630-632)
          639.2
    following
      abortion 639.2
      ectopic or molar pregnancy
          639.2
    obstetrical trauma 665.5
  uterus — see Injury, internal,
      uterus
  vagina — see Laceration, vagina
  vessel, from catheter 998.2
  vulva, complicating delivery
      664.0
Tear stone 375.57
Teeth, tooth — see also condition
  grinding 306.8
Teething 520.7
  syndrome 520.7
Tegmental syndrome 344.89
Telangiectasia, telangiectasis
      (verrucous) 448.9
  ataxic (cerebellar) 334.8
  familial 448.0
  hemorrhagic, hereditary
      (congenital) (senile) 448.0
  hereditary hemorrhagic 448.0
  retina 362.15
  spider 448.1
Telecanthus (congenital) 743.63

Telescoped bowel or intestine (see
    also Intussusception) 560.0
Teletherapy, adverse effect NEC 990
Telogen effluvium 704.02
Temperature
  body, high (of unknown origin)
      (see also Pyrexia) 780.6
  cold, trauma from 991.9
    newborn 778.2
    specified effect NEC 991.8
  high
    body (of unknown origin) (see
        also Pyrexia) 780.6
    trauma from — see Heat
Temper tantrum (childhood) (see
    also Disturbance, conduct)
    312.1
Temple — see condition
Temporal — see also condition
  lobe syndrome 310.0
**Temporomandibular joint-pain-
    dysfunction syndrome** 524.60
Temporosphenoidal — see condition
Tendency
  bleeding (see also Defect,
      coagulation) 286.9
  homosexual, ego-dystonic 302.0
  paranoid 301.0
  suicide 300.9
Tenderness
  abdominal (generalized)
      (localized) 789.6
  rebound 789.6
  skin 782.0
Tendinitis, tendonitis (see also
    Tenosynovitis) 726.90
  Achilles 726.71
  adhesive 726.90
    shoulder 726.0
  calcific 727.82
    shoulder 726.11
  gluteal 726.5
  patellar 726.64
  peroneal 726.79
  pes anserinus 726.61
  psoas 726.5
  tibialis (anterior) (posterior)
      726.72
  trochanteric 726.5
Tendon — see condition
Tendosynovitis — see Tenosynovitis
Tendovaginitis — see Tenosynovitis
Tenesmus 787.9
  rectal 787.9
  vesical 788.9
Tenia — see Taenia
Teniasis — see Taeniasis
Tennis elbow 726.32
Tenonitis — see also Tenosynovitis
  eye (capsule) 376.04
Tenontosynovitis — see
    Tenosynovitis
Tenontothecitis — see Tenosynovitis
Tenophyte 727.9
Tenosynovitis 727.00
  adhesive 726.90
    shoulder 726.0
  ankle 727.06
  bicipital (calcifying) 726.12
  buttock 727.09
  due to crystals — see Arthritis,
      due to crystals
  elbow 727.09
  finger 727.05
  foot 727.06
  gonococcal 098.51
  hand 727.05
  hip 727.09
  knee 727.09
  radial styloid 727.04
  shoulder 726.10
    adhesive 726.0
  spine 720.1

Tenosynovitis—continued
  supraspinatus 726.10
  toe 727.06
  tuberculous — see Tuberculosis,
      tenosynovitis
  wrist 727.05
Tenovaginitis — see Tenosynovitis
Tension
  arterial, high (see also
      Hypertension) 401.9
    without diagnosis of
        hypertension 796.2
  headache 307.81
  intraocular (elevated) 365.00
  nervous 799.2
  ocular (elevated) 365.00
  pneumothorax 512.0
    iatrogenic 512.1
    postoperative 512.1
    spontaneous 512.0
  premenstrual 625.4
  state 300.9
Tentorium — see condition
Teratencephalus 759.89
Teratism 759.7
Teratoblastoma (malignant)
    (M9080/3) — see Neoplasm,
    by site, malignant
Teratocarcinoma (M9081/3) — see
    also Neoplasm, by site,
    malignant
  liver 155.0
Teratoma (solid) (M9080/1) — see
    also Neoplasm, by site,
    uncertain behavior
  adult (cystic) (M9080/0) — see
      Neoplasm, by site, benign
  and embryonal carcinoma, mixed
      (M9081/3) — see
      Neoplasm, by site,
      malignant
  benign (M9080/0) — see
      Neoplasm, by site, benign
  combined with choriocarcinoma
      (M9101/3) — see
      Neoplasm, by site,
      malignant
  cystic (adult) (M9080/0) — see
      Neoplasm, by site, benign
  differentiated type (M9080/0) —
      see Neoplasm, by site,
      benign
  embryonal (M9080/3) — see also
      Neoplasm, by site,
      malignant
    liver 155.0
  fetal
    sacral, causing fetopelvic
        disproportion 653.7
  immature (M9080/3) — see
      Neoplasm, by site,
      malignant
  liver (M9080/3) 155.0
    adult, benign, cystic,
        differentiated type or
        mature (M9080/0) 211.5
  malignant (M9080/3) — see also
      Neoplasm, by site,
      malignant
    anaplastic type (M9082/3) —
        see Neoplasm, by site,
        malignant
    intermediate type (M9083/3)
        — see Neoplasm, by
        site, malignant
    liver (M9080/3) 155.0
    trophoblastic (M9102/3)
      specified site — see
          Neoplasm, by site,
          malignant
      unspecified site 186.9
    undifferentiated type
        (M9082/3) — see
        Neoplasm, by site,
        malignant

Teratoma—continued
  mature (M9080/0) — see
      Neoplasm, by site, benign
  ovary (M9080/0) 220
    embryonal, immature, or
        malignant (M9080/3)
        183.0
    suprasellar (M9080/3) — see
        Neoplasm, by site,
        malignant
  testis (M9080/3) 186.9
    adult, benign, cystic,
        differentiated type or
        mature (M9080/0) 222.0
    undescended 186.0
Termination
  anomalous — see also
      Malposition, congenital
    portal vein 747.49
    right pulmonary vein 747.42
  pregnancy (legal) (therapeutic)
      (see Abortion, legal) 635.9
    fetus NEC 779.6
    illegal (see also Abortion,
        illegal) 636.9
Ternidens diminutus infestation
    127.7
Terrors, night (child) 307.46
Terry's syndrome 362.21
Tertiary — see condition
Tessellated fundus, retina (tigroid)
    362.89
Test(s)
  AIDS virus V72.6
  allergen V72.7
  bacterial disease NEC (see also
      Screening, by name of
      disease) V74.9
  basal metabolic rate V72.6
  blood-alcohol V70.4
  blood-drug V70.4
  developmental, infant or child
      V20.2
  Dick V74.8
  fertility V26.2
  hearing V72.1
  HIV V72.6
  human immunodeficiency virus
      V72.6
  Kveim V82.8
  laboratory V72.6
    for medicolegal reason V70.4
  Mantoux (for tuberculosis) V74.1
  mycotic organism V75.4
  parasitic agent NEC V75.8
  pregnancy
    positive V22.1
      first pregnancy V22.0
    unconfirmed V72.4
  preoperative V72.84
    cardiovascular V72.81
    respiratory V72.82
    specified NEC V72.83
  sarcoidosis V82.8
  Schick V74.3
  Schultz-Charlton V74.8
  skin, diagnostic
    allergy V72.7
    bacterial agent NEC (see also
        Screening, by name of
        disease) V74.9
    Dick V74.8
    hypersensitivity V72.7
    Kveim V82.8
    Mantoux V74.1
    mycotic organism V75.4
    parasitic agent NEC V75.8
    sarcoidosis V82.8
    Schick V74.3
    Schultz-Charlton V74.8
    tuberculin V74.1
  specified type NEC V72.8
  tuberculin V74.1
  vision V72.0

Test(s)—continued
  Wassermann
    positive (see also Serology for syphilis, positive) 097.1
    false 795.6
Testicle, testicular, testis — see also condition
  feminization (syndrome) 257.8
Tetanus, tetanic (cephalic) (convulsions) 037
  with
    abortion — see Abortion, by type, with sepsis
    ectopic pregnancy (see also categories 633.0-633.9) 639.0
    molar pregnancy (see categories 630-632) 639.0
  following
    abortion 639.0
    ectopic or molar pregnancy 639.0
  inoculation V03.7
    reaction (due to serum) — see Complications, vaccination
  neonatorum 771.3
  puerperal, postpartum, childbirth 670
Tetany, tetanic 781.7
  alkalosis 276.3
  associated with rickets 268.0
  convulsions 781.7
    hysterical 300.11
  functional (hysterical) 300.11
  hyperkinetic 781.7
    hysterical 300.11
  hyperpnea 786.01
    hysterical 300.11
    psychogenic 306.1
  hyperventilation 786.01
    hysterical 300.11
    psychogenic 306.1
  hypocalcemic, neonatal 775.4
  hysterical 300.11
  neonatal 775.4
  parathyroid (gland) 252.1
  parathyroprival 252.1
  postoperative 252.1
  postthyroidectomy 252.1
  pseudotetany 781.7
    hysterical 300.11
    psychogenic 306.1
      specified as conversion reaction 300.11
Tetralogy of Fallot 745.2
Tetraplegia — see Quadriplegia
Thailand hemorrhagic fever 065.4
Thalassanemia 282.4
Thalassemia (alpha) (beta) (disease) (Hb-C) (Hb-D) (Hb-E) (Hb-H) (Hb-I) (Hb-S) (high fetal gene) (high fetal hemoglobin) (intermedia) (major) (minima) (minor) (mixed) (sickle-cell) (trait) (with other hemoglobinopathy) 282.4
Thalassemic variants 282.4
Thaysen-Gee disease (nontropical sprue) 579.0
Thecoma (M8600/0) 220
  malignant (M8600/3) 183.0
Thelarche, precocious 259.1
Thelitis 611.0
  puerperal, postpartum 675.0
Therapeutic — see condition
Therapy V57.9
  blood transfusion, without reported diagnosis V58.2
  breathing V57.0
  chemotherapy V58.1
    fluoride V07.31
    prophylactic NEC V07.39

Therapy—continued
  dialysis (intermittent) (treatment)
    extracorporeal V56.0
    peritoneal V56.8
    renal V56.0
    specified type NEC V56.8
  exercise NEC V57.1
    breathing V57.0
  extracorporeal dialysis (renal) V56.0
  fluoride prophylaxis V07.31
  hemodialysis V56.0
  occupational V57.21
  orthoptic V57.4
  orthotic V57.81
  peritoneal dialysis V56.8
  physical NEC V57.1
  radiation V58.0
  speech V57.3
  vocational V57.22
Thermalgesia 782.0
Thermalgia 782.0
Thermanalgesia 782.0
Thermanesthesia 782.0
Thermic — see condition
Thermography (abnormal) 793.9
  breast 793.8
Thermoplegia 992.0
Thesaurismosis
  amyloid 277.3
  bilirubin 277.4
  calcium 275.4
  cystine 270.0
  glycogen (see also Disease, glycogen storage) 271.0
  kerasin 272.7
  lipoid 272.7
  melanin 255.4
  phosphatide 272.7
  urate 274.9
Thiaminic deficiency 265.1
  with beriberi 265.0
Thibierge-Weissenbach syndrome (cutaneous systemic sclerosis) 710.1
Thickening
  bone 733.99
    extremity 733.99
  breast 611.79
  hymen 623.3
  larynx 478.79
  nail 703.8
    congenital 757.5
  periosteal 733.99
  pluera (see also Pleurisy) 511.0
  skin 782.8
  subepiglottic 478.79
  tongue 529.8
  valve, heart — see Endocarditis
Thiele syndrome 724.6
Thigh — see condition
Thinning vertebra (see also Osteoporosis) 733.00
Thirst, excessive 783.5
  due to deprivation of water 994.3
Thomsen's disease 359.2
Thomson's disease (congenital poikiloderma) 757.33
Thoracic — see also condition
  kidney 753.3
  outlet syndrome 353.0
  stomach — see Hernia, diaphragm
Thoracogastroschisis (congenital) 759.89
Thoracopagus 759.4
Thoracoschisis 756.3
Thorax — see condition
Thorn's syndrome (see also Disease, renal) 593.9

Thornwaldt's, Tornwaldt's
  bursitis (pharyngeal) 478.29
  cyst 478.26
  disease (pharyngeal bursitis) 478.29
Thorson-Biörck syndrome (malignant carcinoid) 259.2
Threadworm (infection) (infestation) 127.4
Threatened
  abortion or miscarriage 640.0
    with subsequent abortion (see also Abortion, spontaneous) 634.9
    affecting fetus 762.1
  labor 644.1
    affecting fetus or newborn 761.8
    premature 644.0
  miscarriage 640.0
    affecting fetus 762.1
  premature
    delivery 644.2
      affecting fetus or newborn 761.8
    labor 644.0
      before 22 completed weeks gestation 640.0
Three-day fever 066.0
Threshers' lung 495.0
Thrix annulata (congenital) 757.4
Throat — see condition
Thrombasthenia (Glanzmann's) (hemorrhagic) (hereditary) 287.1
Thromboangiitis 443.1
  obliterans (general) 443.1
    cerebral 437.1
    vessels
      brain 437.1
      spinal cord 437.1
Thromboarteritis — see Arteritis
Thromboasthenia (Glanzmann's) (hemorrhagic) (hereditary) 287.1
Thrombocytasthenia (Glanzmann's) 287.1
Thrombocythemia (essential) (hemorrhagic) (primary) (M9962/1) 238.7
  idiopathic (M9962/1) 238.7
Thrombocytopathy (dystrophic) (granulopenic) 287.1
Thrombocytopenia, thrombocytopenic 287.5
  with giant hemangioma 287.3
  amegakaryocytic, congenital 287.3
  congenital 287.3
  cyclic 287.3
  dilutional 287.4
  due to
    drugs 287.4
    extracorporeal circulation of blood 287.4
    massive blood transfusion 287.4
    platelet alloimmunization 287.4
  essential 287.3
  hereditary 287.3
  Kasabach-Merritt 287.3
  neonatal, transitory 776.1
    due to
      exchange transfusion 776.1
      idiopathic maternal thrombocytopenia 776.1
      isoimmunization 776.1
  primary 287.3
  puerperal, postpartum 666.3
  purpura (see also Purpura, thrombocytopenic) 287.3
  thrombotic 446.6

Thrombocytopenia, thrombocytopenic —continued
  secondary 287.4
  sex-linked 287.3
Thrombocytosis, essential 289.9
Thromboembolism — see Embolism
Thrombopathy (Bernard-Soulier) 287.1
  constitutional 286.4
  Willebrand-Jürgens (angiohemophilia) 286.4
Thrombopenia (see also Thrombocytopenia) 287.5
Thrombophlebitis 451.9
  antecubital vein 451.82
  antepartum (superficial) 671.2
    affecting fetus or newborn 760.3
    deep 671.3
  arm 451.89
    deep 451.83
    superficial 451.82
  breast, superficial 451.89
  cavernous (venous) sinus — see Thrombophlebitis, intracranial venous sinus
  cephalic vein 451.82
  cerebral (sinus) (vein) 325
    late effect — see category 326
    nonpyogenic 437.6
      in pregnancy or puerperium 671.5
        late effect — see category 438
  due to implanted device — see Complications, due to (presence of) any device, implant or graft classified to 996.0-996.5 NEC
  during or resulting from a procedure NEC 997.2
  femoral 451.11
  femoropopliteal 451.19
  following infusion, perfusion, or transfusion 999.2
  hepatic (vein) 451.89
  idiopathic, recurrent 453.1
  iliac vein 451.81
  iliofemoral 451.11
  intracranial venous sinus (any) 325
    late effect — see category 326
    nonpyogenic 437.6
      in pregnancy or puerperium 671.5
        late effect — see category 438
  jugular vein 451.89
  lateral (venous) sinus — see Thrombophlebitis, intracranial venous sinus
  leg 451.2
    deep (vessels) 451.19
      femoral vein 451.11
      specified vessel NEC 451.19
    superficial (vessels) 451.0
      femoral vein 451.11
  longitudinal (venous) sinus — see Thrombophlebitis, intracranial venous sinus
  lower extremity 451.2
    deep (vessels) 451.19
      femoral vein 451.11
      specified vessel NEC 451.19
    superficial (vessels) 451.0
  migrans, migrating 453.1
  pelvic
    with
      abortion — see Abortion, by type, with sepsis
      ectopic pregnancy — (see also categories 633.0-633.9) 639.0

Thrombophlebitis—continued
　pelvic—continued
　　with—continued
　　　molar pregnancy — (see also categories 630-632) 639.0
　　　following
　　　　abortion 639.0
　　　　ectopic or molar pregnancy 639.0
　　　puerperal 671.4
　popliteal vein 451.19
　portal (vein) 572.1
　postoperative 997.2
　pregnancy (superficial) 671.2
　　affecting fetus or newborn 760.3
　　deep 671.3
　puerperal, postpartum, childbirth (extremities) (superficial) 671.2
　　deep 671.4
　　pelvic 671.4
　　specified site NEC 671.5
　radial vein 451.83
　saphenous (greater) (lesser) 451.0
　sinus (intracranial) — see Thrombophlebitis, intracranial venous sinus
　specified site NEC 451.89
　tibial vein 451.19

Thrombosis, thrombotic (marantic) (multiple) (progressive) (septic) (vein) (vessel) 453.9
　with childbirth or during the puerperium — see Thrombosis, puerperal, postpartum
　antepartum — see Thrombosis, pregnancy
　aorta, aortic 444.1
　　abdominal 444.0
　　bifurcation 444.0
　　saddle 444.0
　　terminal 444.0
　　thoracic 444.1
　　valve — see Endocarditis, aortic
　apoplexy (see also Thrombosis, brain) 434.0
　　late effect — see category 438
　appendix, septic — see Appendicitis, acute ◆
　arteriolar-capillary platelet, disseminated 446.6
　artery, arteries (postinfectional) 444.9
　　auditory, internal 433.8
　　basilar (see also Occlusion, artery, basilar) 433.0
　　carotid (common) (internal) (see also Occlusion, artery, carotid) 433.1
　　　with other precerebral artery 433.3
　　cerebellar (anterior inferior) (posterior inferior) (superior) 433.8
　　cerebral (see also Thrombosis, brain) 434.0
　　choroidal (anterior) 433.8
　　communicating posterior 433.8
　　coronary (see also Infarct, myocardium) 410.9
　　　without myocardial infarction 411.81
　　　due to syphilis 093.89
　　　healed or specified as old 412
　　extremities 444.22
　　　lower 444.22
　　　upper 444.21
　　femoral 444.22
　　hepatic 444.89
　　hypophyseal 433.8

Thrombosis, thrombotic—continued
　artery, arteries—continued
　　meningeal, anterior or posterior 433.8
　　mesenteric (with gangrene) 557.0
　　ophthalmic (see also Occlusion, retina) 362.30
　　pontine 433.8
　　popliteal 444.22
　　precerebral — see Occlusion, artery, precerebral NEC
　　pulmonary 415.1
　　renal 593.81
　　retinal (see also Occlusion, retina) 362.30
　　specified site NEC 444.89
　　spinal, anterior or posterior 433.8
　　traumatic (complication) (early) (see also Injury, blood vessel, by site) 904.9
　　vertebral (see also Occlusion, artery, vertebral) 433.2
　　　with other precerebral artery 433.3
　atrial (endocardial) 424.90
　　due to syphilis 093.89
　auricular (see also Infarct, myocardium) 410.9
　axillary (vein) 453.8
　basilar (artery) (see also Occlusion, artery, basilar) 433.0
　bland NEC 453.9
　brain (artery) (stem) 434.0
　　due to syphilis 094.89
　　late effect — see category 438
　　puerperal, postpartum, childbirth 674.0
　　sinus (see also Thrombosis, intracranial venous sinus) 325
　capillary 448.9
　　arteriolar, generalized 446.6
　cardiac (see also Infarct, myocardium) 410.9
　　due to syphilis 093.89
　　healed or specified as old 412
　　valve — see Endocarditis
　carotid (artery) (common) (internal) (see also Occlusion, artery, carotid) 433.1
　　with other precerebral artery 433.3
　cavernous sinus (venous) — see Thrombosis, intracranial venous sinus
　cerebellar artery (anterior inferior) (posterior inferior) (superior) 433.8
　　late effect — see category 438
　cerebral (arteries) (see also Thrombosis, brain) 434.0
　　late effect — see category 438
　coronary (artery) (see also Infarct, myocardium) 410.9
　　without myocardial infarction 411.81
　　due to syphilis 093.89
　　healed or specified as old 412
　corpus cavernosum 607.82
　cortical (see also Thrombosis, brain) 434.0
　due to (presence of) any device, implant, or graft classifiable to 996.0-996.5 — see Complications, due to (presence of) any device, implant, or graft classified to 996.0-996.5 NEC
　effort 453.8
　endocardial — see Infarct, myocardium

Thrombosis, thrombotic—continued
　eye (see also Occlusion, retina) 362.30
　femoral (vein) (deep) 453.8
　　with inflammation or phlebitis 451.11
　　artery 444.22
　genital organ, male 608.83
　heart (chamber) (see also Infarct, myocardium) 410.9
　hepatic (vein) 453.0
　　artery 444.89
　　infectional or septic 572.1
　iliac (vein) 453.8
　　with inflammation or phlebitis 451.81
　　artery (common) (external) (internal) 444.81
　inflammation, vein — see Thrombophlebitis
　internal carotid artery (see also Occlusion, artery, carotid) 433.1
　　with other precerebral artery 433.3
　intestine (with gangrene) 557.0
　intracranial (see also Thrombosis, brain) 434.0
　　venous sinus (any) 325
　　　nonpyogenic origin 437.6
　　　in pregnancy or puerperium 671.5
　intramural (see also Infarct, myocardium) 410.9
　　without ▼
　　　cardiac condition 429.89
　　　coronary artery disease 429.89
　　　myocardial infarction 429.89 ▲
　　healed or specified as old 412
　jugular (bulb) 453.8
　kidney 593.81
　　artery 593.81
　lateral sinus (venous) — see Thrombosis, intracranial venous sinus
　leg 453.8
　　with inflammation or phlebitis — see Thrombophlebitis
　　deep (vessels) 453.8
　　superficial (vessels) 453.8
　liver (venous) 453.0
　　artery 444.89
　　infectional or septic 572.1
　　portal vein 452
　longitudinal sinus (venous) — see Thrombosis, intracranial venous sinus
　lower extremity — see Thrombosis, leg
　lung 415.1
　marantic, dural sinus 437.6
　meninges (brain) (see also Thrombosis, brain) 434.0
　mesenteric (artery) (with gangrene) 557.0
　　vein (inferior) (superior) 452
　mitral — see Insufficiency, mitral
　mural (heart chamber) (see also Infarct, myocardium) 410.9 ▼
　　without
　　　cardiac condition 429.89
　　　coronary artery disease 429.89
　　　myocardial infarction 429.89 ▲
　　due to syphilis 093.89
　　following myocardial infarction 429.79
　　healed or specified as old 412 ◆
　omentum (with gangrene) 557.0
　ophthalmic (artery) (see also Occlusion, retina) 362.30

Thrombosis, thrombotic—continued
　pampiniform plexus (male) 608.83
　　female 620.8
　parietal (see also Infarct, myocardium) 410.9
　penis, penile 607.82
　peripheral arteries 444.22
　　lower 444.22
　　upper 444.21
　platelet 446.6
　portal 452
　　due to syphilis 093.89
　　infectional or septic 572.1
　precerebral artery — see also Occlusion, artery, precerebral NEC
　pregnancy 671.9
　　deep (vein) 671.3
　　superficial (vein) 671.2
　puerperal, postpartum, childbirth 671.9
　　brain (artery) 674.0
　　venous 671.5
　　cardiac 674.8
　　cerebral (artery) 674.0
　　venous 671.5
　　deep (vein) 671.4
　　intracranial sinus (nonpyogenic) (venous) 671.5
　　pelvic 671.4
　　pulmonary (artery) 673.2
　　specified site NEC 671.5
　　superficial 671.2
　pulmonary (artery) (vein) 415.1
　renal (artery) 593.81
　　vein 453.3
　resulting from presence of shunt or other internal prosthetic device — see Complications, due to (presence of) any device, implant, or graft classified to 996.0-996.5 NEC
　retina, retinal (artery) 362.30
　　arterial branch 362.32
　　central 362.31
　　partial 362.33
　　vein
　　　central 362.35
　　　tributary (branch) 362.36
　scrotum 608.83
　seminal vesicle 608.83
　sigmoid (venous) sinus (see Thrombosis, intracranial venous sinus) 325
　silent NEC 453.9
　sinus, intracranial (venous) (any) (see also Thrombosis, intracranial venous sinus) 325
　softening, brain (see also Thrombosis, brain) 434.0
　specified site NEC 453.8
　spermatic cord 608.83
　spinal cord 336.1
　　due to syphilis 094.89
　　in pregnancy or puerperium 671.5
　　pyogenic origin 324.1
　　late effect — see category 326
　spleen, splenic 289.59
　　artery 444.89
　testis 608.83
　traumatic (complication) (early) (see also Injury, blood vessel, by site) 904.9
　tricuspid — see Endocarditis, tricuspid
　tunica vaginalis 608.83
　umbilical cord (vessels) 663.6
　　affecting fetus or newborn 762.6

Thrombosis, thrombotic—continued
- vas deferens 608.83
- vena cava (inferior) (superior) 453.2

Thrombus — see Thrombosis

Thrush 112.0
- newborn 771.7

Thumb — see also condition
- gamekeeper's 842.12
- sucking (child problem) 307.9

Thygeson's superficial punctate keratitis 370.21

Thymergasia (see also Psychosis, affective) 296.80

Thymitis 254.8

Thymoma (benign) (M8580/0) 212.6
- malignant (M8580/3) 164.0

Thymus, thymic (gland) — see condition

Thyrocele (see also Goiter) 240.9

Thyroglossal — see also condition
- cyst 759.2
- duct, persistent 759.2

Thyroid (body) (gland) — see also condition
- lingual 759.2

Thyroiditis 245.9
- acute (pyogenic) (suppurative) 245.0
  - nonsuppurative 245.0
- autoimmune 245.2
- chronic (nonspecific) (sclerosing) 245.8
  - fibrous 245.3
  - lymphadenoid 245.2
  - lymphocytic 245.2
  - lymphoid 245.2
- complicating pregnancy, childbirth, or puerperium 648.1
- de Quervain's (subacute granulomatous) 245.1
- fibrous (chronic) 245.3
- giant (cell) (follicular) 245.1
- granulomatous (de Quervain's) (subacute) 245.1
- Hashimoto's (struma lymphomatosa) 245.2
- iatrogenic 245.4
- invasive (fibrous) 245.3
- ligneous 245.3
- lymphocytic (chronic) 245.2
- lymphoid 245.2
- lymphomatous 245.2
- pseudotuberculous 245.1
- pyogenic 245.0
- radiation 245.4
- Riedel's (ligneous) 245.3
- subacute 245.1
- suppurative 245.0
- tuberculous (see also Tuberculosis) 017.5
- viral 245.1
- woody 245.3

Thyrolingual duct, persistent 759.2

Thyromegaly 240.9

Thyrotoxic
- crisis or storm (see also Thyrotoxicosis) 242.9
- heart failure (see also Thyrotoxicosis) 242.9 [425.7]

Thyrotoxicosis 242.9

Note — Use the following fifth-digit subclassification with category 242:

0 without mention of thyrotoxic crisis or storm
1 with mention of thyrotoxic crisis or storm

Thyrotoxicosis—continued
- with
  - goiter (diffuse) 242.0
    - adenomatous 242.3
      - multinodular 242.2
      - uninodular 242.1
    - nodular 242.3
      - multinodular 242.2
      - uninodular 242.1
  - infiltrative
    - dermopathy 242.0
    - ophthalmopathy 242.0
  - thyroid acropachy 242.0
- complicating pregnancy, childbirth, or puerperium 648.1
- due to
  - ectopic thyroid nodule 242.4
  - ingestion of (excessive) thyroid material 242.8
  - specified cause NEC 242.8
- factitia 242.8
- heart 242.9 [425.7]
- neonatal (transient) 775.3

TIA (transient ischemic attack) 435.9
- with transient neurologic deficit 435.9
- late effect — see category 438

Tibia vara 732.4

Tic 307.20
- breathing 307.20
- child problem 307.21
- compulsive 307.22
- convulsive 307.20
- degenerative (generalized) (localized) 333.3
- facial 351.8
- douloureux (see also Neuralgia, trigeminal) 350.1
  - atypical 350.2
- habit 307.20
  - chronic (motor or vocal) 307.22 ◆
  - transient of childhood 307.21
- lid 307.20
  - transient of childhood 307.21
- motor-verbal 307.23
- occupational 300.89
- orbicularis 307.20
  - transient of childhood 307.21
- organic origin 333.3
- postchoreic — see Chorea
- psychogenic 307.20
  - compulsive 307.22
- salaam 781.0
- spasm 307.20
  - chronic (motor or vocal) 307.22 ◆
  - transient of childhood 307.21

Tick (-borne) fever NEC 066.1
- American mountain 066.1
- Colorado 066.1
- hemorrhagic NEC 065.3
  - Crimean 065.0
  - Kyasanur Forest 065.2
  - Omsk 065.1
- mountain 066.1
- nonexanthematous 066.1

Tick-bite fever NEC 066.1
- African 087.1
- Colorado (virus) 066.1
- Rocky Mountain 082.0

Tick paralysis 989.5

Tics and spasms, compulsive 307.22

Tietze's disease or syndrome 733.6

Tight, tightness
- anus 564.8
- chest 786.59
- fascia (lata) 728.9
- foreskin (congenital) 605
- hymen 623.3
- introitus (acquired) (congenital) 623.3
- rectal sphincter 564.8

Tight, tightness—continued
- tendon 727.81
  - Achilles (heel) 727.81
- urethral sphincter 598.9

Tilting vertebra 737.9

Timidity, child 313.21

Tinea (intersecta) (tarsi) 110.9
- amiantacea 110.0
- asbestina 110.0
- barbae 110.0
- beard 110.0
- black dot 110.0
- blanca 111.2
- capitis 110.0
- corporis 110.5
- cruris 110.3
- decalvans 704.09
- flava 111.0
- foot 110.4
- furfuracea 111.0
- imbricata (Tokelau) 110.5
- lepothrix 039.0
- manuum 110.2
- microsporic (see also Dermatophytosis) 110.9
- nigra 111.1
- nodosa 111.2
- pedis 110.4
- scalp 110.0
- specified site NEC 110.8
- sycosis 110.0
- tonsurans 110.0
- trichophytic (see also Dermatophytosis) 110.9
- unguium 110.1
- versicolor 111.0

Tingling sensation (see also Disturbance, sensation) 782.0

Tin-miners' lung 503

Tinnitus (aurium) 388.30
- audible 388.32
- objective 388.32
- subjective 388.31

Tipping pelvis 738.6
- with disproportion (fetopelvic) 653.0
  - affecting fetus or newborn 763.1
  - causing obstructed labor 660.1
    - affecting fetus or newborn 763.1

Tiredness 780.7

Tissue — see condition

Tobacco
- abuse (affecting health) NEC (see also Abuse, drugs, nondependent) 305.1
- heart 989.8

Tobias' syndrome (carcinoma, pulmonary apex) (M8010/3) 162.3

Tocopherol deficiency 269.1

Todd's
- cirrhosis — see Cirrhosis, biliary
- paralysis (postepileptic transitory paralysis) 344.8

Toe — see condition

Toilet, artificial opening (see also Attention to, artificial, opening) V55.9

Tokelau ringworm 110.5

Tollwut 071

Tolosa-Hunt syndrome 378.55

Tommaselli's disease
- correct substance properly administered 599.7
- overdose or wrong substance given or taken 961.4

Tongue — see also condition
- worms 134.1

Tongue tie 750.0

Toni-Fanconi syndrome (cystinosis) 270.0

Tonic pupil 379.46

Tonsil — see condition

Tonsillitis (acute) (catarrhal) (croupous) (follicular) (gangrenous) (infective) (lacunar) (lingual) (malignant) (membranous) (phlegmonous) (pneumococcal) (pseudomembranous) (purulent) (septic) (staphylococcal) (subacute) (suppurative) (toxic) (ulcerative) (vesicular) (viral) 463
- with influenza, flu, or grippe 487.1
- chronic 474.0
- diphtheritic (membranous) 032.0
- hypertrophic 474.0
- influenzal 487.1
- parenchymatous 475
- streptococcal 034.0
- tuberculous (see also Tuberculosis) 012.8
- Vincent's 101

Tonsillopharyngitis 465.8

Tooth, teeth — see condition

Toothache 525.9

Topagnosis 782.0

Tophi (gouty) 274.0
- ear 274.81
- heart 274.82
- specified site NEC 274.82

Torn — see Tear, torn

Tornwaldt's bursitis (disease) (pharyngeal bursitis) 478.29
- cyst 478.26

Torpid liver 573.9

Torsion
- accessory tube 620.5
- adnexa (female) 620.5
- aorta (congenital) 747.29
  - acquired 447.1
- appendix epididymis 608.2
- bile duct 576.8
  - with calculus, choledocholithiasis or stones — see Choledocholithiasis
  - congenital 751.69
- bowel, colon, or intestine 560.2
- cervix (see also Malposition, uterus) 621.6
- duodenum 537.3
- dystonia — see Dystonia, torsion
- epididymis 608.2
  - appendix 608.2
- fallopian tube 620.5
- gallbladder (see also Disease, gallbladder) 575.8
  - congenital 751.69
- gastric 537.89
- hydatid of Morgagni (female) 620.5
- kidney (pedicle) 593.89
- Meckel's diverticulum (congenital) 751.0
- mesentery 560.2
- omentum 560.2
- organ or site, congenital NEC — see Anomaly, specified type NEC
- ovary (pedicle) 620.5
  - congenital 752.0
- oviduct 620.5
- penis 607.89
  - congenital 752.8
- renal 593.89
- spasm — see Dystonia, torsion
- spermatic cord 608.2
- spleen 289.59
- testicle, testis 608.2
- tibia 736.89

INDEX TO DISEASES

Torsion—continued
umbilical cord — see Compression, umbilical cord
uterus (see also Malposition, uterus) 621.6

Torticollis (intermittent) (spastic) 723.5
congenital 754.1
  sternomastoid 754.1
due to birth injury 767.8
hysterical 300.11
psychogenic 306.0
  specified as conversion reaction 300.11
rheumatic 723.5
rheumatoid 714.0
spasmodic 333.83
traumatic, current NEC 847.0

Tortuous
artery 447.1
fallopian tube 752.19
organ or site, congenital NEC — see Distortion
renal vessel, congenital 747.62
retina vessel (congenital) 743.58
  acquired 362.17
ureter 593.4
urethra 599.84
vein — see Varicose, vein

Torula, torular (infection) 117.5
histolytica 117.5
lung 117.5

Torulosis 117.5

Torus
mandibularis 526.81
palatinus 526.81

Touch, vitreous 997.9

Touraine's syndrome (hereditary osteo-onychodysplasia) 756.89

Touraine-Solente-Golé syndrome (acropachyderma) 757.39

Tourette's disease (motor-verbal tic) 307.23

Tower skull 756.0
with exophthalmos 756.0

Toxemia 799.8
with
  abortion — see Abortion, by type, with toxemia
bacterial — see Septicemia
biliary (see also Disease, biliary) 576.8
burn — see Burn, by site
congenital NEC 779.8
eclamptic 642.6
  with pre-existing hypertension 642.7
erysipelatous (see also Erysipelas) 035
fatigue 799.8
fetus or newborn NEC 779.8
food (see also Poisoning, food) 005.9
gastric 537.89
gastrointestinal 558.2
intestinal 558.2
kidney (see also Disease, renal) 593.9
lung 518.89
malarial NEC (see also Malaria) 084.6
maternal (of pregnancy), affecting fetus or newborn 760.0
myocardial — see Myocarditis, toxic
of pregnancy (mild) (pre-eclamptic) 642.4
  with
    convulsions 642.6
    pre-existing hypertension 642.7
    affecting fetus or newborn 760.0

Toxemia—continued
of pregnancy—continued
  severe 642.5
  pre-eclamptic — see Toxemia, of pregnancy
puerperal, postpartum — see Toxemia, of pregnancy
pulmonary 518.89
renal (see also Disease, renal) 593.9
septic (see also Septicemia) 038.9
small intestine 558.2
staphylococcal 038.1
  due to food 005.0
stasis 799.8
stomach 537.89
uremic (see also Uremia) 586
urinary 586

Toxemica cerebropathia psychica (nonalcoholic) 294.0
alcoholic 291.1

Toxic (poisoning) — see also condition from drug or poison — see Table of drugs and chemicals
oil syndrome 710.5
shock syndrome 040.89 ◆
thyroid (gland) (see also Thyrotoxicosis) 242.9

Toxicemia — see Toxemia

Toxicity
fava bean 282.2
from drug or poison — see Table of drugs and chemicals

Toxicosis (see also Toxemia) 799.8
capillary, hemorrhagic 287.0

Toxinfection 799.8
gastrointestinal 558.2

Toxocariasis 128.0

Toxoplasma infection, generalized 130.9

Toxoplasmosis (acquired) 130.9
with pneumonia 130.4
congenital, active 771.2
disseminated (multisystemic) 130.8
maternal
  with suspected damage to fetus affecting management of pregnancy 655.4
  affecting fetus or newborn 760.2
  manifest toxoplasmosis in fetus or newborn 771.2
multiple sites 130.8
multisystemic disseminated 130.8
specified site NEC 130.7

Trabeculation, bladder 596.8

Trachea — see condition

Tracheitis (acute) (catarrhal) (infantile) (membranous) (plastic) (pneumococcal) (septic) (suppurative) (viral) 464.10
with
  bronchitis 490
    acute or subacute 466.0
    chronic 491.8
  tuberculosis — see Tuberculosis, pulmonary
laryngitis (acute) 464.20
  with obstruction 464.21
  chronic 476.1
  tuberculous (see also Tuberculosis, larynx) 012.3
obstruction 464.11
chronic 491.8
  with
    bronchitis (chronic) 491.8
    laryngitis (chronic) 476.1

Tracheitis—continued
chronic—continued
  due to external agent — see Condition, respiratory, chronic, due to
diphtheritic (membranous) 032.3
due to external agent — see Inflammation, respiratory, upper, due to
edematous 464.11
influenzal 487.1
streptococcal 034.0
syphilitic 095.8
tuberculous (see also Tuberculosis) 012.8

Trachelitis (nonvenereal) (see also Cervicitis) 616.0
trichomonal 131.09

Tracheobronchial — see condition

Tracheobronchitis (see also Bronchitis) 490
acute or subacute 466.0
  with bronchospasm or obstruction 466.0
chronic 491.8
influenzal 487.1
senile 491.8

Tracheobronchomegaly (congenital) 748.3

Tracheobronchopneumonitis — see Pneumonia, broncho

Tracheocele (external) (internal) 519.1
congenital 748.3

Tracheomalacia 519.1
congenital 748.3

Tracheopharyngitis (acute) 465.8
chronic 478.9
  due to external agent — see Condition, respiratory, chronic, due to
  due to external agent — see Inflammation, respiratory, upper, due to

Tracheostenosis 519.1
congenital 748.3

Tracheostomy
attention to V55.0
complication 519.0
hemorrhage 519.0
malfunctioning 519.0
obstruction 519.0
sepsis 519.0
status V44.0
stenosis 519.0

Trachoma, trachomatous 076.9
active (stage) 076.1
contraction of conjunctiva 076.1
dubium 076.0
healed or late effect 139.1
initial (stage) 076.0
Türck's (chronic catarrhal laryngitis) 476.0

Trachyphonia 784.49

Training
orthoptic V57.4
orthotic V57.81

Train sickness 994.6

Trait
hemoglobin
  abnormal NEC 282.7
    with thalassemia 282.4
  C (see also Disease, hemoglobin, C) 282.7
    with elliptocytosis 282.7
  S (Hb-S) 282.5
Lepore 282.4
  with other abnormal hemoglobin NEC 282.4
paranoid 301.0
sickle-cell 282.5
  with
    elliptocytosis 282.5
    spherocytosis 282.5

Traits, paranoid 301.0

Tramp V60.0

Trance 780.09
hysterical 300.13

Transaminasemia 790.4

Transfusion, blood
donor V59.0
incompatible 999.6
reaction or complication — see Complications, transfusion
syndrome
  fetomaternal 772.0
  twin-to-twin
    blood loss (donor twin) 772.0
    recipient twin 776.4
without reported diagnosis V58.2

Transient — see also condition
alteration of awareness 780.02
blindness 368.12
deafness (ischemic) 388.02
global amnesia 437.7
person (homeless) NEC V60.0

Transitional, lumbosacral joint of vertebra 756.19

Translocation
autosomes NEC 758.5
  13-15 758.1
  16-18 758.2
  21 or 22 758.0
  balanced in normal individual 758.4
D_1 758.1
E_3 758.2
G 758.0
balanced autosomal in normal individual 758.4
chromosomes NEC 758.9
Down's syndrome 758.0

Translucency, iris 364.53

Transmission of chemical substances through the placenta (affecting fetus or newborn) 760.70
alcohol 760.71
anti-infective agents 760.74
cocaine 760.75
"crack" 760.75
diethylstilbestrol [DES] 760.76 ◆
hallucinogenic agents 760.73
medicinal agents NEC 760.79
narcotics 760.72
obstetric anesthetic or analgesic drug 763.5
specified agent NEC 760.79
suspected, affecting management of pregnancy 655.5

Transplant(ed)
bone V42.4
  marrow V42.8
complication NEC (see also Complications, due to (presence of) any device, implant, or graft classified to 996.0-996.5 NEC
  bone marrow 996.85
  corneal graft NEC 996.79
    infection or inflammation 996.69
    reaction 996.51
    rejection 996.51
  organ (failure) (immune or nonimmune cause) (infection) (rejection) 996.80
    bone marrow 996.85
    heart 996.83
    intestines 996.89
    kidney 996.81
    liver 996.82
    lung 996.84
    pancreas 996.86
    specified NEC 996.89
  skin NEC 996.79
    infection or inflammation 996.69
    rejection 996.52

Transplant

Transplant(ed)—*continued*
  cornea V42.5
  hair V50.0
  heart V42.1
    valve V42.2
  intestine V42.8
  kidney V42.0
  liver V42.7
  lung V42.6
  organ V42.9
    specified NEC V42.8
  pancreas V42.8
  skin V42.3
  tissue V42.9
    specified NEC V42.8
Transplants, ovarian, endometrial
  617.1
Transposed — *see* Transposition
Transposition (congenital) — *see also* Malposition, congenital
  abdominal viscera 759.3
  aorta (dextra) 745.11
  appendix 751.5
  arterial trunk 745.10
  colon 751.5
  great vessels (complete) 745.10
    both originating from right ventricle 745.11
    corrected 745.12
    double outlet right ventricle 745.11
    incomplete 745.11
    partial 745.11
    specified type NEC 745.19
  heart 746.87
    with complete transposition of viscera 759.3
  intestine (large) (small) 751.5
  pulmonary veins 747.49
  reversed jejunal (for bypass) (status) V45.3
  stomach 750.7
    with general transposition of viscera 759.3
  teeth, tooth 524.3
  vessels (complete) 745.10
    partial 745.11
  viscera (abdominal) (thoracic) 759.3
Trans-sexualism 302.50
  with
    asexual history 302.51
    heterosexual history 302.53
    homosexual history 302.52
Transverse — *see also* condition
  arrest (deep), in labor 660.3
    affecting fetus or newborn 763.1
  lie 652.3
    before labor, affecting fetus or newborn 761.7
    causing obstructed labor 660.0
      affecting fetus or newborn 763.1
    during labor, affecting fetus or newborn 763.1
Transvestism, transvestitism
  (transvestic fetishism) 302.3 ◆
Trapped placenta (with hemorrhage) 666.0
  without hemorrhage 667.0
Trauma, traumatism (*see also* Injury, by site) 959.9
  birth — *see* Birth, injury NEC
  causing hemorrhage of pregnancy or delivery 641.8
  complicating
    abortion — *see* Abortion, by type, with damage to pelvic organs
    ectopic pregnancy (*see also* categories 633.0-633.9) 639.2
    molar pregnancy (*see also* categories 630-632) 639.2

INDEX TO DISEASES

Trauma, traumatism—*continued*
  during delivery NEC 665.9
  following
    abortion 639.2
    ectopic or molar pregnancy 639.2
  maternal, during pregnancy, affecting fetus or newborn 760.5
  neuroma — *see* Injury, nerve, by site
  previous major, affecting management of pregnancy, childbirth, or puerperium V23.8
  psychic (current) — *see also* Reaction, adjustment
    previous (history) V15.4
  psychologic, previous (affecting health) V15.4
  transient paralysis — *see* Injury, nerve, by site
Traumatic — *see* condition
Treacher Collins' syndrome
  (incomplete facial dysostosis) 756.0
Treitz's hernia — *see* Hernia, Treitz's
Trematode infestation NEC 121.9
Trematodiasis NEC 121.9
Trembles 988.8
Trembling paralysis (*see also* Parkinsonism) 332.0
Tremor 781.0
  essential (benign) 333.1
  familial 333.1
  flapping (liver) 572.8
  hereditary 333.1
  hysterical 300.11
  intention 333.1
  mercurial 985.0
  muscle 728.85
  Parkinson's (*see also* Parkinsonism) 332.0
  psychogenic 306.0
    specified as conversion reaction 300.11
  senilis 797
  specified type NEC 333.1
Trench
  fever 083.1
  foot 991.4
  mouth 101
  nephritis — *see* Nephritis, acute
Treponema pallidum infection (*see also* Syphilis) 097.9
Treponematosis 102.9
  due to
    T. pallidum — *see* Syphilis
    T. pertenue (yaws) (*see also* Yaws) 102.9
Triad
  Kartagener's 759.3
  Reiter's (complete) (incomplete) 099.3
  Saint's (*see also* Hernia, diaphragm) 553.3
Trichiasis 704.2
  cicatricial 704.2
  eyelid 374.05
    with entropion (*see also* Entropion) 374.00
Trichinella spiralis (infection) (infestation) 124
Trichinelliasis 124
Trichinellosis 124
Trichiniasis 124
Trichinosis 124
Trichobezoar 938
  intestine 936
  stomach 935.2
Trichocephaliasis 127.3
Trichocephalosis 127.3
Trichocephalus infestation 127.3

Trichoclasis 704.2
Trichoepithelioma (M8100/0) — *see also* Neoplasm, skin, benign
  breast 217
  genital organ NEC — *see* Neoplasm, by site, benign
  malignant (M8100/3) — *see* Neoplasm, skin, malignant
Trichofolliculoma (M8101/0) — *see* Neoplasm, skin, benign
Tricholemmoma (M8102/0) — *see* Neoplasm, skin, benign
Trichomatosis 704.2
Trichomoniasis 131.9
  bladder 131.09
  cervix 131.09
  intestinal 007.3
  prostate 131.03
  seminal vesicle 131.09
  specified site NEC 131.8
  urethra 131.02
  urogenitalis 131.00
  vagina 131.01
  vulva 131.01
  vulvovaginal 131.01
Trichomycosis 039.0
  axillaris 039.0
  nodosa 111.2
  nodularis 111.2
  rubra 039.0
Trichonocardiosis (axillaris) (palmellina) 039.0
Trichonodosis 704.2
Trichophytid, trichophyton infection
  (*see also* Dermatophytosis) 110.9
Trichophytide — *see* Dermatophytosis
Trichophytobezoar 938
  intestine 936
  stomach 935.2
Trichophytosis — *see* Dermatophytosis
Trichoptilosis 704.2
Trichorrhexis (nodosa) 704.2
Trichosporosis nodosa 111.2
Trichostasis spinulosa (congenital) 757.4
Trichostrongyliasis (small intestine) 127.6
Trichostrongylosis 127.6
Trichostrongylus (instabilis) infection 127.6
Trichotillomania 312.39 ◆
Trichromat, anomalous (congenital) 368.59
Trichromatopsia, anomalous (congenital) 368.59
Trichuriasis 127.3
Trichuris trichiuria (any site) (infection) (infestation) 127.3
Tricuspid (valve) — *see* condition
Trifid — *see also* Accessory
  kidney (pelvis) 753.3
  tongue 750.13
Trigeminal neuralgia (*see also* Neuralgia, trigeminal) 350.1
Trigeminoencephaloangiomatosis 759.6
Trigeminy 427.89
  postoperative 997.1
Trigger finger (acquired) 727.03
  congenital 756.89
Trigonitis (bladder) (chronic) (pseudomembranous) 595.3
  tuberculous (*see also* Tuberculosis) 016.1
Trigonocephaly 756.0
Trihexosidosis 272.7
Trilobate placenta — *see* Placenta, abnormal

Trunk

Trilocular heart 745.8
Tripartita placenta — *see* Placenta, abnormal
Triple — *see also* Accessory
  kidneys 753.3
  uteri 752.2
  X female 758.8
Triplegia 344.89
  congenital or infantile 343.8
Triplet
  affected by maternal complications of pregnancy 761.5
  healthy liveborn — *see* Newborn, multiple
  pregnancy (complicating delivery) NEC 651.1
    with fetal loss and retention of one or more fetus(es) 651.4
Triplex placenta — *see* Placenta, abnormal
Triplication — *see* Accessory
Trismus 781.0
  neonatorum 771.3
  newborn 771.3
Trisomy (syndrome) NEC 758.5
  13 (partial) 758.1
  16-18 758.2
  18 (partial) 758.2
  21 (partial) 758.0
  22 758.0
  autosomes NEC 758.5
  D_1 758.1
  E_3 758.2
  G (group) 758.0
  group D_1 758.1
  group E 758.2
  group G 758.0
Tritanomaly 368.53
Tritanopia 368.53
Troisier-Hanot-Chauffard syndrome (bronze diabetes) 275.0
Trombidiosis 133.8
Trophedema (hereditary) 757.0
  congenital 757.0
Trophoblastic disease (*see also* Hydatidiform mole) 630
  previous, affecting management of pregnancy V23.1
Tropholymphedema 757.0
Trophoneurosis NEC 356.9
  arm NEC 354.9
  disseminated 710.1
  facial 349.89
  leg NEC 355.8
  lower extremity NEC 355.8
  upper extremity NEC 354.9
Tropical — *see also* condition
  maceration feet (syndrome) 991.4
  wet foot (syndrome) 991.4
Trouble — *see also* Disease
  bowel 569.9
  heart — *see* Disease, heart
  intestine 569.9
  kidney (*see also* Disease, renal) 593.9
  nervous 799.2
  sinus (*see also* Sinusitis) 473.9
Trousseau's syndrome (thrombophlebitis migrans) 453.1
Truancy, childhood — *see also* Disturbance, conduct
  socialized 312.2
  undersocialized, unsocialized 312.1
Truncus
  arteriosus (persistent) 745.0
  common 745.0
  communis 745.0
Trunk — *see* condition

Trychophytide — *see* Dermatophytosis
Trypanosoma infestation — *see* Trypanosomiasis
Trypanosomiasis 086.9
  with meningoencephalitis 086.9 *[323.2]*
  African 086.5
    due to Trypanosoma 086.5
      gambiense 086.3
      rhodesiense 086.4
  American 086.2
    with
      heart involvement 086.0
      other organ involvement 086.1
    without mention of organ involvement 086.2
  Brazilian — *see* Trypanosomiasis, American
  Chagas' — *see* Trypanosomiasis, American
  due to Trypanosoma
    cruzi — *see* Trypanosomiasis, American
    gambiense 086.3
    rhodesiense 086.4
  gambiensis, Gambian 086.3
  North American — *see* Trypanosomiasis, American
  rhodesiensis, Rhodesian 086.4
  South American — *see* Trypanosomiasis, American
T-shaped incisors 520.2
Tsutsugamushi fever 081.2
Tube, tubal, tubular — *see also* condition
  ligation, admission for V25.2
Tubercle — *see also* Tuberculosis
  brain, solitary 013.2
  Darwin's 744.29
  epithelioid noncaseating 135
  Ghon, primary infection 010.0
Tuberculid, tuberculide (indurating) (lichenoid) (miliary) (papulonecrotic) (primary) (skin) (subcutaneous) (*see also* Tuberculosis) 017.0
Tuberculoma — *see also* Tuberculosis
  brain (any part) 013.2
  meninges (cerebral) (spinal) 013.1
  spinal cord 013.4
Tuberculosis, tubercular, tuberculous (calcification) (calcified) (caseous) (chromogenic acid-fast bacilli) (congenital) (degeneration) (disease) (fibrocaseous) (fistula) (gangrene) (interstitial) (isolated circumscribed lesions) (necrosis) (parenchymatous) (ulcerative) 011.9

Tuberculosis, tubercular, tuberculous—*continued*

> Note — Use the following fifth-digit subclassification with categories 010-018:
>
> 0 unspecified
> 1 bacteriological or histological examination not done
> 2 bacteriological or histological examination unknown (at present)
> 3 tubercle bacilli found (in sputum) by microscopy
> 4 tubercle bacilli not found (in sputum) by microscopy, but found by bacterial culture
> 5 tubercle bacilli not found by bacteriological exam-ination, but tuberculosis confirmed histologically
> 6 tubercle bacilli not found by bacteriological or histological examination, but tuberculosis confirmed by other methods [inoculation of animals]
>
> For tuberculous conditions specified as late effects or sequelae, see category 137.

  abdomen 014.8
    lymph gland 014.8
  abscess 011.9
    arm 017.9
    bone (*see also* Osteomyelitis, due to, tuberculosis) 015.9 *[730.8]*
      hip 015.1 *[730.85]*
      knee 015.2 *[730.96]*
      sacrum 015.0 *[730.88]*
      specified site NEC 015.7 *[730.88]*
      spinal 015.0 *[730.88]*
      vertebra 015.0 *[730.88]*
    brain 013.3
    breast 017.9
    Cowper's gland 016.5
    dura (mater) 013.8
      brain 013.3
      spinal cord 013.5
    epidural 013.8
      brain 013.3
      spinal cord 013.5
    frontal sinus — *see* Tuberculosis, sinus
    genital organs NEC 016.9
      female 016.7
      male 016.5
    genitourinary NEC 016.9
    gland (lymphatic) — *see* Tuberculosis, lymph gland
    hip 015.1
    iliopsoas 015.0 *[730.88]*
    intestine 014.8
    ischiorectal 014.8
    joint 015.9
      hip 015.1
      knee 015.2
      specified joint NEC 015.8
      vertebral 015.0 *[730.88]*
    kidney 016.0 *[590.81]*
    knee 015.2
    lumbar 015.0 *[730.88]*
    lung 011.2
      primary, progressive 010.8
    meninges (cerebral) (spinal) 013.0

Tuberculosis, tubercular, tuberculous—*continued*
  abscess—*continued*
    pelvic 016.9
      female 016.7
      male 016.5
    perianal 014.8
      fistula 014.8
    perinephritic 016.0 *[590.81]*
    perineum 017.9
    perirectal 014.8
    psoas 015.0 *[730.88]*
    rectum 014.8
    retropharyngeal 012.8
    sacrum 015.0 *[730.88]*
    scrofulous 017.2
    scrotum 016.5
    skin 017.0
      primary 017.0
    spinal cord 013.5
    spine or vertebra (column) 015.0 *[730.88]*
    strumous 017.2
    subdiaphragmatic 014.8
    testis 016.5
    thigh 017.9
    urinary 016.3
      kidney 016.0 *[590.81]*
    uterus 016.7
  accessory sinus — *see* Tuberculosis, sinus
  Addison's disease 017.6
  adenitis (*see also* Tuberculosis, lymph gland) 017.2
  adenoids 012.8
  adenopathy (*see also* Tuberculosis, lymph gland) 017.2
    tracheobronchial 012.1
      primary progressive 010.8
  adherent pericardium 017.9 *[420.0]*
  adnexa (uteri) 016.7
  adrenal (capsule) (gland) 017.6
  air passage NEC 012.8
  alimentary canal 014.8
  anemia 017.9
  ankle (joint) 015.8
    bone 015.5 *[730.87]*
  anus 014.8
  apex (*see also* Tuberculosis, pulmonary) 011.9
  apical (*see also* Tuberculosis, pulmonary) 011.9
  appendicitis 014.8
  appendix 014.8
  arachnoid 013.0
  artery 017.9
  arthritis (chronic) (synovial) 015.9 *[711.40]*
    ankle 015.8 *[730.87]*
    hip 015.1 *[711.45]*
    knee 015.2 *[711.46]*
    specified site NEC 015.8 *[711.48]*
    spine or vertebra (column) 015.0 *[720.81]*
    wrist 015.8 *[730.83]*
  articular — *see* Tuberculosis, joint
  ascites 014.0
  asthma (*see also* Tuberculosis, pulmonary) 011.9
  axilla, axillary 017.2
    gland 017.2
  bilateral (*see also* Tuberculosis, pulmonary) 011.9
  bladder 016.1
  bone (*see also* Osteomyelitis, due to, tuberculosis) 015.9 *[730.8]*
    hip 015.1 *[730.85]*
    knee 015.2 *[730.86]*
    limb NEC 015.5 *[730.88]*
    sacrum 015.0 *[730.88]*
    specified site NEC 015.7 *[730.88]*

Tuberculosis, tubercular, tuberculous—*continued*
  bone—*continued*
    spinal or vertebral column 015.0 *[730.88]*
  bowel 014.8
    miliary 018.9
  brain 013.2
  breast 017.9
  broad ligament 016.7
  bronchi, bronchial, bronchus 011.3
    ectasia, ectasis 011.5
    fistula 011.3
      primary, progressive 010.8
    gland 012.1
      primary, progressive 010.8
    isolated 012.2
    lymph gland or node 012.1
      primary, progressive 010.8
  bronchiectasis 011.5
  bronchitis 011.3
  bronchopleural 012.0
  bronchopneumonia, bronchopneumonic 011.6
  bronchorrhagia 011.3
  bronchotracheal 011.3
    isolated 012.2
  bronchus — *see* Tuberculosis, bronchi
  bronze disease (Addison's) 017.6
  buccal cavity 017.9
  bulbourethral gland 016.5
  bursa (*see also* Tuberculosis, joint) 015.9
  cachexia NEC (*see also* Tuberculosis, pulmonary) 011.9
  cardiomyopathy 017.9 *[425.8]*
  caries (*see also* Tuberculosis, bone) 015.9 *[730.8]*
  cartilage (*see also* Tuberculosis, bone) 015.9 *[730.8]*
    intervertebral 015.0 *[730.88]*
  catarrhal (*see also* Tuberculosis, pulmonary) 011.9
  cecum 014.8
  cellular tissue (primary) 017.0
  cellulitis (primary) 017.0
  central nervous system 013.9
    specified site NEC 013.8
  cerebellum (current) 013.2
  cerebral (current) 013.2
    meninges 013.0
  cerebrospinal 013.6
    meninges 013.0
  cerebrum (current) 013.2
  cervical 017.2
    gland 017.2
    lymph nodes 017.2
  cervicitis (uteri) 016.7
  cervix 016.7
  chest (*see also* Tuberculosis, pulmonary) 011.9
  childhood type or first infection 010.0
  choroid 017.3 *[363.13]*
  choroiditis 017.3 *[363.13]*
  ciliary body 017.3 *[364.11]*
  colitis 014.8
  colliers' 011.4
  colliquativa (primary) 017.0
  colon 014.8
    ulceration 014.8
  complex, primary 010.0
  complicating pregnancy, childbirth, or puerperium 647.3
    affecting fetus or newborn 760.2
  congenital 771.2
  conjunctiva 017.3 *[370.31]*
  connective tissue 017.9
    bone — *see* Tuberculosis, bone
  contact V01.1

Tuberculosis, tubercular, tuberculous—*continued*
converter (tuberculin test) (without disease) 795.5
cornea (ulcer) 017.3 *[370.31]*
Cowper's gland 016.5
coxae 015.1 *[730.85]*
coxalgia 015.1 *[730.85]*
cul-de-sac of Douglas 014.8
curvature, spine 015.0 *[737.40]*
cutis (colliquativa) (primary) 017.0
cyst, ovary 016.6
cystitis 016.1
dacryocystitis 017.3 *[375.32]*
dactylitis 015.5
diarrhea 014.8
diffuse (*see also* Tuberculosis, miliary) 018.9
   lung — *see* Tuberculosis, pulmonary
   meninges 013.0
digestive tract 014.8
disseminated (*see also* Tuberculosis, miliary) 018.9
   meninges 013.0
duodenum 014.8
dura (mater) 013.9
   abscess 013.8
     cerebral 013.3
     spinal 013.5
dysentery 014.8
ear (inner) (middle) 017.4
   bone 015.6
   external (primary) 017.0
   skin (primary) 017.0
elbow 015.8
emphysema — *see* Tuberculosis, pulmonary
empyema 012.0
encephalitis 013.6
endarteritis 017.9
endocarditis (any valve) 017.9 *[424.91]*
endocardium (any valve) 017.9 *[424.91]*
endocrine glands NEC 017.9
endometrium 016.7
enteric, enterica 014.8
enteritis 014.8
enterocolitis 014.8
epididymis 016.4
epididymitis 016.4
epidural abscess 013.8
   brain 013.3
   spinal cord 013.5
epiglottis 012.3
episcleritis 017.3 *[379.00]*
erythema (induratum) (nodosum) (primary) 017.1
esophagus 017.8
Eustachian tube 017.4
exposure to V01.1
exudative 012.0
   primary, progressive 010.1
eye 017.3
   glaucoma 017.3 *[365.62]*
eyelid (primary) 017.0
   lupus 017.0 *[373.4]*
fallopian tube 016.6
fascia 017.9
fauces 012.8
finger 017.9
first infection 010.0
fistula, perirectal 014.8
Florida 011.6
foot 017.9
funnel pelvis 137.3
gallbladder 017.9
galloping (*see also* Tuberculosis, pulmonary) 011.9
ganglionic 015.9
gastritis 017.9
gastrocolic fistula 014.8
gastroenteritis 014.8
gastrointestinal tract 014.8

Tuberculosis, tubercular, tuberculous—*continued*
general, generalized 018.9
   acute 018.0
   chronic 018.8
genital organs NEC 016.9
   female 016.7
   male 016.5
genitourinary NEC 016.9
genu 015.2
glandulae suprarenalis 017.6
glandular, general 017.2
glottis 012.3
grinders' 011.4
groin 017.2
gum 017.9
hand 017.9
heart 017.9 *[425.8]*
hematogenous — *see* Tuberculosis, miliary
hemoptysis (*see also* Tuberculosis, pulmonary) 011.9
hemorrhage NEC (*see also* Tuberculosis, pulmonary) 011.9
hemothorax 012.0
hepatitis 017.9
hilar lymph nodes 012.1
   primary, progressive 010.8
hip (disease) (joint) 015.1
   bone 015.1 *[730.85]*
hydrocephalus 013.8
hydropneumothorax 012.0
hydrothorax 012.0
hypoadrenalism 017.6
hypopharynx 012.8
ileocecal (hyperplastic) 014.8
ileocolitis 014.8
ileum 014.8
iliac spine (superior) 015.0 *[730.88]*
incipient NEC (*see also* Tuberculosis, pulmonary) 011.9
indurativa (primary) 017.1
infantile 017.0
infection NEC 011.9
   without clinical manifestation 010.0
infraclavicular gland 017.2
inguinal gland 017.2
inguinalis 017.2
intestine (any part) 014.8
iris 017.3 *[364.11]*
iritis 017.3 *[364.11]*
ischiorectal 014.8
jaw 015.7 *[730.88]*
jejunum 014.8
joint 015.9
   hip 015.1
   knee 015.2
   specified site NEC 015.8
   vertebral 015.0 *[730.88]*
keratitis 017.3 *[370.31]*
   interstitial 017.3 *[370.59]*
keratoconjunctivitis 017.3 *[370.31]*
kidney 016.0
knee (joint) 015.2
kyphoscoliosis 015.0 *[737.43]*
kyphosis 015.0 *[737.41]*
lacrimal apparatus, gland 017.3
laryngitis 012.3
larynx 012.3
leptomeninges, leptomeningitis (cerebral) (spinal) 013.0
lichenoides (primary) 017.0
linguae 017.9
lip 017.9
liver 017.9
lordosis 015.0 *[737.42]*
lung — *see* Tuberculosis, pulmonary
luposa 017.0
   eyelid 017.0 *[373.4]*
lymphadenitis — *see* Tuberculosis, lymph gland

Tuberculosis, tubercular, tuberculous—*continued*
lymphangitis — *see* Tuberculosis, lymph gland
lymphatic (gland) (vessel) — *see* Tuberculosis, lymph gland
lymph gland or node (peripheral) 017.2
   abdomen 014.8
   bronchial 012.1
     primary, progressive 010.8
   cervical 017.2
   hilar 012.1
     primary, progressive 010.8
   intrathoracic 012.1
     primary, progressive 010.8
   mediastinal 012.1
     primary, progressive 010.8
   mesenteric 014.8
   peripheral 017.2
   retroperitoneal 014.8
   tracheobronchial 012.1
     primary, progressive 010.8
malignant NEC (*see also* Tuberculosis, pulmonary) 011.9
mammary gland 017.9
marasmus NEC (*see also* Tuberculosis, pulmonary) 011.9
mastoiditis 015.6
maternal, affecting fetus or newborn 760.2
mediastinal (lymph) gland or node 012.1
   primary, progressive 010.8
mediastinitis 012.8
   primary, progressive 010.8
mediastinopericarditis 017.9 *[420.0]*
mediastinum 012.8
   primary, progressive 010.8
medulla 013.9
   brain 013.2
   spinal cord 013.4
melanosis, Addisonian 017.6
membrane, brain 013.0
meninges (cerebral) (spinal) 013.0
meningitis (basilar) (brain) (cerebral) (cerebrospinal) (spinal) 013.0
meningoencephalitis 013.0
mesentery, mesenteric 014.8
   lymph gland or node 014.8
miliary (any site) 018.9
   acute 018.0
   chronic 018.8
   specified type NEC 018.8
millstone makers' 011.4
miners' 011.4
moulders' 011.4
mouth 017.9
multiple 018.9
   acute 018.0
   chronic 018.8
muscle 017.9
myelitis 013.6
myocarditis 017.9 *[422.0]*
myocardium 017.9 *[422.0]*
nasal (passage) (sinus) 012.8
nasopharynx 012.8
neck gland 017.2
nephritis 016.0 *[583.81]*
nerve 017.9
nose (septum) 012.8
ocular 017.3
old NEC 137.0
   without residuals V12.01 ◆
omentum 014.8
oophoritis (acute) (chronic) 016.6
optic 017.3 *[377.39]*
   nerve trunk 017.3 *[377.39]*
   papilla, papillae 017.3 *[377.39]*
orbit 017.3
orchitis 016.5 *[608.81]*
organ, specified NEC 017.9

Tuberculosis, tubercular, tuberculous—*continued*
orificialis (primary) 017.0
osseous (*see also* Tuberculosis, bone) 015.9 *[730.8]*
osteitis (*see also* Tuberculosis, bone) 015.9 *[730.8]*
osteomyelitis (*see also* Tuberculosis, bone) 015.9 *[730.8]*
otitis (media) 017.4
ovaritis (acute) (chronic) 016.6
ovary (acute) (chronic) 016.6
oviducts (acute) (chronic) 016.6
pachymeningitis 013.0
palate (soft) 017.9
pancreas 017.9
papulonecrotic (primary) 017.0
parathyroid glands 017.9
paronychia (primary) 017.0
parotid gland or region 017.9
pelvic organ NEC 016.9
   female 016.7
   male 016.5
pelvis (bony) 015.7 *[730.85]*
penis 016.5
peribronchitis 011.3
pericarditis 017.9 *[420.0]*
pericardium 017.9 *[420.0]*
perichondritis, larynx 012.3
perineum 017.9
periostitis (*see also* Tuberculosis, bone) 015.9 *[730.8]*
periphlebitis 017.9
   eye vessel 017.3 *[362.18]*
   retina 017.3 *[362.18]*
perirectal fistula 014.8
peritoneal gland 014.8
peritoneum 014.0
peritonitis 014.0
pernicious NEC (*see also* Tuberculosis, pulmonary) 011.9
pharyngitis 012.8
pharynx 012.8
phlyctenulosis (conjunctiva) 017.3 *[370.31]*
phthisis NEC (*see also* Tuberculosis, pulmonary) 011.9
pituitary gland 017.9
placenta 016.7
pleura, pleural, pleurisy, pleuritis (fibrinous) (obliterative) (purulent) (simple plastic) (with effusion) 012.0
   primary, progressive 010.1
pneumonia, pneumonic 011.6
pneumothorax 011.7
polyserositis 018.9
   acute 018.0
   chronic 018.8
potters' 011.4
prepuce 016.5
primary 010.9
   complex 010.0
   complicated 010.8
     with pleurisy or effusion 010.1
   progressive 010.8
     with pleurisy or effusion 010.1
   skin 017.0
proctitis 014.8
prostate 016.5 *[601.4]*
prostatitis 016.5 *[601.4]*
pulmonaris (*see also* Tuberculosis, pulmonary) 011.9
pulmonary (artery) (incipient) (malignant) (multiple round foci) (pernicious) (reinfection stage) 011.9
   cavitated or with cavitation 011.2
     primary, progressive 010.8
   childhood type or first infection 010.0

Tuberculosis, tubercular, tuberculous—continued
　pulmonary—continued
　　chromogenic acid-fast bacilli 795.3
　　fibrosis or fibrotic 011.4
　　infiltrative 011.0
　　　primary, progressive 010.9
　　nodular 011.1
　　specified NEC 011.8
　　sputum positive only 795.3
　　status following surgical collapse of lung NEC 011.9
　pyelitis 016.0 [590.81]
　pyelonephritis 016.0 [590.81]
　pyemia — see Tuberculosis, miliary
　pyonephrosis 016.0
　pyopneumothorax 012.0
　pyothorax 012.0
　rectum (with abscess) 014.8
　　fistula 014.8
　reinfection stage (see also Tuberculosis, pulmonary) 011.9
　renal 016.0
　renis 016.0
　reproductive organ 016.7
　respiratory NEC (see also Tuberculosis, pulmonary) 011.9
　　specified site NEC 012.8
　retina 017.3 [363.13]
　retroperitoneal (lymph gland or node) 014.8
　　gland 014.8
　retropharyngeal abscess 012.8
　rheumatism 015.9
　rhinitis 012.8
　sacroiliac (joint) 015.8
　sacrum 015.0 [730.88]
　salivary gland 017.9
　salpingitis (acute) (chronic) 016.6
　sandblasters' 011.4
　sclera 017.3 [379.09]
　scoliosis 015.0 [737.43]
　scrofulous 017.2
　scrotum 016.5
　seminal tract or vesicle 016.5 [608.81]
　senile NEC (see also Tuberculosis, pulmonary) 011.9
　septic NEC (see also Tuberculosis, miliary) 018.9
　shoulder 015.8
　　blade 015.7 [730.8]
　sigmoid 014.8
　sinus (accessory) (nasal) 012.8
　　bone 015.7 [730.88]
　　epididymis 016.4
　skeletal NEC (see also Osteomyelitis, due to tuberculosis) 015.9 [730.8]
　skin (any site) (primary) 017.0
　small intestine 014.8
　soft palate 017.9
　spermatic cord 016.5
　spinal
　　column 015.0 [730.88]
　　cord 013.4
　　disease 015.0 [730.88]
　　medulla 013.4
　　membrane 013.0
　　meninges 013.0
　spine 015.0 [730.88]
　spleen 017.7
　splenitis 017.7
　spondylitis 015.0 [720.81]
　spontaneous pneumothorax — see Tuberculosis, pulmonary
　sternoclavicular joint 015.8
　stomach 017.9
　stonemasons' 011.4
　struma 017.2

Tuberculosis, tubercular, tuberculous—continued
　subcutaneous tissue (cellular) (primary) 017.0
　subcutis (primary) 017.0
　subdeltoid bursa 017.9
　submaxillary 017.9
　　region 017.9
　supraclavicular gland 017.2
　suprarenal (capsule) (gland) 017.6
　swelling, joint (see also Tuberculosis, joint) 015.9
　symphysis pubis 015.7 [730.88]
　synovitis 015.9 [727.01]
　　hip 015.1 [727.01]
　　knee 015.2 [727.01]
　　specified site NEC 015.8 [727.01]
　　spine or vertebra 015.0 [727.01]
　systemic — see Tuberculosis, miliary
　tarsitis (eyelid) 017.0 [373.4]
　ankle (bone) 015.5 [730.87]
　tendon (sheath) — see Tuberculosis, tenosynovitis
　tenosynovitis 015.9 [727.01]
　　hip 015.1 [727.01]
　　knee 015.2 [727.01]
　　specified site NEC 015.8 [727.01]
　　spine or vertebra 015.0 [727.01]
　testis 016.5 [608.81]
　throat 012.8
　thymus gland 017.9
　thyroid gland 017.5
　toe 017.9
　tongue 017.9
　tonsil (lingual) 012.8
　tonsillitis 012.8
　trachea, tracheal 012.8
　　gland 012.1
　　　primary, progressive 010.8
　　isolated 012.2
　tracheobronchial 011.3
　　glandular 012.1
　　　primary, progressive 010.8
　　isolated 012.2
　　lymph gland or node 012.1
　　　primary, progressive 010.8
　tubal 016.6
　tunica vaginalis 016.5
　typhlitis 014.8
　ulcer (primary) (skin) 017.0
　　bowel or intestine 014.8
　　specified site NEC — see Tuberculosis, by site
　unspecified site — see Tuberculosis, pulmonary
　ureter 016.3
　urethra, urethral 016.3
　urinary organ or tract 016.3
　　kidney 016.0
　uterus 016.7
　uveal tract 017.3 [363.13]
　uvula 017.9
　vaccination, prophylactic (against) V03.2
　vagina 016.7
　vas deferens 016.5
　vein 017.9
　verruca (primary) 017.0
　verrucosa (cutis) (primary) 017.0
　vertebra (column) 015.0 [730.88]
　vesiculitis 016.5 [608.81]
　viscera NEC 014.8
　vulva 016.7 [616.51]
　wrist (joint) 015.8
　　bone 015.5 [730.83]

Tuberculum
　auriculae 744.29
　occlusal 520.2
　paramolare 520.2

Tuberous sclerosis (brain) 759.5

Tubo-ovarian — see condition

Tuboplasty, after previous sterilization V26.0

Tubotympanitis 381.10

Tularemia 021.9
　with
　　conjunctivitis 021.3
　　pneumonia 021.2
　bronchopneumonic 021.2
　conjunctivitis 021.3
　cryptogenic 021.1
　disseminated 021.8
　enteric 021.1
　generalized 021.8
　glandular 021.8
　intestinal 021.1
　oculoglandular 021.3
　ophthalmic 021.3
　pneumonia 021.2
　pulmonary 021.2
　specified NEC 021.8
　typhoidal 021.1
　ulceroglandular 021.0
　vaccination, prophylactic (against) V03.4

Tularensis conjunctivitis 021.3

Tumefaction — see also Swelling
　liver (see also Hypertrophy, liver) 789.1

Tumor (M8000/1) — see also Neoplasm, by site, unspecified nature
　Abrikossov's (M9580/0) — see also Neoplasm, connective tissue, benign
　　malignant (M9580/3) — see Neoplasm, connective tissue, malignant
　acinar cell (M8550/1) — see Neoplasm, by site, uncertain behavior
　acinic cell (M8550/1) — see Neoplasm, by site, uncertain behavior
　adenomatoid (M9054/0) — see also Neoplasm, by site, benign
　　odontogenic (M9300/0) 213.1
　　upper jaw (bone) 213.0
　adnexal (skin) (M8390/0) — see Neoplasm, skin, benign
　adrenal
　　cortical (benign) (M8370/0) 227.0
　　malignant (M8370/3) 194.0
　　rest (M8671/0) — see Neoplasm, by site, benign
　alpha cell (M8152/0)
　　malignant (M8152/3)
　　　pancreas 157.4
　　　specified site NEC — see Neoplasm, by site, malignant
　　　unspecified site 157.4
　　pancreas 211.7
　　specified site NEC — see Neoplasm, by site, benign
　　unspecified site 211.7
　aneurysmal (see also Aneurysm) 442.9
　aortic body (M8691/1) 237.3
　　malignant (M8691/3) 194.6
　argentaffin (M8241/1) — see Neoplasm, by site, uncertain behavior
　basal cell (M8090/1) — see also Neoplasm, skin, uncertain behavior
　benign (M8000/0) — see Neoplasm, by site, benign

Tumor—continued
　beta cell (M8151/0)
　　malignant (M8151/3)
　　　pancreas 157.4
　　　specified site — see Neoplasm, by site, malignant
　　　unspecified site 157.4
　　pancreas 211.7
　　specified site NEC — see Neoplasm, by site, benign
　　unspecified site 211.7
　blood — see Hematoma
　brenner (M9000/0) 220
　　borderline malignancy (M9000/1) 236.2
　　malignant (M9000/3) 183.0
　　proliferating (M9000/1) 236.2
　Brooke's (M8100/0) — see Neoplasm, skin, benign
　brown fat (M8880/0) — see Lipoma, by site
　Burkitt's (M9750/3) 200.2
　calcifying epithelial odontogenic (M9340/0) 213.1
　　upper jaw (bone) 213.0
　carcinoid (M8240/1) — see Carcinoid
　carotid body (M8692/1) 237.3
　　malignant (M8692/3) 194.5
　Castleman's (mediastinal lymph node hyperplasia) 785.6
　cells (M8001/1) — see also Neoplasm, by site, unspecified nature
　　benign (M8001/0) — see Neoplasm, by site, benign
　　malignant (M8001/3) — see Neoplasm, by site, malignant
　　uncertain whether benign or malignant (M8001/1) — see Neoplasm, by site, uncertain nature
　cervix
　　in pregnancy or childbirth 654.6
　　　affecting fetus or newborn 763.8
　　causing obstructed labor 660.2
　　　affecting fetus or newborn 763.1
　chondromatous giant cell (M9230/0) — see Neoplasm, bone, benign
　chromaffin (M8700/0) — see also Neoplasm, by site, benign
　　malignant (M8700/3) — see Neoplasm, by site, malignant
　Cock's peculiar 706.2
　Codman's (benign chondroblastoma) (M9230/0) — see Neoplasm, bone, benign
　dentigerous, mixed (M9282/0) 213.1
　　upper jaw (bone) 213.0
　dermoid (M9084/0) — see Neoplasm, by site, benign
　　with malignant transformation (M9084/3) 183.0
　desmoid (extra-abdominal) (M8821/1) — see also Neoplasm, connective tissue, uncertain behavior
　　abdominal (M8822/1) — see Neoplasm, connective tissue, uncertain behavior
　embryonal (mixed) (M9080/1) — see also Neoplasm, by site, uncertain behavior
　　liver (M9080/3) 155.0

Tumor—*continued*
- endodermal sinus (M9071/3)
  - specified site — *see* Neoplasm, by site, malignant
  - unspecified site
    - female 183.0
    - male 186.9
- epithelial
  - benign (M8010/0) — *see* Neoplasm, by site, benign
  - malignant (M8010/3) — *see* Neoplasm, by site, malignant
- Ewing's (M9260/3) — *see* Neoplasm, bone, malignant
- fatty — *see* Lipoma
- fetal, causing disproportion 653.7
  - causing obstructed labor 660.1
- fibroid (M8890/0) — *see* Leiomyoma
- G cell (M8153/1)
  - malignant (M8153/3)
    - pancreas 157.4
    - specified site NEC — *see* Neoplasm, by site, malignant
    - unspecified site 157.4
  - specified site — *see* Neoplasm, by site, uncertain behavior
  - unspecified site 235.5
- giant cell (type) (M8003/1) — *see also* Neoplasm, by site, unspecified nature
  - bone (M9250/1) 238.0
    - malignant (M9250/3) — *see* Neoplasm, bone, malignant
  - chondromatous (M9230/0) — *see* Neoplasm, bone, benign
  - malignant (M8003/3) — *see* Neoplasm, by site, malignant
  - peripheral (gingiva) 523.8
  - soft parts (M9251/1) — *see also* Neoplasm, connective tissue, uncertain behavior
    - malignant (M9251/3) — *see* Neoplasm, connective tissue, malignant
  - tendon sheath 727.02
- glomus (M8711/0) — *see also* Hemangioma, by site
  - jugulare (M8690/1) 237.3
    - malignant (M8690/3) 194.6
- gonadal stromal (M8590/1) — *see* Neoplasm, by site, uncertain behavior
- granular cell (M9580/0) — *see also* Neoplasm, connective tissue, benign
  - malignant (M9580/3) — *see* Neoplasm, connective tissue, malignant
- granulosa cell (M8620/1) 236.2
  - malignant (M8620/3) 183.0
- granulosa cell-theca cell (M8621/1) 236.2
  - malignant (M8621/3) 183.0
- Grawitz's (hypernephroma) (M8312/3) 189.0
- hazard-crile (M8350/3) 193
- hemorrhoidal — *see* Hemorrhoids
- hilar cell (M8660/0) 220
- hurthle cell (benign) (M8290/0) 226
  - malignant (M8290/3) 193
- hydatid (*see also* Echinococcus) 122.9
- hypernephroid (M8311/1) — *see also* Neoplasm, by site, uncertain behavior

Tumor—*continued*
- interstitial cell (M8650/1) — *see also* Neoplasm, by site, uncertain behavior
  - benign (M8650/0) — *see* Neoplasm, by site, benign
  - malignant (M8650/3) — *see* Neoplasm, by site, malignant
- islet cell (M8150/0)
  - malignant (M8150/3)
    - pancreas 157.4
    - specified site — *see* Neoplasm, by site, malignant
    - unspecified site 157.4
  - pancreas 211.7
  - specified site NEC — *see* Neoplasm, by site, benign
  - unspecified site 211.7
- juxtaglomerular (M8361/1) 236.91
- Krukenberg's (M8490/6) 198.6
- Leydig cell (M8650/1)
  - benign (M8650/0)
    - specified site — *see* Neoplasm, by site, benign
    - unspecified site
      - female 220
      - male 222.0
  - malignant (M8650/3)
    - specified site — *see* Neoplasm, by site, malignant
    - unspecified site
      - female 183.0
      - male 186.9
  - specified site — *see* Neoplasm, by site, uncertain behavior
  - unspecified site
    - female 236.2
    - male 236.4
- lipid cell, ovary (M8670/0) 220
- lipoid cell, ovary (M8670/0) 220
- lymphomatous, benign (M9590/0) — *see also* Neoplasm, by site, benign
- Malherbe's (M8110/0) — *see* Neoplasm, skin, benign
- malignant (M8000/3) — *see also* Neoplasm, by site, malignant
  - fusiform cell (type) (M8004/3) — *see* Neoplasm, by site, malignant
  - giant cell (type) (M8003/3) — *see* Neoplasm, by site, malignant
  - mixed NEC (M8940/3) — *see* Neoplasm, by site, malignant
  - small cell (type) (M8002/3) — *see* Neoplasm, by site, malignant
  - spindle cell (type) (M8004/3) — *see* Neoplasm, by site, malignant
- mast cell (M9740/1) 238.5
  - malignant (M9740/3) 202.6
- melanotic, neuroectodermal (M9363/0) — *see* Neoplasm, by site, benign
- mesenchymal
  - malignant (M8800/3) — *see* Neoplasm, connective tissue, malignant
  - mixed (M8990/1) — *see* Neoplasm, connective tissue, uncertain behavior

Tumor—*continued*
- mesodermal, mixed (M8951/3) — *see also* Neoplasm, by site, malignant
  - liver 155.0
- mesonephric (M9110/1) — *see also* Neoplasm, by site, uncertain behavior
  - malignant (M9110/3) — *see* Neoplasm, by site, malignant
- metastatic
  - from specified site (M8000/3) — *see* Neoplasm, by site, malignant
  - to specified site (M8000/6) — *see* Neoplasm, by site, malignant, secondary
- mixed NEC (M8940/0) — *see also* Neoplasm, by site, benign
  - malignant (M8940/3) — *see* Neoplasm, by site, malignant
- mucocarcinoid, malignant (M8243/3) — *see* Neoplasm, by site, malignant
- mucoepidermoid (M8430/1) — *see* Neoplasm, by site, uncertain behavior
- Mullerian, mixed (M8950/3) — *see* Neoplasm, by site, malignant
- myoepithelial (M8982/0) — *see* Neoplasm, by site, benign
- neurogenic olfactory (M9520/3) 160.0
- nonencapsulated sclerosing (M8350/3) 193
- odontogenic (M9270/1) 238.0
  - adenomatoid (M9300/0) 213.1
    - upper jaw (bone) 213.0
  - benign (M9270/0) 213.1
    - upper jaw (bone) 213.0
  - calcifying epithelial (M9340/0) 213.1
    - upper jaw (bone) 213.0
  - malignant (M9270/3) 170.1
    - upper jaw (bone) 170.0
  - squamous (M9312/0) 213.1
    - upper jaw (bone) 213.0
- ovarian stromal (M8590/1) 236.2
- ovary
  - in pregnancy or childbirth 654.4
    - affecting fetus or newborn 763.8
    - causing obstructed labor 660.2
      - affecting fetus or newborn 763.1
- pacinian (M9507/0) — *see* Neoplasm, skin, benign
- Pancoast's (M8010/3) 162.3
- papillary — *see* Papilloma
- pelvic, in pregnancy or childbirth 654.9
  - affecting fetus or newborn 763.8
  - causing obstructed labor 660.2
    - affecting fetus or newborn 763.1
- phantom 300.11
- plasma cell (M9731/1) 238.6
  - benign (M9731/0) — *see* Neoplasm, by site, benign
  - malignant (M9731/3) 203.8
- polyvesicular vitelline (M9071/3)
  - specified site — *see* Neoplasm, by site, malignant
  - unspecified site
    - female 183.0
    - male 186.9
- Pott's puffy (*see also* Osteomyelitis) 730.2

Tumor—*continued*
- Rathke's pouch (M9350/1) 237.0
- regaud's (M8082/3) — *see* Neoplasm, nasopharynx, malignant
- rete cell (M8140/0) 222.0
- retinal anlage (M9363/0) — *see* Neoplasm, by site, benign
- Rokitansky's 620.2
- salivary gland type, mixed (M8940/0) — *see also* Neoplasm, by site, benign
  - malignant (M8940/3) — *see* Neoplasm, by site, malignant
- Sampson's 617.1
- Schloffer's (*see also* Peritonitis) 567.2
- Schmincke (M8082/3) — *see* Neoplasm, nasopharynx, malignant
- sebaceous (*see also* Cyst, sebaceous) 706.2
- secondary (M8000/6) — *see* Neoplasm, by site, secondary
- Sertoli cell (M8640/0)
  - with lipid storage (M8641/0)
    - specified site — *see* Neoplasm, by site, benign
    - unspecified site
      - female 220
      - male 222.0
  - specified site — *see* Neoplasm, by site, benign
  - unspecified site
    - female 220
    - male 222.0
- Sertoli-Leydig cell (M8631/0)
  - specified site, — *see* Neoplasm, by site, benign
  - unspecified site
    - female 220
    - male 222.0
- sex cord (-stromal) (M8590/1) — *see* Neoplasm, by site, uncertain behavior
- skin appendage (M8390/0) — *see* Neoplasm, skin, benign
- soft tissue
  - benign (M8800/0) — *see* Neoplasm, connective tissue, benign
  - malignant (M8800/3) — *see* Neoplasm, connective tissue, malignant
- sternomastoid 754.1
- superior sulcus (lung) (pulmonary) (syndrome) (M8010/3) 162.3
- suprasulcus (M8010/3) 162.3
- sweat gland (M8400/1) — *see also* Neoplasm, skin, uncertain behavior
  - benign (M8400/0) — *see* Neoplasm, skin, benign
  - malignant (M8400/3) — *see* Neoplasm, skin, malignant
- syphilitic brain 094.89
  - congenital 090.49
- testicular stromal (M8590/1) 236.4
- theca cell (M8600/0) 220
- theca cell-granulosa cell (M8621/1) 236.2
- theca-lutein (M8610/0) 220
- turban (M8200/0) 216.4

Tumor—continued
  uterus
    in pregnancy or childbirth 654.1
      affecting fetus or newborn 763.8
      causing obstructed labor 660.2
        affecting fetus or newborn 763.1
  vagina
    in pregnancy or childbirth 654.7
      affecting fetus or newborn 763.8
      causing obstructed labor 660.2
        affecting fetus or newborn 763.1
  varicose (see also Varicose, vein) 454.9
  von Recklinghausen's (M9540/1) 237.71
  vulva
    in pregnancy or childbirth 654.8
      affecting fetus or newborn 763.8
      causing obstructed labor 660.2
        affecting fetus or newborn 763.1
  Warthin's (salivary gland) (M8561/0) 210.2
  white — see also Tuberculosis, arthritis
  White-Darier 757.39
  Wilms' (nephroblastoma) (M8960/3) 189.0
  yolk sac (M9071/3)
    specified site — see Neoplasm, by site, malignant
    unspecified site
      female 183.0
      male 186.9

Tumorlet (M8040/1) — see Neoplasm, by site, uncertain behavior
Tungiasis 134.1
Tunica vasculosa lentis 743.39
Tunnel vision 368.45
Turban tumor (M8200/0) 216.4
Türck's trachoma (chronic catarrhal laryngitis) 476.0
Türk's syndrome (ocular retraction syndrome) 378.71
Turner's
  hypoplasia (tooth) 520.4
  syndrome 758.6
  tooth 520.4
Turner-Kieser syndrome (hereditary osteo-onychodysplasia) 756.89
Turner-Varny syndrome 758.6
Turricephaly 756.0
Tussis convulsiva (see also Whooping cough) 033.9
Twin
  affected by maternal complications of pregnancy 761.5
  conjoined 759.4
  healthy liveborn — see Newborn, twin
  pregnancy (complicating delivery) NEC 651.0
    with fetal loss and retention of one fetus 651.3
Twinning, teeth 520.2
Twist, twisted
  bowel, colon, or intestine 560.2
  hair (congenital) 757.4
  mesentery 560.2

Twist, twisted—continued
  omentum 560.2
  organ or site, congenital NEC — see Anomaly, specified type NEC
  ovarian pedicle 620.5
    congenital 752.0
  umbilical cord — see Compression, umbilical cord
Twitch 781.0
Tylosis 700
  buccalis 528.6
  gingiva 523.8
  linguae 528.6
  palmaris et plantaris 757.39
Tympanism 787.3
Tympanites (abdominal) (intestine) 787.3
Tympanitis — see Myringitis
Tympanosclerosis 385.00
  involving
    combined sites NEC 385.09
      with tympanic membrane 385.03
    tympanic membrane 385.01
      with ossicles 385.02
        and middle ear 385.03
Tympanum — see condition
Tympany
  abdomen 787.3
  chest 786.7
Typhlitis (see also Appendicitis) 541
Typhoenteritis 002.0
Typhogastric fever 002.0
Typhoid (abortive) (ambulant) (any site) (fever) (hemorrhagic) (infection) (intermittent) (malignant) (rheumatic) 002.0
  with pneumonia 002.0 [484.8]
  abdominal 002.0
  carrier (suspected) of V02.1
  cholecystitis (current) 002.0
  clinical (Widal and blood test negative) 002.0
  endocarditis 002.0 [421.1]
  inoculation reaction — see Complications, vaccination
  meningitis 002.0 [320.7]
  mesenteric lymph nodes 002.0
  myocarditis 002.0 [422.0]
  osteomyelitis (see also Osteomyelitis, due to, typhoid) 002.0 [730.8]
  perichondritis, larynx 002.0 [478.71]
  pneumonia 002.0 [484.8]
  spine 002.0 [720.81]
  ulcer (perforating) 002.0
  vaccination, prophylactic (against) V03.1
  Widal negative 002.0
Typhomalaria (fever) (see also Malaria) 084.6
Typhomania 002.0
Typhoperitonitis 002.0
Typhus (fever) 081.9
  abdominal, abdominalis 002.0
  African tick 082.1
  amarillic (see also Fever, Yellow) 060.9
  brain 081.9
  cerebral 081.9
  classical 080
  endemic (flea-borne) 081.0
  epidemic (louse-borne) 080
  exanthematic NEC 080
  exanthematicus SAI 080
    brillii SAI 081.1
    Mexicanus SAI 081.0
    pediculo vestimenti causa 080
    typhus murinus 081.0
  flea-borne 081.0
  Indian tick 082.1

Typhus—continued
  Kenya tick 082.1
  louse-borne 080
  Mexican 081.0
    flea-borne 081.0
    louse-borne 080
    tabardillo 080
  mite-borne 081.2
  murine 081.0
  North Asian tick-borne 082.2
  petechial 081.9
  Queensland tick 082.3
  rat 081.0
  recrudescent 081.1
  recurrent (see also Fever, relapsing) 087.9
  São Paulo 082.0
  scrub (China) (India) (Malaya) (New Guinea) 081.2
  shop (of Malaya) 081.0
  Siberian tick 082.2
  tick-borne NEC 082.9
  tropical 081.2
  vaccination, prophylactic (against) V05.8
Tyrosinosis (Medes) (Sakai) 270.2
Tyrosinuria 270.2
Tyrosyluria 270.2

U

Uehlinger's syndrome (acropachyderma) 757.39
Uhl's anomaly or disease (hypoplasia of myocardium, right ventricle) 746.84
Ulcer, ulcerated, ulcerating, ulceration, ulcerative 707.9
  with gangrene 707.9 [785.4]
  abdomen (wall) (see also Ulcer, skin) 707.8
  ala, nose 478.1
  alveolar process 526.5
  amebic (intestine) 006.9
    skin 006.6
  anastomotic — see Ulcer, gastrojejunal
  anorectal 569.41
  antral — see Ulcer, stomach
  anus (sphincter) (solitary) 569.41
    varicose — see Varicose, ulcer, anus
  aphthous (oral) (recurrent) 528.2
    genital organ(s)
      female 616.8
      male 608.89
    mouth 528.2
  arm (see also Ulcer, skin) 707.8
  artery NEC 447.2
    without rupture 447.8
  arteriosclerotic plaque — see Arteriosclerosis, by site
  atrophic NEC — see Ulcer, skin
  Barrett's (chronic peptic ulcer of esophagus) 530.2
  bile duct 576.8
  bladder (solitary) (sphincter) 596.8
    bilharzial (see also Schistosomiasis) 120.9 [595.4]
    submucosal (see also Cystitis) 595.1
    tuberculous (see also Tuberculosis) 016.1
  bleeding NEC — see Ulcer, peptic, with hemorrhage
  bone 730.9
  bowel (see also Ulcer, intestine) 569.82
  breast 611.0
  bronchitis 491.8
  bronchus 519.1
  buccal (cavity) (traumatic) 528.9

Ulcer, ulcerated, ulcerating, ulceration, ulcerative—continued
  burn (acute) — see Ulcer, duodenum
  Buruli 031.1
  buttock (see also Ulcer, skin) 707.8
  decubitus (see also Ulcer, decubitus) 707.0
  cancerous (M8000/3) — see Neoplasm, by site, malignant
  cardia — see Ulcer, stomach
  cardio-esophageal (peptic) 530.2
  cecum (see also Ulcer, intestine) 569.82
  cervix (uteri) (trophic) 622.0
    with mention of cervicitis 616.0
  chancroidal 099.0
  chest (wall) (see also Ulcer, skin) 707.8
  Chiclero 085.4
  chin (pyogenic) (see also Ulcer, skin) 707.8
  chronic (cause unknown) — see also Ulcer, skin
    penis 607.89
  Cochin-China 085.1
  colitis — see Colitis, ulcerative ◆
  colon (see also Ulcer, intestine) 569.82
  conjunctiva (acute) (postinfectional) 372.00
  cornea (infectional) 370.00
    with perforation 370.06
    annular 370.02
    catarrhal 370.01
    central 370.03
    dendritic 054.42
    marginal 370.01
    mycotic 370.05
    phlyctenular, tuberculous (see also Tuberculosis) 017.3 [370.31]
    ring 370.02
    rodent 370.07
    serpent, serpiginous 370.04
    superficial marginal 370.01
    tuberculous (see also Tuberculosis) 017.3 [370.31]
  corpus cavernosum (chronic) 607.89
  crural — see Ulcer, lower extremity
  Curling's — see Ulcer, duodenum
  Cushing's — see Ulcer, peptic
  cystitis (interstitial) 595.1
  decubitus (any site) 707.0
    with gangrene 707.0 [785.4]
  dendritic 054.42
  diabetes, diabetic (mellitus) 250.8 [707.9]
    lower limb 250.8 [707.1]
    specified site NEC 250.8 [707.8]
  Dieulafoy's — see Ulcer, stomach
  due to
    infection NEC — see Ulcer, skin
    radiation, radium — see Ulcer, by site
    trophic disturbance (any region) — see Ulcer, skin
    x-ray — see Ulcer, by site
  duodenum, duodenal (eroded) (peptic) 532.9

Ulcer

Ulcer, ulcerated, ulcerating, ulceration, ulcerative—
continued

> Note — *Use the following fifth-digit subclassification with categories 531-534:*
>
> 0   without mention of obstruction
> 1   with obstruction

  with
    hemorrhage (chronic) 532.4
      and perforation 532.6
    perforation (chronic) 532.5
      and hemorrhage 532.6
  acute 532.3
    with
      hemorrhage 532.0
        and perforation 532.2
      perforation 532.1
        and hemorrhage 532.2
  bleeding (recurrent) — *see* Ulcer, duodenum, with hemorrhage
  chronic 532.7
    with
      hemorrhage 532.4
        and perforation 532.6
      perforation 532.5
        and hemorrhage 532.6
  penetrating — *see* Ulcer, duodenum, with perforation
  perforating — *see* Ulcer, duodenum, with perforation
dysenteric NEC 009.0
elusive 595.1
endocarditis (any valve) (acute) (chronic) (subacute) 421.0
enteritis — *see* Colitis, ulcerative
enterocolitis 556.0
epiglottis 478.79
esophagus (peptic) 530.2
  due to ingestion
    aspirin 530.2
    chemicals 530.2
    medicinal agents 530.2
  fungal 530.2
  infectional 530.2
  varicose (*see also* Varix, esophagus) 456.1
    bleeding (*see also* Varix, esophagus, bleeding) 456.0
eye NEC 360.00
  dendritic 054.42
eyelid (region) 373.01
face (*see also* Ulcer, skin) 707.8
fauces 478.29
Fenwick (-Hunner) (solitary) (*see also* Cystitis) 595.1
fistulous NEC — *see* Ulcer, skin
foot (indolent) (*see also* Ulcer, lower extremity) 707.1
  perforating 707.1
    leprous 030.1
    syphilitic 094.0
  trophic 707.1
  varicose 454.0
    inflamed or infected 454.2
frambesial, initial or primary 102.0
gallbladder or duct 575.8
gall duct 576.8
gangrenous (*see also* Gangrene) 785.4
gastric — *see* Ulcer, stomach
gastrocolic — *see* Ulcer, gastrojejunal

Ulcer, ulcerated, ulcerating, ulceration, ulcerative—
continued

gastroduodenal — *see* Ulcer, peptic
gastroesophageal — *see* Ulcer, stomach
gastrohepatic — *see* Ulcer, stomach
gastrointestinal — *see* Ulcer, gastrojejunal
gastrojejunal (eroded) (peptic) 534.9

> Note — *Use the following fifth-digit subclassification with categories 531-534:*
>
> 0   without mention of obstruction
> 1   with obstruction

  with
    hemorrhage (chronic) 534.4
      and perforation 534.6
    perforation 534.5
      and hemorrhage 534.6
  acute 534.3
    with
      hemorrhage 534.0
        and perforation 534.2
      perforation 534.1
        and hemorrhage 534.2
  bleeding (recurrent) — *see* Ulcer, gastrojejunal, with hemorrhage
  chronic 534.7
    with
      hemorrhage 534.4
        and perforation 534.6
      perforation 534.5
        and hemorrhage 534.6
  penetrating — *see* Ulcer, gastrojejunal, with perforation
  perforating — *see* Ulcer, gastrojejunal, with perforation
gastrojejunocolic — *see* Ulcer, gastrojejunal
genital organ
  female 629.8
  male 608.89
gingiva 523.8
gingivitis 523.1
glottis 478.79
granuloma of pudenda 099.2
groin (*see also* Ulcer, skin) 707.8
gum 523.8
gumma, due to yaws 102.4
hand (*see also* Ulcer, skin) 707.8
hard palate 528.9
heel (*see also* Ulcer, lower extremity) 707.1
  decubitus (*see also* Ulcer, decubitus) 707.0
hemorrhoids 455.8
  external 455.5
  internal 455.2
hip (*see also* Ulcer, skin) 707.8
  decubitus (*see also* Ulcer, decubitus) 707.0
Hunner's 595.1
hypopharynx 478.29
hypopyon (chronic) (subacute) 370.04
hypostaticum — *see* Ulcer, varicose
ileocolitis 556.1
ileum (*see also* Ulcer, intestine) 569.82

Ulcer, ulcerated, ulcerating, ulceration, ulcerative—
continued

intestine, intestinal 569.82
  with perforation 569.83
  amebic 006.9
  duodenal — *see* Ulcer, duodenum
  granulocytopenic (with hemorrhage) 288.0
  marginal 569.82
  perforating 569.83
  small, primary 569.82
  stercoraceous 569.82
  stercoral 569.82
  tuberculous (*see also* Tuberculosis) 014.8
  typhoid (fever) 002.0
  varicose 456.8
ischemic 707.9
  lower extremity (*see also* Ulcer, lower extremity) 707.1
jejunum, jejunal — *see* Ulcer, gastrojejunal
keratitis (*see also* Ulcer, cornea) 370.00
knee — *see* Ulcer, lower extremity
labium (majus) (minus) 616.50
laryngitis (*see also* Laryngitis) 464.0
larynx (aphthous) (contact) 478.79
  diphtheritic 032.3
leg — *see* Ulcer, lower extremity
lip 528.5
Lipschütz's 616.50
lower extremity (atrophic) (chronic) (neurogenic) (perforating) (pyogenic) (trophic) (tropical) 707.1
  with gangrene 707.1 [785.4]
    arteriosclerotic 440.24
  arteriosclerotic 440.23
    with gangrene 440.24
  arteriosclerotic 440.23
    with gangrene 440.24
  decubitus 707.0
    with gangrene 707.0 [785.4]
  varicose 454.0
    inflamed or infected 454.2
luetic — *see* Ulcer, syphilitic
lung 518.89
  tuberculous (*see also* Tuberculosis) 011.2
malignant (M8000/3) — *see* Neoplasm, by site, malignant
marginal NEC — *see* Ulcer, gastrojejunal
meatus (urinarius) 597.89
Meckel's diverticulum 751.0
Meleney's (chronic undermining) 686.2
Mooren's (cornea) 370.07
mouth (traumatic) 528.9
mycobacterial (skin) 031.1
nasopharynx 478.29
navel cord (newborn) 771.4
neck (*see also* Ulcer, skin) 707.8
  uterus 622.0
neurogenic NEC — *see* Ulcer, skin
nose, nasal (infectional) (passage) 478.1
  septum 478.1
    varicose 456.8
  skin — *see* Ulcer, skin
  spirochetal NEC 104.8
oral mucosa (traumatic) 528.9
palate (soft) 528.9
penetrating NEC — *see* Ulcer, peptic, with perforation
penis (chronic) 607.89
peptic (site unspecified) 533.9

Ulcer, ulcerated, ulcerating, ulceration, ulcerative—
continued

> Note — *Use the following fifth-digit subclassification with categories 531-534:*
>
> 0   without mention of obstruction
> 1   with obstruction

  with
    hemorrhage 533.4
      and perforation 533.6
    perforation (chronic) 533.5
      and hemorrhage 533.6
  acute 533.3
    with
      hemorrhage 533.0
        and perforation 533.2
      perforation 533.1
        and hemorrhage 533.2
  bleeding (recurrent) — *see* Ulcer, peptic, with hemorrhage
  chronic 533.7
    with
      hemorrhage 533.4
        and perforation 533.6
      perforation 533.5
        and hemorrhage 533.6
  penetrating — *see* Ulcer, peptic, with perforation
  perforating NEC (*see also* Ulcer, peptic, with perforation) 533.5
  skin 707.9
perineum (*see also* Ulcer, skin) 707.8
peritonsillar 474.8
phagedenic (tropical) NEC — *see* Ulcer, skin
pharynx 478.29
phlebitis — *see* Phlebitis
plaster (*see also* Ulcer, decubitus) 707.0
popliteal space — *see* Ulcer, lower extremity
postpyloric — *see* Ulcer, duodenum
prepuce 607.89
prepyloric — *see* Ulcer, stomach
pressure (*see also* Ulcer, decubitus) 707.0
primary of intestine 569.82
  with perforation 569.83
proctitis 556.2
  with ulcerative sigmoiditis 556.3
prostate 601.8
pseudopeptic — *see* Ulcer, peptic
pyloric — *see* Ulcer, stomach
rectosigmoid 569.82
  with perforation 569.83
rectum (sphincter) (solitary) 569.41
  stercoraceous, stercoral 569.41
  varicose — *see* Varicose, ulcer, anus
retina (*see also* Chorioretinitis) 363.20
rodent (M8090/3) — *see also* Neoplasm, skin, malignant
  cornea 370.07
round — *see* Ulcer, stomach
sacrum (region) (*see also* Ulcer, skin) 707.8
Saemisch's 370.04
scalp (*see also* Ulcer, skin) 707.8
sclera 379.09

Ulcer, ulcerated, ulcerating, ulceration, ulcerative—*continued*
 scrofulous (*see also* Tuberculosis) 017.2
 scrotum 608.89
  tuberculous (*see also* Tuberculosis) 016.5
  varicose 456.4
 seminal vesicle 608.89
 sigmoid 569.82
  with perforation 569.83
 skin (atrophic) (chronic) (neurogenic) (perforating) (pyogenic) (trophic) 707.9
  with gangrene 707.9 [785.4]
  amebic 006.6
  decubitus 707.0
   with gangrene 707.0 [785.4]
  in granulocytopenia 288.0
  lower extremity (*see also* Ulcer, lower extremity) 707.1
   with gangrene 707.1 [785.4]
    arteriosclerotic 440.24
    arteriosclerotic 440.23
     with gangrene 440.24
  mycobacterial 031.1
  syphilitic (early) (secondary) 091.3
  tuberculous (primary) (*see also* Tuberculosis) 017.0
  varicose — *see* Ulcer, varicose
 sloughing NEC — *see* Ulcer, skin
 soft palate 528.9
 solitary, anus or rectum (sphincter) 569.41
 sore throat 462
  streptococcal 034.0
 spermatic cord 608.89
 spine (tuberculous) 015.0 [730.88]
 stasis (leg) (venous) 454.0
  inflamed or infected 454.2
 stercoral, stercoraceous 569.82
  with perforation 569.83
  anus or rectum 569.41
 stoma, stomal — *see* Ulcer, gastrojejunal
 stomach (eroded) (peptic) (round) 531.9

Note — Use the following fifth-digit subclassification with categories 531-534:

 0 *without mention of obstruction*
 1 *with obstruction*

  with
   hemorrhage 531.4
    and perforation 531.6
   perforation (chronic) 531.5
    and hemorrhage 531.6
  acute 531.3
   with
    hemorrhage 531.0
     and perforation 531.2
    perforation 531.1
     and hemorrhage 531.2
   bleeding (recurrent) — *see* Ulcer, stomach, with hemorrhage
  chronic 531.7
   with
    hemorrhage 531.4
     and perforation 531.6
    perforation 531.5
     and hemorrhage 531.6

Ulcer, ulcerated, ulcerating, ulceration, ulcerative—*continued*
 stomach—*continued*
   penetrating — *see* Ulcer, stomach, with perforation
   perforating — *see* Ulcer, stomach, with perforation
  stomatitis 528.0
  stress — *see* Ulcer, peptic
  strumous (tuberculous) (*see also* Tuberculosis) 017.2
  submental (*see also* Ulcer, skin) 707.8
  submucosal, bladder 595.1
  syphilitic (any site) (early) (secondary) 091.3
   late 095.9
   perforating 095.9
    foot 094.0
  testis 608.89
  thigh — *see* Ulcer, lower extremity
  throat 478.29
   diphtheritic 032.0
  toe — *see* Ulcer, lower extremity
  tongue (traumatic) 529.0
  tonsil 474.8
   diphtheritic 032.0
  trachea 519.1
  trophic — *see* Ulcer, skin
  tropical NEC (*see also* Ulcer, skin) 707.9
  tuberculous — *see* Tuberculosis, ulcer
  tunica vaginalis 608.89
  turbinate 730.9
  typhoid (fever) 002.0
   perforating 002.0
  umbilicus (newborn) 771.4
  unspecified site NEC — *see* Ulcer, skin
  urethra (meatus) (*see also* Urethritis) 597.89
  uterus 621.8
   cervix 622.0
    with mention of cervicitis 616.0
   neck 622.0
    with mention of cervicitis 616.0
  vagina 616.8
  valve, heart 421.0
  varicose (lower extremity, any part) 454.0
   anus — *see* Varicose, ulcer, anus
   broad ligament 456.5
   esophagus (*see also* Varix, esophagus) 456.1
    bleeding (*see also* Varix, esophagus, bleeding) 456.0
   inflamed or infected 454.2
   nasal septum 456.8
   perineum 456.6
   rectum — *see* Varicose, ulcer, anus
   scrotum 456.4
   specified site NEC 456.8
   sublingual 456.3
   vulva 456.6
  vas deferens 608.89
  vesical (*see also* Ulcer, bladder) 596.8
  vulva (acute) (infectional) 616.50
   Behçet's syndrome 136.1 [616.51]
   herpetic 054.12
   tuberculous 016.7 [616.51]
  vulvobuccal, recurring 616.50
  x-ray — *see* Ulcer, by site
  yaws 102.4
Ulcerosa scarlatina 034.1

Ulcus — *see also* Ulcer
 cutis tuberculosum (*see also* Tuberculosis) 017.0
 duodeni — *see* Ulcer, duodenum
 durum 091.0
  extragenital 091.2
 gastrojejunale — *see* Ulcer, gastrojejunal
 hypostaticum — *see* Ulcer, varicose
 molle (cutis) (skin) 099.0
 serpens corneae (pneumococcal) 370.04
 ventriculi — *see* Ulcer, stomach
Ulegyria 742.4
Ulerythema
 acneiforma 701.8
 centrifugum 695.4
 ophryogenes 757.4
Ullrich (-Bonnevie) (-Turner) syndrome 758.6
Ullrich-Feichtiger syndrome 759.89
Ulnar — *see* condition
Ulorrhagia 523.8
Ulorrhea 523.8
Umbilicus, umbilical — *see also* condition
 cord necrosis, affecting fetus or newborn 762.6
Unavailability of medical facilities (at) V63.9
 due to
  investigation by social service agency V63.8
  lack of services at home V63.1
  remoteness from facility V63.0
  waiting list V63.2
 home V63.1
 outpatient clinic V63.0
 specified reason NEC V63.8
Uncinaria americana infestion 126.1
Uncinariasis (*see also* Ancylostomiasis) 126.9
Unconscious, unconsciousness 780.09
Underdevelopment — *see also* Undeveloped
 sexual 259.0
Undernourishment 269.9
Undernutrition 269.9
Under observation — *see* Observation
Underweight 783.4
 for gestational age — *see* Light-for-dates
Underwood's disease (sclerema neonatorum) 778.1
Undescended — *see also* Malposition, congenital
 cecum 751.4
 colon 751.4
 testis 752.5
Undetermined diagnosis or cause 799.9
Undeveloped, undevelopment — *see also* Hypoplasia
 brain (congenital) 742.1
 cerebral (congenital) 742.1
 fetus or newborn 764.9
 heart 746.89
 lung 748.5
 testis 257.2
 uterus 259.0
Undiagnosed (disease) 799.9
Undulant fever (*see also* Brucellosis) 023.9
Unemployment, anxiety concerning V62.0
Unequal leg (acquired) (length) 736.81
 congenital 755.30
Unerupted teeth, tooth 520.6

Unextracted dental root 525.3
Unguis incarnatus 703.0
Unicornis uterus 752.3
Unicorporeus uterus 752.3
Uniformis uterus 752.3
Unilateral — *see also* condition
 development, breast 611.8
 organ or site, congenital NEC — *see* Agenesis
 vagina 752.49
Unilateralis uterus 752.3
Unilocular heart 745.8
Uninhibited bladder 596.54
 with cauda equina syndrome 344.61
 neurogenic — *see* Neurogenic, bladder 596.54
Union, abnormal — *see also* Fusion
 divided tendon 727.89
 larynx and trachea 748.3
Universal
 joint, cervix 620.6
 mesentery 751.4
Unknown
 cause of death 799.9
 diagnosis 799.9
Unna's disease (seborrheic dermatitis) 690
Unresponsiveness, adrenocorticotropin (ACTH) 255.4
Unsoundness of mind (*see also* Psychosis) 298.9
Unspecified cause of death 799.9
Unstable
 back NEC 724.9
 colon 569.89
 joint — *see* Instability, joint
 lie 652.0
  affecting fetus or newborn (before labor) 761.7
  causing obstructed labor 660.0
   affecting fetus or newborn 763.1
 lumbosacral joint (congenital) 756.19
  acquired 724.6
 sacroiliac 724.6
 spine NEC 724.9
Untruthfulness, child problem (*see also* Disturbance, conduct) 312.0
Unverricht (-Lundborg) disease, syndrome, or epilepsy 333.2
Unverricht-Wagner syndrome (dermatomyositis) 710.3
Upper respiratory — *see* condition
Upset
 gastric 536.8
  psychogenic 306.4
 gastrointestinal 536.8
  psychogenic 306.4
  virus (*see also* Enteritis, viral) 008.8
 intestinal (large) (small) 564.9
  psychogenic 306.4
 menstruation 626.9
 mental 300.9
 stomach 536.8
  psychogenic 306.4
Urachus — *see also* condition
 patent 753.7
 persistent 753.7
Uratic arthritis 274.0
Urbach's lipoid proteinosis 272.8
Urbach-Oppenheim disease or syndrome (necrobiosis lipoidica diabeticorum) 250.8 [709.3]
Urbach-Wiethe disease or syndrome (lipoid proteinosis) 272.8
Urban yellow fever 060.1

Urea, blood, high — see Uremia
Uremia, uremic (absorption)
    (amaurosis) (amblyopia)
    (aphasia) (apoplexy) (coma)
    (delirium) (dementia) (dropsy)
    (dyspnea) (fever) (intoxication)
    (mania) (paralysis) (poisoning)
    (toxemia) (vomiting) 586
    with
        abortion — see Abortion, by
            type, with renal failure
        ectopic pregnancy (see also
            categories 633.0-633.9)
            639.3
        hypertension (see also
            Hypertension, kidney)
            403.91 ◆
        molar pregnancy (see also
            categories 630-632)
            639.3
    chronic 585
    complicating
        abortion 639.3
        ectopic or molar pregnancy
            639.3
        hypertension (see also
            Hypertension, kidney)
            403.91 ◆
        labor and delivery 669.3
    congenital 779.8
    extrarenal 788.9
    hypertensive (chronic) (see also
        Hypertension, kidney)
        403.91 ◆
    maternal NEC, affecting fetus or
        newborn 760.1
    neuropathy 585 [357.4]
    pericarditis 585 [420.0]
    prerenal 788.9
    pyelitic (see also Pyelitis) 590.80
Ureter, ureteral — see condition
Ureteralgia 788.0
Ureterectasis 593.89
Ureteritis 593.89
    cystica 590.3
    due to calculus 592.1
    gonococcal (acute) 098.19
        chronic or duration of 2
            months or over 098.39
    nonspecific 593.89
Ureterocele (acquired) 593.89
    congenital 753.2
Ureterolith 592.1
Ureterolithiasis 592.1
Ureterostomy status V44.6
    with complication 997.5
Urethra, urethral — see condition
Urethralgia 788.9
Urethritis (abacterial) (acute)
    (allergic) (anterior) (chronic)
    (nonvenereal) (posterior)
    (recurrent) (simple) (subacute)
    (ulcerative) (undifferentiated)
    597.80
    diplococcal (acute) 098.0
        chronic or duration of 2
            months or over 098.2
    due to Trichomonas (vaginalis)
        131.02
    gonococcal (acute) 098.0
        chronic or duration of 2
            months or over 098.2
    nongonococcal (sexually
        transmitted) 099.40
        Chlamydia trachomatis 099.41
        Reiter's 099.3
        specified organism NEC
            099.49 ◆
    nonspecific (sexually transmitted)
        (see also Urethritis,
        nongonococcal) 099.40
    not sexually transmitted 597.80
    Reiter's 099.3

Urethritis—continued
    trichomonal or due to
        Trichomonas (vaginalis)
        131.02
    tuberculous (see also
        Tuberculosis) 016.3
    venereal NEC (see also Urethritis,
        nongonococcal) 099.40
Urethrocele
    female 618.0
        with uterine prolapse 618.4
            complete 618.3
            incomplete 618.2
    male 599.5
Urethrolithiasis 594.2
Urethro-oculoarticular syndrome
    099.3
Urethro-oculosynovial syndrome
    099.3
Urethrorectal — see condition
Urethrorrhagia 599.84
Urethrorrhea 788.7
Urethrostomy status V44.6
    with complication 997.5
Urethrotrigonitis 595.3
Urethrovaginal — see condition
Urhidrosis, uridrosis 705.89
Uric acid
    diathesis 274.9
    in blood 790.6
Uricacidemia 790.6
Uricemia 790.6
Uricosuria 791.9
Urination
    frequent 788.41
    painful 788.1
Urine, urinary — see also condition
    abnormality NEC 788.69
    blood in (see also Hematuria)
        599.7
    discharge, excessive 788.42
    enuresis 788.30
        nonorganic origin 307.6
    extravasation 788.8
    frequency 788.41
    incontinence 788.30
        active 788.30
        female 788.30
            stress 625.6
            and urge 788.33
        male 788.30
            stress 788.32
            and urge 788.33
        mixed (stress and urge) 788.33
        neurogenic 788.39
        nonorganic origin 307.6
        stress (female) 625.6
        male NEC 788.32
    intermittent stream 788.61
    pus in 599.0
    retention or stasis NEC 788.20
        bladder, incomplete emptying
            788.21
        psychogenic 306.53
        specified NEC 788.29
    secretion
        deficient 788.5
        excessive 788.42
        frequency 788.41
    stream
        intermittent 788.61
        slowing 788.62
        splitting 788.61
        weak 788.62
Urinemia — see Uremia
Urinoma NEC 599.9
    bladder 596.8
    kidney 593.89
    renal 593.89
    ureter 593.89
    urethra 599.84
Uroarthritis, infectious 099.3
Urodialysis 788.5

Urolithiasis 592.9
Uronephrosis 593.89
Uropathy 599.9
    obstructive 599.6
Urosepsis 599.0
Urticaria 708.9
    with angioneurotic edema 995.1
        hereditary 277.6
    allergic 708.0
    cholinergic 708.5
    chronic 708.8
    cold, familial 708.2
    dermatographic 708.3
    due to
        cold or heat 708.2
        drugs 708.0
        food 708.0
        inhalants 708.0
        plants 708.8
        serum 999.5
    factitial 708.3
    giant 995.1
        hereditary 277.6
    gigantea 995.1
        hereditary 277.6
    idiopathic 708.1
    larynx 995.1
        hereditary 277.6
    medicamentosa 693.0
        due to drug applied to skin
            692.3
    neonatorum 778.8
    nonallergic 708.1
    papulosa (Hebra) 698.2
    perstans hemorrhagica 757.39
    pigmentosa 757.33
    recurrent periodic 708.8
    serum 999.5
    solare 692.72
    specified type NEC 708.8
    thermal (cold) (heat) 708.2
    vibratory 708.4
Urticarioides acarodermatitis 133.9
Use of
    nonprescribed drugs (see also
        Abuse, drugs,
        nondependent) 305.9
    patent medicines (see also Abuse,
        drugs, nondependent)
        305.9
Usher-Senear disease (pemphigus
    erythematosus) 694.4
Uta 085.5
Uteromegaly 621.2
Uterovaginal — see condition
Uterovesical — see condition
Uterus — see condition
Utriculitis (utriculus prostaticus)
    597.89
Uveal — see condition
Uveitis (anterior) (see also
    Iridocyclitis) 364.3
    acute or subacute 364.00
        due to or associated with
            gonococcal infection
                098.41
            herpes (simplex) 054.44
            zoster 053.22
        primary 364.01
        recurrent 364.02
    secondary (noninfectious)
        364.04
        infectious 364.03
    allergic 360.11
    chronic 364.10
        due to or associated with
            sarcoidosis 135 [364.11]
            tuberculosis (see also
                Tuberculosis) 017.3
                [364.11]

Uveitis—continued
    due to
        operation 360.11
        toxoplasmosis (acquired)
            130.2
            congenital (active) 771.2
    granulomatous 364.10
    heterochromic 364.21
    lens-induced 364.23
    nongranulomatous 364.00
    posterior 363.20
        disseminated — see
            Chorioretinitis,
            disseminated
        focal — see Chorioretinitis,
            focal
    recurrent 364.02
    sympathetic 360.11
    syphilitic (secondary) 091.50
        congenital 090.0 [363.13]
        late 095.8 [363.13]
    tuberculous (see also
        Tuberculosis) 017.3
        [364.11]
Uveoencephalitis 363.22
Uveokeratitis (see also Iridocyclitis)
    364.3
Uveoparotid fever 135
Uveoparotitis 135
Uvula — see condition
Uvulitis (acute) (catarrhal) (chronic)
    (gangrenous) (membranous)
    (suppurative) (ulcerative) 528.3

V

Vaccination
    complication or reaction — see
        Complications, vaccination
    not done (contraindicated) V64.0
        because of patient's decision
            V64.2
    prophylactic (against) V05.9
        arthropod-borne viral
            disease NEC V05.1
            encephalitis V05.0
        chickenpox V05.4
        cholera (alone) V03.0
            with typhoid-paratyphoid
                (cholera + TAB)
                V06.0
        common cold V04.7
        diphtheria (alone) V03.5
            with
                poliomyelitis (DTP+
                    polio) V06.3
                tetanus V06.5 ▼
                pertussis combined
                    (DTP) V06.1 ▲
                typhoid-paratyphoid
                    (DTP + TAB)
                    V06.2
        disease (single) NEC V05.9
            bacterial NEC V03.9
                specified type NEC
                    V03.89 ◆
            combinations NEC V06.9
                specified type NEC
                    V06.8
            specified type NEC V05.8
        encephalitis, viral, arthropod-
            borne V05.0
        Hemophilus influenzae, type B
            [Hib] V03.81 ◆
        hepatitis, viral V05.3
        influenza V04.8
            with ▼
                Streptococcus
                    pneumoniae
                    [pneumococcus]
                    V06.6 ▲
        lileieshmaniasis V05.2
        measles (alone) V04.2
            with mumps-rubella (MMR)
                V06.4

Vaccination — continued
prophylactic — continued
- mumps (alone) V04.6
  - with measles and rubella (MMR) V06.4
- pertussis alone V03.6
- plague V03.3
- poliomyelitis V04.0
  - with diphtheria-tetanus-pertussis (DTP + polio) V06.3
- rabies V04.5
- rubella (alone) V04.3
  - with measles and mumps (MMR) V06.4
- smallpox V04.1
- Streptococcus pneumoniae [pneumococcus] V03.82 ▼
  - with
    - influenza V06.6 ▲
- tetanus toxoid (alone) V03.7
  - with diphtheria [Td] V06.5 ▼
    - with
      - pertussis (DTP) V06.1
        - with poliomyelitis (DTP+polio) V06.3 ▲
- tuberculosis (BCG) V03.2
- tularemia V03.4
- typhoid-paratyphoid (TAB) (alone) V03.1
  - with diphtheria-tetanus-pertussis (TAB + DTP) V06.2
- varicella V05.4
- viral
  - encephalitis, arthropod-borne V05.0
  - hepatitis V05.3
  - yellow fever V04.4

Vaccinia (generalized) 999.0
- congenital 771.2
- conjunctiva 999.3
- eyelids 999.0 [373.5]
- localized 999.3
- nose 999.3
- not from vaccination 051.0
  - eyelid 051.0 [373.5]
- sine vaccinatione 051.0
- without vaccination 051.0

Vacuum
- extraction of fetus or newborn 763.3
- in sinus (accessory) (nasal) (see also Sinusitis) 473.9

Vagabond V60.0

Vagabondage V60.0

Vagabonds' disease 132.1

Vagina, vaginal — see condition

Vaginalitis (tunica) 608.4

Vaginismus (reflex) 625.1
- functional 306.51
- hysterical 300.11
- psychogenic 306.51

Vaginitis (acute) (chronic) (circumscribed) (diffuse) (emphysematous) (Hemophilus vaginalis) (nonspecific) (nonvenereal) (ulcerative) 616.10
- with
  - abortion — see Abortion, by type, with sepsis
  - ectopic pregnancy (see also categories 633.0-633.9) 639.0
  - molar pregnancy (see also categories 630-632) 639.0
- adhesive, congenital 752.49
- atrophic, postmenopausal 627.3

Vaginitis — continued
- blennorrhagic (acute) 098.0
  - chronic or duration of 2 months or over 098.2
- candidal 112.1
- chlamydial 099.53
- complicating pregnancy or puerperium 646.6
  - affecting fetus or newborn 760.8
- congenital (adhesive) 752.49
- due to
  - C. albicans 112.1
  - Trichomonas (vaginalis) 131.01
- following
  - abortion 639.0
  - ectopic or molar pregnancy 639.0
- gonococcal (acute) 098.0
  - chronic or duration of 2 months or over 098.2
- granuloma 099.2
- Monilia 112.1
- mycotic 112.1
- pinworm 127.4 [616.11]
- postirradiation 616.10
- postmenopausal atrophic 627.3
- senile (atrophic) 627.3
- syphilitic (early) 091.0
  - late 095.8
- trichomonal 131.01
- tuberculous (see also Tuberculosis) 016.7
- venereal NEC 099.8

Vagotonia 352.3

Vagrancy V60.0

Vallecula — see condition

Valley fever 114.0

Valsuani's disease (progressive pernicious anemia, puerperal) 648.2

Valve, valvular (formation) — see also condition
- cerebral ventricle (communicating) in situ V45.2
- cervix, internal os 752.49
- colon 751.5
- congenital NEC — see Atresia
- formation, congenital NEC — see Atresia
- heart defect — see Anomaly, heart, valve
- ureter (pelvic junction) (vesical orifice) 753.2
- urethra 753.6

Valvulitis (chronic) (see also Endocarditis) 424.90
- rheumatic (chronic) (inactive) (with chorea) 397.9
  - active or acute (aortic) (mitral) (pulmonary) (tricuspid) 391.1
- syphilitic NEC 093.20
  - aortic 093.22
  - mitral 093.21
  - pulmonary 093.24
  - tricuspid 093.23

Valvulopathy — see Endocarditis

van Bogaert's leukoencephalitis (sclerosing) (subacute) 046.2

van Bogaert-Nijssen (-Peiffer) **disease** 330.0

van Buchem's syndrome (hyperostosis corticalis) 733.3

van Creveld-von Gierke disease (glycogenosis I) 271.0

van den Bergh's disease (enterogenous cyanosis) 289.7

van der Hoeve's syndrome (brittle bones and blue sclera, deafness) 756.51

van der Hoeve-Halbertsma-Waardenburg syndrome (ptosis-epicanthus) 270.2

van der Hoeve-Waardenburg-Gualdi syndrome (ptosis epicanthus) 270.2

Vanillism 692.89

Vanishing lung 492.0

van Neck (-Odelberg) **disease or syndrome** (juvenile osteochondrosis) 732.1

Vapor asphyxia or suffocation NEC 987.9
- specified agent — see Table of drugs and chemicals

Vaquez's disease (M9950/1) 238.4

Vaquez-Osler disease (polycythemia vera) (M9950/1) 238.4

Variance, lethal ball, prosthetic heart valve 996.02

Variants, thalassemic 282.4

Variations in hair color 704.3

Varicella 052.9
- with
  - complication 052.8
    - specified NEC 052.7
  - pneumonia 052.1
  - vaccination and inoculation (prophylactic) V05.4

Varices — see Varix

Varicocele (scrotum) (thrombosed) 456.4
- ovary 456.5
- perineum 456.6
- spermatic cord (ulcerated) 456.4

Varicose
- aneurysm (ruptured) (see also Aneurysm) 442.9
- dermatitis (lower extremity) — see Varicose, vein, inflamed or infected
- eczema — see Varicose, vein
- phlebitis — see Varicose, vein, inflamed or infected
- placental vessel — see Placenta, abnormal
- tumor — see Varicose, vein
- ulcer (lower extremity, any part) 454.0
  - anus 455.8
    - external 455.5
    - internal 455.2
  - esophagus (see also Varix, esophagus) 456.1
    - bleeding (see also Varix, esophagus, bleeding) 456.0
  - inflamed or infected 454.2
  - nasal septum 456.8
  - perineum 456.6
  - rectum — see Varicose, ulcer, anus
  - scrotum 456.4
  - specified site NEC 456.8
- vein (lower extremity) (ruptured) (see also Varix) 454.9
  - with
    - inflammation or infection 454.1
      - ulcerated 454.2
    - stasis dermatitis 454.1
      - with ulcer 454.2
    - ulcer 454.0
      - inflamed or infected 454.2
  - anus — see Hemorrhoids
  - broad ligament 456.5
  - congenital (peripheral) NEC 747.60
    - gastrointestinal 747.61
    - lower limb 747.64
    - renal 747.62
    - specified NEC 747.69
    - upper limb 747.63

Varicose — continued
vein — continued
- esophagus (ulcerated) (see also Varix, esophagus) 456.1
  - bleeding (see also Varix, esophagus, bleeding) 456.0
- inflamed or infected 454.1
  - with ulcer 454.2
- in pregnancy or puerperium 671.0
- vulva or perineum 671.1
- nasal septum (with ulcer) 456.8
- pelvis 456.5
- perineum 456.6
  - in pregnancy, childbirth, or puerperium 671.1
- rectum — see Hemorrhoids
- scrotum (ulcerated) 456.4
- specified site NEC 456.8
- sublingual 456.3
- ulcerated 454.0
  - inflamed or infected 454.2
- umbilical cord, affecting fetus or newborn 762.6
- urethra 456.8
- vulva 456.6
  - in pregnancy, childbirth, or puerperium 671.1
- vessel — see also Varix
- placenta — see Placenta, abnormal

Varicosis, varicosities, varicosity (see also Varix) 454.9

Variola 050.9
- hemorrhagic (pustular) 050.0
- major 050.0
- minor 050.1
- modified 050.2

Varioloid 050.2

Variolosa, purpura 050.0

Varix (lower extremity) (ruptured) 454.9
- with
  - inflammation or infection 454.1
    - with ulcer 454.2
  - stasis dermatitis 454.1
    - with ulcer 454.2
  - ulcer 454.0
    - with inflammation or infection 454.2
- aneurysmal (see also Aneurysm) 442.9
- anus — see Hemorrhoids
- arteriovenous (congenital) (peripheral) NEC 747.60
  - gastrointestinal 747.61
  - lower limb 747.64
  - renal 747.62
  - specified NEC 747.69
  - spinal 747.82
  - upper limb 747.63
- bladder 456.5
- broad ligament 456.5
- congenital (peripheral) NEC 747.60
- esophagus (ulcerated) 456.1
  - bleeding 456.0
  - in
    - cirrhosis of liver 571.5 [456.20]
    - portal hypertension 572.3 [456.20]
- congenital 747.69
  - in
    - cirrhosis of liver 571.5 [456.21]
      - with bleeding 571.5 [456.20]
    - portal hypertension 572.3 [456.21]
      - with bleeding 572.3 [456.20]

Varix—continued
 inflamed or infected 454.1
  ulcerated 454.2
 in pregnancy or puerperium
  671.0
  perineum 671.1
  vulva 671.1
 labia (majora) 456.6
 orbit 456.8
  congenital 747.69
 ovary 456.5
 papillary 448.1
 pelvis 456.5
 perineum 456.6
  in pregnancy or puerperium
   671.1
 pharynx 456.8
 placenta — see Placenta,
  abnormal
 rectum — see Hemorrhoids
 renal papilla 456.8
 retina 362.17
 scrotum (ulcerated) 456.4
 sigmoid colon 456.8
 specified site NEC 456.8
 spinal (cord) (vessels) 456.8
 spleen, splenic (vein) (with
  phlebolith) 456.8
 sublingual 456.3
 ulcerated 454.0
  inflamed or infected 454.2
 umbilical cord, affecting fetus or
  newborn 762.6
 uterine ligament 456.5
 vocal cord 456.8
 vulva 456.6
  in pregnancy, childbirth, or
   puerperium 671.1
Vasa previa 663.5
 affecting fetus or newborn 762.6
 hemorrhage from, affecting fetus
  or newborn 772.0
Vascular — see also condition
 loop on papilla (optic) 743.51
 sheathing, retina 362.13
 spasm 443.9
 spider 448.1
Vascularity, pulmonary, congenital
 747.3
Vascularization
 choroid 362.16
 cornea 370.60
  deep 370.63
  localized 370.61
 retina 362.16
 subretinal 362.16
Vasculitis 447.6
 allergic 287.0
 cryoglobulinemic 273.2
 disseminated 447.6
 kidney 447.8
 nodular 695.2
 retinal 362.10
 rheumatic — see Fever,
  rheumatic
Vas deferens — see condition
Vas deferentitis 608.4
Vasectomy, admission for V25.2
Vasitis 608.4
 nodosa 608.4
 scrotum 608.4
 spermatic cord 608.4
 testis 608.4
 tuberculous (see also
  Tuberculosis) 016.5
 tunica vaginalis 608.4
 vas deferens 608.4
Vasodilation 443.9
Vasomotor — see condition
**Vasoplasty, after previous
 sterilization** V26.0
Vasoplegia, splanchnic (see also
 Neuropathy, peripheral,
 autonomic) 337.9

Vasospasm 443.9
 cerebral (artery) 435.9
  with transient neurologic
   deficit 435.9
 nerve
  arm NEC 354.9
  autonomic 337.9
  brachial plexus 353.0
  cervical plexus 353.2
  leg NEC 355.8
  lower extremity NEC 355.8
  peripheral NEC 355.9
  spinal NEC 355.9
  sympathetic 337.9
  upper extremity NEC 354.9
 peripheral NEC 443.9
 retina (artery) (see also Occlusion,
  retinal, artery) 362.30
Vasospastic — see condition
Vasovagal attack (paroxysmal) 780.2
 psychogenic 306.2
Vater's ampulla — see condition
VATER syndrome 759.89
Vegetation, vegetative
 adenoid (nasal fossa) 474.2
 consciousness (persistent) 780.03
 endocardium (acute) (any valve)
  (chronic) (subacute) 421.0
 heart (mycotic) (valve) 421.0
 state (persistent) 780.03
Veil
 Jackson's 751.4
 over face (causing asphyxia)
  768.9
Vein, venous — see condition
Veldt sore (see also Ulcer, skin)
 707.9
Velpeau's hernia — see Hernia,
 femoral
Venereal
 balanitis NEC 099.8
 bubo 099.1
 disease 099.9
  specified nature or type NEC
   099.8
 granuloma inguinale 099.2
 lymphogranuloma (Durand-
  Nicolas-Favre), any site
  099.1
 salpingitis 098.37
 urethritis (see also Urethritis,
  nongonococcal) 099.40
 vaginitis NEC 099.8
 warts 078.19
Vengefulness, in child (see also
 Disturbance, conduct) 312.0
Venofibrosis 459.89
Venom, venomous
 bite or sting (animal or insect)
  989.5
 poisoning 989.5
Venous — see condition
Ventouse delivery NEC 669.5
 affecting fetus or newborn 763.3
Ventral — see condition
Ventricle, ventricular — see also
 condition
 escape 427.69
 standstill (see also Arrest, cardiac)
  427.5
Ventriculitis, cerebral (see also
 Meningitis) 322.9
Ventriculostomy status V45.2
Verbiest's syndrome (claudicatio
 intermittens spinalis) 435.1
Vernet's syndrome 352.6
Verneuil's disease (syphilitic bursitis)
 095.7
Verruca (filiformis) 078.10
 acuminata (any site) 078.11
 necrogenica (primary) (see also
  Tuberculosis) 017.0
 plana (juvenilis) 078.19

Verruca—continued
 peruana 088.0
 peruviana 088.0
 plantaris 078.19
 seborrheica 702.19
  inflamed 702.11
 senilis 702.0
 tuberculosa (primary) (see also
  Tuberculosis) 017.0
 venereal 078.19
 viral NEC 078.10
Verrucosities (see also Verruca)
 078.10
Verrucous endocarditis (acute) (any
 valve) (chronic) (subacute)
 710.0 [424.91]
 nonbacterial 710.0 [424.91]
Verruga
 peruana 088.0
 peruviana 088.0
Verse's disease (calcinosis
 intervertebralis) 275.4
 [722.90]
Version
 before labor, affecting fetus or
  newborn 761.7
 cephalic (correcting previous
  malposition) 652.1
  affecting fetus or newborn
   763.1
 cervix (see also Malposition,
  uterus) 621.6
 uterus (postinfectional)
  (postpartal, old) (see also
  Malposition, uterus) 621.6
 forward — see Anteversion,
  uterus
 lateral — see Lateroversion,
  uterus
Vertebra, vertebral — see condition
Vertigo 780.4
 auditory 386.19
 aural 386.19
 benign paroxysmal positional
  386.11
 central origin 386.2
 cerebral 386.2
 Dix and Hallpike (epidemic)
  386.12
 endemic paralytic 078.81
 epidemic 078.81
  Dix and Hallpike 386.12
  Gerlier's 078.81
  Pedersen's 386.12
  vestibular neuronitis 386.12
 epileptic — see Epilepsy
 Gerlier's (epidemic) 078.81
 hysterical 300.11
 labyrinthine 386.10
 laryngeal 786.2
 malignant positional 386.2
 Ménière's (see also Disease,
  Ménière's) 386.00
 menopausal 627.2
 otogenic 386.19
 paralytic 078.81
 paroxysmal positional, benign
  386.11
 Pedersen's (epidemic) 386.12
 peripheral 386.19
  specified type NEC 386.19
 positional
  benign paroxysmal 386.11
  malignant 386.2
Verumontanitis (chronic) (see also
 Urethritis) 597.89
Vesania (see also Psychosis) 298.9
Vesical — see condition
Vesicle
 cutaneous 709.8
 seminal — see condition
 skin 709.8
Vesicocolic — see condition
Vesicoperineal — see condition
Vesicorectal — see condition

Vesicourethrorectal — see condition
Vesicovaginal — see condition
Vesicular — see condition
Vesiculitis (seminal) 608.0
 amebic 006.8
 gonorrheal (acute) 098.14
  chronic or duration of 2
   months or over 098.34
 trichomonal 131.09
 tuberculous (see also
  Tuberculosis) 016.5
  [608.81]
Vestibulitis (ear) (see also
 Labyrinthitis) 386.30
 nose (external) 478.1
Vestibulopathy, acute peripheral
 (recurrent) 386.12
Vestige, vestigial — see also
 Persistence
 branchial 744.41
 structures in vitreous 743.51
Vibriosis NEC 027.9
Vidal's disease (lichen simplex
 chronicus) 698.3
Video display tube syndrome 723.8
Vienna type encephalitis 049.8
Villaret's syndrome 352.6
Villous — see condition
Vincent's
 angina 101
 bronchitis 101
 disease 101
 gingivitis 101
 infection (any site) 101
 laryngitis 101
 stomatitis 101
 tonsillitis 101
Vinson-Plummer syndrome
 (sideropenic dysphagia) 280.8
Viosterol deficiency (see also
 Deficiency, calciferol) 268.9
Virchow's disease 733.99
Viremia 790.8
Virilism (adrenal) (female) NEC
 255.2
 with
  3-beta-hydroxysteroid
   dehydrogenase defect
   255.2
  11-hydroxylase defect 255.2
  21-hydroxylase defect 255.2
  adrenal
   hyperplasia 255.2
   insufficiency (congenital)
    255.2
   cortical hyperfunction 255.2
Virilization (female) (suprarenal) (see
 also Virilism) 255.2
 isosexual 256.4
Virulent bubo 099.0
Virus, viral — see also condition
 infection NEC (see also Infection,
  viral) 079.99
 septicemia 079.99
Viscera, visceral — see condition
Visceroptosis 569.89
Visible peristalsis 787.4
Vision, visual
 binocular, suppression 368.31
 blurred, blurring 368.8
  hysterical 300.11
 defect, defective (see also
  Impaired, vision) 369.9
 disorientation (syndrome) 368.16
 disturbance NEC (see also
  Disturbance, vision) 368.9
  hysterical 300.11
 examination V72.0
 field, limitation 368.40
 fusion, with defective steropsis
  368.33
 hallucinations 368.16
 halos 368.16

Vision, visual

Vision, visual—*continued*
  loss 369.9
    both eyes (*see also* Blindness, both eyes) 369.3
    complete (*see also* Blindness, both eyes) 369.00
    one eye 369.8
    sudden 368.16
  low (both eyes) 369.20
    one eye (other eye normal) (*see also* Impaired, vision) 369.70
      blindness, other eye 369.10
  perception, simultaneous without fusion 368.32
  tunnel 368.45
Vitality, lack or want of 780.7
  newborn 779.8
Vitamin deficiency NEC (*see also* Deficiency, vitamin) 269.2
Vitelline duct, persistent 751.0
Vitiligo 709.01 ◆
  due to pinta (carate) 103.2
  eyelid 374.53
  vulva 624.8
Vitium cordis — *see* Disease, heart
Vitreous — *see also* condition
  touch syndrome 997.9
Vocal cord — *see* condition
Vocational rehabilitation V57.22 ◆
Vogt's (Cecile) disease or syndrome 333.7
Vogt-Koyanagi syndrome 364.24
Vogt-Spielmeyer disease (amaurotic familial idiocy) 330.1
Voice
  change (*see also* Dysphonia) 784.49
  loss (*see also* Aphonia) 784.41
Volhard-Fahr disease (malignant nephrosclerosis) 403.00
Volhynian fever 083.1
Volkmann's ischemic contracture or paralysis (complicating trauma) 958.6
Voluntary starvation 307.1
Volvulus (bowel) (colon) (intestine) 560.2
  with
    hernia — *see also* Hernia, by site, with obstruction
    gangrenous — *see* Hernia, by site, with gangrene
    perforation 560.2
  congenital 751.5
  duodenum 537.3
  fallopian tube 620.5
  oviduct 620.5
  stomach (due to absence of gastrocolic ligament) 537.89
Vomiting 787.03 ▼▲
  with nausea 787.01
  allergic 535.4
  asphyxia 933.1
  bilious (cause unknown) 787.0
    following gastrointestinal surgery 564.3
  blood (*see also* Hematemesis) 578.0
  causing asphyxia, choking, or suffocation (*see also* Asphyxia, food) 933.1
  cyclical 536.2
    psychogenic 306.4
  epidemic 078.82
  fecal matter 569.89
  following gastrointestinal surgery 564.3
  functional 536.8
    psychogenic 306.4
  habit 536.2
  hysterical 300.11

Vomiting—*continued*
  nervous 306.4
  neurotic 306.4
  newborn 779.3
  of or complicating pregnancy 643.9
    due to
      organic disease 643.8
      specific cause NEC 643.8
    early — *see* Hyperemesis, gravidarum
    late (after 22 completed weeks of gestation) 643.2
  pernicious or persistent 536.2
    complicating pregnancy — *see* Hyperemesis, gravidarum
  psychogenic 306.4
  physiological 787.0
  psychic 306.4
  psychogenic 307.54
  stercoral 569.89
  uncontrollable 536.2
    psychogenic 306.4
  uremic — *see* Uremia
  winter 078.82
von Bechterew (-Strumpell) disease or syndrome (ankylosing spondylitis) 720.0
von Bezold's abscess 383.01
von Economo's disease (encephalitis lethargica) 049.8
von Eulenburg's disease (congenital paramyotonia) 359.2
von Gierke's disease (glycogenosis I) 271.0
von Gies' joint 095.8
von Graefe's disease or syndrome 378.72
von Hippel (-Lindau) disease or syndrome (retinocerebral angiomatosis) 759.6
von Jaksch's anemia or disease (pseudoleukemia infantum) 285.8
von Recklinghausen's
  disease or syndrome (nerves) (skin) (M9540/1) 237.71
  bones (osteitis fibrosa cystica) 252.0
  tumor (M9540/1) 237.71
von Recklinghausen-Applebaum disease (hemochromatosis) 275.0
von Schroetter's syndrome (intermittent venous claudication) 453.8
von Willebrand (-Jürgens) (-Minot) disease or syndrome (angiohemophilia) 286.4
von Zambusch's disease (lichen sclerosus et atrophicus) 701.0
Voorhoeve's disease or dyschondroplasia 756.4
Vossius' ring 921.3
  late effect 366.21
Voyeurism 302.82
Vrolik's disease (osteogenesis imperfecta) 756.51
Vulva — *see* condition
Vulvismus 625.1
Vulvitis (acute) (allergic) (aphthous) (chronic) (gangrenous) (hypertrophic) (intertriginous) 616.10
  with
    abortion — *see* Abortion, by type, with sepsis
    ectopic pregnancy (*see also* categories 633.0-633.9) 639.0

Vulvitis—*continued*
  with—*continued*
    molar pregnancy (*see also* categories 630-632) 639.0
  adhesive, congenital 752.49
  blennorhagic (acute) 098.0
    chronic or duration of 2 months or over 098.2
  chlamydial 099.53
  complicating pregnancy or puerperium 646.6
  due to Ducrey's bacillus 099.0
  following
    abortion 639.0
    ectopic or molar pregnancy 639.0
  gonococcal (acute) 098.0
    chronic or duration of 2 months or over 098.2
  herpetic 054.11
  leukoplakic 624.0
  monilial 112.1
  puerperal, postpartum, childbirth 646.6
  syphilitic (early) 091.0
    late 095.8
  trichomonal 131.01
Vulvorectal — *see* condition
Vulvovaginitis (*see also* Vulvitis) 616.10
  amebic 006.8
  chlamydial 099.53
  gonococcal (acute) 098.0
    chronic or duration of 2 months or over 098.2
  herpetic 054.11
  monilial 112.1
  trichomonal (Trichomonas vaginalis) 131.01

W

Waardenburg's syndrome 756.89
  meaning ptosis-epicanthus 270.2
Waardenburg-Klein syndrome (ptosis-epicanthus) 270.2
Wagner's disease (colloid milium) 709.3
Wagner (-Unverricht) syndrome (dermatomyositis) 710.3
Waiting list, person on V63.2
  undergoing social agency investigation V63.8
Wakefulness disorder (*see also* Hypersomnia) 780.54
  nonorganic origin 307.43
Waldenström's
  disease (osteochondrosis, capital femoral) 732.1
  hepatitis (lupoid hepatitis) 571.49
  hypergammaglobulinemia 273.0
  macroglobulinemia 273.3
  purpura, hypergammaglobulinemic 273.0
  syndrome (macroglobulinemia) 273.3
Waldenström-Kjellberg syndrome (sideropenic dysphagia) 280.8
Walking
  difficulty 719.7
    psychogenic 307.9
  sleep 307.46
    hysterical 300.13
Wall, abdominal — *see* condition
Wallenberg's syndrome (posterior inferior cerebellar artery) (*see also* Disease, cerebrovascular, acute) 436

Weak, weakness

Wallgren's
  disease (obstruction of splenic vein with collateral circulation) 459.89
  meningitis (*see also* Meningitis, aseptic) 047.9
Wandering
  acetabulum 736.39
  gallbladder 751.69
  kidney, congenital 753.3
  organ or site, congenital NEC — *see* Malposition, congenital
  pacemaker (atrial) (heart) 427.89
  spleen 289.59
Wardrop's disease (with lymphangitis) 681.9
  finger 681.02
  toe 681.11
War neurosis 300.16
Wart (common) (digitate) (filiform) (infectious) (juvenile) (plantar) (viral) 078.10
  external genital organs (venereal) 078.19
  fig 078.19
  Hassall-Henle's (of cornea) 371.41
  Henle's (of cornea) 371.41
  juvenile 078.19
  moist 078.10
  Peruvian 088.0
  plantar 078.19
  prosector (*see also* Tuberculosis) 017.0
  seborrheic 702.19 ▼
    inflamed 702.11 ▲
  senile 702.0
  specified NEC 078.19
  syphilitic 091.3
  tuberculous (*see also* Tuberculosis) 017.0
  venereal (female) (male) 078.19
Warthin's tumor (salivary gland) (M8561/0) 210.2
Washerwoman's itch 692.4
Wassilieff's disease (leptospiral jaundice) 100.0
Wasting
  disease 799.4
    due to malnutrition 261
  extreme (due to malnutrition) 261
  muscular NEC 728.2
  palsy, paralysis 335.21
Water
  clefts 366.12
  deprivation of 994.3
  in joint (*see also* Effusion, joint) 719.0
  intoxication 276.6
  itch 120.3
  lack of 994.3
  loading 276.6
  on
    brain — *see* Hydrocephalus
    chest 511.8
  poisoning 276.6
Waterbrash 787.1
Water-hammer pulse (*see also* Insufficiency, aortic) 424.1
Waterhouse (-Friderichsen) disease or syndrome 036.3
Water-losing nephritis 588.8
Wax in ear 380.4
Waxy
  degeneration, any site 277.3
  disease 277.3
  kidney 277.3 [583.81]
  liver (large) 277.3
  spleen 277.3
Weak, weakness (generalized) 780.7
  arches (acquired) 734
    congenital 754.61
  bladder sphincter 596.59
  congenital 779.8

Weak, weakness—continued
eye muscle — see Strabismus
foot (double) — see Weak, arches
heart, cardiac (see also Failure, heart) 428.9
   congenital 746.9
mind 317
muscle 728.9
myocardium (see also Failure, heart) 428.9
newborn 779.8
pelvic fundus 618.8
pulse 785.9
senile 797
valvular — see Endocarditis

Wear, worn, tooth, teeth
(approximal) (hard tissues) (interproximal) (occlusal) 521.1

Weather, weathered
effects of
  cold NEC 991.9
    specified effect NEC 991.8
  hot (see also Heat) 992.9
skin 692.74

Web, webbed (congenital) — see also Anomaly, specified type NEC
canthus 743.63
digits (see also Syndactylism) 755.10
esophagus 750.3
fingers (see also Syndactylism, fingers) 755.11
larynx (glottic) (subglottic) 748.2
neck (pterygium colli) 744.5
Paterson-Kelly (sideropenic dysphagia) 280.8
popliteal syndrome 756.89
toes (see also Syndactylism, toes) 755.13

Weber's paralysis or syndrome 344.89
Weber-Christian disease or syndrome (nodular nonsuppurative panniculitis) 729.30
Weber-Cockayne syndrome (epidermolysis bullosa) 757.39
Weber-Dimitri syndrome 759.6
Weber-Gubler syndrome 344.89
Weber-Leyden syndrome 344.89
Weber-Osler syndrome (familial hemorrhagic telangiectasia) 448.0
Wedge-shaped or wedging vertebra (see also Osteoporosis) 733.00
Wegener's granulomatosis or syndrome 446.4
Wegner's disease (syphilitic osteochondritis) 090.0
Weight
gain (abnormal) (excessive) 783.1
  during pregnancy 646.1
  insufficient 646.8
less than 1000 grams at birth 765.0
loss (cause unknown) 783.2

Weightlessness 994.9
Weil's disease (leptospiral jaundice) 100.0
Weill-Marchesani syndrome (brachymorphism and ectopia lentis) 759.89
Weingarten's syndrome (tropical eosinophilia) 518.3
Weir Mitchell's disease (erythromelalgia) 443.89
Weiss-Baker syndrome (carotid sinus syncope) 337.0
Weissenbach-Thibierge syndrome (cutaneous systemic sclerosis) 710.1

Wen (see also Cyst, sebaceous) 706.2
Wenckebach's phenomenon, heart block (second degree) 426.13
Werdnig-Hoffmann syndrome (muscular atrophy) 335.0
Werlhof's disease (see also Purpura, thrombocytopenic) 287.3
Werlhof-Wichmann syndrome (see also Purpura, thrombocytopenic) 287.3
Wermer's syndrome or disease (polyendocrine adenomatosis) 258.0
Werner's disease or syndrome (progeria adultorum) 259.8
Werner-His disease (trench fever) 083.1
Werner-Schultz disease (agranulocytosis) 288.0
Wernicke's encephalopathy, disease, or syndrome (superior hemorrhagic polioencephalitis) 265.1
Wernicke-Korsakoff syndrome or psychosis (nonalcoholic) 294.0
alcoholic 291.1
Wernicke-Posadas disease (see also Coccidioidomycosis) 114.9
Wesselsbron fever 066.3
West African fever 084.8
West Nile fever 066.3
Westphal-Strümpell syndrome (hepatolenticular degeneration) 275.1
Wet
brain (alcoholic) (see also Alcoholism) 303.9
feet, tropical (syndrome) (maceration) 991.4
lung (syndrome)
  adult 518.5
  newborn 770.6 ▲
Wharton's duct — see condition
Wheal 709.8
Wheezing 786.09
Whiplash injury or syndrome 847.0
Whipple's disease or syndrome (intestinal lipodystrophy) 040.2
Whipworm 127.3
"Whistling face" syndrome (craniocarpotarsal dystrophy) 759.89
White — see also condition
kidney
  large — see Nephrosis
  small 582.9
leg, puerperal, postpartum, childbirth 671.4
  nonpuerperal 451.19
mouth 112.0
patches of mouth 528.6
sponge nevus of oral mucosa 750.26
spot lesions, teeth 521.0
White's disease (congenital) (keratosis follicularis) 757.39
Whitehead 706.2
Whitlow (with lymphangitis) 681.01
herpetic 054.6
Whitmore's disease or fever (melioidosis) 025
Whooping cough 033.9
with pneumonia 033.9 [484.3]
due to
  Bordetella
    bronchoseptica 033.8
      with pneumonia 033.8 [484.3]
    parapertussis 033.1
      with pneumonia 033.1 [484.3]

Whooping cough—continued
due to—continued
  Bordetella—continued
    pertussis 033.0
      with pneumonia 033.0 [484.3]
  specified organism NEC 033.8
    with pneumonia 033.8 [484.3]
vaccination, prophylactic (against) V03.6
Wichmann's asthma (laryngismus stridulus) 478.75
Widal (-Abrami) syndrome (acquired hemolytic jaundice) 283.9
Widening aorta (see also Aneurysm, aorta) 441.9
ruptured 441.5
Wilkie's disease or syndrome 557.1
Wilkinson-Sneddon disease or syndrome (subcorneal pustular dermatosis) 694.1
Willan's lepra 696.1
Willan-Plumbe syndrome (psoriasis) 696.1
Willebrand (-Jürgens) syndrome or thrombopathy (angiohemophilia) 286.4
Willi-Prader syndrome (hypogenital dystrophy with diabetic tendency) 759.81
Willis' disease (diabetes mellitus) (see also Diabetes) 250.0
Wilms' tumor or neoplasm (nephroblastoma) (M8960/3) 189.0
Wilson's
disease or syndrome (hepatolenticular degeneration) 275.1
hepatolenticular degeneration 275.1
lichen ruber 697.0
Wilson-Brocq disease (dermatitis exfoliativa) 695.89
Wilson-Mikity syndrome 770.7
Window — see also Imperfect, closure aorticopulmonary 745.0
Winged scapula 736.89
Winter — see also condition
vomiting disease 078.82
Wise's disease 696.2
Wiskott-Aldrich syndrome (eczema-thrombocytopenia) 279.12
Withdrawal symptoms, syndrome
alcohol 291.8
  delirium (acute) 291.0
  chronic 291.1
  newborn 760.71
drug or narcotic 292.0
newborn, infant of dependent mother 779.5
steroid NEC
  correct substance properly administered 255.4
  overdose or wrong substance given or taken 962.0
Withdrawing reaction, child or adolescent 313.22
Witts' anemia (achlorhydric anemia) 280.9
Witzelsucht 301.9
Woakes' syndrome (ethmoiditis) 471.1
Wohlfart-Kugelberg-Welander disease 335.11
Woillez' disease (acute idiopathic pulmonary congestion) 518.5
Wolff-Parkinson-White syndrome (anomalous atrioventricular excitation) 426.7

Wolhynian fever 083.1
Wolman's disease (primary familial xanthomatosis) 272.7
Wood asthma 495.8
Woolly, wooly hair (congenital) (nevus) 757.4
Wool-sorters' disease 022.1
Word
blindness (congenital) (developmental) 315.01
  secondary to organic lesion 784.61
deafness (secondary to organic lesion) 784.69
  developmental 315.31
Worm(s) (colic) (fever) (infection) (infestation) (see also Infestation) 128.9
guinea 125.7
in intestine NEC 127.9
Worm-eaten soles 102.3
Worn out (see also Exhaustion) 780.7
"Worried well" V65.5
Wound, open (by cutting or piercing instrument) (by firearms) (cut) (dissection) (incised) (laceration) (penetration) (perforating) (puncture) (with initial hemorrhage, not internal) 879.8

> Note — For fracture with open wound, see Fracture.
>
> For laceration, traumatic rupture, tear or penetrating wound of internal organs, such as heart, lung, liver, kidney, pelvic organs, etc., whether or not accompanied by open wound or fracture in the same region, see Injury, internal.
>
> For contused wound, see Contusion. For crush injury, see Crush. For abrasion, insect bite (nonvenomous), blister, or scratch, see Injury, superficial.
>
> Complicated includes wounds with:
>
>   delayed healing
>   delayed treatment
>   foreign body
>   primary infection
>
> For late effect of open wound, see Late, effect, wound, open, by site.

abdomen, abdominal (external) (muscle) 879.2
  complicated 879.3
  wall (anterior) 879.2
    complicated 879.3
    lateral 879.4
      complicated 879.5
alveolar (process) 873.62
  complicated 873.72
ankle 891.0
  with tendon involvement 891.2
  complicated 891.1
anterior chamber, eye (see also Wound, open, intraocular) 871.9
anus 879.6
  complicated 879.7
arm 884.0
  with tendon involvement 884.2
  complicated 884.1
forearm 881.00
  with tendon involvement 881.20
  complicated 881.10

Wound, open—*continued*
  arm—*continued*
    multiple sites — *see* Wound, open, multiple, upper limb
    upper 880.03
      with tendon involvement 880.23
      complicated 880.13
      multiple sites (with axillary or shoulder regions) 880.09
        with tendon involvement 880.29
        complicated 880.19
  artery — *see* Injury, blood vessel, by site
  auditory
    canal (external) (meatus) 872.02
      complicated 872.12
    ossicles (incus) (malleus) (stapes) 872.62
      complicated 872.72
  auricle, ear 872.01
    complicated 872.11
  axilla 880.02
    with tendon involvement 880.22
    complicated 880.12
      with tendon involvement 880.29
    involving other sites of upper arm 880.09
    complicated 880.19
  back 876.0
    complicated 876.1
  bladder — *see* Injury, internal, bladder
  blood vessel — *see* Injury, blood vessel, by site
  brain — *see* Injury, intracranial, with open intracranial wound
  breast 879.0
    complicated 879.1
  brow 873.42
    complicated 873.52
  buccal mucosa 873.61
    complicated 873.71
  buttock 877.0
    complicated 877.1
  calf 891.0
    with tendon involvement 891.2
    complicated 891.1
  canaliculus lacrimalis 870.8
    with laceration of eyelid 870.2
  canthus, eye 870.8
    laceration — *see* Laceration, eyelid
  cavernous sinus — *see* Injury, intracranial
  cerebellum — *see* Injury, intracranial
  cervical esophagus 874.4
    complicated 874.5
  cervix — *see* Injury, internal, cervix
  cheek(s) (external) 873.41
    complicated 873.51
    internal 873.61
      complicated 873.71
  chest (wall) (external) 875.0
    complicated 875.1
  chin 873.44
    complicated 873.54
  choroid 363.63
  ciliary body (eye) (*see also* Wound, open, intraocular) 871.9
  clitoris 878.8
    complicated 878.9
  cochlea 872.64
    complicated 872.74
  complicated 879.9

Wound, open—*continued*
  conjunctiva — *see* Wound, open, intraocular
  cornea (nonpenetrating) (*see also* Wound, open, intraocular) 871.9
  costal region 875.0
    complicated 875.1
  Descemet's membrane (*see also* Wound, open, intraocular) 871.9
  digit(s)
    foot 893.0
      with tendon involvement 893.2
      complicated 893.1
    hand 883.0
      with tendon involvement 883.2
      complicated 883.1
  drumhead, ear 872.61
    complicated 872.71
  ear 872.8
    canal 872.02
      complicated 872.12
    complicated 872.9
    drum 872.61
      complicated 872.71
    external 872.00
      complicated 872.10
    multiple sites 872.69
      complicated 872.79
    ossicles (incus) (malleus) (stapes) 872.62
      complicated 872.72
    specified part NEC 872.69
      complicated 872.79
  elbow 881.01
    with tendon involvement 881.21
    complicated 881.11
  epididymis 878.2
    complicated 878.3
  epigastric region 879.2
    complicated 879.3
  epiglottis 874.01
    complicated 874.11
  esophagus (cervical) 874.4
    complicated 874.5
    thoracic — *see* Injury, internal, esophagus
  Eustachian tube 872.63
    complicated 872.73
  extremity
    lower (multiple) NEC 894.0
      with tendon involvement 894.2
      complicated 894.1
    upper (multiple) NEC 884.0
      with tendon involvement 884.2
      complicated 884.1
  eye(s) (globe) — *see* Wound, open, intraocular
  eyeball NEC 871.9
    laceration (*see also* Laceration, eyeball) 871.4
    penetrating (*see also* Penetrating wound, eyeball) 871.7
  eyebrow 873.42
    complicated 873.52
  eyelid NEC 870.8
    laceration — *see* Laceration, eyelid
  face 873.40
    complicated 873.50
    multiple sites 873.49
      complicated 873.59
    specified part NEC 873.49
      complicated 873.59
  fallopian tube — *see* Injury, internal, fallopian tube
  finger(s) (nail) (subungual) 883.0
    with tendon involvement 883.2
    complicated 883.1

Wound, open—*continued*
  flank 879.4
    complicated 879.5
  foot (any part except toe(s) alone) 892.0
    with tendon involvement 892.2
    complicated 892.1
  forearm 881.00
    with tendon involvement 881.20
    complicated 881.10
  forehead 873.42
    complicated 873.52
  genital organs (external) NEC 878.8
    complicated 878.9
    internal — *see* Injury, internal, by site
  globe (eye) (*see also* Wound, open, eyeball) 871.9
  groin 879.4
    complicated 879.5
  gum(s) 873.62
    complicated 873.72
  hand (except finger(s) alone) 882.0
    with tendon involvement 882.2
    complicated 882.1
  head NEC 873.8
    with intracranial injury — *see* Injury, intracranial
    due to or associated with skull fracture — *see* Fracture, skull
    complicated 873.9
    scalp — *see* Wound, open, scalp
  heel 892.0
    with tendon involvement 892.2
    complicated 892.1
  high-velocity (grease gun) — *see* Wound, open, complicated, by site
  hip 890.0
    with tendon involvement 890.2
    complicated 890.1
  hymen 878.6
    complicated 878.7
  hypochondrium 879.4
    complicated 879.5
  hypogastric region 879.2
    complicated 879.3
  iliac (region) 879.4
    complicated 879.5
  incidental to
    dislocation — *see* Dislocation, open, by site
    fracture — *see* Fracture, open, by site
    intracranial injury — *see* Injury, intracranial, with open intracranial wound
    nerve injury — *see* Injury, nerve, by site
  inguinal region 879.4
    complicated 879.5
  instep 892.0
    with tendon involvement 892.2
    complicated 892.1
  interscapular region 876.0
    complicated 876.1
  intracranial — *see* Injury, intracranial, with open intracranial wound
  intraocular 871.9
    with
      partial loss (of intraocular tissue) 871.2
      prolapse or exposure (of intraocular tissue) 871.1

Wound, open—*continued*
  intraocular—*continued*
    laceration (*see also* Laceration, eyeball) 871.4
    penetrating 871.7
      with foreign body (nonmagnetic) 871.6
      magnetic 871.5
    without prolapse (of intraocular tissue) 871.0
  iris (*see also* Wound, open, eyeball) 871.9
  jaw (fracture not involved) 873.44
    with fracture — *see* Fracture, jaw
    complicated 873.54
  knee 891.0
    with tendon involvement 891.2
    complicated 891.1
  labium (majus) (minus) 878.4
    complicated 878.5
  lacrimal apparatus, gland, or sac 870.8
    with laceration of eyelid 870.2
  larynx 874.01
    with trachea 874.00
      complicated 874.10
    complicated 874.11
  leg (multiple) 891.0
    with tendon involvement 891.2
    complicated 891.1
    lower 891.0
      with tendon involvement 891.2
      complicated 891.1
    thigh 890.0
      with tendon involvement 890.2
      complicated 890.1
    upper 890.0
      with tendon involvement 890.2
      complicated 890.1
  lens (eye) (alone) (*see also* Cataract, traumatic) 366.20
    with involvement of other eye structures — *see* Wound, open, eyeball
  limb
    lower (multiple) NEC 894.0
      with tendon involvement 894.2
      complicated 894.1
    upper (multiple) NEC 884.0
      with tendon involvement 884.2
      complicated 884.1
  lip 873.43
    complicated 873.53
  loin 876.0
    complicated 876.1
  lumbar region 876.0
    complicated 876.1
  malar region 873.41
    complicated 873.51
  mastoid region 873.49
    complicated 873.59
  mediastinum — *see* Injury, internal, mediastinum
  midthoracic region 875.0
    complicated 875.1
  mouth 873.60
    complicated 873.70
    floor 873.64
      complicated 873.74
    multiple sites 873.69
      complicated 873.79
    specified site NEC 873.69
      complicated 873.79

Wound, open—continued
multiple, unspecified site(s) 879.8

> Note — Multiple open wounds of sites classifiable to the same four-digit category should be classified to that category unless they are in different limbs.
>
> Multiple open wounds of sites classifiable to different four-digit categories, or to different limbs, should be coded separately.

    complicated 879.9
  lower limb(s) (one or both) (sites classifiable to more than one three-digit category in 890 to 893) 894.0
    with tendon involvement 894.2
    complicated 894.1
  upper limb(s) (one or both) (sites classifiable to more than one three-digit category in 880 to 883) 884.0
    with tendon involvement 884.2
    complicated 884.1
  muscle — see Sprain, by site
  nail
    finger(s) 883.0
      complicated 883.1
    thumb 883.0
      complicated 883.1
    toe(s) 893.0
      complicated 893.1
  nape (neck) 874.8
    complicated 874.9
    specified part NEC 874.8
      complicated 874.9
  nasal — see also Wound, open, nose
    cavity 873.22
      complicated 873.32
    septum 873.21
      complicated 873.31
    sinuses 873.23
      complicated 873.33
  nasopharynx 873.22
    complicated 873.32
  neck 874.8
    complicated 874.9
    nape 874.8
      complicated 874.9
    specified part NEC 874.8
      complicated 874.9
  nerve — see Injury, nerve, by site
  nose 873.20
    complicated 873.30
    multiple sites 873.29
      complicated 873.39
    septum 873.21
      complicated 873.31
    sinuses 873.23
      complicated 873.33
  occipital region — see Wound, open, scalp
  ocular NEC 871.9
    adnexa 870.9
      specified region NEC 870.8
    laceration (see also Laceration, ocular) 871.4
    muscle (extraocular) 870.3
      with foreign body 870.4
      eyelid 870.1
    intraocular — see Wound, open, eyeball
    penetrating (see also Penetrating wound, ocular) 871.7
  orbit 870.8
    penetrating 870.3
      with foreign body 870.4
  orbital region 870.9

Wound, open—continued
  ovary — see Injury, internal, pelvic organs
  palate 873.65
    complicated 873.75
  palm 882.0
    with tendon involvement 882.2
    complicated 882.1
  parathyroid (gland) 874.2
    complicated 874.3
  parietal region — see Wound, open, scalp
  pelvic floor or region 879.6
    complicated 879.7
  penis 878.0
    complicated 878.1
  perineum 879.6
    complicated 879.7
  periocular area 870.8
    laceration of skin 870.0
  pharynx 874.4
    complicated 874.5
  pinna 872.01
    complicated 872.11
  popliteal space 891.0
    with tendon involvement 891.2
    complicated 891.1
  prepuce 878.0
    complicated 878.1
  pubic region 879.2
    complicated 879.3
  pudenda 878.8
    complicated 878.9
  rectovaginal septum 878.8
    complicated 878.9
  sacral region 877.0
    complicated 877.1
  sacroiliac region 877.0
    complicated 877.1
  salivary (ducts) (glands) 873.69
    complicated 873.79
  scalp 873.0
    complicated 873.1
  scalpel, fetus or newborn 767.8
  scapular region 880.01
    with tendon involvement 880.21
    complicated 880.11
    involving other sites of upper arm 880.09
      with tendon involvement 880.29
      complicated 880.19
  sclera — (see also Wound, open, intraocular) 871.9
  scrotum 878.2
    complicated 878.3
  seminal vesicle — see Injury, internal, pelvic organs
  shin 891.0
    with tendon involvement 891.2
    complicated 891.1
  shoulder 880.00
    with tendon involvement 880.20
    complicated 880.10
    involving other sites of upper arm 880.09
      with tendon involvement 880.29
      complicated 880.19
  skin NEC 879.8
    complicated 879.9
  skull — see also Injury, intracranial, with open intracranial wound
    with skull fracture — see Fracture, skull
  spermatic cord (scrotal) 878.2
    complicated 878.3
    pelvic region — see Injury, internal, spermatic cord
  spinal cord — see Injury, spinal

Wound, open—continued
  sternal region 875.0
    complicated 875.1
  subconjunctival — see Wound, open, intraocular
  subcutaneous NEC 879.8
    complicated 879.9
  submaxillary region 873.44
    complicated 873.54
  submental region 873.44
    complicated 873.54
  subungual
    finger(s) (thumb) — see Wound, open, finger
    toe(s) — see Wound, open, toe
  supraclavicular region 874.8
    complicated 874.9
  supraorbital 873.42
    complicated 873.52
  temple 873.49
    complicated 873.59
  temporal region 873.49
    complicated 873.59
  testis 878.2
    complicated 878.3
  thigh 890.0
    with tendon involvement 890.2
    complicated 890.1
  thorax, thoracic (external) 875.0
    complicated 875.1
  throat 874.8
    complicated 874.9
  thumb (nail) (subungual) 883.0
    with tendon involvement 883.2
    complicated 883.1
  thyroid (gland) 874.2
    complicated 874.3
  toe(s) (nail) (subungual) 893.0
    with tendon involvement 893.2
    complicated 893.1
  tongue 873.64
    complicated 873.74
  tonsil — see Wound, open, neck
  trachea (cervical region) 874.02
    with larynx 874.00
      complicated 874.10
    complicated 874.12
    intrathoracic — see Injury, internal, trachea
  trunk (multiple) NEC 879.6
    complicated 879.7
    specified site NEC 879.6
      complicated 879.7
  tunica vaginalis 878.2
    complicated 878.3
  tympanic membrane 872.61
    complicated 872.71
  tympanum 872.61
    complicated 872.71
  umbilical region 879.2
    complicated 879.3
  ureter — see Injury, internal, ureter
  urethra — see Injury, internal, urethra
  uterus — see Injury, internal, uterus
  uvula 873.69
    complicated 873.79
  vagina 878.6
    complicated 878.7
  vas deferens — see Injury, internal, vas deferens
  vitreous (humor) 871.2
  vulva 878.4
    complicated 878.5
  wrist 881.02
    with tendon involvement 881.22
    complicated 881.12

Wright's syndrome (hyperabduction) 447.8
  pneumonia 390 [517.1]

Wringer injury — see Crush injury, by site
Wrinkling of skin 701.8
Wrist — see also condition
  drop (acquired) 736.05
Wrong drug (given in error) NEC 977.9
  specified drug or substance — see Table of drugs and chemicals
Wry neck — see also Torticollis
  congenital 754.1
Wuchereria infestation 125.0
  bancrofti 125.0
  Brugia malayi 125.1
  malayi 125.1
Wuchereriasis 125.0
Wuchereriosis 125.0
Wuchernde struma langhans (M8332/3) 193

X

Xanthelasma 272.2
  eyelid 272.2 [374.51]
  palpebrarum 272.2 [374.51]
Xanthelasmatosis (essential) 272.2
Xanthelasmoidea 757.33
Xanthine stones 277.2
Xanthinuria 277.2
Xanthofibroma (M8831/0) — see Neoplasm, connective tissue, benign
Xanthoma(s), xanthomatosis 272.2
  with
    hyperlipoproteinemia
      type I 272.3
      type III 272.2
      type IV 272.1
      type V 272.3
  bone 272.7
  craniohypophyseal 277.8
  cutaneotendinous 272.7
  diabeticorum 250.8 [272.2]
  disseminatum 272.7
  eruptive 272.2
  eyelid 272.2 [374.51]
  familial 272.7
  hereditary 272.7
  hypercholesterinemic 272.0
  hypercholesterolemic 272.0
  hyperlipemic 272.4
  hyperlipidemic 272.4
  infantile 272.7
  joint 272.7
  juvenile 272.7
  multiple 272.7
  multiplex 272.7
  primary familial 272.7
  tendon (sheath) 272.7
  tuberosum 272.2
  tuberous 272.2
  tubo-eruptive 272.2
Xanthosis 709.09
  surgical 998.81
Xenophobia 300.29
Xeroderma (congenital) 757.39
  acquired 701.1
    eyelid 373.33
  eyelid 373.33
  pigmentosum 757.33
  vitamin A deficiency 264.8
Xerophthalmia 372.53
  vitamin A deficiency 264.7
Xerosis
  conjunctiva 372.53
    with Bitôt's spot 372.53
      vitamin A deficiency 264.1
    vitamin A deficiency 264.0
  cornea 371.40
    with corneal ulceration 370.00
      vitamin A deficiency 264.3

Xerosis—continued
    cornea—continued
        vitamin A deficiency 264.2
    cutis 706.8
    skin 706.8
Xerostomia 527.7
Xiphodynia 733.90
Xiphoidalgia 733.90
Xiphoiditis 733.99
Xiphopagus 759.4
XO syndrome 758.6
X-ray
    effects, adverse, NEC 990
    of chest
        for suspected tuberculosis V71.2
        routine V72.5
XXX syndrome 758.8
XXXXY syndrome 758.8
XXY syndrome 758.7
Xyloketosuria 271.8
Xylosuria 271.8
Xylulosuria 271.8
XYY syndrome 758.8

Y

Yawning 786.09
    psychogenic 306.1
Yaws 102.9
    bone or joint lesions 102.6
    butter 102.1
    chancre 102.0
    cutaneous, less than five years after infection 102.2
    early (cutaneous) (macular) (maculopapular) (micropapular) (papular) 102.2
        frambeside 102.2
        skin lesions NEC 102.2
    eyelid 102.9 [373.4]
    ganglion 102.6
    gangosis, gangosa 102.5
    gumma, gummata 102.4
        bone 102.6
    gummatous
        frambeside 102.4
        osteitis 102.6
        periostitis 102.6
    hydrarthrosis 102.6
    hyperkeratosis (early) (late) (palmar) (plantar) 102.3
    initial lesions 102.0
    joint lesions 102.6
    juxta-articular nodules 102.7
    late nodular (ulcerated) 102.4
    latent (without clinical manifestations) (with positive serology) 102.8
    mother 102.0
    mucosal 102.7
    multiple papillomata 102.1
    nodular, late (ulcerated) 102.4
    osteitis 102.6
    papilloma, papillomata (palmar) (plantar) 102.1
    periostitis (hypertrophic) 102.6
    ulcers 102.4
    wet crab 102.1
Yeast infection (see also Candidiasis) 112.9
Yellow
    atrophy (liver) 570
        chronic 571.8
        resulting from administration of blood, plasma, serum, or other biological substance (within 8 months of administration) — see Hepatitis, viral

Yellow—continued
    fever — see Fever, yellow
    jack (see also Fever, yellow) 060.9
    jaundice (see also Jaundice) 782.4
Yersinia septica 027.8

Z

Zagari's disease (xerostomia) 527.7
Zahorsky's disease (exanthema subitum) 057.8
    syndrome (herpangina) 074.0
Zenker's diverticulum (esophagus) 530.6
Ziehen-Oppenheim disease 333.6
Zieve's syndrome (jaundice, hyperlipemia, and hemolytic anemia) 571.1
Zika fever 066.3
Zollinger-Ellison syndrome (gastric hypersecretion with pancreatic islet cell tumor) 251.5
Zona (see also Herpes, zoster) 053.9
Zoophilia (erotica) 302.1
Zoophobia 300.29
Zoster (herpes) (see also Herpes, zoster) 053.9
Zuelzer (-Ogden) anemia or syndrome (nutritional megaloblastic anemia) 281.2
Zygodactyly (see also Syndactylism) 755.10
Zygomycosis 117.7
Zymotic — see condition

TABLE OF DRUGS AND CHEMICALS

VOLUME 2

SECTION 2

SECTION 2

Alphabetic Index to Poisoning and External Causes of Adverse Effects of Drugs and Other Chemical Substances

TABLE OF DRUGS AND CHEMICALS

This table contains a classification of drugs and other chemical substances to identify poisoning states and external causes of adverse effects.

Each of the listed substances in the table is assigned a code according to the poisoning classification (960-989). These codes are used when there is a statement of poisoning, overdose, wrong substance given or taken, or intoxication.

The table also contains a listing of external causes of adverse effects. An adverse effect is a pathologic manifestation due to ingestion or exposure to drugs or other chemical substances (e.g., dermatitis, hypersensitivity reaction, aspirin gastritis). The adverse effect is to be identified by the appropriate code found in Section 1, Index to Diseases and Injuries. An external cause code can then be used to identify the circumstances involved. The table headings pertaining to external causes are defined below:

Accidental poisoning (E850-E869) — accidental overdose of drug, wrong substance given or taken, drug taken inadvertently, accidents in the usage of drugs and biologicals in medical and surgical procedures, and to show external causes of poisonings classifiable to 980-989.

Therapeutic use (E930-E949) — a correct substance properly administered in therapeutic or prophylactic dosage as the external cause of adverse effects.

Suicide attempt (E950-E952) — instances in which self-inflicted injuries or poisonings are involved.

Assault (E961-E962) — injury or poisoning inflicted by another person with the intent to injure or kill.

Undetermined (E980-E982) — to be used when the intent of the poisoning or injury cannot be determined whether it was intentional or accidental.

The American Hospital Formulary Service list numbers are included in the table to help classify new drugs not identified in the table by name. The AHFS list numbers are keyed to the continually revised American Hospital Formulary Service (AHFS).* These listings are found in the table under the main term **Drug.**

Excluded from the table are radium and other radioactive substances. The classification of adverse effects and complications pertaining to these substances will be found in Section 1, Index to Diseases and Injuries, and Section 3, Index to External Causes of Injuries.

Although certain substances are indexed with one or more subentries, the majority are listed according to one use or state. It is recognized that many substances may be used in various ways, in medicine and in industry, and may cause adverse effects whatever the state of the agent (solid, liquid, or fumes arising from a liquid). In cases in which the reported data indicates a use or state not in the table, or which is clearly different from the one listed, an attempt should be made to classify the substance in the form which most nearly expresses the reported facts.

*American Hospital Formulary Service, 2 vol. (Washington, D.C.: American Society of Hospital Pharmacists, 1959–)

TABLE OF DRUGS AND CHEMICALS

Substance	Poisoning	Accident	Therapeutic Use	Suicide Attempt	Assault	Undetermined
1-propanol	980.3	E860.4	—	E950.9	E962.1	E980.9
2-propanol	980.2	E860.3	—	E950.9	E962.1	E980.9
2, 4-D (dichlorophenoxyacetic acid)	989.4	E863.5	—	E950.6	E962.1	E980.7
2, 4-toluene diisocyanate	983.0	E864.0	—	E950.7	E962.1	E980.6
2, 4, 5-T (trichlorophenoxyacetic acid)	989.2	E863.5	—	E950.6	E962.1	E980.7
14-hydroxydihydromorphinone	965.09	E850.2	E935.2	E950.0	E962.0	E980.0
ABOB	961.7	E857	E931.7	E950.4	E962.0	E980.4
Abrus (seed)	988.2	E865.3	—	E950.9	E962.1	E980.9
Absinthe	980.0	E860.1	—	E950.9	E962.1	E980.9
beverage	980.0	E860.0	—	E950.9	E962.1	E980.9
Acenocoumarin, acenocoumarol	964.2	E858.2	E934.2	E950.4	E962.0	E980.4
Acepromazine	969.1	E853.0	E939.1	E950.3	E962.0	E980.3
Acetal	982.8	E862.4	—	E950.9	E962.1	E980.9
Acetaldehyde (vapor)	987.8	E869.8	—	E952.8	E962.2	E982.8
liquid	989.8	E866.8	—	E950.9	E962.1	E980.9
Acetaminophen	965.4	E850.4	E935.4	E950.0	E962.0	E980.0
Acetaminosalol	965.1	E850.3	E935.3	E950.0	E962.0	E980.0
Acetanilid(e)	965.4	E850.4	E935.4	E950.0	E962.0	E980.0
Acetarsol, acetarsone	961.1	E857	E931.1	E950.4	E962.0	E980.4
Acetazolamide	974.2	E858.5	E944.2	E950.4	E962.0	E980.4
Acetic						
acid	983.1	E864.1	—	E950.7	E962.1	E980.6
with sodium acetate (ointment)	976.3	E858.7	E946.3	E950.4	E962.0	E980.4
irrigating solution	974.5	E858.5	E944.5	E950.4	E962.0	E980.4
lotion	976.2	E858.7	E946.2	E950.4	E962.0	E980.4
anhydride	983.1	E864.1	—	E950.7	E962.1	E980.6
ether (vapor)	982.8	E862.4	—	E950.9	E962.1	E980.9
Acetohexamide	962.3	E858.0	E932.3	E950.4	E962.0	E980.4
Acetomenaphthone	964.3	E858.2	E934.3	E950.4	E962.0	E980.4
Acetomorphine	965.01	E850.0	E935.0	E950.0	E962.0	E980.0
Acetone (oils) (vapor)	982.8	E862.4	—	E950.9	E962.1	E980.9
Acetophenazine (maleate)	969.1	E853.0	E939.1	E950.3	E962.0	E980.3
Acetophenetidin	965.4	E850.4	E935.4	E950.0	E962.0	E980.0
Acetophenone	982.0	E862.4	—	E950.9	E962.1	E980.9
Acetorphine	965.09	E850.2	E935.2	E950.0	E962.0	E980.0
Acetosulfone (sodium)	961.8	E857	E931.8	E950.4	E962.0	E980.4
Acetrizoate (sodium)	977.8	E858.8	E947.8	E950.4	E962.0	E980.4
Acetylcarbromal	967.3	E852.2	E937.3	E950.2	E962.0	E980.2
Acetylcholine (chloride)	971.0	E855.3	E941.0	E950.4	E962.0	E980.4
Acetylcysteine	975.5	E858.6	E945.5	E950.4	E962.0	E980.4
Acetyldigitoxin	972.1	E858.3	E942.1	E950.4	E962.0	E980.4
Acetyldihydrocodeine	965.09	E850.2	E935.2	E950.0	E962.0	E980.0
Acetyldihydrocodeinone	965.09	E850.2	E935.2	E950.0	E962.0	E980.0
Acetylene (gas) (industrial)	987.1	E868.1	—	E951.8	E962.2	E981.8
incomplete combustion of — see Carbon monoxide, fuel, utility						
tetrachloride (vapor)	982.3	E862.4	—	E950.9	E962.1	E980.9
Acetyliodosalicylic acid	965.1	E850.3	E935.3	E950.0	E962.0	E980.0
Acetylphenylhydrazine	965.8	E850.8	E935.8	E950.0	E962.0	E980.0
Acetylsalicylic acid	965.1	E850.3	E935.3	E950.0	E962.0	E980.0
Achromycin	960.4	E856	E930.4	E950.4	E962.0	E980.4
ophthalmic preparation	976.5	E858.7	E946.5	E950.4	E962.0	E980.4
topical NEC	976.0	E858.7	E946.0	E950.4	E962.0	E980.4
Acidifying agents	963.2	E858.1	E933.2	E950.4	E962.0	E980.4
Acids (corrosive) NEC	983.1	E864.1	—	E950.7	E962.1	E980.6
Aconite (wild)	988.2	E865.4	—	E950.9	E962.1	E980.9
Aconitine (liniment)	976.8	E858.7	E946.8	E950.4	E962.0	E980.4
Aconitum ferox	988.2	E865.4	—	E950.9	E962.1	E980.9
Acridine	983.0	E864.0	—	E950.7	E962.1	E980.6
vapor	987.8	E869.8	—	E952.8	E962.2	E982.8
Acriflavine	961.9	E857	E931.9	E950.4	E962.0	E980.4
Acrisorcin	976.0	E858.7	E946.0	E950.4	E962.0	E980.4
Acrolein (gas)	987.8	E869.8	—	E952.8	E962.2	E982.8
liquid	989.8	E866.8	—	E950.9	E962.1	E980.9
Actaeu spicata	988.2	E865.4	—	E950.9	E962.1	E980.9
Acterol	961.5	E857	E931.5	E950.4	E962.0	E980.4
ACTH	962.4	E858.0	E932.4	E950.4	E962.0	E980.4
Acthar	962.4	E858.0	E932.4	E950.4	E962.0	E980.4
Actinomycin (C)(D)	960.7	E856	E930.7	E950.4	E962.0	E980.4
Adalin (acetyl)	967.3	E852.2	E937.3	E950.2	E962.0	E980.2
Adenosine (phosphate)	977.8	E858.8	E947.8	E950.4	E962.0	E980.4
Adhesives	989.8	E866.6	—	E950.9	E962.1	E980.9
ADH	962.5	E858.0	E932.5	E950.4	E962.0	E980.4
Adicillin	960.0	E856	E930.0	E950.4	E962.0	E980.4
Adiphenine	975.1	E855.6	E945.1	E950.4	E962.0	E980.4
Adjunct, pharmaceutical	977.4	E858.8	E947.4	E950.4	E962.0	E980.4

TABLE OF DRUGS AND CHEMICALS

Substance	Poisoning	Accident	Therapeutic-Use	Suicide Attempt	Assault	Undetermined
Adrenal (extract, cortex or medulla) (glucocorticoids) (hormones) (mineralocorticoids)	962.0	E858.0	E932.0	E950.4	E962.0	E980.4
ENT agent	976.6	E858.7	E946.6	E950.4	E962.0	E980.4
ophthalmic preparation	976.5	E858.7	E946.5	E950.4	E962.0	E980.4
topical NEC	976.0	E858.7	E946.0	E950.4	E962.0	E980.4
Adrenalin	971.2	E855.5	E941.2	E950.4	E962.0	E980.4
Adrenergic blocking agents	971.3	E855.6	E941.3	E950.4	E962.0	E980.4
Adrenergics	971.2	E855.5	E941.2	E950.4	E962.0	E980.4
Adrenochrome (derivatives)	972.8	E858.3	E942.8	E950.4	E962.0	E980.4
Adrenocorticotropic hormone	962.4	E858.0	E932.4	E950.4	E962.0	E980.4
Adrenocorticotropin	962.4	E858.0	E932.4	E950.4	E962.0	E980.4
Adriamycin	960.7	E856	E930.7	E950.4	E962.0	E980.4
Aerosol spray — see Sprays						
Aerosporin	960.8	E856	E930.8	E950.4	E962.0	E980.4
ENT agent	976.6	E858.7	E946.6	E950.4	E962.0	E980.4
ophthalmic preparation	976.5	E858.7	E946.5	E950.4	E962.0	E980.4
topical NEC	976.0	E858.7	E946.0	E950.4	E962.0	E980.4
Aethusa cynapium	988.2	E865.4	—	E950.9	E962.1	E980.9
Afghanistan black	969.6	E854.1	E939.6	E950.3	E962.0	E980.3
Aflatoxin	989.7	E865.9	—	E950.9	E962.1	E980.9
African boxwood	988.2	E865.4	—	E950.9	E962.1	E980.9
Agar (-agar)	973.3	E858.4	E943.3	E950.4	E962.0	E980.4
Agricultural agent NEC	989.8	E863.9	—	E950.6	E962.1	E980.7
Agrypnal	967.0	E851	E937.0	E950.1	E962.0	E980.1
Air contaminant(s), source or type not specified	987.9	E869.9	—	E952.9	E962.2	E982.9
specified type — see specific substance						
Akee	988.2	E865.4	—	E950.9	E962.1	E980.9
Akrinol	976.0	E858.7	E946.0	E950.4	E962.0	E980.4
Alantolactone	961.6	E857	E931.6	E950.4	E962.0	E980.4
Albamycin	960.8	E856	E930.8	E950.4	E962.0	E980.4
Albumin (normal human serum)	964.7	E858.2	E934.7	E950.4	E962.0	E980.4
Alcohol	980.9	E860.9	—	E950.9	E962.1	E980.9
absolute	980.0	E860.1	—	E950.9	E962.1	E980.9
beverage	980.0	E860.0	E947.8	E950.9	E962.1	E980.9
amyl	980.3	E860.4	—	E950.9	E962.1	E980.9
antifreeze	980.1	E860.2	—	E950.9	E962.1	E980.9
butyl	980.3	E860.4	—	E950.9	E962.1	E980.9
dehydrated	980.0	E860.1	—	E950.9	E962.1	E980.9
beverage	980.0	E860.0	E947.8	E950.9	E862.1	E980.9
denatured	980.0	E860.1	—	E950.9	E962.1	E980.9
deterrents	977.3	E858.8	E947.3	E950.4	E962.0	E980.4
diagnostic (gastric function)	977.8	E858.8	E947.8	E950.4	E962.0	E980.4
ethyl	980.0	E860.1	—	E950.9	E962.1	E980.9
beverage	980.0	E860.0	E947.8	E950.9	E962.1	E980.9
grain	980.0	E860.1	—	E950.9	E962.1	E980.9
beverage	980.0	E860.0	E947.8	E950.9	E962.1	E980.9
industrial	980.9	E860.9	—	E950.9	E962.1	E980.9
isopropyl	980.2	E860.3	—	E950.9	E962.1	E980.9
methyl	980.1	E860.2	—	E950.9	E962.1	E980.9
preparation for consumption	980.0	E860.0	E947.8	E950.9	E962.1	E980.9
propyl	980.3	E860.4	—	E950.9	E962.1	E980.9
secondary	980.2	E860.3	—	E950.9	E962.1	E980.9
radiator	980.1	E860.2	—	E950.9	E962.1	E980.9
rubbing	980.2	E860.3	—	E950.9	E962.1	E980.9
specified type NEC	980.8	E860.8	—	E950.9	E962.1	E980.9
surgical	980.9	E860.9	—	E950.9	E962.1	E980.9
vapor (from any type of alcohol)	987.8	E869.8	—	E952.8	E962.2	E982.8
wood	980.1	E860.2	—	E950.9	E962.1	E980.9
Alcuronium chloride	975.2	E858.6	E945.2	E950.4	E962.0	E980.4
Aldactone	974.4	E858.5	E944.4	E950.4	E962.0	E980.4
Aldicarb	989.3	E863.2	—	E950.6	E962.1	E980.7
Aldomet	972.6	E858.3	E942.6	E950.4	E962.0	E980.4
Aldosterone	962.0	E858.0	E932.0	E950.4	E962.0	E980.4
Aldrin (dust)	989.2	E863.0	—	E950.6	E962.1	E980.7
Algeldrate	973.0	E858.4	E943.0	E950.4	E962.0	E980.4
Alidase	963.4	E858.1	E933.4	E950.4	E962.0	E980.4
Aliphatic thiocyanates	989.0	E866.8	—	E950.9	E962.1	E980.9
Alkaline antiseptic solution (aromatic)	976.6	E858.7	E946.6	E950.4	E962.0	E980.4
Alkalinizing agents (medicinal)	963.3	E858.1	E933.3	E950.4	E962.0	E980.4
Alkalis, caustic	983.2	E864.2	—	E950.7	E962.1	E980.6
Alkalizing agents (medicinal)	963.3	E858.1	E933.3	E950.4	E962.0	E980.4
Alka-seltzer	965.1	E850.3	E935.3	E950.0	E962.0	E980.0
Alkavervir	972.6	E858.3	E942.6	E950.4	E962.0	E980.4
Allegron	969.0	E854.0	E939.0	E950.3	E962.0	E980.3
Allobarbital, allobarbitone	967.0	E851	E937.0	E950.1	E962.0	E980.1
Allopurinol	974.7	E858.5	E944.7	E950.4	E962.0	E980.4

TABLE OF DRUGS AND CHEMICALS

Substance	Poisoning	Accident	Therapeutic-Use	Suicide Attempt	Assault	Undetermined
Allylestrenol	962.2	E858.0	E932.2	E950.4	E962.0	E980.4
Allylisopropylacetylurea	967.8	E852.8	E937.8	E950.2	E962.0	E980.2
Allylisopropylmalonylurea	967.0	E851	E937.0	E950.1	E962.0	E980.1
Allyltribromide	967.3	E852.2	E937.3	E950.2	E962.0	E980.2
Aloe, aloes, aloin	973.1	E858.4	E943.1	E950.4	E962.0	E980.4
Aloxidone	966.0	E855.0	E936.0	E950.4	E962.0	E980.4
Aloxiprin	965.1	E850.3	E935.3	E950.0	E962.0	E980.0
Alpha amylase	963.4	E858.1	E933.4	E950.4	E962.0	E980.4
Alphaprodine (hydrochloride)	965.09	E850.2	E935.2	E950.0	E962.0	E980.0
Alpha tocopherol	963.5	E858.1	E933.5	E950.4	E962.0	E980.4
Alseroxylon	972.6	E858.3	E942.6	E950.4	E962.0	E980.4
Alum (ammonium) (potassium)	983.2	E864.2	—	E950.7	E962.1	E980.6
medicinal (astringent) NEC	976.2	E858.7	E946.2	E950.4	E962.0	E980.4
Aluminium, aluminum (gel) (hydroxide)	973.0	E858.4	E943.0	E950.4	E962.0	E980.4
acetate solution	976.2	E858.7	E946.2	E950.4	E962.0	E980.4
aspirin	965.1	E850.3	E935.3	E950.0	E962.0	E980.0
carbonate	973.0	E858.4	E943.0	E950.4	E962.0	E980.4
glycinate	973.0	E858.4	E943.0	E950.4	E962.0	E980.4
nicotinate	972.2	E858.3	E942.2	E950.4	E962.0	E980.4
ointment (surgical) (topical)	976.3	E858.7	E946.3	E950.4	E962.0	E980.4
phosphate	973.0	E858.4	E943.0	E950.4	E962.0	E980.4
subacetate	976.2	E858.7	E946.2	E950.4	E962.0	E980.4
topical NEC	976.3	E858.7	E946.3	E950.4	E962.0	E980.4
Alurate	967.0	E851	E937.0	E950.1	E962.0	E980.1
Alverine (citrate)	975.1	E858.6	E945.1	E950.4	E962.0	E980.4
Alvodine	965.09	E850.2	E935.2	E950.0	E962.0	E980.0
Amanita phalloides	988.1	E865.5	—	E950.9	E962.1	E980.9
Amantadine (hydrochloride)	966.4	E855.0	E936.4	E950.4	E962.0	E980.4
Ambazone	961.9	E857	E931.9	E950.4	E962.0	E980.4
Ambenonium	971.0	E855.3	E941.0	E950.4	E962.0	E980.4
Ambutonium bromide	971.1	E855.4	E941.1	E950.4	E962.0	E980.4
Ametazole	977.8	E858.8	E947.8	E950.4	E962.0	E980.4
Amethocaine (infiltration) (topical)	968.5	E855.2	E938.5	E950.4	E962.0	E980.4
nerve block (peripheral) (plexus)	968.6	E855.2	E938.6	E950.4	E962.0	E980.4
spinal	968.7	E855.2	E938.7	E950.4	E962.0	E980.4
Amethopterin	963.1	E858.1	E933.1	E950.4	E962.0	E980.4
Amfepramone	977.0	E858.8	E947.0	E950.4	E962.0	E980.4
Amidon	965.02	E850.1	E935.1	E950.0	E962.0	E980.0
Amidopyrine	965.5	E850.5	E935.5	E950.0	E962.0	E980.0
Aminacrine	976.0	E858.7	E946.0	E950.4	E962.0	E980.4
Aminitrozole	961.5	E857	E931.5	E950.4	E962.0	E980.4
Aminoacetic acid	974.5	E858.5	E944.5	E950.4	E962.0	E980.4
Amino acids	974.5	E858.5	E944.5	E950.4	E962.0	E980.4
Aminocaproic acid	964.4	E858.2	E934.4	E950.4	E962.0	E980.4
Aminoethylisothiourium	963.8	E858.1	E933.8	E950.4	E962.0	E980.4
Aminoglutethimide	966.3	E855.0	E936.3	E950.4	E962.0	E980.4
Aminometradine	974.3	E858.5	E944.3	E950.4	E962.0	E980.4
Aminopentamide	971.1	E855.4	E941.1	E950.4	E962.0	E980.4
Aminophenazone	965.5	E850.5	E935.5	E950.0	E962.0	E980.0
Aminophenol	983.0	E864.0	—	E950.7	E962.1	E980.6
Aminophenylpyridone	969.5	E853.8	E939.5	E950.3	E962.0	E980.3
Aminophyllin	975.7	E858.6	E945.7	E950.4	E962.0	E980.4
Aminopterin	963.1	E858.1	E933.1	E950.4	E962.0	E980.4
Aminopyrine	965.5	E850.5	E935.5	E950.0	E962.0	E980.0
Aminosalicylic acid	961.8	E857	E931.8	E950.4	E962.0	E980.4
Amiphenazole	970.1	E854.3	E940.1	E950.4	E962.0	E980.4
Amiquinsin	972.6	E858.3	E942.6	E950.4	E962.0	E980.4
Amisometradine	974.3	E858.5	E944.3	E950.4	E962.0	E980.4
Amitriptyline	969.0	E854.0	E939.0	E950.3	E962.0	E980.3
Ammonia (fumes) (gas) (vapor)	987.8	E869.8	—	E952.8	E962.2	E982.8
liquid (household) NEC	983.2	E861.4	—	E950.7	E962.1	E980.6
spirit, aromatic	970.8	E854.3	E940.8	E950.4	E962.0	E980.4
Ammoniated mercury	976.0	E858.7	E946.0	E950.4	E962.0	E980.4
Ammonium						
carbonate	983.2	E864.2	—	E950.7	E962.1	E980.6
chloride (acidifying agent)	963.2	E858.1	E933.2	E950.4	E962.0	E980.4
expectorant	975.5	E858.6	E945.5	E950.4	E962.0	E980.4
compounds (household) NEC	983.2	E861.4	—	E950.7	E962.1	E980.6
fumes (any usage)	987.8	E869.8	—	E952.8	E962.2	E982.8
industrial	983.2	E864.2	—	E950.7	E962.1	E980.6
ichthyosulfonate	976.4	E858.7	E946.4	E950.4	E962.0	E980.4
mandelate	961.9	E857	E931.9	E950.4	E962.0	E980.4
Amobarbital	967.0	E851	E937.0	E950.1	E962.0	E980.1
Amodiaquin(e)	961.4	E857	E931.4	E950.4	E962.0	E980.4
Amopyroquin(e)	961.4	E857	E931.4	E950.4	E962.0	E980.4
Amphenidone	969.5	E853.8	E939.5	E950.3	E962.0	E980.3

TABLE OF DRUGS AND CHEMICALS

Substance	Poisoning	Accident	Therapeutic Use	Suicide Attempt	Assault	Undetermined
Amphetamine	969.7	E854.2	E939.7	E950.3	E962.0	E980.3
Amphomycin	960.8	E856	E930.8	E950.4	E962.0	E980.4
Amphotericin B	960.1	E856	E930.1	E950.4	E962.0	E980.4
topical	976.0	E858.7	E946.0	E950.4	E962.0	E980.4
Ampicillin	960.0	E856	E930.0	E950.4	E962.0	E980.4
Amprotropine	971.1	E855.4	E941.1	E950.4	E962.0	E980.4
Amygdalin	977.8	E858.8	E947.8	E950.4	E962.0	E980.4
Amyl						
acetate (vapor)	982.8	E862.4	—	E950.9	E962.1	E980.9
alcohol	980.3	E860.4	—	E950.9	E962.1	E980.9
nitrite (medicinal)	972.4	E858.3	E942.4	E950.4	E962.0	E980.4
Amylase (alpha)	963.4	E858.1	E933.4	E950.4	E962.0	E980.4
Amylene hydrate	980.8	E860.8	—	E950.9	E962.1	E980.9
Amylobarbitone	967.0	E851	E937.0	E950.1	E962.0	E980.1
Amylocaine	968.9	E855.2	E938.9	E950.4	E962.0	E980.4
infiltration (subcutaneous)	968.5	E855.2	E938.5	E950.4	E962.0	E980.4
nerve block (peripheral) (plexus)	968.6	E855.2	E938.6	E950.4	E962.0	E980.4
spinal	968.7	E855.2	E938.7	E950.4	E962.0	E980.4
topical (surface)	968.5	E855.2	E938.5	E950.4	E962.0	E980.4
Amytal (sodium)	967.0	E851	E937.0	E950.1	E962.0	E980.1
Analeptics	970.0	E854.3	E940.0	E950.4	E962.0	E980.4
Analgesics	965.9	E850.9	E935.9	E950.0	E962.0	E980.0
aromatic NEC	965.4	E850.4	E935.4	E950.0	E962.0	E980.0
non-narcotic NEC	965.7	E850.7	E935.7	E950.0	E962.0	E980.0
specified NEC	965.8	E850.8	E935.8	E950.0	E962.0	E980.0
Anamirta cocculus	988.2	E865.3	—	E950.9	E962.1	E980.9
Ancillin	960.0	E856	E930.0	E950.4	E962.0	E980.4
Androgens (anabolic congeners)	962.1	E858.0	E932.1	E950.4	E962.0	E980.4
Androstalone	962.1	E858.0	E932.1	E950.4	E962.0	E980.4
Androsterone	962.1	E858.0	E932.1	E950.4	E962.0	E980.4
Anemone pulsatilla	988.2	E865.4	—	E950.9	E962.1	E980.9
Anesthesia, anesthetic (general) NEC	968.4	E855.1	E938.4	E950.4	E962.0	E980.4
block (nerve) (plexus)	968.6	E855.2	E938.6	E950.4	E962.0	E980.4
gaseous NEC	968.2	E855.1	E938.2	E950.4	E962.0	E980.4
halogenated hydrocarbon derivatives NEC	968.2	E855.1	E938.2	E950.4	E962.0	E980.4
infiltration (intradermal) (subcutaneous) (submucosal)	968.5	E855.2	E938.5	E950.4	E962.0	E980.4
intravenous	968.3	E855.1	E938.3	E950.4	E962.0	E980.4
local NEC	968.9	E855.2	E938.9	E950.4	E962.0	E980.4
nerve blocking (peripheral) (plexus)	968.6	E855.2	E938.6	E950.4	E962.0	E980.4
rectal NEC	968.3	E855.1	E938.3	E950.4	E962.0	E980.4
spinal	968.7	E855.2	E938.7	E950.4	E962.0	E980.4
surface	968.5	E855.2	E938.5	E950.4	E962.0	E980.4
topical	968.5	E855.2	E938.5	E950.4	E962.0	E980.4
Aneurine	963.5	E858.1	E933.5	E950.4	E962.0	E980.4
Angio-Conray	977.8	E858.8	E947.8	E950.4	E962.0	E980.4
Angiotensin	971.2	E855.5	E941.2	E950.4	E962.0	E980.4
Anhydrohydroxyprogesterone	962.2	E858.0	E932.2	E950.4	E962.0	E980.4
Anhydron	974.3	E858.5	E944.3	E950.4	E962.0	E980.4
Anileridine	965.09	E850.2	E935.2	E950.0	E962.0	E980.0
Aniline (dye) (liquid)	983.0	E864.0	—	E950.7	E962.1	E980.6
analgesic	965.4	E850.4	E935.4	E950.0	E962.0	E980.0
derivatives, therapeutic NEC	965.4	E850.4	E935.4	E950.0	E962.0	E980.0
vapor	987.8	E869.8	—	E952.8	E962.2	E982.8
Anisindione	964.2	E858.2	E934.2	E950.4	E962.0	E980.4
Anisotropine	971.1	E855.4	E941.1	E950.4	E962.0	E980.4
Anorexic agents	977.0	E858.8	E947.0	E950.4	E962.0	E980.4
Ant (bite) (sting)	989.5	E905.5	—	E950.9	E962.1	E980.9
Antabuse	977.3	E858.8	E947.3	E950.4	E962.0	E980.4
Antacids	973.0	E858.4	E943.0	E950.4	E962.0	E980.4
Antazoline	963.0	E858.1	E933.0	E950.4	E962.0	E980.4
Anthelmintics	961.6	E857	E931.6	E950.4	E962.0	E980.4
Anthralin	976.4	E858.7	E946.4	E950.4	E962.0	E980.4
Anthramycin	960.7	E856	E930.7	E950.4	E962.0	E980.4
Antiadrenergics	971.3	E855.6	E941.3	E950.4	E962.0	E980.4
Antiallergic agents	963.0	E858.1	E933.0	E950.4	E962.0	E980.4
Antianemic agents NEC	964.1	E858.2	E934.1	E950.4	E962.0	E980.4
Antiaris toxicaria	988.2	E865.4	—	E950.9	E962.1	E980.9
Antiarteriosclerotic agents	972.2	E858.3	E942.2	E950.4	E962.0	E980.4
Antiasthmatics	975.7	E858.6	E945.7	E950.4	E962.0	E980.4
Antibiotics	960.9	E856	E930.9	E950.4	E962.0	E980.4
antifungal	960.1	E856	E930.1	E950.4	E962.0	E980.4
antimycobacterial	960.6	E856	E930.6	E950.4	E962.0	E980.4
antineoplastic	960.7	E856	E930.7	E950.4	E962.0	E980.4
cephalosporin (group)	960.5	E856	E930.5	E950.4	E962.0	E980.4
chloramphenicol (group)	960.2	E856	E930.2	E950.4	E962.0	E980.4
macrolides	960.3	E856	E930.3	E950.4	E962.0	E980.4

TABLE OF DRUGS AND CHEMICALS

Substance	Poisoning	Accident	Therapeutic-Use	Suicide Attempt	Assault	Undetermined
Antibiotics—continued						
specified NEC	960.8	E856	E930.8	E950.4	E962.0	E980.4
tetracycline (group)	960.4	E856	E930.4	E950.4	E962.0	E980.4
Anticancer agents NEC	963.1	E858.1	E933.1	E950.4	E962.0	E980.4
antibiotics	960.7	E856	E930.7	E950.4	E962.0	E980.4
Anticholinergics	971.1	E855.4	E941.1	E950.4	E962.0	E980.4
Anticholinesterase (organophosphorus) (reversible)	971.0	E855.3	E941.0	E950.4	E962.0	E980.4
Anticoagulants	964.2	E858.2	E934.2	E950.4	E962.0	E980.4
antagonists	964.5	E858.2	E934.5	E950.4	E962.0	E980.4
Anti-common cold agents NEC	975.6	E858.6	E945.6	E950.4	E962.0	E980.4
Anticonvulsants NEC	966.3	E855.0	E936.3	E950.4	E962.0	E980.4
Antidepressants	969.0	E854.0	E939.0	E950.3	E962.0	E980.3
Antidiabetic agents	962.3	E858.0	E932.3	E950.4	E962.0	E980.4
Antidiarrheal agents	973.5	E858.4	E943.5	E950.4	E962.0	E980.4
Antidiuretic hormone	962.5	E858.0	E932.5	E950.4	E962.0	E980.4
Antidotes NEC	977.2	E858.8	E947.2	E950.4	E962.0	E980.4
Antiemetic agents	963.0	E858.1	E933.0	E950.4	E962.0	E980.4
Antiepilepsy agent NEC	966.3	E855.0	E936.3	E950.4	E962.0	E980.4
Antifertility pills	962.2	E858.0	E932.2	E950.4	E962.0	E980.4
Antiflatulents	973.8	E858.4	E943.8	E950.4	E962.0	E980.4
Antifreeze	989.8	E866.8	—	E950.9	E962.1	E980.9
alcohol	980.1	E860.2	—	E950.9	E962.1	E980.9
ethylene glycol	982.8	E862.4	—	E950.9	E962.1	E980.9
Antifungals (nonmedicinal) (sprays)	989.4	E863.6	—	E950.6	E962.1	E980.7
medicinal NEC	961.9	E857	E931.9	E950.4	E962.0	E980.4
antibiotic	960.1	E856	E930.1	E950.4	E962.0	E980.4
topical	976.0	E858.7	E946.0	E950.4	E962.0	E980.4
Antigastric secretion agents	973.0	E858.4	E943.0	E950.4	E962.0	E980.4
Anthelmintics	961.6	E857	E931.6	E950.4	E962.0	E980.4
Antihemophilic factor (human)	964.7	E858.2	E934.7	E950.4	E962.0	E980.4
Antihistamine	963.0	E858.1	E933.0	E950.4	E962.0	E980.4
Antihypertensive agents NEC	972.6	E858.3	E942.6	E950.4	E962.0	E980.4
Anti-infectives NEC	961.9	E857	E931.9	E950.4	E962.0	E980.4
antibiotics	960.9	E856	E930.9	E950.4	E962.0	E980.4
specified NEC	960.8	E856	E930.8	E950.4	E962.0	E980.4
anthelmintic	961.6	E857	E931.6	E950.4	E962.0	E980.4
antimalarial	961.4	E857	E931.4	E950.4	E962.0	E980.4
antimycobacterial NEC	961.8	E857	E931.8	E950.4	E962.0	E980.4
antibiotics	960.6	E856	E930.6	E950.4	E962.0	E980.4
antiprotozoal NEC	961.5	E857	E931.5	E950.4	E962.0	E980.4
blood	961.4	E857	E931.4	E950.4	E962.0	E980.4
antiviral	961.7	E857	E931.7	E950.4	E962.0	E980.4
arsenical	961.1	E857	E931.1	E950.4	E962.0	E980.4
ENT agents	976.6	E858.7	E946.6	E950.4	E962.0	E980.4
heavy metals NEC	961.2	E857	E931.2	E950.4	E962.0	E980.4
local	976.0	E858.7	E946.0	E950.4	E962.0	E980.4
ophthalmic preparation	976.5	E858.7	E946.5	E950.4	E962.0	E980.4
topical NEC	976.0	E858.7	E946.0	E950.4	E962.0	E980.4
Anti-inflammatory agents (topical)	976.0	E858.7	E946.0	E950.4	E962.0	E980.4
Antiknock (tetraethyl lead)	984.1	E862.1	—	E950.9	E962.1	E980.9
Antilipemics	972.2	E858.3	E942.2	E950.4	E962.0	E980.4
Antimalarials	961.4	E857	E931.4	E950.4	E962.0	E980.4
Antimony (compounds) (vapor) NEC	985.4	E866.2	—	E950.9	E962.1	E980.9
anti-infectives	961.2	E857	E931.2	E950.4	E962.0	E980.4
pesticides (vapor)	985.4	E863.4	—	E950.6	E962.2	E980.7
potassium tartrate	961.2	E857	E931.2	E950.4	E962.0	E980.4
tartrated	961.2	E857	E931.2	E950.4	E962.0	E980.4
Antimuscarinic agents	971.1	E855.4	E941.1	E950.4	E962.0	E980.4
Antimycobacterials NEC	961.8	E857	E931.8	E950.4	E962.0	E980.4
antibiotics	960.6	E856	E930.6	E950.4	E962.0	E980.4
Antineoplastic agents	963.1	E858.1	E933.1	E950.4	E962.0	E980.4
antibiotics	960.7	E856	E930.7	E950.4	E962.0	E980.4
Anti-Parkinsonism agents	966.4	E855.0	E936.4	E950.4	E962.0	E980.4
Antiphlogistics	965.6	E850.6	E935.6	E950.0	E962.0	E980.0
Antiprotozoals NEC	961.5	E857	E931.5	E950.4	E962.0	E980.4
blood	961.4	E857	E931.4	E950.4	E962.0	E980.4
Antipruritics (local)	976.1	E858.7	E946.1	E950.4	E962.0	E980.4
Antipsychotic agents NEC	969.3	E853.8	E939.3	E950.3	E962.0	E980.3
Antipyretics	965.9	E850.9	E935.9	E950.0	E962.0	E980.0
specified NEC	965.8	E850.8	E935.8	E950.0	E962.0	E980.0
Antipyrine	965.5	E850.5	E935.5	E950.0	E962.0	E980.0
Antirabies serum (equine)	979.9	E858.8	E949.9	E950.4	E962.0	E980.4
Antirheumatics	965.6	E850.6	E935.6	E950.0	E962.0	E980.0
Antiseborrheics	976.4	E858.7	E946.4	E950.4	E962.0	E980.4
Antiseptics (external) (medicinal)	976.0	E858.7	E946.0	E950.4	E962.0	E980.4
Antistine	963.0	E858.1	E933.0	E950.4	E962.0	E980.4

TABLE OF DRUGS AND CHEMICALS

Substance	Poisoning	Accident	Therapeutic-Use	Suicide Attempt	Assault	Undetermined
Antithyroid agents	962.8	E858.0	E932.8	E950.4	E962.0	E980.4
Antitoxin, any	979.9	E858.8	E949.9	E950.4	E962.0	E980.4
Antituberculars	961.8	E857	E931.8	E950.4	E962.0	E980.4
antibiotics	960.6	E856	E930.6	E950.4	E962.0	E980.4
Antitussives	975.4	E858.6	E945.4	E950.4	E962.0	E980.4
Antivaricose agents (sclerosing)	972.7	E858.3	E942.7	E950.4	E962.0	E980.4
Antivenin (crotaline) (spider-bite)	979.9	E858.8	E949.9	E950.4	E962.0	E980.4
Antivert	963.0	E858.1	E933.0	E950.4	E962.0	E980.4
Antivirals NEC	961.7	E857	E931.7	E950.4	E962.0	E980.4
Ant poisons — see Pesticides						
Antrol	989.4	E863.4	—	E950.6	E962.1	E980.7
fungicide	989.4	E863.6	—	E950.6	E962.1	E980.7
Apomorphine hydrochloride (emetic)	973.6	E858.4	E943.6	E950.4	E962.0	E980.4
Appetite depressants, central	977.0	E858.8	E947.0	E950.4	E962.0	E980.4
Apresoline	972.6	E858.3	E942.6	E950.4	E962.0	E980.4
Aprobarbital, aprobarbitone	967.0	E851	E937.0	E950.1	E962.0	E980.1
Apronalide	967.8	E852.8	E937.8	E950.2	E962.0	E980.2
Aqua fortis	983.1	E864.1	—	E950.7	E962.1	E980.6
Arachis oil (topical)	976.3	E858.7	E946.3	E950.4	E962.0	E980.4
cathartic	973.2	E858.4	E943.2	E950.4	E962.0	E980.4
Aralen	961.4	E857	E931.4	E950.4	E962.0	E980.4
Arginine salts	974.5	E858.5	E944.5	E950.4	E962.0	E980.4
Argyrol	976.0	E858.7	E946.0	E950.4	E962.0	E980.4
ENT agent	976.6	E858.7	E946.6	E950.4	E962.0	E980.4
ophthalmic preparation	976.5	E858.7	E946.5	E950.4	E962.0	E980.4
Aristocort	962.0	E858.0	E932.0	E950.4	E962.0	E980.4
ENT agent	976.6	E858.7	E946.6	E950.4	E962.0	E980.4
ophthalmic preparation	976.5	E858.7	E946.5	E950.4	E962.0	E980.4
topical NEC	976.0	E858.7	E946.0	E950.4	E962.0	E980.4
Aromatics, corrosive	983.0	E864.0	—	E950.7	E962.1	E980.6
disinfectants	983.0	E861.4	—	E950.7	E962.1	E980.6
Arsenate of lead (insecticide)	985.1	E863.4	—	E950.8	E962.1	E980.8
herbicide	985.1	E863.5	—	E950.8	E962.1	E980.8
Arsenic, arsenicals (compounds) (dust) (fumes) (vapor) NEC	985.1	E866.3	—	E950.8	E962.1	E980.8
anti-infectives	961.1	E857	E931.1	E950.4	E962.0	E980.4
pesticide (dust) (fumes)	985.1	E863.4	—	E950.8	E962.1	E980.8
Arsine (gas)	985.1	E866.3	—	E950.8	E962.1	E980.8
Arsphenamine (silver)	961.1	E857	E931.1	E950.4	E962.0	E980.4
Arsthinol	961.1	E857	E931.1	E950.4	E962.0	E980.4
Artane	971.1	E855.4	E941.1	E950.4	E962.0	E980.4
Arthropod (venomous) NEC	989.5	E905.5	—	E950.9	E962.1	E980.9
Ascaridole	961.6	E857	E931.6	E950.4	E962.0	E980.4
Ascorbic acid	963.5	E858.1	E933.5	E950.4	E962.0	E980.4
Asiaticoside	976.0	E858.7	E946.0	E950.4	E962.0	E980.4
Aspidium (oleoresin)	961.6	E857	E931.6	E950.4	E962.0	E980.4
Aspirin	965.1	E850.3	E935.3	E950.0	E962.0	E980.0
Astringents (local)	976.2	E858.7	E946.2	E950.4	E962.0	E980.4
Atabrine	961.3	E857	E931.3	E950.4	E962.0	E980.4
Ataractics	969.5	E853.8	E939.5	E950.3	E962.0	E980.3
Atonia drug, intestinal	973.3	E858.4	E943.3	E950.4	E962.0	E980.4
Atophan	974.7	E858.5	E944.7	E950.4	E962.0	E980.4
Atropine	971.1	E855.4	E941.1	E950.4	E962.0	E980.4
Attapulgite	973.5	E858.4	E943.5	E950.4	E962.0	E980.4
Attenuvax	979.4	E858.8	E949.4	E950.4	E962.0	E980.4
Aureomycin	960.4	E856	E930.4	E950.4	E962.0	E980.4
ophthalmic preparation	976.5	E858.7	E946.5	E950.4	E962.0	E980.4
topical NEC	976.0	E858.7	E946.0	E950.4	E962.0	E980.4
Aurothioglucose	965.6	E850.6	E935.6	E950.0	E962.0	E980.0
Aurothioglycanide	965.6	E850.6	E935.6	E950.0	E962.0	E980.0
Aurothiomalate	965.6	E850.6	E935.6	E950.0	E962.0	E980.0
Automobile fuel	981	E862.1	—	E950.9	E962.1	E980.9
Autonomic nervous system agents NEC	971.9	E855.9	E941.9	E950.4	E962.0	E980.4
Avlosulfon	961.8	E857	E931.8	E950.4	E962.0	E980.4
Avomine	967.8	E852.8	E937.8	E950.2	E962.0	E980.2
Azacyclonol	969.5	E853.8	E939.5	E950.3	E962.0	E980.3
Azapetine	971.3	E855.6	E941.3	E950.4	E962.0	E980.4
Azaribine	963.1	E858.1	E933.1	E950.4	E962.0	E980.4
Azaserine	960.7	E856	E930.7	E950.4	E962.0	E980.4
Azathioprine	963.1	E858.1	E933.1	E950.4	E962.0	E980.4
Azosulfamide	961.0	E857	E931.0	E950.4	E962.0	E980.4
Azulfidine	961.0	E857	E931.0	E950.4	E962.0	E980.4
Azuresin	977.8	E858.8	E947.8	E950.4	E962.0	E980.4
Bacimycin	976.0	E858.7	E946.0	E950.4	E962.0	E980.4
ophthalmic preparation	976.5	E858.7	E946.5	E950.4	E962.0	E980.4

TABLE OF DRUGS AND CHEMICALS

Substance	Poisoning	Accident	Therapeutic-Use	Suicide Attempt	Assault	Undetermined
Bacitracin	960.8	E856	E930.8	E950.4	E962.0	E980.4
ENT agent	976.6	E858.7	E946.6	E950.4	E962.0	E980.4
ophthalmic preparation	976.5	E858.7	E946.5	E950.4	E962.0	E980.4
topical NEC	976.0	E858.7	E946.0	E950.4	E962.0	E980.4
Baking soda	963.3	E858.1	E933.3	E950.4	E962.0	E980.4
BAL	963.8	E858.1	E933.8	E950.4	E962.0	E980.4
Bamethan (sulfate)	972.5	E858.3	E942.5	E950.4	E962.0	E980.4
Bamipine	963.0	E858.1	E933.0	E950.4	E962.0	E980.4
Baneberry	988.2	E865.4	—	E950.9	E962.1	E980.9
Banewort	988.2	E865.4	—	E950.9	E962.1	E980.9
Barbenyl	967.0	E851	E937.0	E950.1	E962.0	E980.1
Barbital, barbitone	967.0	E851	E937.0	E950.1	E962.0	E980.1
Barbiturates, barbituric acid	967.0	E851	E937.0	E950.1	E962.0	E980.1
anesthetic (intravenous)	968.3	E855.1	E938.3	E950.4	E962.0	E980.4
Barium (carbonate) (chloride) (sulfate)	985.8	E866.4	—	E950.9	E962.1	E980.9
diagnostic agent	977.8	E858.8	E947.8	E950.4	E962.0	E980.4
pesticide	985.8	E863.4	—	E950.6	E962.1	E980.7
rodenticide	985.8	E863.7	—	E950.6	E962.1	E980.7
Barrier cream	976.3	E858.7	E946.3	E950.4	E962.0	E980.4
Battery acid or fluid	983.1	E864.1	—	E950.7	E962.1	E980.6
Bay rum	980.8	E860.8	—	E950.9	E962.1	E980.9
BCG vaccine	978.0	E858.8	E948.0	E950.4	E962.0	E980.4
Bearsfoot	988.2	E865.4	—	E950.9	E962.1	E980.9
Beclamide	966.3	E855.0	E936.3	E950.4	E962.0	E980.4
Bee (sting) (venom)	989.5	E905.3	—	E950.9	E962.1	E980.9
Belladonna (alkaloids)	971.1	E855.4	E941.1	E950.4	E962.0	E980.4
Bemegride	970.0	E854.3	E940.0	E950.4	E962.0	E980.4
Benactyzine	969.8	E855.8	E939.8	E950.3	E962.0	E980.3
Benadryl	963.0	E858.1	E933.0	E950.4	E962.0	E980.4
Bendrofluazide	974.3	E858.5	E944.3	E950.4	E962.0	E980.4
Bendroflumethiazide	974.3	E858.5	E944.3	E950.4	E962.0	E980.4
Benemid	974.7	E858.5	E944.7	E950.4	E962.0	E980.4
Benethamine penicillin G	960.0	E856	E930.0	E950.4	E962.0	E980.4
Benisone	976.0	E858.7	E946.0	E950.4	E962.0	E980.4
Benoquin	976.8	E858.7	E946.8	E950.4	E962.0	E980.4
Benoxinate	968.5	E855.2	E938.5	E950.4	E962.0	E980.4
Bentonite	976.3	E858.7	E946.3	E950.4	E962.0	E980.4
Benzalkonium (chloride)	976.0	E858.7	E946.0	E950.4	E962.0	E980.4
ophthalmic preparation	976.5	E858.7	E946.5	E950.4	E962.0	E980.4
Benzamidosalicylate (calcium)	961.8	E857	E931.8	E950.4	E962.0	E980.4
Benzathine penicillin	960.0	E856	E930.0	E950.4	E962.0	E980.4
Benzcarbimine	963.1	E858.1	E933.1	E950.4	E962.0	E980.4
Benzedrex	971.2	E855.5	E941.2	E950.4	E962.0	E980.4
Benzedrine (amphetamine)	969.7	E854.2	E939.7	E950.3	E962.0	E980.3
Benzene (acetyl) (dimethyl) (methyl) (solvent) (vapor)	982.0	E862.4	—	E950.9	E962.1	E980.9
hexachloride (gamma) (insecticide) (vapor)	989.2	E863.0	—	E950.6	E962.1	E980.7
Benzethonium	976.0	E858.7	E946.0	E950.4	E962.0	E980.4
Benzhexol (chloride)	966.4	E855.0	E936.4	E950.4	E962.0	E980.4
Benzilonium	971.1	E855.4	E941.1	E950.4	E962.0	E980.4
Benzin(e) — see Ligroin						
Benziodarone	972.4	E858.3	E942.4	E950.4	E962.0	E980.4
Benzocaine	968.5	E855.2	E938.5	E950.4	E962.0	E980.4
Benzodiapin	969.4	E853.2	E939.4	E950.3	E962.0	E980.3
Benzodiazepines (tranquilizers) NEC	969.4	E853.2	E939.4	E950.3	E962.0	E980.3
Benzoic acid (with salicylic acid) (anti-infective)	976.0	E858.7	E946.0	E950.4	E962.0	E980.4
Benzoin	976.3	E858.7	E946.3	E950.4	E962.0	E980.4
Benzol (vapor)	982.0	E862.4	—	E950.9	E962.1	E980.9
Benzomorphan	965.09	E850.2	E935.2	E950.0	E962.0	E980.0
Benzonatate	975.4	E858.6	E945.4	E950.4	E962.0	E980.4
Benzothiadiazides	974.3	E858.5	E944.3	E950.4	E962.0	E980.4
Benzoylpas	961.8	E857	E931.8	E950.4	E962.0	E980.4
Benzperidol	969.5	E853.8	E939.5	E950.3	E962.0	E980.3
Benzphetamine	977.0	E858.8	E947.0	E950.4	E962.0	E980.4
Benzpyrinium	971.0	E855.3	E941.0	E950.4	E962.0	E980.4
Benzquinamide	963.0	E858.1	E933.0	E950.4	E962.0	E980.4
Benzthiazide	974.3	E858.5	E944.3	E950.4	E962.0	E980.4
Benztropine	971.1	E855.4	E941.1	E950.4	E962.0	E980.4
Benzyl						
acetate	982.8	E862.4	—	E950.9	E962.1	E980.9
benzoate (anti-infective)	976.0	E858.7	E946.0	E950.4	E962.0	E980.4
morphine	965.09	E850.2	E935.2	E950.0	E962.0	E980.0
penicillin	960.0	E856	E930.0	E950.4	E962.0	E980.4
Bephenium hydroxynapthoate	961.6	E857	E931.6	E950.4	E962.0	E980.4
Bergamot oil	989.8	E866.8	—	E950.9	E962.1	E980.9
Berries, poisonous	988.2	E865.3	—	E950.9	E962.1	E980.9
Beryllium (compounds) (fumes)	985.3	E866.4	—	E950.9	E962.1	E980.9

TABLE OF DRUGS AND CHEMICALS

Substance	Poisoning	Accident	Therapeutic-Use	Suicide Attempt	Assault	Undetermined
Beta-carotene	976.3	E858.7	E946.3	E950.4	E962.0	E980.4
Beta-Chlor	967.1	E852.0	E937.1	E950.2	E962.0	E980.2
Betamethasone	962.0	E858.0	E932.0	E950.4	E962.0	E980.4
topical	976.0	E858.7	E946.0	E950.4	E962.0	E980.4
Betazole	977.8	E858.8	E947.8	E950.4	E962.0	E980.4
Bethanechol	971	E855.3	E941.0	E950.4	E962.0	E980.4
Bethanidine	972.6	E858.3	E942.6	E950.4	E962.0	E980.4
Betula oil	976.3	E858.7	E946.3	E950.4	E962.0	E980.4
Bhang	969.6	E854.1	E939.6	E950.3	E962.0	E980.3
Bialamicol	961.5	E857	E931.5	E950.4	E962.0	E980.4
Bichloride of mercury — see Mercury, chloride						
Bichromates (calcium) (crystals) (potassium) (sodium)	983.9	E864.3	—	E950.7	E962.1	E980.6
fumes	987.8	E869.8	—	E952.8	E962.2	E982.8
Biguanide derivatives, oral	962.3	E858.0	E932.3	E950.4	E962.0	E980.4
Biligrafin	977.8	E858.8	E947.8	E950.4	E962.0	E980.4
Bilopaque	977.8	E858.8	E947.8	E950.4	E962.0	E980.4
Bioflavonoids	972.8	E858.3	E942.8	E950.4	E962.0	E980.4
Biological substance NEC	979.9	E858.8	E949.9	E950.4	E962.0	E980.4
Biperiden	966.4	E855.0	E936.4	E950.4	E962.0	E980.4
Bisacodyl	973.1	E858.4	E943.1	E950.4	E962.0	E980.4
Bishydroxycoumarin	964.2	E858.2	E934.2	E950.4	E962.0	E980.4
Bismarsen	961.1	E857	E931.1	E950.4	E962.0	E980.4
Bismuth (compounds) NEC	985.8	E866.4	—	E950.9	E962.1	E980.9
anti-infectives	961.2	E857	E931.2	E950.4	E962.0	E980.4
subcarbonate	973.5	E858.4	E943.5	E950.4	E962.0	E980.4
sulfarsphenamine	961.1	E857	E931.1	E950.4	E962.0	E980.4
Bithionol	961.6	E857	E931.6	E950.4	E962.0	E980.4
Bitter almond oil	989.0	E866.8	—	E950.9	E962.1	E980.9
Bittersweet	988.2	E865.4	—	E950.9	E962.1	E930.9
Black						
flag	989.4	E863.4	—	E950.6	E962.1	E980.7
henbane	988.2	E865.4	—	E950.9	E962.1	E980.9
leaf (40)	989.4	E863.4	—	E950.6	E962.1	E980.7
widow spider (bite)	989.5	E905.1	—	E950.9	E962.1	E980.9
antivenin	979.9	E858.8	E949.9	E950.4	E962.0	E980.4
Blast furnace gas (carbon monoxide from)	986	E868.8	—	E952.1	E962.2	E982.1
Bleach NEC	983.9	E864.3	—	E950.7	E962.1	E980.6
Bleaching solutions	983.9	E864.3	—	E950.7	E962.1	E980.6
Bleomycin (sulfate)	960.7	E856	E930.7	E950.4	E962.0	E980.4
Blockain	968.9	E855.2	E938.9	E950.4	E962.0	E980.4
infiltration (subcutaneous)	968.5	E855.2	E938.5	E950.4	E962.0	E980.4
nerve block (peripheral) (plexus)	968.6	E855.2	E938.6	E950.4	E962.0	E980.4
topical (surface)	968.5	E855.2	E938.5	E950.4	E962.0	E980.4
Blood (derivatives) (natural) (plasma) (whole)	964.7	E858.2	E934.7	E950.4	E962.0	E980.4
affecting agent	964.9	E858.2	E934.9	E950.4	E962.0	E980.4
specified NEC	964.8	E858.2	E934.8	E950.4	E962.0	E980.4
substitute (macromolecular)	964.8	E858.2	E934.8	E950.4	E962.0	E980.4
Blue velvet	965.09	E850.2	E935.2	E950.0	E962.0	E980.0
Bone meal	989.8	E866.5	—	E950.9	E962.1	E980.9
Bonine	963.0	E858.1	E933.0	E950.4	E962.0	E980.4
Boracic acid	976.0	E858.7	E946.0	E950.4	E962.0	E980.4
ENT agent	976.6	E858.7	E946.6	E950.4	E962.0	E980.4
ophthalmic preparation	976.5	E858.7	E946.5	E950.4	E962.0	E980.4
Borate (cleanser) (sodium)	989.6	E861.3	—	E950.9	E962.1	E980.9
Borax (cleanser)	989.6	E861.3	—	E950.9	E962.1	E980.9
Boric acid	976.0	E858.7	E946.0	E950.4	E962.0	E980.4
ENT agent	976.6	E858.7	E946.6	E950.4	E962.0	E980.4
ophthalmic preparation	976.5	E858.7	E946.5	E950.4	E962.0	E980.4
Boron hydride NEC	989.8	E866.8	—	E950.9	E962.1	E980.9
fumes or gas	987.8	E869.8	—	E952.8	E962.2	E982.8
Brake fluid vapor	987.8	E869.8	—	E952.8	E962.2	E982.8
Brass (compounds) (fumes)	985.8	E866.4	—	E950.9	E962.1	E980.9
Brasso	981	E861.3	—	E950.9	E962.1	E980.9
Bretylium (tosylate)	972.6	E858.3	E942.6	E950.4	E962.0	E980.4
Brevital (sodium)	968.3	E855.1	E938.3	E950.4	E962.0	E980.4
British antilewisite	963.8	E858.1	E933.8	E950.4	E962.0	E980.4
Bromal (hydrate)	967.3	E852.2	E937.3	E950.2	E962.0	E980.2
Bromelains	963.4	E858.1	E933.4	E950.4	E962.0	E980.4
Bromides NEC	967.3	E852.2	E937.3	E950.2	E962.0	E980.2
Bromine (vapor)	987.8	E869.8	—	E952.8	E962.2	E982.8
compounds (medicinal)	967.3	E852.2	E937.3	E950.2	E962.0	E980.2
Bromisovalum	967.3	E852.2	E937.3	E950.2	E962.0	E980.2
Bromobenzyl cyanide	987.5	E869.3	—	E952.8	E962.2	E982.8
Bromodiphenhydramine	963.0	E858.1	E933.0	E950.4	E962.0	E980.4
Bromoform	967.3	E852.2	E937.3	E950.2	E962.0	E980.2
Bromophenol blue reagent	977.8	E858.8	E947.8	E950.4	E962.0	E980.4

TABLE OF DRUGS AND CHEMICALS

Substance	Poisoning	Accident	Therapeutic-Use	Suicide Attempt	Assault	Undetermined
Bromosalicylhydroxamic acid	961.8	E857	E931.8	E950.4	E962.0	E980.4
Bromo-seltzer	965.4	E850.4	E935.4	E950.0	E962.0	E980.0
Brompheniramine	963.0	E858.1	E933.0	E950.4	E962.0	E980.4
Bromural	967.3	E852.2	E937.3	E950.2	E962.0	E980.2
Brown spider (bite) (venom)	989.5	E905.1	—	E950.9	E962.1	E980.9
Brucia	988.2	E865.3	—	E950.9	E962.1	E980.9
Brucine	989.1	E863.7	—	E950.6	E962.1	E980.7
Brunswick green — see Copper						
Bryonia (alba) (dioica)	988.2	E865.4	—	E950.9	E962.1	E980.9
Buclizine	969.5	E853.8	E939.5	E950.3	E962.0	E980.3
Bufferin	965.1	E850.3	E935.3	E950.0	E962.0	E980.0
Bufotenine	969.6	E854.1	E939.6	E950.3	E962.0	E980.3
Buphenine	971.2	E855.5	E941.2	E950.4	E962.0	E980.4
Bupivacaine	968.9	E855.2	E938.9	E950.4	E962.0	E980.4
infiltration (subcutaneous)	968.5	E855.2	E938.5	E950.4	E962.0	E980.4
nerve block (peripheral) (plexus)	968.6	E855.2	E938.6	E950.4	E962.0	E980.4
Busulfan	963.1	E858.1	E933.1	E950.4	E962.0	E980.4
Butabarbital (sodium)	967.0	E851	E937.0	E950.1	E962.0	E980.1
Butabarbitone	967.0	E851	E937.0	E950.1	E962.0	E980.1
Butabarpal	967.0	E851	E937.0	E950.1	E962.0	E980.1
Butacaine	968.5	E855.2	E938.5	E950.4	E962.0	E980.4
Butallylonal	967.0	E851	E937.0	E950.1	E962.0	E980.1
Butane (distributed in mobile container)	987.0	E868.0	—	E951.1	E962.2	E981.1
distributed through pipes	987.0	E867	—	E951.0	E962.2	E981.0
incomplete combustion of — see Carbon monoxide, butane						
Butanol	980.3	E860.4	—	E950.9	E962.1	E980.9
Butanone	982.8	E862.4	—	E950.9	E962.1	E980.9
Butaperazine	969.1	E853.0	E939.1	E950.3	E962.0	E980.3
Butazolidin	965.5	E850.5	E935.5	E950.0	E962.0	E980.0
Butethal	967.0	E851	E937.0	E950.1	E962.0	E980.1
Butethamate	971.1	E855.4	E941.1	E950.4	E962.0	E980.4
Buthalitone (sodium)	968.3	E855.1	E938.3	E950.4	E962.0	E980.4
Butisol (sodium)	967.0	E851	E937.0	E950.1	E962.0	E980.1
Butobarbital, butobarbitone	967.0	E851	E937.0	E950.1	E962.0	E980.1
Butriptyline	969.0	E854.0	E939.0	E950.3	E962.0	E980.3
Buttercups	988.2	E865.4	—	E950.9	E962.1	E980.9
Butter of antimony — see Antimony						
Butyl						
acetate (secondary)	982.8	E862.4	—	E950.9	E962.1	E980.9
alcohol	980.3	E860.4	—	E950.9	E962.1	E980.9
carbinol	980.8	E860.8	—	E950.9	E962.1	E980.9
carbitol	982.8	E862.4	—	E950.9	E962.1	E980.9
cellosolve	982.8	E862.4	—	E950.9	E962.1	E980.9
chloral (hydrate)	967.1	E852.0	E937.1	E950.2	E962.0	E980.2
formate	982.8	E862.4	—	E950.9	E962.1	E980.9
scopolammonium bromide	971.1	E855.4	E941.1	E950.4	E962.0	E980.4
Butyn	968.5	E855.2	E938.5	E950.4	E962.0	E980.4
Butyrophenone (-based tranquilizers)	969.2	E853.1	E939.2	E950.3	E962.0	E980.3
Cacodyl, cacodylic acid — see Arsenic						
Cactinomycin	960.7	E856	E930.7	E950.4	E962.0	E980.4
Cade oil	976.4	E858.7	E946.4	E950.4	E962.0	E980.4
Cadmium (chloride) (compounds) (dust) (fumes) (oxide)	985.5	E866.4	—	E950.9	E962.1	E980.9
sulfide (medicinal) NEC	976.4	E858.7	E946.4	E950.4	E962.0	E980.4
Caffeine	969.7	E854.2	E939.7	E950.3	E962.0	E980.3
Calabar bean	988.2	E865.4	—	E950.9	E962.1	E980.9
Caladium seguinium	988.2	E865.4	—	E950.9	E962.1	E980.9
Calamine (liniment) (lotion)	976.3	E858.7	E946.3	E950.4	E962.0	E980.4
Calciferol	963.5	E858.1	E933.5	E950.4	E962.0	E980.4
Calcium (salts) NEC	974.5	E858.5	E944.5	E950.4	E962.0	E980.4
acetylsalicylate	965.1	E850.3	E935.3	E950.0	E962.0	E980.0
benzamidosalicylate	961.8	E857	E931.8	E950.4	E962.0	E980.4
carbaspirin	965.1	E850.3	E935.3	E950.0	E962.0	E980.0
carbimide (citrated)	977.3	E858.8	E947.3	E950.4	E962.0	E980.4
carbonate (antacid)	973.0	E858.4	E943.0	E950.4	E962.0	E980.4
cyanide (citrated)	977.3	E858.8	E947.3	E950.4	E962.0	E980.4
dioctyl sulfosuccinate	973.2	E858.4	E943.2	E950.4	E962.0	E980.4
disodium edathamil	963.8	E858.1	E933.8	E950.4	E962.0	E980.4
disodium edetate	963.8	E858.1	E933.8	E950.4	E962.0	E980.4
EDTA	963.8	E858.1	E933.8	E950.4	E962.0	E980.4
hydrate, hydroxide	983.2	E864.2	—	E950.7	E962.1	E980.6
mandelate	961.9	E857	E931.9	E950.4	E962.0	E980.4
oxide	983.2	E864.2	—	E950.7	E962.1	E980.6
Calomel — see Mercury, chloride						
Caloric agents NEC	974.5	E858.5	E944.5	E950.4	E962.0	E980.4
Calusterone	963.1	E858.1	E933.1	E950.4	E962.0	E980.4
Camoquin	961.4	E857	E931.4	E950.4	E962.0	E980.4

TABLE OF DRUGS AND CHEMICALS

Substance	Poisoning	Accident	Therapeutic-Use	Suicide Attempt	Assault	Undetermined
Camphor (oil)	976.1	E858.7	E946.1	E950.4	E962.0	E980.4
Candeptin	976.0	E858.7	E946.0	E950.4	E962.0	E980.4
Candicidin	976.0	E858.7	E946.0	E950.4	E962.0	E980.4
Cannabinols	969.6	E854.1	E939.6	E950.3	E962.0	E980.3
Cannabis (derivatives) (indica) (sativa)	969.6	E854.1	E939.6	E950.3	E962.0	E980.3
Canned heat	980.1	E860.2	—	E950.9	E962.1	E980.9
Cantharides, cantharidin, cantharis	976.8	E858.7	E946.8	E950.4	E962.0	E980.4
Capillary agents	972.8	E858.3	E942.8	E950.4	E962.0	E980.4
Capreomycin	960.6	E856	E930.6	E950.4	E962.0	E980.4
Captodiame, captodiamine	969.5	E853.8	E939.5	E950.3	E962.0	E980.3
Caramiphen (hydrochloride)	971.1	E855.4	E941.1	E950.4	E962.0	E980.4
Carbachol	971.0	E855.3	E941.0	E950.4	E962.0	E980.4
Carbacrylamine resins	974.5	E858.5	E944.5	E950.4	E962.0	E980.4
Carbamate (sedative)	967.8	E852.8	E937.8	E950.2	E962.0	E980.2
herbicide	989.3	E863.5	—	E950.6	E962.1	E980.7
insecticide	989.3	E863.2	—	E950.6	E962.1	E980.7
Carbamazepine	966.3	E855.0	E936.3	E950.4	E962.0	E980.4
Carbamic esters	967.8	E852.8	E937.8	E950.2	E962.0	E980.2
Carbamide	974.4	E858.5	E944.4	E950.4	E962.0	E980.4
topical	976.8	E858.7	E946.8	E950.4	E962.0	E980.4
Carbamylcholine chloride	971.0	E855.3	E941.0	E950.4	E962.0	E980.4
Carbarsone	961.1	E857	E931.1	E950.4	E962.0	E980.4
Carbaryl	989.3	E863.2	—	E950.6	E962.1	E980.7
Carbaspirin	965.1	E850.3	E935.3	E950.0	E962.0	E980.0
Carbazochrome	972.8	E858.3	E942.8	E950.4	E962.0	E980.4
Carbenicillin	960.0	E856	E930.0	E950.4	E962.0	E980.4
Carbenoxolone	973.8	E858.4	E943.8	E950.4	E962.0	E980.4
Carbetapentane	975.4	E858.6	E945.4	E950.4	E962.0	E980.4
Carbimazole	962.8	E858.0	E932.8	E950.4	E962.0	E980.4
Carbinol	980.1	E860.2	—	E950.9	E962.1	E980.9
Carbinoxamine	963.0	E858.1	E933.0	E950.4	E962.0	E980.4
Carbitol	982.8	E862.4	—	E950.9	E962.1	E980.9
Carbocaine	968.9	E855.2	E938.9	E950.4	E962.0	E980.4
infiltration (subcutaneous)	968.5	E855.2	E938.5	E950.4	E962.0	E980.4
nerve block (peripheral) (plexus)	968.6	E855.2	E938.6	E950.4	E962.0	E980.4
topical (surface)	968.5	E855.2	E938.5	E950.4	E962.0	E980.4
Carbol-fuchsin solution	976.0	E858.7	E946.0	E950.4	E962.0	E980.4
Carbolic acid (see also Phenol)	983.0	E864.0	—	E950.7	E962.1	E980.6
Carbomycin	960.8	E856	E930.8	E950.4	E962.0	E980.4
Carbon						
bisulfide (liquid) (vapor)	982.2	E862.4	—	E950.9	E962.1	E980.9
dioxide (gas)	987.8	E869.8	—	E952.8	E962.2	E982.8
disulfide (liquid) (vapor)	982.2	E862.4	—	E950.9	E962.1	E980.9
monoxide (from incomplete combustion of) (in) NEC	986	E868.9	—	E952.1	E962.2	E982.1
blast furnace gas	986	E868.8	—	E952.1	E962.2	E982.1
butane (distributed in mobile container)	986	E868.0	—	E951.1	E962.2	E981.1
distributed through pipes	986	E867	—	E951.0	E962.2	E981.0
charcoal fumes	986	E868.3	—	E952.1	E962.2	E982.1
coal						
gas (piped)	986	E867	—	E951.0	E962.2	E981.0
solid (in domestic stoves, fireplaces)	986	E868.3	—	E952.1	E962.2	E982.1
coke (in domestic stoves, fireplaces)	986	E868.3	—	E952.1	E962.2	E982.1
exhaust gas (motor) not in transit	986	E868.2	—	E952.0	E962.2	E982.0
combustion engine, any not in watercraft	986	E868.2	—	E952.0	E962.2	E982.0
farm tractor, not in transit	986	E868.2	—	E952.0	E962.2	E982.0
gas engine	986	E868.2	—	E952.0	E962.2	E982.0
motor pump	986	E868.2	—	E952.0	E962.2	E982.0
motor vehicle, not in transit	986	E868.2	—	E952.0	E962.2	E982.0
fuel (in domestic use)	986	E868.3	—	E952.1	E962.2	E982.1
gas (piped)	986	E867	—	E951.0	E962.2	E981.0
in mobile container	986	E868.0	—	E951.1	E962.2	E981.1
utility	986	E868.1	—	E951.8	E962.2	E981.1
in mobile container	986	E868.0	—	E951.1	E962.2	E981.1
piped (natural)	986	E867	—	E951.0	E962.2	E981.0
illuminating gas	986	E868.1	—	E951.8	E962.2	E981.8
industrial fuels or gases, any	986	E868.8	—	E952.1	E962.2	E982.1
kerosene (in domestic stoves, fireplaces)	986	E868.3	—	E952.1	E962.2	E982.1
kiln gas or vapor	986	E868.8	—	E952.1	E962.2	E982.1
motor exhaust gas, not in transit	986	E868.2	—	E952.0	E962.2	E982.0
piped gas (manufactured) (natural)	986	E867	—	E951.0	E962.2	E981.0
producer gas	986	E868.8	—	E952.1	E962.2	E982.1
propane (distributed in mobile container)	986	E868.0	—	E951.1	E962.2	E981.1
distributed through pipes	986	E867	—	E951.0	E962.2	E981.0
specified source NEC	986	E868.8	—	E952.1	E962.2	E982.1
stove gas	986	E868.1	—	E951.8	E962.2	E981.8
piped	986	E867	—	E951.0	E962.2	E981.0

TABLE OF DRUGS AND CHEMICALS

Substance	Poisoning	Accident	Therapeutic-Use	Suicide Attempt	Assault	Undetermined
Carbon—*continued*						
monoxide—*continued*						
utility gas	986	E868.1	—	E951.8	E962.2	E981.8
piped	986	E867	—	E951.0	E962.2	E981.0
water gas	986	E868.1	—	E951.8	E962.2	E981.8
wood (in domestic stoves, fireplaces)	986	E868.3	—	E952.1	E962.2	E982.1
tetrachloride (vapor) NEC	987.8	E869.8	—	E952.8	E962.2	E982.8
liquid (cleansing agent) NEC	982.1	E861.3	—	E950.9	E962.1	E980.9
solvent	982.1	E862.4	—	E950.9	E962.1	E980.9
Carbonic acid (gas)	987.8	E869.8	—	E952.8	E962.2	E982.8
anhydrase inhibitors	974.2	E858.5	E944.2	E950.4	E962.0	E980.4
Carbowax	976.3	E858.7	E946.3	E950.4	E962.0	E980.4
Carbrital	967.0	E851	E937.0	E950.1	E962.0	E980.1
Carbromal (derivatives)	967.3	E852.2	E937.3	E950.2	E962.0	E980.2
Cardiac						
depressants	972.0	E858.3	E942.0	E950.4	E962.0	E980.4
rhythm regulators	972.0	E858.3	E942.0	E950.4	E962.0	E980.4
Cardiografin	977.8	E858.8	E947.8	E950.4	E962.0	E980.4
Cardio-green	977.8	E858.8	E947.8	E950.4	E962.0	E980.4
Cardiotonic glycosides	972.1	E858.3	E942.1	E950.4	E962.0	E980.4
Cardiovascular agents NEC	972.9	E858.3	E942.9	E950.4	E962.0	E980.4
Cardrase	974.2	E858.5	E944.2	E950.4	E962.0	E980.4
Carfusin	976.0	E858.7	E946.0	E950.4	E962.0	E980.4
Carisoprodol	968.0	E855.1	E938.0	E950.4	E962.0	E980.4
Carmustine	963.1	E858.1	E933.1	E950.4	E962.0	E980.4
Carotene	963.5	E858.1	E933.5	E950.4	E962.0	E980.4
Carphenazine (maleate)	969.1	E853.0	E939.1	E950.3	E962.0	E980.3
Carter's Little Pills	973.1	E858.4	E943.1	E950.4	E962.0	E980.4
Cascara (sagrada)	973.1	E858.4	E943.1	E950.4	E962.0	E980.4
Cassava	988.2	E865.4	—	E950.9	E962.1	E980.9
Castellani's paint	976.0	E858.7	E946.0	E950.4	E962.0	E980.4
Castor						
bean	988.2	E865.3	—	E950.9	E962.1	E980.9
oil	973.1	E858.4	E943.1	E950.4	E962.0	E980.4
Caterpillar (sting)	989.5	E905.5	—	E950.9	E962.1	E980.9
Catha (edulis)	970.8	E854.3	E940.8	E950.4	E962.0	E980.4
Cathartics NEC	973.3	E858.4	E943.3	E950.4	E962.0	E980.4
contact	973.1	E858.4	E943.1	E950.4	E962.0	E980.4
emollient	973.2	E858.4	E943.2	E950.4	E962.0	E980.4
intestinal irritants	973.1	E858.4	E943.1	E950.4	E962.0	E980.4
saline	973.3	E858.4	E943.3	E950.4	E962.0	E980.4
Cathomycin	960.8	E856	E930.8	E950.4	E962.0	E980.4
Caustic(s)	983.9	E864.4	—	E950.7	E962.1	E980.6
alkali	983.2	E864.2	—	E950.7	E962.1	E980.6
hydroxide	983.2	E864.2	—	E950.7	E962.1	E980.6
potash	983.2	E864.2	—	E950.7	E962.1	E980.6
soda	983.2	E864.2	—	E950.7	E962.1	E980.6
specified NEC	983.9	E864.3	—	E950.7	E962.1	E980.6
Ceepryn	976.0	E858.7	E946.0	E950.4	E962.0	E980.4
ENT agent	976.6	E858.7	E946.6	E950.4	E962.0	E980.4
lozenges	976.6	E858.7	E946.6	E950.4	E962.0	E980.4
Celestone	962.0	E858	E932.0	E950.4	E962.0	E980.4
topical	976.0	E858.7	E946.0	E950.4	E962.0	E980.4
Cellosolve	982.8	E862.4	—	E950.9	E962.1	E980.9
Cell stimulants and proliferants	976.8	E858.7	E946.8	E950.4	E962.0	E980.4
Cellulose derivatives, cathartic	973.3	E858.4	E943.3	E950.4	E962.0	E980.4
nitrates (topical)	976.3	E858.7	E946.3	E950.4	E962.0	E980.4
Centipede (bite)	989.5	E905.4	—	E950.9	E962.1	E980.9
Central nervous system						
depressants	968.4	E855.1	E938.4	E950.4	E962.0	E980.4
anesthetic (general) NEC	968.4	E855.1	E938.4	E950.4	E962.0	E980.4
gases NEC	968.2	E855.1	E938.2	E950.4	E962.0	E980.4
intravenous	968.3	E855.1	E938.3	E950.4	E962.0	E980.4
barbiturates	967.0	E851	E937.0	E950.1	E962.0	E980.1
bromides	967.3	E852.2	E937.3	E950.2	E962.0	E980.2
cannabis sativa	969.6	E854.1	E939.6	E950.3	E962.0	E980.3
chloral hydrate	967.1	E852.0	E937.1	E950.2	E962.0	E980.2
hallucinogenics	969.6	E854.1	E939.6	E950.3	E962.0	E980.3
hypnotics	967.9	E852.9	E937.9	E950.2	E962.0	E980.2
specified NEC	967.8	E852.8	E937.8	E950.2	E962.0	E980.2
muscle relaxants	968.0	E855.1	E938.0	E950.4	E962.0	E980.4
paraldehyde	967.2	E852.1	E937.2	E950.2	E962.0	E980.2
sedatives	967.9	E852.9	E937.9	E950.2	E962.0	E980.2
mixed NEC	967.6	E852.5	E937.6	E950.2	E962.0	E980.2
specified NEC	967.8	E852.8	E937.8	E950.2	E962.0	E980.2
muscle-tone depressants	968.0	E855.1	E938.0	E950.4	E962.0	E980.4

Substance	Poisoning	Accident	Therapeutic-Use	Suicide Attempt	Assault	Undetermined
Central nervous system—continued						
stimulants	970.9	E854.3	E940.9	E950.4	E962.0	E980.4
amphetamines	969.7	E854.2	E939.7	E950.3	E962.0	E980.3
analeptics	970.0	E854.3	E940.0	E950.4	E962.0	E980.4
antidepressants	969.0	E854.0	E939.0	E950.3	E962.0	E980.3
opiate antagonists	970.1	E854.3	E940.0	E950.4	E962.0	E980.4
specified NEC	970.8	E854.3	E940.8	E950.4	E962.0	E980.4
Cephalexin	960.5	E856	E930.5	E950.4	E962.0	E980.4
Cephaloglycin	960.5	E856	E930.5	E950.4	E962.0	E980.4
Cephaloridine	960.5	E856	E930.5	E950.4	E962.0	E980.4
Cephalosporins NEC	960.5	E856	E930.5	E950.4	E962.0	E980.4
N (adicillin)	960.0	E856	E930.0	E950.4	E962.0	E980.4
Cephalothin (sodium)	960.5	E856	E930.5	E950.4	E962.0	E980.4
Cerbera (odallam)	988.2	E865.4	—	E950.9	E962.1	E980.9
Cerberin	972.1	E858.3	E942.1	E950.4	E962.0	E980.4
Cerebral stimulants	970.9	E854.3	E940.9	E950.4	E962.0	E980.4
psychotherapeutic	969.7	E854.2	E939.7	E950.3	E962.0	E980.3
specified NEC	970.8	E854.3	E940.8	E950.4	E962.0	E980.4
Cetalkonium (chloride)	976.0	E858.7	E946.0	E950.4	E962.0	E980.4
Cetoxime	963.0	E858.1	E933.0	E950.4	E962.0	E980.4
Cetrimide	976.2	E858.7	E946.2	E950.4	E962.0	E980.4
Cetylpyridinium	976.0	E858.7	E946.0	E950.4	E962.0	E980.4
ENT agent	976.6	E858.7	E946.6	E950.4	E962.0	E980.4
lozenges	976.6	E858.7	E946.6	E950.4	E962.0	E980.4
Cevadilla — see Sabadilla						
Cevitamic acid	963.5	E858.1	E933.5	E950.4	E962.0	E980.4
Chalk, precipitated	973.0	E858.4	E943.0	E950.4	E962.0	E980.4
Charcoal						
fumes (carbon monoxide)	986	E868.3	—	E952.1	E962.2	E982.1
industrial	986	E868.8	—	E952.1	E962.2	E982.1
medicinal (activated)	973.0	E858.4	E943.0	E950.4	E962.0	E980.4
Chelating agents NEC	977.2	E858.8	E947.2	E950.4	E962.0	E980.4
Chelidonium majus	988.2	E865.4	—	E950.9	E962.1	E980.9
Chemical substance	989.9	E866.9	—	E950.9	E962.1	E980.9
specified NEC	989.8	E866.8	—	E950.9	E962.1	E980.9
Chenopodium (oil)	961.6	E857	E931.6	E950.4	E962.0	E980.4
Cherry laurel	988.2	E865.4	—	E950.9	E962.1	E980.9
Chiniofon	961.3	E857	E931.3	E950.4	E962.0	E980.4
Chlophedianol	975.4	E858.6	E945.4	E950.4	E962.0	E980.4
Chloral (betaine) (formamide) (hydrate)	967.1	E852.0	E937.1	E950.2	E962.0	E980.2
Chloralamide	967.1	E852.0	E937.1	E950.2	E962.0	E980.2
Chlorambucil	963.1	E858.1	E933.1	E950.4	E962.0	E980.4
Chloramphenicol	960.2	E856	E930.2	E950.4	E962.0	E980.4
ENT agent	976.6	E858.7	E946.6	E950.4	E962.0	E980.4
ophthalmic preparation	976.5	E858.7	E946.5	E950.4	E962.0	E980.4
topical NEC	976.0	E858.7	E946.0	E950.4	E962.0	E980.4
Chlorate(s) (potassium) (sodium) NEC	983.9	E864.3	—	E950.7	E962.1	E980.6
herbicides	989.4	E863.5	—	E950.6	E962.1	E980.7
Chlorcyclizine	963.0	E858.1	E933.0	E950.4	E962.0	E980.4
Chlordan(e) (dust)	989.2	E863.0	—	E950.6	E962.1	E980.7
Chlordantoin	976.0	E858.7	E946.0	E950.4	E962.0	E980.4
Chlordiazepoxide	969.4	E853.2	E939.4	E950.3	E962.0	E980.3
Chloresium	976.8	E858.7	E946.8	E950.4	E962.0	E980.4
Chlorethiazol	967.1	E852.0	E937.1	E950.2	E962.0	E980.2
Chlorethyl — see Ethyl, chloride						
Chloretone	967.1	E852.0	E937.1	E950.2	E962.0	E980.2
Chlorex	982.3	E862.4	—	E950.9	E962.1	E980.9
Chlorhexadol	967.1	E852.0	E937.1	E950.2	E962.0	E980.2
Chlorhexidine (hydrochloride)	976.0	E858.7	E946.0	E950.4	E962.0	E980.4
Chlorhydroxyquinolin	976.0	E858.7	E946.0	E950.4	E962.0	E980.4
Chloride of lime (bleach)	983.9	E864.3	—	E950.7	E962.1	E980.6
Chlorinated						
camphene	989.2	E863.0	—	E950.6	E962.1	E980.7
diphenyl	989.8	E866.8	—	E950.9	E962.1	E980.9
hydrocarbons NEC	989.2	E863.0	—	E950.6	E962.1	E980.7
solvent	982.3	E862.4	—	E950.9	E962.1	E980.9
lime (bleach)	983.9	E864.3	—	E950.7	E962.1	E980.6
naphthalene — see Naphthalene						
pesticides NEC	989.2	E863.0	—	E950.6	E962.1	E980.7
soda — see Sodium, hypochlorite						
Chlorine (fumes) (gas)	987.6	E869.8	—	E952.8	E962.2	E982.8
bleach	983.9	E864.3	—	E950.7	E962.1	E980.6
compounds NEC	983.9	E864.3	—	E950.7	E962.1	E980.6
disinfectant	983.9	E861.4	—	E950.7	E962.1	E980.6
releasing agents NEC	983.9	E864.3	—	E950.7	E962.1	E980.6
Chlorisondamine	972.3	E858.3	E942.3	E950.4	E962.0	E980.4

TABLE OF DRUGS AND CHEMICALS

Substance	Poisoning	Accident	Therapeutic-Use	Suicide Attempt	Assault	Undetermined
Chlormadinone	962.2	E858.0	E932.2	E950.4	E962.0	E980.4
Chlormerodrin	974.0	E858.5	E944.0	E950.4	E962.0	E980.4
Chlormethiazole	967.1	E852.0	E937.1	E950.2	E962.0	E980.2
Chlormethylenecycline	960.4	E856	E930.4	E950.4	E962.0	E980.4
Chlormezanone	969.5	E853.8	E939.5	E950.3	E962.0	E980.3
Chloroacetophenone	987.5	E869.3	—	E952.8	E962.2	E982.8
Chloroaniline	983.0	E864.0	—	E950.7	E962.1	E980.6
Chlorobenzene, chlorobenzol	982.0	E862.4	—	E950.9	E962.1	E980.9
Chlorobutanol	967.1	E852.0	E937.1	E950.2	E962.0	E980.2
Chlorodinitrobenzene	983.0	E864.0	—	E950.7	E962.1	E980.6
dust or vapor	987.8	E869.8	—	E952.8	E962.2	E982.8
Chloroethane — see Ethyl, chloride						
Chloroform (fumes) (vapor)	987.8	E869.8	—	E952.8	E962.2	E982.8
anesthetic (gas)	968.2	E855.1	E938.2	E950.4	E962.0	E980.4
liquid NEC	968.4	E855.1	E938.4	E950.4	E962.0	E980.4
solvent	982.3	E862.4	—	E950.9	E962.1	E980.9
Chloroguanide	961.4	E857	E931.4	E950.4	E962.0	E980.4
Chloromycetin	960.2	E856	E930.2	E950.4	E962.0	E980.4
ENT agent	976.6	E858.7	E946.6	E950.4	E962.0	E980.4
ophthalmic preparation	976.5	E858.7	E946.5	E950.4	E962.0	E980.4
otic solution	976.6	E858.7	E946.6	E950.4	E962.0	E980.4
topical NEC	976.0	E858.7	E946.0	E950.4	E962.0	E980.4
Chloronitrobenzene	983.0	E864.0	—	E950.7	E962.1	E980.6
dust or vapor	987.8	E869.8	—	E952.8	E962.2	E982.8
Chlorophenol	983.0	E864.0	—	E950.7	E962.1	E980.6
Chlorophenothane	989.2	E863.0	—	E950.6	E962.1	E980.7
Chlorophyll (derivatives)	976.8	E858.7	E946.8	E950.4	E962.0	E980.4
Chloropicrin (fumes)	987.8	E869.8	—	E952.8	E962.2	E982.8
fumigant	989.4	E863.8	—	E950.6	E962.1	E980.7
fungicide	989.4	E863.6	—	E950.6	E962.1	E980.7
pesticide (fumes)	989.4	E863.4	—	E950.6	E962.1	E980.7
Chloroprocaine	968.9	E855.2	E938.9	E950.4	E962.0	E980.4
infiltration (subcutaneous)	968.5	E855.2	E938.5	E950.4	E962.0	E980.4
nerve block (peripheral) (plexus)	968.6	E855.2	E938.6	E950.4	E962.0	E980.4
Chloroptic	976.5	E858.7	E946.5	E950.4	E962.0	E980.4
Chloropurine	963.1	E858.1	E933.1	E950.4	E962.0	E980.4
Chloroquine (hydrochloride) (phosphate)	961.4	E857	E931.4	E950.4	E962.0	E980.4
Chlorothen	963.0	E858.1	E933.0	E950.4	E962.0	E980.4
Chlorothiazide	974.3	E858.5	E944.3	E950.4	E962.0	E980.4
Chlorotrianisene	962.2	E858.0	E932.2	E950.4	E962.0	E980.4
Chlorovinyldichloroarsine	985.1	E866.3	—	E950.8	E962.1	E980.8
Chloroxylenol	976.0	E858.7	E946.0	E950.4	E962.0	E980.4
Chlorphenesin (carbamate)	968.0	E855.1	E938.0	E950.4	E962.0	E980.4
topical (antifungal)	976.0	E858.7	E946.0	E950.4	E962.0	E980.4
Chlorpheniramine	963.0	E858.1	E933.0	E950.4	E962.0	E980.4
Chlorphenoxamine	966.4	E855.0	E936.4	E950.4	E962.0	E980.4
Chlorphentermine	977.0	E858.8	E947.0	E950.4	E962.0	E980.4
Chlorproguanil	961.4	E857	E931.4	E950.4	E962.0	E980.4
Chlorpromazine	969.1	E853.0	E939.1	E950.3	E962.0	E980.3
Chlorpropamide	962.3	E858.0	E932.3	E950.4	E962.0	E980.4
Chlorprothixene	969.3	E853.8	E939.3	E950.3	E962.0	E980.3
Chlorquinaldol	976.0	E858.7	E946.0	E950.4	E962.0	E980.4
Chlortetracycline	960.4	E856	E930.4	E950.4	E962.0	E980.4
Chlorthalidone	974.4	E858.5	E944.4	E950.4	E962.0	E980.4
Chlortrianisene	962.2	E858.0	E932.2	E950.4	E962.0	E980.4
Chlor-Trimeton	963.0	E858.1	E933.0	E950.4	E962.0	E980.4
Chlorzoxazone	968.0	E855.1	E938.0	E950.4	E962.0	E980.4
Choke damp	987.8	E869.8	—	E952.8	E962.2	E982.8
Cholebrine	977.8	E858.8	E947.8	E950.4	E962.0	E980.4
Cholera vaccine	978.2	E858.8	E948.2	E950.4	E962.0	E980.4
Cholesterol-lowering agents	972.2	E858.3	E942.2	E950.4	E962.0	E980.4
Cholestyramine (resin)	972.2	E858.3	E942.2	E950.4	E962.0	E980.4
Cholic acid	973.4	E858.4	E943.4	E950.4	E962.0	E980.4
Choline						
dihydrogen citrate	977.1	E858.8	E947.1	E950.4	E962.0	E980.4
salicylate	965.1	E850.3	E935.3	E950.0	E962.0	E980.0
theophyllinate	974.1	E858.5	E944.1	E950.4	E962.0	E980.4
Cholinergics	971.0	E855.3	E941.0	E950.4	E962.0	E980.4
Cholografin	977.8	E858.8	E947.8	E950.4	E962.0	E980.4
Chorionic gonadotropin	962.4	E858.0	E932.4	E950.4	E962.0	E980.4
Chromates	983.9	E864.3	—	E950.7	E962.1	E980.6
dust or mist	987.8	E869.8	—	E952.8	E962.2	E982.8
lead	984.0	E866.0	—	E950.9	E962.1	E980.9
paint	984.0	E861.5	—	E950.9	E962.1	E980.9
Chromic acid	983.9	E864.3	—	E950.7	E962.1	E980.6
dust or mist	987.8	E869.8	—	E952.8	E962.2	E982.8

Substance	Poisoning	Accident	Therapeutic Use	Suicide Attempt	Assault	Undetermined
Chromium	985.6	E866.4	—	E950.9	E962.1	E980.9
compounds — see Chromates						
Chromonar	972.4	E858.3	E942.4	E950.4	E962.0	E980.4
Chromyl chloride	983.9	E864.3	—	E950.7	E962.1	E980.6
Chrysarobin (ointment)	976.4	E858.7	E946.4	E950.4	E962.0	E980.4
Chrysazin	973.1	E858.4	E943.1	E950.4	E962.0	E980.4
Chymar	963.4	E858.1	E933.4	E950.4	E962.0	E980.4
ophthalmic preparation	976.5	E858.7	E946.5	E950.4	E962.0	E980.4
Chymotrypsin	963.4	E858.1	E933.4	E950.4	E962.0	E980.4
ophthalmic preparation	976.5	E858.7	E946.5	E950.4	E962.0	E980.4
Cicuta maculata or virosa	988.2	E865.4	—	E950.9	E962.1	E980.9
Cigarette lighter fluid	981	E862.1	—	E950.9	E962.1	E980.9
Cinchocaine (spinal)	968.7	E855.2	E938.7	E950.4	E962.0	E980.4
topical (surface)	968.5	E855.2	E938.5	E950.4	E962.0	E980.4
Cinchona	961.4	E857	E931.4	E950.4	E962.0	E980.4
Cinchonine alkaloids	961.4	E857	E931.4	E950.4	E962.0	E980.4
Cinchophen	974.7	E858.5	E944.7	E950.4	E962.0	E980.4
Cinnarizine	963.0	E858.1	E933.0	E950.4	E962.0	E980.4
Citanest	968.9	E855.2	E938.9	E950.4	E962.0	E980.4
infiltration (subcutaneous)	968.5	E855.2	E938.5	E950.4	E962.0	E980.4
nerve block (peripheral) (plexus)	968.6	E855.2	E938.6	E950.4	E962.0	E980.4
Citric acid	989.8	E866.8	—	E950.9	E962.1	E980.9
Citrovorum factor	964.1	E858.2	E934.1	E950.4	E962.0	E980.4
Claviceps purpurea	988.2	E865.4	—	E950.9	E962.1	E980.9
Cleaner, cleansing agent NEC	989.8	E861.3	—	E950.9	E962.1	E980.9
of paint or varnish	982.8	E862.9	—	E950.9	E962.1	E980.9
Clematis vitalba	988.2	E865.4	—	E950.9	E962.1	E980.9
Clemizole	963.0	E858.1	E933.0	E950.4	E962.0	E980.4
penicillin	960.0	E856	E930.0	E950.4	E962.0	E980.4
Clidinium	971.1	E855.4	E941.1	E950.4	E962.0	E980.4
Clindamycin	960.8	E856	E930.8	E950.4	E962.0	E980.4
Cliradon	965.09	E850.2	E935.2	E950.0	E962.0	E980.0
Clocortolone	962.0	E858.0	E932.0	E950.4	E962.0	E980.4
Clofedanol	975.4	E858.6	E945.4	E950.4	E962.0	E980.4
Clofibrate	972.2	E858.3	E942.2	E950.4	E962.0	E980.4
Clomethiazole	967.1	E852.0	E937.1	E950.2	E962.0	E980.2
Clomiphene	977.8	E858.8	E947.8	E950.4	E962.0	E980.4
Clonazepam	969.4	E853.2	E939.4	E950.3	E962.0	E980.3
Clonidine	972.6	E858.3	E942.6	E950.4	E962.0	E980.4
Clopamide	974.3	E858.5	E944.3	E950.4	E962.0	E980.4
Clorazepate	969.4	E853.2	E939.4	E950.3	E962.0	E980.3
Clorexolone	974.4	E858.5	E944.4	E950.4	E962.0	E980.4
Clorox (bleach)	983.9	E864.3	—	E950.7	E962.1	E980.6
Clortermine	977.0	E858.8	E947.0	E950.4	E962.0	E980.4
Clotrimazole	976.0	E858.7	E946.0	E950.4	E962.0	E980.4
Cloxacillin	960.0	E856	E930.0	E950.4	E962.0	E980.4
Coagulants NEC	964.5	E858.2	E934.5	E950.4	E962.0	E980.4
Coal (carbon monoxide from) — see also Carbon, monoxide, coal						
oil — see Kerosene						
tar NEC	983.0	E864.0	—	E950.7	E962.1	E980.6
fumes	987.8	E869.8	—	E952.8	E962.2	E982.8
medicinal (ointment)	976.4	E858.7	E946.4	E950.4	E962.0	E980.4
analgesics NEC	965.5	E850.5	E935.5	E950.0	E962.0	E980.0
naphtha (solvent)	981	E862.0	—	E950.9	E962.1	E980.9
Cobalt (fumes) (industrial)	985.8	E866.4	—	E950.9	E962.1	E980.9
Cobra (venom)	989.5	E905.0	—	E950.9	E962.1	E980.9
Coca (leaf)	970.8	E854.3	E940.8	E950.4	E962.0	E980.4
Cocaine (hydrochloride) (salt)	968.5	E855.2	E938.5	E950.4	E962.0	E980.4
Coccidioidin	977.8	E858.8	E947.8	E950.4	E962.0	E980.4
Cocculus indicus	988.2	E865.3	—	E950.9	E962.1	E980.9
Cochineal	989.8	E866.8	—	E950.9	E962.1	E980.9
medicinal products	977.4	E858.8	E947.4	E950.4	E962.0	E980.4
Codeine	965.09	E850.2	E935.2	E950.0	E962.0	E980.0
Coffee	989.8	E866.8	—	E950.9	E962.1	E980.9
Cogentin	971.1	E855.4	E941.1	E950.4	E962.0	E980.4
Coke fumes or gas (carbon monoxide)	986	E868.3	—	E952.1	E962.2	E982.1
industrial use	986	E868.8	—	E952.1	E962.2	E982.1
Colace	973.2	E858.4	E943.2	E950.4	E962.0	E980.4
Colchicine	974.7	E858.5	E944.7	E950.4	E962.0	E980.4
Colchicum	988.2	E865.3	—	E950.9	E962.1	E980.9
Cold cream	976.3	E858.7	E946.3	E950.4	E962.0	E980.4
Colestipol	972.2	E858.3	E942.2	E950.4	E962.0	E980.4
Colistimethate	960.8	E856	E930.8	E950.4	E962.0	E980.4
Colistin	960.8	E856	E930.8	E950.4	E962.0	E980.4
Collagenase	976.8	E858.7	E946.8	E950.4	E962.0	E980.4
Collodion (flexible)	976.3	E858.7	E946.3	E950.4	E962.0	E980.4

Substance	Poisoning	Accident	Therapeutic-Use	Suicide Attempt	Assault	Undetermined
Colocynth	973.1	E858.4	E943.1	E950.4	E962.0	E980.4
Coloring matter — see Dye(s)						
Combustion gas — see Carbon, monoxide						
Compazine	969.1	E853.0	E939.1	E950.3	E962.0	E980.3
Compound						
42 (warfarin)	989.4	E863.7	—	E950.6	E962.1	E980.7
269 (endrin)	989.2	E863.0	—	E950.6	E962.1	E980.7
497 (dieldrin)	989.2	E863.0	—	E950.6	E962.1	E980.7
1080 (sodium fluoroacetate)	989.4	E863.7	—	E950.6	E962.1	E980.7
3422 (parathion)	989.3	E863.1	—	E950.6	E962.1	E980.7
3911 (phorate)	989.3	E863.1	—	E950.6	E962.1	E980.7
3956 (toxaphene)	989.2	E863.0	—	E950.6	E962.1	E980.7
4049 (malathion)	989.3	E863.1	—	E950.6	E962.1	E980.7
4124 (dicapthon)	989.4	E863.4	—	E950.6	E962.1	E980.7
E (cortisone)	962.0	E858.0	E932.0	E950.4	E962.0	E980.4
F (hydrocortisone)	962.0	E858.0	E932.0	E950.4	E962.0	E980.4
Congo red	977.8	E858.8	E947.8	E950.4	E962.0	E980.4
Coniine, conine	965.7	E850.7	E935.7	E950.0	E962.0	E980.0
Conium (maculatum)	988.2	E865.4	—	E950.9	E962.1	E980.9
Conjugated estrogens (equine)	962.2	E858.0	E932.2	E950.4	E962.0	E980.4
Contac	975.6	E858.6	E945.6	E950.4	E962.0	E980.4
Contact lens solution	976.5	E858.7	E946.5	E950.4	E962.0	E980.4
Contraceptives (oral)	962.2	E858.0	E932.2	E950.4	E962.0	E980.4
vaginal	976.8	E858.7	E946.8	E950.4	E962.0	E980.4
Contrast media (roentgenographic)	977.8	E858.8	E947.8	E950.4	E962.0	E980.4
Convallaria majalis	988.2	E865.4	—	E950.9	E962.1	E980.9
Copper (dust) (fumes) (salts) NEC	985.8	E866.4	—	E950.9	E962.1	E980.9
arsenate, arsenite	985.1	E866.3	—	E950.8	E962.1	E980.8
insecticide	985.1	E863.4	—	E950.8	E962.1	E980.8
emetic	973.6	E858.4	E943.6	E950.4	E962.0	E980.4
fungicide	985.8	E863.6	—	E950.6	E962.1	E980.7
insecticide	985.8	E863.4	—	E950.6	E962.1	E980.7
oleate	976.0	E858.7	E946.0	E950.4	E962.0	E980.4
sulfate	983.9	E864.3	—	E950.7	E962.1	E980.6
fungicide	983.9	E863.6	—	E950.7	E962.1	E980.6
cupric	973.6	E858.4	E943.6	E950.4	E962.0	E980.4
cuprous	983.9	E864.3	—	E950.7	E962.1	E980.6
Copperhead snake (bite) (venom)	989.5	E905.0	—	E950.9	E962.1	E980.9
Coral (sting)	989.5	E905.6	—	E950.9	E962.1	E980.9
snake (bite) (venom)	989.5	E905.0	—	E950.9	E962.1	E980.9
Cordran	976.0	E858.7	E946.0	E950.4	E962.0	E980.4
Corn cures	976.4	E858.7	E946.4	E950.4	E962.0	E980.4
Cornhusker's lotion	976.3	E858.7	E946.3	E950.4	E962.0	E980.4
Corn starch	976.3	E858.7	E946.3	E950.4	E962.0	E980.4
Corrosive	983.9	E864.4	—	E950.7	E962.1	E980.6
acids NEC	983.1	E864.1	—	E950.7	E962.1	E980.6
aromatics	983.0	E864.0	—	E950.7	E962.1	E980.6
disinfectant	983.0	E861.4	—	E950.7	E962.1	E980.6
fumes NEC	987.9	E869.9	—	E952.9	E962.2	E982.9
specified NEC	983.9	E864.3	—	E950.7	E962.1	E980.6
sublimate — see Mercury, chloride						
Cortate	962.0	E858.0	E932.0	E950.4	E962.0	E980.4
Cort-Dome	962.0	E858.0	E932.0	E950.4	E962.0	E980.4
ENT agent	976.6	E858.7	E946.6	E950.4	E962.0	E980.4
ophthalmic preparation	976.5	E858.7	E946.5	E950.4	E962.0	E980.4
topical NEC	976.0	E858.7	E946.0	E950.4	E962.0	E980.4
Cortef	962.0	E858.0	E932.0	E950.4	E962.0	E980.4
ENT agent	976.6	E858.7	E946.6	E950.4	E962.0	E980.4
ophthalmic preparation	976.5	E858.7	E946.5	E950.4	E962.0	E980.4
topical NEC	976.0	E858.7	E946.0	E950.4	E962.0	E980.4
Corticosteroids (fluorinated)	962.0	E858.0	E932.0	E950.4	E962.0	E980.4
ENT agent	976.6	E858.7	E946.6	E950.4	E962.0	E980.4
ophthalmic preparation	976.5	E858.7	E946.5	E950.4	E962.0	E980.4
topical NEC	976.0	E858.7	E946.0	E950.4	E962.0	E980.4
Corticotropin	962.4	E858.0	E932.4	E950.4	E962.0	E980.4
Cortisol	962.0	E858.0	E932.0	E950.4	E962.0	E980.4
ENT agent	976.6	E858.7	E946.6	E950.4	E962.0	E980.4
ophthalmic preparation	976.5	E858.7	E946.5	E950.4	E962.0	E980.4
topical NEC	976.0	E858.7	E946.0	E950.4	E962.0	E980.4
Cortisone derivatives (acetate)	962.0	E858.0	E932.0	E950.4	E962.0	E980.4
ENT agent	976.6	E858.7	E946.6	E950.4	E962.0	E980.4
ophthalmic preparation	976.5	E858.7	E946.5	E950.4	E962.0	E980.4
topical NEC	976.0	E858.7	E946.0	E950.4	E962.0	E980.4
Cortogen	962.0	E858.0	E932.0	E950.4	E962.0	E980.4
ENT agent	976.6	E858.7	E946.6	E950.4	E962.0	E980.4
ophthalmic preparation	976.5	E858.7	E946.5	E950.4	E962.0	E980.4

Substance	Poisoning	Accident	Therapeutic Use	Suicide Attempt	Assault	Undetermined
Cortone	962.0	E858.0	E932.0	E950.4	E962.0	E980.4
ENT agent	976.6	E858.7	E946.6	E950.4	E962.0	E980.4
ophthalmic preparation	976.5	E858.7	E946.5	E950.4	E962.0	E980.4
Cortril	962.0	E858.0	E932.0	E950.4	E962.0	E980.4
ENT agent	976.6	E858.7	E946.6	E950.4	E962.0	E980.4
ophthalmic preparation	976.5	E858.7	E946.5	E950.4	E962.0	E980.4
topical NEC	976.0	E858.7	E946.0	E950.4	E962.0	E980.4
Cosmetics	989.8	E866.7	—	E950.9	E962.1	E980.9
Cosyntropin	977.8	E858.8	E947.8	E950.4	E962.0	E980.4
Cotarnine	964.5	E858.2	E934.5	E950.4	E962.0	E980.4
Cottonseed oil	976.3	E858.7	E946.3	E950.4	E962.0	E980.4
Cough mixtures (antitussives)	975.4	E858.6	E945.4	E950.4	E962.0	E980.4
containing opiates	965.09	E850.2	E935.2	E950.0	E962.0	E980.0
expectorants	975.5	E858.6	E945.5	E950.4	E962.0	E980.4
Coumadin	964.2	E858.2	E934.2	E950.4	E962.0	E980.4
rodenticide	989.4	E863.7	—	E950.6	E962.1	E980.7
Coumarin	964.2	E858.2	E934.2	E950.4	E962.0	E980.4
Coumetarol	964.2	E858.2	E934.2	E950.4	E962.0	E980.4
Cowbane	988.2	E865.4	—	E950.9	E962.1	E980.9
Cozyme	963.5	E858.1	E933.5	E950.4	E962.0	E980.4
Creolin	983.0	E864.0	—	E950.7	E962.1	E980.6
disinfectant	983.0	E861.4	—	E950.7	E962.1	E980.6
Creosol (compound)	983.0	E864.0	—	E950.7	E962.1	E980.6
Creosote (beechwood) (coal tar)	983.0	E864.0	—	E950.7	E962.1	E980.6
medicinal (expectorant)	975.5	E858.6	E945.5	E950.4	E962.0	E980.4
syrup	975.5	E858.6	E945.5	E950.4	E962.0	E980.4
Cresol	983.0	E864.0	—	E950.7	E962.1	E980.6
disinfectant	983.0	E861.4	—	E950.7	E962.1	E980.6
Cresylic acid	983.0	E864.0	—	E950.7	E962.1	E980.6
Cropropamide	965.7	E850.7	E935.7	E950.0	E962.0	E980.0
with crotethamide	970.0	E854.3	E940.0	E950.4	E962.0	E980.4
Crotamiton	976.0	E858.7	E946.0	E950.4	E962.0	E980.4
Crotethamide	965.7	E850.7	E935.7	E950.0	E962.0	E980.0
with cropropamide	970.0	E854.3	E940.0	E950.4	E962.0	E980.4
Croton (oil)	973.1	E858.4	E943.1	E950.4	E962.0	E980.4
chloral	967.1	E852.0	E937.1	E950.2	E962.0	E980.2
Crude oil	981	E862.1	—	E950.9	E962.1	E980.9
Cryogenine	965.8	E850.8	E935.8	E950.0	E962.0	E980.0
Cryolite (pesticide)	989.4	E863.4	—	E950.6	E962.1	E980.7
Cryptenamine	972.6	E858.3	E942.6	E950.4	E962.0	E980.4
Crystal violet	976.0	E858.7	E946.0	E950.4	E962.0	E980.4
Cuckoopint	988.2	E865.4	—	E950.9	E962.1	E980.9
Cumetharol	964.2	E858.2	E934.2	E950.4	E962.0	E980.4
Cupric sulfate	973.6	E858.4	E943.6	E950.4	E962.0	E980.4
Cuprous sulfate	983.9	E864.3	—	E950.7	E962.1	E980.6
Curare, curarine	975.2	E858.6	E945.2	E950.4	E962.0	E980.4
Cyanic acid — see Cyanide(s)						
Cyanide(s) (compounds) (hydrogen) (potassium) (sodium) NEC	989.0	E866.8	—	E950.9	E962.1	E980.9
dust or gas (inhalation) NEC	987.7	E869.8	—	E952.8	E962.2	E982.8
fumigant	989.0	E863.8	—	E950.6	E962.1	E980.7
mercuric — see Mercury						
pesticide (dust) (fumes)	989.0	E863.4	—	E950.6	E962.1	E980.7
Cyanocobalamin	964.1	E858.2	E934.1	E950.4	E962.0	E980.4
Cyanogen (chloride) (gas) NEC	987.8	E869.8	—	E952.8	E962.2	E982.8
Cyclaine	968.5	E855.2	E938.5	E950.4	E962.0	E980.4
Cyclamen europaeum	988.2	E865.4	—	E950.9	E962.1	E980.9
Cyclandelate	972.5	E858.3	E942.5	E950.4	E962.0	E980.4
Cyclazocine	965.09	E850.2	E935.2	E950.0	E962.0	E980.0
Cyclizine	963.0	E858.1	E933.0	E950.4	E962.0	E980.4
Cyclobarbital, cyclobarbitone	967.0	E851	E937.0	E950.1	E962.0	E980.1
Cycloguanil	961.4	E857	E931.4	E950.4	E962.0	E980.4
Cyclohexane	982.0	E862.4	—	E950.9	E962.1	E980.9
Cyclohexanol	980.8	E860.8	—	E950.9	E962.1	E980.9
Cyclohexanone	982.8	E862.4	—	E950.9	E962.1	E980.9
Cyclomethycaine	968.5	E855.2	E938.5	E950.4	E962.0	E980.4
Cyclopentamine	971.2	E855.5	E941.2	E950.4	E962.0	E980.4
Cyclopenthiazide	974.3	E858.5	E944.3	E950.4	E962.0	E980.4
Cyclopentolate	971.1	E855.4	E941.1	E950.4	E962.0	E980.4
Cyclophosphamide	963.1	E858.1	E933.1	E950.4	E962.0	E980.4
Cyclopropane	968.2	E855.1	E938.2	E950.4	E962.0	E980.4
Cycloserine	960.6	E856	E930.6	E950.4	E962.0	E980.4
Cyclothiazide	974.3	E858.5	E944.3	E950.4	E962.0	E980.4
Cycrimine	966.4	E855.0	E936.4	E950.4	E962.0	E980.4
Cymarin	972.1	E858.3	E942.1	E950.4	E962.0	E980.4
Cyproheptadine	963.0	E858.1	E933.0	E950.4	E962.0	E980.4
Cyprolidol	969.0	E854.0	E939.0	E950.3	E962.0	E980.3

TABLE OF DRUGS AND CHEMICALS

Substance	Poisoning	Accident	Therapeutic-Use	Suicide Attempt	Assault	Undetermined
Cytarabine	963.1	E858.1	E933.1	E950.4	E962.0	E980.4
Cytisus						
laburnum	988.2	E865.4	—	E950.9	E962.1	E980.9
scoparius	988.2	E865.4	—	E950.9	E962.1	E980.9
Cytomel	962.7	E858.0	E932.7	E950.4	E962.0	E980.4
Cytosine (antineoplastic)	963.1	E858.1	E933.1	E950.4	E962.0	E980.4
Cytoxan	963.1	E858.1	E933.1	E950.4	E962.0	E980.4
Dacarbazine	963.1	E858.1	E933.1	E950.4	E962.0	E980.4
Dactinomycin	960.7	E856	E930.7	E950.4	E962.0	E980.4
DADPS	961.8	E857	E931.8	E950.4	E962.0	E980.4
Dakin's solution (external)	976.0	E858.7	E946.0	E950.4	E962.0	E980.4
Dalmane	969.4	E853.2	E939.4	E950.3	E962.0	E980.3
DAM	977.2	E858.8	E947.2	E950.4	E962.0	E980.4
Danilone	964.2	E858.2	E934.2	E950.4	E962.0	E980.4
Danthron	973.1	E858.4	E943.1	E950.4	E962.0	E980.4
Dantrolene	975.2	E858.6	E945.2	E950.4	E962.0	E980.4
Daphne (gnidium) (mezereum)	988.2	E865.4	—	E950.9	E962.1	E980.9
berry	988.2	E865.3	—	E950.9	E962.1	E980.9
Dapsone	961.8	E857	E931.8	E950.4	E962.0	E980.4
Daraprim	961.4	E857	E931.4	E950.4	E962.0	E980.4
Darnel	988.2	E865.3	—	E950.9	E962.1	E980.9
Darvon	965.8	E850.8	E935.8	E950.0	E962.0	E980.0
Daunorubicin	960.7	E856	E930.7	E950.4	E962.0	E980.4
DBI	962.3	E858.0	E932.3	E950.4	E962.0	E980.4
D-Con (rodenticide)	989.4	E863.7	—	E950.6	E962.1	E980.7
DDS	961.8	E857	E931.8	E950.4	E962.0	E980.4
DDT	989.2	E863.0	—	E950.6	E962.1	E980.7
Deadly nightshade	988.2	E865.4	—	E950.9	E962.1	E980.9
berry	988.2	E865.3	—	E950.9	E962.1	E980.9
Deanol	969.7	E854.2	E939.7	E950.3	E962.0	E980.3
Debrisoquine	972.6	E858.3	E942.6	E950.4	E962.0	E980.4
Decaborane	989.8	E866.8	—	E950.9	E962.1	E980.9
fumes	987.8	E869.8	—	E952.8	E962.2	E982.8
Decadron	962.0	E858.0	E932.0	E950.4	E962.0	E980.4
ENT agent	976.6	E858.7	E946.6	E950.4	E962.0	E980.4
ophthalmic preparation	976.5	E858.7	E946.5	E950.4	E962.0	E980.4
topical NEC	976.0	E858.7	E946.0	E950.4	E962.0	E980.4
Decahydronaphthalene	982.0	E862.4	—	E950.9	E962.1	E980.9
Decalin	982.0	E862.4	—	E950.9	E962.1	E980.9
Decamethonium	975.2	E858.6	E945.2	E950.4	E962.0	E980.4
Decholin	973.4	E858.4	E943.4	E950.4	E962.0	E980.4
sodium (diagnostic)	977.8	E858.8	E947.8	E950.4	E962.0	E980.4
Declomycin	960.4	E856	E930.4	E950.4	E962.0	E980.4
Deferoxamine	963.8	E858.1	E933.8	E950.4	E962.0	E980.4
Dehydrocholic acid	973.4	E858.4	E943.4	E950.4	E962.0	E980.4
DeKalin	982.0	E862.4	—	E950.9	E962.1	E980.9
Delalutin	962.2	E858.0	E932.2	E950.4	E962.0	E980.4
Delphinium	988.2	E865.3	—	E950.9	E962.1	E980.9
Deltasone	962.0	E858.0	E932.0	E950.4	E962.0	E980.4
Deltra	962.0	E858.0	E932.0	E950.4	E962.0	E980.4
Delvinal	967.0	E851	E937.0	E950.1	E962.0	E980.1
Demecarium (bromide)	971.0	E855.3	E941.0	E950.4	E962.0	E980.4
Demeclocycline	960.4	E856	E930.4	E950.4	E962.0	E980.4
Demecolcine	963.1	E858.1	E933.1	E950.4	E962.0	E980.4
Demelanizing agents	976.8	E858.7	E946.8	E950.4	E962.0	E980.4
Demerol	965.09	E850.2	E935.2	E950.0	E962.0	E980.0
Demethylchlortetracycline	960.4	E856	E930.4	E950.4	E962.0	E980.4
Demethyltetracycline	960.4	E856	E930.4	E950.4	E962.0	E980.4
Demeton	989.3	E863.1	—	E950.6	E962.1	E980.7
Demulcents	976.3	E858.7	E946.3	E950.4	E962.0	E980.4
Demulen	962.2	E858.0	E932.2	E950.4	E962.0	E980.4
Denatured alcohol	980.0	E860.1	—	E950.9	E962.1	E980.9
Dendrid	976.5	E858.7	E946.5	E950.4	E962.0	E980.4
Dental agents, topical	976.7	E858.7	E946.7	E950.4	E962.0	E980.4
Deodorant spray (feminine hygiene)	976.8	E858.7	E946.8	E950.4	E962.0	E980.4
Deoxyribonuclease	963.4	E858.1	E933.4	E950.4	E962.0	E980.4
Depressants						
appetite, central	977.0	E858.8	E947.0	E950.4	E962.0	E980.4
cardiac	972.0	E858.3	E942.0	E950.4	E962.0	E980.4
central nervous system (anesthetic)	968.4	E855.1	E938.4	E950.4	E962.0	E980.4
psychotherapeutic	969.5	E853.9	E939.5	E950.3	E962.0	E980.3
Dequalinium	976.0	E858.7	E946.0	E950.4	E962.0	E980.4
Dermolate	976.2	E858.7	E946.2	E950.4	E962.0	E980.4
DES	962.2	E858.0	E932.2	E950.4	E962.0	E980.4
Desenex	976.0	E858.7	E946.0	E950.4	E962.0	E980.4
Deserpidine	972.6	E858.3	E942.6	E950.4	E962.0	E980.4

TABLE OF DRUGS AND CHEMICALS

Substance	Poisoning	Accident	Therapeutic-Use	Suicide Attempt	Assault	Undetermined
Desipramine	969.0	E854.0	E939.0	E950.3	E962.0	E980.3
Deslanoside	972.1	E858.3	E942.1	E950.4	E962.0	E980.4
Desocodeine	965.09	E850.2	E935.2	E950.0	E962.0	E980.0
Desomorphine	965.09	E850.2	E935.2	E950.0	E962.0	E980.0
Desonide	976.0	E858.7	E946.0	E950.4	E962.0	E980.4
Desoxycorticosterone derivatives	962.0	E858.0	E932.0	E950.4	E962.0	E980.4
Desoxyephedrine	969.7	E854.2	E939.7	E950.3	E962.0	E980.3
DET	969.6	E854.1	E939.6	E950.3	E962.0	E980.3
Detergents (ingested) (synthetic)	989.6	E861.0	—	E950.9	E962.1	E980.9
external medication	976.2	E858.7	E946.2	E950.4	E962.0	E980.4
Deterrent, alcohol	977.3	E858.8	E947.3	E950.4	E962.0	E980.4
Detrothyronine	962.7	E858.0	E932.7	E950.4	E962.0	E980.4
Dettol (external medication)	976.0	E858.7	E946.0	E950.4	E962.0	E980.4
Dexamethasone	962.0	E858.0	E932.0	E950.4	E962.0	E980.4
ENT agent	976.6	E858.7	E946.6	E950.4	E962.0	E980.4
ophthalmic preparation	976.5	E858.7	E946.5	E950.4	E962.0	E980.4
topical NEC	976.0	E858.7	E946.0	E950.4	E962.0	E980.4
Dexamphetamine	969.7	E854.2	E939.7	E950.3	E962.0	E980.3
Dexedrine	969.7	E854.2	E939.7	E950.3	E962.0	E980.3
Dexpanthenol	963.5	E858.1	E933.5	E950.4	E962.0	E980.4
Dextran	964.8	E858.2	E934.8	E950.4	E962.0	E980.4
Dextriferron	964.0	E858.2	E934.0	E950.4	E962.0	E980.4
Dextroamphetamine	969.7	E854.2	E939.7	E950.3	E962.0	E980.3
Dextro calcium pantothenate	963.5	E858.1	E933.5	E590.4	E962.0	E980.4
Dextromethorphan	975.4	E858.6	E945.4	E950.4	E962.0	E980.4
Dextromoramide	965.09	E850.2	E935.2	E950.0	E962.0	E980.0
Dextro pantothenyl alcohol	963.5	E858.1	E933.5	E950.4	E962.0	E980.4
topical	976.8	E858.7	E946.8	E950.4	E962.0	E980.4
Dextropropoxyphene (hydrochloride)	965.8	E850.8	E935.8	E950.0	E962.0	E980.0
Dextrorphan	965.09	E850.2	E935.2	E950.0	E962.0	E980.0
Dextrose NEC	974.5	E858.5	E944.5	E950.4	E962.0	E980.4
Dextrothyroxin	962.7	E858.0	E932.7	E950.4	E962.0	E980.4
DFP	971.0	E855.3	E941.0	E950.4	E962.0	E980.4
DHE-45	972.9	E858.3	E942.9	E950.4	E962.0	E980.4
Diabinese	962.3	E858.0	E932.3	E950.4	E962.0	E980.4
Diacetyl monoxime	977.2	E858.8	E947.2	E950.4	E962.0	E980.4
Diacetylmorphine	965.01	E850.0	E935.0	E950.0	E962.0	E980.0
Diagnostic agents	977.8	E858.8	E947.8	E950.4	E962.0	E980.4
Dial (soap)	976.2	E858.7	E946.2	E950.4	E962.0	E980.4
sedative	967.0	E851	E937.0	E950.1	E962.0	E980.1
Diallylbarbituric acid	967.0	E851	E937.0	E950.1	E962.0	E980.1
Diaminodiphenylsulfone	961.8	E857	E931.8	E950.4	E962.0	E980.4
Diamorphine	965.01	E850.0	E935.0	E950.0	E962.0	E980.0
Diamox	974.2	E858.5	E944.2	E950.4	E962.0	E980.4
Diamthazole	976.0	E858.7	E946.0	E950.4	E962.0	E980.4
Diaphenylsulfone	961.8	E857	E931.8	E950.4	E962.0	E980.4
Diasone (sodium)	961.8	E857	E931.8	E950.4	E962.0	E980.4
Diazepam	969.4	E853.2	E939.4	E950.3	E962.0	E980.3
Diazinon	989.3	E863.1	—	E950.6	E962.1	E980.7
Diazomethane (gas)	987.8	E869.8	—	E952.8	E962.2	E982.8
Diazoxide	972.5	E858.3	E942.5	E950.4	E962.0	E980.4
Dibenamine	971.3	E855.6	E941.3	E950.4	E962.0	E980.4
Dibenzheptropine	963.0	E858.1	E933	E950.4	E962.0	E980.4
Dibenzyline	971.3	E855.6	E941.3	E950.4	E962.0	E980.4
Diborane (gas)	987.8	E869.8	—	E952.8	E962.2	E982.8
Dibromomannitol	963.1	E858.1	E933.1	E950.4	E962.0	E980.4
Dibucaine (spinal)	968.7	E855.2	E938.7	E950.4	E962.0	E980.4
topical (surface)	968.5	E855.2	E938.5	E950.4	E962.0	E980.4
Dibunate sodium	975.4	E858.6	E945.4	E950.4	E962.0	E980.4
Dibutoline	971.1	E855.4	E941.1	E950.4	E962.0	E980.4
Dicapthon	989.4	E863.4	—	E950.6	E962.1	E980.7
Dichloralphenazone	967.1	E852.0	E937.1	E950.2	E962.0	E980.2
Dichlorodifluoromethane	987.4	E869.2	—	E952.8	E962.2	E982.8
Dichloroethane	982.3	E862.4	—	E950.9	E962.1	E980.9
Dichloroethylene	982.3	E862.4	—	E950.9	E962.1	E980.9
Dichloroethyl sulfide	987.8	E869.8	—	E952.8	E962.2	E982.8
Dichlorohydrin	982.3	E862.4	—	E950.9	E962.1	E980.9
Dichloromethane (solvent) (vapor)	982.3	E862.4	—	E950.9	E962.1	E980.9
Dichlorophen(e)	961.6	E857	E931.6	E950.4	E962.0	E980.4
Dichlorphenamide	974.2	E858.5	E944.2	E950.4	E962.0	E980.4
Dichlorvos	989.3	E863.1	—	E950.6	E962.1	E980.7
Dicoumarin, dicumarol	964.2	E858.2	E934.2	E950.4	E962.0	E980.4
Dicyanogen (gas)	987.8	E869.8	—	E952.8	E962.2	E982.8
Dicyclomine	971.1	E855.4	E941.1	E950.4	E962.0	E980.4
Dieldrin (vapor)	989.2	E863.0	—	E950.6	E962.1	E980.7
Dienestrol	962.2	E858.0	E932.2	E950.4	E962.0	E980.4

TABLE OF DRUGS AND CHEMICALS

Substance	Poisoning	Accident	Therapeutic-Use	Suicide Attempt	Assault	Undetermined
Dietetics	977.0	E858.8	E947.0	E950.4	E962.0	E980.4
Diethazine	966.4	E855.0	E936.4	E950.4	E962.0	E980.4
Diethyl						
barbituric acid	967.0	E851	E937.0	E950.1	E962.0	E980.1
carbamazine	961.6	E857	E931.6	E950.4	E962.0	E980.4
carbinol	980.8	E860.8	—	E950.9	E962.1	E980.9
carbonate	982.8	E862.4	—	E950.9	E962.1	E980.9
ether (vapor) — see Ether(s)						
propion	977.0	E858.8	E947.0	E950.4	E962.0	E980.4
stilbestrol	962.2	E858.0	E932.2	E950.4	E962.0	E980.4
Diethylene						
dioxide	982.8	E862.4	—	E950.9	E962.1	E980.9
glycol (monoacetate) (monoethyl ether)	982.8	E862.4	—	E950.9	E962.1	E980.9
Diethylsulfone-diethylmethane	967.8	E852.8	E937.8	E950.2	E962.0	E980.2
Difencloxazine	965.09	E850.2	E935.2	E950.0	E962.0	E980.0
Diffusin	963.4	E858.1	E933.4	E950.4	E962.0	E980.4
Diflos	971.0	E855.3	E941.0	E950.4	E962.0	E980.4
Digestants	973.4	E858.4	E943.4	E950.4	E962.0	E980.4
Digitalin(e)	972.1	E858.3	E942.1	E950.4	E962.0	E980.4
Digitalis glycosides	972.1	E858.3	E942.1	E950.4	E962.0	E980.4
Digitoxin	972.1	E858.3	E942.1	E950.4	E962.0	E980.4
Digoxin	972.1	E858.3	E942.1	E950.4	E962.0	E980.4
Dihydrocodeine	965.09	E850.2	E935.2	E950.0	E962.0	E980.0
Dihydrocodeinone	965.09	E850.2	E935.2	E950.0	E962.0	E980.0
Dihydroergocristine	972.9	E858.3	E942.9	E950.4	E962.0	E980.4
Dihydroergotamine	972.9	E858.3	E942.9	E950.4	E962.0	E980.4
Dihydroergotoxine	972.9	E858.3	E942.9	E950.4	E962.0	E980.4
Dihydrohydroxycodeinone	965.09	E850.2	E935.2	E950.0	E962.0	E980.0
Dihydrohydroxymorphinone	965.09	E850.2	E935.2	E950.0	E962.0	E980.0
Dihydroisocodeine	965.09	E850.2	E935.2	E950.0	E962.0	E980.0
Dihydromorphine	965.09	E850.2	E935.2	E950.0	E962.0	E980.0
Dihydromorphinone	965.09	E850.2	E935.2	E950.0	E962.0	E980.0
Dihydrostreptomycin	960.6	E856	E930.6	E950.4	E962.0	E980.4
Dihydrotachysterol	962.6	E858.0	E932.6	E950.4	E962.0	E980.4
Dihydroxyanthraquinone	973.1	E858.4	E943.1	E950.4	E962.0	E980.4
Dihydroxycodeinone	965.09	E850.2	E935.2	E950.0	E962.0	E980.0
Diiodohydroxyquin	961.3	E857	E931.3	E950.4	E962.0	E980.4
topical	976.0	E858.7	E946.0	E950.4	E962.0	E980.4
Diiodohydroxyquinoline	961.3	E857	E931.3	E950.4	E962.0	E980.4
Dilantin	966.1	E855.0	E936.1	E950.4	E962.0	E980.4
Dilaudid	965.09	E850.2	E935.2	E950.0	E962.0	E980.0
Diloxanide	961.5	E857	E931.5	E950.4	E962.0	E980.4
Dimefline	970.0	E854.3	E940.0	E950.4	E962.0	E980.4
Dimenhydrinate	963.0	E858.1	E933.0	E950.4	E962.0	E980.4
Dimercaprol	963.8	E858.1	E933.8	E950.4	E962.0	E980.4
Dimercaptopropanol	963.8	E858.1	E933.8	E950.4	E962.0	E980.4
Dimetane	963.0	E858.1	E933.0	E950.4	E962.0	E980.4
Dimethicone	976.3	E858.7	E946.3	E950.4	E962.0	E980.4
Dimethindene	963.0	E858.1	E933.0	E950.4	E962.0	E980.4
Dimethisoquin	968.5	E855.2	E938.5	E950.4	E962.0	E980.4
Dimethisterone	962.2	E858.0	E932.2	E950.4	E962.0	E980.4
Dimethoxanate	975.4	E858.6	E945.4	E950.4	E962.0	E980.4
Dimethyl						
arsine, arsinic acid — see Arsenic						
carbinol	980.2	E860.3	—	E950.9	E962.1	E980.9
diguanide	962.3	E858.0	E932.3	E950.4	E962.0	E980.4
ketone	982.8	E862.4	—	E950.9	E962.1	E980.9
vapor	987.8	E869.8	—	E952.8	E962.2	E982.8
meperidine	965.09	E850.2	E935.2	E950.0	E962.0	E980.0
parathion	989.3	E863.1	—	E950.6	E962.1	E980.7
polysiloxane	973.8	E858.4	E943.8	E950.4	E962.0	E980.4
sulfate (fumes)	987.8	E869.8	—	E952.8	E962.2	E982.8
liquid	983.9	E864.3	—	E950.7	E962.1	E980.6
sulfoxide NEC	982.8	E862.4	—	E950.9	E962.1	E980.9
medicinal	976.4	E858.7	E946.4	E950.4	E962.0	E980.4
triptamine	969.6	E854.1	E939.6	E950.4	E962.0	E980.3
tubocurarine	975.2	E858.6	E945.2	E950.4	E962.0	E980.4
Dindevan	964.2	E858.2	E934.2	E950.4	E962.0	E980.4
Dinitro (-ortho-) cresol (herbicide) (spray)	989.4	E863.5	—	E950.6	E962.1	E980.7
insecticide	989.4	E863.4	—	E950.6	E962.1	E980.7
Dinitrobenzene	983.0	E864.0	—	E950.7	E962.1	E980.6
vapor	987.8	E869.8	—	E952.8	E962.2	E982.8
Dinitro-orthocresol (herbicide)	989.4	E863.5	—	E950.6	E962.1	E980.7
insecticide	989.4	E863.4	—	E950.6	E962.1	E980.7
Dinitrophenol (herbicide) (spray)	989.4	E863.5	—	E950.6	E962.1	E980.7
insecticide	989.4	E863.4	—	E950.6	E962.1	E980.7

Substance	Poisoning	Accident	Therapeutic-Use	Suicide Attempt	Assualt	Undetermined
Dinoprost	975.0	E858.6	E945.0	E950.4	E962.0	E980.4
Dioctyl sulfosuccinate (calcium) (sodium)	973.2	E858.4	E943.2	E950.4	E962.0	E980.4
Diodoquin	961.3	E857	E931.3	E950.4	E962.0	E980.4
Dione derivatives NEC	966.3	E855.0	E936.3	E950.4	E962.0	E980.4
Dionin	965.09	E850.2	E935.2	E950.0	E962.0	E980.0
Dioxane	982.8	E862.4	—	E950.9	E962.1	E980.9
Dioxyline	972.5	E858.3	E942.5	E950.4	E962.0	E980.4
Dipentene	982.8	E862.4	—	E950.9	E962.1	E980.9
Diphemanil	971.1	E855.4	E941.1	E950.4	E962.0	E980.4
Diphenadione	964.2	E858.2	E934.2	E950.4	E962.0	E980.4
Diphenhydramine	963.0	E858.1	E933.0	E950.4	E962.0	E980.4
Diphenidol	963.0	E858.1	E933.0	E950.4	E962.0	E980.4
Diphenoxylate	973.5	E858.4	E943.5	E950.4	E962.0	E980.4
Diphenylchloroarsine	985.1	E866.3	—	E950.8	E962.1	E980.8
Diphenylhydantoin (sodium)	966.1	E855.0	E936.1	E950.4	E962.0	E980.4
Diphenylpyraline	963.0	E858.1	E933.0	E950.4	E962.0	E980.4
Diphtheria						
antitoxin	979.9	E858.8	E949.9	E950.4	E962.0	E980.4
toxoid	978.5	E858.8	E948.5	E950.4	E962.0	E980.4
with tetanus toxoid	978.9	E858.8	E948.9	E950.4	E962.0	E980.4
with pertussis component	978.6	E858.8	E948.6	E950.4	E962.0	E980.4
vaccine	978.5	E858.8	E948.5	E950.4	E962.0	E980.4
Dipipanone	965.09	E850.2	E935.2	E950.0	E962.0	E980.0
Diplovax	979.5	E858.8	E949.5	E950.4	E962.0	E980.4
Diprophylline	975.1	E858.6	E945.1	E950.4	E962.0	E980.4
Dipyridamole	972.4	E858.3	E942.4	E950.4	E962.0	E980.4
Dipyrone	965.5	E850.5	E935.5	E950.0	E962.0	E980.0
Diquat	989.4	E863.5	—	E950.6	E962.1	E980.7
Disinfectant NEC	983.9	E861.4	—	E950.7	E962.1	E980.6
alkaline	983.2	E861.4	—	E950.7	E962.1	E980.6
aromatic	983.0	E861.4	—	E950.7	E962.1	E980.6
Disipal	966.4	E855.0	E936.4	E950.4	E962.0	E980.4
Disodium edetate	963.8	E858.1	E933.8	E950.4	E962.0	E980.4
Disulfamide	974.4	E858.5	E944.4	E950.4	E962.0	E980.4
Disulfanilamide	961.0	E857	E931.0	E950.4	E962.0	E980.4
Disulfiram	977.3	E858.8	E947.3	E950.4	E962.0	E980.4
Dithiazanine	961.6	E857	E931.6	E950.4	E962.0	E980.4
Dithioglycerol	963.8	E858.1	E933.8	E950.4	E962.0	E980.4
Dithranol	976.4	E858.7	E946.4	E950.4	E962.0	E980.4
Diucardin	974.3	E858.5	E944.3	E950.4	E962.0	E980.4
Diupres	974.3	E858.5	E944.3	E950.4	E962.0	E980.4
Diuretics NEC	974.4	E858.5	E944.4	E950.4	E962.0	E980.4
carbonic acid anhydrase inhibitors	974.2	E858.5	E944.2	E950.4	E962.0	E980.4
mercurial	974.0	E858.5	E944.0	E950.4	E962.0	E980.4
osmotic	974.4	E858.5	E944.4	E950.4	E962.0	E980.4
purine derivatives	974.1	E858.5	E944.1	E950.4	E962.0	E980.4
saluretic	974.3	E858.5	E944.3	E950.4	E962.0	E980.4
Diuril	974.3	E858.5	E944.3	E950.4	E962.0	E980.4
Divinyl ether	968.2	E855.1	E938.2	E950.4	E962.0	E980.4
D-lysergic acid diethylamide	969.6	E854.1	E939.6	E950.3	E962.0	E980.3
DMCT	960.4	E856	E930.4	E950.4	E962.0	E980.4
DMSO	982.8	E862.4	—	E950.9	E962.1	E980.9
DMT	969.6	E854.1	E939.6	E950.3	E962.0	E980.3
DNOC	989.4	E863.5	—	E950.6	E962.1	E980.7
DOCA	962.0	E858.0	E932.0	E950.4	E962.0	E980.4
Dolophine	965.02	E850.1	E935.1	E950.0	E962.0	E980.0
Doloxene	965.8	E850.8	E935.8	E950.0	E962.0	E980.0
DOM	969.6	E854.1	E939.6	E950.3	E962.0	E980.3
Domestic gas — see Gas, utility						
Domiphen (bromide) (lozenges)	976.6	E858.7	E946.6	E950.4	E962.0	E980.4
Dopa (levo)	966.4	E855.0	E936.4	E950.4	E962.0	E980.4
Dopamine	971.2	E855.5	E941.2	E950.4	E962.0	E980.4
Doriden	967.5	E852.4	E937.5	E950.2	E962.0	E980.2
Dormiral	967.0	E851	E937.0	E950.1	E962.0	E980.1
Dormison	967.8	E852.8	E937.8	E950.2	E962.0	E980.2
Dornase	963.4	E858.1	E933.4	E950.4	E962.0	E980.4
Dorsacaine	968.5	E855.2	E938.5	E950.4	E962.0	E980.4
Doxapram	970.0	E854.3	E940.0	E950.4	E962.0	E980.4
Doxepin	969.0	E854.0	E939.0	E950.3	E962.0	E980.3
Doxorubicin	960.7	E856	E930.7	E950.4	E962.0	E980.4
Doxycycline	960.4	E856	E930.4	E950.4	E962.0	E980.4
Doxylamine	963.0	E858.1	E933.0	E950.4	E962.0	E980.4
Dramamine	963.0	E858.1	E933.0	E950.4	E962.0	E980.4
Drano (drain cleaner)	983.2	E864.2	—	E950.7	E962.1	E980.6
Dromoran	965.09	E850.2	E935.2	E950.0	E962.0	E980.0
Dromostanolone	962.1	E858.0	E932.1	E950.4	E962.0	E980.4

TABLE OF DRUGS AND CHEMICALS

Substance	Poisoning	Accident	Therapeutic Use	Suicide Attempt	Assault	Undetermined
Droperidol	969.2	E853.1	E939.2	E950.3	E962.0	E980.3
Drug	977.9	E858.9	E947.9	E950.5	E962.0	E980.5
specified NEC	977.8	E858.8	E947.8	E950.4	E962.0	E980.4
AHFS List						
4:00 antihistamine drugs	963.0	E858.1	E933.0	E950.4	E962.0	E980.4
8:04 amebacides	961.5	E857	E931.5	E950.4	E962.0	E980.4
arsenical anti-infectives	961.1	E857	E931.1	E950.4	E962.0	E980.4
quinoline derivatives	961.3	E857	E931.3	E950.4	E962.0	E980.4
8:08 anthelmintics	961.6	E857	E931.6	E950.4	E962.0	E980.4
quinoline derivatives	961.3	E857	E931.3	E950.4	E962.0	E980.4
8:12.04 antifungal antibiotics	960.1	E856	E930.1	E950.4	E962.0	E980.4
8:12.06 cephalosporins	960.5	E856	E930.5	E950.4	E962.0	E980.4
8:12.08 chloramphenicol	960.2	E856	E930.2	E950.4	E962.0	E980.4
8:12.12 erythromycins	960.3	E856	E930.3	E950.4	E962.0	E980.4
8:12.16 penicillins	960.0	E856	E930.0	E950.4	E962.0	E980.4
8:12.20 streptomycins	960.6	E856	E930.6	E950.4	E962.0	E980.4
8:12.24 tetracyclines	960.4	E856	E930.4	E950.4	E962.0	E980.4
8:12.28 other antibiotics	960.8	E856	E930.8	E950.4	E962.0	E980.4
antimycobacterial	960.6	E856	E930.6	E950.4	E962.0	E980.4
macrolides	960.3	E856	E930.3	E950.4	E962.0	E980.4
8:16 antituberculars	961.8	E857	E931.8	E950.4	E962.0	E980.4
antibiotics	960.6	E856	E930.6	E950.4	E962.0	E980.4
8:18 antivirals	961.7	E857	E931.7	E950.4	E962.0	E980.4
8:20 plasmodicides (antimalarials)	961.4	E857	E931.4	E950.4	E962.0	E980.4
8:24 sulfonamides	961.0	E857	E931.0	E950.4	E962.0	E980.4
8:26 sulfones	961.8	E857	E931.8	E950.4	E962.0	E980.4
8:28 treponemicides	961.2	E857	E931.2	E950.4	E962.0	E980.4
8:32 trichomonacides	961.5	E857	E931.5	E950.4	E962.0	E980.4
quinoline derivatives	961.3	E857	E931.3	E950.4	E962.0	E980.4
nitrofuran derivatives	961.9	E857	E931.9	E950.4	E962.0	E980.4
8:36 urinary germicides	961.9	E857	E931.9	E950.4	E962.0	E980.4
quinoline derivatives	961.3	E857	E931.3	E950.4	E962.0	E980.4
8:40 other anti-infectives	961.9	E857	E931.9	E950.4	E962.0	E980.4
10:00 antineoplastic agents	963.1	E858.1	E933.1	E950.4	E962.0	E980.4
antibiotics	960.7	E856	E930.7	E950.4	E962.0	E980.4
progestogens	962.2	E858.0	E932.2	E950.4	E962.0	E980.4
12:04 parasympathomimetic (cholinergic) agents	971.0	E855.3	E941.0	E950.4	E962.0	E980.4
12:08 parasympatholytic (cholinergic-blocking) agents	971.1	E855.4	E941.1	E950.4	E962.0	E980.4
12:12 Sympathomimetic (adrenergic) agents	971.2	E855.5	E941.2	E950.4	E962.0	E980.4
12:16 sympatholytic (adrenergic-blocking) agents	971.3	E855.6	E941.3	E950.4	E962.0	E980.4
12:20 skeletal muscle relaxants						
central nervous system muscletone depressants	968.0	E855.1	E938.0	E950.4	E962.0	E980.4
myoneural blocking agents	975.2	E858.6	E945.2	E950.4	E962.0	E980.4
16:00 blood derivatives	964.7	E858.2	E934.7	E950.4	E962.0	E980.4
20:04 antianemia drugs	964.1	E858.2	E934.1	E950.4	E962.0	E980.4
20:04.04 iron preparations	964.0	E858.2	E934.0	E950.4	E962.0	E980.4
20:04.08 liver and stomach preparations	964.1	E858.2	E934.1	E950.4	E962.0	E980.4
20:12.04 anticoagulants	964.2	E858.2	E934.2	E950.4	E962.0	E980.4
20:12.08 antiheparin agents	964.5	E858.2	E934.5	E950.4	E962.0	E980.4
20:12.12 coagulants	964.5	E858.2	E934.5	E950.4	E962.0	E980.4
20:12.16 hemostatics NEC	964.5	E858.2	E934.5	E950.4	E962.0	E980.4
capillary active drugs	972.8	E858.3	E942.8	E950.4	E962.0	E980.4
24:04 cardiac drugs	972.9	E858.3	E942.9	E950.4	E962.0	E980.4
cardiotonic agents	972.1	E858.3	E942.1	E950.4	E962.0	E980.4
rhythm regulators	972.0	E858.3	E942.0	E950.4	E962.0	E980.4
24:06 antilipemic agents	972.2	E858.3	E942.2	E950.4	E962.0	E980.4
thyroid derivatives	962.7	E858.0	E932.7	E950.4	E962.0	E980.4
24:08 hypotensive agents	972.6	E858.3	E942.6	E950.4	E962.0	E980.4
adrenergic blocking agents	971.3	E855.6	E941.3	E950.4	E962.0	E980.4
ganglion blocking agents	972.3	E858.3	E942.3	E950.4	E962.0	E980.4
vasodilators	972.5	E858.3	E942.5	E950.4	E962.0	E980.4
24:12 vasodilating agents NEC	972.5	E858.3	E942.5	E950.4	E962.0	E980.4
coronary	972.4	E858.3	E942.4	E950.4	E962.0	E980.4
nicotinic acid derivatives	972.2	E858.3	E942.2	E950.4	E962.0	E980.4
24:16 sclerosing agents	972.7	E858.3	E942.7	E950.4	E962.0	E980.4
28:04 general anesthetics	968.4	E855.1	E938.4	E950.4	E962.0	E980.4
gaseous anesthetics	968.2	E855.1	E938.2	E950.4	E962.0	E980.4
halothane	968.1	E855.1	E938.1	E950.4	E962.0	E980.4
intravenous anesthetics	968.3	E855.1	E938.3	E950.4	E962.0	E980.4
28:08 analgesics and antipyretics	965.9	E850.9	E935.9	E950.0	E962.0	E980.0
antirheumatics	965.6	E850.6	E935.6	E950.0	E962.0	E980.0
aromatic analgesics	965.4	E850.4	E935.4	E950.0	E962.0	E980.0
non-narcotic NEC	965.7	E850.7	E935.7	E950.0	E962.0	E980.0
opium alkaloids	965.00	E850.2	E935.2	E950.0	E962.0	E980.0
heroin	965.01	E850.0	E935.0	E950.0	E962.0	E980.0
methadone	965.02	E850.1	E935.1	E950.0	E962.0	E980.0

TABLE OF DRUGS AND CHEMICALS

Substance	Poisoning	Accident	Therapeutic-Use	Suicide Attempt	Assault	Undetermined
Drug—*continued*						
28:08 analgesics and antipyretics—*continued*						
opium alkaloids—*continued*						
specified type NEC	965.09	E850.2	E935.2	E950.0	E962.0	E980.0
pyrazole derivatives	965.5	E850.5	E935.5	E950.0	E962.0	E980.0
salicylates	965.1	E850.3	E935.3	E950.0	E962.0	E980.0
specified NEC	965.8	E850.8	E935.8	E950.0	E962.0	E980.0
28:10 narcotic antagonists	970.1	E854.3	E940.1	E950.4	E962.0	E980.4
28:12 anticonvulsants	966.3	E855.0	E936.3	E950.4	E962.0	E980.4
barbiturates	967.0	E851	E937.0	E950.1	E962.0	E980.1
benzodiazepine-based tranquilizers	969.4	E853.4	E939.4	E950.3	E962.0	E980.3
bromides	967.3	E852.2	E937.3	E950.2	E962.0	E980.2
hydantoin derivatives	966.1	E855.0	E936.1	E950.4	E962.0	E980.4
oxazolidine (derivatives)	966.0	E855.0	E936.0	E950.4	E962.0	E980.4
succinimides	966.2	E855.0	E936.2	E950.4	E962.0	E980.4
28:16.04 antidepressants	969.0	E854.0	E939.0	E950.3	E962.0	E980.3
28:16.08 tranquilizers	969.5	E853.9	E939.5	E950.3	E962.0	E980.3
benzodiazepine-based	969.4	E853.2	E939.4	E950.3	E962.0	E980.3
butyrophenone-based	969.2	E853.1	E939.2	E950.3	E962.0	E980.3
major NEC	969.3	E853.8	E939.3	E950.3	E962.0	E980.3
phenothiazine-based	969.1	E853.0	E939.1	E950.3	E962.0	E980.3
28:16.12 other psychotherapeutic agents	969.8	E855.8	E939.8	E950.3	E962.0	E980.3
28:20 respiratory and cerebral stimulants	970.9	E854.3	E940.9	E950.4	E962.0	E980.4
analeptics	970.0	E854.3	E940.0	E950.4	E962.0	E980.4
anorexigenic agents	977.0	E858.8	E947.0	E950.4	E962.0	E980.4
psychostimulants	969.7	E854.2	E939.7	E950.3	E962.0	E980.3
specified NEC	970.8	E854.3	E940.8	E950.4	E962.0	E980.4
28:24 sedatives and hypnotics	967.9	E852.9	E937.9	E950.2	E962.0	E980.2
barbiturates	967.0	E851	E937.0	E950.1	E962.0	E980.1
benzodiazepine-based tranquilizers	969.4	E853.2	E939.4	E950.3	E962.0	E980.3
chloral hydrate (group)	967.1	E852.0	E937.1	E950.2	E962.0	E980.2
glutethamide group	967.5	E852.4	E937.5	E950.2	E962.0	E980.2
intravenous anesthetics	968.3	E855.1	E938.3	E950.4	E962.0	E980.4
methaqualone (compounds)	967.4	E852.3	E937.4	E950.2	E962.0	E980.2
paraldehyde	967.2	E852.1	E937.2	E950.2	E962.0	E980.2
phenothiazine-based tranquilizers	969.1	E853.0	E939.1	E950.3	E962.0	E980.3
specified NEC	967.8	E852.8	E937.8	E950.2	E962.0	E980.2
thiobarbiturates	968.3	E855.1	E938.3	E950.4	E962.0	E980.4
tranquilizer NEC	969.5	E853.9	E939.5	E950.3	E962.0	E980.3
36:04 to 36:88 diagnostic agents	977.8	E858.8	E947.8	E950.4	E962.0	E980.4
40:00 electrolyte, caloric, and water balance agents NEC	974.5	E858.5	E944.5	E950.4	E962.0	E980.4
40:04 acidifying agents	963.2	E858.1	E933.2	E950.4	E962.0	E980.4
40:08 alkalinizing agents	963.3	E858.1	E933.3	E950.4	E962.0	E980.4
40:10 ammonia detoxicants	974.5	E858.5	E944.5	E950.4	E962.0	E980.4
40:12 replacement solutions	974.5	E858.5	E944.5	E950.4	E962.0	E980.4
plasma expanders	964.8	E858.2	E934.8	E950.4	E962.0	E980.4
40:16 sodium-removing resins	974.5	E858.5	E944.5	E950.4	E962.0	E980.4
40:18 potassium-removing resins	974.5	E858.5	E944.5	E950.4	E962.0	E980.4
40:20 caloric agents	974.5	E858.5	E944.5	E950.4	E962.0	E980.4
40:24 salt and sugar substitutes	974.5	E858.5	E944.5	E950.4	E962.0	E980.4
40:28 diuretics NEC	974.4	E858.5	E944.4	E950.4	E962.0	E980.4
carbonic acid anhydrase inhibitors	974.2	E858.5	E944.2	E950.4	E962.0	E980.4
mercurials	974.0	E858.5	E944.0	E950.4	E962.0	E980.4
purine derivatives	974.1	E858.5	E944.1	E950.4	E962.0	E980.4
saluretics	974.3	E858.5	E944.3	E950.4	E962.0	E980.4
thiazides	974.3	E858.5	E944.3	E950.4	E962.0	E980.4
40:36 irrigating solutions	974.5	E858.5	E944.5	E950.4	E962.0	E980.4
40:40 uricosuric agents	974.7	E858.5	E944.7	E950.4	E962.0	E980.4
44:00 enzymes	963.4	E858.1	E933.4	E950.4	E962.0	E980.4
fibrinolysis-affecting agents	964.4	E858.2	E934.4	E950.4	E962.0	E980.4
gastric agents	973.4	E858.4	E943.4	E950.4	E962.0	E980.4
48:00 expectorants and cough preparations						
antihistamine agents	963.0	E858.1	E933.0	E950.4	E962.0	E980.4
antitussives	975.4	E858.6	E945.4	E950.4	E962.0	E980.4
codeine derivatives	965.09	E850.2	E935.2	E950.0	E962.0	E980.0
expectorants	975.5	E858.6	E945.5	E950.4	E962.0	E980.4
narcotic agents NEC	965.09	E850.2	E935.2	E950.0	E962.0	E980.0
52:04 anti-infectives (EENT)						
ENT agent	976.6	E858.7	E946.6	E950.4	E962.0	E980.4
ophthalmic preparation	976.5	E858.7	E946.5	E950.4	E962.0	E980.4
52:04.04 antibiotics (EENT)						
ENT agent	976.6	E858.7	E946.6	E950.4	E962.0	E980.4
ophthalmic preparation	976.5	E858.7	E946.5	E950.4	E962.0	E980.4
52:04.06 antivirals (EENT)						
ENT agent	976.6	E858.7	E946.6	E950.4	E962.0	E980.4
ophthalmic preparation	976.5	E858.7	E946.5	E950.4	E962.0	E980.4

TABLE OF DRUGS AND CHEMICALS

Substance	Poisoning	Accident	Therapeutic-Use	Suicide Attempt	Assault	Undetermined
Drug—continued						
52:04.08 sulfonamides (EENT)						
ENT agent	976.6	E858.7	E946.6	E950.4	E962.0	E980.4
ophthalmic preparation	976.5	E858.7	E946.5	E950.4	E962.0	E980.4
52:04.12 miscellaneous anti-infectives (EENT)						
ENT agent	976.6	E858.7	E946.6	E950.4	E962.0	E980.4
ophthalmic preparation	976.5	E858.7	E946.5	E950.4	E962.0	E980.4
52:08 anti-inflammatory agents (EENT)						
ENT agent	976.6	E858.7	E946.6	E950.4	E962.0	E980.4
ophthalmic preparation	976.5	E858.7	E946.5	E950.4	E962.0	E980.4
52:10 carbonic anhydrase inhibitors	974.2	E858.5	E944.2	E950.4	E962.0	E980.4
52:12 contact lens solutions	976.5	E858.7	E946.5	E950.4	E962.0	E980.4
52:16 local anesthetics (EENT)	968.5	E855.2	E938.5	E950.4	E962.0	E980.4
52:20 miotics	971.0	E855.3	E941.0	E950.4	E962.0	E980.4
52:24 mydriatics						
adrenergics	971.2	E855.5	E941.2	E950.4	E962.0	E980.4
anticholinergics	971.1	E855.4	E941.1	E950.4	E962.0	E980.4
antimuscarinics	971.1	E855.4	E941.1	E950.4	E962.0	E980.4
parasympatholytics	971.1	E855.4	E941.1	E950.4	E962.0	E980.4
spasmolytics	971.1	E855.4	E941.1	E950.4	E962.0	E980.4
sympathomimetics	971.2	E855.5	E941.2	E950.4	E962.0	E980.4
52:28 mouth washes and gargles	976.6	E858.7	E946.6	E950.4	E962.0	E980.4
52:32 vasoconstrictors (ENT)	971.2	E855.5	E941.2	E950.4	E962.0	E980.4
52:36 unclassified agents (EENT)						
ENT agent	976.6	E858.7	E946.6	E950.4	E962.0	E980.4
ophthalmic preparation	976.5	E858.7	E946.5	E950.4	E962.0	E980.4
56:04 antacids and adsorbents	973.0	E858.4	E943.0	E950.4	E962.0	E980.4
56:08 antidiarrhea agents	973.5	E858.4	E943.5	E950.4	E962.0	E980.4
56:10 antiflatulents	973.8	E858.4	E943.8	E950.4	E962.0	E980.4
56:12 cathartics NEC	973.3	E858.4	E943.3	E950.4	E962.0	E980.4
emollients	973.2	E858.4	E943.2	E950.4	E962.0	E980.4
irritants	973.1	E858.4	E943.1	E950.4	E962.0	E980.4
56:16 digestants	973.4	E858.4	E943.4	E950.4	E962.0	E980.4
56:20 emetics and antiemetics						
antiemetics	963.0	E858.1	E933.0	E950.4	E962.0	E980.4
emetics	973.6	E858.4	E943.6	E950.4	E962.0	E980.4
56:24 lipotropic agents	977.1	E858.8	E947.1	E950.4	E962.0	E980.4
56:40 miscellaneous G.I. drugs	973.8	E858.4	E943.8	E950.4	E962.0	E980.4
60:00 gold compounds	965.6	E850.6	E935.6	E950.0	E962.0	E980.0
64:00 heavy metal antagonists	963.8	E858.1	E933.8	E950.4	E962.0	E980.4
68:04 adrenals	962.0	E858.0	E932.0	E950.4	E962.0	E980.4
68:08 androgens	962.1	E858.0	E932.1	E950.4	E962.0	E980.4
68:12 contraceptives, oral	962.2	E858.0	E932.2	E950.4	E962.0	E980.4
68:16 estrogens	962.2	E858.0	E932.2	E950.4	E962.0	E980.4
68:18 gonadotropins	962.4	E858.0	E932.4	E950.4	E962.0	E980.4
68:20 insulins and antidiabetic agents	962.3	E858.0	E932.3	E950.4	E962.0	E980.4
68:20.08 insulins	962.3	E858.0	E932.3	E950.4	E962.0	E980.4
68:24 parathyroid	962.6	E858.0	E932.6	E950.4	E962.0	E980.4
68:28 pituitary (posterior)	962.5	E858.0	E932.5	E950.4	E962.0	E980.4
anterior	962.4	E858.0	E932.4	E950.4	E962.0	E980.4
68:32 progestogens	962.2	E858.0	E932.2	E950.4	E962.0	E980.4
68:34 other corpus luteum						
hormones NEC	962.2	E858.0	E932.2	E950.4	E962.0	E980.4
68:36 thyroid and antithyroid						
antithyroid	962.8	E858.0	E932.8	E950.4	E962.0	E980.4
thyroid (derivatives)	962.7	E858.0	E932.7	E950.4	E962.0	E980.4
72:00 local anesthetics NEC	968.9	E855.2	E938.9	E950.4	E962.0	E980.4
topical (surface)	968.5	E855.2	E938.5	E950.4	E962.0	E980.4
infiltration (intradermal) (subcutaneous) (submucosal)	968.5	E855.2	E938.5	E950.4	E962.0	E980.4
nerve blocking (peripheral) (plexus) (regional)	968.6	E855.2	E938.6	E950.4	E962.0	E980.4
spinal	968.7	E855.2	E938.7	E950.4	E962.0	E980.4
76:00 oxytocics	975.0	E858.6	E945.0	E950.4	E962.0	E980.4
78:00 radioactive agents	990	—	—	—	—	—
80:04 serums NEC	979.9	E858.8	E949.9	E950.4	E962.0	E980.4
immune gamma globulin (human)	964.6	E858.2	E934.6	E950.4	E962.0	E980.4
80:08 toxoids NEC	978.8	E858.8	E948.8	E950.4	E962.0	E980.4
diphtheria	978.5	E858.8	E948.5	E950.4	E962.0	E980.4
and tetanus	978.9	E858.8	E948.9	E950.4	E962.0	E980.4
with pertussis component	978.6	E858.8	E948.6	E950.4	E962.0	E980.4
tetanus	978.4	E858.8	E948.4	E950.4	E962.0	E980.4
and diphtheria	978.9	E858.8	E948.9	E950.4	E962.0	E980.4
with pertussis component	978.6	E858.8	E948.6	E950.4	E962.0	E980.4

TABLE OF DRUGS AND CHEMICALS

Substance	Poisoning	External Cause (E-Code)				
		Accident	Therapeutic-Use	Suicide Attempt	Assault	Undetermined
Drug—continued						
80:12 vaccines	979.9	E858.8	E949.9	E950.4	E962.0	E980.4
bacterial NEC	978.8	E858.8	E948.8	E950.4	E962.0	E980.4
with						
other bacterial components	978.9	E858.8	E948.9	E950.4	E962.0	E980.4
pertussis component	978.6	E858.8	E948.6	E950.4	E962.0	E980.4
viral and rickettsial components	979.7	E858.8	E949.7	E950.4	E962.0	E980.4
rickettsial NEC	979.6	E858.8	E949.6	E950.4	E962.0	E980.4
with						
bacterial component	979.7	E858.8	E949.7	E950.4	E962.0	E980.4
pertussis component	978.6	E858.8	E948.6	E950.4	E962.0	E980.4
viral component	979.7	E858.8	E949.7	E950.4	E962.0	E980.4
viral NEC	979.6	E858.8	E949.6	E950.4	E962.0	E980.4
with						
bacterial component	979.7	E858.8	E949.7	E950.4	E962.0	E980.4
pertussis component	978.6	E858.8	E948.6	E950.4	E962.0	E980.4
rickettsial component	979.7	E858.8	E949.7	E950.4	E962.0	E980.4
84:04.04 antibiotics (skin and mucous membrane)	976.0	E858.7	E946.0	E950.4	E962.0	E980.4
84:04.08 fungicides (skin and mucous membrane)	976.0	E858.7	E946.0	E950.4	E962.0	E980.4
84:04.12 scabicides and pediculicides (skin and mucous membrane)	976.0	E858.7	E946.0	E950.4	E962.0	E980.4
84:04.16 miscellaneous local anti-infectives (skin and mucous membrane)	976.0	E858.7	E946.0	E950.4	E962.0	E980.4
84:06 anti-inflammatory agents (skin and mucous membrane)	976.0	E858.7	E946.0	E950.4	E962.0	E980.4
84:08 antipruritics and local anesthetics						
antipruritics	976.1	E858.7	E946.1	E950.4	E962.0	E980.4
local anesthetics	968.5	E855.2	E938.5	E950.4	E962.0	E980.4
84:12 astringents	976.2	E858.7	E946.2	E950.4	E962.0	E980.4
84:16 cell stimulants and proliferants	976.8	E858.7	E946.8	E950.4	E962.0	E980.4
84:20 detergents	976.2	E858.7	E946.2	E950.4	E962.0	E980.4
84:24 emollients, demulcents, and protectants	976.3	E858.7	E946.3	E950.4	E962.0	E980.4
84:28 keratolytic agents	976.4	E858.7	E946.4	E950.4	E962.0	E980.4
84:32 keratoplastic agents	976.4	E858.7	E946.4	E950.4	E962.0	E980.4
84:36 miscellaneous agents (skin and mucous membrane)	976.8	E858.7	E946.8	E950.4	E962.0	E980.4
86:00 spasmolytic agents	975.1	E858.6	E945.1	E950.4	E962.0	E980.4
antiasthmatics	975.7	E858.6	E945.7	E950.4	E962.0	E980.4
papaverine	972.5	E858.3	E942.5	E950.4	E962.0	E980.4
theophylline	974.1	E858.5	E944.1	E950.4	E962.0	E980.4
88:04 vitamin A	963.5	E858.1	E933.5	E950.4	E962.0	E980.4
88:08 vitamin B complex	963.5	E858.1	E933.5	E950.4	E962.0	E980.4
hematopoietic vitamin	964.1	E858.2	E934.1	E950.4	E962.0	E980.4
nicotinic acid derivatives	972.2	E858.3	E942.2	E950.4	E962.0	E980.4
88:12 vitamin C	963.5	E858.1	E933.5	E950.4	E962.0	E980.4
88:16 vitamin D	963.5	E858.1	E933.5	E950.4	E962.0	E980.4
88:20 vitamin E	963.5	E858.1	E933.5	E950.4	E962.0	E980.4
88:24 vitamin K activity	964.3	E858.2	E934.3	E950.4	E962.0	E980.4
88:28 multivitamin preparations	963.5	E858.1	E933.5	E950.4	E962.0	E980.4
92:00 unclassified therapeutic agents	977.8	E858.8	E947.8	E950.4	E962.0	E980.4
Duboisine	971.1	E855.4	E941.1	E950.4	E962.0	E980.4
Dulcolax	973.1	E858.4	E943.1	E950.4	E962.0	E980.4
Duponol (C) (EP)	976.2	E858.7	E946.2	E950.4	E962.0	E980.4
Durabolin	962.1	E858.0	E932.1	E950.4	E962.0	E980.4
Dyclone	968.5	E855.2	E938.5	E950.4	E962.0	E980.4
Dyclonine	968.5	E855.2	E938.5	E950.4	E962.0	E980.4
Dydrogesterone	962.2	E858.0	E932.2	E950.4	E962.0	E980.4
Dyes NEC	989.8	E866.8	—	E950.9	E962.1	E980.9
diagnostic agents	977.8	E858.8	E947.8	E950.4	E962.0	E980.4
pharmaceutical NEC	977.4	E858.8	E947.4	E950.4	E962.0	E980.4
Dyfols	971.0	E855.3	E941.0	E950.4	E962.0	E980.4
Dymelor	962.3	E858.0	E932.3	E950.4	E962.0	E980.4
Dynamite	989.8	E866.8	—	E950.9	E962.1	E980.9
fumes	987.8	E869.8	—	E952.8	E962.2	E982.8
Dyphylline	975.1	E858.6	E945.1	E950.4	E962.0	E980.4
Ear preparations	976.6	E858.7	E946.6	E950.4	E962.0	E980.4
Echothiopate, ecothiopate	971.0	E855.3	E941.0	E950.4	E962.0	E980.4
Ectylurea	967.8	E852.8	E937.8	E950.2	E962.0	E980.2
Edathamil disodium	963.8	E858.1	E933.8	E950.4	E962.0	E980.4
Edecrin	974.4	E858.5	E944.4	E950.4	E962.0	E980.4
Edetate, disodium (calcium)	963.8	E858.1	E933.8	E950.4	E962.0	E980.4
Edrophonium	971.0	E855.3	E941.0	E950.4	E962.0	E980.4
Elase	976.8	E858.7	E946.8	E950.4	E962.0	E980.4
Elaterium	973.1	E858.4	E943.1	E950.4	E962.0	E980.4
Elder	988.2	E865.4	—	E950.9	E962.1	E980.9
berry (unripe)	988.2	E865.3	—	E950.9	E962.1	E980.9
Electrolytes NEC	974.5	E858.5	E944.5	E950.4	E962.0	E980.4
Electrolytic agent NEC	974.5	E858.5	E944.5	E950.4	E962.0	E980.4
Embramine	963.0	E858.1	E933.0	E950.4	E962.0	E980.4
Emetics	973.6	E858.4	E943.6	E950.4	E962.0	E980.4

TABLE OF DRUGS AND CHEMICALS

Substance	Poisoning	Accident	Therapeutic-Use	Suicide Attempt	Assault	Undetermined
Emetine (hydrochloride)	961.5	E857	E931.5	E950.4	E962.0	E980.4
Emollients	976.3	E858.7	E946.3	E950.4	E962.0	E980.4
Emylcamate	969.5	E853.8	E939.5	E950.3	E962.0	E980.3
Encyprate	969.0	E854.0	E939.0	E950.3	E962.0	E980.3
Endocaine	968.5	E855.2	E938.5	E950.4	E962.0	E980.4
Endrin	989.2	E863.0	—	E950.6	E962.1	E980.7
Enflurane	968.2	E855.1	E938.2	E950.4	E962.0	E980.4
Enovid	962.2	E858.0	E932.2	E950.4	E962.0	E980.4
ENT preparations (anti-infectives)	976.6	E858.7	E946.6	E950.4	E962.0	E980.4
Enzodase	963.4	E858.1	E933.4	E950.4	E962.0	E980.4
Enzymes NEC	963.4	E858.1	E933.4	E950.4	E962.0	E980.4
Epanutin	966.1	E855.0	E936.1	E950.4	E962.0	E980.4
Ephedra (tincture)	971.2	E855.5	E941.2	E950.4	E962.0	E980.4
Ephedrine	971.2	E855.5	E941.2	E950.4	E962.0	E980.4
Epiestriol	962.2	E858.0	E932.2	E950.4	E962.0	E980.4
Epinephrine	971.2	E855.5	E941.2	E950.4	E962.0	E980.4
Epsom sait	973.3	E858.4	E943.3	E950.4	E962.0	E980.4
Equanil	969.5	E853.8	E939.5	E950.3	E962.0	E980.3
Equisetum (diuretic)	974.4	E858.5	E944.4	E950.4	E962.0	E980.4
Ergometrine	975.0	E858.6	E945.0	E950.4	E962.0	E980.4
Ergonovine	975.0	E858.6	E945.0	E950.4	E962.0	E980.4
Ergot NEC	988.2	E865.4	—	E950.9	E962.1	E980.9
medicinal (alkaloids)	975.0	E858.6	E945.0	E950.4	E962.0	E980.4
Ergotamine (tartrate) (for migraine) NEC	972.9	E858.3	E942.9	E950.4	E962.0	E980.4
Ergotrate	975.0	E858.6	E945.0	E950.4	E962.0	E980.4
Erythrityl tetranitrate	972.4	E858.3	E942.4	E950.4	E962.0	E980.4
Erythrol tetranitrate	972.4	E858.3	E942.4	E950.4	E962.0	E980.4
Erythromycin	960.3	E856	E930.3	E950.4	E962.0	E980.4
ophthalmic preparation	976.5	E858.7	E946.5	E950.4	E962.0	E980.4
topical NEC	976.0	E858.7	E946.0	E950.4	E962.0	E980.4
Eserine	971.0	E855.3	E941.0	E950.4	E962.0	E980.4
Eskabarb	967.0	E851	E937.0	E950.1	E962.0	E980.1
Eskalith	969.8	E855.8	E939.8	E950.3	E962.0	E980.3
Estradiol (cypionate) (dipropionate) (valerate)	962.2	E858.0	E932.2	E950.4	E962.0	E980.4
Estriol	962.2	E858.0	E932.2	E950.4	E962.0	E980.4
Estrogens (with progestogens)	962.2	E858.0	E932.2	E950.4	E962.0	E980.4
Estrone	962.2	E858.0	E932.2	E950.4	E962.0	E980.4
Etafedrine	971.2	E855.5	E941.2	E950.4	E962.0	E980.4
Ethacrynate sodium	974.4	E858.5	E944.4	E950.4	E962.0	E980.4
Ethacrynic acid	974.4	E858.5	E944.4	E950.4	E962.0	E980.4
Ethambutol	961.8	E857	E931.8	E950.4	E962.0	E980.4
Ethamide	974.2	E858.5	E944.2	E950.4	E962.0	E980.4
Ethamivan	970.0	E854.3	E940.0	E950.4	E962.0	E980.4
Ethamsylate	964.5	E858.2	E934.5	E950.4	E962.0	E980.4
Ethanol	980.0	E860.1	—	E950.9	E962.1	E980.9
beverage	980.0	E860.0	—	E950.9	E962.1	E980.9
Ethchlorvynol	967.8	E852.8	E937.8	E950.2	E962.0	E980.2
Ethebenecid	974.7	E858.5	E944.7	E950.4	E962.0	E980.4
Ether(s) (diethyl) (ethyl) (vapor)	987.8	E869.8	—	E952.8	E962.2	E982.8
anesthetic	968.2	E855.1	E938.2	E950.4	E962.0	E980.4
petroleum — see Ligroin						
solvent	982.8	E862.4	—	E950.9	E962.1	E980.9
Ethidine chloride (vapor)	987.8	E869.8	—	E952.8	E962.2	E982.8
liquid (solvent)	982.3	E862.4	—	E950.9	E962.1	E980.9
Ethinamate	967.8	E852.8	E937.8	E950.2	E962.0	E980.2
Ethinylestradiol	962.2	E858.0	E932.2	E950.4	E962.0	E980.4
Ethionamide	961.8	E857	E931.8	E950.4	E962.0	E980.4
Ethisterone	962.2	E858.0	E932.2	E950.4	E962.0	E980.4
Ethobral	967.0	E851	E937.0	E950.1	E962.0	E980.1
Ethocaine (infiltration) (topical)	968.5	E855.2	E938.5	E950.4	E962.0	E980.4
nerve block (peripheral) (plexus)	968.6	E855.2	E938.6	E950.4	E962.0	E980.4
spinal	968.7	E855.2	E938.7	E950.4	E962.0	E980.4
Ethoheptazine (citrate)	965.7	E850.7	E935.7	E950.0	E962.0	E980.0
Ethopropazine	966.4	E855.0	E936.4	E950.4	E962.0	E980.4
Ethosuximide	966.2	E855.0	E936.2	E950.4	E962.0	E980.4
Ethotoin	966.1	E855.0	E936.1	E950.4	E962.0	E980.4
Ethoxazene	961.9	E857	E931.9	E950.4	E962.0	E980.4
Ethoxzolamide	974.2	E858.5	E944.2	E950.4	E962.0	E980.4
Ethyl						
acetate (vapor)	982.8	E862.4	—	E950.9	E962.1	E980.9
alcohol	980.0	E860.1	—	E950.9	E962.1	E980.9
beverage	980.0	E860.0	—	E950.9	E962.1	E980.9
aldehyde (vapor)	987.8	E869.8	—	E952.8	E962.2	E982.8
liquid	989.8	E866.8	—	E950.9	E962.1	E980.9
aminobenzoate	968.5	E855.2	E938.5	E950.4	E962.0	E980.4
biscoumacetate	964.2	E858.2	E934.2	E950.4	E962.0	E980.4

Substance	Poisoning	Accident	Therapeutic Use	Suicide Attempt	Assault	Undetermined
Ethyl—*continued*						
bromide (anesthetic)	968.2	E855.1	E938.2	E950.4	E962.0	E980.4
carbamate (antineoplastic)	963.1	E858.1	E933.1	E950.4	E962.0	E980.4
carbinol	980.3	E860.4	—	E950.9	E962.1	E980.9
chaulmoograte	961.8	E857	E931.8	E950.4	E962.0	E980.4
chloride (vapor)	987.8	E869.8	—	E952.8	E962.2	E982.8
anesthetic (local)	968.5	E855.2	E938.5	E950.4	E962.0	E980.4
inhaled	968.2	E855.1	E938.2	E950.4	E962.0	E980.4
solvent	982.3	E862.4	—	E950.9	E962.1	E980.9
estranol	962.1	E858.0	E932.1	E950.4	E962.0	E980.4
ether — *see* Ether(s)						
formate (solvent) NEC	982.8	E862.4	—	E950.9	E962.1	E980.9
iodoacetate	987.5	E869.3	—	E952.8	E962.2	E982.8
lactate (solvent) NEC	982.8	E862.4	—	E950.9	E962.1	E980.9
methylcarbinol	980.8	E860.8	—	E950.9	E962.1	E980.9
morphine	965.09	E850.2	E935.2	E950.0	E962.0	E980.0
Ethylene (gas)	987.1	E869.8	—	E952.8	E962.2	E982.8
anesthetic (general)	968.2	E855.1	E938.2	E950.4	E962.0	E980.4
chlorohydrin (vapor)	982.3	E862.4	—	E950.9	E962.1	E980.9
dichloride (vapor)	982.3	E862.4	—	E950.9	E962.1	E980.9
glycol(s) (any) (vapor)	982.8	E862.4	—	E950.9	E962.1	E980.9
Ethylidene						
chloride NEC	982.3	E862.4	—	E950.9	E962.1	E980.9
diethyl ether	982.8	E862.4	—	E950.9	E962.1	E980.9
Ethynodiol	962.2	E858.0	E932.2	E950.4	E962.0	E980.4
Etidocaine	968.9	E855.2	E938.9	E950.4	E962.0	E980.4
infiltration (subcutaneous)	968.5	E855.2	E938.5	E950.4	E962.0	E980.4
nerve (peripheral) (plexus)	968.6	E855.2	E938.6	E950.4	E962.0	E980.4
Etilfen	967.0	E851	E937.0	E950.1	E962.0	E980.1
Etomide	965.7	E850.7	E935.7	E950.0	E962.0	E980.0
Etorphine	965.09	E850.2	E935.2	E950.0	E962.0	E980.0
Etoval	967.0	E851	E937.0	E950.1	E962.0	E980.1
Etryptamine	969.0	E854.0	E939.0	E950.3	E962.0	E980.3
Eucaine	968.5	E855.2	E938.5	E950.4	E962.0	E980.4
Eucalyptus (oil) NEC	975.5	E858.6	E945.5	E950.4	E962.0	E980.4
Eucatropine	971.1	E855.4	E941.1	E950.4	E962.0	E980.4
Eucodal	965.09	E850.2	E935.2	E950.0	E962.0	E980.0
Euneryl	967.0	E851	E937.0	E950.1	E962.0	E980.1
Euphthalmine	971.1	E855.4	E941.1	E950.4	E962.0	E980.4
Eurax	976.0	E858.7	E946.0	E950.4	E962.0	E980.4
Euresol	976.4	E858.7	E946.4	E950.4	E962.0	E980.4
Euthroid	962.7	E858.0	E932.7	E950.4	E962.0	E980.4
Evans blue	977.8	E858.8	E947.8	E950.4	E962.0	E980.4
Evipal	967.0	E851	E937.0	E950.1	E962.0	E980.1
sodium	968.3	E855.1	E938.3	E950.4	E962.0	E980.4
Evipan	967.0	E851	E937.0	E950.1	E962.0	E980.1
sodium	968.3	E855.1	E938.3	E950.4	E962.0	E980.4
Exalgin	965.4	E850.4	E935.4	E950.0	E962.0	E980.0
Excipients, pharmaceutical	977.4	E858.8	E947.4	E950.4	E962.0	E980.4
Exhaust gas — *see* Carbon, monoxide						
Ex-Lax (phenolphthalein)	973.1	E858.4	E943.1	E950.4	E962.0	E980.4
Expectorants	975.5	E858.6	E945.5	E950.4	E962.0	E980.4
External medications (skin) (mucous membrane)	976.9	E858.7	E946.9	E950.4	E962.0	E980.4
dental agent	976.7	E858.7	E946.7	E950.4	E962.0	E980.4
ENT agent	976.6	E858.7	E946.6	E950.4	E962.0	E980.4
ophthalmic preparation	976.5	E858.7	E946.5	E950.4	E962.0	E980.4
specified NEC	976.8	E858.7	E946.8	E950.4	E962.0	E980.4
Eye agents (anti-infective)	976.5	E858.7	E946.5	E950.4	E962.0	E980.4
Factor IX complex (human)	964.5	E858.2	E934.5	E950.4	E962.0	E980.4
Fecal softeners	973.2	E858.4	E943.2	E950.4	E962.0	E980.4
Fenbutrazate	977.0	E858.8	E947.0	E950.4	E962.0	E980.4
Fencamfamin	970.8	E854.3	E940.8	E950.4	E962.0	E980.4
Fenfluramine	977.0	E858.8	E947.0	E950.4	E962.0	E980.4
Fenoprofen	965.6	E850.6	E935.6	E950.0	E962.0	E980.0
Fentanyl	965.09	E850.2	E935.2	E950.0	E962.0	E980.0
Fentazin	969.1	E853.0	E939.1	E950.3	E962.0	E980.3
Fenticlor, fentichlor	976.0	E858.7	E946.0	E950.4	E962.0	E980.4
Fer de lance (bite) (venom)	989.5	E905.0	—	E950.9	E962.1	E980.9
Ferric — *see* Iron						
Ferrocholinate	964.0	E858.2	E934.0	E950.4	E962.0	E980.4
Ferrous fumarate, gluconate, lactate, salt NEC, sulfate (medicinal)	964.0	E858.2	E934.0	E950.4	E962.0	E980.4
Ferrum — *see* Iron						
Fertilizers NEC	989.8	E866.5	—	E950.9	E962.1	E980.4
with herbicide mixture	989.4	E863.5	—	E950.6	E962.1	E980.7
Fibrinogen (human)	964.7	E858.2	E934.7	E950.4	E962.0	E980.4
Fibrinolysin	964.4	E858.2	E934.4	E950.4	E962.0	E980.4

TABLE OF DRUGS AND CHEMICALS

Substance	Poisoning	Accident	Therapeutic-Use	Suicide Attempt	Assault	Undetermined
Fibrinolysis-affecting agents	964.4	E858.2	E934.4	E950.4	E962.0	E980.4
Filix mas	961.6	E857	E931.6	E950.4	E962.0	E980.4
Fiorinal	965.1	E850.3	E935.3	E950.0	E962.0	E980.0
Fire damp	987.1	E869.8	—	E952.8	E962.2	E982.8
Fish, nonbacterial or noxious	988.0	E865.2	—	E950.9	E962.1	E980.9
shell	988.0	E865.1	—	E950.9	E962.1	E980.9
Flagyl	961.5	E857	E931.5	E950.4	E962.0	E980.4
Flavoxate	975.1	E858.6	E945.1	E950.4	E962.0	E980.4
Flaxedil	975.2	E858.6	E945.2	E950.4	E962.0	E980.4
Flaxseed (medicinal)	976.3	E858.7	E946.3	E950.4	E962.0	E980.4
Florantyrone	973.4	E858.4	E943.4	E950.4	E962.0	E980.4
Floraquin	961.3	E857	E931.3	E950.4	E962.0	E980.4
Florinef	962.0	E858.0	E932.0	E950.4	E962.0	E980.4
ENT agent	976.6	E858.7	E946.6	E950.4	E962.0	E980.4
ophthalmic preparation	976.5	E858.7	E946.5	E950.4	E962.0	E980.4
topical NEC	976.0	E858.7	E946.0	E950.4	E962.0	E980.4
Flowers of sulfur	976.4	E858.7	E946.4	E950.4	E962.0	E980.4
Floxuridine	963.1	E858.1	E933.1	E950.4	E962.0	E980.4
Flucytosine	961.9	E857	E931.9	E950.4	E962.0	E980.4
Fludrocortisone	962.0	E858.0	E932.0	E950.4	E962.0	E980.4
ENT agent	976.6	E858.7	E946.6	E950.4	E962.0	E980.4
ophthalmic preparation	976.5	E858.7	E946.5	E950.4	E962.0	E980.4
topical NEC	976.0	E858.7	E946.0	E950.4	E962.0	E980.4
Flumethasone	976.0	E858.7	E946.0	E950.4	E962.0	E980.4
Flumethiazide	974.3	E858.5	E944.3	E950.4	E962.0	E980.4
Flumidin	961.7	E857	E931.7	E950.4	E962.0	E980.4
Fluocinolone	976.0	E858.7	E946.0	E950.4	E962.0	E980.4
Fluocortolone	962.0	E858.0	E932.0	E950.4	E962.0	E980.4
Fluohydrocortisone	962.0	E858.0	E932.0	E950.4	E962.0	E980.4
ENT agent	976.6	E858.7	E946.6	E950.4	E962.0	E980.4
ophthalmic preparation	976.5	E858.7	E946.5	E950.4	E962.0	E980.4
topical NEC	976.0	E858.7	E946.0	E950.4	E962.0	E980.4
Fluonid	976.0	E858.7	E946.0	E950.4	E962.0	E980.4
Fluopromazine	969.1	E853.0	E939.1	E950.3	E962.0	E980.3
Fluoracetate	989.4	E863.7	—	E950.6	E962.1	E980.7
Fluorescein (sodium)	977.8	E858.8	E947.8	E950.4	E962.0	E980.4
Fluoride(s) (pesticides) (sodium) NEC	989.4	E863.4	—	E950.6	E962.1	E980.7
hydrogen — see Hydrofluoric acid						
medicinal	976.7	E858.7	E946.7	E950.4	E962.0	E980.4
not pesticide NEC	983.9	E864.4	—	E950.7	E962.1	E980.6
stannous	976.7	E858.7	E946.7	E950.4	E962.0	E980.4
Fluorinated corticosteroids	962.0	E858.0	E932.0	E950.4	E962.0	E980.4
Fluorine (compounds) (gas)	987.8	E869.8	—	E952.8	E962.2	E982.8
salt — see Fluoride(s)						
Fluoristan	976.7	E858.7	E946.7	E950.4	E962.0	E980.4
Fluoroacetate	989.4	E863.7	—	E950.6	E962.1	E980.7
Fluorodeoxy uridine	963.1	E858.1	E933.1	E950.4	E962.0	E980.4
Fluorometholone (topical) NEC	976.0	E858.7	E946.0	E950.4	E962.0	E980.4
ophthalmic preparation	976.5	E858.7	E946.5	E950.4	E962.0	E980.4
Fluorouracil	963.1	E858.1	E933.1	E950.4	E962.0	E980.4
Fluothane	968.1	E855.1	E938.1	E950.4	E962.0	E980.4
Fluoxymesterone	962.1	E858.0	E932.1	E950.4	E962.0	E980.4
Fluphenazine	969.1	E853.0	E939.1	E950.3	E962.0	E980.3
Fluprednisolone	962.0	E858.0	E932.0	E950.4	E962.0	E980.4
Flurandrenolide	976.0	E858.7	E946.0	E950.4	E962.0	E980.4
Flurazepam (hydrochloride)	969.4	E853.2	E939.4	E950.3	E962.0	E980.3
Flurobate	976.0	E858.7	E946.0	E950.4	E962.0	E980.4
Flurothyl	969.8	E855.8	E939.8	E950.3	E962.0	E980.3
Fluroxene	968.2	E855.1	E938.2	E950.4	E962.0	E980.4
Folacin	964.1	E858.2	E934.1	E950.4	E962.0	E980.4
Folic acid	964.1	E858.2	E934.1	E950.4	E962.0	E980.4
Follicle stimulating hormone	962.4	E858.0	E932.4	E950.4	E962.0	E980.4
Food, foodstuffs, nonbacterial or noxious	988.9	E865.9	—	E950.9	E962.1	E980.9
berries, seeds	988.2	E865.3	—	E950.9	E962.1	E980.9
fish	988.0	E865.2	—	E950.9	E962.1	E980.9
mushrooms	988.1	E865.5	—	E950.9	E962.1	E980.9
plants	988.2	E865.9	—	E950.9	E962.1	E980.9
specified type NEC	988.2	E865.4	—	E950.9	E962.1	E980.9
shellfish	988.0	E865.1	—	E950.9	E962.1	E980.9
specified NEC	988.8	E865.8	—	E950.9	E962.1	E980.9
Fool's parsley	988.2	E865.4	—	E950.9	E962.1	E980.9
Formaldehyde (solution)	989.8	E861.4	—	E950.9	E962.1	E980.9
fungicide	989.4	E863.6	—	E950.6	E962.1	E980.7
gas or vapor	987.8	E869.8	—	E952.8	E962.2	E982.8

TABLE OF DRUGS AND CHEMICALS

Substance	Poisoning	Accident	Therapeutic Use	Suicide Attempt	Assault	Undetermined
Formalin	989.8	E861.4	—	E950.9	E962.1	E980.9
fungicide	989.4	E863.6	—	E950.6	E962.1	E980.7
vapor	987.8	E869.8	—	E952.8	E962.2	E982.8
Formic acid	983.1	E864.1	—	E950.7	E962.1	E980.6
vapor	987.8	E869.8	—	E952.8	E962.2	E982.8
Fowler's solution	985.1	E866.3	—	E950.8	E962.1	E980.8
Foxglove	988.2	E865.4	—	E950.9	E962.1	E980.9
Fox green	977.8	E858.8	E947.8	E950.4	E962.0	E980.4
Framycetin	960.8	E856	E930.8	E950.4	E962.0	E980.4
Frangula (extract)	973.1	E858.4	E943.1	E950.4	E962.0	E980.4
Frei antigen	977.8	E858.8	E947.8	E950.4	E962.0	E980.4
Freons	987.4	E869.2	—	E952.8	E962.2	E982.8
Fructose	974.5	E858.5	E944.5	E950.4	E962.0	E980.4
Frusemide	974.4	E858.5	E944.4	E950.4	E962.0	E980.4
FSH	962.4	E858.0	E932.4	E950.4	E962.0	E980.4
Fuel						
automobile	981	E862.1	—	E950.9	E962.1	E980.9
exhaust gas, not in transit	986	E868.2	—	E952.0	E962.2	E982.0
vapor NEC	987.1	E869.8	—	E952.8	E962.2	E982.8
gas (domestic use) — see also Carbon, monoxide, fuel						
utility	987.1	E868.1	—	E951.8	E962.2	E981.8
incomplete combustion of — see Carbon, monoxide, fuel, utility in mobile container	987.0	E868.0	—	E951.1	E962.2	E981.1
piped (natural)	987.1	E867	—	E951.0	E962.2	E981.0
industrial, incomplete combustion	986	E868.3	—	E952.1	E962.2	E982.1
Fugillin	960.8	E856	E930.8	E950.4	E962.0	E980.4
Fulminate of mercury	985.0	E866.1	—	E950.9	E962.1	E980.9
Fulvicin	960.1	E856	E930.1	E950.4	E962.0	E980.4
Fumadil	960.8	E856	E930.8	E950.4	E962.0	E980.4
Fumagillin	960.8	E856	E930.8	E950.4	E962.0	E980.4
Fumes (from)	987.9	E869.9	—	E952.9	E962.2	E982.9
carbon monoxide — see Carbon, monoxide						
charcoal (domestic use)	986	E868.3	—	E952.1	E962.2	E982.1
chloroform — see Chloroform						
coke (in domestic stoves, fireplaces)	986	E868.3	—	E952.1	E962.2	E982.1
corrosive NEC	987.8	E869.8	—	E952.8	E962.2	E982.8
ether — see Ether(s)						
freons	987.4	E869.2	—	E952.8	E962.2	E982.8
hydrocarbons	987.1	E869.8	—	E952.8	E962.2	E982.8
petroleum (liquefied)	987.0	E868.0	—	E951.1	E962.2	E981.1
distributed through pipes (pure or mixed with air)	987.0	E867	—	E951.0	E962.2	E981.0
lead — see Lead						
metals — see specified metal						
nitrogen dioxide	987.2	E869.0	—	E952.8	E962.2	E982.8
pesticides — see Pesticides						
petroleum (liquefied)	987.0	E868.0	—	E951.1	E962.2	E981.1
distributed through pipes (pure or mixed with air)	987.0	E867	—	E951.0	E962.2	E981.0
polyester	987.8	E869.8	—	E952.8	E962.2	E982.8
specified source other (see also substance specified)	987.8	E869.8	—	E952.8	E962.2	E982.8
sulfur dioxide	987.3	E869.1	—	E952.8	E962.2	E982.8
Fumigants	989.4	E863.8	—	E950.6	E962.1	E980.7
Fungi, noxious, used as food	988.1	E865.5	—	E950.9	E962.1	E980.9
Fungicides (see also Antifungals)	989.4	E863.6	—	E950.6	E962.1	E980.7
Fungizone	960.1	E856	E930.1	E950.4	E962.0	E980.4
topical	976.0	E858.7	E946.0	E950.4	E962.0	E980.4
Furacin	976.0	E858.7	E946.0	E950.4	E962.0	E980.4
Furadantin	961.9	E857	E931.9	E950.4	E962.0	E980.4
Furazolidone	961.9	E857	E931.9	E950.4	E962.0	E980.4
Furnace (coal burning) (domestic), gas from	986	E868.3	—	E952.1	E962.2	E982.1
industrial	986	E868.8	—	E952.1	E962.2	E982.1
Furniture polish	989.8	E861.2	—	E950.9	E962.1	E980.9
Furosemide	974.4	E858.5	E944.4	E950.4	E962.0	E980.4
Furoxone	961.9	E857	E931.9	E950.4	E962.0	E980.4
Fusel oil (amyl) (butyl) (propyl)	980.3	E860.4	—	E950.9	E962.1	E980.9
Fusidic acid	960.8	E856	E930.8	E950.4	E962.0	E980.4
Gallamine	975.2	E858.6	E945.2	E950.4	E962.0	E980.4
Gallotannic acid	976.2	E858.7	E946.2	E950.4	E962.0	E980.4
Gamboge	973.1	E858.4	E943.1	E950.4	E962.0	E980.4
Gamimune	964.6	E858.2	E934.6	E950.4	E962.0	E980.4
Gamma-benzene hexachloride (vapor)	989.2	E863.0	—	E950.6	E962.1	E980.7
Gamma globulin	964.6	E858.2	E934.6	E950.4	E962.0	E980.4
Gamulin	964.6	E858.2	E934.6	E950.4	E962.0	E980.4
Ganglionic blocking agents	972.3	E858.3	E942.3	E950.4	E962.0	E980.4
Ganja	969.6	E854.1	E939.6	E950.3	E962.0	E980.3

TABLE OF DRUGS AND CHEMICALS

Substance	Poisoning	Accident	Therapeutic-Use	Suicide Attempt	Assualt	Undetermined
Garamycin	960.8	E856	E930.8	E950.4	E962.0	E980.4
ophthalmic preparation	976.5	E858.7	E946.5	E950.4	E962.0	E980.4
topical NEC	976.0	E858.7	E946.0	E950.4	E962.0	E980.4
Gardenal	967.0	E851	E937.0	E950.1	E962.0	E980.1
Gardepanyl	967.0	E851	E937.0	E950.1	E962.0	E980.1
Gas	987.9	E869.9	—	E952.9	E962.2	E982.9
acetylene	987.1	E868.1	—	E951.8	E962.2	E981.8
incomplete combustion of — see Carbon, monoxide, fuel, utility						
air contaminants, source or type not specified	987.9	E869.9	—	E952.9	E962.2	E982.9
anesthetic (general) NEC	968.2	E855.1	E938.2	E950.4	E962.0	E980.4
blast furnace	986	E868.8	—	E952.1	E962.2	E982.1
butane — see Butane						
carbon monoxide — see Carbon, monoxide						
chlorine	987.6	E869.8	—	E952.8	E962.2	E982.8
coal — see Carbon, monoxide, coal						
cyanide	987.7	E869.8	—	E952.8	E962.2	E982.8
dicyanogen	987.8	E869.8	—	E952.8	E962.2	E982.8
domestic — see Gas, utility						
exhaust — see Carbon, monoxide, exhaust gas						
from wood- or coal-burning stove or fireplace	986	E868.3	—	E952.1	E962.2	E982.1
fuel (domestic use) — see also Carbon, monoxide, fuel						
industrial use	986	E868.8	—	E952.1	E962.2	E982.1
utility	987.1	E868.1	—	E951.8	E962.2	E981.8
incomplete combustion of — see Carbon, monoxide, fuel, utility						
in mobile container	987.0	E868.0	—	E951.1	E962.2	E981.1
piped (natural)	987.1	E867	—	E951.0	E962.2	E981.0
garage	986	E868.2	—	E952.0	E962.2	E982.0
hydrocarbon NEC	987.1	E869.8	—	E952.8	E962.2	E982.8
incomplete combustion of — see Carbon, monoxide, fuel, utility						
liquefied (mobile container)	987.0	E868.0	—	E951.1	E962.2	E981.1
piped	987.0	E867	—	E951.0	E962.2	E981.0
hydrocyanic acid	987.7	E869.8	—	E952.8	E962.2	E982.8
illuminating — see Gas, utility						
incomplete combustion, any — see Carbon, monoxide						
kiln	986	E868.8	—	E952.1	E962.2	E982.1
lacrimogenic	987.5	E869.3	—	E952.8	E962.2	E982.8
marsh	987.1	E869.8	—	E952.8	E962.2	E982.8
motor exhaust, not in transit	986	E868.8	—	E952.1	E962.2	E982.1
mustard — see Mustard, gas						
natural	987.1	E867	—	E951.0	E962.2	E981.0
nerve (war)	987.9	E869.9	—	E952.9	E962.2	E982.9
oils	981	E862.1	—	E950.9	E962.1	E980.9
petroleum (liquefied) (distributed in mobile containers)	987.0	E868.0	—	E951.1	E962.2	E981.1
piped (pure or mixed with air)	987.0	E867	—	E951.1	E962.2	E981.1
piped (manufactured) (natural) NEC	987.1	E867	—	E951.0	E962.2	E981.0
producer	986	E868.8	—	E952.1	E962.2	E982.1
propane — see Propane						
refrigerant (freon)	987.4	E869.2	—	E952.8	E962.2	E982.8
not freon	987.9	E869.9	—	E952.9	E962.2	E982.9
sewer	987.8	E869.8	—	E952.8	E962.2	E982.8
specified source NEC (see also substance specified)	987.8	E869.8	—	E952.8	E962.2	E982.8
stove — see Gas, utility						
tear	987.5	E869.3	—	E952.8	E962.2	E982.8
utility (for cooking, heating, or lighting) (piped) NEC	987.1	E868.1	—	E951.8	E962.2	E981.8
incomplete combustion of — see Carbon, monoxide, fuel, utilty						
in mobile container	987.0	E868.0	—	E951.1	E962.2	E981.1
piped (natural)	987.1	E867	—	E951.0	E962.2	E981.0
water	987.1	E868.1	—	E951.8	E962.2	E981.8
incomplete combustion of — see Carbon, monoxide, fuel, utility						
Gaseous substance — see Gas						
Gasoline, gasolene	981	E862.1	—	E950.9	E962.1	E980.9
vapor	987.1	E869.8	—	E952.8	E962.2	E982.8
Gastric enzymes	973.4	E858.4	E943.4	E950.4	E962.0	E980.4
Gastrografin	977.8	E858.8	E947.8	E950.4	E962.0	E980.4
Gastrointestinal agents	973.9	E858.4	E943.9	E950.4	E962.0	E980.4
specified NEC	973.8	E858.4	E943.8	E950.4	E962.0	E980.4
Gaultheria procumbens	988.2	E865.4	—	E950.9	E962.1	E980.9
Gelatin (intravenous)	964.8	E858.2	E934.8	E950.4	E962.0	E980.4
absorbable (sponge)	964.5	E858.2	E934.5	E950.4	E962.0	E980.4
Gelfilm	976.8	E858.7	E946.8	E950.4	E962.0	E980.4
Gelfoam	964.5	E858.2	E934.5	E950.4	E962.0	E980.4
Gelsemine	970.8	E854.3	E940.8	E950.4	E962.0	E980.4
Gelsemium (sempervirens)	988.2	E865.4	—	E950.9	E962.1	E980.9
Gemonil	967.0	E851	E937.0	E950.1	E962.0	E980.1

Substance	Poisoning	Accident	Therapeutic Use	Suicide Attempt	Assault	Undetermined
Gentamicin	960.8	E856	E930.8	E950.4	E962.0	E980.4
ophthalmic preparation	976.5	E858.7	E946.5	E950.4	E962.0	E980.4
topical NEC	976.0	E858.7	E946.0	E950.4	E962.0	E980.4
Gentian violet	976.0	E858.7	E946.0	E950.4	E962.0	E980.4
Gexane	976.0	E858.7	E946.0	E950.4	E962.0	E980.4
Gila monster (venom)	989.5	E905.0	—	E950.9	E962.1	E980.9
Ginger, Jamaica	989.8	E866.8	—	E950.9	E962.1	E980.9
Gitalin	972.1	E858.3	E942.1	E950.4	E962.0	E980.4
Gitoxin	972.1	E858.3	E942.1	E950.4	E962.0	E980.4
Glandular extract (medicinal) NEC	977.9	E858.9	E947.9	E950.5	E962.0	E980.5
Glaucarubin	961.5	E857	E931.5	E950.4	E962.0	E980.4
Globin zinc insulin	962.3	E858.0	E932.3	E950.4	E962.0	E980.4
Glucagon	962.3	E858.0	E932.3	E950.4	E962.0	E980.4
Glucochloral	967.1	E852.0	E937.1	E950.2	E962.0	E980.2
Glucocorticoids	962.0	E858.0	E932.0	E950.4	E962.0	E980.4
Glucose	974.5	E858.5	E944.5	E950.4	E962.0	E980.4
oxidase reagent	977.8	E858.8	E947.8	E950.4	E962.0	E980.4
Glucosulfone sodium	961.8	E857	E931.8	E950.4	E962.0	E980.4
Glue(s)	989.8	E866.6	—	E950.9	E962.1	E980.9
Glutamic acid (hydrochloride)	973.4	E858.4	E943.4	E950.4	E962.0	E980.4
Glutathione	963.8	E858.1	E933.8	E950.4	E962.0	E980.4
Glutethimide (group)	967.5	E852.4	E937.5	E950.2	E962.0	E980.2
Glycerin (lotion)	976.3	E858.7	E946.3	E950.4	E962.0	E980.4
Glycerol (topical)	976.3	E858.7	E946.3	E950.4	E962.0	E980.4
Glyceryl						
guaiacolate	975.5	E858.6	E945.5	E950.4	E962.0	E980.4
triacetate (topical)	976.0	E858.7	E946.0	E950.4	E962.0	E980.4
trinitrate	972.4	E858.3	E942.4	E950.4	E962.0	E980.4
Glycine	974.5	E858.5	E944.5	E950.4	E962.0	E980.4
Glycobiarsol	961.1	E857	E931.1	E950.4	E962.0	E980.4
Glycols (ether)	982.8	E862.4	—	E950.9	E962.1	E980.9
Glycopyrrolate	971.1	E855.4	E941.1	E950.4	E962.0	E980.4
Glymidine	962.3	E858.0	E932.3	E950.4	E962.0	E980.4
Gold (compounds) (salts)	965.6	E850.6	E935.6	E950.0	E962.0	E980.0
Golden sulfide of antimony	985.4	E866.2	—	E950.9	E962.1	E980.9
Goldylocks	988.2	E865.4	—	E950.9	E962.1	E980.9
Gonadal tissue extract	962.9	E858.0	E932.9	E950.4	E962.0	E980.4
female	962.2	E858.0	E932.2	E950.4	E962.0	E980.4
male	962.1	E858.0	E932.1	E950.4	E962.0	E980.4
Gonadotropin	962.4	E858.0	E932.4	E950.4	E962.0	E980.4
Grain alcohol	980.0	E860.1	—	E950.9	E962.1	E980.9
beverage	980.0	E860.0	—	E950.9	E962.1	E980.9
Gramicidin	960.8	E856	E930.8	E950.4	E962.0	E980.4
Gratiola officinalis	988.2	E865.4	—	E950.9	E962.1	E980.9
Grease	989.8	E866.8	—	E950.9	E962.1	E980.9
Green hellebore	988.2	E865.4	—	E950.9	E962.1	E980.9
Green soap	976.2	E858.7	E946.2	E950.4	E962.0	E980.4
Grifulvin	960.1	E856	E930.1	E950.4	E962.0	E980.4
Griseofulvin	960.1	E856	E930.1	E950.4	E962.0	E980.4
Growth hormone	962.4	E858.0	E932.4	E950.4	E962.0	E980.4
Guaiacol	975.5	E858.6	E945.5	E950.4	E962.0	E980.4
Guaiac reagent	977.8	E858.8	E947.8	E950.4	E962.0	E980.4
Guaifenesin	975.5	E858.6	E945.5	E950.4	E962.0	E980.4
Guaiphenesin	975.5	E858.6	E945.5	E950.4	E962.0	E980.4
Guanatol	961.4	E857	E931.4	E950.4	E962.0	E980.4
Guanethidine	972.6	E858.3	E942.6	E950.4	E962.0	E980.4
Guano	989.8	E866.5	—	E950.9	E962.1	E980.9
Guanochlor	972.6	E858.3	E942.6	E950.4	E962.0	E980.4
Guanoctine	972.6	E858.3	E942.6	E950.4	E962.0	E980.4
Guanoxan	972.6	E858.3	E942.6	E950.4	E962.0	E980.4
Hair treatment agent NEC	976.4	E858.7	E946.4	E950.4	E962.0	E980.4
Halcinonide	976.0	E858.7	E946.0	E950.4	E962.0	E980.4
Halethazole	976.0	E858.7	E946.0	E950.4	E962.0	E980.4
Hallucinogens	969.6	E854.1	E939.6	E950.3	E962.0	E980.3
Haloperidol	969.2	E853.1	E939.2	E950.3	E962.0	E980.3
Haloprogin	976.0	E858.7	E946.0	E950.4	E962.0	E980.4
Halotex	976.0	E858.7	E946.0	E950.4	E962.0	E980.4
Halothane	968.1	E855.1	E938.1	E950.4	E962.0	E980.4
Halquinols	976.0	E858.7	E946.0	E950.4	E962.0	E980.4
Harmonyl	972.6	E858.3	E942.6	E950.4	E962.0	E980.4
Hartmann's solution	974.5	E858.5	E944.5	E950.4	E962.0	E980.4
Hashish	969.6	E854.1	E939.6	E950.3	E962.0	E980.3
Hawaiian wood rose seeds	969.6	E854.1	E939.6	E950.3	E962.0	E980.3
Headache cures, drugs, powders NEC	977.9	E858.9	E947.9	E950.5	E962.0	E980.5
Heavenly Blue (morning glory)	969.6	E854.1	E939.6	E950.3	E962.0	E980.3

TABLE OF DRUGS AND CHEMICALS

Substance	Poisoning	Accident	Therapeutic-Use	Suicide Attempt	Assault	Undetermined
Heavy metal						
antagonists	963.8	E858.1	E933.8	E950.4	E962.0	E980.4
anti-infectives	961.2	E857	E931.2	E950.4	E962.0	E980.4
Hedaquinium	976.0	E858.7	E946.0	E950.4	E962.0	E980.4
Hedge hyssop	988.2	E865.4	—	E950.9	E962.1	E980.9
Heet	976.8	E858.7	E946.8	E950.4	E962.0	E980.4
Helenin	961.6	E857	E931.6	E950.4	E962.0	E980.4
Hellebore (black) (green) (white)	988.2	E865.4	—	E950.9	E962.1	E980.9
Hemlock	988.2	E865.4	—	E950.9	E962.1	E980.9
Hemostatics	964.5	E858.2	E934.5	E950.4	E962.0	E980.4
capillary active drugs	972.8	E858.3	E942.8	E950.4	E962.0	E980.4
Henbane	988.2	E865.4	—	E950.9	E962.1	E980.9
Heparin (sodium)	964.2	E858.2	E934.2	E950.4	E962.0	E980.4
Heptabarbital, heptabarbitone	967.0	E851	E937.0	E950.1	E962.0	E980.1
Heptachlor	989.2	E863.0	—	E950.6	E962.1	E980.7
Heptalgin	965.09	E850.2	E935.2	E950.0	E962.0	E980.0
Herbicides	989.4	E863.5	—	E950.6	E962.1	E980.7
Heroin	965.01	E850.0	E935.0	E950.0	E962.0	E980.0
Herplex	976.5	E858.7	E946.5	E950.4	E962.0	E980.4
HES	964.8	E858.2	E934.8	E950.4	E962.0	E980.4
Hetastarch	964.8	E858.2	E934.8	E950.4	E962.0	E980.4
Hexachlorocyclohexane	989.2	E863.0	—	E950.6	E962.1	E980.7
Hexachlorophene	976.2	E858.7	E946.2	E950.4	E962.0	E980.4
Hexadimethrine (bromide)	964.5	E858.2	E934.5	E950.4	E962.0	E980.4
Hexafluorenium	975.2	E858.6	E945.2	E950.4	E962.0	E980.4
Hexa-germ	976.2	E858.7	E946.2	E950.4	E962.0	E980.4
Hexahydrophenol	980.8	E860.8	—	E950.9	E962.1	E980.9
Hexalin	980.8	E860.8	—	E950.9	E962.1	E980.9
Hexamethonium	972.3	E858.3	E942.3	E950.4	E962.0	E980.4
Hexamethyleneamine	961.9	E857	E931.9	E950.4	E962.0	E980.4
Hexamine	961.9	E857	E931.9	E950.4	E962.0	E980.4
Hexanone	982.8	E862.4	—	E950.9	E962.1	E980.9
Hexapropymate	967.8	E852.8	E937.8	E950.2	E962.0	E980.2
Hexestrol	962.2	E858.0	E932.2	E950.4	E962.0	E980.4
Hexethal (sodium)	967.0	E851	E937.0	E950.1	E962.0	E980.1
Hexetidine	976.0	E858.7	E946.0	E950.4	E962.0	E980.4
Hexobarbital, hexobarbitone	967.0	E851	E937.0	E950.1	E962.0	E980.1
sodium (anesthetic)	968.3	E855.1	E938.3	E950.4	E962.0	E980.4
soluble	968.3	E855.1	E938.3	E950.4	E962.0	E980.4
Hexocyclium	971.1	E855.4	E941.1	E950.4	E962.0	E980.4
Hexoestrol	962.2	E858.0	E932.2	E950.4	E962.0	E980.4
Hexone	982.8	E862.4	—	E950.9	E962.1	E980.9
Hexylcaine	968.5	E855.2	E938.5	E950.4	E962.0	E980.4
Hexylresorcinol	961.6	E857	E931.6	E950.4	E962.0	E980.4
Hinkle's pills	973.1	E858.4	E943.1	E950.4	E962.0	E980.4
Histalog	977.8	E858.8	E947.8	E950.4	E962.0	E980.4
Histamine (phosphate)	972.5	E858.3	E942.5	E950.4	E962.0	E980.4
Histoplasmin	977.8	E858.8	E947.8	E950.4	E962.0	E980.4
Holly berries	988.2	E865.3	—	E950.9	E962.1	E980.9
Homatropine	971.1	E855.4	E941.1	E950.4	E962.0	E980.4
Homo-tet	964.6	E858.2	E934.6	E950.4	E962.0	E980.4
Hormones (synthetic substitute) NEC	962.9	E858.0	E932.9	E950.4	E962.0	E980.4
adrenal cortical steroids	962.0	E858.0	E932.0	E950.4	E962.0	E980.4
antidiabetic agents	962.3	E858.0	E932.3	E950.4	E962.0	E980.4
follicle stimulating	962.4	E858.0	E932.4	E950.4	E962.0	E980.4
gonadotropic	962.4	E858.0	E932.4	E950.4	E962.0	E980.4
growth	962.4	E858.0	E932.4	E950.4	E962.0	E980.4
ovarian (substitutes)	962.2	E858.0	E932.2	E950.4	E962.0	E980.4
parathyroid (derivatives)	962.6	E858.0	E932.6	E950.4	E962.0	E980.4
pituitary (posterior)	962.5	E858.0	E932.5	E950.4	E962.0	E980.4
anterior	962.4	E858.0	E932.4	E950.4	E962.0	E980.4
thyroid (derivative)	962.7	E858.0	E932.7	E950.4	E962.0	E980.4
Hornet (sting)	989.5	E905.3	—	E950.9	E962.1	E980.9
Horticulture agent NEC	989.4	E863.9	—	E950.6	E962.1	E980.7
Hyaluronidase	963.4	E858.1	E933.4	E950.4	E962.0	E980.4
Hyazyme	963.4	E858.1	E933.4	E950.4	E962.0	E980.4
Hycodan	965.09	E850.2	E935.2	E950.0	E962.0	E980.0
Hydantoin derivatives	966.1	E855.0	E936.1	E950.4	E962.0	E980.4
Hydeltra	962.0	E858.0	E932.0	E950.4	E962.0	E980.4
Hydergine	971.3	E855.6	E941.3	E950.4	E962.0	E980.4
Hydrabamine penicillin	960.0	E856	E930.0	E950.4	E962.0	E980.4
Hydralazine, hydrallazine	972.6	E858.3	E942.6	E950.4	E962.0	E980.4
Hydrargaphen	976.0	E858.7	E946.0	E950.4	E962.0	E980.4
Hydrazine	983.9	E864.3	—	E950.7	E962.1	E980.6
Hydriodic acid	975.5	E858.6	E945.5	E950.4	E962.0	E980.4

TABLE OF DRUGS AND CHEMICALS

Substance	Poisoning	Accident	Therapeutic-Use	Suicide Attempt	Assault	Undetermined
Hydrocarbon gas	987.1	E869.8	—	E952.8	E962.2	E982.8
incomplete combustion of — see Carbon, monoxide, fuel, utility						
liquefied (mobile container)	987.0	E868.0	—	E951.1	E962.2	E981.1
piped (natural)	987.0	E867	—	E951.0	E962.2	E981.0
Hydrochloric acid (liquid)	983.1	E864.1	—	E950.7	E962.1	E980.6
medicinal	973.4	E858.4	E943.4	E950.4	E962.0	E980.4
vapor	987.8	E869.8	—	E952.8	E962.2	E982.8
Hydrochlorothiazide	974.3	E858.5	E944.3	E950.4	E962.0	E980.4
Hydrocodone	965.09	E850.2	E935.2	E950.0	E962.0	E980.0
Hydrocortisone	962.0	E858.0	E932.0	E950.4	E962.0	E980.4
ENT agent	976.6	E858.7	E946.6	E950.4	E962.0	E980.4
ophthalmic preparation	976.5	E858.7	E946.5	E950.4	E962.0	E980.4
topical NEC	976.0	E858.7	E946.0	E950.4	E962.0	E980.4
Hydrocortone	962.0	E858.0	E932.0	E950.4	E962.0	E980.4
ENT agent	976.6	E858.7	E946.6	E950.4	E962.0	E980.4
ophthalmic preparation	976.5	E858.7	E946.5	E950.4	E962.0	E980.4
topical NEC	976.0	E858.7	E946.0	E950.4	E962.0	E980.4
Hydrocyanic acid — see Cyanide(s)						
Hydroflumethiazide	974.3	E858.5	E944.3	E950.4	E962.0	E980.4
Hydrofluoric acid (liquid)	983.1	E864.1	—	E950.7	E962.1	E980.6
vapor	987.8	E869.8	—	E952.8	E962.2	E982.8
Hydrogen	987.8	E869.8	—	E952.8	E962.2	E982.8
arsenide	985.1	E866.3	—	E950.8	E962.1	E980.8
arseniureted	985.1	E866.3	—	E950.8	E962.1	E980.8
cyanide (salts)	989.0	E866.8	—	E950.9	E962.1	E980.9
gas	987.7	E869.8	—	E952.8	E962.2	E982.8
fluoride (liquid)	983.1	E864.1	—	E950.7	E962.1	E980.6
vapor	987.8	E869.8	—	E952.8	E962.2	E982.8
peroxide (solution)	976.6	E858.7	E946.6	E950.4	E962.0	E980.4
phosphureted	987.8	E869.8	—	E952.8	E962.2	E982.8
sulfide (gas)	987.8	E869.8	—	E952.8	E962.2	E982.8
arseniureted	985.1	E866.3	—	E950.8	E962.1	E980.8
sulfureted	987.8	E869.8	—	E952.8	E962.2	E982.8
Hydromorphinol	965.09	E850.2	E935.2	E950.0	E962.0	E980.0
Hydromorphinone	965.09	E850.2	E935.2	E950.0	E962.0	E980.0
Hydromorphone	965.09	E850.2	E935.2	E950.0	E962.0	E980.0
Hydromox	974.3	E858.5	E944.3	E950.4	E962.0	E980.4
Hydrophilic lotion	976.3	E858.7	E946.3	E950.4	E962.0	E980.4
Hydroquinone	983.0	E864.0	—	E950.7	E962.1	E980.6
vapor	987.8	E869.8	—	E952.8	E962.2	E982.8
Hydrosulfuric acid (gas)	987.8	E869.8	—	E952.8	E962.2	E982.8
Hydrous wool fat (lotion)	976.3	E858.7	E946.3	E950.4	E962.0	E980.4
Hydroxide, caustic	983.2	E864.2	—	E950.7	E962.1	E980.6
Hydroxocobalamin	964.1	E858.2	E934.1	E950.4	E962.0	E980.4
Hydroxyamphetamine	971.2	E855.5	E941.2	E950.4	E962.0	E980.4
Hydroxychloroquine	961.4	E857	E931.4	E950.4	E962.0	E980.4
Hydroxydihydrocodeinone	965.09	E850.2	E935.2	E950.0	E962.0	E980.0
Hydroxyethyl starch	964.8	E858.2	E934.8	E950.4	E962.0	E980.4
Hydroxyphenamate	969.5	E853.8	E939.5	E950.3	E962.0	E980.3
Hydroxyphenylbutazone	965.5	E850.5	E935.5	E950.0	E962.0	E980.0
Hydroxyprogesterone	962.2	E858.0	E932.2	E950.4	E962.0	E980.4
Hydroxyquinoline derivatives	961.3	E857	E931.3	E950.4	E962.0	E980.4
Hydroxystilbamidine	961.5	E857	E931.5	E950.4	E962.0	E980.4
Hydroxyurea	963.1	E858.1	E933.1	E950.4	E962.0	E980.4
Hydroxyzine	969.5	E853.8	E939.5	E950.3	E962.0	E980.3
Hyoscine (hydrobromide)	971.1	E855.4	E941.1	E950.4	E962.0	E980.4
Hyoscyamine	971.1	E855.4	E941.1	E950.4	E962.0	E980.4
Hyoscyamus (albus) (niger)	988.2	E865.4	—	E950.9	E962.1	E980.9
Hypaque	977.8	E858.8	E947.8	E950.4	E962.0	E980.4
Hypertussis	964.6	E858.2	E934.6	E950.4	E962.0	E980.4
Hypnotics NEC	967.9	E852.9	E937.9	E950.2	E962.0	E980.2
Hypochlorites — see Sodium, hypochlorite						
Hypotensive agents NEC	972.6	E858.3	E942.6	E950.4	E962.0	E980.4
Ibufenac	965.6	E850.6	E935.6	E950.0	E962.0	E980.0
Ibuprofen	965.6	E850.6	E935.6	E950.0	E962.0	E980.0
ICG	977.8	E858.8	E947.8	E950.4	E962.0	E980.4
Ichthammol	976.4	E858.7	E946.4	E950.4	E962.0	E980.4
Ichthyol	976.4	E858.7	E946.4	E950.4	E962.0	E980.4
Idoxuridine	976.5	E858.7	E946.5	E950.4	E962.0	E980.4
IDU	976.5	E858.7	E946.5	E950.4	E962.0	E980.4
Iletin	962.3	E858.0	E932.3	E950.4	E962.0	E980.4
Ilex	988.2	E865.4	—	E950.9	E962.1	E980.9
Illuminating gas — see Gas, utility						
Ilopan	963.5	E858.1	E933.5	E950.4	E962.0	E980.4

TABLE OF DRUGS AND CHEMICALS

Substance	Poisoning	Accident	Therapeutic-Use	Suicide Attempt	Assault	Undetermined
Ilotycin	960.3	E856	E930.3	E950.4	E962.0	E980.4
ophthalmic preparation	976.5	E858.7	E946.5	E950.4	E962.0	E980.4
topical NEC	976.0	E858.7	E946.0	E950.4	E962.0	E980.4
Imipramine	969.0	E854.0	E939.0	E950.3	E962.0	E980.3
Immu-G	964.6	E858.2	E934.6	E950.4	E962.0	E980.4
Immuglobin	964.6	E858.2	E934.6	E950.4	E962.0	E980.4
Immune serum globulin	964.6	E858.2	E934.6	E950.4	E962.0	E980.4
Immunosuppressive agents	963.1	E858.1	E933.1	E950.4	E962.0	E980.4
Immu-tetanus	964.6	E858.2	E934.6	E950.4	E962.0	E980.4
Indandione (derivatives)	964.2	E858.2	E934.2	E950.4	E962.0	E980.4
Inderal	972.0	E858.3	E942.0	E950.4	E962.0	E980.4
Indian						
hemp	969.6	E854.1	E939.6	E950.3	E962.0	E980.3
tobacco	988.2	E865.4	—	E950.9	E962.1	E980.9
Indigo carmine	977.8	E858.8	E947.8	E950.4	E962.0	E980.4
Indocin	965.6	E850.6	E935.6	E950.0	E962.0	E980.0
Indocyanine green	977.8	E858.8	E947.8	E950.4	E962.0	E980.4
Indomethacin	965.6	E850.6	E935.6	E950.0	E962.0	E980.0
Industrial						
alcohol	980.9	E860.9	—	E950.9	E962.1	E980.9
fumes	987.8	E869.8	—	E952.8	E962.2	E982.8
solvents (fumes) (vapors)	982.8	E862.9	—	E950.9	E962.1	E980.9
Influenza vaccine	979.6	E858.8	E949.6	E950.4	E962.0	E982.8
Ingested substances NEC	989.9	E866.9	—	E950.9	E962.1	E980.9
INH (isoniazid)	961.8	E857	E931.8	E950.4	E962.0	E980.4
Inhalation, gas (noxious) — see Gas						
Ink	989.8	E866.8	—	E950.9	E962.1	E980.9
Innovar	967.6	E852.5	E937.6	E950.2	E962.0	E980.2
Inositol niacinate	972.2	E858.3	E942.2	E950.4	E962.0	E980.4
Inproquone	963.1	E858.1	E933.1	E950.4	E962.0	E980.4
Insect (sting), venomous	989.5	E905.5	—	E950.9	E962.1	E980.9
Insecticides (see also Pesticides)	989.4	E863.4	—	E950.6	E962.1	E980.7
chlorinated	989.2	E863.0	—	E950.6	E962.1	E980.7
mixtures	989.4	E863.3	—	E950.6	E962.1	E980.7
organochlorine (compounds)	989.2	E863.0	—	E950.6	E962.1	E980.7
organophosphorus (compounds)	989.3	E863.1	—	E950.6	E962.1	E980.7
Insular tissue extract	962.3	E858.0	E932.3	E950.4	E962.0	E980.4
Insulin (amorphous) (globin) (isophane) (Lente) (NPH) (protamine) (Semilente) (Ultralente) (zinc)	962.3	E858.0	E932.3	E950.4	E962.0	E980.4
Intranarcon	968.3	E855.1	E938.3	E950.4	E962.0	E980.4
Inulin	977.8	E858.8	E947.8	E950.4	E962.0	E980.4
Invert sugar	974.5	E858.5	E944.5	E950.4	E962.0	E980.4
Iodide NEC (see also Iodine)	976.0	E858.7	E946.0	E950.4	E962.0	E980.4
mercury (ointment)	976.0	E858.7	E946.0	E950.4	E962.0	E980.4
methylate	976.0	E858.7	E946.0	E950.4	E962.0	E980.4
potassium (expectorant) NEC	975.5	E858.6	E945.5	E950.4	E962.0	E980.4
Iodinated glycerol	975.5	E858.6	E945.5	E950.4	E962.0	E980.4
Iodine (antiseptic, external) (tincture) NEC	976.0	E858.7	E946.0	E950.4	E962.0	E980.4
diagnostic	977.8	E858.8	E947.8	E950.4	E962.0	E980.4
for thyroid conditions (antithyroid)	962.8	E858.0	E932.8	E950.4	E962.0	E980.4
vapor	987.8	E869.8	—	E952.8	E962.2	E982.8
Iodized oil	977.8	E858.8	E947.8	E950.4	E962.0	E980.4
Iodobismitol	961.2	E857	E931.2	E950.4	E962.0	E980.4
Iodochlorhydroxyquin	961.3	E857	E931.3	E950.4	E962.0	E980.4
topical	976.0	E858.7	E946.0	E950.4	E962.0	E980.4
Iodoform	976.0	E858.7	E946.0	E950.4	E962.0	E980.4
Iodopanoic acid	977.8	E858.8	E947.8	E950.4	E962.0	E980.4
Iodophthalein	977.8	E858.8	E947.8	E950.4	E962.0	E980.4
Ion exchange resins	974.5	E858.5	E944.5	E950.4	E962.0	E980.4
Iopanoic acid	977.8	E858.8	E947.8	E950.4	E962.0	E980.4
Iophendylate	977.8	E858.8	E947.8	E950.4	E962.0	E980.4
Iothiouracil	962.8	E858.0	E932.8	E950.4	E962.0	E980.4
Ipecac	973.6	E858.4	E943.6	E950.4	E962.0	E980.4
Ipecacuanha	973.6	E858.4	E943.6	E950.4	E962.0	E980.4
Ipodate	977.8	E858.8	E947.8	E950.4	E962.0	E980.4
Ipral	967.0	E851	E937.0	E950.1	E962.0	E980.1
Iproniazid	969.0	E854.0	E939.0	E950.3	E962.0	E980.3
Iron (compounds) (medicinal) (preparations)	964.0	E858.2	E934.0	E950.4	E962.0	E980.4
dextran	964.0	E858.2	E934.0	E950.4	E962.0	E980.4
nonmedicinal (dust) (fumes) NEC	985.8	E866.4	—	E950.9	E962.1	E980.9
Irritant drug	977.9	E858.9	E947.9	E950.5	E962.0	E980.5
Ismelin	972.6	E858.3	E942.6	E950.4	E962.0	E980.4
Isoamyl nitrite	972.4	E858.3	E942.4	E950.4	E962.0	E980.4
Isobutyl acetate	982.8	E862.4	—	E950.9	E962.1	E980.9
Isocarboxazid	969.0	E854.0	E939.0	E950.3	E962.0	E980.3
Isoephedrine	971.2	E855.5	E941.2	E950.4	E962.0	E980.4

TABLE OF DRUGS AND CHEMICALS

Substance	Poisoning	Accident	Therapeutic-Use	Suicide Attempt	Assault	Undetermined
Isoetharine	971.2	E855.5	E941.2	E950.4	E962.0	E980.4
Isofluorophate	971.0	E855.3	E941.0	E950.4	E962.0	E980.4
Isoniazid (INH)	961.8	E857	E931.8	E950.4	E962.0	E980.4
Isopentaquine	961.4	E857	E931.4	E950.4	E962.0	E980.4
Isophane insulin	962.3	E858.0	E932.3	E950.4	E962.0	E980.4
Isopregnenone	962.2	E858.0	E932.2	E950.4	E962.0	E980.4
Isoprenaline	971.2	E855.5	E941.2	E950.4	E962.0	E980.4
Isopropamide	971.1	E855.4	E941.1	E950.4	E962.0	E980.4
Isopropanol	980.2	E860.3	—	E950.9	E962.1	E980.9
topical (germicide)	976.0	E858.7	E946.0	E950.4	E962.0	E980.4
Isopropyl						
acetate	982.8	E862.4	—	E950.9	E962.1	E980.9
alcohol	980.2	E860.3	—	E950.9	E962.1	E980.9
topical (germicide)	976.0	E858.7	E946.0	E950.4	E962.0	E980.4
ether	982.8	E862.4	—	E950.9	E962.1	E980.9
Isoproterenol	971.2	E855.5	E941.2	E950.4	E962.0	E980.4
Isosorbide dinitrate	972.4	E858.3	E942.4	E950.4	E962.0	E980.4
Isothipendyl	963.0	E858.1	E933.0	E950.4	E962.0	E980.4
Isoxazolyl penicillin	960.0	E856	E930.0	E950.4	E962.0	E980.4
Isoxsuprine hydrochloride	972.5	E858.3	E942.5	E950.4	E962.0	E980.4
l-thyroxine sodium	962.7	E858.0	E932.7	E950.4	E962.0	E980.4
Jaborandi (pilocarpus) (extract)	971.0	E855.3	E941.0	E950.4	E962.0	E980.4
Jalap	973.1	E858.4	E943.1	E950.4	E962.0	E980.4
Jamaica						
dogwood (bark)	965.7	E850.7	E935.7	E950.0	E962.0	E980.0
ginger	989.8	E866.8	—	E950.9	E962.1	E980.9
Jatropha	988.2	E865.4	—	E950.9	E962.1	E980.9
curcas	988.2	E865.3	—	E950.9	E962.1	E980.9
Jectofer	964.0	E858.2	E934.0	E950.4	E962.0	E980.4
Jellyfish (sting)	989.5	E905.6	—	E950.9	E962.1	E980.9
Jequirity (bean)	988.2	E865.3	—	E950.9	E962.1	E980.9
Jimson weed	988.2	E865.4	—	E950.9	E962.1	E980.9
seeds	988.2	E865.3	—	E950.9	E962.1	E980.9
Juniper tar (oil) (ointment)	976.4	E858.7	E946.4	E950.4	E962.0	E980.4
Kallikrein	972.5	E858.3	E942.5	E950.4	E962.0	E980.4
Kanamycin	960.6	E856	E930.6	E950.4	E962.0	E980.4
Kantrex	960.6	E856	E930.6	E950.4	E962.0	E980.4
Kaolin	973.5	E858.4	E943.5	E950.4	E962.0	E980.4
Karaya (gum)	973.3	E858.4	E943.3	E950.4	E962.0	E980.4
Kemithal	968.3	E855.1	E938.3	E950.4	E962.0	E980.4
Kenacort	962.0	E858.0	E932.0	E950.4	E962.0	E980.4
Keratolytics	976.4	E858.7	E946.4	E950.4	E962.0	E980.4
Keratoplastics	976.4	E858.7	E946.4	E950.4	E962.0	E980.4
Kerosene, kerosine (fuel) (solvent) NEC	981	E862.4	—	E950.9	E962.1	E980.9
insecticide	981	E863.4	—	E950.6	E962.1	E980.7
vapor	987.1	E869.8	—	E952.8	E962.2	E982.8
Ketamine	968.3	E855.1	E938.3	E950.4	E962.0	E980.4
Ketobemidone	965.09	E850.2	E935.2	E950.0	E962.0	E980.0
Ketols	982.8	E862.4	—	E950.9	E962.1	E980.9
Ketone oils	982.8	E862.4	—	E950.9	E962.1	E980.9
Kiln gas or vapor (carbon monoxide)	986	E868.8	—	E952.1	E962.2	E982.1
Konsyl	973.3	E858.4	E943.3	E950.4	E962.0	E980.4
Kosam seed	988.2	E865.3	—	E950.9	E962.1	E980.9
Krait (venom)	989.5	E905.0	—	E950.9	E962.1	E980.9
Kwell (insecticide)	989.2	E863.0	—	E950.6	E962.1	E980.7
anti-infective (topical)	976.0	E858.7	E946.0	E950.4	E962.0	E980.4
Laburnum (flowers) (seeds)	988.2	E865.3	—	E950.9	E962.1	E980.9
leaves	988.2	E865.4	—	E950.9	E962.1	E980.9
Lacquers	989.8	E861.6	—	E950.9	E962.1	E980.9
Lacrimogenic gas	987.5	E869.3	—	E952.8	E962.2	E982.8
Lactic acid	983.1	E864.1	—	E950.7	E962.1	E980.6
Lactobacillus acidophilus	973.5	E858.4	E943.5	E950.4	E962.0	E980.4
Lactoflavin	963.5	E858.1	E933.5	E950.4	E962.0	E980.4
Lactuca (virosa) (extract)	967.8	E852.8	E937.8	E950.2	E962.0	E980.2
Lactucarium	967.8	E852.8	E937.8	E950.2	E962.0	E980.2
Laevulose	974.5	E858.5	E944.5	E950.4	E962.0	E980.4
Lanatoside(C)	972.1	E858.3	E942.1	E950.4	E962.0	E980.4
Lanolin (lotion)	976.3	E858.7	E946.3	E950.4	E962.0	E980.4
Largactil	969.1	E853.0	E939.1	E950.3	E962.0	E980.3
Larkspur	988.2	E865.3	—	E950.9	E962.1	E980.9
Laroxyl	969.0	E854.0	E939.0	E950.3	E962.0	E980.3
Lasix	974.4	E858.5	E944.4	E950.4	E962.0	E980.4
Lathyrus (seed)	988.2	E865.3	—	E950.9	E962.1	E980.9
Laudanum	965.09	E850.2	E935.2	E950.0	E962.0	E980.0
Laudexium	975.2	E858.6	E945.2	E950.4	E962.0	E980.4
Laurel, black or cherry	988.2	E865.4	—	E950.9	E962.1	E980.9

TABLE OF DRUGS AND CHEMICALS

Substance	Poisoning	Accident	Therapeutic-Use	Suicide Attempt	Assault	Undetermined
Laurolinium	976.0	E858.7	E946.0	E950.4	E962.0	E980.4
Lauryl sulfoacetate	976.2	E858.7	E946.2	E950.4	E962.0	E980.4
Laxatives NEC	973.3	E858.4	E943.3	E950.4	E962.0	E980.4
emollient	973.2	E858.4	E943.2	E950.4	E962.0	E980.4
L-dopa	966.4	E855.0	E936.4	E950.4	E962.0	E980.4
Lead (dust) (fumes) (vapor) NEC	984.9	E866.0	—	E950.9	E962.1	E980.9
acetate (dust)	984.1	E866.0	—	E950.9	E962.1	E980.9
anti-infectives	961.2	E857	E931.2	E950.4	E962.0	E980.4
antiknock compound (tetraethyl)	984.1	E862.1	—	E950.9	E962.1	E980.9
arsenate, arsenite (dust) (insecticide) (vapor)	985.1	E863.4	—	E950.8	E962.1	E980.8
herbicide	985.1	E863.5	—	E950.8	E962.1	E980.8
carbonate	984.0	E866.0	—	E950.9	E962.1	E980.9
paint	984.0	E861.5	—	E950.9	E962.1	E980.9
chromate	984.0	E866.0	—	E950.9	E962.1	E980.9
paint	984.0	E861.5	—	E950.9	E962.1	E980.9
dioxide	984.0	E866.0	—	E950.9	E962.1	E980.9
inorganic (compound)	984.0	E866.0	—	E950.9	E962.1	E980.9
paint	984.0	E861.5	—	E950.9	E962.1	E980.9
iodide	984.0	E866.0	—	E950.9	E962.1	E980.9
pigment (paint)	984.0	E861.5	—	E950.9	E962.1	E980.9
monoxide (dust)	984.0	E866.0	—	E950.9	E962.1	E980.9
paint	984.0	E861.5	—	E950.9	E962.1	E980.9
organic	984.1	E866.0	—	E950.9	E962.1	E980.9
oxide	984.0	E866.0	—	E950.9	E962.1	E980.9
paint	984.0	E861.5	—	E950.9	E962.1	E980.9
paint	984.0	E861.5	—	E950.9	E962.1	E980.9
salts	984.0	E866.0	—	E950.9	E962.1	E980.9
specified compound NEC	984.8	E866.0	—	E950.9	E962.1	E980.9
tetra-ethyl	984.1	E862.1	—	E950.9	E962.1	E980.9
Lebanese red	969.6	E854.1	E939.6	E950.3	E962.0	E980.3
Lente Iletin (insulin)	962.3	E858.0	E932.3	E950.4	E962.0	E980.4
Leptazol	970.0	E854.3	E940.0	E950.4	E962.0	E980.4
Leritine	965.09	E850.2	E935.2	E950.0	E962.0	E980.0
Letter	962.7	E858.0	E932.7	E950.4	E962.0	E980.4
Lettuce opium	967.8	E852.8	E937.8	E950.2	E962.0	E980.2
Leucovorin (factor)	964.1	E858.2	E934.1	E950.4	E962.0	E980.4
Leukeran	963.1	E858.1	E933.1	E950.4	E962.0	E980.4
Levallorphan	970.1	E854.3	E940.1	E950.4	E962.0	E980.4
Levanil	967.8	E852.8	E937.8	E950.2	E962.0	E980.2
Levarterenol	971.2	E855.5	E941.2	E950.4	E962.0	E980.4
Levodopa	966.4	E855.0	E936.4	E950.4	E962.0	E980.4
Levo-dromoran	965.09	E850.2	E935.2	E950.0	E962.0	E980.0
Levoid	962.7	E858.0	E932.7	E950.4	E962.0	E980.4
Levo-iso-methadone	965.02	E850.1	E935.1	E950.0	E962.0	E980.0
Levomepromazine	967.8	E852.8	E937.8	E950.2	E962.0	E980.2
Levoprome	967.8	E852.8	E937.8	E950.2	E962.0	E980.2
Levopropoxyphene	975.4	E858.6	E945.4	E950.4	E962.0	E980.4
Levorphan, levophanol	965.09	E850.2	E935.2	E950.0	E962.0	E980.0
Levothyroxine (sodium)	962.7	E858.0	E932.7	E950.4	E962.0	E980.4
Levsin	971.1	E855.4	E941.1	E950.4	E962.0	E980.4
Levulose	974.5	E858.5	E944.5	E950.4	E962.0	E980.4
Lewisite (gas)	985.1	E866.3	—	E950.8	E962.1	E980.8
Librium	969.4	E853.2	E939.4	E950.3	E962.0	E980.3
Lidex	976.0	E858.7	E946.0	E950.4	E962.0	E980.4
Lidocaine (infiltration) (topical)	968.5	E855.2	E938.5	E950.4	E962.0	E980.4
nerve block (peripheral) (plexus)	968.6	E855.2	E938.6	E950.4	E962.0	E980.4
spinal	968.7	E855.2	E938.7	E950.4	E962.0	E980.4
Lighter fluid	981	E862.1	—	E950.9	E962.1	E980.9
Lignocaine (infiltration) (topical)	968.5	E855.2	E938.5	E950.4	E962.0	E980.4
nerve block (peripheral) (plexus)	968.6	E855.2	E938.6	E950.4	E962.0	E980.4
spinal	968.7	E855.2	E938.7	E950.4	E962.0	E980.4
Ligroin(e) (solvent)	981	E862.0	—	E950.9	E962.1	E980.9
vapor	987.1	E869.8	—	E952.8	E962.2	E982.8
Ligustrum vulgare	988.2	E865.3	—	E950.9	E962.1	E980.9
Lily of the valley	988.2	E865.4	—	E950.9	E962.1	E980.9
Lime (chloride)	983.2	E864.2	—	E950.7	E962.1	E980.6
solution, sulferated	976.4	E858.7	E946.4	E950.4	E962.0	E980.4
Limonene	982.8	E862.4	—	E950.9	E962.1	E980.9
Lincomycin	960.8	E856	E930.8	E950.4	E962.0	E980.4
Lindane (insecticide) (vapor)	989.2	E863.0	—	E950.6	E962.1	E980.7
anti-infective (topical)	976.0	E858.7	E946.0	E950.4	E962.0	E980.4
Liniments NEC	976.9	E858.7	E946.9	E950.4	E962.0	E980.4
Linoleic acid	972.2	E858.3	E942.2	E950.4	E962.0	E980.4
Liothyronine	962.7	E858.0	E932.7	E950.4	E962.0	E980.4
Liotrix	962.7	E858.0	E932.7	E950.4	E962.0	E980.4
Lipancreatin	973.4	E858.4	E943.4	E950.4	E962.0	E980.4

Substance	Poisoning	Accident	Therapeutic-Use	Suicide Attempt	Assault	Undetermined
Lipo-Lutin	962.2	E858.0	E932.2	E950.4	E962.0	E980.4
Lipotropic agents	977.1	E858.8	E947.1	E950.4	E962.0	E980.4
Liquefied petroleum gases	987.0	E868.0	—	E951.1	E962.2	E981.1
piped (pure or mixed with air)	987.0	E867	—	E951.0	E962.2	E981.0
Liquid						
petrolatum	973.2	E858.4	E943.2	E950.4	E962.0	E980.4
substance	989.9	E866.9	—	E950.9	E962.1	E980.9
specified NEC	989.8	E866.8	—	E950.9	E962.1	E980.9
Lirugen	979.4	E858.8	E949.4	E950.4	E962.0	E980.4
Lithane	969.8	E855.8	E939.8	E950.3	E962.0	E980.3
Lithium	985.8	E866.4	—	E950.9	E962.1	E980.9
carbonate	969.8	E855.8	E939.8	E950.3	E962.0	E980.3
Lithonate	969.8	E855.8	E939.8	E950.3	E962.0	E980.3
Liver (extract) (injection) (preparations)	964.1	E858.2	E934.1	E950.4	E962.0	E980.4
Lizard (bite) (venom)	989.5	E905.0	—	E950.9	E962.1	E980.9
LMD	964.8	E858.2	E934.8	E950.4	E962.0	E980.4
Lobelia	988.2	E865.4	—	E950.9	E962.1	E980.9
Lobeline	970.0	E854.3	E940.0	E950.4	E962.0	E980.4
Locorten	976.0	E858.7	E946.0	E950.4	E962.0	E980.4
Lolium temulentum	988.2	E865.3	—	E950.9	E962.1	E980.9
Lomotil	973.5	E858.4	E943.5	E950.4	E962.0	E980.4
Lomustine	963.1	E858.1	E933.1	E950.4	E962.0	E980.4
Lophophora williamsii	969.6	E854.1	E939.6	E950.3	E962.0	E980.3
Lorazepam	969.4	E853.2	E939.4	E950.3	E962.0	E980.3
Lotions NEC	976.9	E858.7	E946.9	E950.4	E962.0	E980.4
Lotusate	967.0	E851	E937.0	E950.1	E962.0	E980.1
Lowila	976.2	E858.7	E946.2	E950.4	E962.0	E980.4
Loxapine	969.3	E853.8	E939.3	E950.3	E962.0	E980.3
Lozenges (throat)	976.6	E858.7	E946.6	E950.4	E962.0	E980.4
LSD (25)	969.6	E854.1	E939.6	E950.3	E962.0	E980.3
Lubricating oil NEC	981	E862.2	—	E950.9	E962.1	E980.9
Lucanthone	961.6	E857	E931.6	E950.4	E962.0	E980.4
Luminal	967.0	E851	E937.0	E950.1	E962.0	E980.1
Lung irritant (gas) NEC	987.9	E869.9	—	E952.9	E962.2	E982.9
Lutocylol	962.2	E858.0	E932.2	E950.4	E962.0	E980.4
Lutromone	962.2	E858.0	E932.2	E950.4	E962.0	E980.4
Lututrin	975.0	E858.6	E945.0	E950.4	E962.0	E980.4
Lye (concentrated)	983.2	E864.2	—	E950.7	E962.1	E980.6
Lygranum (skin test)	977.8	E858.8	E947.8	E950.4	E962.0	E980.4
Lymecycline	960.4	E856	E930.4	E950.4	E962.0	E980.4
Lymphogranuloma venereum antigen	977.8	E858.8	E947.8	E950.4	E962.0	E980.4
Lynestrenol	962.2	E858.0	E932.2	E950.4	E962.0	E980.4
Lyovac Sodium Edecrin	974.4	E858.5	E944.4	E950.4	E962.0	E980.4
Lypressin	962.5	E858.0	E932.5	E950.4	E962.0	E980.4
Lysergic acid (amide) (diethylamide)	969.6	E854.1	E939.6	E950.3	E962.0	E980.3
Lysergide	969.6	E854.1	E939.6	E950.3	E962.0	E980.3
Lysine vasopressin	962.5	E858.0	E932.5	E950.4	E962.0	E980.4
Lysol	983.0	E864.0	—	E950.7	E962.1	E980.6
Lytta (vitatta)	976.8	E858.7	E946.8	E950.4	E962.0	E980.4
Mace	987.5	E869.3	—	E952.8	E962.2	E982.8
Macrolides (antibiotics)	960.3	E856	E930.3	E950.4	E962.0	E980.4
Mafenide	976.0	E858.7	E946.0	E950.4	E962.0	E980.4
Magaldrate	973.0	E858.4	E943.0	E950.4	E962.0	E980.4
Magic mushroom	969.6	E854.1	E939.6	E950.3	E962.0	E980.3
Magnamycin	960.8	E856	E930.8	E950.4	E962.0	E980.4
Magnesia magma	973.0	E858.4	E943.0	E950.4	E962.0	E980.4
Magnesium (compounds) (fumes) NEC	985.8	E866.4	—	E950.9	E962.1	E980.9
antacid	973.0	E858.4	E943.0	E950.4	E962.0	E980.4
carbonate	973.0	E858.4	E943.0	E950.4	E962.0	E980.4
cathartic	973.3	E858.4	E943.3	E950.4	E962.0	E980.4
citrate	973.3	E858.4	E943.3	E950.4	E962.0	E980.4
hydroxide	973.0	E858.4	E943.0	E950.4	E962.0	E980.4
oxide	973.0	E858.4	E943.0	E950.4	E962.0	E980.4
sulfate (oral)	973.3	E858.4	E943.3	E950.4	E962.0	E980.4
intravenous	966.3	E855.0	E936.3	E950.4	E962.0	E980.4
trisilicate	973.0	E858.4	E943.0	E950.4	E962.0	E980.4
Malathion (insecticide)	989.3	E863.1	—	E950.6	E962.1	E980.7
Male fern (oleoresin)	961.6	E857	E931.6	E950.4	E962.0	E980.4
Mandelic acid	961.9	E857	E931.9	E950.4	E962.0	E980.4
Manganese compounds (fumes) NEC	985.2	E866.4	—	E950.9	E962.1	E980.9
Mannitol (diuretic) (medicinal) NEC	974.4	E858.5	E944.4	E950.4	E962.0	E980.4
hexanitrate	972.4	E858.3	E942.4	E950.4	E962.0	E980.4
mustard	963.1	E858.1	E933.1	E950.4	E962.0	E980.4
Mannomustine	963.1	E858.1	E933.1	E950.4	E962.0	E980.4
MAO inhibitors	969.0	E854.0	E939.0	E950.3	E962.0	E980.3
Mapharsen	961.1	E857	E931.1	E950.4	E962.0	E980.4

TABLE OF DRUGS AND CHEMICALS

Substance	Poisoning	Accident	Therapeutic-Use	Suicide Attempt	Assault	Undetermined
Marcaine	968.9	E855.2	E938.9	E950.4	E962.0	E980.4
infiltration (subcutaneous)	968.5	E855.2	E938.5	E950.4	E962.0	E980.4
nerve block (peripheral) (plexus)	968.6	E855.2	E938.6	E950.4	E962.0	E980.4
Marezine	963.0	E858.1	E933.0	E950.4	E962.0	E980.4
Marihuana, marijuana (derivatives)	969.6	E854.1	E939.6	E950.3	E962.0	E980.3
Marine animals or plants (sting)	989.5	E905.6	—	E950.9	E962.1	E980.9
Marplan	969.0	E854.0	E939.0	E950.3	E962.0	E980.3
Marsh gas	987.1	E869.8	—	E952.8	E962.2	E982.8
Marsilid	969.0	E854.0	E939.0	E950.3	E962.0	E980.3
Matulane	963.1	E858.1	E933.1	E950.4	E962.0	E980.4
Mazindol	977.0	E858.8	E947.0	E950.4	E962.0	E980.4
Meadow saffron	988.2	E865.3	—	E950.9	E962.1	E980.9
Measles vaccine	979.4	E858.8	E949.4	E950.4	E962.0	E980.4
Meat, noxious or nonbacterial	988.8	E865.0	—	E950.9	E962.1	E980.9
Mebanazine	969.0	E854.0	E939.0	E950.3	E962.0	E980.3
Mebaral	967.0	E851	E937.0	E950.1	E962.0	E980.1
Mebendazole	961.6	E857	E931.6	E950.4	E962.0	E980.4
Mebeverine	975.1	E858.6	E945.1	E950.4	E962.0	E980.4
Mebhydroline	963.0	E858.1	E933.0	E950.4	E962.0	E980.4
Mebrophenhydramine	963.0	E858.1	E933.0	E950.4	E962.0	E980.4
Mebutamate	969.5	E853.8	E939.5	E950.3	E962.0	E980.3
Mecamylamine (chloride)	972.3	E858.3	E942.3	E950.4	E962.0	E980.4
Mechlorethamine hydrochloride	963.1	E858.1	E933.1	E950.4	E962.0	E980.4
Meclizene (hydrochloride)	963.0	E858.1	E933.0	E950.4	E962.0	E980.4
Meclofenoxate	970.0	E854.3	E940.0	E950.4	E962.0	E980.4
Meclozine (hydrochloride)	963.0	E858.1	E933.0	E950.4	E962.0	E980.4
Medazepam	969.5	E853.2	E939.4	E950.3	E962.0	E980.3
Medicine, medicinal substance	977.9	E858.9	E947.9	E950.5	E962.0	E980.5
specified NEC	977.8	E858.8	E947.8	E950.4	E962.0	E980.4
Medinal	967.0	E851	E937.0	E950.1	E962.0	E980.1
Medomin	967.0	E851	E937.0	E950.1	E962.0	E980.1
Medroxyprogesterone	962.2	E858.0	E932.2	E950.4	E962.0	E980.4
Medrysone	976.5	E858.7	E946.5	E950.4	E962.0	E980.4
Mefenamic acid	965.7	E850.7	E935.7	E950.0	E962.0	E980.0
Megahallucinogen	969.6	E854.1	E939.6	E950.3	E962.0	E980.3
Megestrol	962.2	E858.0	E932.2	E950.4	E962.0	E980.4
Meglumine	977.8	E858.8	E947.8	E950.4	E962.0	E980.4
Meladinin	976.3	E858.7	E946.3	E950.4	E962.0	E980.4
Melanizing agents	976.3	E858.7	E946.3	E950.4	E962.0	E980.4
Melarsoprol	961.1	E857	E931.1	E950.4	E962.0	E980.4
Melia azedarach	988.2	E865.3	—	E950.9	E962.1	E980.9
Mellaril	969.1	E853.0	E939.1	E950.3	E962.0	E980.3
Meloxine	976.3	E858.7	E946.3	E950.4	E962.0	E980.4
Melphalan	963.1	E858.1	E933.1	E950.4	E962.0	E980.4
Menadiol sodium diphosphate	964.3	E858.2	E934.3	E950.4	E962.0	E980.4
Menadione (sodium bisulfite)	964.3	E858.2	E934.3	E950.4	E962.0	E980.4
Menaphthone	964.3	E858.2	E934.3	E950.4	E962.0	E980.4
Meningococcal vaccine	978.8	E858.8	E948.8	E950.4	E962.0	E980.4
Menningovax-C	978.8	E858.8	E948.8	E950.4	E962.0	E980.4
Menotropins	962.4	E858.0	E932.4	E950.4	E962.0	E980.4
Menthol NEC	976.1	E858.7	E946.1	E950.4	E962.0	E980.4
Mepacrine	961.3	E857	E931.3	E950.4	E962.0	E980.4
Meparfynol	967.8	E852.8	E937.8	E950.2	E962.0	E980.2
Mepazine	969.1	E853.0	E939.1	E950.3	E962.0	E980.3
Mepenzolate	971.1	E855.4	E941.1	E950.4	E962.0	E980.4
Meperidine	965.09	E850.2	E935.2	E950.0	E962.0	E980.0
Mephenamin(e)	966.4	E855.0	E936.4	E950.4	E962.0	E980.4
Mephenesin (carbamate)	968.0	E855.1	E938.0	E950.4	E962.0	E980.4
Mephenoxalone	969.5	E853.8	E939.5	E950.3	E962.0	E980.3
Mephentermine	971.2	E855.5	E941.2	E950.4	E962.0	E980.4
Mephenytoin	966.1	E855.0	E936.1	E950.4	E962.0	E980.4
Mephobarbital	967.0	E851	E937.0	E950.1	E962.0	E980.1
Mepiperphenidol	971.1	E855.4	E941.1	E950.4	E962.0	E980.4
Mepivacaine	968.9	E855.2	E938.9	E950.4	E962.0	E980.4
infiltration (subcutaneous)	968.5	E855.2	E938.5	E950.4	E962.0	E980.4
nerve block (peripheral) (plexus)	968.6	E855.2	E938.6	E950.4	E962.0	E980.4
topical (surface)	968.5	E855.2	E938.5	E950.4	E962.0	E980.4
Meprednisone	962.0	E858.0	E932.0	E950.4	E962.0	E980.4
Meprobam	969.5	E853.8	E939.5	E950.3	E962.0	E980.3
Meprobamate	969.5	E853.8	E939.5	E950.3	E962.0	E980.3
Mepyramine (maleate)	963.0	E858.1	E933.0	E950.4	E962.0	E980.4
Meralluride	974.0	E858.5	E944.0	E950.4	E962.0	E980.4
Merbaphen	974.0	E858.5	E944.0	E950.4	E962.0	E980.4
Merbromin	976.0	E858.7	E946.0	E950.4	E962.0	E980.4
Mercaptomerin	974.0	E858.5	E944.0	E950.4	E962.0	E980.4
Mercaptopurine	963.1	E858.1	E933.1	E950.4	E962.0	E980.4

TABLE OF DRUGS AND CHEMICALS

Substance	Poisoning	External Cause (E-Code) Accident	Therapeutic-Use	Suicide Attempt	Assault	Undetermined
Mercumatilin	974.0	E858.5	E944.0	E950.4	E962.0	E980.4
Mercuramide	974.0	E858.5	E944.0	E950.4	E962.0	E980.4
Mercuranin	976.0	E858.7	E946.0	E950.4	E962.0	E980.4
Mercurochrome	976.0	E858.7	E946.0	E950.4	E962.0	E980.4
Mercury, mercuric, mercurous (compounds) (cyanide) (fumes)						
(nonmedicinal) (vapor) NEC	985.0	E866.1	—	E950.9	E962.1	E980.9
ammoniated	976.0	E858.7	E946.0	E950.4	E962.0	E980.4
anti-infective	961.2	E857	E931.2	E950.4	E962.0	E980.4
topical	976.0	E858.7	E946.0	E950.4	E962.0	E980.4
chloride (antiseptic) NEC	976.0	E858.7	E946.0	E950.4	E962.0	E980.4
fungicide	985.0	E863.6	—	E950.6	E962.1	E980.7
diuretic compounds	974.0	E858.5	E944.0	E950.4	E962.0	E980.4
fungicide	985.0	E863.6	—	E950.6	E962.1	E980.7
organic (fungicide)	985.0	E863.6	—	E950.6	E962.1	E980.7
Merethoxylline	974.0	E858.5	E944.0	E950.4	E962.0	E980.4
Mersalyl	974.0	E858.5	E944.0	E950.4	E962.0	E980.4
Merthiolate (topical)	976.0	E858.7	E946.0	E950.4	E962.0	E980.4
ophthalmic preparation	976.5	E858.7	E946.5	E950.4	E962.0	E980.4
Meruvax	979.4	E858.8	E949.4	E950.4	E962.0	E980.4
Mescal buttons	969.6	E854.1	E939.6	E950.3	E962.0	E980.3
Mescaline (salts)	969.6	E854.1	E939.6	E950.3	E962.0	E980.3
Mesoridazine besylate	969.1	E853.0	E939.1	E950.3	E962.0	E980.3
Mestanolone	962.1	E858.0	E932.1	E950.4	E962.0	E980.4
Mestranol	962.2	E858.0	E932.2	E950.4	E962.0	E980.4
Metacresylacetate	976.0	E858.7	E946.0	E950.4	E962.0	E980.4
Metaldehyde (snail killer) NEC	989.4	E863.4	—	E950.6	E962.1	E980.7
Metals (heavy) (nonmedicinal) NEC	985.9	E866.4	—	E950.9	E962.1	E980.9
dust, fumes, or vapor NEC	985.9	E866.4	—	E950.9	E962.1	E980.9
light NEC	985.9	E866.4	—	E950.9	E962.1	E980.9
dust, fumes, or vapor NEC	985.9	E866.4	—	E950.9	E962.1	E980.9
pesticides (dust) (vapor)	985.9	E863.4	—	E950.6	E962.1	E980.7
Metamucil	973.3	E858.4	E943.3	E950.4	E962.0	E980.4
Metaphen	976.0	E858.7	E946.0	E950.4	E962.0	E980.4
Metaproterenol	975.1	E858.6	E945.1	E950.4	E962.0	E980.4
Metaraminol	972.8	E858.3	E942.8	E950.4	E962.0	E980.4
Metaxalone	968.0	E855.1	E938.0	E950.4	E962.0	E980.4
Metformin	962.3	E858.0	E932.3	E950.4	E962.0	E980.4
Methacycline	960.4	E856	E930.4	E950.4	E962.0	E980.4
Methadone	965.02	E850.1	E935.1	E950.0	E962.0	E980.0
Methallenestril	962.2	E858.0	E932.2	E950.4	E962.0	E980.4
Methamphetamine	969.7	E854.2	E939.7	E950.3	E962.0	E980.3
Methandienone	962.1	E858.0	E932.1	E950.4	E962.0	E980.4
Methandriol	962.1	E858.0	E932.1	E950.4	E962.0	E980.4
Methandrostenolone	962.1	E858.0	E932.1	E950.4	E962.0	E980.4
Methane gas	987.1	E869.8	—	E952.8	E962.2	E982.8
Methanol	980.1	E860.2	—	E950.9	E962.1	E980.9
vapor	987.8	E869.8	—	E952.8	E962.2	E982.8
Methantheline	971.1	E855.4	E941.1	E950.4	E962.0	E980.4
Methaphenilene	963.0	E858.1	E933.0	E950.4	E962.0	E980.4
Methapyrilene	963.0	E858.1	E933.0	E950.4	E962.0	E980.4
Methaqualone (compounds)	967.4	E852.3	E937.4	E950.2	E962.0	E980.2
Metharbital, metharbitone	967.0	E851	E937.0	E950.1	E962.0	E980.1
Methazolamide	974.2	E858.5	E944.2	E950.4	E962.0	E980.4
Methdilazine	963.0	E858.1	E933.0	E950.4	E962.0	E980.4
Methedrine	969.7	E854.2	E939.7	E950.3	E962.0	E980.3
Methenamine (mandelate)	961.9	E857	E931.9	E950.4	E962.0	E980.4
Methenolone	962.1	E858.0	E932.1	E950.4	E962.0	E980.4
Methergine	975.0	E858.6	E945.0	E950.4	E962.0	E980.4
Methiacil	962.8	E858.0	E932.8	E950.4	E962.0	E980.4
Methicillin (sodium)	960.0	E856	E930.0	E950.4	E962.0	E980.4
Methimazole	962.8	E858.0	E932.8	E950.4	E962.0	E980.4
Methionine	977.1	E858.8	E947.1	E950.4	E962.0	E980.4
Methisazone	961.7	E857	E931.7	E950.4	E962.0	E980.4
Methitural	967.0	E851	E937.0	E950.1	E962.0	E980.1
Methixene	971.1	E855.4	E941.1	E950.4	E962.0	E980.4
Methobarbital, methobarbitone	967.0	E851	E937.0	E950.1	E962.0	E980.1
Methocarbamol	968.0	E855.1	E938.0	E950.4	E962.0	E980.4
Methohexital, methohexitone (sodium)	968.3	E855.1	E938.3	E950.4	E962.0	E980.4
Methoin	966.1	E855.0	E936.1	E950.4	E962.0	E980.4
Methopholine	965.7	E850.7	E935.7	E950.0	E962.0	E980.0
Methorate	975.4	E858.6	E945.4	E950.4	E962.0	E980.4
Methoserpidine	972.6	E858.3	E942.6	E950.4	E962.0	E980.4
Methotrexate	963.1	E858.1	E933.1	E950.4	E962.0	E980.4
Methotrimeprazine	967.8	E852.8	E937.8	E950.2	E962.0	E980.2
Methoxa-Dome	976.3	E858.7	E946.3	E950.4	E962.0	E980.4
Methoxamine	971.2	E855.5	E941.2	E950.4	E962.0	E980.4

TABLE OF DRUGS AND CHEMICALS

Substance	Poisoning	Accident	Therapeutic-Use	Suicide Attempt	Assault	Undetermined
Methoxsalen	976.3	E858.7	E946.3	E950.4	E962.0	E980.4
Methoxybenzyl penicillin	960.0	E856	E930.0	E950.4	E962.0	E980.4
Methoxychlor	989.2	E863.0	—	E950.6	E962.1	E980.7
Methoxyflurane	968.2	E855.1	E938.2	E950.4	E962.0	E980.4
Methoxyphenamine	971.2	E855.5	E941.2	E950.4	E962.0	E980.4
Methoxypromazine	969.1	E853.0	E939.1	E950.3	E962.0	E980.3
Methoxypsoralen	976.3	E858.7	E946.3	E950.4	E962.0	E980.4
Methscopolamine (bromide)	971.1	E855.4	E941.1	E950.4	E962.0	E980.4
Methsuximide	966.2	E855.0	E936.2	E950.4	E962.0	E980.4
Methyclothiazide	974.3	E858.5	E944.3	E950.4	E962.0	E980.4
Methyl						
acetate	982.8	E862.4	—	E950.9	E962.1	E980.9
acetone	982.8	E862.4	—	E950.9	E962.1	E980.9
alcohol	980.1	E860.2	—	E950.9	E962.1	E980.9
amphetamine	969.7	E854.2	E939.7	E950.3	E962.0	E980.3
androstanolone	962.1	E858.0	E932.1	E950.4	E962.0	E980.4
atropine	971.1	E855.4	E941.1	E950.4	E962.0	E980.4
benzene	982.0	E862.4	—	E950.9	E962.1	E980.9
bromide (gas)	987.8	E869.8	—	E952.8	E962.2	E982.8
fumigant	987.8	E863.8	—	E950.6	E962.2	E980.7
butanol	980.8	E860.8	—	E950.9	E962.1	E980.9
carbinol	980.1	E860.2	—	E950.9	E962.1	E980.9
cellosolve	982.8	E862.4	—	E950.9	E962.1	E980.9
cellulose	973.3	E858.4	E943.3	E950.4	E962.0	E980.4
chloride (gas)	987.8	E869.8	—	E952.8	E962.2	E982.8
cyclohexane	982.8	E862.4	—	E950.9	E962.1	E980.9
cyclohexanone	982.8	E862.4	—	E950.9	E962.1	E980.9
dihydromorphinone	965.09	E850.2	E935.2	E950.0	E962.0	E980.0
ergometrine	975.0	E858.6	E945.0	E950.4	E962.0	E980.4
ergonovine	975.0	E858.6	E945.0	E950.4	E962.0	E980.4
ethyl ketone	982.8	E862.4	—	E950.9	E962.1	E980.9
hydrazine	983.9	E864.3	—	E950.7	E962.1	E980.6
isobutyl ketone	982.8	E862.4	—	E950.9	E962.1	E980.9
morphine NEC	965.09	E850.2	E935.2	E950.0	E962.0	E980.0
parafynol	967.8	E852.8	E937.8	E950.2	E962.0	E980.2
parathion	989.3	E863.1	—	E950.6	E962.1	E980.7
pentynol NEC	967.8	E852.8	E937.8	E950.2	E962.0	E980.2
peridol	969.2	E853.1	E939.2	E950.3	E962.0	E980.3
phenidate	969.7	E854.2	E939.7	E950.3	E962.0	E980.3
prednisolone	962.0	E858.0	E932.0	E950.4	E962.0	E980.4
ENT agent	976.6	E858.7	E946.6	E950.4	E962.0	E980.4
ophthalmic preparation	976.5	E858.7	E946.5	E950.4	E962.0	E980.4
topical NEC	976.0	E858.7	E946.0	E950.4	E962.0	E980.4
propylcarbinol	980.8	E860.8	—	E950.9	E962.1	E980.9
rosaniline NEC	976.0	E858.7	E946.0	E950.4	E962.0	E980.4
salicylate NEC	976.3	E858.7	E946.3	E950.4	E962.0	E980.4
sulfate (fumes)	987.8	E869.8	—	E952.8	E962.2	E982.8
liquid	983.9	E864.3	—	E950.7	E962.1	E980.6
sulfonal	967.8	E852.8	E937.8	E950.2	E962.0	E980.2
testosterone	962.1	E858.0	E932.1	E950.4	E962.0	E980.4
thiouracil	962.8	E858.0	E932.8	E950.4	E962.0	E980.4
Methylated spirit	980.0	E860.1	—	E950.9	E962.1	E980.9
Methyldopa	972.6	E858.3	E942.6	E950.4	E962.0	E980.4
Methylene						
blue	961.9	E857	E931.9	E950.4	E962.0	E980.4
chloride or dichloride (solvent) NEC	982.3	E862.4	—	E950.9	E962.1	E980.9
Methylhexabital	967.0	E851	E937.0	E950.1	E962.0	E980.1
Methylparaben (ophthalmic)	976.5	E858.7	E946.5	E950.4	E962.0	E980.4
Methyprylon	967.5	E852.4	E937.5	E950.2	E962.0	E980.2
Methysergide	971.3	E855.6	E941.3	E950.4	E962.0	E980.4
Metoclopramide	963.0	E858.1	E933.0	E950.4	E962.0	E980.4
Metofoline	965.7	E850.7	E935.7	E950.0	E962.0	E980.0
Metopon	965.09	E850.2	E935.2	E950.0	E962.0	E980.0
Metronidazole	961.5	E857	E931.5	E950.4	E962.0	E980.4
Metycaine	968.9	E855.2	E938.9	E950.4	E962.0	E980.4
infiltration (subcutaneous)	968.5	E855.2	E938.5	E950.4	E962.0	E980.4
nerve block (peripheral) (plexus)	968.6	E855.2	E938.6	E950.4	E962.0	E980.4
topical (surface)	968.5	E855.2	E938.5	E950.4	E962.0	E980.4
Metyrapone	977.8	E858.8	E947.8	E950.4	E962.0	E980.4
Mevinphos	989.3	E863.1	—	E950.6	E962.1	E980.7
Mezereon (berries)	988.2	E865.3	—	E950.9	E962.1	E980.9
Micatin	976.0	E858.7	E946.0	E950.4	E962.0	E980.4
Miconazole	976.0	E858.7	E946.0	E950.4	E962.0	E980.4
Midol	965.1	E850.3	E935.3	E950.0	E962.0	E980.0
Milk of magnesia	973.0	E858.4	E943.0	E950.4	E962.0	E980.4
Millipede (tropical) (venomous)	989.5	E905.4	—	E950.9	E962.1	E980.9

Substance	Poisoning	Accident	Therapeutic-Use	Suicide Attempt	Assault	Undetermined
Miltown	969.5	E853.8	E939.5	E950.3	E962.0	E980.3
Mineral						
oil (medicinal)	973.2	E858.4	E943.2	E950.4	E962.0	E980.4
nonmedicinal	981	E862.1	—	E950.9	E962.1	E980.9
topical	976.3	E858.7	E946.3	E950.4	E962.0	E980.4
salts NEC	974.6	E858.5	E944.6	E950.4	E962.0	E980.4
spirits	981	E862.0	—	E950.9	E962.1	E980.9
Minocycline	960.4	E856	E930.4	E950.4	E962.0	E980.4
Mithramycin (antineoplastic)	960.7	E856	E930.7	E950.4	E962.0	E980.4
Mitobronitol	963.1	E858.1	E933.1	E950.4	E962.0	E980.4
Mitomycin (antineoplastic)	960.7	E856	E930.7	E950.4	E962.0	E980.4
Mitotane	963.1	E858.1	E933.1	E950.4	E962.0	E980.4
Moderil	972.6	E858.3	E942.6	E950.4	E962.0	E980.4
Molindone	969.3	E853.8	E939.3	E950.3	E962.0	E980.3
Monistat	976.0	E858.7	E946.0	E950.4	E962.0	E980.4
Monkshood	988.2	E865.4	—	E950.9	E962.1	E980.9
Monoamine oxidase inhibitors	969.0	E854.0	E939.0	E950.3	E962.0	E980.3
Monochlorobenzene	982.0	E862.4	—	E950.9	E962.1	E980.9
Monosodium glutamate	989.8	E866.8	—	E950.9	E962.1	E980.9
Monoxide, carbon — see Carbon, monoxide						
Moperone	969.2	E853.1	E939.2	E950.3	E962.0	E980.3
Morning glory seeds	969.6	E854.1	E939.6	E950.3	E962.0	E980.3
Moroxydine (hydrochloride)	961.7	E857	E931.7	E950.4	E962.0	E980.4
Morphazinamide	961.8	E857	E931.8	E950.4	E962.0	E980.4
Morphinans	965.09	E850.2	E935.2	E950.0	E962.0	E980.0
Morphine NEC	965.09	E850.2	E935.2	E950.0	E962.0	E980.0
antagonists	970.1	E854.3	E940.1	E950.4	E962.0	E980.4
Morpholinylethylmorphine	965.09	E850.2	E935.2	E950.0	E962.0	E980.0
Morrhuate sodium	972.7	E858.3	E942.7	E950.4	E962.0	E980.4
Moth balls (see also Pesticides)	989.4	E863.4	—	E950.6	E962.1	E980.7
naphthalene	983.0	E863.4	—	E950.7	E962.1	E980.6
Motor exhaust gas — see Carbon, monoxide, exhaust gas						
Mouth wash	976.6	E858.7	E946.6	E950.4	E962.0	E980.4
Mucolytic agent	975.5	E858.6	E945.5	E950.4	E962.0	E980.4
Mucomyst	975.5	E858.6	E945.5	E950.4	E962.0	E980.4
Mucous membrane agents (external)	976.9	E858.7	E946.9	E950.4	E962.0	E980.4
specified NEC	976.8	E858.7	E946.8	E950.4	E962.0	E980.4
Mumps						
immune globulin (human)	964.6	E858.2	E934.6	E950.4	E962.0	E980.4
skin test antigen	977.8	E858.8	E947.8	E950.4	E962.0	E980.4
vaccine	979.6	E858.8	E949.6	E950.4	E962.0	E980.4
Mumpsvax	979.6	E858.8	E949.6	E950.4	E962.0	E980.4
Muriatic acid — see Hydrochloric acid						
Muscarine	971.0	E855.3	E941.0	E950.4	E962.0	E980.4
Muscle affecting agents NEC	975.3	E858.6	E945.3	E950.4	E962.0	E980.4
oxytocic	975.0	E858.6	E945.0	E950.4	E962.0	E980.4
relaxants	975.3	E858.6	E945.3	E950.4	E962.0	E980.4
central nervous system	968.0	E855.1	E938.0	E950.4	E962.0	E980.4
skeletal	975.2	E858.6	E945.2	E950.4	E962.0	E980.4
smooth	975.1	E858.6	E945.1	E950.4	E962.0	E980.4
Mushrooms, noxious	988.1	E865.5	—	E950.9	E962.1	E980.9
Mussel, noxious	988.0	E865.1	—	E950.9	E962.1	E980.9
Mustard (emetic)	973.6	E858.4	E943.6	E950.4	E962.0	E980.4
gas	987.8	E869.8	—	E952.8	E962.2	E982.8
nitrogen	963.1	E858.1	E933.1	E950.4	E962.0	E980.4
Mustine	963.1	E858.1	E933.1	E950.4	E962.0	E980.4
M-vac	979.4	E858.8	E949.4	E950.4	E962.0	E980.4
Mycifradin	960.8	E856	E930.8	E950.4	E962.0	E980.4
topical	976.0	E858.7	E946.0	E950.4	E962.0	E980.4
Mycitracin	960.8	E856	E930.8	E950.4	E962.0	E980.4
ophthalmic preparation	976.5	E858.7	E946.5	E950.4	E962.0	E980.4
Mycostatin	960.1	E856	E930.1	E950.4	E962.0	E980.4
topical	976.0	E858.7	E946.0	E950.4	E962.0	E980.4
Mydriacyl	971.1	E855.4	E941.1	E950.4	E962.0	E980.4
Myelobromal	963.1	E858.1	E933.1	E950.4	E962.0	E980.4
Myleran	963.1	E858.1	E933.1	E950.4	E962.0	E980.4
Myochrysin(e)	965.6	E850.6	E935.6	E950.0	E962.0	E980.0
Myoneural blocking agents	975.2	E858.6	E945.2	E950.4	E962.0	E980.4
Myristica fragrans	988.2	E865.3	—	E950.9	E962.1	E980.9
Myristicin	988.2	E865.3	—	E950.9	E962.1	E980.9
Mysoline	966.3	E855.0	E936.3	E950.4	E962.0	E980.4
Nafcillin (sodium)	960.0	E856	E930.0	E950.4	E962.0	E980.4
Nalidixic acid	961.9	E857	E931.9	E950.4	E962.0	E980.4
Nalorphine	970.1	E854.3	E940.1	E950.4	E962.0	E980.4
Naloxone	970.1	E854.3	E940.1	E950.4	E962.0	E980.4
Nandrolone (decanoate) (phenproprioate)	962.1	E858.0	E932.1	E950.4	E962.0	E980.4

TABLE OF DRUGS AND CHEMICALS

Substance	Poisoning	Accident	Therapeutic-Use	Suicide Attempt	Assault	Undetermined
Naphazoline	971.2	E855.5	E941.2	E950.4	E962.0	E980.4
Naphtha (painter's) (petroleum)	981	E862.0	—	E950.9	E962.1	E980.9
solvent	981	E862.0	—	E950.9	E962.1	E980.9
vapor	987.1	E869.8	—	E952.8	E962.2	E982.8
Naphthalene (chlorinated)	983.0	E864.0	—	E950.7	E962.1	E980.6
insecticide or moth repellent	983.0	E863.4	—	E950.7	E962.1	E980.6
vapor	987.8	E869.8	—	E952.8	E962.2	E982.8
Naphthol	983.0	E864.0	—	E950.7	E962.1	E980.6
Naphthylamine	983.0	E864.0	—	E950.7	E962.1	E980.6
Naproxen	965.6	E850.6	E935.6	E950.0	E962.0	E980.0
Narcotic (drug)	967.9	E852.9	E937.9	E950.2	E962.0	E980.2
analgesic NEC	965.8	E850.8	E935.8	E950.0	E962.0	E980.0
antagonist	970.1	E854.3	E940.1	E950.4	E962.0	E980.4
specified NEC	967.8	E852.8	E937.8	E950.2	E962.0	E980.2
Narcotine	975.4	E858.6	E945.4	E950.4	E962.0	E980.4
Nardil	969.0	E854.0	E939.0	E950.3	E962.0	E980.3
Natrium cyanide — see Cyanide(s)						
Natural						
blood (product)	964.7	E858.2	E934.7	E950.4	E962.0	E980.4
gas (piped)	987.1	E867	—	E951.0	E962.2	E981.0
incomplete combustion	986	E867	—	E951.0	E962.2	E981.0
Nealbarbital, nealbarbitone	967.0	E851	E937.0	E950.1	E962.0	E980.1
Nectadon	975.4	E858.6	E945.4	E950.4	E962.0	E980.4
Nematocyst (sting)	989.5	E905.6	—	E950.9	E962.1	E980.9
Nembutal	967.0	E851	E937.0	E950.1	E962.0	E980.1
Neoarsphenamine	961.1	E857	E931.1	E950.4	E962.0	E980.4
Neocinchophen	974.7	E858.5	E944.7	E950.4	E962.0	E980.4
Neomycin	960.8	E856	E930.8	E950.4	E962.0	E980.4
ENT agent	976.6	E858.7	E946.6	E950.4	E962.0	E980.4
ophthalmic preparation	976.5	E858.7	E946.5	E950.4	E962.0	E980.4
topical NEC	976.0	E858.7	E946.0	E950.4	E962.0	E980.4
Neonal	967.0	E851	E937.0	E950.1	E962.0	E980.1
Neoprontosil	961.0	E857	E931.0	E950.4	E962.0	E980.4
Neosalvarsan	961.1	E857	E931.1	E950.4	E962.0	E980.4
Neosilversalvarsan	961.1	E857	E931.1	E950.4	E962.0	E980.4
Neosporin	960.8	E856	E930.8	E950.4	E962.0	E980.4
ENT agent	976.6	E858.7	E946.6	E950.4	E962.0	E980.4
opthalmic preparation	976.5	E858.7	E946.5	E950.4	E962.0	E980.4
topical NEC	976.0	E858.7	E946.0	E950.4	E962.0	E980.4
Neostigmine	971.0	E855.3	E941.0	E950.4	E962.0	E980.4
Neraval	967.0	E851	E937.0	E950.1	E962.0	E980.1
Neravan	967.0	E851	E937.0	E950.1	E962.0	E980.1
Nerium oleander	988.2	E865.4	—	E950.9	E962.1	E980.9
Nerve gases (war)	987.9	E869.9	—	E952.9	E962.2	E982.9
Nesacaine	968.9	E855.2	E938.9	E950.4	E962.0	E980.4
infiltration (subcutaneous)	968.5	E855.2	E938.5	E950.4	E962.0	E980.4
nerve block (peripheral) (plexus)	968.6	E855.2	E938.6	E950.4	E962.0	E980.4
Neurobarb	967.0	E851	E937.0	E950.1	E962.0	E980.1
Neuroleptics NEC	969.3	E853.8	E939.3	E950.3	E962.0	E980.3
Neutral spirits	980.0	E860.1	—	E950.9	E962.1	E980.9
beverage	980.0	E860.0	—	E950.9	E962.1	E980.9
Niacin, niacinamide	972.2	E858.3	E942.2	E950.4	E962.0	E980.4
Nialamide	969.0	E854.0	E939.0	E950.3	E962.0	E980.3
Nickle (carbonyl) (compounds) (fumes) (tetracarbonyl) (vapor)	985.8	E866.4	—	E950.9	E962.1	E980.9
Niclosamide	961.6	E857	E931.6	E950.4	E962.0	E980.4
Nicomorphine	965.09	E850.2	E935.2	E950.0	E962.0	E980.0
Nicotinamide	972.2	E858.3	E942.2	E950.4	E962.0	E980.4
Nicotine (insecticide) (spray) (sulfate) NEC	989.4	E863.4	—	E950.6	E962.1	E980.7
not insecticide	989.8	E866.8	—	E950.9	E962.1	E980.9
Nicotinic acid (derivatives)	972.2	E858.3	E942.2	E950.4	E962.0	E980.4
Nicotinyl alcohol	972.2	E858.3	E942.2	E950.4	E962.0	E980.4
Nicoumalone	964.2	E858.2	E934.2	E950.4	E962.0	E980.4
Nifenazone	965.5	E850.5	E935.5	E950.0	E962.0	E980.0
Nifuraldezone	961.9	E857	E931.9	E950.4	E962.0	E980.4
Nightshade (deadly)	988.2	E865.4	—	E950.9	E962.1	E980.9
Nikethamide	970.0	E854.3	E940.0	E950.4	E962.0	E980.4
Nilstat	960.1	E856	E930.1	E950.4	E962.0	E980.4
topical	976.0	E858.7	E946.0	E950.4	E962.0	E980.4
Niridazole	961.6	E857	E931.6	E950.4	E962.0	E980.4
Nisentil	965.09	E850.2	E935.2	E950.0	E962.0	E980.0
Nitrates	972.4	E858.3	E942.4	E950.4	E962.0	E980.4
Nitrazepam	969.4	E853.2	E939.4	E950.3	E962.0	E980.3
Nitric						
acid (liquid)	983.1	E864.1	—	E950.7	E962.1	E980.6
vapor	987.8	E869.8	—	E952.8	E962.2	E982.8
oxide (gas)	987.2	E869.0	—	E952.8	E962.2	E982.8

Substance	Poisoning	Accident	Therapeutic-Use	Suicide Attempt	Assault	Undetermined
Nitrite, amyl (medicinal) (vapor)	972.4	E858.3	E942.4	E950.4	E962.0	E980.4
Nitroaniline	983.0	E864.0	—	E950.7	E962.1	E980.6
vapor	987.8	E869.8	—	E952.8	E962.2	E982.8
Nitrobenzene, nitrobenzol	983.0	E864.0	—	E950.7	E962.1	E980.6
vapor	987.8	E869.8	—	E952.8	E962.2	E982.8
Nitrocellulose	976.3	E858.7	E946.3	E950.4	E962.0	E980.4
Nitrofuran derivatives	961.9	E857	E931.9	E950.4	E962.0	E980.4
Nitrofurantoin	961.9	E857	E931.9	E950.4	E962.0	E980.4
Nitrofurazone	976.0	E858.7	E946.0	E950.4	E962.0	E980.4
Nitrogen (dioxide) (gas) (oxide)	987.2	E869.0	—	E952.8	E962.2	E982.8
mustard (antineoplastic)	963.1	E858.1	E933.1	E950.4	E962.0	E980.4
Nitroglycerin, nitroglycerol (medicinal)	972.4	E858.3	E942.4	E950.4	E962.0	E980.4
nonmedicinal	989.8	E866.8	—	E950.9	E962.1	E980.9
fumes	987.8	E869.8	—	E952.8	E962.2	E982.8
Nitrohydrochloric acid	983.1	E864.1	—	E950.7	E962.1	E980.6
Nitromersol	976.0	E858.7	E946.0	E950.4	E962.0	E980.4
Nitronaphthalene	983.0	E864.0	—	E950.7	E962.2	E980.6
Nitrophenol	983.0	E864.0	—	E950.7	E962.2	E980.6
Nitrothiazol	961.6	E857	E931.6	E950.4	E962.0	E980.4
Nitrotoluene, nitrotoluol	983.0	E864.0	—	E950.7	E962.1	E980.6
vapor	987.8	E869.8	—	E952.8	E962.2	E982.8
Nitrous	968.2	E855.1	E938.2	E950.4	E962.0	E980.4
acid (liquid)	983.1	E864.1	—	E950.7	E962.1	E980.6
fumes	987.2	E869.0	—	E952.8	E962.2	E982.8
oxide (anesthetic) NEC	968.2	E855.1	E938.2	E950.4	E962.0	E980.4
Nitrozone	976.0	E858.7	E946.0	E950.4	E962.0	E980.4
Noctec	967.1	E852.0	E937.1	E950.2	E962.0	E980.2
Noludar	967.5	E852.4	E937.5	E950.2	E962.0	E980.2
Noptil	967.0	E851	E937.0	E950.1	E962.0	E980.1
Noradrenalin	971.2	E855.5	E941.2	E950.4	E962.0	E980.4
Noramidopyrine	965.5	E850.5	E935.5	E950.0	E962.0	E980.0
Norepinephrine	971.2	E855.5	E941.2	E950.4	E962.0	E980.4
Norethandrolone	962.1	E858.0	E932.1	E950.4	E962.0	E980.4
Norethindrone	962.2	E858.0	E932.2	E950.4	E962.0	E980.4
Norethisterone	962.2	E858.0	E932.2	E950.4	E962.0	E980.4
Norethynodrel	962.2	E858.0	E932.2	E950.4	E962.0	E980.4
Norlestrin	962.2	E858.0	E932.2	E950.4	E962.0	E980.4
Norlutin	962.2	E858.0	E932.2	E950.4	E962.0	E980.4
Normorphine	965.09	E850.2	E935.2	E950.0	E962.0	E980.0
Nortriptyline	969.0	E854.0	E939.0	E950.3	E962.0	E980.3
Noscapine	975.4	E858.6	E945.4	E950.4	E962.0	E980.4
Nose preparations	976.6	E858.7	E946.6	E950.4	E962.0	E980.4
Novobiocin	960.8	E856	E930.8	E950.4	E962.0	E980.4
Novocain (infiltration) (topical)	968.5	E855.2	E938.5	E950.4	E962.0	E980.4
nerve block (peripheral) (plexus)	968.6	E855.2	E938.6	E950.4	E962.0	E980.4
spinal	968.7	E855.2	E938.7	E950.4	E962.0	E980.4
Noxythiolin	961.9	E857	E931.9	E950.4	E962.0	E980.4
NPH Iletin (insulin)	962.3	E858.0	E932.3	E950.4	E962.0	E980.4
Numorphan	965.09	E850.2	E935.2	E950.0	E962.0	E980.0
Nunol	967.0	E851	E937.0	E950.1	E962.0	E980.1
Nupercaine (spinal anesthetic)	968.7	E855.2	E938.7	E950.4	E962.0	E980.4
topical (surface)	968.5	E855.2	E938.5	E950.4	E962.0	E980.4
Nutmeg oil (liniment)	976.3	E858.7	E946.3	E950.4	E962.0	E980.4
Nux vomica	989.1	E863.7	—	E950.6	E962.1	E980.7
Nydrazid	961.8	E857	E931.8	E950.4	E962.0	E980.4
Nylidrin	971.2	E855.5	E941.2	E950.4	E962.0	E980.4
Nystatin	960.1	E856	E930.1	E950.4	E962.0	E980.4
topical	976.0	E858.7	E946.0	E950.4	E962.0	E980.4
Nytol	963.0	E858.2	E934.2	E950.4	E962.0	E980.4
Oblivion	967.8	E852.8	E937.8	E950.2	E962.0	E980.2
Octyl nitrite	972.4	E858.3	E942.4	E950.4	E962.0	E980.4
Oestradiol (cypionate) (dipropionate) (valerate)	962.2	E858.0	E932.2	E950.4	E962.0	E980.4
Oestriol	962.2	E858.0	E932.2	E950.4	E962.0	E980.4
Oestrone	962.2	E858.0	E932.2	E950.4	E962.0	E980.4
Oil (of) NEC	989.8	E866.8	—	E950.9	E962.1	E980.9
bitter almond	989.0	E866.8	—	E950.9	E962.1	E980.9
camphor	976.1	E858.7	E946.1	E950.4	E962.0	E980.4
colors	989.8	E861.6	—	E950.9	E962.1	E980.9
fumes	987.8	E869.8	—	E952.8	E962.2	E982.8
lubricating	981	E862.2	—	E950.9	E962.1	E980.9
specified source, other — see substance specified						
vitriol (liquid)	983.1	E864.1	—	E950.7	E962.1	E980.6
fumes	987.8	E869.8	—	E952.8	E962.2	E982.8
wintergreen (bitter) NEC	976.3	E858.7	E946.3	E950.4	E962.0	E980.4
Ointments NEC	976.9	E858.7	E946.9	E950.4	E962.0	E980.4

TABLE OF DRUGS AND CHEMICALS

Substance	Poisoning	Accident	Therapeutic-Use	Suicide Attempt	Assault	Undetermined
Oleander	988.2	E865.4	—	E950.9	E962.1	E980.9
Oleandomycin	960.3	E856	E930.3	E950.4	E962.0	E980.4
Oleovitamin A	963.5	E858.1	E933.5	E950.4	E962.0	E980.4
Oleum ricini	973.1	E858.4	E943.1	E950.4	E962.0	E980.4
Olive oil (medicinal) NEC	973.2	E858.4	E943.2	E950.4	E962.0	E980.4
OMPA	989.3	E863.1	—	E950.6	E962.1	E980.7
Oncovin	963.1	E858.1	E933.1	E950.4	E962.0	E980.4
Ophthaine	968.5	E855.2	E938.5	E950.4	E962.0	E980.4
Ophthetic	968.5	E855.2	E938.5	E950.4	E962.0	E980.4
Opiates, opioids, opium NEC	965.00	E850.2	E935.2	E950.0	E962.0	E980.0
antagonists	970.1	E854.3	E940.1	E950.4	E962.0	E980.4
Oracon	962.2	E858.0	E932.2	E950.4	E962.0	E980.4
Oragrafin	977.8	E858.8	E947.8	E950.4	E962.0	E980.4
Oral contraceptives	962.2	E858.0	E932.2	E950.4	E962.0	E980.4
Orciprenaline	975.1	E858.6	E945.1	E950.4	E962.0	E980.4
Organidin	975.5	E858.6	E945.5	E950.4	E962.0	E980.4
Organophosphates	989.3	E863.1	—	E950.6	E962.1	E980.7
Orimune	979.5	E858.8	E949.5	E950.4	E962.0	E980.4
Orinase	962.3	E858.0	E932.3	E950.4	E962.0	E980.4
Orphenadrine	966.4	E855.0	E936.4	E950.4	E962.0	E980.4
Ortal (sodium)	967.0	E851	E937.0	E950.1	E962.0	E980.1
Orthoboric acid	976.0	E858.7	E946.0	E950.4	E962.0	E980.4
ENT agent	976.6	E858.7	E946.6	E950.4	E962.0	E980.4
ophthalmic preparation	976.5	E858.7	E946.5	E950.4	E962.0	E980.4
Orthocaine	968.5	E855.2	E938.5	E950.4	E962.0	E980.4
Ortho-Novum	962.2	E858.0	E932.2	E950.4	E962.0	E980.4
Orthotolidine (reagent)	977.8	E858.8	E947.8	E950.4	E962.0	E980.4
Osmic acid (liquid)	983.1	E864.1	—	E950.7	E962.1	E980.6
fumes	987.8	E869.8	—	E952.8	E962.2	E982.8
Osmotic diuretics	974.4	E858.5	E944.4	E950.4	E962.0	E980.4
Ouabain	972.1	E858.3	E942.1	E950.4	E962.0	E980.4
Ovarian hormones (synthetic substitutes)	962.2	E858.0	E932.2	E950.4	E962.0	E980.4
Ovral	962.2	E858.0	E932.2	E950.4	E962.0	E980.4
Ovulation suppressants	962.2	E858.0	E932.2	E950.4	E962.0	E980.4
Ovulen	962.2	E858.0	E932.2	E950.4	E962.0	E980.4
Oxacillin (sodium)	960.0	E856	E930.0	E950.4	E962.0	E980.4
Oxalic acid	983.1	E864.1	—	E950.7	E962.1	E980.6
Oxanamide	969.5	E853.8	E939.5	E950.3	E962.0	E980.3
Oxandrolone	962.1	E858.0	E932.1	E950.4	E962.0	E980.4
Oxazepam	969.4	E853.2	E939.4	E950.3	E962.0	E980.3
Oxazolidine derivatives	966.0	E855.0	E936.0	E950.4	E962.0	E980.4
Ox bile extract	973.4	E858.4	E943.4	E950.4	E962.0	E980.4
Oxedrine	971.2	E855.5	E941.2	E950.4	E962.0	E980.4
Oxeladin	975.4	E858.6	E945.4	E950.4	E962.0	E980.4
Oxethazaine NEC	968.5	E855.2	E938.5	E950.4	E962.0	E980.4
Oxidizing agents NEC	983.9	E864.3	—	E950.7	E962.1	E980.6
Oxolinic acid	961.3	E857	E931.3	E950.4	E962.0	E980.4
Oxophenarsine	961.1	E857	E931.1	E950.4	E962.0	E980.4
Oxsoralen	976.3	E858.7	E946.3	E950.4	E962.0	E980.4
Oxtriphylline	975.7	E858.6	E945.7	E950.4	E962.0	E980.4
Oxybuprocaine	968.5	E855.2	E938.5	E950.4	E962.0	E980.4
Oxybutynin	975.1	E858.6	E945.1	E950.4	E962.0	E980.4
Oxycodone	965.09	E850.2	E935.2	E950.0	E962.0	E980.0
Oxygen	987.8	E869.8	—	E952.8	E962.2	E982.8
Oxylone	976.0	E858.7	E946.0	E950.4	E962.0	E980.4
ophthalmic preparation	976.5	E858.7	E946.5	E950.4	E962.0	E980.4
Oxymesterone	962.1	E858.0	E932.1	E950.4	E962.0	E980.4
Oxymetazoline	971.2	E855.5	E941.2	E950.4	E962.0	E980.4
Oxymetholone	962.1	E858.0	E932.1	E950.4	E962.0	E980.4
Oxymorphone	965.09	E850.2	E935.2	E950.0	E962.0	E980.0
Oxypertine	969.0	E854.0	E939.0	E950.3	E962.0	E980.3
Oxyphenbutazone	965.5	E850.5	E935.5	E950.0	E962.0	E980.0
Oxyphencyclimine	971.1	E855.4	E941.1	E950.4	E962.0	E980.4
Oxyphenisatin	973.1	E858.4	E943.1	E950.4	E962.0	E980.4
Oxyphenonium	971.1	E855.4	E941.1	E950.4	E962.0	E980.4
Oxyquinoline	961.3	E857	E931.3	E950.4	E962.0	E980.4
Oxytetracycline	960.4	E856	E930.4	E950.4	E962.0	E980.4
Oxytocics	975.0	E858.6	E945.0	E950.4	E962.0	E980.4
Oxytocin	975.0	E858.6	E945.0	E950.4	E962.0	E980.4
Ozone	987.8	E869.8	—	E952.8	E962.2	E982.8
PABA	976.3	E858.7	E946.3	E950.4	E962.0	E980.4
Packed red cells	964.7	E858.2	E934.7	E950.4	E962.0	E980.4
Paint NEC	989.8	E861.6	—	E950.9	E962.1	E980.9
cleaner	982.8	E862.9	—	E950.9	E962.1	E980.9
fumes NEC	987.8	E869.8	—	E952.8	E962.1	E982.8
lead (fumes)	984.0	E861.5	—	E950.9	E962.1	E980.9

TABLE OF DRUGS AND CHEMICALS

Substance	Poisoning	Accident	Therapeutic-Use	Suicide Attempt	Assault	Undetermined
Paint—continued						
solvent NEC	982.8	E862.9	—	E950.9	E962.1	E980.9
stripper	982.8	E862.9	—	E950.9	E962.1	E980.9
Palfium	965.09	E850.2	E935.2	E950.0	E962.0	E980.0
Paludrine	961.4	E857	E931.4	E950.4	E962.0	E980.4
PAM	977.2	E855.8	E947.2	E950.4	E962.0	E980.4
Pamaquine (naphthoate)	961.4	E857	E931.4	E950.4	E962.0	E980.4
Pamprin	965.1	E850.3	E935.3	E950.0	E962.0	E980.0
Panadol	965.4	E850.4	E935.4	E950.0	E962.0	E980.0
Pancreatic dornase (mucolytic)	963.4	E858.1	E933.4	E950.4	E962.0	E980.4
Pancreatin	973.4	E858.4	E943.4	E950.4	E962.0	E980.4
Pancrelipase	973.4	E858.4	E943.4	E950.4	E962.0	E980.4
Pangamic acid	963.5	E858.1	E933.5	E950.4	E962.0	E980.4
Panthenol	963.5	E858.1	E933.5	E950.4	E962.0	E980.4
topical	976.8	E858.7	E946.8	E950.4	E962.0	E980.4
Pantopaque	977.8	E858.8	E947.8	E950.4	E962.0	E980.4
Pantopon	965.00	E850.2	E935.2	E950.0	E962.0	E980.0
Pantothenic acid	963.5	E858.1	E933.5	E950.4	E962.0	E980.4
Panwarfin	964.2	E858.2	E934.2	E950.4	E962.0	E980.4
Papain	973.4	E858.4	E943.4	E950.4	E962.0	E980.4
Papaverine	972.5	E858.3	E942.5	E950.4	E962.0	E980.4
Para-aminobenzoic acid	976.3	E858.7	E946.3	E950.4	E962.0	E980.4
Para-aminophenol derivatives	965.4	E850.4	E935.4	E950.0	E962.0	E980.0
Para-aminosalicylic acid (derivatives)	961.8	E857	E931.8	E950.4	E962.0	E980.4
Paracetaldehyde (medicinal)	967.2	E852.1	E937.2	E950.2	E962.0	E980.2
Paracetamol	965.4	E850.4	E935.4	E950.0	E962.0	E980.0
Paracodin	965.09	E850.2	E935.2	E950.0	E962.0	E980.0
Paradione	966.0	E855	E936.0	E950.4	E962.0	E980.4
Paraffin(s) (wax)	981	E862.3	—	E950.9	E962.1	E980.9
liquid (medicinal)	973.2	E858.4	E943.2	E950.4	E962.0	E980.4
nonmedicinal (oil)	981	E962.1	—	E950.9	E962.1	E980.9
Paraldehyde (medicinal)	967.2	E852.1	E937.2	E950.2	E962.0	E980.2
Paramethadione	966.0	E855	E936.0	E950.4	E962.0	E980.4
Paramethasone	962.0	E858.0	E932.0	E950.4	E962.0	E980.4
Paraquat	989.4	E863.5	—	E950.6	E962.1	E980.7
Parasympatholytics	971.1	E855.4	E941.1	E950.4	E962.0	E980.4
Parasympathomimetics	971.0	E855.5	E941.0	E950.4	E962.0	E980.4
Parathion	989.3	E863.1	—	E950.6	E962.1	E980.7
Parathormone	962.6	E858.0	E932.6	E950.4	E962.0	E980.4
Parathyroid (derivatives)	962.6	E858.0	E932.6	E950.4	E962.0	E980.4
Paratyphoid vaccine	978.1	E858.8	E948.1	E950.4	E962.0	E980.4
Paredrine	971.2	E855.5	E941.2	E950.4	E962.0	E980.4
Paregoric	965.00	E850.2	E935.2	E950.0	E962.0	E980.0
Pargyline	972.3	E858.3	E942.3	E950.4	E962.0	E980.4
Paris green	985.1	E866.3	—	E950.8	E962.1	E980.8
insecticide	985.1	E863.4	—	E950.8	E962.1	E980.8
Parnate	969.0	E854.0	E939.0	E950.3	E962.0	E980.3
Paromomycin	960.8	E856	E930.8	E950.4	E962.0	E980.4
Paroxypropione	963.1	E858.1	E933.1	E950.4	E962.0	E980.4
Parzone	965.09	E850.2	E935.2	E950.0	E962.0	E980.0
PAS	961.8	E857	E931.8	E950.4	E962.0	E980.4
PCP (pentachlorophenol)	989.4	E863.6	—	E950.6	E962.1	E980.7
herbicide	989.4	E863.5	—	E950.6	E962.1	E980.7
insecticide	989.4	E863.4	—	E950.6	E962.1	E980.7
phencyclidine	968.3	E855.1	E938.3	E950.4	E962.0	E980.4
Peach kernel oil (emulsion)	973.2	E858.4	E943.2	E950.4	E962.0	E980.4
Peanut oil (emulsion) NEC	973.2	E858.4	E943.2	E950.4	E962.0	E980.4
topical	976.3	E858.7	E946.3	E950.4	E962.0	E980.4
Pearly Gates (morning glory seeds)	969.6	E854.1	E939.6	E950.3	E962.0	E980.3
Pecazine	969.1	E853.0	E939.1	E950.3	E962.0	E980.3
Pecilocin	960.1	E856	E930.1	E950.4	E962.0	E980.4
Pectin (with kaolin) NEC	973.5	E858.4	E943.5	E950.4	E962.0	E980.4
Pelletierine tannate	961.6	E857	E931.6	E950.4	E962.0	E980.4
Pemoline	969.7	E854.2	E939.7	E950.3	E962.0	E980.3
Pempidine	972.3	E858.3	E942.3	E950.4	E962.0	E980.4
Penamecillin	960.0	E856	E930.0	E950.4	E962.0	E980.4
Penethamate hydriodide	960.0	E856	E930.0	E950.4	E962.0	E980.4
Penicillamine	963.8	E858.1	E933.8	E950.4	E962.0	E980.4
Penicillin (any type)	960.0	E856	E930.0	E950.4	E962.0	E980.4
Penicillinase	963.4	E858.1	E933.4	E950.4	E962.0	E980.4
Pentachlorophenol (fungicide)	989.4	E863.6	—	E950.6	E962.1	E980.7
herbicide	989.4	E863.5	—	E950.6	E962.1	E980.7
insecticide	989.4	E863.4	—	E950.6	E962.1	E980.7
Pentaerythritol	972.4	E858.3	E942.4	E950.4	E962.0	E980.4
chloral	967.1	E852.0	E937.1	E950.2	E962.0	E980.2
tetranitrate NEC	972.4	E858.3	E942.4	E950.4	E962.0	E980.4

Substance	Poisoning	Accident	Therapeutic Use	Suicide Attempt	Assault	Undetermined
Pentagastrin	977.8	E858.8	E947.8	E950.4	E962.0	E980.4
Pentalin	982.3	E862.4	—	E950.9	E962.1	E980.9
Pentamethonium (bromide)	972.3	E858.3	E942.3	E950.4	E962.0	E980.4
Pentamidine	961.5	E857	E931.5	E950.4	E962.0	E980.4
Pentanol	980.8	E860.8	—	E950.9	E962.1	E980.9
Pentaquine	961.4	E857	E931.4	E950.4	E962.0	E980.4
Pentazocine	965.8	E850.8	E935.8	E950.0	E962.0	E980.0
Penthienate	971.1	E855.4	E941.1	E950.4	E962.0	E980.4
Pentobarbital, pentobarbitone (sodium)	967.0	E851	E937.0	E950.1	E962.0	E980.1
Pentolinium (tartrate)	972.3	E858.3	E942.3	E950.4	E962.0	E980.4
Pentothal	968.3	E855.1	E938.3	E950.4	E962.0	E980.4
Pentylenetetrazol	970.0	E854.3	E940.0	E950.4	E962.0	E980.4
Pentylsalicylamide	961.8	E857	E931.8	E950.4	E962.0	E980.4
Pepsin	973.4	E858.4	E943.4	E950.4	E962.0	E980.4
Peptavlon	977.8	E858.8	E947.8	E950.4	E962.0	E980.4
Percaine (spinal)	968.7	E855.2	E938.7	E950.4	E962.0	E980.4
topical (surface)	968.5	E855.2	E938.5	E950.4	E962.0	E980.4
Perchloroethylene (vapor)	982.3	E862.4	—	E950.9	E962.1	E980.9
medicinal	961.6	E857	E931.6	E950.4	E962.0	E980.4
Percodan	965.09	E850.2	E935.2	E950.0	E962.0	E980.0
Percogesic	965.09	E850.2	E935.2	E950.0	E962.0	E980.0
Percorten	962.0	E858.0	E932.0	E950.4	E962.0	E980.4
Pergonal	962.4	E858.0	E932.4	E950.4	E962.0	E980.4
Perhexiline	972.4	E858.3	E942.4	E950.4	E962.0	E980.4
Periactin	963.0	E858.1	E933.0	E950.4	E962.0	E980.4
Periclor	967.1	E852.0	E937.1	E950.2	E962.0	E980.2
Pericyazine	969.1	E853.0	E939.1	E950.3	E962.0	E980.3
Peritrate	972.4	E858.3	E942.4	E950.4	E962.0	E980.4
Permanganates NEC	983.9	E864.3	—	E950.7	E962.1	E980.6
potassium (topical)	976.0	E858.7	E946.0	E950.4	E962.0	E980.4
Pernocton	967.0	E851	E937.0	E950.1	E962.0	E980.1
Pernoston	967.0	E851	E937.0	E950.1	E962.0	E980.1
Peronin(e)	965.09	E850.2	E935.2	E950.0	E962.0	E980.0
Perphenazine	969.1	E853.0	E939.1	E950.3	E962.0	E980.3
Pertofrane	969.0	E854	E939.0	E950.3	E962.0	E980.3
Pertussis						
immune serum (human)	964.6	E858.2	E934.6	E950.4	E962.0	E980.4
vaccine (with diphtheria toxoid) (with tetanus toxoid)	978.6	E858.8	E948.6	E950.4	E962.0	E980.4
Peruvian balsam	976.8	E858.7	E946.8	E950.4	E962.0	E980.4
Pesticides (dust) (fumes) (vapor)	989.4	E863.4	—	E950.6	E962.1	E980.7
arsenic	985.1	E863.4	—	E950.8	E962.1	E980.8
chlorinated	989.2	E863.0	—	E950.6	E962.1	E980.7
cyanide	989.0	E863.4	—	E950.6	E962.1	E980.7
kerosene	981	E863.4	—	E950.6	E962.1	E980.7
mixture (of compounds)	989.4	E863.3	—	E950.6	E962.1	E980.7
naphthalene	983.0	E863.4	—	E950.7	E962.1	E980.6
organochlorine (compounds)	989.2	E863.0	—	E950.6	E962.1	E980.7
petroleum (distillate) (products) NEC	981	E863.4	—	E950.6	E962.1	E980.7
specified ingredient NEC	989.4	E863.4	—	E950.6	E962.1	E980.7
strychnine	989.1	E863.4	—	E950.6	E962.1	E980.7
thallium	985.8	E863.7	—	E950.6	E962.1	E980.7
Pethidine (hydrochloride)	965.09	E850.2	E935.2	E950.0	E962.0	E980.0
Petrichloral	967.1	E852.0	E937.1	E950.2	E962.0	E980.2
Petrol	981	E862.1	—	E950.9	E962.1	E980.9
vapor	987.1	E869.8	—	E952.8	E962.2	E982.8
Petrolatum (jelly) (ointment)	976.3	E858.7	E946.3	E950.4	E962.0	E980.4
hydrophilic	976.3	E858.7	E946.3	E950.4	E962.0	E980.4
liquid	973.2	E858.4	E943.2	E950.4	E962.0	E980.4
topical	976.3	E858.7	E946.3	E950.4	E962.0	E980.4
nonmedicinal	981	E862.1	—	E950.9	E962.1	E980.9
Petroleum (cleaners) (fuels) (products) NEC	981	E862.1	—	E950.9	E962.1	E980.9
benzin(e) — see Ligroin						
ether — see Ligroin						
jelly — see Petrolatum						
naphtha — see Ligroin						
pesticide	981	E863.4	—	E950.6	E962.1	E980.7
solids	981	E862.3	—	E950.9	E962.1	E980.9
solvents	981	E862.0	—	E950.9	E962.1	E980.9
vapor	987.1	E869.8	—	E952.8	E962.2	E982.8
Peyote	969.6	E854.1	E939.6	E950.3	E962.0	E980.3
Phanodorm, phanodorn	967.0	E851	E937.0	E950.1	E962.0	E980.1
Phanquinone, phanquone	961.5	E857	E931.5	E950.4	E962.0	E980.4
Pharmaceutical excipient or adjunct	977.4	E858.8	E947.4	E950.4	E962.0	E980.4
Phenacemide	966.3	E855.0	E936.3	E950.4	E962.0	E980.4
Phenacetin	965.4	E850.4	E935.4	E950.0	E962.0	E980.0
Phenadoxone	965.09	E850.2	E935.2	E950.0	E962.0	E980.0

TABLE OF DRUGS AND CHEMICALS

Substance	Poisoning	Accident	Therapeutic-Use	Suicide Attempt	Assault	Undetermined
Phenaglycodol	969.5	E853.8	E939.5	E950.3	E962.0	E980.3
Phenantoin	966.1	E855.0	E936.1	E950.4	E962.0	E980.4
Phenaphthazine reagent	977.8	E858.8	E947.8	E950.4	E962.0	E980.4
Phenazocine	965.09	E850.2	E935.2	E950.0	E962.0	E980.0
Phenazone	965.5	E850.5	E935.5	E950.0	E962.0	E980.0
Phenazopyridine	976.1	E858.7	E946.1	E950.4	E962.0	E980.4
Phenbenicillin	960.0	E856	E930.0	E950.4	E962.0	E980.4
Phenbutrazate	977.0	E858.8	E947.0	E950.4	E962.0	E980.4
Phencyclidine	968.3	E855.1	E938.3	E950.4	E962.0	E980.4
Phendimetrazine	977.0	E858.8	E947.0	E950.4	E962.0	E980.4
Phenelzine	969.0	E854.0	E939.0	E950.3	E962.0	E980.3
Phenergan	967.8	E852.8	E937.8	E950.2	E962.0	E980.2
Phenethicillin (potassium)	960.0	E856	E930.0	E950.4	E962.0	E980.4
Phenetsal	965.1	E850.3	E935.3	E950.0	E962.0	E980.0
Pheneturide	966.3	E855.0	E936.3	E950.4	E962.0	E980.4
Phenformin	962.3	E858.0	E932.3	E950.4	E962.0	E980.4
Phenglutarimide	971.1	E855.4	E941.1	E950.4	E962.0	E980.4
Phenicarbazide	965.8	E850.8	E935.8	E950.0	E962.0	E980.0
Phenindamine (tartrate)	963.0	E858.1	E933.0	E950.4	E962.0	E980.4
Phenindione	964.2	E858.2	E934.2	E950.4	E962.0	E980.4
Pheniprazine	969.0	E854.0	E939.0	E950.3	E962.0	E980.3
Pheniramine (maleate)	963.0	E858.1	E933.0	E950.4	E962.0	E980.4
Phenmetrazine	977.0	E858.8	E947.0	E950.4	E962.0	E980.4
Phenobal	967.0	E851	E937.0	E950.1	E962.0	E980.1
Phenobarbital	967.0	E851	E937.0	E950.1	E962.0	E980.1
Phenobarbitone	967.0	E851	E937.0	E950.1	E962.0	E980.1
Phenoctide	976.0	E858.7	E946.0	E950.4	E962.0	E980.4
Phenol (derivatives) NEC	983.0	E864.0	—	E950.7	E962.1	E980.6
disinfectant	983.0	E864.0	—	E950.7	E962.1	E980.6
pesticide	989.4	E863.4	—	E950.6	E962.1	E980.7
red	977.8	E858.8	E947.8	E950.4	E962.0	E980.4
Phenolphthalein	973.1	E858.4	E943.1	E950.4	E962.0	E980.4
Phenolsulfonphthalein	977.8	E858.8	E947.8	E950.4	E962.0	E980.4
Phenomorphan	965.09	E850.2	E935.2	E950.0	E962.0	E980.0
Phenonyl	967.0	E851	E937.0	E950.1	E962.0	E980.1
Phenoperidine	965.09	E850.2	E935.2	E950.0	E962.0	E980.0
Phenoquin	974.7	E858.5	E944.7	E950.4	E962.0	E980.4
Phenothiazines (tranquilizers) NEC	969.1	E853.0	E939.1	E950.3	E962.0	E980.3
insecticide	989.3	E863.4	—	E950.6	E962.1	E980.7
Phenoxybenzamine	971.3	E855.6	E941.3	E950.4	E962.0	E980.4
Phenoxymethyl penicillin	960.0	E856	E930.0	E950.4	E962.0	E980.4
Phenprocoumon	964.2	E858.2	E934.2	E950.4	E962.0	E980.4
Phensuximide	966.2	E855.0	E936.2	E950.4	E962.0	E980.4
Phentermine	977.0	E858.8	E947.0	E950.4	E962.0	E980.4
Phentolamine	971.3	E855.6	E941.3	E950.4	E962.0	E980.4
Phenyl						
butazone	965.5	E850.5	E935.5	E950.0	E962.0	E980.0
enediamine	983.0	E864.0	—	E950.7	E962.1	E980.6
hydrazine	983.0	E864.0	—	E950.7	E962.1	E980.6
antineoplastic	963.1	E858.1	E933.1	E950.4	E962.0	E980.4
mercuric compounds — see Mercury						
salicylate	976.3	E858.7	E946.3	E950.4	E962.0	E980.4
Phenylephrin	971.2	E855.5	E941.2	E950.4	E962.0	E980.4
Phenylethylbiguanide	962.3	E858.0	E932.3	E950.4	E962.0	E980.4
Phenylpropanolamine	971.2	E855.5	E941.2	E950.4	E962.0	E980.4
Phenylsulfthion	989.3	E863.1	—	E950.6	E962.1	E980.7
Phenyramidol, phenyramidon	965.7	E850.7	E935.7	E950.0	E962.0	E980.0
Phenytoin	966.1	E855.0	E936.1	E950.4	E962.0	E980.4
pHisoHex	976.2	E858.7	E946.2	E950.4	E962.0	E980.4
Pholcodine	965.09	E850.2	E935.2	E950.0	E962.0	E980.0
Phorate	989.3	E863.1	—	E950.6	E962.1	E980.7
Phosdrin	989.3	E863.1	—	E950.6	E962.1	E980.7
Phosgene (gas)	987.8	E869.8	—	E952.8	E962.2	E982.8
Phosphate (tricresyl)	989.8	E866.8	—	E950.9	E962.1	E980.9
organic	989.3	E863.1	—	E950.6	E962.1	E980.7
solvent	982.8	E862.4	—	E950.9	E926.1	E980.9
Phosphine	987.8	E869.8	—	E952.8	E962.2	E982.8
fumigant	987.8	E863.8	—	E950.6	E962.2	E980.7
Phospholine	971.0	E855.5	E941.0	E950.4	E962.0	E980.4
Phosphoric acid	983.1	E864.1	—	E950.7	E962.1	E980.6
Phosphorus (compounds) NEC	983.9	E864.3	—	E950.7	E962.1	E980.6
rodenticide	983.9	E863.7	—	E950.7	E962.1	E980.6
Phthalimidoglutarimide	967.8	E852.8	E937.8	E950.2	E962.0	E980.2
Phthalylsulfathiazole	961.0	E857	E931.0	E950.4	E962.0	E980.4
Phylloquinone	964.3	E858.2	E934.3	E950.4	E962.0	E980.4
Physeptone	965.02	E850.1	E935.1	E950.0	E962.0	E980.0

Substance	Poisoning	Accident	Therapeutic Use	Suicide Attempt	Assault	Undetermined
Physostigma venenosum	988.2	E865.4	—	E950.9	E962.1	E980.9
Physostigmine	971.0	E855.3	E941.0	E950.4	E962.0	E980.4
Phytolacca decandra	988.2	E865.4	—	E950.9	E962.1	E980.9
Phytomenadione	964.3	E858.2	E934.3	E950.4	E962.0	E980.4
Phytonadione	964.3	E858.2	E934.3	E950.4	E962.0	E980.4
Picric (acid)	983.0	E864.0	—	E950.7	E962.1	E980.6
Picrotoxin	970.0	E854.3	E940.0	E950.4	E962.0	E980.4
Pilocarpine	971.0	E855.3	E941.0	E950.4	E962.0	E980.4
Pilocarpus (jaborandi) extract	971.0	E855.3	E941.0	E950.4	E962.0	E980.4
Pimaricin	960.1	E856	E930.1	E950.4	E962.0	E980.4
Piminodine	965.09	E850.2	E935.2	E950.0	E962.0	E980.0
Pine oil, pinesol (disinfectant)	983.9	E861.4	—	E950.7	E962.1	E980.6
Pinkroot	961.6	E857	E931.6	E950.4	E962.0	E980.4
Pipadone	965.09	E850.2	E935.2	E950.0	E962.0	E980.0
Pipamazine	963.0	E858.1	E933.0	E950.4	E962.0	E980.4
Pipazethate	975.4	E858.6	E945.4	E950.4	E962.0	E980.4
Pipenzolate	971.1	E855.4	E941.1	E950.4	E962.0	E980.4
Piperacetazine	969.1	E853.0	E939.1	E950.3	E962.0	E980.3
Piperazine NEC	961.6	E857	E931.6	E950.4	E962.0	E980.4
estrone sulfate	962.2	E858.0	E932.2	E950.4	E962.0	E980.4
Piper cubeba	988.2	E865.4	—	E950.9	E962.1	E980.9
Piperidione	975.4	E858.6	E945.4	E950.4	E962.0	E980.4
Piperidolate	971.1	E855.4	E941.1	E950.4	E962.0	E980.4
Piperocaine	968.9	E855.2	E938.9	E950.4	E962.0	E980.4
infiltration (subcutaneous)	968.5	E855.2	E938.5	E950.4	E962.0	E980.4
nerve block (peripheral) (plexus)	968.6	E855.2	E938.6	E950.4	E962.0	E980.4
topical (surface)	968.5	E855.2	E938.5	E950.4	E962.0	E980.4
Pipobroman	963.1	E858.1	E933.1	E950.4	E962.0	E980.4
Pipradrol	970.8	E854.3	E940.8	E950.4	E962.0	E980.4
Piscidia (bark) (erythrina)	965.7	E850.7	E935.7	E950.0	E962.0	E980.0
Pitch	983.0	E864.0	—	E950.7	E962.1	E980.6
Pitkin's solution	968.7	E855.2	E938.7	E950.4	E962.0	E980.4
Pitocin	975.0	E858.6	E945.0	E950.4	E962.0	E980.4
Pitressin (tannate)	962.5	E858.0	E932.5	E950.4	E962.0	E980.4
Pituitary extracts (posterior)	962.5	E858.0	E932.5	E950.4	E962.0	E980.4
anterior	962.4	E858.0	E932.4	E950.4	E962.0	E980.4
Pituitrin	962.5	E858.0	E932.5	E950.4	E962.0	E980.4
Placental extract	962.9	E858.0	E932.9	E950.4	E962.0	E980.4
Placidyl	967.8	E852.8	E937.8	E950.2	E962.0	E980.2
Plague vaccine	978.3	E858.8	E948.3	E950.4	E962.0	E980.4
Plant foods or fertilizers NEC	989.8	E866.5	—	E950.9	E962.1	E980.9
mixed with herbicides	989.4	E863.5	—	E950.6	E962.1	E980.7
Plants, noxious, used as food	988.2	E865.9	—	E950.9	E962.1	E980.9
berries and seeds	988.2	E865.3	—	E950.9	E962.1	E980.9
specified type NEC	988.2	E865.4	—	E950.9	E962.1	E980.9
Plasma (blood)	964.7	E858.2	E934.7	E950.4	E962.0	E980.4
expanders	964.8	E858.2	E934.8	E950.4	E962.0	E980.4
Plasmanate	964.7	E858.2	E934.7	E950.4	E962.0	E980.4
Plegicil	969.1	E853.0	E939.1	E950.3	E962.0	E980.3
Podophyllin	976.4	E858.7	E946.4	E950.4	E962.0	E980.4
Podophyllum resin	976.4	E858.7	E946.4	E950.4	E962.0	E980.4
Poison NEC	989.9	E866.9	—	E950.9	E962.1	E980.9
Poisonous berries	988.2	E865.3	—	E950.9	E962.1	E980.9
Pokeweed (any part)	988.2	E865.4	—	E950.9	E962.1	E980.9
Poldine	971.1	E855.4	E941.1	E950.4	E962.0	E980.4
Poliomyelitis vaccine	979.5	E858.8	E949.5	E950.4	E962.0	E980.4
Poliovirus vaccine	979.5	E858.8	E949.5	E950.4	E962.0	E980.4
Polish (car) (floor) (furniture) (metal) (silver)	989.8	E861.2	—	E950.9	E962.1	E980.9
abrasive	989.8	E861.3	—	E950.9	E962.1	E980.9
porcelain	989.8	E861.3	—	E950.9	E962.1	E980.9
Poloxalkol	973.2	E858.4	E943.2	E950.4	E962.0	E980.4
Polyaminostyrene resins	974.5	E858.5	E944.5	E950.4	E962.0	E980.4
Polycycline	960.4	E856	E930.4	E950.4	E962.0	E980.4
Polyester resin hardener	982.8	E862.4	—	E950.9	E962.1	E980.9
fumes	987.8	E869.8	—	E952.8	E962.2	E982.8
Polyestradiol (phosphate)	962.2	E858.0	E932.2	E950.4	E962.0	E980.4
Polyethanolamine alkyl sulfate	976.2	E858.7	E946.2	E950.4	E962.0	E980.4
Polyethylene glycol	976.3	E858.7	E946.3	E950.4	E962.0	E980.4
Polyferose	964.0	E858.2	E934.0	E950.4	E962.0	E980.4
Polymyxin B	960.8	E856	E930.8	E950.4	E962.0	E980.4
ENT agent	976.6	E858.7	E946.6	E950.4	E962.0	E980.4
ophthalmic preparation	976.5	E858.7	E946.5	E950.4	E962.0	E980.4
topical NEC	976.0	E858.7	E946.0	E950.4	E962.0	E980.4
Polynoxylin(e)	976.0	E858.7	E946.0	E950.4	E962.0	E980.4
Polyoxymethyleneurea	976.0	E858.7	E946.0	E950.4	E962.0	E980.4
Polytetrafluoroethylene (inhaled)	987.8	E869.8	—	E952.8	E962.2	E982.8

TABLE OF DRUGS AND CHEMICALS

	\multicolumn{6}{c}{External Cause (E-Code)}
Substance	Poisoning	Accident	Therapeutic Use	Suicide Attempt	Assault	Undetermined
Polythiazide	974.3	E858.5	E944.3	E950.4	E962.0	E980.4
Polyvinylpyrrolidone	964.8	E858.2	E934.8	E950.4	E962.0	E980.4
Pontocaine (hydrochloride) (infiltration) (topical)	968.5	E855.2	E938.5	E950.4	E962.0	E980.4
nerve block (peripheral) (plexus)	968.6	E855.2	E938.6	E950.4	E962.0	E980.4
spinal	968.7	E855.2	E938.7	E950.4	E962.0	E980.4
Pot	969.6	E854.1	E939.6	E950.3	E962.0	E980.3
Potash (caustic)	983.2	E864.2	—	E950.7	E962.1	E980.6
Potassic saline injection (lactated)	974.5	E858.5	E944.5	E950.4	E962.0	E980.4
Potassium (salts) NEC	974.5	E858.5	E944.5	E950.4	E962.0	E980.4
aminosalicylate	961.8	E857	E931.8	E950.4	E962.0	E980.4
arsenite (solution)	985.1	E866.3	—	E950.8	E962.1	E980.8
bichromate	983.9	E864.3	—	E950.7	E962.1	E980.6
bisulfate	983.9	E864.3	—	E950.7	E962.1	E980.6
bromide (medicinal) NEC	967.3	E852.2	E937.3	E950.2	E962.0	E980.2
carbonate	983.2	E864.2	—	E950.7	E962.1	E980.6
chlorate NEC	983.9	E864.3	—	E950.7	E962.1	E980.6
cyanide — see Cyanide						
hydroxide	983.2	E864.2	—	E950.7	E962.1	E980.6
iodide (expectorant) NEC	975.5	E858.6	E945.5	E950.4	E962.0	E980.4
nitrate	989.8	E866.8	—	E950.9	E962.1	E980.9
oxalate	983.9	E864.3	—	E950.7	E962.1	E980.6
perchlorate NEC	977.8	E858.8	E947.8	E950.4	E962.0	E980.4
antithyroid	962.8	E858.0	E932.8	E950.4	E962.0	E980.4
permanganate	976.0	E858.7	E946.0	E950.4	E962.0	E980.4
nonmedicinal	983.9	E864.3	—	E950.7	E962.1	E980.6
Povidone-iodine (anti-infective) NEC	976.0	E858.7	E946.0	E950.4	E962.0	E980.4
Practolol	972.0	E858.3	E942.0	E950.4	E962.0	E980.4
Pralidoxime (chloride)	977.2	E858.8	E947.2	E950.4	E962.0	E980.4
Pramoxine	968.5	E855.2	E938.5	E950.4	E962.0	E980.4
Prazosin	972.6	E858.3	E942.6	E950.4	E962.0	E980.4
Prednisolone	962.0	E858.0	E932.0	E950.4	E962.0	E980.4
ENT agent	976.6	E858.7	E946.6	E950.4	E962.0	E980.4
ophthalmic preparation	976.5	E858.7	E946.5	E950.4	E962.0	E980.4
topical NEC	976.0	E858.7	E946.0	E950.4	E962.0	E980.4
Prednisone	962.0	E858.0	E932.0	E950.4	E962.0	E980.4
Pregnanediol	962.2	E858.0	E932.2	E950.4	E962.0	E980.4
Pregneninolone	962.2	E858.0	E932.2	E950.4	E962.0	E980.4
Preludin	977.0	E858.8	E947.0	E950.4	E962.0	E980.4
Premarin	962.2	E858.0	E932.2	E950.4	E962.0	E980.4
Prenylamine	972.4	E858.3	E942.4	E950.4	E962.0	E980.4
Preparation H	976.8	E858.7	E946.8	E950.4	E962.0	E980.4
Preservatives	989.8	E866.8	—	E950.9	E962.1	E980.9
Pride of China	988.2	E865.3	—	E950.9	E962.1	E980.9
Prilocaine	968.9	E855.2	E938.9	E950.4	E962.0	E980.4
infiltration (subcutaneous)	968.5	E855.2	E938.5	E950.4	E962.0	E980.4
nerve block (peripheral) (plexus)	968.6	E855.2	E938.6	E950.4	E962.0	E980.4
Primaquine	961.4	E857	E931.4	E950.4	E962.0	E980.4
Primidone	966.3	E855.0	E936.3	E950.4	E962.0	E980.4
Primula (veris)	988.2	E865.4	—	E950.9	E962.1	E980.9
Prinadol	965.09	E850.2	E935.2	E950.0	E962.0	E980.0
Priscol, Priscoline	971.3	E855.6	E941.3	E950.4	E962.0	E980.4
Privet	988.2	E865.4	—	E950.9	E962.1	E980.9
Privine	971.2	E855.5	E941.2	E950.4	E962.0	E980.4
Pro-Banthine	971.1	E855.4	E941.1	E950.4	E962.0	E980.4
Probarbitol	967.0	E851	E937.0	E950.1	E962.0	E980.1
Probenecid	974.7	E858.5	E944.7	E950.4	E962.0	E980.4
Procainamide (hydrochloride)	972.0	E858.3	E942.0	E950.4	E962.0	E980.4
Procaine (hydrochloride) (infiltration) (topical)	968.5	E855.2	E938.5	E950.4	E962.0	E980.4
nerve block (peripheral) (plexus)	968.6	E855.2	E938.6	E950.4	E962.0	E980.4
penicillin G	960.0	E856	E930.0	E950.4	E962.0	E980.4
spinal	968.7	E855.2	E938.7	E950.4	E962.0	E980.4
Procalmidol	969.5	E853.8	E939.5	E950.3	E962.0	E980.3
Procarbazine	963.1	E858.1	E933.1	E950.4	E962.0	E980.4
Prochlorperazine	969.1	E853.0	E939.1	E950.3	E962.0	E980.3
Procyclidine	966.4	E855.0	E936.4	E950.4	E962.0	E980.4
Producer gas	986	E868.8	—	E952.1	E962.2	E982.1
Profenamine	966.4	E855.0	E936.4	E950.4	E962.0	E980.4
Profenil	975.1	E858.6	E945.1	E950.4	E962.0	E980.4
Progesterones	962.2	E858.0	E932.2	E950.4	E962.0	E980.4
Progestin	962.2	E858.0	E932.2	E950.4	E962.0	E980.4
Progestogens (with estrogens)	962.2	E858.0	E932.2	E950.4	E962.0	E980.4
Progestone	962.2	E858.0	E932.2	E950.4	E962.0	E980.4
Proguanil	961.4	E857	E931.4	E950.4	E962.0	E980.4
Prolactin	962.4	E858.0	E932.4	E950.4	E962.0	E980.4
Proloid	962.7	E858.0	E932.7	E950.4	E962.0	E980.4
Proluton	962.2	E858.0	E932.2	E950.4	E962.0	E980.4

Substance	Poisoning	Accident	Therapeutic Use	Suicide Attempt	Assault	Undetermined
Promacetin	961.8	E857	E931.8	E950.4	E962.0	E980.4
Promazine	969.1	E853.0	E939.1	E950.3	E962.0	E980.3
Promedol	965.09	E850.2	E935.2	E950.0	E962.0	E980.0
Promethazine	967.8	E852.8	E937.8	E950.2	E962.0	E980.2
Promin	961.8	E857	E931.8	E950.4	E962.0	E980.4
Pronestyl (hydrochloride)	972.0	E858.3	E942.0	E950.4	E962.0	E980.4
Pronetalol, pronethalol	972.0	E858.3	E942.0	E950.4	E962.0	E980.4
Prontosil	961.0	E857	E931.0	E950.4	E962.0	E980.4
Propamidine isethionate	961.5	E857	E931.5	E950.4	E962.0	E980.4
Propanal (medicinal)	967.8	E852.8	E937.8	E950.2	E962.0	E980.2
Propane (gas) (distributed in mobile container)	987.0	E868.0	—	E951.1	E962.2	E981.1
distributed through pipes	987.0	E867	—	E951.0	E962.2	E981.0
incomplete combustion of — see Carbon monoxide, Propane						
Propanidid	968.3	E855.1	E938.3	E950.4	E962.0	E980.4
Propanol	980.3	E860.4	—	E950.9	E962.1	E980.9
Propantheline	971.1	E855.4	E941.1	E950.4	E962.0	E980.4
Proparacaine	968.5	E855.2	E938.5	E950.4	E962.0	E980.4
Propatyl nitrate	972.4	E858.3	E942.4	E950.4	E962.0	E980.4
Propicillin	960.0	E856	E930.0	E950.4	E962.0	E980.4
Propiolactone (vapor)	987.8	E869.8	—	E952.8	E962.2	E982.8
Propiomazine	967.8	E852.8	E937.8	E950.2	E962.0	E980.2
Propionaldehyde (medicinal)	967.8	E852.8	E937.8	E950.2	E962.0	E980.2
Propionate compound	976.0	E858.7	E946.0	E950.4	E962.0	E980.4
Propion gel	976.0	E858.7	E946.0	E950.4	E962.0	E980.4
Propitocaine	968.9	E855.2	E938.9	E950.4	E962.0	E980.4
infiltration (subcutaneous)	968.5	E855.2	E938.5	E950.4	E962.0	E980.4
nerve block (peripheral) (plexus)	968.6	E855.2	E938.6	E950.4	E962.0	E980.4
Propoxur	989.3	E863.2	—	E950.6	E962.1	E980.7
Propoxycaine	968.9	E855.2	E938.9	E950.4	E962.0	E980.4
infiltration (subcutaneous)	968.5	E855.2	E938.5	E950.4	E962.0	E980.4
nerve block (peripheral) (plexus)	968.6	E855.2	E938.6	E950.4	E962.0	E980.4
topical (surface)	968.5	E855.2	E938.5	E950.4	E962.0	E980.4
Propoxyphene (hydrochloride)	965.8	E850.8	E935.8	E950.0	E962.0	E980.0
Propranolol	972.0	E858.3	E942.0	E950.4	E962.0	E980.4
Propyl						
alcohol	980.3	E860.4	—	E950.9	E962.1	E980.9
carbinol	980.3	E860.4	—	E950.9	E962.1	E980.9
hexadrine	971.2	E855.5	E941.2	E950.4	E962.0	E980.4
iodone	977.8	E858.8	E947.8	E950.4	E962.0	E980.4
thiouracil	962.8	E858.0	E932.8	E950.4	E962.0	E980.4
Propylene	987.1	E869.8	—	E952.8	E962.2	E982.8
Propylparaben (ophthalmic)	976.5	E858.7	E946.5	E950.4	E962.0	E980.4
Proscillaridin	972.1	E858.3	E942.1	E950.4	E962.0	E980.4
Prostaglandins	975.0	E858.6	E945.0	E950.4	E962.0	E980.4
Prostigmin	971.0	E855.3	E941.0	E950.4	E962.0	E980.4
Protamine (sulfate)	964.5	E858.2	E934.5	E950.4	E962.0	E980.4
zinc insulin	962.3	E858.0	E932.3	E950.4	E962.0	E980.4
Protectants (topical)	976.3	E858.7	E946.3	E950.4	E962.0	E980.4
Protein hydrolysate	974.5	E858.5	E944.5	E950.4	E962.0	E980.4
Prothionamide	961.8	E857	E931.8	E950.4	E962.0	E980.4
Prothipendyl	969.5	E853.8	E939.5	E950.3	E962.0	E980.3
Protokylol	971.2	E855.5	E941.2	E950.4	E962.0	E980.4
Protopam	977.2	E858.8	E947.2	E950.4	E962.0	E980.4
Protoveratrine(s) (A) (B)	972.6	E858.3	E942.6	E950.4	E962.0	E980.4
Protriptyline	969.0	E854.0	E939.0	E950.3	E962.0	E980.3
Provera	962.2	E858.0	E932.2	E950.4	E962.0	E980.4
Provitamin A	963.5	E858.1	E933.5	E950.4	E962.0	E980.4
Proxymetacaine	968.5	E855.2	E938.5	E950.4	E962.0	E980.4
Proxyphylline	975.1	E858.6	E945.1	E950.4	E962.0	E980.4
Prunus						
laurocerasus	988.2	E865.4	—	E950.9	E962.1	E980.9
virginiana	988.2	E865.4	—	E950.9	E962.1	E980.9
Prussic acid	989.0	E866.8	—	E950.9	E962.1	E980.9
vapor	987.7	E869.8	—	E952.8	E962.2	E982.8
Pseudoephedrine	971.2	E855.5	E941.2	E950.4	E962.0	E980.4
Psilocin	969.6	E854.1	E939.6	E950.3	E962.0	E980.3
Psilocybin	969.6	E854.1	E939.6	E950.3	E962.0	E980.3
PSP	977.8	E858.8	E947.8	E950.4	E962.0	E980.4
Psychedelic agents	969.6	E854.1	E939.6	E950.3	E962.0	E980.3
Psychodysleptics	969.6	E854.1	E939.6	E950.3	E962.0	E980.3
Psychostimulants	969.7	E854.2	E939.7	E950.3	E962.0	E980.3
Psychotherapeutic agents	969.9	E855.9	E939.9	E950.3	E962.0	E980.3
antidepressants	969.0	E854.0	E939.0	E950.3	E962.0	E980.3
specified NEC	969.8	E855.8	E939.8	E950.3	E962.0	E980.3
tranquilizers NEC	969.5	E853.9	E939.5	E950.3	E962.0	E980.3
Psychotomimetic agents	969.6	E854.1	E939.6	E950.3	E962.0	E980.3

Psychotropic agents — TABLE OF DRUGS AND CHEMICALS — Replacement solutions

		External Cause (E-Code)				
Substance	Poisoning	Accident	Therapeutic-Use	Suicide Attempt	Assault	Undetermined
Psychotropic agents	969.9	E855.9	E939.9	E950.3	E962.0	E980.3
specified NEC	969.8	E855.8	E939.8	E950.3	E962.0	E980.3
Psyllium	973.3	E858.4	E943.3	E950.4	E962.0	E980.4
Pteroylglutamic acid	964.1	E858.2	E934.1	E950.4	E962.0	E980.4
Pteroyltriglutamate	963.1	E858.1	E933.1	E950.4	E962.0	E980.4
PTFE	987.8	E869.8	—	E952.8	E962.2	E982.8
Pulsatilla	988.2	E865.4	—	E950.9	E962.1	E980.9
Purex (bleach)	983.9	E864.3	—	E950.7	E962.1	E980.6
Purine diuretics	974.1	E858.5	E944.1	E950.4	E962.0	E980.4
Purinethol	963.1	E858.1	E933.1	E950.4	E962.0	E980.4
PVP	964.8	E858.2	E934.8	E950.4	E962.0	E980.4
Pyrabital	965.7	E850.7	E935.7	E950.0	E962.0	E980.0
Pyramidon	965.5	E850.5	E935.5	E950.0	E962.0	E980.0
Pyrantel (pamoate)	961.6	E857	E931.6	E950.4	E962.0	E980.4
Pyrathiazine	963.0	E858.1	E933.0	E950.4	E962.0	E980.4
Pyrazinamide	961.8	E857	E931.8	E950.4	E962.0	E980.4
Pyrazinoic acid (amide)	961.8	E857	E931.8	E950.4	E962.0	E980.4
Pyrazole (derivatives)	965.5	E850.5	E935.5	E950.0	E962.0	E980.0
Pyrazolone (analgesics)	965.5	E850.5	E935.5	E950.0	E962.0	E980.0
Pyrethrins, pyrethrum	989.4	E863.4	—	E950.6	E962.1	E980.7
Pyribenzamine	963.0	E858.1	E933.0	E950.4	E962.0	E980.4
Pyridine (liquid) (vapor)	982.0	E862.4	—	E950.9	E962.1	E980.9
aldoxime chloride	977.2	E858.8	E947.2	E950.4	E962.0	E980.4
Pyridium	976.1	E858.7	E946.1	E950.4	E962.0	E980.4
Pyridostigmine	971.0	E855.3	E941.0	E950.4	E962.0	E980.4
Pyridoxine	963.5	E858.1	E933.5	E950.4	E962.0	E980.4
Pyrilamine	963.0	E858.1	E933.0	E950.4	E962.0	E980.4
Pyrimethamine	961.4	E857	E931.4	E950.4	E962.0	E980.4
Pyrogallic acid	983.0	E864.0	—	E950.7	E962.1	E980.6
Pyroxylin	976.3	E858.7	E946.3	E950.4	E962.0	E980.4
Pyrrobutamine	963.0	E858.1	E933.0	E950.4	E962.0	E980.4
Pyrrocaine	968.5	E855.2	E938.5	E950.4	E962.0	E980.4
Pyrvinium (pamoate)	961.6	E857	E931.6	E950.4	E962.0	E980.4
PZI	962.3	E858.0	E932.3	E950.4	E962.0	E980.4
Quaalude	967.4	E852.3	E937.4	E950.2	E962.0	E980.2
Quaternary ammonium derivatives	971.1	E855.4	E941.1	E950.4	E962.0	E980.4
Quicklime	983.2	E864.2	—	E950.7	E962.1	E980.6
Quinacrine	961.3	E857	E931.3	E950.4	E962.0	E980.4
Quinaglute	972.0	E858.3	E942.0	E950.4	E962.0	E980.4
Quinalbarbitone	967.0	E851	E937.0	E950.1	E962.0	E980.1
Quinestradiol	962.2	E858.0	E932.2	E950.4	E962.0	E980.4
Quinethazone	974.3	E858.5	E944.3	E950.4	E962.0	E980.4
Quinidine (gluconate) (polygalacturonate) (salts) (sulfate)	972.0	E858.3	E942.0	E950.4	E962.0	E980.4
Quinine	961.4	E857	E931.4	E950.4	E962.0	E980.4
Quiniobine	961.3	E857	E931.3	E950.4	E962.0	E980.4
Quinolines	961.3	E857	E931.3	E950.4	E962.0	E980.4
Quotane	968.5	E855.2	E938.5	E950.4	E962.0	E980.4
Rabies						
immune globulin (human)	964.6	E858.2	E934.6	E950.4	E962.0	E980.4
vaccine	979.1	E858.8	E949.1	E950.4	E962.0	E980.4
Racemoramide	965.09	E850.2	E935.2	E950.0	E962.0	E980.0
Racemorphan	965.09	E850.2	E935.2	E950.0	E962.0	E980.0
Radiator alcohol	980.1	E860.2	—	E950.9	E962.1	E980.9
Radio-opaque (drugs) (materials)	977.8	E858.8	E947.8	E950.4	E962.0	E980.4
Ranunculus	988.2	E865.4	—	E950.9	E962.1	E980.9
Rat poison	989.4	E863.7	—	E950.6	E962.1	E980.7
Rattlesnake (venom)	989.5	E905.0	—	E950.9	E962.1	E980.9
Raudixin	972.6	E858.3	E942.6	E950.4	E962.0	E980.4
Rautensin	972.6	E858.3	E942.6	E950.4	E962.0	E980.4
Rautina	972.6	E858.3	E942.6	E950.4	E962.0	E980.4
Rautotal	972.6	E858.3	E942.6	E950.4	E962.0	E980.4
Rauwiloid	972.6	E858.3	E942.6	E950.4	E962.0	E980.4
Rauwoldin	972.6	E858.3	E942.6	E950.4	E962.0	E980.4
Rauwolfia (alkaloids)	972.6	E858.3	E942.6	E950.4	E962.0	E980.4
Realgar	985.1	E866.3	—	E950.8	E962.1	E980.8
Red cells, packed	964.7	E858.2	E934.7	E950.4	E962.0	E980.4
Reducing agents, industrial NEC	983.9	E864.3	—	E950.7	E962.1	E980.6.
Refrigerant gas (freon)	987.4	E869.2	—	E952.8	E962.2	E982.8
not freon	987.9	E869.9	—	E952.9	E962.2	E982.9
Regroton	974.4	E858.5	E944.4	E950.4	E962.0	E980.4
Rela	968.0	E855.1	E938.0	E950.4	E962.0	E980.4
Relaxants, skeletal muscle (autonomic)	975.2	E858.6	E945.2	E950.4	E962.0	E980.4
central nervous system	968.0	E855.1	E938.0	E950.4	E962.0	E980.4
Renese	974.3	E858.5	E944.3	E950.4	E962.0	E980.4
Renografin	977.8	E858.8	E947.8	E950.4	E962.0	E980.4
Replacement solutions	974.5	E858.5	E944.5	E950.4	E962.0	E980.4

TABLE OF DRUGS AND CHEMICALS

Substance	Poisoning	Accident	Therapeutic-Use	Suicide Attempt	Assault	Undetermined
Rescinnamine	972.6	E858.3	E942.6	E950.4	E962.0	E980.4
Reserpine	972.6	E858.3	E942.6	E950.4	E962.0	E980.4
Resorcin, resorcinol	976.4	E858.7	E946.4	E950.4	E962.0	E980.4
Respaire	975.5	E858.6	E945.5	E950.4	E962.0	E980.4
Respiratory agents NEC	975.8	E858.6	E945.8	E950.4	E962.0	E980.4
Retinoic acid	976.8	E858.7	E946.8	E950.4	E962.0	E980.4
Retinol	963.5	E858.1	E933.5	E950.4	E962.0	E980.4
Rh$_o$ (D) immune globulin (human)	964.6	E858.2	E934.6	E950.4	E962.0	E980.4
Rhodine	965.1	E850.3	E935.3	E950.0	E962.0	E980.0
RhoGAM	964.6	E858.2	E934.6	E950.4	E962.0	E980.4
Riboflavin	963.5	E858.1	E933.5	E950.4	E962.0	E980.4
Ricin	989.8	E866.8	—	E950.9	E962.1	E980.9
Ricinus communis	988.2	E865.3	—	E950.9	E962.1	E980.9
Rickettsial vaccine NEC	979.6	E858.8	E949.6	E950.4	E962.0	E980.4
with viral and bacterial vaccine	979.7	E858.8	E949.7	E950.4	E962.0	E980.4
Rifampin	960.6	E856	E930.6	E950.4	E962.0	E980.4
Rimifon	961.8	E857	E931.8	E950.4	E962.0	E980.4
Ringer's injection (lactated)	974.5	E858.5	E944.5	E950.4	E962.0	E980.4
Ristocetin	960.8	E856	E930.8	E950.4	E962.0	E980.4
Ritalin	969.7	E854.2	E939.7	E950.3	E962.0	E980.3
Roach killers — see Pesticides						
Rocky Mountain spotted fever vaccine	979.6	E858.8	E949.6	E950.4	E962.0	E980.4
Rodenticides	989.4	E863.7	—	E950.6	E962.1	E980.7
Rolaids	973.0	E858.4	E943.0	E950.4	E962.0	E980.4
Rolitetracycline	960.4	E856	E930.4	E950.4	E962.0	E980.4
Romilar	975.4	E858.6	E945.4	E950.4	E962.0	E980.4
Rose water ointment	976.3	E858.7	E946.3	E950.4	E962.0	E980.4
Rotenone	989.4	E863.7	—	E950.6	E962.1	E980.7
Rotoxamine	963.0	E858.1	E933.0	E950.4	E962.0	E980.4
Rough-on-rats	989.4	E863.7	—	E950.6	E962.1	E980.7
Rubbing alcohol	980.2	E860.3	—	E950.9	E962.1	E980.9
Rubella virus vaccine	979.4	E858.8	E949.4	E950.4	E962.0	E980.4
Rubelogen	979.4	E858.8	E949.4	E950.4	E962.0	E980.4
Rubeovax	979.4	E858.8	E949.4	E950.4	E962.0	E980.4
Rubidomycin	960.7	E856	E930.7	E950.4	E962.0	E980.4
Rue	988.2	E865.4	—	E950.9	E962.1	E980.9
Ruta	988.2	E865.4	—	E950.9	E962.1	E980.9
Sabadilla (medicinal)	976.0	E858.7	E946.0	E950.4	E962.0	E980.4
pesticide	989.4	E863.4	—	E950.6	E962.1	E980.7
Sabin oral vaccine	979.5	E858.8	E949.5	E950.4	E962.0	E980.4
Saccharated iron oxide	964.0	E858.2	E934.0	E950.4	E962.0	E980.4
Saccharin	974.5	E858.5	E944.5	E950.4	E962.0	E980.4
Safflower oil	972.2	E858.3	E942.2	E950.4	E962.0	E980.4
Salicylamide	965.1	E850.3	E935.3	E950.0	E962.0	E980.0
Salicylate(s)	965.1	E850.3	E935.3	E950.0	E962.0	E980.0
methyl	976.3	E858.7	E946.3	E950.4	E962.0	E980.4
theobromine calcium	974.1	E858.5	E944.1	E950.4	E962.0	E980.4
Salicylazosulfapyridine	961.0	E857	E931.0	E950.4	E962.0	E980.4
Salicylhydroxamic acid	976.0	E858.7	E946.0	E950.4	E962.0	E980.4
Salicylic acid (keratolytic) NEC	976.4	E858.7	E946.4	E950.4	E962.0	E980.4
congeners	965.1	E850.3	E935.3	E950.0	E962.0	E980.0
salts	965.1	E850.3	E935.3	E950.0	E962.0	E980.0
Saliniazid	961.8	E857	E931.8	E950.4	E962.0	E980.4
Salol	976.3	E858.7	E946.3	E950.4	E962.0	E980.4
Salt (substitute) NEC	974.5	E858.5	E944.5	E950.4	E962.0	E980.4
Saluretics	974.3	E858.5	E944.3	E950.4	E962.0	E980.4
Saluron	974.3	E858.5	E944.3	E950.4	E962.0	E980.4
Salvarsan 606 (neosilver) (silver)	961.1	E857	E931.1	E950.4	E962.0	E980.4
Sambucus canadensis	988.2	E865.4	—	E950.9	E962.1	E980.9
berry	988.2	E865.3	—	E950.9	E962.1	E980.9
Sandril	972.6	E858.3	E942.6	E950.4	E962.0	E980.4
Sanguinaria canadensis	988.2	E865.4	—	E950.9	E962.1	E980.9
Saniflush (cleaner)	983.9	E861.3	—	E950.7	E962.1	E980.6
Santonin	961.6	E857	E931.6	E950.4	E962.0	E980.4
Santyl	976.8	E858.7	E946.8	E950.4	E962.0	E980.4
Sarkomycin	960.7	E856	E930.7	E950.4	E962.0	E980.4
Saroten	969.0	E854.0	E939.0	E950.3	E962.0	E980.3
Saturnine — see Lead						
Savin (oil)	976.4	E858.7	E946.4	E950.4	E962.0	E980.4
Scammony	973.1	E858.4	E943.1	E950.4	E962.0	E980.4
Scarlet red	976.8	E858.7	E946.8	E950.4	E962.0	E980.4
Scheele's green	985.1	E866.3	—	E950.8	E962.1	E980.8
insecticide	985.1	E863.4	—	E950.6	E962.1	E980.8
Schradan	989.3	E863.1	—	E950.6	E962.1	E980.7
Schweinfurt(h) green	985.1	E866.3	—	E950.8	E962.1	E980.8
insecticide	985.1	E863.4	—	E950.8	E962.1	E980.8

Substance	Poisoning	Accident	Therapeutic Use	Suicide Attempt	Assault	Undetermined
Scilla — see Squill						
Sclerosing agents	972.7	E858.3	E942.7	E950.4	E962.0	E980.4
Scopolamine	971.1	E855.4	E941.1	E950.4	E962.0	E980.4
Scouring powder	989.8	E861.3	—	E950.9	E962.1	E980.9
Sea						
anemone (sting)	989.5	E905.6	—	E950.9	E962.1	E980.9
cucumber (sting)	989.5	E905.6	—	E950.9	E962.1	E980.9
snake (bite) (venom)	989.5	E905.0	—	E950.9	E962.1	E980.9
urchin spine (puncture)	989.5	E905.6	—	E950.9	E962.1	E980.9
Secbutabarbital	967.0	E851	E937.0	E950.1	E962.0	E980.1
Secbutabarbitone	967.0	E851	E937.0	E950.1	E962.0	E980.1
Secobarbital	967.0	E851	E937.0	E950.1	E962.0	E980.1
Seconal	967.0	E851	E937.0	E950.1	E962.0	E980.1
Secretin	977.8	E858.8	E947.8	E950.4	E962.0	E980.4
Sedatives, nonbarbiturate	967.9	E852.9	E937.9	E950.2	E962.0	E980.2
specified NEC	967.8	E852.8	E937.8	E950.2	E962.0	E980.2
Sedormid	967.8	E852.8	E937.8	E950.2	E962.0	E980.2
Seed (plant)	988.2	E865.3	—	E950.9	E962.1	E980.9
disinfectant or dressing	989.8	E866.5	—	E950.9	E962.1	E980.9
Selenium (fumes) NEC	985.8	E866.4	—	E950.9	E962.1	E980.9
disulfide or sulfide	976.4	E858.7	E946.4	E950.4	E962.0	E980.4
Selsun	976.4	E858.7	E946.4	E950.4	E962.0	E980.4
Senna	973.1	E858.4	E943.1	E950.4	E962.0	E980.4
Septisol	976.2	E858.7	E946.2	E950.4	E962.0	E980.4
Serax	969.4	E853.2	E939.4	E950.3	E962.0	E980.3
Serenesil	967.8	E852.8	E937.8	E950.2	E962.0	E980.2
Serenium (hydrochloride)	961.9	E857	E931.9	E950.4	E962.0	E980.4
Sernyl	968.3	E855.1	E938.3	E950.4	E962.0	E980.4
Serotonin	977.8	E858.8	E947.8	E950.4	E962.0	E980.4
Serpasil	972.6	E858.3	E942.6	E950.4	E962.0	E980.4
Sewer gas	987.8	E869.8	—	E952.8	E962.2	E982.8
Shampoo	989.6	E861.0	—	E950.9	E962.1	E980.9
Shellfish, nonbacterial or noxious	988.0	E865.1	—	E950.9	E962.1	E980.9
Silicones NEC	989.8	E866.8	E947.8	E950.9	E962.1	E980.9
Silvadene	976.0	E858.7	E946.0	E950.4	E962.0	E980.4
Silver (compound) (medicinal) NEC	976.0	E858.7	E946.0	E950.4	E962.0	E980.4
anti-infectives	976.0	E858.7	E946.0	E950.4	E962.0	E980.4
arsphenamine	961.1	E857	E931.1	E950.4	E962.0	E980.4
nitrate	976.0	E858.7	E946.0	E950.4	E962.0	E980.4
ophthalmic preparation	976.5	E858.7	E946.5	E950.4	E962.0	E980.4
toughened (keratolytic)	976.4	E858.7	E946.4	E950.4	E962.0	E980.4
nonmedicinal (dust)	985.8	E866.4	—	E950.9	E962.1	E980.9
protein (mild) (strong)	976.0	E858.7	E946.0	E950.4	E962.0	E980.4
salvarsan	961.1	E857	E931.1	E950.4	E962.0	E980.4
Simethicone	973.8	E858.4	E943.8	E950.4	E962.0	E980.4
Sinequan	969.0	E854.0	E939.0	E950.3	E962.0	E980.3
Singoserp	972.6	E858.3	E942.6	E950.4	E962.0	E980.4
Sintrom	964.2	E858.2	E934.2	E950.4	E962.0	E980.4
Sitosterols	972.2	E858.3	E942.2	E950.4	E962.0	E980.4
Skeletal muscle relaxants	975.2	E858.6	E945.2	E950.4	E962.0	E980.4
Skin						
agents (external)	976.9	E858.7	E946.9	E950.4	E962.0	E980.4
specified NEC	976.8	E858.7	E946.8	E950.4	E962.0	E980.4
test antigen	977.8	E858.8	E947.8	E950.4	E962.0	E980.4
Sleep-eze	963.0	E858.1	E933.0	E950.4	E962.0	E980.4
Sleeping draught (drug) (pill) (tablet)	967.9	E852.9	E937.9	E950.2	E962.0	E980.4
Smallpox vaccine	979.0	E858.8	E949.0	E950.4	E962.0	E980.4
Smelter fumes NEC	985.9	E866.4	—	E950.9	E962.1	E980.9
Smog	987.3	E869.1	—	E952.8	E962.2	E982.8
Smoke NEC	987.9	E869.9	—	E952.9	E962.2	E982.9
Smooth muscle relaxant	975.1	E858.6	E945.1	E950.4	E962.0	E980.4
Snail killer	989.4	E863.4	—	E950.6	E962.1	E980.7
Snake (bite) (venom)	989.5	E905.0	—	E950.9	E962.1	E980.9
Snuff	989.8	E866.8	—	E950.9	E962.1	E980.9
Soap (powder) (product)	989.6	E861.1	—	E950.9	E962.1	E980.9
medicinal, soft	976.2	E858.7	E946.2	E950.4	E962.0	E980.4
Soda (caustic)	983.2	E864.2	—	E950.7	E962.1	E980.6
bicarb	963.3	E858.1	E933.3	E950.4	E962.0	E980.4
chlorinated — see Sodium, hypochlorite						
Sodium						
acetosulfone	961.8	E857	E931.8	E950.4	E962.0	E980.4
acetrizoate	977.8	E858.8	E947.8	E950.4	E962.0	E980.4
amytal	967.0	E851	E937.0	E950.1	E962.0	E980.1
arsenate — see Arsenic						
bicarbonate	963.3	E858.1	E933.3	E950.4	E962.0	E980.4
bichromate	983.9	E864.3	—	E950.7	E962.1	E980.6

Substance	Poisoning	Accident	Therapeutic Use	Suicide Attempt	Assault	Undetermined
Sodium—continued						
biphosphate	963.2	E858.1	E933.2	E950.4	E962.0	E980.4
bisulfate	983.9	E864.3	—	E950.7	E962.1	E980.6
borate (cleanser)	989.6	E861.3	—	E950.9	E962.1	E980.9
bromide NEC	967.3	E852.2	E937.3	E950.2	E962.0	E980.2
cacodylate (nonmedicinal) NEC	978.8	E858.8	E948.8	E950.4	E962.0	E980.4
anti-infective	961.1	E857	E931.1	E950.4	E962.0	E980.4
herbicide	989.4	E863.5	—	E950.6	E962.1	E980.7
calcium edetate	963.8	E858.1	E933.8	E950.4	E962.0	E980.4
carbonate NEC	983.2	E864.2	—	E950.7	E962.1	E980.6
chlorate NEC	983.9	E864.3	—	E950.7	E962.1	E980.6
herbicide	983.9	E863.5	—	E950.7	E962.1	E980.6
chloride NEC	974.5	E858.5	E944.5	E950.4	E962.0	E980.4
chromate	983.9	E864.3	—	E950.7	E962.1	E980.6
citrate	963.3	E858.1	E933.3	E950.4	E962.0	E980.4
cyanide — see Cyanide(s)						
cyclamate	974.5	E858.5	E944.5	E950.4	E962.0	E980.4
diatrizoate	977.8	E858.8	E947.8	E950.4	E962.0	E980.4
dibunate	975.4	E858.6	E945.4	E950.4	E962.0	E980.4
dioctyl sulfosuccinate	973.2	E858.4	E943.2	E950.4	E962.0	E980.4
edetate	963.8	E858.1	E933.8	E950.4	E962.0	E980.4
ethacrynate	974.4	E858.5	E944.4	E950.4	E962.0	E980.4
fluoracetate (dust) (rodenticide)	989.4	E863.7	—	E950.6	E962.1	E980.7
fluoride — see Fluoride(s)						
free salt	974.5	E858.5	E944.5	E950.4	E962.0	E980.4
glucosulfone	961.8	E857	E931.8	E950.4	E962.0	E980.4
hydroxide	983.2	E864.2	—	E950.7	E962.1	E980.6
hypochlorite (bleach) NEC	983.9	E864.3	—	E950.7	E962.1	E980.6
disinfectant	983.9	E861.4	—	E950.7	E962.1	E980.6
medicinal (anti-infective) (external)	976.0	E858.7	E946.0	E950.4	E962.0	E980.4
vapor	987.8	E869.8	—	E952.8	E962.2	E982.8
hyposulfite	976.0	E858.7	E946.0	E950.4	E962.0	E980.4
indigotindisulfonate	977.8	E858.8	E947.8	E950.4	E962.0	E980.4
iodide	977.8	E858.8	E947.8	E950.4	E962.0	E980.4
iothalamate	977.8	E858.8	E947.8	E950.4	E962.0	E980.4
iron edetate	964.0	E858.2	E934.0	E950.4	E962.0	E980.4
lactate	963.3	E858.1	E933.3	E950.4	E962.0	E980.4
lauryl sulfate	976.2	E858.7	E946.2	E950.4	E962.0	E980.4
L-triiodothyronine	962.7	E858.0	E932.7	E950.4	E962.0	E980.4
metrizoate	977.8	E858.8	E947.8	E950.4	E962.0	E980.4
monofluoracetate (dust) (rodenticide)	989.4	E863.7	—	E950.6	E962.1	E980.7
morrhuate	972.7	E858.3	E942.7	E950.4	E962.0	E980.4
nafcillin	960.0	E856	E930.0	E950.4	E962.0	E980.4
nitrate (oxidizing agent)	983.9	E864.3	—	E950.7	E962.1	E980.6
nitrite (medicinal)	972.4	E858.3	E942.4	E950.4	E962.0	E980.4
nitroferricyanide	972.6	E858.3	E942.6	E950.4	E962.0	E980.4
nitroprusside	972.6	E858.3	E942.6	E950.4	E962.0	E980.4
para-aminohippurate	977.8	E858.8	E947.8	E950.4	E962.0	E980.4
perborate (nonmedicinal) NEC	989.8	E866.8	—	E950.9	E962.1	E980.9
medicinal	976.6	E858.7	E946.6	E950.4	E962.0	E980.4
soap	989.6	E861.1	—	E950.9	E962.1	E980.9
percarbonate — see Sodium, perborate						
phosphate	973.3	E858.4	E943.3	E950.4	E962.0	E980.4
polystyrene sulfonate	974.5	E858.5	E944.5	E950.4	E962.0	E980.4
propionate	976.0	E858.7	E946.0	E950.4	E962.0	E980.4
psylliate	972.7	E858.3	E942.7	E950.4	E962.0	E980.4
removing resins	974.5	E858.5	E944.5	E950.4	E962.0	E980.4
salicylate	965.1	E850.3	E935.3	E950.0	E962.0	E980.0
sulfate	973.3	E858.4	E943.3	E950.4	E962.0	E980.4
sulfoxone	961.8	E857	E931.8	E950.4	E962.0	E980.4
tetradecyl sulfate	972.7	E858.3	E942.7	E950.4	E962.0	E980.4
thiopental	968.3	E855.1	E938.3	E950.4	E962.0	E980.4
thiosalicylate	965.1	E850.3	E935.3	E950.0	E962.0	E980.0
thiosulfate	976.0	E858.7	E946.0	E950.4	E962.0	E980.4
tolbutamide	977.8	E858.8	E947.8	E950.4	E962.0	E980.4
tyropanoate	977.8	E858.8	E947.8	E950.4	E962.0	E980.4
Solanine	977.8	E858.8	E947.8	E950.4	E962.0	E980.4
Solanum dulcamara	988.2	E865.4	—	E950.9	E962.1	E980.9
Solapsone	961.8	E857	E931.8	E950.4	E962.0	E980.4
Solasulfone	961.8	E857	E931.8	E950.4	E962.0	E980.4
Soldering fluid	983.1	E864.1	—	E950.7	E962.1	E980.6
Solid substance	989.9	E866.9	—	E950.9	E962.1	E980.9
specified NEC	989.9	E866.8	—	E950.9	E962.1	E980.9
Solvents, industrial	982.8	E862.9	—	E950.9	E962.1	E980.9
naphtha	981	E862.0	—	E950.9	E962.1	E980.9
petroleum	981	E862.0	—	E950.9	E962.1	E980.9

TABLE OF DRUGS AND CHEMICALS

Substance	Poisoning	Accident	Therapeutic-Use	Suicide Attempt	Assault	Undetermined
Solvents, industrial—continued						
specified NEC	982.8	E862.4	—	E950.9	E962.1	E980.9
Soma	968.0	E855.1	E938.0	E950.4	E962.0	E980.4
Somatotropin	962.4	E858.0	E932.4	E950.4	E962.0	E980.4
Sominex	963.0	E858.1	E933.0	E950.4	E962.0	E980.4
Somnos	967.1	E852.2	E937.1	E950.2	E962.0	E980.2
Somonal	967.0	E851	E937.0	E950.1	E962.0	E980.1
Soneryl	967.0	E851	E937.0	E950.1	E962.0	E980.1
Soothing syrup	977.9	E858.9	E947.9	E950.5	E962.0	E980.5
Sopor	967.4	E852.2	E937.4	E950.2	E962.0	E980.2
Soporific drug	967.9	E852.9	E937.9	E950.2	E962.0	E980.2
specified type NEC	967.8	E852.8	E937.8	E950.2	E962.0	E980.2
Sorbitol NEC	977.4	E858.8	E947.4	E950.4	E962.0	E980.4
Sotradecol	972.7	E858.3	E942.7	E950.4	E962.0	E980.4
Spacoline	975.1	E858.6	E945.1	E950.4	E962.0	E980.4
Spanish fly	976.8	E858.7	E946.8	E950.4	E962.0	E980.4
Sparine	969.1	E853.0	E939.1	E950.3	E962.0	E980.3
Sparteine	975.0	E858.6	E945.0	E950.4	E962.0	E980.4
Spasmolytics	975.1	E858.6	E945.1	E950.4	E962.0	E980.4
anticholinergics	971.1	E855.4	E941.1	E950.4	E962.0	E980.4
Spectinomycin	960.8	E856	E930.8	E950.4	E962.0	E980.4
Speed	969.7	E854.2	E939.7	E950.3	E962.0	E980.3
Spermicides	976.8	E858.7	E946.8	E950.4	E962.0	E980.4
Spider (bite) (venom)	989.5	E905.1	—	E950.9	E962.1	E980.9
antivenin	979.9	E858.8	E949.9	E950.4	E962.0	E980.4
Spigelia (root)	961.6	E857	E931.6	E950.4	E962.0	E980.4
Spiperone	969.2	E853.1	E939.2	E950.3	E962.0	E980.3
Spiramycin	960.3	E856	E930.3	E950.4	E962.0	E980.4
Spirilene	969.5	E853.8	E939.5	E950.3	E962.0	E980.3
Spirit(s) (neutral) NEC	980.0	E860.1	—	E950.9	E962.1	E980.9
beverage	980.0	E860.0	—	E950.9	E962.1	E980.9
industrial	980.9	E860.9	—	E950.9	E962.1	E980.9
mineral	981	E862.0	—	E950.9	E962.1	E980.9
of salt — see Hydrochloric acid						
surgical	980.9	E860.9	—	E950.9	E962.1	E980.9
Spironolactone	974.4	E858.5	E944.4	E950.4	E962.0	E980.4
Sponge, absorbable (gelatin)	964.5	E858.2	E934.5	E950.4	E962.0	E980.4
Sporostacin	976.0	E858.7	E946.0	E950.4	E962.0	E980.4
Sprays (aerosol)	989.8	E866.8	—	E950.9	E962.1	E980.9
cosmetic	989.8	E866.7	—	E950.9	E962.1	E980.9
medicinal NEC	977.9	E858.9	E947.9	E950.5	E962.0	E980.5
pesticides — see Pesticides						
specified content — see substance specified						
Spurge flax	988.2	E865.4	—	E950.9	E962.1	E980.9
Spurges	988.2	E865.4	—	E950.9	E962.1	E980.9
Squill (expectorant) NEC	975.5	E858.6	E945.5	E950.4	E962.0	E980.4
rat poison	989.4	E863.7	—	E950.6	E962.1	E980.7
Squirting cucumber (cathartic)	973.1	E858.4	E943.1	E950.4	E962.0	E980.4
Stains	989.8	E866.8	—	E950.9	E962.1	E980.9
Stannous — see also Tin						
fluoride	976.7	E858.7	E946.7	E950.4	E962.0	E980.4
Stanolone	962.1	E858.0	E932.1	E950.4	E962.0	E980.4
Stanozolol	962.1	E858.0	E932.1	E950.4	E962.0	E980.4
Staphisagria or stavesacre (pediculicide)	976.0	E858.7	E946.0	E950.4	E962.0	E980.4
Stelazine	969.1	E853.0	E939.1	E950.3	E962.0	E980.3
Stemetil	969.1	E853.0	E939.1	E950.3	E962.0	E980.3
Sterculia (cathartic) (gum)	973.3	E858.4	E943.3	E950.4	E962.0	E980.4
Sternutator gas	987.8	E869.8	—	E952.8	E962.2	E982.8
Steroids NEC	962.0	E858.0	E932.0	E950.4	E962.0	E980.4
ENT agent	976.6	E858.7	E946.6	E950.4	E962.0	E980.4
ophthalmic preparation	976.5	E858.7	E946.5	E950.4	E962.0	E980.4
topical NEC	976.0	E858.7	E946.0	E950.4	E962.0	E980.4
Stibine	985.8	E866.4	—	E950.9	E962.1	E980.9
Stibophen	961.2	E857	E931.2	E950.4	E962.0	E980.4
Stilbamide, stilbamidine	961.5	E857	E931.5	E950.4	E962.0	E980.4
Stilbestrol	962.2	E858.0	E932.2	E950.4	E962.0	E980.4
Stimulants (central nervous system)	970.9	E854.3	E940.9	E950.4	E962.0	E980.4
analeptics	970.0	E854.3	E940.0	E950.4	E962.0	E980.4
opiate antagonist	970.1	E854.3	E940.1	E950.4	E962.0	E980.4
psychotherapeutic NEC	969.0	E854.0	E939.0	E950.3	E962.0	E980.3
specified NEC	970.8	E854.3	E940.8	E950.4	E962.0	E980.4
Storage batteries (acid) (cells)	983.1	E864.1	—	E950.7	E962.1	E980.6
Stovaine	968.9	E855.2	E938.9	E950.4	E962.0	E980.4
infiltration (subcutaneous)	968.5	E855.2	E938.5	E950.4	E962.0	E980.4
nerve block (peripheral) (plexus)	968.6	E855.2	E938.6	E950.4	E962.0	E980.4
spinal	968.7	E855.2	E938.7	E950.4	E962.0	E980.4

Substance	Poisoning	Accident	Therapeutic-Use	Suicide Attempt	Assault	Undetermined
Stovaine—continued						
topical (surface)	968.5	E855.2	E938.5	E950.4	E962.0	E980.4
Stovarsal	961.1	E857	E931.1	E950.4	E962.0	E980.4
Stove gas — see Gas, utility						
Stoxil	976.5	E858.7	E946.5	E950.4	E962.0	E980.4
STP	969.6	E854.1	E939.6	E950.3	E962.0	E980.3
Stramonium (medicinal) NEC	971.1	E855.4	E941.1	E950.4	E962.0	E980.4
natural state	988.2	E865.4	—	E950.9	E962.1	E980.9
Streptodornase	964.4	E858.2	E934.4	E950.4	E962.0	E980.4
Streptoduocin	960.6	E856	E930.6	E950.4	E962.0	E980.4
Streptokinase	964.4	E858.2	E934.4	E950.4	E962.0	E980.4
Streptomycin	960.6	E856	E930.6	E950.4	E962.0	E980.4
Streptozocin	960.7	E856	E930.7	E950.4	E962.0	E980.4
Stripper (paint) (solvent)	982.8	E862.9	—	E950.9	E962.1	E980.9
Strobane	989.2	E863.0	—	E950.6	E962.1	E980.7
Strophanthin	972.1	E858.3	E942.1	E950.4	E962.0	E980.4
Strophanthus hispidus or kombe	988.2	E865.4	—	E950.9	E962.1	E980.9
Strychnine (rodenticide) (salts)	989.1	E863.7	—	E950.6	E962.1	E980.7
medicinal NEC	970.8	E854.3	E940.8	E950.4	E962.0	E980.4
Strychnos (ignatii) — see Strychnine						
Styramate	968.0	E855.1	E938.0	E950.4	E962.0	E980.4
Styrene	983.0	E864.0	—	E950.7	E962.1	E980.6
Succinimide (anticonvulsant)	966.2	E855.0	E936.2	E950.4	E962.0	E980.4
mercuric — see Mercury						
Succinylcholine	975.2	E858.6	E945.2	E950.4	E962.0	E980.4
Succinylsulfathiazole	961.0	E857	E931.0	E950.4	E962.0	E980.4
Sucrose	974.5	E858.5	E944.5	E950.4	E962.0	E980.4
Sulfacetamide	961.0	E857	E931.0	E950.4	E962.0	E980.4
ophthalmic preparation	976.5	E858.7	E946.5	E950.4	E962.0	E980.4
Sulfachlorpyridazine	961.0	E857	E931.0	E950.4	E962.0	E980.4
Sulfacytine	961.0	E857	E931.0	E950.4	E962.0	E980.4
Sulfadiazine	961.0	E857	E931.0	E950.4	E962.0	E980.4
silver (topical)	976.0	E858.7	E946.0	E950.4	E962.0	E980.4
Sulfadimethoxine	961.0	E857	E931.0	E950.4	E962.0	E980.4
Sulfadimidine	961.0	E857	E931.0	E950.4	E962.0	E980.4
Sulfaethidole	961.0	E857	E931.0	E950.4	E962.0	E980.4
Sulfafurazole	961.0	E857	E931.0	E950.4	E962.0	E980.4
Sulfaguanidine	961.0	E857	E931.0	E950.4	E962.0	E980.4
Sulfamerazine	961.0	E857	E931.0	E950.4	E962.0	E980.4
Sulfameter	961.0	E857	E931.0	E950.4	E962.0	E980.4
Sulfamethizole	961.0	E857	E931.0	E950.4	E962.0	E980.4
Sulfamethoxazole	961.0	E857	E931.0	E950.4	E962.0	E980.4
Sulfamethoxydiazine	961.0	E857	E931.0	E950.4	E962.0	E980.4
Sulfamethoxypyridazine	961.0	E857	E931.0	E950.4	E962.0	E980.4
Sulfamethylthiazole	961.0	E857	E931.0	E950.4	E962.0	E980.4
Sulfamylon	976.0	E858.7	E946.0	E950.4	E962.0	E980.4
Sulfan blue (diagnostic dye)	977.8	E858.8	E947.8	E950.4	E962.0	E980.4
Sulfanilamide	961.0	E857	E931.0	E950.4	E962.0	E980.4
Sulfanilylguanidine	961.0	E857	E931.0	E950.4	E962.0	E980.4
Sulfaphenazole	961.0	E857	E931.0	E950.4	E962.0	E980.4
Sulfaphenylthiazole	961.0	E857	E931.0	E950.4	E962.0	E980.4
Sulfaproxyline	961.0	E857	E931.0	E950.4	E962.0	E980.4
Sulfapyridine	961.0	E857	E931.0	E950.4	E962.0	E980.4
Sulfapyrimidine	961.0	E857	E931.0	E950.4	E962.0	E980.4
Sulfarsphenamine	961.1	E857	E931.1	E950.4	E962.0	E980.4
Sulfasalazine	961.0	E857	E931.0	E950.4	E962.0	E980.4
Sulfasomizole	961.0	E857	E931.0	E950.4	E962.0	E980.4
Sulfasuxidine	961.0	E857	E931.0	E950.4	E962.0	E980.4
Sulfinpyrazone	974.7	E858.5	E944.7	E950.4	E962.0	E980.4
Sulfisoxazole	961.0	E857	E931.0	E950.4	E962.0	E980.4
ophthalmic preparation	976.5	E858.7	E946.5	E950.4	E962.0	E980.4
Sulfomyxin	960.8	E856	E930.8	E950.4	E962.0	E980.4
Sulfonal	967.8	E852.8	E937.8	E950.2	E962.0	E980.2
Sulfonamides (mixtures)	961.0	E857	E931.0	E950.4	E962.0	E980.4
Sulfones	961.8	E857	E931.8	E950.4	E962.0	E980.4
Sulfonethylmethane	967.8	E852.8	E937.8	E950.2	E962.0	E980.2
Sulfonmethane	967.8	E852.8	E937.8	E950.2	E962.0	E980.2
Sulfonphthal, sulfonphthol	977.8	E858.8	E947.8	E950.4	E962.0	E980.4
Sulfonylurea derivatives, oral	962.3	E858.0	E932.3	E950.4	E962.0	E980.4
Sulfoxone	961.8	E857	E931.8	E950.4	E962.0	E980.4
Sulfur, sulfureted, sulfuric, sulfurous, sulfuryl (compounds) NEC	989.8	E866.8	—	E950.9	E962.1	E980.9
acid	983.1	E864.1	—	E950.7	E962.1	E980.6
dioxide	987.3	E869.1	—	E952.8	E962.2	E982.8
ether — see Ether(s)						
hydrogen	987.8	E869.8	—	E952.8	E962.2	E982.8
medicinal (keratolytic) (ointment) NEC	976.4	E858.7	E946.4	E950.4	E962.0	E980.4

Substance	Poisoning	Accident	Therapeutic-Use	Suicide Attempt	Assault	Undetermined
Sulfur, sulfureted, sulfuric, sulfurous, sulfuryl —continued						
pesticide (vapor)	989.4	E863.4	—	E950.6	E962.1	E980.7
vapor NEC	987.8	E869.8	—	E952.8	E962.2	E982.8
Sulkowitch's reagent	977.8	E858.8	E947.8	E950.4	E962.0	E980.4
Sulph — see also Sulf-						
Sulphadione	961.8	E857	E931.8	E950.4	E962.0	E980.4
Sulthiame, sultiame	966.3	E855.0	E936.3	E950.4	E962.0	E980.4
Superinone	975.5	E858.6	E945.5	E950.4	E962.0	E980.4
Suramin	961.5	E857	E931.5	E950.4	E962.0	E980.4
Surfacaine	968.5	E855.2	E938.5	E950.4	E962.0	E980.4
Surital	968.3	E855.1	E938.3	E950.4	E962.0	E980.4
Sutilains	976.8	E858.7	E946.8	E950.4	E962.0	E980.4
Suxamethonium (bromide) (chloride) (iodide)	975.2	E858.6	E945.2	E950.4	E962.0	E980.4
Suxethonium (bromide)	975.2	E858.6	E945.2	E950.4	E962.0	E980.4
Sweet oil (birch)	976.3	E858.7	E946.3	E950.4	E962.0	E980.4
Sym-dichloroethyl ether	982.3	E862.4	—	E950.9	E962.1	E980.9
Sympatholytics	971.3	E855.6	E941.3	E950.4	E962.0	E980.4
Sympathomimetics	971.2	E855.5	E941.2	E950.4	E962.0	E980.4
Synalar	976.0	E858.7	E946.0	E950.4	E962.0	E980.4
Synthroid	962.7	E858.0	E932.7	E950.4	E962.0	E980.4
Syntocinon	975.0	E858.6	E945.0	E950.4	E962.0	E950.4
Syrosingopine	972.6	E858.3	E942.6	E950.4	E962.0	E980.4
Systemic agents (primarily)	963.9	E858.1	E933.9	E950.4	E962.0	E980.4
specified NEC	963.8	E858.1	E933.8	E950.4	E962.0	E980.4
Tablets (see also specified substance)	977.9	E858.9	E947.9	E950.5	E962.0	E980.5
Tace	962.2	E858.0	E932.2	E950.4	E962.0	E980.4
Tacrine	971.0	E855.3	E941.0	E950.4	E962.0	E980.4
Talbutal	967.0	E851	E937.0	E950.1	E962.0	E980.1
Talc	976.3	E858.7	E946.3	E950.4	E962.0	E980.4
Talcum	976.3	E858.7	E946.3	E950.4	E962.0	E980.4
Tandearil, tanderil	965.5	E850.5	E935.5	E950.0	E962.0	E980.0
Tannic acid	983.1	E864.1	—	E950.7	E962.1	E980.6
medicinal (astringent)	976.2	E858.7	E946.2	E950.4	E962.0	E980.4
Tannin — see Tannic acid						
Tansy	988.2	E865.4	—	E950.9	E962.1	E980.9
TAO	960.3	E856	E930.3	E950.4	E962.0	E980.4
Tapazole	962.8	E858.0	E932.8	E950.4	E962.0	E980.4
Tar NEC	983.0	E864.0	—	E950.7	E962.1	E980.6
camphor — see Naphthalene						
fumes	987.8	E869.8	—	E952.8	E962.2	E982.8
Taractan	969.3	E853.8	E939.3	E950.3	E962.0	E980.3
Tarantula (venomous)	989.5	E905.1	—	E950.9	E962.1	E980.9
Tartar emetic (anti-infective)	961.2	E857	E931.2	E950.4	E962.0	E980.4
Tartaric acid	983.1	E864.1	—	E950.7	E962.1	E980.6
Tartrated antimony (anti-infective)	961.2	E857	E931.2	E950.4	E962.0	E980.4
TCA — see Trichloroacetic acid						
TDI	983.0	E864.0	—	E950.7	E962.1	E980.6
vapor	987.8	E869.8	—	E952.8	E962.2	E982.8
Tear gas	987.5	E869.3	—	E952.8	E962.2	E982.8
Teclothiazide	974.3	E858.5	E944.3	E950.4	E962.0	E980.4
Tegretol	966.3	E855.0	E936.3	E950.4	E962.0	E980.4
Telepaque	977.8	E858.8	E947.8	E950.4	E962.0	E980.4
Tellurium	985.8	E866.4	—	E950.9	E962.1	E980.9
fumes	985.8	E866.4	—	E950.9	E962.1	E980.9
TEM	963.1	E858.1	E933.1	E950.4	E962.0	E980.4
TEPA	963.1	E858.1	E933.1	E950.4	E962.0	E980.4
TEPP	989.3	E863.1	—	E950.6	E962.1	E980.7
Terbutaline	971.2	E855.5	E941.2	E950.4	E962.0	E980.4
Teroxalene	961.6	E857	E931.6	E950.4	E962.0	E980.4
Terpin hydrate	975.5	E858.6	E945.5	E950.4	E962.0	E980.4
Terramycin	960.4	E856	E930.4	E950.4	E962.0	E980.4
Tessalon	975.4	E858.6	E945.4	E950.4	E962.0	E980.4
Testosterone	962.1	E858.0	E932.1	E950.4	E962.0	E980.4
Tetanus (vaccine)	978.4	E858.8	E948.4	E950.4	E962.0	E980.4
antitoxin	979.9	E858.8	E949.9	E950.4	E962.0	E980.4
immune globulin (human)	964.6	E858.2	E934.6	E950.4	E962.0	E980.4
toxoid	978.4	E858.8	E948.4	E950.4	E962.0	E980.4
with diphtheria toxoid	978.9	E858.8	E948.9	E950.4	E962.0	E980.4
with pertussis	978.6	E858.8	E948.6	E950.4	E962.0	E980.4
Tetrabenazine	969.5	E853.8	E939.5	E950.3	E962.0	E980.3
Tetracaine (infiltration) (topical)	968.5	E855.2	E938.5	E950.4	E962.0	E980.4
nerve block (peripheral) (plexus)	968.6	E855.2	E938.6	E950.4	E962.0	E980.4
spinal	968.7	E855.2	E938.7	E950.4	E962.0	E980.4
Tetrachlorethylene — see Tetrachloroethylene						
Tetrachlormethiazide	974.3	E858.5	E944.3	E950.4	E962.0	E980.4

TABLE OF DRUGS AND CHEMICALS

Substance	Poisoning	Accident	Therapeutic-Use	Suicide Attempt	Assault	Undetermined
Tetrachloroethane (liquid) (vapor)	982.3	E862.4	—	E950.9	E962.1	E980.9
paint or varnish	982.3	E861.6	—	E950.9	E962.1	E980.9
Tetrachloroethylene (liquid) (vapor)	982.3	E862.4	—	E950.9	E962.1	E980.9
medicinal	961.6	E857	E931.6	E950.4	E962.0	E980.4
Tetrachloromethane — see Carbon, tetrachloride						
Tetracycline	960.4	E856	E930.4	E950.4	E962.0	E980.4
ophthalmic preparation	976.5	E858.7	E946.5	E950.4	E962.0	E980.4
topical NEC	976.0	E858.7	E946.0	E950.4	E962.0	E980.4
Tetraethylammonium chloride	972.3	E858.3	E942.3	E950.4	E962.0	E980.4
Tetraethyl lead (antiknock compound)	984.1	E862.1	—	E950.9	E962.1	E980.9
Tetraethyl pyrophosphate	989.3	E863.1	—	E950.6	E962.1	E980.7
Tetraethylthiuram disulfide	977.3	E858.8	E947.3	E950.4	E962.0	E980.4
Tetrahydroaminoacridine	971.0	E855.3	E941.0	E950.4	E962.0	E980.4
Tetrahydrocannabinol	969.6	E854.1	E939.6	E950.3	E962.0	E980.3
Tetrahydronaphthalene	982.0	E862.4	—	E950.9	E962.1	E980.9
Tetrahydrozoline	971.2	E855.5	E941.2	E950.4	E962.0	E980.4
Tetralin	982.0	E862.4	—	E950.9	E962.1	E980.9
Tetramethylthiuram (disulfide) NEC	989.4	E863.6	—	E950.6	E962.1	E980.7
medicinal	976.2	E858.7	E946.2	E950.4	E962.0	E980.4
Tetronal	967.8	E852.8	E937.8	E950.2	E962.0	E980.2
Tetryl	983.0	E864.0	—	E950.7	E962.1	E980.6
Thalidomide	967.8	E852.8	E937.8	E950.2	E962.0	E980.2
Thallium (compounds) (dust) NEC	985.8	E866.4	—	E950.9	E962.1	E980.9
pesticide (rodenticide)	985.8	E863.7	—	E950.6	E962.1	E980.7
THC	969.6	E854.1	E939.6	E950.3	E962.0	E980.3
Thebacon	965.09	E850.2	E935.2	E950.0	E962.0	E980.0
Thebaine	965.09	E850.2	E935.2	E950.0	E962.0	E980.0
Theobromine (calcium salicylate)	974.1	E858.5	E944.1	E950.4	E962.0	E980.4
Theophylline (diuretic)	974.1	E858.5	E944.1	E950.4	E962.0	E980.4
ethylenediamine	975.7	E858.6	E945.7	E950.4	E962.0	E980.4
Thiabendazole	961.6	E857	E931.6	E950.4	E962.0	E980.4
Thialbarbital, thialbarbitone	968.3	E855.1	E938.3	E950.4	E962.0	E980.4
Thiamine	963.5	E858.1	E933.5	E950.4	E962.0	E980.4
Thiamylal (sodium)	968.3	E855.1	E938.3	E950.4	E962.0	E980.4
Thiazesim	969.0	E854.0	E939.0	E950.3	E962.0	E980.3
Thiazides (diuretics)	974.3	E858.5	E944.3	E950.4	E962.0	E980.4
Thiethylperazine	963.0	E858.1	E933.0	E950.4	E962.0	E980.4
Thimerosal (topical)	976.0	E858.7	E946.0	E950.4	E962.0	E980.4
ophthalmic preparation	976.5	E858.7	E946.5	E950.4	E962.0	E980.4
Thioacetazone	961.8	E857	E931.8	E950.4	E962.0	E980.4
Thiobarbiturates	968.3	E855.1	E938.3	E950.4	E962.0	E980.4
Thiobismol	961.2	E857	E931.2	E950.4	E962.0	E980.4
Thiocarbamide	962.8	E858.0	E932.8	E950.4	E962.0	E980.4
Thiocarbarsone	961.1	E857	E931.1	E950.4	E962.0	E980.4
Thiocarlide	961.8	E857	E931.8	E950.4	E962.0	E980.4
Thioguanine	963.1	E858.1	E933.1	E950.4	E962.0	E980.4
Thiomercaptomerin	974.0	E858.5	E944.0	E950.4	E962.0	E980.4
Thiomerin	974.0	E858.5	E944.0	E950.4	E962.0	E980.4
Thiopental, thiopentone (sodium)	968.3	E855.1	E938.3	E950.4	E962.0	E980.4
Thiopropazate	969.1	E853.0	E939.1	E950.3	E962.0	E980.3
Thioproperazine	969.1	E853.0	E939.1	E950.3	E962.0	E980.3
Thioridazine	969.1	E853.0	E939.1	E950.3	E962.0	E980.3
Thio-TEPA, thiotepa	963.1	E858.1	E933.1	E950.4	E962.0	E980.4
Thiothixene	969.3	E853.8	E939.3	E950.3	E962.0	E980.3
Thiouracil	962.8	E858.0	E932.8	E950.4	E962.0	E980.4
Thiourea	962.8	E858.0	E932.8	E950.4	E962.0	E980.4
Thiphenamil	971.1	E855.4	E941.1	E950.4	E962.0	E980.4
Thiram NEC	989.4	E863.6	—	E950.6	E962.1	E980.7
medicinal	976.2	E858.7	E946.2	E950.4	E962.0	E980.4
Thonzylamine	963.0	E858.1	E933.0	E950.4	E962.0	E980.4
Thorazine	969.1	E853.0	E939.1	E950.3	E962.0	E980.3
Thornapple	988.2	E865.4	—	E950.9	E962.1	E980.9
Throat preparation (lozenges) NEC	976.6	E858.7	E946.6	E950.4	E962.0	E980.4
Thrombin	964.5	E858.2	E934.5	E950.4	E962.0	E980.4
Thrombolysin	964.4	E858.2	E934.4	E950.4	E962.0	E980.4
Thymol	983.0	E864.0	—	E950.7	E962.1	E980.6
Thymus extract	962.9	E858.0	E932.9	E950.4	E962.0	E980.4
Thyroglobulin	962.7	E858.0	E932.7	E950.4	E962.0	E980.4
Thyroid (derivatives) (extract)	962.7	E858.0	E932.7	E950.4	E962.0	E980.4
Thyrolar	962.7	E858.0	E932.7	E950.4	E962.0	E980.4
Thyrothrophin, thyrotropin	977.8	E858.8	E947.8	E950.4	E962.0	E980.4
Thyroxin(e)	962.7	E858.0	E932.7	E950.4	E962.0	E980.4
Tigan	963.0	E858.1	E933.0	E950.4	E962.0	E980.4
Tigloidine	968.0	E855.1	E938.0	E950.4	E962.0	E980.4
Tin (chloride) (dust) (oxide) NEC	985.8	E866.4	—	E950.9	E962.1	E980.9
anti-infectives	961.2	E857	E931.2	E950.4	E962.0	E980.4

TABLE OF DRUGS AND CHEMICALS

Substance	Poisoning	Accident	Therapeutic-Use	Suicide Attempt	Assault	Undetermined
Tinactin	976.0	E858.7	E946.0	E950.4	E962.0	E980.4
Tincture, iodine — see Iodine						
Tindal	969.1	E853.0	E939.1	E950.3	E962.0	E980.3
Titanium (compounds) (vapor)	985.8	E866.4	—	E950.9	E962.1	E980.9
ointment	976.3	E858.7	E946.3	E950.4	E962.0	E980.4
Titroid	962.7	E858.0	E932.7	E950.4	E962.0	E980.4
TMTD — see Tetramethylthiuram disulfide						
TNT	989.8	E866.8	—	E950.9	E962.1	E980.9
fumes	987.8	E869.8	—	E952.8	E962.2	E982.8
Toadstool	988.1	E865.5	—	E950.9	E962.1	E980.9
Tobacco NEC	989.8	E866.8	—	E950.9	E962.1	E980.9
Indian	988.2	E865.4	—	E950.9	E962.1	E980.9
smoke, second-hand	987.8	E869.4	—	—	—	— ◆
Tocopherol	963.5	E858.1	E933.5	E950.4	E962.0	E980.4
Tocosamine	975.0	E858.6	E945.0	E950.4	E962.0	E980.4
Tofranil	969.0	E854.0	E939.0	E950.3	E962.0	E980.3
Toilet deodorizer	989.8	E866.8	—	E950.9	E962.1	E980.9
Tolazamide	962.3	E858.0	E932.3	E950.4	E962.0	E980.4
Tolazoline	971.3	E855.6	E941.3	E950.4	E962.0	E980.4
Tolbutamide	962.3	E858.0	E932.3	E950.4	E962.0	E980.4
sodium	977.8	E858.8	E947.8	E950.4	E962.0	E980.4
Tolmetin	965.6	E856.0	E935.6	E950.0	E962.0	E980.0
Tolnaftate	976.0	E858.7	E946.0	E950.4	E962.0	E980.4
Tolpropamine	976.1	E858.7	E946.1	E950.4	E962.0	E980.4
Tolserol	968.0	E855.1	E938.0	E950.4	E962.0	E980.4
Toluene (liquid) (vapor)	982.0	E862.4	—	E950.9	E962.1	E980.9
diisocyanate	983.0	E864.0	—	E950.7	E962.1	E980.6
Toluidine	983.0	E864.0	—	E950.7	E962.1	E980.6
vapor	987.8	E869.8	—	E952.8	E962.2	E982.8
Toluol (liquid) (vapor)	982.0	E862.4	—	E950.9	E962.1	E980.9
Tolylene-2,4-diisocyanate	983.0	E864.0	—	E950.7	E962.1	E980.6
Tonics, cardiac	972.1	E858.3	E942.1	E950.4	E962.0	E980.4
Toxaphene (dust) (spray)	989.2	E863.0	—	E950.6	E962.1	E980.7
Toxoids NEC	978.8	E858.8	E948.8	E950.4	E962.0	E980.4
Tractor fuel NEC	981	E862.1	—	E950.9	E962.1	E980.9
Tragacanth	973.3	E858.4	E943.3	E950.4	E962.0	E980.4
Tramazoline	971.2	E855.5	E941.2	E950.4	E962.0	E980.4
Tranquilizers	969.5	E853.9	E939.5	E950.3	E962.0	E980.3
benzodiazepine-based	969.4	E853.2	E939.4	E950.3	E962.0	E980.3
butyrophenone-based	969.2	E853.1	E939.2	E950.3	E962.0	E980.3
major NEC	969.3	E853.8	E939.3	E950.3	E962.0	E980.3
phenothiazine-based	969.1	E853.0	E939.1	E950.3	E962.0	E980.3
specified NEC	969.5	E853.8	E939.5	E950.3	E962.0	E980.3
Trantoin	961.9	E857	E931.9	E950.4	E962.0	E980.4
Tranxene	969.4	E853.2	E939.4	E950.3	E962.0	E980.3
Tranylcypromine (sulfate)	969.0	E854.0	E939.0	E950.3	E962.0	E980.3
Trasentine	975.1	E858.6	E945.1	E950.4	E962.0	E980.4
Travert	974.5	E858.5	E944.5	E950.4	E962.0	E980.4
Trecator	961.8	E857	E931.8	E950.4	E962.0	E980.4
Tretinoin	976.8	E858.7	E946.8	E950.4	E962.0	E980.4
Triacetin	976.0	E858.7	E946.0	E950.4	E962.0	E980.4
Triacetyloleandomycin	960.3	E856	E930.3	E950.4	E962.0	E980.4
Triamcinolone	962.0	E858.0	E932.0	E950.4	E962.0	E980.4
ENT agent	976.6	E858.7	E946.6	E950.4	E962.0	E980.4
ophthalmic preparation	976.5	E858.7	E946.5	E950.4	E962.0	E980.4
topical NEC	976.0	E858.7	E946.0	E950.4	E962.0	E980.4
Triamterene	974.4	E858.5	E944.4	E950.4	E962.0	E980.4
Triaziquone	963.1	E858.1	E933.1	E950.4	E962.0	E980.4
Tribromacetaldehyde	967.3	E852.2	E937.3	E950.2	E962.0	E980.2
Tribromoethanol	968.2	E855.1	E938.2	E950.4	E962.0	E980.4
Tribromomethane	967.3	E852.2	E937.3	E950.2	E962.0	E980.2
Trichlorethane	982.3	E862.4	—	E950.9	E962.1	E980.9
Trichlormethiazide	974.3	E858.5	E944.3	E950.4	E962.0	E980.4
Trichloroacetic acid	983.1	E864.1	—	E950.7	E962.1	E980.6
medicinal (keratolytic)	976.4	E858.7	E946.4	E950.4	E962.0	E980.4
Trichloroethanol	967.1	E852.0	E937.1	E950.2	E962.0	E980.2
Trichloroethylene (liquid) (vapor)	982.3	E862.4	—	E950.9	E962.1	E980.9
anesthetic (gas)	968.2	E855.1	E938.2	E950.4	E962.0	E980.4
Trichloroethyl phosphate	967.1	E852.0	E937.1	E950.2	E962.0	E980.2
Trichlorofluoromethane NEC	987.4	E869.2	—	E952.8	E962.2	E982.8
Trichlorotriethylamine	963.1	E858.1	E933.1	E950.4	E962.0	E980.4
Trichomonacides NEC	961.5	E857	E931.5	E950.4	E962.0	E980.4
Trichomycin	960.1	E856	E930.1	E950.4	E962.0	E980.4
Triclofos	967.1	E852.0	E937.1	E950.2	E962.0	E980.2
Tricresyl phosphate	989.8	E866.8	—	E950.9	E962.1	E980.9
solvent	982.8	E862.4	—	E950.9	E962.1	E980.9

Substance	Poisoning	Accident	Therapeutic Use	Suicide Attempt	Assault	Undetermined
Tricyclamol	966.4	E855.0	E936.4	E950.4	E962.0	E980.4
Tridesilon	976.0	E858.7	E946.0	E950.4	E962.0	E980.4
Tridihexethyl	971.1	E855.4	E941.1	E950.4	E962.0	E980.4
Tridione	966.0	E855.0	E936.0	E950.4	E962.0	E980.4
Triethanolamine NEC	983.2	E864.2	—	E950.7	E962.1	E980.6
detergent	983.2	E861.0	—	E950.7	E962.1	E980.6
trinitrate	972.4	E858.3	E942.4	E950.4	E962.0	E980.4
Triethanomelamine	963.1	E858.1	E933.1	E950.4	E962.0	E980.4
Triethylene melamine	963.1	E858.1	E933.1	E950.4	E962.0	E980.4
Triethylenephosphoramide	963.1	E858.1	E933.1	E950.4	E962.0	E980.4
Triethylenethiophosphoramide	963.1	E858.1	E933.1	E950.4	E962.0	E980.4
Trifluoperazine	969.1	E853.0	E939.1	E950.3	E962.0	E980.3
Trifluperidol	969.2	E853.1	E939.2	E950.3	E962.0	E980.3
Triflupromazine	969.1	E853.0	E939.1	E950.3	E962.0	E980.3
Trihexyphenidyl	971.1	E855.4	E941.1	E950.4	E962.0	E980.4
Triiodothyronine	962.7	E858.0	E932.7	E950.4	E962.0	E980.4
Trilene	968.2	E855.1	E938.2	E950.4	E962.0	E980.4
Trimeprazine	963.0	E858.1	E933.0	E950.4	E962.0	E980.4
Trimetazidine	972.4	E858.3	E942.4	E950.4	E962.0	E980.4
Trimethadione	966.0	E855.0	E936.0	E950.4	E962.0	E980.4
Trimethaphan	972.3	E858.3	E942.3	E950.4	E962.0	E980.4
Trimethidinium	972.3	E858.3	E942.3	E950.4	E962.0	E980.4
Trimethobenzamide	963.0	E858.1	E933.0	E950.4	E962.0	E980.4
Trimethylcarbinol	980.8	E860.8	—	E950.9	E962.1	E980.9
Trimethylpsoralen	976.3	E858.7	E946.3	E950.4	E962.0	E980.4
Trimeton	963.0	E858.1	E933.0	E950.4	E962.0	E980.4
Trimipramine	969.0	E854.0	E939.0	E950.3	E962.0	E980.3
Trimustine	963.1	E858.1	E933.1	E950.4	E962.0	E980.4
Trinitrin	972.4	E858.3	E942.4	E950.4	E962.0	E980.4
Trinitrophenol	983.0	E864.0	—	E950.7	E962.1	E980.6
Trinitrotoluene	989.8	E866.8	—	E950.9	E962.1	E980.9
fumes	987.8	E869.8	—	E952.8	E962.2	E982.8
Trional	967.8	E852.8	E937.8	E950.2	E962.0	E980.2
Trioxide of arsenic — see Arsenic						
Trioxsalen	976.3	E858.7	E946.3	E950.4	E962.0	E980.4
Tripelennamine	963.0	E858.1	E933.0	E950.4	E962.0	E980.4
Triperidol	969.2	E853.1	E939.2	E950.3	E962.0	E980.3
Triprolidine	963.0	E858.1	E933.0	E950.4	E962.0	E980.4
Trisoralen	976.3	E858.7	E946.3	E950.4	E962.0	E980.4
Troleandomycin	960.3	E856	E930.3	E950.4	E962.0	E980.4
Trolnitrate (phosphate)	972.4	E858.3	E942.4	E950.4	E962.0	E980.4
Trometamol	963.3	E858.1	E933.3	E950.4	E962.0	E980.4
Tromethamine	963.3	E858.1	E933.3	E950.4	E962.0	E980.4
Tronothane	968.5	E855.2	E938.5	E950.4	E962.0	E980.4
Tropicamide	971.1	E855.4	E941.1	E950.4	E962.0	E980.4
Troxidone	966.0	E855.0	E936.0	E950.4	E962.0	E980.4
Tryparsamide	961.1	E857	E931.1	E950.4	E962.0	E980.4
Trypsin	963.4	E858.1	E933.4	E950.4	E962.0	E980.4
Tryptizol	969.0	E854.0	E939.0	E950.3	E962.0	E980.3
Tuaminoheptane	971.2	E855.5	E941.2	E950.4	E962.0	E980.4
Tuberculin (old)	977.8	E858.8	E947.8	E950.4	E962.0	E980.4
Tubocurare	975.2	E858.6	E945.2	E950.4	E962.0	E980.4
Tubocurarine	975.2	E858.6	E945.2	E950.4	E962.0	E980.4
Turkish green	969.6	E854.1	E939.6	E950.3	E962.0	E980.3
Turpentine (spirits of) (liquid) (vapor)	982.8	E862.4	—	E950.9	E962.1	E980.9
Tybamate	969.5	E853.8	E939.5	E950.3	E962.0	E980.3
Tyloxapol	975.5	E858.6	E945.5	E950.4	E962.0	E980.4
Tymazoline	971.2	E855.5	E941.2	E950.4	E962.0	E980.4
Typhoid vaccine	978.1	E858.8	E948.1	E950.4	E962.0	E980.4
Typhus vaccine	979.2	E858.8	E949.2	E950.4	E962.0	E980.4
Tyrothricin	976.0	E858.7	E946.0	E950.4	E962.0	E980.4
ENT agent	976.6	E858.7	E946.6	E950.4	E962.0	E980.4
ophthalmic preparation	976.5	E858.7	E946.5	E950.4	E962.0	E980.4
Undecenoic acid	976.0	E858.7	E946.0	E950.4	E962.0	E980.4
Undecylenic acid	976.0	E858.7	E946.0	E950.4	E962.0	E980.4
Unna's boot	976.3	E858.7	E946.3	E950.4	E962.0	E980.4
Uracil mustard	963.1	E858.1	E933.1	E950.4	E962.0	E980.4
Uramustine	963.1	E858.1	E933.1	E950.4	E962.0	E980.4
Urari	975.2	E858.6	E945.2	E950.4	E962.0	E980.4
Urea	974.4	E858.5	E944.4	E950.4	E962.0	E980.4
topical	976.8	E858.7	E946.8	E950.4	E962.0	E980.4
Urethan(e) (antineoplastic)	963.1	E858.1	E933.1	E950.4	E962.0	E980.4
Urginea (maritima) (scilla) — see Squill						
Uric acid metabolism agents NEC	974.7	E858.5	E944.7	E950.4	E962.0	E980.4
Urokinase	964.4	E858.2	E934.4	E950.4	E962.0	E980.4
Urokon	977.8	E858.8	E947.8	E950.4	E962.0	E980.4

Substance	Poisoning	Accident	Therapeutic-Use	Suicide Attempt	Assault	Undetermined
Urotropin	961.9	E857	E931.9	E950.4	E962.0	E980.4
Urtica	988.2	E865.4	—	E950.9	E962.1	E980.9
Utility gas — see Gas, utility						
Vaccine NEC	979.9	E858.8	E949.9	E950.4	E962.0	E980.4
bacterial NEC	978.8	E858.8	E948.8	E950.4	E962.0	E980.4
with						
other bacterial component	978.9	E858.8	E948.9	E950.4	E962.0	E980.4
pertussis component	978.6	E858.8	E948.6	E950.4	E962.0	E980.4
viral-rickettsial component	979.7	E858.8	E949.7	E950.4	E962.0	E980.4
mixed NEC	978.9	E858.8	E948.9	E950.4	E962.0	E980.4
BCG	978.0	E858.8	E948.0	E950.4	E962.0	E980.4
cholera	978.2	E858.8	E948.2	E950.4	E962.0	E980.4
diphtheria	978.5	E858.8	E948.5	E950.4	E962.0	E980.4
influenza	979.6	E858.8	E949.6	E950.4	E962.0	E980.4
measles	979.4	E858.8	E949.4	E950.4	E962.0	E980.4
meningococcal	978.8	E858.8	E948.8	E950.4	E962.0	E980.4
mumps	979.6	E858.8	E949.6	E950.4	E962.0	E980.4
paratyphoid	978.1	E858.8	E948.1	E950.4	E962.0	E980.4
pertussis (with diphtheria toxoid) (with tetanus toxoid)	978.6	E858.8	E948.6	E950.4	E962.0	E980.4
plague	978.3	E858.8	E948.3	E950.4	E962.0	E980.4
poliomyelitis	979.5	E858.8	E949.5	E950.4	E962.0	E980.4
poliovirus	979.5	E858.8	E949.5	E950.4	E962.0	E980.4
rabies	979.1	E858.8	E949.1	E950.4	E962.0	E980.4
rickettsial NEC	979.6	E858.8	E949.6	E950.4	E962.0	E980.4
with						
bacterial component	979.7	E858.8	E949.7	E950.4	E962.0	E980.4
pertussis component	978.6	E858.8	E948.6	E950.4	E962.0	E980.4
viral component	979.7	E858.8	E949.7	E950.4	E962.0	E980.4
Rocky mountain spotted fever	979.6	E858.8	E949.6	E950.4	E962.0	E980.4
rubella virus	979.4	E858.8	E949.4	E950.4	E962.0	E980.4
sabin oral	979.5	E858.8	E949.5	E950.4	E962.0	E980.4
smallpox	979.0	E858.8	E949.0	E950.4	E962.0	E980.4
tetanus	978.4	E858.8	E948.4	E950.4	E962.0	E980.4
typhoid	978.1	E858.8	E948.1	E950.4	E962.0	E980.4
typhus	979.2	E858.8	E949.2	E950.4	E962.0	E980.4
viral NEC	979.6	E858.8	E949.6	E950.4	E962.0	E980.4
with						
bacterial component	979.7	E858.8	E949.7	E950.4	E962.0	E980.4
pertussis component	978.6	E858.8	E948.6	E950.4	E962.0	E980.4
rickettsial component	979.7	E858.8	E949.7	E950.4	E962.0	E980.4
yellow fever	979.3	E858.8	E949.3	E950.4	E962.0	E980.4
Vaccinia immune globulin (human)	964.6	E858.2	E934.6	E950.4	E962.0	E980.4
Vaginal contraceptives	976.8	E858.7	E946.8	E950.4	E962.0	E980.4
Valethamate	971.1	E855.4	E941.1	E950.4	E962.0	E980.4
Valisone	976.0	E858.7	E946.0	E950.4	E962.0	E980.4
Valium	969.4	E853.2	E939.4	E950.3	E962.0	E980.3
Valmid	967.8	E852.8	E937.8	E950.2	E962.0	E980.2
Vanadium	985.8	E866.4	—	E950.9	E962.1	E980.9
Vancomycin	960.8	E856	E930.8	E950.4	E962.0	E980.4
Vapor (see also Gas)	987.9	E869.9	—	E952.9	E962.2	E982.9
kiln (carbon monoxide)	986	E868.8	—	E952.1	E962.2	E982.1
lead — see Lead						
specified source NEC (see also specific substance)	987.8	E869.8	—	E952.8	E962.2	E982.8
Varidase	964.4	E858.2	E934.4	E950.4	E962.0	E980.4
Varnish	989.8	E861.6	—	E950.9	E962.1	E980.9
cleaner	982.8	E862.9	—	E950.9	E962.1	E980.9
Vaseline	976.3	E858.7	E946.3	E950.4	E962.0	E980.4
Vasodilan	972.5	E858.3	E942.5	E950.4	E962.0	E980.4
Vasodilators NEC	972.5	E858.3	E942.5	E950.4	E962.0	E980.4
coronary	972.4	E858.3	E942.4	E950.4	E962.0	E980.4
Vasopressin	962.5	E858.0	E932.5	E950.4	E962.0	E980.4
Vasopressor drugs	962.5	E858.0	E932.5	E950.4	E962.0	E980.4
Venom, venomous (bite) (sting)	989.5	E905.9	—	E950.9	E962.1	E980.9
arthropod NEC	989.5	E905.9	—	E950.9	E962.1	E980.9
bee	989.5	E905.3	—	E950.9	E962.1	E980.9
centipede	989.5	E905.4	—	E950.9	E962.1	E980.9
hornet	989.5	E905.3	—	E950.9	E962.1	E980.9
lizard	989.5	E905.0	—	E950.9	E962.1	E980.9
marine animals or plants	989.5	E905.6	—	E950.9	E962.1	E980.9
millipede (tropical)	989.5	E905.4	—	E950.9	E962.1	E980.9
plant NEC	989.5	E905.7	—	E950.9	E962.1	E980.9
marine	989.5	E905.6	—	E950.9	E962.1	E980.9
scorpion	989.5	E905.2	—	E950.9	E962.1	E980.9
snake	989.5	E905.0	—	E950.9	E962.1	E980.9
specified NEC	989.5	E905.8	—	E950.9	E962.1	E980.9

TABLE OF DRUGS AND CHEMICALS

Substance	Poisoning	Accident	Therapeutic-Use	Suicide Attempt	Assault	Undetermined
Venom, venomous—*continued*	989.5	E905.1	—	E950.9	E962.1	E980.9
spider	989.5	E905.3	—	E950.9	E962.1	E980.9
wasp	967.0	E851	E937.0	E950.1	E962.0	E980.1
Veramon						
Veratrum						
album	988.2	E865.4	—	E950.9	E962.1	E980.9
alkaloids	972.6	E858.3	E942.6	E950.4	E962.0	E980.4
viride	988.2	E865.4	—	E950.9	E962.1	E980.9
Verdigris (*see also* Copper)	985.8	E866.4	—	E950.9	E962.1	E980.9
Veronal	967.0	E851	E937.0	E950.1	E962.0	E980.1
Veroxil	961.6	E857	E931.6	E950.4	E962.0	E980.4
Versidyne	965.7	E850.7	E935.7	E950.0	E962.0	E980.0
Vienna						
green	985.1	E866.3	—	E950.8	E962.1	E980.8
insecticide	985.1	E863.4	—	E950.6	E962.1	E980.7
red	989.8	E866.8	—	E950.9	E962.1	E980.9
pharmaceutical dye	977.4	E858.8	E947.4	E950.4	E962.0	E980.4
Vinbarbital, vinbarbitone	967.0	E851	E937.0	E950.1	E962.0	E980.1
Vinblastine	963.1	E858.1	E933.1	E950.4	E962.0	E980.4
Vincristine	963.1	E858.1	E933.1	E950.4	E962.0	E980.4
Vinesthene, vinethene	968.2	E855.1	E938.2	E950.4	E962.0	E980.4
Vinyl						
bital	967.0	E851	E937.0	E950.1	E962.0	E980.1
ether	968.2	E855.1	E938.2	E950.4	E962.0	E980.4
Vioform	961.3	E857	E931.3	E950.4	E962.0	E980.4
topical	976.0	E858.7	E946.0	E930.4	E962.0	E980.4
Viomycin	960.6	E856	E930.6	E950.4	E962.0	E980.4
Viosterol	963.5	E858.1	E933.5	E950.4	E962.0	E980.4
Viper (venom)	989.5	E905.0	—	E950.9	E962.1	E980.9
Viprynium (embonate)	961.6	E857	E931.6	E950.4	E962.0	E980.4
Virugon	961.7	E857	E931.7	E950.4	E962.0	E980.4
Visine	976.5	E858.7	E946.5	E950.4	E962.0	E980.4
Vitamins NEC	963.5	E858.1	E933.5	E950.4	E962.0	E980.4
B_{12}	964.1	E858.2	E934.1	E950.4	E962.0	E980.4
hematopoietic	964.1	E858.2	E934.1	E950.4	E962.0	E980.4
K	964.3	E858.2	E934.3	E950.4	E962.0	E980.4
Vleminckx's solution	976.4	E858.7	E946.4	E950.4	E962.0	E980.4
Warfarin (potassium) (sodium)	964.2	E858.2	E934.2	E950.4	E962.0	E980.4
rodenticide	989.4	E863.7	—	E950.6	E962.1	E980.7
Wasp (sting)	989.5	E905.3	—	E950.9	E962.1	E980.9
Water						
balance agents NEC	974.5	E858.5	E944.5	E950.4	E962.0	E980.4
gas	987.1	E868.1	—	E951.8	E962.2	E981.8
incomplete combustion of — *see* Carbon, monoxide, fuel, utility						
hemlock	988.2	E865.4	—	E950.9	E962.1	E980.9
moccasin (venom)	989.5	E905.0	—	E950.9	E962.1	E980.9
Wax (paraffin) (petroleum)	981	E862.3	—	E950.9	E962.1	E980.9
automobile	989.8	E861.2	—	E950.9	E962.1	E980.9
floor	981	E862.0	—	E950.9	E962.1	E980.9
Weed killers NEC	989.4	E863.5	—	E950.6	E962.1	E980.7
Welldorm	967.1	E852.0	E937.1	E950.2	E962.0	E980.2
White						
arsenic — *see* Arsenic						
hellebore	988.2	E865.4	—	E950.9	E962.1	E980.9
lotion (keratolytic)	976.4	E858.7	E946.4	E950.4	E962.0	E980.4
spirit	981	E862.0	—	E950.9	E962.1	E980.9
Whitewashes	989.8	E861.6	—	E950.9	E962.1	E980.9
Whole blood	964.7	E858.2	E934.7	E950.4	E962.0	E980.4
Wild						
black cherry	988.2	E865.4	—	E950.9	E962.1	E980.9
poisonous plants NEC	988.2	E865.4	—	E950.9	E962.1	E980.9
Window cleaning fluid	989.8	E861.3	—	E950.9	E962.1	E980.9
Wintergreen (oil)	976.3	E858.7	E946.3	E950.4	E962.0	E980.4
Witch hazel	976.2	E858.7	E946.2	E950.4	E962.0	E980.4
Wood						
alcohol	980.1	E860.2	—	E950.9	E962.1	E980.9
spirit	980.1	E860.2	—	E950.9	E962.1	E980.9
Woorali	975.2	E858.6	E945.2	E950.4	E962.0	E980.4
Wormseed, American	961.6	E857	E931.6	E950.4	E962.0	E980.4
Xanthine diuretics	974.1	E858.5	E944.1	E950.4	E962.0	E980.4
Xanthocillin	960.0	E856	E930.0	E950.4	E962.0	E980.4
Xanthotoxin	976.3	E858.7	E946.3	E950.4	E962.0	E980.4
Xylene (liquid) (vapor)	982.0	E862.4	—	E950.9	E962.1	E980.9
Xylocaine (infiltration) (topical)	968.5	E855.2	E938.5	E950.4	E962.0	E980.4
nerve block (peripheral) (plexus)	968.6	E855.2	E938.6	E950.4	E962.0	E980.4
spinal	968.7	E855.2	E938.7	E950.4	E962.0	E980.4

Substance	Poisoning	Accident	Therapeutic-Use	Suicide Attempt	Assualt	Undetermined
Xylol (liquid) (vapor)	982.0	E862.4	—	E950.9	E962.1	E980.9
Xylometazoline	971.2	E855.5	E941.2	E950.4	E962.0	E980.4
Yellow						
fever vaccine	979.3	E858.8	E949.3	E950.4	E962.0	E980.4
jasmine	988.2	E865.4	—	E950.9	E962.1	E980.9
Yew	988.2	E865.4	—	E950.9	E962.1	E980.9
Zactane	965.7	E850.7	E935.7	E950.0	E962.0	E980.0
Zaroxolyn	974.3	E858.5	E944.3	E950.4	E962.0	E980.4
Zephiran (topical)	976.0	E858.7	E946.0	E950.4	E962.0	E980.4
ophthalmic preparation	976.5	E858.7	E946.5	E950.4	E962.0	E980.4
Zerone	980.1	E860.2	—	E950.9	E962.1	E980.9
Zinc (compounds) (fumes) (salts) (vapor) NEC	985.8	E866.4	—	E950.9	E962.1	E980.9
anti-infectives	976.0	E858.7	E946.0	E950.4	E962.0	E980.4
antivaricose	972.7	E858.3	E942.7	E950.4	E962.0	E980.4
bacitracin	976.0	E858.7	E946.0	E950.4	E962.0	E980.4
chloride	976.2	E858.7	E946.2	E950.4	E962.0	E980.4
gelatin	976.3	E858.7	E946.3	E950.4	E962.0	E980.4
oxide	976.3	E858.7	E946.3	E950.4	E962.0	E980.4
peroxide	976.0	E858.7	E946.0	E950.4	E962.0	E980.4
pesticides	985.8	E863.4	—	E950.6	E962.1	E980.7
phosphide (rodenticide)	985.8	E863.7	—	E950.6	E962.1	E980.7
stearate	976.3	E858.7	E946.3	E950.4	E962.0	E980.4
sulfate (antivaricose)	972.7	E858.3	E942.7	E950.4	E962.0	E980.4
ENT agent	976.6	E858.7	E946.6	E950.4	E962.0	E980.4
ophthalmic solution	976.5	E858.7	E946.5	E950.4	E962.0	E980.4
topical NEC	976.0	E858.7	E946.0	E950.4	E962.0	E980.4
undecylenate	976.0	E858.7	E946.0	E950.4	E962.0	E980.4
Zoxazolamine	968.0	E855.1	E938.0	E950.4	E962.0	E980.4
Zygadenus (venenosus)	988.2	E865.4	—	E950.9	E962.1	E980.9

INDEX TO EXTERNAL CAUSES

VOLUME 2

SECTION 3

SECTION 3

Alphabetic Index to External Causes of Injury and Poisoning (E Code)

This section contains the index to the codes which classify environmental events, circumstances, and other conditions as the cause of injury and other adverse effects. Where a code from the section Supplementary Classification of External Causes of Injury and Poisoning (E800-E998) is applicable, it is intended that the E code shall be used in addition to a code from the main body of the classification, Chapters 1 to 17.

The alphabetic index to the E codes is organized by main terms which describe the *accident, circumstance, event,* or specific *agent* which caused the injury or other adverse effect.

> *Note — Transport accidents (E800-E848) include accidents involving:*
> *aircraft and spacecraft (E840-E845)*
> *watercraft (E830-E838)*
> *motor vehicle (E810-E825)*
> *railway (E800-E807)*
> *other road vehicles (E826-E829)*
>
> *For definitions and examples related to transport accidents — see Volume 1 code categories E800-E848.*
>
> *The fourth-digit subdivisions for use with categories E800-E848 to identify the injured person are found in Volume 2, on pp. 402-406.*
>
> *For identifying the place in which an accident or poisoning occurred (circumstances classifiable to categories E850-E869 and E880-E928) — see the listing in this section under "Accident, occurring."*

See the Table of Drugs and Chemicals (Section 2 of this volume) for identifying the specific agent involved in drug overdose or a wrong substance given or taken in error, and for intoxication or poisoning by a drug or other chemical substance.

The specific adverse effect, reaction, or localized toxic effect to a correct drug or substance properly administered in therapeutic or prophylactic dosage should be classified according to the nature of the adverse effect (e.g., allergy, dermatitis, tachycardia) listed in Section 1 of this volume.

Abandonment

Abandonment
  causing exposure to weather
      conditions — *see* Exposure
  child, with intent to injure or kill
      E968.4
  helpless person, infant, newborn
      E904.0
    with intent to injure or kill
      E968.4

Abortion, criminal, injury to child
  E968.8

Abuse, child E967.9
  by
    parent(s) E967.0
    specified person(s), except
      parents E967.1
    unspecified person E967.9

Accident (to) E928.9
  aircraft (in transit) (powered) E841
    at landing, take-off E840
    due to, caused by cataclysm
      — *see* categories E908,
      E909
    late effect of E929.1
    unpowered (*see also* Collision,
      aircraft, unpowered)
      E842
    while alighting, boarding E843
  amphibious vehicle
    on
      land — *see* Accident,
        motor vehicle
      water — *see* Accident,
        watercraft
  animal, ridden NEC E828
  animal-drawn vehicle NEC E827
  balloon (*see also* Collision,
    aircraft, unpowered) E842
  caused by, due to
    abrasive wheel (metalworking)
      E919.3
    animal NEC E906.9
      being ridden (in sport or
        transport) E828
    avalanche NEC E909
    band saw E919.4
    bench saw E919.4
    bore, earth-drilling or mining
      (land) (seabed) E919.1
    bulldozer E919.7
    cataclysmic
      earth surface movement or
        eruption E909
      storm E908
    chain
      hoist E919.2
        agricultural operations
          E919.0
        mining operations
          E919.1
      saw E920.1
    circular saw E919.4
    cold (excessive) (*see also* Cold,
      exposure to) E901.9
    combine E919.0
    conflagration — *see*
      Conflagration
    corrosive liquid, substance
      NEC E924.1
    cotton gin E919.8
    crane E919.2
      agricultural operations
        E919.0
      mining operations E919.1
    cutting or piercing instrument
      (*see also* Cut) E920.9
    dairy equipment E919.8
    derrick E919.2
      agricultural operations
        E919.0
      mining operations E919.1
    drill E920.1
      earth (land) (seabed) E919.1
      hand (powered) E920.1
        not powered E920.4
      metalworking E919.3
      woodworking E919.4

Accident—*continued*
  caused by, due to—*continued*
    earth(-)
      drilling machine E919.1
      moving machine E919.7
      scraping machine E919.7
    electric
      current (*see also* Electric
        shock) E925.9
      motor — *see also* Accident,
        machine, by type of
        machine
        current (of) — *see*
          Electric shock
    elevator (building) (grain)
      E919.2
      agricultural operations
        E919.0
      mining operations E919.1
    environmental factors NEC
      E928.9
    excavating machine E919.7
    explosive material (*see also*
      Explosion) E923.9
    farm machine E919.0
    fire, flames — *see also* Fire
      conflagration — *see*
        Conflagration
    firearm missile — *see* Shooting
    forging (metalworking)
      machine E919.3
    forklift (truck) E919.2
      agricultural operations
        E919.0
      mining operations E919.1
    gas turbine E919.5
    harvester E919.0
    hay derrick, mower, or rake
      E919.0
    heat (excessive) (*see also* Heat)
      E900.9
    hoist (*see also* Accident,
      caused by, due to, lift)
      E919.2
      chain — *see* Accident,
        caused by, due to,
        chain
      shaft E919.1
    hot
      liquid E924.0
        caustic or corrosive
          E924.1
      object (not producing fire
        or flames) E924.8
      substance E924.9
        caustic or corrosive
          E924.1
        liquid (metal) NEC
          E924.0
        specified type NEC
          E924.8
    ignition — *see* Ignition
    internal combustion engine
      E919.5
    landslide NEC E909
    lathe (metalworking) E919.3
      turnings E920.8
      woodworking E919.4
    lift, lifting (appliances) E919.2
      agricultural operations
        E919.0
      mining operations E919.1
      shaft E919.1
    lightning NEC E907
    machine, machinery — *see*
      also Accident, machine
      drilling, metal E919.3
      manufacturing, for
        manufacture of
        beverages E919.8
        clothing E919.8
        foodstuffs E919.8
        paper E919.8
        textiles E919.8
      milling, metal E919.3
      moulding E919.4
      power press, metal E919.3

Accident—*continued*
  caused by, due to—*continued*
    machine, machinery—
      continued
      printing E919.8
      rolling mill, metal E919.3
      sawing, metal E919.3
      specified type NEC E919.8
      spinning E919.8
      weaving E919.8
    natural factor NEC E928.9
    overhead plane E919.4
    plane E920.4
      overhead E919.4
    powered
      hand tool NEC E920.1
      saw E919.4
        hand E920.1
    printing machine E919.8
    pulley (block) E919.2
      agricultural operations
        E919.0
      mining operations E919.1
      transmission E919.6
    radial saw E919.4
    radiation — *see* Radiation
    reaper E919.0
    road scraper E919.7
      when in transport under its
        own power — *see*
        categories E810-E825
    roller coaster E919.8
    sander E919.4
    saw E920.4
      band E919.4
      bench E919.4
      chain E920.1
      circular E919.4
      hand E920.4
        powered E920.1
      powered, except hand
        E919.4
      radial E919.4
    sawing machine, metal E919.3
    shaft
      hoist E919.1
      lift E919.1
      transmission E919.6
    shears E920.4
      hand E920.4
        powered E920.1
      mechanical E919.3
    shovel E920.4
      steam E919.7
    spinning machine E919.8
    steam — *see also* Burning,
      steam
      engine E919.5
      shovel E919.7
    thresher E919.0
    thunderbolt NEC E907
    tractor E919.0
      when in transport under its
        own power — *see*
        categories E810-E825
    transmission belt, cable, chain,
      gear, pinion, pulley,
      shaft E919.6
    turbine (gas) (water driven)
      E919.5
    under-cutter E919.1
    weaving machine E919.8
    winch E919.2
      agricultural operations
        E919.0
      mining operations E919.1
  diving E883.0
    with insufficient air supply
      E913.2
  glider (hang) (*see also* Collision,
    aircraft, unpowered) E842
  hovercraft
    on
      land — *see* Accident,
        motor vehicle
      water — *see* Accident,
        watercraft

Accident—*continued*
  ice yacht (*see also* Accident,
    vehicle NEC) E848
  in
    medical, surgical procedure
      as, or due to misadventure
        — *see* Misadventure
      causing an abnormal
        reaction or later
        complication without
        mention of
        misadventure — *see*
        Reaction, abnormal
  kite carrying a person (*see also*
    Collision, aircraft,
    unpowered) E842
  land yacht (*see also* Accident,
    vehicle NEC) E848
  late effect of — *see* Late effect
  launching pad E845
  machine, machinery (*see also*
    Accident, caused by, due
    to, by specific type of
    machine) E919.9
    agricultural including animal-
      powered E919.0
    earth-drilling E919.1
    earth moving or scraping
      E919.7
    excavating E919.7
    involving transport under own
      power on highway or
      transport vehicle — *see*
      categories E810-E825,
      E840-E845
    lifting (appliances) E919.2
    metalworking E919.3
    mining E919.1
    prime movers, except electric
      motors E919.5
      electric motors — *see*
        Accident, machine,
        by specific type of
        machine
    recreational E919.8
    specified type NEC E919.8
    transmission E919.6
    watercraft (deck) (engine
      room) (galley) (laundry)
      (loading) E836
    woodworking or forming
      E919.4
  motor vehicle (on public
    highway) (traffic) E819
    due to cataclysm — *see*
      categories E908, E909
    involving
      collision (*see also* Collision,
        motor vehicle) E812
      nontraffic, not on public
        highway — *see*
        categories E820-E825
      not involving collision — *see*
        categories E816-E819
  nonmotor vehicle NEC E829
  nonroad — *see* Accident,
    vehicle NEC
  road, except pedal cycle,
    animal-drawn vehicle,
    or animal being ridden
    E829
  nonroad vehicle NEC — *see*
    Accident, vehicle NEC
  not elsewhere classifiable
    involving
      cable car (not on rails) E847
        on rails E829
      coal car in mine E846
      hand truck — *see* Accident,
        vehicle NEC
      logging car E846
      sled(ge), meaning snow or ice
        vehicle E848
      tram, mine or quarry E846

Accident—continued
  nonmotor vehicle NEC—continued
   truck
    mine or quarry E846
    self-propelled, industrial E846
    station baggage E846
   tub, mine or quarry E846
   vehicle NEC E848
    snow and ice E848
    used only on industrial premises E846
   wheelbarrow E848
  occurring (at) (in)
   apartment E849.0
   baseball field, diamond E849.4
   construction site, any E849.3
   dock E849.8
    yard E849.3
   dormitory E849.7
   factory (building) (premises) E849.3
   farm E849.1
    buildings E849.1
    house E849.0
   football field E849.4
   forest E849.8
   garage (place of work) E849.3
    private (home) E849.0
   gravel pit E849.2
   gymnasium E849.4
   highway E849.5
   home (private) (residential) E849.0
    institutional E849.7
   hospital E849.7
   hotel E849.6
   house (private) (residential) E849.0
    movie E849.6
    public E849.6
   institution, residential E849.7
   jail E849.7
   mine E849.2
   motel E849.6
   movie house E849.6
   office (building) E849.6
   orphanage E849.7
   park (public) E849.4
    mobile home E849.8
    trailer E849.8
   parking lot or place E849.8
   place
    industrial NEC E849.3
    parking E849.8
    public E849.8
     specified place NEC E849.5
    recreational NEC E849.4
    sport NEC E849.4
   playground (park) (school) E849.4
   prison E849.6
   public building NEC E849.6
   quarry E849.2
   railway
    line NEC E849.8
    yard E849.3
   residence
    home (private) E849.0
    resort (beach) (lake) (mountain) (seashore) (vacation) E849.4
   restaurant E849.6
   sand pit E849.2
   school (building) (private) (public) (state) E849.6
    reform E849.7
    riding E849.4
   seashore E849.8
    resort E849.4
   shop (place of work) E849.3
    commercial E849.6
   skating rink E849.4
   sports palace E849.4

Accident—continued
  occurring (at) (in)—continued
   stadium E849.4
   store E849.6
   street E849.5
   swimming pool (public) E849.4
    private home or garden E849.0
   tennis court E849.4
   theatre, theater E849.6
   trailer court E849.8
   tunnel E849.8
    under construction E849.2
   warehouse E849.3
   yard
    dock E849.3
    industrial E849.3
    private (home) E849.0
    railway E849.3
  off-road type motor vehicle (not on public highway) NEC E821
   on public highway — see catagories E810-E819
  pedal cycle E826
  railway E807
   due to cataclysm — see categories E908, E909
   involving
    burning by engine, locomotive, train (see also Explosion, railway engine) E803
    collision (see also Collision, railway) E800
    derailment (see also Derailment, railway) E802
    explosion (see also Explosion, railway engine) E803
    fall (see also Fall, from, railway rolling stock) E804
    fire (see also Explosion, railway engine) E803
    hitting by, being struck by object falling in, on, from, rolling stock, train, vehicle E806
    rolling stock, train, vehicle E805
    overturning, railway rolling stock, train, vehicle (see also Derailment, railway) E802
    running off rails, railway (see also Derailment, railway) E802
    specified circumstances NEC E806
    train or vehicle hit by
     avalanche E909
     falling object (earth, rock, tree) E806
      due to cataclysm — see categories E908, E909
     landslide E909
  ski(ing) E885
   jump E884.9
   lift or tow (with chair or gondola) E847
  snow vehicle, motor driven (not on public highway) E820
   on public highway — see catagories E810-E819
  spacecraft E845
  specified cause NEC E928.8
  street car E829
  traffic NEC E819

Accident—continued
  vehicle NEC (with pedestrian) E848
   battery powered
    airport passenger vehicle E846
    truck (baggage) (mail) E846
   powered commercial or industrial (with other vehicle or object within commercial or industrial premises) E846
  watercraft E838
   with
    drowning or submersion resulting from
     accident other than to watercraft E832
     accident to watercraft E830
    injury, except drowning or submersion, resulting from
     accident other than to watercraft — see categories E833-E838
     accident to watercraft E831
   due to, caused by cataclysm — see categories E908, E909
   machinery E836
Acid throwing E961
Acosta syndrome E902.0
Aeroneurosis E902.1
Aero-otitis media — see Effects of, air pressure
Aerosinusitis — see Effects of, air pressure
After-effect, late — see Late effect
Air
  blast in war operations E933
  embolism (traumatic) NEC E928.9
   in
    infusion or transfusion E874.1
    perfusion E874.2
   sickness E903
Alpine sickness E902.0
Altitude sickness — see Effects of, air pressure
Anaphylactic shock, anaphylaxis (see also Table of drugs and chemicals) E947.9
  due to bite or sting (venomous) — see Bite, venomous
Andes disease E902.0
Apoplexy
  heat — see Heat
Arachnidism E905.1
Arson E968.0
Asphyxia, asphyxiation
  by
   chemical in war operations E997.2
   explosion — see Explosion
   food (bone) (regurgitated food) (seed) E911
   foreign object, exccpt food E912
   fumes in war operations E997.2
   gas — see also Table of drugs and chemicals
    in war operations E997.2
   legal
    execution E978
    intervention (tear) E972
   tear E972
   mechanical means (see also Suffocation) E913.9

Asphyxia, asphyxiation—continued
  from
   conflagration — see Conflagration
   fire — see also Fire
    in war operations E990.9
   ignition — see Ignition
Aspiration
  foreign body — see Foreign body, aspiration
  mucus, not of newborn (with asphyxia, obstruction respiratory passage, suffocation) E912
  phlegm (with asphyxia, obstruction respiratory passage, suffocation) E912
  vomitus (with asphyxia, obstruction respiratory passage, suffocation) (see also Foreign body, aspiration, food) E911
Assassination (attempt) (see also Assault) E968.9
Assault (homicidal) (by) (in) E968.9
  acid E961
   swallowed E962.1
  bite (of human being) E968.8
  bomb ((placed in) car or house) E965.8
   antipersonnel E965.5
   letter E965.7
   petrol E965.7
  brawl (hand) (fists) (foot) E960.0
  burning, burns (by fire) E968.0
   acid E961
    swallowed E962.1
   caustic, corrosive substance E961
    swallowed E962.1
   chemical from swallowing caustic, corrosive substance NEC E962.1
   hot liquid E968.3
    scalding E968.3
   vitriol E961
    swallowed E962.1
  caustic, corrosive substance E961
   swallowed E962.1
  cut, any part of body E966
  dagger E966
  drowning E964
  explosive(s) E965.9
   bomb (see also Assault, bomb) E965.8
   dynamite E965.8
  fight (hand) (fists) (foot) E960.0
   with weapon E968.9
    blunt or thrown E968.2
    cutting or piercing E966
    firearm — see Shooting, homicide
  fire E968.0
  firearm(s) — see Shooting, homicide
  garrotting E963
  gunshot (wound) — see Shooting, homicide
  hanging E963
  injury NEC E968.9
   to child due to criminal abortion E968.8
  knife E966
  late effect of E969
  ligature E963
  poisoning E962.9
   drugs or medicinals E962.0
   gas(es) or vapors, except drugs and medicinals E962.2
   solid or liquid substances, except drugs and medicinals E962.1
  puncture, any part of body E966
  pushing
   before moving object, train, vehicle E968.8
   from high place E968.1

Assault —continued
  rape E960.1
  scalding E968.3
  shooting — see Shooting, homicide
  stab, any part of body E966
  strangulation E963
  submersion E964
  suffocation E963
  violence NEC E968.9
  vitriol E961
    swallowed E962.1
  weapon E968.9
    blunt or thrown E968.2
    cutting or piercing E966
    firearm — see Shooting, homicide
  wound E968.9
    cutting E966
    gunshot — see Shooting, homicide
    knife E966
    piercing E966
    puncture E966
    stab E966
Attack by animal NEC E906.9
Avalanche E909
  falling on or hitting
    motor vehicle (in motion) (on public highway) E909
    railway train E909
Aviators' disease E902.1

B

Barotitis, barodontalgia, barosinusitis, barotrauma (otitic) (sinus) — see Effects of, air pressure
Battered
  baby or child (syndrome) — see Abuse, child
  person other than baby or child — see Assault
Bayonet wound (see also Cut, by bayonet) E920.3
  in
    legal intervention E974
    war operations E995
Bean in nose E912
Bed set on fire NEC E898.0
Beheading (by guillotine)
  homicide E966
  legal execution E978
Bending, injury in E927
Bends E902.0
Bite
  animal (nonvenomous) NEC E906.3
    venomous NEC E905.9
    arthropod (nonvenomous) NEC E906.4
      venomous — see Sting
  black widow spider E905.1
  cat E906.3
  centipede E905.4
  cobra E905.0
  copperhead snake E905.0
  coral snake E905.0
  dog E906.0
  fer de lance E905.0
  gila monster E905.0
  human being E968.8
  insect (nonvenomous) E906.4
    venomous — see Sting
  krait E905.0
  late effect of — see Late effect
  lizard E906.2
    venomous E905.0
  mamba E905.0
  marine animal
    nonvenomous E906.3
      snake E906.2

Bite—continued
  marine animal—continued
    venomous E905.6
      snake E905.0
  millipede E906.4
    venomous E905.4
  moray eel E906.3
  rat E906.1
  rattlesnake E905.0
  rodent, except rat E906.3
  serpent — see Bite, snake
  shark E906.3
  snake (venomous) E905.0
    nonvenomous E906.2
    sea E905.0
  spider E905.1
    nonvenomous E906.4
  tarantula (venomous) E905.1
  venomous NEC E905.9
    by specific animal — see category E905
  viper E905.0
  water moccasin E905.0
Blast (air) in war operations E993
  from nuclear explosion E996
  underwater E992
Blizzard E908
Blow E928.9
  by law-enforcing agent, police (on duty) E975
    with blunt object (baton) (nightstick) (stave) (truncheon) E973
Blowing up (see also Explosion) E923.9
Brawl (hand) (fists) (foot) E960.0
Breakage (accidental)
  cable of cable car not on rails E847
  ladder (causing fall) E881.0
  part (any) of
    animal-drawn vehicle E827
    ladder (causing fall) E881.0
    motor vehicle
      in motion (on public highway) E818
      not on public highway E825
    nonmotor road vehicle, except animal-drawn vehicle or pedal cycle E829
    off-road type motor vehicle (not on public highway) NEC E821
      on public highway E818
    pedal cycle E826
    scaffolding (causing fall) E881.1
    snow vehicle, motor-driven (not on public highway) E820
      on public highway E818
    vehicle NEC — see Accident, vehicle
Broken
  glass, injury by E920.8
  power line (causing electric shock) E925.1
Bumping against, into (accidentally)
  object (moving) (projected) (stationary) E917.9
    with fall E888
    caused by crowd (with fall) E917.1
    in
      running water E917.2
      sports E917.0
  person(s) E917.9
    with fall E886.9
      in sports E886.0
    as, or caused by, a crowd (with fall) E917.1
    in sports E917.0
      with fall E886.0

Burning, burns (accidental) (by) (from) (on) E899
  acid (any kind) E924.1
    swallowed — see Table of drugs and chemicals
  bedclothes (see also Fire, specified NEC) E898.0
  blowlamp (see also Fire, specified NEC) E898.1
  blowtorch (see also Fire, specified NEC) E898.1
  boat, ship, watercraft — see categories E830, E831, E837
  bonfire (controlled) E897
    uncontrolled E892
  candle (see also Fire, specified NEC) E898.1
  caustic liquid, substance E924.1
    swallowed — see Table of drugs and chemicals
  chemical E924.1
    from swallowing caustic, corrosive substance — see Table of drugs and chemicals
    in war operations E997.2
  cigar(s) or cigarette(s) (see also Fire, specified NEC) E898.1
  clothes, clothing, nightdress — see Ignition, clothes
    with conflagration — see Conflagration
  conflagration — see Conflagration
  corrosive liquid, substance E924.1
    swallowed — see Table of drugs and chemicals
  electric current (see also Electric shock) E925.9
  fire, flames (see also Fire) E899
  flare, Verey pistol E922.8
  heat
    from appliance (electrical) E924.8
    in local application, or packing during medical or surgical procedure E873.5
  homicide (attempt) (see also Assault, burning) E968.0
  hot
    liquid E924.0
      caustic or corrosive E924.1
    object (not producing fire or flames) E924.8
    substance E924.9
      caustic or corrosive E924.1
      liquid (metal) NEC E924.0
      specified type NEC E924.8
  ignition — see also Ignition
    clothes, clothing, nightdress — see also Ignition, clothes
      with conflagration — see Conflagration
    highly inflammable material (benzine) (fat) (gasoline) (kerosene) (paraffin) (petrol) E894
  inflicted by other person
    stated as
      homicidal, intentional (see also Assault, burning) E968.0
      undetermined whether accidental or intentional (see also Burn, stated as undetermined whether accidental or intentional) E988.1
  internal, from swallowed caustic, corrosive liquid, substance — see Table of drugs and chemicals

Burning, burns—continued
  in war operations (from fire-producing device or conventional weapon) E990.9
    from nuclear explosion E996
    petrol bomb E990.9
  lamp (see also Fire, specified NEC) E898.1
  late effect of NEC E929.4
  lighter (cigar) (cigarette) (see also Fire, specified NEC) E898.1
  lightning E907
  liquid (boiling) (hot) (molten) E924.0
    caustic, corrosive (external) E924.1
      swallowed — see Table of drugs and chemicals
  local application of externally applied substance in medical or surgical care E873.5
  machinery — see Accident, machine
  matches (see also Fire, specified NEC) E898.1
  medicament, externally applied E873.5
  metal, molten E924.0
  object (hot) E924.8
    producing fire or flames — see Fire
  pipe (smoking) (see also Fire, specified NEC) E898.1
  radiation — see Radiation
  railway engine, locomotive, train (see also Explosion, railway engine) E803
  self-inflicted (unspecified whether accidental or intentional) E988.1
    caustic or corrosive substance NEC E988.7
    stated as intentional, purposeful E958.1
      caustic or corrosive substance NEC E958.7
    stated as undetermined whether accidental or intentional E988.1
      caustic or corrosive substance NEC E988.7
  steam E924.0
    pipe E924.8
  substance (hot) E924.9
    boiling or molten E924.0
    caustic, corrosive (external) E924.1
      swallowed — see Table of drugs and chemicals
  suicidal (attempt) NEC E958.1
    caustic substance E958.7
    late effect of E959
  therapeutic misadventure
    overdose of radiation E873.2
  torch, welding (see also Fire, specified NEC) E898.1
  trash fire (see also Burning, bonfire) E897
  vapor E924.0
  vitriol E924.1
  x-rays E926.3
    in medical, surgical procedure — see Misadventure, failure, in dosage, radiation
Butted by animal E906.8

C

Cachexia, lead or saturnine E866.0
  from pesticide NEC (see also Table of drugs and chemicals) E863.4

| Caisson disease | INDEX TO EXTERNAL CAUSES | Collision |

Caisson disease E902.2
Capital punishment (any means) E978
Car sickness E903
Casualty (not due to war) NEC E928.9
 war (see also War operations) E995
Cat
 bite E906.3
 scratch E906.8
Cataclysmic (any injury)
 earth surface movement or eruption E909
 storm or flood resulting from storm E908
Catching fire — see Ignition
Caught
 between
  objects (moving) (stationary and moving) E918
   and machinery — see Accident, machine
 by cable car, not on rails E847
 in
  machinery (moving parts of) — see, Accident, machine
  object E918
Cave-in (causing asphyxia, suffocation (by pressure)) (see also Suffocation, due to, cave-in) E913.3
 with injury other than asphyxia or suffocation E916
  with asphyxia or suffocation (see also Suffocation, due to, cave-in) E913.3
 struck or crushed by E916
  with asphyxia or suffocation (see also Suffocation, due to, cave-in) E913.3
Change(s) in air pressure — see also Effects of, air pressure
 sudden, in aircraft (ascent) (descent) (causing aeroneurosis or aviators' disease) E902.1
Chilblains E901.0
 due to manmade conditions E901.1
Choking (on) (any object except food or vomitus) E912
 apple E911
 bone E911
 food, any type (regurgitated) E911
 mucus or phlegm E912
 seed E911
Civil insurrection — see War operations
Cloudburst (any injury) E908
Cold, exposure to (accidental) (excessive) (extreme) (place) E901.9
 causing chilblains or immersion foot E901.0
 due to
  manmade conditions E901.1
  specified cause NEC E901.8
  weather (conditions) E901.0
 late effect of NEC E929.5
 self-inflicted (undetermined whether accidental or intentional) E988.3
  suicidal E958.3
 suicide E958.3
Colic, lead, painter's, or saturnine — see category E866
Collapse
 building E916
  burning E891.8
  private E890.8
 due to heat — see Heat

Collapse—continued
 machinery — see Accident, machine
 postoperative NEC E878.9
 structure, burning NEC E891.8
Collision (accidental)

Note — In the case of collisions between different types of vehicles, persons and objects, priority in classification is in the following order:

    Aircraft
    Watercraft
    Motor vehicle
    Railway vehicle
    Pedal Cycle
    Animal-drawn vehicle
    Animal being ridden
    Streetcar or other nonmotor road vehicle
    Other vehicle
    Pedestrian or person using pedestrian conveyance
    Object (except where falling from or set in motion by vehicle etc. listed above)

In the listing below, the combinations are listed only under the vehicle etc. having priority. For definitions, see Volume 1, page 247.

 aircraft (with object or vehicle) (fixed) (movable) (moving) E841
  with
   person (while landing, taking off) (without accident to aircraft) E844
   powered (in transit) (with unpowered aircraft) E841
   while landing, taking off E840
   unpowered E842
   while landing, taking off E840
 animal being ridden (in sport or transport) E828
  and
   animal (being ridden) (herded) (unattended) E828
   nonmotor road vehicle, except pedal cycle or animal-drawn vehicle E828
   object (fallen) (fixed) (movable) (moving) not falling from or set in motion by vehicle of higher priority E828
   pedestrian (conveyance or vehicle) E828
 animal-drawn vehicle E827
  and
   animal (being ridden) (herded) (unattended) E827
   nonmotor road vehicle, except pedal cycle E827

Collision—continued
 animal-drawn vehicle—continued
  and—continued
   object (fallen) (fixed) (movable) (moving) not falling from or set in motion by vehicle of higher priority E827
   pedestrian (conveyance or vehicle) E827
   streetcar E827
 motor vehicle (on public highway) (traffic accident) E812
  after leaving, running off, public highway (without antecedent collision) (without re-entry) E816
   with antecedent collision on public highway — see categories E810-E815
   with re-entrance collision with another motor vehicle E811
  and
   abutment (bridge) (overpass) E815
   animal (herded) (unattended) E815
    carrying person, property E813
   animal-drawn vehicle E813
   another motor vehicle (abandoned) (disabled) (parked) (stalled) (stopped) E812
    with, involving re-entrance (on same roadway) (across median strip) E811
   any object, person, or vehicle off the public highway resulting from a noncollision motor vehicle nontraffic accident E816
   avalanche, fallen or not moving E815
   falling E909
   boundary fence E815
   culvert E815
   fallen
    stone E815
    tree E815
    guard post or guard rail E815
    inter-highway divider E815
    landslide, fallen or not moving E815
    moving E909
   machinery (road) E815
   nonmotor road vehicle NEC E813
   object (any object, person, or vehicle off the public highway resulting from a noncollision motor vehicle nontraffic accident) E815
    off, normally not on, public highway resulting from a noncollision motor vehicle traffic accident E816
   pedal cycle E813
   pedestrian (conveyance) E814
   person (using pedestrian conveyance) E814
   post or pole (lamp) (light) (signal) (telephone) (utility) E815

Collision—continued
 and—continued
  fallen—continued
   railway rolling stock, train, vehicle E810
   safety island E815
   street car E813
   traffic signal, sign, or marker (temporary) E815
   tree E815
   tricycle E813
   wall of cut made for road E815
  due to cataclysm — see categories E908, E909
  not on public highway, nontraffic accident E822
  and
   animal (carrying person, property) (herded) (unattended) E822
   animal-drawn vehicle E822
   another motor vehicle (moving), except off-road motor vehicle E822
    stationary E823
   avalanche, fallen, not moving E823
    moving E909
   landslide, fallen, not moving E823
    moving E909
   nonmotor vehicle (moving) E822
    stationary E823
   object (fallen) (normally) (fixed) (movable but not in motion) (stationary) E823
    moving, except when falling from, set in motion by, aircraft or cataclysm E822
   pedal cycle (moving) E822
    stationary E823
   pedestrian (conveyance) E822
   person (using pedestrian conveyance) E822
   railway rolling stock, train, vehicle (moving) E822
    stationary E823
   road vehicle (any) (moving) E822
    stationary E823
   tricycle (moving) E822
    stationary E823
  off-road type motor vehicle (not on public highway) E821
  and
   animal (being ridden) (-drawn vehicle) E821
   another off-road motor vehicle, except snow vehicle E821
   other motor vehicle, not on public highway E821
   other object or vehicle NEC, fixed or movable, not set in motion by aircraft, motor vehicle on highway, or snow vehicle, motor driven E821
   pedal cycle E821
   pedestrian (conveyance) E821
   railway train E821

Collision

Collision—continued
  off-road type motor vehicle—continued
    on public highway — see Collision, motor vehicle
  pedal cycle E826
    and
      animal (carrying person, property) (herded) (unherded) E826
      animal-drawn vehicle E826
      another pedal cycle E826
      nonmotor road vehicle E826
      object (fallen) (fixed) (movable) (moving) not falling from or set in motion by aircraft, motor vehicle, or railway train NEC E826
      pedestrian (conveyance) E826
      person (using pedestrian conveyance) E826
      street car E826
  pedestrian(s) (conveyance) E917.9
    with fall E886.9
      in sports E886.0
    and
      crowd, human stampede (with fall) E917.1
      machinery — see Accident, machine
      object (fallen) (moving) (projected) (stationary) not falling from or set in motion by any vehicle classifiable to E800-E848 E917.9
        with fall E888
      caused by a crowd E917.1
      in
        running water E917.2
          with drowning or submersion — see Submersion
        sports E917.0
      vehicle, nonmotor, nonroad E848
      in
        running water E917.2
          with drowning or submersion — see Submersion
        sports E917.0
          with fall E886.0
    person(s) (using pedestrian conveyance) (see also Collision, pedestrian) E917.9
  railway (rolling stock) (train) (vehicle) (with (subsequent) derailment, explosion, fall or fire) E800
    with antecedent derailment E802
    and
      animal (carrying person) (herded) (unattended) E801
      another railway train or vehicle E800
      buffers E801
      fallen tree on railway E801
      farm machinery, nonmotor (in transport) (stationary) E801
      gates E801
      nonmotor vehicle E801

Collision—continued
  pedestrian(s) —continued
    railway —continued
      and—continued
        object (fallen) (fixed) (movable) (moving) not falling from, set in motion by, aircraft or motor vehicle NEC E801
        pedal cycle E801
        pedestrian (conveyance) E805
        person (using pedestrian conveyance) E805
        platform E801
        rock on railway E801
        street car E801
    snow vehicle, motor-driven (not on public highway) E820
      and
        animal (being ridden) (-drawn vehicle) E820
        another off-road motor vehicle E820
        other motor vehicle, not on public highway E820
        other object or vehicle NEC, fixed or movable, not set in motion by aircraft or motor vehicle on highway E820
        pedal cycle E820
        pedestrian (conveyance) E820
        railway train E820
      on public highway — see Collision, motor vehicle
  street car(s) E829
    and
      animal, herded, not being ridden, unattended E829
      nonmotor road vehicle NEC E829
      object (fallen) (fixed) (movable) (moving) not falling from or set in motion by aircraft, animal-drawn vehicle, animal being ridden, motor vehicle, pedal cycle, or railway train E829
      pedestrian (conveyance) E829
      person (using pedestrian conveyance) E829
  vehicle
    animal-drawn — see Collision, animal-drawn vehicle
    motor — see Collision, motor vehicle

Collision—continued
  vehicle—continued
    nonmotor
      nonroad E848
        and
          another nonmotor, nonroad vehicle E848
          object (fallen) (fixed) (movable) (moving) not falling from or set in motion by aircraft, animal-drawn vehicle, animal being ridden, motor vehicle, nonmotor road vehicle, pedal cycle, railway train, or streetcar E848
      road, except animal being ridden, animal-drawn vehicle, or pedal cycle E829
        and
          animal, herded, not being ridden, unattended E829
          another nonmotor road vehicle, except animal being ridden, animal-drawn vehicle, or pedal cycle E829
          object (fallen) (fixed) (movable) (moving) not falling from or set in motion by, aircraft, animal-drawn vehicle, animal being ridden, motor vehicle, pedal cycle, or railway train E829
          pedestrian (conveyance) E829
          person (using pedestrian conveyance) E829
          vehicle, nonmotor, nonroad E829
  watercraft E838
    and
      person swimming or water skiing E838
    causing
      drowning, submersion E830
      injury except drowning, submersion E831

Combustion, spontaneous — see Ignition

Complication of medical or surgical procedure or treatment
  as an abnormal reaction — see Reaction, abnormal
  delayed, without mention of misadventure — see Reaction, abnormal
  due to misadventure — see Misadventure

Compression
  divers' squeeze E902.2
  trachea by
    food E911
    foreign body, except food E912

Crushed

Conflagration
  building or structure, except private dwelling (barn) (church) (convalescent or residential home) (factory) (farm outbuilding) (hospital) (hotel) (institution (educational) (domitory) (residential)) (school) (shop) (store) (theatre) E891.9
    with or causing (injury due to)
      accident or injury NEC E891.9
        specified circumstance NEC E891.8
      burns, burning E891.3
      carbon monoxide E891.2
      fumes E891.2
        polyvinylchloride (PVC) or similar material E891.1
      smoke E891.2
      causing explosion E891.0
  not in building or structure E892
  private dwelling (apartment) (boarding house) (camping place) (caravan) (farmhouse) (home (private)) (house) (lodging house) (private garage) (rooming house) (tenement) E890.9
    with or causing (injury due to)
      accident or injury NEC E890.9
        specified circumstance NEC E890.8
      burns, burning E890.3
      carbon monoxide E890.2
      fumes E890.2
        polyvinylchloride (PVC) or similar material E890.1
      smoke E890.2
      causing explosion E890.0

Contact with
  dry ice E901.1
  liquid air, hydrogen, nitrogen E901.1

Cramp(s)
  Heat — see Heat
  swimmers (see also category E910) E910.2
    not in recreation or sport E910.3

Cranking (car) (truck) (bus) (engine), injury by E917.9

Crash
  aircraft (in transit) (powered) E841
    at landing, take-off E840
    in war operations E994
    on runway NEC E840
    stated as
      homicidal E968.8
      suicidal E968.8
      undetermined whether accidental or intentional E988.6
    unpowered E842
    glider E842
  motor vehicle — see also Accident, motor vehicle
    homicidal E968.8
    suicidal E958.5
    undetermined whether accidental or intentional E988.5

Crushed (accidentally) E928.9
  between
    boat(s), ship(s), watercraft (and dock or pier) (without accident to watercraft) E838
      after accident to, or collision, watercraft E831

Crushed—*continued*
  between—*continued*
    objects (moving) (stationary and moving) E918
    by
      avalanche NEC E909
      boat, ship, watercraft after accident to, collision, watercraft E831
      cave-in E916
        with asphyxiation or suffocation (see also Suffocation, due to, cave-in) E913.3
      crowd, human stampede E917.1
      falling
        aircraft (see also Accident, aircraft) E841
          in war operations E994
        earth, material E916
          with asphyxiation or suffocation (see also Suffocation, due to, cave-in) E913.3
        object E916
          on ship, watercraft E838
            while loading, unloading watercraft E838
      landslide NEC E909
      lifeboat after abandoning ship E831
      machinery — see Accident, machine
      railway rolling stock, train, vehicle (part of) E805
      street car E829
      vehicle NEC — see Accident, vehicle NEC
  in
    machinery — see Accident, machine
    object E918
    transport accident — see categories E800-E848
  late effect of NEC E929.9
Cut, cutting (any part of body) (accidental) E920.9
  by
    arrow E920.8
    axe E920.4
    bayonet (see also Bayonet wound) E920.3
    blender E920.2
    broken glass E920.8
    can opener E920.4
      powered E920.2
    chisel E920.4
    circular saw E919.4
    cutting or piercing instrument — see also category E920
    late effect of E929.8
    dagger E920.3
    dart E920.8
    drill — see Accident, caused by drill
    edge of stiff paper E920.8
    electric
      beater E920.2
      fan E920.2
      knife E920.2
      mixer E920.2
    fork E920.4
    garden fork E920.4
    hand saw or tool (not powered) E920.4
      powered E920.1
    hedge clipper E920.4
      powered E920.1
    hoe E920.4
    ice pick E920.4
    knife E920.3
      electric E920.2
    lathe turnings E920.8

Cut, cutting—*continued*
  by—*continued*
    lawn mower E920.4
      powered E920.0
        riding E919.8
    machine — see Accident, machine
    meat
      grinder E919.8
      slicer E919.8
    nails E920.8
    needle E920.4
    object, edged, pointed, sharp — see category E920
    paper cutter E920.4
    piercing instrument — see also category E920
      late effect of E929.8
    pitchfork E920.4
    powered
      can opener E920.2
      garden cultivator E920.1
        riding E919.8
      hand saw E920.1
      hand tool NEC E920.1
      hedge clipper E920.1
      household appliance or implement E920.2
      lawn mower (hand) E920.0
        riding E919.8
      rivet gun E920.1
      staple gun E920.1
    rake E920.4
    saw
      circular E919.4
      hand E920.4
    scissors E920.4
    screwdriver E920.4
    sewing machine (electric) (powered) E920.2
      not powered E920.4
    shears E920.4
    shovel E920.4
    spade E920.4
    splinters E920.8
    sword E920.3
    tin can lid E920.8
    wood slivers E920.8
  homicide (attempt) E966
  inflicted by other person
    stated as
      intentional, homicidal E966
      undetermined whether accidental or intentional E986
    late effect of NEC E929.8
  legal
    execution E978
    intervention E974
  self-inflicted (unspecified whether accidental or intentional) E986
    stated as intentional, purposeful E956
  stated as undetermined whether accidental or intentional E986
  suicidal (attempt) E956
  war operations E995
Cyclone (any injury) E908

D

Death due to injury occurring one year or more previous — see Late effect
Decapitation (accidental circumstances) NEC E928.9
  homicidal E966
  legal execution (by guillotine) E978
Deprivation — see also Privation
  homicidal intent E968.4

Derailment (accidental)
  railway (rolling stock) (train) (vehicle) (with subsequent collision) E802
    with
      collision (antecedent) (see also Collision, railway) E800
      explosion (subsequent) (without antecedent collision) E802
        antecedent collision E803
      fall (without collision (antecedent)) E802
      fire (without collision (antecedent)) E802
    street car E829
Descent
  parachute (voluntary) (without accident to aircraft) E844
    due to accident to aircraft — see categories E840-E842
Desertion
  child, with intent to injure or kill E968.4
  helpless person, infant, newborn E904.0
    with intent to injure or kill E968.4
Destitution — see Privation
Disability, late effect or sequela of injury — see Late effect
Disease
  Andes E902.0
  aviators' E902.1
  caisson E902.2
  range E902.0
Divers' disease, palsy, paralysis, squeeze E902.0
Dog bite E906.0
Dragged by
  cable car (not on rails) E847
    on rails E829
  motor vehicle (on highway) E814
    not on highway, nontraffic accident E825
  street car E829
Drinking poison (accidental) — see Table of drugs and chemicals
Drowning — see Submersion
Dust in eye E914

E

Earth falling (on) (with asphyxia or suffocation (by pressure)) (see also Suffocation, due to, cave-in) E913.3
  as, or due to, a cataclysm (involving any transport vehicle) — see categories E908, E909
  not due to cataclysmic action E913.3
    motor vehicle (in motion) (on public highway) E810
      not on public highway E825
    nonmotor road vehicle NEC E829
    pedal cycle E826
    railway rolling stock, train, vehicle E806
    street car E829
  struck or crushed by E916
    with asphyxiation or suffocation E913.3
    with injury other than asphyxia, suffocation E916
Earthquake (any injury) E909

Effect(s) (adverse) of
  air pressure E902.9
    at high altitude E902.9
      in aircraft E902.1
      residence or prolonged visit (causing conditions classifiable to E902.0) E902.0
    due to
      diving E902.2
      specified cause NEC E902.8
    in aircraft E902.1
  cold, excessive (exposure to) (see also Cold, exposure to) E901.9
  heat (excessive) (see also Heat) E900.9
  hot
    place — see Heat
    weather E900.0
  insulation — see Heat
  late — see Late effect of
  motion E903
  nuclear explosion or weapon in war operations (blast) (fireball) (heat) (radiation) (direct) (secondary) E996
  radiation — see Radiation
  travel E903
Electric shock, electrocution (accidental) (from exposed wire, faulty appliance, high voltage cable, live rail, open socket) (by) (in) E925.9
  appliance or wiring
    domestic E925.0
    factory E925.2
    farm (building) E925.8
    house E925.0
  home E925.0
  industrial (conductor) (control apparatus) (transformer) E925.2
  outdoors E925.8
  public building E925.8
  residential institution E925.8
  school E925.8
  specified place NEC E925.8
  caused by other person
    stated as
      intentional, homicidal E968.8
      undetermined whether accidental or intentional E988.4
  electric power generating plant, distribution station E925.1
  homicidal (attempt) E968.8
  legal execution E978
  lightning E907
  machinery E925.9
    domestic E925.0
    factory E925.2
    farm E925.8
    home E925.0
  misadventure in medical or surgical procedure
    in electroshock therapy E873.4
  self-inflicted (undetermined whether accidental or intentional) E988.4
    stated as intentional E958.4
    stated as undetermined whether accidental or intentional E988.4
  suicidal (attempt) E958.4
  transmission line E925.1
Electrocution — see Electric shock
Embolism
  air (traumatic) NEC — see Air, embolism
Encephalitis
  lead or saturnine E866.0
    from pesticide NEC E863.4

Entanglement
   in
      bedclothes, causing suffocation E913.0
      wheel of pedal cycle E826

Entry of foreign body, material, any — *see* Foreign body

Execution, legal (any method) E978

Exhaustion
   cold — *see* Cold, exposure to
   due to excessive exertion E927
   heat — *see* Heat

Explosion (accidental) (in) (of) (on) E923.9
   acetylene E923.2
   aerosol can E921.8
   aircraft (in transit) (powered) E841
      at landing, take-off E840
      in war operations E994
      unpowered E842
   air tank (compressed) (in machinery) E921.1
   anesthetic gas in operating theatre E923.2
   automobile tire NEC E921.8
      causing transport accident — *see* categories E810-E825
   blasting (cap) (materials) E923.1
   boiler (machinery), not on transport vehicle E921.0
      steamship — *see* Explosion, watercraft
   bomb E923.8
      in war operations E993
         after cessation of hostilities E998
         atom, hydrogen or nuclear E996
         injury by fragments from E991.9
            antipersonnel bomb E991.3
   butane E923.2
   caused by
      other person
         stated as
            intentional, homicidal — *see* Assault, explosive
            undetermined whether accidental or homicidal E985.5
   coal gas E923.2
   detonator E923.1
   dyamite E923.1
   explosive (material) NEC E923.9
      gas(es) E923.2
      missile E923.8
         in war operations E993
            injury by fragments from E991.9
               antipersonnel bomb E991.3
      used in blasting operations E923.1
   fire-damp E923.2
   fireworks E923.0
   gas E923.2
      cylinder (in machinery) E921.1
         pressure tank (in machinery) E921.1
      gasoline (fumes) (tank) not in moving motor vehicle E923.2
      grain store (military) (munitions) E923.8
   grenade E923.8
      in war operations E993
         injury by fragments from E991.9
   homicide (attempt) — *see* Assault, explosive
   hot water heater, tank (in machinery) E921.0
   in mine (of explosive gases) NEC E923.2

Explosion—*continued*
   late effect of NEC E929.8
   machinery — *see also* Accident, machine
      pressure vessel — *see* Explosion, pressure vessel
   methane E923.2
   missile E923.8
      in war operations E993
         injury by fragments from E991.9
   motor vehicle (part of)
      in motion (on public highway) E818
      not on public highway E825
   munitions (dump) (factory) E923.8
      in war operations E993
   of mine E923.8
      in war operations
         after cessation of hostilities E998
         at sea or in harbor E992
         land E993
            after cessation of hostilities E998
            injury by fragments from E991.9
         marine E992
   own weapons in war operations E993
      injury by fragments from E991.9
         antipersonnel bomb E991.3
   pressure
      cooker E921.8
      gas tank (in machinery) E921.1
      vessel (in machinery) E921.9
         on transport vehicle — *see* categories E800-E848
         specified type NEC E921.8
   propane E923.2
   railway engine, locomotive, train (boiler) (with subsequent collision, derailment, fall) E803
      with
         collision (antecedent) (*see also* Collision, railway) E800
         derailment (antecedent) E802
         fire (without antecedent collision or derailment) E803
   secondary fire resulting from — *see* Fire
   self-inflicted (unspecified whether accidental or intentional) E985.5
      stated as intentional, purposeful E955.5
   shell (artillery) E923.8
      in war operations E993
         injury by fragments from E991.9
   stated as undetermined whether caused accidentally or purposely inflicted E985.5
   steam or water lines (in machinery) E921.0
   suicide (attempted) E955.5
   torpedo E923.8
      in war operations E992
   transport accident — *see* categories E800-E848
   war operations — *see* War operations, explosion
   watercraft (boiler) E837
      causing drowning, submersion (after jumping from watercraft) E830

Exposure (weather) (conditions) (rain) (wind) E904.3
   with homicidal intent E968.4
   excessive E904.3
      cold (*see also* Cold, exposure to) E901.9
         self-inflicted — *see* Cold, exposure to, self-inflicted
      heat (*see also* Heat) E900.9
   helpless person, infant, newborn due to abandonment or neglect E904.0
   noise E928.1
   prolonged in deep-freeze unit or refrigerator E901.1
   radiation — *see* Radiation
   resulting from transport accident — *see* categories E800-E848
   smoke from, due to
      fire — *see* Fire
      tobacco, second-hand E869.4
   vibration E928.2

F

Fall, falling (accidental) E888
   building E916
      burning E891.8
         private E890.8
   down
      escalator E880.0
      ladder E881.0
         in boat, ship, watercraft E833
      staircase E880.9
      stairs, steps — *see* Fall, from, stairs
   earth (with asphyxia or suffocation (by pressure)) (*see also* Earth, falling) E913.3
   from, off
      aircraft (at landing, take-off) (in-transit) (while alighting, boarding) E843
         resulting from accident to aircraft — *see* categories E840-E842
      animal (in sport or transport) E828
      animal-drawn vehicle E827
      balcony E882
      bed E884.2
      bicycle E826
      boat, ship, watercraft (into water) E832
         after accident to, collision, fire on E830
         and subsequently struck by (part of) boat E831
         and subsequently struck by (part of) boat E838
         burning, crushed, sinking E830
            and subsequently struck by (part of) boat E831
      bridge E882
      building E882
         burning E891.8
            private E890.8
      bunk in boat, ship, watercraft E834
         due to accident to watercraft E831
      cable car (not on rails) E847
         on rails E829
      car — *see* Fall from motor vehicle
      chair E884.2
      cliff E884.1

Fall, falling—*continued*
   from, off—*continued*
      elevation aboard ship E834
         due to accident to ship E831
      embankment E884.9
      escalator E880.0
      flagpole E882
      furniture NEC E884.9
      gangplank (into water) (*see also* Fall, from, boat) E832
         to dock, dock E834
      hammock on ship E834
         due to accident to watercraft E831
      haystack E884.9
      high place NEC E884.9
         stated as undetermined whether accidental or intentional — *see* Jumping, from, high place
      horse (in sport or transport) E828
      ladder E881.0
         in boat, ship, watercraft E833
         due to accident to watercraft E831
      machinery — *see also* Accident, machine
         not in operation E884.9
      motor vehicle (in motion) (on public highway) E818
         not on public highway E825
            stationary, except while alighting, boarding, entering, leaving E884.9
            while alighting, boarding, entering, leaving E824
         stationary, except while alighting, boarding, entering, leaving E884.9
         while alighting, boarding, entering, leaving, except off-road type motor vehicle E817
         off-road type — *see* Fall, from, off-road type motor vehicle
      nonmotor road vehicle (while alighting, boarding) NEC E829
         stationary, except while alighting, boarding, entering, leaving E884.9
      off road type motor vehicle (not on public highway) NEC E821
         on public highway E818
            while alighting, boarding, entering, leaving E817
      snow vehicle — *see* Fall from snow vehicle, motor-driven
      one
         deck to another on ship E834
            due to accident to ship E831

Fall, falling | INDEX TO EXTERNAL CAUSES | Fire

Fall, falling—continued
  from, off—continued
    one—continued
      level to another NEC
        E884.9
      boat, ship, or watercraft
        E834
        due to accident to
          watercraft
          E831
    pedal cycle E826
    playground equipment E884.0
    railway rolling stock, train,
      vehicle, (while alighting,
      boarding) E804
      with
        collision (see also
          Collision, railway)
          E800
        derailment (see also
          Derailment,
          railway) E802
        explosion (see also
          Explosion, railway
          engine) E803
    rigging (aboard ship) E834
      due to accident to
        watercraft E831
    scaffolding E881.1
    snow vehicle, motor-driven
      (not on public highway)
      E820
      on public highway E818
      while alighting,
        boarding,
        entering, leaving
        E817
    stairs, step E880.9
      boat, ship, watercraft E833
        due to accident to
          watercraft E831
      motor bus, motor vehicle
        — see Fall, from,
        motor vehicle, while
        alighting, boarding
      street car E829
    stationary vehicle NEC E884.9
    stepladder E881.0
    street car (while boarding,
      alighting) E829
      stationary, except while
        boarding or alighting
        E884.9
    structure NEC E882
      burning E891.8
    table E884.9
    tower E882
    tree E884.9
    turret E882
    vehicle NEC — see also
      Accident, vehicle NEC
      stationary E884.9
    viaduct E882
    wall E882
    window E882
  in, on
    aircraft (at landing, take-off)
      (in-transit) E843
      resulting from accident to
        aircraft — see
        categories E840-E842
    boat, ship, watercraft E835
      due to accident to
        watercraft E831
      one level to another NEC
        E834
      on ladder, stairs E833
    cutting or piercing instrument
      or machine — see Cut
    deck (of boat, ship, watercraft)
      E835
      due to accident to
        watercraft E831
    escalator E880.0
    gangplank E835
    glass, broken E920.8
    knife — see Cut, knife

Fall, falling—continued
  in, on—continued
    ladder E881.0
      in boat, ship, watercraft
        E833
        due to accident to
          watercraft E831
    object, edged, pointed or
      sharp — see Cut
    pitchfork E920.4
    railway rolling stock, train,
      vehicle (while alighting,
      boarding) E804
      with
        collision (see also
          Collision, railway)
          E800
        derailment (see also
          Derailment,
          railway) E802
        explosion (see also
          Explosion, railway
          engine) E803
    scaffolding E881.1
    scissors E920.4
    staircase, stairs, steps (see also
      Fall, from, stairs) E880.9
    street car E829
    water transport (see also Fall,
      in, boat) E835
  into
    cavity E883.9
    dock E883.9
      from boat, ship, watercraft
        (see also Fall, from,
        boat) E832
    hold (of ship) E834
      due to accident to
        watercraft E831
    hole E883.9
    manhole E883.2
    moving part of machinery —
      see Accident, machine
    opening in surface NEC
      E883.9
    pit E883.9
    quarry E883.9
    shaft E883.9
    storm drain E883.2
    tank E883.9
    water (with drowning or
      submersion) E910.9
    well E883.1
  late effect of NEC E929.3
  object (see also Hit by, object,
    falling) E916
  over
    animal E885
    cliff E884.1
    embankment E884.9
    small object E885
  overboard (see also Fall, from,
    boat) E832
  rock E916
  same level NEC E888
    aircraft (any kind) E843
      resulting from accident to
        aircraft — see
        categories E840-E842
    boat, ship, watercraft E835
      due to accident to,
        collision, watercraft
        E831
    from
      collision, pushing, shoving,
        by or with other
        person(s) E886.9
        as, or caused by, a
          crowd E917.1
        in sports E886.0
      slipping stumbling, tripping
        E885
  snowslide E916
    as avalanche E909
  stone E916

Fall, falling—continued
  through
    hatch (on ship) E834
      due to accident to
        watercraft E831
    roof E882
    window E882
  timber E916
  while alighting from, boarding,
    entering, leaving
    aircraft (any kind) E843
    motor bus, motor vehicle —
      see Fall, from, motor
      vehicle, while alighting,
      boarding
    nonmotor road vehicle NEC
      E829
    railway train E804
    street car E829
Fallen on by
  animal (horse) (not being ridden)
    E906.8
    being ridden (in sport or
      transport) E828
Fell or jumped from high place, so stated — see Jumping, from, high place
Felo-de-se (see also Suicide) E958.9
Fever
  heat — see Heat
  thermic — see Heat
Fight (hand) (fist) (foot) (see also Assault, fight) E960.0
Fire (accidental) (caused by great heat from appliance (electrical), hot object or hot substance) (secondary, resulting from explosion) E899
  conflagration — see Conflagration
  controlled, normal (in brazier, fireplace, furnace, or stove) (charcoal) (coal) (coke) (electric) (gas) (wood)
    bonfire E897
    brazier, not in building or
      structure E897
    in building or structure, except
      private dwelling (barn)
      (church) (convalescent
      or residential home)
      (factory) (farm
      outbuilding) (hospital)
      (hotel) (institution
      (educational) (dormitory)
      (residential)) (private
      garage) (school) (shop)
      (store) (theatre) E896
    in private dwelling (apartment)
      (boarding house)
      (camping place)
      (caravan) (farmhouse)
      (home (private)) (house)
      (lodging house)
      (rooming house)
      (tenement) E895
    not in building or structure
      E897
    trash E897
  forest (uncontrolled) E892
  grass (uncontrolled) E892
  hay (uncontrolled) E892
  homicide (attempt) E968.0
    late effect of E969
  in, of, on, starting in
    aircraft (in transit) (powered)
      E841
    at landing, take-off E840
    stationary E892
    unpowered (balloon)
      (glider) E842
    balloon E842
    boat, ship, watercraft — see
      categories E830, E831,
      E837

Fire—continued
  in, of, on, starting in—continued
    building or structure, except
      private dwelling (barn)
      (church) (convalescent
      or residential home)
      (factory) (farm
      outbuilding) (hospital)
      (hotel) (institution
      (educational) (dormitory)
      (residential)) (school)
      (shop) (store) (theatre)
      (see also Conflagration,
      building or structure,
      except private dwelling)
      E891.9
    forest (uncontrolled) E892
    glider E842
    grass (uncontrolled) E892
    hay (uncontrolled) E892
    lumber (uncontrolled) E892
    machinery — see Accident,
      machine
    mine (uncontrolled) E892
    motor vehicle (in motion) (on
      public highway) E818
      not on public highway
        E825
      stationary E892
    prairie (uncontrolled) E892
    private dwelling (apartment)
      (boarding house)
      (camping place)
      (caravan) (farmhouse)
      (home (private)) (house)
      (lodging house) (private
      garage) (rooming house)
      (tenement) (see also
      Conflagration, private
      dwelling) E890.9
    railway rolling stock, train,
      vehicle (see also
      Explosion, railway
      engine) E803
      stationary E892
    room NEC E898.1
    street car (in motion) E829
      stationary E892
    transport vehicle, stationary
      NEC E892
    tunnel (uncontrolled) E892
    war operations (by fire-
      producing device or
      conventional weapon)
      E990.9
      from nuclear explosion
        E996
      petrol bomb E990.0
  late effect of NEC E929.4
  lumber (uncontrolled) E892
  mine (uncontrolled) E892
  prairie (uncontrolled) E892
  self-inflicted (unspecified whether
    accidental or intentional)
    E988.1
    stated as intentional,
      purposeful E958.1
  specified NEC E898.1
    with
      conflagration — see
        Conflagration
      ignition (of)
        clothing — see Ignition,
          clothes
        highly inflammable
          material (benzine)
          (fat) (gasoline)
          (kerosene)
          (paraffin) (petrol)
          E894
  started by other person
    stated as
      with intent to injure or kill
        E968.0
      undetermined whether or
        not with intent to
        injure or kill E988.1

Fire—continued
    suicide (attempted) E958.1
        late effect of E959
    tunnel (uncontrolled) E892
Fireball effects from nuclear explosion in war operations E996
Fireworks (explosion) E923.0
Flash burns from explosion (see also Explosion) E923.9
Flood (any injury) (resulting from storm) E908
    caused by collapse of dam or manmade structure E909
Forced landing (aircraft) E840
Foreign body, object or material
    (entrance into (accidental))
    air passage (causing injury) E915
        with asphyxia, obstruction, suffocation E912
            food or vomitus E911
        nose (with asphyxia, obstruction, suffocation) E912
        causing injury without asphyxia, obstruction, suffocation E915
    alimentary canal (causing injury) (with obstruction) E915
        with asphyxia, obstruction respiratory passage, suffocation E912
            food E911
        mouth E915
            with asphyxia, obstruction, suffocation E912
                food E911
        pharynx E915
            with asphyxia, obstruction, suffocation E912
                ood E911
    aspiration (with asphyxia, obstruction respiratory passage, suffocation) E912
        causing injury without asphyxia, obstruction respiratory passage, suffocation E915
            food (regurgitated) (vomited) E911
        causing injury without asphyxia, obstruction respiratory passage, suffocation E915
        mucus (not of newborn) E912
        phlegm E912
    bladder (causing injury or obstruction) E915
    bronchus, bronchi — see Foreign body, air passages
    conjunctival sac E914
    digestive system — see Foreign body, alimentary canal
    ear (causing injury or obstruction) E915
    esophagus (causing injury or obstruction) (see also Foreign body, alimentary canal) E915
    eye (any part) E914
    eyelid E914
    hairball (stomach) (with obstruction) E915
    ingestion — see Foreign body, alimentary canal
    inhalation — see Foreign body, aspiration
    intestine (causing injury or obstruction) E915
    iris E914
    lacrimal apparatus E914
    larynx — see Foreign body, air passage
    late effect of NEC E929.8

Foreign body, object or material—continued
    lung — see Foreign body, air passage
    mouth — see Foreign body, alimentary canal, mouth
    nasal passage — see Foreign body, air passage, nose
    nose — see Foreign body, air passage, nose
    ocular muscle E914
    operation wound (left in) — see Misadventure, foreign object
    orbit E914
    pharynx — see Foreign body, alimentary canal, pharynx
    rectum (causing injury or obstruction) E915
    stomach (hairball) (causing injury or obstruction) E915
    tear ducts or glands E914
    trachea — see Foreign body, air passage
    urethra (causing injury or obstruction) E915
    vagina (causing injury or obstruction) E915
Found dead, injured
    from exposure (to) — see Exposure
    on
        public highway E819
        railway right of way E807
Fracture (circumstances unknown or unspecified) E887
    due to specified external means — see manner of accident
    late effect of NEC E929.3
    occuring in water transport NEC E835
Freezing — see Cold, exposure to
Frostbite E901.0
    due to manmade conditions E901.1
Frozen — see Cold, exposure to

G

Garrotting, homicidal (attempted) E963
Gored E906.8
Gunshot wound (see also Shooting) E922.9

H

Hailstones, injury by E904.3
Hairball (stomach) (with obstruction) E915
Hanged himself (see also Hanging, self-inflicted) E983.0
Hang gliding E842
Hanging (accidental) E913.8
    caused by other person
        in accidental circumstances E913.8
        stated as
            intentional, homicidal E963
            undetermined whether accidental or intentional E983.0
    homicide (attempt) E963
    in bed or cradle E913.0
    legal execution E978
    self-inflicted (unspecified whether accidental or intentional) E983.0
        in accidental circumstances E913.8
        stated as intentional, purposeful E953.0

Hanging—continued
    stated as undetermined whether accidental or intentional E983.0
    suicidal (attempt) E953.0
Heat (apoplexy) (collapse) (cramps) (effects of) (excessive) (exhaustion) (fever) (prostration) (stroke) E900.9
    due to
        manmade conditions (as listed in E900.1, except boat, ship, watercraft) E900.1
        weather (conditions) E900.0
    from
        electric heating appartus causing burning E924.8
        nuclear explosion in war operations E996
    generated in, boiler, engine, evaporator, fire room of boat, ship, watercraft E838
    inappropriate in local application or packing in medical or surgical procedure E873.5
    late effect of NEC E989
Hemorrhage
    delayed following medical or surgical treatment without mention of misadventure — see Reaction, abnormal
    during medical or surgical treatment as misadventure — see Misadventure, cut
High
    altitude, effects E902.9
    level of radioactivity, effects — see Radiation
    pressure effects — see also Effects of, air pressure
        from rapid descent in water (causing caisson or divers' disease, palsy, or paralysis) E902.2
    temperature, effects — see Heat
Hit, hitting (accidental) by
    aircraft (propeller) (without accident to aircraft) E844
        unpowered E842
    avalanche E909
    being thrown against object in or part of
        motor vehicle (in motion) (on public highway) E818
            not on public highway E825
        nonmotor road vehicle NEC E829
        street car E829
    boat, ship, watercraft
        after fall from watercraft E838
        damaged, involved in accident E831
        while swimming, water skiing E838
    bullet (see also Shooting) E922.9
        from air gun E917.9
        in war operations E991.2
            rubber E991.0
    flare, Very pistol (see also Shooting) E922.8
    hailstones E904.3
    landslide E909
    law-enforcing agent (on duty) E975
        with blunt object (baton) (night stick) (stave) (truncheon) E973
    machine — see Accident, machine
    missile
        firearm (see also Shooting) E922.9
        in war operations — see War operations, missile

Hit, hitting—continued
    motor vehicle (on public highway) (traffic accident) E814
        not on public highway, nontraffic accident E822
    nonmotor road vehicle NEC E829
    object
        falling E916
            from, in, on
                aircraft E844
                    due to accident to aircraft — see categories E840-E842
                    unpowered E842
                boat, ship, watercraft E838
                    due to accident to watercraft E831
                building E916
                    burning E891.8
                        private E890.8
                cataclysmic
                  earth surface movement or eruption E909
                  storm E908
                cave-in E916
                  with asphyxiation or suffocation (see also Suffocation, due to, cave-in) E913.3
                earthquake E909
                motor vehicle (in motion) (on public highway) E818
                  not on public highway E825
                      stationary E916
                nonmotor road vehicle NEC E829
                pedal cycle E826
                railway rolling stock, train, vehicle E806
                street car E829
                structure, burning NEC E891.8
                vehicle, stationary E916
        moving NEC — see Striking against, object
        projected NEC — see Striking against, object
        set in motion by
            compressed air or gas, spring, striking, throwing — see Striking against, object
            explosion — see Explosion
        thrown into, on, or towards
            motor vehicle (in motion) (on public highway) E818
                not on public highway E825
            nonmotor road vehicle NEC E829
            pedal cycle E826
            strect car E829
    off-road type motor vehicle (not on public highway) E821
        on public highway E814
    other person(s) E917.9
        with blunt or thrown object E917.9
            in sports E917.0
        intentionally, homicidal E968.2
        as, or caused by, a crowd (with fall) E917.1
        in sports E917.0

Hit, hitting—*continued*
   pedal cycle E826
   police (on duty) E975
      with blunt object (baton)
         (nightstick) (stave)
         (truncheon) E973
   railway, rolling stock, train,
      vehicle (part of) E805
   shot — *see* Shooting
   snow vehicle, motor-driven (not
      on public highway) E820
      on public highway E814
   street car E829
   vehicle NEC — *see* Accident,
      vehicle NEC
Homicide, homicidal (attempt)
   (justifiable) (*see also* Assault)
   E968.9
Hot
   liquid, object, substance,
      accident caused by — *see*
      also Accident, caused by,
      hot, by type of substance
      late effect of E929.8
   place, effects — *see* Heat
   weather, effects E900.0
Humidity, causing problem E904.3
Hunger E904.1
   resulting from
      abandonment or neglect
      E904.0
      transport accident — *see*
      categories E800-E848
Hurricane (any injury) E908
Hypobarism, hypobaropathy — *see*
   Effects of, air pressure
Hypothermia — *see* Cold, exposure
   to

I

Ictus
   caloris — *see* Heat
   solaris E900.0
Ignition (accidental)
   anesthetic gas in operating
      theatre E923.2
   bedclothes
      with
         conflagration — *see*
         Conflagration
         ignition (of)
           clothing — *see* Ignition,
           clothes
           highly inflammable
              material (benzine)
              (fat) (gasoline)
              (kerosene)
              (paraffin) (petrol)
              E894
   benzine E894
   clothes, clothing (from controlled
      fire) (in building) E893.9
      with conflagration — *see*
         Conflagration
      from
         bonfire E893.2
         highly inflammable
           material E894
         sources or material as listed
           in E893.8
         trash fire E893.2
         uncontrolled fire — *see*
           Conflagration
      in
         private dwelling E893.0
         specified building or
           structure, except
           private dwelling
           E893.1
      not in building or structure
         E893.2
   explosive material — *see*
      Explosion

Ignition—*continued*
   fat E894
   gasoline E894
   kerosene E894
   material
      explosive — *see* Explosion
      highly inflammable E894
         with conflagration — *see*
         Conflagration
         with explosion E923.2
   nightdress — *see* Ignition, clothes
   paraffin E894
   petrol E894
Immersion — *see* Submersion
Implantation of quills of porcupine
   E906.8
Inanition (from) E904.9
   hunger — *see* Lack of, food
   resulting from homicidal intent
      E968.4
   thirst — *see* Lack of, water
Inattention after, at birth E904.0
   homicidal, infanticidal intent
      E968.4
Infanticide (*see also* Assault)
Ingestion
   foreign body (causing injury)
      (with obstruction) — *see*
      Foreign body, alimentary
      canal
   poisonous substance NEC — *see*
      Table of drugs and
      chemicals
Inhalation
   excessively cold substance,
      manmade E901.1
   foreign body — *see* Foreign body,
      aspiration
   liquid air, hydrogen, nitrogen
      E901.1
   mucus, not of newborn (with
      asphyxia, obstruction
      respiratory passage,
      suffocation) E912
   phlegm (with asphyxia,
      obstruction respiratory
      passage, suffocation) E912
   poisonous gas — *see* Table of
      drugs and chemicals
   smoke from, due to
      fire — *see* Fire
      tobacco, second-hand
         E869.4
   vomitus (with asphyxia,
      obstruction respiratory
      passage, suffocation) E911
Injury, injured (accidental(ly)) NEC
   E928.9
   by, caused by, from
      air rifle (B-B gun) E917.9
      animal (not being ridden) NEC
         E906.9
         being ridden (in sport or
           transport) E828
      assult (*see also* Assault) E968.9
      avalanche E909
      bayonet (*see also* Bayonet
         wound) E920.3
      being thrown against some
         part of, or object in
         motor vehicle (in motion)
           (on public highway)
           E818
           not on public highway
              E825
           nonmotor road vehicle
              NEC E829
           off-road motor vehicle NEC
              E821
           railway train E806
           snow vehicle, motor-driven
              E820
           street car E829
      bending E927
      broken glass E920.8
      bullet — *see* Shooting

Injury, injured—*continued*
   by, caused by, from—*continued*
      cave-in (*see also* Suffocation,
         due to, cave-in) E913.3
         earth surface movement or
           eruption E909
         storm E908
         without asphyxiation or
           suffocation E916
      cloudburst E908
      cutting or piercing instrument
         (*see also* Cut) E920.9
      cyclone E908
      earthquake E909
      electric current (*see also*
         Electric shock) E925.9
      explosion (*see also* Explosion)
         E923.9
      fire — *see* Fire
      flare, Very pistol E922.8
      flood E908
      foreign body — *see* Foreign
         body
      hailstones E904.3
      hurricane E908
      landslide E909
      law-enforcing agent, police, in
         course of legal
         intervention — *see*
         Legal intervention
      lightning E907
      live rail or live wire — *see*
         Electric shock
      machinery — *see also*
         Accident, machine
         aircraft, without accident to
           aircraft E844
         boat, ship, watercraft (deck)
           (engine room)
           (galley) (laundry)
           (loading) E836
      missile
         explosive E923.8
         firearm — *see* Shooting
         in war operations — *see*
           War operations,
           missile
      moving part of motor vehicle
         (in motion) (on public
         highway) E818
         not on public highway,
           nontraffic accident
           E825
         while alighting, boarding,
           entering, leaving —
           see Fall, from, motor
           vehicle, while
           alighting, boarding
      nail E920.8
      needle (hypodermic) (sewing)
         E920.4[f73]
      noise E928.1
      object
         fallen on
           motor vehicle (in
              motion) (on
              public highway)
              E818
           not on public
              highway E825
      falling — *see* Hit by,
         object, falling
      radiation — *see* Radiation
      railway rolling stock, train,
         vehicle (part of) E805
         door or window E806
      rotating propeller, aircraft
         E844
      rough landing of off-road type
         motor vehicle (after
         leaving ground or rough
         terrain) E821
      snow vehicle E820
      saber (*see also* Wound, saber)
         E920.3
      shot — *see* Shooting
      sound waves E928.1

Injury, injured—*continued*
   by, caused by, from—*continued*
      splinter or sliver, wood E920.8
      straining E927
      street car (door) E829
      suicide (attempt) E958.9
      sword E920.3
      third rail — *see* Electric shock
      thunderbolt E907
      tidal wave E909
         caused by storm E908
      tornado E908
      torrential rain E908
      twisting E927
      vehicle NEC — *see* Accident,
         vehicle NEC
      vibration E928.2
      volcanic eruption E909
      weapon burst, in war
         operations E993
      weightlessness (in spacecraft,
         real or simulated)
         E928.0
      wood splinter or sliver E920.8
   due to
      civil insurrection — *see* War
         operations
         occurring after cessation of
           hostilities E998
      war operations — *see* War
         operations
         occurring after cessation of
           hostilities E998
   homicidal (*see also* Assault)
      E968.9
   in, on
      civil insurrection — *see* War
         operations
      fight E960.0
      parachute descent (voluntary)
         (without accident to
         aircraft) E844
         with accident to aircraft —
           see categories E840-
           E842
      public highway E819
      railway right of way E807
      war operations — *see* War
         operations
   inflicted (by)
      in course of arrest (attempted),
         suppression of
         disturbance,
         maintenance of order,
         by law enforcing agents
         — *see* Legal
         intervention
      law-enforcing agent (on duty)
         — *see* Legal
         intervention
      other person
         stated as
           accidental E928.9
           homicidal, intentional
              — *see* Assault
           undetermined whether
              accidental or
              intentional — *see*
              Injury, stated as
              undetermined
      police (on duty) — *see* Legal
         intervention
   late effect of E929.9
   purposely (inflicted) by other
      person(s) — *see* Assault
   self-inflicted (unspecified whether
      accidental or intentional)
      E988.9
      stated as
         accidental E928.9
         intentionally, purposely
           E958.9
   specified cause NEC E928.8

Injury, injured—continued
stated as
undetermined whether
accidentally or
purposely inflicted (by)
E988.9
cut (any part of body) E986
cutting or piercing
instrument
(classifiable to E920)
E986
drowning E984
explosive(s) (missile)
E985.5
falling from high place
E987.9
manmade structure,
except residential
E987.1
natural site E987.2
residential premises E987.0
hanging E983.0
knife E986
late effect of E989
puncture (any part of body)
E986
shooting — see Shooting,
stated as undetermined
whether accidental or
intentional
specified means NEC E988.8
stab (any part of body) E986
strangulation — see
Suffocation, stated as
undetermined whether
accidental or intentional
submersion E984
suffocation — see Suffocation,
stated as undetermined
whether accidental or
intentional
to child due to criminal abortion
E968.8
Insufficient nourishment — see also
Lack of, food
homicidal intent E968.4
Insulation, effects — see Heat
Interruption of respiration by
food lodged in esophagus E911
foreign body, except food, in
esophagus E912
Intervention, legal — see Legal
intervention
Intoxication, drug or poison — see
Table of drugs and chemicals
Irradiation — see Radiation

J

Jammed (accidentally)
between objects (moving)
(stationary and moving)
E918
in object E918
**Jumped or fell from high place, so
stated** — see Jumping, from,
high place, stated as
in undetermined circumstances
Jumping
before train, vehicle or other
moving object (unspecified
whether accidental or
intentional) E988.0
stated as
intentional, purposeful
E958.0
suicidal (attempt) E958.0
from
aircraft
by parachute (voluntarily)
(without accident to
aircraft) E844

Jumping—continued
from—continued
aircraft—continued
due to accident to aircraft
— see categories
E840-E842
boat, ship, watercraft (into
water)
after accident to, fire on,
watercraft E830
and subsequently struck
by (part of) boat
E831
burning, crushed, sinking
E830
and subsequently struck
by (part of) boat
E831
voluntarily, without
accident (to boat)
with injury other
than drowning or
submersion E883.0
building
burning E891.8
private E890.8
cable car (not on rails) E847
on rails E829
high place
in accidental circumstances
or in sport — see
categories E880-E884
stated as
with intent to injure self
E957.9
man-made structures
NEC E957.1
natural sites E957.2
residential premises
E957.0
in undetermined
circumstances
E987.9
man-made structures
NEC E987.1
natural sites E987.2
residential premises
E987.0
suicidal (attempt) E957.9
man-made structures
NEC E957.1
natural sites E957.1
residential premises
E957.0
motor vehicle (in motion) (on
public highway) — see
Fall, from, motor vehicle
nonmotor road vehicle NEC
E829
street car E829
structure, burning NEC E891.8
into water
with injury other than
drowning or submersion
E883.0
drowning or submersion —
see Submersion
from, off, watercraft — see
Jumping, from, boat
Justifiable homicide — see Assault

K

Kicked by
animal E906.8
person(s) (accidentally) E917.9
with intent to injure or kill
E960.0
as, or caused by a crowd (with
fall) E917.1
in fight E960.0
in sports (with fall) E917.0
Kicking against
object (moving) (projected)
(stationary) E917.9
in sports E917.0

Kicking against—continued
person — see Striking against,
person
Killed, killing (accidentally) NEC (see
also Injury) E928.9
in
action — see War operations
brawl, fight (hand) (fists) (foot)
E960.0
by weapon — see also
Assault
cutting, piercing E966
firearm — see Shooting,
homicide
self
stated as
accident E928.9
suicide — see Suicide
unspecified whether
accidental or suicidal
E988.9
Knocked down (accidentally) (by)
NEC E928.9
animal (not being ridden) E906.8
being ridden (in sport or
transport) E828
blast from explosion (see also
Explosion) E923.9
crowd, human stampede E917.1
late effect of — see Late effect
person (accidentally) E917.9
in brawl, fight E960.0
in sports E917.0
transport vehicle — see vehicle
involved under Hit by
while boxing E917.0

L

Laceration NEC E928.9
Lack of
air (refrigerator or closed place),
suffocation by E913.2
care (helpless person) (infant)
(newborn) E904.0
homicidal intent E968.4
food except as result of transport
accident E904.1
helpless person, infant,
newborn due to
abandonment or neglect
E904.0
water except as result of transport
accident E904.2
helpless person, infant,
newborn due to
abandonment or neglect
E904.0
Landslide E909
falling on, hitting
motor vehicle (any) (in motion)
(on or off public
highway) E909
railway rolling stock, train,
vehicle E909
Late effect of
accident NEC (accident
classifiable to E928.9)
E929.9
specified NEC (accident
classifiable to E910-
E928.8) E929.8
assault E969
fall, accidental (accident
classifiable to E880-E888)
E929.3
fire, accident caused by (accident
classifiable to E890-E899)
E929.4
homicide, attempt (any means)
E969
injury undetermined whether
accidentally or purposely
inflicted (injury classifiable
to E980-E988) E989

Late effect of—continued
legal intervention (injury
classifiable to E970-E976)
E977
medical or surgical procedure,
test or therapy
as, or resulting in, or from
abnormal or delayed
reaction or
complication — see
Reaction, abnormal
misadventure — see
Misadventure
motor vehicle accident (accident
classifiable to E810-E825)
E929.0
natural or environmental factor,
accident due to (accident
classifiable to E900-E909)
E929.5
poisoning, accidental (accident
classifiable to E850-E858,
E860-E869) E929.2
suicide, attempt (any means)
E959
transport accident NEC (accident
classifiable to E800-E807,
E826-E838, E840-E848)
E929.1
war operations, injury due to
(injury classifiable to E990-
E998) E999
Launching pad accident E845
Legal
execution, any method E978
intervention (by) (injury from)
E976
baton E973
bayonet E974
blow E975
blunt object (baton)
(nightstick) (stave)
(truncheon) E973
cutting or piercing instrument
E974
dynamite E971
execution, any method E973
explosive(s) (shell) E971
firearm(s) E970
gas (asphyxiation) (poisoning)
(tear) E972
grenade E971
late effect of E977
machine gun E970
manhandling E975
mortar bomb E971
nightstick E973
revolver E970
rifle E970
specified means NEC E975
stabbing E974
stave E973
truncheon E973
Lifting, injury in E927
Lightning (shock) (stroke) (struck by)
E907
Liquid (noncorrosive) in eye E914
corrosive E924.1
Loss of control
motor vehicle (on public
highway) (without
antecedent collision) E816
with
antecedent collision on
public highway —
see Collision, motor
vehicle
involving any object,
person or vehicle
not on public
highway E816
on public highway —
see Collision,
motor vehicle

Loss of control—continued
  motor vehicle—continued
    not on public highway,
      nontraffic accident E825
      with antecedent collision
        — see Collision,
        motor vehicle, not
        on public highway
    off-road type motor vehicle
      (not on public highway)
      E821
    on public highway — see
      Loss of control,
      motor vehicle
    snow vehicle, motor-driven
      (not on public highway)
      E820
      on public highway — see
        Loss of control,
        motor vehicle

Lost at sea E832
  with accident to watercraft E830
  in war operations E995

Low
  pressure, effects — see Effects of,
    air pressure
  temperature, effects — see Cold,
    exposure to

Lying before train, vehicle or other moving object (unspecified whether accidental or intentional) E988.0
  stated as intentional, purposeful, suicidal (attempt) E958.0

Lynching (see also Assault) E968.9

M

Malfunction, atomic power plant in water transport E838

Mangled (accidentally) NEC E928.9

Manhandling (in brawl, fight) E960.0
  legal intervention E975

Manslaughter (nonaccidental) — see Assault

Marble in nose E912

Mauled by animal E906.8

Medical procedure, complication of
  delayed or as an abnormal reaction
    without mention of misadventure — see Reaction, abnormal
  due to or as a result of misadventure — see Misadventure

Minamata disease E865.2

Misadventure(s) to patient(s) during surgical or medical care E876.9
  contaminated blood, fluid, drug or biological substance (presence of agents and toxins as listed in E875) E875.9
    administered (by) NEC E875.9
      infusion E875.0
      injection E875.1
      specified means NEC E875.2
      transfusion E875.0
      vaccination E875.1
  cut, cutting, puncture, perforation or hemorrhage (accidental) (inadvertent) (inappropriate) (during) E870.9
    aspiration of fluid or tissue (by puncture or catheterization, except heart) E870.5
      biopsy E870.8
        needle (aspirating) E870.5
      blood sampling E870.5

Misadventure(s) to patient(s) during surgical or medical care—continued
  cut, cutting, puncture, perforation or hemorrhage—continued
    catheterization E870.5
      heart E870.6
    dialysis (kidney) E870.2
    endoscopic examination E870.4
    enema E870.7
    infusion E870.1
    injection E870.3
    lumbar puncture E870.5
    needle biopsy E870.5
    paracentesis, abdominal E870.5
    perfusion E870.2
    specified procedure NEC E870.8
    surgical operation E870.0
    thoracentesis E870.5
    transfusion E870.1
    vaccination E870.3
  excessive amount of blood or other fluid during transfusion or infusion E873.0
  failure
    in dosage E873.9
      electroshock therapy E873.4
      inappropriate temperature (too hot or too cold) in local application and packing E873.5
      infusion
        excessive amount of fluid E873.0
        incorrect dilution of fluid E873.1
      insulin-shock therapy E873.4
      nonadministration of necessary drug or medicinal E873.6
      overdose — see also Overdose
        radiation, in therapy E873.2
      radiation
        inadvertent exposure of patient (receiving radiation for test or therapy) E873.3
        not receiving radiation for test or therapy — see Radiation
        overdose E873.2
      specified procedure NEC E873.8
      transfusion
        excessive amount of blood E873.0
    mechanical, of instrument or apparatus (during procedure) E874.9
      aspiration of fluid or tissue (by puncture or catheterization, except of heart) E874.4
        biopsy E874.8
          needle (aspirating) E874.4
        blood sampling E874.4
        catheterization E874.4
          heart E874.5
        dialysis (kidney) E874.2
        endoscopic examination E874.3
        enema E874.8

Misadventure(s) to patient(s) during surgical or medical care—continued
  failure—continued
    mechanical, of instrument or apparatus—continued
      infusion E874.1
      injection E874.8
      lumbar puncture E874.4
      needle biopsy E874.4
      paracentesis, abdominal E874.4
      perfusion E874.2
      specified procedure NEC E874.8
      surgical operation E874.0
      thoracentesis E874.4
      transfusion E874.1
      vaccination E874.8
    sterile precautions (during procedure) E872.9
      aspiration of fluid or tissue (by puncture or catheterization, except heart) E872.5
      biopsy E872.8
        needle (aspirating) E872.5
      blood sampling E872.5
      catheterization E872.5
        heart E872.6
      dialysis (kidney) E872.2
      endoscopic examination E872.4
      enema E872.8
      infusion E872.1
      injection E872.3
      lumbar puncture E872.5
      needle biopsy E872.5
      paracentesis, abdominal E872.5
      perfusion E872.2
      removal of catheter or packing E872.8
      specified procedure NEC E872.8
      surgical operation E872.0
      thoracentesis E872.5
      transfusion E872.1
      vaccination E872.3
    suture or ligature during surgical procedure E876.2
    to introduce or to remove tube or instrument E876.4
      foreign object left in body — see Misadventure, foreign object
  foreign object left in body (during procedure) E871.9
    aspiration of fluid or tissue (by puncture or catheterization, except heart) E871.5
    biopsy E871.8
      needle (aspirating) E871.5
    blood sampling E871.5
    catheterization E871.5
      heart E871.6
    dialysis (kidney) E871.2
    endoscopic examination E871.4
    enema E871.8
    infusion E871.1
    injection E871.3
    lumbar puncture E871.5
    needle biopsy E871.5
    paracentesis, abdominal E871.5
    perfusion E871.2
    removal of catheter or packing E871.7
    specified procedure NEC E871.8
    surgical operation E871.0

Misadventure(s) to patient(s) during surgical or medical care—continued
  foreign object left in body—continued
    thoracentesis E871.5
    transfusion E871.1
    vaccination E871.3
  hemorrhage — see Misadventure, cut
  inadvertent exposure of patient to radiation (being received for test or therapy) E873.3
  inappropriate
    operation performed E876.5
    temperature (too hot or too cold) in local application or packing E873.5
  infusion — see also Misadventure, by specific type, infusion
    excessive amount of fluid E873.0
    incorrect dilution of fluid E873.1
    wrong fluid E876.1
  mismatched blood in transfusion E876.0
  nonadministration of necessary drug or medicinal E873.6
  overdose — see also Overdose
    radiation, in therapy E873.2
  perforation — see Misadventure, cut
  performance of inappropriate operation E876.5
  puncture — see Misadventure, cut
  specified type NEC E876.8
    failure
      suture or ligature during surgical operation E876.2
      to introduce or to remove tube or instrument E876.4
    foreign object left in body E871.9
    infusion of wrong fluid E876.1
    performance of inappropriate operation E876.5
    transfusion of mismatched blood E876.0
    wrong
      fluid in infusion E876.1
      placement of endotracheal tube during anesthetic procedure E876.3
  transfusion — see also Misadventure, by specific type, transfusion
    excessive amount of blood E873.0
    mismatched blood E876.0
  wrong
    drug given in error — see Table of drugs and chemicals
    fluid in infusion E876.1
    placement of endotracheal tube during anesthetic procedure E876.3

Motion (effects) E903
  sickness E903

Mountain sickness E902.0

Mucus aspiration or inhalation, not of newborn (with asphyxia, obstruction respiratory passage, suffocation) E912

Mudslide of cataclysmic nature E909

Murder (attempt) (see also Assault) E968.9

N

Nail, injury by E920.8
Needlestick E920.4
Neglect — *see also* Privation
   criminal E968.4
   homicidal intent E968.4
Noise (causing injury) (pollution) E928.1

O

Object
   falling
      from, in, on, hitting
         aircraft E844
            due to accident to aircraft — *see* categories E840-E842
         machinery — *see also* Accident, machine
            not in operation E916
         motor vehicle (in motion) (on public highway) E818
            not on public highway E825
            stationary E916
         nonmotor road vehicle NEC E829
         pedal cycle E826
         person E916
         railway rolling stock, train, vehicle E806
         street car E829
         watercraft E838
            due to accident to watercraft E831
   set in motion by
      accidental explosion of pressure vessel — *see* category E921
      firearm — *see* category E922
      machine(ry) — *see* Accident, machine
      transport vehicle — *see* categories E800-E848
   thrown from, in, on, towards
      aircraft E844
      cable car (not on rails) E847
         on rails E829
      motor vehicle (in motion) (on public highway) E818
         not on public highway E825
      nonmotor road vehicle NEC E829
      pedal cycle E826
      street car E829
      vehicle NEC — *see* Accident, vehicle NEC
Obstruction
   air passages, larynx, respiratory passages
      by
         external means NEC — *see* Suffocation
         food, any type (regurgitated) (vomited) E911
         material or object, except food E912
         mucus E912
         phlegm E912
         vomitus E911

Obstruction—*continued*
   digestive tract, except mouth or pharynx
      by
         food, any type E915
         foreign body (any) E915
   esophagus
      food E911
      foreign body, except food E912
      without asphyxia or obstruction of respiratory passage E915
   mouth or pharynx
      by
         food, any type E911
         material or object, except food E912
   respiration — *see* Obstruction, air passages
Oil in eye E914
Overdose
   anesthetic (drug) — *see* Table of drugs and chemicals
   drug — *see* Table of drugs and chemicals
Overexertion (lifting) (pulling) (pushing) E927
Overexposure (accidental) (to)
   cold (*see also* Cold, exposure to) E901.9
      due to manmade conditions E901.1
   heat (*see also* Heat) E900.9
   radiation — *see* Radiation
   radioactivity — *see* Radiation
   sun, except sunburn E900.0
   weather — *see* Exposure
   wind — *see* Exposure
Overheated (*see also* Heat) E900.9
Overlaid E913.0
Overturning (accidental)
   animal-drawn vehicle E827
   boat, ship, watercraft
      causing
         drowning, submersion E830
         injury except drowning, submersion E831
   machinery — *see* Accident, machine
   motor vehicle (*see also* Loss of control, motor vehicle) E816
      with antecedent collision on public highway — *see* Collision, motor vehicle
      not on public highway, nontraffic accident E825
         with antecedent collision — *see* Collision, motor vehicle, not on public highway
   nonmotor road vehicle NEC E829
   off-road type motor vehicle — *see* Loss of control, off-road type motor vehicle
   pedal cycle E826
   railway rolling stock, train, vehicle (*see also* Derailment, railway) E802
   street car E829
   vehicle NEC — *see* Accident, vehicle NEC

P

Palsy, divers' E902.2
Parachuting (voluntary) (without accident to aircraft) E844
   due to accident to aircraft — *see* categories E840-E842
Paralysis
   divers' E902.2
   lead or saturnine E866.0
      from pesticide NEC E863.4
Pecked by bird E906.8
Phlegm aspiration or inhalation (with asphyxia, obstruction respiratory passage, suffocation) E912
Piercing (*see also* Cut) E920.9
Pinched
   between objects (moving) (stationary and moving) E918
   in object E918
Pinned under
   machine(ry) — *see* Accident, machine
Place of occurrence of accident — *see* Accident (to), occurring (at) (in)
Plumbism E866.0
   from insecticide NEC E863.4
Poisoning (accidental) (by) — *see also* Table of drugs and chemicals
   carbon monoxide
      generated by
         aircraft in transit E844
         motor vehicle
            in motion (on public highway) E818
            not on public highway E825
         watercraft (in transit) (not in transit) E838
   caused by injection of poisons or toxins into or through skin by plant thorns, spines, or other mechanism E905.7
      marine or sea plants E905.6
   fumes or smoke due to
      conflagration — *see* Conflagration
      explosion or fire — *see* Fire
      ignition — *see* Ignition
   gas
      in legal intervention E972
      legal execution, by E978
      on watercraft E838
      used as anesthetic — *see* Table of drugs and chemicals
   in war operations E997.2
   late effect of — *see* Late effect
   legal
      execution E978
      intervention
         by gas E972
Pressure, external, causing asphyxia, suffocation (*see also* Suffocation) E913.9
Privation E904.9
   food (*see also* Lack of, food) E904.1
   helpless person, infant, newborn due to abandonment or neglect E904.0
   late effect of NEC E929.5
   resulting from transport accident — *see* categories E800-E848
   water (*see also* Lack of, water) E904.2
Projected objects, striking against or struck by — *see* Striking against, object

Prolonged stay in
   high altitude (causing conditions as listed in E902.0) E902.0
   weightless environment E928.0
Prostration
   heat — *see* Heat
Pulling, injury in E927
Puncture, puncturing (*see also* Cut) E920.9
   by
      plant thorns or spines E920.8
         toxic reaction E905.7
            marine or sea plants E905.6
      sea-urchin spine E905.6
Pushing (injury in) (overexertion) E927
   by other person(s) (accidental) E917.9
      as, or caused by, a crowd, human stampede (with fall) E917.1
      before moving vehicle or object
         stated as
            intentional, homicidal E968.8
            undetemined whether accidental or intentional E988.8
      from
         high place
            in accidental circumstances — *see* categories E880-E884
            stated as
                intentional, homicidal E968.1
                undetermined whether accidental or intentional E987.9
         man-made structure, except residential E987.1
         natural site E987.2
         residential E987.0
      motor vehicle (*see also* Fall, from, motor vehicle) E818
      stated as
         intentional, homicidal E968.8
         undetermined whether accidental or intentional E988.8
   in sports E917.0
      with fall E886.0
   with fall E886.9
      in sports E886.0

R

Radiation (exposure to) E926.9
   abnormal reaction to medical test or therapy E879.2
   arc lamps E926.2
   atomic power plant (malfunction) NEC E926.9
      in water transport E838
   electromagnetic, ionizing E926.3
   gamma rays E926.3
   in
      war operations (from or following nuclear explosion) (direct) (secondary) E996
      laser(s) E997.0
      water transport E838

Radiation

Radiation—continued
  inadvertent exposure of patient
    (receiving test or therapy)
    E873.3
  infrared (heaters and lamps)
    E926.1
    excessive heat E900.1
  ionized, ionizing (particles,
    artificially accelerated)
    E926.8
    electromagnetic E926.3
  isotopes, radioactive — see
    Radiation, radioactive
    isotopes
  laser(s) E926.4
    in war operations E997.0
    misadventure in medical care
      — see Misadventure,
      failure, in dosage,
      radiation
  late effect of NEC E929.8
    excessive heat from — see
      Heat
  light sources (visible) (ultraviolet)
    E926.2
  misadventure in medical or
    surgical procedure — see
    Misadventure, failure, in
    dosage, radiation
  overdose (in medical or surgical
    procedure) E873.2
  radar E926.0
  radioactive isotopes E926.5
    atomic power plant
      malfunction E926.5
    in water transport E838
    misadventure in medical or
      surgical treatment — see
      Misadventure, failure, in
      dosage, radiation
  radiobiologicals — see Radiation,
    radioactive isotopes
  radiofrequency E926.0
  radiopharmaceuticals — see
    Radiation, radioactive
    isotopes
  radium NEC E926.9
  sun E926.2
    excessive heat from E900.0
  welding arc or torch E926.2
    excessive heat from E900.1
  x-rays (hard) (soft) E926.3
    misadventure in medical or
      surgical treatment — see
      Misadventure, failure, in
      dosage, radiation
Rape E960.1
Reaction, abnormal to or following
  (medical or surgical
    procedure) E879.9
  amputation (of limbs) E878.5
  anastomosis (arteriovenous)
    (blood vessel)
    (gastrojejunal) (skin)
    (tendon) (natural, artificial
    material, tissue) E878.2
    external stoma, creation of
      E878.3
  aspiration (of fluid) E879.4
    tissue E879.8
  biopsy E879.8
  blood
    sampling E879.7
    transfusion
      procedure E879.8
  bypass — see Reaction,
    abnormal, anastomosis
  catheterization
    cardiac E879.0
    urinary E879.6
  colostomy E878.3
  cystostomy E878.3
  dialysis (kidney) E879.1
  drugs or biologicals — see Table
    of drugs and chemicals
  duodenostomy E878.3
  electroshock therapy E879.3

Reaction, abnormal to or following
  —continued
  formation of external stoma
    E878.3
  gastrostomy E878.3
  graft — see Reaction, abnormal,
    anastomosis
  hypothermia E879.8
  implant, implantation (of)
    artificial
      internal device (cardiac
        pacemaker)
        (electrodes in brain)
        (heart valve
        prosthesis)
        (orthopedic) E878.1
      material or tissue (for
        anastomosis or
        bypass) E878.2
        with creation of external
          stoma E878.3
    natural tissues (for anastomosis
      or bypass) E878.2
      as transplantion — see
        Reaction, abnormal,
        transplant
      with creation of external
        stoma E878.3
  infusion
    procedure E879.8
  injection
    procedure E879.8
  insertion of gastric or duodenal
    sound E879.5
  insulin-shock therapy E879.3
  lumbar puncture E879.4
  perfusion E879.1
  procedures other than surgical
    operation (see also
    Reaction, abnormal, by
    specific type of procedure)
    E879.9
    specified procedure NEC
      E879.8
  radiological procedure or therapy
    E879.2
  removal of organ (partial) (total)
    NEC E878.6
    with
      anastomosis, bypass or
        graft E878.2
      formation of external stoma
        E878.3
      implant of artificial internal
        device E878.1
      transplant
        partial organ E878.4
        whole organ E878.0
  sampling
    blood E879.7
    fluid NEC E879.4
    tissue E879.8
  shock therapy E879.3
  surgical operation (see also
    Reaction, abnormal, by
    specified type of operation)
    E878.9
    restorative NEC E878.4
      with
        anastomosis, bypass or
          graft E878.2
        fomation of external
          stoma E878.3
        implant(ation) — see
          Reaction,
          abnormal, implant
        transplant(ation) — see
          Reaction,
          abnormal,
          transplant
        specified operation NEC
          E878.8
  thoracentesis E879.4
  transfusion
    procedure E879.8

Reaction, abnormal to or following
  —continued
  transplant, transplantation (heart)
    (kidney) (liver) E878.0
    partial organ E878.4
  ureterostomy E878.3
  vaccination E879.8
Reduction in
  atmospheric pressure — see also
    Effects of, air pressure
    while surfacing from
      deep water diving causing
        caisson or divers'
        disease, palsy or
        paralysis E902.2
      underground E902.8
Residual (effect) — see Late effect
Rock falling on or hitting
  (accidentally) motor vehicle
    (in motion) (on public
    highway) E818
    not on public highway E825
  nonmotor road vehicle NEC E829
  pedal cycle E826
  person E916
  railway rolling stock, train,
    vehicle E806
Running off, away
  animal (being ridden) (in sport or
    transport) E829
    not being ridden E906.8
  animal-drawn vehicle E827
  rails, railway (see also
    Derailment) E802
  roadway
    motor vehicle (without
      antecedent collision)
      E816
      nontraffic accident E825
        with antecedent
          collision — see
          Collision, motor
          vehicle, not on
          public highway
      with
        antecedent collision —
          see Collision
          motor vehicle
        subsequent collision
          involving any object,
          person or
          vehicle not on
          public
          highway E816
          on public highway
          E811
    nonmotor road vehicle NEC
      E829
    pedal cycle E826
Run over (accidentally) (by)
  animal (not being ridden) E906.8
    being ridden (in sport or
      transport) E828
  animal-drawn vehicle E827
  machinery — see Accident,
    machine
  motor vehicle (on public
    highway) — see Hit by,
    motor vehicle
  nonmotor road vehicle NEC E829
  railway train E805
  street car E829
  vehicle NEC E848

S

Saturnism E866.0
  from insecticide NEC E863.4
Scald, scalding (accidental) (by)
  (from) (in) E924.0
  acid — see Scald, caustic
  caustic or corrosive liquid,
    substance E924.1
    swallowed — see Table of
      drugs and chemicals

Scald, scalding—continued
  homicide (attempt) — see Assault,
    burning
  inflicted by other person
    stated as
      intentional or homicidal
        E968.3
      undetermined whether
        accidental or
        intentional E988.2
  late effect of NEC E929.8
  liquid (boiling) (hot) E924.0
  local application of externally
    applied substance in
    medical or surgical care
    E873.5
  molten metal E924.0
  self-inflicted (unspecified whether
    accidental or intentional)
    E988.2
    stated as intentional,
      purposeful E958.2
    stated as undetermined whether
      accidental or intentional
      E988.2
  steam E924.0
  transport accident — see
    catagories E800-E848
  vapor E924.0
Scratch, cat E906.8
Sea
  sickness E903
Self-mutilation — see Suicide
Shock
  anaphylactic (see also Table of
    drugs and chemicals)
    E947.9
    due to
      bite (venomous) — see
        Bite, venomous NEC
      sting — see Sting
  electric (see also Electric shock)
    E925.9
    from electric appliance or current
      (see also Electric shock)
      E925.9
Shooting, shot (accidental(ly))
  E922.9
  hand gun (pistol) (revolver)
    E922.0
  himself (see also Shooting, self-
    inflicted) E985.4
    hand gun (pistol) (revolver)
      E985.0
    military firearm, except hand
      gun E985.3
      hand gun (pistol) (revolver)
        E985.0
    rifle (hunting) E985.2
      military E985.3
    shotgun (automatic) E985.1
    specified firearm NEC E985.4
    Verey pistol E985.4
  homicide (attempt) E965.4
    hand gun (pistol) (revolver)
      E965.0
    military firearm, except hand
      gun E965.3
      hand gun (pistol) (revolver)
        E965.0
    rifle (hunting) E965.2
      military E965.3
    shotgun (automatic) E965.1
    specified firearm NEC E965.4
    Verey pistol E965.4
  inflicted by other person
    in accidental circumstances
      E922.9
      hand gun (pistol) (revolver)
        E922.0
      military firearm, except
        hand gun E922.3
        hand gun (pistol)
          (revolver) E922.0
      rifle (hunting) E922.2
        military E922.3

Shooting, shot—continued
  inflicted by other person—continued
    in accidental circumstances—continued
      shotgun (automatic) E922.1
      specified firearm NEC E922.8
      Verey pistol E922.8
    stated as
      intentional, homicidal E965.4
        hand gun (pistol) (revolver) E965.0
        military firearm, except hand gun E965.3
          hand gun (pistol) (revolver) E965.0
        rifle (hunting) E965.2
          military E965.3
        shotgun (automatic) E965.1
        specified firearm E965.4
        Verey pistol E965.4
      undetermined whether accidental or intentional E985.4
        hand gun (pistol) (revolver) E985.0
        military firearm, except hand gun E985.3
          hand gun (pistol) (revolver) E985.0
        rifle (hunting) E985.2
        shotgun (automatic) E985.1
        specified firearm NEC E985.4
        Verey pistol E985.4
  in war operations — see War operations, shooting
  legal
    execution E978
    intervention E970
  military firearm, except hand gun E922.3
    hand gun (pistol) (revolver) E922.0
    rifle (hunting) E922.2
      military E922.3
  self-inflicted (unspecified whether accidental or intentional) E985.4
    hand gun (pistol) (revolver) E985.0
    military firearm, except hand gun E985.3
      hand gun (pistol) (revolver) E985.0
    rifle (hunting) E985.2
      military E985.3
    shotgun (automatic) E985.1
    specified firearm NEC E985.4
    stated as
      accidental E922.9
        hand gun (pistol) (revolver) E922.0
        military firearm, except hand gun E922.3
          hand gun (pistol) (revolver) E922.0
        rifle (hunting) E922.2
          military E922.3
        shotgun (automatic) E922.1
        specified firearm NEC E922.8
        Verey pistol E922.8
      intentional, purposeful E955.4
        hand gun (pistol) (revolver) E955.0

Shooting, shot—continued
  self-inflicted—continued
    stated as—continued
      intentional, purposeful—continued
        military firearm, except hand gun E955.3
          hand gun (pistol) (revolver) E955.0
        rifle (hunting) E955.2
          military E955.3
        shotgun (automatic) E955.1
        specified firearm NEC E955.4
        Verey pistol E955.4
      shotgun (automatic) E922.1
      specified firearm NEC E922.8
      stated as undetermined whether accidental or intentional E985.4
        hand gun (pistol) (revolver) E985.0
        military firearm, except hand gun E985.3
          hand gun (pistol) (revolver) E985.0
        rifle (hunting) E985.2
          military E985.3
        shotgun (automatic) E985.1
        specified firearm NEC E985.4
        Verey pistol E985.4
      suicidal (attempt) E955.4
        hand gun (pistol) (revolver) E955.0
        military firearm, except hand gun E955.3
          hand gun (pistol) (revolver) E955.0
        rifle (hunting) E955.2
          military E955.3
        shotgun (automatic) E955.1
        specified firearm NEC E955.4
        Verey pistol E955.4
      Verey pistol E922.8

Shoving (accidentally) by other person (see also Pushing by other person) E917.9

Sickness
  air E903
  alpine E902.0
  car E903
  motion E903
  mountain E902.0
  sea E903
  travel E903

Sinking (accidental)
  boat, ship, watercraft (causing drowning, submersion) E830
    causing injury except drowning, submersion E831

Siriasis E900.0

Skydiving E844

Slashed wrists (see also Cut, self-inflicted) E986

Slipping (accidental)
  on
    deck (of boat, ship, watercraft) (icy) (oily) (wet) E835
    ice E885
    ladder of ship E833
      due to accident to watercraft E831
    mud E885
    oil E885
    snow E885
    stairs of ship E833
      due to accident to watercraft E831
    surface
      slippery E885
      wet E885

Sliver, wood, injury by E920.8

Smothering, smothered (see also Suffocation) E913.9

Solid substance in eye (any part) or adnexa E914

Sound waves (causing injury) E928.1

Splinter, injury by E920.8

Stab, stabbing E966
  accidental — see Cut

Starvation E904.1
  helpless person, infant, newborn — see Lack of food
  homicidal intent E968.4
  late effect of NEC E929.5
  resulting from accident connected with transport — see catagories E800-E848

Stepped on
  by
    animal (not being ridden) E906.8
      being ridden (in sport or transport) E828
    crowd E917.1
    person E917.9
      in sports E917.0
  in sports E917.0

Stepping on
  object (moving) (projected) (stationary) E917.9
    with fall E888
    in sports E917.0
  person E917.9
    by crowd E917.1
    in sports E917.0

Sting E905.9
  ant E905.5
  bee E905.3
  caterpillar E905.5
  coral E905.6
  hornet E905.3
  insect NEC E905.5
  jellyfish E905.6
  marine animal or plant E905.6
  nematocysts E905.6
  scorpion E905.2
  sea anemone E905.6
  sea cucumber E905.6
  wasp E905.3
  yellow jacket E905.3

Storm (causing flood) E908

Straining, injury in E927

Strangling — see Suffocation

Strangulation — see Suffocation

Strenuous movements (in recreational or other activities) E927

Striking against
  bottom (when jumping or diving into water) E883.0
  object (moving) (projected) (stationary) E917.9
    with fall E888
      caused by crowd (with fall) E917.1
    in
      running water E917.2
        with drowning or submersion — see Submersion
      sports E917.0
  person(s) E917.9
    with fall E886.9
      in sports E886.0
    as, or caused by, a crowd E917.1
      in sports E917.0
        with fall E886.0

Stroke
  heat — see Heat
  lightning E907

Struck by — see also Hit by
  lightning E907
  thunderbolt E907

Stumbling over animal, carpet, curb, rug or (small) object (with fall) E885
  without fall — see Striking against, object

Submersion (accidental) E910.8
  boat, ship, watercraft (causing drowning, submersion) E830
    causing injury except drowning, submersion E831
  by other person
    in accidental circumstances — see category E910
    intentional, homicidal E964
    stated as undetermined whether due to accidental or intentional E984
  due to
    accident
      machinery — see Accident, machine
      to boat, ship, watercraft E830
      transport — see categories E800-E848
    avalanche E909
    cataclysmic
      earth surface movement or eruption E909
      storm E908
    cloudburst E908
    cyclone E908
    fall
      from
        boat, ship, watercraft (not involved in accident) E832
          burning, crushed E830
          involved in accident, collision E830
        gangplank (into water) E832
        overboard NEC E832
    flood E908
    hurricane E908
    jumping into water E910.8
      from boat, ship, watercraft
        burning, crushed, sinking E830
        involved in accident, collision E830
        not involved in accident, for swim E910.2
      in recreational activity (without diving equipment) E910.2
        with or using diving equipment E910.1
      to rescue another person E910.3
  homicide (attempt) E964
  in
    bathtub E910.4
    specified activity, not sport, transport or recreational E910.3
    sport or recreational activity (without diving equipment) E910.2
      with or using diving equipment E910.1
    water skiing E910.0
  swimming pool NEC E910.8
  war operations E995
  water transport E832
    due to accident to boat, ship, watercraft E830
  landslide E909
    overturning boat, ship, watercraft E909
    sinking boat, ship, watercraft E909

Submersion—continued
  landslide—continued
    submersion boat, ship, watercraft E909
    tidal wave E909
      caused by storm E908
    torrential rain E908
  late effect of NEC E929.8
  quenching tank E910.8
  self-inflicted (unspecified whether accidental or intentional) E984
    in accidental circumstances — see category E910
    stated as intentional, purposeful E954
    stated as undetermined whether accidental or intentional E984
  suicidal (attempted) E954
  while
    attempting rescue of another person E910.3
    engaged in
      marine salvage E910.3
      underwater construction or repairs E910.3
    fishing, not from boat E910.2
    hunting, not from boat E910.2
    ice skating E910.2
    pearl diving E910.3
    placing fishing nets E910.3
    playing in water E910.2
    scuba diving E910.1
      nonrecreational E910.3
    skin diving E910.1
    snorkel diving E910.2
    spear fishing underwater E910.1
    surfboarding E910.2
    swimming (swimming pool) E910.2
    wading (in water) E910.2
    water skiing E910.0

Sucked
  into
    jet (aircraft) E844

Suffocation (accidental) (by external means) (by pressure) (mechanical) E913.9
  caused by other person
    in accidental circumstances — see category E913
    stated as
      intentional, homicidal E963
      undetermined whether accidental or intentional E983.9
        by, in
          hanging E983.0
          plastic bag E983.1
          specified means NEC E983.8
  due to, by
    avalanche E909
    bedclothes E913.0
    bib E913.0
    blanket E913.0
    cave-in E913.3
    caused by cataclysmic earth surface movement or eruption E909
    conflagration — see Conflagration
    explosion — see Explosion
    falling earth, other substance E913.3
    fire — see Fire
    food, any type (ingestion) (inhalation) (regurgitated) (vomited) E911

Suffocation—continued
  due to, by—continued
    foreign body, except food (ingestion) (inhalation) E912
    ignition — see Ignition
    landslide E909
    machine(ry) — see Accident, machine
    material, object except food entering by nose or mouth, ingested, inhaled E912
    mucus (aspiration) (inhalation), not of newborn E912
    phlegm (aspiration) (inhalation) E912
    pillow E913.0
    plastic bag — see Suffocation, in, plastic bag
    sheet (plastic) E913.0
    specified means NEC E913.8
    vomitus (aspiration) (inhalation) E911
  homicidal (attempt) E963
  in
    airtight enclosed place E913.2
    baby carriage E913.0
    bed E913.0
    closed place E913.2
    cot, cradle E913.0
    perambulator E913.0
    plastic bag (in accidental circumstances) E913.1
      homicidal, purposely inflicted by other person E963
      self-inflicted (unspecified whether accidental or intentional) E983.1
        in accidental circumstances E913.1
        intentional, suicidal E953.1
        stated as undetermined whether accidentally or purposely inflicted E983.1
      suicidal, purposely self-inflicted E953.1
    refrigerator E913.2
  self-inflicted — see also Suffocation, stated as undetermined whether accidental or intentional E953.9
    in accidental circumstances — see category E913
    stated as intentional, purposeful — see Suicide, suffocation
    stated as undetermined whether accidental or intentional E983.9
      by, in
        hanging E983.0
        plastic bag E983.1
        specified means NEC E983.8
  suicidal — see Suicide, suffocation

Suicide, suicidal (attempted) (by) E958.9
  burning, burns E958.1
  caustic substance E958.7
    poisoning E950.7
    swallowed E950.7
  cold, extreme E958.3
  cut (any part of body) E956
  cutting or piercing instrument (classifiable to E920) E956
  drowning E954
  electrocution E958.4
  explosive(s) (classifiable to E923) E955.5

Suicide, suicidal—continued
  fire E958.1
  firearm (classifiable to E922) — see Shooting, suicidal
  hanging E953.0
  jumping
    before moving object, train, vehicle E958.0
    from high place — see Jumping, from, high place, stated as, suicidal
  knife E956
  late effect of E959
  motor vehicle, crashing of E958.5
  poisoning — see Table of drugs and chemicals
  puncture (any part of body) E956
  scald E958.2
  shooting — see Shooting, suicidal
  specified means NEC E958.8
  stab (any part of body) E956
  strangulation — see Suicide, suffocation
  submersion E954
  suffocation E953.9
    by, in
      hanging E953.0
      plastic bag E953.1
      specified means NEC E953.8
  wound NEC E958.9

Sunburn E926.2
Sunstroke E900.0
Supersonic waves (causing injury) E928.1
Surgical procedure, complication of
  delayed or as an abnormal reaction without mention of misadventure — see Reaction, abnormal
  due to or as a result of misadventure — see Misadventure

Swallowed, swallowing
  foreign body — see Foreign body, alimentary canal
  poison — see Table of drugs and chemicals
  substance
    caustic — see Table of drugs and chemicals
    corrosive — see Table or drugs and chemicals
    poisonous — see Table of drugs and chemicals

Swimmers cramp (see also category E910) E910.2
  not in recreation or sport E910.3

Syndrome, battered
  baby or child — see Abuse, child
  wife — see Assault

T

Tackle in sport E886.0
Thermic fever E900.9
Thermoplegia E900.9
Thirst — see also Lack of water
  resulting from accident connected with transport — see categories E800-E848
Thrown (accidently)
  against object in or part of vehicle
    by motion of vehicle
      aircraft E844
      boat, ship, watercraft E838
      motor vehicle (on public highway) E818
        not on public highway E825

Thrown—continued
  against object in or part of vehicle—continued
    by motion of vehicle—continued
      motor vehicle—continued
        off-road type (not on public highway) E821
        on public highway E818
        snow vehicle E820
          on public highway E818
      nonmotor road vehicle NEC E829
      railway rolling stock, train, vehicle E806
      street car E829
  from
    animal (being ridden) (in sport or transport) E828
    high place, homicide (attempt) E968.1
    machinery — see Accident, machine
    vehicle NEC — see Accident, vehicle NEC
  off — see Thrown, from
  overboard (by motion of boat, ship, watercraft) E832
    by accident to boat, ship, watercraft E830

Thunderbolt NEC E907
Tidal wave (any injury) E909
  caused by storm E908
Took
  overdose of drug — see Table of drugs and chemicals
  poison — see Table of drugs and chemicals
Tornado (any injury) E908
Torrential rain (any injury) E908
Traffic accident NEC E819
Trampled by animal E906.8
  being ridden (in sport or transport) E828
Trapped (accidently)
  between
    objects (moving) (stationary and moving) E918
  by
    door of
      elevator E918
      motor vehicle (on public highway) (while alighting, boarding) — see Fall, from, motor vehicle, while alighting
      railway train (underground) E806
      street car E829
      subway train E806
  in object E918
Travel (effects) E903
  sickness E903
Tree
  falling on or hitting E916
    motor vehicle (in motion) (on public highway) E818
      not on public highway E825
    nonmotor road vehicle NEC E829
    pedal cycle E826
    person E916
    railway rolling stock, train, vehicle E806
    street car E829
Trench foot E901.0

Tripping over animal, carpet, curb, rug, or small object (with fall) E885
  without fall — *see* Striking against, object
Twisting, injury in E927

V

Violence, nonaccidental (*see also* Assault) E968.9
Volcanic eruption (any injury) E909
Vomitus in air passages (with asphyxia, obstruction or suffocation) E911

W

War operations (during hostilities) (injury) (by) (in) E995
  after cessation of hostilities, injury due to E998
  air blast E993
  aircraft burned, destroyed, exploded, shot down E994
  asphyxia from
    chemical E997.2
    fire, conflagration (caused by fire producing device or conventional weapon) E990.9
      from nuclear explosion E996
    petrol bomb E990.0
    fumes E997.2
    gas E997.2
  battle wound NEC E995
  bayonet E995
  biological warfare agents E997.1
  blast (air) (effects) E993
    from nuclear explosion E996
    underwater E992
  bomb (mortar) (explosion) E993
    after cessation of hostilities E998
    fragments, injury by E991.9
      antipersonnel E991.3
  bullet(s) (from carbine, machine gun, pistol, rifle, shotgun) E991.2
    rubber E991.0
  burn from
    chemical E997.2
    fire, conflagration (caused by fire-producing device or conventional weapon) E990.9
      from nuclear explosion E996
    petrol bomb E990.0
    gas E997.2
  burning aircraft E994
  chemical E997.2
  chlorine E997.2
  conventional warfare, specified from NEC E995
  crushing by falling aircraft E994
  depth charge E992
  destruction of aircraft E994
  disability as sequela one year or more after injury E999
  drowning E995
  effect (direct) (secondary) nuclear weapon E996
  explosion (artillery shell) (breech block) (cannon shell) E993
    after cessation of hostilities of bomb, mine placed in war E998
    aircraft E994

War operations—*continued*
  explosion—*continued*
    bomb (mortar) E993
      atom E996
      hydrogen E996
      injury by fragments from E991.9
        antipersonnel E991.3
      nuclear E996
    depth charge E992
      injury by fragments from E991.9
      antipersonnel E991.3
    marine weapon E992
    mine
      at sea or in harbor E992
      land E993
        injury by fragments from E991.9
      marine E992
    munitions (accidental) (being used in war) (dump) (factory) E993
    nuclear (weapon) E996
    own weapons (accidental) E993
      injury by fragments from E991.9
        antipersonnel E991.3
    sea-based artillery shell E992
    torpedo E992
  exposure to ionizing radiation from nuclear explosion E996
  falling aircraft E994
  fire or fire-producing device E990.9
    petrol bomb E990.0
  fireball effects from nuclear explosion E996
  fragments from
    antipersonnel bomb E991.3
    artillery shell, bomb NEC, grenade, guided missile, land mine, rocket, shell, shrapnel E991.9
  fumes E997.2
  gas E997.2
  grenade (explosion) E993
    fragments, injury by E991.9
  guided missile (explosion) E993
    fragments, injury by E991.9
    nuclear E996
  heat from nuclear explosion E996
  injury due to, but occurring after cessation of hostilities E998
  lacrimator (gas) (chemical) E997.2
  land mine (explosion) E993
    after cessation of hostilities E998
    fragments, injury by E991.9
  laser(s) E997.0
  late effcct of E999
  lewisite E997.2
  lung irritant (chemical) (fumes) (gas) E997.2
  marine mine E992
  mine
    after cessation of hostilities E998
    at sea E992
    in harbor E992
    land (explosion) E993
      fragments, injury by E991.9
    marine E992
  missile (guided) (explosion) E993
    fragments, injury by E991.9
    marine E992
    nuclear E996
  mortar bomb (explosion) E993
    fragments, injury by E991.9
  mustard gas E997.2
  nerve gas E997.2
  phosgene E997.2
  poisoning (chemical) (fumes) (gas) E997.2

War operations—*continued*
  radiation, ionizing from nuclear explosion E996
  rocket (explosion) E993
    fragments, injury by E991.9
  saber, sabre E995
  screening smoke E997.8
  shell (aircraft) (artillery) (cannon) (land based) (explosion) E993
    fragments, injury by E991.9
    sea-based E992
  shooting E991.2
    after cessation of hostilities E998
    bullet(s) E991.2
      rubber E991.0
    pellet(s) (rifle) E991.1
  shrapnel E991.9
  submersion E995
  torpedo E992
  unconventional warfare, except by nuclear weapon E997.9
    biological (warfare) E997.1
    gas, fumes, chemicals E997.2
    laser(s) E997.0
    specified type NEC E997.8
  underwater blast E992
  vesicant (chemical) (fumes) (gas) E997.2
  weapon burst E993
Washed
  away by flood — *see* Flood
  away by tidal wave — *see* Tidal wave
  off road by storm (transport vehicle) E908
  overboard E832
Weather exposure — *see also* Exposure
  cold E901.0
  hot E900.0
Weightlessness (causing injury) (effects of) (in spacecraft, real or simulated) E928.0
Wound (accidental) NEC (*see also* Injury) E928.9
  battle (*see also* War operations) E995
  bayonet E920.3
    in
      legal intervention E974
      war operations E995
  gunshot — *see* Shooting
  incised — *see* Cut
  saber, sabre E920.3
    in war operations E995
      categories 633.0-633.9) 639.3

INDEX TO EXTERNAL CAUSES

Fourth Digit Subdivisions for the External Cause (E) Code

Railway Accidents (E800-E807)

The following fourth-digit subdivisions are for use with categories E800-E807 to identify the injured person:

.0 **Railway employee**
Any person who by virtue of his employment in connection with a railway, whether by the railway company or not, is at increased risk of involvement in a railway accident, such as:

catering staff on train	postal staff on train
driver	railway fireman
guard	shunter
porter	sleeping car attendant

.1 **Passenger on railway**
Any authorized person traveling on a train, except a railway employee

> **EXCLUDES** intending passenger waiting at station (.8)
> unauthorized rider on railway vehicle (.8)

.2 **Pedestrian**
See definition (r), Vol. 1, page 248

.3 **Pedal cyclist**
See definition (p), Vol. 1, page 248

.8 **Other specified person**
Intending passenger waiting at station
Unauthorized rider on railway vehicle

.9 **Unspecified person**

Motor Vehicle Traffic and Nontraffic Accidents (E810-E825)

The following fourth-digit subdivisions are for use with categories E810-E819 and E820-E825 to identify the injured person:

.0 **Driver of motor vehicle other than motorcycle**
See definition (1), Vol. 1, page 248

.1 **Passenger in motor vehicle other than motorcycle**
See definition (1), Vol. 1, page 248

.2 **Motorcyclist**
See definition (1), Vol. 1, page 248

.3 **Passenger on motorcycle**
See definition (1), Vol. 1, page 248

.4 **Occupant of streetcar**

.5 **Rider of animal; occupant of animal-drawn vehicle**

.6 **Pedal cyclist**
See definition (p), Vol. 1, page 248

.7 **Pedestrian**
See definition (r), Vol. 1, page 248

.8 **Other specified person**
Occupant of vehicle other than above
Person in railway train involved in accident
Unauthorized rider of motor vehicle

.9 **Unspecified person**

INDEX TO EXTERNAL CAUSES

Other Road Vehicle Accidents (E826-E829)

(animal-drawn vehicle, streetcar, pedal cycle, and other nonmotor road vehicle accidents)

The following fourth-digit subdivisions are for use with categories E826-E829 to identify the injured person:

.0 **Pedestrian**
See definition (r), Vol. 1, page 248

.1 **Pedal cyclist** (does not apply to codes E827, E828, E829)
See definition (p), Vol. 1, page 248

.2 **Rider of animal** (does not apply to code E829)

.3 **Occupant of animal-drawn vehicle** (does not apply to codes E828, E829)

.4 **Occupant of streetcar**

.8 **Other specified person**

.9 **Unspecified person**

Water Transport Accidents (E830-E838)

The following fourth-digit subdivisions are for use with categories E830-E838 to identify the injured person:

.0 **Occupant of small boat, unpowered**

.1 **Occupant of small boat, powered**
See definition (t), Vol. 1, page 248
EXCLUDES water skier (.4)

.2 **Occupant of other watercraft — crew**
Persons:
    engaged in operation of watercraft
    providing passenger services [cabin attendants, ship's physician, catering personnel]
    working on ship during voyage in other capacity [musician in band, operators of shops and beauty parlors]

.3 **Occupant of other watercraft — other than crew**
Passenger
Occupant of lifeboat, other than crew, after abandoning ship

.4 **Water skier**

.5 **Swimmer**

.6 **Dockers, stevedores**
Longshoreman employed on the dock in loading and unloading ships

.8 **Other specified person**
Immigration and custom officials on board ship
Persons:
    accompanying passenger or member of crew visiting boat
Pilot (guiding ship into port)

.9 **Unspecified person**

INDEX TO EXTERNAL CAUSES

Air and Space Transport Accidents (E840-E845)

The following fourth-digit subdivisions are for use with categories E840-E845 to identify the injured person:

.0 **Occupant of spacecraft**

.1 **Occupant of military aircraft, any**
   Crew
   Passenger (civilian) (military)
   Troops
   in military aircraft [air force] [army] [national guard] [navy]

   EXCLUDES occupants of aircraft operated under jurisdiction of police departments (.5)
   parachutist (.7)

.2 **Crew of commercial aircraft (powered) in surface to surface transport**

.3 **Other occupant of commercial aircraft (powered) in surface to surface transport**
   Flight personnel:
      not part of crew
      on familiarization flight
   Passenger on aircraft

.4 **Occupant of commercial aircraft (powered) in surface to air transport**
   Occupant [crew] [passenger] of aircraft (powered) engaged in activities, such as:
      air drops of emergency supplies
      air drops of parachutists, except from military craft
      crop dusting
      lowering of construction material [bridge or telephone pole]
      sky writing

.5 **Occupant of other powered aircraft**
   Occupant [crew] [passenger] of aircraft (powered) engaged in activities, such as:
      aerial spraying (crops) (fire retardants)
      aerobatic flying
      aircraft racing
      rescue operation
      storm surveillance
      traffic suveillance
   Occupant of private plane NOS

.6 **Occupant of unpowered aircraft, except parachutist**
   Occupant of aircraft classifiable to E842

.7 **Parachutist (military) (other)**
   Person making voluntary descent
   EXCLUDES person making descent after accident to aircraft (.1-.6)

.8 **Ground crew, airline employee**
   Persons employed at airfields (civil) (military) or launching pads, not occupants of aircraft

.9 **Other person**

1. INFECTIOUS AND PARASITIC DISEASES (001-139)

Note: Categories for "late effects" of infectious and parasitic diseases are to be found at 137-139.

INCLUDES diseases generally recognized as communicable or transmissible as well as a few diseases of unknown but possibly infectious origin

EXCLUDES acute respiratory infections (460-466)
carrier or suspected carrier of infectious organism (V02.0-V02.9)
certain localized infections
influenza (487.0-487.8)

INTESTINAL INFECTIOUS DISEASES (001-009)

EXCLUDES helminthiases (120.0-129)

- **001 Cholera**
  - 001.0 Due to Vibrio cholerae
  - 001.1 Due to Vibrio cholerae el tor
  - ◆ 001.9 Cholera, unspecified
- **002 Typhoid and paratyphoid fevers**
  - 002.0 Typhoid fever
    Typhoid (fever) (infection) [any site]
  - 002.1 Paratyphoid fever A
  - 002.2 Paratyphoid fever B
  - 002.3 Paratyphoid fever C
  - ◆ 002.9 Paratyphoid fever, unspecified
- **003 Other salmonella infections**
  INCLUDES infection or food poisoning by Salmonella [any serotype]
  - 003.0 Salmonella gastroenteritis
    Salmonellosis
  - 003.1 Salmonella septicemia
  - ● 003.2 Localized salmonella infections
    - ◆ 003.20 Localized salmonella infection, unspecified
    - 003.21 Salmonella meningitis
    - 003.22 Salmonella pneumonia
    - 003.23 Salmonella arthritis
    - 003.24 Salmonella osteomyelitis
    - ◆ 003.29 Other
  - ◆ 003.8 Other specified salmonella infections
  - ◆ 003.9 Salmonella infection, unspecified
- **004 Shigellosis**
  INCLUDES bacillary dysentery
  - 004.0 Shigella dysenteriae
    Infection by group A Shigella (Schmitz) (Shiga)
  - 004.1 Shigella flexneri
    Infection by group B Shigella
  - 004.2 Shigella boydii
    Infection by group C Shigella
  - 004.3 Shigella sonnei
    Infection by group D Shigella
  - ◆ 004.8 Other specified shigella infections
  - ◆ 004.9 Shigellosis, unspecified
- **005 Other food poisoning (bacterial)**
  EXCLUDES salmonella infections (003.0-003.9)
  toxic effect of:
    food contaminants (989.7)
    noxious foodstuffs (988.0-988.9)
  - 005.0 Staphylococcal food poisoning
    Staphylococcal toxemia specified as due to food
  - 005.1 Botulism
    Food poisoning due to Clostridium botulinum
  - 005.2 Food poisoning due to Clostridium perfringens [C. welchii]
    Enteritis necroticans
  - 005.3 Food poisoning due to other Clostridia
  - 005.4 Food poisoning due to Vibrio parahaemolyticus
  - 005.8 Other bacterial food poisoning
    Food poisoning due to Bacillus cereus
    EXCLUDES salmonella food poisoning (003.0-003.9)
  - ◆ 005.9 Food poisoning, unspecified
- **006 Amebiasis**
  INCLUDES infection due to Entamoeba histolytica
  EXCLUDES amebiasis due to organisms other than Entamoeba histolytica (007.8)
  - 006.0 Acute amebic dysentery without mention of abscess
    Acute amebiasis
  - 006.1 Chronic intestinal amebiasis without mention of abscess
    Chronic: Chronic:
      amebiasis   amebic dysentery
  - 006.2 Amebic nondysenteric colitis
  - 006.3 Amebic liver abscess
    Hepatic amebiasis
  - 006.4 Amebic lung abscess
    Amebic abscess of lung (and liver)
  - 006.5 Amebic brain abscess
    Amebic abscess of brain (and liver) (and lung)
  - 006.6 Amebic skin ulceration
    Cutaneous amebiasis
  - ◆ 006.8 Amebic infection of other sites
    Amebic: Ameboma
      appendicitis
      balanitis
    EXCLUDES specific infections by free-living amebae (136.2)
  - ◆ 006.9 Amebiasis, unspecified
    Amebiasis NOS
- **007 Other protozoal intestinal diseases**
  INCLUDES protozoal: protozoal:
                colitis   dysentery
                diarrhea
  - 007.0 Balantidiasis
    Infection by Balantidium coli
  - 007.1 Giardiasis
    Infection by Giardia lamblia
    Lambliasis
  - 007.2 Coccidiosis
    Infection by Isospora belli and Isospora hominis
    Isosporiasis
  - 007.3 Intestinal trichomoniasis
  - ◆ 007.8 Other specified protozoal intestinal diseases
    Amebiasis due to organisms other than Entamoeba histolytica
  - ◆ 007.9 Unspecified protozoal intestinal disease
    Flagellate diarrhea
    Protozoal dysentery NOS
- **008 Intestinal infections due to other organisms**
  INCLUDES any condition classifiable to 009.0-009.3 with mention of the responsible organisms
  EXCLUDES food poisoning by these organisms (005.0-005.9)
  - ● 008.0 Escherichia coli [E. coli]
    - ◆ 008.00 E. coli, unspecified
      E. coli enteritis NOS
    - 008.01 Enteropathogenic E. coli
    - 008.02 Enterotoxigenic E. coli
    - 008.03 Enteroinvasive E. coli
    - 008.04 Enterohemorrhagic E. coli
    - ◆ 008.09 Other intestinal E. coli infections
  - 008.1 Arizona group of paracolon bacilli
  - 008.2 Aerobacter aerogenes
    Enterobacter aeogenes
  - 008.3 Proteus (mirabilis) (morganii)
  - ● 008.4 Other specified bacteria
    - 008.41 Staphylococcus
      Staphylococcal enterocolitis
    - 008.42 Pseudomonas
    - 008.43 Campylobacter
    - 008.44 Yersinia enterocolitica
    - 008.45 Clostridium difficile
      Pseudomembranous colitis
    - ◆ 008.46 Other anaerobes
      Anaerobic enteritis NOS
      Gram-negative anaerobes
      Bacteroides (fragilis)
    - ◆ 008.47 Other gram-negative bacteria
      Gram-negative enteritis NOS
      EXCLUDES gram-negative anaerobes (008.46)
    - ◆ 008.49 Other
  - ◆ 008.5 Bacterial enteritis, unspecified
  - ● 008.6 Enteritis due to specified virus
    - 008.61 Rotavirus
    - 008.62 Adenovirus
    - 008.63 Norwalk virus
      Norwalk-like agent

● Additional digits required   ◆ Nonspecific code   ■ Not a primary diagnosis   Volume 1 — 1

- **008.64 Other small round viruses [SRVs]**
  Small round virus NOS
- **008.65 Calcivirus**
- **008.66 Astrovirus**
- **008.67 Enterovirus NEC**
  Coxsackievirus
  Echovirus
  EXCLUDES *poliovirus enteritis (045.0-045.9)*
- **008.69 Other viral enteritis**
  Torovirus

008.8 Other organism, not elsewhere classified
Viral:
  enteritis NOS
  gastroenteritis
EXCLUDES *influenza with involvement of gastrointestinal tract (487.8)*

009 Ill-defined intestinal infections
EXCLUDES *diarrheal disease or intestinal infection due to specified organism (001.0-008.8)*
diarrhea following gastrointestinal surgery (564.4)
intestinal malabsorption (579.0-579.9)
other noninfectious gastroenteritis and colitis (558.1-558.9)
regional enteritis (555.0-555.9)
ulcerative colitis (556)

- **009.0 Infectious colitis, enteritis, and gastroenteritis**
  Colitis ⎫
  Enteritis ⎬ septic
  Gastroenteritis ⎭
  Dysentery:
    NOS
    catarrhal
    hemorrhagic
- **009.1 Colitis, enteritis, and gastroenteritis of presumed infectious origin**
  EXCLUDES *colitis NOS (558.9)*
  enteritis NOS (558.9)
  gastroenteritis NOS (558.9)
- **009.2 Infectious diarrhea**
  Diarrhea: Infectious diarrheal
    dysenteric   disease NOS
    epidemic
- **009.3 Diarrhea of presumed infectious origin**
  EXCLUDES *diarrhea NOS (558.9)*

TUBERCULOSIS (010-018)
INCLUDES infection by Mycobacterium tuberculosis (human) (bovine)
EXCLUDES *congenital tuberculosis (771.2)*
late effects of tuberculosis (137.0-137.4)

The following fifth-digit subclassification is for use with categories 010-018:
- 0 unspecified
- 1 bacteriological or histological examination not done
- 2 bacteriological or histological examination unknown (at present)
- 3 tubercle bacilli found (in sputum) by microscopy
- 4 tubercle bacilli not found (in sputum) by microscopy, but found by bacterial culture
- 5 tubercle bacilli not found by bacteriological examination, but tuberculosis confirmed histologically
- 6 tubercle bacilli not found by bacteriologicalor histological examination but tuberculosis confirmed by other methods [inoculation of animals]

010 Primary tuberculous infection
EXCLUDES *nonspecific reaction to tuberculin skin test without active tuberculosis (795.5)*
positive PPD (795.5)
positive tuberculin skin test without active tuberculosis (795.5)
- **010.0 Primary tuberculous complex**
- **010.1 Tuberculous pleurisy in primary progressive tuberculosis**
- **010.8 Other primary progressive tuberculosis**
  EXCLUDES *tuberculous erythema nodosum (017.1)*
- **010.9 Primary tuberculous infection, unspecified**

011 Pulmonary tuberculosis
Use additional code, if desired, to identify any associated silicosis (502)
- **011.0 Tuberculosis of lung, infiltrative**
- **011.1 Tuberculosis of lung, nodular**
- **011.2 Tuberculosis of lung with cavitation**
- **011.3 Tuberculosis of bronchus**
  EXCLUDES *isolated bronchial tuberculosis (012.2)*
- **011.4 Tuberculous fibrosis of lung**
- **011.5 Tuberculous bronchiectasis**
- **011.6 Tuberculous pneumonia [any form]**
- **011.7 Tuberculous pneumothorax**
- **011.8 Other specified pulmonary tuberculosis**
- **011.9 Pulmonary tuberculosis, unspecified**
  Respiratory tuberculosis NOS
  Tuberculosis of lung NOS

012 Other respiratory tuberculosis
EXCLUDES *respiratory tuberculosis, unspecified (011.9)*
- **012.0 Tuberculous pleurisy**
  Tuberculous empyema   Tuberculosis of pleura
  Tuberculous hydrothorax
  EXCLUDES *pleurisy with effusion without mention of cause (511.9)*
  tuberculous pleurisy in primary progressive tuberculosis (010.1)
- **012.1 Tuberculosis of intrathoracic lymph nodes**
  Tuberculosis of lymph nodes: Tuberculous
    hilar   tracheobronchial
    mediastinal   adenopathy
    tracheobronchial
  EXCLUDES *that specified as primary (010.0-010.9)*
- **012.2 Isolated tracheal or bronchial tuberculosis**
- **012.3 Tuberculous laryngitis**
  Tuberculosis of glottis
- **012.8 Other specified respiratory tuberculosis**
  Tuberculosis of: Tuberculosis of:
    mediastinum   nose (septum)
    nasopharynx   sinus [any nasal]

013 Tuberculosis of meninges and central nervous system
- **013.0 Tuberculous meningitis**
  Tuberculosis of
    meninges (cerebral) (spinal)
  Tuberculous:
    leptomeningitis
    meningoencephalitis
  EXCLUDES *tuberculoma of meninges (013.1)*
- **013.1 Tuberculoma of meninges**
- **013.2 Tuberculoma of brain**
  Tuberculosis of brain (current disease)
- **013.3 Tuberculous abscess of brain**
- **013.4 Tuberculoma of spinal cord**
- **013.5 Tuberculous abscess of spinal cord**
- **013.6 Tuberculous encephalitis or myelitis**
- **013.8 Other specified tuberculosis of central nervous system**
- **013.9 Unspecified tuberculosis of central nervous system**
  Tuberculosis of central nervous system NOS

014 Tuberculosis of intestines, peritoneum, and mesenteric glands
- **014.0 Tuberculous peritonitis**
  Tuberculous ascites
- **014.8 Other**
  Tuberculosis (of):   Tuberculous enteritis
    anus
    intestine (large) (small)
    mesenteric glands
    rectum
    retroperitoneal (lymph nodes)

015 Tuberculosis of bones and joints
Use additional code, if desired, to identify manifestation, as:
  tuberculous: tuberculous:
    arthropathy (711.4)   osteomyelitis (730.8)
    necrosis of bone (730.8) synovitis (727.01)
    osteitis (730.8)   tenosynovitis (727.01)

INFECTIOUS AND PARASITIC DISEASES

- ● 015.0 **Vertebral column**
  Pott's disease
  Use additional code, if desired, to identify manifestation, as:
  curvature of spine [Pott's] (737.4)
  kyphosis (737.4)
  spondylitis (720.81)
- ● 015.1 **Hip**
- ● 015.2 **Knee**
- ● 015.5 **Limb bones**
  Tuberculous dactylitis
- ● 015.6 **Mastoid**
  Tuberculous mastoiditis
- ◆ 015.7 **Other specified bone**
- ◆ 015.8 **Other specified joint**
- ◆ 015.9 **Tuberculosis of unspecified bones and joints**
- ● 016 **Tuberculosis of genitourinary system**
  - ● 016.0 **Kidney**
    Renal tuberculosis
    Use additional code, if desired, to identify manifestation, as:
    tuberculous:
    nephropathy (583.81)
    pyelitis (590.81)
    pyelonephritis (590.81)
  - ● 016.1 **Bladder**
  - ● 016.2 **Ureter**
  - ◆ 016.3 **Other urinary organs**
  - ● 016.4 **Epididymis**
  - ◆ 016.5 **Other male genital organs**
    Use additional code, if desired, to identify manifestation, as:
    tuberculosis of:
    prostate (601.4)
    seminal vesicle (608.81)
    testis (608.81)
  - ● 016.6 **Tuberculous oophoritis and salpingitis**
  - ◆ 016.7 **Other female genital organs**
    Tuberculous:
    cervicitis
    endometritis
  - ◆ 016.9 **Genitourinary tuberculosis, unspecified**
- ● 017 **Tuberculosis of other organs**
  - ● 017.0 **Skin and subcutaneous cellular tissue**
    Lupus: Tuberculosis:
      exedens   cutis
      vulgaris   lichenoides
    Scrofuloderma   papulonecrotica
    Tuberculosis: verrucosa cutis
      colliquativa
    EXCLUDES *lupus erythematosus (695.4)*
    disseminated (710.0)
    lupus NOS (710.0)
    nonspecific reaction to tuberculin skin test without active tuberculosis (795.5)
    positive PPD (795.5)
    positive tuberculin skin test without active tuberculosis (795.5)
  - ● 017.1 **Erythema nodosum with hypersensitivity reaction in tuberculosis**
    Bazin's disease
    Erythema:
      induratum
      nodosum, tuberculous
    Tuberculosis indurativa
    EXCLUDES *erythema nodosum NOS (695.2)*
  - ● 017.2 **Peripheral lymph nodes**
    Scrofula
    Scrofulous abscess
    Tuberculous adenitis
    EXCLUDES *tuberculosis of lymph nodes:*
    bronchial and mediastinal (012.1)
    mesenteric and retroperitoneal (014.8)
    tuberculous tracheobronchial adenopathy (012.1)
  - ● 017.3 **Eye**
    Use additional code, if desired, to identify manifestation, as:
    tuberculous:
    chorioretinitis, disseminated (363.13)
    episcleritis (379.09)
    interstitial keratitis (370.59)
    iridocyclitis, chronic (364.11)
    keratoconjunctivitis (phlyctenular) (370.31)
  - ● 017.4 **Ear**
    Tuberculosis of ear
    Tuberculous otitis media
    EXCLUDES *tuberculous mastoiditis (015.6)*
  - ● 017.5 **Thyroid gland**
  - ● 017.6 **Adrenal glands**
    Addison's disease, tuberculous
  - ● 017.7 **Spleen**
  - ● 017.8 **Esophagus**
  - ◆ 017.9 **Other specified organs**
    Use additional code, if desired, to identify manifestation, as:
    tuberculosis of:
    endocardium [any valve] (424.91)
    myocardium (422.0)
    pericardium (420.0)
- ● 018 **Miliary tuberculosis**
  INCLUDES *tuberculosis:*
  disseminated
  generalized
  miliary, whether of a single specified site, multiple sites, or unspecified site
  polyserositis
  - ● 018.0 **Acute miliary tuberculosis**
  - ◆ 018.8 **Other specified miliary tuberculosis**
  - ◆ 018.9 **Miliary tuberculosis, unspecified**

ZOONOTIC BACTERIAL DISEASES (020-027)

- ● 020 **Plague**
  INCLUDES *infection by Yersinia [Pasteurella] pestis*
  - 020.0 **Bubonic**
  - 020.1 **Cellulocutaneous**
  - 020.2 **Septicemic**
  - 020.3 **Primary pneumonic**
  - 020.4 **Secondary pneumonic**
  - ◆ 020.5 **Pneumonic, unspecified**
  - ◆ 020.8 **Other specified types of plague**
    Abortive plague
    Ambulatory plague
    Pestis minor
  - ◆ 020.9 **Plague, unspecified**
- ● 021 **Tularemia**
  INCLUDES *deerfly fever*
  infection by Francisella [Pasteurella] tularensis
  rabbit fever
  - 021.0 **Ulceroglandular tularemia**
  - 021.1 **Enteric tularemia**
    Tularemia:
      cryptogenic
      intestinal
      typhoidal
  - 021.2 **Pulmonary tularemia**
    Bronchopneumonic tularemia
  - 021.3 **Oculoglandular tularemia**
  - ◆ 021.8 **Other specified tularemia**
    Tularemia:
      generalized or disseminated
      glandular
  - ◆ 021.9 **Unspecified tularemia**
- ● 022 **Anthrax**
  - 022.0 **Cutaneous anthrax**
    Malignant pustule
  - 022.1 **Pulmonary anthrax**
    Respiratory anthrax   Wool-sorters' disease
  - 022.2 **Gastrointestinal anthrax**
  - 022.3 **Anthrax septicemia**
  - ◆ 022.8 **Other specified manifestations of anthrax**
  - ◆ 022.9 **Anthrax, unspecified**

TABULAR LIST

- **023 Brucellosis**
  - INCLUDES: fever: Malta, Mediterranean, undulant
  - 023.0 Brucella melitensis
  - 023.1 Brucella abortus
  - 023.2 Brucella suis
  - 023.3 Brucella canis
  - ◆ 023.8 Other brucellosis
    - Infection by more than one organism
  - ◆ 023.9 Brucellosis, unspecified
- 024 Glanders
  - Infection by:
    - Actinobacillus mallei
    - Farcy
    - Malleomyces mallei
    - Malleus
    - Pseudomonas mallei
- 025 Melioidosis
  - Infection by:
    - Malleomyces pseudomallei
    - Pseudomonas pseudomallei
    - Whitmore's bacillus
    - Pseudoglanders
- **026 Rat-bite fever**
  - 026.0 Spirillary fever
    - Rat-bite fever due to Spirillum minor [S. minus]
    - Sodoku
  - 026.1 Streptobacillary fever
    - Epidemic arthritic erythema
    - Haverhill fever
    - Rat-bite fever due to Streptobacillus moniliformis
  - ◆ 026.9 Unspecified rat-bite fever
- 027 Other zoonotic bacterial diseases
  - 027.0 Listeriosis
    - Infection / Septicemia by Listeria monocytogenes
    - Use additional code, if desired, to identify manifestation, as meningitis (320.7)
    - EXCLUDES: congenital listeriosis (771.2)
  - 027.1 Erysipelothrix infection
    - Erysipeloid (of Rosenbach)
    - Infection / Septicemia by Erysipelothrix insidiosa [E. rhusiopathiae]
  - 027.2 Pasteurellosis
    - Pasteurella pseudotuberculosis infection
    - Mesenteric adenitis / Septic infection (cat bite) (dog bite) by Pasteurella multocida [P. septica]
    - EXCLUDES: infection by:
      - Francisella [Pasteurella] tularensis (021.0-021.9)
      - Yersinia [Pasteurella] pestis (020.0-020.9)
  - ◆ 027.8 Other specified zoonotic bacterial diseases
  - ◆ 027.9 Unspecified zoonotic bacterial disease

OTHER BACTERIAL DISEASES (030-041)

EXCLUDES: bacterial venereal diseases (098.0-099.9)
bartonellosis (088.0)

- **030 Leprosy**
  - INCLUDES: Hansen's disease
  - infection by Mycobacterium leprae
  - 030.0 Lepromatous [type L]
    - Lepromatous leprosy (macular) (diffuse) (infiltrated) (nodular) (neuritic)
  - 030.1 Tuberculoid [type T]
    - Tuberculoid leprosy (macular) (maculoanesthetic) (major) (minor) (neuritic)
  - 030.2 Indeterminate [group I]
    - Indeterminate [uncharacteristic] leprosy (macular) (neuritic)
  - 030.3 Borderline [group B]
    - Borderline or dimorphous leprosy (infiltrated) (neuritic)
  - ◆ 030.8 Other specified leprosy
  - ◆ 030.9 Leprosy, unspecified
- **031 Diseases due to other mycobacteria**
  - 031.0 Pulmonary
    - Infection by Mycobacterium:
      - avium
      - intracellulare [Battey bacillus]
      - kansasii
    - Battey disease
  - 031.1 Cutaneous
    - Buruli ulcer
    - Infection by Mycobacterium:
      - marinum [M. balnei]
      - ulcerans
  - ◆ 031.8 Other specified mycobacterial diseases
  - ◆ 031.9 Unspecified diseases due to mycobacteria
    - Atypical mycobacterium infection NOS
- **032 Diphtheria**
  - INCLUDES: infection by Corynebacterium diphtheriae
  - 032.0 Faucial diphtheria
    - Membranous angina, diphtheritic
  - 032.1 Nasopharyngeal diphtheria
  - 032.2 Anterior nasal diphtheria
  - 032.3 Laryngeal diphtheria
    - Laryngotracheitis, diphtheritic
  - ● 032.8 Other specified diphtheria
    - 032.81 Conjunctival diphtheria
      - Pseudomembranous diphtheritic conjunctivitis
    - 032.82 Diphtheritic myocarditis
    - 032.83 Diphtheritic peritonitis
    - 032.84 Diphtheritic cystitis
    - 032.85 Cutaneous diphtheria
    - ◆ 032.89 Other
  - ◆ 032.9 Diphtheria, unspecified
- **033 Whooping cough**
  - INCLUDES: pertussis
  - Use additional code, if desired, to identify any associated pneumonia (484.3)
  - 033.0 Bordetella pertussis [B. pertussis]
  - 033.1 Bordetella parapertussis [B. parapertussis]
  - ◆ 033.8 Whooping cough due to other specified organism
    - Bordetella bronchiseptica [B. bronchiseptica]
  - ◆ 033.9 Whooping cough, unspecified organism
- **034 Streptococcal sore throat and scarlet fever**
  - 034.0 Streptococcal sore throat
    - Septic: angina, sore throat
    - Streptococcal: angina, laryngitis, pharyngitis, tonsillitis
  - 034.1 Scarlet fever
    - Scarlatina
    - EXCLUDES: parascarlatina (057.8)
- 035 Erysipelas
  - EXCLUDES: postpartum or puerperal erysipelas (670)
- **036 Meningococcal infection**
  - 036.0 Meningococcal meningitis
    - Cerebrospinal fever (meningococcal)
    - Meningitis: cerebrospinal, epidemic
  - 036.1 Meningococcal encephalitis
  - 036.2 Meningococcemia
    - Meningococcal septicemia
  - 036.3 Waterhouse-Friderichsen syndrome, meningococcal
    - Meningococcal hemorrhagic adrenalitis
    - Meningococcic adrenal syndrome
    - Waterhouse-Friderichsen syndrome NOS
  - ● 036.4 Meningococcal carditis
    - ◆ 036.40 Meningococcal carditis, unspecified
    - 036.41 Meningococcal pericarditis
    - 036.42 Meningococcal endocarditis
    - 036.43 Meningococcal myocarditis
  - ● 036.8 Other specified meningococcal infections
    - 036.81 Meningococcal optic neuritis
    - 036.82 Meningococcal arthropathy
    - ◆ 036.89 Other
  - ◆ 036.9 Meningococcal infection, unspecified
    - Meningococcal infection NOS
- 037 Tetanus
  - EXCLUDES: tetanus:
    - complicating:
      - abortion (634-638 with .0, 639.0)
      - ectopic or molar pregnancy (639.0)
    - neonatorum (771.3)
    - puerperal (670)

INFECTIOUS AND PARASITIC DISEASES

- **038 Septicemia**
    - **EXCLUDES** *bacteremia (790.7)*
        during labor (659.3)
        following ectopic or molar pregnancy (639.0)
        following infusion, injection, transfusion, or vaccination (999.3)
        postoperative (998.5)
        postpartum, puerperal (670)
        that complicating abortion (634-638 with .0, 639.0)
    - 038.0 Streptococcal septicemia
    - 038.1 Staphylococcal septicemia
    - 038.2 Pneumococcal septicemia
    - 038.3 Septicemia due to anaerobes
        Septicemia due to bacteroides
        - **EXCLUDES** *gas gangrene (040.0)*
            that due to anaerobic streptococci (038.0)
    - 038.4 Septicemia due to other gram-negative organisms
        - ◆ 038.40 Gram-negative organism, unspecified
            Gram-negative septicemia NOS
        - 038.41 Hemophilus influenzae [H. influenzae]
        - 038.42 Escherichia coli [E. coli]
        - 038.43 Pseudomonas
        - 038.44 Serratia
        - ◆ 038.49 Other
    - ◆ 038.8 Other specified septicemias
        - **EXCLUDES** *septicemia (due to):*
            anthrax (022.3)
            gonococcal (098.89)
            herpetic (054.5)
            meningococcal (036.2)
            septicemic plague (020.2)
    - ◆ 038.9 Unspecified septicemia
        Septicemia NOS
        - **EXCLUDES** *bacteremia NOS (790.7)*
- **039 Actinomycotic infections**
    - **INCLUDES** actinomycotic mycetoma
        infection by Actinomycetales, such as species of Actinomyces, Actinomadura, Nocardia, Streptomyces
        maduromycosis (actinomycotic)
        schizomycetoma (actinomycotic)
    - 039.0 Cutaneous
        Erythrasma
        Trichomycosis axillaris
    - 039.1 Pulmonary
        Thoracic actinomycosis
    - 039.2 Abdominal
    - 039.3 Cervicofacial
    - 039.4 Madura foot
        - **EXCLUDES** *madura foot due to mycotic infection (117.4)*
    - ◆ 039.8 Of other specified sites
    - ◆ 039.9 Of unspecified site
        Actinomycosis NOS
        Maduromycosis NOS
        Nocardiosis NOS
- **040 Other bacterial diseases**
    - **EXCLUDES** *bacteremia NOS (790.7)*
        bacterial infection NOS (041.9)
    - 040.0 Gas gangrene
        Gas bacillus infection or gangrene
        Infection by Clostridium:
            histolyticum
            oedematiens
            perfringens [welchii]
            septicum
            sordellii
        Malignant edema
        Myonecrosis, clostridial
        Myositis, clostridial
    - 040.1 Rhinoscleroma
    - 040.2 Whipple's disease
        Intestinal lipodystrophy
    - 040.3 Necrobacillosis
    - ●◆ 040.8 Other specified bacterial diseases
        - 040.81 Tropical pyomyositis
        - ◆ 040.89 Other

- **041 Bacterial infection in conditions classified elsewhere and of unspecified site**
    Note: This category is provided to be used as an additional code where it is desired to identify the bacterial agent in diseases classified elsewhere. This category will also be used to classify bacterial infections of unspecified nature or site.
    - **EXCLUDES** *bacteremia NOS (790.7)*
        septicemia (038.0-038.9)
    - ● 041.0 Streptococcus
        - ◆ 041.00 Streptococcus, unspecified
        - 041.01 Group A
        - 041.02 Group B
        - 041.03 Group C
        - 041.04 Group D
        - 041.05 Group G
        - ◆ 041.09 Other Streptococcus
    - ● 041.1 Staphylococcus
        - ◆ 041.10 Staphylococcus, unspecified
        - 041.11 Staphylococcus aureus
        - ◆ 041.19 Other Staphylococcus
    - 041.2 Pneumococcus
    - 041.3 Friedländer's bacillus
        Infection by Klebsiella pneumoniae
    - 041.4 Escherichia coli [E. coli]
    - 041.5 Hemophilus influenzae [H. influenzae]
    - 041.6 Proteus (mirabilis) (morganii)
    - 041.7 Pseudomonas
    - ● 041.8 Other specified bacterial infections
        - 041.81 Mycoplasma
            Eaton's agent
            Pleuropneumonia-like organisms [PPLO]
        - 041.82 Bacillus fragilis
        - 041.83 Clostridium perfringens
        - ◆ 041.84 Other anaerobes
            Gram-negative anaerobes
            Bacteroides (fragilis)
        - ◆ 041.85 Other gram-negative organisms
            Aerobacter aerogenes
            Gram-negative bacteria NOS
            Mima polymorpha
            Serratia
            - **EXCLUDES** *gram-negative anaerobes (041.84)*
        - ◆ 041.89 Other specified bacteria
    - ◆ 041.9 Bacterial infection, unspecified

HUMAN IMMUNODEFICIENCY VIRUS (HIV) INFECTION (042) ▼

- 042 Human immunodeficiency virus [HIV] disease
    Acquired immune deficiency syndrome
    Acquired immunodeficiency syndrome
    AIDS
    AIDS-like syndrome
    AIDS-related complex
    ARC
    HIV infection, symptomatic
    Use additional code(s) to identify all manifestations of HIV.
    Use additional code, if desired, to identify HIV-2 infection (079.53)
    - **EXCLUDES** *asymptomatic HIV infection status (V08)*
        exposure to HIV virus (V01.7)
        nonspecific serologic evidence of HIV (795.71) ▲

POLIOMYELITIS AND OTHER NON-ARTHROPOD-BORNE VIRAL DISEASES OF CENTRAL NERVOUS SYSTEM (045-049)

- **045 Acute poliomyelitis**
    - **EXCLUDES** *late effects of acute poliomyelitis (138)*
    The following fifth-digit subclassification is for use with category 045:
    - ◆ 0 poliovirus, unspecified type
    - 1 poliovirus type I
    - 2 poliovirus type II
    - 3 poliovirus type III
    - ● 045.0 Acute paralytic poliomyelitis specified as bulbar
        Infantile paralysis (acute)
        Poliomyelitis (acute) (anterior) } specified as bulbar

        Polioencephalitis (acute) (bulbar)
        Polioencephalomyelitis (acute) (anterior) (bulbar)

● Additional digits required   ◆ Nonspecific code   ■ Not a primary diagnosis

- ◆● 045.1 Acute poliomyelitis with other paralysis
  - Paralysis:
    - acute atrophic, spinal
    - infantile, paralytic
  - Poliomyelitis (acute) } with paralysis except bulbar
    - anterior
    - epidemic
- ● 045.2 Acute nonparalytic poliomyelitis
  - Poliomyelitis (acute) } specified as nonparalytic
    - anterior
    - epidemic
- ◆● 045.9 Acute poliomyelitis, unspecified
  - Infantile paralysis
  - Poliomyelitis (acute) } unspecified whether paralytic or nonparalytic
    - anterior
    - epidemic
- ● 046 Slow virus infection of central nervous system
  - 046.0 Kuru
  - 046.1 Jakob-Creutzfeldt disease
    - Subacute spongiform encephalopathy
  - 046.2 Subacute sclerosing panencephalitis
    - Dawson's inclusion body encephalitis
    - Van Bogaert's sclerosing leukoencephalitis
  - 046.3 Progressive multifocal leukoencephalopathy
    - Multifocal leukoencephalopathy NOS
  - ◆ 046.8 Other specified slow virus infection of central nervous system
  - ◆ 046.9 Unspecified slow virus infection of central nervous system
- ● 047 Meningitis due to enterovirus
  - **INCLUDES** meningitis:
    - abacterial
    - aseptic
    - viral
  - **EXCLUDES** meningitis due to:
    - adenovirus (049.1)
    - arthropod-borne virus (060.0-066.9)
    - leptospira (100.81)
    - virus of:
      - herpes simplex (054.72)
      - herpes zoster (053.0)
      - lymphocytic choriomeningitis (049.0)
      - mumps (072.1)
      - poliomyelitis (045.0-045.9) any other infection specifically classified elsewhere
  - 047.0 Coxsackievirus
  - 047.1 ECHO virus
    - Meningo-eruptive syndrome
  - ◆ 047.8 Other specified viral meningitis
  - ◆ 047.9 Unspecified viral meningitis
    - Viral meningitis NOS
- ◆ 048 Other enterovirus diseases of central nervous system
  - Boston exanthem
- ● 049 Other non-arthropod-borne viral diseases of central nervous system
  - **EXCLUDES** late effects of viral encephalitis (139.0)
  - 049.0 Lymphocytic choriomeningitis
    - Lymphocytic:
      - meningitis (serous) (benign)
      - meningoencephalitis (serous) (benign)
  - 049.1 Meningitis due to adenovirus
  - ◆ 049.8 Other specified non-arthropod-borne viral diseases of central nervous system
    - Encephalitis:
      - acute:
        - inclusion body
        - necrotizing
      - von Economo's disease
    - Encephalitis:
      - epidemic
      - lethargica
      - Rio Bravo
  - ◆ 049.9 Unspecified non-arthropod-borne viral diseases of central nervous system
    - Viral encephalitis NOS

VIRAL DISEASES ACCOMPANIED BY EXANTHEM (050-057)

EXCLUDES arthropod-borne viral diseases (060.0-066.9)
Boston exanthem (048)

- ● 050 Smallpox
  - 050.0 Variola major
    - Hemorrhagic (pustular) smallpox
    - Malignant smallpox
    - Purpura variolosa
  - 050.1 Alastrim
    - Variola minor
  - 050.2 Modified smallpox
    - Varioloid
  - ◆ 050.9 Smallpox, unspecified
- ● 051 Cowpox and paravaccinia
  - 051.0 Cowpox
    - Vaccinia not from vaccination
    - **EXCLUDES** vaccinia (generalized) (from vaccination) (999.0)
  - 051.1 Pseudocowpox
    - Milkers' node
  - 051.2 Contagious pustular dermatitis
    - Ecthyma contagiosum
    - Orf
  - ◆ 051.9 Paravaccinia, unspecified
- ● 052 Chickenpox
  - 052.0 Postvaricella encephalitis
    - Postchickenpox encephalitis
  - 052.1 Varicella (hemorrhagic) pneumonitis
  - ◆ 052.7 With other specified complications
  - ◆ 052.8 With unspecified complication
  - 052.9 Varicella without mention of complication
    - Chickenpox NOS
    - Varicella NOS
- ● 053 Herpes zoster
  - **INCLUDES** shingles
    zona
  - 053.0 With meningitis
  - ● 053.1 With other nervous system complications
    - ◆ 053.10 With unspecified nervous system complication
    - 053.11 Geniculate herpes zoster
      - Herpetic geniculate ganglionitis
    - 053.12 Postherpetic trigeminal neuralgia
    - 053.13 Postherpetic polyneuropathy
    - ◆ 053.19 Other
  - ● 053.2 With ophthalmic complications
    - 053.20 Herpes zoster dermatitis of eyelid
      - Herpes zoster ophthalmicus
    - 053.21 Herpes zoster keratoconjunctivitis
    - 053.22 Herpes zoster iridocyclitis
    - ◆ 053.29 Other
  - ● 053.7 With other specified complications
    - 053.71 Otitis externa due to herpes zoster
    - ◆ 053.79 Other
  - ◆ 053.8 With unspecified complication
  - 053.9 Herpes zoster without mention of complication
    - Herpes zoster NOS
- ● 054 Herpes simplex
  - **EXCLUDES** congenital herpes simplex (771.2)
  - 054.0 Eczema herpeticum
    - Kaposi's varicelliform eruption
  - ● 054.1 Genital herpes
    - ◆ 054.10 Genital herpes, unspecified
      - Herpes progenitalis
    - 054.11 Herpetic vulvovaginitis
    - 054.12 Herpetic ulceration of vulva
    - 054.13 Herpetic infection of penis
    - ◆ 054.19 Other
  - 054.2 Herpetic gingivostomatitis
  - 054.3 Herpetic meningoencephalitis
    - Herpes encephalitis
    - Simian B disease
  - 054.4 With ophthalmic complications
    - ◆ 054.40 With unspecified ophthalmic complication
    - 054.41 Herpes simplex dermatitis of eyelid
    - 054.42 Dendritic keratitis
    - 054.43 Herpes simplex disciform keratitis
    - 054.44 Herpes simplex iridocyclitis
    - ◆ 054.49 Other
  - 054.5 Herpetic septicemia
  - 054.6 Herpetic whitlow
    - Herpetic felon

INFECTIOUS AND PARASITIC DISEASES

- ● **054.7 With other specified complications**
  - 054.71 Visceral herpes simplex
  - 054.72 Herpes simplex meningitis
  - 054.73 Herpes simplex otitis externa
  - ◆ 054.79 Other
- ◆ **054.8 With unspecified complication**
- **054.9 Herpes simplex without mention of complication**
- ● **055 Measles**
  - **INCLUDES** morbilli
  - rubeola
  - **055.0 Postmeasles encephalitis**
  - **055.1 Postmeasles pneumonia**
  - **055.2 Postmeasles otitis media**
  - **055.7 With other specified complications**
    - 055.71 Measles keratoconjunctivitis
    - Measles keratitis
  - ◆ 055.79 Other
  - ◆ **055.8 With unspecified complication**
  - **055.9 Measles without mention of complication**
- ● **056 Rubella**
  - **INCLUDES** German measles
  - **EXCLUDES** congenital rubella (771.0)
  - ● **056.0 With neurological complications**
    - ◆ 056.00 With unspecified neurological complication
    - 056.01 Encephalomyelitis due to rubella
      - Encephalitis } due to rubella
      - Meningoencephalitis
    - ◆ 056.09 Other
  - ● **056.7 With other specified complications**
    - 056.71 Arthritis due to rubella
    - ◆ 056.79 Other
  - ◆ **056.8 With unspecified complications**
  - **056.9 Rubella without mention of complication**
- ● **057 Other viral exanthemata**
  - **057.0 Erythema infectiosum [fifth disease]**
  - **057.8 Other specified viral exanthemata**
    - Dukes (-Filatow) disease
    - Exanthema subitum [sixth disease]
    - Fourth disease
    - Parascarlatina
    - Pseudoscarlatina
    - Roseola infantum
  - ◆ **057.9 Viral exanthem, unspecified**

ARTHROPOD-BORNE VIRAL DISEASES (060-066)

Use additional code, if desired, to identify any associated meningitis (321.2)

EXCLUDES late effects of viral encephalitis (139.0)

- ● **060 Yellow fever**
  - **060.0 Sylvatic**
    - Yellow fever: jungle
    - Yellow fever: sylvan
  - **060.1 Urban**
  - ◆ **060.9 Yellow fever, unspecified**
- **061 Dengue**
  - Breakbone fever
  - **EXCLUDES** hemorrhagic fever caused by dengue virus (065.4)
- ● **062 Mosquito-borne viral encephalitis**
  - **062.0 Japanese encephalitis**
    - Japanese B encephalitis
  - **062.1 Western equine encephalitis**
  - **062.2 Eastern equine encephalitis**
    - **EXCLUDES** Venezuelan equine encephalitis (066.2)
  - **062.3 St. Louis encephalitis**
  - **062.4 Australian encephalitis**
    - Australian arboencephalitis
    - Australian X disease
    - Murray Valley encephalitis
  - **062.5 California virus encephalitis**
    - Encephalitis:
      - California
      - La Crosse
    - Tahyna fever
  - ◆ **062.8 Other specified mosquito-borne viral encephalitis**
    - Encephalitis by Ilheus virus
  - ◆ **062.9 Mosquito-borne viral encephalitis, unspecified**
- ● **063 Tick-borne viral encephalitis**
  - **INCLUDES** diphasic meningoencephalitis
  - **063.0 Russian spring-summer [taiga] encephalitis**
  - **063.1 Louping ill**
  - **063.2 Central European encephalitis**
  - ◆ **063.8 Other specified tick-borne viral encephalitis**
    - Langat encephalitis
    - Powassan encephalitis
  - ◆ **063.9 Tick-borne viral encephalitis, unspecified**
- **064 Viral encephalitis transmitted by other and unspecified arthropods**
  - Arthropod-borne viral encephalitis, vector unknown
  - Negishi virus encephalitis
  - **EXCLUDES** viral encephalitis NOS (049.9)
- ● **065 Arthropod-borne hemorrhagic fever**
  - **065.0 Crimean hemorrhagic fever [CHF Congo virus]**
    - Central Asian hemorrhagic fever
  - **065.1 Omsk hemorrhagic fever**
  - **065.2 Kyasanur Forest disease**
  - ◆ **065.3 Other tick-borne hemorrhagic fever**
  - **065.4 Mosquito-borne hemorrhagic fever**
    - Chikungunya hemorrhagic fever
    - Dengue hemorrhagic fever
    - **EXCLUDES** Chikungunya fever (066.3)
    - dengue (061)
    - yellow fever (060.0-060.9)
  - ◆ **065.8 Other specified arthropod-borne hemorrhagic fever**
    - Mite-borne hemorrhagic fever
  - ◆ **065.9 Arthropod-borne hemorrhagic fever, unspecified**
    - Arbovirus hemorrhagic fever NOS
- ● **066 Other arthropod-borne viral diseases**
  - **066.0 Phlebotomus fever**
    - Changuinola fever
    - Sandfly fever
  - **066.1 Tick-borne fever**
    - Nairobi sheep disease
    - Tick fever:
      - American mountain
      - Colorado
    - Tick fever:
      - Kemerovo
      - Quaranfil
  - **066.2 Venezuelan equine fever**
    - Venezuelan equine encephalitis
  - ◆ **066.3 Other mosquito-borne fever**
    - Fever (viral):
      - Bunyamwera
      - Bwamba
      - Chikungunya
      - Guama
      - Mayaro
      - Mucambo
      - O'nyong-nyong
    - Fever (viral):
      - Oropouche
      - Pixuna
      - Rift valley
      - Ross river
      - Wesselsbron
      - West Nile
      - Zika
    - **EXCLUDES** dengue (061)
    - yellow fever (060.0-060.9)
  - ◆ **066.8 Other specified arthropod-borne viral diseases**
    - Chandipura fever
    - Piry fever
  - ◆ **066.9 Arthropod-borne viral disease, unspecified**
    - Arbovirus infection NOS

OTHER DISEASES DUE TO VIRUSES AND CHLAMYDIAE (070-079)

- ● **070 Viral hepatitis**
  - **INCLUDES** viral hepatitis (acute) (chronic) ◆
  - **EXCLUDES** cytomegalic inclusion virus hepatitis (078.5)
  - **070.0 Viral hepatitis A with hepatic coma**
  - **070.1 Viral hepatitis A without mention of hepatic coma**
    - Infectious hepatitis

  The following fifth-digit subclassification is for use with categories 070.2 and 070.3: ▼
  - ◆ 0 acute or unspecified, without mention of hepatitis delta
  - ◆ 1 acute or unspecified, with hepatitis delta
  - 2 chronic, without mention of hepatitis delta
  - 3 chronic, with hepatitis delta

  - ● **070.2 Viral hepatitis B with hepatic coma**
  - ● **070.3 Viral hepatitis B without mention of hepatic coma**
    - Serum hepatitis
  - ● **070.4 Other specified viral hepatitis with hepatic coma**
    - ◆ 070.41 Acute or unspecified hepatitis C with hepatic coma
    - 070.42 Hepatitis delta without mention of active hepatitis B disease with hepatic coma
      - Hepatitis delta with hepatitis B carrier state
    - 070.43 Hepatitis E with hepatic coma
    - 070.44 Chronic hepatitis C with hepatic coma ▲

● Additional digits required ◆ Nonspecific code ■ Not a primary diagnosis

- 070.49 Other specified viral hepatitis with hepatic coma ▼
- 070.5 Other specified viral hepatitis without mention of hepatic coma
  - 070.51 Acute or unspecified hepatitis C without mention of hepatic coma
  - 070.52 Hepatitis delta without mention of active hepatititis B disease or hepatic coma
  - 070.53 Hepatitis E without mention of hepatic coma
  - 070.54 Chronic hepatitis C without mention of hepatic coma
  - 070.59 Other specified viral hepatitis without mention of hepatic coma ▲
- 070.6 Unspecified viral hepatitis with hepatic coma
- 070.9 Unspecified viral hepatitis without mention of hepatic coma
  - Viral hepatitis NOS

071 Rabies
Hydrophobia   Lyssa

072 Mumps
- 072.0 Mumps orchitis
- 072.1 Mumps meningitis
- 072.2 Mumps encephalitis
  - Mumps meningoencephalitis
- 072.3 Mumps pancreatitis
- 072.7 Mumps with other specified complications
  - 072.71 Mumps hepatitis
  - 072.72 Mumps polyneuropathy
  - 072.79 Other
- 072.8 Mumps with unspecified complication
- 072.9 Mumps without mention of complication
  - Epidemic parotitis   Infectious parotitis

073 Ornithosis
INCLUDES parrot fever
psittacosis
- 073.0 With pneumonia
  - Lobular pneumonitis due to ornithosis
- 073.7 With other specified complications
- 073.8 With unspecified complication
- 073.9 Ornithosis, unspecified

074 Specific diseases due to Coxsackievirus
EXCLUDES *Coxsackievirus:*
  infection NOS (079.2)
  meningitis (047.O)
- 074.0 Herpangina
  - Vesicular pharyngitis
- 074.1 Epidemic pleurodynia
  - Bornholm disease   Epidemic:
  - Devil's grip   myalgia
                                       myositis
- 074.2 Coxsackie carditis
  - 074.20 Coxsackie carditis, unspecified
  - 074.21 Coxsackie pericarditis
  - 074.22 Coxsackie endocarditis
  - 074.23 Coxsackie myocarditis
    - Aseptic myocarditis of newborn
- 074.3 Hand, foot, and mouth disease
  - Vesicular stomatitis and exanthem
- 074.8 Other specified diseases due to Coxsackie virus
  - Acute lymphonodular pharyngitis

075 Infectious mononucleosis
Glandular fever
Monocytic angina
Pfeiffer's disease

076 Trachoma
EXCLUDES *late effect of trachoma (139.1)*
- 076.0 Initial stage
  - Trachoma dubium
- 076.1 Active stage
  - Granular conjunctivitis (trachomatous)
  - Trachomatous
    - follicular conjunctivitis
    - pannus
- 076.9 Trachoma, unspecified
  - Trachoma NOS

077 Other diseases of conjunctiva due to viruses and Chlamydiae
EXCLUDES *ophthalmic complications of viral diseases classified elsewhere*
- 077.0 Inclusion conjunctivitis
  - Paratrachoma
  - Swimming pool conjunctivitis
  - **EXCLUDES** *inclusion blennorrhea (neonatal) (771.6)*
- 077.1 Epidemic keratoconjunctivitis
  - Shipyard eye
- 077.2 Pharyngoconjunctival fever
  - Viral pharyngoconjunctivitis
- 077.3 Other adenoviral conjunctivitis
  - Acute adenoviral follicular conjunctivitis
- 077.4 Epidemic hemorrhagic conjunctivitis
  - Apollo:
    - conjunctivitis
    - disease
  - Conjunctivitis due to enterovirus type 70
  - Hemorrhagic conjunctivitis (acute) (epidemic)
- 077.8 Other viral conjunctivitis
  - Newcastle conjunctivitis
- 077.9 Unspecified diseases of conjunctiva due to viruses and Chlamydiae
  - 077.98 Due to Chlamydiae
  - 077.99 Due to viruses
    - Viral conjunctivitis NOS

078 Other diseases due to viruses and Chlamydiae
EXCLUDES *viral infection NOS (079.0-079.9)*
viremia NOS (790.8)
- 078.0 Molluscum contagiosum
- 078.1 Viral warts
  - 078.10 Viral warts, unspecified
    - Condyloma NOS   Verruca:
    - Verruca: vulgaris
      - NOS   Warts (infectious)
  - 078.11 Condyloma acuminatum
  - 078.19 Other specified viral warts
    - Genital warts NOS   Verruca:
    - Verruca: plantaris
      - plana
- 078.2 Sweating fever
  - Miliary fever   Sweating disease
- 078.3 Cat-scratch disease
  - Benign lymphoreticulosis (of inoculation)
  - Cat-scratch fever
- 078.4 Foot and mouth disease
  - Aphthous fever
  - Epizootic:
    - aphthae
    - stomatitis
- 078.5 Cytomegaloviral disease
  - Cytomegalic inclusion disease
  - Salivary gland virus disease
  - Use additional code, if desired, to identify manifestation, as:
    - cytomegalic inclusion virus:
      - hepatitis (573.1)
      - pneumonia (484.1)
  - **EXCLUDES** *congenital cytomegalovirus infection (771.1)*
- 078.6 Hemorrhagic nephrosonephritis
  - Hemorrhagic fever:
    - epidemic
    - Korean
    - Russian
    - with renal syndrome
- 078.7 Arenaviral hemorrhagic fever
  - Hemorrhagic fever: Hemorrhagic fever:
    - Argentine   Junin virus
    - Bolivian   Machupo virus
- 078.8 Other specified diseases due to viruses and Chlamydiae
  - **EXCLUDES** *epidemic diarrhea (009.2)*
  lymphogranuloma venereum (099.1)
  - 078.81 Epidemic vertigo
  - 078.82 Epidemic vomiting syndrome
    - Winter vomiting disease
  - 078.88 Other specified diseases due to Chlamydiae
  - 078.89 Other specified diseases due to viruses
    - Epidemic cervical myalgia
    - Marburg disease
    - Tanapox

INFECTIOUS AND PARASITIC DISEASES

- **079 Viral and chlamydial infection in conditions classified elsewhere and of unspecified site**
  Note: This category is provided to be used as an additional code where it is desired to identify the viral agent in diseases classifiable elsewhere. This category will also be used to classify virus infection of unspecified nature or site.
  - 079.0 Adenovirus
  - 079.1 ECHO virus
  - 079.2 Coxsackievirus
  - 079.3 Rhinovirus
  - 079.4 Human papilloma virus
  - **079.5 Retrovirus**
    EXCLUDES human immunodeficiency virus, type 1 [HIV-1] (042-044)
    human T-cell lymphotrophic virus, type III [HTLV-III] (042-044)
    lymphadenopathy-associated virus [LAV] (042-044)
    - ◆ 079.50 Retrovirus, unspecified
    - 079.51 Human T-cell lymphotrophic virus, type I [HTLV-I]
    - 079.52 Human T-cell lymphotrophic virus, type II [HTLV-II]
    - 079.53 Human immunodeficiency virus, type 2 [HIV-2]
    - 079.59 Other specified retrovirus
  - **079.8 Other specified viral and chlamydial infection**
    - 079.88 Other specified chlamydial infection
    - 079.89 Other specified viral infection
  - **079.9 Unspecified viral and chlamydial infections**
    EXCLUDES viremia NOS (790.8)
    - ◆ 079.98 Unspecified chlamydial infection
      Chlamydial infections NOS
    - ◆ 079.99 Unspecified viral infection
      Viral infections NOS

RICKETTSIOSES AND OTHER ARTHROPOD-BORNE DISEASES (080-088)

EXCLUDES arthropod-borne viral diseases (060.0-066.9)

- 080 Louse-borne [epidemic] typhus
  Typhus (fever):   Typhus (fever):
    classical   exanthematic NOS
    epidemic   louse-borne
- **081 Other typhus**
  - 081.0 Murine [endemic] typhus
    Typhus (fever):   Typhus (fever):
      endemic   flea-borne
  - 081.1 Brill's disease
    Brill-Zinsser disease
    Recrudescent typhus (fever)
  - 081.2 Scrub typhus
    Japanese river fever   Mite-borne typhus
    Kedani fever   Tsutsugamushi
  - ◆ 081.9 Typhus, unspecified
    Typhus (fever) NOS
- **082 Tick-borne rickettsioses**
  - 082.0 Spotted fevers
    Rocky mountain spotted fever
    Sao Paulo fever
  - 082.1 Boutonneuse fever
    African tick typhus   Marseilles fever
    India tick typhus   Mediterranean tick fever
    Kenya tick typhus
  - 082.2 North Asian tick fever
    Siberian tick typhus
  - 082.3 Queensland tick typhus
  - ◆ 082.8 Other specified tick-borne rickettsioses
    Lone star fever
  - ◆ 082.9 Tick-borne rickettsiosis, unspecified
    Tick-borne typhus NOS
- **083 Other rickettsioses**
  - 083.0 Q fever
  - 083.1 Trench fever
    Quintan fever   Wolhynian fever
  - 083.2 Rickettsialpox
    Vesicular rickettsiosis
  - ◆ 083.8 Other specified rickettsioses
  - ◆ 083.9 Rickettsiosis, unspecified

- **084 Malaria**
  Note: Subcategories 084.0-084.6 exclude the listed conditions with mention of pernicious complications (084.8-084.9).
  EXCLUDES congenital malaria (771.2)
  - 084.0 Falciparum malaria [malignant tertian]
    Malaria (fever):
      by Plasmodium falciparum
      subtertian
  - 084.1 Vivax malaria [benign tertian]
    Malaria (fever) by Plasmodium vivax
  - 084.2 Quartan malaria
    Malaria (fever) by Plasmodium malariae
    Malariae malaria
  - 084.3 Ovale malaria
    Malaria (fever) by Plasmodium ovale
  - ◆ 084.4 Other malaria
    Monkey malaria
  - 084.5 Mixed malaria
    Malaria (fever) by more than one parasite
  - ◆ 084.6 Malaria, unspecified
    Malaria (fever) NOS
  - 084.7 Induced malaria
    Therapeutically induced malaria
    EXCLUDES accidental infection from syringe, blood transfusion, etc. (084.0-084.6, above, according to parasite species)
    transmission from mother to child during delivery (771.2)
  - 084.8 Blackwater fever
    Hemoglobinuric: Malarial hemoglobinuria
      fever (bilious)
      malaria
  - ◆ 084.9 Other pernicious complications of malaria
    Algid malaria
    Cerebral malaria
    Use additional code, if desired, to identify complication, as:
    malarial:
      hepatitis (573.2)
      nephrosis (581.81)
- **085 Leishmaniasis**
  - 085.0 Visceral [kala-azar]
    Dumdum fever   Leishmaniasis:
    Infection by Leishmania: dermal, post-kala-azar
      donovani   Mediterranean
      infantum   visceral (Indian)
  - 085.1 Cutaneous, urban
    Aleppo boil
    Baghdad boil
    Delhi boil
    Infection by Leishmania tropica (minor)
    Leishmaniasis, cutaneous:
      dry form
      late
      recurrent
      ulcerating
    Oriental sore
  - 085.2 Cutaneous, Asian desert
    Infection by Leishmania   Leishmaniasis, cutaneous:
      tropica major   rural
    Leishmaniasis, cutaneous: wet form
      acute necrotizing   zoonotic form
  - 085.3 Cutaneous, Ethiopian
    Infection by Leishmania ethiopica
    Leishmaniasis, cutaneous:
      diffuse
      lepromatous
  - 085.4 Cutaneous, American
    Chiclero ulcer
    Infection by Leishmania mexicana
    Leishmaniasis tegumentaria diffusa
  - 085.5 Mucocutaneous (American)
    Espundia
    Infection by Leishmania braziliensis
    Uta
  - ◆ 085.9 Leishmaniasis, unspecified

● Additional digits required   ◆ Nonspecific code   ■ Not a primary diagnosis

- **086 Trypanosomiasis**
  Use additional code, if desired, to identify manifestations, as:
  trypanosomiasis:
  encephalitis (323.2)
  meningitis (321.3)
  - **086.0 Chagas' disease with heart involvement**
    American trypanosomiasis } with heart
    Infection by Trypanosoma cruzi } involve-
    Any condition classifiable to 086.2 } ment
  - **086.1 Chagas' disease with other organ involvement**
    American trypanoso-
    miasis
    Infection by
    Trypanosoma
    Brace:cruzi } with involvement of organ other than heart
    Any condition classi-
    fiable to 086.2
  - **086.2 Chagas' disease without mention of organ involvement**
    American trypanosomiasis
    Infection by Trypanosoma cruzi
  - **086.3 Gambian trypanosomiasis**
    Gambian sleeping sickness
    Infection by Trypanosoma gambiense
  - **086.4 Rhodesian trypanosomiasis**
    Infection by Trypanosoma rhodesiense
    Rhodesian sleeping sickness
  - ◆ **086.5 African trypanosomiasis, unspecified**
    Sleeping sickness NOS
  - ◆ **086.9 Trypanosomiasis, unspecified**
- **087 Relapsing fever**
  INCLUDES recurrent fever
  - **087.0 Louse-borne**
  - **087.1 Tick-borne**
  - ◆ **087.9 Relapsing fever, unspecified**
- **088 Other arthropod-borne diseases**
  - **088.0 Bartonellosis**
    Carrión's disease   Verruga peruana
    Oroya fever
  - ◆ **088.8 Other specified arthropod-borne diseases**
    - **088.81 Lyme disease**
      Erythema chronicum migrans
    - **088.82 Babesiosis**
      Babesiasis
    - ◆ **088.89 Other**
  - ◆ **088.9 Arthropod-borne disease, unspecified**

SYPHILIS AND OTHER VENEREAL DISEASES (090-099)

EXCLUDES nonvenereal endemic syphilis (104.0)
urogenital trichomoniasis (131.0)

- **090 Congenital syphilis**
  - **090.0 Early congenital syphilis, symptomatic**
    Congenital syphilitic: Syphilitic (congenital):
    choroiditis   epiphysitis
    coryza (chronic)   osteochondritis
    hepatomegaly   pemphigus
    mucous patches
    periostitis
    splenomegaly
    Any congenital syphilitic condition specified as early or
    manifest less than two years after birth
  - **090.1 Early congenital syphilis, latent**
    Congenital syphilis without clinical manifestations, with
    positive serological reaction and negative spinal fluid
    test, less than two years after birth
  - ◆ **090.2 Early congenital syphilis, unspecified**
    Congenital syphilis NOS, less than two years after birth
  - **090.3 Syphilitic interstitial keratitis**
    Syphilitic keratitis:
    parenchymatous
    punctata profunda
    EXCLUDES interstitial keratitis NOS (370.50)
  - ● **090.4 Juvenile neurosyphilis**
    Use additional code, if desired, to identify any associated
    mental disorder
  - ◆ **090.40 Juvenile neurosyphilis, unspecified**
    Congenital neurosyphilis   Juvenile:
    Dementia paralytica   general paresis
    juvenilis   tabes
                                taboparesis
  - **090.41 Congenital syphilitic encephalitis**
  - **090.42 Congenital syphilitic meningitis**
  - ◆ **090.49 Other**
  - ◆ **090.5 Other late congenital syphilis, symptomatic**
    Gumma due to congenital syphilis
    Hutchinson's teeth
    Syphilitic saddle nose
    Any congenital syphilitic condition specified as late or
    manifest two years or more after birth
  - **090.6 Late congenital syphilis, latent**
    Congenital syphilis without clinical manifestations, with
    positive serological reaction and negative spinal fluid
    test, two years or more after birth
  - ◆ **090.7 Late congenital syphilis, unspecified**
    Congenital syphilis NOS, two years or more after birth
  - ◆ **090.9 Congenital syphilis, unspecified**
- **091 Early syphilis, symptomatic**
  EXCLUDES early cardiovascular syphilis (093.0-093.9)
  early neurosyphilis (094.0-094.9)
  - **091.0 Genital syphilis (primary)**
    Genital chancre
  - **091.1 Primary anal syphilis**
  - ◆ **091.2 Other primary syphilis**
    Primary syphilis of: Primary syphilis of:
    breast   lip
    fingers   tonsils
  - **091.3 Secondary syphilis of skin or mucous membranes**
    Condyloma latum   Secondary syphilis of:
    Secondary syphilis of: pharynx
    anus   skin
    tonsils   tonsils
    mouth   vulva
    vulva
  - **091.4 Adenopathy due to secondary syphilis**
    Syphilitic adenopathy (secondary)
    Syphilitic lymphadenitis (secondary)
  - ● **091.5 Uveitis due to secondary syphilis**
    - ◆ **091.50 Syphilitic uveitis, unspecified**
    - **091.51 Syphilitic chorioretinitis (secondary)**
    - **091.52 Syphilitic iridocyclitis (secondary)**
  - ● **091.6 Secondary syphilis of viscera and bone**
    - **091.61 Secondary syphilitic periostitis**
    - **091.62 Secondary syphilitic hepatitis**
      Secondary syphilis of liver
    - ◆ **091.69 Other viscera**
  - **091.7 Secondary syphilis, relapse**
    Secondary syphilis, relapse (treated) (untreated)
  - ● **091.8 Other forms of secondary syphilis**
    - **091.81 Acute syphilitic meningitis (secondary)**
    - **091.82 Syphilitic alopecia**
    - ◆ **091.89 Other**
  - ◆ **091.9 Unspecified secondary syphilis**
- **092 Early syphilis, latent**
  INCLUDES syphilis (acquired) without clinical
  manifestations, with positive
  serological reaction and negative
  spinal fluid test, less than two years
  after infection
  - **092.0 Early syphilis, latent, serological relapse after treatment**
  - ◆ **092.9 Early syphilis, latent, unspecified**
- **093 Cardiovascular syphilis**
  - **093.0 Aneurysm of aorta, specified as syphilitic**
    Dilatation of aorta, specified as syphilitic
  - **093.1 Syphilitic aortitis**
  - ● **093.2 Syphilitic endocarditis**
    - ◆ **093.20 Valve, unspecified**
      Syphilitic ostial coronary disease
    - **093.21 Mitral valve**
    - **093.22 Aortic valve**
      Syphilitic aortic incompetence or stenosis
    - **093.23 Tricuspid valve**
    - **093.24 Pulmonary valve**

INFECTIOUS AND PARASITIC DISEASES

- **093.8 Other specified cardiovascular syphilis**
  - 093.81 Syphilitic pericarditis
  - 093.82 Syphilitic myocarditis
  - ◆ 093.89 Other
- ◆ 093.9 Cardiovascular syphilis, unspecified
- **094 Neurosyphilis**
  - Use additional code, if desired, to identify any associated mental disorder
  - 094.0 Tabes dorsalis
    - Locomotor ataxia (progressive)
    - Posterior spinal sclerosis (syphilitic)
    - Tabetic neurosyphilis
    - Use additional code, if desired, to identify manifestation, as: neurogenic arthropathy [Charcot's joint disease] (713.5)
  - 094.1 General paresis
    - Dementia paralytica
    - General paralysis (of the insane) (progressive)
    - Paretic neurosyphilis
    - Taboparesis
  - 094.2 Syphilitic meningitis
    - Meningovascular syphilis
    - EXCLUDES acute syphilitic meningitis (secondary) (091.81)
  - 094.3 Asymptomatic neurosyphilis
  - **094.8 Other specified neurosyphilis**
    - 094.81 Syphilitic encephalitis
    - 094.82 Syphilitic Parkinsonism
    - 094.83 Syphilitic disseminated retinochoroiditis
    - 094.84 Syphilitic optic atrophy
    - 094.85 Syphilitic retrobulbar neuritis
    - 094.86 Syphilitic acoustic neuritis
    - 094.87 Syphilitic ruptured cerebral aneurysm
    - ◆ 094.89 Other
  - ◆ 094.9 Neurosyphilis, unspecified
    - Gumma (syphilitic) of central nervous system NOS
- **095 Other forms of late syphilis, with symptoms**
  - INCLUDES gumma (syphilitic)
    - syphilis, late, tertiary, or unspecified stage
  - 095.0 Syphilitic episcleritis
  - 095.1 Syphilis of lung
  - 095.2 Syphilitic peritonitis
  - 095.3 Syphilis of liver
  - 095.4 Syphilis of kidney
  - 095.5 Syphilis of bone
  - 095.6 Syphilis of muscle
    - Syphilitic myositis
  - 095.7 Syphilis of synovium, tendon, and bursa
    - Syphilitic: bursitis
    - Syphilitic: synovitis
  - ◆ 095.8 Other specified forms of late symptomatic syphilis
    - EXCLUDES cardiovascular syphilis (093.0-093.9)
    - neurosyphilis (094.0-094.9)
  - ◆ 095.9 Late symptomatic syphilis, unspecified
- 096 Late syphilis, latent
  - Syphilis (acquired) without clinical manifestations, with positive serological reaction and negative spinal fluid test, two years or more after infection
- **097 Other and unspecified syphilis**
  - ◆ 097.0 Late syphilis, unspecified
  - ◆ 097.1 Latent syphilis, unspecified
    - Positive serological reaction for syphilis
  - ◆ 097.9 Syphilis, unspecified
    - Syphilis (acquired) NOS
    - EXCLUDES syphilis NOS causing death under two years of age (090.9)
- **098 Gonococcal infections**
  - 098.0 Acute, of lower genitourinary tract
    - Gonococcal: Bartholinitis (acute)
    - urethritis (acute)
    - vulvovaginitis (acute)
    - Gonorrhea (acute): NOS
    - genitourinary (tract) NOS
  - **098.1 Acute, of upper genitourinary tract**
    - ◆ 098.10 Gonococcal infection (acute) of upper genitourinary tract, site unspecified
    - 098.11 Gonococcal cystitis (acute)
      - Gonorrhea (acute) of bladder
    - 098.12 Gonococcal prostatitis (acute)
    - 098.13 Gonococcal epididymo-orchitis (acute)
      - Gonococcal orchitis (acute)
    - 098.14 Gonococcal seminal vesiculitis (acute)
      - Gonorrhea (acute) of seminal vesicle
    - 098.15 Gonococcal cervicitis (acute)
      - Gonorrhea (acute) of cervix
    - 098.16 Gonococcal endometritis (acute)
      - Gonorrhea (acute) of uterus
    - 098.17 Gonococcal salpingitis, specified as acute
    - ◆ 098.19 Other
  - 098.2 Chronic, of lower genitourinary tract
    - Gonococcal: Bartholinitis, urethritis, vulvovaginitis
    - Gonorrhea: NOS, genitourinary (tract)
    - specified as chronic or with duration of two months or more
  - **098.3 Chronic, of upper genitourinary tract**
    - INCLUDES any condition classifiable to 098.1 stated as chronic or with a duration of two months or more
    - ◆ 098.30 Chronic gonococcal infection of upper genitourinary tract, site unspecified
    - 098.31 Gonococcal cystitis, chronic
      - Any condition classifiable to 098.11, specified as chronic
      - Gonorrhea of bladder, chronic
    - 098.32 Gonococcal prostatitis, chronic
      - Any condition classifiable to 098.12, specified as chronic
    - 098.33 Gonococcal epididymo-orchitis, chronic
      - Any condition classifiable to 098.13, specified as chronic
      - Chronic gonococcal orchitis
    - 098.34 Gonococcal seminal vesiculitis, chronic
      - Any condition classifiable to 098.14, specified as chronic
      - Gonorrhea of seminal vesicle, chronic
    - 098.35 Gonococcal cervicitis, chronic
      - Any condition classifiable to 098.15, specified as chronic
      - Gonorrhea of cervix, chronic
    - 098.36 Gonococcal endometritis, chronic
      - Any condition classifiable to 098.16, specified as chronic
    - 098.37 Gonococcal salpingitis (chronic)
    - ◆ 098.39 Other
  - **098.4 Gonococcal infection of eye**
    - 098.40 Gonococcal conjunctivitis (neonatorum)
      - Gonococcal ophthalmia (neonatorum)
    - 098.41 Gonococcal iridocyclitis
    - 098.42 Gonococcal endophthalmia
    - 098.43 Gonococcal keratitis
    - ◆ 098.49 Other
  - **098.5 Gonococcal infection of joint**
    - 098.50 Gonococcal arthritis
      - Gonococcal infection of joint NOS
    - 098.51 Gonococcal synovitis and tenosynovitis
    - 098.52 Gonococcal bursitis
    - 098.53 Gonococcal spondylitis
    - ◆ 098.59 Other
      - Gonococcal rheumatism
  - 098.6 Gonococcal infection of pharynx
  - 098.7 Gonococcal infection of anus and rectum
    - Gonococcal proctitis
  - **098.8 Gonococcal infection of other specified sites**
    - 098.81 Gonococcal keratosis (blennorrhagica)
    - 098.82 Gonococcal meningitis
    - 098.83 Gonococcal pericarditis
    - 098.84 Gonococcal endocarditis
    - ◆ 098.85 Other gonococcal heart disease

● Additional digits required ◆ Nonspecific code ■ Not a primary diagnosis

098.86 Gonococcal peritonitis
◆ 098.89 Other
Gonococcemia
● 099 Other venereal diseases
  099.0 Chancroid
    Bubo (inguinal):
      chancroidal
      due to Hemophilus
      ducreyi
    Chancre:
      Ducrey's
    Chancre:
      simple
      soft
    Ulcus molle (cutis) (skin)
  099.1 Lymphogranuloma venereum
    Climatic or tropical bubo
    (Durand-) Nicolas-Favre disease
    Esthiomene
    Lymphogranuloma inguinale
  099.2 Granuloma inguinale
    Donovanosis
    Granuloma pudendi (ulcerating)
    Granuloma venereum
    Pudendal ulcer
  099.3 Reiter's disease
    Reiter's syndrome
  ● 099.4 Other nongonococcal urethritis [NGU]
    ◆ 099.40 Unspecified
      Nonspecific urethritis
    099.41 Chlamydia trachomatis
    ◆ 099.49 Other specified organism
  ● 099.5 Other venereal diseases due to Chlamydia trachomatis
    EXCLUDES *Chlamydia trachomatis infection of conjunctiva (076.0-076.9, 077.0, 077.9)*
    Lymphogranuloma venereum (099.1)
    ◆ 099.50 Unspecified site
    099.51 Pharynx
    099.52 Anus and rectum
    099.53 Lower genitourinary sites
      EXCLUDES *urethra (099.41)*
      Use additional code, if desired, to specify site of infection, such as: cervix (616.0) vagina and vulva (616.11) bladder (595.4)
    ◆ 099.54 Other genitourinary sites
      Use additional code, if desired to specify site of infection, such as: testis and epididymis (604.91) pelvic inflammatory disease NOS (614.9)
    ◆ 099.55 Unspecified genitourinary site
    099.56 Peritoneum
      Perihepatitis
    ◆ 099.59 Other specified site
  ◆ 099.8 Other specified venereal diseases
  ◆ 099.9 Venereal disease, unspecified

OTHER SPIROCHETAL DISEASES (100-104)

● 100 Leptospirosis
  100.0 Leptospirosis icterohemorrhagica
    Leptospiral or spirochetal jaundice (hemorrhagic)
    Weil's disease
  ● 100.8 Other specified leptospiral infections
    100.81 Leptospiral meningitis (aseptic)
    ◆ 100.89 Other
      Fever:
        Fort Bragg
        pretibial
        swamp
      Infection by Leptospira:
        australis
        bataviae
        pyrogenes
  ◆ 100.9 Leptospirosis, unspecified
  101 Vincent's angina
    Acute necrotizing ulcerative:
      gingivitis
      stomatitis
    Fusospirochetal pharyngitis
    Spirochetal stomatitis
    Trench mouth
    Vincent's:
      gingivitis
      infection [any site]
● 102 Yaws
  INCLUDES frambesia
  pian

102.0 Initial lesions
  Chancre of yaws
  Frambesia, initial or primary
  Initial frambesial ulcer
  Mother yaw
102.1 Multiple papillomata and wet crab yaws
  Butter yaws
  Frambesioma
  Pianoma
  Plantar or palmar papilloma of yaws
◆ 102.2 Other early skin lesions
  Early yaws (cutaneous) (macular) (papular) (maculopapular) (micropapular)
  Frambeside of early yaws
  Cutaneous yaws, less than five years after infection
102.3 Hyperkeratosis
  Ghoul hand
  Hyperkeratosis, palmar or plantar (early) (late) due to yaws
  Worm-eaten soles
102.4 Gummata and ulcers
  Nodular late yaws (ulcerated)
  Gummatous frambeside
102.5 Gangosa
  Rhinopharyngitis mutilans
102.6 Bone and joint lesions
  Goundou
  Gumma, bone
  Gummatous osteitis or periostitis
  } of yaws (late)

  Hydrarthrosis
  Osteitis
  Periostitis (hypertrophic)
  } of yaws (early) (late)
◆ 102.7 Other manifestations
  Juxta-articular nodules of yaws
  Mucosal yaws
102.8 Latent yaws
  Yaws without clinical manifestations, with positive serology
◆ 102.9 Yaws, unspecified
● 103 Pinta
  103.0 Primary lesions
    Chancre (primary)
    Papule (primary)
    Pintid
    } of pinta [carate]
  103.1 Intermediate lesions
    Erythematous plaques
    Hyperchromic lesions
    Hyperkeratosis
    } of pinta [carate]
  103.2 Late lesions
    Cardiovascular lesions
    Skin lesions:
      achromic
      cicatricial
      dyschromic
    Vitiligo
    } of pinta [carate]
  103.3 Mixed lesions
    Achromic and hyperchromic skin lesions of pinta [carate]
  ◆ 103.9 Pinta, unspecified
● 104 Other spirochetal infection
  104.0 Nonvenereal endemic syphilis
    Bejel
    Njovera
  ◆ 104.8 Other specified spirochetal infections
    EXCLUDES *relapsing fever (087.0-087.9)*
    syphilis (090.0-097.9)
  ◆ 104.9 Spirochetal infection, unspecified

MYCOSES (110-118)

EXCLUDES *infection by Actinomycetales, such as species of Actinomyces, Actinomadura, Nocardia, Streptomyces (039.0-039.9)*

● 110 Dermatophytosis
  INCLUDES infection by species of Epidermophyton, Microsporum, and Trichophyton
  tinea, any type except those in 111

INFECTIOUS AND PARASITIC DISEASES

- **110.0** **Of scalp and beard**
  - Kerion
  - Sycosis, mycotic
  - Trichophytic tinea [black dot tinea], scalp
- **110.1** **Of nail**
  - Dermatophytic onychia
  - Onychomycosis
  - Tinea unguium
- **110.2** **Of hand**
  - Tinea manuum
- **110.3** **Of groin and perianal area**
  - Dhobie itch
  - Eczema marginatum
  - Tinea cruris
- **110.4** **Of foot**
  - Athlete's foot
  - Tinea pedis
- **110.5** **Of the body**
  - Herpes circinatus
  - Tinea imbricata [Tokelau]
- **110.6** **Deep seated dermatophytosis**
  - Granuloma trichophyticum
  - Majocchi's granuloma
- ◆ **110.8** **Of other specified sites**
- ◆ **110.9** **Of unspecified site**
  - Favus NOS
  - Microsporic tinea NOS
  - Ringworm NOS
- ● **111** **Dermatomycosis, other and unspecified**
  - **111.0** **Pityriasis versicolor**
    - Infection by Malassezia [Pityrosporum] furfur
    - Tinea flava
    - Tinea versicolor
  - **111.1** **Tinea nigra**
    - Infection by Cladosporium species
    - Keratomycosis nigricans
    - Microsporosis nigra
    - Pityriasis nigra
    - Tinea palmaris nigra
  - **111.2** **Tinea blanca**
    - Infection by Trichosporon (beigelii) cutaneum
    - White piedra
  - **111.3** **Black piedra**
    - Infection by Piedraia hortai
  - ◆ **111.8** **Other specified dermatomycoses**
  - ◆ **111.9** **Dermatomycosis, unspecified**
- ● **112** **Candidiasis**
  - **INCLUDES** infection by Candida species moniliasis
  - **EXCLUDES** neonatal monilial infection (771.7)
  - **112.0** **Of mouth**
    - Thrush (oral)
  - **112.1** **Of vulva and vagina**
    - Candidal vulvovaginitis
    - Monilial vulvovaginitis
  - **112.2** **Of other urogenital sites**
    - Candidal balanitis
  - **112.3** **Of skin and nails**
    - Candidal intertrigo
    - Candidal onychia
    - Candidal perionyxis [paronychia]
  - **112.4** **Of lung**
    - Candidal pneumonia
  - **112.5** **Disseminated**
    - Systemic candidiasis
  - ● **112.8** **Of other specified sites**
    - **112.81** Candidal endocarditis
    - **112.82** Candidal otitis externa
      - Otomycosis in moniliasis
    - **112.83** Candidal meningitis
    - **112.84** Candidal esophagitis
    - **112.85** Candidal enteritis
    - ◆ **112.89** Other
  - ◆ **112.9** **Of unspecified site**
- ● **114** **Coccidioidomycosis**
  - **INCLUDES** infection by Coccidioides (immitis)
  - Posada-Wernicke disease
  - **114.0** **Primary coccidioidomycosis (pulmonary)**
    - Acute pulmonary coccidioidomycosis
    - Coccidioidomycotic pneumonitis
    - Desert rheumatism
    - Pulmonary coccidioidomycosis
    - San Joaquin Valley fever
  - **114.1** **Primary extrapulmonary coccidioidomycosis**
    - Chancriform syndrome
    - Primary cutaneous coccidioidomycosis
  - **114.2** **Coccidioidal meningitis**
  - ◆ **114.3** **Other forms of progressive coccidioidomycosis**
    - Coccidioidal granuloma
    - Disseminated coccidioidomycosis
  - **114.4** **Chronic pulmonary coccidioidomycosis**
  - ◆ **114.5** **Pulmonary coccidioidomycosis, unspecified**
  - ◆ **114.9** **Coccidioidomycosis, unspecified**
- ● **115** **Histoplasmosis**
  - The following fifth-digit subclassification is for use with category 115:
    - 0 without mention of manifestation
    - 1 meningitis
    - 2 retinitis
    - 3 pericarditis
    - 4 endocarditis
    - 5 pneumonia
    - ◆ 9 other
  - ● **115.0** **Infection by Histoplasma capsulatum**
    - American histoplasmosis
    - Darling's disease
    - Reticuloendothelial cytomycosis
    - Small form histoplasmosis
  - ● **115.1** **Infection by Histoplasma duboisii**
    - African histoplasmosis
    - Large form histoplasmosis
  - ◆● **115.9** **Histoplasmosis, unspecified**
    - Histoplasmosis NOS
- ● **116** **Blastomycotic infection**
  - **116.0** **Blastomycosis**
    - Blastomycotic dermatitis
    - Chicago disease
    - Cutaneous blastomycosis
    - Disseminated blastomycosis
    - Gilchrist's disease
    - Infection by Blastomyces [Ajellomyces] dermatitidis
    - North American blastomycosis
    - Primary pulmonary blastomycosis
  - **116.1** **Paracoccidioidomycosis**
    - Brazilian blastomycosis
    - Infection by Paracoccidioides [Blastomyces] brasiliensis
    - Lutz-Splendore-Almeida disease
    - Mucocutaneous-lymphangitic paracoccidioidomycosis
    - Pulmonary paracoccidioidomycosis
    - South American blastomycosis
    - Visceral paracoccidioidomycosis
  - **116.2** **Lobomycosis**
    - Infections by Loboa [Blastomyces] loboi
    - Keloidal blastomycosis
    - Lobo's disease
- ● **117** **Other mycoses**
  - **117.0** **Rhinosporidiosis**
    - Infection by Rhinosporidium seeberi
  - **117.1** **Sporotrichosis**
    - Cutaneous sporotrichosis
    - Disseminated sporotrichosis
    - Infection by Sporothrix [Sporotrichum] schenckii
    - Lymphocutaneous sporotrichosis
    - Pulmonary sporotrichosis
    - Sporotrichosis of the bones
  - **117.2** **Chromoblastomycosis**
    - Chromomycosis
    - Infection by Cladosporidium carrionii, Fonsecaea compactum, Fonsecaea pedrosoi, Phialophora verrucosa
  - **117.3** **Aspergillosis**
    - Infection by Aspergillus species, mainly A. fumigatus, A. flavus group, A. terreus group
  - **117.4** **Mycotic mycetomas**
    - Infection by various genera and species of Ascomycetes and Deuteromycetes, such as Acremonium [Cephalosporium] falciforme, Neotestudina rosatii, Madurella grisea, Madurella mycetomii, Pyrenochaeta romeroi, Zopfia [Leptosphaeria] senegalensis
    - Madura foot, mycotic
    - Maduromycosis, mycotic
    - **EXCLUDES** actinomycotic mycetomas (039.0-039.9)
  - **117.5** **Cryptococcosis**
    - Busse-Buschke's disease
    - European cryptococcosis
    - Infection by Cryptococcus neoformans
    - Pulmonary cryptococcosis
    - Systemic cryptococcosis
    - Torula

● Additional digits required   ◆ Nonspecific code   ■ Not a primary diagnosis

117.6	**Allescheriosis [Petriellidosis]**	
	Infections by Allescheria [Petriellidium] boydii [Monosporium apiospermum]	
	EXCLUDES *mycotic mycetoma (117.4)*	
117.7	**Zygomycosis [Phycomycosis or Mucormycosis]**	
	Infection by species of Absidia, Basidiobolus, Conidiobolus, Cunninghamella, Entomophthora, Mucor, Rhizopus, Saksenaea	
117.8	**Infection by dematiacious fungi, [Phaehyphomycosis]**	
	Infection by dematiacious fungi, such as Cladosporium trichoides [bantianum], Dreschlera hawaiiensis, Phialophora gougerotii, Phialophora jeanselmi	
◆ 117.9	**Other and unspecified mycoses**	
118	**Opportunistic mycoses**	
	Infection of skin, subcutaneous tissues, and/or organs by a wide variety of fungi generally considered to be pathogenic to compromised hosts only (e.g., infection by species of Alternaria, Dreschlera, Fusarium)	

HELMINTHIASES (120-129)

● **120 Schistosomiasis [bilharziasis]**
  120.0 **Schistosoma haematobium**
    Vesical schistosomiasis NOS
  120.1 **Schistosoma mansoni**
    Intestinal schistosomiasis NOS
  120.2 **Schistosoma japonicum**
    Asiatic schistosomiasis NOS   Katayama disease or fever
  120.3 **Cutaneous**
    Cercarial dermatitis   Schistosome dermatitis
    Infection by cercariae   Swimmers' itch
      of Schistosoma
  ◆ 120.8 **Other specified schistosomiasis**
    Infection by Schistosoma: Infection by Schistosoma:
      bovis   spindale
      intercalatum   Schistosomiasis chestermani
      mattheii
  ◆ 120.9 **Schistosomiasis, unspecified**
    Blood flukes NOS   Hemic distomiasis

● **121 Other trematode infections**
  121.0 **Opisthorchiasis**
    Infection by:
      cat liver fluke
      Opisthorchis (felineus) (tenuicollis) (viverrini)
  121.1 **Clonorchiasis**
    Biliary cirrhosis due to clonorchiasis
    Chinese liver fluke disease
    Hepatic distomiasis due to Clonorchis sinensis
    Oriental liver fluke disease
  121.2 **Paragonimiasis**
    Infection by Paragonimus
    Lung fluke disease (oriental)
    Pulmonary distomiasis
  121.3 **Fascioliasis**
    Infection by Fasciola: Liver flukes NOS
      gigantica   Sheep liver fluke infection
      hepatica
  121.4 **Fasciolopsiasis**
    Infection by Fasciolopsis (buski)
    Intestinal distomiasis
  121.5 **Metagonimiasis**
    Infection by Metagonimus yokogawai
  121.6 **Heterophyiasis**
    Infection by:
      Heterophyes heterophyes
      Stellantchasmus falcatus
  ◆ 121.8 **Other specified trematode infections**
    Infection by:
      Dicrocoelium dendriticum
      Echinostoma ilocanum
      Gastrodiscoides hominis
  ◆ 121.9 **Trematode infection, unspecified**
    Distomiasis NOS   Fluke disease NOS

● **122 Echinococcosis**
  INCLUDES echinococciasis
              hydatid disease
              hydatidosis
  122.0 **Echinococcus granulosus infection of liver**
  122.1 **Echinococcus granulosus infection of lung**
  122.2 **Echinococcus granulosus infection of thyroid**
  ◆ 122.3 **Echinococcus granulosus infection, other**
  ◆ 122.4 **Echinococcus granulosus infection, unspecified**
  122.5 **Echinococcus multilocularis infection of liver**
  ◆ 122.6 **Echinococcus multilocularis infection, other**
  ◆ 122.7 **Echinococcus multilocularis infection, unspecified**
  ◆ 122.8 **Echinococcosis, unspecified, of liver**
  ◆ 122.9 **Echinococcosis, other and unspecified**

● **123 Other cestode infection**
  123.0 **Taenia solium infection, intestinal form**
    Pork tapeworm (adult) (infection)
  123.1 **Cysticercosis**
    Cysticerciasis
    Infection by Cysticercus cellulosae [larval form of Taenia solium]
  123.2 **Taenia saginata infection**
    Beef tapeworm (infection)
    Infection by Taeniarhynchus saginatus
  ◆ 123.3 **Taeniasis, unspecified**
  123.4 **Diphyllobothriasis, intestinal**
    Diphyllobothrium (adult) (latum) (pacificum) infection
    Fish tapeworm (infection)
  123.5 **Sparganosis [larval diphyllobothriasis]**
    Infection by:
      Diphyllobothrium larvae
      Sparganum (mansoni) (proliferum)
      Spirometra larvae
  123.6 **Hymenolepiasis**
    Dwarf tapeworm (infection)
    Hymenolepis (diminuta) (nana) infection
    Rat tapeworm (infection)
  ◆ 123.8 **Other specified cestode infection**
    Diplogonoporus (grandis) ⎫
    Dipylidium (caninum)   ⎬ infection
    Dog tapeworm (infection) ⎭
  ◆ 123.9 **Cestode infection, unspecified**
    Tapeworm (infection) NOS

  124 **Trichinosis**
    Trichinella spiralis
    Trichinellosis infection
    Trichiniasis

● **125 Filarial infection and dracontiasis**
  125.0 **Bancroftian filariasis**
    Chyluria   ⎫
    Elephantiasis   ⎪
    Infection   ⎬ due to Wuchereria bancrofti
    Lymphadenitis   ⎪
    Lymphangitis   ⎪
    Wuchereriasis   ⎭

  125.1 **Malayan filariasis**
    Brugia filariasis ⎫
    Chyluria   ⎪
    Elephantiasis   ⎬ due to Brugia [Wuchereria] malayi
    Infection   ⎪
    Lymphadenitis   ⎪
    Lymphangitis   ⎭

  125.2 **Loiasis**
    Eyeworm disease of Africa   Loa loa infection
  125.3 **Onchocerciasis**
    Onchocerca volvulus infection
    Onchocercosis
  125.4 **Dipetalonemiasis**
    Infection by:
      Acanthocheilonema perstans
      Dipetalonema perstans
  125.5 **Mansonella ozzardi infection**
    Filariasis ozzardi
  ◆ 125.6 **Other specified filariasis**
    Dirofilaria infection
    Infection by:
      Acanthocheilonema streptocerca
      Dipetalonema streptocerca
  125.7 **Dracontiasis**
    Guinea-worm infection
    Infection by Dracunculus medinensis
  ◆ 125.9 **Unspecified filariasis**

INFECTIOUS AND PARASITIC DISEASES

- ● **126 Ancylostomiasis and necatoriasis**
  - INCLUDES: cutaneous larva migrans due to Ancylostoma
    - hookworm (disease) (infection)
    - uncinariasis
  - 126.0 Ancylostoma duodenale
  - 126.1 Necator americanus
  - 126.2 Ancylostoma braziliense
  - 126.3 Ancylostoma ceylanicum
  - ◆ 126.8 Other specified Ancylostoma
  - ◆ 126.9 Ancylostomiasis and necatoriasis, unspecified
    - Creeping eruption NOS
    - Cutaneous larva migrans NOS
- ● **127 Other intestinal helminthiases**
  - 127.0 Ascariasis
    - Ascaridiasis
    - Infection by Ascaris lumbricoides
    - Roundworm infection
  - 127.1 Anisakiasis
    - Infection by Anisakis larva
  - 127.2 Strongyloidiasis
    - Infection by Strongyloides stercoralis
    - EXCLUDES: trichostrongyliasis (127.6)
  - 127.3 Trichuriasis
    - Infection by Trichuris trichiuria
    - Trichocephaliasis
    - Whipworm (disease) (infection)
  - 127.4 Enterobiasis
    - Infection by Enterobius vermicularis
    - Oxyuriasis
    - Oxyuris vermicularis infection
    - Pinworm (disease) (infection)
    - Threadworm infection
  - 127.5 Capillariasis
    - Infection by Capillaria philippinensis
    - EXCLUDES: infection by Capillaria hepatica (128.8)
  - 127.6 Trichostrongyliasis
    - Infection by Trichostrongylus species
  - ◆ 127.7 Other specified intestinal helminthiasis
    - Infection by:
      - Oesophagostomum apiostomum and related species
      - Ternidens diminutus
      - Other specified intestinal helminth
      - Physalopteriasis
  - 127.8 Mixed intestinal helminthiasis
    - Infection by intestinal helminths classified to more than one of the categories 120.0-127.7
    - Mixed helminthiasis NOS
  - ◆ 127.9 Intestinal helminthiasis, unspecified
- ● **128 Other and unspecified helminthiases**
  - 128.0 Toxocariasis
    - Larva migrans visceralis
    - Toxocara (canis) (cati) infection
    - Visceral larva migrans syndrome
  - 128.1 Gnathostomiasis
    - Infection by Gnathostoma spinigerum and related species
  - ◆ 128.8 Other specified helminthiasis
    - Infection by:
      - Angiostrongylus cantonensis
      - Capillaria hepatica
      - other specified helminth
  - ◆ 128.9 Helminth infection, unspecified
    - Helminthiasis NOS
    - Worms NOS
- ◆ **129 Intestinal parasitism, unspecified**

OTHER INFECTIOUS AND PARASITIC DISEASES (130–136)

- ● **130 Toxoplasmosis**
  - INCLUDES: infection by toxoplasma gondii
    - toxoplasmosis (acquired)
  - EXCLUDES: congenital toxoplasmosis (771.2)
  - 130.0 Meningoencephalitis due to toxoplasmosis
    - Encephalitis due to acquired toxoplasmosis
  - 130.1 Conjunctivitis due to toxoplasmosis
  - 130.2 Chorioretinitis due to toxoplasmosis
    - Focal retinochoroiditis due to acquired toxoplasmosis
  - 130.3 Myocarditis due to toxoplasmosis
  - 130.4 Pneumonitis due to toxoplasmosis
  - 130.5 Hepatitis due to toxoplasmosis
  - ◆ 130.7 Toxoplasmosis of other specified sites
  - 130.8 Multisystemic disseminated toxoplasmosis
    - Toxoplasmosis of multiple sites
  - ◆ 130.9 Toxoplasmosis, unspecified
- ● **131 Trichomoniasis**
  - INCLUDES: infection due to Trichomonas (vaginalis)
  - ● 131.0 Urogenital trichomoniasis
    - ◆ 131.00 Urogenital trichomoniasis, unspecified
      - Fluor (vaginalis) } trichomonal or due to Trichomonas (vaginalis)
      - Leukorrhea (vaginalis)
    - 131.01 Trichomonal vulvovaginitis
      - Vaginitis, trichomonal or due to Trichomonas (vaginalis)
    - 131.02 Trichomonal urethritis
    - 131.03 Trichomonal prostatitis
    - ◆ 131.09 Other
  - ◆ 131.8 Other specified sites
    - EXCLUDES: intestinal (007.3)
  - ◆ 131.9 Trichomoniasis, unspecified
- ● **132 Pediculosis and phthirus infestation**
  - 132.0 Pediculus capitis [head louse]
  - 132.1 Pediculus corporis [body louse]
  - 132.2 Phthirus pubis [pubic louse]
    - Pediculus pubis
  - 132.3 Mixed infestation
    - Infestation classifiable to more than one of the categories 132.0-132.2
  - ◆ 132.9 Pediculosis, unspecified
- ● **133 Acariasis**
  - 133.0 Scabies
    - Infestation by Sarcoptes scabiei
    - Norwegian scabies
    - Sarcoptic itch
  - ◆ 133.8 Other acariasis
    - Chiggers
    - Infestation by:
      - Demodex folliculorum
      - Trombicula
  - ◆ 133.9 Acariasis, unspecified
    - Infestation by mites NOS
- ● **134 Other infestation**
  - 134.0 Myiasis
    - Infestation by:
      - Dermatobia (hominis)
      - fly larvae
      - Gasterophilus (intestinalis)
      - maggots
      - Oestrus ovis
  - ◆ 134.1 Other arthropod infestation
    - Infestation by:
      - chigoe
      - sand flea
      - Tunga penetrans
      - Jigger disease
      - Scarabiasis
      - Tungiasis
  - 134.2 Hirudiniasis
    - Hirudiniasis (external) (internal)
    - Leeches (aquatic) (land)
  - ◆ 134.8 Other specified infestations
  - ◆ 134.9 Infestation, unspecified
    - Infestation (skin) NOS
    - Skin parasites NOS
- **135 Sarcoidosis**
  - Besnier-Boeck-Schaumann disease
  - Lupoid (miliary) of Boeck
  - Lupus pernio (Besnier)
  - Lymphogranulomatosis, benign (Schaumann's)
  - Sarcoid (any site):
    - NOS
    - Boeck
    - Darier-Roussy
  - Uveoparotid fever
- ● **136 Other and unspecified infectious and parasitic diseases**
  - 136.0 Ainhum
    - Dactylolysis spontanea
  - 136.1 Behçet's syndrome

● Additional digits required ◆ Nonspecific code ■ Not a primary diagnosis

- **136.2 Specific infections by free-living amebae**
  Meningoencephalitis due to Naegleria
- **136.3 Pneumocystosis**
  Pneumonia due to Pneumocystis carinii
- **136.4 Psorospermiasis**
- **136.5 Sarcosporidiosis**
  Infection by Sarcocystis lindemanni
- ◆ **136.8 Other specified infectious and parasitic diseases**
  Candiru infestation
- ◆ **136.9 Unspecified infectious and parasitic diseases**
  Infectious disease NOS
  Parasitic disease NOS

LATE EFFECTS OF INFECTIOUS AND PARASITIC DISEASES (137-139)

● **137 Late effects of tuberculosis**
  Note: This category is to be used to indicate conditions classifiable to 010-018 as the cause of late effects, which are themselves classified elsewhere. The "late effects" include those specified as such, as sequelae, or as due to old or inactive tuberculosis, without evidence of active disease.
- ◆ **137.0 Late effects of respiratory or unspecified tuberculosis**
- **137.1 Late effects of central nervous system tuberculosis**
- **137.2 Late effects of genitourinary tuberculosis**
- **137.3 Late effects of tuberculosis of bones and joints**
- ◆ **137.4 Late effects of tuberculosis of other specified organs**

138 Late effects of acute poliomyelitis
  Note: This category is to be used to indicate conditions classifiable to 045 as the cause of late effects, which are themselves classified elsewhere. The "late effects" include conditions specified as such, or as sequelae, or as due to old or inactive poliomyelitis, without evidence of active disease.

● **139 Late effects of other infectious and parasitic diseases**
  Note: This category is to be used to indicate conditions classifiable to categories 001-009, 020-041, 046-136 as the cause of late effects, which are themselves classified elsewhere. The "late effects" include conditions specified as such; they also include sequela of diseases classifiable to the above categories if there is evidence that the disease itself is no longer present.
- **139.0 Late effects of viral encephalitis**
  Late effects of conditions classifiable to 049.8-049.9, 062-064
- **139.1 Late effects of trachoma**
  Late effects of conditions classifiable to 076
- ◆ **139.8 Late effects of other and unspecified infectious and parasitic diseases**

2. NEOPLASMS (140-239)

Notes:
1. Content
   This chapter contains the following broad groups:
   - 140-195   Malignant neoplasms, stated or presumed to be primary, of specified sites, except of lymphatic and hematopoietic tissue
   - 196-198   Malignant neoplasms, stated or presumed to be secondary, of specified sites
   - 199   Malignant neoplasms, without specification of site
   - 200-208   Malignant neoplasms, stated or presumed to be primary, of lymphatic and hematopoietic tissue
   - 210-229   Benign neoplasms
   - 230-234   Carcinoma in situ
   - 235-238   Neoplasms of uncertain behavior [see Note, page 29]
   - 239   Neoplasms of unspecified nature
2. Functional activity
   All neoplasms are classified in this chapter, whether or not functionally active. An additional code from Chapter 3 may be used, if desired, to identify such functional activity associated with any neoplasm, e.g.:
   catecholamine-producing malignant pheochromocytoma of adrenal:
   code 194.0, additional code 255.6
   basophil adenoma of pituitary with Cushing's syndrome:
   code 227.3, additional code 255.0

3. Morphology [Histology]
   For those wishing to identify the histological type of neoplasms, a comprehensive coded nomenclature, which comprises the morphology rubrics of the ICD-Oncology, is given on pages 207-210.
4. Malignant neoplasms overlapping site boundaries
   Categories 140-195 are for the classification of primary malignant neoplasms according to their point of origin. A malignant neoplasm that overlaps two or more subcategories within a three-digit rubric and whose point of origin cannot be determined should be classified to the subcategory .8 "Other." For example, "carcinoma involving tip and ventral surface of tongue" should be assigned to 141.8. On the other hand, "carcinoma of tip of tongue, extending to involve the ventral surface" should be coded to 141.2, as the point of origin, the tip, is known. Three subcategories (149.8, 159.8, 165.8) have been provided for malignant neoplasms that overlap the boundaries of three-digit rubrics within certain systems. Overlapping malignant neoplasms that cannot be classified as indicated above should be assigned to the appropriate subdivision of category 195 (Malignant neoplasm of other and ill-defined sites).

MALIGNANT NEOPLASM OF LIP, ORAL CAVITY, AND PHARYNX (140-149)

EXCLUDES   carcinoma in situ (230.0)

● **140 Malignant neoplasm of lip**
  EXCLUDES   skin of lip (173.0)
- **140.0 Upper lip, vermilion border**
  Upper lip: Upper lip:
    NOS   lipstick area
    external
- **140.1 Lower lip, vermilion border**
  Lower lip: Lower lip:
    NOS   lipstick area
    external
- **140.3 Upper lip, inner aspect**
  Upper lip: Upper lip:
    buccal aspect   mucosa
    frenulum   oral aspect
- **140.4 Lower lip, inner aspect**
  Lower lip: Lower lip:
    buccal aspect   mucosa
    frenulum   oral aspect
- ◆ **140.5 Lip, unspecified, inner aspect**
  Lip, not specified whether upper or lower:
    buccal aspect
    frenulum
    mucosa
    oral aspect
- **140.6 Commissure of lip**
  Labial commissure
- ◆ **140.8 Other sites of lip**
  Malignant neoplasm of contiguous or overlapping sites of lip whose point of origin cannot be determined
- ◆ **140.9 Lip, unspecified, vermilion border**
  Lip, not specified as upper or lower:
    NOS
    external
    lipstick area

● **141 Malignant neoplasm of tongue**
- **141.0 Base of tongue**
  Dorsal surface of base of tongue
  Fixed part of tongue NOS
- **141.1 Dorsal surface of tongue**
  Anterior two-thirds of tongue, dorsal surface
  Dorsal tongue NOS
  Midline of tongue
  EXCLUDES   dorsal surface of base of tongue (141.0)
- **141.2 Tip and lateral border of tongue**
- **141.3 Ventral surface of tongue**
  Anterior two-thirds of tongue, ventral surface
  Frenulum linguae
- ◆ **141.4 Anterior two-thirds of tongue, part unspecified**
  Mobile part of tongue NOS
- **141.5 Junctional zone**
  Border of tongue at junction of fixed and mobile parts at insertion of anterior tonsillar pillar
- **141.6 Lingual tonsil**

- ◆ **141.8** Other sites of tongue
  Malignant neoplasm of contiguous or overlapping sites of tongue whose point of origin cannot be determined
- ◆ **141.9** Tongue, unspecified
  Tongue NOS
- ● **142** Malignant neoplasm of major salivary glands
  INCLUDES salivary ducts
  EXCLUDES malignant neoplasm of minor salivary glands:
  NOS (145.9)
  buccal mucosa (145.0)
  soft palate (145.3)
  tongue (141.0-141.9)
  tonsil, palatine (146.0)
  - **142.0** Parotid gland
  - **142.1** Submandibular gland
    Submaxillary gland
  - **142.2** Sublingual gland
  - ◆ **142.8** Other major salivary glands
    Malignant neoplasm of contiguous or overlapping sites of salivary glands and ducts whose point of origin cannot be determined
  - ◆ **142.9** Salivary gland, unspecified
    Salivary gland (major) NOS
- ● **143** Malignant neoplasm of gum
  INCLUDES alveolar (ridge) mucosa
  gingiva (alveolar) (marginal)
  interdental papillae
  EXCLUDES malignant odontogenic neoplasms (170.0-170.1)
  - **143.0** Upper gum
  - **143.1** Lower gum
  - ◆ **143.8** Other sites of gum
    Malignant neoplasm of contiguous or overlapping sites of gum whose point of origin cannot be determined
  - ◆ **143.9** Gum, unspecified
- ● **144** Malignant neoplasm of floor of mouth
  - **144.0** Anterior portion
    Anterior to the premolar-canine junction
  - **144.1** Lateral portion
  - ◆ **144.8** Other sites of floor of mouth
    Malignant neoplasm of contiguous or overlapping sites of floor of mouth whose point of origin cannot be determined
  - ◆ **144.9** Floor of mouth, part unspecified
- ● **145** Malignant neoplasm of other and unspecified parts of mouth
  EXCLUDES mucosa of lips (140.0-140.9)
  - **145.0** Cheek mucosa
    Buccal mucosa   Cheek, inner aspect
  - **145.1** Vestibule of mouth
    Buccal sulcus (upper) (lower)
    Labial sulcus (upper) (lower)
  - **145.2** Hard palate
  - **145.3** Soft palate
    EXCLUDES nasopharyngeal [posterior] [superior] surface of soft palate (147.3)
  - **145.4** Uvula
  - ◆ **145.5** Palate, unspecified
    Junction of hard and soft palate
    Roof of mouth
  - **145.6** Retromolar area
  - ◆ **145.8** Other specified parts of mouth
    Malignant neoplasm of contiguous or overlapping sites of mouth whose point of origin cannot be determined
  - ◆ **145.9** Mouth, unspecified
    Buccal cavity NOS
    Minor salivary gland, unspecified site
    Oral cavity NOS
- ● **146** Malignant neoplasm of oropharynx
  - **146.0** Tonsil
    Tonsil: Tonsil:
    NOS   palatine
    faucial
    EXCLUDES lingual tonsil (141.6)
    pharyngeal tonsil (147.1)
  - **146.1** Tonsillar fossa
  - **146.2** Tonsillar pillars (anterior) (posterior)
    Faucial pillar   Palatoglossal arch
    Glossopalatine fold Palatopharyngeal arch
  - **146.3** Vallecula
    Anterior and medial surface of the pharyngoepiglottic fold
  - **146.4** Anterior aspect of epiglottis
    Epiglottis, free border [margin]
    Glossoepiglottic fold(s)
    EXCLUDES epiglottis:
    NOS (161.1)
    suprahyoid portion (161.1)
  - **146.5** Junctional region
    Junction of the free margin of the epiglottis, the aryepiglottic fold, and the pharyngoepiglottic fold
  - **146.6** Lateral wall of oropharynx
  - **146.7** Posterior wall of oropharynx
  - ◆ **146.8** Other specified sites of oropharynx
    Branchial cleft
    Malignant neoplasm of contiguous or overlapping sites of oropharynx whose point of origin cannot be determined
  - ◆ **146.9** Oropharynx, unspecified
- ● **147** Malignant neoplasm of nasopharynx
  - **147.0** Superior wall
    Roof of nasopharynx
  - **147.1** Posterior wall
    Adenoid   Pharyngeal tonsil
  - **147.2** Lateral wall
    Fossa of Rosenmüller   Pharyngeal recess
    Opening of auditory tube
  - **147.3** Anterior wall
    Floor of nasopharynx
    Nasopharyngeal [posterior] [superior] surface of soft palate
    Posterior margin of nasal septum and choanae
  - ◆ **147.8** Other specified sites of nasopharynx
    Malignant neoplasm of contiguous or overlapping sites of nasopharynx whose point of origin cannot be determined
  - ◆ **147.9** Nasopharynx, unspecified
    Nasopharyngeal wall NOS
- ● **148** Malignant neoplasm of hypopharynx
  - **148.0** Postcricoid region
  - **148.1** Pyriform sinus
    Pyriform fossa
  - **148.2** Aryepiglottic fold, hypopharyngeal aspect
    Aryepiglottic fold or interarytenoid fold:
    NOS
    marginal zone
    EXCLUDES aryepiglottic fold or interarytenoid fold, laryngeal aspect (161.1)
  - **148.3** Posterior hypopharyngeal wall
  - ◆ **148.8** Other specified sites of hypopharynx
    Malignant neoplasm of contiguous or overlapping sites of hypopharynx whose point of origin cannot be determined
  - ◆ **148.9** Hypopharynx, unspecified
    Hypopharyngeal wall NOS   Hypopharynx NOS
- ● **149** Malignant neoplasm of other and ill-defined sites within the lip, oral cavity, and pharynx
  - ◆ **149.0** Pharynx, unspecified
  - **149.1** Waldeyer's ring
  - ◆ **149.8** Other
    Malignant neoplasms of lip, oral cavity, and pharynx whose point of origin cannot be assigned to any one of the categories 140-148
    EXCLUDES "book leaf" neoplasm [ventral surface of tongue and floor of mouth] (145.8)
  - ◆ **149.9** Ill-defined

MALIGNANT NEOPLASM OF DIGESTIVE ORGANS AND PERITONEUM (150-159)

EXCLUDES carcinoma in situ (230.1-230.9)

- ● **150** Malignant neoplasm of esophagus
  - **150.0** Cervical esophagus
  - **150.1** Thoracic esophagus
  - **150.2** Abdominal esophagus
    EXCLUDES adenocarcinoma (151.0)
    cardio-esophageal junction (151.0)
  - **150.3** Upper third of esophagus
    Proximal third of esophagus
  - **150.4** Middle third of esophagus

TABULAR LIST

- **150.5 Lower third of esophagus**
  Distal third of esophagus
  EXCLUDES adenocarcinoma (151.0)
  cardio-esophageal junction (151.0)
- ◆ **150.8 Other specified part**
  Malignant neoplasm of contiguous or overlapping sites of esophagus whose point of origin cannot be determined
- ◆ **150.9 Esophagus, unspecified**

● **151 Malignant neoplasm of stomach**
- **151.0 Cardia**
  Cardiac orifice   Cardio-esophageal junction
  EXCLUDES squamous cell carcinoma (150.2, 150.5)
- **151.1 Pylorus**
  Prepylorus   Pyloric canal
- **151.2 Pyloric antrum**
  Antrum of stomach NOS
- **151.3 Fundus of stomach**
- **151.4 Body of stomach**
- ◆ **151.5 Lesser curvature, unspecified**
  Lesser curvature, not classifiable to 151.1-151.4
- ◆ **151.6 Greater curvature, unspecified**
  Greater curvature, not classifiable to 151.0-151.4
- ◆ **151.8 Other specified sites of stomach**
  Anterior wall, not classifiable to 151.0-151.4
  Posterior wall, not classifiable to 151.0-151.4
  Malignant neoplasm of contiguous or overlapping sites of stomach whose point of origin cannot be determined
- ◆ **151.9 Stomach, unspecified**
  Carcinoma ventriculi   Gastric cancer

● **152 Malignant neoplasm of small intestine, including duodenum**
- **152.0 Duodenum**
- **152.1 Jejunum**
- **152.2 Ileum**
  EXCLUDES ileocecal valve (153.4)
- **152.3 Meckel's diverticulum**
- ◆ **152.8 Other specified sites of small intestine**
  Duodenojejunal junction
  Malignant neoplasm of contiguous or overlapping sites of small intestine whose point of origin cannot be determined
- ◆ **152.9 Small intestine, unspecified**

● **153 Malignant neoplasm of colon**
- **153.0 Hepatic flexure**
- **153.1 Transverse colon**
- **153.2 Descending colon**
  Left colon
- **153.3 Sigmoid colon**
  Sigmoid (flexure)
  EXCLUDES rectosigmoid junction (154.0)
- **153.4 Cecum**
  Ileocecal valve
- **153.5 Appendix**
- **153.6 Ascending colon**
  Right colon
- **153.7 Splenic flexure**
- ◆ **153.8 Other specified sites of large intestine**
  Malignant neoplasm of contiguous or overlapping sites of colon whose point of origin cannot be determined
  EXCLUDES ileocecal valve (153.4)
  rectosigmoid junction (154.0)
- ◆ **153.9 Colon, unspecified**
  Large intestine NOS

● **154 Malignant neoplasm of rectum, rectosigmoid junction, and anus**
- **154.0 Rectosigmoid junction**
  Colon with rectum   Rectosigmoid (colon)
- **154.1 Rectum**
  Rectal ampulla
- **154.2 Anal canal**
  Anal sphincter
  EXCLUDES skin of anus (172.5, 173.5)
- ◆ **154.3 Anus, unspecified**
  EXCLUDES anus:
  margin (172.5, 173.5)
  skin (172.5, 173.5)
  perianal skin (172.5, 173.5)
- ◆ **154.8 Other**
  Anorectum
  Cloacogenic zone
  Malignant neoplasm of contiguous or overlapping sites of rectum, rectosigmoid junction, and anus whose point of origin cannot be determined

● **155 Malignant neoplasm of liver and intrahepatic bile ducts**
- **155.0 Liver, primary**
  Carcinoma:
  liver, specified as primary
  hepatocellular
  liver cell
  Hepatoblastoma
- **155.1 Intrahepatic bile ducts**
  Canaliculi biliferi
  Interlobular:
  bile ducts
  biliary canals
  Intrahepatic:
  biliary passages
  canaliculi
  gall duct
  EXCLUDES hepatic duct (156.1)
- ◆ **155.2 Liver, not specified as primary or secondary**

● **156 Malignant neoplasm of gallbladder and extrahepatic bile ducts**
- **156.0 Gallbladder**
- **156.1 Extrahepatic bile ducts**
  Biliary duct or passage NOS   Hepatic duct
  Common bile duct   Sphincter of Oddi
  Cystic duct
- **156.2 Ampulla of Vater**
- ◆ **156.8 Other specified sites of gallbladder and extrahepatic bile ducts**
  Malignant neoplasm of contiguous or overlapping sites of gallbladder and extrahepatic bile ducts whose point of origin cannot be determined
- ◆ **156.9 Biliary tract, part unspecified**
  Malignant neoplasm involving both intrahepatic and extrahepatic bile ducts

● **157 Malignant neoplasm of pancreas**
- **157.0 Head of pancreas**
- **157.1 Body of pancreas**
- **157.2 Tail of pancreas**
- **157.3 Pancreatic duct**
  Duct of:
  Santorini
  Wirsung
- **157.4 Islets of Langerhans**
  Islets of Langerhans, any part of pancreas
  Use additional code, if desired, to identify any functional activity
- ◆ **157.8 Other specified sites of pancreas**
  Ectopic pancreatic tissue
  Malignant neoplasm of contiguous or overlapping sites of pancreas whose point of origin cannot be determined
- ◆ **157.9 Pancreas, part unspecified**

● **158 Malignant neoplasm of retroperitoneum and peritoneum**
- **158.0 Retroperitoneum**
  Periadrenal tissue   Perirenal tissue
  Perinephric tissue   Retrocecal tissue
- ◆ **158.8 Specified parts of peritoneum**
  Cul-de-sac (of Douglas)
  Mesentery
  Mesocolon
  Omentum
  Peritoneum:
  parietal
  pelvic
  Rectouterine pouch
  Malignant neoplasm of contiguous or overlapping sites of retroperitoneum and peritoneum whose point of origin cannot be determined
- ◆ **158.9 Peritoneum, unspecified**

● **159 Malignant neoplasm of other and ill-defined sites within the digestive organs and peritoneum**
- ◆ **159.0 Intestinal tract, part unspecified**
  Intestine NOS

- **159.1 Spleen, not elsewhere classified**

    Angiosarcoma } of spleen
    Fibrosarcoma

    EXCLUDES Hodgkin's disease (201.0-201.9)
    lymphosarcoma (200.1)
    reticulosarcoma (200.0)

- **159.8 Other sites of digestive system and intra-abdominal organs**

    Malignant neoplasm of digestive organs and peritoneum whose point of origin cannot be assigned to any one of the categories 150-158

    EXCLUDES anus and rectum (154.8)
    cardio-esophageal junction (151.0)
    colon and rectum (154.0)

- **159.9 Ill-defined**

    Alimentary canal or tract NOS
    Gastrointestinal tract NOS

    EXCLUDES abdominal NOS (195.2)
    intra-abdominal NOS (195.2)

MALIGNANT NEOPLASM OF RESPIRATORY AND INTRATHORACIC ORGANS (160-165)

EXCLUDES carcinoma in situ (231.0-231.9)

● **160 Malignant neoplasm of nasal cavities, middle ear, and accessory sinuses**

  160.0 Nasal cavities

    Cartilage of nose   Septum of nose
    Conchae, nasal   Vestibule of nose
    Internal nose

    EXCLUDES nasal bone (170.0)
    nose NOS (195.0)
    olfactory bulb (192.0)
    posterior margin of septum and choanae (147.3)
    skin of nose (172.3, 173.3)
    turbinates (170.0)

  160.1 Auditory tube, middle ear, and mastoid air cells

    Antrum tympanicum   Tympanic cavity
    Eustachian tube

    EXCLUDES auditory canal (external) (172.2, 173.2)
    bone of ear (meatus) (170.0)
    cartilage of ear (171.0)
    ear (external) (skin) (172.2, 173.2)

  160.2 Maxillary sinus

    Antrum (Highmore) (maxillary)

  160.3 Ethmoidal sinus
  160.4 Frontal sinus
  160.5 Sphenoidal sinus
- **160.8 Other**

    Malignant neoplasm of contiguous or overlapping sites of nasal cavities, middle ear, and accessory sinuses whose point of origin cannot be determined

- **160.9 Accessory sinus, unspecified**

● **161 Malignant neoplasm of larynx**

  161.0 Glottis

    Intrinsic larynx
    Laryngeal commissure (anterior) (posterior)
    True vocal cord
    Vocal cord NOS

  161.1 Supraglottis

    Aryepiglottic fold or interarytenoid fold, laryngeal aspect
    Epiglottis (suprahyoid portion) NOS
    Extrinsic larynx
    False vocal cords
    Posterior (laryngeal) surface of epiglottis
    Ventricular bands

    EXCLUDES anterior aspect of epiglottis (146.4)
    aryepiglottic fold or interarytenoid fold:
    NOS (148.2)
    hypopharyngeal aspect (148.2)
    marginal zone (148.2)

  161.2 Subglottis
  161.3 Laryngeal cartilages

    Cartilage: Cartilage:
    arytenoid   cuneiform
    cricoid   thyroid

- **161.8 Other specified sites of larynx**

    Malignant neoplasm of contiguous or overlapping sites of larynx whose point of origin cannot be determined

- **161.9 Larynx, unspecified**

● **162 Malignant neoplasm of trachea, bronchus, and lung**

  162.0 Trachea

    Cartilage } of trachea
    Mucosa

  162.2 Main bronchus

    Carina
    Hilus of lung

  162.3 Upper lobe, bronchus or lung
  162.4 Middle lobe, bronchus or lung
  162.5 Lower lobe, bronchus or lung
- **162.8 Other parts of bronchus or lung**

    Malignant neoplasm of contiguous or overlapping sites of bronchus or lung whose point of origin cannot be determined

- **162.9 Bronchus and lung, unspecified**

● **163 Malignant neoplasm of pleura**

  163.0 Parietal pleura
  163.1 Visceral pleura
- **163.8 Other specified sites of pleura**

    Malignant neoplasm of contiguous or overlapping sites of pleura whose point of origin cannot be determined

- **163.9 Pleura, unspecified**

● **164 Malignant neoplasm of thymus, heart, and mediastinum**

  164.0 Thymus
  164.1 Heart

    Endocardium
    Epicardium
    Myocardium
    Pericardium

    EXCLUDES great vessels (171.4)

  164.2 Anterior mediastinum
  164.3 Posterior mediastinum
- **164.8 Other**

    Malignant neoplasm of contiguous or overlapping sites of thymus, heart, and mediastinum whose point of origin cannot be determined

- **164.9 Mediastinum, part unspecified**

● **165 Malignant neoplasm of other and ill-defined sites within the respiratory system and intrathoracic organs**

  165.0 Upper respiratory tract, part unspecified
- **165.8 Other**

    Malignant neoplasm of respiratory and intrathoracic organs whose point of origin cannot be assigned to any one of the categories 160-164

- **165.9 Ill-defined sites within the respiratory system**

    Respiratory tract NOS

    EXCLUDES intrathoracic NOS (195.1)
    thoracic NOS (195.1)

MALIGNANT NEOPLASM OF BONE, CONNECTIVE TISSUE, SKIN, AND BREAST (170-176)

EXCLUDES carcinoma in situ:
breast (233.0)
skin (232.0-232.9)

● **170 Malignant neoplasm of bone and articular cartilage**

  INCLUDES cartilage (articular) (joint)
  periosteum

  EXCLUDES bone marrow NOS (202.9)
  cartilage:
  ear (171.0)
  eyelid (171.0)
  larynx (161.3)
  nose (160.0)
  synovia (171.0-171.9)

170.0 Bones of skull and face, except mandible
Bone:
- ethmoid
- frontal
- malar
- nasal
- occipital

Bone:
- orbital
- parietal
- sphenoid
- temporal
- zygomatic

Maxilla (superior)
Turbinate
Upper jaw bone
Vomer

EXCLUDES: carcinoma, any type except intraosseous or odontogenic:
maxilla, maxillary (sinus) (160.2)
upper jaw bone (143.0)
jaw bone (lower) (170.1)

170.1 Mandible
Inferior maxilla
Jaw bone NOS
Lower jaw bone

EXCLUDES: carcinoma, any type except intraosseous or odontogenic:
jaw bone NOS (143.9)
lower (143.1)
upper jaw bone (170.0)

170.2 Vertebral column, excluding sacrum and coccyx
Spinal column   Vertebra
Spine

EXCLUDES: sacrum and coccyx (170.6)

170.3 Ribs, sternum, and clavicle
Costal cartilage   Xiphoid process
Costovertebral joint

170.4 Scapula and long bones of upper limb
Acromion   Radius
Bones NOS of upper limb   Ulna
Humerus

170.5 Short bones of upper limb
Carpal   Pisiform
Cuneiform, wrist   Scaphoid (of hand)
Metacarpal   Semilunar or lunate
Navicular, of hand   Trapezium
Phalanges of hand   Trapezoid
Unciform

170.6 Pelvic bones, sacrum, and coccyx
Coccygeal vertebra   Pubic bone
Ilium   Sacral vertebra
Ischium

170.7 Long bones of lower limb
Bones NOS of lower limb   Fibula
Femur   Tibia

170.8 Short bones of lower limb
Astragalus [talus]   Navicular (of ankle)
Calcaneus   Patella
Cuboid   Phalanges of foot
Cuneiform, ankle   Tarsal
Metatarsal

◆ **170.9 Bone and articular cartilage, site unspecified**

● **171 Malignant neoplasm of connective and other soft tissue**

INCLUDES:
- blood vessel
- bursa
- fascia
- fat
- ligament, except uterine
- muscle
- peripheral, sympathetic, and parasympathetic nerves and ganglia
- synovia
- tendon (sheath)

EXCLUDES: cartilage (of):
articular (170.0-170.9)
larynx (161.3)
nose (160.0)
connective tissue:
breast (174.0-175.9)
internal organs—code to malignant neoplasm of the site [e.g., leiomyosarcoma of stomach, 151.9]
heart (164.1)
uterine ligament (183.4)

171.0 Head, face, and neck
Cartilage of:
ear
eyelid

171.2 Upper limb, including shoulder
Arm   Forearm
Finger   Hand

171.3 Lower limb, including hip
Foot   Thigh
Leg   Toe
Popliteal space

171.4 Thorax
Axilla
Diaphragm
Great vessels

EXCLUDES: heart (164.1)
mediastinum (164.2-164.9)
thymus (164.0)

171.5 Abdomen
Abdominal wall
Hypochondrium

EXCLUDES: peritoneum (158.8)
retroperitoneum (158.0)

171.6 Pelvis
Buttock   Inguinal region
Groin   Perineum

EXCLUDES: pelvic peritoneum (158.8)
retroperitoneum (158.0)
uterine ligament, any (183.3-183.5)

◆ **171.7 Trunk, unspecified**
Back NOS
Flank NOS

◆ **171.8 Other specified sites of connective and other soft tissue**
Malignant neoplasm of contiguous or overlapping sites of connective tissue whose point of origin cannot be determined

◆ **171.9 Connective and other soft tissue, site unspecified**

● **172 Malignant melanoma of skin**

INCLUDES: melanocarcinoma
melanoma (skin) NOS

EXCLUDES: skin of genital organs (184.0-184.9, 187.1-187.9)
sites other than skin—code to malignant neoplasm of the site

172.0 Lip

EXCLUDES: vermilion border of lip (140.0-140.1, 140.9)

172.1 Eyelid, including canthus

172.2 Ear and external auditory canal
Auricle (ear)   External [acoustic] meatus
Auricular canal, external Pinna

◆ **172.3 Other and unspecified parts of face**
Cheek (external)   Forehead
Chin   Nose, external
Eyebrow   Temple

172.4 Scalp and neck

172.5 Trunk, except scrotum
Axilla   Perianal skin
Breast   Perineum
Buttock
Groin

EXCLUDES: anal canal (154.2)
anus NOS (154.3)
scrotum (187.7)

172.6 Upper limb, including shoulder
Arm   Forearm
Finger   Hand

172.7 Lower limb, including hip
Ankle   Leg
Foot   Popliteal area
Heel   Thigh
Knee   Toe

◆ **172.8 Other specified sites of skin**
Malignant melanoma of contiguous or overlapping sites of skin whose point of origin cannot be determined

◆ **172.9 Melanoma of skin, site unspecified**

NEOPLASMS

- **173 Other malignant neoplasm of skin**
    - INCLUDES: malignant neoplasm of:
        - sebaceous glands
        - sudoriferous, sudoriparous glands
        - sweat glands
    - EXCLUDES:
        - Kaposi's sarcoma (176.0-176.9)
        - malignant melanoma of skin (172.0-172.9)
        - skin of genital organs (184.0-184.9, 187.1-187.9)
    - **173.0 Skin of lip**
        - EXCLUDES: vermilion border of lip (140.0-140.1, 140.9)
    - **173.1 Eyelid, including canthus**
        - EXCLUDES: cartilage of eyelid (171.0)
    - **173.2 Skin of ear and external auditory canal**
        - Auricle (ear)
        - Auricular canal, external
        - External meatus
        - Pinna
        - EXCLUDES: cartilage of ear (171.0)
    - ◆ **173.3 Skin of other and unspecified parts of face**
        - Cheek, external
        - Chin
        - Eyebrow
        - Forehead
        - Nose, external
        - Temple
    - **173.4 Scalp and skin of neck**
    - **173.5 Skin of trunk, except scrotum**
        - Axillary fold
        - Perianal skin
        - Skin of:
            - abdominal wall
            - anus
            - back
            - breast
        - Skin of:
            - buttock
            - chest wall
            - groin
            - perineum
        - Umbilicus
        - EXCLUDES:
            - anal canal (154.2)
            - anus NOS (154.3)
            - skin of scrotum (187.7)
    - **173.6 Skin of upper limb, including shoulder**
        - Arm
        - Finger
        - Forearm
        - Hand
    - **173.7 Skin of lower limb, including hip**
        - Ankle
        - Foot
        - Heel
        - Knee
        - Leg
        - Popliteal area
        - Thigh
        - Toe
    - ◆ **173.8 Other specified sites of skin**
        - Malignant neoplasm of contiguous or overlapping sites of skin whose point of origin cannot be determined
    - ◆ **173.9 Skin, site unspecified**
- **174 Malignant neoplasm of female breast**
    - INCLUDES: breast (female)
        - connective tissue
        - soft parts
        - Paget's disease of:
            - breast
            - nipple
    - EXCLUDES: skin of breast (172.5, 173.5)
    - **174.0 Nipple and areola**
    - **174.1 Central portion**
    - **174.2 Upper-inner quadrant**
    - **174.3 Lower-inner quadrant**
    - **174.4 Upper-outer quadrant**
    - **174.5 Lower-outer quadrant**
    - **174.6 Axillary tail**
    - ◆ **174.8 Other specified sites of female breast**
        - Ectopic sites
        - Inner breast
        - Lower breast
        - Malignant neoplasm of contiguous or overlapping sites of breast whose point of origin cannot be determined
        - Midline of breast
        - Outer breast
        - Upper breast
    - ◆ **174.9 Breast (female), unspecified**
- **175 Malignant neoplasm of male breast**
    - EXCLUDES: skin of breast (172.5, 173.5)
    - **175.0 Nipple and areola**
    - ◆ **175.9 Other and unspecified sites of male breast**
        - Ectopic breast tissue, male

- **176 Kaposi's sarcoma**
    - **176.0 Skin**
    - **176.1 Soft tissue**
        - INCLUDES:
            - blood vessel
            - connective tissue
            - fascia
            - ligament
            - lymphatic(s) NEC
            - muscle
        - EXCLUDES: lymph glands and nodes (176.5)
    - **176.2 Palate**
    - **176.3 Gastrointestinal sites**
    - **176.4 Lung**
    - **176.5 Lymph nodes**
    - ◆ **176.8 Other specified sites**
        - INCLUDES: oral cavity NEC
    - ◆ **176.9 Unspecified**
        - Viscera NOS

MALIGNANT NEOPLASM OF GENITOURINARY ORGANS (179-189)
- EXCLUDES: carcinoma in situ (233.1-233.9)
- ◆ **179 Malignant neoplasm of uterus, part unspecified**
- **180 Malignant neoplasm of cervix uteri**
    - INCLUDES: invasive malignancy [carcinoma]
    - EXCLUDES: carcinoma in situ (233.1)
    - **180.0 Endocervix**
        - Cervical canal NOS
        - Endocervical canal
        - Endocervical gland
    - **180.1 Exocervix**
    - ◆ **180.8 Other specified sites of cervix**
        - Cervical stump
        - Squamocolumnar junction of cervix
        - Malignant neoplasm of contiguous or overlapping sites of cervix uteri whose point of origin cannot be determined
    - ◆ **180.9 Cervix uteri, unspecified**
- **181 Malignant neoplasm of placenta**
    - Choriocarcinoma NOS
    - Chorioepithelioma NOS
    - EXCLUDES:
        - chorioadenoma (destruens) (236.1)
        - hydatidiform mole (630)
            - malignant (236.1)
        - invasive mole (236.1)
        - male choriocarcinoma NOS (186.0-186.9)
- **182 Malignant neoplasm of body of uterus**
    - EXCLUDES: carcinoma in situ (233.2)
    - **182.0 Corpus uteri, except isthmus**
        - Cornu
        - Endometrium
        - Fundus
        - Myometrium
    - **182.1 Isthmus**
        - Lower uterine segment
    - ◆ **182.8 Other specified sites of body of uterus**
        - Malignant neoplasm of contiguous or overlapping sites of body of uterus whose point of origin cannot be determined
        - EXCLUDES: uterus NOS (179)
- **183 Malignant neoplasm of ovary and other uterine adnexa**
    - EXCLUDES: Douglas' cul-de-sac (158.8)
    - **183.0 Ovary**
        - Use additional code, if desired, to identify any functional activity
    - **183.2 Fallopian tube**
        - Oviduct
        - Uterine tube
    - **183.3 Broad ligament**
        - Mesovarium
        - Parovarian region
    - **183.4 Parametrium**
        - Uterine ligament NOS
        - Uterosacral ligament
    - **183.5 Round ligament**
    - ◆ **183.8 Other specified sites of uterine adnexa**
        - Tubo-ovarian
        - Utero-ovarian
        - Malignant neoplasm of contiguous or overlapping sites of ovary and other uterine adnexa whose point of origin cannot be determined
    - ◆ **183.9 Uterine adnexa, unspecified**

- **184** Malignant neoplasm of other and unspecified female genital organs
  - EXCLUDES   carcinoma in situ (233.3)
  - **184.0** Vagina
    - Gartner's duct
    - Vaginal vault
  - **184.1** Labia majora
    - Greater vestibular [Bartholin's] gland
  - **184.2** Labia minora
  - **184.3** Clitoris
  - ◆ **184.4** Vulva, unspecified
    - External female genitalia NOS
    - Pudendum
  - ◆ **184.8** Other specified sites of female genital organs
    - Malignant neoplasm of contiguous or overlapping sites of female genital organs whose point of origin cannot be determined
  - ◆ **184.9** Female genital organ, site unspecified
    - Female genitourinary tract NOS
- **185** Malignant neoplasm of prostate
  - EXCLUDES   seminal vesicles (187.8)
- **186** Malignant neoplasm of testis
  - Use additional code, if desired, to identify any functional activity
  - **186.0** Undescended testis
    - Ectopic testis
    - Retained testis
  - ◆ **186.9** Other and unspecified testis
    - Testis:
      - NOS
      - descended
      - scrotal
- **187** Malignant neoplasm of penis and other male genital organs
  - **187.1** Prepuce
    - Foreskin
  - **187.2** Glans penis
  - **187.3** Body of penis
    - Corpus cavernosum
  - ◆ **187.4** Penis, part unspecified
    - Skin of penis NOS
  - **187.5** Epididymis
  - **187.6** Spermatic cord
    - Vas deferens
  - **187.7** Scrotum
    - Skin of scrotum
  - ◆ **187.8** Other specified sites of male genital organs
    - Seminal vesicle
    - Tunica vaginalis
    - Malignant neoplasm of contiguous or overlapping sites of penis and other male genital organs whose point of origin cannot be determined
  - ◆ **187.9** Male genital organ, site unspecified
    - Male genital organ or tract NOS
- **188** Malignant neoplasm of bladder
  - EXCLUDES   carcinoma in situ (233.7)
  - **188.0** Trigone of urinary bladder
  - **188.1** Dome of urinary bladder
  - **188.2** Lateral wall of urinary bladder
  - **188.3** Anterior wall of urinary bladder
  - **188.4** Posterior wall of urinary bladder
  - **188.5** Bladder neck
    - Internal urethral orifice
  - **188.6** Ureteric orifice
  - **188.7** Urachus
  - ◆ **188.8** Other specified sites of bladder
    - Malignant neoplasm of contiguous or overlapping sites of bladder whose point of origin cannot be determined
  - ◆ **188.9** Bladder, part unspecified
    - Bladder wall NOS
- **189** Malignant neoplasm of kidney and other and unspecified urinary organs
  - **189.0** Kidney, except pelvis
    - Kidney NOS
    - Kidney parenchyma
  - **189.1** Renal pelvis
    - Renal calyces
    - Ureteropelvic junction
  - **189.2** Ureter
    - EXCLUDES   ureteric orifice of bladder (188.6)
  - **189.3** Urethra
    - EXCLUDES   urethral orifice of bladder (188.5)
  - **189.4** Paraurethral glands
- ◆ **189.8** Other specified sites of urinary organs
  - Malignant neoplasm of contiguous or overlapping sites of kidney and other urinary organs whose point of origin cannot be determined
- ◆ **189.9** Urinary organ, site unspecified
  - Urinary system NOS

MALIGNANT NEOPLASM OF OTHER AND UNSPECIFIED SITES (190-199)

EXCLUDES   carcinoma in situ (234.0-234.9)

- **190** Malignant neoplasm of eye
  - EXCLUDES   carcinoma in situ (234.0)
    - eyelid (skin) (172.1, 173.1)
    - cartilage (171.0)
    - optic nerve (192.0)
    - orbital bone (170.0)
  - **190.0** Eyeball, except conjunctiva, cornea, retina, and choroid
    - Ciliarybody
    - Sclera
    - Crystalline lens
    - Uveal tract
    - Iris
  - **190.1** Orbit
    - Connective tissue of orbit
    - Extraocular muscle
    - Retrobulbar
    - EXCLUDES   bone of orbit (170.0)
  - **190.2** Lacrimal gland
  - **190.3** Conjunctiva
  - **190.4** Cornea
  - **190.5** Retina
  - **190.6** Choroid
  - **190.7** Lacrimal duct
    - Lacrimal sac
    - Nasolacrimal duct
  - ◆ **190.8** Other specified sites of eye
    - Malignant neoplasm of contiguous or overlapping sites of eye whose point of origin cannot be determined
  - ◆ **190.9** Eye, part unspecified
- **191** Malignant neoplasm of brain
  - EXCLUDES   cranial nerves (192.0)
    - retrobulbar area (190.1)
  - **191.0** Cerebrum, except lobes and ventricles
    - Basal ganglia
    - Globus pallidus
    - Cerebral cortex
    - Hypothalamus
    - Corpus striatum
    - Thalamus
  - **191.1** Frontal lobe
  - **191.2** Temporal lobe
    - Hippocampus
    - Uncus
  - **191.3** Parietal lobe
  - **191.4** Occipital lobe
  - **191.5** Ventricles
    - Choroid plexus
    - Floor of ventricle
  - **191.6** Cerebellum NOS
    - Cerebellopontine angle
  - **191.7** Brain stem
    - Cerebral peduncle
    - Midbrain
    - Medulla oblongata
    - Pons
  - ◆ **191.8** Other parts of brain
    - Corpus callosum
    - Tapetum
    - Malignant neoplasm of contiguous or overlapping sites of brain whose point of origin cannot be determined
  - ◆ **191.9** Brain, unspecified
    - Cranial fossa NOS
- **192** Malignant neoplasm of other and unspecified parts of nervous system
  - EXCLUDES   peripheral, sympathetic, and parasympathetic nerves and ganglia (171.0-171.9)
  - **192.0** Cranial nerves
    - Olfactory bulb
  - **192.1** Cerebral meninges
    - Dura (mater)
    - Falx (cerebelli) (cerebri)
    - Meninges NOS
    - Tentorium
  - **192.2** Spinal cord
    - Cauda equina
  - **192.3** Spinal meninges

NEOPLASMS

- ◆ **192.8 Other specified sites of nervous system**
  Malignant neoplasm of contiguous or overlapping sites of other parts of nervous system whose point of origin cannot be determined
- ◆ **192.9 Nervous system, part unspecified**
  Nervous system (central) NOS
  EXCLUDES: meninges NOS (192.1)

193 Malignant neoplasm of thyroid gland
  Sipple's syndrome
  Thyroglossal duct
  Use additional code, if desired, to identify any functional activity

● **194 Malignant neoplasm of other endocrine glands and related structures**
  Use additional code, if desired, to identify any functional activity
  EXCLUDES: islets of Langerhans (157.4)
  ovary (183.0)
  testis (186.0-186.9)
  thymus (164.0)

- **194.0 Adrenal gland**
  Adrenal cortex   Suprarenal gland
  Adrenal medulla
- **194.1 Parathyroid gland**
- **194.3 Pituitary gland and craniopharyngeal duct**
  Craniobuccal pouch   Rathke's pouch
  Hypophysis   Sella turcica
- **194.4 Pineal gland**
- **194.5 Carotid body**
- **194.6 Aortic body and other paraganglia**
  Coccygeal body   Para-aortic body
  Glomus jugulare
- ◆ **194.8 Other**
  Pluriglandular involvement NOS
  Note: If the sites of multiple involvements are known, they should be coded separately.
- ◆ **194.9 Endocrine gland, site unspecified**

● **195 Malignant neoplasm of other and ill-defined sites**
  INCLUDES: malignant neoplasms of contiguous sites, not elsewhere classified, whose point of origin cannot be determined
  EXCLUDES: malignant neoplasm:
  lymphatic and hematopoietic tissue (200.0-208.9)
  secondary sites (196.0-198.8)
  unspecified site (199.0-199.1)

- **195.0 Head, face, and neck**
  Cheek NOS   Nose NOS
  Jaw NOS   Supraclavicular region NOS
- **195.1 Thorax**
  Axilla   Intrathoracic NOS
  Chest (wall) NOS
- **195.2 Abdomen**
  Intra-abdominal NOS
- **195.3 Pelvis**
  Groin
  Inguinal region NOS
  Presacral region
  Sacrococcygeal region
  Sites overlapping systems within pelvis, as:
  rectovaginal (septum)
  rectovesical (septum)
- **195.4 Upper limb**
- **195.5 Lower limb**
- ◆ **195.8 Other specified sites**
  Back NOS
  Flank NOS
  Trunk NOS

● **196 Secondary and unspecified malignant neoplasm of lymph nodes**
  EXCLUDES: any malignant neoplasm of lymph nodes, specified as primary (200.0-202.9)
  Hodgkin's disease (201.0-201.9)
  lymphosarcoma (200.1)
  reticulosarcoma (200.0)
  other forms of lymphoma (202.0-202.9)

- **196.0 Lymph nodes of head, face, and neck**
  Cervical   Scalene
  Cervicofacial   Supraclavicular
- **196.1 Intrathoracic lymph nodes**
  Bronchopulmonary   Mediastinal
  Intercostal   Tracheobronchial
- **196.2 Intra-abdominal lymph nodes**
  Intestinal   Retroperitoneal
  Mesenteric
- **196.3 Lymph nodes of axilla and upper limb**
  Brachial   Infraclavicular
  Epitrochlear   Pectoral
- **196.5 Lymph nodes of inguinal region and lower limb**
  Femoral   Popliteal
  Groin   Tibial
- **196.6 Intrapelvic lymph nodes**
  Hypogastric   Obturator
  Iliac   Parametrial
- ◆ **196.8 Lymph nodes of multiple sites**
- ◆ **196.9 Site unspecified**
  Lymph nodes NOS

● **197 Secondary malignant neoplasm of respiratory and digestive systems**
  EXCLUDES: lymph node metastasis (196.0-196.9)

- **197.0 Lung**
  Bronchus
- **197.1 Mediastinum**
- **197.2 Pleura**
- ◆ **197.3 Other respiratory organs**
  Trachea
- **197.4 Small intestine, including duodenum**
- **197.5 Large intestine and rectum**
- **197.6 Retroperitoneum and peritoneum**
- **197.7 Liver, specified as secondary**
- ◆ **197.8 Other digestive organs and spleen**

● **198 Secondary malignant neoplasm of other specified sites**
  EXCLUDES: lymph node metastasis (196.0-196.9)

- **198.0 Kidney**
- ◆ **198.1 Other urinary organs**
- **198.2 Skin**
  Skin of breast
- **198.3 Brain and spinal cord**
- ◆ **198.4 Other parts of nervous system**
  Meninges (cerebral) (spinal)
- **198.5 Bone and bone marrow**
- **198.6 Ovary**
- **198.7 Adrenal gland**
  Suprarenal gland
- ● **198.8 Other specified sites**
  - **198.81 Breast**
    EXCLUDES: skin of breast (198.2)
  - **198.82 Genital organs**
  - ◆ **198.89 Other**
    EXCLUDES: retroperitoneal lymph nodes (196.2)

● **199 Malignant neoplasm without specification of site**

- **199.0 Disseminated**
  Carcinomatosis ⎫
  Generalized: ⎬ unspecified site
  cancer   ⎪ (primary)
  malignancy   ⎪ (secondary)
  Multiple cancer ⎭

- ◆ **199.1 Other**
  Cancer   ⎫ unspecified site
  Carcinoma   ⎬ (primary)
  Malignancy ⎭ (secondary)

● Additional digits required   ◆ Nonspecific code   ▌ Not a primary diagnosis

MALIGNANT NEOPLASM OF LYMPHATIC AND HEMATOPOIETIC TISSUE (200-208)

EXCLUDES secondary neoplasm of:
  bone marrow (198.5)
  spleen (197.8)
secondary and unspecified neoplasm of lymph nodes (196.0-196.9)

The following fifth-digit subclassification is for use with categories 200-202:
- 0 unspecified site, extranodal and solid organ sites
- 1 lymph nodes of head, face, and neck
- 2 intrathoracic lymph nodes
- 3 intra-abdominal lymph nodes
- 4 lymph nodes of axilla and upper limb
- 5 lymph nodes of inguinal region and lower limb
- 6 intrapelvic lymph nodes
- 7 spleen
- 8 lymph nodes of multiple sites

200 Lymphosarcoma and reticulosarcoma

200.0 Reticulosarcoma
Lymphoma (malignant):
  histiocytic (diffuse):
    nodular
    pleomorphic cell type
    reticulum cell type
Reticulum cell sarcoma:
  NOS
  pleomorphic cell type

200.1 Lymphosarcoma
Lymphoblastoma (diffuse)
Lymphoma (malignant):
  lymphoblastic (diffuse)
  lymphocytic (cell type) (diffuse)
  lymphosarcoma type
Lymphosarcoma:
  NOS
  diffuse NOS
  lymphoblastic (diffuse)
  lymphocytic (diffuse)
  prolymphocytic

EXCLUDES lymphosarcoma:
  follicular or nodular (202.0)
  mixed cell type (200.8)
  lymphosarcoma cell leukemia (207.8)

200.2 Burkitt's tumor or lymphoma
Malignant lymphoma, Burkitt's type

200.8 Other named variants
Lymphoma (malignant):
  lymphoplasmacytoid type
  mixed lymphocytic-histiocytic (diffuse)
Lymphosarcoma, mixed cell type (diffuse)
Reticulolymphosarcoma (diffuse)

201 Hodgkin's disease

201.0 Hodgkin's paragranuloma
201.1 Hodgkin's granuloma
201.2 Hodgkin's sarcoma
201.4 Lymphocytic-histiocytic predominance
201.5 Nodular sclerosis
Hodgkin's disease, nodular sclerosis:
  NOS
  cellular phase

201.6 Mixed cellularity
201.7 Lymphocytic depletion
Hodgkin's disease, lymphocytic depletion:
  NOS
  diffuse fibrosis
  reticular type

201.9 Hodgkin's disease, unspecified
Hodgkin's:
  disease NOS
  lymphoma NOS
Malignant:
  lymphogranuloma
  lymphogranulomatosis

202 Other malignant neoplasms of lymphoid and histiocytic tissue

202.0 Nodular lymphoma
Brill-Symmers disease
Lymphoma:
  follicular (giant)
  lymphocytic, nodular
Lymphosarcoma:
  follicular (giant)
  nodular
Reticulosarcoma, follicular or nodular

202.1 Mycosis fungoides
202.2 Sézary's disease
202.3 Malignant histiocytosis
Histiocytic medullary reticulosis
Malignant:
  reticuloendotheliosis
  reticulosis

202.4 Leukemic reticuloendotheliosis
Hairy-cell leukemia

202.5 Letterer-Siwe disease
Acute:
  differentiated progressive histiocytosis
  histiocytosis X (progressive)
  infantile reticuloendotheliosis
  reticulosis of infancy

EXCLUDES Hand-Schüller-Christian disease (277.8)
  histiocytosis (acute) (chronic) (277.8)
  histiocytosis X (chronic) (277.8)

202.6 Malignant mast cell tumors
Malignant:
  mastocytoma
  mastocytosis
Mast cell sarcoma
Systemic tissue mast cell disease

EXCLUDES mast cell leukemia (207.8)

202.8 Other lymphomas
Lymphoma (malignant):
  NOS
  diffuse

EXCLUDES benign lymphoma (229.0)

202.9 Other and unspecified malignant neoplasms of lymphoid and histiocytic tissue
Malignant neoplasm of bone marrow NOS

203 Multiple myeloma and immunoproliferative neoplasms

The following fifth-digit subclassification is for use with category 203:
- 0 without mention of remission
- 1 in remission

203.0 Multiple myeloma
Kahler's disease
Myelomatosis

EXCLUDES solitary myeloma (238.6)

203.1 Plasma cell leukemia
Plasmacytic leukemia

203.8 Other immunoproliferative neoplasms

204 Lymphoid leukemia

INCLUDES leukemia:
  lymphatic
  lymphoblastic
  lymphocytic
  lymphogenous

The following fifth-digit subclassification is for use with category 204:
- 0 without mention of remission
- 1 in remission

204.0 Acute
EXCLUDES acute exacerbation of chronic lymphoid leukemia (204.1)

204.1 Chronic
204.2 Subacute
204.8 Other lymphoid leukemia
Aleukemic leukemia:
  lymphatic
  lymphocytic
  lymphoid

204.9 Unspecified lymphoid leukemia

205 Myeloid leukemia

INCLUDES leukemia:
  granulocytic
  myeloblastic
  myelocytic
  myelogenous
  myelomonocytic
  myelosclerotic
  myelosis

The following fifth-digit subclassification is for use with category 205:
- 0 without mention of remission
- 1 in remission

205.0 Acute
Acute promyelocytic leukemia

EXCLUDES acute exacerbation of chronic myeloid leukemia (205.1)

205.1 Chronic
Eosinophilic leukemia
Neutrophilic leukemia

205.2 Subacute
205.3 Myeloid sarcoma
Chloroma
Granulocytic sarcoma

NEOPLASMS

- ◆● **205.8** Other myeloid leukemia
  - Aleukemic leukemia: granulocytic, myelogenous
  - Aleukemic leukemia: myeloid
  - Aleukemic myelosis
- ◆● **205.9** Unspecified myeloid leukemia
- ● **206** Monocytic leukemia
  - INCLUDES leukemia: histiocytic, monoblastic, monocytoid

  The following fifth-digit subclassification is for use with category 206:
  - 0 without mention of remission
  - 1 in remission

  - ● **206.0** Acute
    - EXCLUDES acute exacerbation of chronic monocytic leukemia (206.1)
  - ● **206.1** Chronic
  - ● **206.2** Subacute
  - ◆● **206.8** Other monocytic leukemia
    - Aleukemic:
      - monocytic leukemia
      - monocytoid leukemia
  - ◆● **206.9** Unspecified monocytic leukemia
- ● **207** Other specified leukemia
  - EXCLUDES leukemic reticuloendotheliosis (202.4)
    - plasma cell leukemia (203.1)

  The following fifth-digit subclassification is for use with category 207:
  - 0 without mention of remission
  - 1 in remission

  - ● **207.0** Acute erythremia and erythroleukemia
    - Acute erythremic myelosis
    - Di Guglielmo's disease
    - Erythremic myelosis
  - ● **207.1** Chronic erythremia
    - Heilmeyer-Schöner disease
  - ● **207.2** Megakaryocytic leukemia
    - Megakaryocytic myelosis
    - Thrombocytic leukemia
  - ◆● **207.8** Other specified leukemia
    - Lymphosarcoma cell leukemia
- ● **208** Leukemia of unspecified cell type

  The following fifth-digit subclassification is for use with category 208:
  - 0 without mention of remission
  - 1 in remission

  - ◆● **208.0** Acute
    - Acute leukemia NOS
    - Blast cell leukemia
    - Stem cell leukemia
    - EXCLUDES acute exacerbation of chronic unspecified leukemia (208.1)
  - ◆● **208.1** Chronic
    - Chronic leukemia NOS
  - ◆● **208.2** Subacute
    - Subacute leukemia NOS
  - ◆● **208.8** Other leukemia of unspecified cell type
  - ◆● **208.9** Unspecified leukemia
    - Leukemia NOS

BENIGN NEOPLASMS (210-229)

- ● **210** Benign neoplasm of lip, oral cavity, and pharynx
  - EXCLUDES cyst (of):
    - jaw (526.0-526.2, 526.89)
    - oral soft tissue (528.4)
    - radicular (522.8)

  - **210.0** Lip
    - Frenulum labii
    - Lip (inner aspect) (mucosa) (vermilion border)
    - EXCLUDES labial commissure (210.4)
      - skin of lip (216.0)
  - **210.1** Tongue
    - Lingual tonsil
  - **210.2** Major salivary glands
    - Gland: parotid, sublingual
    - Gland: submandibular
    - EXCLUDES benign neoplasms of minor salivary glands:
      - NOS (210.4)
      - buccal mucosa (210.4)
      - lips (210.0)
      - palate (hard) (soft) (210.4)
      - tongue (210.1)
      - tonsil, palatine (210.5)
  - **210.3** Floor of mouth
  - ◆ **210.4** Other and unspecified parts of mouth
    - Gingiva
    - Gum (upper) (lower)
    - Labial commissure
    - Oral cavity NOS
    - Oral mucosa
    - Palate (hard) (soft)
    - Uvula
    - EXCLUDES benign odontogenic neoplasms of bone (213.0-213.1)
      - developmental odontogenic cysts (526.0)
      - mucosa of lips (210.0)
      - nasopharyngeal [posterior] [superior] surface of soft palate (210.7)
  - **210.5** Tonsil
    - Tonsil (faucial) (palatine)
    - EXCLUDES lingual tonsil (210.1)
      - pharyngeal tonsil (210.7)
      - tonsillar:
        - fossa (210.6)
        - pillars (210.6)
  - ◆ **210.6** Other parts of oropharynx
    - Branchial cleft or vestiges
    - Epiglottis, anterior aspect
    - Fauces NOS
    - Mesopharynx NOS
    - Tonsillar: fossa, pillars
    - Vallecula
    - EXCLUDES epiglottis:
      - NOS (212.1)
      - suprahyoid portion (212.1)
  - **210.7** Nasopharynx
    - Adenoid tissue
    - Lymphadenoid tissue
    - Pharyngeal tonsil
    - Posterior nasal septum
  - **210.8** Hypopharynx
    - Arytenoid fold
    - Laryngopharynx
    - Postcricoid region
    - Pyriform fossa
  - ◆ **210.9** Pharynx, unspecified
    - Throat NOS
- ● **211** Benign neoplasm of other parts of digestive system
  - **211.0** Esophagus
  - **211.1** Stomach
    - Body, Cardia, Fundus } of stomach
    - Cardiac orifice
    - Pylorus
  - **211.2** Duodenum, jejunum, and ileum
    - Small intestine NOS
    - EXCLUDES ampulla of Vater (211.5)
      - ileocecal valve (211.3)
  - **211.3** Colon
    - Appendix
    - Cecum
    - Ileocecal valve
    - Large intestine NOS
    - EXCLUDES rectosigmoid junction (211.4)
  - **211.4** Rectum and anal canal
    - Anal canal or sphincter
    - Anus NOS
    - Rectosigmoid junction
    - EXCLUDES anus:
      - margin (216.5)
      - skin (216.5)
      - perianal skin (216.5)
  - **211.5** Liver and biliary passages
    - Ampulla of Vater
    - Common bile duct
    - Cystic duct
    - Gallbladder
    - Hepatic duct
    - Sphincter of Oddi
  - **211.6** Pancreas, except islets of Langerhans

	211.7	**Islets of Langerhans**
		Islet cell tumor
		Use additional code, if desired, to identify any functional activity
	211.8	**Retroperitoneum and peritoneum**
		Mesentery Omentum
		Mesocolon Retroperitoneal tissue
◆	**211.9**	**Other and unspecified site**
		Alimentary tract NOS Intestine NOS
		Digestive system NOS Spleen, not elsewhere classified
		Gastrointestinal tract NOS
		Intestinal tract NOS

● **212 Benign neoplasm of respiratory and intrathoracic organs**

212.0 Nasal cavities, middle ear, and accessory sinuses
Cartilage of nose
Eustachian tube
Nares
Septum of nose
Sinus:
  ethmoidal
  frontal
  maxillary
  sphenoidal

EXCLUDES auditory canal (external) (216.2)
bone of:
  ear (213.0)
  nose [turbinates] (213.0)
cartilage of ear (215.0)
ear (external) (skin) (216.2)
nose NOS (229.8)
  skin (216.3)
olfactory bulb (225.1)
polyp of:
  accessory sinus (471.8)
  ear (385.30-385.35)
  nasal cavity (471.0)
  posterior margin of septum and choanae (210.7)

212.1 Larynx
Cartilage:
  arytenoid
  cricoid
  cuneiform
  thyroid
Epiglottis (suprahyoid portion) NOS
Glottis
Vocal cords (false) (true)

EXCLUDES epiglottis, anterior aspect (210.6)
polyp of vocal cord or larynx (478.4)

212.2 Trachea
212.3 Bronchus and lung
  Carina Hilus of lung
212.4 Pleura
212.5 Mediastinum
212.6 Thymus
212.7 Heart
  EXCLUDES great vessels (215.4)
◆ **212.8 Other specified sites**
◆ **212.9 Site unspecified**
  Respiratory organ NOS
  Upper respiratory tract NOS
  EXCLUDES intrathoracic NOS (229.8)
  thoracic NOS (229.8)

● **213 Benign neoplasm of bone and articular cartilage**
  INCLUDES cartilage (articular) (joint)
  periosteum
  EXCLUDES cartilage of:
    ear (215.0)
    eyelid (215.0)
    larynx (212.1)
    nose (212.0)
  exostosis NOS (726.91)
  synovia (215.0-215.9)

213.0 Bones of skull and face
  EXCLUDES lower jaw bone (213.1)
213.1 Lower jaw bone
213.2 Vertebral column, excluding sacrum and coccyx
213.3 Ribs, sternum, and clavicle
213.4 Scapula and long bones of upper limb
213.5 Short bones of upper limb
213.6 Pelvic bones, sacrum, and coccyx
213.7 Long bones of lower limb
213.8 Short bones of lower limb
◆ **213.9 Bone and articular cartilage, site unspecified**

● **214 Lipoma**
  INCLUDES angiolipoma
  fibrolipoma
  hibernoma
  lipoma (fetal) (infiltrating) (intramuscular)
  myelolipoma
  myxolipoma

214.0 Skin and subcutaneous tissue of face
◆ **214.1 Other skin and subcutaneous tissue**
214.2 Intrathoracic organs
214.3 Intra-abdominal organs
214.4 Spermatic cord
◆ **214.8 Other specified sites**
◆ **214.9 Lipoma, unspecified site**

● **215 Other benign neoplasm of connective and other soft tissue**
  INCLUDES blood vessel
  bursa
  fascia
  ligament
  muscle
  peripheral, sympathetic, and parasympathetic nerves and ganglia
  synovia
  tendon (sheath)
  EXCLUDES cartilage:
    articular (213.0-213.9)
    larynx (212.1)
    nose (212.0)
  connective tissue of:
    breast (217)
    internal organ, except lipoma and hemangioma— code to benign neoplasm of the site
  lipoma (214.0-214.9)

215.0 Head, face, and neck
215.2 Upper limb, including shoulder
215.3 Lower limb, including hip
215.4 Thorax
  EXCLUDES heart (212.7)
  mediastinum (212.5)
  thymus (212.6)
215.5 Abdomen
  Abdominal wall Hypochondrium
215.6 Pelvis
  Buttock Inguinal region
  Groin Perineum
  EXCLUDES uterine:
    leiomyoma (218.0-218.9)
    ligament, any (221.0)
◆ **215.7 Trunk, unspecified**
  Back NOS Flank NOS
◆ **215.8 Other specified sites**
◆ **215.9 Site unspecified**

● **216 Benign neoplasm of skin**
  INCLUDES blue nevus
  dermatofibroma
  hydrocystoma
  pigmented nevus
  syringoadenoma
  syringoma
  EXCLUDES skin of genital organs (221.0-222.9)

216.0 Skin of lip
  EXCLUDES vermilion border of lip (210.0)
216.1 Eyelid, including canthus
  EXCLUDES cartilage of eyelid (215.0)
216.2 Ear and external auditory canal
  Auricle (ear) External meatus
  Auricular canal, external Pinna
  EXCLUDES cartilage of ear (215.0)
◆ **216.3 Skin of other and unspecified parts of face**
  Cheek, external
  Eyebrow
  Nose, external
  Temple
216.4 Scalp and skin of neck

NEOPLASMS

216.5 Skin of trunk, except scrotum
- Axillary fold
- Perianal skin
- Skin of:
  - abdominal wall
  - anus
  - back
  - breast
- Skin of:
  - buttock
  - chest wall
  - groin
  - perineum
  - Umbilicus

EXCLUDES anal canal (211.4)
anus NOS (211.4)
skin of scrotum (222.4)

216.6 Skin of upper limb, including shoulder
216.7 Skin of lower limb, including hip
◆ **216.8 Other specified sites of skin**
◆ **216.9 Skin, site unspecified**

217 Benign neoplasm of breast
- Breast (male) (female)
  - connective tissue
  - glandular tissue
  - soft parts

EXCLUDES adenofibrosis (610.2)
benign cyst of breast (610.0)
fibrocystic disease (610.1)
skin of breast (216.5)

● **218 Uterine leiomyoma**
INCLUDES fibroid (bleeding) (uterine)
uterine:
  fibromyoma
  myoma

218.0 Submucous leiomyoma of uterus
218.1 Intramural leiomyoma of uterus
- Interstitial leiomyoma of uterus
218.2 Subserous leiomyoma of uterus
◆ **218.9 Leiomyoma of uterus, unspecified**

● **219 Other benign neoplasm of uterus**
219.0 Cervix uteri
219.1 Corpus uteri
- Endometrium
- Fundus
- Myometrium

◆ **219.8 Other specified parts of uterus**
◆ **219.9 Uterus, part unspecified**

220 Benign neoplasm of ovary
Use additional code, if desired, to identify any functional activity (256.0-256.1)

EXCLUDES cyst:
corpus albicans (620.2)
corpus luteum (620.1)
endometrial (617.1)
follicular (atretic) (620.0)
graafian follicle (620.0)
ovarian NOS (620.2)
retention (620.2)

● **221 Benign neoplasm of other female genital organs**
INCLUDES adenomatous polyp
benign teratoma

EXCLUDES cyst:
epoophoron (752.11)
fimbrial (752.11)
Gartner's duct (752.11)
parovarian (752.11)

221.0 Fallopian tube and uterine ligaments
- Oviduct
- Parametruim
- Uterine ligament (broad) (round) (uterosacral)
- Uterine tube

221.1 Vagina
221.2 Vulva
- Clitoris
- External female genitalia NOS
- Greater vestibular [Bartholin's] gland
- Labia (majora) (minora)
- Pudendum

EXCLUDES Bartholin's (duct) (gland) cyst (616.2)

◆ **221.8 Other specified sites of female genital organs**
◆ **221.9 Female genital organ, site unspecified**
- Female genitourinary tract NOS

● **222 Benign neoplasm of male genital organs**
222.0 Testis
Use additional code, if desired, to identify any functional activity

222.1 Penis
- Corpus cavernosum
- Glans penis
- Prepuce

222.2 Prostate
EXCLUDES adenomatous hyperplasia of prostate (600)
prostatic:
  adenoma (600)
  enlargement (600)
  hypertrophy (600)

222.3 Epididymis
222.4 Scrotum
- Skin of scrotum

◆ **222.8 Other specified sites of male genital organs**
- Seminal vesicle
- Spermatic cord

◆ **222.9 Male genital organ, site unspecified**
- Male genitourinary tract NOS

● **223 Benign neoplasm of kidney and other urinary organs**
223.0 Kidney, except pelvis
- Kidney NOS

EXCLUDES renal:
calyces (223.1)
pelvis (223.1)

223.1 Renal pelvis
223.2 Ureter
EXCLUDES ureteric orifice of bladder (223.3)

223.3 Bladder
● **223.8 Other specified sites of urinary organs**
223.81 Urethra
EXCLUDES urethral orifice of bladder (223.3)
◆ **223.89 Other**

◆ **223.9 Urinary organ, site unspecified**
- Urinary system NOS

● **224 Benign neoplasm of eye**
EXCLUDES cartilage of eyelid (215.0)
eyelid (skin) (216.1)
optic nerve (225.1)
orbital bone (213.0)

224.0 Eyeball, except conjunctiva, cornea, retina, and choroid
- Ciliarybody
- Iris
- Sclera
- Uveal tract

224.1 Orbit
EXCLUDES bone of orbit (213.0)

224.2 Lacrimal gland
224.3 Conjunctiva
224.4 Cornea
224.5 Retina
EXCLUDES hemangioma of retina (228.03)

224.6 Choroid
224.7 Lacrimal duct
- Lacrimal sac
- Nasolacrimal duct

◆ **224.8 Other specified parts of eye**
◆ **224.9 Eye, part unspecified**

● **225 Benign neoplasm of brain and other parts of nervous system**
EXCLUDES hemangioma (228.02)
neurofibromatosis (237.7)
peripheral, sympathetic, and parasympathetic nerves and ganglia (215.0-215.9)
retrobulbar (224.1)

225.0 Brain
225.1 Cranial nerves
225.2 Cerebral meninges
- Meninges NOS
- Meningioma (cerebral)

225.3 Spinal cord
- Cauda equina

225.4 Spinal meninges
- Spinal meningioma

◆ **225.8 Other specified sites of nervous system**
◆ **225.9 Nervous system, part unspecified**
- Nervous system (central) NOS

EXCLUDES meninges NOS (225.2)

● Additional digits required   ◆ Nonspecific code   ▌Not a primary diagnosis

226 Benign neoplasm of thyroid glands
Use additional code, if desired, to identify any functional activity

● **227 Benign neoplasm of other endocrine glands and related structures**
Use additional code, if desired, to identify any functional activity
EXCLUDES   ovary (220)
pancreas (211.6)
testis (222.0)

- 227.0 **Adrenal gland**
  Suprarenal gland
- 227.1 **Parathyroid gland**
- 227.3 **Pituitary gland and craniopharyngeal duct (pouch)**
  Craniobuccal pouch   Rathke's pouch
  Hypophysis   Sella turcica
- 227.4 **Pineal gland**
  Pineal body
- 227.5 **Carotid body**
- 227.6 **Aortic body and other paraganglia**
  Coccygeal body
  Glomus jugulare
  Para-aortic body
- ◆ 227.8 **Other**
- ◆ 227.9 **Endocrine gland, site unspecified**

● **228 Hemangioma and lymphangioma, any site**
INCLUDES   angioma (benign) (cavernous) (congenital) NOS
cavernous nevus
glomus tumor
hemangioma (benign) (congenital)
EXCLUDES   benign neoplasm of spleen, except hemangioma and lymphangioma (211.9)
glomus jugulare (227.6)
nevus:
  NOS (216.0-216.9)
  blue or pigmented (216.0-216.9)
  vascular (757.32)

- ● 228.0 **Hemangioma, any site**
  - ◆ 228.00 Of unspecified site
  -   228.01 Of skin and subcutaneous tissue
  -   228.02 Of intracranial structures
  -   228.03 Of retina
  -   228.04 Of intra-abdominal structures
      Peritoneum   Retroperitoneal tissue
  - ◆ 228.09 Of other sites
      Systemic angiomatosis
- 228.1 **Lymphangioma, any site**
  Congenital lymphangioma   Lymphatic nevus

● **229 Benign neoplasm of other and unspecified sites**
- 229.0 **Lymph nodes**
  EXCLUDES   lymphangioma (228.1)
- ◆ 229.8 **Other specified sites**
  Intrathoracic NOS
  Thoracic NOS
- ◆ 229.9 **Site unspecified**

CARCINOMA IN SITU (230-234)

INCLUDES   Bowen's disease
erythroplasia
Queyrat's erythroplasia
EXCLUDES   leukoplakia—see Alphabetic Index

● **230 Carcinoma in situ of digestive organs**
- 230.0 **Lip, oral cavity, and pharynx**
  Gingiva   Oropharynx
  Hypopharynx   Salivary gland or duct
  Mouth [any part] Tongue
  Nasopharynx
  EXCLUDES   aryepiglottic fold or interarytenoid fold, laryngeal aspect (231.0)
  epiglottis:
    NOS (231.0)
    suprahyoid portion (231.0)
  skin of lip (232.0)
- 230.1 **Esophagus**
- 230.2 **Stomach**
  Body ⎫
  Cardia ⎬ of stomach
  Fundus ⎭
  Cardiac orifice
  Pylorus
- 230.3 **Colon**
  Appendix   Ileocecal valve
  Cecum   Large intestine NOS
  EXCLUDES   rectosigmoid junction (230.4)
- 230.4 **Rectum**
  Rectosigmoid junction
- 230.5 **Anal canal**
  Anal sphincter
- ◆ 230.6 **Anus, unspecified**
  EXCLUDES   anus:
    margin (232.5)
    skin (232.5)
  perianal skin (232.5)
- ◆ 230.7 **Other and unspecified parts of intestine**
  Duodenum   Jejunum
  Ileum   Small intestine NOS
  EXCLUDES   ampulla of Vater (230.8)
- 230.8 **Liver and biliary system**
  Ampulla of Vater   Gallbladder
  Common bile duct   Hepatic duct
  Cystic duct   Sphincter of Oddi
- ◆ 230.9 **Other and unspecified digestive organs**
  Digestive organ NOS   Pancreas
  Gastrointestinal tract NOS Spleen

● **231 Carcinoma in situ of respiratory system**
- 231.0 **Larynx**
  Cartilage: Epiglottis:
    arytenoid   NOS
    cricoid   posterior surface
    cuneiform   suprahyoid portion
    thyroid   Vocal cords (false) (true)
  EXCLUDES   aryepiglottic fold or interarytenoid fold:
    NOS (230.0)
    hypopharyngeal aspect (230.0)
    marginal zone (230.0)
- 231.1 **Trachea**
- 231.2 **Bronchus and lung**
  Carina
  Hilus of lung
- ◆ 231.8 **Other specified parts of respiratory system**
  Accessory sinuses   Nasal cavities
  Middle ear   Pleura
  EXCLUDES   ear (external) (skin) (232.2)
  nose NOS (234.8)
  skin (232.3)
- ◆ 231.9 **Respiratory system, part unspecified**
  Respiratory organ NOS

● **232 Carcinoma in situ of skin**
INCLUDES   pigment cells
- 232.0 **Skin of lip**
  EXCLUDES   vermilion border of lip (230.0)
- 232.1 **Eyelid, including canthus**
- 232.2 **Ear and external auditory canal**
- ◆ 232.3 **Skin of other and unspecified parts of face**
- 232.4 **Scalp and skin of neck**
- 232.5 **Skin of trunk, except scrotum**
  Anus, margin   Skin of:
  Axillary fold   breast
  Perianal skin   buttock
  Skin of: chest wall
    abdominal wall   groin
    anus   perineum
    back   Umbilicus
  EXCLUDES   anal canal (230.5)
  anus NOS (230.6)
  skin of genital organs (233.3, 233.5-233.6)
- 232.6 **Skin of upper limb, including shoulder**
- 232.7 **Skin of lower limb, including hip**
- ◆ 232.8 **Other specified sites of skin**
- ◆ 232.9 **Skin, site unspecified**

● **233 Carcinoma in situ of breast and genitourinary system**
- 233.0 **Breast**
  EXCLUDES   Paget's disease (174.0-174.9)
  skin of breast (232.5)
- 233.1 **Cervix uteri**
- ◆ 233.2 **Other and unspecified parts of uterus**
- ◆ 233.3 **Other and unspecified female genital organs**

- 233.4 Prostate
- 233.5 Penis
- ◆ 233.6 Other and unspecified male genital organs
- 233.7 Bladder
- ◆ 233.9 Other and unspecified urinary organs
- ● 234 Carcinoma in situ of other and unspecified sites
  - 234.0 Eye
    - EXCLUDES: cartilage of eyelid (234.8)
      - eyelid (skin) (232.1)
      - optic nerve (234.8)
      - orbital bone (234.8)
  - ◆ 234.8 Other specified sites
    - Endocrine gland [any]
  - ◆ 234.9 Site unspecified
    - Carcinoma in situ NOS

NEOPLASMS OF UNCERTAIN BEHAVIOR (235-238)

Note: Categories 235–238 classify by site certain histomorphologically well-defined neoplasms, the subsequent behavior of which cannot be predicted from the present appearance.

- ● 235 Neoplasm of uncertain behavior of digestive and respiratory systems
  - 235.0 Major salivary glands
    - Gland:
      - parotid
      - sublingual
      - submandibular
    - EXCLUDES: minor salivary glands (235.1)
  - 235.1 Lip, oral cavity, and pharynx
    - Gingiva
    - Hypopharynx
    - Minor salivary glands
    - Mouth
    - Nasopharynx
    - Oropharynx
    - Tongue
    - EXCLUDES: aryepiglottic fold or interarytenoid fold, laryngeal aspect (235.6)
      - epiglottis:
        - NOS (235.6)
        - suprahyoid portion (235.6)
      - skin of lip (238.2)
  - 235.2 Stomach, intestines, and rectum
  - 235.3 Liver and biliary passages
    - Ampulla of Vater
    - Bile ducts [any]
    - Gallbladder
    - Liver
  - 235.4 Retroperitoneum and peritoneum
  - ◆ 235.5 Other and unspecified digestive organs
    - Anal:
      - canal
      - sphincter
    - Anus NOS
    - Esophagus
    - Pancreas
    - Spleen
    - EXCLUDES: anus:
      - margin (238.2)
      - skin (238.2)
      - perianal skin (238.2)
  - 235.6 Larynx
    - EXCLUDES: aryepiglottic fold or interarytenoid fold:
      - NOS (235.1)
      - hypopharyngeal aspect (235.1)
      - marginal zone (235.1)
  - 235.7 Trachea, bronchus, and lung
  - 235.8 Pleura, thymus, and mediastinum
  - ◆ 235.9 Other and unspecified respiratory organs
    - Accessory sinuses
    - Middle ear
    - Nasal cavities
    - Respiratory organ NOS
    - EXCLUDES: ear (external) (skin) (238.2)
      - nose (238.8)
      - skin (238.2)
- ● 236 Neoplasm of uncertain behavior of genitourinary organs
  - 236.0 Uterus
  - 236.1 Placenta
    - Chorioadenoma (destruens)
    - Invasive mole
    - Malignant hydatid(iform) mole
  - 236.2 Ovary
    - Use additional code, if desired, to identify any functional activity
  - ◆ 236.3 Other and unspecified female genital organs
  - 236.4 Testis
    - Use additional code, if desired, to identify any functional activity
  - 236.5 Prostate
  - ◆ 236.6 Other and unspecified male genital organs
  - 236.7 Bladder
  - ● 236.9 Other and unspecified urinary organs
    - ◆ 236.90 Urinary organ, unspecified
    - 236.91 Kidney and ureter
    - ◆ 236.99 Other
- ● 237 Neoplasm of uncertain behavior of endocrine glands and nervous system
  - 237.0 Pituitary gland and craniopharyngeal duct
    - Use additional code, if desired, to identify any functional activity
  - 237.1 Pineal gland
  - 237.2 Adrenal gland
    - Suprarenal gland
    - Use additional code, if desired, to identify any functional activity
  - 237.3 Paraganglia
    - Aortic body
    - Carotid body
    - Coccygeal body
    - Glomus jugulare
  - ◆ 237.4 Other and unspecified endocrine glands
    - Parathyroid gland
    - Thyroid gland
  - 237.5 Brain and spinal cord
  - 237.6 Meninges
    - Meninges:
      - NOS
      - cerebral
      - spinal
  - ● 237.7 Neurofibromatosis
    - von Recklinghausen's disease
    - ◆ 237.70 Neurofibromatosis, unspecified
    - 237.71 Neurofibromatosis, Type 1 [von Recklinghausen's disease]
    - 237.72 Neurofibromatosis, Type 2 [acoustic neurofibromatosis]
  - ◆ 237.9 Other and unspecified parts of nervous system
    - Cranial nerves
    - EXCLUDES: peripheral, sympathetic, and parasympathetic nerves and ganglia (238.1)
- ● 238 Neoplasm of uncertain behavior of other and unspecified sites and tissues
  - 238.0 Bone and articular cartilage
    - EXCLUDES: cartilage:
      - ear (238.1)
      - eyelid (238.1)
      - larynx (235.6)
      - nose (235.9)
      - synovia (238.1)
  - ◆ 238.1 Connective and other soft tissue
    - Peripheral, sympathetic, and parasympathetic nerves and ganglia
    - EXCLUDES: cartilage (of):
      - articular (238.0)
      - larynx (235.6)
      - nose (235.9)
      - connective tissue of breast (238.3)
  - 238.2 Skin
    - EXCLUDES: anus NOS (235.5)
      - skin of genital organs (236.3, 236.6)
      - vermilion border of lip (235.1)
  - 238.3 Breast
    - EXCLUDES: skin of breast (238.2)
  - 238.4 Polycythemia vera
  - 238.5 Histiocytic and mast cells
    - Mast cell tumor NOS
    - Mastocytoma NOS
  - 238.6 Plasma cells
    - Plasmacytoma NOS
    - Solitary myeloma

- **238.7 Other lymphatic and hematopoietic tissues**
  Disease:
    lymphoproliferative (chronic) NOS
    myeloproliferative (chronic) NOS
  Idiopathic thrombocythemia
  Megakaryocytic myelosclerosis
  Myelodysplastic syndrome
  Myelosclerosis with myeloid metaplasia
  Panmyelosis (acute)
  EXCLUDES myelfibrosis (289.8)
  myelosclerosis NOS (289.8)
  myelosis:
    NOS (205.9)
    megakaryocytic (207.2)

- **238.8 Other specified sites**
  Eye
  Heart
  EXCLUDES eyelid (skin) (238.2)
  cartilage (238.1)

- **238.9 Site unspecified**

NEOPLASMS OF UNSPECIFIED NATURE (239)

- **239 Neoplasms of unspecified nature**
  Note: Category 239 classifies by site neoplasms of unspecified morphology and behavior. The term "mass," unless otherwise stated, is not to be regarded as a neoplastic growth.
  INCLUDES "growth" NOS
  neoplasm NOS
  new growth NOS
  tumor NOS

  - **239.0 Digestive system**
    EXCLUDES anus:
      margin (239.2)
      skin (239.2)
      perianal skin (239.2)
  - **239.1 Respiratory system**
  - **239.2 Bone, soft tissue, and skin**
    EXCLUDES anal canal (239.0)
    anus NOS (239.0)
    bone marrow (202.9)
    cartilage:
      larynx (239.1)
      nose (239.1)
    connective tissue of breast (239.3)
    skin of genital organs (239.5)
    vermilion border of lip (239.0)
  - **239.3 Breast**
    EXCLUDES skin of breast (239.2)
  - **239.4 Bladder**
  - **239.5 Other genitourinary organs**
  - **239.6 Brain**
    EXCLUDES cerebral meninges (239.7)
    cranial nerves (239.7)
  - **239.7 Endocrine glands and other parts of nervous system**
    EXCLUDES peripheral, sympathetic, and parasympathetic nerves and ganglia (239.2)
  - **239.8 Other specified sites**
    EXCLUDES eyelid (skin) (239.2)
    cartilage (239.2)
    great vessels (239.2)
    optic nerve (239.7)
  - **239.9 Site unspecified**

3. ENDOCRINE, NUTRITIONAL AND METABOLIC DISEASES, AND IMMUNITY DISORDERS (240-279)

EXCLUDES endocrine and metabolic disturbances specific to the fetus and newborn (775.0-775.9)

Note: All neoplasms, whether functionally active or not, are classified in Chapter 2. Codes in Chapter 3 (i.e., 242.8, 246.0, 251-253, 255-259) may be used, if desired, to identify such functional activity associated with any neoplasm, or by ectopic endocrine tissue.

DISORDERS OF THYROID GLAND (240-246)

- **240 Simple and unspecified goiter**
  - **240.0 Goiter, specified as simple**
    Any condition classifiable to 240.9, specified as simple
  - **240.9 Goiter, unspecified**
    Enlargement of thyroid
    Goiter or struma:
      NOS
      diffuse colloid
      endemic
    Goiter or struma:
      hyperplastic
      nontoxic (diffuse)
      parenchymatous
      sporadic
    EXCLUDES congenital (dyshormonogenic) goiter (246.1)

- **241 Nontoxic nodular goiter**
  EXCLUDES adenoma of thyroid (226)
  cystadenoma of thyroid (226)
  - **241.0 Nontoxic uninodular goiter**
    Thyroid nodule   Uninodular goiter (nontoxic)
  - **241.1 Nontoxic multinodular goiter**
    Multinodular goiter (nontoxic)
  - **241.9 Unspecified nontoxic nodular goiter**
    Adenomatous goiter
    Nodular goiter (nontoxic) NOS
    Struma nodosa (simplex)

- **242 Thyrotoxicosis with or without goiter**
  EXCLUDES neonatal thyrotoxicosis (775.3)
  The following fifth-digit subclassification is for use with category 242:
    0 without mention of thyrotoxic crisis or storm
    1 with mention of thyrotoxic crisis or storm
  - **242.0 Toxic diffuse goiter**
    Basedow's disease
    Exophthalmic or toxic goiter NOS
    Graves' disease
    Primary thyroid hyperplasia
  - **242.1 Toxic uninodular goiter**
    Thyroid nodule ⎫
    Uninodular goiter ⎬ toxic or with hyperthyroidism
  - **242.2 Toxic multinodular goiter**
    Secondary thyroid hyperplasia
  - **242.3 Toxic nodular goiter, unspecified**
    Adenomatous goiter ⎫
    Nodular goiter ⎬ toxic or with hyperthyroidism
    Struma nodosa ⎭
    Any condition classifiable to 241.9 specified as toxic or with hyperthyroidism
  - **242.4 Thyrotoxicosis from ectopic thyroid nodule**
  - **242.8 Thyrotoxicosis of other specified origin**
    Overproduction of thyroid-stimulating hormone [TSH]
    Thyrotoxicosis:
      factitia
      from ingestion of excessive thyroid material
    Use additional E code, if desired, to identify cause, if drug-induced
  - **242.9 Thyrotoxicosis without mention of goiter or other cause**
    Hyperthyroidism NOS
    Thyrotoxicosis NOS

- **243 Congenital hypothyroidism**
  Congenital thyroid insufficiency
  Cretinism (athyrotic) (endemic)
  Use additional code, if desired, to identify associated mental retardation
  EXCLUDES congenital (dyshormonogenic) goiter (246.1)

- **244 Acquired hypothyroidism**
  INCLUDES athyroidism (acquired)
  hypothyroidism (acquired)
  myxedema (adult) (juvenile)
  thyroid (gland) insufficiency (acquired)

ENDOCRINE, NUTRITIONAL AND METABOLIC, IMMUNITY

- 244.0 Postsurgical hypothyroidism
- ◆ 244.1 Other postablative hypothyroidism
  Hypothyroidism following therapy, such as irradiation
- 244.2 Iodine hypothyroidism
  Hypothyroidism resulting from administration or ingestion of iodide
  Use additional E code, if desired, to identify drug
- ◆ 244.3 Other iatrogenic hypothyroidism
  Hypothyroidism resulting from:
  P-aminosalicylic acid [PAS]
  Phenylbutazone
  Resorcinol
  Iatrogenic hypothyroidism NOS
  Use additional E code, if desired, to identify drug
- ◆ 244.8 Other specified acquired hypothyroidism
  Secondary hypothyroidism NEC
- ◆ 244.9 Unspecified hypothyroidism
  Hypothyroidism } primary or NOS
  Myxedema

● 245 Thyroiditis
- 245.0 Acute thyroiditis
  Abscess of thyroid
  Thyroiditis:
    nonsuppurative, acute
    pyogenic
    suppurative
  Use additional code, if desired, to identify organism
- 245.1 Subacute thyroiditis
  Thyroiditis: Thyroiditis:
    de Quervain's   granulomatous
    giant cell   viral
- 245.2 Chronic lymphocytic thyroiditis
  Hashimoto's disease   Thyroiditis:
  Struma lymphomatosa   autoimmune
                           lymphocytic (chronic)
- 245.3 Chronic fibrous thyroiditis
  Struma fibrosa   Thyroiditis:
  Thyroiditis: ligneous
    invasive (fibrous)   Riedel's
- 245.4 Iatrogenic thyroiditis
  Use additional code, if desired, to identify cause
- ◆ 245.8 Other and unspecified chronic thyroiditis
  Chronic thyroiditis:
    NOS
    nonspecific
- ◆ 245.9 Thyroiditis, unspecified
  Thyroiditis NOS

● 246 Other disorders of thyroid
- 246.0 Disorders of thyrocalcitonin secretion
  Hypersecretion of calcitonin or thyrocalcitonin
- 246.1 Dyshormonogenic goiter
  Congenital (dyshormonogenic) goiter
  Goiter due to enzyme defect in synthesis of thyroid hormone
  Goitrous cretinism (sporadic)
- 246.2 Cyst of thyroid
  EXCLUDES cystadenoma of thyroid (226)
- 246.3 Hemorrhage and infarction of thyroid
- ◆ 246.8 Other specified disorders of thyroid
  Abnormality of thyroid-binding globulin
  Atrophy of thyroid
  Hyper-TBG-nemia
  Hypo-TBG-nemia
- ◆ 246.9 Unspecified disorder of thyroid

DISEASES OF OTHER ENDOCRINE GLANDS (250-259)

● 250 Diabetes mellitus
  EXCLUDES gestational diabetes (648.8)
  hyperglycemia NOS (790.6)
  neonatal diabetes mellitus (775.1)
  nonclinical diabetes (790.2)
  that complicating pregnancy, childbirth, or the puerperium (648.0)

  The following fifth-digit subclassification is for use with category 250:
  0 type II [non-insulin dependent type] [NIDDM type] [adult-onset type] or unspecified type, not stated as uncontrolled
  1 type I [insulin dependent type] [IDDM] [juvenile type], not stated as uncontrolled
  2 type II [non-insulin dependent type] [NIDDM type] [adult-onset type] or unspecified type, uncontrolled
  3 type I [insulin dependent type] [IDDM] [juvenile type], uncontrolled

● 250.0 Diabetes mellitus without mention of complication
  Diabetes mellitus without mention of complication or manifestation classifiable to 250.1-250.9
  Diabetes (mellitus) NOS
● 250.1 Diabetes with ketoacidosis
  Diabetic:
    acidosis } without mention of coma
    ketosis
● 250.2 Diabetes with hyperosmolarity
  Hyperosmolar (nonketotic) coma
● 250.3 Diabetes with other coma
  Diabetic coma (with ketoacidosis)
  Diabetic hypoglycemic coma
  Insulin coma NOS
  EXCLUDES diabetes with hyperosmolar coma (250.2)
● 250.4 Diabetes with renal manifestations
  Use additional code, if desired, to identify manifestation, as:
  diabetic:
    nephropathy NOS (583.81)
    nephrosis (581.81)
    intercapillary glomerulosclerosis (581.81)
    Kimmelstiel-Wilson syndrome (581.81)
● 250.5 Diabetes with ophthalmic manifestations
  Use additional code, if desired, to identify manifestation, as:
  diabetic:
    blindness (369.00-369.9)
    cataract (366.41)
    glaucoma (365.44)
    retinal edema (362.83)
    retinopathy (362.01-362.02)
● 250.6 Diabetes with neurological manifestations
  Use additional code, if desired, to identify manifestation, as:
  diabetic:
    amyotrophy (358.1)
    mononeuropathy (354.0-355.9)
    neurogenic arthropathy (713.5)
    peripheral autonomic neuropathy (337.1)
    polyneuropathy (357.2)
● 250.7 Diabetes with peripheral circulatory disorders
  Use additional code, if desired, to identify manifestation, as:
  diabetic:
    gangrene (785.4)
    peripheral angiopathy (443.81)
◆● 250.8 Diabetes with other specified manifestations
  Diabetic hypoglycemia
  Hypoglycemic shock
  Use additional code, if desired, to identify manifestation, as:
    diabetic bone changes (731.8)
  Use additional E code, if desired, to identify cause, if drug-induced.
  EXCLUDES intercurrent infections in diabetic patients
◆● 250.9 Diabetes with unspecified complication

● Additional digits required   ◆ Nonspecific code   ▌Not a primary diagnosis

251 Other disorders of pancreatic internal secretion

251.0 Hypoglycemic coma
Iatrogenic hyperinsulinism
Non-diabetic insulin coma
Use additional E code, if desired, to identify cause, if drug-induced
EXCLUDES hypoglycemic coma in diabetes mellitus (250.3)

251.1 Other specified hypoglycemia
Hyperinsulinism:
  NOS
  ectopic
  functional
Hyperplasia of pancreatic islet beta cells NOS
EXCLUDES hypoglycemia:
  in diabetes mellitus (250.8)
  in infant of diabetic mother (775.0)
  neonatal hypoglycemia (775.6)
  hypoglycemic coma (251.0)
Use additional E code, if desired, to identify cause, if drug-induced.

251.2 Hypoglycemia, unspecified
Hypoglycemia:
  NOS
  reactive
  spontaneous
EXCLUDES hypoglycemia:
  with coma (251.0)
  in diabetes mellitus (250.8)
  leucine-induced (270.3)

251.3 Postsurgical hypoinsulinemia
Hypoinsulinemia following complete or partial pancreatectomy
Postpancreatectomy hyperglycemia

251.4 Abnormality of secretion of glucagon
Hyperplasia of pancreatic islet alpha cells with glucagon excess

251.5 Abnormality of secretion of gastrin
Hyperplasia of pancreatic alpha cells with gastrin excess
Zollinger-Ellison syndrome

251.8 Other specified disorders of pancreatic internal secretion

251.9 Unspecified disorder of pancreatic internal secretion
Islet cell hyperplasia NOS

252 Disorders of parathyroid gland

252.0 Hyperparathyroidism
Hyperplasia of parathyroid
Osteitis fibrosa cystica generalisata
von Recklinghausen's disease of bone
EXCLUDES ectopic hyperparathyroidism (259.3)
  secondary hyperparathyroidism (of renal origin) (588.8)

252.1 Hypoparathyroidism
Parathyroiditis (autoimmune)
Tetany:
  parathyroid
  parathyroprival
EXCLUDES pseudohypoparathyroidism (275.4)
  pseudopseudohypoparathyroidism (275.4)
  tetany NOS (781.7)
  transitory neonatal hypoparathyroidism (775.4)

252.8 Other specified disorders of parathyroid gland
Cyst
Hemorrhage of parathyroid gland

252.9 Unspecified disorder of parathyroid gland

253 Disorders of the pituitary gland and its hypothalamic control
INCLUDES the listed conditions whether the disorder is in the pituitary or the hypothalamus
EXCLUDES Cushing's syndrome (255.0)

253.0 Acromegaly and gigantism
Overproduction of growth hormone

253.1 Other and unspecified anterior pituitary hyperfunction
Forbes-Albright syndrome
EXCLUDES overproduction of:
  ACTH (255.3)
  thyroid-stimulating hormone [TSH] (242.8)

253.2 Panhypopituitarism
Cachexia, pituitary
Necrosis of pituitary (postpartum)
Pituitary insufficiency NOS
Sheehan's syndrome
Simmonds' disease
EXCLUDES iatrogenic hypopituitarism (253.7)

253.3 Pituitary dwarfism
Isolated deficiency of (human) growth hormone [HGH]
Lorain-Levi dwarfism

253.4 Other anterior pituitary disorders
Isolated or partial deficiency of an anterior pituitary hormone, other than growth hormone
Prolactin deficiency

253.5 Diabetes insipidus
Vasopressin deficiency
EXCLUDES nephrogenic diabetes insipidus (588.1)

253.6 Other disorders of neurohypophysis
Syndrome of inappropriate secretion of antidiuretic hormone [ADH]
EXCLUDES ectopic antidiuretic hormone secretion (259.3)

253.7 Iatrogenic pituitary disorders
Hypopituitarism:
  hormone-induced
  hypophysectomy-induced
Hypopituitarism:
  postablative
  radiotherapy-induced
Use additional E code, if desired, to identify cause

253.8 Other disorders of the pituitary and other syndromes of diencephalohypophyseal origin
Abscess of pituitary
Adiposogenital dystrophy
Cyst of Rathke's pouch
Fröhlich's syndrome
EXCLUDES craniopharyngioma (237.0)

253.9 Unspecified
Dyspituitarism

254 Diseases of thymus gland
EXCLUDES aplasia or dysplasia with immunodeficiency (279.2)
  hypoplasia with immunodeficiency (279.2)
  myastheniagravis (358.0)

254.0 Persistent hyperplasia of thymus
Hypertrophy of thymus

254.1 Abscess of thymus

254.8 Other specified diseases of thymus gland
Atrophy
Cyst of thymus
EXCLUDES thymoma (212.6)

254.9 Unspecified disease of thymus gland

255 Disorders of adrenal glands
INCLUDES the listed conditions whether the basic disorder is in the adrenals or is pituitary-induced

255.0 Cushing's syndrome
Adrenal hyperplasia due to excess ACTH
Cushing's syndrome:
  NOS
  iatrogenic
  idiopathic
  pituitary-dependent
Ectopic ACTH syndrome
Iatrogenic syndrome of excess cortisol
Overproduction of cortisolf
Use additional E code, if desired, to identify cause, if drug-induced
EXCLUDES congenital adrenal hyperplasia (255.2)

255.1 Hyperaldosteronism
Aldosteronism (primary) (secondary)
Bartter's syndrome
Conn's syndrome

255.2 Adrenogenital disorders
Achard-Thiers syndrome
Adrenogenital syndromes, virilizing or feminizing, whether acquired or associated with congenital adrenal hyperplasia consequent on inborn enzyme defects in hormone synthesis
Congenital adrenal hyperplasia
Female adrenal pseudohermaphroditism
Male:
  macrogenitosomia praecox
  sexual precocity with adrenal hyperplasia
Virilization (female) (suprarenal)
EXCLUDES adrenal hyperplasia due to excess ACTH (255.0)
  isosexual virilization (256.4)

ENDOCRINE, NUTRITIONAL AND METABOLIC, IMMUNITY

- ◆ 255.3 **Other corticoadrenal overactivity**
  - Acquired benign adrenal androgenic overactivity
  - Overproduction of ACTH
- 255.4 **Corticoadrenal insufficiency**
  - Addisonian crisis
  - Addison's disease NOS
  - Adrenal:
    - atrophy (autoimmune)
    - calcification
  - Adrenal:
    - crisis
    - hemorrhage
    - infarction
    - insufficiency NOS
  - EXCLUDES tuberculous Addison's disease (017.6)
- ◆ 255.5 **Other adrenal hypofunction**
  - Adrenal medullary insufficiency
  - EXCLUDES Waterhouse-Friderichsen syndrome (meningococcal) (036.3)
- 255.6 **Medulloadrenal hyperfunction**
  - Catecholamine secretion by pheochromocytoma
- ◆ 255.8 **Other specified disorders of adrenal glands**
  - Abnormality of cortisol-binding globulin
- ◆ 255.9 **Unspecified disorder of adrenal glands**
- ● 256 **Ovarian dysfunction**
  - 256.0 **Hyperestrogenism**
  - ◆ 256.1 **Other ovarian hyperfunction**
    - Hypersecretion of ovarian androgens
  - 256.2 **Postablative ovarian failure**
    - Ovarian failure:
      - iatrogenic
      - postirradiation
      - postsurgical
  - 256.3 **Other ovarian failure**
    - Premature menopause NOS
    - Primary ovarian failure
  - 256.4 **Polycystic ovaries**
    - Isosexual virilization
    - Stein-Leventhal syndrome
  - ◆ 256.8 **Other ovarian dysfunction**
  - ◆ 256.9 **Unspecified ovarian dysfunction**
- ● 257 **Testicular dysfunction**
  - 257.0 **Testicular hyperfunction**
    - Hypersecretion of testicular hormones
  - 257.1 **Postablative testicular hypofunction**
    - Testicular hypofunction:
      - iatrogenic
      - postirradiation
      - postsurgical
  - ◆ 257.2 **Other testicular hypofunction**
    - Defective biosynthesis of testicular androgen
    - Eunuchoidism:
      - NOS
      - hypogonadotropic
    - Failure:
      - Leydig's cell, adult
      - seminiferous tubule, adult
    - Testicular hypogonadism
    - EXCLUDES azoospermia (606.0)
  - ◆ 257.8 **Other testicular dysfunction**
    - Goldberg-Maxwell syndrome
    - Male pseudohermaphroditism with testicular feminization
    - Testicular feminization
  - ◆ 257.9 **Unspecified testicular dysfunction**
- ● 258 **Polyglandular dysfunction and related disorders**
  - 258.0 **Polyglandular activity in multiple endocrine adenomatosis**
    - Wermer's syndrome
  - ◆ 258.1 **Other combinations of endocrine dysfunction**
    - Lloyd's syndrome
    - Schmidt's syndrome
  - ◆ 258.8 **Other specified polyglandular dysfunction**
  - ◆ 258.9 **Polyglandular dysfunction, unspecified**
- ● 259 **Other endocrine disorders**
  - 259.0 **Delay in sexual development and puberty, not elsewhere classified**
    - Delayed puberty
  - 259.1 **Precocious sexual development and puberty, not elsewhere classified**
    - Sexual precocity:
      - NOS
      - constitutional
    - Sexual precocity:
      - cryptogenic
      - idiopathic
  - 259.2 **Carcinoid syndrome**
    - Hormone secretion by carcinoid tumors
  - 259.3 **Ectopic hormone secretion, not elsewhere classified**
    - Ectopic:
      - antidiuretic hormone secretion [ADH]
      - hyperparathyroidism
    - EXCLUDES ectopic ACTH syndrome (255.0)
  - 259.4 **Dwarfism, not elsewhere classified**
    - Dwarfism:
      - NOS
      - constitutional
    - EXCLUDES dwarfism:
      - achondroplastic (756.4)
      - intrauterine (759.7)
      - nutritional (263.2)
      - pituitary (253.3)
      - renal (588.0)
      - progeria (259.8)
  - ◆ 259.8 **Other specified endocrine disorders**
    - Pineal gland dysfunction
    - Progeria
    - Werner's syndrome
  - ◆ 259.9 **Unspecified endocrine disorder**
    - Disturbance:
      - endocrine NOS
      - hormone NOS
    - Infantilism NOS

NUTRITIONAL DEFICIENCIES (260-269)

EXCLUDES deficiency anemias (280.0-281.9)

- 260 **Kwashiorkor**
  - Nutritional edema with dyspigmentation of skin and hair
- 261 **Nutritional marasmus**
  - Nutritional atrophy
  - Severe calorie deficiency
  - Severe malnutrition NOS
- ● 262 **Other severe, protein-calorie malnutrition**
  - Nutritional edema without mention of dyspigmentation of skin and hair
- ● 263 **Other and unspecified protein-calorie malnutrition**
  - 263.0 **Malnutrition of moderate degree**
  - 263.1 **Malnutrition of mild degree**
  - 263.2 **Arrested development following protein-calorie malnutrition**
    - Nutritional dwarfism
    - Physical retardation due to malnutrition
  - ◆ 263.8 **Other protein-calorie malnutrition**
  - ◆ 263.9 **Unspecified protein-calorie malnutrition**
    - Dystrophy due to malnutrition
    - Malnutrition (calorie) NOS
    - EXCLUDES nutritional deficiency NOS (269.9)
- ● 264 **Vitamin A deficiency**
  - 264.0 **With conjunctival xerosis**
  - 264.1 **With conjunctival xerosis and Bitot's spot**
    - Bitot's spot in the young child
  - 264.2 **With corneal xerosis**
  - 264.3 **With corneal ulceration and xerosis**
  - 264.4 **With keratomalacia**
  - 264.5 **With night blindness**
  - 264.6 **With xerophthalmic scars of cornea**
  - 264.7 **Other ocular manifestations of vitamin A deficiency**
    - Xerophthalmia due to vitamin A deficiency
  - ◆ 264.8 **Other manifestations of vitamin A deficiency**
    - Follicular keratosis | due to vitamin A
    - Xeroderma | deficiency
  - ◆ 264.9 **Unspecified vitamin A deficiency**
    - Hypovitaminosis A NOS
- ● 265 **Thiamine and niacin deficiency states**
  - 265.0 **Beriberi**
  - ◆ 265.1 **Other and unspecified manifestations of thiamine deficiency**
    - Other vitamin B_1 deficiency states
  - 265.2 **Pellagra**
    - Deficiency:
      - niacin (-tryptophan)
      - nicotinamide
      - nicotinic acid
    - Deficiency:
      - vitamin PP
      - Pellagra (alcoholic)
- ● 266 **Deficiency of B-complex components**
  - 266.0 **Ariboflavinosis**
    - Riboflavin [vitamin B_2] deficiency

● Additional digits required   ◆ Nonspecific code   ∎ Not a primary diagnosis

266.1 Vitamin B$_6$ deficiency
Deficiency:
 pyridoxal
 pyridoxamine
 pyridoxine
Vitamin B$_6$ deficiency syndrome
EXCLUDES *vitamin B$_6$-responsive sideroblastic anemia (285.0)*

● **266.2 Other B-complex deficiencies**
Deficiency:
 cyanocobalamin
 folic acid
Deficiency:
 vitamin B$_{12}$
EXCLUDES *combined system disease with anemia (281.0-281.1)*
deficiency anemias (281.0-281.9)
subacute degeneration of spinal cord with anemia (281.0-281.1)

266.9 Unspecified vitamin B deficiency

267 Ascorbic acid deficiency
Deficiency of vitamin C
Scurvy
EXCLUDES *scorbutic anemia (281.8)*

● **268 Vitamin D deficiency**
EXCLUDES *vitamin D-resistant:*
 osteomalacia (275.3)
 rickets (275.3)

268.0 Rickets, active
EXCLUDES *celiac rickets (579.0)*
renal rickets (588.0)

268.1 Rickets, late effect
Any condition specified as due to rickets and stated to be a late effect or sequela of rickets
Use additional code, if desired, to identify the nature of late effect

◆ **268.2 Osteomalacia, unspecified**
◆ **268.9 Unspecified vitamin D deficiency**
Avitaminosis D

● **269 Other nutritional deficiencies**

269.0 Deficiency of vitamin K
EXCLUDES *deficiency of coagulation factor due to vitamin K deficiency (286.7)*
vitamin K deficiency of newborn (776.0)

◆ **269.1 Deficiency of other vitamins**
Deficiency:
 vitamin E
 vitamin P

◆ **269.2 Unspecified vitamin deficiency**
Multiple vitamin deficiency NOS

269.3 Mineral deficiency, not elsewhere classified
Deficiency:
 calcium, dietary
 iodine
EXCLUDES *deficiency:*
 calcium NOS (275.4)
 potassium (276.8)
 sodium (276.1)

◆ **269.8 Other nutritional deficiency**
EXCLUDES *failure to thrive (783.4)*
feeding problems (783.3)
newborn (779.3)

◆ **269.9 Unspecified nutritional deficiency**

OTHER METABOLIC AND IMMUNITY DISORDERS (270-279)
Use additional code, if desired, to identify any associated mental retardation

● **270 Disorders of amino-acid transport and metabolism**
EXCLUDES *abnormal findings without manifest disease (790.0-796.9)*
disorders of purine and pyrimidine metabolism (277.1-277.2)
gout (274.0-274.9)

270.0 Disturbances of amino-acid transport
Cystinosis
Cystinuria
Fanconi (-de Toni) (-Debré) syndrome
Glycinuria (renal)
Hartnup disease

270.1 Phenylketonuria [PKU]
Hyperphenylalaninemia

◆ **270.2 Other disturbances of aromatic amino-acid metabolism**
Albinism
Alkaptonuria
Alkaptonuric ochronosis
Disturbances of metabolism of tyrosine and tryptophan
Homogentisic acid defects
Hydroxykynureninuria
Hypertyrosinemia
Indicanuria
Kynureninase defects
Oasthouse urine disease
Ochronosis
Tyrosinosis
Tyrosinuria
Waardenburg syndrome
EXCLUDES *vitamin B$_6$-deficiency syndrome (266.1)*

270.3 Disturbances of branched-chain amino-acid metabolism
Disturbances of metabolism of leucine, isoleucine, and valine
Hypervalinemia
Intermittent branched-chain ketonuria
Leucine-induced hypoglycemia
Leucinosis
Maple syrup urine disease

270.4 Disturbances of sulphur-bearing amino-acid metabolism
Cystathioninemia
Cystathioninuria
Disturbances of metabolism of methionine, homocystine, and cystathionine
Homocystinuria
Hypermethioninemia
Methioninemia

270.5 Disturbances of histidine metabolism
Carnosinemia
Histidinemia
Hyperhistidinemia
Imidazole aminoaciduria

270.6 Disorders of urea cycle metabolism
Argininosuccinic aciduria
Citrullinemia
Disorders of metabolism of ornithine, citrulline, argininosuccinic acid, arginine, and ammonia
Hyperammonemia
Hyperornithinemia

◆ **270.7 Other disturbances of straight-chain amino-acid metabolism**
Glucoglycinuria
Glycinemia (with methyl-malonic acidemia)
Hyperglycinemia
Hyperlysinemia
Other disturbances of metabolism of glycine, threonine, serine, glutamine, and lysine
Pipecolic acidemia
Saccharopinuria

◆ **270.8 Other specified disorders of amino-acid metabolism**
Alaninemia
Ethanolaminuria
Glycoprolinuria
Hydroxyprolinemia
Hyperprolinemia
Iminoacidopathy
Prolinemia
Prolinuria
Sarcosinemia

◆ **270.9 Unspecified disorder of amino-acid metabolism**

● **271 Disorders of carbohydrate transport and metabolism**
EXCLUDES *abnormality of secretion of glucagon (251.4)*
diabetes mellitus (250.0-250.9)
hypoglycemia NOS (251.2)
mucopolysaccharidosis (277.5)

271.0 Glycogenosis
Amylopectinosis
Glucose-6-phosphatase deficiency
Glycogen storage disease
McArdle's disease
Pompe's disease
von Gierke's disease

271.1 Galactosemia
Galactose-1-phosphate uridyl transferase deficiency
Galactosuria

271.2 Hereditary fructose intolerance
Essential benign fructosuria
Fructosemia

271.3 Intestinal disaccharidase deficiencies and disaccharide malabsorption
Intolerance or malabsorption (congenital) (of):
 glucose-galactose
 lactose
 sucrose-isomaltose

271.4 Renal glycosuria
Renal diabetes

◆ **271.8 Other specified disorders of carbohydrate transport and metabolism**
Essential benign pentosuria
Fucosidosis
Glycolic aciduria
Hyperoxaluria (primary)
Mannosidosis
Oxalosis
Xylosuria
Xylulosuria

ENDOCRINE, NUTRITIONAL AND METABOLIC, IMMUNITY

- ◆ **271.9** Unspecified disorder of carbohydrate transport and metabolism
- ● **272 Disorders of lipoid metabolism**
  - EXCLUDES: *localized cerebral lipidoses (330.1)*
  - **272.0 Pure hypercholesterolemia**
    - Familial hypercholesterolemia
    - Fredrickson Type IIa hyperlipoproteinemia
    - Hyperbetalipoproteinemia
    - Hyperlipidemia, Group A
    - Low-density-lipoid-type [LDL] hyperlipoproteinemia
  - **272.1 Pure hyperglyceridemia**
    - Endogenous hyperglyceridemia
    - Fredrickson Type IV hyperlipoproteinemia
    - Hyperlipidemia, Group B
    - Hyperprebetalipoproteinemia
    - Hypertriglyceridemia, essential
    - Very-low-density-lipoid-type [VLDL] hyperlipoproteinemia
  - **272.2 Mixed hyperlipidemia**
    - Broad- or floating-betalipoproteinemia
    - Fredrickson Type IIb or III hyperlipoproteinemia
    - Hypercholesterolemia with endogenous hyperglyceridemia
    - Hyperbetalipoproteinemia with prebetalipoproteinemia
    - Tubo-eruptive xanthoma
    - Xanthoma tuberosum
  - **272.3 Hyperchylomicronemia**
    - Bürger-Grütz syndrome
    - Fredrickson type I or V hyperlipoproteinemia
    - Hyperlipidemia, Group D
    - Mixed hyperglyceridemia
  - ◆ **272.4 Other and unspecified hyperlipidemia**
    - Alpha-lipoproteinemia
    - Combined hyperlipidemia
    - Hyperlipidemia NOS
    - Hyperlipoproteinemia NOS
  - **272.5 Lipoprotein deficiencies**
    - Abetalipoproteinemia
    - Bassen-Kornzweig syndrome
    - High-density lipoid deficiency
    - Hypoalphalipoproteinemia
    - Hypobetalipoproteinemia (familial)
  - **272.6 Lipodystrophy**
    - Barraquer-Simons disease
    - Progressive lipodystrophy
    - Use additional E code, if desired, to identify cause, if iatrogenic
    - EXCLUDES: *intestinal lipodystrophy (040.2)*
  - **272.7 Lipidoses**
    - Chemically-induced lipidosis
    - Disease:
      - Anderson's
      - Fabry's
      - Gaucher's
      - I cell [mucolipidosis I]
      - lipid storage NOS
      - Niemann-Pick
      - pseudo-Hurler's or mucolipdosis III
    - Disease:
      - triglyceride storage, Type I or II
      - Wolman's or triglyceride storage, Type III
    - Mucolipidosis II
    - Primary familial xanthomatosis
    - EXCLUDES: *cerebral lipidoses (330.1)*
      Tay-Sachs disease (330.1)
  - ◆ **272.8 Other disorders of lipoid metabolism**
    - Hoffa's disease or liposynovitis prepatellaris
    - Launois-Bensaude's lipomatosis
    - Lipoid dermatoarthritis
  - ◆ **272.9 Unspecified disorder of lipoid metabolism**
- ● **273 Disorders of plasma protein metabolism**
  - EXCLUDES: *agammaglobulinemia and hypogammaglobulinemia (279.0-279.2)*
    coagulation defects (286.0-286.9)
    hereditary hemolytic anemias (282.0-282.9)
  - **273.0 Polyclonal hypergammaglobulinemia**
    - Hypergammaglobulinemic purpura:
      - benign primary
      - Waldenström's
  - **273.1 Monoclonal paraproteinemia**
    - Benign monoclonal hypergammaglobulinemia [BMH]
    - Monoclonal gammopathy:
      - NOS
      - associated with lymphoplasmacytic dyscrasias
      - benign
    - Paraproteinemia:
      - benign (familial)
      - secondary to malignant or inflammatory disease
  - ◆ **273.2 Other paraproteinemias**
    - Cryoglobulinemic:
      - purpura
      - vasculitis
    - Mixed cryoglobulinemia
  - **273.3 Macroglobulinemia**
    - Macroglobulinemia (idiopathic) (primary)
    - Waldenström's macroglobulinemia
  - ◆ **273.8 Other disorders of plasma protein metabolism**
    - Abnormality of transport protein
    - Bisalbuminemia
  - ◆ **273.9 Unspecified disorder of plasma protein metabolism**
- ● **274 Gout**
  - EXCLUDES: *lead gout (984.0-984.9)*
  - **274.0 Gouty arthropathy**
  - ● **274.1 Gouty nephropathy**
    - ◆ **274.10** Gouty nephropathy, unspecified
    - **274.11** Uric acid nephrolithiasis
    - ◆ **274.19** Other
  - ● **274.8 Gout with other specified manifestations**
    - **274.81** Gouty tophi of ear
    - ◆ **274.82** Gouty tophi of other sites
      - Gouty tophi of heart
    - ◆ **274.89** Other
      - Use additional code, if desired, to identify manifestations, as:
        - gouty:
          - iritis (364.11)
          - neuritis (357.4)
  - ◆ **274.9 Gout, unspecified**
- ● **275 Disorders of mineral metabolism**
  - EXCLUDES: *abnormal findings without manifest disease (790.0-796.9)*
  - **275.0 Disorders of iron metabolism**
    - Bronzed diabetes
    - Hemochromatosis
    - Pigmentary cirrhosis (of liver)
    - EXCLUDES: *anemia:*
      iron deficiency (280.0-280.9)
      sideroblastic (285.0)
  - **275.1 Disorders of copper metabolism**
    - Hepatolenticular degeneration
    - Wilson's disease
  - **275.2 Disorders of magnesium metabolism**
    - Hypermagnesemia
    - Hypomagnesemia
  - **275.3 Disorders of phosphorus metabolism**
    - Familial hypophosphatemia
    - Hypophosphatasia
    - Vitamin D-resistant:
      - osteomalacia
      - rickets
  - **275.4 Disorders of calcium metabolism**
    - Calcinosis
    - Hypercalcemia
    - Hypercalcinuria
    - Nephrocalcinosis
    - Pseudohypoparathyroidism
    - Pseudopseudohypoparathryoidism
    - EXCLUDES: *parathyroid disorders (252.0-252.9)*
      vitamin D deficiency (268.0-268.9)
  - ◆ **275.8 Other specified disorders of mineral metabolism**
  - ◆ **275.9 Unspecified disorder of mineral metabolism**
- ● **276 Disorders of fluid, electrolyte, and acid-base balance**
  - EXCLUDES: *diabetes insipidus (253.5)*
    familial periodic paralysis (359.3)

● Additional digits required ◆ Nonspecific code ■ Not a primary diagnosis

276.0 Hyperosmolality and/or hypernatremia
Sodium [Na] excess
Sodium [Na] overload

276.1 Hyposmolality and/or hyponatremia
Sodium [Na] deficiency

276.2 Acidosis
Acidosis:
  NOS
  lactic
Acidosis:
  metabolic
  respiratory
EXCLUDES *diabetic acidosis (250.1)*

276.3 Alkalosis
Alkalosis:
  NOS
  metabolic
  respiratory

276.4 Mixed acid-base balance disorder
Hypercapnia with mixed acid-base disorder

276.5 Volume depletion
Dehydration
Depletion of volume of plasma or extracellular fluid
Hypovolemia
EXCLUDES *hypovolemic shock:*
  postoperative (998.0)
  traumatic (958.4)

276.6 Fluid overload
Fluid retention
EXCLUDES *ascites (789.5)*
  localized edema (782.3)

276.7 Hyperpotassemia
Hyperkalemia
Potassium [K]:
  excess
Potassium [K]:
  intoxication
  overload

276.8 Hypopotassemia
Hypokalemia
Potassium [K] deficiency

◆ **276.9 Electrolyte and fluid disorders not elsewhere classified**
Electrolyte imbalance
Hyperchloremia
Hypochloremia
EXCLUDES *electrolyte imbalance:*
  associated with hyperemesis gravidarum (643.1)
  complicating labor and delivery (669.0)
  following abortion and ectopic or molar pregnancy (634-638 with .4, 639.4)

● **277 Other and unspecified disorders of metabolism**

● **277.0 Cystic fibrosis**
Fibrocystic disease of the pancreas
Mucoviscidosis
  277.00 Without mention of meconium ileus
  277.01 With meconium ileus
    Meconium:
      ileus (of newborn)
      obstruction of intestine in mucoviscidosis

277.1 Disorders of porphyrin metabolism
Hematoporphyria
Hematoporphyrinuria
Hereditary coproporphyria
Porphyria
Porphyrinuria
Protocoproporphyria
Protoporphyria
Pyrroloporphyria

◆ **277.2 Other disorders of purine and pyrimidine metabolism**
Hypoxanthine-guanine-phosphoribosyltransferase deficiency [HG-PRT deficiency]
Lesch-Nyhan syndrome
Xanthinuria
EXCLUDES *gout (274.0-274.9)*
  orotic aciduric anemia (281.4)

277.3 Amyloidosis
Amyloidosis:
  NOS
  inherited systemic
  nephropathic
  neuropathic (Portuguese) (Swiss)
  secondary
Benign paroxysmal peritonitis
Familial Mediterranean fever
Hereditary cardiac amyloidosis

277.4 Disorders of bilirubin excretion
Hyperbilirubinemia:
  congenital
  constitutional
Syndrome:
  Crigler-Najjar
Syndrome:
  Dubin-Johnson
  Gilbert's
  Rotor's
EXCLUDES *hyperbilirubinemias specific to the perinatal period (774.0-774.7)*

277.5 Mucopolysaccharidosis
Gargoylism
Hunter's syndrome
Hurler's syndrome
Lipochondrodystrophy
Maroteaux-Lamy syndrome
Morquio-Brailsford disease
Osteochondrodystrophy
Sanfilippo's syndrome
Scheie's syndrome

◆ **277.6 Other deficiencies of circulating enzymes**
Alpha 1-antitrypsin deficiency
Hereditary angioedema

◆ **277.8 Other specified disorders of metabolism**
Hand-Schüller-Christian disease
Histiocytosis (acute) (chronic)
Histiocytosis X (chronic)
EXCLUDES *histiocytosis:*
  acute differentiated progressive (202.5)
  X, acute (progressive) (202.5)

◆ **277.9 Unspecified disorder of metabolism**
Enzymopathy NOS

● **278 Obesity and other hyperalimentation**
EXCLUDES *hyperalimentation NOS (783.6)*
  poisoning by vitamins NOS (963.5)
  polyphagia (783.6)

278.0 Obesity
EXCLUDES *adiposogenital dystrophy (253.8)*
  obesity of endocrine origin NOS (259.9)

278.1 Localized adiposity
Fat pad

278.2 Hypervitaminosis A

278.3 Hypercarotinemia

278.4 Hypervitaminosis D

◆ **278.8 Other hyperalimentation**

● **279 Disorders involving the immune mechanism**

● **279.0 Deficiency of humoral immunity**
  ◆ **279.00 Hypogammaglobulinemia, unspecified**
    Agammaglobulinemia NOS
  279.01 Selective IgA immunodeficiency
  279.02 Selective IgM immunodeficiency
  ◆ **279.03 Other selective immunoglobulin deficiencies**
    Selective deficiency of IgG
  279.04 Congenital hypogammaglobulinemia
    Agammaglobulinemia:
      Bruton's type
      X-linked
  279.05 Immunodeficiency with increased IgM
    Immunodeficiency with hyper-IgM:
      autosomal recessive
      X-linked
  279.06 Common variable immunodeficiency
    Dysgammaglobulinemia (acquired) (congenital) (primary)
    Hypogammaglobulinemia:
      acquired primary
      congenital non-sex-linked
      sporadic
  ◆ **279.09 Other**
    Transient hypogammaglobulinemia of infancy

● **279.1 Deficiency of cell-mediated immunity**
  ◆ **279.10 Immunodeficiency with predominant T-cell defect, unspecified**
  279.11 DiGeorge's syndrome
    Pharyngeal pouch syndrome
    Thymic hypoplasia
  279.12 Wiskott-Aldrich syndrome
  279.13 Nezelof's syndrome
    Cellular immunodeficiency with abnormal immunoglobulin deficiency
  ◆ **279.19 Other**
    EXCLUDES *ataxia-telangiectasia (334.8)*

279.2 Combined immunity deficiency
Agammaglobulinemia:
- autosomal recessive
- Swiss-type
- x-linked recessive

Severe combined immuno-deficiency [SCID]

Thymic:
- alymphoplasia
- aplasia or dysplasia with immunodeficiency

EXCLUDES *thymic hypoplasia (279.11)*

279.3 Unspecified immunity deficiency
279.4 Autoimmune disease, not elsewhere classified
Autoimmune disease NOS

EXCLUDES *transplant failure or rejection (996.80-996.89)*

279.8 Other specified disorders involving the immune mechanism
Single complement [C_1-C_9] deficiency or dysfunction

279.9 Unspecified disorder of immune mechanism

4. DISEASES OF THE BLOOD AND BLOOD-FORMING ORGANS (280-289)

EXCLUDES *anemia complicating pregnancy or the puerperium (648.2)*

280 Iron deficiency anemias
INCLUDES anemia:
- asiderotic
- hypochromic-microcytic
- sideropenic

EXCLUDES *familial microcytic anemia (282.4)*

280.0 Secondary to blood loss (chronic)
Normocytic anemia due to blood loss

EXCLUDES *acute posthemorrhagic anemia (285.1)*

280.1 Secondary to inadequate dietary iron intake
280.8 Other specified iron deficiency anemias
- Paterson-Kelly syndrome
- Plummer-Vinson syndrome
- Sideropenic dysphagia

280.9 Iron deficiency anemia, unspecified
Anemia:
- achlorhydric
- chlorotic
- idiopathic hypochromic
- iron [Fe] deficiency NOS

281 Other deficiency anemias
281.0 Pernicious anemia
Anemia:
- Addison's
- Biermer's
- congenital pernicious

Congenital intrinsic factor [Castle's] deficiency

EXCLUDES *combined system disease without mention of anemia (266.2)*
subacute degeneration of spinal cord without mention of anemia (266.2)

281.1 Other vitamin B_{12} deficiency anemia
Anemia:
- vegan's
- vitamin B_{12} deficiency (dietary)
- due to selective vitamin B_{12} malabsorption with proteinuria

Syndrome:
- Imerslund's
- Imerslund-Gräsbeck

EXCLUDES *combined system disease without mention of anemia (266.2)*
subacute degeneration of spinal cord without mention of anemia (266.2)

281.2 Folate-deficiency anemia
Congenital folate malabsorption
Folate or folic acid deficiency anemia:
- NOS
- dietary
- drug-induced

Goat's milk anemia
Nutritional megaloblastic anemia (of infancy)
Use additional E code, if desired, to identify drug

281.3 Other specified megaloblastic anemias not elsewhere classified
Combined B_{12} and folate-deficiency anemia
Refractory megaloblastic anemia

281.4 Protein-deficiency anemia
Amino-acid-deficiency anemia

281.8 Anemia associated with other specified nutritional deficiency
Scorbutic anemia

281.9 Unspecified deficiency anemia
Anemia:
- dimorphic
- macrocytic
- megaloblastic NOS
- nutritional NOS
- simple chronic

282 Hereditary hemolytic anemias
282.0 Hereditary spherocytosis
- Acholuric (familial) jaundice
- Congenital hemolytic anemia (spherocytic)
- Congenital spherocytosis
- Minkowski-Chauffard syndrome
- Spherocytosis (familial)

EXCLUDES *hemolytic anemia of newborn (773.0-773.5)*

282.1 Hereditary elliptocytosis
- Elliptocytosis (congenital)
- Ovalocytosis (congenital) (hereditary)

282.2 Anemias due to disorders of glutathione metabolism
Anemia:
- 6-phosphogluconic dehydrogenase deficiency
- enzyme deficiency, drug-induced
- erythrocytic glutathione deficiency
- glucose-6-phosphate dehydrogenase [G-6-PD] deficiency
- glutathione-reductase deficiency
- hemolytic nonspherocytic (hereditary), type I

Disorder of pentose phosphate pathway
Favism

282.3 Other hemolytic anemias due to enzyme deficiency
Anemia:
- hemolytic nonspherocytic (hereditary), type II
- hexokinase deficiency
- pyruvate kinase [PK] deficiency
- triosephosphate isomerase deficiency

282.4 Thalassemias
- Cooley's anemia
- Hereditary leptocytosis
- Mediterranean anemia (with other hemoglobinopathy)
- Microdrepanocytosis
- Sickle-cell thalassemia
- Thalassemia (alpha) (beta) (intermedia) (minima) (minor) (mixed) (trait) (with other hemoglobinopathy)
- Thalassemia-Hb-S disease

EXCLUDES *sickle-cell:*
anemia (282.60-282.69)
trait (282.5)

282.5 Sickle-cell trait
- Hb-AS genotype
- Hemoglobin S [Hb-S] trait
- Heterozygous:
  - hemoglobin S
  - Hb-S

EXCLUDES *that with other hemoglobinopathy (282.60-282.69)*
that with thalassemia (282.4)

282.6 Sickle-cell anemia
EXCLUDES *sickle-cell thalassemia (282.4)*
sickle-cell trait (282.5)

282.60 Sickle-cell anemia, unspecified
282.61 Hb-S disease without mention of crisis
282.62 Hb-S disease with mention of crisis
Sickle-cell crisis NOS
282.63 Sickle-cell/Hb-C disease
Hb-S/Hb-C disease
282.69 Other
Disease:
- Hb-S/Hb-D
- Hb-S/Hb-E
- sickle-cell/Hb-D
- sickle-cell/Hb-E

- **282.7 Other hemoglobinopathies**
  Abnormal hemoglobin NOS
  Congenital Heinz-body anemia
  Disease:
    Hb-Bart's
    hemoglobin C [Hb-C]
    hemoglobin D [Hb-D]
    hemoglobin E [Hb-E]
    hemoglobin Zurich [Hb-Zurich]
  Hemoglobinopathy NOS
  Hereditary persistence of fetal hemoglobin [HPFH]
  Unstable hemoglobin hemolytic disease
  EXCLUDES *familial polycythemia (289.6)*
  hemoglobin M [Hb-M] disease (289.7)
  high-oxygen-affinity hemoglobin (289.0)
- **282.8 Other specified hereditary hemolytic anemias**
  Stomatocytosis
- **282.9 Hereditary hemolytic anemia, unspecified**
  Hereditary hemolytic anemia NOS

● **283 Acquired hemolytic anemias**
- **283.0 Autoimmune hemolytic anemias**
  Autoimmune hemolytic disease (cold type)(warm type)
  Chronic cold hemagglutinin disease
  Cold agglutinin diseaseor hemoglobinuria
  Hemolytic anemia:
    cold type (secondary) (symptomatic)
    drug-induced
    warm type (secondary) (symptomatic)
  Use additional E code, if desired, to identify cause, if drug-induced
  EXCLUDES *Evans' syndrome (287.3)*
  hemolytic disease of newborn (773.0-773.5)
- **283.1 Non-autoimmune hemolytic anemias**
  Use additional E code, if desired, to identify cause
  - **283.10 Non-autoimmune hemolytic anemia, unspecified**
  - **283.11 Hemolytic-uremic syndrome**
  - **283.19 Other non-autoimmune hemolytic anemias**
    Hemolytic anemia:
      mechanical
      microangiopathic
      toxic
- **283.2 Hemoglobinuria due to hemolysis from external causes**
  Acute intravascular hemolysis
  Hemoglobinuria:
    from exertion
    march
    paroxysmal (cold) (nocturnal)
    due to other hemolysis
  Marchiafava-Micheli syndrome
  Use additional E code, if desired, to identify cause
- **283.9 Acquired hemolytic anemia, unspecified**
  Acquired hemolytic anemia NOS
  Chronic idiopathic hemolytic anemia

● **284 Aplastic anemia**
- **284.0 Constitutional aplastic anemia**
  Aplasia, (pure) red cell:
    congenital
    of infants
    primary
  Blackfan-Diamond syndrome
  Familial hypoplastic anemia
  Fanconi's anemia
  Pancytopenia with malformations
- **284.8 Other specified aplastic anemias**
  Aplastic anemia (due to):
    chronic systemic disease
    drugs
    infection
    radiation
    toxic (paralytic)
  Pancytopenia (acquired)
  Red cell aplasia (acquired) (adult) (pure) (with thymoma)
  Use additional E code, if desired, to identify cause
- **284.9 Aplastic anemia, unspecified**
  Anemia:
    aplastic (idiopathic) NOS
    aregenerative
    hypoplastic NOS
  Anemia:
    nonregenerative
    refractory
    Medullary hypoplasia

● **285 Other and unspecified anemias**
- **285.0 Sideroblastic anemia**
  Anemia:
    hypochromic with iron loading
    sideroachrestic
    sideroblastic
      acquired
      congenital
      hereditary
      primary
      refractory
      secondary (drug-induced) (due to disease)
      sex-linked hypochromic
      vitamin B_6-responsive
  Pyridoxine-responsive (hypochromic) anemia
  Use additional E code, if desired, to identify cause, if drug induced
- **285.1 Acute posthemorrhagic anemia**
  Anemia due to acute blood loss
  EXCLUDES *anemia due to chronic blood loss (280.0)*
  blood loss anemia NOS (280.0)
- **285.8 Other specified anemias**
  Anemia:
    dyserythropoietic (congenital)
    dyshematopoietic (congenital)
    leukoerythroblastic
    von Jaksch's
  Infantile pseudoleukemia
- **285.9 Anemia, unspecified**
  Anemia:
    NOS
    essential
    normocytic, not due
      to blood loss
  Anemia:
    profound
    progressive
    secondary
  Oligocythemia
  EXCLUDES *anemia (due to):*
  blood loss:
    acute (285.1)
    chronic or unspecified (280.0)
  iron deficiency (280.0-280.9)

● **286 Coagulation defects**
- **286.0 Congenital factor VIII disorder**
  Antihemophilic globulin [AHG] deficiency
  Factor VIII (functional) deficiency
  Hemophilia:
    NOS
    A
    classical
    familial
    hereditary
  Subhemophilia
  EXCLUDES *factor VIII deficiency with vascular defect (286.4)*
- **286.1 Congenital factor IX disorder**
  Christmas disease
  Deficiency:
    factor IX (functional)
    plasma thromboplastin component [PTC]
  Hemophilia B
- **286.2 Congenital factor XI deficiency**
  Hemophilia C
  Plasma thromboplastin antecedent [PTA] deficiency
  Rosenthal's disease
- **286.3 Congenital deficiency of other clotting factors**
  Congenital afibrinogenemia
  Deficiency:
    AC globulin factor:
      I [fibrinogen]
      II [prothrombin]
      V [labile]
      VII [stable]
      X [Stuart-Prower]
      XII [Hageman]
      XIII [fibrin stabilizing]
    Laki-Lorand factor
    proaccelerin
  Disease
    Owren's
    Stuart-Prower
  Dysfibrinogenemia
    (congenital)
  Dysprothrombinemia
    (constitutional)
  Hypoproconvertinemia
  Hypoprothrombinemia
    (hereditary)
  Parahemophilia

INFECTIOUS AND PARASITIC DISEASES

286.4 **von Willebrand's disease**
Angiohemophilia (A) (B)
Constitutional thrombopathy
Factor VIII deficiency with vascular defect
Pseudohemophilia type B
Vascular hemophilia
von Willebrand's (-Jürgens') disease
EXCLUDES factor VIII deficiency:
NOS (286.0)
with functional defect (286.0)
hereditary capillary fragility (287.8)

286.5 **Hemorrhagic disorder due to circulating anticoagulants**
Antithrombinemia
Antithromboplastinemia
Antithromboplastinogenemia
Hyperheparinemia
Increase in:
anti-VIIIa
anti-IXa
anti-Xa
anti-XIa
antithrombin
Systemic lupus erythematosus [SLE] inhibitor
Use additional Ecode, if desired, to identify cause, if drug induced

286.6 **Defibrination syndrome**
Afibrinogenemia, acquired
Consumption coagulopathy
Diffuse or disseminated intravascular coagulation [DIC syndrome]
Fibrinolytic hemorrhage, acquired
Hemorrhagic fibrinogenolysis
Pathologic fibrinolysis
Purpura:
fibrinolytic
fulminans
EXCLUDES that complicating:
abortion (634-638 with .1, 639.1)
pregnancy or the puerperium (641.3, 666.3)
disseminated intravascular coagulation in newborn (776.2)

286.7 **Acquired coagulation factor deficiency**
Deficiency of coagulation factor due to:
liver disease
vitamin K deficiency
Hypoprothrombinemia, acquired
EXCLUDES vitamin K deficiency of newborn (776.0)
Use additional E code, if desired, to identify cause, if drug induced

◆ **286.9** **Other and unspecified coagulation defects**
Defective coagulation NOS
Deficiency, coagulation factor NOS
Delay, coagulation
Disorder:
coagulation
hemostasis
EXCLUDES abnormal coagulation profile (790.92)
hemorrhagic disease of newborn (776.0)
that complicating:
abortion (634-638 with .1, 639.1)
pregnancy or the puerperium (641.3, 666.3)

● **287** **Purpura and other hemorrhagic conditions**
EXCLUDES hemorrhagic thrombocythemia (238.7)
purpura fulminans (286.6)

287.0 **Allergic purpura**
Peliosis rheumatica
Purpura:
anaphylactoid
autoimmune
Henoch's
nonthrombocytopenic:
hemorrhagic
idiopathic
Purpura:
rheumatica
Schönlein-Henoch
vascular
Vasculitis, allergic
EXCLUDES hemorrhagic purpura (287.3)
purpura annularis telangiectodes (709.1)

287.1 **Qualitative platelet defects**
Thrombasthenia (hemorrhagic) (hereditary)
Thrombocytasthenia
Thrombocytopathy (dystrophic)
Thrombopathy (Bernard-Soulier)
EXCLUDES von Willebrand's disease (286.4)

◆ **287.2** **Other nonthrombocytopenic purpuras**
Purpura:
NOS
senile
Purpura:
simplex

287.3 **Primary thrombocytopenia**
Evans' syndrome
Megakaryocytic hypoplasia
Purpura, thrombocytopenic
congenital
hereditary
idiopathic
Throbocytopenia:
congenital
hereditary
primary
Tidal platelet dysgenesis
EXCLUDES thrombotic thrombocytopenic purpura (446.6)
transient thrombocytopenia of newborn (776.1)

287.4 **Secondary thrombocytopenia**
Posttransfusion purpura
Thrombocytopenia (due to):
dilutional
drugs
extracorporeal circulation of blood
platelet alloimmunization
Use additional E code, if desired, to identify cause
EXCLUDES transient thrombocytopenia of newborn (776.1)

◆ **287.5** **Thrombocytopenia, unspecified**
◆ **287.8** **Other specified hemorrhagic conditions**
Capillary fragility (hereditary)
Vascular pseudohemophilia

◆ **287.9** **Unspecified hemorrhagic conditions**
Hemorrhagic diathesis (familial)

● **288** **Diseases of white blood cells**
EXCLUDES leukemia (204.0-208.9)

288.0 **Agranulocytosis**
Infantile genetic agranulo-cytosis
Kostmann's syndrome
Neutropenia:
NOS
cyclic
Neutropenia:
drug-induced
immune
periodic
toxic
Neutropenic splenomegaly
Use additional E code, if desired, to identify drug or other cause
EXCLUDES transitory neonatal neutropenia (776.7)

288.1 **Functional disorders of polymorphonuclear neutrophils**
Chronic (childhood) granulomatous disease
Congenital dysphagocytosis
Job's syndrome
Lipochrome histiocytosis (familial)
Progressive septic granulomatosis

288.2 **Genetic anomalies of leukocytes**
Anomaly (granulation) (granulocyte) or syndrome:
Alder's (-Reilly)
Chédiak-Steinbrinck (-Higashi)
Jordan's
May-Hegglin
Pelger-Huet
Hereditary:
hypersegmentation
hyposegmentation
leukomelanopathy

288.3 **Eosinophilia**
Eosinophilia
allergic
hereditary
idiopathic
Eosinophilia
secondary
Eosinophilic leukocytosis
EXCLUDES Löffler's syndrome (518.3)
pulmonary eosinophilia (518.3)

◆ **288.8** **Other specified disease of white blood cells**
Leukemoid reaction
lymphocytic
monocytic
myelocytic
Leukocytosis
Lymphocytopenia
Lymphocytosis (symptomatic)
Lymphopenia
Monocytosis (symptomatic)
Plasmacytosis
EXCLUDES immunity disorders (279.0-279.9)

● Additional digits required   ◆ Nonspecific code   ■ Not a primary diagnosis

288.9

- ◆ **288.9** Unspecified disease of white blood cells
- ● **289** Other diseases of blood and blood-forming organs
  - **289.0** Polycythemia, secondary
    - High-oxygen-affinity hemoglobin
    - Polycythemia:
      - acquired
      - benign
      - due to:
        - fall in plasma volume
        - high altitude
        - emotional
    - Polycythemia:
      - erythropoietin
      - hypoxemic
      - nephrogenous
      - relative
      - spurious
      - stress
    - EXCLUDES polycythemia:
      - neonatal (776.4)
      - primary (238.4)
      - vera (238.4)
  - **289.1** Chronic lymphadenitis
    - Chronic:
      - adenitis
      - lymphadenitis } any lymph node, except mesenteric
    - EXCLUDES acute lymphadenitis (683)
      - mesenteric (289.2)
      - enlarged glands NOS (785.6)
  - ◆ **289.2** Nonspecific mesenteric lymphadenitis
    - Mesenteric lymphadenitis (acute) (chronic)
  - ◆ **289.3** Lymphadenitis, unspecified, except mesenteric
  - **289.4** Hypersplenism
    - "Big spleen" syndrome
    - Dyssplenism
    - Hypersplenia
    - EXCLUDES primary splenic neutropenia (288.0)
  - ● **289.5** Other diseases of spleen
    - ◆ **289.50** Disease of spleen, unspecified
    - **289.51** Chronic congestive splenomegaly
    - ◆ **289.59** Other
      - Lien migrans
      - Perisplenitis
      - Splenic:
        - abscess
        - atrophy
        - cyst
      - Splenic:
        - fibrosis
        - infarction
        - rupture, nontraumatic
      - Splenitis
      - Wandering spleen
      - EXCLUDES bilharzial splenic fibrosis (120.0-120.9)
        - hepatolienal fibrosis (571.5)
        - splenomegaly NOS (789.2)
  - **289.6** Familial polycythemia
    - Familial:
      - benign polycythemia
      - erythrocytosis
  - **289.7** Methemoglobinemia
    - Congenital NADH [DPNH]-methemoglobin-reductase deficiency
    - Hemoglobin M [Hb-M] disease
    - Methemoglobinemia:
      - NOS
      - acquired (with sulfhemoglobinemia)
      - hereditary
      - toxic
    - Stokvis' disease
    - Sulfhemoglobinemia
    - Use additional E code, if desired, to identify cause
  - ◆ **289.8** Other specified diseases of blood and blood-forming organs
    - Hypergammaglobulinemia
    - Myelofibrosis
    - Pseudocholinesterase deficiency
  - ◆ **289.9** Unspecified diseases of blood and blood-forming organs
    - Blood dyscrasia NOS
    - Erythroid hyperplasia

5. MENTAL DISORDERS (290-319)

In the *International Classification of Diseases, 9th Revision* (ICD-9), the corresponding Chapter V, "Mental Disorders," includes a glossary which defines the contents of each category. The introduction to Chapter V in ICD-9 indicates that the glossary is intended so that psychiatrists can make the diagnosis based on the descriptions provided rather than from the category titles. Lay coders are instructed to code whatever diagnosis the physician records.

Chapter 5, "Mental Disorders," in ICD-9-CM uses the standard classification format with inclusion and exclusion terms, omitting the glossary as part of the main text.

The mental disorders section of ICD-9-CM has been expanded to incorporate additional psychiatric disorders not listed in ICD-9. The glossary from ICD-9 does not contain all these terms. It now appears in Appendix B, pages 211-220 which also contains descriptions and definitions for the terms added in ICD-9-CM. Some of these were provided by the American Psychiatric Association's Task Force on Nomenclature and Statistics who are preparing the *Diagnostic and Statistical Manual*, Third Edition (DSM-III), and others from *A Psychiatric Glossary*.

The American Psychiatric Association provided invaluable assistance in modifying Chapter 5 of ICD-9-CM to incorporate detail useful to American clinicians and gave permission to use material from the aforementioned sources.

1. Manual of the *International Statistical Classification of Diseases, Injuries, and Causes of Death*, 9th Revision, World Health Organization, Geneva, Switzerland, 1975.
2. American Psychiatric Association, Task Force on Nomenclature and Statistics, Robert L. Spitzer, M.D., Chairman.
3. *A Psychiatric Glossary*, Fourth Edition, American Psychiatric Association, Washington, D.C., 1975.

PSYCHOSES (290-299)

EXCLUDES mental retardation (317-319)

ORGANIC PSYCHOTIC CONDITIONS (290-294)

INCLUDES psychotic organic brain syndrome

EXCLUDES nonpsychotic syndromes of organic etiology (310.0-310.9)
  psychoses classifiable to 295-298 and without impairment of orientation, comprehension, calculation, learning capacity, and judgement, but associated with physical disease, injury, or condition affecting the brain [eg., following childbirth] (295.0-298.8)

- ● **290** Senile and presenile organic psychotic conditions
  - EXCLUDES dementia not classified as senile, presenile, or arteriosclerotic (294.1)
    - psychoses classifiable to 295-298 occurring in the senium without dementia or delirium (295.0-298.8)
    - senility with mental changes of nonpsychotic severity (310.1)
    - transient organic psychotic conditions (293.0-293.9)
  - Use additional code to identify the associated neurological conditions, as:
    - Alzheimer's disease (331.0)
    - Jakob-Creutzfeldt disease (046.1)
    - Pick's disease of the brain (331.1)
  - **290.0** Senile dementia, uncomplicated
    - Senile dementia:
      - NOS
      - simple type
    - EXCLUDES mild memory disturbances, not amounting to dementia, associated with senile brain disease (310.1)
      - senile dementia with:
        - delirium or confusion (290.3)
        - delusional [paranoid] features (290.20)
        - depressive features (290.21)
  - ● **290.1** Presenile dementia
    - Brain syndrome with presenile brain disease
    - Dementia in:
      - Alzheimer's disease
      - Jakob-Creutzfeldt disease
      - Pick's disease of the brain
    - EXCLUDES arteriosclerotic dementia (290.40-290.43)
      - dementia associated with other cerebral conditions (294.1)

290.10 Presenile dementia, uncomplicated
Presenile dementia:
NOS
simple type
290.11 Presenile dementia with delirium
Presenile dementia with acute confusional state
290.12 Presenile dementia with delusional features
Presenile dementia, paranoid type
290.13 Presenile dementia with depressive features
Presenile dementia, depressed type

● **290.2 Senile dementia with delusional or depressive features**
EXCLUDES senile dementia:
NOS (290.0)
with delirium and/or confusion (290.3)
290.20 Senile dementia with delusional features
Senile dementia, paranoid type
Senile psychosis NOS
290.21 Senile dementia with depressive features
290.3 Senile dementia with delirium
Senile dementia with acute confusional state
EXCLUDES senile:
dementia NOS (290.0)
psychosis NOS (290.20)

● **290.4 Arteriosclerotic dementia**
Multi-infarct dementia or psychosis
Use additional code to identify cerebral atherosclerosis (437.0)
EXCLUDES suspected cases with no clear evidence of arteriosclerosis (290.9)
290.40 Arteriosclerotic dementia, uncomplicated
Arteriosclerotic dementia:
NOS
simple type
290.41 Arteriosclerotic dementia with delirium
Arteriosclerotic dementia with acute confusional state
290.42 Arteriosclerotic dementia with delusional features
Arteriosclerotic dementia, paranoid type
290.43 Arteriosclerotic dementia with depressive features
Arteriosclerotic dementia, depressed type

◆ **290.8 Other specified senile psychotic conditions**
Presbyophrenic psychosis
◆ **290.9 Unspecified senile psychotic condition**

● **291 Alcoholic psychoses**
EXCLUDES alcoholism without psychosis (303.0-303.9)
291.0 Alcohol withdrawal delirium
Alcoholic delirium
Delirium tremens
291.1 Alcohol amnestic syndrome
Alcoholic polyneuritic psychosis
Korsakoff's psychosis, alcoholic
Wernicke-Korsakoff syndrome (alcoholic)
◆ **291.2 Other alcoholic dementia**
Alcoholic dementia NOS
Alcoholism associated with dementia NOS
Chronic alcoholic brain syndrome
291.3 Alcohol withdrawal hallucinosis
Alcoholic:
hallucinosis (acute)
psychosis with hallucinosis
EXCLUDES alcohol withdrawal with delirium (291.0)
schizophrenia (295.0-295.9) and paranoid states (297.0-297.9) taking the form of chronic hallucinosis with clear consciousness in an alcoholic
291.4 Idiosyncratic alcohol intoxication
Pathologic:
alcohol intoxication
drunkenness
EXCLUDES acute alcohol intoxication (305.0)
in alcoholism (303.0)
simple drunkenness (305.0)
291.5 Alcoholic jealousy
Alcoholic: Alcoholic:
paranoia   psychosis, paranoid type
EXCLUDES nonalcoholic paranoid states (297.0-297.9)
schizophrenia, paranoid type (295.3)

◆ **291.8 Other specified alcoholic psychosis**
Alcohol:
abstinence syndrome or symptoms
withdrawal syndrome or symptoms
EXCLUDES alcohol withdrawal:
delirium (291.0)
hallucinosis (291.3)
delirium tremens (291.0)
◆ **291.9 Unspecified alcoholic psychosis**
Alcoholic:
mania NOS
psychosis NOS
Alcoholism (chronic) with psychosis

● **292 Drug psychoses**
INCLUDES drug-induced mental disorders
organic brain syndrome associated with consumption of drugs
Use additional code for any associated drug dependence (304.0-304.9)
Use additional E code, if desired, to identify drug
292.0 Drug withdrawal syndrome
Drug:
abstinence syndrome or symptoms
withdrawal syndrome or symptoms
● **292.1 Paranoid and/or hallucinatory states induced by drugs**
292.11 Drug-induced organic delusional syndrome
Paranoid state induced by drugs
292.12 Drug-induced hallucinosis
Hallucinatory state induced by drugs
EXCLUDES states following LSD or other hallucinogens, lasting only a few days or less ["bad trips"] (305.3)
292.2 Pathological drug intoxication
Drug reaction: ⎫
NOS   ⎬ resulting in brief psychotic states
idiosyncratic ⎪
pathologic   ⎭
EXCLUDES expected brief psychotic reactions to hallucinogens ["bad trips"] (305.3)
physiological side-effects of drugs (e.g., dystonias)
● **292.8 Other specified drug-induced mental disorders**
292.81 Drug-induced delirium
292.82 Drug-induced dementia
292.83 Drug-induced amnestic syndrome
292.84 Drug-induced organic affective syndrome
Depressive state induced by drugs
◆ **292.89 Other**
Drug-induced organic personality syndrome
◆ **292.9 Unspecified drug-induced mental disorder**
Organic psychosis NOS due to or associated with drugs

● **293 Transient organic psychotic conditions**
INCLUDES transient organic mental disorders not associated with alcohol or drugs
Use additional code to identify the associated physical or neurological condition
EXCLUDES confusional state or delirium superimposed on senile dementia (290.3)
dementia due to:
alcohol (291.0-291.9)
arteriosclerosis (290.40-290.43)
drugs (292.82)
senility (290.0)
293.0 Acute delirium
Acute:
confusional state
infective psychosis
organic reaction
posttraumatic organic psychosis
psycho-organic syndrome
Acute psychosis associated with endocrine, metabolic, or cerebrovascular disorder
Epileptic:
confusional state
twilight state

● Additional digits required   ◆ Nonspecific code   ■ Not a primary diagnosis

293.1 Subacute delirium
Subacute:
- confusional state
- infective psychosis
- organic reaction
- posttraumatic organic psychosis
- psycho-organic syndrome
- psychosis associated with endocrine or metabolic disorder

● 293.8 Other specified transient organic mental disorders

293.81 Organic delusional syndrome
Transient organic psychotic condition, paranoid type

293.82 Organic hallucinosis syndrome
Transient organic psychotic condition, hallucinatory type

293.83 Organic affective syndrome
Transient organic psychotic condition, depressive type

◆ 293.89 Other

◆ 293.9 Unspecified transient organic mental disorder
Organic psychosis:
- infective NOS
- posttraumatic NOS

Organic psychosis:
- transient NOS
- Psycho-organic syndrome

● 294 Other organic psychotic conditions (chronic)
INCLUDES organic psychotic brain syndromes (chronic), not elsewhere classified

294.0 Amnestic syndrome
Korsakoff's psychosis or syndrome (nonalcoholic)
EXCLUDES alcoholic:
- amnestic syndrome (291.1)
- Korsakoff's psychosis (291.1)

294.1 Dementia in conditions classified elsewhere
Use additional code to identify the underlying physical condition, as:
dementia in:
- cerebral lipidoses (330.1)
- epilepsy (345.0-345.9)
- general paresis [syphilis] (094.1)
- hepatolenticular degeneration (275.1)
- Huntington's chorea (333.4)
- polyarteritis nodosa (446.0)
- syphilis (094.1)

EXCLUDES dementia:
- arteriosclerotic (290.40-290.43)
- presenile (290.10-290.13)
- senile (290.0)
- epileptic psychosis NOS (294.8)

◆ 294.8 Other specified organic brain syndromes (chronic)
Epileptic psychosis NOS
Mixed paranoid and affective organic psychotic states
Use additional code for associated epilepsy (345.0-345.9)
EXCLUDES mild memory disturbances, not amounting to dementia (310.1)

◆ 294.9 Unspecified organic brain syndrome (chronic)
Organic psychosis (chronic)

OTHER PSYCHOSES (295-299)
Use additional code to identify any associated physical disease, injury, or condition affecting the brain with psychoses classifiable to 295-298

● 295 Schizophrenic disorders
INCLUDES schizophrenia of the types described in 295.0-295.9 occurring in children
EXCLUDES childhood type schizophrenia (299.9)
infantile autism (299.0)

The following fifth-digit subclassification is for use with category 295:
- ◆ 0 unspecified
- 1 subchronic
- 2 chronic
- 3 subchronic with acute exacerbation
- 4 chronic with acute exacerbation
- 5 in remission

● 295.0 Simple type
Schizophrenia simplex
EXCLUDES latent schizophrenia (295.5)

● 295.1 Disorganized type
Hebephrenia
Hebephrenic type schizophrenia

● 295.2 Catatonic type
Catatonic (schizophrenia):
- agitation
- excitation
- excited type
- stupor
- withdrawn type

Schizophrenic:
- catalepsy
- catatonia
- flexibilitas cerea

● 295.3 Paranoid type
Paraphrenic schizophrenia
EXCLUDES involutional paranoid state (297.2)
paranoia (297.1)
paraphrenia (297.2)

● 295.4 Acute schizophrenic episode
Oneirophrenia
Schizophreniform:
- attack
- disorder
- psychosis, confusional type

EXCLUDES acute forms of schizophrenia of:
- catatonic type (295.2)
- hebephrenic type (295.1)
- paranoid type (295.3)
- simple type (295.0)
- undifferentiated type (295.8)

● 295.5 Latent schizophrenia
Latent schizophrenic reaction
Schizophrenia:
- borderline
- incipient

Schizophrenia:
- prepsychotic
- prodromal
- pseudoneurotic
- pseudopsychopathic

EXCLUDES schizoid personality (301.20-301.22)

● 295.6 Residual schizophrenia
Chronic undifferentiated schizophrenia
Restzustand (schizophrenic)
Schizophrenic residual state

● 295.7 Schizo-affective type
Cyclic schizophrenia
Mixed schizophrenic and affective psychosis
Schizo-affective psychosis
Schizophreniform psychosis, affective type

◆ ● 295.8 Other specified types of schizophrenia
Acute (undifferentiated) schizophrenia
Atypical schizophrenia
Cenesthopathic schizophrenia
EXCLUDES infantile autism (299.0)

◆ ● 295.9 Unspecified schizophrenia
Schizophrenia:
- NOS
- mixed NOS
- undifferentiated NOS

Schizophrenic reaction NOS
Schizophreniform psychosis NOS

● 296 Affective psychoses
INCLUDES episodic affective disorders
EXCLUDES neurotic depression (300.4)
reactive depressive psychosis (298.0)
reactive excitation (298.1)

The following fifth-digit subclassification is for use with categories 296.0-296.6:
- ◆ 0 unspecified
- 1 mild
- 2 moderate
- 3 severe, without mention of psychotic behavior
- 4 severe, specified as with psychotic behavior
- 5 in partial or unspecified remission
- 6 in full remission

● 296.0 Manic disorder, single episode
Hypomania (mild) NOS
Hypomanic psychosis
Mania (monopolar) NOS
Manic-depressive psychosis or reaction:
- hypomanic
- manic
} single episode or unspecified

EXCLUDES circular type, if there was a previous attack of depression (296.4)

MENTAL DISORDERS

- **296.1 Manic disorder, recurrent episode**
  Any condition classifiable to 296.0, stated to be recurrent
  - EXCLUDES: circular type, if there was a previous attack of depression (296.4)

- **296.2 Major depressive disorder, single episode**
  - Depressive psychosis
  - Endogenous depression
  - Involutional melancholia
  - Manic-depressive psychosis or reaction, depressed type
  - Monopolar depression
  - Psychotic depression

  } single episode or unspecified
  - EXCLUDES:
    - circular type, if previous attack was of manic type (296.5)
    - depression NOS (311)
    - reactive depression (neurotic) (300.4)
    - psychotic (298.0)

- **296.3 Major depressive disorder, recurrent episode**
  Any condition classifiable to 296.2, stated to be recurrent
  - EXCLUDES:
    - circular type, if previous attack was of manic type (296.5)
    - depression NOS (311)
    - reactive depression (neurotic) (300.4)
    - psychotic (298.0)

- **296.4 Bipolar affective disorder, manic**
  - Bipolar disorder, now manic
  - Manic-depressive psychosis, circular type but currently manic
  - EXCLUDES: brief compensatory or rebound mood swings (296.99)

- **296.5 Bipolar affective disorder, depressed**
  - Bipolar disorder, now depressed
  - Manic-depressive psychosis, circular type but currently depressed
  - EXCLUDES: brief compensatory or rebound mood swings (296.99)

- **296.6 Bipolar affective disorder, mixed**
  - Manic-depressive psychosis, circular type, mixed

- ◆ **296.7 Bipolar affective disorder, unspecified**
  - Atypical bipolar affective disorder NOS
  - Manic-depressive psychosis, circular type, current condition not specified as either manic or depressive

- **296.8 Manic-depressive psychosis, other and unspecified**
  - ◆ **296.80 Manic-depressive psychosis, unspecified**
    - Manic-depressive:
      - reaction NOS
      - syndrome NOS
  - **296.81 Atypical manic disorder**
  - **296.82 Atypical depressive disorder**
  - ◆ **296.89 Other**
    - Manic-depressive psychosis, mixed type

- **296.9 Other and unspecified affective psychoses**
  - EXCLUDES: psychogenic affective psychoses (298.0-298.8)
  - ◆ **296.90 Unspecified affective psychosis**
    - Affective psychosis NOS
    - Melancholia NOS
  - ◆ **296.99 Other specified affective psychoses**
    - Mood swings: brief compensatory
    - Mood swings: rebound

- **297 Paranoid states**
  - INCLUDES: paranoid disorders
  - EXCLUDES:
    - acute paranoid reaction (298.3)
    - alcoholic jealousy or paranoid state (291.5)
    - paranoid schizophrenia (295.3)
  - **297.0 Paranoid state, simple**
  - **297.1 Paranoia**
    - Chronic paranoid psychosis
    - Sander's disease
    - Systematized delusions
    - EXCLUDES: paranoid personality disorder (301.0)
  - **297.2 Paraphrenia**
    - Involutional paranoid state
    - Late paraphrenia
    - Paraphrenia (involutional)
  - **297.3 Shared paranoid disorder**
    - Folie à deux
    - Induced psychosis or paranoid disorder
  - ◆ **297.8 Other specified paranoid states**
    - Paranoia querulans
    - Sensitiver Beziehungswahn
    - EXCLUDES:
      - acute paranoid reaction or state (298.3)
      - senile paranoid state (290.20)
  - ◆ **297.9 Unspecified paranoid state**
    - Paranoid: disorder NOS
    - Paranoid: psychosis NOS
    - Paranoid: reaction NOS
    - Paranoid: state NOS

- **298 Other nonorganic psychoses**
  - INCLUDES: psychotic conditions due to or provoked by:
    - emotional stress
    - environmental factors as major part of etiology
  - **298.0 Depressive type psychosis**
    - Psychogenic depressive psychosis
    - Psychotic reactive depression
    - Reactive depressive psychosis
    - EXCLUDES:
      - manic-depressive psychosis, depressed type (296.2-296.3)
      - neurotic depression (300.4)
      - reactive depression NOS (300.4)
  - **298.1 Excitative type psychosis**
    - Acute hysterical psychosis
    - Psychogenic excitation
    - Reactive excitation
    - EXCLUDES: manic-depressive psychosis, manic type (296.0-296.1)
  - **298.2 Reactive confusion**
    - Psychogenic confusion
    - Psychogenic twilight state
    - EXCLUDES: acute confusional state (293.0)
  - **298.3 Acute paranoid reaction**
    - Acute psychogenic paranoid psychosis
    - Bouffée délirante
    - EXCLUDES: paranoid states (297.0-297.9)
  - **298.4 Psychogenic paranoid psychosis**
    - Protracted reactive paranoid psychosis
  - ◆ **298.8 Other and unspecified reactive psychosis**
    - Brief reactive psychosis NOS
    - Hysterical psychosis
    - Psychogenic psychosis NOS
    - Psychogenic stupor
    - EXCLUDES: acute hysterical psychosis (298.1)
  - ◆ **298.9 Unspecified psychosis**
    - Atypical psychosis
    - Psychosis NOS

- **299 Psychoses with origin specific to childhood**
  - INCLUDES: pervasive developmental disorders
  - EXCLUDES: adult type psychoses occurring in childhood, as:
    - affective disorders (296.0-296.9)
    - manic-depressive disorders (296.0-296.9)
    - schizophrenia (295.0-295.9)

  The following fifth-digit subclassification is for use with category 299:
  - 0 current or active state
  - 1 residual state

  - **299.0 Infantile autism**
    - Childhood autism
    - Infantile psychosis
    - Kanner's syndrome
    - EXCLUDES:
      - disintegrative psychosis (299.1)
      - Heller's syndrome (299.1)
      - schizophrenic syndrome of childhood (299.9)
  - **299.1 Disintegrative psychosis**
    - Heller's syndrome
    - Use additional code to identify any associated neurological disorder
    - EXCLUDES:
      - infantile autism (299.0)
      - schizophrenic syndrome of childhood (299.9)

● Additional digits required ◆ Nonspecific code ■ Not a primary diagnosis

- ◆ ● **299.8** Other specified early childhood psychoses
  - Atypical childhood psychosis
  - Borderline psychosis of childhood
  - **EXCLUDES** simple stereotypies without psychotic disturbance (307.3)
- ◆ ● **299.9** Unspecified
  - Child psychosis NOS
  - Schizophrenia, childhood type NOS
  - Schizophrenic syndrome of childhood NOS
  - **EXCLUDES** schizophrenia of adult type occurring in childhood (295.0-295.9)

NEUROTIC DISORDERS, PERSONALITY DISORDERS, AND OTHER NONPSYCHOTIC MENTAL DISORDERS (300-316)

- ● **300** Neurotic disorders
  - ● **300.0** Anxiety states
    - **EXCLUDES** anxiety in:
      - acute stress reaction (308.0)
      - transient adjustment reaction (309.24)
      - neurasthenia (300.5)
      - psychophysiological disorders (306.0-306.9)
      - separation anxiety (309.21)
    - ◆ **300.00** Anxiety state, unspecified
      - Anxiety:
        - neurosis
        - reaction
        - state (neurotic)
      - Atypical anxiety disorder
    - **300.01** Panic disorder
      - Panic:
        - attack
        - state
    - **300.02** Generalized anxiety disorder
    - ◆ **300.09** Other
  - ● **300.1** Hysteria
    - **EXCLUDES** adjustment reaction (309.0-309.9)
      - anorexia nervosa (307.1)
      - gross stress reaction (308.0-308.9)
      - hysterical personality (301.50-301.59)
      - psychophysiologic disorders (306.0-306.9)
    - ◆ **300.10** Hysteria, unspecified
    - **300.11** Conversion disorder
      - Astasia-abasia, hysterical
      - Conversion hysteria or reaction
      - Hysterical
        - blindness
        - deafness
        - paralysis
    - **300.12** Psychogenic amnesia
      - Hysterical amnesia
    - **300.13** Psychogenic fugue
      - Hysterical fugue
    - **300.14** Multiple personality
      - Dissociative identity disorder ◆
    - ◆ **300.15** Dissociative disorder or reaction, unspecified
    - **300.16** Factitious illness with psychological symptoms
      - Compensation neurosis
      - Ganser's syndrome, hysterical
    - ◆ **300.19** Other and unspecified factitious illness
      - Factitious illness (with physical symptoms) NOS
      - **EXCLUDES** multiple operations or hospital addiction syndrome (301.51)
  - ● **300.2** Phobic disorders
    - **EXCLUDES** anxiety state not associated with a specific situation or object (300.00-300.09)
      - obsessional phobias (300.3)
    - ◆ **300.20** Phobia, unspecified
      - Anxiety-hysteria NOS
      - Phobia NOS
    - **300.21** Agoraphobia with panic attacks
      - Fear of:
        - open spaces
        - streets   } with panic attacks
        - travel
    - **300.22** Agoraphobia without mention of panic attacks
      - Any condition classifiable to 300.21 without mention of panic attacks
  - **300.23** Social phobia
    - Fear of:
      - eating in public
      - public speaking
      - washing in public
  - ◆ **300.29** Other isolated or simple phobias
    - Acrophobia   Claustrophobia
    - Animal phobias   Fear of crowds
  - **300.3** Obsessive-compulsive disorders
    - Anancastic neurosis
    - Compulsive neurosis
    - Obsessional phobia [any]
    - **EXCLUDES** obsessive-compulsive symptoms occurring in:
      - endogenous depression (296.2-296.3)
      - organic states (eg., encephalitis)
      - schizophrenia (295.0-295.9)
  - **300.4** Neurotic depression
    - Anxiety depression   Dysthymic disorder ◆
    - Depression with anxiety   Neurotic depressive state
    - Depressive reaction   Reactive depression
    - **EXCLUDES** adjustment reaction with depressive symptoms (309.0-309.1)
      - depression NOS (311)
      - manic-depressive psychosis, depressed type (296.2-296.3)
      - reactive depressive psychosis (298.0)
  - **300.5** Neurasthenia
    - Fatigue neurosis
    - Nervous debility
    - Psychogenic:
      - asthenia
      - general fatigue
    - Use additional code to identify any associated physical disorder
    - **EXCLUDES** anxiety state (300.00-300.09)
      - neurotic depression (300.4)
      - psychophysiological disorders (306.0-306.9)
      - specific nonpsychotic mental disorders following organic brain damage (310.0-310.9)
  - **300.6** Depersonalization syndrome
    - Depersonalization disorder
    - Derealization (neurotic)
    - Neurotic state with depersonalization episode
    - **EXCLUDES** depersonalization associated with:
      - anxiety (300.00-300.09)
      - depression (300.4)
      - manic-depressive disorder or psychosis (296.0-296.9)
      - schizophrenia (295.0-295.9)
  - **300.7** Hypochondriasis
    - Atypical somatoform disorder
    - Body dysmorphic disorder ◆
    - **EXCLUDES** hypochondriasis in:
      - hysteria (300.10-300.19)
      - manic-depressive psychosis, depressed type (296.2-296.3)
      - neurasthenia (300.5)
      - obsessional disorder (300.3)
      - schizophrenia (295.0-295.9)
  - ● **300.8** Other neurotic disorders
    - **300.81** Somatization disorder
      - Briquet's disorder
    - ◆ **300.89** Other
      - Occupational neurosis, including writers' cramp
      - Psychasthenia
      - Psychasthenic neurosis
  - ◆ **300.9** Unspecified neurotic disorder
    - Neurosis NOS
    - Psychoneurosis NOS
- ● **301** Personality disorders
  - **INCLUDES** character neurosis
  - Use additional code to identify any associated neurosis or psychosis, or physical condition
  - **EXCLUDES** nonpsychotic personality disorder associated with organic brain syndromes (310.0-310.9)

MENTAL DISORDERS

- **301.0 Paranoid personality disorder**
  Fanatic personality
  Paranoid personality (disorder)
  Paranoid traits
  EXCLUDES acute paranoid reaction (298.3)
  alcoholic paranoia (291.5)
  paranoid schizophrenia (295.3)
  paranoid states (297.0-297.9)

- ● **301.1 Affective personality disorder**
  EXCLUDES affective psychotic disorders (296.0-296.9)
  neurasthenia (300.5)
  neurotic depression (300.4)
  - ◆ 301.10 Affective personality disorder, unspecified
  - 301.11 Chronic hypomanic personality disorder
    Chronic hypomanic disorder
    Hypomanic personality
  - 301.12 Chronic depressive personality disorder
    Chronic depressive disorder
    Depressive character or personality
  - 301.13 Cyclothymic disorder
    Cycloid personality
    Cyclothymia ◆
    Cyclothymic personality

- ● **301.2 Schizoid personality disorder**
  EXCLUDES schizophrenia (295.0-295.9)
  - ◆ 301.20 Schizoid personality disorder, unspecified
  - 301.21 Introverted personality
  - 301.22 Schizotypal personality

- **301.3 Explosive personality disorder**
  Aggressive:
    personality
    reaction
  Aggressiveness
  Emotional instability (excessive)
  Pathological emotionality
  Quarrelsomeness
  EXCLUDES dyssocial personality (301.7)
  hysterical neurosis (300.10-300.19)

- **301.4 Compulsive personality disorder**
  Anancastic personality
  Obsessional personality
  EXCLUDES obsessive-compulsive disorder (300.3)
  phobic state (300.20-300.29)

- ● **301.5 Histrionic personality disorder**
  EXCLUDES hysterical neurosis (300.10-300.19)
  - ◆ 301.50 Histrionic personality disorder, unspecified
    Hysterical personality NOS
  - 301.51 Chronic factitious illness with physical symptoms
    Hospital addiction syndrome
    Multiple operations syndrome
    Munchausen syndrome
  - ◆ 301.59 Other histrionic personality disorder
    Personality:
      emotionally unstable
      labile
      psychoinfantile

- **301.6 Dependent personality disorder**
  Asthenic personality
  Inadequate personality
  Passive personality
  EXCLUDES neurasthenia (300.5)
  passive-aggressive personality (301.84)

- **301.7 Antisocial personality disorder**
  Amoral personality
  Asocial personality
  Dyssocial personality
  Personality disorder with predominantly sociopathic or asocial manifestation
  EXCLUDES disturbance of conduct without specifiable personality disorder (312.0-312.9)
  explosive personality (301.3)

- ● **301.8 Other personality disorders**
  - 301.81 Narcissistic personality
  - 301.82 Avoidant personality
  - 301.83 Borderline personality
  - 301.84 Passive-aggressive personality

- ◆ 301.89 Other
  Personality:
    eccentric
    "haltlose" type
    immature
    masochistic
    psychoneurotic
  EXCLUDES psychoinfantile personality (301.59)

- ◆ **301.9 Unspecified personality disorder**
  Pathological personality NOS
  Personality disorder NOS
  Psychopathic:
    constitutional state
    personality (disorder)

- ● **302 Sexual deviations and disorders**
  EXCLUDES sexual disorder manifest in:
    organic brain syndrome (290.0-294.9, 310.0-310.9)
    psychosis (295.0-298.9)

  - 302.0 Ego-dystonic homosexuality
    Ego-dystonic lesbianism
    Homosexual conflict disorder
    EXCLUDES homosexual pedophilia (302.2)
  - 302.1 Zoophilia
    Bestiality
  - 302.2 Pedophilia
  - 302.3 Transvestism
    EXCLUDES trans-sexualism (302.5)
  - 302.4 Exhibitionism
  - ● 302.5 Trans-sexualism
    EXCLUDES transvestism (302.3)
    - ◆ 302.50 With unspecified sexual history
    - 302.51 With asexual history
    - 302.52 With homosexual history
    - 302.53 With heterosexual history
  - 302.6 Disorders of psychosexual identity
    Feminism in boys
    Gender identity disorder of childhood
    EXCLUDES gender identity disorder in adult (302.85)
    homosexuality (302.0)
    trans-sexualism (302.50-302.53)
    transvestism (302.3)
  - ● 302.7 Psychosexual dysfunction
    EXCLUDES impotence of organic origin (607.84)
    normal transient symptoms from ruptured hymen
    transient or occasional failures of erection due to fatigue, anxiety, alcohol, or drugs
    - ◆ 302.70 Psychosexual dysfunction, unspecified
    - 302.71 With inhibited sexual desire
    - 302.72 With inhibited sexual excitement
      Frigidity
      Impotence
    - 302.73 With inhibited female orgasm
    - 302.74 With inhibited male orgasm
    - 302.75 With premature ejaculation
    - 302.76 With functional dyspareunia
      Dyspareunia, psychogenic
    - ◆ 302.79 With other specified psychosexual dysfunctions
  - ● 302.8 Other specified psychosexual disorders
    - 302.81 Fetishism
    - 302.82 Voyeurism
    - 302.83 Sexual masochism
    - 302.84 Sexual sadism
    - 302.85 Gender identity disorder of adolescent or adult life
    - ◆ 302.89 Other
      Nymphomania
      Satyriasis
  - ◆ 302.9 Unspecified psychosexual disorder
    Pathologic sexuality NOS
    Sexual deviation NOS

● Additional digits required   ◆ Nonspecific code   ▌Not a primary diagnosis

303 Alcohol dependence syndrome

Use additional code to identify any associated condition, as:
 alcoholic psychoses (291.0-291.9)
 drug dependence (304.0-304.9)
 physical complications of alcohol, such as:
  cerebral degeneration (331.7)
  cirrhosis of liver (571.2)
  epilepsy (345.0-345.9)
  gastritis (535.3)
  hepatitis (571.1)
  liver damage NOS (571.3)

EXCLUDES *drunkenness NOS (305.0)*

The following fifth-digit subclassification is for use with category 303:
- 0 unspecified
- 1 continuous
- 2 episodic
- 3 in remission

303.0 Acute alcoholic intoxication
 Acute drunkenness in alcoholism

303.9 Other and unspecified alcohol dependence
 Chronic alcoholism
 Dipsomania

304 Drug dependence

EXCLUDES *nondependent abuse of drugs (305.1-305.9)*

The following fifth-digit subclassification is for use with category 304:
- 0 unspecified
- 2 episodic
- 3 in remission

304.0 Opioid type dependence
 Heroin
 Meperidine
 Methadone
 Morphine
 Opium
 Opium alkaloids and their derivatives
 Synthetics with morphine-like effects

304.1 Barbiturate and similarly acting sedative or hypnotic dependence
 Barbiturates
 Nonbarbiturate sedatives and tranquilizers with a similar effect:
  chlordiazepoxide
  diazepam
  glutethimide
  meprobamate
  methaqualone

304.2 Cocaine dependence
 Coca leaves and derivatives

304.3 Cannabis dependence
 Hashish   Marihuana
 Hemp

304.4 Amphetamine and other psychostimulant dependence
 Methylphenidate
 Phenmetrazine

304.5 Hallucinogen dependence
 Dimethyltryptamine [DMT]
 Lysergic acid diethylamide [LSD] and derivatives
 Mescaline
 Psilocybin

304.6 Other specified drug dependence
 Absinthe addiction   Glue sniffing
 EXCLUDES *tobacco dependence (305.1)*

304.7 Combinations of opioid type drug with any other
304.8 Combinations of drug dependence excluding opioid type drug
304.9 Unspecified drug dependence
 Drug addiction NOS   Drug dependence NOS

305 Nondependent abuse of drugs

Note: Includes cases where a person, for whom no other diagnosis is possible, has come under medical care because of the maladaptive effect of a drug on which he is not dependent and that he has taken on his own initiative to the detriment of his health or social functioning.

EXCLUDES
 *alcohol dependence syndrome (303.0-303.9)
 drug dependence (304.0-304.9)
 drug withdrawal syndrome (292.0)
 poisoning by drugs or medicinal substances (960.0-979.9)*

The following fifth-digit subclassification is for use with codes 305.0, 305.2-305.9:
- 0 unspecified
- 1 continuous
- 2 episodic
- 3 in remission

305.0 Alcohol abuse
 Drunkenness NOS
 Excessive drinking of alcohol NOS
 "Hangover" (alcohol)
 Inebriety NOS
 EXCLUDES *acute alcohol intoxication in alcoholism (303.0)
 alcoholic psychoses (291.0-291.9)
 physical complications of alcohol, such as:
  cirrhosis of liver (571.2)
  epilepsy (345.00-345.91)
  gastritis (535.3)*

305.1 Tobacco use disorder
 Tobacco dependence
 EXCLUDES *history of tobacco use (V15.82)*

305.2 Cannabis abuse
305.3 Hallucinogen abuse
 Acute intoxication from hallucinogens ["bad trips"]
 LSD reaction

305.4 Barbiturate and similarly acting sedative or hypnotic abuse
305.5 Opioid abuse
305.6 Cocaine abuse
305.7 Amphetamine or related acting sympathomimetic abuse
305.8 Antidepressant type abuse
305.9 Other, mixed, or unspecified drug abuse
 "Laxative habit"
 Misuse of drugs NOS
 Nonprescribed use of drugs or patent medicinals

306 Physiological malfunction arising from mental factors

INCLUDES psychogenic:
 physical symptoms } not involving
 physiological } tissue
 manifestations } damage

EXCLUDES *hysteria (300.11-300.19)
 physical symptoms secondary to a psychiatric disorder classified elsewhere
 psychic factors associated with physical conditions involving tissue damage classified elsewhere (316)
 specific nonpsychotic mental disorders following organic brain damage (310.0-310.9)*

306.0 Musculoskeletal
 Psychogenic paralysis
 Psychogenic torticollis
 EXCLUDES *Gilles de la Tourette's syndrome (307.23)
 paralysis as hysterical or conversion reaction (300.11)
 tics (307.20-307.22)*

306.1 Respiratory
 Psychogenic:
  air hunger
  cough
  hiccough
  hyperventilation
  yawning
 EXCLUDES *psychogenic asthma (316 and 493.9)*

306.2 Cardiovascular
 Cardiac neurosis
 Cardiovascular neurosis
 Neurocirculatory asthenia
 Psychogenic cardiovascular disorder
 EXCLUDES *psychogenic paroxysmal tachycardia (316 and 427.2)*

306.3 Skin
 Psychogenic pruritus
 EXCLUDES *psychogenic:
  alopecia (316 and 704.00)
  dermatitis (316 and 692.9)
  eczema (316 and 691.8 or 692.9)
  urticaria (316 and 708.0-708.9)*

MENTAL DISORDERS

306.4 Gastrointestinal
Aerophagy
Cyclical vomiting, psychogenic
Diarrhea, psychogenic
Nervous gastritis
Psychogenic dyspepsia
> **EXCLUDES** cyclical vomiting NOS (536.2)
> globus hystericus (300.11)
> mucous colitis (316 and 564.1)
> psychogenic:
>   cardiospasm (316 and 530.0)
>   duodenal ulcer (316 and 532.0-532.9)
>   gastric ulcer (316 and 531.0-531.9)
>   peptic ulcer NOS (316 and 533.0-533.9)
>   vomiting NOS (307.54)

● **306.5 Genitourinary**
> **EXCLUDES** enuresis, psychogenic (307.6)
> frigidity (302.72)
> impotence (302.72)
> psychogenic dyspareunia (302.76)

◆ **306.50** Psychogenic genitourinary malfunction, unspecified
306.51 Psychogenic vaginismus
   Functional vaginismus
306.52 Psychogenic dysmenorrhea
306.53 Psychogenic dysuria
◆ **306.59** Other

306.6 Endocrine
306.7 Organs of special sense
> **EXCLUDES** hysterical blindness or deafness (300.11)
> psychophysical visual disturbances (368.16)

◆ **306.8 Other specified psychophysiological malfunction**
   Bruxism   Teeth grinding

◆ **306.9 Unspecified psychophysiological malfunction**
   Psychophysiologic disorder NOS
   Psychosomatic disorder NOS

● **307 Special symptoms or syndromes, not elsewhere classified**
Note: This category is intended for use if the psychopathology is manifested by a single specific symptom or group of symptoms which is not part of an organic illness or other mental disorder classifiable elsewhere.
> **EXCLUDES** those due to mental disorders classified elsewhere
> those of organic origin

307.0 Stammering and stuttering
> **EXCLUDES** dysphasia (784.5)
> lisping or lalling (307.9)
> retarded development of speech (315.31-315.39)

307.1 Anorexia nervosa
> **EXCLUDES** eating disturbance NOS (307.50)
> feeding problem (783.3)
>   of nonorganic origin (307.59)
> loss of appetite (783.0)
>   of nonorganic origin (307.59)

● **307.2 Tics**
> **EXCLUDES** nail-biting or thumb-sucking (307.9)
> stereotypies occurring in isolation (307.3)
> tics of organic origin (333.3)

◆ **307.20** Tic disorder, unspecified
307.21 Transient tic disorder of childhood
307.22 Chronic motor tic disorder
307.23 Gilles de la Tourette's disorder
   Motor-verbal tic disorder

307.3 Stereotyped repetitive movements
   Body-rocking   Spasmus nutans
   Head banging   Stereotypies NOS
> **EXCLUDES** tics (307.20-307.23)
> of organic origin (333.3)

● **307.4 Specific disorders of sleep of nonorganic origin**
> **EXCLUDES** narcolepsy (347)
> those of unspecified cause (780.50-780.59)

◆ **307.40** Nonorganic sleep disorder, unspecified
307.41 Transient disorder of initiating or maintaining sleep
   Hyposomnia } associated with intermittent
   Insomnia   emotional reactions
   Sleeplessness   or conflicts

307.42 Persistent disorder of initiating or maintaining sleep
   Hyposomnia, insomnia, or sleeplessness associated with:
     anxiety
     conditioned arousal
     depression (major) (minor)
     psychosis

307.43 Transient disorder of initiating or maintaining wakefulness
   Hypersomnia associated with acute or intermittent emotional reactions or conflicts

307.44 Persistent disorder of initiating or maintaining wakefulness
   Hypersomnia associated with depression (major) (minor)

307.45 Phase-shift disruption of 24-hour sleep-wake cycle
   Irregular sleep-wake rhythm, nonorganic origin
   Jet lag syndrome
   Rapid time-zone change
   Shifting sleep-work schedule

307.46 Somnambulism or night terrors

◆ **307.47** Other dysfunctions of sleep stages or arousal from sleep
   Nightmares:
     NOS
     REM-sleep type
   Sleep drunkenness

307.48 Repetitive intrusions of sleep
   Repetitive intrusion of sleep with:
     atypical polysomnographic features
     environmental disturbances
     repeated REM-sleep interruptions

◆ **307.49** Other
   "Short-sleeper"
   Subjective insomnia complaint

● **307.5 Other and unspecified disorders of eating**
> **EXCLUDES** anorexia:
>   nervosa (307-1)
>   of unspecified cause (783.0)
> overeating, of unspecified cause (783.6)
> vomiting:
>   NOS (787.0)
>   cyclical (536.2)
>   psychogenic (306.4)

◆ **307.50** Eating disorder, unspecified
307.51 Bulimia
   Overeating of nonorganic origin
307.52 Pica
   Perverted appetite of nonorganic origin
307.53 Psychogenic rumination
   Regurgitation, of nonorganic origin, of food with reswallowing
> **EXCLUDES** obsessional rumination (300.3)

307.54 Psychogenic vomiting
◆ **307.59** Other
   Infantile feeding disturbances } of nonorganic origin
   Loss of appetite

307.6 Enuresis
   Enuresis (primary) (secondary) of nonorganic origin
> **EXCLUDES** enuresis of unspecified cause (788.3)

307.7 Encopresis
   Encopresis (continuous) (discontinuous) of nonorganic origin
> **EXCLUDES** encopresis of unspecified cause (787.6)

● **307.8 Psychalgia**
◆ **307.80** Psychogenic pain, site unspecified
307.81 Tension headache
> **EXCLUDES** headache:
>   NOS (784.0)
>   migraine (346.0-346.9)

- **307.89 Other**
  Psychogenic backache
  EXCLUDES   pains not specifically attributable to a psychological cause (in):
  back (724.5)
  joint (719.4)
  limb (729.5)
  lumbago (724.2)
  rheumatic (729.0)
- **307.9 Other and unspecified special symptoms or syndromes, not elsewhere classified**
  Hair plucking
  Lalling
  Lisping
  Masturbation
  Nail-biting
  Thumb-sucking

308 Acute reaction to stress
INCLUDES   catastrophic stress
combat fatigue
gross stress reaction (acute)
transient disorders in response to exceptional physical or mental stress which usually subside within hours or days

EXCLUDES   adjustment reaction or disorder (309.0-309.9)
chronic stress reaction (309.1-309.9)

- **308.0 Predominant disturbance of emotions**
  Anxiety
  Emotional crisis } as acute reaction to exceptional [gross] stress
  Panic state
- **308.1 Predominant disturbance of consciousness**
  Fugues as acute reaction to exceptional [gross] stress
- **308.2 Predominant psychomotor disturbance**
  Agitation states } as acute reaction to exceptional [gross] stress
  Stupor
- **308.3 Other acute reactions to stress**
  Acute situational disturbance
  Brief or acute posttraumatic stress disorder
  EXCLUDES   prolonged posttraumatic emotional disturbance (309.81)
- **308.4 Mixed disorders as reaction to stress**
- **308.9 Unspecified acute reaction to stress**

309 Adjustment reaction
INCLUDES   adjustment disorders
reaction (adjustment) to chronic stress
EXCLUDES   acute reaction to major stress (308.0-308.9)
neurotic disorders (300.0-300.9)

- **309.0 Brief depressive reaction**
  Adjustment disorder with depressed mood
  Grief reaction
  EXCLUDES   affective psychoses (296.0-296.9)
  neurotic depression (300.4)
  prolonged depressive reaction (309.1)
  psychogenic depressive psychosis (298.0)
- **309.1 Prolonged depressive reaction**
  EXCLUDES   affective psychoses (296.0-296.9)
  neurotic depression (300.4)
  psychogenic depressive psychosis (298.0)
- **309.2 With predominant disturbance of other emotions**
  - 309.21 Separation anxiety disorder
  - 309.22 Emancipation disorder of adolescence and early adult life
  - 309.23 Specific academic or work inhibition
  - 309.24 Adjustment reaction with anxious mood
  - 309.28 Adjustment reaction with mixed emotional features
    Adjustment reaction with anxiety and depression
  - **309.29 Other**
    Culture shock
- **309.3 With predominant disturbance of conduct**
  Conduct disturbance } as adjustment reaction
  Destructiveness
  EXCLUDES   destructiveness in child (312.9)
  disturbance of conduct NOS (312.9)
  dyssocial behavior without manifest psychiatric disorder (V71.01-V71.02)
  personality disorder with predominantly sociopathic or asocial manifestations (301.7)
- **309.4 With mixed disturbance of emotions and conduct**
- **309.8 Other specified adjustment reactions**
  - 309.81 Prolonged posttraumatic stress disorder
    Chronic posttraumatic stress disorder
    Concentration camp syndrome
    EXCLUDES   posttraumatic brain syndrome:
    nonpsychotic (310.2)
    psychotic (293.0-293.9)
  - 309.82 Adjustment reaction with physical symptoms
  - 309.83 Adjustment reaction with withdrawal
    Elective mutism as adjustment reaction
    Hospitalism (in children) NOS
  - **309.89 Other**
- **309.9 Unspecified adjustment reaction**
  Adaptation reaction NOS
  Adjustment reaction NOS

310 Specific nonpsychotic mental disorders due to organic brain damage
EXCLUDES   neuroses, personality disorders, or other nonpsychotic conditions occurring in a form similar to that seen with functional disorders but in association with a physical condition (300.0-300.9, 301.0-301.9)

- **310.0 Frontal lobe syndrome**
  Lobotomy syndrome
  Postleucotomy syndrome [state]
  EXCLUDES   postcontusion syndrome (310.2)
- **310.1 Organic personality syndrome**
  Cognitive or personality change of other type, of nonpsychotic severity
  Mild memory disturbance
  Organic psychosyndrome of nonpsychotic severity
  Presbyophrenia NOS
  Senility with mental changes of nonpsychotic severity
- **310.2 Postconcussion syndrome**
  Postcontusion syndrome or encephalopathy
  Posttraumatic brain syndrome, nonpsychotic
  Status postcommotio cerebri
  EXCLUDES   frontal lobe syndrome (310.0)
  postencephalitic syndrome (310.8)
  any organic psychotic conditions following head injury (293.0-294.0)
- **310.8 Other specified nonpsychotic mental disorders following organic brain damage**
  Postencephalitic syndrome
  Other focal (partial) organic psychosyndromes
- **310.9 Unspecified nonpsychotic mental disorder following organic brain damage**

311 Depressive disorder, not elsewhere classified
Depressive disorder NOS
Depressive state NOS
Depression NOS
EXCLUDES   acute reaction to major stress with depressive symptoms (308.0)
affective personality disorder (301.10-301.13)
affective psychoses (296.0-296.9)
brief depressive reaction (309.0)
depressive states associated with stressful events (309.0-309.1)
disturbance of emotions specific to childhood and adolescence, with misery and unhappiness (313.1)
mixed adjustment reaction withdepressive symptoms (309.4)
neurotic depression (300.4)
prolonged depressive adjustment reaction (309.1)
psychogenic depressive psychosis (298.0)

312 Disturbance of conduct, not elsewhere classified
EXCLUDES   adjustment reaction with disturbance of conduct (309.3)
drug dependence (304.0-304.9)
dyssocial behavior without manifest psychiatric disorder (V71.01-V71.02)
personality disorder with predominantly sociopathic or asocial manifestations (301.7)
sexual deviations (302.0-302.9)

MENTAL DISORDERS

The following fifth-digit subclassification is for use with categories 312.0-312.2:
- 0 unspecified
- 1 mild
- 2 moderate
- 3 severe

- **312.0** Undersocialized conduct disorder, aggressive type
  - Aggressive outburst
  - Anger reaction
  - Unsocialized aggressive disorder
- **312.1** Undersocialized conduct disorder, unaggressive type
  - Childhood truancy, unsocialized   Tantrums
  - Solitary stealing
- **312.2** Socialized conduct disorder
  - Childhood truancy, socialized
  - Group delinquency
  - EXCLUDES: gang activity without manifest psychiatric disorder (V71.01)
- **312.3** Disorders of impulse control, not elsewhere classified
  - **312.30** Impulse control disorder, unspecified
  - **312.31** Pathological gambling
  - **312.32** Kleptomania
  - **312.33** Pyromania
  - **312.34** Intermittent explosive disorder
  - **312.35** Isolated explosive disorder
  - **312.39** Other
- **312.4** Mixed disturbance of conduct and emotions
  - Neurotic delinquency
  - EXCLUDES: compulsive conduct disorder (312.3)
- **312.8** Other specified disturbances of conduct, not elsewhere classified
  - **312.81** Conduct disorder, childhood onset type
  - **312.82** Conduct disorder, adolescent onset type
  - **312.89** Other conduct disorder
- **312.9** Unspecified disturbance of conduct
  - Delinquency (juvenile)

- **313** Disturbance of emotions specific to childhood and adolescence
  - EXCLUDES: adjustment reaction (309.0-309.9)
    emotional disorder of neurotic type (300.0-300.9)
    masturbation, nail-biting, thumbsucking, and other isolated symptoms (307.0-307.9)
  - **313.0** Overanxious disorder
    - Anxiety and fearfulness } of childhood and
    - Overanxious disorder } adolescence
    - EXCLUDES: abnormal separation anxiety (309.21)
      anxiety states (300.00-300.09)
      hospitalism in children (309.83)
      phobic state (300.20-300.29)
  - **313.1** Misery and unhappiness disorder
    - EXCLUDES: depressive neurosis (300.4)
  - **313.2** Sensitivity, shyness, and social withdrawal disorder
    - EXCLUDES: infantile autism (299.0)
      schizoid personality (301.20-301.22)
      schizophrenia (295.0-295.9)
    - **313.21** Shyness disorder of childhood
      - Sensitivity reaction of childhood or adolescence
    - **313.22** Introverted disorder of childhood
      - Social withdrawal } of childhood or
      - Withdrawal reaction } adolescence
    - **313.23** Elective mutism
      - EXCLUDES: elective mutism as adjustment reaction (309.83)
  - **313.3** Relationship problems
    - Sibling jealousy
    - EXCLUDES: relationship problems associated with aggression, destruction, or other forms of conduct disturbance (312.0-312.9)
  - **313.8** Other or mixed emotional disturbances of childhood or adolescence
    - **313.81** Oppositional disorder
    - **313.82** Identity disorder
    - **313.83** Academic underachievement disorder
    - **313.89** Other
  - **313.9** Unspecified emotional disturbance of childhood or adolescence

- **314** Hyperkinetic syndrome of childhood
  - EXCLUDES: hyperkinesis as symptom of underlying disorder—code the underlying disorder
  - **314.0** Attention deficit disorder
    - **314.00** Without mention of hyperactivity
      - Predominantly inattentive type
    - **314.01** With hyperactivity
      - Combined type
      - Overactivity NOS
      - Predominantly hyperactive/impulsive type
      - Simple disturbance of attention with overactivity
  - **314.1** Hyperkinesis with developmental delay
    - Developmental disorder of hyperkinesis
    - Use additional code to identify any associated neurological disorder
  - **314.2** Hyperkinetic conduct disorder
    - Hyperkinetic conduct disorder without developmental delay
    - EXCLUDES: hyperkinesis with significant delays in specific skills (314.1)
  - **314.8** Other specified manifestations of hyperkinetic syndrome
  - **314.9** Unspecified hyperkinetic syndrome
    - Hyperkinetic reaction of childhood or adolescence NOS
    - Hyperkinetic syndrome NOS

- **315** Specific delays in development
  - EXCLUDES: that due to a neurological disorder (320.0-389.9)
  - **315.0** Specific reading disorder
    - **315.00** Reading disorder, unspecified
    - **315.01** Alexia
    - **315.02** Developmental dyslexia
    - **315.09** Other
      - Specific spelling difficulty
  - **315.1** Specific arithmetical disorder
    - Dyscalculia
  - **315.2** Other specific learning difficulties
    - EXCLUDES: specific arithmetical disorder (315.1)
      specific reading disorder (315.00-315.09)
  - **315.3** Developmental speech or language disorder
    - **315.31** Developmental language disorder
      - Developmental aphasia
      - Word deafness
      - EXCLUDES: acquired aphasia (784.3)
        elective mutism (309.83, 313.0, 313.23)
    - **315.39** Other
      - Developmental articulation disorder
      - Dyslalia
      - EXCLUDES: lisping and lalling (307.9)
        stammering and stuttering (307.0)
  - **315.4** Coordination disorder
    - Clumsiness syndrome
    - Dyspraxia syndrome
    - Specific motor development disorder
  - **315.5** Mixed development disorder
  - **315.8** Other specified delays in development
  - **315.9** Unspecified delay in development
    - Developmental disorder NOS

- **316** Psychic factors associated with diseases classified elsewhere
  - Psychologic factors in physical conditions classified elsewhere
  - Use additional code to identify the associated physical condition, as: psychogenic:
    - asthma (493.9)
    - dermatitis (692.9)
    - duodenal ulcer (532.0-532.9)
    - eczema (691.8, 692.9)
    - gastric ulcer (531.0-531.9)
    - mucous colitis (564.1)
    - paroxysmal tachycardia (427.2)
    - ulcerative colitis (556)
    - urticaria (708.0-708.9)
    - psychosocial dwarfism (259.4)
  - EXCLUDES: physical symptoms and physiological malfunctions, not involving tissue damage, of mental origin (306.0-306.9)

MENTAL RETARDATION (317-319)

317   Mild mental retardation
    Feeble-minded
    High-grade defect
    IQ 50-70
    Mild mental subnormality
    Moron

● **318   Other specified mental retardation**
    318.0   Moderate mental retardation
        Imbecile
        IQ 35-49
        Moderate mental subnormality
    318.1   Severe mental retardation
        IQ 20-34
        Severe mental subnormality
    318.2   Profound mental retardation
        Idiocy
        IQ under 20
        Profound mental subnormality

◆ **319   Unspecified mental retardation**
    Mental deficiency NOS
    Mental subnormality NOS

6. DISEASES OF THE NERVOUS SYSTEM AND SENSE ORGANS (320-389)

INFLAMMATORY DISEASES OF THE CENTRAL NERVOUS SYSTEM (320-326)

● **320   Bacterial meningitis**

    INCLUDES   arachnoiditis
        leptomeningitis
        meningitis   } bacterial
        meningoencephalitis
        meningomyelitis
        pachymeningitis

    320.0   Hemophilus meningitis
        Meningitis due to Hemophilus influenzae [H. influenzae]
    320.1   Pneumococcal meningitis
    320.2   Streptococcal meningitis
    320.3   Staphylococcal meningitis
    320.7   *Meningitis in other bacterial diseases classified elsewhere*
        Code also underlying disease, as:
            actinomycosis (039.8)
            listeriosis (027.0)
            typhoid fever (002.0)
            whooping cough (033.0-033.9)
        EXCLUDES *meningitis (in):*
            epidemic (036.0)
            gonococcal (098.82)
            meningococcal (036.0)
            salmonellosis (003.21)
            syphilis:
                NOS (094.2)
                congenital (090.42)
                meningovascular (094.2)
                secondary (091.81)
            tuberculous (013.0)

● **320.8   Meningitis due to other specified bacteria**
    320.81   Anaerobic meningitis
        Gram-negative anaerobes
        Bacteroides (fragilis)
    320.82   Meningitis due to gram-negative bacteria, not elsewhere classified
        Aerobacter aerogenes
        Escherichia coli [E. coli]
        Friedländer bacillus
        Proteus morganii
        Pseudomonas
        EXCLUDES *gram-negative anaerobes (320.81)*
◆   **320.89   Meningitis due to other specified bacteria**
        Bacillus pyocyaneus
◆ **320.9   Meningitis due to unspecified bacterium**
    Meningitis: Meningitis:
        bacterial NOS   pyogenic NOS
        purulent NOS   suppurative NOS

● **321   Meningitis due to other organisms**

    INCLUDES   arachnoiditis
        leptomeningiti   } due to organisms
        meningitis   other than
        pachymeningitis   bacteria

    321.0   *Cryptococcal meningitis*
        Code also underlying disease (117.5)
◆   **321.1   *Meningitis in other fungal diseases***
        Code also underlying disease (110.0-118)
        EXCLUDES *meningitis in:*
            candidiasis (112.83)
            coccidioidomycosis (114.2)
            histoplasmosis (115.01, 115.11, 115.91)
    321.2   *Meningitis due to viruses not elsewhere classified*
        Code also underlying disease, as:
            meningitis due to arbovirus (060.0-066.9)
        EXCLUDES *meningitis (due to):*
            abacterial (047.0-047.9)
            adenovirus (049.1)
            aseptic NOS (047.9)
            Coxsackie (virus)(047.0)
            ECHO virus (047.1)
            enterovirus (047.0-047.9)
            herpes simplex virus (054.72)
            herpes zoster virus (053.0)
            lymphocytic choriomeningitis virus (049.0)
            mumps (072.1)
            viral NOS (047.9)
            meningo-eruptive syndrome (047.1)
    321.3   *Meningitis due to trypanosomiasis*
        Code also underlying disease (086.0-086.9)
    321.4   *Meningitis in sarcoidosis*
        Code also underlying disease (135)
◆   **321.8   *Meningitis due to other nonbacterial organisms classified elsewhere***
        Code also underlying disease
        EXCLUDES *leptospiral meningitis (100.81)*

● **322   Meningitis of unspecified cause**

    INCLUDES   arachnoiditis
        leptomeningitis   } with no organism
        meningitis   specified as
        pachymeningitis   cause

    322.0   Nonpyogenic meningitis
        Meningitis with clear cerebrospinal fluid
    322.1   Eosinophilic meningitis
    322.2   Chronic meningitis
◆   **322.9   Meningitis, unspecified**

● **323   Encephalitis, myelitis, and encephalomyelitis**

    INCLUDES   acute disseminated encephalomyelitis
        meningoencephalitis, except bacterial
        meningomyelitis, except bacterial
        myelitis (acute):
            ascending
            transverse
    EXCLUDES *bacterial:*
        meningoencephalitis (320.0-320.9)
        meningomyelitis (320.0-320.9)

    323.0   *Encephalitis in viral diseases classified elsewhere*
        Code also underlying disease, as:
            cat-scratch disease (078.3)
            infectious mononucleosis (075)
            ornithosis (073.7)
        EXCLUDES *encephalitis (in):*
            arthropod-borne viral (062.0-064)
            herpes simplex (054.3)
            mumps (072.2)
            poliomyelitis (045.0-045.9)
            rubella (056.01)
            slow virus infections of central nervous system (046.0-046.9)
            other viral diseases of central nervous system (049.8-049.9)
            viral NOS (049.9)

323.1 NERVOUS SYSTEM AND SENSE ORGANS 332.0

■ *323.1* **Encephalitis in rickettsial diseases classified elsewhere**
    Code also underlying disease (080-083.9)
■ *323.2* **Encephalitis in protozoal diseases classified elsewhere**
    Code also underlying disease, as:
        malaria (084.0-084.9)
        trypanosomiasis (086.0-086.9)
■ ◆ *323.4* **Other encephalitis due to infection classified elsewhere**
    Code also underlying disease
    EXCLUDES encephalitis (in):
        meningococcal (036.1)
        syphilis:
            NOS (094.81)
            congenital (090.41)
        toxoplasmosis (130.0)
        tuberculosis (013.6)
        meningoencephalitis due to free-living ameba [Naegleria] (136.2)

323.5 **Encephalitis following immunization procedures**
    Encephalitis   } postimmunization or
    Encephalomyelitis   } postvaccinal
    Use additional E code, if desired, to identify vaccine

■ *323.6* **Postinfectious encephalitis**
    Code also underlying disease
    EXCLUDES encephalitis:
        postchickenpox (052.0)
        postmeasles (055.0)

■ *323.7* **Toxic encephalitis**
    Code also underlying cause, as:
        carbon tetrachloride (982.1)
        hydroxyquinoline derivatives (961.3)
        lead (984.0-984.9)
        mercury (985.0)
        thallium (985.8)

◆ 323.8 **Other causes of encephalitis**
◆ 323.9 **Unspecified cause of encephalitis**
● 324 **Intracranial and intraspinal abscess**
    324.0 **Intracranial abscess**
        Abscess (embolic):
            cerebellar
            cerebral
        Abscess (embolic) of brain [any part]:
            epidural
            extradural
            otogenic
            subdural
        EXCLUDES tuberculous (013.3)
    324.1 **Intraspinal abscess**
        Abscess (embolic) of spinal cord [any part]:
            epidural
            extradural
            subdural
        EXCLUDES tuberculous (013.5)
    ◆ 324.9 **Of unspecified site**
        Extradural or subdural abscess NOS

325 **Phlebitis and thrombophlebitis of intracranial venous sinuses**
    Embolism
    Endophlebitis
    Phlebitis, septic or
        suppurative
    Thrombophlebitis
    Thrombosis
    } of cavernous, lateral, or other intracranial or unspecified intracranial venous sinus

    EXCLUDES that specified as:
        complicating pregnancy, childbirth, or the puerperium (671.5)
        of nonpyogenic origin (437.6)

326 **Late effects of intracranial abscess or pyogenic infection**
    Note: This category is to be used to indicate conditions whose primary classification is to 320-325 [excluding 320.7, 321.0-321.8, 323.0-323.4, 323.6-323.7] as the cause of late effects, themselves classifiable elsewhere. The "late effects" include conditions specified as such, or as sequelae, which may occur at any time after the resolution of the causal condition.
    Use additional code, if desired, to identify condition, as:
        hydrocephalus (331.4)
        paralysis (342.0-342.9, 344.0-344.9)

HEREDITARY AND DEGENERATIVE DISEASES OF THE CENTRAL NERVOUS SYSTEM (330-337)

EXCLUDES hepatolenticular degeneration (275.1)
    multiple sclerosis (340)
    other demyelinating diseases of central nervous system (341.0-341.9)

● 330 **Cerebral degenerations usually manifest in childhood**
    Use additional code, if desired, to identify associated mental retardation
    330.0 **Leukodystrophy**
        Krabbe's disease   Pelizaeus-Merzbacher
        Leukodystrophy   disease
            NOS   Sulfatide lipidosis
            globoid cell
            metachromatic
            sudanophilic
    330.1 **Cerebral lipidoses**
        Amaurotic (familial) idiocy   Disease:
        Disease: Spielmeyer-Vogt
            Batten   Tay-Sachs
            Jansky-Bielschowsky   Gangliosidosis
            Kufs'
    ■ 330.2 **Cerebral degeneration in generalized lipidoses**
        Code also underlying disease, as:
            Fabry's disease (272.7)
            Gaucher's disease (272.7)
            Niemann-Pick disease (272.7)
            sphingolipidosis (272.7)
    ■ ◆ 330.3 **Cerebral degeneration of childhood in other diseases classified elsewhere**
        Code also underlying disease, as:
            Hunter's disease (277.5)
            mucopolysaccharidosis (277.5)
    ◆ 330.8 **Other specified cerebral degenerations in childhood**
        Alpers' disease or gray-matter degeneration
        Infantile necrotizing encephalomyelopathy
        Leigh's disease
        Subacute necrotizing encephalopathy or encephalomyelopathy
    ◆ 330.9 **Unspecified cerebral degeneration in childhood**

● 331 **Other cerebral degenerations**
    331.0 **Alzheimer's disease**
    331.1 **Pick's disease**
    331.2 **Senile degeneration of brain**
        EXCLUDES senility NOS (797)
    331.3 **Communicating hydrocephalus**
        EXCLUDES congenital hydrocephalus (741.0, 742.3)
    331.4 **Obstructive hydrocephalus**
        Acquired hydrocephalus NOS
        EXCLUDES congenital hydrocephalus (741.0, 742.3)
    ■ 331.7 **Cerebral degeneration in diseases classified elsewhere**
        Code also underlying disease, as:
            alcoholism (303.0-303.9)
            beriberi (265.0)
            cerebrovascular disease (430-438)
            congenital hydrocephalus (741.0, 742.3)
            neoplastic disease (140.0-239.9)
            myxedema (244.0-244.9)
            vitamin B_{12} deficiency (266.2)
        EXCLUDES cerebral degeneration in:
            Jakob-Creutzfeldt disease (046.1)
            progressive multifocal leukoencephalopathy (046.3)
            subacute spongiform encephalopathy (046.1)
    ● 331.8 **Other cerebral degeneration**
        331.81 **Reye's syndrome**
        ◆ 331.89 **Other**
            Cerebral ataxia
    ◆ 331.9 **Cerebral degeneration, unspecified**
● 332 **Parkinson's disease**
    332.0 **Paralysis agitans**
        Parkinsonism or Parkinson's disease:
            NOS   primary
            idiopathic

● Additional digits required   ◆ Nonspecific code   ■ Not a primary diagnosis

Volume 1 — 51

332.1 Secondary Parkinsonism
Parkinsonism due to drugs
Use additional E code, if desired, to identify drug, if drug-induced
EXCLUDES Parkinsonism (in):
Huntington's disease (333.4)
progressive supranuclear palsy (333.0)
Shy-Drager syndrome (333.0)
syphilitic (094.82)

● 333 Other extrapyramidal disease and abnormal movement disorders
INCLUDES other forms of extrapyramidal, basal ganglia, or striatopallidal disease
EXCLUDES abnormal movements of head NOS (781.0)

◆ **333.0 Other degenerative diseases of the basal ganglia**
Atrophy or degeneration:
olivopontocerebellar [Déjérine-Thomas syndrome]
pigmentary pallidal [Hallervorden-Spatz disease]
striatonigral
Parkinsonian syndrome associated with:
idiopathic orthostatic hypotension
symptomatic orthostatic hypotension
Progressive supranuclear ophthalmoplegia or palsy
Shy-Drager syndrome

◆ **333.1 Essential and other specified forms of tremor**
Benign essential tremor
Familial tremor
Use additional E code, if desired, to identify drug, if drug-induced
EXCLUDES tremor NOS (781.0)

333.2 Myoclonus
Familial essential myoclonus
Progressive myoclonic epilepsy
Unverricht-Lundborg disease
Use additional E code, if desired, to identify drug, if drug-induced

333.3 Tics of organic origin
EXCLUDES Gilles de la Tourette's syndrome (307.23)
habit spasm (307.22)
tic NOS (307.20)
Use additional E code, if desired, to identify drug, if drug-induced

333.4 Huntington's chorea

◆ **333.5 Other choreas**
Hemiballism(us)
Paroxysmal choreo-athetosis
EXCLUDES Sydenham's or rheumatic chorea (392.0-392.9)
Use additional E code, if desired, to identify drug, if drug-induced

333.6 Idiopathic torsion dystonia
Dystonia:
deformans progressiva
musculorum deformans
(Schwalbe-) Ziehen-Oppenheim disease

333.7 Symptomatic torsion dystonia
Athetoid cerebral palsy [Vogt's disease]
Double athetosis (syndrome)
Use additional E code, if desired, to identify drug, if drug-induced

● **333.8 Fragments of torsion dystonia**
Use additional E code, if desired, to identify drug, if drug-induced
333.81 Blepharospasm
333.82 Orofacial dyskinesia
333.83 Spasmodic torticollis
EXCLUDES torticollis:
NOS (723.5)
hysterical (300.11)
psychogenic (306.0)
333.84 Organic writers' cramp
EXCLUDES pychogenic (300.89)
◆ 333.89 Other

● **333.9 Other and unspecified extrapyramidal diseases and abnormal movement disorders**
◆ 333.90 Unspecified extrapyramidal disease and abnormal movement disorder
333.91 Stiff-man syndrome
333.92 Neuroleptic malignant syndrome ▼
Use additional E code to identify drug
333.93 Benign shuddering attacks ▲
◆ 333.99 Other
Restless legs

● 334 Spinocerebellar disease
EXCLUDES olivopontocerebellar degeneration (333.0)
peroneal muscular atrophy (356.1)

334.0 Friedreich's ataxia
334.1 Hereditary spastic paraplegia
334.2 Primary cerebellar degeneration
Cerebellar ataxia:
Marie's
Sanger-Brown
Dyssynergia cerebellaris myoclonica
Primary cerebellar degeneration:
NOS
hereditary
sporadic

◆ **334.3 Other cerebellar ataxia**
Cerebellar ataxia NOS
Use additional E code, if desired, to identify drug, if drug-induced

▮ **334.4 Cerebellar ataxia in diseases classified elsewhere**
Code also underlying disease, as:
alcoholism (303.0-303.9)
myxedema (244.0-244.9)
neoplastic disease (140.0-239.9)

◆ **334.8 Other spinocerebellar diseases**
Ataxia-telangiectasia [Louis-Bar syndrome]
Corticostriatal-spinal degeneration

◆ **334.9 Spinocerebellar disease, unspecified**

● 335 Anterior horn cell disease
335.0 Werdnig-Hoffmann disease
Infantile spinal muscular atrophy
Progressive muscular atrophy of infancy

● **335.1 Spinal muscular atrophy**
◆ 335.10 Spinal muscular atrophy, unspecified
335.11 Kugelberg-Welander disease
Spinal muscular atrophy:
familial
juvenile
◆ 335.19 Other
Adult spinal muscular atrophy

● **335.2 Motor neuron disease**
335.20 Amyotrophic lateral sclerosis
Motor neuron disease (bulbar) (mixed type)
335.21 Progressive muscular atrophy
Duchenne-Aran muscular atrophy
Progressive muscular atrophy (pure)
335.22 Progressive bulbar palsy
335.23 Pseudobulbar palsy
335.24 Primary lateral sclerosis
◆ 335.29 Other

◆ **335.8 Other anterior horn cell diseases**
◆ **335.9 Anterior horn cell disease, unspecified**

● 336 Other diseases of spinal cord
336.0 Syringomyelia and syringobulbia
336.1 Vascular myelopathies
Acute infarction of spinal cord (embolic) (nonembolic)
Arterial thrombosis of spinal cord
Edema of spinal cord
Hematomyelia
Subacute necrotic myelopathy

▮ **336.2 Subacute combined degeneration of spinal cord in diseases classified elsewhere**
Code also underlying disease, as:
pernicious anemia (281.0)
other vitamin B_{12} deficiency anemia (281.1)
vitamin B_{12} deficiency (266.2)

▮ **336.3 Myelopathy in other diseases classified elsewhere**
Code also underlying disease, as:
myelopathy in neoplastic disease (140.0-239.9)
EXCLUDES myelopathy in:
intervertebral disc disorder (722.70-722.73)
spondylosis (721.1, 721.41-721.42, 721.91)

NERVOUS SYSTEM AND SENSE ORGANS

- ◆ **336.8 Other myelopathy**
  - Myelopathy:
    - drug-induced
    - radiation-induced
  - Use additonal E code, if desired, to identify cause
- ◆ **336.9 Unspecified disease of spinal cord**
  - Cord compression NOS
  - Myelopathy NOS
  - **EXCLUDES** *myelitis (323.0-323.9)*
  - *spinal (canal) stenosis (723.0, 724.00-724.09)*

● **337 Disorders of the autonomic nervous system**
  - **INCLUDES** disorders of peripheral autonomic, sympathetic, parasympathetic, or vegetative system
  - **EXCLUDES** *familial dysautonomia [Riley-Day syndrome] (742.8)*
  - **337.0 Idiopathic peripheral autonomic neuropathy**
    - Carotid sinus syncope or syndrome
    - Cervical sympathetic dystrophy or paralysis
  - ■ *337.1 Peripheral autonomic neuropathy in disorders classified elsewhere*
    - Code also underlying disease, as:
      - amyloidosis (277.3)
      - diabetes (250.6)
  - ● **337.2 Reflex sympathetic dystrophy**
    - ◆ 337.20 Reflex sympathetic dystrophy, unspecified
    - 337.21 Reflex sympathetic dystrophy of the upper limb
    - 337.22 Reflex sympathetic dystrophy of the lower limb
    - ◆ 337.29 Reflex sympathetic dystrophy of other specified site
  - ◆ **337.9 Unspecified disorder of autonomic nervous system**

OTHER DISORDERS OF THE CENTRAL NERVOUS SYSTEM (340-349)

340 Multiple sclerosis
  - Disseminated or multiple sclerosis:
    - NOS
    - brain stem
    - cord
    - generalized

● **341 Other demyelinating diseases of central nervous system**
  - **341.0 Neuromyelitis optica**
  - **341.1 Schilder's disease**
    - Baló's concentric sclerosis
    - Encephalitis periaxialis:
      - concentrica [Baló's]
      - diffusa [Schilder's]
  - ◆ **341.8 Other demyelinating diseases of central nervous system**
    - Central demyelination of corpus callosum
    - Central pontine myelinosis
    - Marchiafava (-Bignami) disease
  - ◆ **341.9 Demyelinating disease of central nervous system, unspecified**

● **342 Hemiplegia and hemiparesis**
  - Note: This category is to be used when hemiplegia (complete) (incomplete) is reported without further specification, or is stated to be old or long-standing but of unspecified cause. The category is also for use in multiple coding to identify these types of hemiplegia resulting from any cause.
  - **EXCLUDES** *congenital (343.1)*
  - *infantile NOS (343.4)*
  - The following fifth-digits are for use with codes 342.0-342.9: ▼
    - ◆ 0 affecting unspecified side
    - 1 affecting dominant side
    - 2 affecting nondominant side ▲
  - ● **342.0 Flaccid hemiplegia**
  - ● **342.1 Spastic hemiplegia**
  - ● **342.8 Other specified hemiplegia** ◆
  - ● **342.9 Hemiplegia, unspecified**

● **343 Infantile cerebral palsy**
  - **INCLUDES** cerebral:
    - palsy NOS
    - spastic infantile paralysis
    - congenital spastic paralysis (cerebral)
    - Little's disease
    - paralysis (spastic) due to birth injury:
      - intracranial
      - spinal
  - **EXCLUDES** *hereditary cerebral paralysis, such as:*
    - *hereditary spastic paraplegia (334.1)*
    - *Vogt's disease (333.7)*
    - *spastic paralysis specified as noncongenital or noninfantile (344.0-344.9)*
  - **343.0 Diplegic**
    - Congenital diplegia
    - Congenital paraplegia
  - **343.1 Hemiplegic**
    - Congenital hemiplegia
    - **EXCLUDES** *infantile hemiplegia NOS (343.4)*
  - **343.2 Quadriplegic**
    - Tetraplegic
  - **343.3 Monoplegic**
  - **343.4 Infantile hemiplegia**
    - Infantile hemiplegia (postnatal) NOS
  - ◆ **343.8 Other specified infantile cerebral palsy**
  - ◆ **343.9 Infantile cerebral palsy, unspecified**
    - Cerebral palsy NOS

● **344 Other paralytic syndromes**
  - Note: This category is to be used when the listed conditions are reported without further specification or are stated to be old or long-standing but of unspecified cause. The category is also for use in multiple coding to identify these conditions resulting from any cause.
  - **INCLUDES** paralysis (complete) (incomplete), except as classifiable to 342 and 343
  - **EXCLUDES** *congenital or infantile cerebral palsy (343.0-343.9)*
    - *hemiplegia (342.0-342.9)*
    - *congenital or infantile (343.1, 343.4)*
  - ● **344.0 Quadriplegia and quadriparesis** ▼
    - ◆ 344.00 Quadriplegia unspecified
    - 344.01 C_1-C_4 complete
    - 344.02 C_1-C_4 incomplete
    - 344.03 C_5-C_7 complete
    - 344.04 C_5-C_7 incomplete
    - ◆ 344.09 Other ▲
  - **344.1 Paraplegia**
    - Paralysis of both lower limbs
    - Paraplegia (lower)
  - **344.2 Diplegia of upper limbs**
    - Diplegia (upper)
    - Paralysis of both upper limbs
  - ● **344.3 Monoplegia of lower limb**
    - Paralysis of lower limb
    - ◆ 344.30 Affecting unspecified side ▼
    - 344.31 Affecting dominant side
    - 344.32 Affecting nondominant side ▲
  - ● **344.4 Monoplegia of upper limb**
    - Paralysis of upper limb
    - ◆ 344.40 Affecting unspecified side ▼
    - 344.41 Affecting dominant side
    - 344.42 Affecting nondominant side ▲
  - ◆ **344.5 Unspecified monoplegia**
  - ● **344.6 Cauda equina syndrome**
    - 344.60 Without mention of neurogenic bladder
    - 344.61 With neurogenic bladder
      - Acontractile bladder
      - Autonomic hyperreflexia of bladder
      - Cord bladder
      - Detrusor hyperreflexia
  - ● **344.8 Other specified paralytic syndromes**
    - 344.81 Locked-in state
    - ◆ 344.89 Other specified paralytic syndrome
  - ◆ **344.9 Paralysis, unspecified**

● **345 Epilepsy**
  - The following fifth-digit subclassification is for use with categories 345.0, .1, .4-.9:
    - 0 without mention of intractable epilepsy
    - 1 with intractableepilepsy
  - **EXCLUDES** *progressive myoclonic epilepsy (333.2)*
  - ● **345.0 Generalized nonconvulsive epilepsy**
    - Absences:
      - atonic
      - typical
    - Minor epilepsy
    - Petit mal
    - Pykno-epilepsy
    - Seizures:
      - akinetic
      - atonic

● Additional digits required ◆ Nonspecific code ■ Not a primary diagnosis

Volume 1 — 53

345.1 Generalized convulsive epilepsy
Epileptic seizures:
  myoclonic
  tonic
  tonic-clonic
Grand mal
Major epilepsy
EXCLUDES convulsions:
  NOS (780.3)
  infantile (780.3)
  newborn (779.0)
  infantile spasms (345.6)

345.2 Petit mal status
Epileptic absence status

345.3 Grand mal status
Status epilepticus NOS
EXCLUDES epilepsia partialis continua (345.7)
  status:
    psychomotor (345.7)
    temporal lobe (345.7)

345.4 Partial epilepsy, with impairment of consciousness
Epilepsy:
  limbic system
  partial:
    secondarily generalized
    with memory and ideational disturbances
  psychomotor
  psychosensory
  temporal lobe
Epileptic automatism

345.5 Partial epilepsy, without mention of impairment of consciousness
Epilepsy:
  Bravais-Jacksonian NOS
  focal (motor) NOS
  Jacksonian NOS
  motor partial
  partial NOS
Epilepsy:
  sensory-induced
  somatomotor
  somatosensory
  visceral
  visual

345.6 Infantile spasms
Hypsarrhythmia
Lightning spasms
Salaam attacks
EXCLUDES salaam tic (781.0)

345.7 Epilepsia partialis continua
Kojevnikov's epilepsy

345.8 Other forms of epilepsy
Epilepsy:
  cursive [running]
  gelastic

345.9 Epilepsy, unspecified
Epileptic convulsions, fits, or seizures NOS
EXCLUDES convulsive seizure or fit NOS (780.3)

346 Migraine
The following fifth-digit subclassification is for use with category 346:
  0 without mention of intractable migraine
  1 with intractable migraine, so stated

346.0 Classical migraine
Migraine preceded or accompanied by transient focal neurological phenomena
Migraine with aura

346.1 Common migraine
Atypical migraine
Sick headache

346.2 Variants of migraine
Cluster headache
Histamine cephalgia
Horton's neuralgia
Migraine:
  abdominal
  basilar
Migraine:
  lower half
  retinal
Neuralgia:
  ciliary
  migrainous

346.8 Other forms of migraine
Migraine:
  hemiplegic
  ophthalmoplegic

346.9 Migraine, unspecified

347 Cataplexy and narcolepsy

348 Other conditions of brain

348.0 Cerebral cysts
Arachnoid cyst
Porencephalic cyst
Porencephaly, acquired
Pseudoporencephaly
EXCLUDES porencephaly (congenital) (742.4)

348.1 Anoxic brain damage
EXCLUDES that occurring in:
  abortion (634-638 with .7, 639.8)
  ectopic or molar pregnancy (639.8)
  labor or delivery (668.2, 669.4)
  that of newborn (767.0, 768.0-768.9, 772.1-772.2)
Use additional E code, if desired, to identify cause

348.2 Benign intracranial hypertension
Pseudotumor cerebri
EXCLUDES hypertensive encephalopathy (437.2)

348.3 Encephalopathy, unspecified

348.4 Compression of brain
Compression | brain (stem)
Herniation |
Posterior fossa compression syndrome

348.5 Cerebral edema

348.8 Other conditions of brain
Cerebral:
  calcification
  fungus

348.9 Unspecified condition of brain

349 Other and unspecified disorders of the nervous system

349.0 Reaction to spinal or lumbar puncture
Headache following lumbar puncture

349.1 Nervous system complications from surgically implanted device
EXCLUDES immediate postoperative complications (997.0)
mechanical complications of nervous system device (996.2)

349.2 Disorders of meninges, not elsewhere classified
Adhesions, meningeal (cerebral) (spinal)
Cyst, spinal meninges

349.8 Other specified disorders of nervous system
349.81 Cerebrospinal fluid rhinorrhea
Pseudomeningocele
EXCLUDES cerebrospinal fluid otorrhea (388.61)
349.82 Toxic encephalopathy
Use additional E code, if desired, to identify cause
349.89 Other

349.9 Unspecified disorders of nervous system
Disorder of nervous system (central) NOS

DISORDERS OF THE PERIPHERAL NERVOUS SYSTEM (350-359)
EXCLUDES diseases of:
  acoustic [8th] nerve (388.5)
  oculomotor [3rd, 4th, 6th] nerves (378.0-378.9)
  optic [2nd] nerve (377.0-377.9)
  peripheral autonomic nerves (337.0-337.9)
neuralgia
neuritis } NOS or "rheumatic" (729.2)
radiculitis
peripheral neuritis in pregnancy (646.4)

350 Trigeminal nerve disorders
INCLUDES disorders of 5th cranial nerve

350.1 Trigeminal neuralgia
Tic douloureux
Trifacial neuralgia
Trigeminal neuralgia NOS
EXCLUDES postherpetic (053.12)

350.2 Atypical face pain

350.8 Other specified trigeminal nerve disorders

350.9 Trigeminal nerve disorder, unspecified

351 Facial nerve disorders
INCLUDES disorders of 7th cranial nerve
EXCLUDES that in newborn (767.5)

351.0 Bell's palsy
Facial palsy

NERVOUS SYSTEM AND SENSE ORGANS

- 351.1 **Geniculate ganglionitis**
  - Geniculate ganglionitis NOS
  - EXCLUDES: herpetic (053.11)
- ◆ 351.8 **Other facial nerve disorders**
  - Facial myokymia
  - Melkersson's syndrome
- ◆ 351.9 **Facial nerve disorder, unspecified**
- ● 352 **Disorders of other cranial nerves**
  - 352.0 **Disorders of olfactory [1st] nerve**
  - 352.1 **Glossopharyngeal neuralgia**
  - ◆ 352.2 **Other disorders of glossopharyngeal [9th] nerve**
  - 352.3 **Disorders of pneumogastric [10th] nerve**
    - Disorders of vagal nerve
    - EXCLUDES: paralysis of vocal cords or larynx (478.30-478.34)
  - 352.4 **Disorders of accessory [11th] nerve**
  - 352.5 **Disorders of hypoglossal [12th] nerve**
  - 352.6 **Multiple cranial nerve palsies**
    - Collet-Sicard syndrome
    - Polyneuritis cranialis
  - ◆ 352.9 **Unspecified disorder of cranial nerves**
- ● 353 **Nerve root and plexus disorders**
  - EXCLUDES: conditions due to:
    - intervertebral disc disorders (722.0-722.9)
    - spondylosis (720.0-721.9)
    - vertebrogenic disorders (723.0-724.9)
  - 353.0 **Brachial plexus lesions**
    - Cervical rib syndrome
    - Costoclavicular syndrome
    - Scalenus anticus syndrome
    - Thoracic outlet syndrome
    - EXCLUDES: brachial neuritis or radiculitis NOS (723.4)
      - that in newborn (767.6)
  - 353.1 **Lumbosacral plexus lesions**
  - 353.2 **Cervical root lesions, not elsewhere classified**
  - 353.3 **Thoracic root lesions, not elsewhere classified**
  - 353.4 **Lumbosacral root lesions, not elsewhere classified**
  - 353.5 **Neuralgic amyotrophy**
    - Parsonage-Aldren-Turner syndrome
  - 353.6 **Phantom limb (syndrome)**
  - ◆ 353.8 **Other nerve root and plexus disorders**
  - ◆ 353.9 **Unspecified nerve root and plexus disorder**
- ● 354 **Mononeuritis of upper limb and mononeuritis multiplex**
  - 354.0 **Carpal tunnel syndrome**
    - Median nerve entrapment
    - Partial thenar atrophy
  - ◆ 354.1 **Other lesion of median nerve**
    - Median nerve neuritis
  - 354.2 **Lesion of ulnar nerve**
    - Cubital tunnel syndrome
    - Tardy ulnar nerve palsy
  - 354.3 **Lesion of radial nerve**
    - Acute radial nerve palsy
  - 354.4 **Causalgia of upper limb**
    - EXCLUDES: causalgia:
      - NOS (355.9)
      - lower limb (355.71)
  - 354.5 **Mononeuritis multiplex**
    - Combinations of single conditions classifiable to 354 or 355
  - ◆ 354.8 **Other mononeuritis of upper limb**
  - ◆ 354.9 **Mononeuritis of upper limb, unspecified**
- ● 355 **Mononeuritis of lower limb and unspecified site**
  - 355.0 **Lesion of sciatic nerve**
    - EXCLUDES: sciatica NOS (724.3)
  - 355.1 **Meralgia paresthetica**
    - Lateral cutaneous femoral nerve of thigh compression or syndrome
  - ◆ 355.2 **Other lesion of femoral nerve**
  - 355.3 **Lesion of lateral popliteal nerve**
    - Lesion of common peroneal nerve
  - 355.4 **Lesion of medial popliteal nerve**
  - 355.5 **Tarsal tunnel syndrome**
  - 355.6 **Lesion of plantar nerve**
    - Morton's metatarsalgia, neuralgia, or neuroma
  - ● 355.7 **Other mononeuritis of lower limb**
    - 355.71 **Causalgia of lower limb**
      - EXCLUDES: causalgia:
        - NOS (355.9)
        - upper limb (354.4)
    - ◆ 355.79 **Other mononeuritis of lower limb**
  - ◆ 355.8 **Mononeuritis of lower limb, unspecified**
  - ◆ 355.9 **Mononeuritis of unspecified site**
    - Causalgia NOS
    - EXCLUDES: causalgia:
      - lower limb (355.71)
      - upper limb (354.4)
- ● 356 **Hereditary and idiopathic peripheral neuropathy**
  - 356.0 **Hereditary peripheral neuropathy**
    - Déjérine-Sottas disease
  - 356.1 **Peroneal muscular atrophy**
    - Charcot-Marie-Tooth disease
    - Neuropathicmuscular atrophy
  - 356.2 **Hereditary sensory neuropathy**
  - 356.3 **Refsum's disease**
    - Heredopathia atactica polyneuritiformis
  - 356.4 **Idiopathic progressive polyneuropathy**
  - ◆ 356.8 **Other specified idiopathic peripheral neuropathy**
    - Supranuclear paralysis
  - ◆ 356.9 **Unspecified**
- ● 357 **Inflammatory and toxic neuropathy**
  - 357.0 **Acute infective polyneuritis**
    - Guillain-Barré syndrome   Postinfectious polyneuritis
  - ■ 357.1 **Polyneuropathy in collagen vascular disease**
    - Code also underlying disease, as:
      - disseminated lupus erythematosus (710.0)
      - polyarteritis nodosa (446.0)
      - rheumatoid arthritis (714.0)
  - ■ 357.2 **Polyneuropathy in diabetes**
    - Code also underlying disease (250.6)
  - ■ 357.3 **Polyneuropathy in malignant disease**
    - Code also underlying disease (140.0-208.9)
  - ■ ◆ 357.4 **Polyneuropathy in other diseases classified elsewhere**
    - Code also underlying disease, as:
      - amyloidosis (277.3)
      - beriberi (265.0)
      - deficiency of B vitamins (266.0-266.9)
      - diphtheria (032.0-032.9)
      - hypoglycemia (251.2)
      - pellagra (265.2)
      - porphyria (277.1)
      - sarcoidosis (I 35)
      - uremia (585)
    - EXCLUDES: polyneuropathy in:
      - herpes zoster (053.13)
      - mumps (072.72)
  - 357.5 **Alcoholic polyneuropathy**
  - 357.6 **Polyneuropathy due to drugs**
    - Use additional E code, if desired, to identify drug
  - ◆ 357.7 **Polyneuropathy due to other toxic agents**
    - Use additional E code, if desired, to identify toxic agent
  - ◆ 357.8 **Other**
  - ◆ 357.9 **Unspecified**
- ● 358 **Myoneural disorders**
  - 358.0 **Myasthenia gravis**
  - ■ 358.1 **Myasthenic syndromes in diseases classified elsewhere**
    - Amyotrophy } from stated cause
    - Eaton-Lambert syndrome } classified elsewhere
    - Code also underlying disease, as:
      - botulism (005.1)
      - diabetes mellitus (250.6)
      - hypothyroidism (244.0-244.9)
      - malignant neoplasm (140.0-208.9)
      - pernicious anemia (281.0)
      - thyrotoxicosis (242.0-242.9)
  - 358.2 **Toxic myoneural disorders**
    - Use additional E code, if desired, to identify toxic agent
  - ◆ 358.8 **Other specified myoneural disorders**
  - ◆ 358.9 **Myoneural disorders, unspecified**
- ● 359 **Muscular dystrophies and other myopathies**
  - EXCLUDES: idiopathic polymyositis (710.4)
  - 359.0 **Congenital hereditary muscular dystrophy**
    - Benign congenital myopathy
    - Central core disease
    - Centronuclear myopathy
    - Myotubular myopathy
    - Nemaline body disease
    - EXCLUDES: arthrogryposis multiplex congenita (754.89)

● Additional digits required   ◆ Nonspecific code   ■ Not a primary diagnosis

359.1 **Hereditary progressive muscular dystrophy**
Muscular dystrophy:
NOS
distal
Duchenne
Erb's
fascioscapulohumeral
Muscular dystrophy:
Gower's
Landouzy-Déjérine
limb-girdle
ocular
oculopharyngeal

359.2 **Myotonic disorders**
Dystrophia myotonica
Eulenburg's disease
Myotonia congenita
Paramyotonia congenita
Steinert's disease
Thomsen's disease

359.3 **Familial periodic paralysis**
Hypokalemic familial periodic paralysis

359.4 **Toxic myopathy**
Use additional E code, if desired, to identify toxic agent

359.5 ***Myopathy in endocrine diseases classified elsewhere***
Code also underlying disease, as:
Addison's disease (255.4)
Cushing's syndrome (255.0)
hypopituitarism (253.2)
myxedema (244.0-244.9)
thyrotoxicosis (242.0-242.9)

359.6 ***Symptomatic inflammatory myopathy in diseases classified elsewhere***
Code also underlying disease, as:
amyloidosis (277.3)
disseminated lupus erythematosus (710.0)
malignant neoplasm (140.0-208.9)
polyarteritis nodosa (446.0)
rheumatoid arthritis (714.0)
sarcoidosis (135)
scleroderma (710.1)
Sjögren's disease (710.2)

359.8 **Other myopathies**
359.9 **Myopathy, unspecified**

DISORDERS OF THE EYE AND ADNEXA (360-379)

360 **Disorders of the globe**
INCLUDES disorders affecting multiple structures of eye

360.0 **Purulent endophthalmitis**
360.00 **Purulent endophthalmitis, unspecified**
360.01 **Acute endophthalmitis**
360.02 **Panophthalmitis**
360.03 **Chronic endophthalmitis**
360.04 **Vitreous abscess**

360.1 **Other endophthalmitis**
360.11 **Sympathetic uveitis**
360.12 **Panuveitis**
360.13 **Parasitic endophthalmitis NOS**
360.14 **Ophthalmia nodosa**
360.19 **Other**
Phacoanaphylactic endophthalmitis

360.2 **Degenerative disorders of globe**
360.20 **Degenerative disorder of globe, unspecified**
360.21 **Progressive high (degenerative) myopia**
Malignant myopia
360.23 **Siderosis**
360.24 **Other metallosis**
Chalcosis
360.29 **Other**
EXCLUDES *xerophthalmia (264.7)*

360.3 **Hypotony of eye**
360.30 **Hypotony, unspecified**
360.31 **Primary hypotony**
360.32 **Ocular fistula causing hypotony**
360.33 **Hypotony associated with other ocular disorders**
360.34 **Flat anterior chamber**

360.4 **Degenerated conditions of globe**
360.40 **Degenerated globe or eye, unspecified**
360.41 **Blind hypotensive eye**
Atrophy of globe
Phthisis bulbi
360.42 **Blind hypertensive eye**
Absolute glaucoma
360.43 **Hemophthalmos, except current injury**
EXCLUDES *traumatic (871.0-871.9, 921.0-921.9)*
360.44 **Leucocoria**

360.5 **Retained (old) intraocular foreign body, magnetic**
EXCLUDES *current penetrating injury with magnetic foreign body (871.5)*
retained (old) foreign body of orbit (376.6)
360.50 **Foreign body, magnetic, intraocular, unspecified**
360.51 **Foreign body, magnetic, in anterior chamber**
360.52 **Foreign body, magnetic, in iris or ciliary body**
360.53 **Foreign body, magnetic, in lens**
360.54 **Foreign body, magnetic, in vitreous**
360.55 **Foreign body, magnetic, in posterior wall**
360.59 **Foreign body, magnetic, in other or multiple sites**

360.6 **Retained (old) intraocular foreign body, nonmagnetic**
Retained (old) foreign body:
NOS
nonmagnetic
EXCLUDES *current penetrating injury with (nonmagnetic) foreign body (871.6)*
retained (old) foreign body in orbit (376.6)
360.60 **Foreign body, intraocular, unspecified**
360.61 **Foreign body in anterior chamber**
360.62 **Foreign body in iris or ciliary body**
360.63 **Foreign body in lens**
360.64 **Foreign body in vitreous**
360.65 **Foreign body in posterior wall**
360.69 **Foreign body in other or multiple sites**

360.8 **Other disorders of globe**
360.81 **Luxation of globe**
360.89 **Other**

360.9 **Unspecified disorder of globe**

361 **Retinal detachments and defects**

361.0 **Retinal detachment with retinal defect**
Rhegmatogenous retinal detachment
EXCLUDES *detachment of retinal pigment epithelium (362.42-362.43)*
retinal detachment (serous) (without defect) (361.2)
361.00 **Retinal detachment with retinal defect, unspecified**
361.01 **Recent detachment, partial, with single defect**
361.02 **Recent detachment, partial, with multiple defects**
361.03 **Recent detachment, partial, with giant tear**
361.04 **Recent detachment, partial, with retinal dialysis**
Dialysis (juvenile) of retina (with detachment)
361.05 **Recent detachment, total or subtotal**
361.06 **Old detachment, partial**
Delimited old retinal detachment
361.07 **Old detachment, total or subtotal**

361.1 **Retinoschisis and retinal cysts**
EXCLUDES *juvenile retinoschisis (362.73)*
microcystoid degeneration of retina (362.62)
parasitic cyst of retina (360.13)
361.10 **Retinoschisis, unspecified**
361.11 **Flat retinoschisis**
361.12 **Bullous retinoschisis**
361.13 **Primary retinal cysts**
361.14 **Secondary retinal cysts**
361.19 **Other**
Pseudocyst of retina

361.2 **Serous retinal detachment**
Retinal detachment without retinal defect
EXCLUDES *central serous retinopathy (362.41)*
retinal pigment epithelium detachment (362.42-362.43)

361.3 **Retinal defects without detachment**
EXCLUDES *chorioretinal scars after surgery for detachment (363.30-363.35)*
peripheral retinal degeneration without defect (362.60-362.66)
361.30 **Retinal defect, unspecified**
Retinal break(s) NOS
361.31 **Round hole of retina without detachment**
361.32 **Horseshoe tear of retina without detachment**
Operculum of retina without mention of detachment
361.33 **Multiple defects of retina without detachment**

361.8 **Other forms of retinal detachment**
361.81 **Traction detachment of retina**
Traction detachment with vitreoretinal organization

- 361.89 Other
- ◆ 361.9 Unspecified retinal detachment
- ● 362 Other retinal disorders
  - EXCLUDES chorioretinal scars (363.30-363.35)
  - chorioretinitis (363.0-363.2)
  - ● 362.0 Diabetic retinopathy
    - Code also diabetes (250.5)
    - ■ 362.01 Background diabetic retinopathy
      - Diabetic retinal microaneurysms
      - Diabetic retinopathy NOS
    - ■ 362.02 Proliferative diabetic retinopathy
  - ● 362.1 Other background retinopathy and retinal vascular changes
    - ◆ 362.10 Background retinopathy, unspecified
    - 362.11 Hypertensive retinopathy
    - 362.12 Exudative retinopathy
      - Coats' syndrome
    - 362.13 Changes in vascular appearance
      - Vascular sheathing of retina
      - Use additional code for any associated atherosclerosis (440.8)
    - 362.14 Retinal microaneurysms NOS
    - 362.15 Retinal telangiectasia
    - 362.16 Retinal neovascularization NOS
      - Neovascularization:
        - choroidal
        - subretinal
    - ◆ 362.17 Other intraretinal microvascular abnormalities
      - Retinal varices
    - 362.18 Retinal vasculitis
      - Eales' disease
      - Retinal:
        - arteritis
        - endarteritis
      - Retinal:
        - perivasculitis
        - phlebitis
  - ● 362.2 Other proliferative retinopathy
    - 362.21 Retrolental fibroplasia
    - ◆ 362.29 Other nondiabetic proliferative retinopathy
  - ● 362.3 Retinal vascular occlusion
    - ◆ 362.30 Retinal vascular occlusion, unspecified
    - 362.31 Central retinal artery occlusion
    - 362.32 Arterial branch occlusion
    - 362.33 Partial arterial occlusion
      - Hollenhorst plaque
      - Retinal microembolism
    - 362.34 Transient arterial occlusion
      - Amaurosis fugax
    - 362.35 Central retinal vein occlusion
    - 362.36 Venous tributary (branch) occlusion
    - 362.37 Venous engorgement
      - Occlusion:
        - incipient } of retinal
        - partial } vein
  - ● 362.4 Separation of retinal layers
    - EXCLUDES retinal detachment (serous) (361.2)
    - rhegmatogenous (361.00-361.07)
    - ◆ 362.40 Retinal layer separation, unspecified
    - 362.41 Central serous retinopathy
    - 362.42 Serous detachment of retinal pigment epithelium
      - Exudative detachment of retinal pigment epithelium
    - 362.43 Hemorrhagic detachment of retinal pigment epithelium
  - ● 362.5 Degeneration of macula and posterior pole
    - EXCLUDES degeneration of optic disc (377.21-377.24)
    - hereditary retinal degeneration [dystrophy] (362.70-362.77)
    - ◆ 362.50 Macular degeneration (senile), unspecified
    - 362.51 Nonexudative senile macular degeneration
      - Senile macular degeneration:
        - atrophic
        - dry
    - 362.52 Exudative senile macular degeneration
      - Kuhnt-Junius degeneration
      - Senile macular degeneration:
        - disciform
        - wet
    - 362.53 Cystoid macular degeneration
    - 362.54 Macular cyst, hole, or pseudohole
    - 362.55 Toxic maculopathy
      - Use additional E code, if desired, to identify drug, if drug induced
    - 362.56 Macular puckering
      - Preretinal fibrosis
    - 362.57 Drusen (degenerative)
  - ● 362.6 Peripheral retinal degenerations
    - EXCLUDES hereditary retinal degeneration [dystrophy] (362.70-362.77)
    - retinal degeneration with retinal defect (361.00-361.07)
    - ◆ 362.60 Peripheral retinal degeneration, unspecified
    - 362.61 Paving stone degeneration
    - 362.62 Microcystoid degeneration
      - Blessig's cysts   Iwanoff's cysts
    - 362.63 Lattice degeneration
      - Palisade degeneration of retina
    - 362.64 Senile reticular degeneration
    - 362.65 Secondary pigmentary degeneration
      - Pseudoretinitis pigmentosa
    - 362.66 Secondary vitreoretinal degenerations
  - ● 362.7 Hereditary retinal dystrophies
    - ◆ 362.70 Hereditary retinal dystrophy, unspecified
    - ■ 362.71 *Retinal dystrophy in systemic or cerebroretinal lipidoses*
      - Code also underlying disease, as:
        - cerebroretinal lipidoses (330.1)
        - systemic lipidoses (272.7)
    - ■◆ 362.72 *Retinal dystrophy in other systemic disorders and syndromes*
      - Code also underlying disease, as:
        - Bassen-Kornzweig syndrome (272.5)
        - Refsum's disease (356.3)
    - 362.73 Vitreoretinal dystrophies
      - Juvenile retinoschisis
    - 362.74 Pigmentary retinal dystrophy
      - Retinal dystrophy, albipunctate
      - Retinitis pigmentosa
    - ◆ 362.75 Other dystrophies primarily involving the sensory retina
      - Progressive cone(-rod) dystrophy
      - Stargardt's disease
    - 362.76 Dystrophies primarily involving the retinal pigment epithelium
      - Fundus flavimaculatus
      - Vitelliform dystrophy
    - 362.77 Dystrophies primarily involving Bruch's membrane
      - Dystrophy:
        - hyaline
        - pseudoinflammatory foveal
      - Hereditary drusen
  - ● 362.8 Other retinal disorders
    - EXCLUDES chorioretinal inflammations (363.0-363.2)
    - chorioretinal scars (363.30-363.35)
    - 362.81 Retinal hemorrhage
      - Hemorrhage:
        - preretinal
        - retinal (deep) (superficial)
        - subretinal
    - 362.82 Retinal exudates and deposits
    - 362.83 Retinal edema
      - Retinal:
        - cotton wool spots
        - edema (localized) (macular) (peripheral)
    - 362.84 Retinal ischemia
    - 362.85 Retinal nerve fiber bundle defects
    - ◆ 362.89 Other retinal disorders
  - ◆ 362.9 Unspecified retinal disorder
- ● 363 Chorioretinal inflammations, scars, and other disorders of choroid
  - ● 363.0 Focal chorioretinitis and focal retinochoroiditis
    - EXCLUDES focal chorioretinitis or retinochoroiditis in:
      - histoplasmosis (115.02, 115.12, 115.92)
      - toxoplasmosis (130.2)
      - congenital infection (771.2)
    - ◆ 363.00 Focal chorioretinitis, unspecified
      - Focal:
        - choroiditis or chorioretinitis NOS
        - retinitis or retinochoroiditis NOS

TABULAR LIST

- 363.01 Focal choroiditis and chorioretinitis, juxtapapillary
- ◆ 363.03 Focal choroiditis and chorioretinitis of other posterior pole
- 363.04 Focal choroiditis and chorioretinitis, peripheral
- 363.05 Focal retinitis and retinochoiroiditis, juxtapapillary
    Neuroretinitis
- 363.06 Focal retinitis and retinochoroiditis, macular or paramacular
- ◆ 363.07 Focal retinitis and retinochoroiditis of other posterior pole
- 363.08 Focal retinitis and retinochoroiditis, peripheral
- ● 363.1 Disseminated chorioretinitis and disseminated retinochoroiditis
    EXCLUDES disseminated choroiditis or chorioretinitis in secondary syphilis (091.51)
    neurosyphilitic disseminated retinitis or retinochoroiditis (094.83)
    retinal (peri)vasculitis (362.18)
    - ◆ 363.10 Disseminated chorioretinitis, unspecified
        Disseminated:
            choroiditis or chorioretinitis NOS
            retinitis or retinochoroiditis NOS
    - 363.11 Disseminated choroiditis and chorioretinitis, posterior pole
    - 363.12 Disseminated choroiditis and chorioretinitis, peripheral
    - 363.13 Disseminated choroiditis and chorioretinitis, generalized
        Use additional code for any underlying disease, as:
            tuberculosis (017.3)
    - 363.14 Disseminated retinitis and retinochoroiditis, metastatic
    - 363.15 Disseminated retinitis and retinochoroiditis, pigment epitheliopathy
        Acute posterior multifocal placoid pigment epitheliopathy
- ● 363.2 Other and unspecified forms of chorioretinitis and retinochoroiditis
    EXCLUDES panophthalmitis (360.02)
    sympathetic uveitis (360.11)
    uveitis NOS (364.3)
    - ◆ 363.20 Chorioretinitis, unspecified
        Choroiditis NOS
        Retinitis NOS
        Uveitis, posterior NOS
    - 363.21 Pars planitis
        Posterior cyclitis
    - 363.22 Harada's disease
- ● 363.3 Chorioretinal scars
    Scar (postinflammatory) (postsurgical) (posttraumatic):
        choroid
        retina
    - ◆ 363.30 Chorioretinal scar, unspecified
    - 363.31 Solar retinopathy
    - ◆ 363.32 Other macular scars
    - ◆ 363.33 Other scars of posterior pole
    - 363.34 Peripheral scars
    - 363.35 Disseminated scars
- ● 363.4 Choroidal degenerations
    - ◆ 363.40 Choroidal degeneration, unspecified
        Choroidal sclerosis NOS
    - 363.41 Senile atrophy of choroid
    - 363.42 Diffuse secondary atrophy of choroid
    - 363.43 Angioid streaks of choroid
- ● 363.5 Hereditary choroidal dystrophies
    Hereditary choroidal atrophy:
        partial [choriocapillaris]
        total [all vessels]
    - ◆ 363.50 Hereditary choroidal dystrophy or atrophy, unspecified
    - 363.51 Circumpapillary dystrophy of choroid, partial
    - 363.52 Circumpapillary dystrophy of choroid, total
        Helicoid dystrophy of choroid
    - 363.53 Central dystrophy of choroid, partial
        Dystrophy, choroidal:
            central areolar
            circinate
    - 363.54 Central choroidal atrophy, total
        Dystrophy, choroidal: Dystrophy, choroidal:
            central gyrate   serpiginous
    - 363.55 Choroideremia
    - ◆ 363.56 Other diffuse or generalized dystrophy, partial
        Diffuse choroidal sclerosis
    - ◆ 363.57 Other diffuse or generalized dystrophy, total
        Generalized gyrate atrophy, choroid
- ● 363.6 Choroidal hemorrhage and rupture
    - ◆ 363.61 Choroidal hemorrhage, unspecified
    - 363.62 Expulsive choroidal hemorrhage
    - 363.63 Choroidal rupture
- ● 363.7 Choroidal detachment
    - ◆ 363.70 Choroidal detachment, unspecified
    - 363.71 Serous choroidal detachment
    - 363.72 Hemorrhagic choroidal detachment
- ◆ 363.8 Other disorders of choroid
- ◆ 363.9 Unspecified disorder of choroid
- ● 364 Disorders of iris and ciliary body
    - ● 364.0 Acute and subacute iridocyclitis
        Anterior uveitis
        Cyclitis   } acute
        Iridocyclitis   } subacute
        Iritis
        EXCLUDES gonococcal (098.41)
        herpes simplex (054.44)
        herpes zoster (053.22)
        - ◆ 364.00 Acute and subacute iridocyclitis, unspecified
        - 364.01 Primary iridocyclitis
        - 364.02 Recurrent iridocyclitis
        - 364.03 Secondary iridocyclitis, infectious
        - 364.04 Secondary iridocyclitis, noninfectious
            Aqueous: Aqueous:
                cells   flare
                fibrin
        - 364.05 Hypopyon
    - ● 364.1 Chronic iridocyclitis
        EXCLUDES posterior cyclitis (363.21)
        - ◆ 364.10 Chronic iridocyclitis, unspecified
        - 364.11 Chronic iridocyclitis in diseases classified elsewhere
            Code also underlying disease, as:
                sarcoidosis (135)
                tuberculosis (017.3)
            EXCLUDES syphilitic iridocyclitis (091.52)
    - ● 364.2 Certain types of iridocyclitis
        EXCLUDES posterior cyclitis (363.21)
        sympathetic uveitis (360.11)
        - 364.21 Fuchs' heterochromic cyclitis
        - 364.22 Glaucomatocyclitic crises
        - 364.23 Lens-induced iridocyclitis
        - 364.24 Vogt-Koyanagi syndrome
    - ◆ 364.3 Unspecified iridocyclitis
        Uveitis NOS
    - ● 364.4 Vascular disorders of iris and ciliary body
        - 364.41 Hyphema
            Hemorrhage of iris or ciliary body
        - 364.42 Rubeosis iridis
            Neovascularization of iris or ciliary body
    - ● 364.5 Degenerations of iris and ciliary body
        - 364.51 Essential or progressive iris atrophy
        - 364.52 Iridoschisis
        - 364.53 Pigmentary iris degeneration
            Acquired heterochromia
            Pigment dispersion syn-   } of iris
                drome
            Translucency
        - 364.54 Degeneration of pupillary margin
            Atrophy of sphincter
            Ectropion of pigment   } of iris
                epithelium
        - 364.55 Miotic cysts of pupillary margin
        - 364.56 Degenerative changes of chamber angle
        - 364.57 Degenerative changes of ciliary body
        - ◆ 364.59 Other iris atrophy
            Iris atrophy (generalized) (sector shaped)

NERVOUS SYSTEM AND SENSE ORGANS

- **364.6** Cysts of iris, ciliary body, and anterior chamber
  - **EXCLUDES** miotic pupillary cyst (364.55)
  - parasitic cyst (360.13)
  - 364.60 Idiopathic cysts
  - 364.61 Implantation cysts
    - Epithelial down-growth, anterior chamber
    - Implantation cysts (surgical) (traumatic)
  - 364.62 Exudative cysts of iris or anterior chamber
  - 364.63 Primary cyst of pars plana
  - 364.64 Exudative cyst of pars plana
- **364.7** Adhesions and disruptions of iris and ciliary body
  - **EXCLUDES** flat anterior chamber (360.34)
  - ◆ 364.70 Adhesions of iris, unspecified
    - Synechiae (iris) NOS
  - 364.71 Posterior synechiae
  - 364.72 Anterior synechiae
  - 364.73 Goniosynechiae
    - Peripheral anterior synechiae
  - 364.74 Pupillary membranes
    - Iris bombé
    - Pupillary:
      - occlusion
      - seclusion
  - 364.75 Pupillary abnormalities
    - Deformed pupil
    - Ectopic pupil
    - Rupture of sphincter, pupil
  - 364.76 Iridodialysis
  - 364.77 Recession of chamber angle
- ◆ **364.8** Other disorders of iris and ciliary body
  - Prolapse of iris NOS
  - **EXCLUDES** prolapse of iris in recent wound (871.1)
- ◆ **364.9** Unspecified disorder of iris and ciliary body

- **365 Glaucoma**
  - **EXCLUDES** blind hypertensive eye [absolute glaucoma] (360.42)
  - congenital glaucoma (743.20-743.22)
  - **365.0** Borderline glaucoma [glaucoma suspect]
    - ◆ 365.00 Preglaucoma, unspecified
    - 365.01 Open angle with borderline findings
      - Open angle with:
        - borderline intraocular pressure
        - cupping of optic discs
    - 365.02 Anatomical narrow angle
    - 365.03 Steroid responders
    - ◆ 365.04 Ocular hypertension
  - **365.1** Open-angle glaucoma
    - ◆ 365.10 Open-angle glaucoma, unspecified
      - Wide-angle glaucoma NOS
    - 365.11 Primary open angle glaucoma
      - Chronic simple glaucoma
    - 365.12 Low tension glaucoma
    - 365.13 Pigmentary glaucoma
    - 365.14 Glaucoma of childhood
      - Infantile or juvenile glaucoma
    - 365.15 Residual stage of open angle glaucoma
  - **365.2** Primary angle-closure glaucoma
    - ◆ 365.20 Primary angle-closure glaucoma, unspecified
    - 365.21 Intermittent angle-closure glaucoma
      - Angle-closure glaucoma:
        - interval
        - subacute
    - 365.22 Acute angle-closure glaucoma
    - 365.23 Chronic angle-closure glaucoma
    - 365.24 Residual stage of angle-closure glaucoma
  - **365.3** Corticosteroid-induced glaucoma
    - 365.31 Glaucomatous stage
    - 365.32 Residual stage
  - **365.4** Glaucoma associated with congenital anomalies, dystrophies, and systemic syndromes
    - ■ 365.41 Glaucoma associated with chamber angle anomalies
      - Code also associated disorder, as:
        - Axenfeld's anomaly (743.44)
        - Rieger's anomaly or syndrome (743.44)
    - ■ 365.42 Glaucoma associated with anomalies of iris
      - Code also associated disorder, as:
        - aniridia (743.45)
        - essential iris atrophy (364.51)
  - ■ 365.43 Glaucoma associated with other anterior segment anomalies
    - Code also associated disorder, as:
      - microcornea (743.41)
  - ■ 365.44 Glaucoma associated with systemic syndromes
    - Code also associated disease, as:
      - neurofibromatosis (237.7)
      - Sturge-Weber (-Dimitri) syndrome (759.6)
  - **365.5** Glaucoma associated with disorders of the lens
    - 365.51 Phacolytic glaucoma
      - Use additional code for associated hypermature cataract (366.18)
    - 365.52 Pseudoexfoliation glaucoma
      - Use additional code for associated pseudoexfoliation of capsule (366.11)
    - ◆ 365.59 Glaucoma associated with other lens disorders
      - Use additional code for associated disorder, as:
        - dislocation of lens (379.33-379.34)
        - spherophakia (743.36)
  - **365.6** Glaucoma associated with other ocular disorders
    - ◆ 365.60 Glaucoma associated with unspecified ocular disorder
    - 365.61 Glaucoma associated with pupillary block
      - Use additional code for associated disorder, as:
        - seclusion of pupil [iris bombé] (364.74)
    - 365.62 Glaucoma associated with ocular inflammations
      - Use additional code for associated disorder, as:
        - glaucomatocyclitic crises (364.22)
        - iridocyclitis (364.0-364.3)
    - 365.63 Glaucoma associated with vascular disorders
      - Use additional code for associated disorder, as:
        - central retinal vein occlusion (362.35)
        - hyphema (364.41)
    - 365.64 Glaucoma associated with tumors or cysts
      - Use additional code for associated disorder, as:
        - benign neoplasm (224.0-224.9)
        - epithelial down-growth (364.61)
        - malignant neoplasm (190.0-190.9)
    - 365.65 Glaucoma associated with ocular trauma
      - Use additional code for associated condition, as:
        - contusion of globe (921.3)
        - recession of chamber angle (364.77)
  - **365.8** Other specified forms of glaucoma
    - 365.81 Hypersecretion glaucoma
    - 365.82 Glaucoma with increased episcleral venous pressure
    - ◆ 365.89 Other specified glaucoma
  - ◆ **365.9** Unspecified glaucoma

- **366 Cataract**
  - **EXCLUDES** congenital cataract (743.30-743.34)
  - **366.0** Infantile, juvenile, and presenile cataract
    - ◆ 366.00 Nonsenile cataract, unspecified
    - 366.01 Anterior subcapsular polar cataract
    - 366.02 Posterior subcapsular polar cataract
    - 366.03 Cortical, lamellar, or zonular cataract
    - 366.04 Nuclear cataract
    - ◆ 366.09 Other and combined forms of nonsenile cataract
  - **366.1** Senile cataract
    - ◆ 366.10 Senile cataract, unspecified
    - 366.11 Pseudoexfoliation of lens capsule
    - 366.12 Incipient cataract
      - Cataract:
        - coronary
        - immature NOS
        - punctate
        - Water clefts
    - 366.13 Anterior subcapsular polar senile cataract
    - 366.14 Posterior subcapsular polar senile cataract
    - 366.15 Cortical senile cataract
    - 366.16 Nuclear sclerosis
      - Cataracta brunescens   Nuclear cataract
    - 366.17 Total or mature cataract
    - 366.18 Hypermature cataract
      - Morgagni cataract
    - ◆ 366.19 Other and combined forms of senile cataract
  - **366.2** Traumatic cataract
    - ◆ 366.20 Traumatic cataract, unspecified
    - 366.21 Localized traumatic opacities
      - Vossius' ring

● Additional digits required   ◆ Nonspecific code   ■ Not a primary diagnosis

- **366.22 Total traumatic cataract**
- **366.23 Partially resolved traumatic cataract**
- ● **366.3 Cataract secondary to ocular disorders**
  - ◆ **366.30 Cataracta complicata, unspecified**
  - **366.31 Glaucomatous flecks (subcapsular)**
    Use additional code for underlying glaucoma (365.0-365.9)
  - **366.32 Cataract in inflammatory disorders**
    Use additional code for underlying condition, as: chronic choroiditis (363.0-363.2)
  - **366.33 Cataract with neovascularization**
    Use additional code for underlying condition, as: chronic iridocyclitis (364.10)
  - **366.34 Cataract in degenerative disorders**
    Sunflower cataract
    Use additional code for underlying condition, as:
    chalcosis (360.24)
    degenerative myopia (360.21)
    pigmentary retinal dystrophy (362.74)
- ● **366.4 Cataract associated with other disorders**
  - ■ **366.41 *Diabetic cataract***
    Code also diabetes (250.5)
  - ■ **366.42 *Tetanic cataract***
    Code also underlying disease, as:
    calcinosis (275.4)
    hypoparathyroidism (252.1)
  - ■ **366.43 *Myotonic cataract***
    Code also underlying disorder (359.2)
  - ■◆ **366.44 *Cataract associated with other syndromes***
    Code also underlying condition, as:
    craniofacial dysostosis (756.0)
    galactosemia (271.1)
  - **366.45 Toxic cataract**
    Drug-induced cataract
    Use additional E code, if desired, to identify drug or other toxic substance
  - ◆ **366.46 Cataract associated with radiation and other physical influences**
    Use additional E code, if desired, to identify cause
- ● **366.5 After-cataract**
  - ◆ **366.50 After-cataract, unspecified**
    Secondary cataract NOS
  - **366.51 Soemmering's ring**
  - ◆ **366.52 Other after-cataract, not obscuring vision**
  - **366.53 After-cataract, obscuring vision**
- ◆ **366.8 Other cataract**
  Calcification of lens
- ◆ **366.9 Unspecified cataract**
- ● **367 Disorders of refraction and accommodation**
  - **367.0 Hypermetropia**
    Far-sightedness
    Hyperopia
  - **367.1 Myopia**
    Near-sightedness
  - ● **367.2 Astigmatism**
    - ◆ **367.20 Astigmatism, unspecified**
    - **367.21 Regular astigmatism**
    - **367.22 Irregular astigmatism**
  - ● **367.3 Anisometropia and aniseikonia**
    - **367.31 Anisometropia**
    - **367.32 Aniseikonia**
  - **367.4 Presbyopia**
  - ● **367.5 Disorders of accommodation**
    - **367.51 Paresis of accommodation**
      Cycloplegia
    - **367.52 Total or complete internal ophthalmoplegia**
    - **367.53 Spasm of accommodation**
  - ● **367.8 Other disorders of refraction and accommodation**
    - **367.81 Transient refractive change**
    - ◆ **367.89 Other**
      Drug-induced ⎫ disorders of refraction and
      Toxic   ⎭ accommodation
  - ◆ **367.9 Unspecified disorder of refraction and accommodation**
- ● **368 Visual disturbances**
  EXCLUDES *electrophysiological disturbances (794.11-794.14)*
  - ● **368.0 Amblyopia ex anopsia**
    - ◆ **368.00 Amblyopia, unspecified**
    - **368.01 Strabismic amblyopia**
      Suppression amblyopia
    - **368.02 Deprivation amblyopia**
    - **368.03 Refractive amblyopia**
  - ● **368.1 Subjective visual disturbances**
    - ◆ **368.10 Subjective visual disturbance, unspecified**
    - **368.11 Sudden visual loss**
    - **368.12 Transient visual loss**
      Concentric fading   Scintillating scotoma
    - **368.13 Visual discomfort**
      Asthenopia   Photophobia
      Eye strain
    - **368.14 Visual distortions of shape and size**
      Macropsia   Micropsia
      Metamorphopsia
    - ◆ **368.15 Other visual distortions and entoptic phenomena**
      Photopsia
      Refractive:
        diplopia
        polyopia
      Visual halos
    - **368.16 Psychophysical visual disturbances**
      Visual:
        agnosia
        disorientation syndrome
        hallucinations
  - **368.2 Diplopia**
    Double vision
  - ● **368.3 Other disorders of binocular vision**
    - ◆ **368.30 Binocular vision disorder, unspecified**
    - **368.31 Suppression of binocular vision**
    - **368.32 Simultaneous visual perception without fusion**
    - **368.33 Fusion with defective stereopsis**
    - **368.34 Abnormal retinal correspondence**
  - ● **368.4 Visual field defects**
    - ◆ **368.40 Visual field defect, unspecified**
    - **368.41 Scotoma involving central area**
      Scotoma:
        central
        centrocecal
        paracentral
    - **368.42 Scotoma of blind spot area**
      Enlarged:
        angioscotoma
        blind spot
      Paracecal scotoma
    - **368.43 Sector or arcuate defects**
      Scotoma:
        arcuate
        Bjerrum
        Seidel
    - ◆ **368.44 Other localized visual field defect**
      Scotoma:
        NOS
        ring
      Visual field defect:
        nasal step
        peripheral
    - **368.45 Generalized contraction or constriction**
    - **368.46 Homonymous bilateral field defects**
      Hemianopsia (altitudinal) (homonymous)
      Quadrant anopia
    - **368.47 Heteronymous bilateral field defects**
      Hemianopsia:
        binasal
        bitemporal
  - ● **368.5 Color vision deficiencies**
    Color blindness
    - **368.51 Protan defect**
      Protanomaly   Protanopia
    - **368.52 Deutan defect**
      Deuteranomaly   Deuteranopia
    - **368.53 Tritan defect**
      Tritanomaly   Tritanopia
    - **368.54 Achromatopsia**
      Monochromatism (cone) (rod)
    - **368.55 Acquired color vision deficiencies**
    - ◆ **368.59 Other color vision deficiencies**

- **368.6 Night blindness**
  - Hemeralopia
  - Nyctalopia
  - ◆ 368.60 Night blindness, unspecified
  - 368.61 Congenital night blindness
    - Hereditary night blindness
    - Oguchi's disease
  - 368.62 Acquired night blindness
    - **EXCLUDES** *that due to vitamin A deficiency (264.5)*
  - 368.63 Abnormal dark adaptation curve
    - Abnormal threshold | of cones or
    - Delayed adaptation | rods
  - ◆ 368.69 Other night blindness
- ◆ **368.8 Other specified visual disturbances**
  - Blurred vision NOS
- ◆ **368.9 Unspecified visual disturbance**
- ● **369 Blindness and low vision**

  Note: Visual impairment refers to a functional limitation of the eye (e.g., limited visual acuity or visual field). It should be distinguished from visual disability, indicating a limitation of the abilities of the individual (e.g., limited reading skills, vocational skills), and from visual handicap, indicating a limitation of personal and socioeconomic independence (e.g., limited mobility, limited employability).

  The levels of impairment defined in the table on page 62 are based on the recommendations of the WHO Study Group on Prevention of Blindness (Geneva, November 6–10, 1972; WHO Technical Report Series 518), and of the International Council of Ophthalmology (1976).

  Note that definitions of blindness vary in different settings.

  For international reporting WHO defines blindness as profound impairment. This definition can be applied to blindness of one eye (369.1, 369.6) and to blindness of the individual (369.0).

  For determination of benefits in the U.S.A., the definition of legal blindness as severe impairment is often used. This definition applies to blindness of the individual only.

  EXCLUDES *correctable impaired vision due to refractive errors (367.0-367.9)*

- ● **369.0 Profound impairment, both eyes**
  - ◆ 369.00 Impairment level not further specified
    - Blindness:
      - NOS according to WHO definition
      - both eyes
  - 369.01 Better eye: total impairment; lesser eye: total impairment
  - ◆ 369.02 Better eye: near-total impairment; lesser eye: not further specified
  - 369.03 Better eye: near-total impairment; lesser eye: total impairment
  - 369.04 Better eye: near-total impairment; lesser eye: near-total impairment
  - ◆ 369.05 Better eye: profound impairment; lesser eye: not further specified
  - 369.06 Better eye: profound impairment; lesser eye: total impairment
  - 369.07 Better eye: profound impairment; lesser eye: near-total impairment
  - 369.08 Better eye: profound impairment; lesser eye: profound impairment
- ● **369.1 Moderate or severe impairment, better eye, profound impairment lesser eye**
  - ◆ 369.10 Impairment level not further specified
    - Blindness, one eye, low vision other eye
  - ◆ 369.11 Better eye: severe impairment; lesser eye: blind, not further specified
  - 369.12 Better eye: severe impairment; lesser eye: total impairment
  - 369.13 Better eye: severe impairment; lesser eye: near-total impairment
  - 369.14 Better eye: severe impairment; lesser eye: profound impairment
  - ◆ 369.15 Better eye: moderate impairment; lesser eye: blind, not further specified
  - 369.16 Better eye: moderate impairment; lesser eye: total impairment
  - 369.17 Better eye: moderate impairment; lesser eye: near-total impairment
  - 369.18 Better eye: moderate impairment; lesser eye: profound impairment
- ● **369.2 Moderate or severe impairment, both eyes**
  - ◆ 369.20 Impairment level not further specified
    - Low vision, both eyes NOS
  - ◆ 369.21 Better eye: severe impairment; lesser eye: not further specified
  - 369.22 Better eye: severe impairment; lesser eye: severe impairment
  - ◆ 369.23 Better eye: moderate impairment; lesser eye: not further specified
  - 369.24 Better eye: moderate impairment; lesser eye: severe impairment
  - 369.25 Better eye: moderate impairment; lesser eye: moderate impairment
- **369.3 Unqualified visual loss, both eyes**
  - **EXCLUDES** *blindness NOS:*
    - *legal [U.S.A. definition] (369.4)*
    - *WHO definition (369.00)*
- **369.4 Legal blindness, as defined in U.S.A.**
  - Blindness NOS according to U.S.A. definition
  - **EXCLUDES** *legal blindness with specification of impairment level (369.01-369.08, 369.11-369.14, 369.21-369.22)*
- ● **369.6 Profound impairment, one eye**
  - ◆ 369.60 Impairment level not further specified
    - Blindness, one eye
  - ◆ 369.61 One eye: total impairment; other eye: not specified
  - 369.62 One eye: total impairment; other eye: near-normal vision
  - 369.63 One eye: total impairment; other eye: normal vision
  - ◆ 369.64 One eye: near-total impairment; other eye: not specified
  - 369.65 One eye: near-total impairment; other eye: near-normal vision
  - 369.66 One eye: near-total impairment; other eye: normal vision
  - ◆ 369.67 One eye: profound impairment; other eye: not specified
  - 369.68 One eye: profound impairment; other eye: near-normal vision
  - ◆ 369.69 One eye: profound impairment; other eye: normal vision
- ● **369.7 Moderate or severe impairment, one eye**
  - ◆ 369.70 Impairment level not further specified
    - Low vision, one eye
  - ◆ 369.71 One eye: severe impairment; other eye: not specified
  - 369.72 One eye: severe impairment; other eye: near-normal vision
  - 369.73 One eye: severe impairment; other eye: normal vision
  - ◆ 369.74 One eye: moderate impairment; other eye: not specified
  - 369.75 One eye: moderate impairment; other eye: near-normal vision
  - 369.76 One eye: moderate impairment; other eye: normal vision
- **369.8 Unqualified visual loss, one eye**
- ◆ **369.9 Unspecified visual loss**

Classification		LEVELS OF VISUAL IMPAIRMENT	Additional descriptors which may be encountered
"legal"	WHO	Visual acuity and/or visual field limitation (whichever is worse)	
LEGAL BLINDNESS (U.S.A.) both eyes	(NEAR-) NORMAL VISION	RANGE OF NORMAL VISION 20/10 20/13 20/16 20/20 20/25 2.0 1.6 1.25 1.0 0.8	
		NEAR-NORMAL VISION 20/30 20/40 20/50 20/60 0.7 0.6 0.5 0.4 0.3	
	LOW VISION	MODERATE VISUAL IMPAIRMENT 20/70 20/80 20/100 20/125 20/160 0.25 0.20 0.16 0.12	Moderate low vision
		SEVERE VISUAL IMPAIRMENT 20/200 20/250 20/320 20/400 0.10 0.08 0.06 0.05 Visual field: 20 degrees or less	Severe low vision, "Legal" blindness
	BLINDNESS (WHO) one or both eyes	PROFOUND VISUAL IMPAIRMENT 20/500 20/630 20/800 20/1000 0.04 0.03 0.025 0.02 Count fingers at: less than 3m (10 ft.) Visual field: 10 degrees or less	Profound low vision, Moderate blindness
		NEAR-TOTAL VISUAL IMPAIRMENT Visual acuity: less than 0.02 (20/1000) Count fingers at: 1m (3 ft.) or less Hand movements: 5m (15 ft.) or less Light projection, light perception Visual field: 5 degrees or less	Severe blindness, Near-total blindness
		TOTAL VISUAL IMPAIRMENT No light perception (NLP)	Total blindness

Visual acuity refers to best achievable acuity with correction.
Non-listed Snellen fractions may be classified by converting to the nearest decimal equivalent, e.g., 10/200 = 0.05, 6/30 = 0.20.
CF (count fingers) without designation of distance, may be classified to profound impairment.
HM (hand motion) without designation of distance, may be classified to near-total impairment.
Visual field measurements refer to the largest field diameter for a 1/100 white test object.

● **370 Keratitis**
- ● **370.0 Corneal ulcer**
  - EXCLUDES *that due to vitamin A deficiency (264.3)*
  - ◆ 370.00 Corneal ulcer, unspecified
  - 370.01 Marginal corneal ulcer
  - 370.02 Ring corneal ulcer
  - 370.03 Central corneal ulcer
  - 370.04 Hypopyon ulcer
    Serpiginous ulcer
  - 370.05 Mycotic corneal ulcer
  - 370.06 Perforated corneal ulcer
  - 370.07 Mooren's ulcer
- ● **370.2 Superficial keratitis without conjunctivitis**
  - EXCLUDES *dendritic [herpes simplex] keratitis (054.42)*
  - ◆ 370.20 Superficial keratitis, unspecified
  - 370.21 Punctate keratitis
    Thygeson's superficial punctate keratitis
  - 370.22 Macular keratitis
    Keratitis: Keratitis:
      areolar   stellate
      nummular   striate
  - 370.23 Filamentary keratitis
  - 370.24 Photokeratitis
    Snow blindness
    Welders' keratitis
- ● **370.3 Certain types of keratoconjunctivitis**
  - 370.31 Phlyctenular keratoconjunctivitis
    Phlyctenulosis
    Use additional code for any associated tuberculosis (017.3)
  - 370.32 Limbar and corneal involvement in vernal conjunctivitis
    Use additional code for vernal conjunctivitis (372.13)
  - ◆ 370.33 Keratoconjunctivitis sicca, not specified as Sjögren's
    EXCLUDES *Sjögren's syndrome (710.2)*
  - 370.34 Exposure keratoconjunctivitis
  - 370.35 Neurotrophic keratoconjunctivitis
- ● **370.4 Other and unspecified keratoconjunctivitis**
  - ◆ 370.40 Keratoconjunctivitis, unspecified
    Superficial keratitis with conjunctivitis NOS
  - ■ *370.44 Keratitis or keratoconjunctivitis in exanthema*
    Code also underlying condition (050.0-052.9)
    EXCLUDES *herpes simplex (054.43)*
    herpes zoster (053.21)
    measles (055.71)
  - ◆ 370.49 Other
    EXCLUDES *epidemic keratoconjunc-tivitis (077.1)*
- ● **370.5 Interstitial and deep keratitis**
  - ◆ 370.50 Interstitial keratitis, unspecified
  - 370.52 Diffuse interstitial keratitis
    Cogan's syndrome
  - 370.54 Sclerosing keratitis
  - 370.55 Corneal abscess
  - ◆ 370.59 Other
    EXCLUDES *disciform herpes simplex keratitis (054.43)*
    syphilitic keratitis (090.3)
- ● **370.6 Corneal neovascularization**
  - ◆ 370.60 Corneal neovascularization, unspecified
  - 370.61 Localized vascularization of cornea
  - 370.62 Pannus (corneal)
  - 370.63 Deep vascularization of cornea
  - 370.64 Ghost vessels (corneal)
- ◆ **370.8 Other forms of keratitis**
- ◆ **370.9 Unspecified keratitis**

● **371 Corneal opacity and other disorders of cornea**
- ● **371.0 Corneal scars and opacities**
  - EXCLUDES *that due to vitamin A deficiency (264.6)*
  - ◆ 371.00 Corneal opacity, unspecified
    Corneal scar NOS
  - 371.01 Minor opacity of cornea
    Corneal nebula
  - 371.02 Peripheral opacity of cornea
    Corneal macula not interfering with central vision

NERVOUS SYSTEM AND SENSE ORGANS

- **371.03 Central opacity of cornea**
  Corneal:
  - leucoma ⎫
  - macula ⎬ interfering with central vision
- **371.04 Adherent leucoma**
- *371.05 Phthisical cornea*
  Code also underlying tuberculosis (017.3)
- ● **371.1 Corneal pigmentations and deposits**
  - ◆ **371.10 Corneal deposit, unspecified**
  - **371.11 Anterior pigmentations**
    Stähli's lines
  - **371.12 Stromal pigmentations**
    Hematocornea
  - **371.13 Posterior pigmentations**
    Krukenberg spindle
  - **371.14 Kayser-Fleischer ring**
  - **371.15 Other deposits associated with metabolic disorders**
  - **371.16 Argentous deposits**
- ● **371.2 Corneal edema**
  - ◆ **371.20 Corneal edema, unspecified**
  - **371.21 Idiopathic corneal edema**
  - **371.22 Secondary corneal edema**
  - **371.23 Bullous keratopathy**
  - **371.24 Corneal edema due to wearing of contact lenses**
- ● **371.3 Changes of corneal membranes**
  - ◆ **371.30 Corneal membrane change, unspecified**
  - **371.31 Folds and rupture of Bowman's membrane**
  - **371.32 Folds in Descemet's membrane**
  - **371.33 Rupture in Descemet's membrane**
- ● **371.4 Corneal degenerations**
  - ◆ **371.40 Corneal degeneration, unspecified**
  - **371.41 Senile corneal changes**
    Arcus senilis   Hassall-Henle bodies
  - **371.42 Recurrent erosion of cornea**
    EXCLUDES Mooren's ulcer (370.07)
  - **371.43 Band-shaped keratopathy**
  - ◆ **371.44 Other calcerous degenerations of cornea**
  - **371.45 Keratomalacia NOS**
    EXCLUDES that due to vitamin A deficiency (264.4)
  - **371.46 Nodular degeneration of cornea**
    Salzmann's nodular dystrophy
  - **371.48 Peripheral degenerations of cornea**
    Marginal degeneration of cornea [Terrien's]
  - ◆ **371.49 Other**
    Discrete colliquative keratopathy
- ● **371.5 Hereditary corneal dystrophies**
  - ◆ **371.50 Corneal dystrophy, unspecified**
  - **371.51 Juvenile epithelial corneal dystrophy**
  - **371.52 Other anterior corneal dystrophies**
    Corneal dystrophy: Corneal dystrophy:
      microscopic cystic   ring-like
  - **371.53 Granular corneal dystrophy**
  - **371.54 Lattice corneal dystrophy**
  - **371.55 Macular corneal dystrophy**
  - ◆ **371.56 Other stromal corneal dystrophies**
    Crystalline corneal dystrophy
  - **371.57 Endothelial corneal dystrophy**
    Combined corneal dystrophy
    Cornea guttata
    Fuchs' endothelial dystrophy
  - ◆ **371.58 Other posterior corneal dystrophies**
    Polymorphous corneal dystrophy
- ● **371.6 Keratoconus**
  - ◆ **371.60 Keratoconus, unspecified**
  - **371.61 Keratoconus, stable condition**
  - **371.62 Keratoconus, acute hydrops**
- ● **371.7 Other corneal deformities**
  - ◆ **371.70 Corneal deformity, unspecified**
  - **371.71 Corneal ectasia**
  - **371.72 Descemetocele**
  - **371.73 Corneal staphyloma**
- ● **371.8 Other corneal disorders**
  - **371.81 Corneal anesthesia and hypoesthesia**
  - **371.82 Corneal disorder due to contact lens**
    EXCLUDES corneal edema (371.24)
  - ◆ **371.89 Other**
- ◆ **371.9 Unspecified corneal disorder**
- ● **372 Disorders of conjunctiva**
  EXCLUDES keratoconjunctivitis (370.3-370.4)
- ● **372.0 Acute conjunctivitis**
  - ◆ **372.00 Acute conjunctivitis, unspecified**
  - **372.01 Serous conjunctivitis, except viral**
    EXCLUDES viral conjunctivitis NOS (077.9)
  - **372.02 Acute follicular conjunctivitis**
    Conjunctival folliculosis NOS
    EXCLUDES conjunctivitis:
      adenoviral (acute follicular) (077.3)
      epidemic hemorrhagic (077.4)
      inclusion (077.0)
      Newcastle (077.8)
      epidemic keratoconjunctivitis (077.1)
      pharyngoconjunctival fever (077.2)
  - ◆ **372.03 Other mucopurulent conjunctivitis**
    Catarrhal conjunctivitis
    EXCLUDES blennorrhea neonatorum (gonococcal) (098.40)
      neonatal conjunctivitis (771.6)
      ophthalmia neonatorum NOS (771.6)
  - **372.04 Pseudomembranous conjunctivitis**
    Membranous conjunctivitis
    EXCLUDES diphtheritic conjunctivitis (032.81)
  - **372.05 Acute atopic conjunctivitis**
- ● **372.1 Chronic conjunctivitis**
  - **372.10 Chronic conjunctivitis, unspecified**
  - **372.11 Simple chronic conjunctivitis**
  - **372.12 Chronic follicular conjunctivitis**
  - **372.13 Vernal conjunctivitis**
  - ◆ **372.14 Other chronic allergic conjunctivitis**
  - *372.15 Parasitic conjunctivitis*
    Code also underlying disease, as:
      filariasis (125.0-125.9)
      mucocutaneous leishmaniasis (085.5)
- ● **372.2 Blepharoconjunctivitis**
  - ◆ **372.20 Blepharoconjunctivitis, unspecified**
  - **372.21 Angular blepharoconjunctivitis**
  - **372.22 Contact blepharoconjunctivitis**
- ● **372.3 Other and unspecified conjunctivitis**
  - ◆ **372.30 Conjunctivitis, unspecified**
  - *372.31 Rosacea conjunctivitis*
    Code also underlying rosacea dermatitis (695.3)
  - *372.33 Conjunctivitis in mucocutaneous disease*
    Code also underlying disease, as:
      erythema multiforme (695.1)
      Reiter's disease (099.3)
    EXCLUDES ocular pemphigoid (694.61)
  - ◆ **372.39 Other**
- ● **372.4 Pterygium**
  EXCLUDES pseudopterygium (372.52)
  - ◆ **372.40 Pterygium, unspecified**
  - **372.41 Peripheral pterygium, stationary**
  - **372.42 Peripheral pterygium, progressive**
  - **372.43 Central pterygium**
  - **372.44 Double pterygium**
  - **372.45 Recurrent pterygium**
- ● **372.5 Conjunctival degenerations and deposits**
  - ◆ **372.50 Conjunctival degeneration, unspecified**
  - **372.51 Pinguecula**
  - **372.52 Pseudopterygium**
  - **372.53 Conjunctival xerosis**
    EXCLUDES conjunctival xerosis due to vitamin A deficiency (264.0, 264.1, 264.7)
  - **372.54 Conjunctival concretions**
  - **372.55 Conjunctival pigmentations**
    Conjunctival argyrosis
  - **372.56 Conjunctival deposits**
- ● **372.6 Conjunctival scars**
  - **372.61 Granuloma of conjunctiva**
  - **372.62 Localized adhesions and strands of conjunctiva**

● Additional digits required   ◆ Nonspecific code   ▌ Not a primary diagnosis

- **372.63** Symblepharon
  - Extensive adhesions of conjunctiva
- **372.64** Scarring of conjunctiva
  - Contraction of eye socket (after enucleation)
- ● **372.7** Conjunctival vascular disorders and cysts
  - **372.71** Hyperemia of conjunctiva
  - **372.72** Conjunctival hemorrhage
    - Hyposphagma
    - Subconjunctival hemorrhage
  - **372.73** Conjunctival edema
    - Chemosis of conjunctiva   Subconjunctival edema
  - **372.74** Vascular abnormalities of conjunctiva
    - Aneurysm(ata) of conjunctiva
  - **372.75** Conjunctival cysts
- ◆ **372.8** Other disorders of conjunctiva
- ◆ **372.9** Unspecified disorder of conjunctiva

● **373** Inflammation of eyelids
- ● **373.0** Blepharitis
  - **EXCLUDES** blepharoconjunctivitis (372.20-372.22)
  - ◆ **373.00** Blepharitis, unspecified
  - **373.01** Ulcerative blepharitis
  - **373.02** Squamous blepharitis
- ● **373.1** Hordeolum and other deep inflammation of eyelid
  - **373.11** Hordeolum externum
    - Hordeolum NOS
    - Stye
  - **373.12** Hordeolum internum
    - Infection of meibomian gland
  - **373.13** Abscess of eyelid
    - Furuncle of eyelid
- **373.2** Chalazion
  - Meibomian (gland) cyst
  - **EXCLUDES** infected meibomian gland (373.12)
- ● **373.3** Noninfectious dermatoses of eyelid
  - **373.31** Eczematous dermatitis of eyelid
  - **373.32** Contact and allergic dermatitis of eyelid
  - **373.33** Xeroderma of eyelid
  - **373.34** Discoid lupus erythematosus of eyelid
- ■ *373.4* Infective dermatitis of eyelid of types resulting in deformity
  - Code also underlying disease, as:
    - leprosy (030.0-030.9)
    - lupus vulgaris (tuberculous) (017.0)
    - yaws (102.0-102.9)
- ■◆ *373.5* Other infective dermatitis of eyelid
  - Code also underlying disease, as:
    - actinomycosis (039.3)
    - impetigo (684)
    - mycotic dermatitis (110.0-111.9)
    - vaccinia (051.0)
    - postvaccination (999.0)
  - **EXCLUDES** herpes:
    - simplex (054.41)
    - zoster (053.20)
- ■ *373.6* Parasitic infestation of eyelid
  - Code also underlying disease, as:
    - leishmaniasis (085.0-085.9)
    - loiasis (125.2)
    - onchocerciasis (125.3)
    - pediculosis (132.0)
- ◆ **373.8** Other inflammations of eyelids
- ◆ **373.9** Unspecified inflammation of eyelid

● **374** Other disorders of eyelids
- ● **374.0** Entropion and trichiasis of eyelid
  - ◆ **374.00** Entropion, unspecified
  - **374.01** Senile entropion
  - **374.02** Mechanical entropion
  - **374.03** Spastic entropion
  - **374.04** Cicatricial entropion
  - **374.05** Trichiasis without entropion
- ● **374.1** Ectropion
  - ◆ **374.10** Ectropion, unspecified
  - **374.11** Senile ectropion
  - **374.12** Mechanical ectropion
  - **374.13** Spastic ectropion
  - **374.14** Cicatricial ectropion
- ● **374.2** Lagophthalmos
  - ◆ **374.20** Lagophthalmos, unspecified
  - **374.21** Paralytic lagophthalmos
  - **374.22** Mechanical lagophthalmos
  - **374.23** Cicatricial lagophthalmos
- ● **374.3** Ptosis of eyelid
  - ◆ **374.30** Ptosis of eyelid, unspecified
  - **374.31** Paralytic ptosis
  - **374.32** Myogenic ptosis
  - **374.33** Mechanical ptosis
  - **374.34** Blepharochalasis
    - Pseudoptosis
- ● **374.4** Other disorders affecting eyelid function
  - **EXCLUDES** blepharoclonus (333.81)
    - blepharospasm (333.81)
    - facial nerve palsy (351.0)
    - third nerve palsy or paralysis (378.51-378.52)
    - tic (psychogenic) (307.20-307.23)
    - organic (333.3)
  - **374.41** Lid retraction or lag
  - **374.43** Abnormal innervation syndrome
    - Jaw-blinking
    - Paradoxical facial movements
  - **374.44** Sensory disorders
  - ◆ **374.45** Other sensorimotor disorders
    - Deficient blink reflex
  - **374.46** Blepharophimosis
    - Ankyloblepharon
- ● **374.5** Degenerative disorders of eyelid and periocular area
  - ◆ **374.50** Degenerative disorder of eyelid, unspecified
  - **374.51** Xanthelasma
    - Xanthoma (planum) (tuberosum) of eyelid
    - Code also underlying condition (272.0-272.9)
  - **374.52** Hyperpigmentation of eyelid
    - Chloasma
    - Dyspigmentation
  - **374.53** Hypopigmentation of eyelid
    - Vitiligo of eyelid
  - **374.54** Hypertrichosis of eyelid
  - **374.55** Hypotrichosis of eyelid
    - Madarosis of eyelid
  - ◆ **374.56** Other degenerative disorders of skin affecting eyelid
- ● **374.8** Other disorders of eyelid
  - **374.81** Hemorrhage of eyelid
    - **EXCLUDES** black eye (921.0)
  - **374.82** Edema of eyelid
    - Hyperemia of eyelid
  - **374.83** Elephantiasis of eyelid
  - **374.84** Cysts of eyelids
    - Sebaceous cyst of eyelid
  - **374.85** Vascular anomalies of eyelid
  - **374.86** Retained foreign body of eyelid
  - **374.87** Dermatochalasis
  - ◆ **374.89** Other disorders of eyelid
- ◆ **374.9** Unspecified disorder of eyelid

● **375** Disorders of lacrimal system
- ● **375.0** Dacryoadenitis
  - ◆ **375.00** Dacryoadenitis, unspecified
  - **375.01** Acute dacryoadenitis
  - **375.02** Chronic dacryoadenitis
  - **375.03** Chronic enlargement of lacrimal gland
- ● **375.1** Other disorders of lacrimal gland
  - **375.11** Dacryops
  - ◆ **375.12** Other lacrimal cysts and cystic degeneration
  - **375.13** Primary lacrimal atrophy
  - **375.14** Secondary lacrimal atrophy
  - ◆ **375.15** Tear film insufficiency, unspecified
    - Dry eye syndrome
  - **375.16** Dislocation of lacrimal gland
- ● **375.2** Epiphora
  - **375.20** Epiphora, unspecified as to cause
  - **375.21** Epiphora due to excess lacrimation
  - **375.22** Epiphora due to insufficient drainage
- ● **375.3** Acute and unspecified inflammation of lacrimal passages
  - **EXCLUDES** neonatal dacryocystitis (771.6)
  - ◆ **375.30** Dacryocystitis, unspecified
  - **375.31** Acute canaliculitis, lacrimal
  - **375.32** Acute dacryocystitis
    - Acute peridacryocystitis
  - **375.33** Phlegmonous dacryocystitis

NERVOUS SYSTEM AND SENSE ORGANS

- ● 375.4 Chronic inflammation of lacrimal passages
  - 375.41 Chronic canaliculitis
  - 375.42 Chronic dacryocystitis
  - 375.43 Lacrimal mucocele
- ● 375.5 Stenosis and insufficiency of lacrimal passages
  - 375.51 Eversion of lacrimal punctum
  - 375.52 Stenosis of lacrimal punctum
  - 375.53 Stenosis of lacrimal canaliculi
  - 375.54 Stenosis of lacrimal sac
  - 375.55 Obstruction of nasolacrimal duct, neonatal
    - **EXCLUDES** congenital anomaly of nasolacrimal duct (743.65)
  - 375.56 Stenosis of nasolacrimal duct, acquired
  - 375.57 Dacryolith
- ● 375.6 Other changes of lacrimal passages
  - 375.61 Lacrimal fistula
  - ◆ 375.69 Other
- ● 375.8 Other disorders of lacrimal system
  - 375.81 Granuloma of lacrimal passages
  - ◆ 375.89 Other
- ◆ 375.9 Unspecified disorder of lacrimal system
- ● 376 Disorders of the orbit
  - ● 376.0 Acute inflammation of orbit
    - ◆ 376.00 Acute inflammation of orbit, unspecified
    - 376.01 Orbital cellulitis
      - Abscess of orbit
    - 376.02 Orbital periostitis
    - 376.03 Orbital osteomyelitis
    - 376.04 Tenonitis
  - ● 376.1 Chronic inflammatory disorders of orbit
    - ◆ 376.10 Chronic inflammation of orbit, unspecified
    - 376.11 Orbital granuloma
      - Pseudotumor (inflammatory) of orbit
    - 376.12 Orbital myositis
    - ■ 376.13 *Parasitic infestation of orbit*
      - Code also underlying disease, as:
        - hydatid infestation of orbit (122.3, 122.6, 122.9)
        - myiasis of orbit (134.0)
  - ● 376.2 *Endocrine exophthalmos*
    - Code also underlying thyroid disorder (242.0-242.9)
    - ■ 376.21 *Thyrotoxic exophthalmos*
    - ■ 376.22 *Exophthalmic ophthalmoplegia*
  - ● 376.3 Other exophthalmic conditions
    - ◆ 376.30 Exophthalmos, unspecified
    - 376.31 Constant exophthalmos
    - 376.32 Orbital hemorrhage
    - 376.33 Orbital edema or congestion
    - 376.34 Intermittent exophthalmos
    - 376.35 Pulsating exophthalmos
    - 376.36 Lateral displacement of globe
  - ● 376.4 Deformity of orbit
    - ◆ 376.40 Deformity of orbit, unspecified
    - 376.41 Hypertelorism of orbit
    - 376.42 Exostosis of orbit
    - 376.43 Local deformities due to bone disease
    - 376.44 Orbital deformities associated with craniofacial deformities
    - 376.45 Atrophy of orbit
    - 376.46 Enlargement of orbit
    - 376.47 Deformity due to trauma or surgery
  - ● 376.5 Enophthalmos
    - ◆ 376.50 Enophthalmos, unspecified as to cause
    - 376.51 Enophthalmos due to atrophy of orbital tissue
    - 376.52 Enophthalmos due to trauma or surgery
  - 376.6 Retained (old) foreign body following penetrating wound of orbit
    - Retrobulbar foreign body
  - ● 376.8 Other orbital disorders
    - 376.81 Orbital cysts
      - Encephalocele of orbit
    - 376.82 Myopathy of extraocular muscles
    - ◆ 376.89 Other
  - ◆ 376.9 Unspecified disorder of orbit
- ● 377 Disorders of optic nerve and visual pathways
  - ● 377.0 Papilledema
    - ◆ 377.00 Papilledema, unspecified
    - 377.01 Papilledema associated with increased intracranial pressure
    - 377.02 Papilledema associated with decreased ocular pressure
    - 377.03 Papilledema associated with retinal disorder
    - 377.04 Foster-Kennedy syndrome
  - ● 377.1 Optic atrophy
    - ◆ 377.10 Optic atrophy, unspecified
    - 377.11 Primary optic atrophy
      - **EXCLUDES** neurosyphilitic optic atrophy (094.84)
    - 377.12 Postinflammatory optic atrophy
    - 377.13 Optic atrophy associated with retinal dystrophies
    - 377.14 Glaucomatous atrophy [cupping] of optic disc
    - 377.15 Partial optic atrophy
      - Temporal pallor of optic disc
    - 377.16 Hereditary optic atrophy
      - Optic atrophy:
        - dominant hereditary
        - Leber's
  - ● 377.2 Other disorders of optic disc
    - 377.21 Drusen of optic disc
    - 377.22 Crater-like holes of optic disc
    - 377.23 Coloboma of optic disc
    - 377.24 Pseudopapilledema
  - ● 377.3 Optic neuritis
    - **EXCLUDES** meningococcal optic neuritis (036.81)
    - ◆ 377.30 Optic neuritis, unspecified
    - 377.31 Optic papillitis
    - 377.32 Retrobulbar neuritis (acute)
      - **EXCLUDES** syphilitic retrobulbar neuritis (094.85)
    - 377.33 Nutritional optic neuropathy
    - 377.34 Toxic optic neuropathy
      - Toxic amblyopia
    - ◆ 377.39 Other
      - **EXCLUDES** ischemic optic neuropathy (377.41)
  - ● 377.4 Other disorders of optic nerve
    - 377.41 Ischemic optic neuropathy
    - 377.42 Hemorrhage in optic nerve sheaths
    - ◆ 377.49 Other
      - Compression of optic nerve
  - ● 377.5 Disorders of optic chiasm
    - 377.51 Associated with pituitary neoplasms and disorders
    - ◆ 377.52 Associated with other neoplasms
    - 377.53 Associated with vascular disorders
    - 377.54 Associated with inflammatory disorders
  - ● 377.6 Disorders of other visual pathways
    - 377.61 Associated with neoplasms
    - 377.62 Associated with vascular disorders
    - 377.63 Associated with inflammatory disorders
  - ● 377.7 Disorders of visual cortex
    - **EXCLUDES** visual:
      - agnosia (368.16)
      - hallucinations (368.16)
      - halos (368.15)
    - 377.71 Associated with neoplasms
    - 377.72 Associated with vascular disorders
    - 377.73 Associated with inflammatory disorders
    - 377.75 Cortical blindness
  - ◆ 377.9 Unspecified disorder of optic nerve and visual pathways
- ● 378 Strabismus and other disorders of binocular eye movements
  - **EXCLUDES** nystagmus and other irregular eye movements (379.50-379.59)
  - ● 378.0 Esotropia
    - Convergent concomitant strabismus
    - **EXCLUDES** intermittent esotropia (378.20-378.22)
    - ◆ 378.00 Esotropia, unspecified
    - 378.01 Monocular esotropia
    - 378.02 Monocular esotropia with A pattern
    - 378.03 Monocular esotropia with V pattern
    - ◆ 378.04 Monocular esotropia with other noncomitancies
      - Monocular esotropia with X or Y pattern
    - 378.05 Alternating esotropia
    - 378.06 Alternating esotropia with A pattern
    - 378.07 Alternating esotropia with V pattern
    - ◆ 378.08 Alternating esotropia with other noncomitancies

● Additional digits required   ◆ Nonspecific code   ■ Not a primary diagnosis

- **378.1** **Exotropia**
  Divergent concomitant strabismus
  EXCLUDES intermittent exotropia (378.20, 378.23-378.24)
  - 378.10 Exotropia, unspecified
  - 378.11 Monocular exotropia
  - 378.12 Monocular exotropia with A pattern
  - 378.13 Monocular exotropia with V pattern
  - 378.14 Monocular exotropia with other noncomitancies
    Monocular exotropia with X or Y pattern
  - 378.15 Alternating exotropia
  - 378.16 Alternating exotropia with A pattern
  - 378.17 Alternating exotropia with V pattern
  - 378.18 Alternating exotropia with other noncomitancies
    Alternating exotropia with X or Y pattern
- **378.2** **Intermittent heterotropia**
  EXCLUDES vertical heterotropia (intermittent) (378.31)
  - 378.20 Intermittent heterotropia, unspecified
    Intermittent: esotropia NOS
    Intermittent: exotropia NOS
  - 378.21 Intermittent esotropia, monocular
  - 378.22 Intermittent esotropia, alternating
  - 378.23 Intermittent exotropia, monocular
  - 378.24 Intermittent exotropia, alternating
- **378.3** **Other and unspecified heterotropia**
  - 378.30 Heterotropia, unspecified
  - 378.31 Hypertropia
    Vertical heterotropia (constant) (intermittent)
  - 378.32 Hypotropia
  - 378.33 Cyclotropia
  - 378.34 Monofixation syndrome
    Microtropia
  - 378.35 Accommodative component in esotropia
- **378.4** **Heterophoria**
  - 378.40 Heterophoria, unspecified
  - 378.41 Esophoria
  - 378.42 Exophoria
  - 378.43 Vertical heterophoria
  - 378.44 Cyclophoria
  - 378.45 Alternating hyperphoria
- **378.5** **Paralytic strabismus**
  - 378.50 Paralytic strabismus, unspecified
  - 378.51 Third or oculomotor nerve palsy, partial
  - 378.52 Third or oculomotor nerve palsy, total
  - 378.53 Fourth or trochlear nerve palsy
  - 378.54 Sixth or abducens nerve palsy
  - 378.55 External ophthalmoplegia
  - 378.56 Total ophthalmoplegia
- **378.6** **Mechanical strabismus**
  - 378.60 Mechanical strabismus, unspecified
  - 378.61 Brown's (tendon) sheath syndrome
  - 378.62 Mechanical strabismus from other musculofascial disorders
  - 378.63 Limited duction associated with other conditions
- **378.7** **Other specified strabismus**
  - 378.71 Duane's syndrome
  - 378.72 Progressive external ophthalmoplegia
  - 378.73 Strabismus in other neuromuscular disorders
- **378.8** **Other disorders of binocular eye movements**
  EXCLUDES nystagmus (379.50-379.56)
  - 378.81 Palsy of conjugate gaze
  - 378.82 Spasm of conjugate gaze
  - 378.83 Convergence insufficiency or palsy
  - 378.84 Convergence excess or spasm
  - 378.85 Anomalies of divergence
  - 378.86 Internuclear ophthalmoplegia
  - 378.87 Other dissociated deviation of eye movements
    Skew deviation
  - 378.9 Unspecified disorder of eye movements
    Ophthalmoplegia NOS
    Strabismus NOS

379 Other disorders of eye

- **379.0** **Scleritis and episcleritis**
  EXCLUDES syphilitic episcleritis (095.0)
  - 379.00 Scleritis, unspecified
    Episcleritis NOS
  - 379.01 Episcleritis periodica fugax
  - 379.02 Nodular episcleritis
  - 379.03 Anterior scleritis
  - 379.04 Scleromalacia perforans
  - 379.05 Scleritis with corneal involvement
    Scleroperikeratitis
  - 379.06 Brawny scleritis
  - 379.07 Posterior scleritis
    Sclerotenonitis
  - 379.09 Other
    Scleral abscess
- **379.1** **Other disorders of sclera**
  EXCLUDES blue sclera (743.47)
  - 379.11 Scleral ectasia
    Scleral staphyloma NOS
  - 379.12 Staphyloma posticum
  - 379.13 Equatorial staphyloma
  - 379.14 Anterior staphyloma, localized
  - 379.15 Ring staphyloma
  - 379.16 Other degenerative disorders of sclera
  - 379.19 Other
- **379.2** **Disorders of vitreous body**
  - 379.21 Vitreous degeneration
    Vitreous: cavitation detachment
    Vitreous: liquefaction
  - 379.22 Crystalline deposits in vitreous
    Asteroid hyalitis
    Synchysis scintillans
  - 379.23 Vitreous hemorrhage
  - 379.24 Other vitreous opacities
    Vitreous floaters
  - 379.25 Vitreous membranes and strands
  - 379.26 Vitreous prolapse
  - 379.29 Other disorders of vitreous
    EXCLUDES vitreous abscess (360.04)
- **379.3** **Aphakia and other disorders of lens**
  EXCLUDES after-cataract (366.50-366.53)
  - 379.31 Aphakia
  - 379.32 Subluxation of lens
  - 379.33 Anterior dislocation of lens
  - 379.34 Posterior dislocation of lens
  - 379.39 Other disorders of lens
- **379.4** **Anomalies of pupillary function**
  - 379.40 Abnormal pupillary function, unspecified
  - 379.41 Anisocoria
  - 379.42 Miosis (persistent), not due to miotics
  - 379.43 Mydriasis (persistent), not due to mydriatics
  - 379.45 Argyll Robertson pupil, atypical
    Argyll Robertson phenomenon or pupil, nonsyphilitic
    EXCLUDES Argyll Robertson pupil (syphilitic) (094.89)
  - 379.46 Tonic pupillary reaction
    Adie's pupil or syndrome
  - 379.49 Other
    Hippus
    Pupillary paralysis
- **379.5** **Nystagmus and other irregular eye movements**
  - 379.50 Nystagmus, unspecified
  - 379.51 Congenital nystagmus
  - 379.52 Latent nystagmus
  - 379.53 Visual deprivation nystagmus
  - 379.54 Nystagmus associated with disorders of the vestibular system
  - 379.55 Dissociated nystagmus
  - 379.56 Other forms of nystagmus
  - 379.57 Deficiencies of saccadic eye movements
    Abnormal optokinetic response
  - 379.58 Deficiencies of smooth pursuit movements
  - 379.59 Other irregularities of eye movements
    Opsoclonus
- **379.8** Other specified disorders of eye and adnexa
- **379.9** **Unspecified disorder of eye and adnexa**
  - 379.90 Disorder of eye, unspecified
  - 379.91 Pain in or around eye
  - 379.92 Swelling or mass of eye
  - 379.93 Redness or discharge of eye
  - 379.99 Other ill-defined disorders of eye
    EXCLUDES blurred vision NOS (368.8)

DISEASES OF THE EAR AND MASTOID PROCESS (380-389)

- **380 Disorders of external ear**
  - **380.0 Perichondritis of pinna**
    Perichondritis of auricle
    - 380.00 Perichondritis of pinna, unspecified
    - 380.01 Acute perichondritis of pinna
    - 380.02 Chronic perichondritis of pinna
  - **380.1 Infective otitis externa**
    - 380.10 Infective otitis externa, unspecified
      Otitis externa (acute): Otitis externa (acute):
        NOS   hemorrhagica
        circumscribed   infective NOS
        diffuse
    - 380.11 Acute infection of pinna
      - EXCLUDES furuncular otitis externa (680.0)
    - 380.12 Acute swimmers' ear
      Beach ear Tank ear
    - 380.13 Other acute infections of external ear
      Code also underlying disease, as:
        erysipelas (035)
        impetigo (684)
        seborrheicdermatitis (690)
      - EXCLUDES herpes simplex (054.73)
        herpes zoster (053.71)
    - 380.14 Malignant otitis externa
    - 380.15 Chronic mycotic otitis externa
      Code also underlying disease, as:
        aspergillosis (117.3)
        otomycosis NOS (111.9)
      - EXCLUDES candidal otitis externa (112.82)
    - 380.16 Other chronic infective otitis externa
      Chronic infective otitis externa NOS
  - **380.2 Other otitis externa**
    - 380.21 Cholesteatoma of external ear
      Keratosis obturans of external ear (canal)
      - EXCLUDES cholesteatoma NOS (385.30-385.35)
        postmastoidectomy (383.32)
    - 380.22 Other acute otitis externa
      Acute otitis externa: Acute otitis externa:
        actinic   eczematoid
        chemical   reactive
        contact
    - 380.23 Other chronic otitis externa
      Chronic otitis externa NOS
  - **380.3 Noninfectious disorders of pinna**
    - 380.30 Disorder of pinna, unspecified
    - 380.31 Hematoma of auricle or pinna
    - 380.32 Acquired deformities of auricle or pinna
      - EXCLUDES cauliflower ear (738.7)
    - 380.39 Other
      - EXCLUDES gouty tophi of ear (274.81)
  - 380.4 Impacted cerumen
    Wax in ear
  - **380.5 Acquired stenosis of external ear canal**
    Collapse of external ear canal
    - 380.50 Acquired stenosis of external ear canal, unspecified as to cause
    - 380.51 Secondary to trauma
    - 380.52 Secondary to surgery
    - 380.53 Secondary to inflammation
  - **380.8 Other disorders of external ear**
    - 380.81 Exostosis of external ear canal
    - 380.89 Other
  - 380.9 Unspecified disorder of external ear
- **381 Nonsuppurative otitis media and Eustachian tube disorders**
  - **381.0 Acute nonsuppurative otitis media**
    Acute tubotympanic catarrh
    Otitis media, acute or subacute:
      catarrhal
      exudative
      transudative
      with effusion
    - EXCLUDES otitic barotrauma (993.0)
    - 381.00 Acute nonsuppurative otitis media, unspecified
    - 381.01 Acute serous otitis media
      Acute or subacute secretory otitis media
    - 381.02 Acute mucoid otitis media
      Acute or subacute seromucinous otitis media
      Blue drum syndrome
    - 381.03 Acute sanguinous otitis media
    - 381.04 Acute allergic serous otitis media
    - 381.05 Acute allergic mucoid otitis media
    - 381.06 Acute allergic sanguinous otitis media
  - **381.1 Chronic serous otitis media**
    Chronic tubotympanic catarrh
    - 381.10 Chronic serous otitis media, simple or unspecified
    - 381.19 Other
      Serosanguinous chronic otitis media
  - **381.2 Chronic mucoid otitis media**
    Glue ear
    - EXCLUDES adhesive middle ear disease (385.10-385.19)
    - 381.20 Chronic mucoid otitis media, simple or unspecified
    - 381.29 Other
      Mucosanguinous chronic otitis media
  - 381.3 Other and unspecified chronic nonsuppurative otitis media
    Otitis media, chronic: Otitis media, chronic:
      allergic   seromucinous
      exudative   transudative
      secretory   with effusion
  - 381.4 Nonsuppurative otitis media, not specified as acute or chronic
    Otitis media: Otitis media:
      allergic   seromucinous
      catarrhal   serous
      exudative   transudative
      mucoid   with effusion
      secretory
  - **381.5 Eustachian salpingitis**
    - 381.50 Eustachian salpingitis, unspecified
    - 381.51 Acute Eustachian salpingitis
    - 381.52 Chronic Eustachian salpingitis
  - **381.6 Obstruction of Eustachian tube**
    Stenosis } of Eustachian tube
    Stricture
    - 381.60 Obstruction of Eustachian tube, unspecified
    - 381.61 Osseous obstruction of Eustachian tube
      Obstruction of Eustachian tube from cholesteatoma, polyp, or other osseous lesion
    - 381.62 Intrinsic cartilagenous obstruction of Eustachian tube
    - 381.63 Extrinsic cartilagenous obstruction of Eustachian tube
      Compression of Eustachian tube
  - 381.7 Patulous Eustachian tube
  - **381.8 Other disorders of Eustachian tube**
    - 381.81 Dysfunction of Eustachian tube
    - 381.89 Other
  - 381.9 Unspecified Eustachian tube disorder
- **382 Suppurative and unspecified otitis media**
  - **382.0 Acute suppurative otitis media**
    Otitis media, acute:
      necrotizing NOS
      purulent
    - 382.00 Acute suppurative otitis media without spontaneous rupture of ear drum
    - 382.01 Acute suppurative otitis media with spontaneous rupture of ear drum
    - 382.02 Acute suppurative otitis media in diseases classified elsewhere
      Code also underlying disease, as:
        influenza (487.8)
        scarlet fever (034.1)
      - EXCLUDES postmeasles otitis (055.2)
  - 382.1 Chronic tubotympanic suppurative otitis media
    Benign chronic suppu-
      rative otitis
      media } (with anterior perforation of ear drum)
    Chronic tubotympanic
      disease

- Additional digits required   ◆ Nonspecific code   ▮ Not a primary diagnosis

- **382.2 Chronic atticoantral suppurative otitis media**
  - Chronic atticoantral disease
  - Persistent mucosal disease
  } (with posterior or superior marginal perforation of ear drum)
- ◆ **382.3 Unspecified chronic suppurative otitis media**
  - Chronic purulent otitis media
  - EXCLUDES tuberculous otitis media (017.4)
- ◆ **382.4 Unspecified suppurative otitis media**
  - Purulent otitis media NOS
- ◆ **382.9 Unspecified otitis media**
  - Otitis media:
    - NOS
    - acute NOS
    - chronic NOS

● **383 Mastoiditis and related conditions**
  - ● **383.0 Acute mastoiditis**
    - Abscess of mastoid
    - Empyema of mastoid
    - **383.00 Acute mastoiditis without complications**
    - **383.01 Subperiosteal abscess of mastoid**
    - ◆ **383.02 Acute mastoiditis with other complications**
      - Gradenigo's syndrome
  - **383.1 Chronic mastoiditis**
    - Caries of mastoid
    - Fistula of mastoid
    - EXCLUDES tuberculous mastoiditis (015.6)
  - ● **383.2 Petrositis**
    - Coalescing osteitis
    - Inflammation
    - Osteomyelitis
    } of petrous bone
    - ◆ **383.20 Petrositis, unspecified**
    - **383.21 Acute petrositis**
    - **383.22 Chronic petrositis**
  - ● **383.3 Complications following mastoidectomy**
    - ◆ **383.30 Postmastoidectomy complication, unspecified**
    - **383.31 Mucosal cyst of postmastoidectomy cavity**
    - **383.32 Recurrent cholesteatoma of postmastoidectomy cavity**
    - **383.33 Granulations of postmastoidectomy cavity**
      - Chronic inflammation of postmastoidectomy cavity
  - ● **383.8 Other disorders of mastoid**
    - **383.81 Postauricular fistula**
    - ◆ **383.89 Other**
  - ◆ **383.9 Unspecified mastoiditis**

● **384 Other disorders of tympanic membrane**
  - ● **384.0 Acute myringitis without mention of otitis media**
    - ◆ **384.00 Acute myringitis, unspecified**
      - Acute tympanitis NOS
    - **384.01 Bullous myringitis**
      - Myringitis bullosa hemorrhagica
    - ◆ **384.09 Other**
  - **384.1 Chronic myringitis without mention of otitis media**
    - Chronic tympanitis
  - ● **384.2 Perforation of tympanic membrane**
    - Perforation of ear drum:
      - NOS
      - persistent posttraumatic
      - postinflammatory
    - EXCLUDES traumatic perforation [current injury] (872.61)
    - ◆ **384.20 Perforation of tympanic membrane, unspecified**
    - **384.21 Central perforation of tympanic membrane**
    - **384.22 Attic perforation of tympanic membrane**
      - Pars flaccida
    - ◆ **384.23 Other marginal perforation of tympanic membrane**
    - **384.24 Multiple perforations of tympanic membrane**
    - **384.25 Total perforation of tympanic membrane**
  - ● **384.8 Other specified disorders of tympanic membrane**
    - **384.81 Atrophic flaccid tympanic membrane**
      - Healed perforation of ear drum
    - **384.82 Atrophic nonflaccid tympanic membrane**
  - ◆ **384.9 Unspecified disorder of tympanic membrane**

● **385 Other disorders of middle ear and mastoid**
  - EXCLUDES mastoiditis (383.0-383.9)
  - ● **385.0 Tympanosclerosis**
    - ◆ **385.00 Tympanosclerosis, unspecified as to involvement**
    - **385.01 Tympanosclerosis involving tympanic membrane only**
    - **385.02 Tympanosclerosis involving tympanic membrane and ear ossicles**
    - **385.03 Tympanosclerosis involving tympanic membrane, ear ossicles, and middle ear**
    - ◆ **385.09 Tympanosclerosis involving other combination of structures**
  - ● **385.1 Adhesive middle ear disease**
    - Adhesive otitis
    - Otitis media:
      - chronic adhesive
      - fibrotic
    - EXCLUDES glue ear (381.20-381.29)
    - ◆ **385.10 Adhesive middle ear disease, unspecified as to involvement**
    - **385.11 Adhesions of drum head to incus**
    - **385.12 Adhesions of drum head to stapes**
    - **385.13 Adhesions of drum head to promontorium**
    - ◆ **385.19 Other adhesions and combinations**
  - ● **385.2 Other acquired abnormality of ear ossicles**
    - **385.21 Impaired mobility of malleus**
      - Ankylosis of malleus
    - ◆ **385.22 Impaired mobility of other ear ossicles**
      - Ankylosis of ear ossicles, except malleus
    - **385.23 Discontinuity or dislocation of ear ossicles**
    - **385.24 Partial loss or necrosis of ear ossicles**
  - ● **385.3 Cholesteatoma of middle ear and mastoid**
    - Cholesterosis
    - Epidermosis
    - Keratosis
    - Polyp
    } of (middle) ear
    - EXCLUDES cholesteatoma:
      - external ear canal (380.21)
      - recurrent of postmastoidectomy cavity (383.32)
    - ◆ **385.30 Cholesteatoma, unspecified**
    - **385.31 Cholesteatoma of attic**
    - **385.32 Cholesteatoma of middle ear**
    - **385.33 Cholesteatoma of middle ear and mastoid**
    - **385.35 Diffuse cholesteatosis**
  - ● **385.8 Other disorders of middle ear and mastoid**
    - **385.82 Cholesterin granuloma**
    - **385.83 Retained foreign body of middle ear**
    - ◆ **385.89 Other**
  - ◆ **385.9 Unspecified disorder of middle ear and mastoid**

● **386 Vertiginous syndromes and other disorders of vestibular system**
  - EXCLUDES vertigo NOS (780.4)
  - ● **386.0 Ménière's disease**
    - Endolymphatic hydrops
    - Lermoyez's syndrome
    - Ménière's syndrome or vertigo
    - ◆ **386.00 Ménière's disease, unspecified**
      - Ménière's disease (active)
    - **386.01 Active Ménière's disease, cochleovestibular**
    - **386.02 Active Ménière's disease, cochlear**
    - **386.03 Active Ménière's disease, vestibular**
    - **386.04 Inactive Ménière's disease**
      - Ménière's disease in remission
  - ● **386.1 Other and unspecified peripheral vertigo**
    - EXCLUDES epidemic vertigo (078.81)
    - ◆ **386.10 Peripheral vertigo, unspecified**
    - **386.11 Benign paroxysmal positional vertigo**
      - Benign paroxysmal positional nystagmus
    - **386.12 Vestibular neuronitis**
      - Acute (and recurrent) peripheral vestibulopathy
    - ◆ **386.19 Other**
      - Aural vertigo
      - Otogenic vertigo
  - **386.2 Vertigo of central origin**
    - Central positional nystagmus
    - Malignant positional vertigo
  - ● **386.3 Labyrinthitis**
    - ◆ **386.30 Labyrinthitis, unspecified**

CIRCULATORY SYSTEM

- 386.31 Serous labyrinthitis
  - Diffuse labyrinthitis
- 386.32 Circumscribed labyrinthitis
  - Focal labyrinthitis
- 386.33 Suppurative labyrinthitis
  - Purulent labyrinthitis
- 386.34 Toxic labyrinthitis
- 386.35 Viral labyrinthitis
- ● 386.4 Labyrinthine fistula
  - ◆ 386.40 Labyrinthine fistula, unspecified
  - 386.41 Round window fistula
  - 386.42 Oval window fistula
  - 386.43 Semicircular canal fistula
  - 386.48 Labyrinthine fistula of combined sites
- ● 386.5 Labyrinthine dysfunction
  - ◆ 386.50 Labyrinthine dysfunction, unspecified
  - 386.51 Hyperactive labyrinth, unilateral
  - 386.52 Hyperactive labyrinth, bilateral
  - 386.53 Hypoactive labyrinth, unilateral
  - 386.54 Hypoactive labyrinth, bilateral
  - 386.55 Loss of labyrinthine reactivity, unilateral
  - 386.56 Loss of labyrinthine reactivity, bilateral
  - 386.58 Other forms and combinations
- ◆ 386.8 Other disorders of labyrinth
- ◆ 386.9 Unspecified vertiginous syndromes and labyrinthine disorders
- ● 387 Otosclerosis
  - **INCLUDES** otospongiosis
  - 387.0 Otosclerosis involving oval window, nonobliterative
  - 387.1 Otosclerosis involving oval window, obliterative
  - 387.2 Cochlear otosclerosis
    - Otosclerosis involving:
      - otic capsule
      - round window
  - ◆ 387.8 Other otosclerosis
  - ◆ 387.9 Otosclerosis, unspecified
- ● 388 Other disorders of ear
  - ● 388.0 Degenerative and vascular disorders of ear
    - ◆ 388.00 Degenerative and vascular disorders, unspecified
    - 388.01 Presbyacusis
    - 388.02 Transient ischemic deafness
  - ● 388.1 Noise effects on inner ear
    - ◆ 388.10 Noise effects on inner ear, unspecified
    - 388.11 Acoustic trauma (explosive) to ear
      - Otitic blast injury
    - 388.12 Noise-induced hearing loss
  - ◆ 388.2 Sudden hearing loss, unspecified
  - ● 388.3 Tinnitus
    - ◆ 388.30 Tinnitus, unspecified
    - 388.31 Subjective tinnitus
    - 388.32 Objective tinnitus
  - ● 388.4 Other abnormal auditory perception
    - ◆ 388.40 Abnormal auditory perception, unspecified
    - 388.41 Diplacusis
    - 388.42 Hyperacusis
    - 388.43 Impairment of auditory discrimination
    - 388.44 Recruitment
  - 388.5 Disorders of acoustic nerve
    - Acoustic neuritis
    - Degeneration / Disorder } of acoustic or eighth nerve
    - **EXCLUDES** acoustic neuroma (225.1)
      - syphilitic acoustic neuritis (094.86)
  - ● 388.6 Otorrhea
    - ◆ 388.60 Otorrhea, unspecified
      - Discharging ear NOS
    - 388.61 Cerebrospinal fluid otorrhea
      - **EXCLUDES** cerebrospinal fluid rhinorrhea (349.81)
    - ◆ 388.69 Other
      - Otorrhagia
  - ● 388.7 Otalgia
    - ◆ 388.70 Otalgia, unspecified
      - Earache NOS
    - 388.71 Otogenic pain
    - 388.72 Referred pain
  - ◆ 388.8 Other disorders of ear
- ◆ 388.9 Unspecified disorder of ear
- ● 389 Hearing loss
  - ● 389.0 Conductive hearing loss
    - Conductive deafness
    - ◆ 389.00 Conductive hearing loss, unspecified
    - 389.01 Conductive hearing loss, external ear
    - 389.02 Conductive hearing loss, tympanic membrane
    - 389.03 Conductive hearing loss, middle ear
    - 389.04 Conductive hearing loss, inner ear
    - 389.08 Conductive hearing loss of combined types
  - ● 389.1 Sensorineural hearing loss
    - Perceptive hearing loss or deafness
    - **EXCLUDES** abnormal auditory perception (388.40-388.44)
      - psychogenic deafness (306.7)
    - ◆ 389.10 Sensorineural hearing loss, unspecified
    - 389.11 Sensory hearing loss
    - 389.12 Neural hearing loss
    - 389.14 Central hearing loss
    - 389.18 Sensorineural hearing loss of combined types
  - 389.2 Mixed conductive and sensorineural hearing loss
    - Deafness or hearing loss of type classifiable to 389.0 with type classifiable to 389.1
  - 389.7 Deaf mutism, not elsewhere classifiable
    - Deaf, nonspeaking
  - ◆ 389.8 Other specified forms of hearing loss
  - ◆ 389.9 Unspecified hearing loss
    - Deafness NOS

7. DISEASES OF THE CIRCULATORY SYSTEM (390-459)

ACUTE RHEUMATIC FEVER (390-392)

- 390 Rheumatic fever without mention of heart involvement
  - Arthritis, rheumatic, acute or subacute
  - Rheumatic fever (active) (acute)
  - Rheumatism, articular, acute or subacute
  - **EXCLUDES** that with heart involvement (391.0-391.9)
- ● 391 Rheumatic fever with heart involvement
  - **EXCLUDES** chronic heart diseases of rheumatic origin (393.0-398.9) unless rheumatic fever is also present or there is evidence of recrudescence or activity of the rheumatic process
  - 391.0 Acute rheumatic pericarditis
    - Rheumatic:
      - fever (active) (acute) with pericarditis
      - pericarditis (acute)
    - Any condition classifiable to 390 with pericarditis
    - **EXCLUDES** that not specified as rheumatic (420.0-420.9)
  - 391.1 Acute rheumatic endocarditis
    - Rheumatic:
      - endocarditis, acute
      - fever (active) (acute) with endocarditis or valvulitis
      - valvulitis acute
    - Any condition classifiable to 390 with endocarditis or valvulitis
  - 391.2 Acute rheumatic myocarditis
    - Rheumatic fever (active) (acute) with myocarditis
    - Any condition classifiable to 390 with myocarditis
  - ◆ 391.8 Other acute rheumatic heart disease
    - Rheumatic:
      - fever (active) (acute) with other or multiple types of heart involvement
      - pancarditis, acute
    - Any condition classifiable to 390 with other or multiple types of heart involvement
  - ◆ 391.9 Acute rheumatic heart disease, unspecified
    - Rheumatic:
      - carditis, acute
      - fever (active) (acute) with unspecified type of heart involvement
      - heart disease, active or acute
    - Any condition classifiable to 390 with unspecified type of heart involvement
- ● 392 Rheumatic chorea
  - **INCLUDES** Sydenham's chorea
  - **EXCLUDES** chorea:
    - NOS (333.5)
    - Huntington's (333.4)

392.0 With heart involvement
Rheumatic chorea with heart involvement of any type classifiable to 391

392.9 Without mention of heart involvement

CHRONIC RHEUMATIC HEART DISEASE (393-398)

393 Chronic rheumatic pericarditis
Adherent pericardium, rheumatic
Chronic rheumatic:
  mediastinopericarditis
  myopericarditis
EXCLUDES pericarditis NOS or not specified as rheumatic (423.0-423.9)

● 394 Diseases of mitral valve
EXCLUDES that with aortic valve involvement (396.0-396.9)

394.0 Mitral stenosis
Mitral (valve):   Mitral (valve):
  obstruction (rheumatic)   stenosis NOS

394.1 Rheumatic mitral insufficiency
Rheumatic mitral:
  incompetence
  regurgitation
EXCLUDES that not specified as rheumatic (424.0)

394.2 Mitral stenosis with insufficiency
Mitral stenosis with incompetence or regurgitation

◆ 394.9 Other and unspecified mitral valve diseases
Mitral (valve):   Mitral (valve):
  disease (chronic)   failure

● 395 Diseases of aortic valve
EXCLUDES that not specified as rheumatic (424.1)
that with mitral valve involvement (396.0-396.9)

395.0 Rheumatic aortic stenosis
Rheumatic aortic (valve) obstruction

395.1 Rheumatic aortic insufficiency
Rheumatic aortic:
  incompetence
  regurgitation

395.2 Rheumatic aortic stenosis with insufficiency
Rheumatic aortic stenosis with incompetence or regurgitation

◆ 395.9 Other and unspecified rheumatic aortic diseases
Rheumatic aortic (valve) disease

● 396 Diseases of mitral and aortic valves
INCLUDES involvement of both mitral and aortic valves, whether specified as rheumatic or not

396.0 Mitral valve stenosis and aortic valve stenosis
Atypical aortic (valve) stenosis
Mitral and aortic (valve) obstruction (rheumatic)

396.1 Mitral valve stenosis and aortic valve insufficiency

396.2 Mitral valve insufficiency and aortic valve stenosis

396.3 Mitral valve insufficiency and aortic valve insufficiency
Mitral and aortic (valve):
  incompetence
  regurgitation

396.8 Multiple involvement of mitral and aortic valves
Stenosis and insufficiency of mitral or aortic valve with stenosis or insufficiency, or both, of the other valve

◆ 396.9 Mitral and aortic valve diseases, unspecified

● 397 Diseases of other endocardial structures

397.0 Diseases of tricuspid valve
Tricuspid (valve) (rheumatic):   Tricuspid (valve) (rheumatic):
  disease   regurgitation
  insufficiency   stenosis
  obstruction

397.1 Rheumatic diseases of pulmonary valve
EXCLUDES that not specified as rheumatic (424.3)

◆ 397.9 Rheumatic diseases of endocardium, valve unspecified
Rheumatic:
  endocarditis (chronic)
  valvulitis (chronic)
EXCLUDES that not specified as rheumatic (424.90-424.99)

● 398 Other rheumatic heart disease

398.0 Rheumatic myocarditis
Rheumatic degeneration of myocardium
EXCLUDES myocarditis not specified as rheumatic (429.0)

● 398.9 Other and unspecified rheumatic heart diseases

◆ 398.90 Rheumatic heart disease, unspecified
Rheumatic:
  carditis
  heart disease NOS
EXCLUDES carditis not specified as rheumatic (429.89)
heart disease NOS not specified as rheumatic (429.9)

398.91 Rheumatic heart failure (congestive)
Rheumatic left ventricular failure

◆ 398.99 Other

HYPERTENSIVE DISEASE (401-405)

EXCLUDES that complicating pregnancy, childbirth, or the puerperium (642.0-642.9)
that involving coronary vessels (410.00-414.9)

● 401 Essential hypertension
INCLUDES high blood pressure
hyperpiesia
hyperpiesis
hypertension (arterial) (essential) (primary) (systemic)
hypertensive vascular:
  degeneration
  disease
EXCLUDES elevated blood pressure without diagnosis of hypertension (796.2)
pulmonary hypertension (416.0-416.9)
that involving vessels of:
  brain (430-438)
  eye (362.11)

401.0 Malignant
401.1 Benign
◆ 401.9 Unspecified

● 402 Hypertensive heart disease
INCLUDES hypertensive:
  cardiomegaly
  cardiopathy
  cardiovascular disease
  heart (disease) (failure)
any condition classifiable to 428, 429.0-429.3, 429.8, 429.9 due to hypertension

● 402.0 Malignant
402.00 Without congestive heart failure
402.01 With congestive heart failure

● 402.1 Benign
402.10 Without congestive heart failure
402.11 With congestive heart failure

● 402.9 Unspecified
◆ 402.90 Without congestive heart failure
◆ 402.91 With congestive heart failure

● 403 Hypertensive renal disease
The following fifth-digit subclassification is for use with category 403:
  0 without mention of renal failure
  1 with renal failure
INCLUDES arteriolar nephritis
arteriosclerosis of:
  kidney
  renal arterioles
arteriosclerotic nephritis (chronic) (interstitial)
hypertensive:
  nephropathy
  renal failure
  uremia (chronic)
nephrosclerosis
renal sclerosis with hypertension
any condition classifiable to 585, 586, or 587 with any condition classifiable to 401
EXCLUDES acute renal failure (584.5-584.9)
renal disease stated as not due to hypertension
renovascular hypertension (405.0-405.9 with fifth-digit 1)

● 403.0 Malignant
● 403.1 Benign
◆ ● 403.9 Unspecified

CIRCULATORY SYSTEM

- **404 Hypertensive heart and renal disease**
  The following fifth-digit subclassification is for use with category 404:
  - 0 without mention of congestive heart failure or renal failure
  - 1 with congestive heart failure
  - 2 with renal failure
  - 3 with congestive heart failure and renal failure

  INCLUDES disease:
  cardiorenal
  cardiovascular renal
  any condition classifiable to 402 with any condition classifiable to 403

  - **404.0** Malignant
  - **404.1** Benign
  - **404.9** Unspecified

- **405 Secondary hypertension**
  - **405.0** Malignant
    - 405.01 Renovascular
    - 405.09 Other
  - **405.1** Benign
    - 405.11 Renovascular
    - 405.19 Other
  - **405.9** Unspecified
    - 405.91 Renovascular
    - 405.99 Other

ISCHEMIC HEART DISEASE (410-414)

INCLUDES that with mention of hypertension
Use additional code, if desired, to identify presence of hypertension (401.0-405.9)

- **410 Acute myocardial infarction**
  The following fifth-digit subclassification is for use with category 410:
  - 0 episode of care unspecified
    Use when the source document does not contain sufficient information for the assignment of fifth digit 1 or 2.
  - 1 initial episode of care
    Use fifth-digit 1 to designate the first episode of care (regardless of facility site) for a newly diagnosed myocardial infarction. The fifth-digit 1 is assigned regardless of the number of times a patient may be transferred during the initial episode of care.
  - 2 subsequent episode of care
    Use fifth-digit 2 to designate an episode of care following the initial episode when the patient is admitted for further observation, evaluation or treatment for a myocardial infarction that has received initial treatment, but is still less than 8 weeks old.

  INCLUDES cardiac infarction
  coronary (artery):
  embolism
  occlusion
  rupture
  thrombosis
  infarction of heart, myocardium, or ventricle
  rupture of heart, myocardium, or ventricle
  any condition classifiable to 414.1-414.9 specified as acute or with a stated duration of 8 weeks or less

  - **410.0** Of anterolateral wall
  - **410.1** Of other anterior wall
    Infarction:
    anterior (wall) NOS
    anteroapical
    anteroseptal
    (with contiguous portion of intraventricular septum)
  - **410.2** Of inferolateral wall
  - **410.3** Of inferoposterior wall
  - **410.4** Of other inferior wall
    Infarction:
    diaphragmatic wall
    inferior (wall) NOS
    (with contiguous portion of intraventricular septum)
  - **410.5** Of other lateral wall
    Infarction:
    apical-lateral
    basal-lateral
    Infarction:
    high lateral
    posterolateral
  - **410.6** True posterior wall infarction
    Infarction:
    posterobasal
    Infarction:
    strictly posterior
  - **410.7** Subendocardial infarction
    Nontransmural infarction
  - **410.8** Of other specified sites
    Infarction of:
    atrium
    papillarymuscle
    septum alone
  - **410.9** Unspecified site
    Acute myocardial infarction NOS
    Coronary occlusion NOS

- **411 Other acute and subacute forms of ischemic heart disease**
  - **411.0** Postmyocardial infarction syndrome
    Dressler's syndrome
  - **411.1** Intermediate coronary syndrome
    Impending infarction   Preinfarction syndrome
    Preinfarction angina   Unstable angina
    EXCLUDES angina (pectoris) (413.9)
    decubitus (413.0)
  - **411.8** Other
    - **411.81** Coronary occlusion without myocardial infarction
      Coronary (artery):
      embolism
      occlusion
      thrombosis
      } without or not resulting in myocardial infarction
    - **411.89** Other
      Coronary insufficiency (acute)
      Subendocardial ischemia

- **412 Old myocardial infarction**
  Healed myocardial infarction
  Past myocardial infarction diagnosed on ECG [EKG] or other special investigation, but currently presenting no symptoms

- **413 Angina pectoris**
  - **413.0** Angina decubitus
    Nocturnal angina
  - **413.1** Prinzmetal angina
    Variant angina pectoris
  - **413.9** Other and unspecified angina pectoris
    Angina:
    NOS
    cardiac
    of effort
    Anginal syndrome
    Status anginosus
    Stenocardia
    Syncope anginosa
    EXCLUDES preinfarction angina (411.1)

- **414 Other forms of chronic ischemic heart disease**
  EXCLUDES arteriosclerotic cardiovascular disease [ASCVD] (429.2)
  cardiovascular:
  arteriosclerosis or sclerosis (429.2)
  degeneration or disease (429.2)
  - **414.0** Coronary atherosclerosis
    Arteriosclerotic heart disease [ASHD]
    Atherosclerotic heart disease
    Coronary (artery):
    arteriosclerosis
    arteritis or endarteritis
    atheroma
    sclerosis
    stricture
    EXCLUDES embolism of graft (996.72) ▼
    occlusion NOS
    thrombus
    - **414.00** Of unspecified vessel
    - **414.01** Of native coronary artery
    - **414.02** Of autologous vein bypass graft
    - **414.03** Of nonautologous biological bypass graft ▲
  - **414.1** Aneurysm of heart
    - **414.10** Of heart (wall)
      Aneurysm (arteriovenous):
      mural
      ventricular
    - **414.11** Of coronary vessels
      Aneurysm (arteriovenous) of coronary vessels

● Additional digits required   ◆ Nonspecific code   ■ Not a primary diagnosis

- ◆ **414.19 Other**
  Arteriovenous fistula, acquired, of heart
- ◆ **414.8 Other specified forms of chronic ischemic heart disease**
  Chronic coronary insufficiency
  Ischemia, myocardial (chronic)
  Any condition classifiable to 410 specified as chronic, or presenting with symptoms after 8 weeks from date of infarction
  EXCLUDES *coronary insufficiency (acute) (411.89)*
- ◆ **414.9 Chronic ischemic heart disease, unspecified**
  Ischemic heart disease NOS

DISEASES OF PULMONARY CIRCULATION (415-417)

● **415 Acute pulmonary heart disease**
- **415.0 Acute cor pulmonale**
  EXCLUDES *cor pulmonale NOS (416.9)*
- **415.1 Pulmonary embolism and infarction**
  Pulmonary (artery) (vein):
    apoplexy
    embolism
    infarction (hemorrhagic)
    thrombosis
  EXCLUDES *that complicating:*
    abortion (634-638 with .6, 639.6)
    ectopic or molar pregnancy (639.6)
    pregnancy, childbirth, or the puerperium (673.0-673.8)

● **416 Chronic pulmonary heart disease**
- **416.0 Primary pulmonary hypertension**
  Idiopathic pulmonary arteriosclerosis
  Pulmonary hypertension (essential) (idiopathic) (primary)
- **416.1 Kyphoscoliotic heart disease**
- ◆ **416.8 Other chronic pulmonary heart diseases**
  Pulmonary hypertension, secondary
- ◆ **416.9 Chronic pulmonary heart disease, unspecified**
  Chronic cardiopulmonary disease
  Cor pulmonale (chronic) NOS

● **417 Other diseases of pulmonary circulation**
- **417.0 Arteriovenous fistula of pulmonary vessels**
  EXCLUDES *congenital arteriovenous fistula (747.3)*
- **417.1 Aneurysm of pulmonary artery**
  EXCLUDES *congenital aneurysm (747.3)*
- ◆ **417.8 Other specified diseases of pulmonary circulation**
  Pulmonary:
    arteritis
    endarteritis
  Rupture } of pulmonary vessel
  Stricture
- ◆ **417.9 Unspecified disease of pulmonary circulation**

OTHER FORMS OF HEART DISEASE (420-429)

● **420 Acute pericarditis**
  INCLUDES acute:
    mediastinopericarditis
    myopericarditis
    pericardial effusion
    pleuropericarditis
    pneumopericarditis
  EXCLUDES *acute rheumatic pericarditis (391.0)*
    postmyocardial infarction syndrome [Dressler's] (411.0)
- ◆ **420.0 Acute pericarditis in diseases classified elsewhere**
  Code also underlying disease, as:
    actinomycosis (039.8)
    amebiasis (006.8)
    nocardiosis (039.8)
    tuberculosis (017.9)
    uremia (585)
  EXCLUDES *pericarditis (acute) (in):*
    Coxsackie (virus) (074.21)
    gonococcal (098.83)
    histoplasmosis (115.0-115.9 with fifth-digit 3)
    meningococcal infection (036.41)
    syphilitic (093.81)

● **420.9 Other and unspecified acute pericarditis**
- ◆ **420.90 Acute pericarditis, unspecified**
  Pericarditis (acute):
    NOS
    infective NOS
    sicca
- **420.91 Acute idiopathic pericarditis**
  Pericarditis, acute: Pericarditis, acute:
    benign   viral
    nonspecific
- ◆ **420.99 Other**
  Pericarditis (acute):
    pneumococcal
    purulent
    staphylococcal
    streptococcal
    suppurative
  Pneumopyopericardium
  Pyopericardium
  EXCLUDES *pericarditis in diseases classified elsewhere (420.0)*

● **421 Acute and subacute endocarditis**
- **421.0 Acute and subacute bacterial endocarditis**
  Endocarditis (acute) (chronic) (subacute):
    bacterial
    infective NOS
    lenta
    malignant
    purulent
    septic
    ulcerative
    vegetative
  Infective aneurysm
  Subacute bacterial endocarditis [SBE]
  Use additional code, if desired, to identify infectious organism [e.g., Streptococcus 041.0, Staphylococcus 041.1]
- ◆ **421.1 *Acute and subacute infective endocarditis in diseases classified elsewhere***
  Code also underlying disease, as:
    blastomycosis (116.0)
    Q fever (083.0)
    typhoid (fever) (002.0)
  EXCLUDES *endocarditis (in):*
    Coxsackie (virus) (074.22)
    gonococcal (098.84)
    histoplasmosis (115.0-115.9 with fifth-digit 4)
    meningococcal infection (036.42)
    monilial (112.81)
- ◆ **421.9 Acute endocarditis, unspecified**
  Endocarditis
  Myoendocarditis } acute or subacute
  Periendocarditis
  EXCLUDES *acute rheumatic endocarditis (391.1)*

● **422 Acute myocarditis**
  EXCLUDES *acute rheumatic myocarditis (391.2)*
- ◆ **422.0 *Acute myocarditis in diseases classified elsewhere***
  Code also underlying disease, as:
    myocarditis (acute):
      influenzal (487.8)
      tuberculous (017.9)
  EXCLUDES *myocarditis (acute) (due to):*
    aseptic, of newborn (074.23)
    Coxsackie (virus) (074.23)
    diphtheritic (032.82)
    meningococcal infection (036.43)
    syphilitic (093.82)
    toxoplasmosis (130.3)
● **422.9 Other and unspecified acute myocarditis**
- ◆ **422.90 Acute myocarditis, unspecified**
  Acute or subacute (interstitial) myocarditis
- **422.91 Idiopathic myocarditis**
  Myocarditis (acute or subacute):
    Fiedler's
    giant cell
    isolated (diffuse) (granulomatous)
    nonspecific granulomatous

CIRCULATORY SYSTEM

422.92 Septic myocarditis
Myocarditis, acute or subacute:
- pneumococcal
- staphylococcal

Use additional code, if desired, to identify infectious organism [e.g., Staphylococcus 041.1]

EXCLUDES myocarditis, acute or subacute:
- in bacterial diseases classified elsewhere (422.0)
- streptococcal (391.2)

422.93 Toxic myocarditis
422.99 Other

423 Other diseases of pericardium
EXCLUDES that specified as rheumatic (393)

423.0 Hemopericardium
423.1 Adhesive pericarditis
- Adherent pericardium
- Fibrosis of pericardium
- Milk spots
- Pericarditis:
  - adhesive
  - obliterative
- Soldiers' patches

423.2 Constrictive pericarditis
- Concato's disease
- Pick's disease of heart (and liver)

423.8 Other specified diseases of pericardium
- Calcification of pericardium
- Fistula of pericardium

423.9 Unspecified disease of pericardium

424 Other diseases of endocardium
EXCLUDES
- bacterial endocarditis (421.0-421.9)
- rheumatic endocarditis (391.1, 394.0-397.9)
- syphilitic endocarditis (093.20-093.24)

424.0 Mitral valve disorders
Mitral (valve):
- incompetence
- insufficiency
- regurgitation

NOS of specified cause, except rheumatic

EXCLUDES mitral (valve):
- disease (394.9)
- failure (394.9)
- stenosis (394.0)
- the listed conditions:
  - specified as rheumatic (394.1)
  - unspecified as to cause but with mention of:
    - diseases of aortic valve (396.0-396.9)
    - mitral stenosis or obstruction (394.2)

424.1 Aortic valve disorders
Aortic (valve):
- incompetence
- insufficiency
- regurgitation
- stenosis

NOS of specified cause, except rheumatic

EXCLUDES
- hypertrophic subaortic stenosis (425.1)
- that specified as rheumatic (395.0-395.9)
- that of unspecified cause but with mention of diseases of mitral valve (396.0-396.9)

424.2 Tricuspid valve disorders, specified as nonrheumatic
Tricuspid valve:
- incompetence
- insufficiency
- regurgitation
- stenosis

of specified cause, except rheumatic

EXCLUDES rheumatic or of unspecified cause (397.0)

424.3 Pulmonary valve disorders
Pulmonic:
- incompetence NOS
- insufficiency NOS
Pulmonic:
- regurgitation NOS
- stenosis NOS

EXCLUDES that specified as rheumatic (397.1)

424.9 Endocarditis, valve unspecified

424.90 Endocarditis, valve unspecified, unspecified cause
Endocarditis (chronic):
- NOS
- nonbacterial thrombotic

Valvular:
- incompetence
- insufficiency
- regurgitation
- stenosis

of unspecified valve, unspecified cause

Valvulitis (chronic)

424.91 Endocarditis in diseases classified elsewhere
Code also underlying disease as:
- atypical verrucous endocarditis [Libman-Sacks] (710.0)
- disseminated lupus erythematosus (710.0)
- tuberculosis (017.9)

EXCLUDES syphilitic (093.20-093.24)

424.99 Other
Any condition classifiable to 424.90 with specified cause, except rheumatic

EXCLUDES
- endocardial fibroelastosis (425.3)
- that specified as rheumatic (397.9)

425 Cardiomyopathy
INCLUDES myocardiopathy

EXCLUDES cardiomyopathy arising during pregnancy or the puerperium (674.8)

425.0 Endomyocardial fibrosis
425.1 Hypertrophic obstructive cardiomyopathy
Hypertrophic subaortic stenosis (idiopathic)

425.2 Obscure cardiomyopathy of Africa
- Becker's disease
- Idiopathic mural endomyocardial disease

425.3 Endocardial fibroelastosis
Elastomyofibrosis

425.4 Other primary cardiomyopathies
Cardiomyopathy:
- NOS
- congestive
- constrictive
- familial
- hypertrophic

Cardiomyopathy:
- idiopathic
- nonobstructive
- obstructive
- restrictive
- Cardiovascular collagenosis

425.5 Alcoholic cardiomyopathy
425.7 Nutritional and metabolic cardiomyopathy
Code also underlying disease, as:
- amyloidosis (277.3)
- beriberi (265.0)
- cardiac glycogenosis (271.0)
- mucopolysaccharidosis (277.5)
- thyrotoxicosis (242.0-242.9)

EXCLUDES gouty tophi of heart (274.82)

425.8 Cardiomyopathy in other diseases classified elsewhere
Code also underlying disease, as:
- Friedreich's ataxia (334.0)
- myotonia atrophica (359.2)
- progressive muscular dystrophy (359.1)
- sarcoidosis (135)

EXCLUDES cardiomyopathy in Chagas' disease (086.0)

425.9 Secondary cardiomyopathy, unspecified

426 Conduction disorders
426.0 Atrioventricular block, complete
Third degree atrioventricular block

426.1 Atrioventricular block, other and unspecified
426.10 Atrioventricular block, unspecified
Atrioventricular [AV] block (incomplete) (partial)

426.11 First degree atrioventricular block
- Incomplete atrioventricular block, first degree
- Prolonged P-R interval NOS

426.12 Mobitz (type) II atrioventricular block
Incomplete atrioventricular block:
- Mobitz (type) II
- second degree, Mobitz (type) II

426.13 Other second degree atrioventricular block
Incomplete atrioventricular block:
- Mobitz (type) I [Wenckebach's]
- second degree:
  - NOS
  - Mobitz (type) I
  - with 2:1 atrioventricular response [block]
- Wenckebach's phenomenon

426.2 Left bundle branch hemiblock
Block:
- left anterior fascicular
- left posterior fascicular

426.3 Other left bundle branch block
Left bundle branch block:
- NOS
- anterior fascicular with posterior fascicular
- complete
- main stem

426.4 Right bundle branch block

426.5 Bundle branch block, other and unspecified

426.50 Bundle branch block, unspecified
426.51 Right bundle branch block and left posterior fascicular block
426.52 Right bundle branch block and left anterior fascicular block
426.53 Other bilateral bundle branch block
Bifascicular block NOS
Bilateral bundle branch block NOS
Right bundle branch with left bundle branch block (incomplete) (main stem)
426.54 Trifascicular block

426.6 Other heart block
Intraventricular block:
- NOS
- diffuse
- myofibrillar

Sinoatrial block
Sinoauricular block

426.7 Anomalous atrioventricular excitation
Atrioventricular conduction:
- accelerated
- accessory
- pre-excitation

Ventricular pre-excitation
Wolff-Parkinson-White syndrome

426.8 Other specified conduction disorders
426.81 Lown-Ganong-Levine syndrome
Syndrome of short P-R interval, normal QRS complexes, and supraventricular tachycardias
426.89 Other
Dissociation:
- atrioventricular [AV]
- interference
- isorhythmic

Nonparoxysmal AV nodal tachycardia

426.9 Conduction disorder, unspecified
Heart block NOS
Stokes-Adams syndrome

427 Cardiac dysrhythmias
EXCLUDES that complicating:
- abortion (634-638 with .7, 639.8)
- ectopic or molar pregnancy (639.8)
- labor or delivery (668.1, 669.4)

427.0 Paroxysmal supraventricular tachycardia
Paroxysmal tachycardia:
- atrial [PAT]
- atrioventricular [AV]

Paroxysmal tachycardia:
- nodaljunctional

427.1 Paroxysmal ventricular tachycardia
Ventricular tachycardia (paroxysmal)

427.2 Paroxysmal tachycardia, unspecified
Bouveret-Hoffmann syndrome
Paroxysmal tachycardia:
- NOS
- essential

427.3 Atrial fibrillation and flutter
427.31 Atrial fibrillation
427.32 Atrial flutter

427.4 Ventricular fibrillation and flutter
427.41 Ventricular fibrillation
427.42 Ventricular flutter

427.5 Cardiac arrest
Cardiorespiratory arrest

427.6 Premature beats
427.60 Premature beats, unspecified
Ectopic beats
Extrasystoles
Extrasystolic arrhythmia
Premature contractions or systoles NOS

427.61 Supraventricular premature beats
Atrial premature beats, contractions, or systoles

427.69 Other
Ventricular premature beats, contractions, or systoles

427.8 Other specified cardiac dysrhythmias
427.81 Sinoatrial node dysfunction
Sinus bradycardia:
- persistent
- severe

Syndrome:
- sick sinus
- tachycardia-bradycardia

EXCLUDES sinus bradycardia NOS (427.89)

427.89 Other
Rhythm disorder:
- coronary sinus
- ectopic
- nodal

Wandering (atrial) pacemaker

EXCLUDES
- carotid sinus syncope (337.0)
- reflex bradycardia (337.0)
- tachycardia NOS (785.0)

427.9 Cardiac dysrhythmia, unspecified
Arrhythmia (cardiac) NOS

428 Heart failure
EXCLUDES
- following cardiac surgery (429.4)
- rheumatic (398.91)
- that complicating:
  - abortion (634-638 with .7, 639.8)
  - ectopic or molar pregnancy (639.8)
  - labor or delivery (668.1, 669.4)
- that due to hypertension (402.0-402.9 with fifth-digit 1)

428.0 Congestive heart failure
Congestive heart disease
Right heart failure (secondary to left heart failure)

428.1 Left heart failure
Acute edema of lung
Acute pulmonary edema
} with heart disease NOS or heart failure

Cardiac asthma
Left ventricular failure

428.9 Heart failure, unspecified
Cardiac failure NOS
Heart failure NOS
Myocardial failure NOS
Weak heart

429 Ill-defined descriptions and complications of heart disease

429.0 Myocarditis, unspecified
Myocarditis:
- NOS
- chronic (interstitial)
- fibroid
- senile
} (with mention of arteriosclerosis)

Use additional code, if desired, to identify presence of arteriosclerosis

EXCLUDES
- acute or subacute (422.0-422.9)
- rheumatic (398.0)
- acute (391.2)
- that due to hypertension (402.0-402.9)

429.1 Myocardial degeneration
Degeneration of heart or myocardium:
- fatty
- mural
- muscular

Myocardial:
- degeneration
- disease
} (with mention of arteriosclerosis)

Use additional code, if desired, to identify presence of arteriosclerosis

EXCLUDES that due to hypertension (402.0-402.9)

CIRCULATORY SYSTEM

◆ **429.2 Cardiovascular disease, unspecified**
  Arteriosclerotic cardiovascular disease [ASCVD]
  Cardiovascular arteriosclerosis
  Cardiovascular:
    degeneration ⎫
    disease   ⎬ (with mention of arte-
    sclerosis   ⎭   riosclerosis)
  Use additional code, if desired, to identify presence of arteriosclerosis
  EXCLUDES *that due to hypertension (402.0-402.9)*

429.3 Cardiomegaly
  Cardiac:
    dilatation
    hypertrophy
  Ventricular dilatation
  EXCLUDES *that due to hypertension (402.0-402.9)*

429.4 Functional disturbances following cardiac surgery
  Cardiac insuffi- ⎫ following cardiac
    ciency   ⎬   surgery or due
  Heart failure   ⎭   to prosthesis
  Postcardiotomy syndrome
  Postvalvulotomy syndrome
  EXCLUDES *cardiac failure in the immediate postoperative period (997.1)*

429.5 Rupture of chordae tendineae
429.6 Rupture of papillary muscle
● **429.7 Certain sequelae of myocardial infarction, not elsewhere classified**
  Use additional code to identify the associated myocardial infarction:
  with onset of 8 weeks or less (410.00-410.92)
  with onset of more than 8 weeks (414.8)
  EXCLUDES *congenital defects of heart (745, 746)*
    coronary aneurysm (414.11)
    disorders of papillary muscle (429.6, 429.81)
    postmyocardial infarction syndrome (411.0)
    rupture of chordae tendineae (429.5)

  429.71 Acquired cardiac septal defect
    EXCLUDES *acute septal infarction (410.00-410.92)*

  ◆ **429.79 Other**
    Mural thrombus (atrial) (ventricular), acquired, following myocardial infarction

● **429.8 Other ill-defined heart diseases**
  ◆ **429.81 Other disorders of papillary muscle**
    Papillary muscle:
      atrophy
      degeneration
      dysfunction
      incompetence
      incoordination
      scarring
  429.82 Hyperkinetic heart disease
  ◆ **429.89 Other**
    Carditis
    EXCLUDES *that due to hypertension (402.0-402.9)*

◆ **429.9 Heart disease, unspecified**
  Heart disease (organic) NOS
  Morbus cordis NOS
  EXCLUDES *that due to hypertension (402.0-402.9)*

CEREBROVASCULAR DISEASE (430-438)

INCLUDES with mention of hypertension (conditions classifiable to 401-405)
Use additional code, if desired, to identify presence of hypertension
EXCLUDES *any condition classifiable to 430-434, 436, 437 occurring during pregnancy, childbirth, or the puerperium, or specified as puerperal (674.0)*

430 Subarachnoid hemorrhage
  Meningeal hemorrhage
  Ruptured:
    berry aneurysm
    (congenital) cerebral aneurysm NOS
  EXCLUDES *syphilitic ruptured cerebral aneurysm (094.87)*

431 Intracerebral hemorrhage
  Hemorrhage (of):   Hemorrhage (of):
    basilar   internal capsule
    bulbar   intrapontine
    cerebellar   pontine
    cerebral   subcortical
    cerebromeningeal   ventricular
    cortical
  Rupture of blood vessel in brain

● **432 Other and unspecified intracranial hemorrhage**
  432.0 Nontraumatic extradural hemorrhage
    Nontraumatic epidural hemorrhage
  432.1 Subdural hemorrhage
    Subdural hematoma, nontraumatic
  ◆ **432.9 Unspecified intracranial hemorrhage**
    Intracranial hemorrhage NOS

● **433 Occlusion and stenosis of precerebral arteries**
  The following fifth-digit subclassification is for use with category 433:
    0 without mention of cerebral infarction
    1 with cerebral infarction
  INCLUDES embolism   ⎫
                narrowing ⎬ of basilar, carotid, and
                obstruction ⎬ vertebral arteries
                thrombosis ⎭
  EXCLUDES *insufficiency NOS of precerebral arteries (435.0-435.9)*

  ● **433.0 Basilar artery**
  ● **433.1 Carotid artery**
  ● **433.2 Vertebral artery**
  ● **433.3 Multiple and bilateral**
  ◆● **433.8 Other specified precerebral artery**
  ◆● **433.9 Unspecified precerebral artery**
    Precerebral artery NOS

● **434 Occlusion of cerebral arteries**
  The following fifth-digit subclassification is for use with category 434:
    0 without mention of cerebral infarction
    1 with cerebral infarction
  ● **434.0 Cerebral thrombosis**
    Thrombosis of cerebral arteries
  ● **434.1 Cerebral embolism**
  ◆● **434.9 Cerebral artery occlusion, unspecified**

● **435 Transient cerebral ischemia**
  INCLUDES cerebrovascular insufficiency (acute) with transient focal neurological signs and symptoms
    insufficiency of basilar, carotid, and vertebral arteries
    spasm of cerebral arteries
  EXCLUDES *acute cerebrovascular insufficiency NOS (437.1)*
    that due to any condition classifiable to 433 (433.0-433.9)
  435.0 Basilar artery syndrome
  435.1 Vertebral artery syndrome
  435.2 Subclavian steal syndrome
  ◆ **435.8 Other specified transient cerebral ischemias**
  ◆ **435.9 Unspecified transient cerebral ischemia**
    Impending cerebrovascular accident
    Intermittent cerebral ischemia
    Transient ischemic attack [TIA]

436 Acute, but ill-defined, cerebrovascular disease
  Apoplexy, apoplectic: Cerebral seizure
    NOS   Cerebrovascular accident
    attack   [CVA] NOS
    cerebral   Stroke
    seizure
  EXCLUDES *any condition classifiable to categories 430-435*

● **437 Other and ill-defined cerebrovascular disease**
  437.0 Cerebral atherosclerosis
    Atheroma of cerebral arteries
    Cerebral arteriosclerosis
  ◆ **437.1 Other generalized ischemic cerebrovascular disease**
    Acute cerebrovascular insufficiency NOS
    Cerebral ischemia (chronic)
  437.2 Hypertensive encephalopathy
  437.3 Cerebral aneurysm, nonruptured
  437.4 Cerebral arteritis
  437.5 Moyamoya disease
  437.6 Nonpyogenic thrombosis of intracranial venous sinus
    EXCLUDES *pyogenic (325)*

	437.7	Transient global amnesia
◆	437.8	Other
◆	437.9	Unspecified
		Cerebrovascular disease or lesion NOS

438 Late effects of cerebrovascular disease
   Note: This category is to be used to indicate conditions in 430-437 as the cause of late effects, themselves classifiable elsewhere. The "late effects" include conditions specified as such, as sequelae, which may occur at any time after the onset of the causal condition.
   Code also sequelae:
      aphasia (784.3)
      dysphasia (784.5)
      hemiplegia (342.0-342.9)
      paralysis (344.0-344.9)

DISEASES OF ARTERIES, ARTERIOLES, AND CAPILLARIES (440-448)

● 440 Atherosclerosis
   INCLUDES arteriolosclerosis
      arteriosclerosis (obliterans) (senile)
      arteriosclerotic vascular disease
      atheroma
      degeneration:
         arterial
         arteriovascular
         vascular
      endarteritis deformans or obliterans
      senile:
         arteritis
         endarteritis
   440.0 Of aorta
   440.1 Of renal artery
      EXCLUDES atherosclerosis of renal arterioles (403.00-403.91)
   ● 440.2 Of native arteries of the extremities ▼
      EXCLUDES atherosclerosis of bypass graft of the extremities (440.30-440.32) ▲
      ◆ 440.20 Atherosclerosis of the extremities, unspecified
      440.21 Atherosclerosis of the extremities with intermittent claudication
      440.22 Atherosclerosis of the extremities with rest pain
         Includes any condition classifiable to 440.21 ◆
      440.23 Atherosclerosis of the extremities with ulceration
         Includes any condition classifiable to 440.21 and 440.22 ◆
      440.24 Atherosclerosis of the extremities with gangrene
         Includes any condition classifiable to 440.21, 440.22, and 440.23
      ◆ 440.29 Other
   ● 440.3 Of bypass graft of extremities ▼
      EXCLUDES atherosclerosis of native arteries of the extremities (440.21-440.24)
         embolism [occlusion NOS] [thrombus] of graft (996.74)
      ◆ 440.30 Of unspecified graft
      440.31 Of autologous vein bypass graft
      440.32 Of nonautologous biological bypass graft ▲
   ◆ 440.8 Of other specified arteries
      EXCLUDES basilar (433.0)
         carotid (433.1)
         cerebral (437.0)
         coronary (414.0)
         mesenteric (557.1)
         precerebral (433.0-433.9)
         pulmonary (416.0)
         vertebral (433.2)
   ◆ 440.9 Generalized and unspecified atherosclerosis
      Arteriosclerotic vascular disease NOS
      EXCLUDES arteriosclerotic cardiovascular disease [ASCVD] (429.2)

● 441 Aortic aneurysm
   EXCLUDES syphilitic aortic aneurysm (093.0)
      traumatic aortic aneurysm (901.0, 902.0)
   ● 441.0 Dissecting aneurysm [any part] ▼
      ◆ 441.00 Unspecified site
      441.01 Thoracic ▲

   441.02 Abdominal ▼
   441.03 Thoracoabdominal ▲
   441.1 Thoracic aneurysm, ruptured
   441.2 Thoracic aneurysm without mention of rupture
   441.3 Abdominal aneurysm, ruptured
   441.4 Abdominal aneurysm without mention of rupture
   ◆ 441.5 Aortic aneurysm of unspecified site, ruptured
      Rupture of aorta NOS
   441.6 Thoracoabdominal aneurysm, ruptured
   441.7 Thoracoabdominal aneurysm, without mention of rupture
   ◆ 441.9 Aortic aneurysm of unspecified site without mention of rupture
      Aneurysm
      Dilatation   } of aorta
      Hyaline necrosis

● 442 Other aneurysm
   INCLUDES aneurysm (ruptured) (cirsoid) (false) (varicose)
      aneurysmal varix
   EXCLUDES arteriovenous aneurysm or fistula:
      acquired (447.0)
      congenital (747.6)
      traumatic (900.0-904.9)
   442.0 Of artery of upper extremity
   442.1 Of renal artery
   442.2 Of iliac artery
   442.3 Of artery of lower extremity
      Aneurysm:
         femoral
         popliteal   } artery
   ● 442.8 Of other specified artery
      442.81 Artery of neck
         Aneurysm of carotid artery (common) (external) (internal)
      442.82 Subclavian artery
      442.83 Splenic artery
      ◆ 442.84 Other visceral artery
         Aneurysm:
            celiac
            gastroduodenal
            gastroepiploic   } artery
            hepatic
            pancreaticoduodenal
            superior mesenteric
      ◆ 442.89 Other
         Aneurysm:
            mediastinal } artery
            spinal
         EXCLUDES cerebral (nonruptured) (437.3)
            ruptured (430)
            coronary (414.11)
            heart (414.10)
            pulmonary (417.1)
   ◆ 442.9 Of unspecified site
● 443 Other peripheral vascular disease
   443.0 Raynaud's syndrome
      Raynaud's:
         disease
         phenomenon (secondary)
      Use additional code, if desired, to identify gangrene (785.4)
   443.1 Thromboangiitis obliterans [Buerger's disease]
      Presenile gangrene
   ● 443.8 Other specified peripheral vascular diseases
      ◆ 443.81 Peripheral angiopathy in diseases classified elsewhere
         Code also underlying disease, as:
            diabetes mellitus (250.7)
      ◆ 443.89 Other
         Acrocyanosis   Erythrocyanosis
         Acroparesthesia: Erythromelalgia
            simple [Schultze's type]
            vasomotor [Nothnagel's type]
         EXCLUDES chilblains (991.5)
            frostbite (991.0-991.3)
            immersion foot (991.4)

CIRCULATORY SYSTEM

- ◆ **443.9 Peripheral vascular disease, unspecified**
  Intermittent claudication NOS
  Peripheral:
   angiopathy NOS
   vascular disease NOS
  Spasm of artery
  EXCLUDES Atherosclerosis of the arteries of the extremities (440.20-440.22)
   spasm of cerebral artery (435.0-435.9)

● **444 Arterial embolism and thrombosis**
  INCLUDES infarction:
   embolic
   thrombotic
   occlusion
  EXCLUDES that complicating:
   abortion (634-638 with .6, 639.6)
   ectopic or molar pregnancy (639.6)
   pregnancy, childbirth, or the pueperium (673.0-673.8)

- **444.0 Of abdominal aorta**
  Aortic bifurcation syndrome
  Aortoiliacobstruction
  Leriche's syndrome
  Saddle embolus
- **444.1 Of thoracic aorta**
  Embolism or thrombosis of aorta (thoracic)
● **444.2 Of arteries of the extremities**
  - **444.21 Upper extremity**
  - **444.22 Lower extremity**
    Arterial embolism or thrombosis:
     femoral
     peripheral NOS
     popliteal
    EXCLUDES iliofemoral (444.81)
● **444.8 Of other specified artery**
  - **444.81 Iliac artery**
  - ◆ **444.89 Other**
    EXCLUDES basilar (433.0)
     carotid (433.1)
     cerebral (434.0-434.9)
     coronary (410.00-410.92)
     mesenteric (557.0)
     ophthalmic (362.30-362.34)
     precerebral (433.0-433.9)
     pulmonary (415.1)
     renal (593.81)
     retinal (362.30-362.34)
     vertebral (433.2)
- ◆ **444.9 Of unspecified artery**

● **446 Polyarteritis nodosa and allied conditions**
- **446.0 Polyarteritis nodosa**
  Disseminated necrotizing periarteritis
  Necrotizing angiitis
  Panarteritis (nodosa)
  Periarteritis (nodosa)
- **446.1 Acute febrile mucocutaneous lymph node syndrome [MCLS]**
  Kawasaki disease
● **446.2 Hypersensitivity angiitis**
  EXCLUDES antiglomerular basement membrane disease without pulmonary hemorrhage (583.89)
  - ◆ **446.20 Hypersensitivity angiitis, unspecified**
  - **446.21 Goodpasture's syndrome**
    Antiglomerular basement membrane antibody-mediatednephritis with pulmonary hemorrhage
    Use additional code, if desired, to identify renal disease (583.81)
  - ◆ **446.29 Other specified hypersensitivity angiitis**
- **446.3 Lethal midline granuloma**
  Malignant granuloma of face
- **446.4 Wegener's granulomatosis**
  Necrotizing respiratory granulomatosis
  Wegener's syndrome
- **446.5 Giant cell arteritis**
  Cranial arteritis   Temporal arteritis
  Horton's disease

- **446.6 Thrombotic microangiopathy**
  Moschcowitz's syndrome
  Thrombotic thrombocytopenic purpura
- **446.7 Takayasu's disease**
  Aortic arch arteritis   Pulseless disease

● **447 Other disorders of arteries and arterioles**
- **447.0 Arteriovenous fistula, acquired**
  Arteriovenous aneurysm, acquired
  EXCLUDES cerebrovascular (437.3)
   coronary (414.19)
   pulmonary (417.0)
   surgically created arteriovenous shunt or fistula:
    complication (996.1, 996.61-996.62)
    status or presence (V45.1)
   traumatic (900.0-904.9)
- **447.1 Stricture of artery**
- **447.2 Rupture of artery**
  Erosion
  Fistula, except arteriovenous } of artery
  Ulcer
  EXCLUDES traumatic rupture of artery (900.0-904.9)
- **447.3 Hyperplasia of renal artery**
  Fibromuscular hyperplasia of renal artery
- **447.4 Celiac artery compression syndrome**
  Celiac axis syndrome   Marable's syndrome
- **447.5 Necrosis of artery**
- ◆ **447.6 Arteritis, unspecified**
  Aortitis NOS
  Endarteritis NOS
  EXCLUDES arteritis, endarteritis:
   aortic arch (446.7)
   cerebral (437.4)
   coronary (414.0)
   deformans (440.0-440.9)
   obliterans (440.0-440.9)
   pulmonary (417.8)
   senile (440.0-440.9)
  polyarteritis NOS (446.0)
  syphilitic aortitis (093.1)
- ◆ **447.8 Other specified disorders of arteries and arterioles**
  Fibromuscular hyperplasia of arteries, except renal
- ◆ **447.9 Unspecified disorders of arteries and arterioles**

● **448 Disease of capillaries**
- **448.0 Hereditary hemorrhagic telangiectasia**
  Rendu-Osler-Weber disease
- **448.1 Nevus, non-neoplastic**
  Nevus: Nevus:
   araneus   spider
   senile   stellar
  EXCLUDES neoplastic (216.0-216.9)
   port wine (757.32)
   strawberry (757.32)
- ◆ **448.9 Other and unspecified capillary diseases**
  Capillary:
   hemorrhage
   hyperpermeability
   thrombosis
  EXCLUDES capillary fragility (hereditary) (287.8)

DISEASES OF VEINS AND LYMPHATICS, AND OTHER DISEASES OF CIRCULATORY SYSTEM (451-459)

● **451 Phlebitis and thrombophlebitis**
  INCLUDES endophlebitis
   inflammation, vein
   periphlebitis
   suppurative phlebitis
  Use additional E code, if desired, to identify drug, if drug-induced
  EXCLUDES that complicating:
   abortion (634-638 with .7, 639.8)
   ectopic or molar pregnancy (639.8)
   pregnancy, childbirth, or the puerperium (671.0-671.9)
  that due to or following:
   implant or catheter device (996.61-996.62)
   infusion, perfusion, or transfusion (999.2)

451.0 Of superficial vessels of lower extremities
Saphenous vein (greater) (lesser)
● 451.1 Of deep vessels of lower extremities
451.11 Femoral vein (deep) (superficial)
◆ 451.19 Other
Femoropopliteal vein
Popliteal vein
Tibial vein
◆ 451.2 Of lower extremities, unspecified
● 451.8 Of other sites
EXCLUDES intracranial venous sinus (325)
nonpyogenic (437.6)
portal (vein) (572.1)
451.81 Iliac vein
451.82 Of superficial veins of upper extremities
Antecubital vein
Basilic vein
Cephalic vein
451.83 Of deep veins of upper extremities
Brachial vein
Radial vein
Ulnar vein
◆ 451.84 Of upper extremities, unspecified
◆ 451.89 Other
Axillary vein
Jugular vein
Subclavian vein
Thrombophlebitis of breast (Mondor's disease)
◆ 451.9 Of unspecified site
452 Portal vein thrombosis
Portal (vein) obstruction
EXCLUDES hepatic vein thrombosis (453.0)
phlebitis of portal vein (572.1)
● 453 Other venous embolism and thrombosis
EXCLUDES that complicating:
abortion (634-638 with .7, 639.8)
ectopic or molar pregnancy (639.8)
pregnancy, childbirth, or the puerperium (671.0-671.9)
that with inflammation, phlebitis, and thrombophlebitis (451.0-451.9)
453.0 Budd-Chiari syndrome
Hepatic vein thrombosis
453.1 Thrombophlebitis migrans
453.2 Of vena cava
453.3 Of renal vein
◆ 453.8 Of other specified veins
EXCLUDES cerebral (434.0-434.9)
coronary (410.00-410.92)
intracranial venous sinus (325)
nonpyogenic (437.6)
mesenteric (557.0)
portal (452)
precerebral (433.0-433.9)
pulmonary (415.1)
◆ 453.9 Of unspecified site
Embolism of vein
Thrombosis (vein)
● 454 Varicose veins of lower extremities
EXCLUDES that complicating pregnancy, childbirth, or the puerperium (671.0)
454.0 With ulcer
Varicose ulcer (lower extremity, any part)
Varicose veins with ulcer of lower extremity [any part] or of unspecified site
Any condition classifiable to 454.9 with ulcer or specified as ulcerated
454.1 With inflammation
Stasis dermatitis
Varicose veins with inflammation of lower extremity [any part] or of unspecified site
Any condition classifiable to 454.9 with inflammation or specified as inflamed
454.2 With ulcer and inflammation
Varicose veins with ulcer and inflammation of lower extremity [any part] or of unspecified site
Any condition classifiable to 454.9 with ulcer and inflammation

454.9 Without mention of ulcer or inflammation
Phlebectasiaa } of lower extremity [any
Varicose veins } part] or of unspeci-
Varix } fied site
● 455 Hemorrhoids
INCLUDES hemorrhoids (anus) (rectum)
piles
varicose veins, anus or rectum
EXCLUDES that complicating pregnancy, childbirth, or the puerperium (671.8)
455.0 Internal hemorrhoids without mention of complication
455.1 Internal thrombosed hemorrhoids
◆ 455.2 Internal hemorrhoids with other complication
Internal hemorrhoids: Internal hemorrhoids:
bleeding strangulated
prolapsed ulcerated
455.3 External hemorrhoids without mention of complication
455.4 External thrombosed hemorrhoids
◆ 455.5 External hemorrhoids with other complication
External hemorrhoids: External hemorrhoids:
bleeding strangulated
prolapsed ulcerated
◆ 455.6 Unspecified hemorrhoids without mention of complication
Hemorrhoids NOS
◆ 455.7 Unspecified thrombosed hemorrhoids
Thrombosed hemorrhoids, unspecified whether internal or external
◆ 455.8 Unspecified hemorrhoids with other complication
Hemorrhoids, unspecified whether internal or external:
bleeding
prolapsed
strangulated
ulcerated
455.9 Residual hemorrhoidal skin tags
Skin tags, anus or rectum
● 456 Varicose veins of other sites
456.0 Esophageal varices with bleeding
456.1 Esophageal varices without mention of bleeding
● 456.2 Esophageal varices in diseases classified elsewhere
Code also underlying cause, as:
cirrhosis of liver (571.0-571.9)
portal hypertension (572.3)
■ 456.20 With bleeding
■ 456.21 Without mention of bleeding
456.3 Sublingual varices
456.4 Scrotal varices
Varicocele
456.5 Pelvic varices
Varices of broad ligament
456.6 Vulval varices
Varices of perineum
EXCLUDES that complicating pregnancy, childbirth, or the puerperium (671.1)
◆ 456.8 Varices of other sites
Varicose veins of nasal septum (with ulcer)
EXCLUDES placental varices (656.7)
retinal varices (362.17)
varicose ulcer of unspecified site (454.0)
varicose veins of unspecified site (454.9)
● 457 Noninfectious disorders of lymphatic channels
457.0 Postmastectomy lymphedema syndrome
Elephantiasis } due to mastectomy
Obliteration of lymphatic vessel }
◆ 457.1 Other lymphedema
Elephantiasis (nonfilarial) NOS
Lymphangiectasis
Lymphedema:
acquired (chronic)
praecox
secondary
Obliteration, lymphatic vessel
EXCLUDES elephantiasis (nonfilarial):
congenital (757.0)
eyelid (374.83)
vulva (624.8)

457.2 **Lymphangitis**
Lymphangitis:
NOS
chronic
subacute
EXCLUDES: acute lymphangitis (682.0-682.9)

◆ **457.8** **Other noninfectious disorders of lymphatic channels**
Chylocele (nonfilarial)
Chylous:
ascites
cyst
Lymph node or vessel:
fistula
infarction
rupture
EXCLUDES: chylocele:
filarial (125.0-125.9)
tunica vaginalis (nonfilarial) (608.84)

◆ **457.9** **Unspecified noninfectious disorder of lymphatic channels**

● **458** **Hypotension**
INCLUDES: hypopiesis
EXCLUDES: cardiovascular collapse (785.50)
maternal hypotension syndrome (669.2)
shock (785.50-785.59)
Shy-Drager syndrome (333.0)

458.0 **Orthostatic hypotension**
Hypotension:
orthostatic (chronic)
postural

458.1 **Chronic hypotension**
Permanent idiopathic hypotension

◆ **458.9** **Hypotension, unspecified**
Hypotension (arterial) NOS

● **459** **Other disorders of circulatory system**
◆ **459.0** **Hemorrhage, unspecified**
Rupture of blood vessel NOS
Spontaneous hemorrhage NEC
EXCLUDES: hemorrhage:
gastrointestinal NOS (578.9)
in newborn NOS (772.9)
secondary or recurrent following trauma (958.2)
traumatic rupture of blood vessel (900.0-904.9)

459.1 **Postphlebitic syndrome**
459.2 **Compression of vein**
Stricture of vein
Vena cava syndrome (inferior) (superior)

● **459.8** **Other specified disorders of circulatory system**
◆ **459.81** **Venous (peripheral) insufficiency, unspecified**
Chronic venous insufficiency NOS
◆ **459.89** **Other**
Collateral circulation (venous), any site
Phlebosclerosis
Venofibrosis

◆ **459.9** **Unspecified circulatory system disorder**

8. DISEASES OF THE RESPIRATORY SYSTEM (460-519)
Use additional code, if desired, to identify infectious organism

ACUTE RESPIRATORY INFECTIONS (460-466)
EXCLUDES: pneumonia and influenza (480.0-487.8)

460 **Acute nasopharyngitis [common cold]**
Coryza (acute)
Nasal catarrh, acute
Nasopharyngitis:
NOS
acute
Nasopharyngitis:
infective NOS
Rhinitis:
acute
infective
EXCLUDES: nasopharyngitis, chronic (472.2)
pharyngitis:
acute or unspecified (462)
chronic (472.1)
rhinitis:
allergic (477.0-477.9)
chronic or unspecified (472.0)
sore throat:
acute or unspecified (462)
chronic (472.1)

● **461** **Acute sinusitis**
INCLUDES: abscess
empyema
infection
inflammation
suppuration
⎫ acute, of sinus (accessory)
⎬ (nasal)
⎭
EXCLUDES: chronic or unspecified sinusitis (473.0-473.9)

461.0 **Maxillary**
Acute antritis
461.1 **Frontal**
461.2 **Ethmoidal**
461.3 **Sphenoidal**
◆ **461.8** **Other acute sinusitis**
Acute pansinusitis
◆ **461.9** **Acute sinusitis, unspecified**
Acute sinusitis NOS

462 **Acute pharyngitis**
Acute sore throat NOS
Pharyngitis (acute):
NOS
gangrenous
infective
phlegmonous
pneumococcal
Pharyngitis (acute):
staphylococcal
suppurative
ulcerative
Sore throat (viral) NOS
Viral pharyngitis
EXCLUDES: abscess:
peritonsillar [quinsy] (475)
pharyngeal NOS (478.29)
retropharyngeal (478.24)
chronic pharyngitis (472.1)
infectious mononucleosis (075)
that specified as (due to):
Coxsackie (virus) (074.0)
gonococcus (098.6)
herpes simplex (054.79)
influenza (487.1)
septic (034.0)
streptococcal (034.0)

463 **Acute tonsillitis**
Tonsillitis (acute):
NOS
follicular
gangrenous
infective
pneumococcal
Tonsillitis (acute):
septic
staphylococcal
suppurative
ulcerative
viral
EXCLUDES: chronic tonsillitis (474.0)
hypertrophy of tonsils (474.1)
peritonsillar abscess [quinsy] (475)
sore throat:
acute or NOS (462)
septic (034.0)
streptococcal tonsillitis (034.0)

● **464** **Acute laryngitis and tracheitis**
EXCLUDES: that associated with influenza (487.1)
that due to Streptococcus (034.0)

464.0 **Acute laryngitis**
Laryngitis (acute):
NOS
edematous
Hemophilus influenzae [H. influenzae]
pneumococcal
septic
suppurative
ulcerative
EXCLUDES: chronic laryngitis (476.0-476.1)
influenzal laryngitis (487.1)

● **464.1** **Acute tracheitis**
Tracheitis (acute):
NOS
catarrhal
viral
EXCLUDES: chronic tracheitis (491.8)
464.10 **Without mention of obstruction**
464.11 **With obstruction**

464.2 TABULAR LIST 478.29

- **464.2 Acute laryngotracheitis**
    Laryngotracheitis (acute)
    Tracheitis (acute) with laryngitis (acute)
    EXCLUDES *chronic laryngotracheitis (476.1)*
    - 464.20 Without mention of obstruction
    - 464.21 With obstruction
- **464.3 Acute epiglottitis**
    Viral epiglottitis
    EXCLUDES *epiglottitis, chronic (476.1)*
    - 464.30 Without mention of obstruction
    - 464.31 With obstruction
  - 464.4 Croup
        Croup syndrome
- **465 Acute upper respiratory infections of multiple or unspecified sites**
    EXCLUDES upper respiratory infection due to:
        influenza (487.1)
        Streptococcus (034.0)
    - 465.0 Acute laryngopharyngitis
  - ◆ 465.8 Other multiple sites
        Multiple URI
  - ◆ 465.9 Unspecified site
        Acute URI NOS
        Upper respiratory infection (acute)
- **466 Acute bronchitis and bronchiolitis**
    INCLUDES that with:
        bronchospasm
        obstruction
    - 466.0 Acute bronchitis
        Bronchitis, acute   Bronchitis, acute
            or subacute: or subacute:
            fibrinous   viral
            membranous   with tracheitis
            pneumococcal   Croupous bronchitis
            purulent   Tracheobronchitis, acute
            septic
    - 466.1 Acute bronchiolitis
        Bronchiolitis (acute)
        Capillary pneumonia

OTHER DISEASES OF THE UPPER RESPIRATORY TRACT (470-478)

- 470 **Deviated nasal septum**
    Deflected septum (nasal) (acquired)
    EXCLUDES *congenital (754.0)*
- **471 Nasal polyps**
    EXCLUDES *adenomatous polyps (212.0)*
    - 471.0 Polyp of nasal cavity
        Polyp: Polyp:
            choanal   nasopharyngeal
    - 471.1 Polypoid sinus degeneration
        Woakes' syndrome or ethmoiditis
  - ◆ 471.8 Other polyp of sinus
        Polyp of sinus: Polyp of sinus:
            accessory   maxillary
            ethmoidal   sphenoidal
  - ◆ 471.9 Unspecified nasal polyp
        Nasal polyp NOS
- **472 Chronic pharyngitis and nasopharyngitis**
    - 472.0 Chronic rhinitis
        Ozena   Rhinitis:
        Rhinitis: hypertrophic
            NOS   obstructive
            atrophic   purulent
            granulomatous   ulcerative
        EXCLUDES *allergic rhinitis (477.0-477.9)*
    - 472.1 Chronic pharyngitis
        Chronic sore throat   Pharyngitis:
        Pharyngitis: granular (chronic)
            atrophic   hypertrophic
    - 472.2 Chronic nasopharyngitis
        EXCLUDES *acute or unspecified nasopharyngitis (460)*
- 473 **Chronic sinusitis**
    INCLUDES   abscess
                   empyema   (chronic) of sinus (accessory) (nasal)
                   infection
                   suppuration

    EXCLUDES *acute sinusitis (461.0-461.9)*

  - 473.0 Maxillary
        Antritis (chronic)
  - 473.1 Frontal
  - 473.2 Ethmoidal
        EXCLUDES *Woakes' ethmoiditis (471.1)*
  - 473.3 Sphenoidal
  - ◆ 473.8 Other chronic sinusitis
        Pansinusitis (chronic)
  - ◆ 473.9 Unspecified sinusitis (chronic)
        Sinusitis (chronic) NOS
- **474 Chronic disease of tonsils and adenoids**
    - 474.0 Chronic tonsillitis
        EXCLUDES *acute or unspecified tonsillitis (463)*
  - **474.1 Hypertrophy of tonsils and adenoids**
        Enlargement
        Hyperplasia   } of tonsils or adenoids
        Hypertrophy
        - 474.10 Tonsils with adenoids
        - 474.11 Tonsils alone
        - 474.12 Adenoids alone
    - 474.2 Adenoid vegetations
  - ◆ 474.8 Other chronic disease of tonsils and adenoids
        Amygdalolith
        Calculus, tonsil
        Cicatrix of tonsil (and adenoid)
        Tonsillar tag
        Ulcer, tonsil
  - ◆ 474.9 Unspecified chronic disease of tonsils and adenoids
        Disease (chronic) of tonsils (and adenoids)
  - 475 Peritonsillar abscess
        Abscess of tonsil
        Peritonsillar cellulitis
        Quinsy
        EXCLUDES tonsillitis:
            acute or NOS (463)
            chronic (474.0)
- 476 **Chronic laryngitis and laryngotracheitis**
    - 476.0 Chronic laryngitis
        Laryngitis:
            catarrhal
            hypertrophic
            sicca
    - 476.1 Chronic laryngotracheitis
        Laryngitis, chronic, with tracheitis (chronic)
        Tracheitis, chronic, with laryngitis
        EXCLUDES *chronic tracheitis (491.8)*
            laryngitis and tracheitis, acute or unspecified (464.0-464.4)
- **477 Allergic rhinitis**
    INCLUDES   allergic rhinitis (nonseasonal) (seasonal)
                   hay fever
                   spasmodic rhinorrhea
    EXCLUDES *allergic rhinitis with asthma (bronchial) (493.0)*
    - 477.0 Due to pollen
        Pollinosis
  - ◆ 477.8 Due to other allergen
  - ◆ 477.9 Cause unspecified
- **478 Other diseases of upper respiratory tract**
    - 478.0 Hypertrophy of nasal turbinates
  - ◆ 478.1 Other diseases of nasal cavity and sinuses
        Abscess
        Necrosis   } of nose (septum)
        Ulcer

        Cyst or mucocele of sinus (nasal)
        Rhinolith
        EXCLUDES *varicose ulcer of nasal septum (456.8)*
  - **478.2 Other diseases of pharynx, not elsewhere classified**
    - ◆ 478.20 Unspecified disease of pharynx
        - 478.21 Cellulitis of pharynx or nasopharynx
        - 478.22 Parapharyngeal abscess
        - 478.24 Retropharyngeal abscess
        - 478.25 Edema of pharynx or nasopharynx
        - 478.26 Cyst of pharynx or nasopharynx
    - ◆ 478.29 Other
        Abscess of pharynx or nasopharynx
        EXCLUDES *ulcerative pharyngitis (462)*

RESPIRATORY SYSTEM

- ● 478.3 Paralysis of vocal cords or larynx
  - ◆ 478.30 Paralysis, unspecified
    - Laryngoplegia
    - Paralysis of glottis
  - 478.31 Unilateral, partial
  - 478.32 Unilateral, complete
  - 478.33 Bilateral, partial
  - 478.34 Bilateral, complete
- 478.4 Polyp of vocal cord or larynx
  - EXCLUDES adenomatous polyps (212.1)
- ◆ 478.5 Other diseases of vocal cords
  - Abscess
  - Cellulitis
  - Granuloma } of vocal cords
  - Leukoplakia
  - Chorditis (fibrinous) (nodosa) (tuberosa)
  - Singers' nodes
- 478.6 Edema of larynx
  - Edema (of):
    - glottis
    - subglottic
    - supraglottic
- ● 478.7 Other diseases of larynx, not elsewhere classified
  - ◆ 478.70 Unspecified disease of larynx
  - 478.71 Cellulitis and perichondritis of larynx
  - 478.74 Stenosis of larynx
  - 478.75 Laryngeal spasm
    - Laryngismus (stridulus)
  - ◆ 478.79 Other
    - Abscess
    - Necrosis
    - Obstruction } of larynx
    - Pachyderma
    - Ulcer
    - EXCLUDES ulcerative laryngitis (464.0)
- ◆ 478.8 Upper respiratory tract hypersensitivity reaction, site unspecified
  - EXCLUDES hypersensitivity reaction of lower respiratory tract, as:
    - extrinsic allergic alveolitis (495.0-495.9)
    - pneumoconiosis (500-505)
- ◆ 478.9 Other and unspecified diseases of upper respiratory tract
  - Abscess
  - Cicatrix } of trachea

PNEUMONIA AND INFLUENZA (480-487)

EXCLUDES pneumonia:
- allergic or eosinophilic (518.3)
- aspiration:
  - NOS (507.0)
  - newborn (770.1)
  - solids and liquids (507.0-507.8)
- congenital (770.0)
- lipoid (507.1)
- passive (514)
- postoperative (997.3)
- rheumatic (390)

- ● 480 Viral pneumonia
  - 480.0 Pneumonia due to adenovirus
  - 480.1 Pneumonia due to respiratory syncytial virus
  - 480.2 Pneumonia due to parainfluenza virus
  - ◆ 480.8 Pneumonia due to other virus not elsewhere classified
    - EXCLUDES congenital rubella pneumonitis (771.0)
      - influenza with pneumonia, any form (487.0)
      - pneumonia complicating viral diseases classified elsewhere (484.1-484.8)
  - ◆ 480.9 Viral pneumonia, unspecified
- 481 Pneumococcal pneumonia [Streptococcus pneumoniae pneumonia]
  - Lobar pneumonia, organism unspecified
- ● 482 Other bacterial pneumonia
  - 482.0 Pneumonia due to Klebsiella pneumoniae
  - 482.1 Pneumonia due to Pseudomonas
  - 482.2 Pneumonia due to Hemophilus influenzae [H. influenzae]
  - ● 482.3 Pneumonia due to Streptococcus
    - EXCLUDES Streptococcus pneumoniae (481)
    - ◆ 482.30 Streptococcus, unspecified
    - 482.31 Group A
    - 482.32 Group B
    - ◆ 482.39 Other Streptococcus
  - 482.4 Pneumonia due to Staphylococcus
  - ● 482.8 Pneumonia due to other specified bacteria
    - EXCLUDES pneumonia, complicating infectious disease classified elsewhere (484.1-484.8)
    - 482.81 Anaerobes
      - Gram-negative anaerobes
      - Bacteroides (melaninogenicus)
    - 482.82 Escherichia coli [E. coli]
    - ◆ 482.83 Other gram-negative bacteria
      - Gram-negative pneumonia NOS
      - Proteus
      - Serratia marcescens
      - EXCLUDES gram-negative anaerobes (482.81)
    - ◆ 482.89 Other specified bacteria
  - ◆ 482.9 Bacterial pneumonia unspecified
- ● 483 Pneumonia due to other specified organism
  - 483.0 Mycoplasma pneumoniae
    - Eaton's agent
    - pleuropneumonia-like organism [PPLO]
  - ◆ 483.8 Other specified organism
- ● 484 Pneumonia in infectious diseases classified elsewhere
  - EXCLUDES influenza with pneumonia, any form (487.0)
  - ■ 484.1 Pneumonia in cytomegalic inclusion disease
    - Code also underlying disease (078.5)
  - ■ 484.3 Pneumonia in whooping cough
    - Code also underlying disease (033.0-033.9)
  - ■ 484.5 Pneumonia in anthrax
    - Code also underlying disease (022.1)
  - ■ 484.6 Pneumonia in aspergillosis
    - Code also underlying disease (117.3)
  - ■ ◆ 484.7 Pneumonia in other systemic mycoses
    - Code also underlying disease
    - EXCLUDES pneumonia in:
      - candidiasis (112.4)
      - coccidioidomycosis (114.0)
      - histoplasmosis (115.0-115.9 with fifth-digit 5)
  - ■ 484.8 Pneumonia in other infectious diseases classified elsewhere
    - Code also underlying disease, as:
      - Q fever (083.0)
      - typhoid fever (002.0)
    - EXCLUDES pneumonia in:
      - actinomycosis (039.1)
      - measles (055.1)
      - nocardiosis (039.1)
      - ornithosis (073.0)
      - Pneumocystis carinii (136.3)
      - salmonellosis (003.22)
      - toxoplasmosis (130.4)
      - tuberculosis (011.6)
      - tularemia (021.2)
      - varicella (052.1)
- ◆ 485 Bronchopneumonia, organism unspecified
  - Bronchopneumonia: Pneumonia:
    - hemorrhagic   lobular
    - terminal   segmental
  - Pleurobronchopneumonia
  - EXCLUDES bronchiolitis (acute) (466.1)
    - chronic (491.8)
    - lipoid pneumonia (507.1)
- ◆ 486 Pneumonia, organism unspecified
  - EXCLUDES hypostatic or passive pneumonia (514)
    - influenza with pneumonia, any form (487.0)
    - inhalation or aspiration pneumonia due to foreign materials (507.0-507.8)
    - pneumonitis due to fumes and vapors (506.0)
- ● 487 Influenza
  - EXCLUDES Hemophilus influenzae [H. influenzae]:
    - infection NOS (041.5)
    - laryngitis (464.0)
    - meningitis (320.0)
    - pneumonia (482.2)

● Additional digits required   ◆ Nonspecific code   ■ Not a primary diagnosis

| 487.0 | TABULAR LIST | 495.7 |

- 487.0 **With pneumonia**
  Influenza with pneumonia, any form
  Influenzal:
    bronchopneumonia
    pneumonia
◆ 487.1 **With other respiratory manifestations**
  Influenza NOS
  Influenzal:
    laryngitis
    pharyngitis
    respiratory infection (upper) (acute)
◆ 487.8 **With other manifestations**
  Encephalopathy due to influenza
  Influenza with involvement of gastrointestinal tract
  EXCLUDES "intestinal flu" [viral gastroenteritis] (008.8)

CHRONIC OBSTRUCTIVE PULMONARY DISEASE AND ALLIED CONDITIONS (490-496)

◆ **490 Bronchitis, not specified as acute or chronic**
  Bronchitis NOS:
    catarrhal
    with tracheitis NOS
  Tracheobronchitis NOS
  EXCLUDES bronchitis:
    allergic NOS (493.9)
    asthmatic NOS (493.9)
    due to fumes and vapors (506.0)

● **491 Chronic bronchitis**
  EXCLUDES chronic obstructive asthma (493.2)
  491.0 **Simple chronic bronchitis**
    Catarrhal bronchitis, chronic
    Smokers' cough
  491.1 **Mucopurulent chronic bronchitis**
    Bronchitis (chronic) (recurrent):
      fetid
      mucopurulent
      purulent
● 491.2 **Obstructive chronic bronchitis**
    Bronchitis:
      asthmatic, chronic
      emphysematous
      obstructive (chronic) (diffuse)
    Bronchitis with:
      chronic airway obstruction
      emphysema
    EXCLUDES asthmatic bronchitis (acute) NOS (493.9)
      chronic obstructive asthma (].2)
    491.20 **Without mention of acute exacerbation**
      Chronic asthmatic bronchitis
      Emphysema with chronic bronchitis
    491.21 **With acute exacerbation**
      Acute bronchitis with chronic obstructive pulmonary disease [COPD]
      Acute and chronic obstructive bronchitis
      Chronic asthmatic bronchitis with acute exacerbation
      Emphysema with both acute and chronic bronchitis
◆ 491.8 **Other chronic bronchitis**
    Chronic:
      tracheitis
      tracheobronchitis
◆ 491.9 **Unspecified chronic bronchitis**
● **492 Emphysema**
  492.0 **Emphysematous bleb**
    Giant bullous emphysema
    Ruptured emphysematous bleb
    Tension pneumatocele
    Vanishing lung

◆ 492.8 **Other emphysema**
    Emphysema (lung or   MacLeod's syndrome
      pulmonary):   Swyer-James syndrome
      NOS   Unilateral hyperlucent lung
      centriacinar
      centrilobular
      obstructive
      panacinar
      panlobular
      unilateral
      vesicular
    EXCLUDES emphysema:
      with both acute and chronic bronchitis (491.21)
      with chronic bronchitis (491.2)
      compensatory (518.2)
      due to fumes and vapors (506.4)
      interstitial (518.1)
        newborn (770.2)
      mediastinal (518.1)
      surgical (subcutaneous) (998.81)   ◆
      traumatic (958.7)
● **493 Asthma**
  The following fifth-digit subclassification is for use with category 493:
    0 without mention of status asthmaticus
    1 with status asthmaticus
● 493.0 **Extrinsic asthma**
    Asthma:
      allergic with stated cause
      atopic
      childhood
      hay
      platinum
    Hay fever with asthma
    EXCLUDES asthma:
      allergic NOS (].9)
      detergent (507.8)
      miners' (500)
      wood (495.8)
● 493.1 **Intrinsic asthma**
    Late-onset asthma
● 493.2 **Chronic obstructive asthma**
    Asthma with chronic obstructive pulmonary disease [COPD]
    EXCLUDES chronic asthmatic bronchitis (491.2)
      chronic obstructive bronchitis (491.2)
◆ ● 493.9 **Asthma, unspecified**
    Asthma (bronchial) (allergic NOS)
    Bronchitis:
      allergic
      asthmatic
494 Bronchiectasis
    Bronchiectasis (fusiform) (postinfectious) (recurrent)
    Bronchiolectasis
    EXCLUDES congenital (748.61)
      tuberculous bronchiectasis (current disease) (011.5)
● **495 Extrinsic allergic alveolitis**
    INCLUDES allergic alveolitis and pneumonitis due to inhaled organic dust particles of fungal, thermophilic actinomycete, or other origin
  495.0 **Farmers' lung**
  495.1 **Bagassosis**
  495.2 **Bird-fanciers' lung**
    Budgerigar-fanciers' disease or lung
    Pigeon-fanciers' disease or lung
  495.3 **Suberosis**
    Cork-handlers' disease or lung
  495.4 **Malt workers' lung**
    Alveolitis due to Aspergillus clavatus
  495.5 **Mushroom workers' lung**
  495.6 **Maple bark-strippers' lung**
    Alveolitis due to Cryptostroma corticale
  495.7 **"Ventilation" pneumonitis**
    Allergic alveolitis due to fungal, thermophilic actinomycete, and other organisms growing in ventilation [air conditioning] systems

RESPIRATORY SYSTEM

◆ **495.8 Other specified allergic alveolitis and pneumonitis**
Cheese-washers' lung
Coffee workers' lung
Fish-meal workers' lung
Furriers' lung
Grain-handlers' disease or lung
Pituitary snuff-takers' disease
Sequoiosis or red-cedar asthma
Wood asthma

◆ **495.9 Unspecified allergic alveolitis and pneumonitis**
Alveolitis, allergic (extrinsic)
Hypersensitivity pneumonitis

◆ **496 Chronic airway obstruction, not elsewhere classified**
Note: This code is not to be used with any code from categories 491-493
Chronic:
nonspecific lung disease
obstructive lung disease
obstructive pulmonary disease [COPD] NOS
EXCLUDES chronic obstructive lung disease [COPD] specified (as) (with):
allergic alveolitis (495.0-495.9)
asthma (.2)
bronchiectasis (494)
bronchitis (491.20-491.21)
with emphysema (491.20-491.21)
emphysema (492.0-492.8)

PNEUMOCONIOSES AND OTHER LUNG DISEASES DUE TO EXTERNAL AGENTS (500-508)

500 Coal workers' pneumoconiosis
Anthracosilicosis   Coal workers' lung
Anthracosis   Miner's asthma
Black lung disease

501 Asbestosis

◆ **502 Pneumoconiosis due to other silica or silicates**
Pneumoconiosis due to talc
Silicotic fibrosis (massive) of lung
Silicosis (simple) (complicated)

◆ **503 Pneumoconiosis due to other inorganic dust**
Aluminosis (of lung)   Graphite fibrosis (of lung)
Bauxite fibrosis (of lung)   Siderosis
Berylliosis   Stannosis

◆ **504 Pneumonopathy due to inhalation of other dust**
Byssinosis   Flax-dressers' disease
Cannabinosis
EXCLUDES allergic alveolitis (495.0-495.9)
asbestosis (501)
bagassosis (495.1)
farmers' lung (495.0)

◆ **505 Pneumoconiosis, unspecified**

● **506 Respiratory conditions due to chemical fumes and vapors**
Use additional E code, if desired, to identify cause

506.0 **Bronchitis and pneumonitis due to fumes and vapors**
Chemical bronchitis (acute)

506.1 **Acute pulmonary edema due to fumes and vapors**
Chemical pulmonary edema (acute)
EXCLUDES acute pulmonary edema NOS (518.4)
chronic or unspecified pulmonary edema (514)

506.2 **Upper respiratory inflammation due to fumes and vapors**

◆ 506.3 **Other acute and subacute respiratory conditions due to fumes and vapors**

506.4 **Chronic respiratory conditions due to fumes and vapors**
Emphysema (diffuse) (chronic)
Obliterative bronchiolitis (chronic) (subacute) } due to inhalation of chemical fumes and vapors
Pulmonary fibrosis (chronic)

◆ 506.9 **Unspecified respiratory conditions due to fumes and vapors**
Silo-fillers' disease

● **507 Pneumonitis due to solids and liquids**
EXCLUDES fetal aspiration pneumonitis (770.1)

507.0 **Due to inhalation of food or vomitus**
Aspiration pneumonia (due to):
NOS
food (regurgitated)
gastric secretions
milk
saliva
vomitus

507.1 **Due to inhalation of oils and essences**
Lipoid pneumonia (exogenous)
EXCLUDES endogenous lipoid pneumonia (516.8)

◆ 507.8 **Due to other solids and liquids**
Detergent asthma

● **508 Respiratory conditions due to other and unspecified external agents**
Use additional E code, if desired, to identify cause

508.0 **Acute pulmonary manifestations due to radiation**
Radiation pneumonitis

508.1 **Chronic and other pulmonary manifestations due to radiation**
Fibrosis of lung following radiation

◆ 508.8 **Respiratory conditions due to other specified external agents**

◆ 508.9 **Respiratory conditions due to unspecified external agent**

OTHER DISEASES OF RESPIRATORY SYSTEM (510-519)

● **510 Empyema**
Use additional code, if desired, to identify infectious organism (041.0-041.9)
EXCLUDES abscess of lung (513.0)

510.0 **With fistula**
Fistula: Fistula:
bronchocutaneous   mediastinal
bronchopleural   pleural
hepatopleural   thoracic
Any condition classifiable to 510.9 with fistula

510.9 **Without mention of fistula**
Abscess: Pleurisy:
pleura   septic
thorax   seropurulent
Empyema (chest) (lung)   suppurative
(pleura)   Pyopneumothorax
Fibrinopurulent pleurisy   Pyothorax
Pleurisy:
purulent

● **511 Pleurisy**
EXCLUDES malignant pleural effusion (197.2) ◆
pleurisy with mention of tuberculosis, current disease (012.0)

511.0 **Without mention of effusion or current tuberculosis**
Adhesion, lung or pleura   Pleurisy:
Calcification of pleura   NOS
Pleurisy (acute) (sterile): pneumococcal
diaphragmatic   staphylococcal
fibrinous   streptococcal
interlobar   Thickening of pleura

◆ 511.1 **With effusion, with mention of a bacterial cause other than tuberculosis**
Pleurisy with effusion (exudative) (serous):
pneumococcal
staphylococcal
streptococcal
other specified nontuberculous bacterial cause

◆ 511.8 **Other specified forms of effusion, except tuberculous**
Encysted pleurisy   Hydropneumothorax
Hemopneumothorax   Hydrothorax
Hemothorax
EXCLUDES traumatic (860.2-860.5)

◆ 511.9 **Unspecified pleural effusion**
Pleural effusion NOS   Pleurisy:
Pleurisy: serous
exudative   with effusion NOS
serofibrinous

● **512 Pneumothorax**

512.0 **Spontaneous tension pneumothorax**

512.1 **Iatrogenic pneumothorax** ▼
Postoperative pneumothorax ▲

● Additional digits required   ◆ Nonspecific code   ▌ Not a primary diagnosis

- **512.8 Other spontaneous pneumothorax**
  - Pneumothorax:
    - NOS
    - acute
  - Pneumothorax:
    - chronic
  - **EXCLUDES** pneumothorax:
    - congenital (770.2)
    - traumatic (860.0-860.1, 860.4-860.5)
    - tuberculous, current disease (011.7)

- **513 Abscess of lung and mediastinum**
  - **513.0 Abscess of lung**
    - Abscess (multiple) of lung
    - Gangrenous or necrotic pneumonia
    - Pulmonary gangrene or necrosis
  - **513.1 Abscess of mediastinum**

- **514 Pulmonary congestion and hypostasis**
  - Hypostatic:
    - bronchopneumonia
    - pneumonia
  - Passive pneumonia
  - Pulmonary congestion (chronic) (passive)
  - Pulmonary edema:
    - NOS
    - chronic
  - **EXCLUDES** acute pulmonary edema:
    - NOS (518.4)
    - with mention of heart disease or failure (428.1)

- **515 Postinflammatory pulmonary fibrosis**
  - Cirrhosis of lung
  - Fibrosis of lung (atrophic) (confluent) (massive) (perialveolar) (peribronchial)
  - Induration of lung
  - } chronic or unspecified

- **516 Other alveolar and parietoalveolar pneumonopathy**
  - **516.0 Pulmonary alveolar proteinosis**
  - **516.1 Idiopathic pulmonary hemosiderosis**
    - Essential brown induration of lung
    - Code also underlying disease (275.0)
  - **516.2 Pulmonary alveolar microlithiasis**
  - **516.3 Idiopathic fibrosing alveolitis**
    - Alveolar capillary block
    - Diffuse (idiopathic) (interstitial) pulmonary fibrosis
    - Hamman-Rich syndrome
  - **516.8 Other specified alveolar and parietoalveolar pneumonopathies**
    - Endogenous lipoid pneumonia
    - Interstitial pneumonia (desquamative) (lymphoid)
    - **EXCLUDES** lipoid pneumonia, exogenous or unspecified (507.1)
  - **516.9 Unspecified alveolar and parietoalveolar pneumonopathy**

- **517 Lung involvement in conditions classified elsewhere**
  - **EXCLUDES** rheumatoid lung (714.81)
  - **517.1 Rheumatic pneumonia**
    - Code also underlying disease (390)
  - **517.2 Lung involvement in systemic sclerosis**
    - Code also underlying disease (710.1)
  - **517.8 Lung involvement in other diseases classified elsewhere**
    - Code also underlying disease, as:
      - amyloidosis (277.3)
      - polymyositis (710.4)
      - sarcoidosis (135)
      - Sjögren's disease (710.2)
      - systemic lupus erythematosus (710.0)
    - **EXCLUDES** syphilis (095.1)

- **518 Other diseases of lung**
  - **518.0 Pulmonary collapse**
    - Atelectasis
    - Collapse of lung
    - Middle lobe syndrome
    - **EXCLUDES** atelectasis:
      - congenital (partial) (770.5)
      - primary (770.4)
      - tuberculous, current disease (011.8)
  - **518.1 Interstitial emphysema**
    - Mediastinal emphysema
    - **EXCLUDES** surgical (subcutaneous) emphysema (998.81)
      - that in fetus or newborn (770.2)
      - traumatic emphysema (958.7)

- **518.2 Compensatory emphysema**
- **518.3 Pulmonary eosinophilia**
  - Eosinophilic asthma
  - Löffler's syndrome
  - Pneumonia:
    - allergic
    - eosinophilic
  - Tropical eosinophilia
- **518.4 Acute edema of lung, unspecified**
  - Acute pulmonary edema NOS
  - Pulmonary edema, postoperative
  - **EXCLUDES** pulmonary edema:
    - acute, with mention of heart disease or failure (428.1)
    - chronic or unspecified (514)
    - due to external agents (506.0-508.9)
- **518.5 Pulmonary insufficiency following trauma and surgery**
  - Adult respiratory distress syndrome
  - Pulmonary insufficiency following:
    - shock
    - surgery
    - trauma
  - Shock lung
  - **EXCLUDES** adult respiratory distress syndrome associated with other conditions (518.82)
    - pneumonia:
      - aspiration (507.0)
      - hypostatic (514)
    - respiratory failure in other conditions (518.81)

- **518.8 Other diseases of lung**
  - **518.81 Respiratory failure**
    - Respiratory failure:
      - NOS
      - acute
      - acute and chronic (acute-on-chronic)
      - chronic
    - **EXCLUDES** acute respiratory distress (518.82)
      - respiratory arrest (799.1)
      - respiratory failure, newborn (770.8)
  - **518.82 Other pulmonary insufficiency, not elsewhere classified**
    - Acute respiratory distress
    - Acute respiratory insufficiency
    - Adult respiratory distress syndrome NEC
    - **EXCLUDES** adult respiratory distress syndrome associated with trauma and surgery (518.5)
      - pulmonary insufficiency following trauma and surgery (518.5)
      - respiratory distress:
        - NOS (786.09)
        - newborn (770.8)
        - syndrome, newborn (769)
      - shock lung (518.5)
  - **518.89 Other diseases of lung, not elsewhere classified**
    - Broncholithiasis
    - Calcification of lung
    - Lung disease NOS
    - Pulmolithiasis

- **519 Other diseases of respiratory system**
  - **519.0 Tracheostomy complication**
    - Hemorrhage from
    - Sepsis of } tracheostomy stoma
    - Tracheal stenosis
    - Tracheoesophageal fistula } following tracheostomy
    - Tracheostomy:
      - hemorrhage
      - obstruction
      - sepsis
  - **519.1 Other diseases of trachea and bronchus, not elsewhere classified**
    - Calcification
    - Stenosis
    - Ulcer } of bronchus or trachea

519.2　Mediastinitis
◆ 519.3　Other diseases of mediastinum, not elsewhere classified
　　　　Fibrosis
　　　　Hernia　　　　} of mediastinum
　　　　Retraction

519.4　Disorders of diaphragm
　　　　Diaphragmitis　　　　Relaxation of diaphragm
　　　　Paralysis of diaphragm
　　　　EXCLUDES congenital defect of diaphragm (756.6)
　　　　　　diaphragmatic hernia (551-553 with .3)
　　　　　　congenital (756.6)

◆ 519.8　Other diseases of respiratory system, not elsewhere classified
◆ 519.9　Unspecified disease of respiratory system
　　　　Respiratory disease (chronic) NOS

9. DISEASES OF THE DIGESTIVE SYSTEM (520-579)

DISEASES OF ORAL CAVITY, SALIVARY GLANDS, AND JAWS (520-529)

● 520　Disorders of tooth development and eruption

520.0　Anodontia
　　　　Absence of teeth (complete) (congenital) (partial)
　　　　Hypodontia
　　　　Oligodontia
　　　　EXCLUDES acquired absence of teeth (525.1)

520.1　Supernumerary teeth
　　　　Distomolar　　　　Paramolar
　　　　Fourth molar　　　Supplemental teeth
　　　　Mesiodens
　　　　EXCLUDES supernumerary roots (520.2)

520.2　Abnormalities of size and form
　　　　Concrescence
　　　　Fusion　　　　} of teeth
　　　　Gemination

　　　　Dens evaginatus　　　Microdontia
　　　　Dens in dente　　　　Peg-shaped [conical] teeth
　　　　Dens invaginatus　　Supernumerary roots
　　　　Enamel pearls　　　　Taurodontism
　　　　Macrodontia　　　　Tuberculum paramolare
　　　　EXCLUDES that due to congenital syphilis (090.5)
　　　　　　tuberculum Carabelli, which is regarded as a normal variation

520.3　Mottled teeth
　　　　Dental fluorosis
　　　　Mottling of enamel
　　　　Nonfluoride enamel opacities

520.4　Disturbances of tooth formation
　　　　Aplasia and hypoplasia of cementum
　　　　Dilaceration of tooth
　　　　Enamel hypoplasia (neonatal) (postnatal) (prenatal)
　　　　Horner's teeth
　　　　Hypocalcification of teeth
　　　　Regional odontodysplasia
　　　　Turner's tooth
　　　　EXCLUDES Hutchinson's teeth and mulberry molars in congenital syphilis (090.5)
　　　　　　mottled teeth (520.3)

520.5　Hereditary disturbances in tooth structure, not elsewhere classified
　　　　Amelogenesis
　　　　Dentinogenesis　　} imperfecta
　　　　Odontogenesis

　　　　Dentinal dysplasia
　　　　Shell teeth

520.6　Disturbances in tooth eruption
　　　　Teeth:　　　　　　　Tooth eruption:
　　　　　embedded　　　　　　late
　　　　　impacted　　　　　　obstructed
　　　　　natal　　　　　　　　premature
　　　　　neonatal
　　　　　primary [deciduous]:
　　　　　　persistent
　　　　　　shedding, premature
　　　　EXCLUDES exfoliation of teeth (attributable to disease of surrounding tissues) (525.0-525.1)
　　　　　　impacted or embedded teeth with abnormal position of such teeth or adjacent teeth (524.3)

520.7　Teething syndrome
◆ 520.8　Other specified disorders of tooth development and eruption
　　　　Color changes during tooth formation
　　　　Pre-eruptive color changes
　　　　EXCLUDES posteruptive color changes (521.7)
◆ 520.9　Unspecified disorder of tooth development and eruption

● 521　Diseases of hard tissues of teeth

521.0　Dental caries
　　　　Caries (of):
　　　　　arrested
　　　　　cementum
　　　　　dentin (acute) (chronic)
　　　　　enamel (acute) (chronic) (incipient)
　　　　Infantile melanodontia
　　　　Odontoclasia
　　　　White spot lesions of teeth

521.1　Excessive attrition
　　　　Approximal wear
　　　　Occlusal wear

521.2　Abrasion
　　　　Abrasion:
　　　　　dentifrice
　　　　　habitual
　　　　　occupational　　} of teeth
　　　　　ritual
　　　　　traditional
　　　　Wedge defect NOS

521.3　Erosion
　　　　Erosion of teeth:　　　Erosion of teeth:
　　　　　NOS　　　　　　　　　idiopathic
　　　　　due to:　　　　　　　occupational
　　　　　　medicine
　　　　　　persistent vomiting

521.4　Pathological resorption
　　　　Internal granuloma of pulp
　　　　Resorption of tooth or root (external) (internal)

521.5　Hypercementosis
　　　　Cementation hyperplasia

521.6　Ankylosis of teeth

521.7　Posteruptive color changes
　　　　Staining [discoloration] of teeth:
　　　　　NOS
　　　　　due to:
　　　　　　drugs
　　　　　　metals
　　　　　　pulpal bleeding
　　　　EXCLUDES accretions [deposits] on teeth (523.6)
　　　　　　pre-eruptive color changes (520.8)

◆ 521.8　Other specified diseases of hard tissues of teeth
　　　　Irradiated enamel　　Sensitive dentin
◆ 521.9　Unspecified disease of hard tissues of teeth

● 522　Diseases of pulp and periapical tissues

522.0　Pulpitis
　　　　Pulpal:
　　　　　abscess
　　　　　polyp
　　　　Pulpitis:
　　　　　acute
　　　　　chronic (hyperplastic) (ulcerative)
　　　　　suppurative

522.1　Necrosis of the pulp
　　　　Pulp gangrene

522.2　Pulp degeneration
　　　　Denticles
　　　　Pulp calcifications
　　　　Pulp stones

522.3　Abnormal hard tissue formation in pulp
　　　　Secondary or irregular dentin

522.4　Acute apical periodontitis of pulpal origin

522.5　Periapical abscess without sinus
　　　　Abscess:
　　　　　dental
　　　　　dentoalveolar
　　　　EXCLUDES periapical abscess with sinus (522.7)

522.6　Chronic apical periodontitis
　　　　Apical or periapical granuloma
　　　　Apical periodontitis NOS

522.7 Periapical abscess with sinus
Fistula:
- alveolar process
- dental

522.8 Radicular cyst
Cyst:
- apical (periodontal)
- periapical

Cyst:
- radiculodental
- residual radicular

EXCLUDES lateral developmental or lateral periodontal cyst (526.0)

◆ 522.9 Other and unspecified diseases of pulp and periapical tissues

● 523 Gingival and periodontal diseases

523.0 Acute gingivitis
EXCLUDES acute necrotizing ulcerative gingivitis (101)
herpetic gingivostomatitis (054.2)

523.1 Chronic gingivitis
Gingivitis (chronic):
- NOS
- desquamative
- hyperplastic

Gingivitis (chronic):
- simple marginal
- ulcerative
- Gingivostomatitis

EXCLUDES herpetic gingivostomatitis (054.2)

523.2 Gingival recession
Gingival recession (generalized) (localized) (postinfective) (postoperative)

523.3 Acute periodontitis
Acute:
- pericementitis
- pericoronitis

Paradontal abscess
Periodontal abscess

EXCLUDES acute apical periodontitis (522.4)
periapical abscess (522.5, 522.7)

523.4 Chronic periodontitis
- Alveolar pyorrhea
- Chronic pericoronitis
- Pericementitis (chronic)
- Periodontitis:
  - NOS

Periodontitis:
- complex
- simplex

EXCLUDES chronic apical periodontitis (522.6)

523.5 Periodontosis

523.6 Accretions on teeth
Dental calculus:
- subgingival
- supragingival

Deposits on teeth:
- betel

Deposits on teeth:
- materia alba
- soft
- tartar
- tobacco

◆ 523.8 Other specified periodontal diseases
Giant cell:
- epulis
- peripheral granuloma

Gingival:
- cysts
- enlargement NOS
- fibromatosis

Gingival polyp
Periodontal lesions due to traumatic occlusion
Peripheral giant cell granuloma

EXCLUDES leukoplakia of gingiva (528.6)

◆ 523.9 Unspecified gingival and periodontal disease

● 524 Dentofacial anomalies, including malocclusion

● 524.0 Major anomalies of jaw size
EXCLUDES hemifacial atrophy or hypertrophy (754.0)
unilateral condylar hyperplasia or hypoplasia of mandible (526.89)

- ◆ 524.00 Unspecified anomaly
- 524.01 Maxillary hyperplasia
- 524.02 Mandibular hyperplasia
- 524.03 Maxillary hypoplasia
- 524.04 Mandibular hypoplasia
- 524.05 Macrogenia
- 524.06 Microgenia
- 524.09 Other specified anomaly

● 524.1 Anomalies of relationship of jaw to cranial base
- ◆ 524.10 Unspecified anomaly
  - prognathism
  - retrognathism
- 524.11 Maxillary asymmetry
- ◆ 524.12 Other jaw asymmetry
- ◆ 524.19 Other specified anomaly

524.2 Anomalies of dental arch relationship
- Crossbite (anterior) (posterior)
- Disto-occlusion
- Mesio-occlusion
- Midline deviation
- Open bite (anterior) (posterior)
- Overbite (excessive)
  - deep
  - horizontal
  - vertical
- Overjet
- Posterior lingual occlusion of mandibular teeth
- Soft tissue impingement

EXCLUDES hemifacial atrophy or hypertrophy (754.0)
unilateral condylar hyperplasia or hypoplasia of mandible (526.89)

524.3 Anomalies of tooth position
- Crowding
- Diastema
- Displacement
- Rotation
- Spacing, abnormal
- Transposition

of tooth, teeth

Impacted or embedded teeth with abnormal position of such teeth or adjacent teeth

◆ 524.4 Malocclusion, unspecified

524.5 Dentofacial functional abnormalities
- Abnormal jaw closure
- Malocclusion due to:
  - abnormal swallowing
  - mouth breathing
  - tongue, lip, or finger habits

● 524.6 Temporomandibular joint disorders
EXCLUDES current temporomandibular joint:
dislocation (830.0-830.1)
strain (848.1)

- ◆ 524.60 Temporomandibular joint disorders, unspecified
  Temporomandibular joint-pain-dysfunction syndrome [TMJ]
- 524.61 Adhesions and ankylosis (bony or fibrous)
- 524.62 Arthralgia of temporomandibular joint
- 524.63 Articular disc disorder (reducing or non-reducing)
- ◆ 524.69 Other specified temporomandibular joint disorders

● 524.7 Dental alveolar anomalies
- ◆ 524.70 Unspecified alveolar anomaly
- 524.71 Alveolar maxillary hyperplasia
- 524.72 Alveolar mandibular hyperplasia
- 524.73 Alveolar maxillary hypoplasia
- 524.74 Alveolar mandibular hypoplasia
- ◆ 524.79 Other specified alveolar anomaly

◆ 524.8 Other specified dentofacial anomalies
◆ 524.9 Unspecified dentofacial anomalies

● 525 Other diseases and conditions of the teeth and supporting structures

525.0 Exfoliation of teeth due to systemic causes
525.1 Loss of teeth due to accident, extraction, or local periodontal disease
Acquired absence of teeth

525.2 Atrophy of edentulous alveolar ridge
525.3 Retained dental root
525.8 Other specified disorders of the teeth and supporting structures
- Enlargement of alveolar ridge NOS
- Irregular alveolar process

◆ 525.9 Unspecified disorder of the teeth and supporting structures

● 526 Diseases of the jaws

526.0 Developmental odontogenic cysts
Cyst:
- dentigerous
- eruption
- follicular
- lateral developmental

Cyst:
- lateral periodontal
- primordial
- Keratocyst

EXCLUDES radicular cyst (522.8)

526.1 Fissural cysts of jaw
Cyst:
- globulomaxillary
- incisor canal
- median anterior maxillary

Cyst:
- median palatal
- nasopalatine
- palatine of papilla

EXCLUDES cysts of oral soft tissues (528.4)

- **526.2** **Other cysts of jaws**
  - Cyst of jaw:
    - NOS
    - aneurysmal
  - Cyst of jaw:
    - hemorrhagic
    - traumatic
- **526.3** **Central giant cell (reparative) granuloma**
  - **EXCLUDES** peripheral giant cell granuloma (523.8)
- **526.4** **Inflammatory conditions**
  - Abscess
  - Osteitis
  - Osteomyelitis (neonatal)
  - Periostitis
  } of jaw (acute) (chronic) (suppurative)
  - Sequestrum of jaw bone
  - **EXCLUDES** alveolar osteitis (526.5)
- **526.5** **Alveolitis of jaw**
  - Alveolar osteitis
  - Dry socket
- **526.8** **Other specified diseases of the jaws**
  - **526.81** Exostosis of jaw
    - Torus mandibularis
    - Torus palatinus
  - **526.89** Other
    - Cherubism
    - Fibrous dysplasia
    - Latent bone cyst
    - Osteoradionecrosis
    } of jaw(s)
    - Unilateral condylar hyperplasia or hypoplasia of mandible
- **526.9** **Unspecified disease of the jaws**
- **527** **Diseases of the salivary glands**
  - **527.0** Atrophy
  - **527.1** Hypertrophy
  - **527.2** Sialoadenitis
    - Parotitis:
      - NOS
      - allergic
      - toxic
    - Sialoangitis
    - Sialodochitis
    - **EXCLUDES** epidemic or infectious parotitis (072.0-072.9)
      - uveoparotid fever (135)
  - **527.3** Abscess
  - **527.4** Fistula
    - **EXCLUDES** congenital fistula of salivary gland (750.24)
  - **527.5** Sialolithiasis
    - Calculus
    - Stone
    } of salivary gland or duct
    - Sialodocholithiasis
  - **527.6** Mucocele
    - Mucous:
      - extravasation cyst of salivary gland
      - retention cyst of salivary gland
    - Ranula
  - **527.7** Disturbance of salivary secretion
    - Hyposecretion
    - Ptyalism
    - Sialorrhea
    - Xerostomia
  - **527.8** Other specified diseases of the salivary glands
    - Benign lymphoepithelial lesion of salivary gland
    - Sialectasia
    - Sialosis
    - Stenosis
    - Stricture
    } of salivary duct
  - **527.9** Unspecified disease of the salivary glands
- **528** **Diseases of the oral soft tissues, excluding lesions specific for gingiva and tongue**
  - **528.0** Stomatitis
    - Stomatitis:
      - NOS
      - ulcerative
    - Vesicular stomatitis
    - **EXCLUDES** stomatitis:
      - acute necrotizing ulcerative (101)
      - aphthous (528.2)
      - gangrenous (528.1)
      - herpetic (054.2)
      - Vincent's (101)
  - **528.1** Cancrum oris
    - Gangrenous stomatitis
    - Noma
  - **528.2** Oral aphthae
    - Aphthous stomatitis
    - Canker sore
    - Periadenitis mucosa necrotica recurrens
    - Recurrent aphthous ulcer
    - Stomatitis herpetiformis
    - **EXCLUDES** herpetic stomatitis (054.2)
  - **528.3** Cellulitis and abscess
    - Cellulitis of mouth (floor)
    - Ludwig's angina
    - Oral fistula
    - **EXCLUDES** abscess of tongue (529.0)
      - cellulitis or abscess of lip (528.5)
      - fistula (of):
        - dental (522.7)
        - lip (528.5)
      - gingivitis (523.0-523.1)
  - **528.4** Cysts
    - Dermoid cyst
    - Epidermoid cyst
    - Epstein's pearl
    - Lymphoepithelial cyst
    - Nasoalveolar cyst
    - Nasolabial cyst
    } of mouth
    - **EXCLUDES** cyst:
      - gingiva (523.8)
      - tongue (529.8)
  - **528.5** Diseases of lips
    - Abscess
    - Cellulitis
    - Fistula
    - Hypertrophy
    } of lip(s)
    - Cheilitis:
      - NOS
      - angular
    - Cheilodynia
    - Cheilosis
    - **EXCLUDES** actinic cheilitis (692.79)
      - congenital fistula of lip (750.25)
      - leukoplakia of lips (528.6)
  - **528.6** Leukoplakia of oral mucosa, including tongue
    - Leukokeratosis of oral mucosa
    - Leukoplakia of:
      - gingiva
      - lips
      - tongue
    - **EXCLUDES** carcinoma in situ (230.0, 232.0)
      - leukokeratosis nicotina palati (528.7)
  - **528.7** Other disturbances of oral epithelium, including tongue
    - Erythroplakia
    - Focal epithelial hyperplasia
    - Leukoedema
    } of mouth or tongue
    - Leukokeratosis nicotina palati
    - **EXCLUDES** carcinoma in situ (230.0, 232.0)
      - leukokeratosis NOS (702)
  - **528.8** Oral submucosal fibrosis, including of tongue
  - **528.9** Other and unspecified diseases of the oral soft tissues
    - Cheek and lip biting
    - Denture sore mouth
    - Denture stomatitis
    - Melanoplakia
    - Papillary hyperplasia of palate
    - Eosinophilic granuloma
    - Irritative hyperplasia
    - Pyogenic granuloma
    - Ulcer (traumatic)
    } of oral mucosa

- **529 Diseases and other conditions of the tongue**
  - **529.0 Glossitis**
    - Abscess } of tongue
    - Ulceration (traumatic) } of tongue
    - EXCLUDES glossitis:
      - benign migratory (529.1)
      - Hunter's (529.4)
      - median rhomboid (529.2)
      - Moeller's (529.4)
  - **529.1 Geographic tongue**
    - Benign migratory glossitis
    - Glossitis areata exfoliativa
  - **529.2 Median rhomboid glossitis**
  - **529.3 Hypertrophy of tongue papillae**
    - Black hairy tongue
    - Coated tongue
    - Hypertrophy of foliate papillae
    - Lingua villosa nigra
  - **529.4 Atrophy of tongue papillae**
    - Bald tongue
    - Glazed tongue
    - Glossitis:
      - Hunter's
      - Moeller's
    - Glossodynia exfoliativa
    - Smooth atrophic tongue
  - **529.5 Plicated tongue**
    - Fissured } tongue
    - Furrowed } tongue
    - Scrotal } tongue
    - EXCLUDES fissure of tongue, congenital (750.13)
  - **529.6 Glossodynia**
    - Glossopyrosis
    - Painful tongue
    - EXCLUDES glossodynia exfoliativa (529.4)
  - ◆ **529.8 Other specified conditions of the tongue**
    - Atrophy
    - Crenated
    - Enlargement } (of) tongue
    - Hypertrophy
    - Glossocele
    - Glossoptosis
    - EXCLUDES erythroplasia of tongue (528.7)
      - leukoplakia of tongue (528.6)
      - macroglossia (congenital) (750.15)
      - microglossia (congenital) (750.16)
      - oral submucosal fibrosis (528.8)
  - ◆ **529.9 Unspecified condition of the tongue**

DISEASES OF ESOPHAGUS, STOMACH, AND DUODENUM (530-537)

- **530 Diseases of esophagus**
  - EXCLUDES esophageal varices (456.0-456.2)
  - **530.0 Achalasia and cardiospasm**
    - Achalasia (of cardia)
    - Aperistalsis of esophagus
    - Megaesophagus
    - EXCLUDES congenital cardiospasm (750.7)
  - **530.1 Esophagitis**
    - Abscess of esophagus
    - Esophagitis:
      - NOS
      - chemical
    - Esophagitis:
      - peptic
      - postoperative
      - regurgitant
    - Use additional E code, if desired, to identify cause, if induced by chemical
    - EXCLUDES tuberculous esophagitis (017.8)
    - ◆ **530.10 Esophagitis, unspecified**
    - **530.11 Reflux esophagitis**
    - ◆ **530.19 Other esophagitis**
  - **530.2 Ulcer of esophagus**
    - Ulcer of esophagus
      - fungal
      - peptic
    - Ulcer of esophagus due to ingestion of:
      - aspirin
      - chemicals
      - medicines
    - Use additional E code, if desired, to identify cause, if induced by chemical or drug
  - **530.3 Stricture and stenosis of esophagus**
    - Compression of esophagus
    - Obstruction of esophagus
    - EXCLUDES congenital stricture of esophagus (750.3)
  - **530.4 Perforation of esophagus**
    - Rupture of esophagus
    - EXCLUDES traumatic perforation of esophagus (862.22, 862.32, 874.4-874.5)
  - **530.5 Dyskinesia of esophagus**
    - Corkscrew esophagus
    - Curling esophagus
    - Esophagospasm
    - Spasm of esophagus
    - EXCLUDES cardiospasm (530.0)
  - **530.6 Diverticulum of esophagus, acquired**
    - Diverticulum, acquired:
      - epiphrenic
      - pharyngoesophageal
      - pulsion
      - subdiaphragmatic
    - Diverticulum, acquired:
      - traction
      - Zenker's (hypopharyngeal)
    - Esophageal pouch, acquired
    - Esophagocele, acquired
    - EXCLUDES congenital diverticulum of esophagus (750.4)
  - **530.7 Gastroesophageal laceration-hemorrhage syndrome**
    - Mallory-Weiss syndrome
  - **530.8 Other specified disorders of esophagus**
    - **530.81 Esophageal reflux**
      - Gastroesophageal reflux
      - EXCLUDES reflux esophagitis (530.11)
    - **530.82 Esophageal hemorrhage**
      - EXCLUDES hemorrhage due to esophageal varices (456.0-456.2)
    - **530.83 Esophageal leukoplakia**
    - **530.84 Tracheoesophageal fistula**
      - EXCLUDES congenital tracheoesophageal fistula (750.3)
    - ◆ **530.89 Other**
      - EXCLUDES Paterson-Kelly syndrome (280.8)
  - ◆ **530.9 Unspecified disorder of esophagus**
- **531 Gastric ulcer**
  - INCLUDES ulcer (peptic):
    - prepyloric
    - pylorus
    - stomach
  - Use additional E code, if desired, to identify drug, if drug-induced
  - EXCLUDES peptic ulcer NOS (533.0-533.9)
  - The following fifth-digit subclassification is for use with category 531:
    - 0 without mention of obstruction
    - 1 with obstruction
  - **531.0 Acute with hemorrhage**
  - **531.1 Acute with perforation**
  - **531.2 Acute with hemorrhage and perforation**
  - **531.3 Acute without mention of hemorrhage or perforation**
  - **531.4 Chronic or unspecified with hemorrhage**
  - **531.5 Chronic or unspecified with perforation**
  - **531.6 Chronic or unspecified with hemorrhage and perforation**
  - **531.7 Chronic without mention of hemorrhage or perforation**
  - ◆ **531.9 Unspecified as acute or chronic, without mention of hemorrhage or perforation**
- **532 Duodenal ulcer**
  - INCLUDES erosion (acute) of duodenum
    - ulcer (peptic):
      - duodenum
      - postpyloric
  - Use additional E code, if desired, to identify drug, if drug-induced
  - EXCLUDES peptic ulcer NOS (533.0-533.9)
  - The following fifth-digit subclassification is for use with category 532:
    - 0 without mention of obstruction
    - 1 with obstruction
  - **532.0 Acute with hemorrhage**
  - **532.1 Acute with perforation**
  - **532.2 Acute with hemorrhage and perforation**
  - **532.3 Acute without mention of hemorrhage or perforation**
  - **532.4 Chronic or unspecified with hemorrhage**
  - **532.5 Chronic or unspecified with perforation**
  - **532.6 Chronic or unspecified with hemorrhage and perforation**
  - **532.7 Chronic without mention of hemorrhage or perforation**
  - ◆ **532.9 Unspecified as acute or chronic, without mention of hemorrhage or perforation**

DIGESTIVE SYSTEM

● **533 Peptic ulcer, site unspecified**
  INCLUDES gastroduodenal ulcer NOS
  peptic ulcer NOS
  stress ulcer NOS
  Use additional E code, if desired, to identify drug, if drug-induced
  EXCLUDES peptic ulcer:
  duodenal (532.0-532.9)
  gastric (531.0-531.9)
  The following fifth-digit subclassification is for use with category 533:
  0 without mention of obstruction
  1 with obstruction
  ● 533.0 Acute with hemorrhage
  ● 533.1 Acute with perforation
  ● 533.2 Acute with hemorrhage and perforation
  ● 533.3 Acute without mention of hemorrhage and perforation
  ● 533.4 Chronic or unspecified with hemorrhage
  ● 533.5 Chronic or unspecified with perforation
  ● 533.6 Chronic or unspecified with hemorrhage and perforation
  ● 533.7 Chronic without mention of hemorrhage or perforation
  ◆● 533.9 Unspecified as acute or chronic, without mention of hemorrhage or perforation

● **534 Gastrojejunal ulcer**
  INCLUDES ulcer (peptic) or erosion:
  anastomotic
  gastrocolic
  gastrointestinal
  gastrojejunal
  jejunal
  marginal
  stomal
  EXCLUDES primary ulcer of small intestine (569.82)
  The following fifth-digit subclassification is for use with category 534:
  0 without mention of obstruction
  1 with obstruction
  ● 534.0 Acute with hemorrhage
  ● 534.1 Acute with perforation
  ● 534.2 Acute with hemorrhage and perforation
  ● 534.3 Acute without mention of hemorrhage or perforation
  ● 534.4 Chronic or unspecified with hemorrhage
  ● 534.5 Chronic or unspecified with perforation
  ● 534.6 Chronic or unspecified with hemorrhage and perforation
  ● 534.7 Chronic without mention of hemorrhage or perforation
  ◆● 534.9 Unspecified as acute or chronic, without mention of hemorrhage or perforation

● **535 Gastritis and duodenitis**
  The following fifth-digit subclassification is for use with category 535
  0 without mention of hemorrhage
  1 with hemorrhage
  ● 535.0 Acute gastritis
  ● 535.1 Atrophic gastritis
  Gastritis:
  atrophic-hyperplastic
  Gastritis:
  chronic (atrophic)
  ● 535.2 Gastric mucosal hypertrophy
  Hypertrophic gastritis
  ● 535.3 Alcoholic gastritis
  ◆● 535.4 Other specified gastritis
  Erosion:
  gastric
  pylorus
  stomach
  Gastritis:
  allergic
  Gastritis:
  bile induced
  irritant
  superficial
  toxic
  ◆● 535.5 Unspecified gastritis and gastroduodenitis
  ● 535.6 Duodenitis

● **536 Disorders of function of stomach**
  EXCLUDES functional disorders of stomach specified as psychogenic (306.4)
  536.0 Achlorhydria
  536.1 Acute dilatation of stomach
  Acute distention of stomach
  536.2 Persistent vomiting
  Habit vomiting
  Persistent vomiting [not of pregnancy]
  Uncontrollable vomiting
  EXCLUDES excessive vomiting in pregnancy (643.0-643.9)
  vomiting NOS (787.0)
  536.3 Gastroparesis ◆
  ◆ 536.8 Dyspepsia and other specified disorders of function of stomach
  Achylia gastrica
  Hourglass contraction of stomach
  Hyperacidity
  Hyperchlorhydria
  Hypochlorhydria
  Indigestion
  EXCLUDES achlorhydria (536.0)
  heartburn (787.1)
  ◆ 536.9 Unspecified functional disorder of stomach
  Functional gastrointestinal:
  disorder
  disturbance
  Functional gastrointestinal:
  irritation

● **537 Other disorders of stomach and duodenum**
  537.0 Acquired hypertrophic pyloric stenosis
  Constriction
  Obstruction
  Stricture
  } of pylorus, acquired or adult
  EXCLUDES congenital or infantile pyloric stenosis (750.5)
  537.1 Gastric diverticulum
  EXCLUDES congenital diverticulum of stomach (750.7)
  537.2 Chronic duodenal ileus
  ◆ 537.3 Other obstruction of duodenum
  Cicatrix
  Stenosis
  Stricture
  Volvulus
  } of duodenum
  EXCLUDES congenital obstruction of duodenum (751.1)
  537.4 Fistula of stomach or duodenum
  Gastrocolic fistula Gastrojejunocolic fistula
  537.5 Gastroptosis
  537.6 Hourglass stricture or stenosis of stomach
  Cascade stomach
  EXCLUDES congenital hourglass stomach (750.7)
  hourglass contraction of stomach (536.8)
  ● 537.8 Other specified disorders of stomach and duodenum
  537.81 Pylorospasm
  EXCLUDES congenital pylorospasm (750.5)
  537.82 Angiodysplasia of stomach and duodenum (without mention of hemorrhage)
  537.83 Angiodysplasia of stomach and duodenum with hemorrhage
  ◆ 537.89 Other
  Gastric or duodenal:
  prolapse
  rupture
  Intestinal metaplasia of gastric mucosa
  Passive congestion of stomach
  EXCLUDES diverticula of duodenum (562.00-562.01)
  gastrointestinal hemorrhage (578.0-578.9)
  ◆ 537.9 Unspecified disorder of stomach and duodenum

APPENDICITIS (540-543)

● **540 Acute appendicitis**
  540.0 With generalized peritonitis
  EXCLUDES acute appendicitis with peritoneal abscess (540.1) ◆
  Appendicitis (acute):
  fulminating
  gangrenous
  obstructive
  Cecitis (acute)
  } with:
  perforation
  peritonitis (generalized)
  rupture
  Rupture of appendix
  540.1 With peritoneal abscess ◆
  with generalized peritonitis
  Abscess of appendix
  540.9 Without mention of peritonitis
  Acute:
  appendicitis:
  fulminating
  gangrenous
  inflamed
  obstructive
  cecitis
  } without mention of perforation, peritonitis, or rupture

● Additional digits required ◆ Nonspecific code ▌ Not a primary diagnosis

- **541** Appendicitis, unqualified
- **542** Other appendicitis
  - Appendicitis:
    - chronic
    - recurrent
    - relapsing
    - subacute
  - **EXCLUDES** hyperplasia (lymphoid) of appendix (543.0)
- **543** Other diseases of appendix
  - **543.0** Hyperplasia of appendix (lymphoid)
  - **543.9** Other and unspecified diseases of appendix
    - Appendicular or appendiceal:
      - colic
      - concretion
      - fistula
    - Diverticulum } of appendix
    - Fecalith
    - Intussusception
    - Mucocele
    - Stercolith

HERNIA OF ABDOMINAL CAVITY (550-553)

INCLUDES hernia:
- acquired
- congenital, except diaphragmatic or hiatal

- **550** Inguinal hernia
  - **INCLUDES** bubonocele
    - inguinal hernia (direct) (double) (indirect) (oblique) (sliding)
    - scrotal hernia
  - The following fifth-digit subclassification is for use with category 550:
    - **0** unilateral or unspecified (not specified as recurrent)
      - Unilateral NOS
    - **1** unilateral or unspecified, recurrent
    - **2** bilateral (not specified as recurrent)
      - Bilateral NOS
    - **3** bilateral, recurrent
  - **550.0** Inguinal hernia, with gangrene
    - Inguinal hernia with gangrene (and obstruction)
  - **550.1** Inguinal hernia, with obstruction, without mention of gangrene
    - Inguinal hernia with mention of incarceration, irreducibility, or strangulation
  - **550.9** Inguinal hernia, without mention of obstruction or gangrene
    - Inguinal hernia NOS
- **551** Other hernia of abdominal cavity, with gangrene
  - **INCLUDES** that with gangrene (and obstruction)
  - **551.0** Femoral hernia with gangrene
    - **551.00** Unilateral or unspecified (not specified as recurrent)
      - Femoral hernia NOS with gangrene
    - **551.01** Unilateral or unspecified, recurrent
    - **551.02** Bilateral (not specified as recurrent)
    - **551.03** Bilateral, recurrent
  - **551.1** Umbilical hernia with gangrene
    - Parumbilical hernia specified as gangrenous
  - **551.2** Ventral hernia with gangrene
    - **551.20** Ventral, unspecified, with gangrene
    - **551.21** Incisional, with gangrene
      - Hernia:
        - postoperative } specified as gangrenous
        - recurrent, ventral
    - **551.29** Other
      - Epigastric hernia specified as gangrenous
  - **551.3** Diaphragmatic hernia with gangrene
    - Hernia:
      - hiatal (esophageal)
      - (sliding)
      - paraesophageal
      - Thoracic stomach } specified as gangrenous
    - **EXCLUDES** congenital diaphragmatic hernia (756.6)
  - **551.8** Hernia of other specified sites, with gangrene
    - Any condition classifiable to 553.8 if specified as gangrenous
  - **551.9** Hernia of unspecified site, with gangrene
    - Any condition classifiable to 553.9 if specified as gangrenous

- **552** Other hernia of abdominal cavity, with obstruction, but without mention of gangrene
  - **EXCLUDES** that with mention of gangrene (551.0-551.9)
  - **552.0** Femoral hernia with obstruction
    - Femoral hernia specified as incarcerated, irreducible, strangulated, or causing obstruction
    - **552.00** Unilateral or unspecified (not specified as recurrent)
    - **552.01** Unilateral or unspecified, recurrent
    - **552.02** Bilateral (not specified as recurrent)
    - **552.03** Bilateral, recurrent
  - **552.1** Umbilical hernia with obstruction
    - Parumbilical hernia specified as incarcerated, irreducible, strangulated, or causing obstruction
  - **552.2** Ventral hernia with obstruction
    - Ventral hernia specified as incarcerated, irreducible, strangulated, or causing obstruction
    - **552.20** Ventral, unspecified, with obstruction
    - **552.21** Incisional, with obstruction
      - Hernia:
        - postoperative
        - recurrent,
        - ventral
      - } specified as incarcerated, irreducible, strangulated, or causing obstruction
    - **552.29** Other
      - Epigastric hernia specified as incarcerated, irreducible, strangulated, or causing obstruction
  - **552.3** Diaphragmatic hernia with obstruction
    - Hernia:
      - hiatal (esophageal)
      - (sliding)
      - paraesophageal
      - Thoracic stomach
      - } specified as incarcerated, irreducible, strangulated, or causing obstruction
    - **EXCLUDES** congenital diaphragmatic hernia (756.6)
  - **552.8** Hernia of other specified sites, with obstruction
    - Any condition classifiable to 553.8 if specified as incarcerated, irreducible, strangulated, or causing obstruction
  - **552.9** Hernia of unspecified site, with obstruction
    - Any condition classifiable to 553.9 if specified as incarcerated, irreducible, strangulated, or causing obstruction
- **553** Other hernia of abdominal cavity without mention of obstruction or gangrene
  - **EXCLUDES** the listed conditions with mention of:
    - gangrene (and obstruction) (551.0-551.9)
    - obstruction (552.0-552.9)
  - **553.0** Femoral hernia
    - **553.00** Unilateral or unspecified (not specified as recurrent)
      - Femoral hernia NOS
    - **553.01** Unilateral or unspecified, recurrent
    - **553.02** Bilateral (not specified as recurrent)
    - **553.03** Bilateral, recurrent
  - **553.1** Umbilical hernia
    - Parumbilical hernia
  - **553.2** Ventral hernia
    - **553.20** Ventral, unspecified
    - **553.21** Incisional
      - Hernia:
        - postoperative
        - recurrent, ventral
    - **553.29** Other
      - Hernia:
        - epigastric
        - spigelian
  - **553.3** Diaphragmatic hernia
    - Hernia:
      - hiatal (esophageal) (sliding)
      - paraesophageal
      - Thoracic stomach
    - **EXCLUDES** congenital:
      - diaphragmatic hernia (756.6)
      - hiatal hernia (750.6)
      - esophagocele (530.6)

DIGESTIVE SYSTEM

- ◆ **553.8 Hernia of other specified sites**
  - Hernia:
    - ischiatic
    - ischiorectal
    - lumbar
    - obturator
    - pudendal
  - Hernia:
    - retroperitoneal
    - sciatic
  - Other abdominal hernia of specified site
  - **EXCLUDES** vaginal enterocele (618.6)
- ◆ **553.9 Hernia of unspecified site**
  - Enterocele
  - Epiplocele
  - Hernia:
    - NOS
    - interstitial
  - Hernia:
    - intestinal
    - intra-abdominal
  - Rupture (nontraumatic)
  - Sarcoepiplocele

NONINFECTIOUS ENTERITIS AND COLITIS (555-558)

- ● **555 Regional enteritis**
  - **INCLUDES** Crohn's disease
  - Granulomatous enteritis
  - **EXCLUDES** ulcerative colitis (556)
  - **555.0 Small intestine**
    - Ileitis:
      - regional
      - segmental
      - terminal
    - Regional enteritis or Crohn's disease of:
      - duodenum
      - ileum
      - jejunum
  - **555.1 Large intestine**
    - Colitis:
      - granulmatous
      - regional
      - transmural
    - Regional enteritis or Crohn's disease of:
      - colon
      - large bowel
      - rectum
  - **555.2 Small intestine with large intestine**
    - Regional ileocolitis
  - ◆ **555.9 Unspecified site**
    - Crohn's disease NOS   Regional enteritis NOS
- ● **556 Ulcerative colitis**
  - **556.0 Ulcerative (chronic) enterocolitis**
  - **556.1 Ulcerative (chronic) ileocolitis**
  - **556.2 Ulcerative (chronic) proctitis**
  - **556.3 Ulcerative (chronic) proctosigmoiditis**
  - **556.4 Pseudopolyposis of colon**
  - **556.5 Left-sided ulcerative (chronic) colitis**
  - **556.6 Universal ulcerative (chronic) colitis**
    - Pancolitis
  - ◆ **556.8 Other ulcerative colitis**
  - ◆ **556.9 Ulcerative colitis, unspecified**
    - Ulcerative enteritis NOS
- ● **557 Vascular insufficiency of intestine**
  - **EXCLUDES** necrotizing enterocolitis of the newborn (777.5)
  - **557.0 Acute vascular insufficiency of intestine**
    - Acute:
      - hemorrhagic enterocolitis
      - ischemic colitis, enteritis, or enterocolitis
      - massive necrosis of intestine
    - Bowel infarction
    - Embolism of mesenteric artery
    - Fulminant enterocolitis
    - Hemorrhagic necrosis of intestine
    - Intestinal gangrene
    - Intestinal infarction (acute) (agnogenic) (hemorrhagic) (nonocclusive)
    - Mesenteric infarction (embolic) (thrombotic)
    - Terminal hemorrhagic enteropathy
    - Thrombosis of mesenteric artery
  - **557.1 Chronic vascular insufficiency of intestine**
    - Angina, abdominal
    - Chronic ischemic colitis, enteritis, or enterocolitis
    - Ischemic stricture of intestine
    - Mesenteric:
      - angina
      - artery syndrome (superior)
      - vascular insufficiency
  - ◆ **557.9 Unspecified vascular insufficiency of intestine**
    - Alimentary pain due to vascular insufficiency
    - Ischemic colitis, enteritis, or enterocolitis NOS

- ● **558 Other noninfectious gastroenteritis and colitis**
  - **EXCLUDES** infectious:
    - colitis, enteritis, or gastroenteritis (009.0-009.1)
    - diarrhea (009.2-009.3)
  - **558.1 Gastroenteritis and colitis due to radiation**
    - Radiation enterocolitis
  - **558.2 Toxic gastroenteritis and colitis**
    - Use additional E code, if desired, to identify cause
  - ◆ **558.9 Other and unspecified noninfectious gastroenteritis and colitis**
    - Colitis
    - Diarrhea
    - Enteritis
    - Gastroenteritis   } NOS, allergic, dietetic, or noninfectious
    - Ileitis
    - Jejunitis
    - Sigmoiditis

OTHER DISEASES OF INTESTINES AND PERITONEUM (560-569)

- ● **560 Intestinal obstruction without mention of hernia**
  - **EXCLUDES** duodenum (537.2-537.3)
    - inguinal hernia with obstruction (550.1)
    - intestinal obstruction complicating hernia (552.0-552.9)
    - mesenteric:
      - embolism (557.0)
      - infarction (557.0)
      - thrombosis (557.0)
    - neonatal intestinal obstruction (277.01, 777.1-777.2, 777.4)
  - **560.0 Intussusception**
    - Intussusception (colon) (intestine) (rectum)
    - Invagination of intestine or colon
    - **EXCLUDES** intussusception of appendix (543.9)
  - **560.1 Paralytic ileus**
    - Adynamic ileus
    - Ileus (of intestine) (of bowel) (of colon)
    - Paralysis of intestine or colon
    - **EXCLUDES** gallstone ileus (560.31)
  - **560.2 Volvulus**
    - Knotting
    - Strangulation
    - Torsion   } of intestine, bowel, or colon
    - Twist
  - ● **560.3 Impaction of intestine**
    - ◆ **560.30 Impaction of intestine, unspecified**
      - Impaction of colon
    - **560.31 Gallstone ileus**
      - Obstruction of intestine by gallstone
    - ◆ **560.39 Other**
      - Concretion of intestine   Fecal impaction
      - Enterolith
  - ● **560.8 Other specified intestinal obstruction**
    - **560.81 Intestinal or peritoneal adhesions with obstruction**
      - **EXCLUDES** adhesions without obstruction (568.0)
    - ◆ **560.89 Other**
      - Mural thickening causing obstruction
      - **EXCLUDES** ischemic stricture of intestine (557.1)
  - ◆ **560.9 Unspecified intestinal obstruction**
    - Enterostenosis
    - Obstruction
    - Occlusion
    - Stenosis   } of intestine or colon
    - Stricture
    - **EXCLUDES** congenital stricture or stenosis of intestine (751.1-751.2)
- ● **562 Diverticula of intestine**
  - Use additional code, if desired, to identify any associated: peritonitis (567.0-567.9)
  - **EXCLUDES** congenital diverticulum of colon (751.5)
    - diverticulum of appendix (543.9)
    - Meckel's diverticulum (751.0)

562.0 TABULAR LIST 569.0

- **562.0 Small intestine**
  - **562.00 Diverticulosis of small intestine (without mention of hemorrhage)**
    Diverticulosis:
    - duodenum ⎫
    - ileum   ⎬ without mention of diverticulitis
    - jejunum ⎭
  - **562.01 Diverticulitis of small intestine (without mention of hemorrhage)**
    Diverticulitis (with diverticulosis):
    - duodenum
    - ileum
    - jejunum
    - small intestine
  - **562.02 Diverticulosis of small intestine with hemorrhage**
  - **562.03 Diverticulitis of small intestine with hemorrhage**
- **562.1 Colon**
  - **562.10 Diverticulosis of colon (without mention of hemorrhage)**
    Diverticulosis:
    - NOS ⎫
    - intestine (large) ⎬ without mention of diverticulitis
    - Diverticular disease (colon) ⎭
  - **562.11 Diverticulitis of colon (without mention of hemorrhage)**
    Diverticulitis (with diverticulosis):
    - NOS
    - colon
    - intestine (large)
  - **562.12 Diverticulosis of colon with hemorrhage**
  - **562.13 Diverticulitis of colon with hemorrhage**

- **564 Functional digestive disorders, not elsewhere classified**
  - **EXCLUDES** functional disorders of stomach (536.0-536.9)
    those specified as psychogenic (306.4)
  - **564.0 Constipation**
  - **564.1 Irritable colon**
    - Colitis:
      - adaptive
      - membranous
      - mucous
    - Enterospasm
    - Irritable bowel syndrome
    - Spastic colon
  - **564.2 Postgastric surgery syndromes**
    - Dumping syndrome
    - Jejunal syndrome
    - Postgastrectomy syndrome
    - Postvagotomy syndrome
    - **EXCLUDES** malnutrition following gastrointestinal surgery (579.3)
      postgastrojejunostomy ulcer (534.0-534.9)
  - **564.3 Vomiting following gastrointestinal surgery**
    Vomiting (bilious) following gastrointestinal surgery
  - **564.4 Other postoperative functional disorders**
    Diarrhea following gastrointestinal surgery
    - **EXCLUDES** colostomy and enterostomy malfunction (569.6)
  - **564.5 Functional diarrhea**
    - **EXCLUDES** diarrhea:
      - NOS (558.9)
      - psychogenic (306.4)
  - **564.6 Anal spasm**
    Proctalgia fugax
  - **564.7 Megacolon, other than Hirschsprung's**
    Dilatation of colon
    - **EXCLUDES** megacolon:
      - congenital [Hirschsprung's] (751.3)
      - toxic (556)
  - **564.8 Other specified functional disorders of intestine**
    Atony of colon
    - **EXCLUDES** malabsorption (579.0-579.9)
  - **564.9 Unspecified functional disorder of intestine**

- **565 Anal fissure and fistula**
  - **565.0 Anal fissure**
    Tear of anus, nontraumatic
    - **EXCLUDES** traumatic (863.89, 863.99)
  - **565.1 Anal fistula**
    Fistula:
    - anorectal
    - rectal
    - rectum to skin
    - **EXCLUDES** fistula of rectum to internal organs—see Alphabetic Index
      ischiorectal fistula (566)
      rectovaginal fistula (619.1)

- **566 Abscess of anal and rectal regions**
  - Abscess:
    - ischiorectal
    - perianal
    - perirectal
  - Cellulitis:
    - anal
  - Cellulitis:
    - perirectal
    - rectal
  - Ischiorectal fistula

- **567 Peritonitis**
  - **EXCLUDES** peritonitis:
    - benign paroxysmal (277.3)
    - pelvic, female (614.5, 614.7)
    - periodic familial (277.3)
    - puerperal (670)
    - with or following:
      - abortion (634-638 with .0, 639.0)
      - appendicitis (540.0-540.1)
      - ectopic or molar pregnancy (639.0)
  - **567.0 Peritonitis in infectious diseases classified elsewhere**
    Code also underlying disease
    - **EXCLUDES** peritonitis:
      - gonococcal (098.86)
      - syphilitic (095.2)
      - tuberculous (014.0)
  - **567.1 Pneumococcal peritonitis**
  - **567.2 Other suppurative peritonitis**
    - Abscess (of):
      - abdominopelvic
      - mesenteric
      - omentum
      - peritoneum
      - retrocecal
      - retroperitoneal
      - subdiaphragmatic
    - Abscess (of):
      - subhepatic
      - subphrenic
    - Peritonitis (acute):
      - general
      - pelvic, male
      - subphrenic
      - suppurative
  - **567.8 Other specified peritonitis**
    - Chronic proliferative peritonitis
    - Fat necrosis of peritoneum
    - Mesenteric saponification
    - Peritonitis due to:
      - bile
      - urine
    - **EXCLUDES** peritonitis (postoperative):
      - chemical (998.7)
      - due to talc (998.7)
  - **567.9 Unspecified peritonitis**
    Peritonitis:
    - NOS
    - of unspecified cause

- **568 Other disorders of peritoneum**
  - **568.0 Peritoneal adhesions**
    - Adhesions (of):
      - abdominal (wall)
      - diaphragm
      - intestine
      - male pelvis
    - Adhesions (of):
      - mesenteric
      - omentum
      - stomach
      - Adhesive bands
    - **EXCLUDES** adhesions:
      - pelvic, female (614.6)
      - with obstruction:
        - duodenum (537.3)
        - intestine (560.81)
  - **568.8 Other specified disorders of peritoneum**
    - **568.81 Hemoperitoneum (nontraumatic)**
    - **568.82 Peritoneal effusion (chronic)**
      - **EXCLUDES** ascites NOS (789.5)
    - **568.89 Other**
      Peritoneal:
      - cyst
      - granuloma
  - **568.9 Unspecified disorder of peritoneum**

- **569 Other disorders of intestine**
  - **569.0 Anal and rectal polyp**

DIGESTIVE SYSTEM

569.1 **Rectal prolapse**
  Procidentia:
    anus (sphincter)
    rectum (sphincter)
  Proctoptosis
  Prolapse:
    anal canal
    rectal mucosa
  EXCLUDES prolapsed hemorrhoids (455.2, 455.5)

569.2 **Stenosis of rectum and anus**
  Stricture of anus (sphincter)

569.3 **Hemorrhage of rectum and anus**
  EXCLUDES gastrointestinal bleeding NOS (578.9)
    melena (578.1)

● **569.4** **Other specified disorders of rectum and anus**
  569.41 **Ulcer of anus and rectum**
    Solitary ulcer } of anus (sphincter) or rectum (sphincter)
    Stercoral ulcer
  569.42 **Anal or rectal pain**
  ◆ **569.49** **Other**
    Granuloma } of rectum (sphincter)
    Rupture
    Hypertrophy of anal papillae
    Proctitis NOS
    EXCLUDES fistula of rectum to:
      internal organs—see Alphabetic Index
      skin (565.1)
      hemorrhoids (455.0-455.9)
      incontinence of sphincter ani (787.6)

569.5 **Abscess of intestine**
  EXCLUDES appendiceal abscess (540.1)

569.6 **Colostomy and enterostomy malfunction**

● **569.8** **Other specified disorders of intestine**
  569.81 **Fistula of intestine, excluding rectum and anus**
    Fistula:
      abdominal wall
      enterocolic
    Fistula:
      enteroenteric
      ileorectal
    EXCLUDES fistula of intestine to internal organs—see Alphabetic Index
      persistent postoperative fistula (998.6)
  569.82 **Ulceration of intestine**
    Primary ulcer of intestine
    Ulceration of colon
    EXCLUDES that with perforation (569.83)
  569.83 **Perforation of intestine**
  569.84 **Angiodysplasia of intestine (without mention of hemorrhage)**
  569.85 **Angiodysplasia of intestine with hemorrhage**
  ◆ **569.89** **Other**
    Enteroptosis
    Granuloma } of intestine
    Prolapse
    Pericolitis
    Perisigmoiditis
    Visceroptosis
    EXCLUDES gangrene of intestine, mesentery, or omentum (557.0)
      hemorrhage of intestine NOS (578.9)
      obstruction of intestine (560.0-560.9)

◆ **569.9** **Unspecified disorder of intestine**

OTHER DISEASES OF DIGESTIVE SYSTEM (570-579)

570 **Acute and subacute necrosis of liver**
  Acute hepatic failure
  Acute or subacute hepatitis, not specified as infective
  Necrosis of liver (acute) (diffuse) (massive) (subacute)
  Parenchymatous degeneration of liver
  Yellow atrophy (liver) (acute) (subacute)
  EXCLUDES icterus gravis of newborn (773.0-773.2)
    serum hepatitis (070.2-070.3)
    that with:
      abortion (634-638 with .7, 639.8)
      ectopic or molar pregnancy (639.8)
      pregnancy, childbirth, or the puerperium (646.7)
      viral hepatitis (070.0-070.9)

● **571** **Chronic liver disease and cirrhosis**
  571.0 **Alcoholic fatty liver**
  571.1 **Acute alcoholic hepatitis**
    Acute alcoholic liver disease
  571.2 **Alcoholic cirrhosis of liver**
    Florid cirrhosis
    Laennec's cirrhosis (alcoholic)
  ◆ **571.3** **Alcoholic liver damage, unspecified**
  ● **571.4** **Chronic hepatitis**
    EXCLUDES viral hepatitis (acute) (chronic) (070.0-070.9)
    ◆ **571.40** **Chronic hepatitis, unspecified**
    571.41 **Chronic persistent hepatitis**
    ◆ **571.49** **Other**
      Chronic hepatitis:
        active
        aggressive
      Recurrent hepatitis
  571.5 **Cirrhosis of liver without mention of alcohol**
    Cirrhosis of liver:
      NOS
      cryptogenic
      macronodular
      micronodular
      posthepatitic
    Cirrhosis of liver:
      postnecrotic
      Healed yellow atrophy (liver)
      Portal cirrhosis
  571.6 **Biliary cirrhosis**
    Chronic nonsuppurative destructive cholangitis
    Cirrhosis:
      cholangitic
      cholestatic
  ◆ **571.8** **Other chronic nonalcoholic liver disease**
    Chronic yellow atrophy (liver)
    Fatty liver, without mention of alcohol
  ◆ **571.9** **Unspecified chronic liver disease without mention of alcohol**

● **572** **Liver abscess and sequelae of chronic liver disease**
  572.0 **Abscess of liver**
    EXCLUDES amebic liver abscess (006.3)
  572.1 **Portal pyemia**
    Phlebitis of portal vein
    Portal thrombophlebitis
    Pylephlebitis
    Pylethrombophlebitis
  572.2 **Hepatic coma**
    Hepatic encephalopathy
    Hepatocerebral intoxication
    Portal-systemic encephalopathy
  572.3 **Portal hypertension**
  572.4 **Hepatorenal syndrome**
    EXCLUDES that following delivery (674.8)
  ◆ **572.8** **Other sequelae of chronic liver disease**

● **573** **Other disorders of liver**
  EXCLUDES amyloid or lardaceous degeneration of liver (277.3)
    congenital cystic disease of liver (751.62)
    glycogen infiltration of liver (271.0)
    hepatomegaly NOS (789.1)
    portal vein obstruction (452)
  573.0 **Chronic passive congestion of liver**
  ■ **573.1** **Hepatitis in viral diseases classified elsewhere**
    Code also underlying disease as:
      Coxsackie virus disease (074.8)
      cytomegalic inclusion virus disease (078.5)
      infectious mononucleosis (075)
    EXCLUDES hepatitis (in):
      mumps (072.71)
      viral (070.0-070.9)
      yellow fever (060.0-060.9)

● Additional digits required ◆ Nonspecific code ■ Not a primary diagnosis Volume 1 — 93

573.2 Hepatitis in other infectious diseases classified elsewhere
Code also underlying disease, as:
malaria (084.9)

EXCLUDES hepatitis in:
late syphilis (095.3)
secondary syphilis (091.62)
toxoplasmosis (130.5)

573.3 Hepatitis, unspecified
Toxic (noninfectious) hepatitis
Use additional E code, if desired, to identify cause

573.4 Hepatic infarction

573.8 Other specified disorders of liver
Hepatoptosis

573.9 Unspecified disorder of liver

574 Cholelithiasis
The following fifth-digit subclassification is for use with category 574:
0 without mention of obstruction
1 with obstruction

574.0 Calculus of gallbladder with acute cholecystitis
Biliary calculus
Calculus of cystic duct } with acute cholecystitis
Cholelithiasis
Any condition classifiable to 574.2 with acute cholecystitis

574.1 Calculus of gallbladder with other cholecystitis
Biliary calculus
Calculus of cystic duct } with cholecystitis
Cholelithiasis
Cholecystitis with cholelithiasis NOS
Any condition classifiable to 574.2 with cholecystitis (chronic)

574.2 Calculus of gallbladder without mention of cholecystitis
Biliary:
 calculus NOS
 colic NOS
 Calculus of cystic duct
Cholelithiasis NOS
Colic (recurrent) of gallbladder
Gallstone (impacted)

574.3 Calculus of bile duct with acute cholecystitis
Calculus of bile duct [any]
Choledocholithiasis } with acute cholecystitis
Any condition classifiable to 574.5 with acute cholecystitis

574.4 Calculus of bile duct with other cholecystitis
Calculus of bile duct [any]
Choledocholithiasis } with cholecystitis (chronic)
Any condition classifiable to 574.5 with cholecystitis (chronic)

574.5 Calculus of bile duct without mention of cholecystitis
Calculus of:
 bile duct [any]
 common duct
 hepatic duct
Choledocholithiasis
Hepatic:
 colic (recurrent)
 lithiasis

575 Other disorders of gallbladder

575.0 Acute cholecystitis
Abscess of gallbladder
Angiocholecystitis
Cholecystitis:
 emphysematous (acute)
 gangrenous
 suppurative
Empyema of gallbladder
Gangrene of gallbladder
} without mention of calculus

EXCLUDES that with:
choledocholithiasis (574.3)
cholelithiasis (574.0)

575.1 Other cholecystitis
Cholecystitis:
 NOS
 chronic
} without mention of calculus

EXCLUDES that with:
choledocholithiasis (574.4)
cholelithiasis (574.1)

575.2 Obstruction of gallbladder
Occlusion
Stenosis
Stricture
} of cystic duct or gallbladder without mention of calculus

EXCLUDES that with calculus (574.0-574.2 with fifth-digit 1)

575.3 Hydrops of gallbladder
Mucocele of gallbladder

575.4 Perforation of gallbladder
Rupture of cystic duct or gallbladder

575.5 Fistula of gallbladder
Fistula:
 cholecystoduodenal
 cholecystoenteric

575.6 Cholesterolosis of gallbladder
Strawberry gallbladder

575.8 Other specified disorders of gallbladder
Adhesions
Atrophy
Cyst
Hypertrophy
Nonfunctioning
Ulcer
} (of) cystic duct or gallbladder

Biliary dyskinesia

EXCLUDES nonvisualization of gallbladder (793.3)

575.9 Unspecified disorder of gallbladder

576 Other disorders of biliary tract

EXCLUDES that involving the:
cystic duct (575.0-575.9)
gallbladder (575.0-575.9)

576.0 Postcholecystectomy syndrome

576.1 Cholangitis
Cholangitis:
 NOS
 acute
 ascending
 chronic
 primary
Cholangitis:
 recurrent
 sclerosing
 secondary
 stenosing
 suppurative

576.2 Obstruction of bile duct
Occlusion
Stenosis
Stricture
} of bile duct, except cystic duct, without mention of calculus

EXCLUDES congenital (751.61)
that with calculus (574.3-574.5 with fifth-digit 1)

576.3 Perforation of bile duct
Rupture of bile duct, except cystic duct

576.4 Fistula of bile duct
Choledochoduodenal fistula

576.5 Spasm of sphincter of Oddi

576.8 Other specified disorders of biliary tract
Adhesions
Atrophy
Cyst
Hypertrophy
Stasis
Ulcer
} of bile duct [any]

EXCLUDES congenital choledochal cyst (751.69)

576.9 Unspecified disorder of biliary tract

577 Diseases of pancreas

577.0 Acute pancreatitis
Abscess of pancreas
Necrosis of pancreas:
 acute
 infective
Pancreatitis:
 NOS
Pancreatitis:
 acute (recurrent)
 apoplectic
 hemorrhagic
 subacute
 suppurative

EXCLUDES mumps pancreatitis (072.3)

577.1 Chronic pancreatitis
Chronic pancreatitis:
 NOS
 infectious
 interstitial
Pancreatitis:
 painless
 recurrent
 relapsing

577.2 Cyst and pseudocyst of pancreas

577.8 Other specified diseases of pancreas
Atrophy
Calculus
Cirrhosis
Fibrosis
} of pancreas

Pancreatic:
  infantilism
  necrosis:
    NOS
    aseptic
    fat
Pancreatolithiasis

EXCLUDES fibrocystic disease of pancreas (277.00-277.01)
islet cell tumor of pancreas (211.7)
pancreatic steatorrhea (579.4)

577.9 Unspecified disease of pancreas

578 Gastrointestinal hemorrhage
EXCLUDES that with mention of:
angiodysplasia of stomach and duodenum (537.83)
angiodysplasia of intestine (569.85)
diverticulitis, intestine:
  large (562.13)
  small (562.03)
diverticulosis, intestine:
  large (562.12)
  small (562.02)
gastritis and duodenitis (535.0-535.6)
ulcer:
  duodenum (532.0-532.9)
  gastric (531.0-531.9)
  gastrojejunal (534.0-534.9)
  peptic (533.0-533.9)

578.0 Hematemesis
Vomiting of blood

578.1 Blood in stool
Melena
EXCLUDES melena of the newborn (772.4, 777.3)
occult blood (792.1)

578.9 Hemorrhage of gastrointestinal tract, unspecified
Gastric hemorrhage
Intestinal hemorrhage

579 Intestinal malabsorption
579.0 Celiac disease
Celiac:
  crisis
  infantilism
  rickets
Gee (-Herter) disease
Gluten enteropathy
Idiopathic steatorrhea
Nontropical sprue

579.1 Tropical sprue
Sprue:
  NOS
  tropical
Tropical steatorrhea

579.2 Blind loop syndrome
Postoperative blind loop syndrome

579.3 Other and unspecified postsurgical nonabsorption
Hypoglycemia
Malnutrition
} following gastrointestinal surgery

579.4 Pancreatic steatorrhea

579.8 Other specified intestinal malabsorption
Enteropathy:
  exudative
  protein-losing
Steatorrhea (chronic)

579.9 Unspecified intestinal malabsorption
Malabsorption syndrome NOS

10. DISEASES OF THE GENITOURINARY SYSTEM (580-629)

NEPHRITIS, NEPHROTIC SYNDROME, AND NEPHROSIS (580-589)

EXCLUDES hypertensive renal disease (403.00-403.91)

580 Acute glomerulonephritis
INCLUDES acute nephritis

580.0 With lesion of proliferative glomerulonephritis
Acute (diffuse) proliferative glomerulonephritis
Acute poststreptococcal glomerulonephritis

580.4 With lesion of rapidly progressive glomerulonephritis
Acute nephritis with lesion of necrotizing glomerulitis

580.8 With other specified pathological lesion in kidney
580.81 Acute glomerulonephritis in diseases classified elsewhere
Code also underlying disease, as:
  infectious hepatitis (070.0-070.9)
  mumps (072.79)
  subacute bacterial endocarditis (421.0)
  typhoid fever (002.0)

580.89 Other
Glomerulonephritis, acute, with lesion of:
  exudative nephritis
  interstitial (diffuse) (focal) nephritis

580.9 Acute glomerulonephritis with unspecified pathological lesion in kidney
Glomerulonephritis:
  NOS
  hemorrhagic
Nephritis
Nephropathy
} specified as acute

581 Nephrotic syndrome
581.0 With lesion of proliferative glomerulonephritis

581.1 With lesion of membranous glomerulonephritis
Epimembranous nephritis
Idiopathic membranous glomerular disease
Nephrotic syndrome with lesion of:
  focal glomerulosclerosis
  sclerosing membranous glomerulonephritis
  segmental hyalinosis

581.2 With lesion of membranoproliferative glomerulonephritis
Nephrotic syndrome with lesion (of):
  endothelial
  hypocomplementemic
  persistent
  lobular
  mesangiocapillary
  mixed membranous
    and proliferative
} glomerulonephritis

581.3 With lesion of minimal change glomerulonephritis
Foot process disease
Lipoid nephrosis
Minimal change:
  glomerular disease
Minimal change:
  glomerulitis
  nephrotic syndrome

581.8 With other specified pathological lesion in kidney
581.81 Nephrotic syndrome in diseases classified elsewhere
Code also underlying disease, as:
  amyloidosis (277.3)
  diabetes mellitus (250.4)
  malaria (084.9)
  polyarteritis (446.0)
  systemic lupus erythematosus (710.0)
EXCLUDES nephrosis in epidemic hemorrhagic fever (078.6)

581.89 Other
Glomerulonephritis with edema and lesion of:
  exudative nephritis
  interstitial (diffuse) (focal) nephritis

581.9 Nephrotic syndrome with unspecified pathological lesion in kidney
Glomerulonephritis with edema NOS
Nephritis:
  nephrotic NOS
  with edema NOS
Nephrosis NOS
Renal disease with edema NOS

● **582 Chronic glomerulonephritis**
  INCLUDES chronic nephritis
  582.0 With lesion of proliferative glomerulonephritis
   Chronic (diffuse) proliferative glomerulonephritis
  582.1 With lesion of membranous glomerulonephritis
   Chronic glomerulonephritis:
    membranous
    sclerosing
   Focal glomerulosclerosis
   Segmental hyalinosis
  582.2 With lesion of membranoproliferative glomerulonephritis
   Chronic glomerulonephritis:
    endothelial
    hypocomplementemic persistent
    lobular
    membranoproliferative
    mesangiocapillary
    mixed membranous and proliferative
  582.4 With lesion of rapidly progressive glomerulonephritis
   Chronic nephritis with lesion of necrotizing glomerulitis
  ● **582.8 With other specified pathological lesion in kidney**
   582.81 Chronic glomerulonephritis in diseases classified elsewhere
    Code also underlying disease, as:
     amyloidosis (277.3)
     systemic lupus erythematosus (710.0)
   ◆ **582.89 Other**
    Chronic glomerulonephritis with lesion of:
     exudative nephritis
     interstitial (diffuse) (focal) nephritis
  ◆ **582.9 Chronic glomerulonephritis with unspecified pathological lesion in kidney**
   Glomerulonephritis:
    NOS
    hemorrhagic   } specified as chronic
    Nephritis
    Nephropathy

● **583 Nephritis and nephropathy, not specified as acute or chronic**
  INCLUDES "renal disease" so stated, not specified as acute or chronic but with stated pathology or cause
  583.0 With lesion of proliferative glomerulonephritis
   Proliferative: Proliferative
    glomerulonephritis   nephritis NOS
    (diffuse) NOS   nephropathy NOS
  583.1 With lesion of membranous glomerulonephritis
   Membranous:
    glomerulonephritis NOS
    nephritis NOS
   Membranous nephropathy NOS
  583.2 With lesion of membranoproliferative glomerulonephritis
   Membranoproliferative:
    glomerulonephritis NOS
    nephritis NOS
    nephropathy NOS
   Nephritis NOS, with lesion of:
    hypocomplementemic
    persistent
    lobular   } glomerulonephritis
    mesangiocapillary
    mixed membranous
    and proliferative
  583.4 With lesion of rapidly progressive glomerulonephritis
   Necrotizing or rapidly progressive:
    glomerulitis NOS
    glomerulonephritis NOS
    nephritis NOS
    nephropathy NOS
   Nephritis, unspecified, with lesion of necrotizing glomerulitis
  583.6 With lesion of renal cortical necrosis
   Nephritis NOS   } with (renal) cortical
   Nephropathy NOS   } necrosis
   Renal cortical necrosis NOS
  583.7 With lesion of renal medullary necrosis
   Nephritis NOS   } with (renal) medullary
   Nephropathy NOS   } [papillary] necrosis

● **583.8 With other specified pathological lesion in kidney**
   583.81 Nephritis and nephropathy, not specified as acute or chronic, in diseases classified elsewhere
    Code also underlying disease, as:
     amyloidosis (277.3)
     diabetes mellitus (250.4)
     gonococcal infection (098.19)
     Goodpasture's syndrome (446.21)
     systemic lupus erythematosus (710.0)
     tuberculosis (016.0)
    EXCLUDES gouty nephropathy (274.10)
             syphilitic nephritis (095.4)
   ◆ **583.89 Other**
    Glomerulitis
    Glomerulonephritis } with lesion of:
    Nephritis   } exudative nephritis
    Nephropathy   } interstitial nephritis
    Renal disease
  ◆ **583.9 With unspecified pathological lesion in kidney**
    Glomerulitis
    Glomerulonephritis } NOS
    Nephritis
    Nephropathy
    EXCLUDES nephropathy complicating pregnancy, labor, or the puerperium (642.0-642.9, 646.2)
             renal disease NOS with no stated cause (593.9)

● **584 Acute renal failure**
  EXCLUDES following labor and delivery (669.3)
           posttraumatic (958.5)
           that complicating:
            abortion (634-638 with .3, 639.3)
            ectopic or molar pregnancy (639.3)
  584.5 With lesion of tubular necrosis
   Lower nephron nephrosis
   Renal failure with (acute) tubular necrosis
   Tubular necrosis:
    NOS
    acute
  584.6 With lesion of renal cortical necrosis
  584.7 With lesion of renal medullary [papillary] necrosis
   Necrotizing renal papillitis
  ◆ **584.8 With other specified pathological lesion in kidney**
  ◆ **584.9 Acute renal failure, unspecified**

585 Chronic renal failure
  Chronic uremia
  Use additional code, if desired, to identify manifestation as:
   uremic:
    neuropathy (357.4)
    pericarditis (420.0)
  EXCLUDES that with any condition classifiable to 401 (403.0-403.9 with fifth-digit 1)

● **586 Renal failure, unspecified**
  Uremia NOS
  EXCLUDES following labor and delivery (669.3)
           posttraumatic renal failure (958.5)
           that complicating:
            abortion (634-638 with .3, 639.3)
            ectopic or molar pregnancy (639.3)
           uremia:
            extrarenal (788.9)
            prerenal (788.9)
           with any condition classifiable to 401 (403.0-403.9 with fifth-digit 1)

◆ **587 Renal sclerosis, unspecified**
  Atrophy of kidney
  Contracted kidney
  Renal:
   cirrhosis
   fibrosis
  EXCLUDES nephrosclerosis (arteriolar) (arteriosclerotic) (403.00-403.92)
           with hypertension (403.00-403.92)

GENITOURINARY SYSTEM

● **588 Disorders resulting from impaired renal function**
- **588.0 Renal osteodystrophy**
  - Azotemic osteodystrophy
  - Phosphate-losing tubular disorders
  - Renal:
    - dwarfism
    - infantilism
    - rickets
- **588.1 Nephrogenic diabetes insipidus**
  - EXCLUDES: diabetes insipidus NOS (253.5)
- ◆ **588.8 Other specified disorders resulting from impaired renal function**
  - Hypokalemic nephropathy
  - Secondary hyperparathyroidism (of renal origin)
  - EXCLUDES: secondary hypertension (405.0-405.9)
- ◆ **588.9 Unspecified disorder resulting from impaired renal function**

● **589 Small kidney of unknown cause**
- **589.0 Unilateral small kidney**
- **589.1 Bilateral small kidneys**
- ◆ **589.9 Small kidney, unspecified**

OTHER DISEASES OF URINARY SYSTEM (590-599)

EXCLUDES: conditions classifiable to 590, 595, 597, 599.0 complicating:
- abortion (634-638 with .7, 639.8)
- ectopic or molar pregnancy (639.8)
- pregnancy, childbirth, or the puerperium (646.6)

● **590 Infections of kidney**
Use additional code, if desired, to identify organism, such as Escherichia coli [E. coli] (041.4)
- ● **590.0 Chronic pyelonephritis**
  - Chronic pyelitis
  - Chronic pyonephrosis
  - Code also any associated vesicoureteral reflux (593.70-593.73)
  - **590.00 Without lesion of renal medullary necrosis**
  - **590.01 With lesion of renal medullary necrosis**
- ● **590.1 Acute pyelonephritis**
  - Acute pyelitis
  - Acute pyonephrosis
  - **590.10 Without lesion of renal medullary necrosis**
  - **590.11 With lesion of renal medullary necrosis**
- **590.2 Renal and perinephric abscess**
  - Abscess:
    - kidney
    - nephritic
  - Abscess:
    - perirenal
  - Carbuncle of kidney
- **590.3 Pyeloureteritis cystica**
  - Infection of renal pelvis and ureter
  - Ureteritis cystica
- ● **590.8 Other pyelonephritis or pyonephrosis, not specified as acute or chronic**
  - ◆ **590.80 Pyelonephritis, unspecified**
    - Pyelitis NOS
    - Pyelonephritis NOS
    - EXCLUDES: calculous pyelonephritis (592.9)
  - ■ **590.81 Pyelitis or pyelonephritis in diseases classified elsewhere**
    - Code also underlying disease, as:
      - tuberculosis (016.0)
- ◆ **590.9 Infection of kidney, unspecified**
  - EXCLUDES: urinary tract infection NOS (599.0)

591 Hydronephrosis
- Hydrocalycosis
- Hydronephrosis
- Hydroureteronephrosis
- EXCLUDES: congenital hydronephrosis (753.2)
  - hydroureter (593.5)

● **592 Calculus of kidney and ureter**
- EXCLUDES: nephrocalcinosis (275.4)
- **592.0 Calculus of kidney**
  - Nephrolithiasis NOS   Staghorn calculus
  - Renal calculus or stone   Stone in kidney
  - EXCLUDES: uric acid nephrolithiasis (274.11)
- **592.1 Calculus of ureter**
  - Ureteric stone   Ureterolithiasis
- ◆ **592.9 Urinary calculus, unspecified**
  - Calculous pyelonephritis

● **593 Other disorders of kidney and ureter**
- **593.0 Nephroptosis**
  - Floating kidney
  - Mobile kidney
- **593.1 Hypertrophy of kidney**
- **593.2 Cyst of kidney, acquired**
  - Cyst (multiple) (solitary) of kidney, not congenital
  - Peripelvic (lymphatic) cyst
  - EXCLUDES: calyceal or pyelogenic cyst of kidney (591)
    - congenital cyst of kidney (753.1)
    - polycystic (disease of) kidney (753.1)
- **593.3 Stricture or kinking of ureter**
  - Angulation | of ureter (post-
  - Constriction | operative)
  - Stricture of pelviureteric junction
- ◆ **593.4 Other ureteric obstruction**
  - Idiopathic retroperitoneal fibrosis
  - Occlusion NOS of ureter
  - EXCLUDES: that due to calculus (592.1)
- **593.5 Hydroureter**
  - EXCLUDES: congenital hydroureter (753.2)
    - hydroureteronephrosis (591)
- **593.6 Postural proteinuria**
  - Benign postural proteinuria
  - Orthostatic proteinuria
  - EXCLUDES: proteinuria NOS (791.0)
- **593.7 Vesicoureteral reflux**
  - Use additional code to identify:
    - chronic pyelonephritis (590.00-590.01)
    - renal agenesis (753.0)
    - renal dysplasia (753.15)
  - ◆ **593.70 Unspecified or without reflux nephropathy**
  - **593.71 With reflux nephropathy, unilateral**
  - **593.72 With reflux nephropathy, bilateral**
  - ◆ **593.73 With reflux nephropathy NOS**
- ● **593.8 Other specified disorders of kidney and ureter**
  - **593.81 Vascular disorders of kidney**
    - Renal (artery):   Renal (artery):
      - embolism   thrombosis
      - hemorrhage   Renal infarction
  - **593.82 Ureteral fistula**
    - Intestinoureteral fistula
    - EXCLUDES: fistula between ureter and female genital tract (619.0)
  - ◆ **593.89 Other**
    - Adhesions, kidney   Polyp of ureter
      or ureter   Pyelectasia
    - Periureteritis
    - EXCLUDES: tuberculosis of ureter (016.2)
      - ureteritis cystica (590.3)
- ◆ **593.9 Unspecified disorder of kidney and ureter**
  - Renal disease NOS
  - Salt-losing nephritis or syndrome
  - EXCLUDES: cystic kidney disease (753.1)
    - nephropathy, so stated (583.0-583.9)
    - renal disease:
      - acute (580.0-580.9)
      - arising in pregnancy or the puerperium (642.1-642.2, 642.4-642.7, 646.2)
      - chronic (582.0-582.9)
      - not specified as acute or chronic, but with stated pathology or cause (583.0-583.9)

● **594 Calculus of lower urinary tract**
- **594.0 Calculus in diverticulum of bladder**
- ◆ **594.1 Other calculus in bladder**
  - Urinary bladder stone
  - EXCLUDES: staghorn calculus (592.0)
- **594.2 Calculus in urethra**
- ◆ **594.8 Other lower urinary tract calculus**
- ◆ **594.9 Calculus of lower urinary tract, unspecified**
  - EXCLUDES: calculus of urinary tract NOS (592.9)

● **595 Cystitis**
- EXCLUDES: prostatocystitis (601.3)
- Use additional code, if desired, to identify organism, such as Escherichia coli [E. coli] (041.4)

TABULAR LIST

595.0 Acute cystitis
  EXCLUDES trigonitis (595.3)
595.1 Chronic interstitial cystitis
  Hunner's ulcer
  Panmural fibrosis of bladder
  Submucous cystitis
◆ **595.2** Other chronic cystitis
  Chronic cystitis NOS
  Subacute cystitis
  EXCLUDES trigonitis (595.3)
595.3 Trigonitis
  Follicular cystitis
  Trigonitis (acute) (chronic)
  Urethrotrigonitis
595.4 Cystitis in diseases classified elsewhere
  Code also underlying disease, as:
    actinomycosis (039.8)
    amebiasis (006.8)
    bilharziasis (120.0-120.9)
    Echinococcus infestation (122.3, 122.6)
  EXCLUDES cystitis:
    diphtheritic (032.84)
    gonococcal (098.11, 098.31)
    monilial (112.2)
    trichomonal (131.09)
    tuberculous (016.1)
● **595.8** Other specified types of cystitis
  595.81 Cystitis cystica
  595.82 Irradiation cystitis
    Use additional E code, if desired, to identify cause
  ◆ **595.89** Other
    Abscess of bladder
    Cystitis:
      bullous
      emphysematous
      glandularis
◆ **595.9** Cystitis, unspecified
● **596** Other disorders of bladder
  Use additional code, if desired, to identify urinary incontinence (625.6, 788.30-788.39)
  596.0 Bladder neck obstruction
    Contracture (acquired)
    Obstruction (acquired) } of bladder neck or vesicourethral orifice
    Stenosis (acquired)
    EXCLUDES congenital (753.6)
  596.1 Intestinovesical fistula
    Fistula: Fistula:
      enterovesical   vesicoenteric
      vesicocolic   vesicorectal
  596.2 Vesical fistula, not elsewhere classified
    Fistula: Fistula:
      bladder NOS   vesicocutaneous
      urethrovesical   vesicoperineal
    EXCLUDES fistula between bladder and female genital tract (619.0)
  596.3 Diverticulum of bladder
    Diverticulitis   } of bladder
    Diverticulum (acquired) (false)
    EXCLUDES that with calculus in diverticulum of bladder (594.0)
  596.4 Atony of bladder
    High compliance bladder
    Hypotonicity } of bladder
    Inertia
    EXCLUDES neurogenic bladder (596.54)
● **596.5** Other functional disorders of bladder
    EXCLUDES cauda equina syndrome with neurogenic bladder (344.61)
  596.51 Hypertonicity of bladder
    Hyperactivity
  596.52 Low bladder compliance
  596.53 Paralysis of bladder

  596.54 Neurogenic bladder NOS
  596.55 Detrusor sphincter dyssynergia
  ◆ **596.59** Other functional disorder of bladder
    Detrusor instability
  596.6 Rupture of bladder, nontraumatic
  596.7 Hemorrhage into bladder wall
    Hyperemia of bladder
    EXCLUDES acute hemorrhagic cystitis (595.0)
  ◆ **596.8** Other specified disorders of bladder
    Bladder: Bladder:
      calcified   hemorrhage
      contracted   hypertrophy
    EXCLUDES cystocele, female (618.0, 618.2-618.4)
      hernia or prolapse of bladder, female (618.0, 618.2-618.4)
  ◆ **596.9** Unspecified disorder of bladder
● **597** Urethritis, not sexually transmitted, and urethral syndrome
    EXCLUDES nonspecific urethritis, so stated (099.4)
  597.0 Urethral abscess
    Abscess: Abscess of:
      periurethral   Cowper's gland
      urethral (gland) Littré's gland
    Abscess of: Periurethral cellulitis
      bulbourethral gland
    EXCLUDES urethral caruncle (599.3)
● **597.8** Other urethritis
  ◆ **597.80** Urethritis, unspecified
  597.81 Urethral syndrome NOS
  ◆ **597.89** Other
    Adenitis, Skene's glands
    Cowperitis
    Meatitis, urethral
    Ulcer, urethra (meatus)
    Verumontanitis
    EXCLUDES trichomonal (131.02)
● **598** Urethral stricture
  Use additional code, if desired, to identify urinary incontinence (625.6, 788.30-788.39)
  INCLUDES pinhole meatus
    stricture of urinary meatus
  EXCLUDES congenital stricture of urethra and urinary meatus (753.6)
● **598.0** Urethral stricture due to infection
  ◆ **598.00** Due to unspecified infection
  598.01 Due to infective diseases classified elsewhere
    Code also underlying disease, as:
      gonococcal infection (098.2)
      schistosomiasis (120.0-120.9)
      syphilis (095.8)
  598.1 Traumatic urethral stricture
    Stricture of urethra:
      late effect of injury
      postobstetric
    EXCLUDES postoperative following surgery on genitourinary tract (598.2)
  598.2 Postoperative urethral stricture
    Postcatheterization stricture of urethra
  ◆ **598.8** Other specified causes of urethral stricture
  ◆ **598.9** Urethral stricture, unspecified
● **599** Other disorders of urethra and urinary tract
  ◆ **599.0** Urinary tract infection, site not specified
    Bacteriuria
    Pyuria
    Use additional code, if desired, to identify organism, such as Escherichia coli [E. coli] (041.4)
  599.1 Urethral fistula
    Fistula:
      urethroperineal
      urethrorectal
    Urinary fistula NOS
    EXCLUDES fistula:
      urethroscrotal (608.89)
      urethrovaginal (619.0)
      urethrovesicovaginal (619.0)
  599.2 Urethral diverticulum
  599.3 Urethral caruncle
    Polyp of urethra

GENITOURINARY SYSTEM

599.4 Urethral false passage

599.5 Prolapsed urethral mucosa
Prolapse of urethra
Urethrocele
EXCLUDES: urethrocele, female (618.0, 618.2-618.4)

◆ **599.6 Urinary obstruction, unspecified**
Use additional code, if desired, to identify urinary incontinence (625.6, 788.30-788.39)
Obstructive uropathy NOS
Urinary (tract) obstruction NOS
EXCLUDES: obstructive nephropathy NOS (593.89)

599.7 Hematuria
Hematuria (benign) (essential)
EXCLUDES: hemoglobinuria (791.2)

● **599.8 Other specified disorders of urethra and urinary tract**
Use additional code, if desired, to identify urinary incontinence (625.6, 788.30-788.39), if present
599.81 Urethral hypermobility
599.82 Intrinsic (urethral) spincter deficiency [ISD]
599.83 Urethral instability
◆ **599.84** Other specified disorders of urethra
Rupture of urethra (nontraumatic)
Urethral:
  cyst
  granuloma
◆ **599.89** Other specified disorders of urinary tract
EXCLUDES: symptoms and other conditions classifiable to 788.0-788.2, 788.4-788.9, 791.0-791.9

◆ **599.9 Unspecified disorder of urethra and urinary tract**

DISEASES OF MALE GENITAL ORGANS (600-608)

600 Hyperplasia of prostate
Use additional code, if desired, to identify urinary incontinence (788.30-788.39)

Adenofibromatous hypertrophy
Adenoma (benign)
Enlargement (benign)
Fibroadenoma   } of prostate
Fibroma
Hypertrophy (benign)
Myoma

Median bar (prostate)
Prostatic obstruction NOS
EXCLUDES: benign neoplasms of prostate (222.2)

● **601 Inflammatory diseases of prostate**
Use additional code, if desired, to identify organism, such as Staphylococcus (041.1), or Streptococcus (041.0)
601.0 Acute prostatitis
601.1 Chronic prostatitis
601.2 Abscess of prostate
601.3 Prostatocystitis
▌ **601.4** *Prostatitis in diseases classified elsewhere*
Code also underlying disease, as:
  actinomycosis (039.8)
  blastomycosis (116.0)
  syphilis (095.8)
  tuberculosis (016.5)
EXCLUDES: prostatitis:
  gonococcal (098.12, 098.32)
  monilial (112.2)
  trichomonal (131.03)
◆ **601.8** Other specified inflammatory diseases of prostate
Prostatitis:
  cavitary
  diverticular
  granulomatous
◆ **601.9** Prostatitis, unspecified
Prostatitis NOS

● **602 Other disorders of prostate**
602.0 Calculus of prostate
Prostatic stone
602.1 Congestion or hemorrhage of prostate
602.2 Atrophy of prostate

◆ **602.8** Other specified disorders of prostate
Fistula
Infarction   } of prostate
Stricture
Periprostatic adhesions

◆ **602.9** Unspecified disorder of prostate

● **603 Hydrocele**
INCLUDES: hydrocele of spermatic cord, testis, or tunica vaginalis
EXCLUDES: congenital (778.6)
603.0 Encysted hydrocele
603.1 Infected hydrocele
Use additional code, if desired, to identify organism
◆ **603.8** Other specified types of hydrocele
◆ **603.9** Hydrocele, unspecified

● **604 Orchitis and epididymitis**
Use additional code, if desired, to identify organism, such as Escherichia coli [E. coli] (041.4), Staphylococcus (041.1), or Streptococcus (041.0)
604.0 Orchitis, epididymitis, and epididymo-orchitis, with abscess
Abscess of epididymis or testis
● **604.9** Other orchitis, epididymitis, and epididymo-orchitis, without mention of abscess
◆ **604.90** Orchitis and epididymitis, unspecified
▌ **604.91** *Orchitis and epididymitis in diseases classified elsewhere*
Code also underlying disease, as:
  diphtheria (032.89)
  filariasis (125.0-125.9)
  syphilis (095.8)
EXCLUDES: orchitis:
  gonococcal (098.13, 098.33)
  mumps (072.0)
  tuberculous (016.5)
  tuberculous epididymitis (016.4)
◆ **604.99** Other

605 Redundant prepuce and phimosis
Adherent prepuce   Phimosis (congenital)
Paraphimosis   Tight foreskin

● **606 Infertility, male**
606.0 Azoospermia
Absolute infertility
Infertility due to:
  germinal (cell) aplasia
  spermatogenic arrest (complete)
606.1 Oligospermia
Infertility due to:
  germinal cell desquamation
  hypospermatogenesis
  incomplete spermatogenic arrest
606.8 Infertility due to extratesticular causes
Infertility due to: Infertility due to:
  drug therapy   radiation
  infection   systemic disease
  obstruction of efferent
    ducts
◆ **606.9** Male infertility, unspecified

● **607 Disorders of penis**
EXCLUDES: phimosis (605)
607.0 Leukoplakia of penis
Kraurosis of penis
EXCLUDES: carcinoma in situ of penis (233.5)
  erythroplasia of Queyrat (233.5)
607.1 Balanoposthitis
Balanitis
Use additional code, if desired, to identify organism
◆ **607.2** Other inflammatory disorders of penis
Abscess
Boil   } of corpus
Carbuncle   cavernosum
Cellulitis   or penis

Cavernitis (penis)
Use additional code, if desired, to identify organism
EXCLUDES: herpetic infection (054.13)
607.3 Priapism
Painful erection

● Additional digits required   ◆ Nonspecific code   ▌ Not a primary diagnosis   Volume 1 — 99

- **607.8 Other specified disorders of penis**
  - 607.81 Balanitis xerotica obliterans
    - Induratio penis plastica
  - 607.82 Vascular disorders of penis
    - Embolism ⎫
    - Hematoma (nontraumatic) ⎬ of corpus cavernosum or penis
    - Hemorrhage ⎪
    - Thrombosis ⎭
  - 607.83 Edema of penis
  - 607.84 Impotence of organic origin
    - **EXCLUDES** nonorganic or unspecified (302.72)
  - ◆ 607.89 Other
    - Atrophy ⎫
    - Fibrosis ⎬ of corpus cavernosum or penis
    - Hypertrophy ⎪
    - Ulcer (chronic) ⎭
- ◆ **607.9 Unspecified disorder of penis**
- ● **608 Other disorders of male genital organs**
  - 608.0 Seminal vesiculitis
    - Abscess ⎫ of seminal vesicle
    - Cellulitis ⎭
    - Vesiculitis (seminal)
    - Use additional code, if desired, to identify organism
    - **EXCLUDES** gonococcal infection (098.14, 098.34)
  - 608.1 Spermatocele
  - 608.2 Torsion of testis
    - Torsion of:
      - epididymis
      - spermatic cord
      - testicle
  - 608.3 Atrophy of testis
  - ◆ 608.4 Other inflammatory disorders of male genital organs
    - Abscess ⎫
    - Boil ⎬ of scrotum, spermatic cord, testis [except abscess], tunica vaginalis, or vas deferens
    - Carbuncle ⎪
    - Cellulitis ⎭
    - Vasitis
    - Use additional code, if desired, to identify organism
    - **EXCLUDES** abscess of testis (604.0)
  - ● 608.8 Other specified disorders of male genital organs
    - ▌ 608.81 Disorders of male genital organs in diseases classified elsewhere
      - Code also underlying disease, as:
        - filariasis (125.0-125.9)
        - tuberculosis (016.5)
    - 608.83 Vascular disorders
      - Hematoma (nontraumatic) ⎫
      - Hemorrhage ⎬ of seminal vesicle, spermatic cord, testis, scrotum, tunica vaginalis, or vas deferens
      - Thrombosis ⎭
      - Hematocele NOS, male
    - 608.84 Chylocele of tunica vaginalis
    - 608.85 Stricture
      - Stricture of:
        - spermatic cord
        - tunica vaginalis
        - vas deferens
    - 608.86 Edema
    - ◆ 608.89 Other
      - Atrophy ⎫
      - Fibrosis ⎬ of seminal vesicle, spermatic cord, testis, scrotum, tunica vaginalis, or vas deferens
      - Hypertrophy ⎪
      - Ulcer ⎭
      - **EXCLUDES** atrophy of testis (608.3)
- ◆ **608.9 Unspecified disorder of male genital organs**

DISORDERS OF BREAST (610-611)

- ● **610 Benign mammary dysplasias**
  - 610.0 Solitary cyst of breast
    - Cyst (solitary) of breast
  - 610.1 Diffuse cystic mastopathy
    - Chronic cystic mastitis
    - Cystic breast
    - Fibrocystic disease of breast
  - 610.2 Fibroadenosis of breast
    - Fibroadenosis of breast: Fibroadenosis of breast:
      - NOS   diffuse
      - chronic   periodic
      - cystic   segmental
  - 610.3 Fibrosclerosis of breast
  - 610.4 Mammary duct ectasia
    - Comedomastitis   Mastitis:
    - Duct ectasia   periductal
                                plasma cel
  - ◆ 610.8 Other specified benign mammary dysplasias
    - Mazoplasia
    - Sebaceous cyst of breast
  - ◆ 610.9 Benign mammary dysplasia, unspecified
- ● **611 Other disorders of breast**
  - **EXCLUDES** that associated with lactation or the puerperium (675.0-676.9)
  - 611.0 Inflammatory disease of breast
    - Abscess (acute) (chronic) (nonpuerperal) of:
      - areola
      - breast
    - Mammillary fistula
    - Mastitis (acute) (subacute) (nonpuerperal):
      - NOS
      - infective
      - retromammary
      - submammary
    - **EXCLUDES** carbuncle of breast (680.2)
      - chronic cystic mastitis (610.1)
      - neonatal infective mastitis (771.5)
      - thrombophlebitis of breast [Mondor's disease] (451.89)
  - 611.1 Hypertrophy of breast
    - Gynecomastia
    - Hypertrophy of breast:
      - NOS
      - massive pubertal
  - 611.2 Fissure of nipple
  - 611.3 Fat necrosis of breast
    - Fat necrosis (segmental) of breast
  - 611.4 Atrophy of breast
  - 611.5 Galactocele
  - 611.6 Galactorrhea not associated with childbirth
  - ● 611.7 Signs and symptoms in breast
    - 611.71 Mastodynia
      - Pain in breast
    - 611.72 Lump or mass in breast
    - ◆ 611.79 Other
      - Induration of breast
      - Inversion of nipple
      - Nipple discharge
      - Retraction of nipple
  - ◆ 611.8 Other specified disorders of breast
    - Hematoma (nontraumatic) ⎫ of breast
    - Infarction ⎭
    - Occlusion of breast duct
    - Subinvolution of breast (postlactational) (postpartum)
  - ◆ 611.9 Unspecified breast disorder

INFLAMMATORY DISEASE OF FEMALE PELVIC ORGANS (614-616)

Use additional code, if desired, to identify organism, such as Staphylococcus (041.1), or Streptococcus (041.0)

EXCLUDES that associated with pregnancy, abortion, childbirth, or the puerperium (630-676.9)

- ● **614 Inflammatory disease of ovary, fallopian tube, pelvic cellular tissue, and peritoneum**
  - **EXCLUDES** endometritis (615.0-615.9)
    - major infection following delivery (670)
    - that complicating:
      - abortion (634-638 with .0, 639.0)
      - ectopic or molar pregnancy (639.0)
      - pregnancy or labor (646.6)
  - 614.0 Acute salpingitis and oophoritis
    - Any condition classifiable to 614.2, specified as acute or subacute

GENITOURINARY SYSTEM

614.1 Chronic salpingitis and oophoritis
Hydrosalpinx
Salpingitis:
  follicularis
  isthmica nodosa
Any condition classifiable to 614.2, specified as chronic

◆ 614.2 Salpingitis and oophoritis not specified as acute, subacute, or chronic
Abscess (of):　　　　　　Perisalpingitis
  fallopian tube
  ovary
  tubo-ovarian
Oophoritis　　　　　　Tubo-ovarian inflammatory
Perioophoritis　　　　　　disease

Pyosalpinx
Salpingitis
Salpingo-oophoritis

EXCLUDES gonococcal infection (chronic) (098.37)
　　　　　　acute (098.17)
　　　　　　tuberculous (016.6)

614.3 Acute parametritis and pelvic cellulitis
Acute inflammatory pelvic disease
Any condition classifiable to 614.4, specified as acute

614.4 Chronic or unspecified parametritis and pelvic cellulitis
Abscess (of):
  broad ligament
  parametrium   } chronic or NOS
  pelvis, female
  pouch of Douglas

Chronic inflammatory pelvic disease
Pelvic cellulitis, female
EXCLUDES tuberculous (016.7)

614.5 Acute or unspecified pelvic peritonitis, female
614.6 Pelvic peritoneal adhesions, female
Adhesions:
  peritubal
  tubo-ovarian
Use additional code, if desired, to identify any associated infertility (628.2)

◆ 614.7 Other chronic pelvic peritonitis, female
EXCLUDES tuberculous (016.7)

◆ 614.8 Other specified inflammatory disease of female pelvic organs and tissues
◆ 614.9 Unspecified inflammatory disease of female pelvic organs and tissues
Pelvic infection or inflammation, female NOS
Pelvic inflammatory disease [PID]

● 615 Inflammatory diseases of uterus, except cervix
EXCLUDES following delivery (670)
　　　　　　hyperplastic endometritis (621.3)
　　　　　　that complicating:
　　　　　　　abortion (634-638 with .0, 639.0)
　　　　　　　ectopic or molar pregnancy (639.0)
　　　　　　　pregnancy or labor (646.6)

615.0 Acute
Any condition classifiable to 615.9, specified as acute or subacute

615.1 Chronic
Any condition classifiable to 615.9, specified as chronic

◆ 615.9 Unspecified inflammatory disease of uterus
Endometritis
Endomyometritis
Metritis
Myometritis
Perimetritis
Pyometra
Uterine abscess

● 616 Inflammatory disease of cervix, vagina, and vulva
EXCLUDES that complicating:
　　　　　　abortion (634-638 with .0, 639.0)
　　　　　　ectopic or molar pregnancy (639.0)
　　　　　　pregnancy, childbirth, or the puerperium (646.6)

616.0 Cervicitis and endocervicitis
Cervicitis　　　} with or without mention of
Endocervicitis　　　erosion or ectropion
Nabothian (gland) cyst or follicle
EXCLUDES erosion or ectropion without mention of cervicitis (622.0)

● 616.1 Vaginitis and vulvovaginitis
◆ 616.10 Vaginitis and vulvovaginitis, unspecified
Vaginitis:
  NOS
  postirradiation
Vulvitis NOS
Vulvovaginitis NOS
Use additional code, if desired, to identify organism, such as Escherichiacoli [E. coli] (041.4), Staphylococcus (041.1), or Streptococcus (041.0)
EXCLUDES noninfective leukorrhea (623.5)
　　　　　　postmenopausal or senile vaginitis (627.3)

■ 616.11 Vaginitis and vulvovaginitis in diseases classified elsewhere
Code also underlying disease, as:
  pinworm vaginitis (127.4)
EXCLUDES herpetic vulvovaginitis (054.11)
　　　　　　monilial vulvotaginitis (112.1)
　　　　　　trichomonal vaginitis or vulvovaginitis (131.01)

616.2 Cyst of Bartholin's gland
Bartholin's duct cyst
616.3 Abscess of Bartholin's gland
Vulvovaginal gland abscess

◆ 616.4 Other abscess of vulva
Abscess　　　}
Carbuncle　　} of vulva
Furuncle　　　}

● 616.5 Ulceration of vulva
◆ 616.50 Ulceration of vulva, unspecified
Ulcer NOS of vulva
■ 616.51 Ulceration of vulva in diseases classified elsewhere
Code also underlying disease, as:
  Behcet's syndrome (136.1)
  tuberculosis (016.7)
EXCLUDES vulvar ulcer (in):
　　　　　　gonococcal (098.0)
　　　　　　herpes simplex (054.12)
　　　　　　syphilitic (091.0)

◆ 616.8 Other specified inflammatory diseases of cervix, vagina, and vulva
Caruncle, vagina or labium
Ulcer, vagina
EXCLUDES noninflammatory disorders of:
　　　　　　cervix (622.0-622.9)
　　　　　　vagina (623.0-623.9)
　　　　　　vulva (624.0-624.9)

◆ 616.9 Unspecified inflammatory disease of cervix, vagina, and vulva

OTHER DISORDERS OF FEMALE GENITAL TRACT (617-629)

● 617 Endometriosis
617.0 Endometriosis of uterus
Adenomyosis
Endometriosis:
  cervix
  internal
  myometrium
EXCLUDES stromal endometriosis (236.0)

617.1 Endometriosis of ovary
Chocolate cyst of ovary
Endometrial cystoma of ovary
617.2 Endometriosis of fallopian tube
617.3 Endometriosis of pelvic peritoneum
Endometriosis:　　　　Endometriosis:
  broad ligament　　　　parametrium
  cul-de-sac (Douglas')　　round ligament
617.4 Endometriosis of rectovaginal septum and vagina

617.5   **Endometriosis of intestine**
Endometriosis:
- appendix
- colon
- rectum

617.6   **Endometriosis in scar of skin**

◆ **617.8**   **Endometriosis of other specified sites**
Endometriosis:
- bladder
- lung
- umbilicus
- vulva

◆ **617.9**   **Endometriosis, site unspecified**

● **618**   **Genital prolapse**
Use additional code, if desired, to identify urinary incontinence (625.6, 788.31, 788.33-788.39)

EXCLUDES   that complicating pregnancy, labor, or delivery (654.4)

618.0   **Prolapse of vaginal walls without mention of uterine prolapse**

Cystocele
Cystourethrocele
Proctocele, female   } without mention of uterine prolapse
Rectocele
Urethrocele, female
Vaginal prolapse

EXCLUDES   that with uterine prolapse (618.2-618.4)
enterocele (618.6)
vaginal vault prolapse following hysterectomy (618.5)

618.1   **Uterine prolapse without mention of vaginal wall prolapse**
Descensus uteri
Uterine prolapse:
- NOS
- complete
- first degree
- second degree
- third degree

EXCLUDES   that with mention of cystocele, urethrocele, or rectocele (618.2-618.4)

618.2   **Uterovaginal prolapse, incomplete**

618.3   **Uterovaginal prolapse, complete**

◆ **618.4**   **Uterovaginal prolapse, unspecified**

618.5   **Prolapse of vaginal vault after hysterectomy**

618.6   **Vaginal enterocele, congenital or acquired**
Pelvic enterocele, congenital or acquired

618.7   **Old laceration of muscles of pelvic floor**

◆ **618.8**   **Other specified genital prolapse**
Incompetence or weakening of pelvic fundus
Relaxation of vaginal outlet or pelvis

◆ **618.9**   **Unspecified genital prolapse**

● **619**   **Fistula involving female genital tract**

EXCLUDES   vesicorectal and intestinovesical fistula (596.1)

619.0   **Urinary-genital tract fistula, female**
Fistula:
- cervicovesical
- ureterovaginal
- urethrovaginal
- urethrovesicovaginal
- uteroureteric
- uterovesical
- vesicocervicovaginal
- vesicovaginal

619.1   **Digestive-genital tract fistula, female**
Fistula:
- intestinouterine
- intestinovaginal
- rectovaginal
- rectovulval
- sigmoidovaginal
- uterorectal

619.2   **Genital tract-skin fistula, female**
Fistula:
- uterus to abdominal wall
- vaginoperineal

◆ **619.8**   **Other specified fistulas involving female genital tract**
Fistula:
- cervix
- cul-de-sac (Douglas')
- uterus
- vagina

◆ **619.9**   **Unspecified fistula involving female genital tract**

● **620**   **Noninflammatory disorders of ovary, fallopian tube, and broad ligament**

EXCLUDES   hydrosalpinx (614.1)

620.0   **Follicular cyst of ovary**
Cyst of graafian follicle

620.1   **Corpus luteum cyst or hematoma**
Corpus luteum hemorrhage or rupture
Lutein cyst

◆ **620.2**   **Other and unspecified ovarian cyst**

Cyst:
- NOS
- corpus albicans
- retention NOS } of ovary
- serous
- theca-lutein

Simple cystoma of ovary

EXCLUDES   cystadenoma (benign) (serous) (220)
developmental cysts (752.0)
neoplastic cysts (220)
polycystic ovaries (256.4)
Stein-Leventhal syndrome (256.4)

620.3   **Acquired atrophy of ovary and fallopian tube**
Senile involution of ovary

620.4   **Prolapse or hernia of ovary and fallopian tube**
Displacement of ovary and fallopian tube
Salpingocele

620.5   **Torsion of ovary, ovarian pedicle, or fallopian tube**
Torsion:
- accessory tube
- hydatid of Morgagni

620.6   **Broad ligament laceration syndrome**
Masters-Allen syndrome

620.7   **Hematoma of broad ligament**
Hematocele, broad ligament

◆ **620.8**   **Other noninflammatory disorders of ovary, fallopian tube, and broad ligament**

Cyst
Polyp   } of broad ligament or fallopian tube

Infarction
Rupture   } of ovary or fallopian tube

Hematosalpinx

EXCLUDES   hematosalpinx in ectopic pregnancy (639.2)
peritubal adhesions (614.6)
torsion of ovary, ovarian pedicle, or fallopian tube (620.5)

◆ **620.9**   **Unspecified noninflammatory disorder of ovary, fallopian tube, and broad ligament**

● **621**   **Disorders of uterus, not elsewhere classified**

621.0   **Polyp of corpus uteri**
Polyp:
- endometrium
- uterus NOS

EXCLUDES   cervical polyp NOS (622.7)

621.1   **Chronic subinvolution of uterus**

EXCLUDES   puerperal (674.8)

621.2   **Hypertrophy of uterus**
Bulky or enlarged uterus

EXCLUDES   puerperal (674.8)

621.3   **Endometrial cystic hyperplasia**
Hyperplasia (adenomatous) (cystic) (glandular) of endometrium

621.4   **Hematometra**
Hemometra

EXCLUDES   that in congenital anomaly (752.2-752.3)

621.5   **Intrauterine synechiae**
Adhesions of uterus
Band(s) of uterus

GENITOURINARY SYSTEM

621.6 Malposition of uterus

Anteversion
Retroflexion } of uterus
Retroversion

EXCLUDES: malposition complicating pregnancy, labor, or delivery (654.3-654.4)
prolapse of uterus (618.1-618.4)

621.7 Chronic inversion of uterus

EXCLUDES: current obstetrical trauma (665.2)
prolapse of uterus (618.1-618.4)

◆ **621.8 Other specified disorders of uterus, not elsewhere classified**

Atrophy, acquired
Cyst
Fibrosis NOS } of uterus
Old laceration (postpartum)
Ulcer

EXCLUDES: bilharzial fibrosis (120.0-120.9)
endometriosis (617.0)
fistulas (619.0-619.8)
inflammatory diseases (615.0-615.9)

◆ **621.9 Unspecified disorder of uterus**

● **622 Noninflammatory disorders of cervix**

EXCLUDES: abnormality of cervix complicating pregnancy, labor, or delivery (654.5-654.6)
fistula (619.0-619.8)

622.0 Erosion and ectropion of cervix

Eversion } of cervix
Ulcer

EXCLUDES: that in chronic cervicitis (616.0)

622.1 Dysplasia of cervix (uteri)

Anaplasia of cervix
Cervical atypism

EXCLUDES: carcinoma in situ of cervix (233.1)
cervical intraepithelial neoplasia III [CIN III] (233.1)

622.2 Leukoplakia of cervix (uteri)

EXCLUDES: carcinoma in situ of cervix (233.1)

622.3 Old laceration of cervix

Adhesions
Band(s) } of cervix
Cicatrix (postpartum)

EXCLUDES: current obstetrical trauma (665.3)

622.4 Stricture and stenosis of cervix

Atresia (acquired)
Contracture } of cervix
Occlusion

Pinpoint os uteri

EXCLUDES: congenital (752.49)
that complicating labor (654.6)

622.5 Incompetence of cervix

EXCLUDES: complicating pregnancy (654.5)
that affecting fetus or newborn (761.0)

622.6 Hypertrophic elongation of cervix

622.7 Mucous polyp of cervix

Polyp NOS of cervix

EXCLUDES: adenomatous polyp of cervix (219.0)

◆ **622.8 Other specified noninflammatory disorders of cervix**

Atrophy (senile)
Cyst
Fibrosis } of cervix
Hemorrhage

EXCLUDES: endometriosis (617.0)
fistula (619.0-619.8)
inflammatory diseases (616.0)

◆ **622.9 Unspecified noninflammatory disorder of cervix**

● **623 Noninflammatory disorders of vagina**

EXCLUDES: abnormality of vagina complicating pregnancy, labor, or delivery (654.7)
congenital absence of vagina (752.49)
congenital diaphragm or bands (752.49)
fistulas involving vagina (619.0-619.8)

623.0 Dysplasia of vagina

EXCLUDES: carcinoma in situ of vagina (233.3)

623.1 Leukoplakia of vagina

623.2 Stricture or atresia of vagina

Adhesions (postoperative) (postradiation) of vagina
Occlusion of vagina
Stenosis, vagina
Use additional E code, if desired, to identify any external cause

EXCLUDES: congenital atresia or stricture (752.49)

623.3 Tight hymenal ring

Rigid hymen
Tight hymenal ring } acquired or congenital
Tight introitus

EXCLUDES: imperforate hymen (752.42)

623.4 Old vaginal laceration

EXCLUDES: old laceration involving muscles of pelvic floor (618.7)

623.5 Leukorrhea, not specified as infective

Leukorrhea NOS of vagina
Vaginal discharge NOS

EXCLUDES: trichomonal (131.00)

623.6 Vaginal hematoma

EXCLUDES: current obstetrical trauma (665.7)

623.7 Polyp of vagina

◆ **623.8 Other specified noninflammatory disorders of vagina**

Cyst } of vagina
Hemorrhage

◆ **623.9 Unspecified noninflammatory disorder of vagina**

● **624 Noninflammatory disorders of vulva and perineum**

EXCLUDES: abnormality of vulva and perineum complicating pregnancy, labor, or delivery (654.8)
condyloma acuminatum (078.1)
fistulas involving:
  perineum — see Alphabetic Index
  vulva (619.0-619.8)
vulvar varices (456.6)
vulvar involvement in skin conditions (690-709.9)

624.0 Dystrophy of vulva

Kraurosis } of vulva
Leukoplakia

EXCLUDES: carcinoma in situ of vulva (233.3)

624.1 Atrophy of vulva

624.2 Hypertrophy of clitoris

EXCLUDES: that in endocrine disorders (255.2, 256.1)

624.3 Hypertrophy of labia

Hypertrophy of vulva NOS

624.4 Old laceration or scarring of vulva

624.5 Hematoma of vulva

EXCLUDES: that complicating delivery (664.5)

624.6 Polyp of labia and vulva

◆ **624.8 Other specified noninflammatory disorders of vulva and perineum**

Cyst
Edema } of vulva
Stricture

◆ **624.9 Unspecified noninflammatory disorder of vulva and perineum**

● **625 Pain and other symptoms associated with female genital organs**

625.0 Dyspareunia

EXCLUDES: psychogenic dyspareunia (302.76)

625.1 Vaginismus

Colpospasm
Vulvismus

EXCLUDES: psychogenic vaginismus (306.51)

625.2 Mittelschmerz

Intermenstrual pain
Ovulation pain

625.3 Dysmenorrhea

Painful menstruation

EXCLUDES: psychogenic dysmenorrhea (306.52)

● Additional digits required ◆ Nonspecific code ■ Not a primary diagnosis

625.4 Premenstrual tension syndromes
Menstrual:
migraine
molimen
Premenstrual tension NOS

625.5 Pelvic congestion syndrome
Congestion-fibrosis syndrome
Taylor's syndrome

625.6 Stress incontinence, female
EXCLUDES *mixed incontinence (788.33)*
stress incontinence, male (788.32)

◆ **625.8 Other specified symptoms associated with female genital organs**

◆ **625.9 Unspecified symptom associated with female genital organs**

● **626 Disorders of menstruation and other abnormal bleeding from female genital tract**
EXCLUDES *menopausal and premenopausal bleeding (627.0)*
pain and other symptoms associated with menstrual cycle (625.2-625.4)
postmenopausal bleeding (627.1)

626.0 Absence of menstruation
Amenorrhea (primary) (secondary)

626.1 Scanty or infrequent menstruation
Hypomenorrhea
Oligomenorrhea

626.2 Excessive or frequent menstruation
Heavy periods
Menometrorrhagia
Menorrhagia
Plymenorrhea
EXCLUDES *premenopausal(627.0)*
that in puberty (626.3)

626.3 Puberty bleeding
Excessive bleeding associated with onset of menstrual periods
Pubertal menorrhagia

626.4 Irregular menstrual cycle
Irregular:
bleeding NOS
menstruation
Irregular:
periods

626.5 Ovulation bleeding
Regular intermenstrual bleeding

626.6 Metrorrhagia
Bleeding unrelated to menstrual cycle
Irregular intermenstrual bleeding

626.7 Postcoital bleeding

◆ **626.8 Other**
Dysfunctional or functional uterine hemorrhage NOS
Menstruation:
retained
suppression of

◆ **626.9 Unspecified**

● **627 Menopausal and postmenopausal disorders**

627.0 Premenopausal menorrhagia
Excessive bleeding associated with onset of menopause
Menorrhagia:
climacteric
menopausal
preclimacteric

627.1 Postmenopausal bleeding

627.2 Menopausal or female climacteric states
Symptoms, such as flushing, sleeplessness, headache, lack of concentration, associated with the menopause

627.3 Postmenopausal atrophic vaginitis
Senile (atrophic) vaginitis

627.4 States associated with artificial menopause
Postartificial menopause syndromes
Any condition classifiable to 627.1, 627.2, or 627.3 which follows induced menopause

◆ **627.8 Other specified menopausal and postmenopausal disorders**
EXCLUDES *premature menopause NOS (256.3)*

◆ **627.9 Unspecified menopausal and postmenopausal disorder**

● **628 Infertility, female**
INCLUDES primary and secondary sterility

628.0 Associated with anovulation
Anovulatory cycle
Use additional code for any associated Stein-Leventhal syndrome (256.4)

▮ ***628.1 Of pituitary-hypothalamic origin***
Code also underlying cause, as:
adiposogenital dystrophy (253.8)
anterior pituitary disorder (253.0-253.4)

628.2 Of tubal origin
Infertility associated with congenital anomaly of tube
Tubal:
block
occlusion
stenosis
Use additional code for any associated peritubal adhesions (614.6)

628.3 Of uterine origin
Infertility associated with congenital anomaly of uterus
Nonimplantation
Use additional code for any associated tuberculous endometritis (016.7)

628.4 Of cervical or vaginal origin
Infertility associated with:
anomaly of cervical mucus
congenital structural anomaly
dysmucorrhea

◆ **628.8 Of other specified origin**

◆ **628.9 Of unspecified origin**

● **629 Other disorders of female genital organs**

629.0 Hematocele, female, not elsewhere classified
EXCLUDES *hematocele or hematoma:*
broad ligament (620.7)
fallopian tube (620.8)
that associated with ectopic pregnancy (633.0-633.9)
uterus (621.4)
vagina (623.6)
vulva (624.5)

629.1 Hydrocele, canal of Nuck
Cyst of canal of Nuck (acquired)
EXCLUDES *congenital (752.41)*

◆ **629.8 Other specified disorders of female genital organs**

◆ **629.9 Unspecified disorder of female genital organs**
Habitual aborter without current pregnancy

11. COMPLICATIONS OF PREGNANCY, CHILDBIRTH, AND THE PUERPERIUM (630-676)

ECTOPIC AND MOLAR PREGNANCY (630-633)

630 Hydatidiform mole
Trophoblastic disease NOS
Vesicularmole
EXCLUDES *chorioadenoma (destruens) (236.1)*
chorionepithelioma (181)
malignant hydatidiform mole (236.1)

◆ **631 Other abnormal product of conception**
Blighted ovum
Mole:
NOS
carneous
Mole:
fleshy
stone

632 Missed abortion
Early fetal death before completion of 22 weeks' gestation with retention of dead fetus
Retained products of conception, not following spontaneous or induced abortion or delivery
EXCLUDES *failed induced abortion (638.0-638.9)*
fetal death (intrauterine) (late) (656.4)
missed delivery (656.4)
that with abnormal product of conception (630, 631)

● **633 Ectopic pregnancy**
INCLUDES ruptured ectopic pregnancy

633.0 Abdominal pregnancy
Intraperitoneal pregnancy

633.1 Tubal pregnancy
Fallopian pregnancy
Rupture of (fallopian) tube due to pregnancy
Tubal abortion

633.2 Ovarian pregnancy

◆ **633.8 Other ectopic pregnancy**
Pregnancy:
cervical
combined
cornual
Pregnancy:
intraligamentous
mesometric
mural

◆ **633.9 Unspecified ectopic pregnancy**

PREGNANCY, CHILDBIRTH, AND THE PUERPERIUM

OTHER PREGNANCY WITH ABORTIVE OUTCOME (634-639)

The following fourth-digit subdivisions are for use with categories 634-638:

.0 Complicated by genital tract and pelvic infection
Endometritis
Salpingo-oophoritis
Sepsis NOS
Septicemia NOS
Any condition classifiable to 639.0, with condition classifiable to 634-638
> EXCLUDES urinary tract infection (634-638 with .7)

.1 Complicated by delayed or excessive hemorrhage
Afibrinogenemia
Defibrination syndrome
Intravascular hemolysis
Any condition classifiable to 639.1, with condition classifiable to 634-638

.2 Complicated by damage to pelvic organs and tissues
Laceration, perforation, or tear of:
  bladder
  uterus
Any condition classifiable to 639.2, with condition classifiable to 634-638

.3 Complicated by renal failure
Oliguria
Uremia
Any condition classifiable to 639.3, with condition classifiable to 634-638

.4 Complicated by metabolic disorder
Electrolyte imbalance with conditions classifiable to 634-638

.5 Complicated by shock
Circulatory collapse
Shock (postoperative) (septic)
Any condition classifiable to 639.5, with condition classifiable to 634-638

.6 Complicated by embolism
Embolism:
  NOS
  amniotic fluid
  pulmonary
Any condition classifiable to 639.6, with condition classifiable to 634-638

♦ .7 With other specified complications
Cardiac arrest or failure
Urinary tract infection
Any condition classifiable to 639.8, with condition classifiable to 634-638

♦ .8 With unspecified complication

.9 Without mention of complication

● **634 Spontaneous abortion**
Requires fifth-digit to identify stage:
  ♦ 0 unspecified
  1 incomplete
  2 complete
> INCLUDES miscarriage
> spontaneous abortion

- ● 634.0 Complicated by genital tract and pelvic infection
- ● 634.1 Complicated by delayed or excessive hemorrhage
- ● 634.2 Complicated by damage to pelvic organs or tissues
- ● 634.3 Complicated by renal failure
- ● 634.4 Complicated by metabolic disorder
- ● 634.5 Complicated by shock
- ● 634.6 Complicated by embolism
- ♦ ● 634.7 With other specified complications
- ♦ ● 634.8 With unspecified complication
- ● 634.9 Without mention of complication

● **635 Legally induced abortion**
Requires fifth-digit to identify stage:
  ♦ 0 unspecified
  1 incomplete
  2 complete
> INCLUDES abortion or termination of pregnancy:
> elective
> legal
> therapeutic
> EXCLUDES menstrual extraction or regulation (V25.3)

- ● 635.0 Complicated by genital tract and pelvic infection
- ● 635.1 Complicated by delayed or excessive hemorrhage
- ● 635.2 Complicated by damage to pelvic organs or tissues
- ● 635.3 Complicated by renal failure
- ● 635.4 Complicated by metabolic disorder
- ● 635.5 Complicated by shock
- ● 635.6 Complicated by embolism
- ♦ ● 635.7 With other specified complications
- ♦ ● 635.8 With unspecified complication
- ● 635.9 Without mention of complication

● **636 Illegally induced abortion**
Requires fifth-digit to identify stage:
  ♦ 0 unspecified
  1 incomplete
  2 complete
> INCLUDES abortion:
> criminal
> illegal
> self-induced

- ● 636.0 Complicated by genital tract and pelvic infection
- ● 636.1 Complicated by delayed or excessive hemorrhage
- ● 636.2 Complicated by damage to pelvic organs or tissues
- ● 636.3 Complicated by renal failure
- ● 636.4 Complicated by metabolic disorder
- ● 636.5 Complicated by shock
- ● 636.6 Complicated by embolism
- ♦ ● 636.7 With other specified complications
- ♦ ● 636.8 With unspecified complication
- ● 636.9 Without mention of complication

● **637 Unspecified abortion**
Requires fifth-digit to identify stage:
  ♦ 0 unspecified
  1 incomplete
  2 complete
> INCLUDES abortion NOS
> retained products of conception following abortion, not classifiable elsewhere

- ♦ ● 637.0 Complicated by genital tract and pelvic infection
- ♦ ● 637.1 Complicated by delayed or excessive hemorrhage
- ♦ ● 637.2 Complicated by damage to pelvic organs or tissues
- ♦ ● 637.3 Complicated by renal failure
- ♦ ● 637.4 Complicated by metabolic disorder
- ♦ ● 637.5 Complicated by shock
- ♦ ● 637.6 Complicated by embolism
- ♦ ● 637.7 With other specified complications
- ♦ ● 637.8 With unspecified complication
- ♦ ● 637.9 Without mention of complication

● **638 Failed attempted abortion**
> INCLUDES failure of attempted induction of (legal) abortion
> EXCLUDES incomplete abortion (634.0-637.9)

- 638.0 Complicated by genital tract and pelvic infection
- 638.1 Complicated by delayed or excessive hemorrhage
- 638.2 Complicated by damage to pelvic organs or tissues
- 638.3 Complicated by renal failure
- 638.4 Complicated by metabolic disorder
- 638.5 Complicated by shock
- 638.6 Complicated by embolism
- ♦ 638.7 With other specified complications
- ♦ 638.8 With unspecified complication
- 638.9 Without mention of complication

● **639 Complications following abortion and ectopic and molar pregnancies**

Note: This category is provided for use when it is required to classify separately the complications classifiable to the fourth-digit level in categories 634-638; for example:

a) when the complication itself was responsible for an episode of medical care, the abortion, ectopic or molar pregnancy itself having been dealt with at a previous episode

b) when these conditions are immediate complications of ectopic or molar pregnancies classifiable to 630-633 where they cannot be identified at fourth-digit level.

● Additional digits required   ♦ Nonspecific code   ▮ Not a primary diagnosis

639.0   **Genital tract and pelvic infection**

       Endometritis
       Parametritis
       Pelvic peritonitis
       Salpingitis
       Salpingo-oophoritis   } following conditions classifiable to 630-638
       Sepsis NOS
       Septicemia NOS

       EXCLUDES   *urinary tract infection (639.8)*

639.1   **Delayed or excessive hemorrhage**

       Afibrinogenemia
       Defibrination syndrome   } following conditions classifiable to 630-638
       Intravascular hemolysis

639.2   **Damage to pelvic organs and tissues**

       Laceration, perforation, or tear of:
         bladder
         bowel
         broad ligament   } following conditions classifiable to 630-638
         cervix
         periurethral tissue
         uterus
         vagina

639.3   **Renal failure**

       Oliguria
       Renal:
         failure (acute)
         shutdown   } following conditions classifiable to 630-638
         tubular necrosis
       Uremia

639.4   **Metabolic disorders**

       Electrolyte imbalance following conditions classifiable to 630-638

639.5   **Shock**

       Circulatory collapse   } following conditions classifiable to 630-638
       Shock (postoperative) (septic)

639.6   **Embolism**

       Embolism:
         NOS
         air
         amniotic fluid
         blood-clot   } following conditions classifiable to 630-638
         fat
         pulmonary
         pyemic
         septic
         soap

◆ **639.8**   **Other specified complications following abortion or ectopic and molar pregnancy**

       Acute yellow atrophy or necrosis of liver
       Cardiac arrest or failure   } following conditions classifiable to 630-638
       Cerebral anoxia
       Urinary tract infection

◆ **639.9**   **Unspecified complication following abortion or ectopic and molar pregnancy**

       Complication(s) not further specified following conditions classifiable to 630-638

COMPLICATIONS MAINLY RELATED TO PREGNANCY (640-648)

INCLUDES   the listed conditions even if they arose or were present during labor, delivery, or the puerperium

The following fifth-digit subclassification is for use with categories 640-648 to denote the current episode of care. Valid fifth-digits are in [brackets] under each code.

◆   **0**   unspecified as to episode of care or not applicable
    1   delivered, with or without mention of antepartum condition

       Antepartum condition with delivery

       Delivery NOS
       Intrapartum obstetric condition   } (with mention of antepartum complication during current episode of care)
       Pregnancy, delivered

    2   delivered, with mention of postpartum complication

       Delivery with mention of puerperal complication during current episode of care

    3   antepartum condition or complication

       Antepartum obstetric condition, not delivered during the current episode of care

    4   postpartum condition or complication

       Postpartum or puerperal obstetric condition or complication following delivery that occurred:
         during previous episode of care
         outside hospital, with subsequent admission for observation or care

● **640**   **Hemorrhage in early pregnancy**

       INCLUDES   hemorrhage before completion of 22 weeks' gestation

   ● **640.0**   **Threatened abortion**
     [0,1,3]

◆ ● **640.8**   **Other specified hemorrhage in early pregnancy**
     [0,1,3]

◆ ● **640.9**   **Unspecified hemorrhage in early pregnancy**
     [0,1,3]

● **641**   **Antepartum hemorrhage, abruptio placentae, and placenta previa**

   ● **641.0**   **Placenta previa without hemorrhage**
     [0,1,3]

       Low implantation of placenta
       Placenta previa noted: } without hemorrhage
         during pregnancy
         before labor (and delivered by cesarean delivery)

   ● **641.1**   **Hemorrhage from placenta previa**
     [0,1,3]

       Low-lying placenta
       Placenta previa   } NOS or with hemorrhage (intrapartum)
         incomplete
         marginal
         partial
         total

       EXCLUDES   *hemorrhage from vasa previa (663.5)*

   ● **641.2**   **Premature separation of placenta**
     [0,1,3]

       Ablatio placentae
       Abruptio placentae
       Accidental antepartum hemorrhage
       Couvelaire uterus
       Detachment of placenta (premature)
       Premature separation of normally implanted placenta

   ● **641.3**   **Antepartum hemorrhage associated with coagulation defects**
     [0,1,3]

       Antepartum or intrapartum hemorrhage associated with:
         afibrinogenemia
         hyperfibrinolysis
         hypofibrinogenemia

◆ ● **641.8**   **Other antepartum hemorrhage**
     [0,1,3]

       Antepartum or intrapartum hemorrhage associated with:
         trauma
         uterine leiomyoma

◆ ● **641.9**   **Unspecified antepartum hemorrhage**
     [0,1,3]

       Hemorrhage:
         antepartum NOS
         intrapartum NOS
         of pregnancy NOS

PREGNANCY, CHILDBIRTH, AND THE PUERPERIUM

- **642 Hypertension complicating pregnancy, childbirth, and the puerperium**
  - **642.0** [0-4] **Benign essential hypertension complicating pregnancy, childbirth, and the puerperium**
    - Hypertension:
      - benign essential
      - chronic NOS
      - essential
      - pre-existing NOS
    - } specified as complicating, or as a reason for obstetric care during pregnancy, childbirth, or the puerperium
  - **642.1** [0-4] **Hypertension secondary to renal disease, complicating pregnancy, childbirth, and the puerperium**
    - Hypertension secondary to renal disease, specified as complicating, or as a reason for obstetric care during pregnancy, childbirth, or the puerperium
  - ◆ **642.2** [0-4] **Other pre-existing hypertension complicating pregnancy, childbirth, and the puerperium**
    - Hypertensive:
      - heart and renal disease
      - heart disease
      - renal disease
      - Malignant hypertension
    - } specified as complicating, or as a reason for obstetric care during pregnancy, childbirth, or the puerperium
  - **642.3** [0-4] **Transient hypertension of pregnancy**
    - Gestational hypertension
    - Transient hypertension, so described, in pregnancy, childbirth, or the puerperium
  - **642.4** [0-4] **Mild or unspecified pre-eclampsia**
    - Hypertension in pregnancy, childbirth, or the puerperium, not specified as pre-existing, with either albuminuria or edema, or both; mild or unspecified
    - Pre-eclampsia:
      - NOS
      - mild
    - Toxemia (pre-eclamptic):
      - NOS
      - mild
    - **EXCLUDES** albuminuria in pregnancy, without mention of hypertension (646.2)
      edema in pregnancy, without mention of hypertension (646.1)
  - **642.5** [0-4] **Severe pre-eclampsia**
    - Hypertension in pregnancy, childbirth, or the puerperium, not specified as pre-existing, with either albuminuria or edema, or both; specified as severe
    - Pre-eclampsia, severe
    - Toxemia (pre-eclamptic), severe
  - **642.6** [0-4] **Eclampsia**
    - Toxemia:
      - eclamptic
      - with convulsions
  - **642.7** [0-4] **Pre-eclampsia or eclampsia superimposed on pre-existing hypertension**
    - Conditions classifiable to 642.4-642.6, with conditions classifiable to 642.0-642.2
  - ◆ **642.9** [0-4] **Unspecified hypertension complicating pregnancy, childbirth, or the puerperium**
    - Hypertension NOS, without mention of albuminuria or edema, complicating pregnancy, childbirth, or the puerperium
- **643 Excessive vomiting in pregnancy**
  - **INCLUDES** hyperemesis
    vomiting:
      persistent
      vicious
    } arising during pregnancy
  - hyperemesis gravidarum
  - **643.0** [0,1,3] **Mild hyperemesis gravidarum**
    - Hyperemesis gravidarum, mild or unspecified, starting before the end of the 22nd week of gestation
  - **643.1** [0,1,3] **Hyperemesis gravidarum with metabolic disturbance**
    - Hyperemesis gravidarum, starting before the end of the 22nd week of gestation, with metabolic disturbance, such as:
      - carbohydrate depletion
      - dehydration
      - electrolyte imbalance
  - **643.2** [0,1,3] **Late vomiting of pregnancy**
    - Excessive vomiting starting after 22 completed weeks of gestation
  - ◆ **643.8** [0,1,3] **Other vomiting complicating pregnancy**
    - Vomiting due to organic disease or other cause, specified as complicating pregnancy, or as a reason for obstetric care during pregnancy
    - Use additional code, if desired, to specify cause
  - ◆ **643.9** [0,1,3] **Unspecified vomiting of pregnancy**
    - Vomiting as a reason for care during pregnancy, length of gestation unspecified
- **644 Early or threatened labor**
  - **644.0** [0,3] **Threatened premature labor**
    - Premature labor after 22 weeks, but before 37 completed weeks of gestation without delivery
    - **EXCLUDES** that occurring before 22 completed weeks of gestation (640.0)
  - ◆ **644.1** [0,3] **Other threatened labor**
    - False labor:
      - NOS
      - after 37 completed weeks of gestation
    - Threatened labor NOS
    - } without delivery
  - **644.2** [0,1] **Early onset of delivery**
    - Onset (spontaneous) of delivery
    - Premature labor with onset of delivery
    - } before 37 completed weeks of gestation
- **645 Prolonged pregnancy**
  - [0,1,3] Post-term pregnancy
    Pregnancy which has advanced beyond 42 weeks of gestation
    Use 0 as fourth-digit for this category
- **646 Other complications of pregnancy, not elsewhere classified**
  - **646.0** [0,1,3] **Papyraceous fetus**
  - **646.1** [0-4] **Edema or excessive weight gain in pregnancy, without mention of hypertension**
    - Gestational edema   Maternal obesity syndrome
    - **EXCLUDES** that with mention of hypertension (642.0-642.9)
  - ◆ **646.2** [0-4] **Unspecified renal disease in pregnancy, without mention of hypertension**
    - Albuminuria
    - Nephropathy NOS
    - Renal disease NOS
    - Uremia
    - } in pregnancy or the puerperium, without mention of hypertension
    - Gestational proteinuria
    - **EXCLUDES** that with mention of hypertension (642.0-642.9)
  - **646.3** [0,1,3] **Habitual aborter**
    - **EXCLUDES** with current abortion (634.0-634.9)
      without current pregnancy (629.9)
  - **646.4** [0-4] **Peripheral neuritis in pregnancy**
  - **646.5** [0-4] **Asymptomatic bacteriuria in pregnancy**
  - **646.6** [0-4] **Infections of genitourinary tract in pregnancy**
    - Conditions classifiable to 590, 595, 597, 599.0, 616 complicating pregnancy, childbirth, or the puerperium
    - Conditions classifiable to 614-615 complicating pregnancy or labor
    - **EXCLUDES** major puerperal infection (670)
  - **646.7** [0,1,3] **Liver disorders in pregnancy**
    - Acute yellow atrophy of liver (obstetric) (true)
    - Icterus gravis
    - Necrosis of liver
    - } of pregnancy
    - **EXCLUDES** hepatorenal syndrome following delivery (674.8)
  - ◆ **646.8** [0-4] **Other specified complications of pregnancy**
    - Fatigue during pregnancy
    - Herpes gestationis
    - Insufficient weight gain of pregnancy

● Additional digits required   ◆ Nonspecific code   ■ Not a primary diagnosis

- **646.9 Unspecified complication of pregnancy**
  [0,1,3]
- **647 Infectious and parasitic conditions in the mother classifiable elsewhere, but complicating pregnancy, childbirth, or the puerperium**
  - INCLUDES: the listed conditions when complicating the pregnant state, aggravated by the pregnancy, or when a main reason for obstetric care
  - EXCLUDES: those conditions in the mother known or suspected to have affected the fetus (655.0-655.9)
  - **647.0 Syphilis**
    [0-4] Conditions classifiable to 090-097
  - **647.1 Gonorrhea**
    [0-4] Conditions classifiable to 098
  - **647.2 Other venereal diseases**
    [0-4] Conditions classifiable to 099
  - **647.3 Tuberculosis**
    [0-4] Conditions classifiable to 010-018
  - **647.4 Malaria**
    [0-4] Conditions classifiable to 084
  - **647.5 Rubella**
    [0-4] Conditions classifiable to 056
  - **647.6 Other viral diseases**
    [0-4] Conditions classifiable to 042 and 050-079, except 056
  - **647.8 Other specified infectious and parasitic diseases**
    [0-4]
  - **647.9 Unspecified infection or infestation**
    [0-4]
- **648 Other current conditions in the mother classifiable elsewhere, but complicating pregnancy, childbirth, or the puerperium**
  - INCLUDES: the listed conditions when complicating the pregnant state, aggravated by the pregnancy, or when a main reason for obstetric care
  - EXCLUDES: those conditions in the mother known or suspected to have affected the fetus (655.0-665.9)
  - **648.0 Diabetes mellitus**
    [0-4] Conditions classifiable to 250
    - EXCLUDES: gestational diabetes (648.8)
  - **648.1 Thyroid dysfunction**
    [0-4] Conditions classifiable to 240-246
  - **648.2 Anemia**
    [0-4] Conditions classifiable to 280-285
  - **648.3 Drug dependence**
    [0-4] Conditions classifiable to 304
  - **648.4 Mental disorders**
    [0-4] Conditions classifiable to 290-303, 305-316, 317-319
  - **648.5 Congenital cardiovascular disorders**
    [0-4] Conditions classifiable to 745-747
  - **648.6 Other cardiovascular diseases**
    [0-4] Conditions classifiable to 390-398, 410-429, 440-459
    - EXCLUDES: cerebrovascular disorders in the puerperium (674.0)
    - venous complications (671.0-671.9)
  - **648.7 Bone and joint disorders of back, pelvis, and lower limbs**
    [0-4] Conditions classifiable to 720-724, and those classifiable to 711-719 or 725-738, specified as affecting the lower limbs
  - **648.8 Abnormal glucose tolerance**
    [0-4] Conditions classifiable to 790.2
    Gestational diabetes
  - **648.9 Other current conditions classifiable elsewhere**
    [0-4] Nutritional deficiencies [conditions classifiable to 260-269]

NORMAL DELIVERY, AND OTHER INDICATIONS FOR CARE IN PREGNANCY, LABOR, AND DELIVERY (650-659)

The following fifth-digit subclassification is for use with categories 651-659 to denote the current episode of care. Valid fifth-digits are in [brackets] under each code.

- 0 unspecified as to episode of care or not applicable
- 1 delivered, with or without mention of antepartum condition
- 2 delivered, with mention of postpartum complication
- 3 antepartum condition or complication
- 4 postpartum condition or complication

- **650 Delivery in a completely normal case**
  Delivery without abnormality or complication classifiable elsewhere in categories 630-676, and with spontaneous cephalic delivery, without mention of fetal manipulation [e.g., rotation, version] or instrumentation [forceps]
  - EXCLUDES: breech delivery (assisted) (spontaneous) NOS (652.2)
    delivery by vacuum extractor, forceps, cesarean section, or breech extraction, without specified complication (669.5-669.7)
- **651 Multiple gestation**
  - **651.0 Twin pregnancy**
    [0,1,3]
  - **651.1 Triplet pregnancy**
    [0,1,3]
  - **651.2 Quadruplet pregnancy**
    [0,1,3]
  - **651.3 Twin pregnancy with fetal loss and retention of one fetus**
    [0,1,3]
  - **651.4 Triplet pregnancy with fetal loss and retention of one or more fetus(es)**
    [0,1,3]
  - **651.5 Quadruplet pregnancy with fetal loss and retention of one or more fetus(es)**
    [0,1,3]
  - **651.6 Other multiple pregnancy with fetal loss and retention of one or more fetus(es)**
    [0,1,3]
  - **651.8 Other specified multiple gestation**
    [0,1,3]
  - **651.9 Unspecified multiple gestation**
    [0,1,3]
- **652 Malposition and malpresentation of fetus**
  Code also any associated obstructed labor (660.0)
  - **652.0 Unstable lie**
    [0,1,3]
  - **652.1 Breech or other malpresentation successfully converted to cephalic presentation**
    [0,1,3] Cephalic version NOS
  - **652.2 Breech presentation without mention of version**
    [0,1,3] Breech delivery (assisted) (spontaneous) NOS
  - **652.3 Transverse or oblique presentation**
    [0,1,3] Oblique lie
    Transverse lie
    - EXCLUDES: transverse arrest of fetal head (660.3)
  - **652.4 Face or brow presentation**
    [0,1,3] Mentum presentation
  - **652.5 High head at term**
    [0,1,3] Failure of head to enter pelvic brim
  - **652.6 Multiple gestation with malpresentation of one fetus or more**
    [0,1,3]
  - **652.7 Prolapsed arm**
    [0,1,3]
  - **652.8 Other specified malposition or malpresentation**
    [0,1,3] Compound presentation
  - **652.9 Unspecified malposition or malpresentation**
    [0,1,3]
- **653 Disproportion**
  Code also any associated obstructed labor (660.1)
  - **653.0 Major abnormality of bony pelvis, not further specified**
    [0,1,3] Pelvic deformity NOS
  - **653.1 Generally contracted pelvis**
    [0,1,3] Contracted pelvis NOS
  - **653.2 Inlet contraction of pelvis**
    [0,1,3] Inlet contraction (pelvis)
  - **653.3 Outlet contraction of pelvis**
    [0,1,3] Outlet contraction (pelvis)
  - **653.4 Fetopelvic disproportion**
    [0,1,3] Cephalopelvic disproportion NOS
    Disproportion of mixed maternal and fetal origin, with normally formed fetus
  - **653.5 Unusually large fetus causing disproportion**
    [0,1,3] Disproportion of fetal origin with normally formed fetus
    Fetal disproportion NOS
    - EXCLUDES: that when the reason for medical care was concern for the fetus (656.6)
  - **653.6 Hydrocephalic fetus causing disproportion**
    [0,1,3]
    - EXCLUDES: that when the reason for medical care was concern for the fetus (655.0)

PREGNANCY, CHILDBIRTH, AND THE PUERPERIUM

- ◆ ● **653.7** Other fetal abnormality causing disproportion
  [0,1,3]
  - Conjoined twins
  - Fetal:
    - ascites
    - hydrops
    - myelomeningocele
    - sacral teratoma
    - tumor
- ◆ ● **653.8** Disproportion of other origin
  [0,1,3] **EXCLUDES** shoulder (girdle) dystocia (660.4)
- ◆ ● **653.9** Unspecified disproportion
  [0,1,3]
- ● **654** Abnormality of organs and soft tissues of pelvis
  - **INCLUDES** the listed conditions during pregnancy, childbirth, or the puerperium
  - Code also any associated obstructed labor (660.2)
  - ● **654.0** Congenital abnormalities of uterus
    [0-4] Double uterus   Uterus bicornis
  - ● **654.1** Tumors of body of uterus
    [0-4] Uterine fibroids
  - ● **654.2** Previous cesarean delivery
    [0,1,3] Uterine scar from previous cesarean delivery
  - ● **654.3** Retroverted and incarcerated gravid uterus
    [0-4]
  - ◆ ● **654.4** Other abnormalities in shape or position of gravid uterus and
    [0-4] of neighboring structures
    - Cystocele   Prolapse of gravid uterus
    - Pelvic floor repair Rectocele
    - Pendulous abdomen   Rigid pelvic floor
  - ● **654.5** Cervical incompetence
    [0-4] Presence of Shirodkar suture with or without mention of cervical incompetence
  - ◆ ● **654.6** Other congenital or acquired abnormality of cervix
    [0-4]
    - Cicatricial cervix   Rigid cervix (uteri)
    - Polyp of cervix   Stenosis or stricture of cervix
    - Previous surgery to cervix   Tumor of cervix
  - ● **654.7** Congenital or acquired abnormality of vagina
    [0-4]
    - Previous surgery to vagina
    - Septate vagina
    - Stenosis of vagina (acquired) (congenital)
    - Stricture of vagina
    - Tumor of vagina
  - ● **654.8** Congenital or acquired abnormality of vulva
    [0-4]
    - Fibrosis of perineum   Rigid perineum
    - Persistent hymen   Tumor of vulva
    - Previous surgery to perineum or vulva
    - **EXCLUDES** varicose veins of vulva (671.1)
  - ◆ ● **654.9** Other and unspecified
    [0-4] Uterine scar NEC
- ● **655** Known or suspected fetal abnormality affecting management of mother
  - **INCLUDES** the listed conditions in the fetus as a reason for observation or obstetrical care of the mother, or for termination of pregnancy
  - ● **655.0** Central nervous system malformation in fetus
    [0,1,3] Fetal or suspected fetal:
    - anencephaly
    - hydrocephalus
    - spina bifida (with myelomeningocele)
  - ● **655.1** Chromosomal abnormality in fetus
    [0,1,3]
  - ● **655.2** Hereditary disease in family possibly affecting fetus
    [0,1,3]
  - ● **655.3** Suspected damage to fetus from viral disease in the mother
    [0,1,3] Suspected damage to fetus from maternal rubella
  - ◆ ● **655.4** Suspected damage to fetus from other disease in the mother
    [0,1,3] Suspected damage to fetus from maternal:
    - alcohol addiction
    - listeriosis
    - toxoplasmosis
  - ● **655.5** Suspected damage to fetus from drugs
    [0,1,3] **EXCLUDES** fetal distress in labor and delivery due to drug administration (656.3)
  - ● **655.6** Suspected damage to fetus from radiation
    [0,1,3]
- ◆ ● **655.8** Other known or suspected fetal abnormality, not elsewhere
  [0,1,3] classified
  - Suspected damage to fetus from:
    - environmental toxins
    - intrauterine contraceptive device
- ◆ ● **655.9** Unspecified
  [0,1,3]
- ● **656** Other fetal and placental problems affecting management of mother
  - ● **656.0** Fetal-maternal hemorrhage
    [0,1,3] Leakage (microscopic) of fetal blood into maternal circulation
  - ● **656.1** Rhesus isoimmunization
    [0,1,3] Anti-D [Rh] antibodies
    Rh incompatibility
  - ◆ ● **656.2** Isoimmunization from other and unspecified blood-group
    [0,1,3] incompatibility
    ABO isoimmunization
  - ● **656.3** Fetal distress
    [0,1,3] Abnormal fetal:
    - acid-base balance
    - heart rate or rhythm
    Fetal:
    - acidemia
    - bradycardia
    - tachycardia
    Meconium in liquor
  - ● **656.4** Intrauterine death
    [0,1,3] Fetal death:
    - NOS
    - after completion of 22 weeks' gestation
    - late
    Missed delivery
    EXCLUDES missed abortion (632)
  - ● **656.5** Poor fetal growth
    [0,1,3]
    - "Light-for-dates"
    - "Placental insufficiency"
    - "Small-for-dates"
  - ● **656.6** Excessive fetal growth
    [0,1,3] "Large-for-dates"
  - ◆ ● **656.7** Other placental conditions
    [0,1,3]
    - Abnormal placenta
    - Placental infarct
    EXCLUDES placental polyp (674.4)
    placentitis (658.4)
  - ◆ ● **656.8** Other specified fetal and placental problems
    [0,1,3] Lithopedian
  - ◆ ● **656.9** Unspecified fetal and placental problem
- ● **657** Polyhydramnios
  [0,1,3] Hydramnios
  Use 0 as fourth-digit for this category
- ● **658** Other problems associated with amniotic cavity and membranes
  EXCLUDES amniotic fluid embolism (673.1)
  - ● **658.0** Oligohydramnios
    [0,1,3] Oligohydramnios without mention of rupture of membranes
  - ● **658.1** Premature rupture of membranes
    [0,1,3] Rupture of amniotic sac less than 24 hours prior to the onset of labor
  - ● **658.2** Delayed delivery after spontaneous or unspecified rupture of
    [0,1,3] membranes
    Prolonged rupture of membranes NOS
    Rupture of amniotic sac 24 hours or more prior to the onset of labor
  - ● **658.3** Delayed delivery after artificial rupture of membranes
    [0,1,3]
  - ● **658.4** Infection of amniotic cavity
    [0,1,3]
    - Amnionitis
    - Chorioamnionitis
    - Membranitis
    - Placentitis
  - ◆ ● **658.8** Other
    [0,1,3]
    - Amnion nodosum
    - Amniotic cyst
  - ◆ ● **658.9** Unspecified
    [0,1,3]

● Additional digits required   ◆ Nonspecific code   ■ Not a primary diagnosis

- **659** Other indications for care or intervention related to labor and delivery, not elsewhere classified
  - **659.0** Failed mechanical induction
    [0,1,3] Failure of induction of labor by surgical or other instrumental methods
  - **659.1** Failed medical or unspecified induction
    [0,1,3] Failed induction NOS
    Failure of induction of labor by medical methods, such as oxytocic drugs
  - **659.2** Maternal pyrexia during labor, unspecified
    [0,1,3]
  - **659.3** Generalized infection during labor
    [0,1,3] Septicemia during labor
  - **659.4** Grand multiparity
    [0,1,3]

    EXCLUDES supervision only, in pregnancy (V23.3)
    without current pregnancy (V61.5)
  - **659.5** Elderly primigravida
    [0,1,3] **EXCLUDES** supervision only, in pregnancy (V23.8)
  - **659.6** Other advanced maternal age
    [0,1,3] **EXCLUDES** elderly primigravida 659.5
  - **659.8** Other specified indications for care or intervention related to labor and delivery
    [0,1,3]
  - **659.9** Unspecified indication for care or intervention related to labor and delivery
    [0,1,3]

COMPLICATIONS OCCURRING MAINLY IN THE COURSE OF LABOR AND DELIVERY (660-669)

The following fifth-digit subclassification is for use with categories 660-669 to denote the current episode of care. Valid fifth-digits are in [brackets] under each code.

- 0 unspecified as to episode of care or not applicable
- 1 delivered, with or without mention of antepartum condition
- 2 delivered, with mention of postpartum complication
- 3 antepartum condition or complication
- 4 postpartum condition or complication

- **660** Obstructed labor
  - **660.0** Obstruction caused by malposition of fetus at onset of labor
    [0,1,3] Any condition classifiable to 652, causing obstruction during labor
    Use additional code from 652.0-652.9, if desired, to identify condition
  - **660.1** Obstruction by bony pelvis
    [0,1,3] Any condition classifiable to 653, causing obstruction during labor
    Use additional code from 653.0-653.9, if desired, to identify condition
  - **660.2** Obstruction by abnormal pelvic soft tissues
    [0,1,3] Prolapse of anterior lip of cervix
    Any condition classifiable to 654, causing obstruction during labor
    Use additional code from 654.0-654.9, if desired, to identify condition
  - **660.3** Deep transverse arrest and persistent occipitoposterior position
    [0,1,3]
  - **660.4** Shoulder (girdle) dystocia
    [0,1,3] Impacted shoulders
  - **660.5** Locked twins
    [0,1,3]
  - **660.6** Failed trial of labor, unspecified
    [0,1,3] Failed trial of labor, without mention of condition or suspected condition
  - **660.7** Failed forceps or vacuum extractor, unspecified
    [0,1,3] Application of ventouse or forceps, without mention of condition
  - **660.8** Other causes of obstructed labor
    [0,1,3]
  - **660.9** Unspecified obstructed labor
    [0,1,3] Dystocia:
    NOS
    fetal NOS
    maternal NOS

- **661** Abnormality of forces of labor
  - **661.0** Primary uterine inertia
    [0,1,3] Failure of cervical dilation
    Hypotonic uterine dysfunction, primary
    Prolonged latent phase of labor
  - **661.1** Secondary uterine inertia
    [0,1,3] Arrested active phase of labor
    Hypotonic uterine dysfunction, secondary
  - **661.2** Other and unspecified uterine inertia
    [0,1,3] Atony of uterus   Poor contractions
    Desultory labor   Slow slope active phase
    Irregular labor   of labor
  - **661.3** Precipitate labor
    [0,1,3]
  - **661.4** Hypertonic, incoordinate, or prolonged uterine contractions
    [0,1,3] Cervical spasm
    Contraction ring (dystocia)
    Dyscoordinate labor
    Hourglass contraction of uterus
    Hypertonic uterine dysfunction
    Incoordinate uterine action
    Retraction ring (Bandl's) (pathological)
    Tetanic contractions
    Uterine dystocia NOS
    Uterine spasm
  - **661.9** Unspecified abnormality of labor
    [0,1,3]

- **662** Long labor
  - **662.0** Prolonged first stage
    [0,1,3]
  - **662.1** Prolonged labor, unspecified
    [0,1,3]
  - **662.2** Prolonged second stage
    [0,1,3]
  - **662.3** Delayed delivery of second twin, triplet, etc.
    [0,1,3]

- **663** Umbilical cord complications
  - **663.0** Prolapse of cord
    [0,1,3] Presentation of cord
  - **663.1** Cord around neck, with compression
    [0,1,3] Cord tightly around neck
  - **663.2** Other and unspecified cord entanglement, with compression
    [0,1,3] Entanglement of cords of twins in mono-amniotic sac
    Knot in cord (with compression)
  - **663.3** Other and unspecified cord entanglement, without mention of compression
    [0,1,3]
  - **663.4** Short cord
    [0,1,3]
  - **663.5** Vasa previa
    [0,1,3] Velamentous insertion of umbilical cord
  - **663.6** Vascular lesions of cord
    [0,1,3] Bruising of cord   Thrombosis of vessels of
    Hematoma of cord   cord
  - **663.8** Other umbilical cord complications
    [0,1,3]
  - **663.9** Unspecified umbilical cord complication
    [0,1,3]

- **664** Trauma to perineum and vulva during delivery
  INCLUDES damage from instruments
  that from extension of episiotomy
  - **664.0** First-degree perineal laceration
    [0,1,4] Perineal laceration, rupture, or tear involving:
    fourchette
    hymen
    labia
    skin
    vagina
    vulva
  - **664.1** Second-degree perineal laceration
    [0,1,4] Perineal laceration, rupture, or tear (following episiotomy) involving:
    pelvic floor
    perineal muscles
    vaginal muscles
    EXCLUDES that involving anal sphincter (664.2)
  - **664.2** Third-degree perineal laceration
    [0,1,4] Perineal laceration, rupture, or tear (following episiotomy) involving:
    anal sphincter
    rectovaginal septum
    sphincter NOS
    EXCLUDES that with anal or rectal mucosal laceration (664.3)

664.3 PREGNANCY, CHILDBIRTH, AND THE PUERPERIUM 671.2

- ● **664.3** **Fourth-degree perineal laceration**
  [0,1,4]   Perineal laceration, rupture, or tear as classifiable to 664.2 and involving also:
  anal mucosa
  rectal mucosa
- ◆ ● **664.4** **Unspecified perineal laceration**
  [0,1,4]   Central laceration
- ● **664.5** **Vulval and perineal hematoma**
  [0,1,4]
- ◆ ● **664.8** **Other specified trauma to perineum and vulva**
  [0,1,4]
- ◆ ● **664.9** **Unspecified trauma to perineum and vulva**
  [0,1,4]
- ● **665** **Other obstetrical trauma**
  INCLUDES   damage from instruments
  - ● **665.0** **Rupture of uterus before onset of labor**
    [0,1,3]
  - ● **665.1** **Rupture of uterus during labor**
    [0,1]   Rupture of uterus NOS
  - ● **665.2** **Inversion of uterus**
    [0,2,4]
  - ● **665.3** **Laceration of cervix**
    [0,1,4]
  - ● **665.4** **High vaginal laceration**
    [0,1,4]   Laceration of vaginal wall or sulcus without mention of perineal laceration
  - ◆ ● **665.5** **Other injury to pelvic organs**
    [0,1,4]   Injury to:
    bladder
    urethra
  - ● **665.6** **Damage to pelvic joints and ligaments**
    [0,1,4]   Avulsion of inner symphyseal cartilage
    Damage to coccyx
    Separation of symphysis (pubis)
  - ● **665.7** **Pelvic hematoma**
    [0,1,2,4]   Hematoma of vagina
  - ◆ ● **665.8** **Other specified obstetrical trauma**
    [0-4]
  - ◆ ● **665.9** **Unspecified obstetrical trauma**
    [0-4]
- ● **666** **Postpartum hemorrhage**
  - ● **666.0** **Third-stage hemorrhage**
    [0,2,4]   Hemorrhage associated with retained, trapped, or adherent placenta
    Retained placenta NOS
  - ◆ ● **666.1** **Other immediate postpartum hemorrhage**
    [0,2,4]   Hemorrhage within the first 24 hours following delivery of placenta
    Postpartum hemorrhage (atonic) NOS
  - ● **666.2** **Delayed and secondary postpartum hemorrhage**
    [0,2,4]   Hemorrhage:
    after the first 24 hours following delivery
    associated with retained portions of placenta or membranes
    Postpartum hemorrhage specified as delayed or secondary
    Retained products of conception NOS, following delivery
  - ● **666.3** **Postpartum coagulation defects**
    [0,2,4]   Postpartum:
    afibrinogenemia
    fibrinolysis
- ● **667** **Retained placenta or membranes, without hemorrhage**
  - ● **667.0** **Retained placenta without hemorrhage**
    [0,2,4]   Placenta accreta
    Retained placenta: } without
    NOS   hemorrhage
    total
  - ● **667.1** **Retained portions of placenta or membranes, without hemorrhage**
    [0,2,4]   Retained products of conception following delivery, without hemorrhage
- ● **668** **Complications of the administration of anesthetic or other sedation in labor and delivery**
  INCLUDES   complications arising from the administration of a general or local anesthetic, analgesic, or other sedation in labor and delivery
  EXCLUDES   reaction to spinal or lumbar puncture (349.0)
  spinal headache (349.0)

- ● **668.0** **Pulmonary complications**
  [0-4]   Inhalation [aspiration] of
  stomach contents or   } following anesthesia or
  secretions   other sedation in
  Mendelson's syndrome   labor or delivery
  Pressure collapse of lung
- ● **668.1** **Cardiac complications**
  [0-4]   Cardiac arrest or failure following anesthesia or other sedation in labor and delivery
- ● **668.2** **Central nervous system complications**
  [0-4]   Cerebral anoxia following anesthesia or other sedation in labor and delivery
- ◆ ● **668.8** **Other complications of anesthesia or other sedation in labor and delivery**
  [0-4]
- ◆ ● **668.9** **Unspecified complication of anesthesia and other sedation**
  [0-4]
- ● **669** **Other complications of labor and delivery, not elsewhere classified**
  - ● **669.0** **Maternal distress**
    [0-4]   Metabolic disturbance in labor and delivery
  - ● **669.1** **Shock during or following labor and delivery**
    [0-4]   Obstetric shock
  - ● **669.2** **Maternal hypotension syndrome**
    [0-4]
  - ● **669.3** **Acute renal failure following labor and delivery**
    [0,2,4]
  - ◆ ● **669.4** **Other complications of obstetrical surgery and procedures**
    [0-4]   Cardiac: } following cesarean or other
    arrest   obstetrical surgery or
    failure   procedure, including delivery
    Cerebral anoxia   NOS ◆
    EXCLUDES   complications of obstetrical surgical wounds (674.1-674.3)
  - ● **669.5** **Forceps or vacuum extractor delivery without mention of indication**
    [0,1]   Delivery by ventouse, without mention of indication
  - ● **669.6** **Breech extraction, without mention of indication**
    [0,1]   **EXCLUDES**   breech delivery NOS (652.2)
  - ● **669.7** **Cesarean delivery, without mention of indication**
    [0,1]
  - ◆ ● **669.8** **Other complications of labor and delivery**
    [0-4]
  - ◆ ● **669.9** **Unspecified complication of labor and delivery**
    [0-4]

COMPLICATIONS OF THE PUERPERIUM (670-676)

Note: Categories 671 and 673-676 include the listed conditions even if they occur during pregnancy or childbirth.
The following fifth-digit subclassification is for use with categories 670-676 to denote the current episode of care. Valid fifth-digits are in [brackets] under each code.

- ◆ 0 unspecified as to episode of care or not applicable
- 1 delivered, with or without mention of antepartum condition
- 2 delivered, with mention of postpartum complication
- 3 antepartum condition or complication
- 4 postpartum condition or complication

- ● **670** **Major puerperal infection**
  [0,2,4]   Puerperal: Puerperal:
  endometritis   peritonitis
  fever   pyemia
  pelvic: salpingitis
  cellulitis   septicemia
  sepsis
  EXCLUDES   infection following abortion (639.0)
  minor genital tract infection following delivery (646.6)
  urinary tract infection following delivery (646.6)
  Use 0 as fourth-digit for this category
- ● **671** **Venous complications in pregnancy and the puerperium**
  - ● **671.0** **Varicose veins of legs**
    [0-4]   Varicose veins NOS
  - ● **671.1** **Varicose veins of vulva and perineum**
    [0-4]
  - ● **671.2** **Superficial thrombophlebitis**
    [0-4]   Thrombophlebitis (superficial)

● Additional digits required   ◆ Nonspecific code   ■ Not a primary diagnosis   Volume 1 — 111

- **671.3 Deep phlebothrombosis, antepartum**
  [0,1,3]   Deep-vein thrombosis, antepartum
- **671.4 Deep phlebothrombosis, postpartum**
  [0,2,4]   Deep-vein thrombosis, postpartum
  Pelvic thrombophlebitis, postpartum
  Phlegmasia alba dolens (puerperal)
- **671.5 Other phlebitis and thrombosis**
  [0-4]   Cerebral venous thrombosis
  Thrombosis of intracranial venous sinus
- **671.8 Other venous complications**
  [0-4]   Hemorrhoids
- **671.9 Unspecified venous complication**
  [0-4]   Phlebitis NOS
  Thrombosis NOS

- **672 Pyrexia of unknown origin during the puerperium**
  [0,2,4]   Puerperal pyrexia NOS
  Use 0 as fourth-digit for this category

- **673 Obstetrical pulmonary embolism**
  INCLUDES pulmonary emboli in pregnancy, childbirth, or the puerperium, or specified as puerperal
  EXCLUDES embolism following abortion (639.6)
  - **673.0 Obstetrical air embolism**
    [0-4]
  - **673.1 Amniotic fluid embolism**
    [0-4]
  - **673.2 Obstetrical blood-clot embolism**
    Puerperal pulmonary embolism NOS
  - **673.3 Obstetrical pyemic and septic embolism**
    [0-4]
  - **673.8 Other pulmonary embolism**
    [0-4]   Fat embolism

- **674 Other and unspecified complications of the puerperium, not elsewhere classified**
  - **674.0 Cerebrovascular disorders in the puerperium**
    [0-4]   Any condition classifiable to 430-434, 436-437 occurring during pregnancy, childbirth, or the puerperium, or specified as puerperal
    EXCLUDES intracranial venous sinus thrombosis (671.5)
  - **674.1 Disruption of cesarean wound**
    [0,2,4]   Dehiscence or disruption of uterine wound
  - **674.2 Disruption of perineal wound**
    [0,2,4]   Breakdown of perineum   Disruption of wound of:
    Disruption of wound of: perineal laceration
    episiotomy   Secondary perineal tear
  - **674.3 Other complications of obstetrical surgical wounds**
    [0,2,4]   Hematoma
    Hemorrhage } of cesarean section or perineal wound
    Infection
    EXCLUDES damage from instruments in delivery (664.0-665.9)
  - **674.4 Placental polyp**
    [0,2,4]
  - **674.8 Other**
    [0,2,4]   Hepatorenal syndrome, following delivery
    Postpartum:
    cardiomyopathy
    subinvolution of uterus
    uterine hypertrophy
  - **674.9 Unspecified**
    [0,2,4]   Sudden death of unknown cause during the puerperium

- **675 Infections of the breast and nipple associated with childbirth**
  INCLUDES the listed conditions during pregnancy, childbirth, or the puerperium
  - **675.0 Infections of nipple**
    [0-4]   Abscess of nipple
  - **675.1 Abscess of breast**
    [0-4]   Abscess: Mastitis:
    mammary   purulent
    subareolar   retromammary
    submammary   submammary
  - **675.2 Nonpurulent mastitis**
    [0-4]   Lymphangitis of breast
    Mastitis:
    NOS
    interstitial
    parenchymatous
  - **675.8 Other specified infections of the breast and nipple**
    [0-4]
  - **675.9 Unspecified infection of the breast and nipple**
    [0-4]

- **676 Other disorders of the breast associated with childbirth and disorders of lactation**
  INCLUDES the listed conditions during pregnancy, the puerperium, or lactation
  - **676.0 Retracted nipple**
    [0-4]
  - **676.1 Cracked nipple**
    [0-4]   Fissure of nipple
  - **676.2 Engorgement of breasts**
    [0-4]
  - **676.3 Other and unspecified disorder of breast**
    [0-4]
  - **676.4 Failure of lactation**
    [0-4]   Agalactia
  - **676.5 Suppressed lactation**
    [0-4]
  - **676.6 Galactorrhea**
    [0-4]   EXCLUDES galactorrhea not associated with childbirth (611.6)
  - **676.8 Other disorders of lactation**
    [0-4]   Galactocele
  - **676.9 Unspecified disorder of lactation**
    [0-4]

- **677 Late effect of complication of pregnancy, childbirth, and the puerperium**
  Note: This category is to be used to indicate conditions in 632-648.9 and 651-676.9 as the cause of the late effect, themselves classifiable elsewhere. The "late effects" include conditions specified as such, or as sequelae, which may occur at any time after puerperium.
  Code also any sequelae

12. DISEASES OF THE SKIN AND SUBCUTANEOUS TISSUE (680-709)

INFECTIONS OF SKIN AND SUBCUTANEOUS TISSUE (680-686)

EXCLUDES certain infections of skin classified under "Infectious and Parasitic Diseases," such as:
erysipelas (035)
erysipeloid of Rosenbach (027.1)
herpes:
simplex (054.0-054.9)
zoster (053.0-053.9)
molluscum contagiosum (078.0)
viral warts (078.1)

- **680 Carbuncle and furuncle**
  INCLUDES boil
  furunculosis
  - **680.0 Face**
    Ear [any part]   Nose (septum)
    Face [any part, except eye]   Temple (region)
    EXCLUDES eyelid (373.13)
    lacrimal apparatus (375.31)
    orbit (376.01)
  - **680.1 Neck**
  - **680.2 Trunk**
    Abdominal wall   Flank
    Back [any part, except   Groin
    buttocks]   Pectoral region
    Breast   Perineum
    Chest wall   Umbilicus
    EXCLUDES buttocks (680.5)
    external genital organs:
    female (616.4)
    male (607.2, 608.4)
  - **680.3 Upper arm and forearm**
    Arm [any part, except   Axilla
    hand]   Shoulder
  - **680.4 Hand**
    Finger [any]   Wrist
    Thumb

SKIN AND SUBCUTANEOUS TISSUE

- 680.5 **Buttock**
  - Anus
  - Gluteal region
- 680.6 **Leg, except foot**
  - Ankle
  - Hip
  - Knee
  - Thigh
- 680.7 **Foot**
  - Heel
  - Toe
- ◆ 680.8 **Other specified sites**
  - Head [any part, except face]
  - Scalp
  - **EXCLUDES** external genital organs:
    - female (616.4)
    - male (607.2, 608.4)
- ◆ 680.9 **Unspecified site**
  - Boil NOS
  - Carbuncle NOS
  - Furuncle NOS

● 681 **Cellulitis and abscess of finger and toe**
  - **INCLUDES** that with lymphangitis
  - Use additional code, if desired, to identify organism, such as Staphylococcus (041.1)
  - ● 681.0 **Finger**
    - 681.00 Cellulitis and abscess, unspecified
    - 681.01 Felon
      - Pulp abscess
      - Whitlow
      - **EXCLUDES** herpetic whitlow (054.6)
    - 681.02 Onychia and paronychia of finger
      - Panaritium } of finger
      - Perionychia }
  - ● 681.1 **Toe**
    - ◆ 681.10 Cellulitis and abscess, unspecified
    - 681.11 Onychia and paronychia of toe
      - Panaritium } of toe
      - Perionychia }
  - ◆ 681.9 **Cellulitis and abscess of unspecified digit**
    - Infection of nail NOS

● 682 **Other cellulitis and abscess**
  - **INCLUDES** abscess (acute)
    - cellulitis (diffuse) } (with lymph-angitis) except of finger or toe
    - lymphangitis, acute
  - Use additional code, if desired, to identify organism, such as Staphylococcus (041.1)
  - **EXCLUDES** lymphangitis (chronic) (subacute) (457.2)
  - 682.0 **Face**
    - Cheek, external
    - Chin
    - Forehead
    - Nose, external
    - Submandibular
    - Temple (region)
    - **EXCLUDES** ear [any part] (380.10-380.16)
      - eyelid (373.13)
      - lacrimal apparatus (375.31)
      - lip (528.5)
      - mouth (528.3)
      - nose (internal) (478.1)
      - orbit (376.01)
  - 682.1 **Neck**
  - 682.2 **Trunk**
    - Abdominal wall
    - Back [any part, except buttock]
    - Chest wall
    - Flank
    - Groin
    - Pectoral region
    - Perineum
    - Umbilicus, except newborn
    - **EXCLUDES** anal and rectal regions (566)
      - breast:
        - NOS (611.0)
        - puerperal (675.1)
      - external genital organs:
        - female (616.3-616.4)
        - male (604.0, 607.2, 608.4)
      - umbilicus, newborn (771.4)
  - 682.3 **Upper arm and forearm**
    - Arm [any part, except hand]
    - Axilla
    - Shoulder
    - **EXCLUDES** hand (682.4)
  - 682.4 **Hand, except fingers and thumb**
    - Wrist
    - **EXCLUDES** finger and thumb (681.00-681.02)
  - 682.5 **Buttock**
    - Gluteal region
    - **EXCLUDES** anal and rectal regions (566)
  - 682.6 **Leg, except foot**
    - Ankle
    - Hip
    - Knee
    - Thigh
  - 682.7 **Foot, except toes**
    - Heel
    - **EXCLUDES** toe (681.10-681.11)
  - ◆ 682.8 **Other specified sites**
    - Head [except face]
    - Scalp
    - **EXCLUDES** face (682.0)
  - ◆ 682.9 **Unspecified site**
    - Abscess NOS
    - Cellulitis NOS
    - Lymphangitis, acute NOS
    - **EXCLUDES** lymphangitis NOS (457.2)

683 **Acute lymphadenitis**
  - Abscess (acute)
  - Adenitis, acute } lymph gland or node, except mesenteric
  - Lymphadenitis, acute
  - Use additional code, if desired, to identify organism, such as Staphylococcus (041.1)
  - **EXCLUDES** enlarged glands NOS (785.6)
    - lymphadenitis:
      - chronic or subacute, except mesenteric (289.1)
      - mesenteric (acute) (chronic) (subacute) (289.2)
      - unspecified (289.3)

684 **Impetigo**
  - Impetiginization of other dermatoses
  - Impetigo (contagiosa) [any site] [any organism]:
    - bullous
    - circinate
    - neonatorum
    - simplex
  - Pemphigus neonatorum
  - **EXCLUDES** impetigo herpetiformis (694.3)

● 685 **Pilonidal cyst**
  - **INCLUDES** fistula } coccygeal or pilonidal
    - sinus
  - 685.0 **With abscess**
  - 685.1 **Without mention of abscess**

● 686 **Other local infections of skin and subcutaneous tissue**
  - Use additional code, if desired, to identify any infectious organism (041.0-041.8)
  - 686.0 **Pyoderma**
    - Dermatitis:
      - purulent
      - septic
    - Dermatitis:
      - suppurative
  - 686.1 **Pyogenic granuloma**
    - Granuloma:
      - septic
      - suppurative
      - telangiectaticum
    - **EXCLUDES** pyogenic granuloma of oral mucosa (528.9)
  - ◆ 686.8 **Other specified local infections of skin and subcutaneous tissue**
    - Bacterid (pustular)
    - Dermatitis vegetans
    - Ecthyma
    - Perlèche
    - **EXCLUDES** dermatitis infectiosa eczematoides (690)
      - panniculitis (729.30-729.39)
  - ◆ 686.9 **Unspecified local infection of skin and subcutaneous tissue**
    - Fistula of skin NOS
    - Skin infection NOS
    - **EXCLUDES** fistula to skin from internal organs — see Alphabetic Index

OTHER INFLAMMATORY CONDITIONS OF SKIN AND SUBCUTANEOUS TISSUE (690-698)

EXCLUDES panniculitis (729.30-729.39)

690 Erythematosquamous dermatosis
Dandruff
Dermatitis infectiosa eczematoides
Parakeratosis
Pityriasis:
  capitis
  simplex
Seborrhea sicca
Seborrheic:
  dermatitis
  eczema

EXCLUDES eczematous dermatitis of eyelid (373.31)
parakeratosis variegata (696.2)
psoriasis (696.0-696.1)
seborrheic keratosis (702)

● **691 Atopic dermatitis and related conditions**

691.0 Diaper or napkin rash
Ammonia dermatitis
Diaper or napkin:
  dermatitis
Psoriasiform napkin eruption
Diaper or napkin:
  erythema
  rash

◆ **691.8 Other atopic dermatitis and related conditions**
Atopic dermatitis
Besnier's prurigo
Eczema:
  atopic
  flexural
  infantile (acute) (chronic)
  intrinsic (allergic)
Neurodermatitis:
  atopic
  diffuse (of Brocq)

● **692 Contact dermatitis and other eczema**

INCLUDES dermatitis:
  NOS
  contact
  occupational
  venenata
eczema (acute) (chronic):
  NOS
  allergic
  erythematous
  occupational

EXCLUDES allergy NOS (995.3)
contact dermatitis of eyelids (373.32)
dermatitis due to substances taken internally (693.0-693.9)
eczema of external ear (380.22)
perioral dermatitis (695.3)
urticarial reactions (708.0-708.9, 995.1)

692.0 Due to detergents
692.1 Due to oils and greases
692.2 Due to solvents
Dermatitis due to solvents of:
  chlorocompound
  cyclohexane
  ester   } group
  glycol
  hydrocarbon
  ketone

692.3 Due to drugs and medicines in contact with skin
Dermatitis (allergic) (contact) due to:
  arnica
  fungicides
  iodine
  keratolytics
  mercurials
Dermatitis (allergic) (contact) due to:
  neomycin
  pediculocides
  phenols
  scabicides
  any drug applied to skin
Dermatitis medicamentosa due to drug applied to skin
Use additional E code, if desired, to identify drug

EXCLUDES allergy NOS due to drugs (995.2)
dermatitis due to ingested drugs (693.0)
dermatitis medicamentosa NOS (693.0)

◆ **692.4 Due to other chemical products**
Dermatitis due to:
  acids
  adhesive plaster
  alkalis
  caustics
  dichromate
Dermatitis due to:
  insecticide
  nylon
  plastic
  rubber

692.5 Due to food in contact with skin
Dermatitis, contact, due to:
  cereals
  fish
  flour
Dermatitis, contact, due to:
  fruit
  meat
  milk

EXCLUDES dermatitis due to:
dyes (692.89)
ingested foods (693.1)
preservatives (692.89)

692.6 Due to plants [except food]
Dermatitis due to:
  lacquer tree [Rhus verniciflua]
  poison:
    ivy [Rhus toxicodendron]
    oak [Rhus diversiloba]
    sumac [Rhus venenata]
    vine [Rhus radicans]
  primrose [Primula]
  ragweed [Senecio jacobae]
  other plants in contact with the skin

EXCLUDES allergy NOS due to pollen (477.0)
nettle rash (708.8)

● **692.7 Due to solar radiation**
◆ **692.70 Unspecified dermatitis due to sun**
692.71 Sunburn
692.72 Acute dermatitis due to solar radiation
Berlogue dermatitis
Photoallergic response
Phototoxic response
Polymorphus light eruption
Acute solar skin damage NOS

EXCLUDES sunburn (692.71)
Use additional E code, if desired, to identify substance, if substance induced

692.73 Actinic reticuloid and actinic granuloma
◆ **692.74 Other chronic dermatitis due to solar radiation**
solar elastosis
chronic solar skin damage NOS

EXCLUDES actinic [solar] keratosis (702.0)

◆ **692.79 Other dermatitis due to solar radiation**
Solar skin damage NOS
Hydroa aestivale
Photodermatitis   } (due to sun)
Photosensitiveness

● **692.8 Due to other specified agents**
692.81 Dermatitis due to cosmetics
◆ **692.82 Dermatitis due to other radiation**
infrared rays   ultraviolet rays
light   x-rays
radiation NOS

EXCLUDES solar radiation (692.70-692.79)

692.83 Dermatitis due to metals
jewelry
◆ **692.89 Other**
Dermatitis due to:
  cold weather
  dyes
  furs
  hot weather
  preservatives
  ultraviolet rays, except from sun

EXCLUDES allergy NOS due to animal hair, dander (animal), or dust (477.8)
sunburn (692.71)

◆ **692.9 Unspecified cause**
Dermatitis:
  NOS
  contact NOS
  venenata NOS
Eczema NOS

● **693 Dermatitis due to substances taken internally**

EXCLUDES adverse effect NOS of drugs and medicines (995.2)
allergy NOS (995.3)
contact dermatitis (692.0-692.9)
urticarial reactions (708.0-708.9, 995.1)

693.0 Due to drugs and medicines
Dermatitis medicamentosa NOS
Use additional E code, if desired, to identify drug
EXCLUDES that due to drugs in contact with skin (692.3)

693.1 Due to food
693.8 Due to other specified substances taken internally
693.9 Due to unspecified substance taken internally
EXCLUDES dermatitis NOS (692.9)

694 Bullous dermatoses

694.0 Dermatitis herpetiformis
Dermatosis herpetiformis
Duhring's disease
Hydroa herpetiformis
EXCLUDES herpes gestationis (646.8)
dermatitis herpetiformis:
juvenile (694.2)
senile (694.5)

694.1 Subcorneal pustular dermatosis
Sneddon-Wilkinson disease or syndrome

694.2 Juvenile dermatitis herpetiformis
Juvenile pemphigoid

694.3 Impetigo herpetiformis

694.4 Pemphigus
Pemphigus:
 NOS
 erythematosus
 foliaceus
Pemphigus:
 malignant
 vegetans
 vulgaris
EXCLUDES pemphigus neonatorum (684)

694.5 Pemphigoid
Benign pemphigus NOS
Bullous pemphigoid
Herpes circinatus bullosus
Senile dermatitis herpetiformis

694.6 Benign mucous membrane pemphigoid
Cicatricial pemphigoid
Mucosynechial atrophic bullous dermatitis
694.60 Without mention of ocular involvement
694.61 With ocular involvement
Ocular pemphigus

694.8 Other specified bullous dermatoses
EXCLUDES herpes gestationis (646.8)

694.9 Unspecified bullous dermatoses

695 Erythematous conditions

695.0 Toxic erythema
Erythema venenatum

695.1 Erythema multiforme
Erythema iris
Herpes iris
Lyell's syndrome
Scalded skin syndrome
Stevens-Johnson syndrome
Toxic epidermal necrolysis

695.2 Erythema nodosum
EXCLUDES tuberculous erythema nodosum (017.1)

695.3 Rosacea
Acne:
 erythematosa
 rosacea
Perioral dermatitis
Rhinophyma

695.4 Lupus erythematosus
Lupus:
 erythematodes (discoid)
 erythematosus (discoid), not disseminated
EXCLUDES lupus (vulgaris) NOS (017.0)
systemic [disseminated] lupus erythematosus (710.0)

695.8 Other specified erythematous conditions
695.81 Ritter's disease
Dermatitis exfoliativa neonatorum
695.89 Other
Erythema intertrigo
Intertrigo
Pityriasis rubra (Hebra)
EXCLUDES mycotic intertrigo (111.0-111.9)

695.9 Unspecified erythematous condition
Erythema NOS
Erythroderma (secondary)

696 Psoriasis and similar disorders

696.0 Psoriatic arthropathy
696.1 Other psoriasis
Acrodermatitis continua
Dermatitis repens
Psoriasis:
 NOS
 any type, except arthropathic
EXCLUDES psoriatic arthropathy (696.0)

696.2 Parapsoriasis
Parakeratosis variegata
Parapsoriasis lichenoides chronica
Pityriasis lichenoides et varioliformis

696.3 Pityriasis rosea
Pityriasis circinata (et maculata)

696.4 Pityriasis rubra pilaris
Devergie's disease   Lichen ruber acuminatus
EXCLUDES pityriasis rubra (Hebra) (695.89)

696.5 Other and unspecified pityriasis
Pityriasis:
 NOS
 alba
 streptogenes
EXCLUDES pityriasis:
 simplex (690)
 versicolor (111.0)

696.8 Other

697 Lichen
EXCLUDES lichen:
 obtusus corneus (698.3)
 pilaris (congenital) (757.39)
 ruber acuminatus (696.4)
 sclerosus et atrophicus (701.0)
 scrofulosus (017.0)
 simplex chronicus (698.3)
 spinulosus (congenital) (757.39)
 urticatus (698.2)

697.0 Lichen planus
Lichen:
 planopilaris
Lichen:
 ruber planus

697.1 Lichen nitidus
Pinkus' disease

697.8 Other lichen, not elsewhere classified
Lichen:
 ruber moniliforme
Lichen:
 striata

697.9 Lichen, unspecified

698 Pruritus and related conditions
EXCLUDES pruritus specified as psychogenic (306.3)

698.0 Pruritus ani
Perianal itch

698.1 Pruritus of genital organs

698.2 Prurigo
Lichen urticatus
Prurigo:
 NOS
 Hebra's
Prurigo:
 mitis
 simplex
Urticaria papulosa (Hebra)
EXCLUDES prurigo nodularis (698.3)

698.3 Lichenification and lichen simplex chronicus
Hyde's disease
Neurodermatitis (circumscripta) (local)
Prurigo nodularis
EXCLUDES neurodermatitis, diffuse (of Brocq) (691.8)

698.4 Dermatitis factitia [artefacta]
Dermatitis ficta
Neurotic excoriation
Use additional code, if desired, to identify any associated mental disorder

698.8 Other specified pruritic conditions
Pruritus:
 hiemalis
 senilis
Winter itch

698.9 Unspecified pruritic disorder
Itch NOS
Pruritus NOS

OTHER DISEASES OF SKIN AND SUBCUTANEOUS TISSUE (700-709)

EXCLUDES conditions confined to eyelids (373.0-374.9)
congenital conditions of skin, hair, and nails (757.0-757.9)

700 Corns and callosities
Callus
Clavus

● 701 Other hypertrophic and atrophic conditions of skin
EXCLUDES dermatomyositis (710.3)
hereditary edema of legs (757.0)
scleroderma (generalized) (710.1)

701.0 Circumscribed scleroderma
Addison's keloid
Dermatosclerosis, localized
Lichen sclerosus et atrophicus
Morphea
Scleroderma, circumscribed or localized

701.1 Keratoderma, acquired
Acquired:
 ichthyosis
 keratoderma palmaris et plantaris
Elastosis perforans serpiginosa
Hyperkeratosis:
 NOS
 follicularis in cutem penetrans
 palmoplantaris climacterica
Keratoderma:
 climactericum
 tylodes, progressive
Keratosis (blennorrhagica)
EXCLUDES Darier's disease [keratosis follicularis] (congenital) (757.39)
keratosis:
 arsenical (692.4)
 gonococcal (098.81)

701.2 Acquired acanthosis nigricans
Keratosis nigricans

701.3 Striae atrophicae
Atrophic spots of skin
Atrophoderma maculatum
Atrophy blanche (of Milian)
Degenerative colloid atrophy
Senile degenerative atrophy
Striae distensae

701.4 Keloid scar
Cheloid   Keloid
Hypertrophic scar

◆ **701.5 Other abnormal granulation tissue**
Excessive granulation

◆ **701.8 Other specified hypertrophic and atrophic conditions of skin**
Acrodermatitis atrophicans chronica
Atrophia cutis senilis
Atrophoderma neuriticum
Confluent and reticulate papillomatosis
Cutis laxa senilis
Elastosis senilis
Folliculitis ulerythematosa reticulata
Gougerot-Carteaud syndrome or disease

◆ **701.9 Unspecified hypertrophic and atrophic conditions of skin**
Atrophoderma

● 702 Other dermatoses
EXCLUDES carcinoma in situ (232.0-232.9)

702.0 Actinic keratosis

● **702.1 Seborrheic keratosis**
702.11 Inflamed seborrheic keratosis ▼
◆ **702.19 Other seborrheic keratosis**
Seborrheic keratosis NOS ▲

◆ **702.8 Other specified dermatoses**

● 703 Diseases of nail
EXCLUDES congenital anomalies (757.5)
onychia and paronychia (681.02, 681.11)

703.0 Ingrowing nail
Ingrowing nail with infection
Unguis incarnatus
EXCLUDES infection, nail NOS (681.9)

◆ **703.8 Other specified diseases of nail**
Dystrophia unguium   Onychauxis
Hypertrophy of nail   Onychogryposis
Koilonychia   Onycholysis
Leukonychia (punctata) (striata)

◆ **703.9 Unspecified disease of nail**

● 704 Diseases of hair and hair follicles
EXCLUDES congenital anomalies (757.4)

● **704.0 Alopecia**
EXCLUDES madarosis (374.55)
syphilitic alopecia (091.82)

◆ **704.00 Alopecia, unspecified**
Baldness
Loss of hair

704.01 Alopecia areata
Ophiasis

704.02 Telogen effluvium

◆ **704.09 Other**
Folliculitis decalvans
Hypotrichosis:
 NOS
 postinfectional NOS
Pseudopelade

704.1 Hirsutism
Hypertrichosis:
 NOS
 lanuginosa, acquired
Polytrichia
EXCLUDES hypertrichosis of eyelid (374.54)

704.2 Abnormalities of the hair
Atrophic hair   Trichiasis:
Clastothrix   NOS
Fragilitas crinium   cicatrical
                        Trichorrhexis (nodosa)
EXCLUDES trichiasis of eyelid (374.05)

704.3 Variations in hair color
Canities (premature)   Poliosis:
Grayness, hair (premature) NOS
Heterochromia of hair   circumscripta, acquired

◆ **704.8 Other specified diseases of hair and hair follicles**
Folliculitis: Seborrhea capitis
 NOS   Sycosis:
 abscedens et suffodiens NOS
 pustular   barbae [not parasitic]
Perifolliculitis: lupoid
 NOS   vulgaris
 capitis abscedens et suffodiens
 scalp

◆ **704.9 Unspecified disease of hair and hair follicles**

● 705 Disorders of sweat glands

705.0 Anhidrosis
Hypohidrosis
Oligohidrosis

705.1 Prickly heat
Heat rash
Miliaria rubra (tropicalis)
Sudamina

● **705.8 Other specified disorders of sweat glands**

705.81 Dyshidrosis
Cheiropompholyx
Pompholyx

705.82 Fox-Fordyce disease

705.83 Hidradenitis
Hidradenitis suppurativa

◆ **705.89 Other**
Bromhidrosis   Granulosis rubra nasi
Chromhidrosis   Urhidrosis
EXCLUDES hidrocystoma (216.0-216.9)
hyperhidrosis (780.8)

◆ **705.9 Unspecified disorder of sweat glands**
Disorder of sweat glands NOS

● 706 Diseases of sebaceous glands

706.0 Acne varioliformis
Acne:
 frontalis
 necrotica

◆ **706.1** Other acne
　　Acne:　　　　　　　　Acne:
　　　NOS　　　　　　　　vulgaris
　　　conglobata　　　　　Blackhead
　　　cystic　　　　　　　Comedo
　　　pustular
　　EXCLUDES　acne rosacea (695.3)

706.2 Sebaceous cyst
　　Atheroma, skin　　　Wen
　　Keratin cyst

706.3 Seborrhea
　　EXCLUDES　seborrhea:
　　　　　　　capitis (704.8)
　　　　　　　sicca (690)
　　　　　　seborrheic keratosis (702)

◆ **706.8** Other specified diseases of sebaceous glands
　　Asteatosis (cutis)
　　Xerosis cutis

◆ **706.9** Unspecified disease of sebaceous glands

● **707** Chronic ulcer of skin
　　EXCLUDES　skin infections (680.0-686.9)
　　　　　specific infections classified under "Infectious and
　　　　　　Parasitic Diseases" (001.0-136.9)
　　　　　varicose ulcer (454.0, 454.2)

707.0 Decubitus ulcer
　　Bed sore　　　　　　Plaster ulcer
　　Decubitus ulcer [any site]　Pressure ulcer

707.1 Ulcer of lower limbs, except decubitus
　　Ulcer, chronic:
　　　neurogenic　} of lower limb
　　　trophic
　　EXCLUDES　that with atherosclerosis of the extremities
　　　　　　(440.23)

◆ **707.8** Chronic ulcer of other specified sites
　　Ulcer, chronic:
　　　neurogenic　} of other specified sites
　　　trophic

◆ **707.9** Chronic ulcer of unspecified site
　　Chronic ulcer NOS　　Tropical ulcer NOS
　　Trophic ulcer NOS　　Ulcer of skin NOS

● **708** Urticaria
　　EXCLUDES　edema:
　　　　　　　angioneurotic (995.1)
　　　　　　　Quincke's (995.1)
　　　　　hereditary angioedema (277.6)
　　　　　urticaria:
　　　　　　　giant (995.1)
　　　　　　　papulosa (Hebra) (698.2)
　　　　　　　pigmentosa (juvenile) (congenital) (757.33)

708.0 Allergic urticaria
708.1 Idiopathic urticaria
708.2 Urticaria due to cold and heat
　　Thermal urticaria
708.3 Dermatographic urticaria
　　Dermatographia　　　Factitial urticaria
708.4 Vibratory urticaria
708.5 Cholinergic urticaria
◆ **708.8** Other specified urticaria
　　Nettle rash
　　Urticaria:
　　　chronic
　　　recurrent periodic
◆ **708.9** Urticaria, unspecified
　　Hives NOS

● **709** Other disorders of skin and subcutaneous tissue
　● **709.0** Dyschromia
　　EXCLUDES　albinism (270.2)
　　　　　　pigmented nevus (216.0-216.9)
　　　　　　that of eyelid (374.52-374.53)
　　◆ **709.00** Dyschromia, unspecified
　　　709.01 Vitiligo
　　◆ **709.09** Other
　709.1 Vascular disorders of skin
　　Angioma serpiginosum
　　Purpura (primary) annularis telangiectodes

709.2 Scar conditions and fibrosis of skin
　　Adherent scar (skin)　　Fibrosis, skin NOS
　　Cicatrix　　　　　　　Scar NOS
　　Disfigurement (due to scar)
　　EXCLUDES　keloid scar (701.4)

709.3 Degenerative skin disorders
　　Calcinosis:　　　　　　Degeneration, skin
　　　circumscripta　　　　Deposits, skin
　　　cutis　　　　　　　　Senile dermatosis NOS
　　Colloid milium　　　　Subcutaneous calcification

709.4 Foreign body granuloma of skin and subcutaneous tissue
　　EXCLUDES　that of muscle (728.82)

◆ **709.8** Other specified disorders of skin
　　Epithelial hyperplasia　Vesicular eruption
　　Menstrual dermatosis

◆ **709.9** Unspecified disorder of skin and subcutaneous tissue
　　Dermatosis NOS

13. DISEASES OF THE MUSCULOSKELETAL SYSTEM AND CONNECTIVE TISSUE (710-739)

The following fifth-digit subclassification is for use with categories 711-712, 715-716, 718-719, and 730:

◆ **0** site unspecified
　1 shoulder region
　　　Acromioclavicular　}
　　　Glenohumeral　　　} joint(s)
　　　Sternoclavicular　　}
　　　Clavicle
　　　Scapula
　2 upper arm
　　　Elbow joint
　　　Humerus
　3 forearm
　　　Radius
　　　Ulna
　　　Wrist joint
　4 hand
　　　Carpus
　　　Metacarpus
　　　Phalanges [fingers]
　5 pelvic region and thigh
　　　Buttock
　　　Femur
　　　Hip (joint)
　6 lower leg
　　　Fibula　　　　　Patella
　　　Knee joint　　　Tibia
　7 ankle and foot
　　　Ankle joint　　　Phalanges, foot
　　　Digits [toes]　　Tarsus
　　　Metatarsus　　　Other joints in foot
◆ **8** other specified sites
　　　Head　　　　　　Skull
　　　Neck　　　　　　Trunk
　　　Ribs　　　　　　Vertebral column
◆ **9** multiple sites

ARTHROPATHIES AND RELATED DISORDERS (710-719)
　　EXCLUDES　disorders of spine (720.0-724.9)

● **710** Diffuse diseases of connective tissue
　　INCLUDES　all collagen diseases whose effects are not mainly
　　　　　　　confined to a single system
　　Use additional code, if desired, to identify manifestation, as:
　　　lung involvement (517.8)
　　　myopathy (359.6)
　　EXCLUDES　those affecting mainly the cardiovascular system, i.e.,
　　　　　　　polyarteritis nodosa and allied conditions
　　　　　　　(446.0-446.7)

710.0 Systemic lupus erythematosus
　　Disseminated lupus erythematosus
　　Libman-Sacks disease
　　Use additional code, if desired, to identify manifestation, as:
　　　endocarditis (424.91)
　　　nephritis (583.81)
　　　　chronic (582.81)
　　　　nephrotic syndrome (581.81)
　　EXCLUDES　lupus erythematosus (discoid) NOS (695.4)

710.1 Systemic sclerosis
- Acrosclerosis
- CRST syndrome
- Progressive systemic sclerosis
- Scleroderma

EXCLUDES circumscribed scleroderma (701.0)

710.2 Sicca syndrome
- Keratoconjunctivitis sicca
- Sjögren's disease

710.3 Dermatomyositis
- Poikilodermatomyositis
- Polymyositis with skin involvement

710.4 Polymyositis

710.5 Eosinophilia myalgia syndrome
- Toxic oil syndrome
- Use additional E code, if desired, to identify drug, if drug induced

710.8 Other specified diffuse diseases of connective tissue
- Multifocal fibrosclerosis (idiopathic) NEC
- Systemic fibrosclerosing syndrome

710.9 Unspecified diffuse connective tissue disease
- Collagen disease NOS

711 Arthropathy associated with infections

INCLUDES arthritis, arthropathy, polyarthritis, polyarthropathy associated with conditions classifiable below

EXCLUDES rheumatic fever (390)

The following fifth-digit subclassification is for use with category 711; valid digits are in [brackets] under each code.
- 0 site unspecified
- 1 shoulder region
- 2 upper arm
- 3 forearm
- 4 hand
- 5 pelvic region and thigh
- 6 lower leg
- 7 ankle and foot
- 8 other specified sites
- 9 multiple sites

711.0 Pyogenic arthritis
[0-9]
Arthritis or polyarthritis (due to):
- coliform [Escherichia coli]
- Hemophilus influenzae [H. influenzae]
- pneumococcal
- Pseudomonas
- staphylococcal
- streptococcal

Pyarthrosis

Use additional code, if desired, to identify infectious organism (041.0-041.8)

711.1 Arthropathy associated with Reiter's disease and nonspecific urethritis
[0-9]
Code also underlying disease as:
- nonspecific urethritis (099.4)
- Reiter's disease (099.3)

711.2 Arthropathy in Behçet's syndrome
[0-9] Code also underlying disease (136.1)

711.3 Postdysenteric arthropathy
[0-9]
Code also underlying disease as:
- dysentery (009.0)
- enteritis, infectious (008.0-009.3)
- paratyphoid fever (002.1-002.9)
- typhoid fever (002.0)

EXCLUDES salmonella arthritis (003.23)

711.4 Arthropathy associated with other bacterial diseases
[0-9]
Code also underlying disease as:
- diseases classifiable to 010-040, 090-099, except as in 711.1, 711.3, and 713.5
- leprosy (030.0-030.9)
- tuberculosis (015.0-015.9)

EXCLUDES gonococcal arthritis (098.50)
meningococcal arthritis (036.82)

711.5 Arthropathy associated with other viral diseases
[0-9]
Code also underlying disease as:
- diseases classifiable to 045-049, 050-079, 480, 487
- O'nyong nyong (066.3)

EXCLUDES that due to rubella (056.71)

711.6 Arthropathy associated with mycoses
[0-9] Code also underlying disease (110.0-118)

711.7 Arthropathy associated with helminthiasis
[0-9] Code also underlying disease as:
- filariasis (125.0-125.9)

711.8 Arthropathy associated with other infectious and parasitic diseases
[0-9]
Code also underlying disease as:
- diseases classifiable to 080-088, 100-104, 130-136

EXCLUDES arthropathy associated with sarcoidosis (713.7)

711.9 Unspecified infective arthritis
[0-9] Infective arthritis or polyarthritis (acute) (chronic) (subacute) NOS

712 Crystal arthropathies

INCLUDES crystal-induced arthritis and synovitis

EXCLUDES gouty arthropathy (274.0)

The following fifth-digit subclassification is for use with category 712; valid digits are in [brackets] under each code. See page 117 for definitions:
- 0 site unspecified
- 1 shoulder region
- 2 upper arm
- 3 forearm
- 4 hand
- 5 pelvic region and thigh
- 6 lower leg
- 7 ankle and foot
- 8 other specified sites
- 9 multiple sites

712.1 Chondrocalcinosis due to dicalcium phosphate crystals
[0-9] Chondrocalcinosis due to dicalcium phosphate crystals (with other crystals)
Code also underlying disease (275.4)

712.2 Chondrocalcinosis due to pyrophosphate crystals
[0-9] Code also underlying disease (275.4)

712.3 Chondrocalcinosis, unspecified
[0-9] Code also underlying disease (275.4)

712.8 Other specified crystal arthropathies
[0-9]

712.9 Unspecified crystal arthropathy
[0-9]

713 Arthropathy associated with other disorders classified elsewhere

INCLUDES arthritis, arthropathy, polyarthritis, polyarthropathy associated with conditions classifiable below

713.0 Arthropathy associated with other endocrine and metabolic disorders
Code also underlying disease as:
- acromegaly (253.0)
- hemochromatosis (275.0)
- hyperparathyroidism (252.0)
- hypogammaglobulinemia (279.00-279.09)
- hypothyroidism (243-244.9)
- lipoid metabolism disorder (272.0-272.9)
- ochronosis (270.2)

EXCLUDES arthropathy associated with:
- amyloidosis (713.7)
- crystal deposition disorders, except gout (712.1-712.9)
- diabetic neuropathy (713.5)
- gouty arthropathy (274.0)

713.1 Arthropathy associated with gastrointestinal conditions other than infections
Code also underlying disease as:
- regional enteritis (555.0-555.9)
- ulcerative colitis (556)

713.2 Arthropathy associated with hematological disorders
Code also underlying disease as:
- hemoglobinopathy (282.4-282.7)
- hemophilia (286.0-286.2)
- leukemia (204.0-208.9)
- malignant reticulosis (202.3)
- multiple myelomatosis (203.0)

EXCLUDES arthropathy associated with Henoch-Schönlein purpura (713.6)

■ 713.3 Arthropathy associated with dermatological disorders
Code also underlying disease as:
erythema multiforme (695.1)
erythema nodosum (695.2)
EXCLUDES psoriatic arthropathy (696.0)

■ 713.4 Arthropathy associated with respiratory disorders
Code also underlying disease as:
diseases classifiable to 490-519
EXCLUDES arthropathy associated with respiratory infections (711.0, 711.4-711.8)

■ 713.5 Arthropathy associated with neurological disorders
Charcot's arthropathy | associated with diseases
Neuropathic arthritis | classifiable elsewhere

Code also underlying disease as:
neuropathic joint disease [Charcot's joints]:
NOS (094.0)
diabetic (250.6)
syringomyelic (336.0)
tabetic [syphilitic] (094.0)

■ 713.6 Arthropathy associated with hypersensitivity reaction
Code also underlying disease as:
Henoch (-Schönlein) purpura (287.0)
serum sickness (999.5)
EXCLUDES allergic arthritis NOS (716.2)

■ ◆ 713.7 Other general diseases with articular involvement
Code also underlying disease as:
amyloidosis (277.3)
familial Mediterranean fever (277.3)
sarcoidosis (135)

■ ◆ 713.8 Arthropathy associated with other conditions classifiable elsewhere
Code also underlying disease as:
conditions classifiable elsewhere except as in 711.1-711.8, 712, and 713.0-713.7

● 714 Rheumatoid arthritis and other inflammatory polyarthropathies
EXCLUDES rheumatic fever (390)
rheumatoid arthritis of spine NOS (720.0)

714.0 Rheumatoid arthritis
Arthritis or polyarthritis:
atrophic
rheumatic (chronic)
Use additional code, if desired, to identify manifestation, as:
myopathy (359.6)
polyneuropathy (357.1)
EXCLUDES juvenile rheumatoid arthritis NOS (714.30)

714.1 Felty's syndrome
Rheumatoid arthritis with splenoadenomegaly and leukopenia

◆ 714.2 Other rheumatoid arthritis with visceral or systemic involvement
Rheumatoid carditis

● 714.3 Juvenile chronic polyarthritis
◆ 714.30 Polyarticular juvenile rheumatoid arthritis, chronic or unspecified
Juvenile rheumatoid arthritis NOS
Still's disease
714.31 Polyarticular juvenile rheumatoid arthritis, acute
714.32 Pauciarticular juvenile rheumatoid arthritis
714.33 Monoarticular juvenile rheumatoid arthritis

714.4 Chronic postrheumatic arthropathy
Chronic rheumatoid nodular fibrositis
Jaccoud's syndrome

● 714.8 Other specified inflammatory polyarthropathies
714.81 Rheumatoid lung
Caplan's syndrome
Diffuse interstitial rheumatoid disease of lung
Fibrosing alveolitis, rheumatoid
◆ 714.89 Other

◆ 714.9 Unspecified inflammatory polyarthropathy
Inflammatory polyarthropathy or polyarthritis NOS
EXCLUDES polyarthropathy NOS (716.5)

● 715 Osteoarthrosis and allied disorders
Note: Localized, in the subcategories below, includes bilateral involvement of the same site.
INCLUDES arthritis or polyarthritis:
degenerative
hypertrophic
degenerative joint disease
osteoarthritis
EXCLUDES Marie-Strümpell spondylitis (720.0)
osteoarthrosis [osteoarthritis] of spine (721.0-721.9)

The following fifth-digit subclassification is for use with category 715; valid digits are in [brackets] under each code. See page 117 for definitions:
◆ 0 site unspecified
1 shoulder region
2 upper arm
3 forearm
4 hand
5 pelvic region and thigh
6 lower leg
7 ankle and foot
◆ 8 other specified sites
◆ 9 multiple sites

● 715.0 Osteoarthrosis, generalized
[0,4,9]
Degenerative joint disease, involving multiple joints
Primary generalized hypertrophic osteoarthrosis

● 715.1 Osteoarthrosis, localized, primary
[0-8] Localized osteoarthropathy, idiopathic

● 715.2 Osteoarthrosis, localized, secondary
[0-8] Coxae malum senilis

◆ 715.3 Osteoarthrosis, localized, not specified whether primary or secondary
[0-8]
Otto's pelvis

◆ 715.8 Osteoarthrosis involving, or with mention of more than one site, but not specified as generalized
[0,9]

◆ 715.9 Osteoarthrosis, unspecified whether generalized or localized
[0-8]

● 716 Other and unspecified arthropathies
EXCLUDES cricoarytenoid arthropathy (478.79)

The following fifth-digit subclassification is for use with category 716; valid digits are in [brackets] under each code. See page 117 for definitions:
◆ 0 site unspecified
1 shoulder region
2 upper arm
3 forearm
4 hand
5 pelvic region and thigh
6 lower leg
7 ankle and foot
◆ 8 other specified sites
◆ 9 multiple sites

● 716.0 Kaschin-Beck disease
[0-9] Endemic polyarthritis

● 716.1 Traumatic arthropathy
[0-9]

● 716.2 Allergic arthritis
[0-9] **EXCLUDES** arthritis associated with Henoch-Schönlein purpura or serum sickness (713.6)

● 716.3 Climacteric arthritis
[0-9] Menopausal arthritis

● 716.4 Transient arthropathy
[0-9] **EXCLUDES** palindromic rheumatism (719.3)

◆ ● 716.5 Unspecified polyarthropathy or polyarthritis
[0-9]

◆ ● 716.6 Unspecified monoarthritis
[0-8] Coxitis

◆ ● 716.8 Other specified arthropathy
[0-9]

◆ ● 716.9 Arthropathy, unspecified
[0-9]
Arthritis
Arthropathy } (acute) (chronic) (subacute)

Articular rheumatism (chronic)
Inflammation of joint NOS

● **717 Internal derangement of knee**
 INCLUDES: degeneration, rupture, old, tear, old } of articular cartilage or meniscus of knee
 EXCLUDES: acute derangement of knee (836.0-836.6)
 ankylosis (718.5)
 contracture (718.4)
 current injury (836.0-836.6)
 deformity (736.4-736.6)
 recurrent dislocation (718.3)

 717.0 Old bucket handle tear of medial meniscus
 Old bucket handle tear of unspecified cartilage
 717.1 Derangement of anterior horn of medial meniscus
 717.2 Derangement of posterior horn of medial meniscus
 ◆ 717.3 Other and unspecified derangement of medial meniscus
 Degeneration of internal semilunar cartilage
 ● 717.4 Derangement of lateral meniscus
 ◆ 717.40 Derangement of lateral meniscus, unspecified
 717.41 Bucket handle tear of lateral meniscus
 717.42 Derangement of anterior horn of lateral meniscus
 717.43 Derangement of posterior horn of lateral meniscus
 ◆ 717.49 Other
 717.5 Derangement of meniscus, not elsewhere classified
 Congenital discoid meniscus
 Cyst of semilunar cartilage
 Derangement of semilunar cartilage NOS
 717.6 Loose body in knee
 Joint mice, knee
 Rice bodies, knee (joint)
 717.7 Chondromalacia of patella
 Chondromalacia patellae
 Degeneration [softening] of articular cartilage of patella
 ● 717.8 Other internal derangement of knee
 717.81 Old disruption of lateral collateral ligament
 717.82 Old disruption of medial collateral ligament
 717.83 Old disruption of anterior cruciate ligament
 717.84 Old disruption of posterior cruciate ligament
 ◆ 717.85 Old disruption of other ligaments of knee
 Capsular ligament of knee
 ◆ 717.89 Other
 Old disruption of ligaments of knee NOS
 ◆ 717.9 Unspecified internal derangement of knee
 Derangement NOS of knee

● **718 Other derangement of joint**
 EXCLUDES: current injury (830.0-848.9)
 jaw (524.6)
 The following fifth-digit subclassification is for use with category 718; valid digits are in [brackets] under each code. See page 117 for definitions:
 ◆ 0 site unspecified
 1 shoulder region
 2 upper arm
 3 forearm
 4 hand
 5 pelvic region and thigh
 6 lower leg
 7 ankle and foot
 ◆ 8 other specified sites
 ◆ 9 multiple sites

 ● 718.0 Articular cartilage disorder
 [0-5,7-9] Meniscus:
 disorder
 rupture, old
 tear, old
 Old rupture of ligament(s) of joint NOS
 EXCLUDES: articular cartilage disorder:
 in ochronosis (270.2)
 knee (717.0-717.9)
 chondrocalcinosis (275.4)
 metastatic calcification (275.4)
 ● 718.1 Loose body in joint
 [0-5,7-9] Joint mice
 EXCLUDES: knee (717.6)
 ● 718.2 Pathological dislocation
 [0-9] Dislocation or displacement of joint, not recurrent and not current injury
 Spontaneous dislocation (joint)

 ● 718.3 Recurrent dislocation of joint
 [0-9]
 ● 718.4 Contracture of joint
 [0-9]
 ● 718.5 Ankylosis of joint
 [0-9] Ankylosis of joint (fibrous) (osseous)
 EXCLUDES: spine (724.9)
 stiffness of joint without mention of ankylosis (719.5)
 ◆ ● 718.6 Unspecified intrapelvic protrusion of acetabulum
 [0-5] Protrusio acetabuli, unspecified
 ◆ ● 718.8 Other joint derangement, not elsewhere classified
 [0-9] Flail joint (paralytic)   Instability of joint
 EXCLUDES: deformities classifiable to 736 (736.0-736.9)
 ● 718.9 Unspecified derangement of joint
 [0-5,7-9]
 EXCLUDES: knee (717.9)

● **719 Other and unspecified disorders of joint**
 EXCLUDES: jaw (524.6)
 The following fifth-digit subclassification is for use with category 719; valid digits are in [brackets] under each code. See page 117 for definitions:
 ◆ 0 site unspecified
 1 shoulder region
 2 upper arm
 3 forearm
 4 hand
 5 pelvic region and thigh
 6 lower leg
 7 ankle and foot
 ◆ 8 other specified sites
 ◆ 9 multiple sites

 ● 719.0 Effusion of joint
 [0-9] Hydrarthrosis
 Swelling of joint, with or without pain
 EXCLUDES: intermittent hydrarthrosis (719.3)
 ● 719.1 Hemarthrosis
 [0-9] EXCLUDES: current injury (840.0-848.9)
 that in hemophilia (286.0-286.2)
 ● 719.2 Villonodular synovitis
 [0-9]
 ● 719.3 Palindromic rheumatism
 [0-9] Hench-Rosenberg syndrome
 Intermittent hydrarthrosis
 ● 719.4 Pain in joint
 [0-9] Arthralgia
 ● 719.5 Stiffness of joint, not elsewhere classified
 [0-9]
 ◆ ● 719.6 Other symptoms referable to joint
 [0-9] Joint crepitus
 Snapping hip
 ● 719.7 Difficulty in walking
 [0,5-9] EXCLUDES: abnormality of gait (781.2)
 ◆ ● 719.8 Other specified disorders of joint
 [0-9] Calcification of joint
 Fistula of joint
 EXCLUDES: temporomandibular joint-pain-dysfunction syndrome [Costen's syndrome] (524.6)
 ◆ ● 719.9 Unspecified disorder of joint
 [0-9]

DORSOPATHIES (720-724)
 EXCLUDES: curvature of spine (737.0-737.9)
 osteochondrosis of spine (juvenile) (732.0)
 adult (732.8)

● **720 Ankylosing spondylitis and other inflammatory spondylopathies**
 720.0 Ankylosing spondylitis
 Rheumatoid arthritis of spine NOS
 Spondylitis:
 Marie-Strümpell
 rheumatoid
 720.1 Spinal enthesopathy
 Disorder of peripheral ligamentous or muscular attachments of spine
 Romanus lesion
 720.2 Sacroiliitis, not elsewhere classified
 Inflammation of sacroiliac joint NOS

- **720.8** Other inflammatory spondylopathies
  - **720.81** *Inflammatory spondylopathies in diseases classified elsewhere*
    - Code also underlying disease as:
      - tuberculosis (015.0)
  - ◆ **720.89** Other
- ◆ **720.9** Unspecified inflammatory spondylopathy
  - Spondylitis NOS
- ● **721** Spondylosis and allied disorders
  - **721.0** Cervical spondylosis without myelopathy
    - Cervical or cervicodorsal:
      - arthritis
      - osteoarthritis
      - spondylarthritis
  - **721.1** Cervical spondylosis with myelopathy
    - Anterior spinal artery compression syndrome
    - Spondylogenic compression of cervical spinal cord
    - Vertebral artery compression syndrome
  - **721.2** Thoracic spondylosis without myelopathy
    - Thoracic:
      - arthritis
      - osteoarthritis
      - spondylarthritis
  - **721.3** Lumbosacral spondylosis without myelopathy
    - Lumbar or lumbosacral: Lumbar or lumbosacral:
      - arthritis   spondylarthritis
      - osteoarthritis
  - ● **721.4** Thoracic or lumbar spondylosis with myelopathy
    - **721.41** Thoracic region
      - Spondylogenic compression of thoracic spinal cord
    - **721.42** Lumbar region
      - Spondylogenic compression of lumbar spinal cord
  - **721.5** Kissing spine
    - Baastrup's syndrome
  - **721.6** Ankylosing vertebral hyperostosis
  - **721.7** Traumatic spondylopathy
    - Kümmell's disease or spondylitis
  - ◆ **721.8** Other allied disorders of spine
  - ● **721.9** Spondylosis of unspecified site
    - **721.90** Without mention of myelopathy
      - Spinal:
        - arthritis (deformans) (degenerative) (hypertrophic)
        - osteoarthritis NOS
      - Spondylarthrosis NOS
    - **721.91** With myelopathy
      - Spondylogenic compression of spinal cord NOS
- ● **722** Intervertebral disc disorders
  - **722.0** Displacement of cervical intervertebral disc without myelopathy
    - Neuritis (brachial) or radiculitis due to displacement or rupture of cervical intervertebral disc
    - Any condition classifiable to 722.2 of the cervical or cervicothoracic intervertebral disc
  - ● **722.1** Displacement of thoracic or lumbar intervertebral disc without myelopathy
    - **722.10** Lumbar intervertebral disc without myelopathy
      - Lumbago or sciatica due to displacement of intervertebral disc
      - Neuritis or radiculitis due to displacement or rupture of lumbar intervertebral disc
      - Any condition classifiable to 722.2 of the lumbar or lumbosacral intervertebral disc
    - **722.11** Thoracic intervertebral disc without myelopathy
      - Any condition classifiable to 722.2 of thoracic intervertebral disc
  - ◆ **722.2** Displacement of intervertebral disc, site unspecified, without myelopathy
    - Discogenic syndrome NOS
    - Herniation of nucleus pulposus NOS
    - Intervertebral disc NOS:
      - extrusion
      - prolapse
      - protrusion
      - rupture
    - Neuritis or radiculitis due to displacement or rupture of intervertebral disc
- ● **722.3** Schmorl's nodes
  - ◆ **722.30** Unspecified region
  - **722.31** Thoracic region
  - **722.32** Lumbar region
  - ◆ **722.39** Other
- **722.4** Degeneration of cervical intervertebral disc
  - Degeneration of cervicothoracic intervertebral disc
- ● **722.5** Degeneration of thoracic or lumbar intervertebral disc
  - **722.51** Thoracic or thoracolumbar intervertebral disc
  - **722.52** Lumbar or lumbosacral intervertebral disc
- ◆ **722.6** Degeneration of intervertebral disc, site unspecified
  - Degenerative disc disease NOS
  - Narrowing of intervertebral disc or space NOS
- ● **722.7** Intervertebral disc disorder with myelopathy
  - ◆ **722.70** Unspecified region
  - **722.71** Cervical region
  - **722.72** Thoracic region
  - **722.73** Lumbar region
- ● **722.8** Postlaminectomy syndrome
  - ◆ **722.80** Unspecified region
  - **722.81** Cervical region
  - **722.82** Thoracic region
  - **722.83** Lumbar region
- ● **722.9** Other and unspecified disc disorder
  - Calcification of intervertebral cartilage or disc
  - Discitis
  - ◆ **722.90** Unspecified region
  - **722.91** Cervical region
  - **722.92** Thoracic region
  - **722.93** Lumbar region
- ● **723** Other disorders of cervical region
  - EXCLUDES conditions due to:
    - intervertebral disc disorders (722.0-722.9)
    - spondylosis (721.0-721.9)
  - **723.0** Spinal stenosis in cervical region
  - **723.1** Cervicalgia
    - Pain in neck
  - **723.2** Cervicocranial syndrome
    - Barré-Liéou syndrome
    - Posterior cervical sympathetic syndrome
  - **723.3** Cervicobrachial syndrome (diffuse)
  - **723.4** Brachial neuritis or radiculitis NOS
    - Cervical radiculitis
    - Radicular syndrome of upper limbs
  - ◆ **723.5** Torticollis, unspecified
    - Contracture of neck
    - EXCLUDES congenital (754.1)
      - due to birth injury (767.8)
      - hysterical (300.11)
      - psychogenic (306.0)
      - spasmodic (333.83)
      - traumatic, current (847.0)
  - **723.6** Panniculitis specified as affecting neck
  - **723.7** Ossification of posterior longitudinal ligament in cervical region
  - ◆ **723.8** Other syndromes affecting cervical region
    - Cervical syndrome NEC
    - Klippel's disease
  - ◆ **723.9** Unspecified musculoskeletal disorders and symptoms referable to neck
    - Cervical (region) disorder NOS
- ● **724** Other and unspecified disorders of back
  - EXCLUDES collapsed vertebra (code to cause, e.g., osteoporosis, 733.00-733.09)
    - conditions due to:
      - intervertebral disc disorders (722.0-722.9)
      - spondylosis (721.0-721.9)
  - ● **724.0** Spinal stenosis, other than cervical
    - ◆ **724.00** Spinal stenosis, unspecified region
    - **724.01** Thoracic region
    - **724.02** Lumbar region
    - ◆ **724.09** Other
  - **724.1** Pain in thoracic spine
  - **724.2** Lumbago
    - Low back pain
    - Low back syndrome
    - Lumbalgia

- **724.3 Sciatica**
  Neuralgia or neuritis of sciatic nerve
  EXCLUDES specified lesion of sciatic nerve (355.0)
- ◆ **724.4 Thoracic or lumbosacral neuritis or radiculitis, unspecified**
  Radicular syndrome of lower limbs
- ◆ **724.5 Backache, unspecified**
  Vertebrogenic (pain) syndrome NOS
- **724.6 Disorders of sacrum**
  Ankylosis / Instability lumbosacral or sacroiliac (joint)
- ● **724.7 Disorders of coccyx**
  - ◆ 724.70 Unspecified disorder of coccyx
  - 724.71 Hypermobility of coccyx
  - ◆ 724.79 Other
    Coccygodynia
- ◆ **724.8 Other symptoms referable to back**
  Ossification of posterior longitudinal ligament NOS
  Panniculitis specified as sacral or affecting back
- ◆ **724.9 Other unspecified back disorders**
  Ankylosis of spine NOS
  Compression of spinal nerve root NEC
  Spinal disorder NOS
  EXCLUDES sacroiliitis (720.2)

RHEUMATISM, EXCLUDING THE BACK (725-729)
INCLUDES disorders of muscles and tendons and their attachments, and of other soft tissues

- **725 Polymyalgia rheumatica**
- ● **726 Peripheral enthesopathies and allied syndromes**
  Note: Enthesopathies are disorders of peripheral ligamentous or muscular attachments.
  EXCLUDES spinal enthesopathy (720.1)
  - **726.0 Adhesive capsulitis of shoulder**
  - ● **726.1 Rotator cuff syndrome of shoulder and allied disorders**
    - ◆ 726.10 Disorders of bursae and tendons in shoulder region, unspecified
      Rotator cuff syndrome NOS
      Supraspinatus syndrome NOS
    - 726.11 Calcifying tendinitis of shoulder
    - 726.12 Bicipital tenosynovitis
    - ◆ 726.19 Other specified disorders
      EXCLUDES complete rupture of rotator cuff, nontraumatic (727.61)
  - ◆ **726.2 Other affections of shoulder region, not elsewhere classified**
    Periarthritis of shoulder
    Scapulohumeral fibrositis
  - ● **726.3 Enthesopathy of elbow region**
    - ◆ 726.30 Enthesopathy of elbow, unspecified
    - 726.31 Medial epicondylitis
    - 726.32 Lateral epicondylitis
      Epicondylitis NOS
      Golfers' elbow
      Tennis elbow
    - 726.33 Olecranon bursitis
      Bursitis of elbow
    - ◆ 726.39 Other
  - **726.4 Enthesopathy of wrist and carpus**
    Bursitis of hand or wrist
    Periarthritis of wrist
  - **726.5 Enthesopathy of hip region**
    Bursitis of hip   Psoas tendinitis
    Gluteal tendinitis   Trochanteric tendinitis
    Iliac crest spur
  - ● **726.6 Enthesopathy of knee**
    - ◆ 726.60 Enthesopathy of knee, unspecified
      Bursitis of knee NOS
    - 726.61 Pes anserinus tendinitis or bursitis
    - 726.62 Tibial collateral ligament bursitis
      Pellegrini-Stieda syndrome
    - 726.63 Fibular collateral ligament bursitis
    - 726.64 Patellar tendinitis
    - 726.65 Prepatellar bursitis
    - ◆ 726.69 Other
      Bursitis:
        infrapatellar
        subpatellar
  - ● **726.7 Enthesopathy of ankle and tarsus**
    - ◆ 726.70 Enthesopathy of ankle and tarsus, unspecified
      Metatarsalgia NOS
      EXCLUDES Morton's metatarsalgia (355.6)
    - 726.71 Achilles bursitis or tendinitis
    - 726.72 Tibialis tendinitis
      Tibialis (anterior) (posterior) tendinitis
    - 726.73 Calcaneal spur
    - ◆ 726.79 Other
      Peroneal tendinitis
  - ◆ **726.8 Other peripheral enthesopathies**
  - ● **726.9 Unspecified enthesopathy**
    - ◆ 726.90 Enthesopathy of unspecified site
      Capsulitis NOS
      Periarthritis NOS
      Tendinitis NOS
    - ◆ 726.91 Exostosis of unspecified site
      Bone spur NOS
- ● **727 Other disorders of synovium, tendon, and bursa**
  - ● **727.0 Synovitis and tenosynovitis**
    - ◆ 727.00 Synovitis and tenosynovitis, unspecified
      Synovitis NOS
      Tenosynovitis NOS
    - ■ 727.01 Synovitis and tenosynovitis in diseases classified elsewhere
      Code also underlying disease as:
        tuberculosis (015.0-015.9)
      EXCLUDES crystal-induced (275.4)
                gonococcal (098.51)
                gouty (274.0)
                syphilitic (095.7)
    - 727.02 Giant cell tumor of tendon sheath
    - 727.03 Trigger finger (acquired)
    - 727.04 Radial styloid tenosynovitis
      de Quervain's disease
    - ◆ 727.05 Other tenosynovitis of hand and wrist
    - 727.06 Tenosynovitis of foot and ankle
    - ◆ 727.09 Other
  - 727.1 Bunion
  - ◆ **727.2 Specific bursitides often of occupational origin**
    Beat: Miners':
      elbow   elbow
      hand   knee
      knee
    Chronic crepitant synovitis of wrist
  - ◆ **727.3 Other bursitis**
    Bursitis NOS
    EXCLUDES bursitis:
      gonococcal (098.52)
      subacromial (726.19)
      subcoracoid (726.19)
      subdeltoid (726.19)
      syphilitic (095.7)
      "frozen shoulder" (726.0)
  - ● **727.4 Ganglion and cyst of synovium, tendon, and bursa**
    - ◆ 727.40 Synovial cyst, unspecified
      EXCLUDES that of popliteal space (727.51)
    - 727.41 Ganglion of joint
    - 727.42 Ganglion of tendon sheath
    - ◆ 727.43 Ganglion, unspecified
    - ◆ 727.49 Other
      Cyst of bursa
  - ● **727.5 Rupture of synovium**
    - ◆ 727.50 Rupture of synovium, unspecified
    - 727.51 Synovial cyst of popliteal space
      Baker's cyst (knee)
    - ◆ 727.59 Other
  - ● **727.6 Rupture of tendon, nontraumatic**
    - ◆ 727.60 Nontraumatic rupture of unspecified tendon
    - 727.61 Complete rupture of rotator cuff
    - 727.62 Tendons of biceps (long head)
    - 727.63 Extensor tendons of hand and wrist
    - 727.64 Flexor tendons of hand and wrist
    - 727.65 Quadriceps tendon
    - 727.66 Patellar tendon
    - 727.67 Achilles tendon
    - ◆ 727.68 Other tendons of foot and ankle
    - ◆ 727.69 Other

MUSCULOSKELETAL SYSTEM AND CONNECTIVE TISSUE

- **727.8** **Other disorders of synovium, tendon, and bursa**
  - **727.81** **Contracture of tendon (sheath)**
    - Short Achilles tendon (acquired)
  - **727.82** **Calcium deposits in tendon and bursa**
    - Calcification of tendon NOS
    - Calcific tendinitis NOS
    - EXCLUDES: *peripheral ligamentous or muscular attachments (726.0-726.9)*
  - ◆ **727.89** **Other**
    - Abscess of bursa or tendon
    - EXCLUDES: *xanthomatosis localized to tendons (272.7)*
- ◆ **727.9** **Unspecified disorder of synovium, tendon, and bursa**
- ● **728** **Disorders of muscle, ligament, and fascia**
  - EXCLUDES: *enthesopathies (726.0-726.9)*
  - *muscular dystrophies (359.0-359.1)*
  - *myoneural disorders (358.0-358.9)*
  - *myopathies (359.2-359.9)*
  - *old disruption of ligaments of knee (717.81-717.89)*
  - **728.0** **Infective myositis**
    - Myositis:
      - purulent
      - suppurative
    - EXCLUDES: *myositis:*
      - *epidemic (074.1)*
      - *interstitial (728.81)*
      - *syphilitic (095.6)*
      - *tropical (040.81)*
  - ● **728.1** **Muscular calcification and ossification**
    - ◆ **728.10** **Calcification and ossification, unspecified**
      - Massive calcification (paraplegic)
    - **728.11** **Progressive myositis ossificans**
    - **728.12** **Traumatic myositis ossificans**
      - Myositis ossificans (circumscripta)
    - **728.13** **Postoperative heterotopic calcification**
    - ◆ **728.19** **Other**
      - Polymyositis ossificans
  - **728.2** **Muscular wasting and disuse atrophy, not elsewhere classified**
    - Amyotrophia NOS
    - Myofibrosis
    - EXCLUDES: *neuralgic amyotrophy (353.5)*
    - *progressive muscular atrophy (335.0-335.9)*
  - ◆ **728.3** **Other specific muscle disorders**
    - Arthrogryposis
    - Immobility syndrome (paraplegic)
    - EXCLUDES: *arthrogryposis multiplex congenita (754.89)*
    - *stiff-man syndrome (333.91)*
  - **728.4** **Laxity of ligament**
  - **728.5** **Hypermobility syndrome**
  - **728.6** **Contracture of palmar fascia**
    - Dupuytren's contracture
  - ● **728.7** **Other fibromatoses**
    - **728.71** **Plantar fascial fibromatosis**
      - Contracture of plantar fascia
      - Plantar fasciitis (traumatic)
    - ◆ **728.79** **Other**
      - Garrod's or knuckle pads
      - Nodular fasciitis
      - Pseudosarcomatous fibromatosis (proliferative) (subcutaneous)
  - ● **728.8** **Other disorders of muscle, ligament, and fascia**
    - **728.81** **Interstitial myositis**
    - **728.82** **Foreign body granuloma of muscle**
      - Talc granuloma of muscle
    - **728.83** **Rupture of muscle, nontraumatic**
    - **728.84** **Diastasis of muscle**
      - Diastasis recti (abdomen)
      - EXCLUDES: *diastasis recti complicating pregnancy, labor, and delivery (665.8)*
    - **728.85** **Spasm of muscle**
    - ◆ **728.89** **Other**
      - Eosinophilic fasciitis
      - Use additional E code, if desired, to identify drug, if drug induced
  - ◆ **728.9** **Unspecified disorder of muscle, ligament, and fascia**

- ● **729** **Other disorders of soft tissues**
  - EXCLUDES: *acroparesthesia (443.89)*
  - *carpal tunnel syndrome (354.0)*
  - *disorders of the back (720.0-724.9)*
  - *entrapment syndromes (354.0-355.9)*
  - *palindromic rheumatism (719.3)*
  - *periarthritis (726.0-726.9)*
  - *psychogenic rheumatism (306.0)*
  - ◆ **729.0** **Rheumatism, unspecified and fibrositis**
  - ◆ **729.1** **Myalgia and myositis, unspecified**
    - Fibromyositis NOS
  - ◆ **729.2** **Neuralgia, neuritis, and radiculitis, unspecified**
    - EXCLUDES: *brachial radiculitis (723.4)*
    - *cervical radiculitis (723.4)*
    - *lumbosacral radiculitis (724.4)*
    - *mononeuritis (354.0-355.9)*
    - *radiculitis due to intervertebral disc involvement (722.0-722.2, 722.7)*
    - *sciatica (724.3)*
  - ● **729.3** **Panniculitis, unspecified**
    - ◆ **729.30** **Panniculitis, unspecified site**
      - Weber-Christian disease
    - **729.31** **Hypertrophy of fat pad, knee**
      - Hypertrophy of infrapatellar fat pad
    - ◆ **729.39** **Other site**
      - EXCLUDES: *panniculitis specified as (affecting):*
      - *back (724.8)*
      - *neck (723.6)*
      - *sacral (724.8)*
  - ◆ **729.4** **Fasciitis, unspecified**
    - EXCLUDES: *nodular fasciitis (728.79)*
  - **729.5** **Pain in limb**
  - **729.6** **Residual foreign body in soft tissue**
    - EXCLUDES: *foreign body granuloma:*
    - *muscle (728.82)*
    - *skin and subcutaneous tissue (709.4)*
  - ● **729.8** **Other musculoskeletal symptoms referable to limbs**
    - **729.81** **Swelling of limb**
    - **729.82** **Cramp**
    - ◆ **729.89** **Other**
      - EXCLUDES: *abnormality of gait (781.2)*
      - *tetany (781.7)*
      - *transient paralysis of limb (781.4)*
  - ◆ **729.9** **Other and unspecified disorders of soft tissue**
    - Polyalgia

OSTEOPATHIES, CHONDROPATHIES, AND ACQUIRED MUSCULOSKELETAL DEFORMITIES (730-739)

- ● **730** **Osteomyelitis, periostitis, and other infections involving bone**
  - EXCLUDES: *jaw (526.4-526.5)*
  - *petrous bone (383.2)*
  - Use additional code, if desired, to identify organism, such as Staphylococcus (041.1)
  - The following fifth-digit subclassification is for use with category 730; valid digits are in [brackets] under each code. See page 117 for definitions:
    - ◆ 0 site unspecified
    - 1 shoulder region
    - 2 upper arm
    - 3 forearm
    - 4 hand
    - 5 pelvic region and thigh
    - 6 lower leg
    - 7 ankle and foot
    - ◆ 8 other specified sites
    - ◆ 9 multiple sites
  - ● **730.0** **Acute osteomyelitis**
    - [0-9] Abscess of any bone except accessory sinus, jaw, or mastoid
    - Acute or subacute osteomyelitis, with or without mention of periostitis
  - ● **730.1** **Chronic osteomyelitis**
    - [0-9] Brodie's abscess
    - Chronic or old osteomyelitis, with or without mention of periostitis
    - Necrosis (acute) of bone
    - Sequestrum of bone
    - Sclerosing osteomyelitis of Garré
    - EXCLUDES: *aseptic necrosis of bone (733.40-733.49)*

● Additional digits required ◆ Nonspecific code ■ Not a primary diagnosis

Volume 1 — 123

- ● **730.2** **Unspecified osteomyelitis**
  [0-9] Osteitis or osteomyelitis NOS, with or without mention of periostitis
  - ● **730.3** **Periostitis without mention of osteomyelitis**
    [0-9] Abscess of periosteum | without mention of
    Periostosis | osteomyelitis
    > **EXCLUDES** that in secondary syphilis (091.61)
  - ● **730.7** *Osteopathy resulting from poliomyelitis*
    [0-9] Code also underlying disease (045.0-045.9)
  - ● **730.8** *Other infections involving bone in diseases classified elsewhere*
    [0-9] Code also underlying disease as:
    tuberculosis (015.0-015.9)
    typhoid fever (002.0)
    > **EXCLUDES** syphilis of bone NOS (095.5)
  - ● **730.9** **Unspecified infection of bone**
    [0-9]
- ● **731** **Osteitis deformans and osteopathies associated with other disorders classified elsewhere**
  - **731.0** **Osteitis deformans without mention of bone tumor**
    Paget's disease of bone
  - **731.1** *Osteitis deformans in diseases classified elsewhere*
    Code also underlying disease as:
    malignant neoplasm of bone (170.0-170.9)
  - **731.2** **Hypertrophic pulmonary osteoarthropathy**
    Bamberger-Marie disease
  - **731.8** *Other bone involvement in diseases classified elsewhere*
    Code also underlying disease as:
    diabetes mellitus (250.8)
- ● **732** **Osteochondropathies**
  - **732.0** **Juvenile osteochondrosis of spine**
    Juvenile osteochondrosis (of):
    marginal or vertebral epiphysis (of Scheuermann)
    spine NOS
    Vertebral epiphysitis
    > **EXCLUDES** adolescent postural kyphosis (737.0)
  - **732.1** **Juvenile osteochondrosis of hip and pelvis**
    Coxa plana
    Ischiopubic synchondrosis (of van Neck)
    Osteochondrosis (juvenile) of:
    acetabulum
    head of femur (of Legg-Calvé-Perthes)
    iliac crest (of Buchanan)
    symphysis pubis (of Pierson)
    Pseudocoxalgia
  - **732.2** **Nontraumatic slipped upper femoral epiphysis**
    Slipped upper femoral epiphysis NOS
  - **732.3** **Juvenile osteochondrosis of upper extremity**
    Osteochondrosis (juvenile) of:
    capitulum of humerus (of Panner)
    carpal lunate (of Kienbock)
    hand NOS
    head of humerus (of Haas)
    heads of metacarpals (of Mauclaire)
    lower ulna (of Burns)
    radial head (of Brailsford)
    upper extremity NOS
  - **732.4** **Juvenile osteochondrosis of lower extremity, excluding foot**
    Osteochondrosis (juvenile) of:
    lower extremity NOS
    primary patellar center (of Köhler)
    proximal tibia (of Blount)
    secondary patellar center (of Sinding-Larsen)
    tibial tubercle (of Osgood-Schlatter)
    Tibia vara
  - **732.5** **Juvenile osteochondrosis of foot**
    Calcaneal apophysitis
    Epiphysitis, os calcis
    Osteochondrosis (juvenile) of:
    astragalus (of Diaz)
    calcaneum (of Sever)
    foot NOS
    metatarsal
    second (of Freiberg)
    fifth (of Iselin)
    os tibiale externum (of Haglund)
    tarsal navicular (of Köhler)
  - **732.6** **Other juvenile osteochondrosis**
    Apophysitis
    Epiphysitis } specified as juvenile, of other site,
    Osteochondritis } or site NOS
    Osteochondrosis
  - **732.7** **Osteochondritis dissecans**
  - **732.8** **Other specified forms of osteochondropathy**
    Adult osteochondrosis of spine
  - **732.9** **Unspecified osteochondropathy**
    Apophysitis
    Epiphysitis
    Osteochondritis } not specified as adult or juvenile,
    Osteochondrosis } of unspecified site
    NOS
- ● **733** **Other disorders of bone and cartilage**
  > **EXCLUDES** bone spur (726.91)
  > cartilage of, or loose body in, joint (717.0-717.9, 718.0-718.9)
  > giant cell granuloma of jaw (526.3)
  > osteitis fibrosa cystica generalisata (252.0)
  > osteomalacia (268.2)
  > polyostotic fibrous dysplasia of bone (756.54)
  > prognathism, retrognathism (524.1)
  > xanthomatosis localized to bone (272.7)
  - ● **733.0** **Osteoporosis**
    - **733.00** **Osteoporosis, unspecified**
      Wedging of vertebra NOS
    - **733.01** **Senile osteoporosis**
      Postmenopausal osteoporosis
    - **733.02** **Idiopathic osteoporosis**
    - **733.03** **Disuse osteoporosis**
    - **733.09** **Other**
      Drug-induced osteoporosis
      Use additional E code, if desired, to identify drug
  - ● **733.1** **Pathologic fracture**
    Spontaneous fracture
    > **EXCLUDES** traumatic fracture (800-829)
    - **733.10** **Pathologic fracture, unspecified site**
    - **733.11** **Pathologic fracture of humerus**
    - **733.12** **Pathologic fracture of distal radius and ulna**
      Wrist NOS
    - **733.13** **Pathologic fracture of vertebrae**
      Collapse of vertebra NOS
    - **733.14** **Pathologic fracture of neck of femur**
      Femur NOS   Hip NOS
    - **733.15** **Pathologic fracture of other specified part of femur**
    - **733.16** **Pathologic fracture of tibia or fibula**
      Ankle NOS
    - **733.19** **Pathologic fracture of other specified site**
  - ● **733.2** **Cyst of bone**
    - **733.20** **Cyst of bone (localized), unspecified**
    - **733.21** **Solitary bone cyst**
      Unicameral bone cyst
    - **733.22** **Aneurysmal bone cyst**
    - **733.29** **Other**
      Fibrous dysplasia (monostotic)
      > **EXCLUDES** cyst of jaw (526.0-526.2, 526.89)
      > osteitis fibrosa cystica (252.0)
      > polyostotic fibrousdysplasia of bone (756.54)
  - **733.3** **Hyperostosis of skull**
    Hyperostosis interna frontalis
    Leontiasis ossium
  - ● **733.4** **Aseptic necrosis of bone**
    > **EXCLUDES** necrosis of bone NOS (730.1)
    > osteochondropathies (732.0-732.9)
    - **733.40** **Aseptic necrosis of bone, site unspecified**
    - **733.41** **Head of humerus**
    - **733.42** **Head and neck of femur**
      Femur NOS
      > **EXCLUDES** Legg-Calvé-Perthes disease (732.1)
    - **733.43** **Medial femoral condyle**
    - **733.44** **Talus**
    - **733.49** **Other**
  - **733.5** **Osteitis condensans**
    Piriform sclerosis of ilium

MUSCULOSKELETAL SYSTEM AND CONNECTIVE TISSUE

- **733.6 Tietze's disease**
  Costochondral junction syndrome
- **733.7 Algoneurodystrophy**
  Disuse atrophy of bone
  Sudeck's atrophy
- ● **733.8 Malunion and nonunion of fracture**
  - 733.81 Malunion of fracture
  - 733.82 Nonunion of fracture
    Pseudoarthrosis (bone)
- ● **733.9 Other and unspecified disorders of bone and cartilage**
  - ◆ 733.90 Disorder of bone and cartilage, unspecified
  - 733.91 Arrest of bone development or growth
    Epiphyseal arrest
  - 733.92 Chondromalacia
    Chondromalacia:
      NOS
      localized, except patella
      systemic
      tibial plateau
    EXCLUDES *chondromalacia of patella (717.7)*
  - ◆ 733.99 Other
    Diaphysitis
    Hypertrophy of bone
    Relapsing polychondritis

734 Flat foot
  Pes planus (acquired)
  Talipes planus (acquired)
  EXCLUDES *congenital (754.61)*
    rigid flat foot (754.61)
    spastic (everted) flat foot (754.61)

● **735 Acquired deformities of toe**
  EXCLUDES *congenital (754.60-754.69, 755.65-755.66)*
  - 735.0 Hallux valgus (acquired)
  - 735.1 Hallux varus (acquired)
  - 735.2 Hallux rigidus
  - 735.3 Hallux malleus
  - ◆ 735.4 Other hammer toe (acquired)
  - 735.5 Claw toe (acquired)
  - ◆ 735.8 Other acquired deformities of toe
  - ◆ 735.9 Unspecified acquired deformity of toe

● **736 Other acquired deformities of limbs**
  EXCLUDES *congenital (754.3-755.9)*
  - ● 736.0 Acquired deformities of forearm, excluding fingers
    - ◆ 736.00 Unspecified deformity
      Deformity of elbow, forearm, hand, or wrist (acquired) NOS
    - 736.01 Cubitus valgus (acquired)
    - 736.02 Cubitus varus (acquired)
    - 736.03 Valgus deformity of wrist (acquired)
    - 736.04 Varus deformity of wrist (acquired)
    - 736.05 Wrist drop (acquired)
    - 736.06 Claw hand (acquired)
    - 736.07 Club hand, acquired
    - ◆ 736.09 Other
  - 736.1 Mallet finger
  - ● 736.2 Other acquired deformities of finger
    - ◆ 736.20 Unspecified deformity
      Deformity of finger (acquired) NOS
    - 736.21 Boutonniere deformity
    - 736.22 Swan-neck deformity
    - ◆ 736.29 Other
      EXCLUDES *trigger finger (727.03)*
  - ● 736.3 Acquired deformities of hip
    - ◆ 736.30 Unspecified deformity
      Deformity of hip (acquired) NOS
    - 736.31 Coxa valga (acquired)
    - 736.32 Coxa vara (acquired)
    - ◆ 736.39 Other
  - ● 736.4 Genu valgum or varum (acquired)
    - 736.41 Genu valgum (acquired)
    - 736.42 Genu varum (acquired)
  - 736.5 Genu recurvatum (acquired)
  - ◆ 736.6 Other acquired deformities of knee
    Deformity of knee (acquired) NOS
  - ● 736.7 Other acquired deformities of ankle and foot
    EXCLUDES *deformities of toe (acquired) (735.0-735.9)*
      pes planus (acquired) (734)
    - ◆ 736.70 Unspecified deformity of ankle and foot, acquired
    - 736.71 Acquired equinovarus deformity
      Clubfoot, acquired
      EXCLUDES *clubfoot not specified as acquired (754.5-754.7)*
    - 736.72 Equinus deformity of foot, acquired
    - 736.73 Cavus deformity of foot
      EXCLUDES *that with claw foot (736.74)*
    - 736.74 Claw foot, acquired
    - 736.75 Cavovarus deformity of foot, acquired
    - ◆ 736.76 Other calcaneus deformity
    - ◆ 736.79 Other
      Acquired:
        pes | not elsewhere classified
        talipes |
  - ● 736.8 Acquired deformities of other parts of limbs
    - 736.81 Unequal leg length (acquired)
    - ◆ 736.89 Other
      Deformity (acquired):
        arm or leg, not elsewhere classified
        shoulder
  - ◆ 736.9 Acquired deformity of limb, site unspecified

● **737 Curvature of spine**
  EXCLUDES *congenital (754.2)*
  - 737.0 Adolescent postural kyphosis
    EXCLUDES *osteochondrosis of spine (juvenile) (732.0)*
      adult (732.8)
  - ● 737.1 Kyphosis (acquired)
    - 737.10 Kyphosis (acquired) (postural)
    - 737.11 Kyphosis due to radiation
    - 737.12 Kyphosis, postlaminectomy
    - ◆ 737.19 Other
      EXCLUDES *that associated with conditions classifiable elsewhere (737.41)*
  - ● 737.2 Lordosis (acquired)
    - 737.20 Lordosis (acquired) (postural)
    - 737.21 Lordosis, postlaminectomy
    - 737.22 Other postsurgical lordosis
    - ◆ 737.29 Other
      EXCLUDES *that associated with conditions classifiable elsewhere (737.42)*
  - ● 737.3 Kyphoscoliosis and scoliosis
    - 737.30 Scoliosis [and kyphoscoliosis], idiopathic
    - 737.31 Resolving infantile idiopathic scoliosis
    - 737.32 Progressive infantile idiopathic scoliosis
    - 737.33 Scoliosis due to radiation
    - 737.34 Thoracogenic scoliosis
    - ◆ 737.39 Other
      EXCLUDES *that associated with conditions classifiable elsewhere (737.43)*
        that in kyphoscoliotic heart disease (416.1)
  - ● 737.4 Curvature of spine associated with other conditions
    Code also associated condition as:
      Charcot-Marie-Tooth disease (356.1)
      mucopolysaccharidosis (277.5)
      neurofibromatosis (237.7)
      osteitis deformans (731.0)
      osteitis fibrosa cystica (252.0)
      osteoporosis (733.00-733.09)
      poliomyelitis (138)
      tuberculosis [Pott's curvature] (015.0)
    - ∎◆ 737.40 Curvature of spine, unspecified
    - ∎ 737.41 *Kyphosis*
    - ∎ 737.42 *Lordosis*
    - ∎ 737.43 *Scoliosis*
  - ◆ 737.8 Other curvatures of spine
  - ◆ 737.9 Unspecified curvature of spine
    Curvature of spine (acquired) (idiopathic) NOS
    Hunchback, acquired
    EXCLUDES *deformity of spine NOS (738.5)*

● **738 Other acquired deformity**
  EXCLUDES *congenital (754.0-756.9, 758.0-759.9)*
    dentofacial anomalies (524.0-524.9)
  - 738.0 Acquired deformity of nose
    Deformity of nose (acquired)
    Overdevelopment of nasal bones
    EXCLUDES *deflected or deviated nasal septum (470)*

● Additional digits required   ◆ Nonspecific code   ∎ Not a primary diagnosis

738.1 — 743.1

- **738.1** Other acquired deformity of head
  - 738.10 Unspecified deformity
  - 738.11 Zygomatic hyperplasia
  - 738.12 Zygomatic hypoplasia
  - 738.19 Other specified deformity
- 738.2 Acquired deformity of neck
- 738.3 Acquired deformity of chest and rib
  - Deformity:
    - chest (acquired)
    - rib (acquired)
  - Pectus:
    - carinatum, acquired
    - excavatum, acquired
- 738.4 Acquired spondylolisthesis
  - Degenerative spondylolisthesis
  - Spondylolysis, acquired
  - **EXCLUDES** congenital (756.12)
- **738.5** Other acquired deformity of back or spine
  - Deformity of spine NOS
  - **EXCLUDES** curvature of spine (737.0-737.9)
- 738.6 Acquired deformity of pelvis
  - Pelvic obliquity
  - **EXCLUDES** intrapelvic protrusion of acetabulum (718.6)
    that in relation to labor and delivery (653.0-653.4, 653.8-653.9)
- 738.7 Cauliflower ear
- **738.8** Acquired deformity of other specified site
  - Deformity of clavicle
- **738.9** Acquired deformity of unspecified site
- **739** Nonallopathic lesions, not elsewhere classified
  - **INCLUDES** segmental dysfunction
    somatic dysfunction
  - 739.0 Head region
    - Occipitocervical region
  - 739.1 Cervical region
    - Cervicothoracic region
  - 739.2 Thoracic region
    - Thoracolumbar region
  - 739.3 Lumbar region
    - Lumbosacral region
  - 739.4 Sacral region
    - Sacrococcygeal region
    - Sacroiliac region
  - 739.5 Pelvic region
    - Hip region
    - Pubic region
  - 739.6 Lower extremities
  - 739.7 Upper extremities
    - Acromioclavicular region
    - Sternoclavicular region
  - 739.8 Rib cage
    - Costochondral region
    - Costovertebral region
    - Sternochondral region
  - 739.9 Abdomen and other

14. CONGENITAL ANOMALIES (740-759)

- **740** Anencephalus and similar anomalies
  - 740.0 Anencephalus
    - Acrania
    - Amyelencephalus
    - Hemicephaly
    - Hemianencephaly
  - 740.1 Craniorachischisis
  - 740.2 Iniencephaly
- **741** Spina bifida
  - **EXCLUDES** spina bifida occulta (756.17)
  - The following fifth-digit subclassification is for use with category 741:
    - 0 unspecified region
    - 1 cervical region
    - 2 dorsal [thoracic] region
    - 3 lumbar region
  - **741.0** With hydrocephalus
    - Arnold-Chiari syndrome, type II
    - Any condition classifiable to 741.9 with any condition classifiable to 742.3
    - Chiari malformation, type II
  - **741.9** Without mention of hydrocephalus
    - Hydromeningocele (spinal)
    - Hydromyelocele
    - Meningocele (spinal)
    - Meningomyelocele
    - Myelocele
    - Myelocystocele
    - Rachischisis
    - Spina bifida (aperta)
    - Syringomyelocele

- **742** Other congenital anomalies of nervous system
  - 742.0 Encephalocele
    - Encephalocystocele
    - Encephalomyelocele
    - Hydroencephalocele
    - Hydromeningocele, cranial
    - Meningocele, cerebral
    - Meningoencephalocele
  - 742.1 Microcephalus
    - Hydromicrocephaly
    - Micrencephaly
  - 742.2 Reduction deformities of brain
    - Absence
    - Agenesis
    - Aplasia
    - Hypoplasia } of part of brain
    - Agyria
    - Arhinencephaly
    - Holoprosencephaly
    - Microgyria
  - 742.3 Congenital hydrocephalus
    - Aqueduct of Sylvius:
      - anomaly
      - obstruction, congenital
      - stenosis
    - Atresia of foramina of Magendie and Luschka
    - Hydrocephalus in newborn
    - **EXCLUDES** hydrocephalus:
      - acquired (331.3-331.4)
      - due to congenital toxoplasmosis (771.2)
      - with any condition classifiable to 741.9 (741.0)
  - **742.4** Other specified anomalies of brain
    - Congenital cerebral cyst
    - Macroencephaly
    - Macrogyria
    - Megalencephaly
    - Multiple anomalies of brain NOS
    - Porencephaly
    - Ulegyria
  - **742.5** Other specified anomalies of spinal cord
    - 742.51 Diastematomyelia
    - 742.53 Hydromyelia
      - Hydrorhachis
    - **742.59** Other
      - Amyelia
      - Atelomyelia
      - Congenital anomaly of spinal meninges
      - Defective development of cauda equina
      - Hypoplasia of spinal cord
      - Myelatelia
      - Myelodysplasia
  - **742.8** Other specified anomalies of nervous system
    - Agenesis of nerve
    - Displacement of brachial plexus
    - Familial dysautonomia
    - Jaw-winking syndrome
    - Marcus-Gunn syndrome
    - Riley-Day syndrome
    - **EXCLUDES** neurofibromatosis (237.7)
  - **742.9** Unspecified anomaly of brain, spinal cord, and nervous system
    - Anomaly
    - Congenital:
      - disease
      - lesion
    - Deformity
    } of:
      - brain
      - nervous system
      - spinal cord

- **743** Congenital anomalies of eye
  - **743.0** Anophthalmos
    - **743.00** Clinical anophthalmos, unspecified
      - Agenesis
      - Congenital absence } of eye
      - Anophthalmos NOS
    - 743.03 Cystic eyeball, congenital
    - 743.06 Cryptophthalmos
  - **743.1** Microphthalmos
    - Dysplasia
    - Hypoplasia } of eye
    - Rudimentary eye

CONGENITAL ANOMALIES

- ◆ 743.10 Microphthalmos, unspecified
- 743.11 Simple microphthalmos
- 743.12 Microphthalmos associated with other anomalies of eye and adnexa
- ● 743.2 Buphthalmos
  - Glaucoma:
    - congenital
    - newborn
  - Hydrophthalmos
  - **EXCLUDES** glaucoma of childhood (365.14)
  - traumatic glaucoma due to birth injury (767.8)
  - ◆ 743.20 Buphthalmos, unspecified
  - 743.21 Simple buphthalmos
  - ◆ 743.22 Buphthalmos associated with other ocular anomalies
    - Keratoglobus, congenital | associated with
    - Megalocornea | buphthalmos
- ● 743.3 Congenital cataract and lens anomalies
  - **EXCLUDES** infantile cataract (366.00-366.09)
  - ◆ 743.30 Congenital cataract, unspecified
  - 743.31 Capsular and subcapsular cataract
  - 743.32 Cortical and zonular cataract
  - 743.33 Nuclear cataract
  - 743.34 Total and subtotal cataract, congenital
  - 743.35 Congenital aphakia
    - Congenital absence of lens
  - 743.36 Anomalies of lens shape
    - Microphakia
    - Spherophakia
  - 743.37 Congenital ectopic lens
  - ◆ 743.39 Other
- ● 743.4 Coloboma and other anomalies of anterior segment
  - 743.41 Anomalies of corneal size and shape
    - Microcornea
    - **EXCLUDES** that associated with buphthalmos (743.22)
  - 743.42 Corneal opacities, interfering with vision, congenital
  - ◆ 743.43 Other corneal opacities, congenital
  - ◆ 743.44 Specified anomalies of anterior chamber, chamber angle, and related structures
    - Anomaly:
      - Axenfeld's
      - Peters'
      - Rieger's
  - 743.45 Aniridia
  - ◆ 743.46 Other specified anomalies of iris and ciliary body
    - Anisocoria, congenital Coloboma of iris
    - Atresia of pupil   Corectopia
  - ◆ 743.47 Specified anomalies of sclera
  - ◆ 743.48 Multiple and combined anomalies of anterior segment
  - ◆ 743.49 Other
- ● 743.5 Congenital anomalies of posterior segment
  - 743.51 Vitreous anomalies
    - Congenital vitreous opacity
  - 743.52 Fundus coloboma
  - 743.53 Chorioretinal degeneration, congenital
  - 743.54 Congenital folds and cysts of posterior segment
  - 743.55 Congenital macular changes
  - ◆ 743.56 Other retinal changes, congenital
  - ◆ 743.57 Specified anomalies of optic disc
    - Coloboma of optic disc (congenital)
  - 743.58 Vascular anomalies
    - Congenital retinal aneurysm
  - ◆ 743.59 Other
- ● 743.6 Congenital anomalies of eyelids, lacrimal system, and orbit
  - 743.61 Congenital ptosis
  - 743.62 Congenital deformities of eyelids
    - Ablepharon   Congenital:
    - Absence of eyelid   ectropion
    - Accessory eyelid   entropion
  - ◆ 743.63 Other specified congenital anomalies of eyelid
    - Absence, agenesis, of cilia
  - ◆ 743.64 Specified congenital anomalies of lacrimal gland
- ◆ 743.65 Specified congenital anomalies of lacrimal passages
  - Absence, agenesis of:
    - lacrimal apparatus
    - punctum lacrimale
    - Accessory lacrimal canal
- ◆ 743.66 Specified congenital anomalies of orbit
- ◆ 743.69 Other
  - Accessory eye muscles
- ◆ 743.8 Other specified anomalies of eye
  - **EXCLUDES** congenital nystagmus (379.51)
  - ocular albinism (270.2)
  - retinitis pigmentosa (362.74)
- 743.9 Unspecified anomaly of eye
  - Congenital:
    - anomaly NOS   } of eye [any part]
    - deformity NOS }
- ● 744 Congenital anomalies of ear, face, and neck
  - **EXCLUDES** anomaly of:
    - cervical spine (754.2, 756.10-756.19)
    - larynx (748.2-748.3)
    - nose (748.0-748.1)
    - parathyroid gland (759.2)
    - thyroid gland (759.2)
    - cleft lip (749.10-749.25)
- ● 744.0 Anomalies of ear causing impairment of hearing
  - **EXCLUDES** congenital deafness without mention of cause (389.0-389.9)
  - ◆ 744.00 Unspecified anomaly of ear with impairment of hearing
  - 744.01 Absence of external ear
    - Absence of:
      - auditory canal (external)
      - auricle (ear) (with stenosis or atresia of auditory canal)
  - ◆ 744.02 Other anomalies of external ear with impairment of hearing
    - Atresia or stricture of auditory canal (external)
  - 744.03 Anomaly of middle ear, except ossicles
    - Atresia or stricture of osseous meatus (ear)
  - 744.04 Anomalies of ear ossicles
    - Fusion of ear ossicles
  - 744.05 Anomalies of inner ear
    - Congenital anomaly of:
      - membranous labyrinth
      - organ of Corti
  - ◆ 744.09 Other
    - Absence of ear, congenital
  - 744.1 Accessory auricle
    - Accessory tragus   Supernumerary:
    - Polyotia   ear
    - Preauricular appendage   lobule
- ● 744.2 Other specified anomalies of ear
  - **EXCLUDES** that with impairment of hearing (744.00-744.09)
  - 744.21 Absence of ear lobe, congenital
  - 744.22 Macrotia
  - 744.23 Microtia
  - ◆ 744.24 Specified anomalies of Eustachian tube
    - Absence of Eustachian tube
  - ◆ 744.29 Other
    - Bat ear   Prominence of auricle
    - Darwin's tubercle Ridge ear
    - Pointed ear
    - **EXCLUDES** preauricular sinus (744.46)
- ◆ 744.3 Unspecified anomaly of ear
  - Congenital:
    - anomaly NOS   } of ear, not elsewhere
    - deformity NOS } classified
- ● 744.4 Branchial cleft cyst or fistula; preauricular sinus
  - 744.41 Branchial cleft sinus or fistula
    - Branchial:
      - sinus (external) (internal)
      - vestige
  - 744.42 Branchial cleft cyst
  - 744.43 Cervical auricle

- 744.46 Preauricular sinus or fistula
- 744.47 Preauricular cyst
- ◆ 744.49 Other
  - Fistula (of): auricle, congenital
  - Fistula (of): cervicoaural
- 744.5 **Webbing of neck**
  - Pterygium colli
- ● 744.8 **Other specified anomalies of face and neck**
  - 744.81 Macrocheilia
    - Hypertrophy of lip, congenital
  - 744.82 Microcheilia
  - 744.83 Macrostomia
  - 744.84 Microstomia
  - ◆ 744.89 Other
    - **EXCLUDES** congenital fistula of lip (750.25)
      musculoskeletal anomalies (754.0-754.1, 756.0)
- ◆ 744.9 **Unspecified anomalies of face and neck**
  - Congenital:
    - anomaly NOS | of face [any part] or
    - deformity NOS | neck [any part]

● 745 **Bulbus cordis anomalies and anomalies of cardiac septal closure**
- 745.0 **Common truncus**
  - Absent septum | between aorta and pulmonary artery
  - Communication (abnormal) |
  - Aortic septal defect
  - Common aortopulmonary trunk
  - Persistent truncus arteriosus
- ● 745.1 **Transposition of great vessels**
  - 745.10 Complete transposition of great vessels
    - Transposition of great vessels:
      - NOS
      - classical
  - 745.11 Double outlet right ventricle
    - Dextratransposition of aorta
    - Incomplete transposition of great vessels
    - Origin of both great vessels from right ventricle
    - Taussig-Bing syndrome or defect
  - 745.12 Corrected transposition of great vessels
  - ◆ 745.19 Other
- 745.2 **Tetralogy of Fallot**
  - Fallot's pentalogy
  - Ventricular septal defect with pulmonary stenosis or atresia, dextraposition of aorta, and hypertrophy of right ventricle
  - **EXCLUDES** Fallot's triad (746.09)
- 745.3 **Common ventricle**
  - Cor triloculare biatriatum
  - Single ventricle
- 745.4 **Ventricular septal defect**
  - Eisenmenger's defect or complex
  - Gerbo dedefect
  - Interventricular septal defect
  - Left ventricular-right atrial communication
  - Roger's disease
  - **EXCLUDES** common atrioventricular canal type (745.69)
    single ventricle (745.3)
- 745.5 **Ostium secundum type atrial septal defect**
  - Defect:
    - atrium secundum
    - fossa ovalis
  - Patent or persistent:
    - foramen ovale
    - ostium secundum
  - Lutembacher's syndrome
- ● 745.6 **Endocardial cushion defects**
  - ◆ 745.60 Endocardial cushion defect, unspecified type
  - 745.61 Ostium primum defect
    - Persistent ostium primum
  - ◆ 745.69 Other
    - Absence of atrial septum
    - Atrioventricular canal type ventricular septal defect
    - Common atrioventricular canal
    - Common atrium
- 745.7 **Cor biloculare**
  - Absence of atrial and ventricular septa
- ◆ 745.8 **Other**
- ◆ 745.9 **Unspecified defect of septal closure**
  - Septal defect NOS

● 746 **Other congenital anomalies of heart**
  - **EXCLUDES** endocardial fibroelastosis (425.3)
- ● 746.0 **Anomalies of pulmonary valve**
  - **EXCLUDES** infundibular or subvalvular pulmonic stenosis (746.83)
    tetralogy of Fallot (745.2)
  - ◆ 746.00 Pulmonary valve anomaly, unspecified
  - 746.01 Atresia, congenital
    - Congenital absence of pulmonary valve
  - 746.02 Stenosis, congenital
  - ◆ 746.09 Other
    - Congenital insufficiency of pulmonary valve
    - Fallot's triad or trilogy
- 746.1 **Tricuspid atresia and stenosis, congenital**
  - Absence of tricuspid valve
- 746.2 **Ebstein's anomaly**
- 746.3 **Congenital stenosis of aortic valve**
  - Congenital aortic stenosis
  - **EXCLUDES** congenital:
    - subaortic stenosis (746.81)
    - supravalvular aortic stenosis (747.22)
- 746.4 **Congenital insufficiency of aortic valve**
  - Bicuspid aortic valve
  - Congenital aortic insufficiency
- 746.5 **Congenital mitral stenosis**
  - Fused commissure
  - Parachute deformity | of mitral valve
  - Supernumerary cusps
- 746.6 **Congenital mitral insufficiency**
- 746.7 **Hypoplastic left heart syndrome**
  - Atresia, or marked hypoplasia, of aortic orifice or valve, with hypoplasia of ascending aorta and defective development of left ventricle (with mitral valve atresia)
- ● 746.8 **Other specified anomalies of heart**
  - 746.81 Subaortic stenosis
  - 746.82 Cor triatriatum
  - 746.83 Infundibular pulmonic stenosis
    - Subvalvular pulmonic stenosis
  - 746.84 Obstructive anomalies of heart, not elsewhere classified
    - Uhl's disease
  - 746.85 Coronary artery anomaly
    - Anomalous origin or communication of coronary artery
    - Arteriovenous malformation of coronary artery
    - Coronary artery:
      - absence
      - arising from aorta or pulmonary trunk
      - single
  - 746.86 Congenital heart block
    - Complete or incomplete atrioventricular [AV] block
  - 746.87 Malposition of heart and cardiac apex
    - Abdominal heart
    - Dextrocardia
    - Ectopia cordis
    - Levocardia (isolated)
    - Mesocardia
    - **EXCLUDES** dextrocardia with complete transposition of viscera (759.3)
  - ◆ 746.89 Other
    - Atresia | of cardiac vein
    - Hypoplasia |
    - Congenital:
      - cardiomegaly
      - diverticulum, left ventricle
      - pericardial defect
- ◆ 746.9 **Unspecified anomaly of heart**
  - Congenital:
    - anomaly of heart NOS
    - heart disease NOS

● 747 **Other congenital anomalies of circulatory system**
- 747.0 **Patent ductus arteriosus**
  - Patent ductus Botalli
  - Persistent ductus arteriosus

CONGENITAL ANOMALIES

- **747.1 Coarctation of aorta**
  - **747.10 Coarctation of aorta (preductal) (postductal)**
    - Hypoplasia of aortic arch
  - **747.11 Interruption of aortic arch**
- **747.2 Other anomalies of aorta**
  - ◆ **747.20 Anomaly of aorta, unspecified**
  - **747.21 Anomalies of aortic arch**
    - Anomalous origin, right subclavian artery
    - Dextraposition of aorta
    - Double aortic arch
    - Kommerell's diverticulum
    - Overriding aorta
    - Persistent:
      - convolutions, aortic arch
      - right aortic arch
    - Vascular ring
    - EXCLUDES *hypoplasia of aortic arch (747.10)*
  - **747.22 Atresia and stenosis of aorta**
    - Absence ⎫
    - Aplasia ⎬ of aorta
    - Hypoplasia ⎪
    - Stricture ⎭
    - Supra (valvular)-aortic stenosis
    - EXCLUDES *congenital aortic (valvular) stenosis or stricture, so stated (746.3)*
      hypoplasia of aorta in hypoplastic left heart syndrome (746.7)
  - ◆ **747.29 Other**
    - Aneurysm of sinus of Valsalva
    - Congenital:
      - aneurysm ⎱ of aorta
      - dilation ⎰
- **747.3 Anomalies of pulmonary artery**
  - Agenesis ⎫
  - Anomaly ⎪
  - Atresia ⎬ of pulmonary artery
  - Coarctation ⎪
  - Hypoplasia ⎪
  - Stenosis ⎭
  - Pulmonary arteriovenous aneurysm
- **747.4 Anomalies of great veins**
  - ◆ **747.40 Anomaly of great veins, unspecified**
    - Anomaly NOS of:
      - pulmonary veins
      - vena cava
  - **747.41 Total anomalous pulmonary venous connection**
    - Total anomalous pulmonary venous return [TAPVR]:
      - subdiaphragmatic
      - supradiaphragmatic
  - **747.42 Partial anomalous pulmonary venous connection**
    - Partial anomalous pulmonary venous return
  - ◆ **747.49 Other anomalies of great veins**
    - Absence ⎱ of vena cava (inferior)
    - Congenital stenosis ⎰ (superior)
    - Persistent:
      - left posterior cardinal vein
      - left superior vena cava
    - Scimitar syndrome
    - Transposition of pulmonary veins NOS
  - **747.5 Absence or hypoplasia of umbilical artery**
    - Single umbilical artery
- **747.6 Other anomalies of peripheral vascular system**
  - Absence ⎫
  - Anomaly ⎬ of artery or vein, not elsewhere classified
  - Atresia ⎭
  - Arteriovenous aneurysm (peripheral)
  - Arteriovenous malformation of the peripheral vascular system
  - Congenital:
    - aneurysm (peripheral)
    - phlebectasia
    - stricture, artery
    - varix
  - Multiple renal arteries
  - EXCLUDES *anomalies of:*
    cerebral vessels (747.81)
    pulmonary artery (747.3)
    congenital retinal aneurysm (743.58)
    hemangioma (228.00-228.09)
    lymphangioma (228.1)
  - ◆ **747.60 Anomaly of the peripheral vascular system, unspecified site**
  - **747.61 Gastrointestinal vessel anomaly**
  - **747.62 Renal vessel anomaly**
  - **747.63 Upper limb vessel anomaly**
  - **747.64 Lower limb vessel anomaly**
  - ◆ **747.69 Anomalies of other specified sites of peripheral vascular system**
- **747.8 Other specified anomalies of circulatory system**
  - **747.81 Anomalies of cerebrovascular system**
    - Arteriovenous malformation of brain
    - Cerebral arteriovenous aneurysm, congenital
    - Congenital anomalies of cerebral vessels
    - EXCLUDES *ruptured cerebral (arteriovenous) aneurysm (430)*
  - **747.82 Spinal vessel anomaly**
    - Arteriovenous malformation of spinal vessel
  - ◆ **747.89 Other**
    - Aneurysm, congenital, specified site not elsewhere classified
    - EXCLUDES *congenital aneurysm:*
      coronary (746.85)
      peripheral (747.6)
      pulmonary (747.3)
      retinal (743.58)
- ◆ **747.9 Unspecified anomaly of circulatory system**
- **748 Congenital anomalies of respiratory system**
  - EXCLUDES *congenital defect of diaphragm (756.6)*
  - **748.0 Choanal atresia**
    - Atresia ⎱ of nares (anterior)
    - Congenital stenosis ⎰ (posterior)
  - ◆ **748.1 Other anomalies of nose**
    - Absent nose
    - Accessory nose
    - Cleft nose
    - Congenital:
      - deformity of nose
      - notching of tip of nose
      - perforation of wall of nasal sinus
    - Deformity of wall of nasal sinus
    - EXCLUDES *congenital deviation of nasal septum (754.0)*
  - **748.2 Web of larynx**
    - Web of larynx:
      - NOS
      - glottic
      - subglottic

● Additional digits required ◆ Nonspecific code ■ Not a primary diagnosis

748.3 Other anomalies of larynx, trachea, and bronchus
Absence or agenesis of:
- bronchus
- larynx
- trachea

Anomaly (of):
- cricoid cartilage
- epiglottis
- thyroid cartilage
- tracheal cartilage

Atresia (of):
- epiglottis
- glottis
- larynx
- trachea

Cleft thyroid, cartilage, congenital

Congenital:
- dilation, trachea
- stenosis:
  - larynx
  - trachea
  - tracheocele

Diverticulum:
- bronchus
- trachea

Fissure of epiglottis
Laryngocele
Posterior cleft of cricoid cartilage (congenital)
Rudimentary tracheal bronchus
Stridor, laryngeal, congenital

748.4 Congenital cystic lung
Disease, lung:
- cystic, congenital
- polycystic, congenital

Honeycomb lung, congenital

EXCLUDES acquired or unspecified cystic lung (518.89)

748.5 Agenesis, hypoplasia, and dysplasia of lung
Absence of lung (fissures) (lobe)
Aplasia of lung
Hypoplasia of lung (lobe)
Sequestration of lung

748.6 Other anomalies of lung
- **748.60** Anomaly of lung, unspecified
- **748.61** Congenital bronchiectasis
- **748.69** Other
  - Accessory lung (lobe)
  - Azygos lobe (fissure), lung

748.8 Other specified anomalies of respiratory system
Abnormal communication between pericardial and pleural sacs
Anomaly, pleural folds
Atresia of nasopharynx
Congenital cyst of mediastinum

748.9 Unspecified anomaly of respiratory system
Anomaly of respiratory system NOS

749 Cleft palate and cleft lip
749.0 Cleft palate
- **749.00** Cleft palate, unspecified
- **749.01** Unilateral, complete
- **749.02** Unilateral, incomplete
  - Cleft uvula
- **749.03** Bilateral, complete
- **749.04** Bilateral, incomplete

749.1 Cleft lip
Cheiloschisis
Congenital fissure of lip
Harelip
Labium leporinum
- **749.10** Cleft lip, unspecified
- **749.11** Unilateral, complete
- **749.12** Unilateral, incomplete
- **749.13** Bilateral, complete
- **749.14** Bilateral, incomplete

749.2 Cleft palate with cleft lip
Cheilopalatoschisis
- **749.20** Cleft palate with cleft lip, unspecified
- **749.21** Unilateral, complete
- **749.22** Unilateral, incomplete
- **749.23** Bilateral, complete
- **749.24** Bilateral, incomplete
- **749.25** Other combinations

750 Other congenital anomalies of upper alimentary tract
EXCLUDES dentofacial anomalies (524.0-524.9)

750.0 Tongue tie
Ankyloglossia

750.1 Other anomalies of tongue
- **750.10** Anomaly of tongue, unspecified
- **750.11** Aglossia
- **750.12** Congenital adhesions of tongue
- **750.13** Fissure of tongue
  - Bifid tongue
  - Double tongue
- **750.15** Macroglossia
  - Congenital hypertrophy of tongue
- **750.16** Microglossia
  - Hypoplasia of tongue
- **750.19** Other

750.2 Other specified anomalies of mouth and pharynx
- **750.21** Absence of salivary gland
- **750.22** Accessory salivary gland
- **750.23** Atresia, salivary duct
  - Imperforate salivary duct
- **750.24** Congenital fistula of salivary gland
- **750.25** Congenital fistula of lip
  - Congenital (mucus) lip pits
- **750.26** Other specified anomalies of mouth
  - Absence of uvula
- **750.27** Diverticulum of pharynx
  - Pharyngeal pouch
- **750.29** Other specified anomalies of pharynx
  - Imperforate pharynx

750.3 Tracheoesophageal fistula, esophageal atresia and stenosis
Absent esophagus
Atresia of esophagus
Congenital:
- esophageal ring
- stenosis of esophagus
- stricture of esophagus

Congenital fistula:
- esophagobronchial
- esophagotracheal

Imperforate esophagus
Webbed esophagus

750.4 Other specified anomalies of esophagus
Dilatation, congenital
Displacement, congenital
Diverticulum
Duplication
Giant
} (of) esophagus

Esophageal pouch

EXCLUDES congenital hiatus hernia (750.6)

750.5 Congenital hypertrophic pyloric stenosis
Congenital or infantile:
- constriction
- hypertrophy
- spasm
- stenosis
- stricture
} of pylorus

750.6 Congenital hiatus hernia
Displacement of cardia through esophageal hiatus

EXCLUDES congenital diaphragmatic hernia (756.6)

750.7 Other specified anomalies of stomach
Congenital:
- cardiospasm
- hourglass stomach

Displacement of stomach
Diverticulum of stomach, congenital
Duplication of stomach
Megalogastria
Microgastria
Transposition of stomach

750.8 Other specified anomalies of upper alimentary tract

750.9 Unspecified anomaly of upper alimentary tract
Congenital:
- anomaly NOS
- deformity NOS
} of upper alimentary tract [any part, except tongue]

751 Other congenital anomalies of digestive system
751.0 Meckel's diverticulum
Meckel's diverticulum (displaced) (hypertrophic)
Persistent:
- omphalomesenteric duct
- vitelline duct

751.1 Atresia and stenosis of small intestine
Atresia of:
- duodenum
- ileum
- intestine NOS

Congenital:
- absence
- obstruction
- stenosis
- stricture
} of small intestine or intestine NOS

Imperforate jejunum

CONGENITAL ANOMALIES

751.2 Atresia and stenosis of large intestine, rectum, and anal canal
- Absence:
  - anus (congenital)
  - appendix, congenital
  - large intestine, congenital
  - rectum
- Atresia of:
  - anus
  - colon
  - rectum
- Congenital or infantile:
  - obstruction of large intestine
  - occlusion of anus
  - stricture of anus
- Imperforate:
  - anus
  - rectum
- Stricture of rectum, congenital

◆ 751.3 Hirschsprung's disease and other congenital functional disorders of colon
- Aganglionosis
- Congenital dilation of colon
- Congenital megacolon
- Macrocolon

751.4 Anomalies of intestinal fixation
- Congenital adhesions:
  - omental, anomalous
  - peritoneal
  - Jackson's membrane
- Malrotation of colon
- Rotation of cecum or colon:
  - failure of
  - incomplete
  - insufficient
- Universal mesentery

◆ 751.5 Other anomalies of intestine
- Congenital diverticulum, colon
- Dolichocolon
- Duplication of:
  - anus
  - appendix
  - cecum
  - intestine
- Ectopic anus
- Megaloappendix
- Megaloduodenum
- Microcolon
- Persistent cloaca
- Transposition of:
  - appendix
  - colon
  - intestine

● 751.6 Anomalies of gallbladder, bile ducts, and liver
  - **◆ 751.60 Unspecified anomaly of gallbladder, bile ducts, and liver**
  - **751.61 Biliary atresia**
    - Congenital:
      - absence
      - hypoplasia   } of bile duct (common)
      - obstruction } or passage
      - stricture
  - **751.62 Congenital cystic disease of liver**
    - Congenital polycystic disease of liver
    - Fibrocystic disease of liver
  - **◆ 751.69 Other anomalies of gallbladder, bile ducts, and liver**
    - Absence of:
      - gallbladder, congenital
      - liver (lobe)
    - Accessory:
      - hepatic ducts
      - liver
    - Congenital:
      - choledochal cyst
      - hepatomegaly
    - Duplication of:
      - biliary duct
      - cystic duct
      - gallbladder
      - liver
    - Floating:
      - gallbladder
      - liver
    - Intrahepatic gallbladder

751.7 Anomalies of pancreas
- Absence
- Agenesis   } of pancreas
- Hypoplasia
- Accessory pancreas
- Annular pancreas
- Ectopic pancreatic tissue
- Pancreatic heterotopia

  EXCLUDES *diabetes mellitus:*
    congenital (250.0-250.9)
    neonatal (775.1)
    fibrocystic disease of pancreas (277.00-277.01)

◆ 751.8 Other specified anomalies of digestive system
- Absence (complete) (partial) of alimentary tract NOS
- Duplication   } of digestive organs NOS
- Malposition, congenital

  EXCLUDES *congenital diaphragmatic hernia (756.6)*
    congenital hiatus hernia (750.6)

◆ 751.9 Unspecified anomaly of digestive system
- Congenital:
  - anomaly NOS   } of digestive system NOS
  - deformity NOS

● 752 Congenital anomalies of genital organs

  EXCLUDES *syndromes associated with anomalies in the number and form of chromosomes (758.0-758.9)*
    testicular feminization syndrome (257.8)

  752.0 Anomalies of ovaries
  - Absence, congenital
  - Accessory   } (of) ovary
  - Ectopic
  - Streak

  ● 752.1 Anomalies of fallopian tubes and broad ligaments
  - **◆ 752.10 Unspecified anomaly of fallopian tubes and broad ligaments**
  - **752.11 Embryonic cyst of fallopian tubes and broad ligaments**
    - Cyst:
      - epoophoron
      - fimbrial
    - Cyst:
      - Gartner's duct
      - parovarian
  - **◆ 752.19 Other**
    - Absence
    - Accessory   } (of) fallopian tube or broad ligament
    - Atresia

  752.2 Doubling of uterus
  - Didelphic uterus
  - Doubling of uterus [any degree] (associated with doubling of cervix and vagina)

  ◆ 752.3 Other anomalies of uterus
  - Absence, congenital
  - Agenesis   } of uterus
  - Aplasia
  - Bicornuate uterus
  - Uterus unicornis
  - Uterus with only one functioning horn

  ● 752.4 Anomalies of cervix, vagina, and external female genitalia
  - **◆ 752.40 Unspecified anomaly of cervix, vagina, and external female genitalia**
  - **752.41 Embryonic cyst of cervix, vagina, and external female genitalia**
    - Cyst of:
      - canal of Nuck, congenital
      - vagina, embryonal
      - vulva, congenital
  - **752.42 Imperforate hymen**
  - **◆ 752.49 Other anomalies of cervix, vagina, and external female genitalia**
    - Absence   } of cervix, clitoris, vagina, or vulva
    - Agenesis
    - Congenital stenosis or stricture of:
      - cervical canal
      - vagina

      EXCLUDES *double vagina associated with total duplication (752.2)*

  752.5 Undescended testicle
  - Cryptorchism
  - Ectopic testis

  752.6 Hypospadias and epispadias
  - Anaspadias
  - Congenital chordee

  752.7 Indeterminate sex and pseudohermaphroditism
  - Gynandrism
  - Hermaphroditism
  - Ovotestis
  - Pseudohermaphroditism (male) (female)
  - Pure gonadal dysgenesis

    EXCLUDES *pseudohermaphroditism:*
      female, with adrenocortical disorder (255.2)
      male, with gonadal disorder (257.8)
      with specified chromosomal anomaly (758.0-758.9)
      testicular feminization syndrome (257.8)

- **752.8 Other specified anomalies of genital organs**
  - Absence of:
    - penis
    - prostate
    - spermatic cord
    - vas deferens
  - Anorchism
  - Aplasia (congenital) of:
    - prostate
    - round ligament
    - testicle
  - Atresia of:
    - ejaculatory duct
    - vas deferens
  - Curvature of penis (lateral)
  - Fusion of testes
  - Hypoplasia of:
    - penis
    - testis
  - Monorchism
  - Paraspadias
  - Polyorchism

  EXCLUDES congenital hydrocele (778.6)
  phimosis or paraphimosis (605)

- **752.9 Unspecified anomaly of genital organs**
  - Congenital:
    - anomaly NOS | of genital organ, not elsewhere
    - deformity NOS | classified

753 Congenital anomalies of urinary system

- **753.0 Renal agenesis and dysgenesis**
  - Atrophy of kidney:
    - congenital
    - infantile
  - Congenital absence of kidney(s)
  - Hypoplasia of kidney(s)
  - Code also any associated vesicoureteral reflux (593.70-593.73)

- **753.1 Cystic kidney disease**

  EXCLUDES acquired cyst of kidney (593.2)

  - **753.10** Cystic kidney disease, unspecified
  - **753.11** Congenital single renal cyst
  - **753.12** Polycystic kidney, unspecified type
  - **753.13** Polycystic kidney, autosomal dominant
  - **753.14** Polycystic kidney, autosomal recessive
  - **753.15** Renal dysplasia
    - Code also any associated vesicoureteral reflux (593.70-593.73)
  - **753.16** Medullary cystic kidney
    - Nephronopthisis
  - **753.17** Medullary sponge kidney
  - **753.19** Other specified cystic kidney disease
    - Multicystic kidney

- **753.2 Obstructive defects of renal pelvis and ureter**
  - Atresia of ureter
  - Congenital:
    - dilatation of ureter
    - hydronephrosis
    - hydroureter
    - megaloureter
    - occlusion of ureter
  - Congenital:
    - stricture of:
      - ureter
      - ureteropelvic junction
      - ureterovesical orifice
    - ureterocele
    - Impervious ureter

- **753.3 Other specified anomalies of kidney**
  - Accessory kidney
  - Congenital:
    - calculus of kidney
    - displaced kidney
  - Discoid kidney
  - Double kidney with double pelvis
  - Ectopic kidney
  - Fusion of kidneys
  - Giant kidney
  - Horseshoe kidney
  - Hyperplasia of kidney
  - Lobulation of kidney
  - Malrotation of kidney
  - Trifid kidney (pelvis)

- **753.4 Other specified anomalies of ureter**
  - Absent ureter
  - Accessory ureter
  - Deviation of ureter
  - Displaced ureteric orifice
  - Double ureter
  - Ectopic ureter
  - Implantation, anomalous of ureter

- **753.5 Exstrophy of urinary bladder**
  - Ectopia vesicae
  - Extroversion of bladder

- **753.6 Atresia and stenosis of urethra and bladder neck**
  - Congenital obstruction:
    - bladder neck
    - urethra
  - Congenital stricture of:
    - urethra (valvular)
    - urinary meatus
    - vesicourethral orifice
  - Imperforate urinary meatus
  - Impervious urethra
  - Urethral valve formation

- **753.7 Anomalies of urachus**
  - Cyst
  - Fistula } (of) urachus
  - Patent
  - sinus
  - Persistent umbilical sinus

- **753.8 Other specified anomalies of bladder and urethra**
  - Absence, congenital of:
    - bladder
    - urethra
  - Accessory:
    - bladder
    - urethra
  - Congenital:
    - diverticulum of bladder
    - hernia of bladder
  - Congenital urethrorectal fistula
  - Congenital prolapse of:
    - bladder (mucosa)
    - urethra
  - Double:
    - urethra
    - urinary meatus

- **753.9 Unspecified anomaly of urinary system**
  - Congenital:
    - anomaly NOS | of urinary system [any part,
    - deformity NOS | except urachus]

754 Certain congenital musculoskeletal deformities

INCLUDES nonteratogenic deformities which are considered to be due to intrauterine malposition and pressure

- **754.0 Of skull, face, and jaw**
  - Asymmetry of face
  - Compression facies
  - Depressions in skull
  - Deviation of nasal septum, congenital
  - Dolichocephaly
  - Plagiocephaly
  - Potter's facies
  - Squashed or bent nose, congenital

  EXCLUDES dentofacial anomalies (524.0-524.9)
  syphilitic saddle nose (090.5)

- **754.1 Of sternocleidomastoid muscle**
  - Congenital sternomastoid torticollis
  - Congenital wryneck
  - Contracture of sternocleidomastoid (muscle)
  - Sternomastoid tumor

- **754.2 Of spine**
  - Congenital postural:
    - lordosis
    - scoliosis

- **754.3 Congenital dislocation of hip**
  - **754.30** Congenital dislocation of hip, unilateral
    - Congenital dislocation of hip NOS
  - **754.31** Congenital dislocation of hip, bilateral
  - **754.32** Congenital subluxation of hip, unilateral
    - Congenital flexion deformity, hip or thigh
    - Predislocation status of hip at birth
    - Preluxation of hip, congenital
  - **754.33** Congenital subluxation of hip, bilateral
  - **754.35** Congenital dislocation of one hip with subluxation of other hip

- **754.4 Congenital genu recurvatum and bowing of long bones of leg**
  - **754.40** Genu recurvatum
  - **754.41** Congenital dislocation of knee (with genu recurvatum)
  - **754.42** Congenital bowing of femur
  - **754.43** Congenital bowing of tibia and fibula
  - **754.44** Congenital bowing of unspecified long bones of leg

- **754.5 Varus deformities of feet**

  EXCLUDES acquired (736.71, 736.75, 736.79)

  - **754.50** Talipes varus
    - Congenital varus deformity of foot, unspecified
    - Pes varus
  - **754.51** Talipes equinovarus
    - Equinovarus (congenital)
  - **754.52** Metatarsus primus varus
  - **754.53** Metatarsus varus
  - **754.59** Other
    - Talipes calcaneovarus

- **754.6 Valgas deformities of feet**

  EXCLUDES valgus deformity of foot (acquired) (736.79)

  - **754.60** Talipes valgus
    - Congenital valgus deformity of foot, unspecified
  - **754.61** Congenital pes planus
    - Congenital rocker bottom flat foot
    - Flat foot, congenital

    EXCLUDES pes planus (acquired) (734)

CONGENITAL ANOMALIES

- 754.62 **Talipes calcaneovalgus**
- ◆ 754.69 **Other**
    Talipes:
        equinovalgus
        planovalgus
- ● 754.7 **Other deformities of feet**
    EXCLUDES acquired (736.70-736.79)
    - ◆ 754.70 **Talipes, unspecified**
        Congenital deformity of foot NOS
    - 754.71 **Talipes cavus**
        Cavus foot (congenital)
    - ◆ 754.79 **Other**
        Asymmetric talipes
        Talipes:
            calcaneus
            equinus
- ● 754.8 **Other specified nonteratogenic anomalies**
    - 754.81 **Pectus excavatum**
        Congenital funnel chest
    - 754.82 **Pectus carinatum**
        Congenital pigeon chest [breast]
    - ◆ 754.89 **Other**
        Club hand (congenital)
        Congenital:
            deformity of chest wall
            dislocation of elbow
        Generalized flexion contractures of lower limb joints, congenital
        Spade-like hand (congenital)

- ● 755 **Other congenital anomalies of limbs**
    EXCLUDES those deformities classifiable to 754.0-754.8
    - ● 755.0 **Polydactyly**
        - ◆ 755.00 **Polydactyly, unspecified digits**
            Supernumerary digits
        - 755.01 **Of fingers**
            Accessory fingers
        - 755.02 **Of toes**
            Accessory toes
    - ● 755.1 **Syndactyly**
        Symphalangy
        Webbing of digits
        - ◆ 755.10 **Of multiple and unspecified sites**
        - 755.11 **Of fingers without fusion of bone**
        - 755.12 **Of fingers with fusion of bone**
        - 755.13 **Of toes without fusion of bone**
        - 755.14 **Of toes with fusion of bone**
    - ● 755.2 **Reduction deformities of upper limb**
        - ◆ 755.20 **Unspecified reduction deformity of upper limb**
            Ectromelia NOS } of upper limb
            Hemimelia NOS
            Shortening of arm, congenital
        - 755.21 **Transverse deficiency of upper limb**
            Amelia of upper limb
            Congenital absence of:
                fingers, all (complete or partial)
                forearm, including hand and fingers
                upper limb, complete
            Congenital amputation of upper limb
            Transverse hemimelia of upper limb
        - 755.22 **Longitudinal deficiency of upper limb, not elsewhere classified**
            Phocomelia NOS of upper limb
            Rudimentary arm
        - 755.23 **Longitudinal deficiency, combined, involving humerus, radius, and ulna (complete or incomplete)**
            Congenital absence of arm and forearm (complete or incomplete) with or without metacarpal deficiency and/or phalangeal deficiency, incomplete
            Phocomelia, complete, of upper limb
        - 755.24 **Longitudinal deficiency, humeral, complete or partial (with or without distal deficiencies, incomplete)**
            Congenital absence of humerus (with or without absence of some [but not all] distal elements)
            Proximal phocomelia of upper limb
        - 755.25 **Longitudinal deficiency, radioulnar, complete or partial (with or without distal deficiencies, incomplete)**
            Congenital absence of radius and ulna (with or without absence of some [but not all] distal elements)
            Distal phocomelia of upper limb
        - 755.26 **Longitudinal deficiency, radial, complete or partial (with or without distal deficiencies, incomplete)**
            Agenesis of radius
            Congenital absence of radius (with or without absence of some [but not all] distal elements)
        - 755.27 **Longitudinal deficiency, ulnar, complete or partial (with or without distal deficiencies, incomplete)**
            Agenesis of ulna
            Congenital absence of ulna (with or without absence of some [but not all] distal elements)
        - 755.28 **Longitudinal deficiency, carpals or metacarpals, complete or partial (with or without incomplete phalangeal deficiency)**
        - 755.29 **Longitudinal deficiency, phalanges, complete or partial**
            Absence of finger, congenital
            Aphalangia of upper limb, terminal, complete or partial
            EXCLUDES terminal deficiency of all five digits (755.21)
            transverse deficiency of phalanges (755.21)
    - ● 755.3 **Reduction deformities of lower limb**
        - ◆ 755.30 **Unspecified reduction deformity of lower limb**
            Ectromelia NOS } of lower limb
            Hemimelia NOS
            Shortening of leg, congenital
        - 755.31 **Transverse deficiency of lower limb**
            Amelia of lower limb
            Congenital absence of:
                foot
                leg, including foot and toes
                lower limb, complete
                toes, all, complete
            Transverse hemimelia of lower limb
        - 755.32 **Longitudinal deficiency of lower limb, not elsewhere classified**
            Phocomelia NOS of lower limb
        - 755.33 **Longitudinal deficiency, combined, involving femur, tibia, and fibula (complete or incomplete)**
            Congenital absence of thigh and (lower) leg (complete or incomplete) with or without metacarpal deficiency and/or phalangeal deficiency, incomplete
            Phocomelia, complete, of lower limb
        - 755.34 **Longitudinal deficiency, femoral, complete or partial (with or without distal deficiencies, incomplete)**
            Congenital absence of femur (with or without absence of some [but not all] distal elements)
            Proximal phocomelia of lower limb
        - 755.35 **Longitudinal deficiency, tibiofibular, complete or partial (with or without distal deficiencies, incomplete)**
            Congenital absence of tibia and fibula (with or without absence of some [but not all] distal elements)
            Distal phocomelia of lower limb
        - 755.36 **Longitudinal deficiency, tibia, complete or partial (with or without distal deficiencies, incomplete)**
            Agenesis of tibia
            Congenital absence of tibia (with or without absence of some [but not all] distal elements)
        - 755.37 **Longitudinal deficiency, fibular, complete or partial (with or without distal deficiencies, incomplete)**
            Agenesis of fibula
            Congenital absence of fibula (with or without absence of some [but not all] distal elements)

- **755.38** Longitudinal deficiency, tarsals or metatarsals, complete or partial (with or without incomplete phalangeal deficiency)
- **755.39** Longitudinal deficiency, phalanges, complete or partial
   Absence of toe, congenital
   Aphalangia of lower limb, terminal, complete or partial
   EXCLUDES terminal deficiency of all five digits (755.31)
   transverse deficiency of phalanges (755.31)

◆ **755.4** Reduction deformities, unspecified limb
   Absence, congenital (complete or partial) of limb NOS
   Amelia
   Ectromelia
   Hemimelia
   Phocomelia
   } of unspecified limb

● **755.5** Other anomalies of upper limb, including shoulder girdle
   ◆ **755.50** Unspecified anomaly of upper limb
   755.51 Congenital deformity of clavicle
   755.52 Congenital elevation of scapula
      Sprengel's deformity
   755.53 Radioulnar synostosis
   755.54 Madelung's deformity
   755.55 Acrocephalosyndactyly
      Apert's syndrome
   755.56 Accessory carpal bones
   755.57 Macrodactylia (fingers)
   755.58 Cleft hand, congenital
      Lobster-claw hand
   ◆ **755.59** Other
      Cleidocranial dysostosis
      Cubitus:
         valgus, congenital
         varus, congenital
      EXCLUDES club hand (congenital) (754.89)
      congenital dislocation of elbow (754.89)

● **755.6** Other anomalies of lower limb, including pelvic girdle
   ◆ **755.60** Unspecified anomaly of lower limb
   755.61 Coxa valga, congenital
   755.62 Coxa vara, congenital
   ◆ **755.63** Other congenital deformity of hip (joint)
      Congenital anteversion of femur (neck)
      EXCLUDES congenital dislocation of hip (754.30-754.35)
   755.64 Congenital deformity of knee (joint)
      Congenital:
         absence of patella
         genu valgum [knock-knee]
         genu varum [bowleg]
      Rudimentary patella
   755.65 Macrodactylia of toes
   ◆ **755.66** Other anomalies of toes
      Congenital: Congenital:
         hallux valgus   hammer toe
         hallux varus
   755.67 Anomalies of foot, not elsewhere classified
      Astragaloscaphoid synostosis
      Calcaneonavicular bar
      Coalition of calcaneus
      Talonavicular synostosis
      Tarsal coalitions
   ◆ **755.69** Other
      Congenital:
         angulation of tibia
         deformity (of):
            ankle (joint)
            sacroiliac (joint)
         fusion of sacroiliac joint

◆ **755.8** Other specified anomalies of unspecified limb
◆ **755.9** Unspecified anomaly of unspecified limb
   Congenital:
      anomaly NOS   } of unspecified
      deformity NOS } limb
   EXCLUDES reduction deformity of unspecified limb (755.4)

● **756** Other congenital musculoskeletal anomalies
   EXCLUDES those deformities classifiable to 754.0-754.8
   756.0 Anomalies of skull and face bones
      Absence of skull bones   Imperfect fusion of skull
      Acrocephaly   Oxycephaly
      Congenital deformity   Platybasia
         of forehead   Premature closure of
      Craniosynostosis   cranial sutures
      Crouzon's disease   Tower skull
      Hypertelorism   Trigonocephaly
      EXCLUDES acrocephalosyndactyly [Apert's syndrome] (755.55)
         dentofacial anomalies (524.0-524.9)
         skull defects associated with brain anomalies, such as:
            anencephalus (740.0)
            encephalocele (742.0)
            hydrocephalus (742.3)
            microcephalus (742.1)

● **756.1** Anomalies of spine
   ◆ **756.10** Anomaly of spine, unspecified
   756.11 Spondylolysis, lumbosacral region
      Prespondylolisthesis (lumbosacral)
   756.12 Spondylolisthesis
   756.13 Absence of vertebra, congenital
   756.14 Hemivertebra
   756.15 Fusion of spine [vertebra], congenital
   756.16 Klippel-Feil syndrome
   756.17 Spina bifida occulta
      EXCLUDES spina bifida (aperta) (741.0-741.9)
   ◆ **756.19** Other
      Platyspondylia
      Supernumerary vertebra

756.2 Cervical rib
   Supernumerary rib in the cervical region
◆ **756.3** Other anomalies of ribs and sternum
   Congenital absence of: Congenital:
      rib   fissure of sternum
      sternum   fusion of ribs
                                 Sternum bifidum
   EXCLUDES nonteratogenic deformity of chest wall (754.81-754.89)

756.4 Chondrodystrophy
   Achondroplasia   Enchondromatosis
   Chondrodystrophia (fetalis)   Ollier's disease
   Dyschondroplasia
   EXCLUDES lipochondrodystrophy [Hurler's syndrome] (277.5)
      Morquio's disease (277.5)

● **756.5** Osteodystrophies
   ◆ **756.50** Osteodystrophy, unspecified
   756.51 Osteogenesis imperfecta
      Fragilitas ossium
      Osteopsathyrosis
   756.52 Osteopetrosis
   756.53 Osteopoikilosis
   756.54 Polyostotic fibrous dysplasia of bone
   756.55 Chondroectodermal dysplasia
      Ellis-van Creveld syndrome
   756.56 Multiple epiphyseal dysplasia
   ◆ **756.59** Other
      Albright (-McCune)-Sternberg syndrome

756.6 Anomalies of diaphragm
   Absence of diaphragm
   Congenital hernia:
      diaphragmatic
      foramen of Morgagni
   Eventration of diaphragm
   EXCLUDES congenital hiatus hernia (750.6)

756.7 Anomalies of abdominal wall
   Exomphalos   Omphalocele
   Gastroschisis   Prune belly (syndrome)
   EXCLUDES umbilical hernia (551-553 with .1)

● **756.8** Other specified anomalies of muscle, tendon, fascia, and connective tissue
   756.81 Absence of muscle and tendon
      Absence of muscle (pectoral)

CONGENITAL ANOMALIES

- 756.82 Accessory muscle
- 756.83 Ehlers-Danlos syndrome
- ◆ 756.89 **Other**
  - Amyotrophia congenita
  - Congenital shortening of tendon
- ◆ 756.9 **Other and unspecified anomalies of musculoskeletal system**
  - Congenital:
    - anomaly NOS ⎱ of musculoskeletal system, not
    - deformity NOS ⎰ elsewhere classified

● 757 **Congenital anomalies of the integument**
  - INCLUDES: anomalies of skin, subcutaneous tissue, hair, nails, and breast
  - EXCLUDES: hemangioma (228.00-228.09)
    - pigmented nevus (216.0-216.9)
  - 757.0 **Hereditary edema of legs**
    - Congenital lymphedema
    - Hereditary trophedema
    - Milroy's disease
  - 757.1 **Ichthyosis congenita**
    - Congenital ichthyosis
    - Harlequin fetus
    - Ichthyosiform erythroderma
  - 757.2 **Dermatoglyphic anomalies**
    - Abnormal palmar creases
- ● 757.3 **Other specified anomalies of skin**
  - 757.31 Congenital ectodermal dysplasia
  - 757.32 Vascular hamartomas
    - Birthmarks
    - Port-wine stain
    - Strawberry nevus
  - 757.33 Congenital pigmentary anomalies of skin
    - Congenital poikiloderma
    - Urticaria pigmentosa
    - Xeroderma pigmentosum
    - EXCLUDES: albinism (270.2)
  - ◆ 757.39 **Other**
    - Accessory skin tags, congenital
    - Congenital scar
    - Epidermolysis bullosa
    - Keratoderma (congenital)
    - EXCLUDES: pilonidal cyst (685.0-685.1)
- ◆ 757.4 **Specified anomalies of hair**
  - Congenital:
    - alopecia
    - atrichosis
    - beaded hair
  - Congenital:
    - hypertrichosis
    - monilethrix
    - Persistent lanugo
- ◆ 757.5 **Specified anomalies of nails**
  - Anonychia
  - Congenital:
    - clubnail
    - koilonychia
  - Congenital:
    - leukonychia
    - onychauxis
    - pachyonychia
- ◆ 757.6 **Specified anomalies of breast**
  - Absent ⎱
  - Accessory ⎰ breast or nipple
  - Supernumerary
  - Hypoplasia of breast
  - EXCLUDES: absence of pectoral muscle (756.81)
- ◆ 757.8 **Other specified anomalies of the integument**
- ◆ 757.9 **Unspecified anomaly of the integument**
  - Congenital:
    - anomaly NOS ⎱ of integument
    - deformity NOS ⎰

● 758 **Chromosomal anomalies**
  - INCLUDES: syndromes associated with anomalies in the number and form of chromosomes
  - 758.0 **Down's syndrome**
    - Mongolism
    - Translocation Down's syndrome
    - Trisomy:
      - 21 or 22
      - G
  - 758.1 **Patau's syndrome**
    - Trisomy:
      - 13
    - Trisomy:
      - D_1
  - 758.2 **Edwards' syndrome**
    - Trisomy:
      - 18
    - Trisomy:
      - E_3
  - 758.3 **Autosomal deletion syndromes**
    - Antimongolism syndrome
    - Cri-du-chat syndrome
  - 758.4 **Balanced autosomal translocation in normal individual**
- ◆ 758.5 **Other conditions due to autosomal anomalies**
  - Accessory autosomes NEC
  - 758.6 **Gonadal dysgenesis**
    - Ovarian dysgenesis
    - Turner's syndrome
    - XO syndrome
    - EXCLUDES: pure gonadal dysgenesis (752.7)
  - 758.7 **Klinefelter's syndrome**
    - XXY syndrome
- ◆ 758.8 **Other conditions due to sex chromosome anomalies**
  - Additional sex chromosome
  - Sex chromosome mosaicism
  - Syndrome:
    - triple X
    - XXX
    - XYY
- ◆ 758.9 **Conditions due to anomaly of unspecified chromosome**

● 759 **Other and unspecified congenital anomalies**
  - 759.0 **Anomalies of spleen**
    - Aberrant ⎱
    - Absent ⎰ spleen
    - Accessory
    - Congenital splenomegaly
    - Ectopic spleen
    - Lobulation of spleen
  - 759.1 **Anomalies of adrenal gland**
    - Aberrant ⎱
    - Absent ⎰ adrenal gland
    - Accessory
    - EXCLUDES: adrenogenital disorders (255.2)
      - congenital disorders of steroid metabolism (255.2)
- ◆ 759.2 **Anomalies of other endocrine glands**
  - Absent parathyroid gland
  - Accessory thyroid gland
  - Persistent thyroglossal or thyrolingual duct
  - Thyroglossal (duct) cyst
  - EXCLUDES: congenital:
    - goiter (246.1)
    - hypothyroidism (243)
  - 759.3 **Situs inversus**
    - Situs inversus or transversus:
      - abdominalis
      - thoracis
    - Transposition of viscera:
      - abdominal
      - thoracic
    - EXCLUDES: dextrocardia without mention of complete transposition (746.87)
  - 759.4 **Conjoined twins**
    - Craniopagus
    - Dicephalus
    - Pygopagus
    - Thoracopagus
    - Xiphopagus
  - 759.5 **Tuberous sclerosis**
    - Bourneville's disease
    - Epiloia
- ◆ 759.6 **Other hamartoses, not elsewhere classified**
  - Syndrome:
    - Peutz-Jeghers
    - Sturge-Weber (-Dimitri)
    - von Hippel-Lindau
  - EXCLUDES: neurofibromatosis (237.7)
  - 759.7 **Multiple congenital anomalies, so described**
    - Congenital:
      - anomaly, multiple NOS
      - deformity, multiple NOS
- ● 759.8 **Other specified anomalies**
  - 759.81 Prader-Willi syndrome
  - 759.82 Marfan syndrome
  - 759.83 Fragile X syndrome ◆
  - ◆ 759.89 Other
    - Congenital malformation syndromes affecting multiple systems, not elsewhere classified
    - Laurence-Moon-Biedl syndrome
- ◆ 759.9 **Congenital anomaly, unspecified**

● Additional digits required   ◆ Nonspecific code   ▪ Not a primary diagnosis

15. CERTAIN CONDITIONS ORIGINATING IN THE PERINATAL PERIOD (760-779)

INCLUDES conditions which have their origin in the perinatal period even though death or morbidity occurs later

MATERNAL CAUSES OF PERINATAL MORBIDITY AND MORTALITY (760-763)

● **760 Fetus or newborn affected by maternal conditions which may be unrelated to present pregnancy**

INCLUDES the listed maternal conditions only when specified as a cause of mortality or morbidity of the fetus or newborn

EXCLUDES maternal endocrine and metabolic disorders affecting fetus or newborn (775.0-775.9)

760.0 Maternal hypertensive disorders
Fetus or newborn affected by maternal conditions classifiable to 642

760.1 Maternal renal and urinary tract diseases
Fetus or newborn affected by maternal conditions classifiable to 580-599

760.2 Maternal infections
Fetus or newborn affected by maternal infectious disease classifiable to 001-136 and 487, but fetus or newborn not manifesting that disease

EXCLUDES congenital infectious diseases (771.0-771.8)
maternal genital tract and other localized infections (760.8)

◆ **760.3 Other chronic maternal circulatory and respiratory diseases**
Fetus or newborn affected by chronic maternal conditions classifiable to 390-459, 490-519, 745-748

760.4 Maternal nutritional disorders
Fetus or newborn affected by:
maternal disorders classifiable to 260-269
maternal malnutrition NOS

EXCLUDES fetal malnutrition (764.10-764.29)

760.5 Maternal injury
Fetus or newborn affected by maternal conditions classifiable to 800-995

760.6 Surgical operation on mother

EXCLUDES cesarean section for present delivery (763.4)
damage to placenta from amniocentesis, cesarean section, or surgical induction (762.1)
previous surgery to uterus or pelvic organs (763.8)

● **760.7 Noxious influences affecting fetus via placenta or breast milk**
Fetus or newborn affected by noxious substance transmitted via placenta or breast milk

EXCLUDES anesthetic and analgesic drugs administered during labor and delivery (763.5)
drug withdrawal syndrome in newborn (779.5)

◆ **760.70 Unspecified noxious substance**
Fetus or newborn affected by:
Drug NEC

760.71 Alcohol
Fetal alcohol syndrome

760.72 Narcotics
760.73 Hallucinogenic agents
760.74 Anti-infectives
Antibiotics

760.75 Cocaine
760.76 Diethylstilbestrol [DES] ◆
◆ **760.79 Other**
Fetus or newborn affected by:
immune sera ⎫
medicinal agents NEC ⎬ transmitted via placenta or breast milk
toxic substance NEC ⎭

◆ **760.8 Other specified maternal conditions affecting fetus or newborn**
Maternal genital tract and other localized infection affecting fetus or newborn, but fetus or newborn not manifesting that disease

EXCLUDES maternal urinary tract infection affecting fetus or newborn (760.1)

◆ **760.9 Unspecified maternal condition affecting fetus or newborn**

● **761 Fetus or newborn affected by maternal complications of pregnancy**

INCLUDES the listed maternal conditions only when specified as a cause of mortality or morbidity of the fetus or newborn

761.0 Incompetent cervix
761.1 Premature rupture of membranes
761.2 Oligohydramnios

EXCLUDES that due to premature rupture of membranes (761.1)

761.3 Polyhydramnios
Hydramnios (acute) (chronic)

761.4 Ectopic pregnancy
Pregnancy:
abdominal
intraperitoneal
tubal

761.5 Multiple pregnancy
Triplet (pregnancy)
Twin (pregnancy)

761.6 Maternal death
761.7 Malpresentation before labor
Breech presentation ⎫
External version ⎪
Oblique lie ⎬ before labor
Transverse lie ⎪
Unstable lie ⎭

◆ **761.8 Other specified maternal complications of pregnancy affecting fetus or newborn**
Spontaneous abortion, fetus

◆ **761.9 Unspecified maternal complication of pregnancy affecting fetus or newborn**

● **762 Fetus or newborn affected by complications of placenta, cord, and membranes**

INCLUDES the listed maternal conditions only when specified as a cause of mortality or morbidity in the fetus or newborn

762.0 Placenta previa
◆ **762.1 Other forms of placental separation and hemorrhage**
Abruptio placentae
Antepartum hemorrhage
Damage to placenta from amniocentesis, cesarean section, or surgical induction
Maternal blood loss
Premature separation of placenta
Rupture of marginal sinus

◆ **762.2 Other and unspecified morphological and functional abnormalities of placenta**
Placental:
dysfunction
infarction
insufficiency

762.3 Placental transfusion syndromes
Placental and cord abnormality resulting in twin-to-twin or other transplacental transfusion
Use additional code, if desired, to indicate resultant condition in fetus or newborn:
fetal blood loss (772.0)
polycythemia neonatorum (776.4)

762.4 Prolapsed cord
Cord presentation

◆ **762.5 Other compression of umbilical cord**
Cord around neck   Knot in cord
Entanglement of cord   Torsion of cord

◆ **762.6 Other and unspecified conditions of umbilical cord**
Short cord
Thrombosis ⎫
Varices ⎬ of umbilical
Velamentous insertion ⎪ cord
Vasa previa ⎭

EXCLUDES infection of umbilical cord (771.4)
single umbilical artery (747.5)

762.7 Chorioamnionitis
Amnionitis
Membranitis
Placentitis

- ◆ 762.8 Other specified abnormalities of chorion and amnion
- ◆ 762.9 Unspecified abnormality of chorion and amnion
- ● 763 **Fetus or newborn affected by other complications of labor and delivery**

  INCLUDES the listed conditions only when specified as a cause of mortality or morbidity in the fetus or newborn

  - 763.0 **Breech delivery and extraction**
  - ◆ 763.1 **Other malpresentation, malposition, and disproportion during labor and delivery**
    Fetus or newborn affected by:
    abnormality of bony pelvis
    contracted pelvis
    persistent occipitoposterior position
    shoulder presentation
    transverse lie
    conditions classifiable to 652, 653, and 660
  - 763.2 **Forceps delivery**
    Fetus or newborn affected by forceps extraction
  - 763.3 **Delivery by vacuum extractor**
  - 763.4 **Cesarean delivery**

    EXCLUDES placental separation or hemorrhage from cesarean section (762.1)

  - 763.5 **Maternal anesthesia and analgesia**
    Reactions and intoxications from maternal opiates and tranquilizers during labor and delivery

    EXCLUDES drug withdrawal syndrome in newborn (779.5)

  - 763.6 **Precipitate delivery**
    Rapid second stage
  - 763.7 **Abnormal uterine contractions**
    Fetus or newborn affected by:
    contraction ring
    hypertonic labor
    hypotonic uterine dysfunction
    uterine inertia or dysfunction
    conditions classifiable to 661, except 661.3
  - ◆ 763.8 **Other specified complications of labor and delivery affecting fetus or newborn**
    Fetus or newborn affected by:
    abnormality of maternal soft tissues
    destructive operation on live fetus to facilitate delivery
    induction of labor (medical)
    previous surgery to uterus or pelvic organs
    other conditions classifiable to 650-669
    other procedures used in labor and delivery
  - ◆ 763.9 **Unspecified complication of labor and delivery affecting fetus or newborn**

OTHER CONDITIONS ORIGINATING IN THE PERINATAL PERIOD (764-779)

The following fifth-digit subclassification is for use with categories 764-765 to denote birthweight:
- ◆ 0 unspecified [weight]
- 1 less than 500 grams
- 2 500-749 grams
- 3 750-999 grams
- 4 1,000-1,249 grams
- 5 1,250-1,499 grams
- 6 1,500-1,749 grams
- 7 1,750-1,999 grams
- 8 2,000-2,499 grams
- 9 2,500 grams and over

- ● 764 **Slow fetal growth and fetal malnutrition**

  EXCLUDES low birthweight due to short gestation (765.00-765.19)

  - ● 764.0 **"Light-for-dates" without mention of fetal malnutrition**
    Infants underweight for gestational age
    "Small-for-dates"
  - ● 764.1 **"Light-for-dates" with signs of fetal malnutrition**
    Infants "light-for-dates" classifiable to 764.0, who in addition show signs of fetal malnutrition, such as dry peeling skin and loss of subcutaneous tissue
  - ● 764.2 **Fetal malnutrition without mention of "light-for-dates"**
    Infants, not underweight for gestational age, showing signs of fetal malnutrition, such as dry peeling skin and loss of subcutaneous tissue
    Intrauterine malnutrition

- ◆ 764.9 **Fetal growth retardation, unspecified**
  Intrauterine growth retardation
- ● 765 **Disorders relating to short gestation and unspecified low birthweight**

  INCLUDES the listed conditions, without further specification, as causes of mortality, morbidity, or additional care, in fetus or newborn

  EXCLUDES low birthweight due to slow fetal growth and fetal malnutrition (764.00-764.99)

  - ● 765.0 **Extreme immaturity**
    Note: Usually implies a birthweight of less than 1000 grams and/or a gestation of less than 28 completed weeks.
  - ◆ ● 765.1 **Other preterm infants**
    Note: Usually implies a birthweight of 1000-2499 grams and/or a gestation of 28-37 completed weeks.
    Prematurity NOS
    Prematurity or small size, not classifiable to 765.0 or as "light-for-dates" in 764

- ● 766 **Disorders relating to long gestation and high birthweight**

  INCLUDES the listed conditions, without further specification, as causes of mortality, morbidity, or additional care, in fetus or newborn

  - 766.0 **Exceptionally large baby**
    Note: Usually implies a birthweight of 4500 grams or more.
  - ◆ 766.1 **Other "heavy-for-dates" infants**
    Other fetus or infant "heavy-" or "large-for-dates" regardless of period of gestation
  - 766.2 **Post-term infant, not "heavy-for-dates"**
    Fetus or infant with gestation period of 294 days or more [42 or more completed weeks], not "heavy-" or "large-for-dates"
    Postmaturity NOS

- ● 767 **Birth trauma**
  - 767.0 **Subdural and cerebral hemorrhage**
    Subdural and cerebral hemorrhage, whether described as due to birth trauma or to intrapartum anoxia or hypoxia
    Subdural hematoma (localized)
    Tentorial tear
    Use additional code, if desired, to identify cause

    EXCLUDES intraventricular hemorrhage (772.1)
    subarachnoid hemorrhage (772.2)

  - 767.1 **Injuries to scalp**
    Caput succedaneum
    Cephalhematoma
    Chignon (from vacuum extraction)
    Massive epicranial subaponeurotic hemorrhage
  - 767.2 **Fracture of clavicle**
  - ◆ 767.3 **Other injuries to skeleton**
    Fracture of:
    long bones
    skull

    EXCLUDES congenital dislocation of hip (754.30-754.35)
    fracture of spine, congenital (767.4)

  - 767.4 **Injury to spine and spinal cord**
    Dislocation
    Fracture } of spine or spinal cord
    Laceration } due to birth trauma
    Rupture
  - 767.5 **Facial nerve injury**
    Facial palsy
  - 767.6 **Injury to brachial plexus**
    Palsy or paralysis:
    brachial
    Erb (-Duchenne)
    Klumpke (-Déjérine)
  - ◆ 767.7 **Other cranial and peripheral nerve injuries**
    Phrenic nerve paralysis
  - ◆ 767.8 **Other specified birth trauma**
    Eye damage
    Hematoma of:
      liver (subcapsular)
      testes
      vulva
    Rupture of:
      liver
      spleen
    Scalpel wound
    Traumatic glaucoma

    EXCLUDES hemorrhage classifiable to 772.0-772.9

  - ◆ 767.9 **Birth trauma, unspecified**
    Birth injury NOS

● Additional digits required   ◆ Nonspecific code   ▪ Not a primary diagnosis

TABULAR LIST

● **768 Intrauterine hypoxia and birth asphyxia**
Use only when associated with newborn morbidity classifiable elsewhere

◆ **768.0 Fetal death from asphyxia or anoxia before onset of labor or at unspecified time**

768.1 Fetal death from asphyxia or anoxia during labor

768.2 Fetal distress before onset of labor, in liveborn infant
Abnormal fetal heart rate or rhythm
Fetal or intrauterine:
 acidosis
 anoxia or hypoxia
Any condition classifiable to 768.4
} first noted before onset of labor, live-born infant

768.3 Fetal distress first noted during labor, in liveborn infant
Abnormal fetal heart rate or rhythm
Fetal or intrauterine:
 acidosis
 anoxia or hypoxia
Any condition classifiable to 768.4
} first noted during labor or delivery, liveborn infant

◆ **768.4 Fetal distress, unspecified as to time of onset, in liveborn infant**
Abnormal fetal heart rate or rhythm
Fetal or intrauterine:
 acidosis
 anoxia
 asphyxia
 distress
 hypercapnia
 hypoxia
} not stated whether first noted before or after onset of labor, live-born infant

768.5 Severe birth asphyxia
Birth asphyxia with neurologic involvement

768.6 Mild or moderate birth asphyxia
Birth asphyxia (without mention of neurologic involvement)

◆ **768.9 Unspecified birth asphyxia in liveborn infant**
Anoxia
Asphyxia
Hypoxia
} NOS, in live-born infant

769 Respiratory distress syndrome
Cardiorespiratory distress syndrome of newborn
Hyaline membrane disease (pulmonary)
Idiopathic respiratory distress syndrome
[IRDS or RDS] of newborn
Pulmonary hypoperfusion syndrome
EXCLUDES transient tachypnea of newborn (770.6)

● **770 Other respiratory conditions of fetus and newborn**

770.0 Congenital pneumonia
Infective pneumonia acquired prenatally
EXCLUDES pneumonia from infection acquired after birth (480.0-486)

770.1 Meconium aspiration syndrome
Aspiration of contents of birth canal NOS
Meconium aspiration below vocal cords
Pneumonitis:
 fetal aspiration
 meconium

770.2 Interstitial emphysema and related conditions
Pneumomediastinum
Pneumopericardium
Pneumothorax
} originating in the perinatal period

770.3 Pulmonary hemorrhage
Hemorrhage:
 alveolar (lung)
 intra-alveolar (lung)
 massive pulmonary
} originating in the perinatal period

770.4 Primary atelectasis
Pulmonary immaturity NOS

◆ **770.5 Other and unspecified atelectasis**
Atelectasis:
 NOS
 partial
 secondary
Pulmonary collapse
} originating in the perinatal period

770.6 Transitory tachypnea of newborn
Idiopathic tachypnea of newborn
Wet lung syndrome
EXCLUDES respiratory distress syndrome (769)

770.7 Chronic respiratory disease arising in the perinatal period
Bronchopulmonary dysplasia
Interstitial pulmonary fibrosis of prematurity
Wilson-Mikity syndrome

◆ **770.8 Other respiratory problems after birth**
Apneic spells NOS
Cyanotic attacks NOS
Respiratory distress NOS
Respiratory failure NOS
} originating in the perinatal period

◆ **770.9 Unspecified respiratory condition of fetus and newborn**

● **771 Infections specific to the perinatal period**
INCLUDES infections acquired before or during birth or via the umbilicus
EXCLUDES congenital pneumonia (770.0)
congenital syphilis (090.0-090.9)
maternal infectious disease as a cause of mortality or morbidity in fetus or newborn, but fetus or newborn not manifesting the disease (760.2)
ophthalmia neonatorum due to gonococcus (098.40)
other infections acquired after birth (001.0-136.9, 480.0-486, etc.)

771.0 Congenital rubella
Congenital rubella pneumonitis

771.1 Congenital cytomegalovirus infection
Congenital cytomegalic inclusion disease

◆ **771.2 Other congenital infections**
Congenital:
 herpes simplex
 listeriosis
 malaria
Congenital:
 toxoplasmosis
 tuberculosis

771.3 Tetanus neonatorum
Tetanus omphalitis
EXCLUDES hypocalcemic tetany (775.4)

771.4 Omphalitis of the newborn
Infection:
 navel cord
 umbilical stump
EXCLUDES tetanus omphalitis (771.3)

771.5 Neonatal infective mastitis
EXCLUDES noninfective neonatal mastitis (778.7)

771.6 Neonatal conjunctivitis and dacryocystitis
Ophthalmia neonatorum NOS
EXCLUDES ophthalmia neonatorum due to gonococcus (098.40)

771.7 Neonatal Candida infection
Neonatal moniliasis
Thrush in newborn

◆ **771.8 Other infection specific to the perinatal period**
Intra-amniotic infection of fetus:
 NOS
 clostridial
 Escherichia coli [E. coli]
Intrauterine sepsis of fetus
Neonatal urinary tract infection
Septicemia [sepsis] of newborn

● **772 Fetal and neonatal hemorrhage**
EXCLUDES hematological disorders of fetus and newborn (776.0-776.9)

772.0 Fetal blood loss
Fetal blood loss from:
 cut end of co-twin's cord
 placenta
 ruptured cord
 vasa previa
Fetal exsanguination
Fetal hemorrhage into:
 co-twin
 mother's circulation

CERTAIN CONDITIONS ORIGINATING IN THE PERINATAL PERIOD

772.1 Intraventricular hemorrhage
Intraventricular hemorrhage from any perinatal cause

772.2 Subarachnoid hemorrhage
Subarachnoid hemorrhage from any perinatal cause
EXCLUDES subdural and cerebral hemorrhage (767.0)

772.3 Umbilical hemorrhage after birth
Slipped umbilical ligature

772.4 Gastrointestinal hemorrhage
EXCLUDES swallowed maternal blood (777.3)

772.5 Adrenal hemorrhage

772.6 Cutaneous hemorrhage
Bruising
Ecchymoses
Petechiae
Superficial hematoma
} in fetus or newborn

◆ **772.8 Other specified hemorrhage of fetus or newborn**
EXCLUDES hemorrhagic disease of newborn (776.0)
pulmonary hemorrhage (770.3)

◆ **772.9 Unspecified hemorrhage of newborn**

● **773 Hemolytic disease of fetus or newborn, due to isoimmunization**

773.0 Hemolytic disease due to Rh isoimmunization
Anemia
Erythroblastosis (fetalis)
Hemolytic disease (fetus) (newborn)
Jaundice
} due to RH: antibodies, isoimmunization, maternal/fetal incompatibility

Rh hemolytic disease
Rh isoimmunization

773.1 Hemolytic disease due to ABO isoimmunization
ABO hemolytic disease
ABO isoimmunization

Anemia
Erythroblastosis (fetalis)
Hemolytic disease (fetus) (newborn)
Jaundice
} due to ABO: antibodies, isoimmunization, maternal/fetal incompatibility

◆ **773.2 Hemolytic disease due to other and unspecified isoimmunization**
Eythroblastosis (fetalis) (neonatorum) NOS
Hemolytic disease (fetus) (newborn) NOS
Jaundice or anemia due to other and unspecified blood-group incompatibility

773.3 Hydrops fetalis due to isoimmunization
Use additional code, if desired, to identify type of isoimmunization (773.0-773.2)

773.4 Kernicterus due to isoimmunization
Use additional code, if desired, to identify type of isoimmunization (773.0-773.2)

773.5 Late anemia due to isoimmunization

● **774 Other perinatal jaundice**

■ **774.0 Perinatal jaundice from hereditary hemolytic anemias**
Code also underlying disease (282.0-282.9)

◆ **774.1 Perinatal jaundice from other excessive hemolysis**
Fetal or neonatal jaundice from:
bruising
drugs or toxins transmitted from mother
infection
polycythemia
swallowed maternal blood
Use additional code, if desired, to identify cause
EXCLUDES jaundice due to isoimmunization (773.0-773.2)

774.2 Neonatal jaundice associated with preterm delivery
Hyperbilirubinemia of prematurity
Jaundice due to delayed conjugation associated with preterm delivery

● **774.3 Neonatal jaundice due to delayed conjugation from other causes**

◆ **774.30 Neonatal jaundice due to delayed conjugation, cause unspecified**

■ **774.31 Neonatal jaundice due to delayed conjugation in diseases classified elsewhere**
Code also underlying diseases as:
congenital hypothyroidism (243)
Crigler-Najjar syndrome (277.4)
Gilbert's syndrome (277.4)

◆ **774.39 Other**
Jaundice due to delayed conjugation from causes, such as:
breast milk inhibitors
delayed development of conjugating system

774.4 Perinatal jaundice due to hepatocellular damage
Fetal or neonatal hepatitis
Giant cell hepatitis
Inspissated bile syndrome

■ ◆ **774.5 Perinatal jaundice from other causes**
Code also underlying cause as:
congenital obstruction of bile duct (751.61)
galactosemia (271.1)
mucoviscidosis (277.00-277.01)

◆ **774.6 Unspecified fetal and neonatal jaundice**
Icterus neonatorum
Neonatal hyperbilirubinemia (transient)
Physiologic jaundice NOS in newborn
EXCLUDES that in preterm infants (774.2)

774.7 Kernicterus not due to isoimmunization
Bilirubin encephalopathy
Kernicterus of newborn NOS
EXCLUDES kernicterus due to isoimmunization (773.4)

● **775 Endocrine and metabolic disturbances specific to the fetus and newborn**
INCLUDES transitory endocrine and metabolic disturbances caused by the infant's response to maternal endocrine and metabolic factors, its removal from them, or its adjustment to extrauterine existence

775.0 Syndrome of "infant of a diabetic mother"
Maternal diabetes mellitus affecting fetus or newborn (with hypoglycemia)

775.1 Neonatal diabetes mellitus
Diabetes mellitus syndrome in newborn infant

775.2 Neonatal myasthenia gravis

775.3 Neonatal thyrotoxicosis
Neonatal hyperthydroidism (transient)

775.4 Hypocalcemia and hypomagnesemia of newborn
Cow's milk hypocalcemia
Hypocalcemic tetany, neonatal
Neonatal hypoparathyroidism
Phosphate-loading hypocalcemia

◆ **775.5 Other transitory neonatal electrolyte disturbances**
Dehydration, neonatal

775.6 Neonatal hypoglycemia
EXCLUDES infant of mother with diabetes mellitus (775.0)

775.7 Late metabolic acidosis of newborn

◆ **775.8 Other transitory neonatal endocrine and metabolic disturbances**
Amino-acid metabolic disorders described as transitory

◆ **775.9 Unspecified endocrine and metabolic disturbances specific to the fetus and newborn**

● **776 Hematological disorders of fetus and newborn**
INCLUDES disorders specific to the fetus or newborn

776.0 Hemorrhagic disease of newborn
Hemorrhagic diathesis of newborn
Vitamin K deficiency of newborn
EXCLUDES fetal or neonatal hemorrhage (772.0-772.9)

776.1 Transient neonatal thrombocytopenia
Neonatal thrombocytopenia due to:
exchange transfusion
idiopathic maternal thrombocytopenia
isoimmunization

776.2 Disseminated intravascular coagulation in newborn

◆ **776.3 Other transient neonatal disorders of coagulation**
Transient coagulation defect, newborn

776.4 Polycythemia neonatorum
Plethora of newborn
Polycythemia due to:
donor twin transfusion
maternal-fetal transfusion

● Additional digits required ◆ Nonspecific code ■ Not a primary diagnosis

776.5 Congenital anemia
Anemia following fetal blood loss
EXCLUDES anemia due to isoimmunization (773.0-773.2, 773.5)
hereditary hemolytic anemias (282.0-282.9)

776.6 Anemia of prematurity

776.7 Transient neonatal neutropenia
Isoimmune neutropenia
Maternal transfer neutropenia
EXCLUDES congenital neutropenia (nontransient) (288.0)

◆ **776.8 Other specified transient hematological disorders**

◆ **776.9 Unspecified hematological disorder specific to fetus or newborn**

● **777 Perinatal disorders of digestive system**
INCLUDES disorders specific to the fetus and newborn
EXCLUDES intestinal obstruction classifiable to 560.0-560.9

777.1 Meconium obstruction
Congenital fecaliths
Delayed passage of meconium
Meconium ileus NOS ◆
Meconium plug syndrome
EXCLUDES meconium ileus in cystic fibrosis (277.01) ◆

777.2 Intestinal obstruction due to inspissated milk

777.3 Hematemesis and melena due to swallowed maternal blood
Swallowed blood syndrome in newborn
EXCLUDES that not due to swallowed maternal blood (772.4)

777.4 Transitory ileus of newborn
EXCLUDES Hirschsprung's disease (751.3)

777.5 Necrotizing enterocolitis in fetus or newborn
Pseudomembranous enterocolitis in newborn

777.6 Perinatal intestinal perforation
Meconium peritonitis

◆ **777.8 Other specified perinatal disorders of digestive system**

◆ **777.9 Unspecified perinatal disorder of digestive system**

● **778 Conditions involving the integument and temperature regulation of fetus and newborn**

778.0 Hydrops fetalis not due to isoimmunization
Idiopathic hydrops
EXCLUDES hydrops fetalis due to isoimmunization (773.3)

778.1 Sclerema neonatorum
Subcutaneous fat necrosis

778.2 Cold injury syndrome of newborn

◆ **778.3 Other hypothermia of newborn**

◆ **778.4 Other disturbances of temperature regulation of newborn**
Dehydration fever in newborn
Environmentally-induced pyrexia
Hyperthermia in newborn
Transitory fever of newborn

◆ **778.5 Other and unspecified edema of newborn**
Edema neonatorum

778.6 Congenital hydrocele
Congenital hydrocele of tunica vaginalis

778.7 Breast engorgement in newborn
Noninfective mastitis of newborn
EXCLUDES infective mastitis of newborn (771.5)

◆ **778.8 Other specified conditions involving the integument of fetus and newborn**
Urticaria neonatorum
EXCLUDES impetigo neonatorum (684)
pemphigus neonatorum (684)

◆ **778.9 Unspecified condition involving the integument and temperature regulation of fetus and newborn**

● **779 Other and ill-defined conditions originating in the perinatal period**
Fits
Seizures } in newborn

◆ **779.1 Other and unspecified cerebral irritability in newborn**

779.2 Cerebral depression, coma, and other abnormal cerebral signs
CNS dysfunction in newborn NOS

779.3 Feeding problems in newborn
Regurgitation of food
Slow feeding } in newborn
Vomiting

779.4 Drug reactions and intoxications specific to newborn
Gray syndrome from chloramphenicol administration in newborn
EXCLUDES fetal alcohol syndrome (760.71)
reactions and intoxications from maternal opiates and tranquilizers (763.5)

779.5 Drug withdrawal syndrome in newborn
Drug withdrawal syndrome in infant of dependent mother
EXCLUDES fetal alcohol syndrome (760.71)

779.6 Termination of pregnancy (fetus)
Fetal death due to:
induced abortion
termination of pregnancy
EXCLUDES spontaneous abortion (fetus) (761.8)

◆ **779.8 Other specified conditions originating in the perinatal period**

◆ **779.9 Unspecified condition originating in the perinatal period**
Congenital debility NOS
Stillbirth NEC

16. SYMPTOMS, SIGNS, AND ILL-DEFINED CONDITIONS (780-799)

This section includes symptoms, signs, abnormal results of laboratory or other investigative procedures, and ill-defined conditions regarding which no diagnosis classifiable elsewhere is recorded.

Signs and symptoms that point rather definitely to a given diagnosis are assigned to some category in the preceding part of the classification. In general, categories 780-796 include the more ill-defined conditions and symptoms that point with perhaps equal suspicion to two or more diseases or to two or more systems of the body, and without the necessary study of the case to make a final diagnosis. Practically all categories in this group could be designated as "not otherwise specified," or as "unknown etiology," or as "transient." The Alphabetic Index should be consulted to determine which symptoms and signs are to be allocated here and which to more specific sections of the classification; the residual subcategories numbered .9 are provided for other relevant symptoms which cannot be allocated elsewhere in the classification.

The conditions and signs or symptoms included in categories 780-796 consist of: (a) cases for which no more specific diagnosis can be made even after all facts bearing on the case have been investigated; (b) signs or symptoms existing at the time of initial encounter that proved to be transient and whose causes could not be determined; (c) provisional diagnoses in a patient who failed to return for further investigation or care; (d) cases referred elsewhere for investigation or treatment before the diagnosis was made; (e) cases in which a more precise diagnosis was not available for any other reason; (f) certain symptoms which represent important problems in medical care and which it might be desired to classify in addition to a known cause.

SYMPTOMS (780-789)

● **780 General symptoms**

● **780.0 Alteration of consciousness**
EXCLUDES coma:
diabetic (250.2-250.3)
hepatic (572.2)
originating in the perinatal period (779.2)

780.01 Coma
780.02 Transient alteration of awareness
780.03 Persistent vegetative state
◆ **780.09 Other**
Drowsiness   Stupor
Semicoma   Unconsciousness
Somnolence

780.1 Hallucinations
Hallucinations: Hallucinations:
  NOS   olfactory
  auditory   tactile
  gustatory
EXCLUDES those associated with mental disorders, as functional psychoses (295.0-298.9)
organic brain syndromes (290.0-294.9, 310.0-310.9)
visual hallucinations (368.16)

780.2 Syncope and collapse
Blackout   (Near) (Pre) syncope ◆
Fainting   Vasovagal attack
EXCLUDES carotid sinus syncope (337.0)
heat syncope (992.1)
neurocirculatory asthenia (306.2)
orthostatic hypotension (458.0)
shock NOS (785.50)

SYMPTOMS, SIGNS, AND ILL-DEFINED CONDITIONS

780.3 Convulsions
Convulsions:
  NOS
  febrile
  infantile
Convulsive:
  disorder NOS
  seizure NOS
  Fit NOS
  EXCLUDES convulsions:
    epileptic (345.10-345.91)
    in newborn (779.0)

780.4 Dizziness and giddiness
Light-headedness   Vertigo NOS
EXCLUDES Méenière's disease and other specified vertiginous syndromes (386.0-386.9)

● **780.5 Sleep disturbances**
EXCLUDES that of nonorganic origin (307.40-307.49)
◆ **780.50** Sleep disturbance, unspecified
  780.51 Insomnia with sleep apnea
◆ **780.52** Other insomnia
    Insomnia NOS
  780.53 Hypersomnia with sleep apnea
◆ **780.54** Other hypersomnia
    Hypersomnia NOS
  780.55 Disruptions of 24-hour sleep-wake cycle
    Inversion of sleep rhythm
    Irregular sleep-wake rhythm NOS
    Non-24-hour sleep-wake rhythm
  780.56 Dysfunctions associated with sleep stages or arousal from sleep
◆ **780.57** Other and unspecified sleep apnea
◆ **780.59** Other

780.6 Pyrexia of unknown origin
Chills with fever
Fever NOS
Hyperpyrexia NOS
EXCLUDES pyrexia of unknown origin (during):
    in newborn (778.4)
    labor (659.2)
    the puerperium (672)

780.7 Malaise and fatigue
Asthenia NOS   Postviral (asthenic) syndrome
Lethargy   Tiredness
EXCLUDES debility, unspecified (799.3)
    fatigue (during):
      combat (308.0-308.9)
      heat (992.6)
      pregnancy (646.8)
    neurasthenia (300.5)
    senile asthenia (797)

780.8 Hyperhidrosis
Diaphoresis
Excessive sweating

◆ **780.9 Other general symptoms**
Amnesia (retrograde)
Chill(s) NOS
Generalized pain
Hypothermia, not associated with low environmental temperature
EXCLUDES hypothermia:
    NOS (accidental) (991.6)
    due to anesthesia (995.89)
    of newborn (778.2-778.3)
  memory disturbance as part of a pattern of mental disorder

● **781 Symptoms involving nervous and musculoskeletal systems**
EXCLUDES depression NOS (311)
    disorders specifically relating to:
      back (724.0-724.9)
      hearing (388.0-389.9)
      joint (718.0-719.9)
      limb (729.0-729.9)
      neck (723.0-723.9)
      vision (368.0-369.9)
    pain in limb (729.5)

781.0 Abnormal involuntary movements
Abnormal head movements
Fasciculation
Spasms NOS
Tremor NOS
EXCLUDES abnormal reflex (796.1)
    chorea NOS (333.5)
    infantile spasms (345.60-345.61)
    spastic paralysis (342.1, 343.0-344.9)
    specified movement disorders classifiable to 333 (333.0-333.9)
    that of nonorganic origin (307.2-307.3)

781.1 Disturbances of sensation of smell and taste
Anosmia   Parosmia
Parageusia

781.2 Abnormality of gait
Gait: Gait:
  ataxic   spastic
  paralytic   staggering
EXCLUDES ataxia:
    NOS (781.3)
    locomotor (progressive) (094.0)
  difficulty in walking (719.7)

781.3 Lack of coordination
Ataxia NOS   Muscular incoordination
EXCLUDES ataxic gait (781.2)
    cerebellar ataxia (334.0-334.9)
    difficulty in walking (719.7)
    vertigo NOS (780.4)

781.4 Transient paralysis of limb
Monoplegia, transient NOS
EXCLUDES paralysis (342.0-344.9)

781.5 Clubbing of fingers

781.6 Meningismus
Dupré's syndrome   Meningism

781.7 Tetany
Carpopedal spasm
EXCLUDES tetanus neonatorum (771.3)
    tetany:
      hysterical (300.11)
      newborn (hypocalcemic) (775.4)
      parathyroid (252.1)
      psychogenic (306.0)

781.8 Neurologic neglect syndrome ▼
Asomatognosia   Left-sided neglect
Hemi-akinesia   Sensory extinction
Hemi-inattention   Sensory neglect
Hemispatial neglect Visuospatial neglect ▲

◆ **781.9 Other symptoms involving nervous and musculoskeletal systems**
Abnormal posture

● **782 Symptoms involving skin and other integumentary tissue**
EXCLUDES symptoms relating to breast (611.71-611.79)

782.0 Disturbance of skin sensation
Anesthesia of skin   Numbness
Burning or prickling sensation   Paresthesia
Hyperesthesia   Tingling
Hypoesthesia

◆ **782.1 Rash and other nonspecific skin eruption**
Exanthem
EXCLUDES vesicular eruption (709.8)

782.2 Localized superficial swelling, mass, or lump
Subcutaneous nodules
EXCLUDES localized adiposity (278.1)

782.3 Edema
Anasarca
Dropsy
Localized edema NOS
EXCLUDES ascites (789.5)
    edema of:
      newborn NOS (778.5)
      pregnancy (642.0-642.9, 646.1)
    fluid retention (276.6)
    hydrops fetalis (773.3, 778.0)
    hydrothorax (511.8)
    nutritional edema (260, 262)

- **782.4 Jaundice, unspecified, not of newborn**
  - Cholemia NOS
  - Icterus NOS
  - EXCLUDES jaundice in newborn (774.0-774.7)
  - due to isoimmunization (773.0-773.2, 773.4)

- 782.5 **Cyanosis**
  - EXCLUDES newborn (770.8)

- **782.6 Pallor and flushing**
  - 782.61 **Pallor**
  - 782.62 **Flushing**
    - Excessive blushing

- 782.7 **Spontaneous ecchymoses**
  - Petechiae
  - EXCLUDES ecchymosis in fetus or newborn (772.6)
  - purpura (287.0-287.9)

- 782.8 **Changes in skin texture**
  - Induration | of skin
  - Thickening

- ◆ 782.9 **Other symptoms involving skin and integumentary tissues**

- ● 783 **Symptoms concerning nutrition, metabolism, and development**
  - 783.0 **Anorexia**
    - Loss of appetite
    - EXCLUDES anorexia nervosa (307.1)
    - loss of appetite of nonorganic origin (307.59)
  - 783.1 **Abnormal weight gain**
    - EXCLUDES excessive weight gain in pregnancy (646.1)
    - obesity (278.0)
  - 783.2 **Abnormal loss of weight**
  - 783.3 **Feeding difficulties and mismanagement**
    - Feeding problem (elderly) (infant)
    - EXCLUDES feeding disturbance or problems:
      - in newborn (779.3)
      - of nonorganic origin (307.50-307.59)
  - 783.4 **Lack of expected normal physiological development**
    - Delayed milestone   Lack of growth
    - Failure to gain weight Physical retardation
    - Failure to thrive   Short stature
    - EXCLUDES delay in sexual development and puberty (259.0)
    - specific delays in mental development (315.0-315.9)
  - 783.5 **Polydipsia**
    - Excessive thirst
  - 783.6 **Polyphagia**
    - Excessive eating
    - Hyperalimentation NOS
    - EXCLUDES disorders of eating of nonorganic origin (307.50-307.59)
  - ◆ 783.9 **Other symptoms concerning nutrition, metabolism, and development**
    - Hypometabolism
    - EXCLUDES abnormal basal metabolic rate (794.7)
    - dehydration (276.5)
    - other disorders of fluid, electrolyte, and acid-base balance (276.0-276.9)

- ● 784 **Symptoms involving head and neck**
  - EXCLUDES encephalopathy NOS (348.3)
  - specific symptoms involving neck classifiable to 723 (723.0-723.9)
  - 784.0 **Headache**
    - Facial pain   Pain in head NOS
    - EXCLUDES atypical face pain (350.2)
    - migraine (346.0-346.9)
    - tension headache (307.81)
  - 784.1 **Throat pain**
    - EXCLUDES dysphagia (787.2)
    - neck pain (723.1)
    - sore throat (462)
    - chronic (472.1)
  - 784.2 **Swelling, mass, or lump in head and neck**
    - Space-occupying lesion, intracranial NOS
  - 784.3 **Aphasia**
    - EXCLUDES developmental aphasia (315.31)
  - ● 784.4 **Voice disturbance**
    - ◆ 784.40 **Voice disturbance, unspecified**
    - 784.41 **Aphonia**
      - Loss of voice
    - ◆ 784.49 **Other**
      - Change in voice   Hypernasality
      - Dysphonia   Hyponasality
      - Hoarseness
  - ◆ 784.5 **Other speech disturbance**
    - Dysarthria
    - Dysphasia
    - Slurred speech
    - EXCLUDES stammering and stuttering (307.0)
    - that of nonorganic origin (307.0, 307.9)
  - ● 784.6 **Other symbolic dysfunction**
    - EXCLUDES developmental learning delays (315.0-315.9)
    - ◆ 784.60 **Symbolic dysfunction, unspecified**
    - 784.61 **Alexia and dyslexia**
      - Alexia (with agraphia)
    - ◆ 784.69 **Other**
      - Acalculia   Agraphia NOS
      - Agnosia   Apraxia
  - 784.7 **Epistaxis**
    - Hemorrhage from nose
    - Nosebleed
  - 784.8 **Hemorrhage from throat**
    - EXCLUDES hemoptysis (786.3)
  - ◆ 784.9 **Other symptoms involving head and neck**
    - Choking sensation   Mouth breathing
    - Halitosis   Sneezing

- ● 785 **Symptoms involving cardiovascular system**
  - EXCLUDES heart failure NOS (428.9)
  - ◆ 785.0 **Tachycardia, unspecified**
    - Rapid heart beat
    - EXCLUDES paroxysmal tachycardia (427.0-427.2)
  - 785.1 **Palpitations**
    - Awareness of heart beat
    - EXCLUDES specified dysrhythmias (427.0-427.9)
  - 785.2 **Undiagnosed cardiac murmurs**
    - Heart murmurs NOS
  - ◆ 785.3 **Other abnormal heart sounds**
    - Cardiac dullness, increased or decreased
    - Friction fremitus, cardiac
    - Precordial friction
  - 785.4 **Gangrene**
    - Gangrene:
      - NOS
      - spreading cutaneous
    - Phagedena
    - Use additional code for any associated condition, as:
      - diabetes (250.7)
      - Raynaud's syndrome (443.0)
    - EXCLUDES gangrene of certain sites — see Alphabetic Index
    - gangrene with atherosclerosis of the extremities (440.24)
    - gas gangrene (040.0)
  - ● 785.5 **Shock without mention of trauma**
    - ◆ 785.50 **Shock, unspecified**
      - Failure of peripheral circulation
    - 785.51 **Cardiogenic shock**
    - ◆ 785.59 **Other**
      - Shock: Shock:
        - endotoxic   hypovolemic
        - gram-negative   septic
      - EXCLUDES shock (due to):
        - anesthetic (995.4)
        - anaphylactic (995.0)
        - due to serum (999.4)
        - electric (994.8)
        - following abortion (639.5)
        - lightning (994.0)
        - obstetrical (669.1)
        - postoperative (998.0)
        - traumatic (958.4)

SYMPTOMS, SIGNS, AND ILL-DEFINED CONDITIONS

785.6 **Enlargement of lymph nodes**
Lymphadenopathy
"Swollen glands"
EXCLUDES lymphadenitis (chronic) (289.1-289.3)
acute (683)

785.9 **Other symptoms involving cardiovascular system**
Bruit (arterial)   Weak pulse

786 **Symptoms involving respiratory system and other chest symptoms**

786.0 **Dyspnea and respiratory abnormalities**
- **786.00** Respiratory abnormality, unspecified
- **786.01** Hyperventilation
  EXCLUDES hyperventilation, psychogenic (306.1)
- **786.02** Orthopnea
- **786.09** Other
  Apnea
  Cheyne-Stokes respiration
  Respiratory:
    distress
    insufficiency
  Shortness of breath
  Tachypnea
  Wheezing
  EXCLUDES respiratory distress:
    following trauma and surgery (518.5)
    newborn (770.8)
    sleep apnea (780.51, 780.53, 780.57)
    syndrome (newborn) (769)
      adult (518.5)
    respiratory failure (518.81)
      newborn (770.8)
    transitory tachypnea of newborn (770.6)

786.1 **Stridor**
EXCLUDES congenital laryngeal stridor (748.3)

786.2 **Cough**
EXCLUDES cough:
  psychogenic (306.1)
  smokers' (491.0)
  with hemorrhage (786.3)

786.3 **Hemoptysis**
Cough with hemorrhage
Pulmonary hemorrhage NOS
EXCLUDES pulmonary hemorrhage of newborn (770.3)

786.4 **Abnormal sputum**
Abnormal:
  amount
  color
  odor
  Excessive
} (of) sputum

786.5 **Chest pain**
- **786.50** Chest pain, unspecified
- **786.51** Precordial pain
- **786.52** Painful respiration
  Pain:
    anterior chest wall
    pleuritic
  Pleurodynia
  EXCLUDES epidemic pleurodynia (074.1)
- **786.59** Other
  Discomfort
  Pressure
  Tightness
  } in chest
  EXCLUDES pain in breast (611.71)

786.6 **Swelling, mass, or lump in chest**
EXCLUDES lump in breast (611.72)

786.7 **Abnormal chest sounds**
Abnormal percussion, chest   Rales
Friction sounds, chest   Tympany, chest
EXCLUDES wheezing (786.09)

786.8 **Hiccough**
EXCLUDES psychogenic hiccough (306.1)

786.9 **Other symptoms involving respiratory system and chest**
Breath-holding spell

787 **Symptoms involving digestive system**
EXCLUDES constipation (564.0)
diarrhea NOS (558.9)
pylorospasm (537.81)
  congenital (750.5)

787.0 **Nausea and vomiting**
Emesis
EXCLUDES hematemesis NOS (578.0)
vomiting:
  bilious, following gastrointestinal surgery (564.3)
  cyclical (536.2)
    psychogenic (306.4)
  excessive, in pregnancy (643.0-643.9)
  habit (536.2)
  of newborn (779.3)
  psychogenic NOS (307.54)
- **787.01** Nausea with vomiting ▼
- **787.02** Nausea alone
- **787.03** Vomiting alone ▲

787.1 **Heartburn**
Pyrosis
Waterbrash
EXCLUDES dyspepsia or indigestion (536.8)

787.2 **Dysphagia**
Difficulty in swallowing

787.3 **Flatulence, eructation, and gas pain**
Abdominal distention (gaseous)
Bloating
Tympanites (abdominal) (intestinal)
EXCLUDES aerophagy (306.4)

787.4 **Visible peristalsis**
Hyperperistalsis

787.5 **Abnormal bowel sounds**
Absent bowel sounds
Hyperactive bowel sounds

787.6 **Incontinence of feces**
Encopresis NOS
Incontinence of sphincter ani
EXCLUDES that of nonorganic origin (307.7)

787.7 **Abnormal feces**
Bulky stools
EXCLUDES abnormal stool content (792.1)
melena:
  NOS (578.1)
  newborn (772.4, 777.3)

787.9 **Other symptoms involving digestive system**
Change in bowel habits
Tenesmus (rectal)
EXCLUDES gastrointestinal hemorrhage (578.0-578.9)
intestinal obstruction (560.0-560.9)
specific functional digestive disorders:
  esophagus (530.0-530.9)
  stomach and duodenum (536.0-536.9)
  those not elsewhere classified (564.0-564.9)

788 **Symptoms involving urinary system**
EXCLUDES hematuria (599.7)
nonspecific findings on examination of the urine (791.0-791.9)
small kidney of unknown cause (589.0-589.9)
uremia NOS (586)

788.0 **Renal colic**
Colic (recurrent) of:
  kidney
  ureter

788.1 **Dysuria**
Painful urination   Strangury

788.2 **Retention of urine**
- **788.20** Retention of urine, unspecified
- **788.21** Incomplete bladder emptying
- **788.29** Other specified retention of urine

788.3 **Urinary incontinence**
EXCLUDES that of nonorganic origin (307.6)

● Additional digits required   ◆ Nonspecific code   ■ Not a primary diagnosis

- ◆ 788.30 Urinary incontinence, unspecified
  Enuresis NOS
  - 788.31 Urge incontinence
  - 788.32 Stress incontinence, male
    - EXCLUDES stress incontinence, female (625.6)
  - 788.33 Mixed incontinence, (male) (female)
    Urge and stress
  - 788.34 Incontinence without sensory awareness
  - 788.35 Post-void dribbling
  - 788.36 Nocturnal enuresis
  - 788.37 Continuous leakage
  - ◆ 788.39 Other urinary incontinence
- ● 788.4 Frequency of urination and polyuria
  - 788.41 Urinary frequency
    Frequency of micturition
  - 788.42 Polyuria
  - 788.43 Nocturia
- 788.5 Oliguria and anuria
  Deficient secretion of urine
  Suppression of urinary secretion
  - EXCLUDES that complicating:
    abortion (634-638 with .3, 639.3)
    ectopic or molar pregnancy (639.3)
    pregnancy, childbirth, or the puerperium (642.0-642.9, 646.2)
- ● 788.6 Other abnormality of urination
  - 788.61 Splitting of urinary stream
    Intermittent urinary stream
  - 788.62 Slowing of urinary stream
    Weak stream
  - ◆ 788.69 Other
- 788.7 Urethral discharge
  Penile discharge
  Urethrorrhea
- 788.8 Extravasation of urine
- ◆ 788.9 Other symptoms involving urinary system
  Extrarenal uremia   Vesical:
  Vesical: tenesmus
    pain

- ● 789 Other symptoms involving abdomen and pelvis
  - EXCLUDES symptoms referable to genital organs:
    female (625.0-625.9)
    male (607.0-608.9)
    psychogenic (302.70-302.79)

  The following fifth-digit subclassification is to be used for codes 789.0, 789.3, 789.4, 789.6: ▼
  - ◆ 0 Unspecified site
  - 1 Right upper quadrant
  - 2 Left upper quadrant
  - 3 Right lower quadrant
  - 4 Left lower quadrant
  - 5 Periumbilic
  - 6 Epigastric
  - ◆ 7 Generalized
  - ◆ 9 Other specified site
    multiple sites ▲
  - ● 789.0 Abdominal pain
    Abdominal tenderness   Cramps, abdominal
    Colic: Epigastric pain
      NOS   Umbilical pain
      infantile
    - EXCLUDES renal colic (788.0)
  - 789.1 Hepatomegaly
    Enlargement of liver
  - 789.2 Splenomegaly
    Enlargement of spleen
  - ● 789.3 Abdominal or pelvic swelling, mass, or lump
    Diffuse or generalized swelling or mass:
      abdominal NOS
      umbilical
    - EXCLUDES abdominal distention (gaseous) (787.3)
      ascites (789.5)
  - ● 789.4 Abdominal rigidity
  - 789.5 Ascites
    Fluid in peritoneal cavity
  - ● 789.6 Abdominal tenderness
    Rebound tenderness ▼▲

- ◆ 789.9 Other symptoms involving abdomen and pelvis
  Umbilical:
    bleeding
    discharge

NONSPECIFIC ABNORMAL FINDINGS (790-796)
- ● 790 Nonspecific findings on examination of blood
  - EXCLUDES abnormality of:
    platelets (287.0-287.9)
    thrombocytes (287.0-287.9)
    white blood cells (288.0-288.9)
  - 790.0 Abnormality of red blood cells
    Abnormal red cell: Anisocytosis
      morphology NOS   Poikilocytosis
      volume NOS
    - EXCLUDES anemia:
      congenital (776.5)
      newborn, due to isoimmunization (773.0-773.2, 773.5)
      of premature infant (776.6)
      other specified types (280.0-285.9)
      hemoglobin disorders (282.5-282.7)
      polycythemia:
        familial (289.6)
        neonatorum (776.4)
        secondary (289.0)
        vera (238.4)
  - 790.1 Elevated sedimentation rate
  - 790.2 Abnormal glucose tolerance test
    - EXCLUDES that complicating pregnancy, childbirth, or the puerperium (648.8)
  - 790.3 Excessive blood level of alcohol
    Elevated blood-alcohol
  - ◆ 790.4 Nonspecific elevation of levels of transaminase or lactic acid dehydrogenase [LDH]
  - ◆ 790.5 Other nonspecific abnormal serum enzyme levels
    Abnormal serum level of: Abnormal serum level of:
      acid phosphatase   amylase
      alkaline phosphatase   lipase
    - EXCLUDES deficiency of circulating enzymes (277.6)
  - ◆ 790.6 Other abnormal blood chemistry
    Abnormal blood level of: Abnormal blood level of:
      cobalt   magnesium
      copper   mineral
      iron   zinc
      lithium
    - EXCLUDES abnormality of electrolyte or acid-base balance (276.0-276.9)
      hypoglycemia NOS (251.2)
      specific finding indicating abnormality of:
        amino-acid transport and metabolism (270.0-270.9)
        carbohydrate transport and metabolism (271.0-271.9)
        lipid metabolism (272.0-272.9)
      uremia NOS (586)
  - 790.7 Bacteremia
    - EXCLUDES septicemia (038)
    Use additional code, if desired, to identify organism (041)
  - ◆ 790.8 Viremia, unspecified
  - ● 790.9 Other nonspecific findings on examination of blood
    - 790.91 Abnormal arterial blood gases
    - 790.92 Abnormal coagulation profile
      Abnormal or prolonged:
        bleeding time
        coagulation time
        partial thromboplastin time [PTT]
        prothrombintime [PT]
      - EXCLUDES coagulation (hemorrhagic) disorders (286.0-286.9)
    - 790.93 Elevated prostate specific antigen, (PSA)
    - ◆ 790.99 Other
- ● 791 Nonspecific findings on examination of urine
  - EXCLUDES hematuria NOS (599.7)
    specific findings indicating abnormality of:
      amino-acid transport and metabolism (270.0-270.9)
      carbohydrate transport and metabolism (271.0-271.9)

SYMPTOMS, SIGNS, AND ILL-DEFINED CONDITIONS

791.0 Proteinuria
  Albuminuria
  Bence-Jones proteinuria
  EXCLUDES: postural proteinuria (593.6)
  that arising during pregnancy or the puerperium (642.0-642.9, 646.2)

791.1 Chyluria
  EXCLUDES: filarial (125.0-125.9)

791.2 Hemoglobinuria

791.3 Myoglobinuria

791.4 Biliuria

791.5 Glycosuria
  EXCLUDES: renal glycosuria (271.4)

791.6 Acetonuria
  Ketonuria

◆ **791.7 Other cells and casts in urine**

◆ **791.9 Other nonspecific findings on examination of urine**
  Crystalluria
  Elevated urine levels of:
    17-ketosteroids
    catecholamines
  Elevated urine levels of:
    indolacetic acid
    vanillylmandelic acid [VMA]
  Melanuria

● **792 Nonspecific abnormal findings in other body substances**
  EXCLUDES: that in chromosomal analysis (795.2)

792.0 Cerebrospinal fluid

792.1 Stool contents
  Abnormal stool color
  Fat in stool
  Mucus in stool
  Occult stool
  Pus in stool
  EXCLUDES: blood in stool [melena] (578.1)
  newborn (772.4, 777.3)

792.2 Semen
  Abnormal spermatozoa
  EXCLUDES: azoospermia (606.0)
  oligospermia (606.1)

792.3 Amniotic fluid

792.4 Saliva
  EXCLUDES: that in chromosomal analysis (795.2)

◆ **792.9 Other nonspecific abnormal findings in body substances**
  Peritoneal fluid
  Pleural fluid
  Synovial fluid
  Vaginal fluids

● **793 Nonspecific abnormal findings on radiological and other examination of body structure**
  INCLUDES: nonspecific abnormal findings of:
    thermography
    ultrasound examination [echogram]
    x-ray examination
  EXCLUDES: abnormal results of function studies and radioisotope scans (794.0-794.9)

793.0 Skull and head
  EXCLUDES: nonspecific abnormal echoencephalogram (794.01)

793.1 Lung field
  Coin lesion } (of) lung
  Shadow

◆ **793.2 Other intrathoracic organ**
  Abnormal:
    echocardiogram
    heart shadow
  Abnormal:
    ultrasound cardiogram
    Mediastinal shift

793.3 Biliary tract
  Nonvisualization of gallbladder

793.4 Gastrointestinal tract

793.5 Genitourinary organs
  Filling defect:
    bladder
    kidney
  Filling defect:
    ureter

793.6 Abdominal area, including retroperitoneum

793.7 Musculoskeletal system

793.8 Breast
  Abnormal mammogram

◆ **793.9 Other**
  Abnormal:
    placental finding by x-ray or ultrasound method
    radiological findings in skin and subcutaneous tissue
  EXCLUDES: abnormal finding by radioisotope localization of placenta (794.9)

● **794 Nonspecific abnormal results of function studies**
  INCLUDES: radioisotope:
    scans
    uptake studies
    scintiphotography

● **794.0 Brain and central nervous system**
  ◆ **794.00** Abnormal function study, unspecified
  794.01 Abnormal echoencephalogram
  794.02 Abnormal electroencephalogram [EEG]
  ◆ **794.09** Other
    Abnormal brain scan

● **794.1 Peripheral nervous system and special senses**
  ◆ **794.10** Abnormal response to nerve stimulation, unspecified
  794.11 Abnormal retinal function studies
    Abnormal electroretinogram [ERG]
  794.12 Abnormal electro-oculogram [EOG]
  794.13 Abnormal visually evoked potential
  794.14 Abnormal oculomotor studies
  794.15 Abnormal auditory function studies
  794.16 Abnormal vestibular function studies
  794.17 Abnormal electromyogram [EMG]
    EXCLUDES: that of eye (794.14)
  ◆ **794.19** Other

794.2 Pulmonary
  Abnormal lung scan
  Reduced:
    ventilatory capacity
    vital capacity

● **794.3 Cardiovascular**
  ◆ **794.30** Abnormal function study, unspecified
  794.31 Abnormal electrocardiogram [ECG] [EKG]
  ◆ **794.39** Other
    Abnormal:
      ballistocardiogram
      phonocardiogram
      vectorcardiogram

794.4 Kidney
  Abnormal renal function test

794.5 Thyroid
  Abnormal thyroid:
    scan
    uptake

◆ **794.6 Other endocrine function study**

794.7 Basal metabolism
  Abnormal basal metabolic rate [BMR]

794.8 Liver
  Abnormal liver scan

◆ **794.9 Other**
  Bladder
  Pancreas
  Placenta
  Spleen

● **795 Nonspecific abnormal histological and immunological findings**
  EXCLUDES: nonspecific abnormalities of red blood cells (790.0)

◆ **795.0 Nonspecific abnormal Papanicolaou smear of cervix**
  Dyskaryotic cervical smear

◆ **795.1 Nonspecific abnormal Papanicolaou smear of other site**

◆ **795.2 Nonspecific abnormal findings on chromosomal analysis**
  Abnormal karyotype

◆ **795.3 Nonspecific positive culture findings**
  Positive culture findings in:
    nose
    sputum
  Positive culture findings in:
    throat
    wound
  EXCLUDES: that of:
    blood (790.7-790.8)
    urine (599.0)

◆ **795.4 Other nonspecific abnormal histological findings**

◆ **795.5 Nonspecific reaction to tuberculin skin test without active tuberculosis**
  Abnormal result of Mantoux test
  PPD positive
  Tuberculin (skin test):
    positive
    reactor

795.6 False positive serological test for syphilis
  False positive Wassermann reaction

● **795.7 Other nonspecific immunological findings**
  EXCLUDES: isoimmunization, in pregnancy (656.1-656.2)
  affecting fetus or newborn (773.0-773.2)

● Additional digits required ◆ Nonspecific code ▮ Not a primary diagnosis

- **795.71 Nonspecific serologic evidence of human immunodeficiency virus [HIV]**
  Inclusive human immunodeficiency [HIV] test (adult) (infant)
  Note: This code is **only** to be used when a test finding is reported as nonspecific. Asymptomatic positive findings are coded to V08. If any HIV infection symptom or condition is present, see code 042. Negative findings are not coded.
  EXCLUDES: acquired immunodeficiency syndrome [AIDS] (042)
  asymptomatic human immunodeficiency virus, [HIV] infection status (V08)
  HIV infection, symptomatic (042)
  human immunodeficiency virus [HIV] disease (042)
  positive (status) NOS (V08)
- **795.79 Other and unspecified nonspecific immunological findings**
  Raised antibody titer
  Raised level of immunoglobulins

796 Other nonspecific abnormal findings
- **796.0 Nonspecific abnormal toxicological findings**
  Abnormal levels of heavy metals or drugs in blood, urine, or other tissue
  EXCLUDES: excessive blood level of alcohol (790.3)
- **796.1 Abnormal reflex**
- **796.2 Elevated blood pressure reading without diagnosis of hypertension**
  Note: This category is to be used to record an episode of elevated blood pressure in a patient in whom no formal diagnosis of hypertension has been made, or as an incidental finding.
- **796.3 Nonspecific low blood pressure reading**
- **796.4 Other abnormal clinical findings**
- **796.9 Other**

ILL-DEFINED AND UNKNOWN CAUSES OF MORBIDITY AND MORTALITY (797-799)

797 Senility without mention of psychosis
Old age   Senile:
Senescence   debility
Senile asthenia   exhaustion
EXCLUDES: senile psychoses (290.0-290.9)

798 Sudden death, cause unknown
- **798.0 Sudden infant death syndrome**
  Cot death
  Crib death
  Sudden death of nonspecific cause in infancy
- **798.1 Instantaneous death**
- **798.2 Death occurring in less than 24 hours from onset of symptoms, not otherwise explained**
  Death known not to be violent or instantaneous, for which no cause could be discovered
  Died without sign of disease
- **798.9 Unattended death**
  Death in circumstances where the body of the deceased was found and no cause could be discovered
  Found dead

799 Other ill-defined and unknown causes of morbidity and mortality
- **799.0 Asphyxia**
  EXCLUDES: asphyxia (due to):
  carbon monoxide (986)
  inhalation of food or foreign body (932-934.9)
  newborn (768.0-768.9)
  traumatic (994.7)
- **799.1 Respiratory arrest**
  Cardiorespiratory failure
  EXCLUDES: cardiac arrest (427.5)
  failure of peripheral circulation (785.50)
  respiratory distress:
   NOS (786.09)
   acute (518.82)
   following trauma and surgery (518.5)
   newborn (770.8)
   syndrome (newborn) (769)
    adult (following trauma and surgery) (518.5)
    other (518.82)
  respiratory failure (518.81)
   newborn (770.8)
  respiratory insufficiency (786.09)
   acute (518.82)
- **799.2 Nervousness**
  "Nerves"
- **799.3 Debility, unspecified**
  EXCLUDES: asthenia (780.7)
  nervous debility (300.5)
  neurasthenia (300.5)
  senile asthenia (797)
- **799.4 Cachexia**
  Wasting disease
  EXCLUDES: nutritional marasmus (261)
- **799.8 Other ill-defined conditions**
- **799.9 Other unknown and unspecified cause**
  Undiagnosed disease, not specified as to site or system involved
  Unknown cause of morbidity or mortality

17. INJURY AND POISONING (800-999)

Note:

1. The principle of multiple coding of injuries should be followed wherever possible. Combination categories for multiple injuries are provided for use when there is insufficient detail as to the nature of the individual conditions, or for primary tabulation purposes when it is more convenient to record a single code; otherwise, the component injuries should be coded separately.

   Where multiple sites of injury are specified in the titles, the word "with" indicates involvement of both sites, and the word "and" indicates involvement of either or both sites. The word "finger" includes thumb.

2. Categories for "late effect" of injuries are to be found at 905-909.

FRACTURES (800-829)
EXCLUDES: malunion (733.81)
nonunion (733.82)
pathological or spontaneous fracture (733.10-733.19)

The terms "condyle," "coronoid process," "ramus," and "symphysis" indicate the portion of the bone fractured, not the name of the bone involved.

The descriptions "closed" and "open" used in the fourth-digit subdivisions include the following terms:

closed (with or without delayed healing):
comminuted	impacted
depressed	linear
elevated	march
fissured	simple
fracture NOS	slipped epiphysis
greenstick	spiral

open (with or without delayed healing):
compound	puncture
infected	with foreign body
missile	

A fracture not indicated as closed or open should be classified as closed.

FRACTURE OF SKULL (800-804)

The following fifth-digit subclassification is for use with the appropriate codes in categories 800, 801, 803, and 804:

- ◆ 0 unspecified state of consciousness
- 1 with no loss of consciousness
- 2 with brief [less than one hour] loss of consciousness
- 3 with moderate [1-24 hours] loss of consciousness
- 4 with prolonged [more than 24 hours] loss of consciousness and return to pre-existing conscious level
- 5 with prolonged [more than 24 hours] loss of consciousness, without return to pre-existing conscious level
- ◆ 6 with loss of consciousness of unspecified duration
- ◆ 9 with concussion, unspecified

● **800 Fracture of vault of skull**

INCLUDES frontal bone
parietal bone

- ● 800.0 Closed without mention of intracranial injury
- ● 800.1 Closed with cerebral laceration and contusion
- ● 800.2 Closed with subarachnoid, subdural, and extradural hemorrhage
- ◆● 800.3 Closed with other and unspecified intracranial hemorrhage
- ◆● 800.4 Closed with intracranial injury of other and unspecified nature
- ● 800.5 Open without mention of intracranial injury
- ● 800.6 Open with cerebral laceration and contusion
- ● 800.7 Open with subarachnoid, subdural, and extradural hemorrhage
- ◆● 800.8 Open with other and unspecified intracranial hemorrhage
- ◆● 800.9 Open with intracranial injury of other and unspecified nature

● **801 Fracture of base of skull**

INCLUDES fossa: sinus:
    anterior ethmoid
    middle frontal
    posterior sphenoid bone
  occiput bone temporal bone
  orbital roof

- ● 801.0 Closed without mention of intracranial injury
- ● 801.1 Closed with cerebral laceration and contusion
- ● 801.2 Closed with subarachnoid, subdural, and extradural hemorrhage
- ◆● 801.3 Closed with other and unspecified intracranial hemorrhage
- ◆● 801.4 Closed with intracranial injury of other and unspecified nature
- ● 801.5 Open without mention of intracranial injury
- ● 801.6 Open with cerebral laceration and contusion
- ● 801.7 Open with subarachnoid, subdural, and extradural hemorrhage
- ◆● 801.8 Open with other and unspecified intracranial hemorrhage
- ◆● 801.9 Open with intracranial injury of other and unspecified nature

● **802 Fracture of face bones**

- 802.0 Nasal bones, closed
- 802.1 Nasal bones, open
- ● 802.2 Mandible, closed
    Inferior maxilla   Lower jaw (bone)
  - ◆ 802.20 Unspecified site
  - 802.21 Condylar process
  - 802.22 Subcondylar
  - 802.23 Coronoid process
  - ◆ 802.24 Ramus, unspecified
  - 802.25 Angle of jaw
  - 802.26 Symphysis of body
  - 802.27 Alveolar border of body
  - ◆ 802.28 Body, other and unspecified
  - 802.29 Multiple sites
- ● 802.3 Mandible, open
  - ◆ 802.30 Unspecified site
  - 802.31 Condylar process
  - 802.32 Subcondylar
  - 802.33 Coronoid process
  - ◆ 802.34 Ramus, unspecified
  - 802.35 Angle of jaw
  - 802.36 Symphysis of body
  - 802.37 Alveolar border of body
  - ◆ 802.38 Body, other and unspecified
  - 802.39 Multiple sites
- ◆ 802.4 Malar and maxillary bones, closed
    Superior maxilla   Zygoma
    Upper jaw (bone)   Zygomatic arch
- 802.5 Malar and maxillary bones, open
- 802.6 Orbital floor (blow-out), closed
- 802.7 Orbital floor (blow-out), open
- ◆ 802.8 Other facial bones, closed
    Alveolus   Palate
    Orbit:
      NOS
      part other than roof or floor
    EXCLUDES orbital:
      floor (802.6)
      roof (801.0-801.9)
- ◆ 802.9 Other facial bones, open

● **803 Other and unqualified skull fractures**

INCLUDES skull NOS
  skull multiple NOS

- ● 803.0 Closed without mention of intracranial injury
- ● 803.1 Closed with cerebral laceration and contusion
- ● 803.2 Closed with subarachnoid, subdural, and extradural hemorrhage
- ◆● 803.3 Closed with other and unspecified intracranial hemorrhage
- ◆● 803.4 Closed with intracranial injury of other and unspecified nature
- ● 803.5 Open without mention of intracranial injury
- ● 803.6 Open with cerebral laceration and contusion
- ● 803.7 Open with subarachnoid, subdural, and extradural hemorrhage
- ◆● 803.8 Open with other and unspecified intracranial hemorrhage
- ◆● 803.9 Open with intracranial injury of other and unspecified nature

● **804 Multiple fractures involving skull or face with other bones**

- ● 804.0 Closed without mention of intracranial injury
- ● 804.1 Closed with cerebral laceration and contusion
- ● 804.2 Closed with subarachnoid, subdural, and extradural hemorrhage
- ◆● 804.3 Closed with other and unspecified intracranial hemorrhage
- ◆● 804.4 Closed with intracranial injury of other and unspecified nature
- ● 804.5 Open without mention of intracranial injury
- ● 804.6 Open with cerebral laceration and contusion
- ● 804.7 Open with subarachnoid, subdural, and extradural hemorrage
- ◆● 804.8 Open with other and unspecified intracranial hemorrhage
- ◆● 804.9 Open with intracranial injury of other and unspecified nature

FRACTURE OF NECK AND TRUNK (805-809)

● **805 Fracture of vertebral column without mention of spinal cord injury**

INCLUDES neural arch
  spine
  spinous process
  transverse process
  vertebra

The following fifth-digit subclassification is for use with codes 805.0-805.1:

- ◆ 0 cervical vertebra, unspecified level
- 1 first cervical vertebra
- 2 second cervical vertebra
- 3 third cervical vertebra
- 4 fourth cervical vertebra
- 5 fifth cervical vertebra
- 6 sixth cervical vertebra
- 7 seventh cervical vertebra
- ◆ 8 multiple cervical vertebrae

- ● 805.0 Cervical, closed
    Atlas
    Axis
- ● 805.1 Cervical, open
- 805.2 Dorsal [thoracic], closed
- 805.3 Dorsal [thoracic], open
- 805.4 Lumbar, closed
- 805.5 Lumbar, open
- 805.6 Sacrum and coccyx, closed
- 805.7 Sacrum and coccyx, open
- ◆ 805.8 Unspecified, closed
- ◆ 805.9 Unspecified, open

- **806 Fracture of vertebral column with spinal cord injury**

  INCLUDES: any condition classifiable to 805 with:
  complete or incomplete transverse lesion (of cord)
  hematomyelia
  injury to:
  cauda equina
  nerve
  paralysis
  paraplegia
  quadriplegia
  spinal concussion

  - **806.0 Cervical, closed**
    - ◆ 806.00 C_1-C_4 level with unspecified spinal cord injury
      Cervical region NOS with spinal cord injury NOS
    - 806.01 C_1-C_4 level with complete lesion of cord
    - 806.02 C_1-C_4 level with anterior cord syndrome
    - 806.03 C_1-C_4 level with central cord syndrome
    - ◆ 806.04 C_1-C_4 level with other specified spinal cord injury
      C_1-C_4 level with:
      incomplete spinal cord lesion NOS
      posterior cord syndrome
    - ◆ 806.05 C_5-C_7 level with unspecified spinal cord injury
    - 806.06 C_5-C_7 level with complete lesion of cord
    - 806.07 C_5-C_7 level with anterior cord syndrome
    - 806.08 C_5-C_7 level with central cord syndrome
    - ◆ 806.09 C_5-C_7 level with other specified spinal cord injury
      C_5-C_7 level with:
      incomplete spinal cord lesion NOS
      posterior cord syndrome

  - **806.1 Cervical, open**
    - ◆ 806.10 C_1-C_4 level with unspecified spinal cord injury
    - 806.11 C_1-C_4 level with complete lesion of cord
    - 806.12 C_1-C_4 level with anterior cord syndrome
    - 806.13 C_1-C_4 level with central cord syndrome
    - ◆ 806.14 C_1-C_4 level with other specified spinal cord injury
      C_1-C_4 level with:
      incomplete spinal cord lesion NOS
      posterior cord syndrome
    - ◆ 806.15 C_5-C_7 level with unspecified spinal cord injury
    - 806.16 C_5-C_7 level with complete lesion of cord
    - 806.17 C_5-C_7 level with anterior cord syndrome
    - 806.18 C_5-C_7 level with central cord syndrome
    - ◆ 806.19 C_5-C_7 level with other specified spinal cord injury
      C_5-C_7 level with:
      incomplete spinal cord lesion NOS
      posterior cord syndrome

  - **806.2 Dorsal [thoracic], closed**
    - ◆ 806.20 T_1-T_6 level with unspecified spinal cord injury
      Thoracic region NOS with spinal cord injury NOS
    - 806.21 T_1-T_6 level with complete lesion of cord
    - 806.22 T_1-T_6 level with anterior cord syndrome
    - 806.23 T_1-T_6 level with central cord syndrome
    - ◆ 806.24 T_1-T_6 level with other specified spinal cord injury
      T_1-T_6 level with:
      incomplete spinal cord lesion NOS
      posterior cord syndrome
    - ◆ 806.25 T_7-T_{12} level with unspecified spinal cord injury
    - 806.26 T_7-T_{12} level with complete lesion of cord
    - 806.27 T_7-T_{12} level with anterior cord syndrome
    - 806.28 T_7-T_{12} level with central cord syndrome
    - ◆ 806.29 T_7-T_{12} level with other specified spinal cord injury
      T_7-T_{12} level with:
      incomplete spinal cord lesion NOS
      posterior cord syndrome

  - **806.3 Dorsal [thoracic], open**
    - ◆ 806.30 T_1-T_6 level with unspecified spinal cord injury
    - 806.31 T_1-T_6 level with complete lesion of cord
    - 806.32 T_1-T_6 level with anterior cord syndrome
    - 806.33 T_1-T_6 level with central cord syndrome
    - ◆ 806.34 T_1-T_6 level with other specified spinal cord injury
      T_1-T_6 level with:
      incomplete spinal cord lesion NOS
      posterior cord syndrome
    - ◆ 806.35 T_7-T_{12} level with unspecified spinal cord injury
    - 806.36 T_7-T_{12} level with complete lesion of cord
    - 806.37 T_7-T_{12} level with anterior cord syndrome
    - 806.38 T_7-T_{12} level with central cord syndrome
    - ◆ 806.39 T_7-T_{12} level with other specified spinal cord injury
      T_7-T_{12} level with:
      incomplete spinal cord lesion NOS
      posterior cord syndrome

  - 806.4 Lumbar, closed
  - 806.5 Lumbar, open
  - **806.6 Sacrum and coccyx, closed**
    - ◆ 806.60 With unspecified spinal cord injury
    - 806.61 With complete cauda equina lesion
    - ◆ 806.62 With other cauda equina injury
    - ◆ 806.69 With other spinal cord injury
  - **806.7 Sacrum and coccyx, open**
    - ◆ 806.70 With unspecified spinal cord injury
    - 806.71 With complete cauda equina lesion
    - ◆ 806.72 With other cauda equina injury
    - ◆ 806.79 With other spinal cord injury
  - ◆ 806.8 Unspecified, closed
  - ◆ 806.9 Unspecified, open

- **807 Fracture of rib(s), sternum, larynx, and trachea**

  The following fifth-digit subclassification is for use with codes 807.0-807.1:
  - ◆ 0 rib(s), unspecified
  - 1 one rib
  - 2 two ribs
  - 3 three ribs
  - 4 four ribs
  - 5 five ribs
  - 6 six ribs
  - 7 seven ribs
  - 8 eight or more ribs
  - 9 multiple ribs, unspecified

  - **807.0 Rib(s), closed**
  - **807.1 Rib(s), open**
  - 807.2 Sternum, closed
  - 807.3 Sternum, open
  - 807.4 Flail chest
  - 807.5 Larynx and trachea, closed
    Hyoid bone   Trachea
    Thyroid cartilage
  - 807.6 Larynx and trachea, open

- **808 Fracture of pelvis**
  - 808.0 Acetabulum, closed
  - 808.1 Acetabulum, open
  - 808.2 Pubis, closed
  - 808.3 Pubis, open
  - **808.4 Other specified part, closed**
    - 808.41 Ilium
    - 808.42 Ischium
    - ◆ 808.43 Multiple pelvic fractures with disruption of pelvic circle
    - ◆ 808.49 Other
      Innominate bone   Pelvic rim
  - **808.5 Other specified part, open**
    - 808.51 Ilium
    - 808.52 Ischium
    - ◆ 808.53 Multiple pelvic fractures with disruption of pelvic circle
    - ◆ 808.59 Other
  - ◆ 808.8 Unspecified, closed
  - ◆ 808.9 Unspecified, open

- **809 Ill-defined fractures of bones of trunk**

  INCLUDES: bones of trunk with other bones except those of skull and face
  multiple bones of trunk

  EXCLUDES: multiple fractures of:
  pelvic bones alone (808.0-808.9)
  ribs alone (807.0-807.1, 807.4)
  ribs or sternum with limb bones (819.0-819.1, 828.0-828.1)
  skull or face with other bones (804.0-804.9)

  - 809.0 Fracture of bones of trunk, closed
  - 809.1 Fracture of bones of trunk, open

FRACTURE OF UPPER LIMB (810-819)

- **810 Fracture of clavicle**
  - INCLUDES: collar bone
    interligamentous part of clavicle
  - The following fifth-digit subclassification is for use with category 810:
    - ◆ 0 unspecified part
      - Clavicle NOS
    - 1 sternal end of clavicle
    - 2 shaft of clavicle
    - 3 acromial end of clavicle
  - ● 810.0 Closed
  - ● 810.1 Open
- **811 Fracture of scapula**
  - INCLUDES: shoulder blade
  - The following fifth-digit subclassification is for use with category 811:
    - ◆ 0 unspecified part
    - 1 acromial process
      - Acromion (process)
    - 2 coracoid process
    - 3 glenoid cavity and neck of scapula
    - ◆ 9 other
      - Scapula body
  - ● 811.0 Closed
  - ● 811.1 Open
- **812 Fracture of humerus**
  - ● 812.0 Upper end, closed
    - ◆ 812.00 Upper end, unspecified part
      - Proximal end   Shoulder
    - 812.01 Surgical neck
      - Neck of humerus NOS
    - 812.02 Anatomical neck
    - 812.03 Greater tuberosity
    - ◆ 812.09 Other
      - Head   Upper epiphysis
  - ● 812.1 Upper end, open
    - ◆ 812.10 Upper end, unspecified part
    - 812.11 Surgical neck
    - 812.12 Anatomical neck
    - 812.13 Greater tuberosity
    - ◆ 812.19 Other
  - ● 812.2 Shaft or unspecified part, closed
    - ◆ 812.20 Unspecified part of humerus
      - Humerus NOS   Upper arm NOS
    - 812.21 Shaft of humerus
  - ● 812.3 Shaft or unspecified part, open
    - ◆ 812.30 Unspecified part of humerus
    - 812.31 Shaft of humerus
  - ● 812.4 Lower end, closed
    - Distal end of humerus   Elbow
    - ◆ 812.40 Lower end, unspecified part
    - 812.41 Supracondylar fracture of humerus
    - 812.42 Lateral condyle
      - External condyle
    - 812.43 Medial condyle
      - Internal epicondyle
    - ◆ 812.44 Condyle(s), unspecified
      - Articular process NOS
      - Lower epiphysis NOS
    - ◆ 812.49 Other
      - Multiple fractures of lower end
      - Trochlea
  - ● 812.5 Lower end, open
    - ◆ 812.50 Lower end, unspecified part
    - 812.51 Supracondylar fracture of humerus
    - 812.52 Lateral condyle
    - 812.53 Medial condyle
    - ◆ 812.54 Condyle(s), unspecified
    - ◆ 812.59 Other
- **813 Fracture of radius and ulna**
  - ● 813.0 Upper end, closed
    - Proximal end
    - ◆ 813.00 Upper end of forearm, unspecified
    - 813.01 Olecranon process of ulna
    - 813.02 Coronoid process of ulna
    - 813.03 Monteggia's fracture
    - ◆ 813.04 Other and unspecified fractures of proximal end of ulna (alone)
      - Multiple fractures of ulna, upper end
    - 813.05 Head of radius
    - 813.06 Neck of radius
    - ◆ 813.07 Other and unspecified fractures of proximal end of radius (alone)
      - Multiple fractures of radius, upper end
    - 813.08 Radius with ulna, upper end [any part]
  - ● 813.1 Upper end, open
    - ◆ 813.10 Upper end of forearm, unspecified
    - 813.11 Olecranon process of ulna
    - 813.12 Coronoid process of ulna
    - 813.13 Monteggia's fracture
    - ◆ 813.14 Other and unspecified fractures of proximal end of ulna (alone)
    - 813.15 Head of radius
    - 813.16 Neck of radius
    - ◆ 813.17 Other and unspecified fractures of proximal end of radius (alone)
    - 813.18 Radius with ulna, upper end [any part]
  - ● 813.2 Shaft, closed
    - ◆ 813.20 Shaft, unspecified
    - 813.21 Radius (alone)
    - 813.22 Ulna (alone)
    - 813.23 Radius with ulna
  - ● 813.3 Shaft, open
    - ◆ 813.30 Shaft, unspecified
    - 813.31 Radius (alone)
    - 813.32 Ulna (alone)
    - 813.33 Radius with ulna
  - ● 813.4 Lower end, closed
    - Distal end
    - ◆ 813.40 Lower end of forearm, unspecified
    - 813.41 Colles' fracture
      - Smith's fracture
    - ◆ 813.42 Other fractures of distal end of radius (alone)
      - Dupuytren's fracture, radius
      - Radius, lower end
    - 813.43 Distal end of ulna (alone)
      - Ulna: Ulna:
        head   lower epiphysis
        lower end   styloid process
    - 813.44 Radius with ulna, lower end
  - ● 813.5 Lower end, open
    - ◆ 813.50 Lower end of forearm, unspecified
    - 813.51 Colles' fracture
    - ◆ 813.52 Other fractures of distal end of radius (alone)
    - 813.53 Distal end of ulna (alone)
    - 813.54 Radius with ulna, lower end
  - ● 813.8 Unspecified part, closed
    - ◆ 813.80 Forearm, unspecified
    - ◆ 813.81 Radius (alone)
    - ◆ 813.82 Ulna (alone)
    - ◆ 813.83 Radius with ulna
  - ● 813.9 Unspecified part, open
    - ◆ 813.90 Forearm, unspecified
    - ◆ 813.91 Radius (alone)
    - ◆ 813.92 Ulna (alone)
    - ◆ 813.93 Radius with ulna
- **814 Fracture of carpal bone(s)**
  - The following fifth-digit subclassification is for use with category 814:
    - ◆ 0 carpal bone, unspecified
      - Wrist NOS
    - 1 navicular [scaphoid] of wrist
    - 2 lunate [semilunar] bone of wrist
    - 3 triquetral [cuneiform] bone of wrist
    - 4 pisiform
    - 5 trapezium bone [larger multangular]
    - 6 trapezoid bone [smaller multangular]
    - 7 capitate bone [os magnum]
    - 8 hamate [unciform] bone
    - ◆ 9 other
  - ● 814.0 Closed
  - ● 814.1 Open

● Additional digits required   ◆ Nonspecific code   ■ Not a primary diagnosis

- **815 Fracture of metacarpal bone(s)**
  - INCLUDES: hand [except finger]
  - metacarpus
  - The following fifth-digit subclassification is for use with category 815:
    - 0 metacarpal bone(s), site unspecified
    - 1 base of thumb [first] metacarpal
      - Bennett's fracture
    - 2 base of other metacarpal bone(s)
    - 3 shaft of metacarpal bone(s)
    - 4 neck of metacarpal bone(s)
    - 9 multiple sites of metacarpus
  - 815.0 Closed
  - 815.1 Open
- **816 Fracture of one or more phalanges of hand**
  - INCLUDES: finger(s) thumb
  - The following fifth-digit subclassification is for use with category 816:
    - 0 phalanx or phalanges, unspecified
    - 1 middle or proximal phalanx or phalanges
    - 2 distal phalanx or phalanges
    - 3 multiple sites
  - 816.0 Closed
  - 816.1 Open
- **817 Multiple fractures of hand bones**
  - INCLUDES: metacarpal bone(s) with phalanx or phalanges of same hand
  - 817.0 Closed
  - 817.1 Open
- **818 Ill-defined fractures of upper limb**
  - INCLUDES: arm NOS
  - multiple bones of same upper limb
  - EXCLUDES: multiple fractures of:
    - metacarpal bone(s) with phalanx or phalanges (817.0-817.1)
    - phalanges of hand alone (816.0-816.1)
    - radius with ulna (813.0-813.9)
  - 818.0 Closed
  - 818.1 Open
- **819 Multiple fractures involving both upper limbs, and upper limb with rib(s) and sternum**
  - INCLUDES: arm(s) with rib(s) or sternum
  - both arms [any bones]
  - 819.0 Closed
  - 819.1 Open

FRACTURE OF LOWER LIMB (820-829)

- **820 Fracture of neck of femur**
  - 820.0 Transcervical fracture, closed
    - 820.00 Intracapsular section, unspecified
    - 820.01 Epiphysis (separation) (upper)
      - Transepiphyseal
    - 820.02 Midcervical section
      - Transcervical NOS
    - 820.03 Base of neck
      - Cervicotrochanteric section
    - 820.09 Other
      - Head of femur   Subcapital
  - 820.1 Transcervical fracture, open
    - 820.10 Intracapsular section, unspecified
    - 820.11 Epiphysis (separation) (upper)
    - 820.12 Midcervical section
    - 820.13 Base of neck
    - 820.19 Other
  - 820.2 Pertrochanteric fracture, closed
    - 820.20 Trochanteric section, unspecified
      - Trochanter: Trochanter:
      - NOS   lesser
      - greater
    - 820.21 Intertrochanteric section
    - 820.22 Subtrochanteric section
  - 820.3 Pertrochanteric fracture, open
    - 820.30 Trochanteric section, unspecified
    - 820.31 Intertrochanteric section
    - 820.32 Subtrochanteric section
  - 820.8 Unspecified part of neck of femur, closed
    - Hip NOS   Neck of femur NOS
  - 820.9 Unspecified part of neck of femur, open
- **821 Fracture of other and unspecified parts of femur**
  - 821.0 Shaft or unspecified part, closed
    - 821.00 Unspecified part of femur
      - Thigh   Upper leg
      - EXCLUDES: hip NOS (820.8)
    - 821.01 Shaft
  - 821.1 Shaft or unspecified part, open
    - 821.10 Unspecified part of femur
    - 821.11 Shaft
  - 821.2 Lower end, closed
    - Distal end
    - 821.20 Lower end, unspecified part
    - 821.21 Condyle, femoral
    - 821.22 Epiphysis, lower (separation)
    - 821.23 Supracondylar fracture of femur
      - Multiple fractures of lower end
    - 821.29 Other
      - Multiple fractures of lower end
  - 821.3 Lower end, open
    - 821.30 Lower end, unspecified part
    - 821.31 Condyle, femoral
    - 821.32 Epiphysis, lower (separation)
    - 821.33 Supracondylar fracture of femur
    - 821.39 Other
- **822 Fracture of patella**
  - 822.0 Closed
  - 822.1 Open
- **823 Fracture of tibia and fibula**
  - EXCLUDES: Dupuytren's fracture (824.4-824.5)
    - ankle (824.4-824.5)
    - radius (813.42, 813.52)
    - Pott's fracture (824.4-824.5)
    - that involving ankle (824.0-824.9)
  - The following fifth-digit subclassification is for use with category 823:
    - 0 tibia alone
    - 1 fibula alone
    - 2 fibula with tibia
  - 823.0 Upper end, closed
    - Head   Tibia:
    - Proximal end   condyles
    -     tuberosity
  - 823.1 Upper end, open
  - 823.2 Shaft, closed
  - 823.3 Shaft, open
  - 823.8 Unspecified part, closed
    - Lower leg NOS
  - 823.9 Unspecified part, open
- **824 Fracture of ankle**
  - 824.0 Medial malleolus, closed
    - Tibia involving:
      - ankle
      - malleolus
  - 824.1 Medial malleolus, open
  - 824.2 Lateral malleolus, closed
    - Fibula involving:
      - ankle
      - malleolus
  - 824.3 Lateral malleolus, open
  - 824.4 Bimalleolar, closed
    - Dupuytren's fracture, fibula
    - Pott's fracture
  - 824.5 Bimalleolar, open
  - 824.6 Trimalleolar, closed
    - Lateral and medial malleolus with anterior or posterior lip of tibia
  - 824.7 Trimalleolar, open
  - 824.8 Unspecified, closed
    - Ankle NOS
  - 824.9 Unspecified, open
- **825 Fracture of one or more tarsal and metatarsal bones**
  - 825.0 Fracture of calcaneus, closed
    - Heel bone
    - Os calcis
  - 825.1 Fracture of calcaneus, open
  - 825.2 Fracture of other tarsal and metatarsal bones, closed
    - 825.20 Unspecified bone(s) of foot [except toes]
      - Instep
    - 825.21 Astragalus
      - Talus

INJURY AND POISONING

- 825.22 Navicular [scaphoid], foot
- 825.23 Cuboid
- 825.24 Cuneiform, foot
- 825.25 Metatarsal bone(s)
- ◆ 825.29 Other
  - Tarsal with metatarsal bone(s) only
  - **EXCLUDES** calcaneus (825.0)
- ● 825.3 Fracture of other tarsal and metatarsal bones, open
  - 825.30 Unspecified bone(s) of foot [except toes]
  - 825.31 Astragalus
  - 825.32 Navicular [scaphoid], foot
  - 825.33 Cuboid
  - 825.34 Cuneiform, foot
  - 825.35 Metatarsal bone(s)
  - ◆ 825.39 Other
- ● 826 Fracture of one or more phalanges of foot
  - **INCLUDES** toe(s)
  - 826.0 Closed
  - 826.1 Open
- ● 827 Other, multiple, and ill-defined fractures of lower limb
  - **INCLUDES** leg NOS
  - multiple bones of same lower limb
  - **EXCLUDES** multiple fractures of:
    - ankle bones alone (824.4-824.9)
    - phalanges of foot alone (826.0-826.1)
    - tarsal with metatarsal bones (825.29, 825.39)
    - tibia with fibula (823.0-823.9 with fifth-digit 2)
  - 827.0 Closed
  - 827.1 Open
- ● 828 Multiple fractures involving both lower limbs, lower with upper limb, and lower limb(s) with rib(s) and sternum
  - **INCLUDES** arm(s) with leg(s) [any bones]
  - both legs [any bones]
  - leg(s) with rib(s) or sternum
  - 828.0 Closed
  - 828.1 Open
- ● 829 Fracture of unspecified bones
  - ◆ 829.0 Unspecified bone, closed
  - ◆ 829.1 Unspecified bone, open

DISLOCATION (830-839)

INCLUDES displacement
subluxation

EXCLUDES congenital dislocation (754.0-755.8)
pathological dislocation (718.2)
recurrent dislocation (718.3)

The descriptions "closed" and "open," used in the fourth-digit subdivisions, include the following terms:

closed:
complete
dislocation NOS
partial
simple
uncomplicated

open:
compound
infected
with foreign body

A dislocation not indicated as closed or open should be classified as closed.

- ● 830 Dislocation of jaw
  - **INCLUDES** jaw (cartilage) (meniscus)
  - mandible
  - maxilla (inferior)
  - temporomandibular (joint)
  - 830.0 Closed dislocation
  - 830.1 Open dislocation
- ● 831 Dislocation of shoulder
  - **EXCLUDES** sternoclavicular joint (839.61, 839.71)
  - sternum (839.61, 839.71)
  - The following fifth-digit subclassification is for use with category 831:
    - ◆ 0 shoulder, unspecified
      - Humerus NOS
    - 1 anterior dislocation of humerus
    - 2 posterior dislocation of humerus
    - 3 inferior dislocation of humerus
    - 4 acromioclavicular (joint)
      - Clavicle
    - ◆ 9 other
      - Scapula
  - ● 831.0 Closed dislocation
  - 831.1 Open dislocation
- ● 832 Dislocation of elbow
  - The following fifth-digit subclassification is for use with category 832:
    - ◆ 0 elbow unspecified
    - 1 anterior dislocation of elbow
    - 2 posterior dislocation of elbow
    - 3 medial dislocation of elbow
    - 4 lateral dislocation of elbow
    - ◆ 9 other
  - ● 832.0 Closed dislocation
  - ● 832.1 Open dislocation
- ● 833 Dislocation of wrist
  - The following fifth-digit subclassification is for use with category 833:
    - ◆ 0 wrist, unspecified part
      - Carpal (bone)
      - Radius, distal end
    - 1 radioulnar (joint), distal
    - 2 radiocarpal (joint)
    - 3 midcarpal (joint)
    - 4 carpometacarpal (joint)
    - 5 metacarpal (bone), proximal end
    - ◆ 9 other
      - Ulna, distal end
  - ● 833.0 Closed dislocation
  - ● 833.1 Open dislocation
- ● 834 Dislocation of finger
  - **INCLUDES** finger(s)
  - phalanx of hand
  - thumb
  - The following fifth-digit subclassification is for use with category 834:
    - ◆ 0 finger, unspecified part
    - 1 metacarpophalangeal (joint)
      - Metacarpal (bone), distal end
    - 2 interphalangeal (joint), hand
  - ● 834.0 Closed dislocation
  - ● 834.1 Open dislocation
- ● 835 Dislocation of hip
  - The following fifth-digit subclassification is for use with category 835:
    - ◆ 0 dislocation of hip, unspecified
    - 1 posterior dislocation
    - 2 obturator dislocation
    - ◆ 3 other anterior dislocation
  - ● 835.0 Closed dislocation
  - ● 835.1 Open dislocation
- ● 836 Dislocation of knee
  - **EXCLUDES** dislocation of knee:
    - old or pathological (718.2)
    - recurrent (718.3)
    - internal derangement of knee joint (717.0-717.5, 717.8-717.9)
    - old tear of cartilage or meniscus of knee (717.0-717.5, 717.8-717.9)
  - 836.0 Tear of medial cartilage or meniscus of knee, current
    - Bucket handle tear:
      - NOS } current injury
      - medial meniscus
  - 836.1 Tear of lateral cartilage or meniscus of knee, current
  - ◆ 836.2 Other tear of cartilage or meniscus of knee, current
    - Tear of:
      - cartilage (semilunar) } current injury, not specified as
      - meniscus } medial or lateral
  - 836.3 Dislocation of patella, closed
  - 836.4 Dislocation of patella, open
  - ● 836.5 Other dislocation of knee, closed
    - ◆ 836.50 Dislocation of knee, unspecified
    - 836.51 Anterior dislocation of tibia, proximal end
      - Posterior dislocation of femur, distal end
    - 836.52 Posterior dislocation of tibia, proximal end
      - Anterior dislocation of femur, distal end
    - 836.53 Medial dislocation of tibia, proximal end
    - 836.54 Lateral dislocation of tibia, proximal end
    - ◆ 836.59 Other
  - ● 836.6 Other dislocation of knee, open
    - ◆ 836.60 Dislocation of knee, unspecified
    - 836.61 Anterior dislocation of tibia, proximal end

● Additional digits required   ◆ Nonspecific code   ■ Not a primary diagnosis

- **836.62** Posterior dislocation of tibia, proximal end
- **836.63** Medial dislocation of tibia, proximal end
- **836.64** Lateral dislocation of tibia, proximal end
- ◆ **836.69** Other

● **837 Dislocation of ankle**
   INCLUDES: astragalus
   fibula, distal end
   navicular, foot
   scaphoid, foot
   tibia, distal end
   - **837.0** Closed dislocation
   - **837.1** Open dislocation

● **838 Dislocation of foot**
   The following fifth-digit subclassification is for use with category 838:
   - ◆ 0 foot, unspecified
   - 1 tarsal (bone), joint unspecified
   - 2 midtarsal (joint)
   - 3 tarsometatarsal (joint)
   - 4 metatarsal (bone), joint unspecified
   - 5 metatarsophalangeal (joint)
   - 6 interphalangeal (joint), foot
   - ◆ 9 other
      Phalanx of foot
      Toe(s)
   - ● **838.0** Closed dislocation
   - ● **838.1** Open dislocation

● **839 Other, multiple, and ill-defined dislocations**
   - ● **839.0** Cervical vertebra, closed
      Cervical spine
      Neck
      - ◆ **839.00** Cervical vertebra, unspecified
      - **839.01** First cervical vertebra
      - **839.02** Second cervical vertebra
      - **839.03** Third cervical vertebra
      - **839.04** Fourth cervical vertebra
      - **839.05** Fifth cervical vertebra
      - **839.06** Sixth cervical vertebra
      - **839.07** Seventh cervical vertebra
      - ◆ **839.08** Multiple cervical vertebrae
   - ● **839.1** Cervical vertebra, open
      - ◆ **839.10** Cervical vertebra, unspecified
      - **839.11** First cervical vertebra
      - **839.12** Second cervical vertebra
      - **839.13** Third cervical vertebra
      - **839.14** Fourth cervical vertebra
      - **839.15** Fifth cervical vertebra
      - **839.16** Sixth cervical vertebra
      - **839.17** Seventh cervical vertebra
      - ◆ **839.18** Multiple cervical vertebrae
   - ● **839.2** Thoracic and lumbar vertebra, closed
      - **839.20** Lumbar vertebra
      - **839.21** Thoracic vertebra
         Dorsal [thoracic] vertebra
   - ● **839.3** Thoracic and lumbar vertebra, open
      - **839.30** Lumbar vertebra
      - **839.31** Thoracic vertebra
   - ● **839.4** Other vertebra, closed
      - ◆ **839.40** Vertebra, unspecified site
         Spine NOS
      - **839.41** Coccyx
      - **839.42** Sacrum
         Sacroiliac (joint)
      - ◆ **839.49** Other
   - ● **839.5** Other vertebra, open
      - ◆ **839.50** Vertebra, unspecified site
      - **839.51** Coccyx
      - **839.52** Sacrum
      - ◆ **839.59** Other
   - ● **839.6** Other location, closed
      - **839.61** Sternum
         Sternoclavicular joint
      - ◆ **839.69** Other
         Pelvis
   - ● **839.7** Other location, open
      - **839.71** Sternum
      - ◆ **839.79** Other

- ◆ **839.8** Multiple and ill-defined, closed
   Arm
   Back
   Hand
   Multiple locations, except fingers or toes alone
   Other ill-defined locations
   Unspecified location
- ◆ **839.9** Multiple and ill-defined, open

SPRAINS AND STRAINS OF JOINTS AND ADJACENT MUSCLES (840-848)

INCLUDES: avulsion
hemarthrosis
laceration   of:
rupture   joint capsule
sprain   ligament
strain   muscle
tear   tendon

EXCLUDES: laceration of tendon in open wounds (880-884 and 890-894 with .2)

● **840 Sprains and strains of shoulder and upper arm**
   - **840.0** Acromioclavicular (joint) (ligament)
   - **840.1** Coracoclavicular (ligament)
   - **840.2** Coracohumeral (ligament)
   - **840.3** Infraspinatus (muscle) (tendon)
   - **840.4** Rotator cuff (capsule)
   - **840.5** Subscapularis (muscle)
   - **840.6** Supraspinatus (muscle) (tendon)
   - ◆ **840.8** Other specified sites of shoulder and upper arm
   - ◆ **840.9** Unspecified site of shoulder and upper arm
      Arm NOS
      Shoulder NOS

● **841 Sprains and strains of elbow and forearm**
   - **841.0** Radial collateral ligament
   - **841.1** Ulnar collateral ligament
   - **841.2** Radiohumeral (joint)
   - **841.3** Ulnohumeral (joint)
   - ◆ **841.8** Other specified sites of elbow and forearm
   - ◆ **841.9** Unspecified site of elbow and forearm
      Elbow NOS

● **842 Sprains and strains of wrist and hand**
   - ● **842.0** Wrist
      - ◆ **842.00** Unspecified site
      - **842.01** Carpal (joint)
      - **842.02** Radiocarpal (joint) (ligament)
      - ◆ **842.09** Other
         Radioulnar joint, distal
   - ● **842.1** Hand
      - ◆ **842.10** Unspecified site
      - **842.11** Carpometacarpal (joint)
      - **842.12** Metacarpophalangeal (joint)
      - **842.13** Interphalangeal (joint)
      - ◆ **842.19** Other
         Midcarpal (joint)

● **843 Sprains and strains of hip and thigh**
   - **843.0** Iliofemoral (ligament)
   - **843.1** Ischiocapsular (ligament)
   - ◆ **843.8** Other specified sites of hip and thigh
   - ◆ **843.9** Unspecified site of hip and thigh
      Hip NOS
      Thigh NOS

● **844 Sprains and strains of knee and leg**
   EXCLUDES: current tear of cartilage or meniscus of knee (836.0-836.2)
   old tear of cartilage or meniscus of knee (717.0-717.5, 717.8-717.9)
   - **844.0** Lateral collateral ligament of knee
   - **844.1** Medial collateral ligament of knee
   - **844.2** Cruciate ligament of knee
   - **844.3** Tibiofibular (joint) (ligament), superior
   - ◆ **844.8** Other specified sites of knee and leg
   - ◆ **844.9** Unspecified site of knee and leg
      Knee NOS
      Leg NOS

- **845 Sprains and strains of ankle and foot**
  - **845.0 Ankle**
    - ◆ 845.00 Unspecified site
    - 845.01 Deltoid (ligament), ankle
      - Internal collateral (ligament), ankle
    - 845.02 Calcaneofibular (ligament)
    - 845.03 Tibiofibular (ligament), distal
    - ◆ 845.09 Other
      - Achilles tendon
  - **845.1 Foot**
    - ◆ 845.10 Unspecified site
    - 845.11 Tarsometatarsal (joint) (ligament)
    - 845.12 Metatarsophalangeal (joint)
    - 845.13 Interphalangeal (joint), toe
    - ◆ 845.19 Other
- **846 Sprains and strains of sacroiliac region**
  - 846.0 Lumbosacral (joint) (ligament)
  - 846.1 Sacroiliac ligament
  - 846.2 Sacrospinatus (ligament)
  - 846.3 Sacrotuberous (ligament)
  - ◆ 846.8 Other specified sites of sacroiliac region
  - ◆ 846.9 Unspecified site of sacroiliac region
- **847 Sprains and strains of other and unspecified parts of back**
  - EXCLUDES *lumbosacral (846.0)*
  - 847.0 Neck
    - Anterior longitudinal (ligament), cervical
    - Atlanto-axial (joints)
    - Atlanto-occipital (joints)
    - Whiplash injury
    - EXCLUDES *neck injury NOS (959.0)*
    - *thyroid region (848.2)*
  - 847.1 Thoracic
  - 847.2 Lumbar
  - 847.3 Sacrum
    - Sacrococcygeal (ligament)
  - 847.4 Coccyx
  - ◆ 847.9 Unspecified site of back
    - Back NOS
- **848 Other and ill-defined sprains and strains**
  - 848.0 Septal cartilage of nose
  - 848.1 Jaw
    - Temporomandibular (joint) (ligament)
  - 848.2 Thyroid region
    - Cricoarytenoid (joint) (ligament)
    - Cricothyroid (joint) (ligament)
    - Thyroid cartilage
  - 848.3 Ribs
    - INCLUDES Chondrocostal (joint) | without mention of
    - Costal cartilage | injury to sternum
  - **848.4 Sternum**
    - ◆ 848.40 Unspecified site
    - 848.41 Sternoclavicular (joint) (ligament)
    - 848.42 Chondrosternal (joint)
    - ◆ 848.49 Other
      - Xiphoid cartilage
  - 848.5 Pelvis
    - Symphysis pubis
    - EXCLUDES *that in childbirth (665.6)*
  - ◆ 848.8 Other specified sites of sprains and strains
  - ◆ 848.9 Unspecified site of sprain and strain

INTRACRANIAL INJURY, EXCLUDING THOSE WITH SKULL FRACTURE (850-854)

EXCLUDES *intracranial injury with skull fracture (800-801 and 803-804, except .0 and .5)*
nerve injury (950.0-951.9)
open wound of head without intracranial injury (870.0-873.9)
skull fracture alone (800-801 and 803-804 with .0, .5)

The description "with open intracranial wound," used in the fourth-digit subdivisions, includes those specified as open or with mention of infection or foreign body.

The following fifth-digit subclassification is for use with categories 851-854:
- ◆ 0 unspecified state of consciousness
- 1 with no loss of consciousness
- 2 with brief [less than one hour] loss of consciousness
- 3 with moderate [1-24 hours] loss of consciousness
- 4 with prolonged [more than 24 hours] loss of consciousness and return to pre-existing conscious level
- 5 with prolonged [more than 24 hours] loss of consciousness, without return to pre-existing conscious level
- ◆ 6 with loss of consciousness of unspecified duration
- ◆ 9 with concussion, unspecified

- **850 Concussion**
  - INCLUDES commotio cerebri
  - EXCLUDES concussion with:
    - cerebral laceration or contusion (851.0-851.9)
    - cerebral hemorrhage (852-853)
    - head injury NOS (854)
  - 850.0 With no loss of consciousness
    - Concussion with mental confusion or disorientation, without loss of consciousness
  - 850.1 With brief loss of consciousness
    - Loss of consciousness for less than one hour
  - 850.2 With moderate loss of consciousness
    - Loss of consciousness for 1-24 hours
  - 850.3 With prolonged loss of consciousness and return to pre-existing conscious level
    - Loss of consciousness for more than 24 hours with complete recovery
  - 850.4 With prolonged loss of consciousness, without return to pre-existing conscious level
  - ◆ 850.5 With loss of consciousness of unspecified duration
  - ◆ 850.9 Concussion, unspecified
- **851 Cerebral laceration and contusion**
  - ● 851.0 Cortex (cerebral) contusion without mention of open intracranial wound
  - ● 851.1 Cortex (cerebral) contusion with open intracranial wound
  - ● 851.2 Cortex (cerebral) laceration without mention of open intracranial wound
  - ● 851.3 Cortex (cerebral) laceration with open intracranial wound
  - ● 851.4 Cerebellar or brain stem contusion without mention of open intracranial wound
  - ● 851.5 Cerebellar or brain stem contusion with open intracranial wound
  - ● 851.6 Cerebellar or brain stem laceration without mention of open intracranial wound
  - ● 851.7 Cerebellar or brain stem laceration with open intracranial wound
  - ◆ ● 851.8 Other and unspecified cerebral laceration and contusion, without mention of open intracranial wound
    - Brain (membrane) NOS
  - ◆ ● 851.9 Other and unspecified cerebral laceration and contusion, with open intracranial wound
- **852 Subarachnoid, subdural, and extradural hemorrhage, following injury**
  - EXCLUDES *Cerebral contusion or laceration (with hemorrhage) (851.0-851.9)*
  - ● 852.0 Subarachnoid hemorrhage following injury without mention of open intracranial wound
    - Middle meningeal hemorrhage following injury
  - ● 852.1 Subarachnoid hemorrhage following injury with open intracranial wound
  - ● 852.2 Subdural hemorrhage following injury without mention of open intracranial wound
  - ● 852.3 Subdural hemorrhage following injury with open intracranial wound
  - ● 852.4 Extradural hemorrhage following injury without mention of open intracranial wound
    - Epidural hematoma following injury
  - ● 852.5 Extradural hemorrhage following injury with open intracranial wound
- **853 Other and unspecified intracranial hemorrhage following injury**
  - ◆ ● 853.0 Without mention of open intracranial wound
    - Cerebral compression due to injury
    - Intracranial hematoma following injury
    - Traumatic cerebral hemorrhage
  - ◆ ● 853.1 With open intracranial wound

- **854 Intracranial injury of other and unspecified nature**
  INCLUDES: brain injury NOS
  head injury NOS
  - ◆● 854.0 Without mention of open intracranial wound
  - ◆● 854.1 With open intracranial wound

INTERNAL INJURY OF THORAX, ABDOMEN, AND PELVIS (860-869)

INCLUDES: blast injuries
blunt trauma
bruise
concussion injuries (except cerebral)
crushing
hematoma
laceration
puncture
tear
traumatic rupture
} of internal organs

EXCLUDES: concussion NOS (850.0-850.9)
flail chest (807.4)
foreign body entering through orifice (930.0-939.9)
injury to blood vessels (901.0-902.9)

The description "with open wound", used in the fourth-digit subdivisions, includes those with mention of infection or foreign body.

- **● 860 Traumatic pneumothorax and hemothorax**
  - 860.0 Pneumothorax without mention of open wound into thorax
  - 860.1 Pneumothorax with open wound into thorax
  - 860.2 Hemothorax without mention of open wound into thorax
  - 860.3 Hemothorax with open wound into thorax
  - 860.4 Pneumohemothorax without mention of open wound into thorax
  - 860.5 Pneumohemothorax with open wound into thorax
- **● 861 Injury to heart and lung**
  EXCLUDES: injury to blood vessels of thorax (901.0-901.9)
  - ● 861.0 Heart, without mention of open wound into thorax
    - ◆ 861.00 Unspecified injury
    - 861.01 Contusion
      Cardiac contusion   Myocardial contusion
    - 861.02 Laceration without penetration of heart chambers
    - 861.03 Laceration with penetration of heart chambers
  - ● 861.1 Heart, with open wound into thorax
    - ◆ 861.10 Unspecified injury
    - 861.11 Contusion
    - 861.12 Laceration without penetration of heart chambers
    - 861.13 Laceration with penetration of heart chambers
  - ● 861.2 Lung, without mention of open wound into thorax
    - ◆ 861.20 Unspecified injury
    - 861.21 Contusion
    - 861.22 Laceration
  - ● 861.3 Lung, with open wound into thorax
    - ◆ 861.30 Unspecified injury
    - 861.31 Contusion
    - 861.32 Laceration
- **● 862 Injury to other and unspecified intrathoracic organs**
  EXCLUDES: injury to blood vessels of thorax (901.0-901.9)
  - 862.0 Diaphragm, without mention of open wound into cavity
  - 862.1 Diaphragm, with open wound into cavity
  - ● 862.2 Other specified intrathoracic organs, without mention of open wound into cavity
    - 862.21 Bronchus
    - 862.22 Esophagus
    - ◆ 862.29 Other
      Pleura   Thymus gland
  - ● 862.3 Other specified intrathoracic organs, with open wound into cavity
    - 862.31 Bronchus
    - 862.32 Esophagus
    - ◆ 862.39 Other
  - ◆ 862.8 Multiple and unspecified intrathoracic organs, without mention of open wound into cavity
    Crushed chest
    Multiple intrathoracic organs
  - ◆ 862.9 Multiple and unspecified intrathoracic organs, with open wound into cavity

- **● 863 Injury to gastrointestinal tract**
  EXCLUDES: anal sphincter laceration during delivery (664.2)
  bile duct (868.0-868.1 with fifth-digit 2)
  gallbladder (868.0-868.1 with fifth-digit 2)
  - 863.0 Stomach, without mention of open wound into cavity
  - 863.1 Stomach, with open wound into cavity
  - ● 863.2 Small intestine, without mention of open wound into cavity
    - ◆ 863.20 Small intestine, unspecified site
    - 863.21 Duodenum
    - ◆ 863.29 Other
  - ● 863.3 Small intestine, with open wound into cavity
    - ◆ 863.30 Small intestine, unspecified site
    - 863.31 Duodenum
    - ◆ 863.39 Other
  - ● 863.4 Colon or rectum, without mention of open wound into cavity
    - ◆ 863.40 Colon, unspecified site
    - 863.41 Ascending [right] colon
    - 863.42 Transverse colon
    - 863.43 Descending [left] colon
    - 863.44 Sigmoid colon
    - 863.45 Rectum
    - ◆ 863.46 Multiple sites in colon and rectum
    - ◆ 863.49 Other
  - ● 863.5 Colon or rectum, with open wound into cavity
    - ◆ 863.50 Colon, unspecified site
    - 863.51 Ascending [right] colon
    - 863.52 Transverse colon
    - 863.53 Descending [left] colon
    - 863.54 Sigmoid colon
    - 863.55 Rectum
    - ◆ 863.56 Multiple sites in colon and rectum
    - ◆ 863.59 Other
  - ● 863.8 Other and unspecified gastrointestinal sites, without mention of open wound into cavity
    - ◆ 863.80 Gastrointestinal tract, unspecified site
    - 863.81 Pancreas, head
    - 863.82 Pancreas, body
    - 863.83 Pancreas, tail
    - ◆ 863.84 Pancreas, multiple and unspecified sites
    - 863.85 Appendix
    - ◆ 863.89 Other
      Intestine NOS
  - ● 863.9 Other and unspecified gastrointestinal sites, with open wound into cavity
    - ◆ 863.90 Gastrointestinal tract, unspecified site
    - 863.91 Pancreas, head
    - 863.92 Pancreas, body
    - 863.93 Pancreas, tail
    - ◆ 863.94 Pancreas, multiple and unspecified sites
    - 863.95 Appendix
    - ◆ 863.99 Other
- **● 864 Injury to liver**
  The following fifth-digit subclassification is for use with category 864:
  - ◆ 0 unspecified injury
  - 1 hematoma and contusion
  - 2 laceration, minor
    Laceration involving capsule only, or without significant involvement of hepatic parenchyma [i.e., less than 1 cm deep]
  - 3 laceration, moderate
    Laceration involving parenchyma but without major disruption of parenchyma [i.e., less than 10 cm long and less than 3 cm deep]
  - 4 laceration, major
    Laceration with significant disruption of hepatic parenchyma [i.e., 10 cm long and 3 cm deep]
    Multiple moderate lacerations, with or without hematoma
    Stellate lacerations of liver
  - ◆ 5 laceration, unspecified
  - ◆ 9 other
  - ● 864.0 Without mention of open wound into cavity
  - ● 864.1 With open wound into cavity

INJURY AND POISONING

- **865 Injury to spleen**

  The following fifth-digit subclassification is for use with category 865:
  - ◆ 0 unspecified injury
  - 1 hematoma without rupture of capsule
  - 2 capsular tears, without major disruption of parenchyma
  - 3 laceration extending into parenchyma
  - 4 massive parenchymal disruption
  - ◆ 9 other

  - ● 865.0 Without mention of open wound into cavity
  - ● 865.1 With open wound into cavity

- **866 Injury to kidney**

  The following fifth-digit subclassification is for use with category 866:
  - ◆ 0 unspecified injury
  - 1 hematoma without rupture of capsule
  - 2 laceration
  - 3 complete disruption of kidney parenchyma

  - ● 866.0 Without mention of open wound into cavity
  - ● 866.1 With open wound into cavity

- **867 Injury to pelvic organs**

  EXCLUDES injury during delivery (664.0-665.9)

  - 867.0 Bladder and urethra, without mention of open wound into cavity
  - 867.1 Bladder and urethra, with open wound into cavity
  - 867.2 Ureter, without mention of open wound into cavity
  - 867.3 Ureter, with open wound into cavity
  - 867.4 Uterus, without mention of open wound into cavity
  - 867.5 Uterus, with open wound into cavity
  - ◆ 867.6 Other specified pelvic organs, without mention of open wound into cavity

    Fallopian tube   Seminal vesicle
    Ovary   Vas deferens
    Prostate
  - ◆ 867.7 Other specified pelvic organs, with open wound into cavity
  - ◆ 867.8 Unspecified pelvic organ, without mention of open wound into cavity
  - ◆ 867.9 Unspecified pelvic organ, with open wound into cavity

- **868 Injury to other intra-abdominal organs**

  The following fifth-digit subclassification is for use with category 868:
  - ◆ 0 unspecified intra-abdominal organ
  - 1 adrenal gland
  - 2 bile duct and gallbladder
  - 3 peritoneum
  - 4 retroperitoneum
  - ◆ 9 other and multiple intra-abdominal organs

  - ● 868.0 Without mention of open wound into cavity
  - ● 868.1 With open wound into cavity

- **869 Internal injury to unspecified or ill-defined organs**

  INCLUDES internal injury NOS
            multiple internal injury NOS

  - ◆ 869.0 Without mention of open wound into cavity
  - ◆ 869.1 With open wound into cavity

OPEN WOUND (870-897)

INCLUDES animal bite
          avulsion
          cut
          laceration
          puncture wound
          traumatic amputation

EXCLUDES burn (940.0-949.5)
          crushing (925-929.9)
          puncture of internal organs (860.0-869.1)
          superficial injury (910.0-919.9)
          that incidental to:
              dislocation (830.0-839.9)
              fracture (800.0-829.1)
              internal injury (860.0-869.1)
              intracranial injury (851.0-854.1)

The description "complicated" used in the fourth-digit subdivisions includes those with mention of delayed healing, delayed treatment, foreign body, or major infection.

OPEN WOUND OF HEAD, NECK, AND TRUNK (870-879)

- **870 Open wound of ocular adnexa**
  - 870.0 Laceration of skin of eyelid and periocular area
  - 870.1 Laceration of eyelid, full-thickness, not involving lacrimal passages
  - 870.2 Laceration of eyelid involving lacrimal passages
  - 870.3 Penetrating wound of orbit, without mention of foreign body
  - 870.4 Penetrating wound of orbit with foreign body

    EXCLUDES retained (old) foreign body in orbit (376.6)
  - ◆ 870.8 Other specified open wounds of ocular adnexa
  - ◆ 870.9 Unspecified open wound of ocular adnexa

- **871 Open wound of eyeball**

  EXCLUDES 2nd cranial nerve [optic] injury (950.0-950.9)
            3rd cranial nerve [oculomotor] injury (951.0)

  - 871.0 Ocular laceration without prolapse of intraocular tissue
  - 871.1 Ocular laceration with prolapse or exposure of intraocular tissue
  - 871.2 Rupture of eye with partial loss of intraocular tissue
  - 871.3 Avulsion of eye

    Traumatic enucleation
  - ◆ 871.4 Unspecified laceration of eye
  - 871.5 Penetration of eyeball with magnetic foreign body

    EXCLUDES retained (old) magnetic foreign body in globe (360.50-360.59)
  - 871.6 Penetration of eyeball with (nonmagnetic) foreign body

    EXCLUDES retained (old) (nonmagnetic) foreign body in globe (360.60-360.69)
  - ◆ 871.7 Unspecified ocular penetration
  - ◆ 871.9 Unspecified open wound of eyeball

- **872 Open wound of ear**
  - ● 872.0 External ear, without mention of complication
    - ◆ 872.00 External ear, unspecified site
    - 872.01 Auricle, ear

      Pinna
    - 872.02 Auditory canal
  - ● 872.1 External ear, complicated
    - ◆ 872.10 External ear, unspecified site
    - 872.11 Auricle, ear
    - 872.12 Auditory canal
  - 872.6 Other specified parts of ear, without mention of complication
    - 872.61 Ear drum

      Drumhead   Tympanic membrane
    - 872.62 Ossicles
    - 872.63 Eustachian tube
    - 872.64 Cochlea
    - ◆ 872.69 Other and multiple sites
  - ● 872.7 Other specified parts of ear, complicated
    - 872.71 Ear drum
    - 872.72 Ossicles
    - 872.73 Eustachian tube
    - 872.74 Cochlea
    - ◆ 872.79 Other and multiple sites
  - ◆ 872.8 Ear, part unspecified, without mention of complication

    Ear NOS
  - ◆ 872.9 Ear, part unspecified, complicated

- **873 Other open wound of head**

  EXCLUDES that with mention of intracranial injury (851.0-854.1)

  - 873.0 Scalp, without mention of complication
  - 873.1 Scalp, complicated
  - ● 873.2 Nose, without mention of complication
    - ◆ 873.20 Nose, unspecified site
    - 873.21 Nasal septum
    - 873.22 Nasal cavity
    - 873.23 Nasal sinus
    - ◆ 873.29 Multiple sites
  - ● 873.3 Nose, complicated
    - ◆ 873.30 Nose, unspecified site
    - 873.31 Nasal septum
    - 873.32 Nasal cavity
    - 873.33 Nasal sinus
    - ◆ 873.39 Multiple sites
  - ● 873.4 Face, without mention of complication
    - ◆ 873.40 Face, unspecified site
    - 873.41 Cheek
    - 873.42 Forehead

      Eyebrow
    - 873.43 Lip
    - 873.44 Jaw
    - ◆ 873.49 Other and multiple sites
  - ● 873.5 Face, complicated
    - ◆ 873.50 Face, unspecified site
    - 873.51 Cheek

- 873.52 Forehead
- 873.53 Lip
- 873.54 Jaw
  - ◆ 873.59 Other and multiple sites
- ● 873.6 Internal structures of mouth, without mention of complication
  - ◆ 873.60 Mouth, unspecified site
  - 873.61 Buccal mucosa
  - 873.62 Gum (alveolar process)
  - 873.63 Tooth (broken)
  - 873.64 Tongue and floor of mouth
  - 873.65 Palate
  - ◆ 873.69 Other and multiple sites
- ● 873.7 Internal structures of mouth, complicated
  - ◆ 873.70 Mouth, unspecified site
  - 873.71 Buccal mucosa
  - 873.72 Gum (alveolar process)
  - 873.73 Tooth (broken)
  - 873.74 Tongue and floor of mouth
  - 873.75 Palate
  - ◆ 873.79 Other and multiple sites
- ◆ 873.8 Other and unspecified open wound of head without mention of complication
  - Head NOS
- ◆ 873.9 Other and unspecified open wound of head, complicated
- 874 Open wound of neck
  - ● 874.0 Larynx and trachea, without mention of complication
    - 874.00 Larynx with trachea
    - 874.01 Larynx
    - 874.02 Trachea
  - ● 874.1 Larynx and trachea, complicated
    - 874.10 Larynx with trachea
    - 874.11 Larynx
    - 874.12 Trachea
  - 874.2 Thyroid gland, without mention of complication
  - 874.3 Thyroid gland, complicated
  - 874.4 Pharynx, without mention of complication
    - Cervical esophagus
  - 874.5 Pharynx, complicated
  - ◆ 874.8 Other and unspecified parts, without mention of complication
    - Nape of neck   Throat NOS
    - Supraclavicular region
  - ◆ 874.9 Other and unspecified parts, complicated
- ● 875 Open wound of chest (wall)
  - EXCLUDES open wound into thoracic cavity (860.0-862.9)
    traumatic pneumothorax and hemothorax (860.1, 860.3, 860.5)
  - 875.0 Without mention of complication
  - 875.1 Complicated
- ● 876 Open wound of back
  - INCLUDES loin
    lumbar region
  - EXCLUDES open wound into thoracic cavity (860.0-862.9)
    traumatic pneumothorax and hemothorax (860.1, 860.3, 860.5)
  - 876.0 Without mention of complication
  - 876.1 Complicated
- ● 877 Open wound of buttock
  - INCLUDES sacroiliac region
  - 877.0 Without mention of complication
  - 877.1 Complicated
- ● 878 Open wound of genital organs (external), including traumatic amputation
  - EXCLUDES injury during delivery (664.0-665.9)
    internal genital organs (867.0-867.9)
  - 878.0 Penis, without mention of complication
  - 878.1 Penis, complicated
  - 878.2 Scrotum and testes, without mention of complication
  - 878.3 Scrotum and testes, complicated
  - 878.4 Vulva, without mention of complication
    - Labium (majus) (minus)
  - 878.5 Vulva, complicated
  - 878.6 Vagina, without mention of complication
  - 878.7 Vagina, complicated
  - ◆ 878.8 Other and unspecified parts, without mention of complication
  - ◆ 878.9 Other and unspecified parts, complicated

- ● 879 Open wound of other and unspecified sites, except limbs
  - 879.0 Breast, without mention of complication
  - 879.1 Breast, complicated
  - 879.2 Abdominal wall, anterior, without mention of complication
    - Abdominal wall NOS   Pubic region
    - Epigastric region   Umbilical region
    - Hypogastric region
  - 879.3 Abdominal wall, anterior, complicated
  - 879.4 Abdominal wall, lateral, without mention of complication
    - Flank   Iliac (region)
    - Groin   Inguinal region
    - Hypochondrium
  - 879.5 Abdominal wall, lateral, complicated
  - ◆ 879.6 Other and unspecified parts of trunk, without mention of complication
    - Pelvic region   Trunk NOS
    - Perineum
  - ◆ 879.7 Other and unspecified parts of trunk, complicated
  - ◆ 879.8 Open wound(s) (multiple) of unspecified site(s) without mention of complication
    - Multiple open wounds NOS   Open wound NOS
  - ◆ 879.9 Open wound(s) (multiple) of unspecified site(s), complicated

OPEN WOUND OF UPPER LIMB (880-887)

- ● 880 Open wound of shoulder and upper arm
  - The following fifth-digit subclassification is for use with category 880:
    - 0 shoulder region
    - 1 scapular region
    - 2 axillary region
    - 3 upper arm
    - ◆ 9 multiple sites
  - ● 880.0 Without mention of complication
  - ● 880.1 Complicated
  - ● 880.2 With tendon involvement
- ● 881 Open wound of elbow, forearm, and wrist
  - The following fifth-digit subclassification is for use with category 881:
    - 0 forearm
    - 1 elbow
    - 2 wrist
  - ● 881.0 Without mention of complication
  - ● 881.1 Complicated
  - ● 881.2 With tendon involvement
- ● 882 Open wound of hand except finger(s) alone
  - 882.0 Without mention of complication
  - 882.1 Complicated
  - 882.2 With tendon involvement
- ● 883 Open wound of finger(s)
  - INCLUDES fingernail
    thumb (nail)
  - 883.0 Without mention of complication
  - 883.1 Complicated
  - 883.2 With tendon involvement
- ● 884 Multiple and unspecified open wound of upper limb
  - INCLUDES arm NOS
    multiple sites of one upper limb
    upper limb NOS
  - ◆ 884.0 Without mention of complication
  - ◆ 884.1 Complicated
  - ◆ 884.2 With tendon involvement
- ● 885 Traumatic amputation of thumb (complete) (partial)
  - INCLUDES thumb(s) (with finger(s) of either hand)
  - 885.0 Without mention of complication
  - 885.1 Complicated
- ● 886 Traumatic amputation of other finger(s) (complete) (partial)
  - INCLUDES finger(s) of one or both hands, without mention of thumb(s)
  - 886.0 Without mention of complication
  - 886.1 Complicated
- ● 887 Traumatic amputation of arm and hand (complete) (partial)
  - 887.0 Unilateral, below elbow, without mention of complication
  - 887.1 Unilateral, below elbow, complicated
  - 887.2 Unilateral, at or above elbow, without mention of complication
  - 887.3 Unilateral, at or above elbow, complicated
  - ◆ 887.4 Unilateral, level not specified, without mention of complication
  - ◆ 887.5 Unilateral, level not specified, complicated

		887.6	Bilateral [any level], without mention of complication
			One hand and other arm
		887.7	Bilateral [any level], complicated

OPEN WOUND OF LOWER LIMB (890-897)

- **890** Open wound of hip and thigh
  - 890.0 Without mention of complication
  - 890.1 Complicated
  - 890.2 With tendon involvement
- **891** Open wound of knee, leg [except thigh], and ankle
  - **INCLUDES** leg NOS
    multiple sites of leg, except thigh
  - **EXCLUDES** that of thigh (890.0-890.2)
    with multiple sites of lower limb (894.0-894.2)
  - 891.0 Without mention of complication
  - 891.1 Complicated
  - 891.2 With tendon involvement
- **892** Open wound of foot except toe(s) alone
  - **INCLUDES** heel
  - 892.0 Without mention of complication
  - 892.1 Complicated
  - 892.2 With tendon involvement
- **893** Open wound of toe(s)
  - **INCLUDES** toenail
  - 893.0 Without mention of complication
  - 893.1 Complicated
  - 893.2 With tendon involvement
- **894** Multiple and unspecified open wound of lower limb
  - **INCLUDES** lower limb NOS
    multiple sites of one lower limb, with thigh
  - ◆ 894.0 Without mention of complication
  - ◆ 894.1 Complicated
  - ◆ 894.2 With tendon involvement
- **895** Traumatic amputation of toe(s) (complete) (partial)
  - **INCLUDES** toe(s) of one or both feet
  - 895.0 Without mention of complication
  - 895.1 Complicated
- **896** Traumatic amputation of foot (complete) (partial)
  - 896.0 Unilateral, without mention of complication
  - 896.1 Unilateral, complicated
  - 896.2 Bilateral, without mention of complication
    - **EXCLUDES** one foot and other leg (897.6-897.7)
  - 896.3 Bilateral, complicated
- **897** Traumatic amputation of leg(s) (complete) (partial)
  - 897.0 Unilateral, below knee, without mention of complication
  - 897.1 Unilateral, below knee, complicated
  - 897.2 Unilateral, at or above knee, without mention of complication
  - 897.3 Unilateral, at or above knee, complicated
  - ◆ 897.4 Unilateral, level not specified, without mention of complication
  - ◆ 897.5 Unilateral, level not specified, complicated
  - 897.6 Bilateral [any level], without mention of complication
    One foot and other leg
  - 897.7 Bilateral [any level], complicated

INJURY TO BLOOD VESSELS (900-904)

INCLUDES arterial hematoma, avulsion, cut, laceration, rupture, traumatic aneurysm or fistula (arteriovenous) } of blood vessel, secondary to other injuries e.g., fracture or open wound

EXCLUDES accidental puncture or laceration during medical procedure (998.2)
intracranial hemorrhage following injury (851.0-854.1)

- **900** Injury to blood vessels of head and neck
  - **900.0** Carotid artery
    - ◆ 900.00 Carotid artery, unspecified
    - 900.01 Common carotid artery
    - 900.02 External carotid artery
    - 900.03 Internal carotid artery
  - 900.1 Internal jugular vein
  - **900.8** Other specified blood vessels of head and neck
    - 900.81 External jugular vein
      Jugular vein NOS
    - ◆ 900.82 Multiple blood vessels of head and neck
    - ◆ 900.89 Other
  - ◆ 900.9 Unspecified blood vessel of head and neck
- **901** Injury to blood vessels of thorax
  - **EXCLUDES** traumatic hemothorax (860.2-860.5)
  - 901.0 Thoracic aorta
  - 901.1 Innominate and subclavian arteries
  - 901.2 Superior vena cava
  - 901.3 Innominate and subclavian veins
  - **901.4** Pulmonary blood vessels
    - ◆ 901.40 Pulmonary vessel(s), unspecified
    - 901.41 Pulmonary artery
    - 901.42 Pulmonary vein
  - **901.8** Other specified blood vessels of thorax
    - 901.81 Intercostal artery or vein
    - 901.82 Internal mammary artery or vein
    - 901.83 Multiple blood vessels of thorax
    - ◆ 901.89 Other
      Azygos vein   Hemiazygos vein
  - ◆ 901.9 Unspecified blood vessel of thorax
- **902** Injury to blood vessels of abdomen and pelvis
  - 902.0 Abdominal aorta
  - **902.1** Inferior vena cava
    - ◆ 902.10 Inferior vena cava, unspecified
    - 902.11 Hepatic veins
    - ◆ 902.19 Other
  - **902.2** Celiac and mesenteric arteries
    - ◆ 902.20 Celiac and mesenteric arteries, unspecified
    - 902.21 Gastric artery
    - 902.22 Hepatic artery
    - 902.23 Splenic artery
    - ◆ 902.24 Other specified branches of celiac axis
    - 902.25 Superior mesenteric artery (trunk)
    - 902.26 Primary branches of superior mesenteric artery
      Ileocolic artery
    - 902.27 Inferior mesenteric artery
    - ◆ 902.29 Other
  - **902.3** Portal and splenic veins
    - 902.31 Superior mesenteric vein and primary subdivisions
      Ileocolic vein
    - 902.32 Inferior mesenteric vein
    - 902.33 Portal vein
    - 902.34 Splenic vein
    - ◆ 902.39 Other
      Cystic vein   Gastric vein
  - **902.4** Renal blood vessels
    - ◆ 902.40 Renal vessel(s), unspecified
    - 902.41 Renal artery
    - 902.42 Renal vein
    - ◆ 902.49 Other
      Suprarenal arteries
  - **902.5** Iliac blood vessels
    - ◆ 902.50 Iliac vessel(s), unspecified
    - 902.51 Hypogastric artery
    - 902.52 Hypogastric vein
    - 902.53 Iliac artery
    - 902.54 Iliac vein
    - 902.55 Uterine artery
    - 902.56 Uterine vein
    - ◆ 902.59 Other
  - **902.8** Other specified blood vessels of abdomen and pelvis
    - 902.81 Ovarian artery
    - 902.82 Ovarian vein
    - 902.87 Multiple blood vessels of abdomen and pelvis
    - ◆ 902.89 Other
  - ◆ 902.9 Unspecified blood vessel of abdomen and pelvis
- **903** Injury to blood vessels of upper extremity
  - **903.0** Axillary blood vessels
    - ◆ 903.00 Axillary vessel(s), unspecified
    - 903.01 Axillary artery
    - 903.02 Axillary vein
  - 903.1 Brachial blood vessels
  - 903.2 Radial blood vessels
  - 903.3 Ulnar blood vessels
  - 903.4 Palmar artery
  - 903.5 Digital blood vessels

- 903.8 **Other specified blood vessels of upper extremity**
  Multiple blood vessels of upper extremity
- 903.9 **Unspecified blood vessel of upper extremity**
- 904 **Injury to blood vessels of lower extremity and unspecified sites**
  - 904.0 **Common femoral artery**
    Femoral artery above profunda origin
  - 904.1 **Superficial femoral artery**
  - 904.2 **Femoral veins**
  - 904.3 **Saphenous veins**
    Saphenous vein (greater) (lesser)
  - 904.4 **Popliteal blood vessels**
    - 904.40 Popliteal vessel(s), unspecified
    - 904.41 Popliteal artery
    - 904.42 Popliteal vein
  - 904.5 **Tibial blood vessels**
    - 904.50 Tibial vessel(s), unspecified
    - 904.51 Anterior tibial artery
    - 904.52 Anterior tibial vein
    - 904.53 Posterior tibial artery
    - 904.54 Posterior tibial vein
  - 904.6 **Deep plantar blood vessels**
  - 904.7 **Other specified blood vessels of lower extremity**
    Multiple blood vessels of lower extremity
  - 904.8 **Unspecified blood vessel of lower extremity**
  - 904.9 **Unspecified site**
    Injury to blood vessel NOS

LATE EFFECTS OF INJURIES, POISONINGS, TOXIC EFFECTS, AND OTHER EXTERNAL CAUSES (905-909)

Note: These categories are to be used to indicate conditions classifiable to 800-999 as the cause of late effects, which are themselves classified elsewhere. The "late effects" include those specified as such, or as sequelae, which may occur at any time after the acute injury.

- 905 **Late effects of musculoskeletal and connective tissue injuries**
  - 905.0 **Late effect of fracture of skull and face bones**
    Late effect of injury classifiable to 800-804
  - 905.1 **Late effect of fracture of spine and trunk without mention of spinal cord lesion**
    Late effect of injury classifiable to 805, 807-809
  - 905.2 **Late effect of fracture of upper extremities**
    Late effect of injury classifiable to 810-819
  - 905.3 **Late effect of fracture of neck of femur**
    Late effect of injury classifiable to 820
  - 905.4 **Late effect of fracture of lower extremities**
    Late effect of injury classifiable to 821-827
  - 905.5 **Late effect of fracture of multiple and unspecified bones**
    Late effect of injury classifiable to 828-829
  - 905.6 **Late effect of dislocation**
    Late effect of injury classifiable to 830-839
  - 905.7 **Late effect of sprain and strain without mention of tendon injury**
    Late effect of injury classifiable to 840-848, except tendon injury
  - 905.8 **Late effect of tendon injury**
    Late effect of tendon injury due to:
      open wound [injury classifiable to 880-884 with .2, 890-894 with .2]
      sprain and strain [injury classifiable to 840-848]
  - 905.9 **Late effect of traumatic amputation**
    Late effect of injury classifiable to 885-887, 895-897
    EXCLUDES *late amputation stump complication (997.60-997.69)*
- 906 **Late effects of injuries to skin and subcutaneous tissues**
  - 906.0 **Late effect of open wound of head, neck, and trunk**
    Late effect of injury classifiable to 870-879
  - 906.1 **Late effect of open wound of extremities without mention of tendon injury**
    Late effect of injury classifiable to 880-884, 890-894 except .2
  - 906.2 **Late effect of superficial injury**
    Late effect of injury classifiable to 910-919
  - 906.3 **Late effect of contusion**
    Late effect of injury classifiable to 920-924
  - 906.4 **Late effect of crushing**
    Late effect of injury classifiable to 925-929
  - 906.5 **Late effect of burn of eye, face, head, and neck**
    Late effect of injury classifiable to 940-941
  - 906.6 **Late effect of burn of wrist and hand**
    Late effect of injury classifiable to 944
  - 906.7 **Late effect of burn of other extremities**
    Late effect of injury classifiable to 943 or 945
  - 906.8 **Late effect of burns of other specified sites**
    Late effect of injury classifiable to 942, 946-947
  - 906.9 **Late effect of burn of unspecified site**
    Late effect of injury classifiable to 948-949
- 907 **Late effects of injuries to the nervous system**
  - 907.0 **Late effect of intracranial injury without mention of skull fracture**
    Late effect of injury classifiable to 850-854
  - 907.1 **Late effect of injury to cranial nerve**
    Late effect of injury classifiable to 950-951
  - 907.2 **Late effect of spinal cord injury**
    Late effect of injury classifiable to 806, 952
  - 907.3 **Late effect of injury to nerve root(s), spinal plexus(es), and other nerves of trunk**
    Late effect of injury classifiable to 953-954
  - 907.4 **Late effect of injury to peripheral nerve of shoulder girdle and upper limb**
    Late effect of injury classifiable to 955
  - 907.5 **Late effect of injury to peripheral nerve of pelvic girdle and lower limb**
    Late effect of injury classifiable to 956
  - 907.9 **Late effect of injury to other and unspecified nerve**
    Late effect of injury classifiable to 957
- 908 **Late effects of other and unspecified injuries**
  - 908.0 **Late effect of internal injury to chest**
    Late effect of injury classifiable to 860-862
  - 908.1 **Late effect of internal injury to intra-abdominal organs**
    Late effect of injury classifiable to 863-866, 868
  - 908.2 **Late effect of internal injury to other internal organs**
    Late effect of injury classifiable to 867 or 869
  - 908.3 **Late effect of injury to blood vessel of head, neck, and extremities**
    Late effect of injury classifiable to 900, 903-904
  - 908.4 **Late effect of injury to blood vessel of thorax, abdomen, and pelvis**
    Late effect of injury classifiable to 901-902
  - 908.5 **Late effect of foreign body in orifice**
    Late effect of injury classifiable to 930-939
  - 908.6 **Late effect of certain complications of trauma**
    Late effect of complications classifiable to 958
  - 908.9 **Late effect of unspecified injury**
    Late effect of injury classifiable to 959
- 909 **Late effects of other and unspecified external causes**
  - 909.0 **Late effect of poisoning due to drug, medicinal or biological substance**
    Late effect of conditions classifiable to 960-979
    EXCLUDES *late effect of adverse effect of drug, medicinal or biological substance (909.5)*
  - 909.1 **Late effect of toxic effects of nonmedical substances**
    Late effect of conditions classifiable to 980-989
  - 909.2 **Late effect of radiation**
    Late effect of conditions classifiable to 990
  - 909.3 **Late effect of complications of surgical and medical care**
    Late effect of conditions classifiable to 996-999
  - 909.4 **Late effect of certain other external causes**
    Late effect of conditions classifiable to 991-994
  - 909.5 **Late effect of adverse effect of drug, medical or biological substance**
    EXCLUDES *late effect of poisoning due to drug, medical or biological substance (909.0)*
  - 909.9 **Late effect of other and unspecified external causes**
    Late effect of conditions classifiable to 995

SUPERFICIAL INJURY (910-919)

EXCLUDES *burn (blisters) (940.0-949.5)*
contusion (920-924.9)
foreign body:
  granuloma (728.82)
  inadvertently left in operative wound (998.4)
  residual in soft tissue (729.6)
insect bite, venomous (989.5)
open wound with incidental foreign body (870.0-897.7)

INJURY AND POISONING

- **910 Superficial injury of face, neck, and scalp except eye**
  - INCLUDES: cheek, ear, gum, lip, nose, throat
  - EXCLUDES: eye and adnexa (918.0-918.9)
  - 910.0 Abrasion or friction burn without mention of infection
  - 910.1 Abrasion or friction burn, infected
  - 910.2 Blister without mention of infection
  - 910.3 Blister, infected
  - 910.4 Insect bite, nonvenomous, without mention of infection
  - 910.5 Insect bite, nonvenomous, infected
  - 910.6 Superficial foreign body (splinter) without major open wound and without mention of infection
  - 910.7 Superficial foreign body (splinter) without major open wound, infected
  - ◆910.8 Other and unspecified superficial injury of face, neck, and scalp without mention of infection
  - ◆910.9 Other and unspecified superficial injury of face, neck, and scalp, infected

- **911 Superficial injury of trunk**
  - INCLUDES: abdominal wall, anus, back, breast, buttock, chest wall, flank, groin, interscapular region, labium (majus) (minus), penis, perineum, scrotum, testis, vagina, vulva
  - EXCLUDES: hip (916.0-916.9); scapular region (912.0-912.9)
  - 911.0 Abrasion or friction burn without mention of infection
  - 911.1 Abrasion or friction burn, infected
  - 911.2 Blister without mention of infection
  - 911.3 Blister, infected
  - 911.4 Insect bite, nonvenomous, without mention of infection
  - 911.5 Insect bite, nonvenomous, infected
  - 911.6 Superficial foreign body (splinter) without major open wound and without mention of infection
  - 911.7 Superficial foreign body (splinter) without major open wound, infected
  - ◆911.8 Other and unspecified superficial injury of trunk without mention of infection
  - ◆911.9 Other and unspecified superficial injury of trunk, infected

- **912 Superficial injury of shoulder and upper arm**
  - INCLUDES: axilla, scapular region
  - 912.0 Abrasion or friction burn without mention of infection
  - 912.1 Abrasion or friction burn, infected
  - 912.2 Blister without mention of infection
  - 912.3 Blister, infected
  - 912.4 Insect bite, nonvenomous, without mention of infection
  - 912.5 Insect bite, nonvenomous, infected
  - 912.6 Superficial foreign body (splinter) without major open wound and without mention of infection
  - 912.7 Superficial foreign body (splinter) without major open wound, infected
  - ◆912.8 Other and unspecified superficial injury of shoulder and upper arm without mention of infection
  - ◆912.9 Other and unspecified superficial injury of shoulder and upper arm, infected

- **913 Superficial injury of elbow, forearm, and wrist**
  - 913.0 Abrasion or friction burn without mention of infection
  - 913.1 Abrasion or friction burn, infected
  - 913.2 Blister without mention of infection
  - 913.3 Blister, infected
  - 913.4 Insect bite, nonvenomous, without mention of infection
  - 913.5 Insect bite, nonvenomous, infected
  - 913.6 Superficial foreign body (splinter) without major open wound and without mention of infection
  - 913.7 Superficial foreign body (splinter) without major open wound, infected
  - ◆913.8 Other and unspecified superficial injury of elbow, forearm, and wrist without mention of infection
  - ◆913.9 Other and unspecified superficial injury of elbow, forearm, and wrist, infected

- **914 Superficial injury of hand(s) except finger(s) alone**
  - 914.0 Abrasion or friction burn without mention of infection
  - 914.1 Abrasion or friction burn, infected
  - 914.2 Blister without mention of infection
  - 914.3 Blister, infected
  - 914.4 Insect bite, nonvenomous, without mention of infection
  - 914.5 Insect bite, nonvenomous, infected
  - 914.6 Superficial foreign body (splinter) without major open wound and without mention of infection
  - 914.7 Superficial foreign body (splinter) without major open wound, infected
  - ◆914.8 Other and unspecified superficial injury of hand without mention of infection
  - ◆914.9 Other and unspecified superficial injury of hand, infected

- **915 Superficial injury of finger(s)**
  - INCLUDES: fingernail, thumb (nail)
  - 915.0 Abrasion or friction burn without mention of infection
  - 915.1 Abrasion or friction burn, infected
  - 915.2 Blister without mention of infection
  - 915.3 Blister, infected
  - 915.4 Insect bite, nonvenomous, without mention of infection
  - 915.5 Insect bite, nonvenomous, infected
  - 915.6 Superficial foreign body (splinter) without major open wound and without mention of infection
  - 915.7 Superficial foreign body (splinter) without major open wound, infected
  - ◆915.8 Other and unspecified superficial injury of fingers without mention of infection
  - ◆915.9 Other and unspecified superficial injury of fingers, infected

- **916 Superficial injury of hip, thigh, leg, and ankle**
  - 916.0 Abrasion or friction burn without mention of infection
  - 916.1 Abrasion or friction burn, infected
  - 916.2 Blister without mention of infection
  - 916.3 Blister, infected
  - 916.4 Insect bite, nonvenomous, without mention of infection
  - 916.5 Insect bite, nonvenomous, infected
  - 916.6 Superficial foreign body (splinter) without major open wound and without mention of infection
  - 916.7 Superficial foreign body (splinter) without major open wound, infected
  - ◆916.8 Other and unspecified superficial injury of hip, thigh, leg, and ankle without mention of infection
  - ◆916.9 Other and unspecified superficial injury of hip, thigh, leg, and ankle, infected

- **917 Superficial injury of foot and toe(s)**
  - INCLUDES: heel, toenail
  - 917.0 Abrasion or friction burn without mention of infection
  - 917.1 Abrasion or friction burn, infected
  - 917.2 Blister without mention of infection
  - 917.3 Blister, infected
  - 917.4 Insect bite, nonvenomous, without mention of infection
  - 917.5 Insect bite, nonvenomous, infected
  - 917.6 Superficial foreign body (splinter) without major open wound and without mention of infection
  - 917.7 Superficial foreign body (splinter) without major open wound, infected
  - ◆917.8 Other and unspecified superficial injury of foot and toes without mention of infection
  - ◆917.9 Other and unspecified superficial injury of foot and toes, infected

- **918 Superficial injury of eye and adnexa**
  - EXCLUDES: burn (940.0-940.9); foreign body on external eye (930.0-930.9)
  - 918.0 Eyelids and periocular area
    - Abrasion
    - Insect bite
    - Superficial foreign body (splinter)
  - 918.1 Cornea
    - Corneal abrasion
    - Superficial laceration
    - EXCLUDES: corneal injury due to contact lens (371.82) ◆
  - 918.2 Conjunctiva
  - ◆918.9 Other and unspecified superficial injuries of eye
    - Eye (ball) NOS

- **919 Superficial injury of other, multiple, and unspecified sites**
  - EXCLUDES: multiple sites classifiable to the same three-digit category (910.0-918.9)
  - ◆919.0 Abrasion or friction burn without mention of infection
  - ◆919.1 Abrasion or friction burn, infected

● Additional digits required ◆ Nonspecific code ■ Not a primary diagnosis

- 919.2 Blister without mention of infection
- 919.3 Blister, infected
- 919.4 Insect bite, nonvenomous, without mention of infection
- 919.5 Insect bite, nonvenomous, infected
- 919.6 Superficial foreign body (splinter) without major open wound and without mention of infection
- 919.7 Superficial foreign body (splinter) without major open wound, infected
- 919.8 Other and unspecified superficial injury without mention of infection
- 919.9 Other and unspecified superficial injury, infected

CONTUSION WITH INTACT SKIN SURFACE (920-924)

INCLUDES bruise, hematoma } without fracture or open wound

EXCLUDES
- concussion (850.0-850.9)
- hemarthrosis (840.0-848.9)
- internal organs (860.0-869.1)
- that incidental to:
  - crushing injury (925-929.9)
  - dislocation (830.0-839.9)
  - fracture (800.0-829.1)
  - internal injury (860.0-869.1)
  - intracranial injury (850.0-854.1)
  - nerve injury (950.0-957.9)
  - openwound (870.0-897.7)

920 Contusion of face, scalp, and neck except eye(s)
Cheek
Ear (auricle)
Gum
Lip
Mandibular joint area
Nose
Throat

921 Contusion of eye and adnexa
- 921.0 Black eye, not otherwise specified
- 921.1 Contusion of eyelids and periocular area
- 921.2 Contusion of orbital tissues
- 921.3 Contusion of eyeball
- 921.9 Unspecified contusion of eye
  - Injury of eye NOS

922 Contusion of trunk
- 922.0 Breast
- 922.1 Chest wall
- 922.2 Abdominal wall
  - Flank
  - Groin
- 922.3 Back
  - Buttock
  - Interscapular region
  - **EXCLUDES** scapular region (923.01)
- 922.4 Genital organs
  - Labium (majus) (minus)
  - Penis
  - Perineum
  - Scrotum
  - Vulva
  - Vagina
  - Testis
- 922.8 Multiple sites of trunk
- 922.9 Unspecified part
  - Trunk NOS

923 Contusion of upper limb
- 923.0 Shoulder and upper arm
  - 923.00 Shoulder region
  - 923.01 Scapular region
  - 923.02 Axillary region
  - 923.03 Upper arm
  - 923.09 Multiple sites
- 923.1 Elbow and forearm
  - 923.10 Forearm
  - 923.11 Elbow
- 923.2 Wrist and hand(s), except finger(s) alone
  - 923.20 Hand(s)
  - 923.21 Wrist
- 923.3 Finger
  - Fingernail
  - Thumb (nail)
- 923.8 Multiple sites of upper limb
- 923.9 Unspecified part of upper limb
  - Arm NOS

924 Contusion of lower limb and of other and unspecified sites
- 924.0 Hip and thigh
  - 924.00 Thigh
  - 924.01 Hip
- 924.1 Knee and lower leg
  - 924.10 Lower leg
  - 924.11 Knee
- 924.2 Ankle and foot, excluding toe(s)
  - 924.20 Foot
    - Heel
  - 924.21 Ankle
- 924.3 Toe
  - Toenail
- 924.4 Multiple sites of lower limb
- 924.5 Unspecified part of lower limb
  - Leg NOS
- 924.8 Multiple sites, not elsewhere classified
- 924.9 Unspecified site

CRUSHING INJURY (925-929)

EXCLUDES
- concussion (850.0-850.9)
- fractures (800-829)
- internal organs (860.0-869.1)
- that incidental to:
  - internal injury (860.0-869.1)
  - intracranial injury (850.0-854.1)

925 Crushing injury of face, scalp, and neck
Cheek
Ear
Larynx
Pharynx
Throat

- 925.1 Crushing injury of face and scalp
  - Cheek
  - Ear
- 925.2 Crushing injury of neck
  - Larynx
  - Pharynx
  - Throat

926 Crushing injury of trunk
EXCLUDES crush injury of internal organs (860.0-869.1)
- 926.0 External genitalia
  - Labium (majus) (minus)
  - Penis
  - Scrotum
  - Testis
  - Vulva
- 926.1 Other specified sites
  - 926.11 Back
  - 926.12 Buttock
  - 926.19 Other
    - Breast
    - **EXCLUDES** crushing of chest (860.0-862.9)
- 926.8 Multiple sites of trunk
- 926.9 Unspecified site
  - Trunk NOS

927 Crushing injury of upper limb
- 927.0 Shoulder and upper arm
  - 927.00 Shoulder region
  - 927.01 Scapular region
  - 927.02 Axillary region
  - 927.03 Upper arm
  - 927.09 Multiple sites
- 927.1 Elbow and forearm
  - 927.10 Forearm
  - 927.11 Elbow
- 927.2 Wrist and hand(s), except finger(s) alone
  - 927.20 Hand(s)
  - 927.21 Wrist
- 927.3 Finger(s)
- 927.8 Multiple sites of upper limb
- 927.9 Unspecified site
  - Arm NOS

928 Crushing injury of lower limb
- 928.0 Hip and thigh
  - 928.00 Thigh
  - 928.01 Hip
- 928.1 Knee and lower leg
  - 928.10 Lower leg
  - 928.11 Knee
- 928.2 Ankle and foot, excluding toe(s) alone
  - 928.20 Foot
    - Heel
  - 928.21 Ankle
- 928.3 Toe(s)
- 928.8 Multiple sites of lower limb
- 928.9 Unspecified site
  - Leg NOS

INJURY AND POISONING

- **929 Crushing injury of multiple and unspecified sites**
  - EXCLUDES: multiple internal injury NOS (869.0-869.1)
  - **929.0 Multiple sites, not elsewhere classified**
  - **929.9 Unspecified site**

EFFECTS OF FOREIGN BODY ENTERING THROUGH ORIFICE (930-939)

EXCLUDES: foreign body:
- granuloma (728.82)
- inadvertently left in operative wound (998.4, 998.7)
- in open wound (800-839, 851-897)
- residual in soft tissues (729.6)
- superficial without major open wound (910-919 with .6 or .7)

- **930 Foreign body on external eye**
  - EXCLUDES: foreign body in penetrating wound of:
    - eyeball (871.5-871.6)
      - retained (old) (360.5-360.6)
    - ocular adnexa (870.4)
      - retained (old) (376.6)
  - 930.0 Corneal foreign body
  - 930.1 Foreign body in conjunctival sac
  - 930.2 Foreign body in lacrimal punctum
  - **930.8 Other and combined sites**
  - **930.9 Unspecified site**
    - External eye NOS
- 931 Foreign body in ear
  - Auditory canal   Auricle
- 932 Foreign body in nose
  - Nasal sinus   Nostril
- **933 Foreign body in pharynx and larynx**
  - 933.0 Pharynx
    - Nasopharynx   Throat NOS
  - 933.1 Larynx
    - Asphyxia due to foreign body
    - Choking due to:
      - food (regurgitated)
      - phlegm
- **934 Foreign body in trachea, bronchus, and lung**
  - 934.0 Trachea
  - 934.1 Main bronchus
  - **934.8 Other specified parts**
    - Bronchioles   Lung
  - **934.9 Respiratory tree, unspecified**
    - Inhalation of liquid or vomitus, lower respiratory tract NOS
- **935 Foreign body in mouth, esophagus, and stomach**
  - 935.0 Mouth
  - 935.1 Esophagus
  - 935.2 Stomach
- 936 Foreign body in intestine and colon
- 937 Foreign body in anus and rectum
  - Rectosigmoid (junction)
- **938 Foreign body in digestive system, unspecified**
  - Alimentary tract NOS   Swallowed foreign body
- **939 Foreign body in genitourinary tract**
  - 939.0 Bladder and urethra
  - 939.1 Uterus, any part
    - EXCLUDES: intrauterine contraceptive device:
      - complications from (996.32, 996.65)
      - presence of (V45.51)
  - 939.2 Vulva and vagina
  - 939.3 Penis
  - **939.9 Unspecified site**

BURNS (940-949)

INCLUDES: burns from:
- electrical heating appliance
- electricity
- flame
- hot object
- lightning
- radiation
- chemical burns (external) (internal)
- scalds

EXCLUDES: friction burns (910-919 with .0, .1)
sunburn (692.71)

- **940 Burn confined to eye and adnexa**
  - 940.0 Chemical burn of eyelids and periocular area
  - **940.1 Other burns of eyelids and periocular area**
  - 940.2 Alkaline chemical burn of cornea and conjunctival sac
  - 940.3 Acid chemical burn of cornea and conjunctival sac
  - 940.4 Other burn of cornea and conjunctival sac
  - 940.5 Burn with resulting rupture and destruction of eyeball
  - 940.9 Unspecified burn of eye and adnexa
- **941 Burn of face, head, and neck**
  - EXCLUDES: mouth (947.0)
  - The following fifth-digit subclassification is for use with category 941:
    - **0 face and head, unspecified site**
    - 1 ear [any part]
    - 2 eye (with other parts of face, head, and neck)
    - 3 lip(s)
    - 4 chin
    - 5 nose (septum)
    - 6 scalp [any part]
      - Temple (region)
    - 7 forehead and cheek
    - 8 neck
    - **9 multiple sites [except with eye] of face, head, and neck**
  - **941.0 Unspecified degree**
  - **941.1 Erythema [first degree]**
  - **941.2 Blisters, epidermal loss [second degree]**
  - **941.3 Full-thickness skin loss [third degree NOS]**
  - **941.4 Deep necrosis of underlying tissues [deep third degree] without mention of loss of a body part**
  - **941.5 Deep necrosis of underlying tissues [deep third degree] with loss of a body part**
- **942 Burn of trunk**
  - EXCLUDES: scapular region (943.0-943.5 with fifth-digit 6)
  - The following fifth-digit subclassification is for use with category 942:
    - **0 trunk, unspecified site**
    - 1 breast
    - 2 chest wall, excluding breast and nipple
    - 3 abdominal wall
      - Flank   Groin
    - 4 back [any part]
      - Buttock   Interscapular region
    - 5 genitalia
      - Labium (majus) (minus)   Scrotum
      - Penis   Testis
      - Perineum   Vulva
    - **9 other and multiple sites of trunk**
  - **942.0 Unspecified degree**
  - **942.1 Erythema [first degree]**
  - **942.2 Blisters, epidermal loss [second degree]**
  - **942.3 Full-thickness skin loss [third degree NOS]**
  - **942.4 Deep necrosis of underlying tissues [deep third degree] without mention of loss of a body part**
  - **942.5 Deep necrosis of underlying tissues [deep third degree] with loss of a body part**
- **943 Burn of upper limb, except wrist and hand**
  - The following fifth-digit subclassification is for use with category 943:
    - **0 upper limb, unspecified site**
    - 1 forearm
    - 2 elbow
    - 3 upper arm
    - 4 axilla
    - 5 shoulder
    - 6 scapular region
    - **9 multiple sites of upper limb, except wrist and hand**
  - **943.0 Unspecified degree**
  - **943.1 Erythema [first degree]**
  - **943.2 Blisters, epidermal loss [second degree]**
  - **943.3 Full-thickness skin loss [third degree NOS]**
  - **943.4 Deep necrosis of underlying tissues [deep third degree] without mention of loss of a body part**
  - **943.5 Deep necrosis of underlying tissues [deep third degree] with loss of a body part**

944 Burn of wrist(s) and hand(s)

The following fifth-digit subclassification is for use with category 944:
- 0 hand, unspecified site
- 1 single digit [finger (nail)] other than thumb
- 2 thumb (nail)
- 3 two or more digits, not including thumb
- 4 two or more digits including thumb
- 5 palm
- 6 back of hand
- 7 wrist
- 8 multiple sites of wrist(s) and hand(s)

- 944.0 Unspecified degree
- 944.1 Erythema [first degree]
- 944.2 Blisters, epidermal loss [second degree]
- 944.3 Full-thickness skin loss [third degree NOS]
- 944.4 Deep necrosis of underlying tissues [deep third degree] without mention of loss of a body part
- 944.5 Deep necrosis of underlying tissues [deep third degree] with loss of a body part

945 Burn of lower limb(s)

The following fifth-digit subclassification is for use with category 945:
- 0 lower limb [leg], unspecified site
- 1 toe(s) (nail)
- 2 foot
- 3 ankle
- 4 lower leg
- 5 knee
- 6 thigh [any part]
- 9 multiple sites of lower limb(s)

- 945.0 Unspecified degree
- 945.1 Erythema [first degree]
- 945.2 Blisters, epidermal loss [second degree]
- 945.3 Full-thickness skin loss [third degree NOS]
- 945.4 Deep necrosis of underlying tissues [deep third degree] without mention of loss of a body part
- 945.5 Deep necrosis of underlying tissues [deep third degree] with loss of a body part

946 Burns of multiple specified sites

INCLUDES burns of sites classifiable to more than one three-digit category in 940-945

EXCLUDES multiple burns NOS (949.0-949.5)

- 946.0 Unspecified degree
- 946.1 Erythema [first degree]
- 946.2 Blisters, epidermal loss [second degree]
- 946.3 Full-thickness skin loss [third degree NOS]
- 946.4 Deep necrosis of underlying tissues [deep third degree] without mention of loss of a body part
- 946.5 Deep necrosis of underlying tissues [deep third degree] with loss of a body part

947 Burn of internal organs

INCLUDES burns from chemical agents (ingested)

- 947.0 Mouth and pharynx
  Gum   Tongue
- 947.1 Larynx, trachea, and lung
- 947.2 Esophagus
- 947.3 Gastrointestinal tract
  Colon   Small intestine
  Rectum   Stomach
- 947.4 Vagina and uterus
- 947.8 Other specified sites
- 947.9 Unspecified site

948 Burns classified according to extent of body surface involved

Note: This category is to be used when the site of the burn is unspecified, or with categories 940-947 when the site is specified.

The following fifth-digit subclassification is for use with category 948 to indicate the percent of body surface with third degree burn; valid digits are in [brackets] under each code:
- 0 less than 10 percent or unspecified
- 1 10-19%
- 2 20-29%
- 3 30-39%
- 4 40-49%
- 5 50-59%
- 6 60-69%
- 7 70-79%
- 8 80-89%
- 9 90% or more of body surface

- 948.0 [0] Burn [any degree] involving less than 10 percent of body surface
- 948.1 [0-1] 10-19 percent of body surface
- 948.2 [0-2] 20-29 percent of body surface
- 948.3 [0-3] 30-39 percent of body surface
- 948.4 [0-4] 40-49 percent of body surface
- 948.5 [0-5] 50-59 percent of body surface
- 948.6 [0-6] 60-69 percent of body surface
- 948.7 [0-7] 70-79 percent of body surface
- 948.8 [0-8] 80-89 percent of body surface
- 948.9 [0-9] 90 percent or more of body surface

949 Burn, unspecified

INCLUDES burn NOS multiple burns NOS

EXCLUDES burn of unspecified site but with statement of the extent of body surface involved (948.0-948.9)

- 949.0 Unspecified degree
- 949.1 Erythema [first degree]
- 949.2 Blisters, epidermal loss [second degree]
- 949.3 Full-thickness skin loss [third degree NOS]
- 949.4 Deep necrosis of underlying tissues [deep third degree] without mention of loss of a body part
- 949.5 Deep necrosis of underlying tissues [deep third degree] with loss of a body part

INJURY TO NERVES AND SPINAL CORD (950-957)

INCLUDES division of nerve
lesion in continuity
traumatic neuroma
traumatic transient paralysis
(with open wound)

EXCLUDES accidental puncture or laceration during medical procedure (998.2)

950 Injury to optic nerve and pathways
- 950.0 Optic nerve injury
  Second cranial nerve
- 950.1 Injury to optic chiasm
- 950.2 Injury to optic pathways
- 950.3 Injury to visual cortex
- 950.9 Unspecified
  Traumatic blindness NOS

951 Injury to other cranial nerve(s)
- 951.0 Injury to oculomotor nerve
  Third cranial nerve
- 951.1 Injury to trochlear nerve
  Fourth cranial nerve
- 951.2 Injury to trigeminal nerve
  Fifth cranial nerve
- 951.3 Injury to abducens nerve
  Sixth cranial nerve
- 951.4 Injury to facial nerve
  Seventh cranial nerve
- 951.5 Injury to acoustic nerve
  Auditory nerve   Traumatic deafness NOS
  Eighth cranial nerve
- 951.6 Injury to accessory nerve
  Eleventh cranial nerve
- 951.7 Injury to hypoglossal nerve
  Twelfth cranial nerve
- 951.8 Injury to other specified cranial nerves
  Glossopharyngeal [9th cranial] nerve
  Olfactory [1st cranial] nerve
  Pneumogastric [10th cranial] nerve
  Traumatic anosmia NOS
  Vagus [10th cranial] nerve
- 951.9 Injury to unspecified cranial nerve

INJURY AND POISONING

- **952 Spinal cord injury without evidence of spinal bone injury**
  - **952.0 Cervical**
    - ◆ 952.00 C_1-C_4 level with unspecified spinal cord injury
      - Spinal cord injury, cervical region NOS
    - 952.01 C_1-C_4 level with complete lesion of spinal cord
    - 952.02 C_1-C_4 level with anterior cord syndrome
    - 952.03 C_1-C_4 level with central cord syndrome
    - ◆ 952.04 C_1-C_4 level with other specified spinal cord injury
      - Incomplete spinal cord lesion at C_1-C_4 level:
        - NOS
        - with posterior cord syndrome
    - ◆ 952.05 C_5-C_7 level with unspecified spinal cord injury
    - 952.06 C_5-C_7 level with complete lesion of spinal cord
    - 952.07 C_5-C_7 level with anterior cord syndrome
    - 952.08 C_5-C_7 level with central cord syndrome
    - ◆ 952.09 C_5-C_7 level with other specified spinal cord injury
      - Incomplete spinal cord lesion at C_5-C_7 level:
        - NOS
        - with posterior cord syndrome
  - **952.1 Dorsal [thoracic]**
    - ◆ 952.10 T_1-T_6 level with unspecified spinal cord injury
      - Spinal cord injury, thoracic region NOS
    - 952.11 T_1-T_6 level with complete lesion of spinal cord
    - 952.12 T_1-T_6 level with anterior cord syndrome
    - 952.13 T_1-T_6 level with central cord syndrome
    - ◆ 952.14 T_1-T_6 level with other specified spinal cord injury
      - Incomplete spinal cord lesion at T_1-T_6 level:
        - NOS
        - with posterior cord syndrome
    - ◆ 952.15 T_7-T_{12} level with unspecified spinal cord injury
    - 952.16 T_7-T_{12} level with complete lesion of spinal cord
    - 952.17 T_7-T_{12} level with anterior cord syndrome
    - 952.18 T_7-T_{12} level with central cord syndrome
    - ◆ 952.19 T_7-T_{12} level with other specified spinal cord injury
      - Incomplete spinal cord lesion at T_7-T_{12} level:
        - NOS
        - with posterior cord syndrome
  - 952.2 Lumbar
  - 952.3 Sacral
  - 952.4 Cauda equina
  - ◆ 952.8 Multiple sites of spinal cord
  - ◆ 952.9 Unspecified site of spinal cord
- **953 Injury to nerve roots and spinal plexus**
  - 953.0 Cervical root
  - 953.1 Dorsal root
  - 953.2 Lumbar root
  - 953.3 Sacral root
  - 953.4 Brachial plexus
  - 953.5 Lumbosacral plexus
  - ◆ 953.8 Multiple sites
  - ◆ 953.9 Unspecified site
- **954 Injury to other nerve(s) of trunk, excluding shoulder and pelvic girdles**
  - 954.0 Cervical sympathetic
  - ◆ 954.1 Other sympathetic
    - Celiac ganglion or plexus   Splanchnic nerve(s)
    - Inferior mesenteric plexus   Stellate ganglion
  - ◆ 954.8 Other specified nerve(s) of trunk
  - ◆ 954.9 Unspecified nerve of trunk
- **955 Injury to peripheral nerve(s) of shoulder girdle and upper limb**
  - 955.0 Axillary nerve
  - 955.1 Median nerve
  - 955.2 Ulnar nerve
  - 955.3 Radial nerve
  - 955.4 Musculocutaneous nerve
  - 955.5 Cutaneous sensory nerve, upper limb
  - 955.6 Digital nerve
  - ◆ 955.7 Other specified nerve(s) of shoulder girdle and upper limb
  - ◆ 955.8 Multiple nerves of shoulder girdle and upper limb
  - ◆ 955.9 Unspecified nerve of shoulder girdle and upper limb
- **956 Injury to peripheral nerve(s) of pelvic girdle and lower limb**
  - 956.0 Sciatic nerve
  - 956.1 Femoral nerve
  - 956.2 Posterior tibial nerve
  - 956.3 Peroneal nerve
  - 956.4 Cutaneous sensory nerve, lower limb
  - ◆ 956.5 Other specified nerve(s) of pelvic girdle and lower limb
  - ◆ 956.8 Multiple nerves of pelvic girdle and lower limb
  - ◆ 956.9 Unspecified nerve of pelvic girdle and lower limb
- **957 Injury to other and unspecified nerves**
  - 957.0 Superficial nerves of head and neck
  - ◆ 957.1 Other specified nerve(s)
  - ◆ 957.8 Multiple nerves in several parts
    - Multiple nerve injury NOS
  - ◆ 957.9 Unspecified site
    - Nerve injury NOS

CERTAIN TRAUMATIC COMPLICATIONS AND UNSPECIFIED INJURIES (958-959)

- **958 Certain early complications of trauma**
  - **EXCLUDES** adult respiratory distress syndrome (518.5)
    - flail chest (807.4)
    - shock lung (518.5)
    - that occurring during or following medical procedures (996.0-999.9)
  - 958.0 Air embolism
    - Pneumathemia
    - **EXCLUDES** that complicating:
      - abortion (634-638 with .6, 639.6)
      - ectopic or molar pregnancy (639.6)
      - pregnancy, childbirth, or the puerperium (673.0)
  - 958.1 Fat embolism
    - **EXCLUDES** that complicating:
      - abortion (634-638 with .6, 639.6)
      - pregnancy, childbirth, or the puerperium (673.8)
  - 958.2 Secondary and recurrent hemorrhage
  - 958.3 Posttraumatic wound infection, not elsewhere classified
  - 958.4 Traumatic shock
    - Shock (immediate) (delayed) following injury
    - **EXCLUDES** shock:
      - anaphylactic (995.0)
        - due to serum (999.4)
      - anesthetic (995.4)
      - electric (994.8)
      - following abortion (639.5)
      - lightning (994.0)
      - nontraumatic NOS (785.50)
      - obstetric (669.1)
      - postoperative (998.0)
  - 958.5 Traumatic anuria
    - Crush syndrome
    - Renal failure following crushing
    - **EXCLUDES** that due to a medical procedure (997.5)
  - 958.6 Volkmann's ischemic contracture
    - Posttraumatic muscle contracture
  - 958.7 Traumatic subcutaneous emphysema
    - **EXCLUDES** subcutaneous emphysema resulting from a procedure (998.81) ◆
  - ◆ 958.8 Other early complications of trauma
- **959 Injury, other and unspecified**
  - **INCLUDES** injury NOS
  - **EXCLUDES** injury NOS of:
    - blood vessels (900.0-904.9)
    - eye (921.0-921.9)
    - head (854.0-854.1)
    - internal organs (860.0-869.1)
    - intracranial sites (854.1)
    - nerves (950.0-951.9, 953.0-957.9)
    - spinal cord (952.0-952.9)
  - ◆ 959.0 Face and neck
    - Cheek   Mouth
    - Ear   Nose
    - Eyebrow   Throat
    - Lip
  - ◆ 959.1 Trunk
    - Abdominal wall   External genital organs
    - Back   Flank
    - Breast   Groin
    - Buttock   Interscapular region
    - Chest wall   Perineum
    - **EXCLUDES** scapular region (959.2)
  - ◆ 959.2 Shoulder and upper arm
    - Axilla   Scapular region

- 959.3 Elbow, forearm, and wrist
- 959.4 Hand, except finger
- 959.5 Finger
    - Fingernail
    - Thumb (nail)
- 959.6 Hip and thigh
    - Upper leg
- 959.7 Knee, leg, ankle, and foot
- 959.8 Other specified sites, including multiple
    - EXCLUDES: multiple sites classifiable to the same four-digit category (959.0-959.7)
- 959.9 Unspecified site

POISONING BY DRUGS, MEDICINAL AND BIOLOGICAL SUBSTANCES (960-979)

Use additional code to specify the effects of the poisoning

INCLUDES: overdose of these substances
wrong substance given or taken in error

EXCLUDES: adverse effects ["hypersensitivity," "reaction," etc.] of correct substance properly administered. Such cases are to be classified according to the nature of the adverse effect, such as:
- adverse effect NOS (995.2)
- allergic lymphadenitis (289.3)
- aspirin gastritis (535.4)
- blood disorders (280.0-289.9)
- dermatitis:
    - contact (692.0-692.9)
    - due to ingestion (693.0-693.9)
- nephropathy (583.9)
    [The drug giving rise to the adverse effect may be identified by use of categories E930-E949.]
- drug dependence (304.0-304.9)
- drug reaction and poisoning affecting the newborn (760.0-779.9)
- nondependent abuse of drugs (305.0-305.9)
- pathological drug intoxication (292.2)

960 Poisoning by antibiotics

EXCLUDES: antibiotics:
- ear, nose, and throat (976.6)
- eye (976.5)
- local (976.0)

- 960.0 Penicillins
    - Ampicillin
    - Carbenicillin
    - Cloxacillin
    - Penicillin G
- 960.1 Antifungal antibiotics
    - Amphotericin B
    - Griseofulvin
    - Nystatin
    - Trichomycin
    - EXCLUDES: preparations intended for topical use (976.0-976.9)
- 960.2 Chloramphenicol group
    - Chloramphenicol
    - Thiamphenicol
- 960.3 Erythromycin and other macrolides
    - Oleandomycin
    - Spiramycin
- 960.4 Tetracycline group
    - Doxycycline
    - Minocycline
    - Oxytetracycline
- 960.5 Cephalosporin group
    - Cephalexin
    - Cephaloglycin
    - Cephaloridine
    - Cephalothin
- 960.6 Antimycobacterial antibiotics
    - Cycloserine
    - Kanamycin
    - Rifampin
    - Streptomycin
- 960.7 Antineoplastic antibiotics
    - Actinomycin such as:
        - Cactinomycin
        - Dactinomycin
    - Bleomycin
    - Daunorubicin
    - Mitomycin
- 960.8 Other specified antibiotics
- 960.9 Unspecified antibiotic

961 Poisoning by other anti-infectives

EXCLUDES: anti-infectives:
- ear, nose, and throat (976.6)
- eye (976.5)
- local (976.0)

- 961.0 Sulfonamides
    - Sulfadiazine
    - Sulfafurazole
    - Sulfamethoxazole
- 961.1 Arsenical anti-infectives
- 961.2 Heavy metal anti-infectives
    - Compounds of:
        - antimony
        - bismuth
    - Compounds of:
        - lead
        - mercury
    - EXCLUDES: mercurial diuretics (974.0)
- 961.3 Quinoline and hydroxyquinoline derivatives
    - Chiniofon
    - Diiodohydroxyquin
    - EXCLUDES: antimalarial drugs (961.4)
- 961.4 Antimalarials and drugs acting on other blood protozoa
    - Chloroquine
    - Cycloguanil
    - Primaquine
    - Proguanil [chloroguanide]
    - Pyrimethamine
    - Quinine
- 961.5 Other antiprotozoal drugs
    - Emetine
- 961.6 Anthelmintics
    - Hexylresorcinol
    - Piperazine
    - Thiabendazole
- 961.7 Antiviral drugs
    - Methisazone
    - EXCLUDES:
        - amantadine (966.4)
        - cytarabine (963.1)
        - idoxuridine (976.5)
- 961.8 Other antimycobacterial drugs
    - Ethambutol
    - Ethionamide
    - Isoniazid
    - Para-aminosalicylic acid derivatives
    - Sulfones
- 961.9 Other and unspecified anti-infectives
    - Flucytosine
    - Nitrofuran derivatives

962 Poisoning by hormones and synthetic substitutes

EXCLUDES: oxytocic hormones (975.0)

- 962.0 Adrenal cortical steroids
    - Cortisone derivatives
    - Desoxycorticosterone derivatives
    - Fluorinated corticosteroids
- 962.1 Androgens and anabolic congeners
    - Methandriol
    - Nandrolone
    - Oxymetholone
    - Testosterone
- 962.2 Ovarian hormones and synthetic substitutes
    - Contraceptives, oral
    - Estrogens
    - Estrogens and progestogens, combined
    - Progestogens
- 962.3 Insulins and antidiabetic agents
    - Acetohexamide
    - Biguanide derivatives, oral
    - Chlorpropamide
    - Glucagon
    - Insulin
    - Phenformin
    - Sulfonylurea derivatives, oral
    - Tolbutamide
- 962.4 Anterior pituitary hormones
    - Corticotropin
    - Gonadotropin
    - Somatotropin [growth hormone]
- 962.5 Posterior pituitary hormones
    - Vasopressin
    - EXCLUDES: oxytocic hormones (975.0)
- 962.6 Parathyroid and parathyroid derivatives
- 962.7 Thyroid and thyroid derivatives
    - Dextrothyroxin
    - Levothyroxine sodium
    - Liothyronine
    - Thyroglobulin
- 962.8 Antithyroid agents
    - Iodides
    - Thiouracil
    - Thiourea
- 962.9 Other and unspecified hormones and synthetic substitutes

963 Poisoning by primarily systemic agents

- 963.0 Antiallergic and antiemetic drugs
    - Antihistamines
    - Chlorpheniramine
    - Diphenhydramine
    - Diphenylpyraline
    - Thonzylamine
    - Tripelennamine
    - EXCLUDES: phenothiazine-based tranquilizers (969.1)
- 963.1 Antineoplastic and immunosuppressive drugs
    - Azathioprine
    - Busulfan
    - Chlorambucil
    - Cyclophosphamide
    - Cytarabine
    - Fluorouracil
    - Mercaptopurine
    - thio-TEPA
    - EXCLUDES: antineoplastic antibiotics (960.7)
- 963.2 Acidifying agents
- 963.3 Alkalizing agents
- 963.4 Enzymes, not elsewhere classified
    - Penicillinase

INJURY AND POISONING

963.5 **Vitamins, not elsewhere classified**
Vitamin A   Vitamin D
Excludes: nicotinic acid (972.2)
vitamin K (964.3)

◆ **963.8** **Other specified systemic agents**
Heavy metal antagonists

◆ **963.9** **Unspecified systemic agent**

● **964** **Poisoning by agents primarily affecting blood constituents**

964.0 **Iron and its compounds**
Ferric salts
Ferrous sulfate and other ferrous salts

964.1 **Liver preparations and other antianemic agents**
Folic acid

964.2 **Anticoagulants**
Coumarin   Phenindione
Heparin   Warfarin sodium

964.3 **Vitamin K [phytonadione]**

964.4 **Fibrinolysis-affecting drugs**
Aminocaproic acid   Streptokinase
Streptodornase   Urokinase

964.5 **Anticoagulant antagonists and other coagulants**
Hexadimethrine   Protamine sulfate

964.6 **Gamma globulin**

964.7 **Natural blood and blood products**
Blood plasma   Packed red cells
Human fibrinogen   Whole blood
Excludes: transfusion reactions (999.4-999.8)

◆ **964.8** **Other specified agents affecting blood constituents**
Macromolecular blood substitutes
Plasma expanders

◆ **964.9** **Unspecified agent affecting blood constituents**

● **965** **Poisoning by analgesics, antipyretics, and antirheumatics**
Excludes: drug dependence (304.0-304.9)
nondependent abuse (305.0-305.9)

● **965.0** **Opiates and related narcotics**

◆ **965.00** Opium (alkaloids), unspecified

965.01 Heroin
Diacetylmorphine

965.02 Methadone

◆ **965.09** Other
Codeine [methylmorphine]
Meperidine [pethidine]
Morphine

965.1 **Salicylates**
Acetylsalicylic acid [aspirin]   Salicylic acid salts

965.4 **Aromatic analgesics, not elsewhere classified**
Acetanilid   Phenacetin [acetophenetidin]
Paracetamol [acetaminophen]

965.5 **Pyrazole derivatives**
Aminophenazone [aminopyrine]
Phenylbutazone

965.6 **Antirheumatics [antiphlogistics]**
Gold salts   Indomethacin
Excludes: salicylates (965.1)
steroids (962.0-962.9)

◆ **965.7** **Other non-narcotic analgesics**
Pyrabital

◆ **965.8** **Other specified analgesics and antipyretics**
Pentazocine

◆ **965.9** **Unspecified analgesic and antipyretic**

● **966** **Poisoning by anticonvulsants and anti-Parkinsonism drugs**

966.0 **Oxazolidine derivatives**
Paramethadione
Trimethadione

966.1 **Hydantoin derivatives**
Phenytoin

966.2 **Succinimides**
Ethosuximide
Phensuximide

◆ **966.3** **Other and unspecified anticonvulsants**
Primidone
Excludes: barbiturates (967.0)
sulfonamides (961.0)

966.4 **Anti-Parkinsonism drugs**
Amantadine
Ethopropazine [profenamine]
Levodopa [L-dopa]

● **967** **Poisoning by sedatives and hypnotics**
Excludes: drug dependence (304.0-304.9)
nondependent abuse (305.0-305.9)

967.0 **Barbiturates**
Amobarbital [amylobarbitone]
Barbital [barbitone]
Butabarbital [butabarbitone]
Pentobarbital [pentobarbitone]
Phenobarbital [phenobarbitone]
Secobarbital [quinalbarbitone]
Excludes: thiobarbiturate anesthetics (968.3)

967.1 **Chloral hydrate group**

967.2 **Paraldehyde**

967.3 **Bromine compounds**
Bromide   Carbromal (derivatives)

967.4 **Methaqualone compounds**

967.5 **Glutethimide group**

967.6 **Mixed sedatives, not elsewhere classified**

◆ **967.8** **Other sedatives and hypnotics**

◆ **967.9** **Unspecified sedative or hypnotic**
Sleeping:
drug
pill   } NOS
tablet

● **968** **Poisoning by other central nervous system depressants and anesthetics**
Excludes: drug dependence (304.0-304.9)
nondependent abuse (305.0-305.9)

968.0 **Central nervous system muscle-tone depressants**
Chlorphenesin (carbamate)   Methocarbamol
Mephenesin

968.1 **Halothane**

◆ **968.2** **Other gaseous anesthetics**
Ether
Halogenated hydrocarbon derivatives, except halothane
Nitrous oxide

968.3 **Intravenous anesthetics**
Ketamine
Methohexital [methohexitone]
Thiobarbiturates, such as thiopental sodium

◆ **968.4** **Other and unspecified general anesthetics**

968.5 **Surface [topical] and infiltration anesthetics**
Cocaine   Procaine
Lidocaine [lignocaine]   Tetracaine

968.6 **Peripheral nerve- and plexus-blocking anesthetics**

968.7 **Spinal anesthetics**

◆ **968.9** **Other and unspecified local anesthetics**

● **969** **Poisoning by psychotropic agents**
Excludes: drug dependence (304.0-304.9)
nondependent abuse (305.0-305.9)

969.0 **Antidepressants**
Amitriptyline
Imipramine
Monoamine oxidase [MAO] inhibitors

969.1 **Phenothiazine-based tranquilizers**
Chlorpromazine   Prochlorperazine
Fluphenazine   Promazine

969.2 **Butyrophenone-based tranquilizers**
Haloperidol
Spiperone
Trifluperidol

◆ **969.3** **Other antipsychotics, neuroleptics, and major tranquilizers**

969.4 **Benzodiazepine-based tranquilizers**
Chlordiazepoxide   Lorazepam
Diazepam   Medazepam
Flurazepam   Nitrazepam

◆ **969.5** **Other tranquilizers**
Hydroxyzine   Meprobamate

969.6 **Psychodysleptics [hallucinogens]**
Cannabis (derivatives)   Mescaline
Lysergide [LSD]   Psilocin
Marihuana (derivatives)   Psilocybin

969.7 **Psychostimulants**
Amphetamine   Caffeine
Excludes: central appetite depressants (977.0)

◆ **969.8** **Other specified psychotropic agents**

◆ **969.9** **Unspecified psychotropic agent**

- **970 Poisoning by central nervous system stimulants**
  - 970.0 Analeptics
    - Lobeline
    - Nikethamide
  - 970.1 Opiate antagonists
    - Levallorphan
    - Naloxone
    - Nalorphine
  - ◆ 970.8 Other specified central nervous system stimulants
  - ◆ 970.9 Unspecified central nervous system stimulant
- **971 Poisoning by drugs primarily affecting the autonomic nervous system**
  - 971.0 Parasympathomimetics [cholinergics]
    - Acetylcholine
    - Pilocarpine
    - Anticholinesterase:
      - organophosphorus
      - reversible
  - 971.1 Parasympatholytics [anticholinergics and antimuscarinics] and spasmolytics
    - Atropine
    - Quaternary ammonium derivatives
    - Homatropine
    - Hyoscine [scopolamine]
    - **EXCLUDES** *papaverine (972.5)*
  - 971.2 Sympathomimetics [adrenergics]
    - Epinephrine [adrenalin]
    - Levarterenol [noradrenalin]
  - 971.3 Sympatholytics [antiadrenergics]
    - Phenoxybenzamine
    - Tolazolinehydrochloride
  - ◆ 971.9 Unspecified drug primarily affecting autonomic nervous system
- **972 Poisoning by agents primarily affecting the cardiovascular system**
  - 972.0 Cardiac rhythm regulators
    - Practolol
    - Propranolol
    - Procainamide
    - Quinidine
    - **EXCLUDES** *lidocaine (968.5)*
  - 972.1 Cardiotonic glycosides and drugs of similar action
    - Digitalis glycosides
    - Strophantins
    - Digoxin
  - 972.2 Antilipemic and antiarteriosclerotic drugs
    - Clofibrate
    - Nicotinic acid derivatives
  - 972.3 Ganglion-blocking agents
    - Pentamethonium bromide
  - 972.4 Coronary vasodilators
    - Dipyridamole
    - Nitrites
    - Nitrates [nitroglycerin]
  - ◆ 972.5 Other vasodilators
    - Cyclandelate
    - Papaverine
    - Diazoxide
    - **EXCLUDES** *nicotinic acid (972.2)*
  - ◆ 972.6 Other antihypertensive agents
    - Clonidine
    - Rauwolfia alkaloids
    - Guanethidine
    - Reserpine
  - 972.7 Antivaricose drugs, including sclerosing agents
    - Sodium morrhuate
    - Zinc salts
  - 972.8 Capillary-active drugs
    - Adrenochrome derivatives
    - Metaraminol
  - ◆ 972.9 Other and unspecified agents primarily affecting the cardiovascular system
- **973 Poisoning by agents primarily affecting the gastrointestinal system**
  - 973.0 Antacids and antigastric secretion drugs
    - Aluminum hydroxide
    - Magnesium trisilicate
  - 973.1 Irritant cathartics
    - Bisacodyl
    - Phenolphthalein
    - Castor oil
  - 973.2 Emollient cathartics
    - Dioctyl sulfosuccinates
  - ◆ 973.3 Other cathartics, including intestinal atonia drugs
    - Magnesium sulfate
  - 973.4 Digestants
    - Pancreatin
    - Pepsin
    - Papain
  - 973.5 Antidiarrheal drugs
    - Kaolin
    - Pectin
    - **EXCLUDES** *anti-infectives (960.0-961.9)*
  - 973.6 Emetics
  - ◆ 973.8 Other specified agents primarily affecting the gastrointestinal system
  - ◆ 973.9 Unspecified agent primarily affecting the gastrointestinal system
- **974 Poisoning by water, mineral, and uric acid metabolism drugs**
  - 974.0 Mercurial diuretics
    - Chlormerodrin
    - Mersalyl
    - Mercaptomerin
  - 974.1 Purine derivative diuretics
    - Theobromine
    - Theophylline
    - **EXCLUDES** *aminophylline [theophylline ethylenediamine] (975.7)*
    - *caffeine (969.7)*
  - 974.2 Carbonic acid anhydrase inhibitors
    - Acetazolamide
  - 974.3 Saluretics
    - Benzothiadiazides
    - Chlorothiazide group
  - ◆ 974.4 Other diuretics
    - Ethacrynic acid
    - Furosemide
  - 974.5 Electrolytic, caloric, and water-balance agents
  - ◆ 974.6 Other mineral salts, not elsewhere classified
  - 974.7 Uric acid metabolism drugs
    - Allopurinol
    - Probenecid
    - Colchicine
- **975 Poisoning by agents primarily acting on the smooth and skeletal muscles and respiratory system**
  - 975.0 Oxytocic agents
    - Ergot alkaloids
    - Prostaglandins
    - Oxytocin
  - 975.1 Smooth muscle relaxants
    - Adiphenine
    - Metaproterenol [orciprenaline]
    - **EXCLUDES** *papaverine (972.5)*
  - 975.2 Skeletal muscle relaxants
  - ◆ 975.3 Other and unspecified drugs acting on muscles
  - 975.4 Antitussives
    - Dextromethorphan
    - Pipazethate
  - 975.5 Expectorants
    - Acetylcysteine
    - Terpin hydrate
    - Guaifenesin
  - 975.6 Anti-common cold drugs
  - 975.7 Antiasthmatics
    - Aminophylline [theophylline ethylenediamine]
  - ◆ 975.8 Other and unspecified respiratory drugs
- **976 Poisoning by agents primarily affecting skin and mucous membrane, ophthalmological, otorhinolaryngological, and dental drugs**
  - 976.0 Local anti-infectives and anti-inflammatory drugs
  - 976.1 Antipruritics
  - 976.2 Local astringents and local detergents
  - 976.3 Emollients, demulcents, and protectants
  - 976.4 Keratolytics, keratoplastics, other hair treatment drugs and preparations
  - 976.5 Eye anti-infectives and other eye drugs
    - Idoxuridine
  - 976.6 Anti-infectives and other drugs and preparations for ear, nose, and throat
  - 976.7 Dental drugs topically applied
    - **EXCLUDES** *anti-infectives (976.0)*
    - *local anesthetics (968.5)*
  - ◆ 976.8 Other agents primarily affecting skin and mucous membrane
    - Spermicides [vaginal contraceptives]
  - ◆ 976.9 Unspecified agent primarily affecting skin and mucous membrane
- **977 Poisoning by other and unspecified drugs and medicinal substances**
  - 977.0 Dietetics
    - Central appetite depressants
  - 977.1 Lipotropic drugs
  - 977.2 Antidotes and chelating agents, not elsewhere classified
  - 977.3 Alcohol deterrents
  - 977.4 Pharmaceutical excipients
    - Pharmaceutical adjuncts
  - ◆ 977.8 Other specified drugs and medicinal substances
    - Contrast media used for diagnostic x-ray procedures
    - Diagnostic agents and kits
  - ◆ 977.9 Unspecified drug or medicinal substance
- **978 Poisoning by bacterial vaccines**
  - 978.0 BCG
  - 978.1 Typhoid and paratyphoid
  - 978.2 Cholera
  - 978.3 Plague
  - 978.4 Tetanus
  - 978.5 Diphtheria
  - 978.6 Pertussis vaccine, including combinations with a pertussis component
  - ◆ 978.8 Other and unspecified bacterial vaccines
  - 978.9 Mixed bacterial vaccines, except combinations with a pertussis component

INJURY AND POISONING

● **979 Poisoning by other vaccines and biological substances**
    EXCLUDES gamma globulin (964.6)
    979.0 Smallpox vaccine
    979.1 Rabies vaccine
    979.2 Typhus vaccine
    979.3 Yellow fever vaccine
    979.4 Measles vaccine
    979.5 Poliomyelitis vaccine
    ◆ 979.6 Other and unspecified viral and rickettsial vaccines
        Mumps vaccine
    979.7 Mixed viral-rickettsial and bacterial vaccines, except combinations with a pertussis component
        EXCLUDES combinations with a pertussis component (978.6)
    ◆ 979.9 Other and unspecified vaccines and biological substances

TOXIC EFFECTS OF SUBSTANCES CHIEFLY NONMEDICINAL AS TO SOURCE (980-989)

Use additional code to specify the nature of the toxic effect ◆
EXCLUDES burns from chemical agents (ingested) (947.0-947.9)
localized toxic effects indexed elsewhere (001.0-799.9)
respiratory conditions due to external agents (506.0-508.9)

● **980 Toxic effect of alcohol**
    980.0 Ethyl alcohol
        Denatured alcohol   Grain alcohol
        Ethanol
        EXCLUDES acute alcohol intoxication (305.0)
            in alcoholism(303.0)
            drunkenness (simple) (305.0)
            pathological (291.4)
    980.1 Methyl alcohol
        Methanol   Wood alcohol
    980.2 Isopropyl alcohol
        Dimethyl carbinol   Rubbing alcohol
        Isopropanol
    980.3 Fusel oil
        Alcohol: Alcohol:
          amyl   propyl
          butyl
    ◆ 980.8 Other specified alcohols
    ◆ 980.9 Unspecified alcohol
  981 Toxic effect of petroleum products
    Benzine   Petroleum:
    Gasoline   ether
    Kerosene   naphtha
    Paraffin wax   spirit
● **982 Toxic effect of solvents other than petroleum-based**
    982.0 Benzene and homologues
    982.1 Carbon tetrachloride
    982.2 Carbon disulfide
        Carbon bisulfide
    ◆ 982.3 Other chlorinated hydrocarbon solvents
        Tetrachloroethylene
        Trichloroethylene
        EXCLUDES chlorinated hydrocarbon preparations other than solvents (989.2)
    982.4 Nitroglycol
    ◆ 982.8 Other nonpetroleum-based solvents
        Acetone
● **983 Toxic effect of corrosive aromatics, acids, and caustic alkalis**
    983.0 Corrosive aromatics
        Carbolic acid or phenol   Cresol
    983.1 Acids
        Acid: Acid:
          hydrochloric   sulfuric
          nitric
    983.2 Caustic alkalis
        Lye   Sodium hydroxide
        Potassium hydroxide
    ◆ 983.9 Caustic, unspecified
● **984 Toxic effect of lead and its compounds (including fumes)**
    INCLUDES that from all sources except medicinal substances
    984.0 Inorganic lead compounds
        Lead dioxide   Lead salts
    984.1 Organic lead compounds
        Lead acetate   Tetraethyl lead
    ◆ 984.8 Other lead compounds
    ◆ 984.9 Unspecified lead compound
● **985 Toxic effect of other metals**
    INCLUDES that from all sources except medicinal substances
    985.0 Mercury and its compounds
        Minamata disease
    985.1 Arsenic and its compounds
    985.2 Manganese and its compounds
    985.3 Beryllium and its compounds
    985.4 Antimony and its compounds
    985.5 Cadmium and its compounds
    985.6 Chromium
    ◆ 985.8 Other specified metals
        Brass fumes   Iron compounds
        Copper salts   Nickel compounds
    ◆ 985.9 Unspecified metal
  986 Toxic effect of carbon monoxide
    Carbon monoxide from any source
● **987 Toxic effect of other gases, fumes, or vapors**
    987.0 Liquefied petroleum gases
        Butane   Propane
    ◆ 987.1 Other hydrocarbon gas
    987.2 Nitrogen oxides
        Nitrogen dioxide   Nitrous fumes
    987.3 Sulfur dioxide
    987.4 Freon
        Dichloromonofluoromethane
    987.5 Lacrimogenic gas
        Bromobenzyl cyanide   Ethyliodoacetate
        Chloroacetophenone
    987.6 Chlorine gas
    987.7 Hydrocyanic acid gas
    ◆ 987.8 Other specified gases, fumes, or vapors
        Phosgene   Polyester fumes
    ◆ 987.9 Unspecified gas, fume, or vapor
● **988 Toxic effect of noxious substances eaten as food**
    EXCLUDES allergic reaction to food, such as:
        gastroenteritis (558.9)
        rash (692.5, 693.1)
       food poisoning (bacterial) (005.0-005.9)
       toxic effects of food contaminants, such as:
        aflatoxin and other mycotoxin (989.7)
        mercury (985.0)
    988.0 Fish and shellfish
    988.1 Mushrooms
    988.2 Berries and other plants
    ◆ 988.8 Other specified noxious substances eaten as food
    ◆ 988.9 Unspecified noxious substance eaten as food
● **989 Toxic effect of other substances, chiefly nonmedicinal as to source**
    989.0 Hydrocyanic acid and cyanides
        Potassium cyanide
        Sodium cyanide
        EXCLUDES gas and fumes (987.7)
    989.1 Strychnine and salts
    989.2 Chlorinated hydrocarbons
        Aldrin   DDT
        Chlordane   Dieldrin
        EXCLUDES chlorinated hydrocarbon solvents (982.0-982.3)
    989.3 Organophosphate and carbamate
        Carbaryl   Parathion
        Dichlorvos   Phorate
        Malathion   Phosdrin
    ◆ 989.4 Other pesticides, not elsewhere classified
        Mixtures of insecticides
    989.5 Venom
        Bites of venomous snakes, lizards, and spiders
        Tick paralysis
    989.6 Soaps and detergents
    989.7 Aflatoxin and other mycotoxin [food contaminants]
    ◆ 989.8 Other substances, chiefly nonmedicinal as to source
    ◆ 989.9 Unspecified substance, chiefly nonmedicinal as to source

● Additional digits required   ◆ Nonspecific code   ▪ Not a primary diagnosis

OTHER AND UNSPECIFIED EFFECTS OF EXTERNAL CAUSES
(990-995)

◆ **990 Effects of radiation, unspecified**
    Complication of: Radiation sickness
      phototherapy
      radiation therapy
    EXCLUDES specified adverse effects of radiation. Such conditions are to be classified according to the nature of the adverse effect, as:
        burns (940.0-949.5)
        dermatitis (692.7-692.8)
        leukemia (204.0-208.9)
        pneumonia (508.0)
        sunburn (692.71)
    [The type of radiation giving rise to the adverse effect may be identified by use of the E codes.]

● **991 Effects of reduced temperature**
  991.0 Frostbite of face
  991.1 Frostbite of hand
  991.2 Frostbite of foot
  ◆ **991.3** Frostbite of other and unspecified sites
  991.4 Immersion foot
      Trench foot
  991.5 Chilblains
      Erythema pernio   Perniosis
  991.6 Hypothermia
      Hypothermia (accidental)
      EXCLUDES hypothermia following anesthesia (995.89)
          hypothermia not associated with low environmental temperature (780.9)
  ◆ **991.8** Other specified effects of reduced temperature
  ◆ **991.9** Unspecified effect of reduced temperature
      Effects of freezing or excessive cold NOS

● **992 Effects of heat and light**
    EXCLUDES burns (940.0-949.5)
        diseases of sweat glands due to heat (705.0-705.9)
        malignant hyperpyrexia following anesthesia (995.89)
        sunburn (692.71)
  992.0 Heat stroke and sunstroke
      Heat apoplexy   Siriasis
      Heat pyrexia   Thermoplegia
      Ictus solaris
  992.1 Heat syncope
      Heat collapse
  992.2 Heat cramps
  992.3 Heat exhaustion, anhydrotic
      Heat prostration due to water depletion
      EXCLUDES that associated with salt depletion (992.4)
  992.4 Heat exhaustion due to salt depletion
      Heat prostration due to salt (and water) depletion
  ◆ **992.5** Heat exhaustion, unspecified
      Heat prostration NOS
  992.6 Heat fatigue, transient
  992.7 Heat edema
  ◆ **992.8** Other specified heat effects
  ◆ **992.9** Unspecified

● **993 Effects of air pressure**
  993.0 Barotrauma, otitic
      Aero-otitis media
      Effects of high altitude on ears
  993.1 Barotrauma, sinus
      Aerosinusitis
      Effects of high altitude on sinuses
  ◆ **993.2** Other and unspecified effects of high altitude
      Alpine sickness   Hypobaropathy
      Andes disease   Mountain sickness
      Anoxia due to high altitude
  993.3 Caisson disease
      Bends   Decompression sickness
      Compressed-air disease   Divers' palsy or paralysis
  993.4 Effects of air pressure caused by explosion
  ◆ **993.8** Other specified effects of air pressure
  ◆ **993.9** Unspecified effect of air pressure

● **994 Effects of other external causes**
    EXCLUDES certain adverse effects not elsewhere classified (995.0-995.8)

  994.0 Effects of lightning
      Shock from lightning
      Struck by lightning NOS
      EXCLUDES burns (940.0-949.5)
  994.1 Drowning and nonfatal submersion
      Bathing cramp   Immersion
  994.2 Effects of hunger
      Deprivation of food   Starvation
  994.3 Effects of thirst
      Deprivation of water
  994.4 Exhaustion due to exposure
  994.5 Exhaustion due to excessive exertion
      Overexertion
  994.6 Motion sickness
      Air sickness   Travel sickness
      Seasickness
  994.7 Asphyxiation and strangulation
      Suffocation (by):   Suffocation (by):
        bedclothes   plastic bag
        cave-in   pressure
        constriction   strangulation
        mechanical
      EXCLUDES asphyxia from:
        carbon monoxide (986)
        inhalation of food or foreign body (932-934.9)
        other gases, fumes, and vapors (987.0-987.9)
  994.8 Electrocution and nonfatal effects of electric current
      Shock from electric current
      EXCLUDES electric burns (940.0-949.5)
  ◆ **994.9** Other effects of external causes
      Effects of:
        abnormal gravitational [G] forces or states
        weightlessness

● **995 Certain adverse effects not elsewhere classified**
  Note: This category is to be used to identify the effects not elsewhere classifiable of unknown, undetermined, or ill-defined causes. This category may also be used to provide an additional code to identify the effects of conditions classified elsewhere.
    EXCLUDES complications of surgical and medical care (996.0-999.9)
  ◆ **995.0** Other anaphylactic shock
      Allergic shock   ⎫
      Anaphylactic   ⎬ NOS or due to adverse effect of correct medicinal substance properly administered
        reaction   ⎭
      Anaphylaxis
      Code also any underlying condition such as:
        poisoning by drugs, medicinals and biologic substances (960-979)
        toxic effects of substances chiefly nonmedical as to source (980-989)
      Use additional E code, if desired, to identify external cause, such as:
        adverse effects of correct medicinal substance properly administered [E930-E949]
      EXCLUDES anaphylactic reaction to serum (999.4)
        anaphylactic shock due to adverse food reaction (995.60-995.69)
  995.1 Angioneurotic edema
      Giant urticaria
      EXCLUDES urticaria:
        due to serum (999.5)
        other specified (698.2, 708.0-708.9, 757.33)
  ◆ **995.2** Unspecified adverse effect of drug, medicinal and biological substance
      Adverse effect   ⎫
      Allergic reaction   ⎬ (due) to correct medicinal substance properly administered
      Hypersensitivity   ⎭
      Idiosyncrasy
      Drug: Drug:
        hypersensitivity NOS   reaction NOS
      EXCLUDES pathological drug intoxication (292.2)

INJURY AND POISONING

◆ **995.3 Allergy, unspecified**
Allergic reaction NOS
Idiosyncrasy NOS
Hypersensitivity NOS
EXCLUDES allergic reaction NOS to correct medicinal substance properly administered (995.2)
specific types of allergic reaction, such as:
allergic diarrhea (558.9)
dermatitis (691.0-693.9)
hayfever (477.0-477.9)

995.4 Shock due to anesthesia
Shock due to anesthesia in which the correct substance was properly administered
EXCLUDES complications of anesthesia in labor or delivery (668.0-668.9)
overdose or wrong substance given (968.0-969.9)
postoperative shock NOS (998.0)
specified adverse effects of anesthesia classified elsewhere, such as:
anoxic brain damage (348.1)
hepatitis (070.0-070.9), etc.
unspecified adverse effect of anesthesia (995.2)

995.5 Child maltreatment syndrome
Battered baby or child syndrome NOS
Emotional and/or nutritional maltreatment of child

● **995.6 Anaphylactic shock due to adverse food reaction**
  ◆ 995.60 Due to unspecified food
  995.61 Due to peanuts
  995.62 Due to crustaceans
  995.63 Due to fruits and vegetables
  995.64 Due to tree nuts and seeds
  995.65 Due to fish
  995.66 Due to food additives
  995.67 Due to milk products
  995.68 Due to eggs
  ◆ 995.69 Due to other specified food

● **995.8 Other specified adverse effects, not elsewhere classified**
  995.81 Adult maltreatment syndrome
    Abused person NEC
    Battered:
      person syndrome NEC
      spouse
      woman
  ◆ 995.89 Other
    Malignant hyperpyrexia or hypothermia due to anesthesia

COMPLICATIONS OF SURGICAL AND MEDICAL CARE, NOT ELSEWHERE CLASSIFIED (996-999)

EXCLUDES adverse effects of medicinal agents (001.0-799.9, 995.0-995.8)
burns from local applications and irradiation (940.0-949.5)
complications of:
conditions for which the procedure was performed
surgical procedures during abortion, labor, and delivery (630-676.9)
poisoning and toxic effects of drugs and chemicals (960.0-989.9)
postoperative conditions in which no complications are present, such as:
artificial opening status (V44.0-V44.9)
closure of external stoma (V55.0-V55.9)
fitting of prosthetic device (V52.0-V52.9)
specified complications classified elsewhere
anesthetic shock (995.4)
electrolyte imbalance (276.0-276.9)
postlaminectomy syndrome (722.80-722.83)
postmastectomy lymphedema syndrome (457.0)
postoperative psychosis (293.0-293.9)
any other condition classified elsewhere in the Alphabetic Index when described as due to a procedure

● **996 Complications peculiar to certain specified procedures**
INCLUDES complications, not elsewhere classified, in the use of artificial substitutes [e.g., Dacron, metal, Silastic, Teflon] or natural sources [e.g., bone] involving:
anastomosis (internal)
graft (bypass) (patch)
implant
internal device:
catheter
electronic
fixation
prosthetic
reimplant
transplant
EXCLUDES accidental puncture or laceration during procedure (998.2)
complications of internal anastomosis of:
gastrointestinal tract (997.4)
urinary tract (997.5)
other specified complications classified elsewhere, such as:
hemolytic anemia (283.1)
functional cardiac disturbances (429.4)
serum hepatitis (070.2-070.3)

● **996.0 Mechanical complication of cardiac device, implant, and graft**
Breakdown (mechanical)   Obstruction, mechanical
Displacement   Perforation
Leakage   Protrusion
  ◆ 996.00 Unspecified device, implant, and graft
  996.01 Due to cardiac pacemaker (electrode)
  996.02 Due to heart valve prosthesis
  996.03 Due to coronary bypass graft
    EXCLUDES atherosclerosis of graft (414.02, 414.03) ▼
    embolism [occlusion NOS] [thrombus] of graft (996.72)
  996.04 Due to automatic implantable cardiac defibrillator ▲
  996.09 Other

◆ **996.1 Mechanical complication of other vascular device, implant, and graft**
Femoral-popliteal bypass graph   ◆
Mechanical complications involving:
aortic (bifurcation) graft (replacement)
arteriovenous:
  fistula   } surgically created
  shunt
balloon (counterpulsation) device, intra-aortic
carotid artery bypass graft
dialysis catheter
umbrella device, vena cava
EXCLUDES atherosclerosis of biological graft (440.30-440.32) ▼
embolism [occlusion NOS] [thrombus] of (biological) (synthetic) graft (996.74) ▲

996.2 Mechanical complication of nervous system device, implant, and graft
Mechanical complications involving:
dorsal column stimulator
electrodes implanted in brain [brain "pacemaker"]
peripheral nerve graft
ventricular (communicating) shunt

● **996.3 Mechanical complication of genitourinary device, implant, and graft**
  ◆ 996.30 Unspecified device, implant, and graft
  996.31 Due to urethral [indwelling] catheter
  996.32 Due to intrauterine contraceptive device
  ◆ 996.39 Other
    Cystostomy catheter
    Prosthetic reconstruction of vas deferens
    Repair (graft) of ureter without mention of resection
    EXCLUDES complications due to:
    external stoma of urinary tract (997.5)
    internal anastomosis of urinary tract (997.5)

● Additional digits required   ◆ Nonspecific code   ■ Not a primary diagnosis

996.4 Mechanical complication of internal orthopedic device, implant, and graft
　　Mechanical complications involving:
　　　　external (fixation) device utilizing internal screw(s), pin(s) or other methods of fixation
　　　　grafts of bone, cartilage, muscle, or tendon
　　　　internal (fixation) device such as nail, plate, rod, etc.
　　　EXCLUDES complications of external orthopedic device, such as:
　　　　　pressure ulcer due to cast (707.0)

● **996.5** Mechanical complication of other specified prosthetic device, implant, and graft
　　Mechanical complications involving:
　　　prosthetic implant in:　　　prosthetic implant in:
　　　　bile duct　　　　　　　　chin
　　　　breast　　　　　　　　　orbit of eye
　　nonabsorbable surgical material NOS
　　other graft, implant, and internal device, not elsewhere classified

　996.51 Due to corneal graft
◆ **996.52** Due to graft of other tissue, not elsewhere classified
　　Skin graft failure or rejection
　　EXCLUDES sloughing of temporary skin allografts or xenografts (pigskin)—omit code

　996.53 Due to ocular lens prosthesis
　　EXCLUDES contact lenses—code to condition

　996.54 Due to breast prosthesis
　　Breast capsule (prosthesis)
　　Mammary implant

◆ **996.59** Due to other implant and internal device, not elsewhere classified
　　Nonabsorbable surgical material NOS
　　Prosthetic implant in:
　　　bile duct
　　　chin
　　　orbit of eye

● **996.6** Infection and inflammatory reaction due to internal prosthetic device, implant, and graft
　　Infection (causing obstruction)　}　due to (presence of) any device, implant, and graft classifiable to 996.0-996.5
　　Inflammation

◆ **996.60** Due to unspecified device, implant, and graft
　996.61 Due to cardiac device, implant, and graft
　　Cardiac pacemaker or defibrillator:
　　　electrode(s), lead(s)
　　　pulse generator
　　　subcutaneous pocket
　　Coronary artery bypass graft
　　Heart valve prosthesis

◆ **996.62** Due to other vascular device, implant, and graft
　　Arterial graft
　　Arteriovenous fistula or shunt
　　Infusion pump
　　Vascular catheter (arterial) (dialysis) (venous)

　996.63 Due to nervous system device, implant, and graft
　　Electrodes implanted in brain
　　Peripheral nerve graft
　　Spinal canal catheter
　　Ventricular (communicating) shunt (catheter)

　996.64 Due to indwelling urinary catheter
◆ **996.65** Due to other genitourinary device, implant, and graft
　　Intrauterine contraceptive device

　996.66 Due to internal joint prosthesis
◆ **996.67** Due to other internal orthopedic device, implant, and graft
　　Bone growth stimulator (electrode)
　　Internal fixation device (pin) (rod) (screw)

◆ **996.69** Due to other internal prosthetic device, implant, and graft
　　Breast prosthesis　　Prosthetic orbital implant
　　Ocular lens prosthesis

● **996.7** Other complications of internal (biological) (synthetic) prosthetic device, implant, and graft
　　Complication NOS
　　　occlusion NOS
　　Embolism
　　Fibrosis　　　　　　　}　due to (presence of) any device, implant, and graft classifiable to 996.0-996.5
　　Hemorrhage
　　Pain
　　Stenosis
　　Thrombus
　　EXCLUDES transplant rejection (996.8)

◆ **996.70** Due to unspecified device, implant, and graft
　996.71 Due to heart valve prosthesis
◆ **996.72** Due to other cardiac device, implant, and graft
　　Cardiac pacemaker or defibrillator:
　　　electrode(s), lead(s)
　　　subcutaneous pocket
　　Coronary artery bypass (graft)
　　EXCLUDES occlusion due to atherosclerosis (414.02-414.03)

　996.73 Due to renal dialysis device, implant, and graft
◆ **996.74** Due to other vascular device, implant, and graft
　　EXCLUDES occlusion of biological graft due to atherosclerosis (440.30-440.32)

　996.75 Due to nervous system device, implant, and graft
　996.76 Due to genitourinary device, implant, and graft
　996.77 Due to internal joint prosthesis
◆ **996.78** Due to other internal orthopedic device, implant, and graft
◆ **996.79** Due to other internal prosthetic device, implant, and graft

● **996.8** Complications of transplanted organ
　　Transplant failure or rejection
　　Use additional code, if desired, to identify nature of complication, such as:
　　　Cytomegalovirus (CMV) infection (078.5)

◆ **996.80** Transplanted organ, unspecified
　996.81 Kidney
　996.82 Liver
　996.83 Heart
　996.84 Lung
　996.85 Bone marrow
　　Graft-versus-host disease (acute) (chronic)
　996.86 Pancreas
◆ **996.89** Other specified transplanted organ
　　Intestines

● **996.9** Complications of reattached extremity or body part
◆ **996.90** Unspecified extremity
　996.91 Forearm
　996.92 Hand
　996.93 Finger(s)
◆ **996.94** Upper extremity, other and unspecified
　996.95 Foot and toe(s)
◆ **996.96** Lower extremity, other and unspecified
◆ **996.99** Other specified body part

● **997** Complications affecting specified body systems, not elsewhere classified
　　Use additional code to identify complications
　　EXCLUDES the listed conditions when specified as:
　　　causing shock (998.0)
　　　complications of:
　　　　anesthesia:
　　　　　adverse effect (001.0-799.9, 995.0-995.8)
　　　　　in labor or delivery (668.0-668.9)
　　　　　poisoning (968.0-969.9)
　　　　implanted device or graft (996.0-996.9)
　　　　obstetrical procedures (669.0-669.4)
　　　　reattached extremity (996.90-996.96)
　　　　transplanted organ (996.80-996.89)

　997.0 Central nervous system complications
　　Anoxic brain damage　　}　during or resulting from a procedure
　　Cerebral hypoxia

INJURY AND POISONING

997.1 Cardiac complications
Cardiac:
    arrest
    insufficiency
Cardiorespiratory failure
Heart failure
} during or resulting from a procedure

EXCLUDES the listed conditions as long-term effects of cardiac surgery or due to the presence of cardiac prosthetic device (429.4)

997.2 Peripheral vascular complications
Phlebitis or thrombophlebitis during or resulting from a procedure

EXCLUDES the listed conditions due to:
    implant or catheter device (996.62)
    infusion, perfusion, or transfusion (999.2)
    complications affecting internal blood vessels, such as:
        mesenteric artery (997.4)
        renal artery (997.5)

997.3 Respiratory complications
Mendelson's syndrome
Pneumonia (aspiration)
} resulting from a procedure

EXCLUDES iatrogenic [postoperative] pneumothorax (512.1) ◆
    Mendelson's syndrome in labor and delivery (668.0)
    specified complications classified elsewhere, such as:
        adult respiratory distress syndrome (518.5)
        pulmonary edema, postoperative (518.4)
        respiratory insufficiency, acute, postoperative (518.5)
        shock lung (518.5)
        tracheostomy complication (519.0)

997.4 Gastrointestinal complications
Complications of:
    external stoma of gastrointestinal tract, not elsewhere classified
    intestinal (internal) anastomosis and bypass, not elsewhere classified, except that involving urinary tract
Hepatic failure
Hepatorenal syndrome
Intestinal obstruction NOS
} specified as due to a procedure

EXCLUDES specified gastrointestinal complications classified elsewhere, such as:
    blind loop syndrome (579.2)
    colostomy or enterostomy malfunction (569.6)
    gastrojejunal ulcer (534.0-534.9)
    postcholecystectomy syndrome (576.0)
    postgastric surgery syndromes (564.2)

997.5 Urinary complications
Complications of:
    external stoma of urinary tract
    internal anastomosis and bypass of urinary tract, including that involving intestinal tract
Oliguria or anuria
Renal:
    failure (acute)
    insufficiency (acute)
    Tubular necrosis (acute)
} specified as due to procedure

EXCLUDES specified complications classified elsewhere, such as:
    postoperative stricture of:
        ureter (593.3)
        urethra (598.2)

● 997.6 Late amputation stump complication
Use additional code to identify site (V49.60-V49.79) ◆

EXCLUDES phantom limb (syndrome) (353.6)

◆ 997.60 Unspecified complication
997.61 Neuroma of amputation stump
997.62 Infection (chronic)
◆ 997.69 Other

◆ 997.9 Complications affecting other specified body systems, not elsewhere classified
Vitreous touch syndrome

EXCLUDES specified complications classified elsewhere, such as:
    broad ligament laceration syndrome (620.6)
    postartificial menopause syndrome (627.4)
    postoperative stricture of vagina (623.2)

● 998 Other complications of procedures, not elsewhere classified

998.0 Postoperative shock
Collapse NOS
Shock (endotoxic) (hypovolemic) (septic)
} during or resulting from a surgical procedure

EXCLUDES shock:
    anaphylactic due to serum (999.4)
    anesthetic (995.4)
    electric (994.8)
    following abortion (639.5)
    obstetric (669.1)
    traumatic (958.4)

998.1 Hemorrhage or hematoma complicating a procedure
Hemorrhage of any site resulting from a procedure

EXCLUDES hemorrhage due to implanted device or graft (996.70-996.79)
    that complicating cesarean section or puerperal perineal wound (674.3)

998.2 Accidental puncture or laceration during a procedure
Accidental perforation by catheter or other instrument during a procedure on:
    blood vessel
    nerve
    organ

EXCLUDES iatrogenic [postoperative] pneumothorax (512.1) ◆
    puncture or laceration caused by implanted device intentionally left in operation wound (996.0-996.5)
    specified complications classified elsewhere, such as:
        broad ligament laceration syndrome (620.6)
        trauma from instruments during delivery (664.0-665.9)

998.3 Disruption of operation wound
Dehiscence
Rupture
} of operation wound

EXCLUDES disruption of:
    cesarean wound (674.1)
    perineal wound, puerperal (674.2)

998.4 Foreign body accidentally left during a procedure
Adhesions
Obstruction
Perforation
} due to foreign body accidentally left in operative wound or body cavity during a procedure

EXCLUDES obstruction or perforation caused by implanted device intentionally left in body (996.0-996.5)

998.5 Postoperative infection
Abscess:
    intra-abdominal
    stitch
    subphrenic
    wound
Septicemia
} postoperative

EXCLUDES infection due to:
    implanted device (996.60-996.69)
    infusion, perfusion, or transfusion (999.3)
    postoperative obstetrical wound infection (674.3)

998.6 Persistent postoperative fistula

998.7 Acute reaction to foreign substance accidentally left during a procedure
Peritonitis:
    aseptic
Peritonitis:
    chemical

● Additional digits required   ◆ Nonspecific code   ■ Not a primary diagnosis

- **998.8 Other specified complications of procedures, not elsewhere classified**
  - 998.81 Emphysema (subcutaneous) (surgical) resulting from a procedure ▼
  - 998.82 Cataract fragments in eye following cataract surgery
  - ◆ 998.89 Other specified complications ▲
- ◆ **998.9 Unspecified complication of procedure, not elsewhere classified**
  - Postoperative complication NOS
  - EXCLUDES complication NOS of obstetrical, surgery or procedure (669.4)

- ● **999 Complications of medical care, not elsewhere classified**
  - INCLUDES complications, not elsewhere classified, of:
    - dialysis (hemodialysis) (peritoneal) (renal)
    - extracorporeal circulation
    - hyperalimentation therapy
    - immunization
    - infusion
    - inhalation therapy
    - injection
    - inoculation
    - perfusion
    - transfusion
    - vaccination
    - ventilation therapy
  - EXCLUDES specified complications classified elsewhere such as:
    - complications of implanted device (996.0-996.9)
    - contact dermatitis due to drugs (692.3)
    - dementia dialysis (294.8)
      - transient (293.9)
    - dialysis disequilibrium syndrome (276.0-276.9)
    - poisoning and toxic effects of drugs and chemicals (960.0-989.9)
    - postvaccinal encephalitis (323.5)
    - water and electrolyte imbalance (276.0-276.9)

  - **999.0 Generalized vaccinia**
  - **999.1 Air embolism**
    - Air embolism to any site following infusion, perfusion, or transfusion
    - EXCLUDES embolism specified as:
      - complicating:
        - abortion (634-638 with .6, 639.6)
        - ectopic or molar pregnancy (639.6)
        - pregnancy, childbirth, or the puerperium (673.0)
      - due to implanted device (996.7)
      - traumatic (958.0)
  - ◆ **999.2 Other vascular complications**
    - Phlebitis
    - Thromboembolism } following infusion, perfusion, or transfusion
    - Thrombophlebitis
    - EXCLUDES the listed conditions when specified as:
      - due to implanted device (996.72-996.74)
      - postoperative NOS (997.2)
  - ◆ **999.3 Other infection**
    - Infection
    - Sepsis } following infusion, injection, transfusion, or vaccination
    - Septicemia
    - EXCLUDES the listed conditions when specified as:
      - due to implanted device (996.60-996.69)
      - postoperative NOS (998.5)
  - **999.4 Anaphylactic shock due to serum**
    - EXCLUDES shock:
      - allergic NOS (995.0)
      - anaphylactic:
        - NOS (995.0)
        - due to drugs and chemicals (995.0)
  - ◆ **999.5 Other serum reaction**
    - Intoxication by serum   Serum sickness
    - Protein sickness   Urticaria due to serum
    - Serum rash
    - EXCLUDES serum hepatitis (070.2-070.3)
  - **999.6 ABO incompatibility reaction**
    - Incompatible blood transfusion
    - Reaction to blood group incompatibility in infusion or transfusion
  - **999.7 Rh incompatibility reaction**
    - Reactions due to Rh factor in infusion or transfusion
  - ◆ **999.8 Other transfusion reaction**
    - Septic shock due to transfusion
    - Transfusion reaction NOS
    - EXCLUDES postoperative shock (998.0)
  - ◆ **999.9 Other and unspecified complications of medical care, not elsewhere classified**
    - Complications, not elsewhere classified, of:
      - electroshock
      - inhalation } therapy
      - ultrasound
      - ventilation
    - Unspecified misadventure of medical care
    - EXCLUDES unspecified complication of:
      - phototherapy (990)
      - radiation therapy (990)

SUPPLEMENTARY CLASSIFICATION OF FACTORS INFLUENCING HEALTH STATUS AND CONTACT WITH HEALTH SERVICES (V01-V82)

This classification is provided to deal with occasions when circumstances other than a disease or injury classifiable to categories 001-999 (the main part of ICD) are recorded as "diagnoses" or "problems." This can arise mainly in three ways:

a) When a person who is not currently sick encounters the health services for some specific purpose, such as to act as a donor of an organ or tissue, to receive prophylactic vaccination, or to discuss a problem which is in itself not a disease or injury. This will be a fairly rare occurrence among hospital inpatients, but will be relatively more common among hospital outpatients and patients of family practitioners, health clinics, etc.

b) When a person with a known disease or injury, whether it is current or resolving, encounters the health care system for a specific treatment of that disease or injury (e.g., dialysis for renal disease; chemotherapy for malignancy; cast change).

c) When some circumstance or problem is present which influences the person's health status but is not in itself a current illness or injury. Such factors may be elicited during population surveys, when the person may or may not be currently sick, or be recorded as an additional factor to be borne in mind when the person is receiving care for some current illness or injury classifiable to categories 001-999.

In the latter circumstances the V code should be used only as a supplementary code and should not be the one selected for use in primary, single cause tabulations. Examples of these circumstances are a personal history of certain diseases, or a person with an artificial heart valve in situ.

PERSONS WITH POTENTIAL HEALTH HAZARDS RELATED TO COMMUNICABLE DISEASES (V01-V09)

EXCLUDES family history of infectious and parasitic diseases (V18.8)
personal history of infectious and parasitic diseases (V12.0)

- **V01 Contact with or exposure to communicable diseases**
  - V01.0 Cholera
    - Conditions classifiable to 001
  - V01.1 Tuberculosis
    - Conditions classifiable to 010-018
  - V01.2 Poliomyelitis
    - Conditions classifiable to 045
  - V01.3 Smallpox
    - Conditions classifiable to 050
  - V01.4 Rubella
    - Conditions classifiable to 056
  - V01.5 Rabies
    - Conditions classifiable to 071
  - V01.6 Venereal diseases
    - Conditions classifiable to 090-099
  - V01.7 Other viral diseases
    - Conditions classifiable to 042-078, except as above
  - V01.8 Other communicable diseases
    - Conditions classifiable to 001-136, except as above
  - V01.9 Unspecified communicable disease
- **V02 Carrier or suspected carrier of infectious diseases**
  - V02.0 Cholera
  - V02.1 Typhoid
  - V02.2 Amebiasis
  - V02.3 Other gastrointestinal pathogens
  - V02.4 Diphtheria
  - V02.5 Other specified bacterial diseases
    - Bacterial disease:
      - meningococcal
      - staphylococcal
      - streptococcal
  - V02.6 Viral hepatitis
    - Hepatitis Australian-antigen [HAA] [SH] carrier
    - Serum hepatitis carrier
  - V02.7 Gonorrhea
  - V02.8 Other venereal diseases
  - V02.9 Other specified infectious organism

- **V03 Need for prophylactic vaccination and inoculation against bacterial diseases**
  - **EXCLUDES** vaccination not carried out because of contraindication (V64.0)
  vaccines against combinations of diseases (V06.0-V06.9)
  - V03.0 Cholera alone
  - V03.1 Typhoid-paratyphoid alone [TAB]
  - V03.2 Tuberculosis [BCG]
  - V03.3 Plague
  - V03.4 Tularemia
  - V03.5 Diphtheria alone
  - V03.6 Pertussis alone
  - V03.7 Tetanus toxoid alone
  - V03.8 Other specified vaccinations against single bacterial diseases
    - V03.81 Hemophilus influenza, type B [Hib]
    - V03.82 Streptococcus pneumoniae [pneumococcus]
    - V03.89 Other specified vaccination
  - V03.9 Unspecified single bacterial disease
- **V04 Need for prophylactic vaccination and inoculation against certain viral diseases**
  - **EXCLUDES** vaccines against combinations of diseases (V06.0-V06.9)
  - V04.0 Poliomyelitis
  - V04.1 Smallpox
  - V04.2 Measles alone
  - V04.3 Rubella alone
  - V04.4 Yellow fever
  - V04.5 Rabies
  - V04.6 Mumps alone
  - V04.7 Common cold
  - V04.8 Influenza
- **V05 Need for other prophylactic vaccination and inoculation against single diseases**
  - **EXCLUDES** vaccines against combinations of diseases (V06.0-V06.9)
  - V05.0 Arthropod-borne viral encephalitis
  - V05.1 Other arthropod-borne viral diseases
  - V05.2 Leishmaniasis
  - V05.3 Viral hepatitis
  - V05.4 Varicella
    - Chickenpox
  - V05.8 Other specified disease
  - V05.9 Unspecified single disease
- **V06 Need for prophylactic vaccination and inoculation against combinations of diseases**
  - Note: Use additional single vaccination codes from categories V03-V05 to identify any vaccinations not included in a combination code.
  - V06.0 Cholera with typhoid-paratyphoid [cholera+TAB]
  - V06.1 Diphtheria-tetanus-pertussis, combined [DTP]
  - V06.2 Diphtheria-tetanus-pertussis with typhoid-paratyphoid [DTP+TAB]
  - V06.3 Diphtheria-tetanus-pertussis with poliomyelitis [DTP+polio]
  - V06.4 Measles-mumps-rubella [MMR]
  - V06.5 Tetanus-diphtheria [Td]
  - V06.6 Streptococcus pneumoniae [pneumococcus] and influenza
  - V06.8 Other combinations
    - **EXCLUDES** multiple single vaccination codes (V03.0-V05.9)
  - V06.9 Unspecified combined vaccine
- **V07 Need for isolation and other prophylactic measures**
  - **EXCLUDES** prophylactic organ removal (V50.41-V50.49)
  - V07.0 Isolation
    - Admission to protect the individual from his surroundings or for isolation of individual after contact with infectious diseases
  - V07.1 Desensitization to allergens
  - V07.2 Prophylactic immunotherapy
    - Administration of:
      - antivenin
      - immune sera [gamma globulin]
      - RhoGAM
      - tetanus antitoxin

● Additional digits required   ◆ Nonspecific code   ■ Not a primary diagnosis

- **V07.3 Other prophylactic chemotherapy**
  - V07.31 Prophylactic fluoride administration
  - V07.39 Other prophylactic chemotherapy
    - EXCLUDES maintenance chemotherapy following disease (V58.1)
- V07.4 Postmenopausal hormone replacement therapy
- V07.8 Other specified prophylactic measure
- V07.9 Unspecified prophylactic measure
- **V08 Asymptomatic human immunodeficiency virus [HIV] infection status**
  - HIV positive NOS
  - Note: This code is *only* to be used when no HIV infection symptoms or conditions are present. If any HIV infection symptoms or conditions are present, see code 042.
  - EXCLUDES AIDS (042)
    - human immunodeficiency virus [HIV] disease (042)
    - exposure to HIV (V01.7)
    - nonspecific serologic evidence of HIV (795.71)
    - symptomatic human immunodeficiency virus [HIV] infection (042)
- **V09 Infection with drug-resistant microorganisms**
  - Note: This category is intended for use as an additional code for infectious conditions classified elsewhere to indicate the presence of drug-resistance of the infectious organism.
  - V09.0 Infection with microorganisms resistant to penicillins
  - V09.1 Infection with microorganisms resistant to cephalosporins and other B-lactam antibiotics
  - V09.2 Infection with microorganisms resistant to macrolides
  - V09.3 Infection with microorganisms resistant to tetracyclines
  - V09.4 Infection with microorganisms resistant to aminoglycosides
  - V09.5 Infection with microorganisms resistant to quinolones and fluoroquinolones
    - V09.50 Without mention of resistance to multiple quinolones and fluoroquinoles
    - V09.51 With resistance to multiple quinolones and fluoroquinoles
  - V09.6 Infection with microorganisms resistant to sulfonamides
  - V09.7 Infection with microorganisms resistant to other specified antimycobacterial agents
    - EXCLUDES Amikacin (V09.4)
      - Kanamycin (V09.4)
      - Streptomycin [SM] (V09.4)
    - V09.70 Without mention of resistance to multiple antimycobacterial agents
    - V09.71 With resistance to multiple antimycobacterial agents
  - V09.8 Infection with microorganisms resistant to other specified drugs
    - V09.80 Without mention of resistance to multiple drugs
    - V09.81 With resistance to multiple drugs
  - V09.9 Infection with drug-resistant microorganisms, unspecified
    - Drug resistance, NOS
    - V09.90 Without mention of multiple drug resistance
    - V09.91 With multiple drug resistance
      - Multiple drug resistance NOS

PERSONS WITH POTENTIAL HEALTH HAZARDS RELATED TO PERSONAL AND FAMILY HISTORY

EXCLUDES obstetric patients where the possibility that the fetus might be affected is the reason for observation or management during pregnancy (655.0-655.9)

- **V10 Personal history of malignant neoplasm**
  - V10.0 Gastrointestinal tract
    - History of conditions classifiable to 140-159
    - V10.00 Gastrointestinal tract, unspecified
    - V10.01 Tongue
    - V10.02 Other and unspecified oral cavity and pharynx
    - V10.03 Esophagus
    - V10.04 Stomach
    - V10.05 Large intestine
    - V10.06 Rectum, rectosigmoid junction, and anus
    - V10.07 Liver
    - V10.09 Other
  - V10.1 Trachea, bronchus, and lung
    - History of conditions classifiable to 162
    - V10.11 Bronchus and lung
    - V10.12 Trachea
  - V10.2 Other respiratory and intrathoracic organs
    - History of conditions classifiable to 160, 161, 163-165
    - V10.20 Respiratory organ, unspecified
    - V10.21 Larynx
    - V10.22 Nasal cavities, middle ear, and accessory sinuses
    - V10.29 Other
  - V10.3 Breast
    - History of conditions classifiable to 174 and 175
  - V10.4 Genital organs
    - History of conditions classifiable to 179-187
    - V10.40 Female genital organ, unspecified
    - V10.41 Cervix uteri
    - V10.42 Other parts of uterus
    - V10.43 Ovary
    - V10.44 Other female genital organs
    - V10.45 Male genital organ, unspecified
    - V10.46 Prostate
    - V10.47 Testis
    - V10.49 Other male genital organs
  - V10.5 Urinary organs
    - History of conditions classifiable to 188 and 189
    - V10.50 Urinary organ, unspecified
    - V10.51 Bladder
    - V10.52 Kidney
    - V10.59 Other
  - V10.6 Leukemia
    - Conditions classifiable to 204-208
    - EXCLUDES leukemia in remission (204-208)
    - V10.60 Leukemia, unspecified
    - V10.61 Lymphoid leukemia
    - V10.62 Myeloid leukemia
    - V10.63 Monocytic leukemia
    - V10.69 Other
  - V10.7 Other lymphatic and hematopoietic neoplasms
    - EXCLUDES listed conditions in 200-203 in remission
    - V10.71 Lymphosarcoma and reticulosarcoma
    - V10.72 Hodgkin's disease
    - V10.79 Other
  - V10.8 Personal history of malignant neoplasm of other sites
    - History of conditions classifiable to 170-173, 190-195
    - V10.81 Bone
    - V10.82 Malignant melanoma of skin
    - V10.83 Other malignant neoplasm of skin
    - V10.84 Eye
    - V10.85 Brain
    - V10.86 Other parts of nervous system
      - EXCLUDES peripheral sympathetic, and parasympathetic nerves (V10.89)
    - V10.87 Thyroid
    - V10.88 Other endocrine glands and related structures
    - V10.89 Other
  - V10.9 Unspecified personal history of malignant neoplasm
- **V11 Personal history of mental disorder**
  - V11.0 Schizophrenia
    - EXCLUDES that in remission (295.0-295.9 with fifth-digit 5)
  - V11.1 Affective disorders
    - Personal history of manic-depressive psychosis
    - EXCLUDES that in remission (296.0-296.6 with fifth-digit 5, 6)
  - V11.2 Neurosis
  - V11.3 Alcoholism
  - V11.8 Other mental disorders
  - V11.9 Unspecified mental disorder
- **V12 Personal history of certain other diseases**
  - V12.0 Infectious and parasitic diseases
    - V12.00 Unspecified infectious and parasitic disease
    - V12.01 Tuberculosis
    - V12.02 Poliomyelitis
    - V12.03 Malaria
    - V12.09 Other
  - V12.1 Nutritional deficiency

- V12.2 **Endocrine, metabolic, and immunity disorders**
  - EXCLUDES: history of allergy (V14.0-V14.9, V15.0)
- V12.3 **Diseases of blood and blood-forming organs**
- V12.4 **Disorders of nervous system and sense organs**
- V12.5 **Diseases of circulatory system**
  - EXCLUDES: old myocardial infarction (412)
  - postmyocardial infarction syndrome (411.0)
- V12.6 **Diseases of respiratory system**
- ● V12.7 **Diseases of digestive system**
  - ◆ V12.70 Unspecified digestive disease ▼
  - V12.71 Peptic ulcer disease
  - V12.72 Colonic polyps
  - ◆ V12.79 Other ▲
- ● **V13 Personal history of other diseases**
  - ● V13.0 **Disorders of urinary system**
    - ◆ V13.00 Unspecified urinary disorder ▼
    - V13.01 Urinary calculi
    - ◆ V13.09 Other ▲
  - V13.1 **Trophoblastic disease**
    - EXCLUDES: supervision during a current pregnancy (V23.1)
  - ◆ V13.2 **Other genital system and obstetric disorders**
    - EXCLUDES: supervision during a current pregnancy of a woman with poor obstetric history (V23.0-V23.9)
    - habitual aborter (646.3)
    - without current pregnancy (629.9)
  - V13.3 Diseases of skin and subcutaneous tissue
  - V13.4 Arthritis
  - ◆ V13.5 Other musculoskeletal disorders
  - V13.6 Congenital malformations
  - V13.7 Perinatal problems
  - ◆ V13.8 Other specified diseases
  - ◆ V13.9 Unspecified disease
- ● **V14 Personal history of allergy to medicinal agents**
  - V14.0 Penicillin
  - ◆ V14.1 Other antibiotic agent
  - V14.2 Sulfonamides
  - ◆ V14.3 Other anti-infective agent
  - V14.4 Anesthetic agent
  - V14.5 Narcotic agent
  - V14.6 Analgesic agent
  - V14.7 Serum or vaccine
  - ◆ V14.8 Other specified medicinal agents
  - ◆ V14.9 Unspecified medicinal agent
- ● **V15 Other personal history presenting hazards to health**
  - ◆ V15.0 Allergy, other than to medicinal agents
  - V15.1 **Surgery to heart and great vessels**
    - EXCLUDES: replacement by transplant or other means (V42.1-V42.2, V43.2-V43.4)
  - ◆ V15.2 **Surgery to other major organs**
    - EXCLUDES: replacement by transplant or other means (V42.0-V43.8)
  - V15.3 **Irradiation**
    - Previous exposure to therapeutic or other ionizing radiation
  - V15.4 **Psychological trauma**
    - EXCLUDES: history of condition classifiable to 290-316 (V11.0-V11.9)
  - V15.5 Injury
  - V15.6 Poisoning
  - V15.7 **Contraception**
    - EXCLUDES: current contraceptive management (V25.0-V25.4)
    - presence of intrauterine contraceptive device as incidental finding (V45.5)
  - ● V15.8 **Other specified personal history presenting hazards to health**
    - V15.81 Noncompliance with medical treatment ▼
    - V15.82 **History of tobacco use**
      - EXCLUDES: tobacco dependence (305.1) ▲
    - ◆ V15.89 Other
  - ◆ V15.9 Unspecified personal history presenting hazards to health
- ● **V16 Family history of malignant neoplasm**
  - V16.0 **Gastrointestinal tract**
    - Family history of condition classifiable to 140-159
  - V16.1 **Trachea, bronchus, and lung**
    - Family history of condition classifiable to 162
  - ◆ V16.2 **Other respiratory and intrathoracic organs**
    - Family history of condition classifiable to 160-161, 163-165
  - V16.3 **Breast**
    - Family history of condition classifiable to 174
  - V16.4 **Genital organs**
    - Family history of condition classifiable to 179-187
  - V16.5 **Urinary organs**
    - Family history of condition classifiable to 189
  - V16.6 **Leukemia**
    - Family history of condition classifiable to 204-208
  - ◆ V16.7 **Other lymphatic and hematopoietic neoplasms**
    - Family history of condition classifiable to 200-203
  - ◆ V16.8 **Other specified malignant neoplasm**
    - Family history of other condition classifiable to 140-199
  - ◆ V16.9 Unspecified malignant neoplasm
- ● **V17 Family history of certain chronic disabling diseases**
  - V17.0 **Psychiatric condition**
    - EXCLUDES: family history of mental retardation (V18.4)
  - V17.1 Stroke (cerebrovascular)
  - ◆ V17.2 **Other neurological diseases**
    - Epilepsy
    - Huntington's chorea
  - ◆ V17.3 Ischemic heart disease
  - ◆ V17.4 Other cardiovascular diseases
  - V17.5 Asthma
  - ◆ V17.6 Other chronic respiratory conditions
  - V17.7 Arthritis
  - ◆ V17.8 Other musculoskeletal diseases
- ● **V18 Family history of certain other specific conditions**
  - V18.0 Diabetes mellitus
  - ◆ V18.1 Other endocrine and metabolic diseases
  - V18.2 Anemia
  - ◆ V18.3 Other blood disorders
  - V18.4 Mental retardation
  - ◆ V18.5 Digestive disorders
  - V18.6 Kidney diseases
  - ◆ V18.7 Other genitourinary diseases
  - V18.8 Infectious and parasitic diseases
- ● **V19 Family history of other conditions**
  - V19.0 Blindness or visual loss
  - ◆ V19.1 Other eye disorders
  - V19.2 Deafness or hearing loss
  - ◆ V19.3 Other ear disorders
  - V19.4 Skin conditions
  - V19.5 Congenital anomalies
  - V19.6 Allergic disorders
  - V19.7 Consanguinity
  - ◆ V19.8 Other condition

PERSONS ENCOUNTERING HEALTH SERVICES IN CIRCUMSTANCES RELATED TO REPRODUCTION AND DEVELOPMENT (V20-V28)

- ● **V20 Health supervision of infant or child**
  - V20.0 Foundling
  - ◆ V20.1 **Other healthy infant or child receiving care**
    - Medical or nursing care supervision of healthy infant in cases of:
      - maternal illness, physical or psychiatric
      - socioeconomic adverse condition at home
      - too many children at home preventing or interfering with normal care
  - V20.2 **Routine infant or child health check**
    - Developmental testing of infant or child
    - Immunizations appropriate for age ▼
    - Routine vision and hearing testing
    - Use additional code(s) to identify:
      - special screening examination(s) performed (V73.0-V82.9) ▲
    - EXCLUDES: special screening for developmental handicaps (V79.3)
- ● **V21 Constitutional states in development**
  - V21.0 Period of rapid growth in childhood
  - V21.1 Puberty

- **V21.2** Other adolescence
- **V21.8** Other specified constitutional states in development
- **V21.9** Unspecified constitutional state in development

● **V22 Normal pregnancy**
  EXCLUDES *pregnancy examination or test, pregnancy unconfirmed (V72.4)*
- **V22.0** Supervision of normal first pregnancy
- **V22.1** Supervision of other normal pregnancy
- **V22.2** Pregnant state, incidental
  Pregnant state NOS

● **V23 Supervision of high-risk pregnancy**
- **V23.0** Pregnancy with history of infertility
- **V23.1** Pregnancy with history of trophoblastic disease
  Pregnancy with history of:
    hydatidiform mole
    vesicular mole
  EXCLUDES *that without current pregnancy (V13.1)*
- **V23.2** Pregnancy with history of abortion
  Pregnancy with history of conditions classifiable to 634-638
  EXCLUDES habitual aborter:
    care during pregnancy (646.3)
    that without current pregnancy (629.9)
- **V23.3** Grand multiparity
  EXCLUDES *care in relation to labor and delivery (659.4)*
  that without current pregnancy (V61.5)
- ◆ **V23.4** Pregnancy with other poor obstetric history
  Pregnancy with history of other conditions classifiable to 630-676
- ◆ **V23.5** Pregnancy with other poor reproductive history
  Pregnancy with history of stillbirth or neonatal death
- **V23.7** Insufficient prenatal care
  History of little or no prenatal care
- ◆ **V23.8** Other high-risk pregnancy
- ◆ **V23.9** Unspecified high-risk pregnancy

● **V24 Postpartum care and examination**
- **V24.0** Immediately after delivery
  Care and observation in uncomplicated cases
- **V24.1** Lactating mother
  Supervision of lactation
- **V24.2** Routine postpartum follow-up

● **V25 Encounter for contraceptive management**
  ● **V25.0** General counseling and advice
    V25.01 Prescription of oral contraceptives
    ◆ **V25.02** Initiation of other contraceptive measures
      Fitting of diaphragm
      Prescription of foams, creams, or other agents
    ◆ **V25.09** Other
      Family planning advice
  V25.1 Insertion of intrauterine contraceptive device
  V25.2 Sterilization
    Admission for interruption of fallopian tubes or vas deferens
  V25.3 Menstrual extraction
    Menstrual regulation
  ● **V25.4** Surveillance of previously prescribed contraceptive methods
    Checking, reinsertion, or removal of contraceptive device
    Repeat prescription for contraceptive method
    Routine examination in connection with contraceptive maintenance
    EXCLUDES *presence of intrauterine contraceptive device as incidental finding (V45.5)*
    ◆ **V25.40** Contraceptive surveillance, unspecified
    V25.41 Contraceptive pill
    V25.42 Intrauterine contraceptive device
      Checking, reinsertion, or removal of intrauterine device
    V25.43 Implantable subdermal contraceptive
    ◆ **V25.49** Other contraceptive method
  V25.5 Insertion of implantable subdermal contraceptive
  ◆ **V25.8** Other specified contraceptive management
    Postvasectomy sperm count
  ◆ **V25.9** Unspecified contraceptive management

● **V26 Procreative management**
- **V26.0** Tuboplasty or vasoplasty after previous sterilization
- **V26.1** Artificial insemination
- **V26.2** Investigation and testing
  Fallopian insufflation
  Sperm counts
  EXCLUDES *postvasectomy sperm count (V25.8)*
- **V26.3** Genetic counseling
- **V26.4** General counseling and advice
- ◆ **V26.8** Other specified procreative management
- ◆ **V26.9** Unspecified procreative management

● **V27 Outcome of delivery**
  Note: This category is intended for the coding of the outcome of delivery on the mother's record.
- **V27.0** Single liveborn
- **V27.1** Single stillborn
- **V27.2** Twins, both liveborn
- **V27.3** Twins, one liveborn and one stillborn
- **V27.4** Twins, both stillborn
- ◆ **V27.5** Other multiple birth, all liveborn
- ◆ **V27.6** Other multiple birth, some liveborn
- ◆ **V27.7** Other multiple birth, all stillborn
- ◆ **V27.9** Unspecified outcome of delivery

  Single birth } outcome to infant
  Multiple birth } unspecified

● **V28 Antenatal screening**
  EXCLUDES *routine prenatal care (V22.0-V23.9)*
- **V28.0** Screening for chromosomal anomalies by amniocentesis
- **V28.1** Screening for raised alpha-fetoprotein levels in amniotic fluid
- ◆ **V28.2** Other screening based on amniocentesis
- **V28.3** Screening for malformation using ultrasonics
- **V28.4** Screening for fetal growth retardation using ultrasonics
- **V28.5** Screening for isoimmunization
- ◆ **V28.8** Other specified antenatal screening
- ◆ **V28.9** Unspecified antenatal screening

● **V29 Observation and evaluation of newborns and infants for suspected condition not found**
  Note: This category is to be used for newborns, within the neonatal period, (the first 28 days of life) who are suspected of having an abnormal condition resulting from exposure from mother or the birth process, but without signs or symptoms, and, which after examination and observation, is found not to exist. ◆
- **V29.0** Observation for suspected infectious condition
- **V29.1** Observation for suspected neurological condition
- **V29.2** Observation for suspected respiratory condition ◆
- ◆ **V29.8** Observation for other specified suspected condition
- ◆ **V29.9** Observation for unspecified suspected condition

LIVEBORN INFANTS ACCORDING TO TYPE OF BIRTH (V30-V39)

Note: These categories are intended for the coding of liveborn infants who are consuming health care [e.g., crib or bassinet occupancy].

The following fourth-digit subdivisions are for use with categories V30-V39:

  0 Born in hospital
  1 Born before admission to hospital
  2 Born outside hospital and not hospitalized

The following two fifth-digits are for use with the fourth-digit .0, Born in hospital:

  0 delivered without mention of cesarean delivery
  1 delivered by cesarean delivery

● **V30** Single liveborn
● **V31** Twin, mate liveborn
● **V32** Twin, mate stillborn
◆ ● **V33** Twin, unspecified
● **V34** Other multiple, mates all liveborn
● **V35** Other multiple, mates all stillborn
● **V36** Other multiple, mates live- and stillborn
◆ ● **V37** Other multiple, unspecified
◆ ● **V39** Unspecified

PERSONS WITH A CONDITION INFLUENCING THEIR HEALTH STATUS (V40-V49)

Note: These categories are intended for use when these conditions are recorded as "diagnoses" or "problems."

- **V40** Mental and behavioral problems
  - V40.0 Problems with learning
  - V40.1 Problems with communication [including speech]
  - V40.2 Other mental problems
  - V40.3 Other behavioral problems
  - V40.9 Unspecified mental or behavioral problem
- **V41** Problems with special senses and other special functions
  - V41.0 Problems with sight
  - V41.1 Other eye problems
  - V41.2 Problems with hearing
  - V41.3 Other ear problems
  - V41.4 Problems with voice production
  - V41.5 Problems with smell and taste
  - V41.6 Problems with swallowing and mastication
  - V41.7 Problems with sexual function
    - **EXCLUDES** marital problems (V61.1)
      psychosexual disorders (302.0-302.9)
  - V41.8 Other problems with special functions
  - V41.9 Unspecified problem with special functions
- **V42** Organ or tissue replaced by transplant
  - **INCLUDES** homologous or heterologous (animal) (human) transplant organ status
  - V42.0 Kidney
  - V42.1 Heart
  - V42.2 Heart valve
  - V42.3 Skin
  - V42.4 Bone
  - V42.5 Cornea
  - V42.6 Lung
  - V42.7 Liver
  - V42.8 Other specified organ or tissue
    - Intestine
    - Pancreas
  - V42.9 Unspecified organ or tissue
- **V43** Organ or tissue replaced by other means
  - **INCLUDES** replacement of organ by:
    - artificial device
    - mechanical device
    - prosthesis
  - **EXCLUDES** cardiac pacemaker in situ (V45.01)
    fitting and adjustment of prosthetic device (V52.0-V52.9)
    renal dialysis status (V45.1)
  - V43.0 Eye globe
  - V43.1 Lens
    - Pseudophakos
  - V43.2 Heart
  - V43.3 Heart valve
  - V43.4 Blood vessel
  - V43.5 Bladder
  - V43.6 Joint
    - V43.60 Unspecified joint
    - V43.61 Shoulder
    - V43.62 Elbow
    - V43.63 Wrist
    - V43.64 Hip
    - V43.65 Knee
    - V43.66 Ankle
    - V43.69 Other
  - V43.7 Limb
  - V43.8 Other organ or tissue
    - Larynx
- **V44** Artificial opening status
  - **EXCLUDES** artificial openings requiring attention or management (V55.0-V55.9)
  - V44.0 Tracheostomy
  - V44.1 Gastrostomy
  - V44.2 Ileostomy
  - V44.3 Colostomy
  - V44.4 Other artificial opening of gastrointestinal tract
  - V44.5 Cystostomy
  - V44.6 Other artificial opening of urinary tract
    - Nephrostomy
    - Ureterostomy
    - Urethrostomy
  - V44.7 Artificial vagina
  - V44.8 Other artificial opening status
  - V44.9 Unspecified artificial opening status
- **V45** Other postsurgical states
  - **EXCLUDES** aftercare management (V51-V58.9)
    malfunction or other complication — code to condition
  - **V45.0** Cardiac device in situ
    - V45.00 Unspecified cardiac device
    - V45.01 Cardiac pacemaker
    - V45.02 Automatic implantable cardiac defibrillator
    - V45.09 Other specified cardiac device
      - Carotid sinus pacemaker in situ
  - V45.1 Renal dialysis status
    - Patient requiring intermittent renal dialysis
    - Presence of arterial-venous shunt (for dialysis)
    - **EXCLUDES** admission for dialysis treatment or session (V56.0)
  - V45.2 Presence of cerebrospinal fluid drainage device
    - Cerebral ventricle (communicating) shunt, valve, or device in situ
    - **EXCLUDES** malfunction (996.2)
  - V45.3 Intestinal bypass or anastomosis status
  - V45.4 Arthrodesis status
  - **V45.5** Presence of contraceptive device
    - **EXCLUDES** checking, reinsertion, or removal of device (V25.42)
      complication from device (996.32)
      insertion of device (V25.1)
    - V45.51 Intrauterine contraceptive device
    - V45.52 Subdermal contraceptive implant
    - V45.59 Other
  - V45.6 States following surgery of eye and adnexa
    - Cataract extraction
    - Filtering bleb } state following eye surgery
    - Surgical eyelid adhesion
    - **EXCLUDES** aphakia (379.31)
      artificial:
        eye globe (V43.0)
        lens (V43.1)
  - **V45.8** Other postsurgical status
    - V45.81 Aortocoronary bypass status
    - V45.82 Percutaneous transluminal coronary angioplasty status
    - V45.89 Other
      - Presence of neuropacemaker or other electronic device
      - **EXCLUDES** artificial heart valve in situ (V43.3)
        vascular prosthesis in situ (V43.4)
- **V46** Other dependence on machines
  - V46.0 Aspirator
  - V46.1 Respirator
    - Iron lung
  - V46.8 Other enabling machines
    - Hyperbaric chamber
    - Possum [Patient-Operated-Selector-Mechanism]
    - **EXCLUDES** cardiac pacemaker (V45.0)
      kidney dialysis machine (V45.1)
  - V46.9 Unspecified machine dependence
- **V47** Other problems with internal organs
  - V47.0 Deficiencies of internal organs
  - V47.1 Mechanical and motor problems with internal organs
  - V47.2 Other cardiorespiratory problems
    - Cardiovascular exercise intolerance with pain (with):
      - at rest
      - less than ordinary activity
      - ordinary activity
  - V47.3 Other digestive problems
  - V47.4 Other urinary problems
  - V47.5 Other genital problems
  - V47.9 Unspecified

● Additional digits required ◆ Nonspecific code ■ Not a primary diagnosis

- **V48 Problems with head, neck, and trunk**
    - V48.0 Deficiencies of head
        - EXCLUDES: deficiencies of ears, eyelids, and nose (V48.8)
    - V48.1 Deficiencies of neck and trunk
    - V48.2 Mechanical and motor problems with head
    - V48.3 Mechanical and motor problems with neck and trunk
    - V48.4 Sensory problem with head
    - V48.5 Sensory problem with neck and trunk
    - V48.6 Disfigurements of head
    - V48.7 Disfigurements of neck and trunk
    - V48.8 Other problems with head, neck, and trunk
    - V48.9 Unspecified problem with head, neck, or trunk
- **V49 Problems with limbs and other problems**
    - V49.0 Deficiencies of limbs
    - V49.1 Mechanical problems with limbs
    - V49.2 Motor problems with limbs
    - V49.3 Sensory problems with limbs
    - V49.4 Disfigurements of limbs
    - V49.5 Other problems of limbs
    - **V49.6 Upper limb amputation status**
        - V49.60 Unspecified level
        - V49.61 Thumb
        - V49.62 Other finger(s)
        - V49.63 Hand
        - V49.64 Wrist
            - Disarticulation of wrist
        - V49.65 Below elbow
        - V49.66 Above elbow
            - Disarticulation of elbow
        - V49.67 Shoulder
            - Disarticulation of shoulder
    - **V49.7 Lower limb amputation status**
        - V49.70 Unspecified level
        - V49.71 Great toe
        - V49.72 Other toe(s)
        - V49.73 Foot
        - V49.74 Ankle
            - Disarticulation of ankle
        - V49.75 Below knee
        - V49.76 Above knee
            - Disarticulation of knee
        - V49.77 Hip
            - Disarticulation of hip
    - V49.8 Other specified problems influencing health status
    - V49.9 Unspecified

PERSONS ENCOUNTERING HEALTH SERVICES FOR SPECIFIC PROCEDURES AND AFTERCARE (V50-V59)

Note: Categories V51-V58 are intended for use to indicate a reason for care in patients who may have already been treated for some disease or injury not now present, or who are receiving care to consolidate the treatment, to deal with residual states, or to prevent recurrence.

EXCLUDES: follow-up examination for medical surveillance following treatment (V67.0-V67.9)

- **V50 Elective surgery for purposes other than remedying health states**
    - V50.0 Hair transplant
    - V50.1 Other plastic surgery for unacceptable cosmetic appearance
        - Breast augmentation or reduction
        - Face-lift
        - EXCLUDES: plastic surgery following healed injury or operation (V51)
    - V50.2 Routine or ritual circumcision
        - Circumcision in the absence of significant medical indication
    - V50.3 Ear piercing
    - **V50.4 Prophylactic organ removal**
        - EXCLUDES: organ donations (V59.0-V59.9)
            - therapeutic organ removal — code to condition
        - V50.41 Breast
        - V50.42 Ovary
        - V50.49 Other
    - V50.8 Other
    - V50.9 Unspecified
- V51 Aftercare involving the use of plastic surgery
    - Plastic surgery following healed injury or operation
    - Repair of scarred tissue
    - EXCLUDES: cosmetic plastic surgery (V50.1)
        - plastic surgery as treatment for current injury — code to condition
- **V52 Fitting and adjustment of prosthetic device**
    - INCLUDES: removal of device
    - EXCLUDES: malfunction or complication of prosthetic device (996.0-996.7)
        - status only, without need for care (V43.0-V43.8)
    - V52.0 Artificial arm (complete) (partial)
    - V52.1 Artificial leg (complete) (partial)
    - V52.2 Artificial eye
    - V52.3 Dental prosthetic device
    - V52.4 Breast prosthesis
        - EXCLUDES: breast implant (V50.1)
    - V52.8 Other specified prosthetic device
    - V52.9 Unspecified prosthetic device
- **V53 Fitting and adjustment of other device**
    - INCLUDES: removal of device
        - replacement of device
    - EXCLUDES: status only, without need for care (V45.0-V45.8)
    - V53.0 Devices related to nervous system and special senses
        - Auditory } substitution device
        - Visual
        - Neuropacemaker (brain) (peripheral nerve) (spinal cord)
    - V53.1 Spectacles and contact lenses
    - V53.2 Hearing aid
    - **V53.3 Cardiac device**
        - Reprogramming
        - V53.31 Cardiac pacemaker
            - EXCLUDES: mechanical complication of cardiac pacemaker (996.01)
        - V53.32 Automatic implantable cardiac defibrillator
        - V53.39 Other cardiac device
    - V53.4 Orthodontic devices
    - V53.5 Ileostomy or other intestinal appliance
        - EXCLUDES: removal of ileostomy (V55.2)
    - V53.6 Urinary devices
    - V53.7 Orthopedic devices
        - Orthopedic:
            - brace
            - cast
            - corset
            - shoes
    - V53.8 Wheelchair
    - V53.9 Other and unspecified device
- **V54 Other orthopedic aftercare**
    - EXCLUDES: malfunction of internal orthopedic device (996.4)
        - other complication of nonmechanical nature (996.60-996.79)
    - V54.0 Aftercare involving removal of fracture plate or other internal fixation device
        - Removal of:
            - pins
            - plates
            - rods
            - screws
    - V54.8 Other orthopedic aftercare
        - Change, checking, or removal of:
            - Kirschner wire
            - plaster cast
            - splint, external
            - other external fixation or traction device
    - V54.9 Unspecified orthopedic aftercare
- **V55 Attention to artificial openings**
    - INCLUDES: closure
        - passage of sounds or bougies
        - reforming
        - removal or replacement of catheter
        - toilet or cleansing
    - EXCLUDES: complications of external stoma (519.0, 569.6, 997.4, 997.5)
        - status only, without need for care (V44.0-V44.9)

V CODES

- **V55**
  - V55.0 Tracheostomy
  - V55.1 Gastrostomy
  - V55.2 Ileostomy
  - V55.3 Colostomy
  - ◆ V55.4 Other artificial opening of digestive tract
  - V55.5 Cystostomy
  - ◆ V55.6 Other artificial opening of urinary tract
    - Nephrostomy
    - Ureterostomy
    - Urethrostomy
  - V55.7 Artificial vagina
  - ◆ V55.8 Other specified artificial opening
  - ◆ V55.9 Unspecified artificial opening
- ● **V56 Encounter for dialysis**
  - Use additional code to identify the associated condition
  - **INCLUDES** dialysis preparation and treatment
  - **EXCLUDES** dialysis preparation — code to condition
  - V56.0 Extracorporeal dialysis
    - Dialysis (renal) NOS
    - **EXCLUDES** dialysis status (V45.1)
  - ◆ V56.8 Other dialysis
    - Peritoneal dialysis
- ● **V57 Care involving use of rehabilitation procedures**
  - Use additional code to identify underlying condition
  - V57.0 Breathing exercises
  - ◆ V57.1 Other physical therapy
    - Therapeutic and remedial exercises, except breathing
  - ● V57.2 Occupational therapy and vocational rehabilitation
    - V57.21 Encounter for occupational therapy ▼
    - V57.22 Encounter for vocational therapy ▲
  - V57.3 Speech therapy
  - V57.4 Orthoptic training
  - ● V57.8 Other specified rehabilitation procedure
    - V57.81 Orthotic training
      - Gait training in the use of artificial limbs
    - ◆ V57.89 Other
      - Multiple training or therapy
  - ◆ V57.9 Unspecified rehabilitation procedure
- ● **V58 Encounter for other and unspecified procedures and aftercare**
  - **EXCLUDES** convalescence (V66)
  - V58.0 Radiotherapy
    - Encounter or admission for radiotherapy
    - **EXCLUDES** encounter for radioactive implant — code to condition
  - V58.1 Chemotherapy
    - Encounter or admission for chemotherapy
    - **EXCLUDES** prophylactic chemotherapy against disease which has never been present (V03.0-V07.9)
  - V58.2 Blood transfusion, without reported diagnosis
  - V58.3 Attention to surgical dressings and sutures
    - Change of dressings
    - Removal of sutures
  - ● V58.4 Other aftercare following surgery
    - **EXCLUDES** attention to artificial openings (V55.0-V55.9)
    - orthopedic aftercare (V54.0-V54.9)
    - V58.41 Encounter for planned postoperative wound closure ▼
      - **EXCLUDES** disruption of operative wound (998.3)
    - ◆ V58.49 Other specified aftercare following surgery ▲
  - V58.5 Orthodontics
  - ● V58.8 Other specified aftercare
    - V58.81 Encounter for removal of vascular catheter ▼
    - ◆ V58.89 Other specified aftercare ▲
  - V58.9 Unspecified aftercare
- ● **V59 Donors**
  - **EXCLUDES** examination of potential donor (V70.8)
  - V59.0 Blood
  - V59.1 Skin
  - V59.2 Bone
  - V59.3 Bone marrow
  - V59.4 Kidney
  - V59.5 Cornea
  - V59.8 Other specified organ or tissue
  - V59.9 Unspecified organ or tissue

PERSONS ENCOUNTERING HEALTH SERVICES IN OTHER CIRCUMSTANCES (V60-V68)

- ● **V60 Housing, household, and economic circumstances**
  - V60.0 Lack of housing
    - Hobos
    - Social migrants
    - Tramps
    - Transients
    - Vagabonds
  - V60.1 Inadequate housing
    - Lack of heating
    - Restriction of space
    - Technical defects in home preventing adequate care
  - V60.2 Inadequate material resources
    - Economic problem
    - Poverty NOS
  - V60.3 Person living alone
  - V60.4 No other household member able to render care
    - Person requiring care (has) (is):
      - family member too handicapped, ill, or otherwise unsuited to render care
      - partner temporarily away from home
      - temporarily away from usual place of abode
    - **EXCLUDES** holiday relief care (V60.5)
  - V60.5 Holiday relief care
    - Provision of health care facilities to a person normally cared for at home, to enable relatives to take a vacation
  - V60.6 Person living in residential institution
    - Boarding school resident
  - ◆ V60.8 Other specified housing or economic circumstances
  - ◆ V60.9 Unspecified housing or economic circumstance
- ● **V61 Other family circumstances**
  - **INCLUDES** when these circumstances or fear of them, affecting the person directly involved or others, are mentioned as the reason, justified or not, for seeking or receiving medical advice or care
  - V61.0 Family disruption
    - Divorce
    - Estrangement
  - V61.1 Marital problems
    - Marital conflict
    - **EXCLUDES** problems related to:
      - psychosexual disorders (302.0-302.9)
      - sexual function (V41.7)
  - ● V61.2 Parent-child problems
    - V61.20 Parent-child problem, unspecified
      - Concern about behavior of child
      - Parent-child conflict
    - V61.21 Child abuse
      - Child battering
      - Child neglect
      - **EXCLUDES** effect of maltreatment on the child (995.5)
    - ◆ V61.29 Other
      - Problem concerning adopted or foster child
  - V61.3 Problems with aged parents or in-laws
  - ● V61.4 Health problems within family
    - V61.41 Alcoholism in family
    - ◆ V61.49 Other
      - Care of } sick or handicapped person
      - Presence of } in family or household
  - V61.5 Multiparity
  - V61.6 Illegitimacy or illegitimate pregnancy
  - ◆ V61.7 Other unwanted pregnancy
  - ◆ V61.8 Other specified family circumstances
    - Problems with family members NEC
  - ◆ V61.9 Unspecified family circumstance
- ● **V62 Other psychosocial circumstances**
  - **INCLUDES** those circumstances or fear of them, affecting the person directly involved or others, mentioned as the reason, justified or not, for seeking or receiving medical advice or care
  - **EXCLUDES** previous psychological trauma (V15.4)

● Additional digits required   ◆ Nonspecific code   ▌ Not a primary diagnosis

- **V62.0 Unemployment**
  - EXCLUDES: circumstances when main problem is economic inadequacy or poverty (V60.2)
- **V62.1 Adverse effects of work environment**
- **V62.2 Other occupational circumstances or maladjustment**
  - Career choice problem
  - Dissatisfaction with employment
- **V62.3 Educational circumstances**
  - Dissatisfaction with school environment
  - Educational handicap
- **V62.4 Social maladjustment**
  - Cultural deprivation
  - Political, religious, or sex discrimination
  - Social:
    - isolation
    - persecution
- **V62.5 Legal circumstances**
  - Imprisonment
  - Legal investigation
  - Litigation
  - Prosecution
- **V62.6 Refusal of treatment for reasons of religion or conscience**
- **V62.8 Other psychological or physical stress, not elsewhere classified**
  - **V62.81 Interpersonal problems, not elsewhere classified**
  - **V62.82 Bereavement, uncomplicated**
    - EXCLUDES: bereavement as adjustment reaction (309.0)
  - **V62.89 Other**
    - Life circumstance problems
    - Phase of life problems
- **V62.9 Unspecified psychosocial circumstance**
- **V63 Unavailability of other medical facilities for care**
  - **V63.0 Residence remote from hospital or other health care facility**
  - **V63.1 Medical services in home not available**
    - EXCLUDES: no other household member able to render care (V60.4)
  - **V63.2 Person awaiting admission to adequate facility elsewhere**
  - **V63.8 Other specified reasons for unavailability of medical facilities**
    - Person on waiting list undergoing social agency investigation
  - **V63.9 Unspecified reason for unavailability of medical facilities**
- **V64 Persons encountering health services for specific procedures, not carried out**
  - **V64.0 Vaccination not carried out because of contraindication**
  - **V64.1 Surgical or other procedure not carried out because of contraindication**
  - **V64.2 Surgical or other procedure not carried out because of patient's decision**
  - **V64.3 Procedure not carried out for other reasons**
- **V65 Other persons seeking consultation without complaint or sickness**
  - **V65.0 Healthy person accompanying sick person**
    - Boarder
  - **V65.1 Person consulting on behalf of another person**
    - Advice or treatment for nonattending third party
    - EXCLUDES: concern (normal) about sick person in family (V61.41-V61.49)
  - **V65.2 Person feigning illness**
    - Malingerer
    - Peregrinating patient
  - **V65.3 Dietary surveillance and counseling**
    - Dietary surveillance and counseling (in):
      - NOS
      - colitis
      - diabetes mellitus
      - food allergies or intolerance
      - gastritis
      - hypercholesterolemia
      - hypoglycemia
      - obesity
  - **V65.4 Other counseling, not elsewhere classified**
    - Health:
      - advice
      - education
      - instruction
    - EXCLUDES: counseling (for):
      - contraception (V25.40-V25.49)
      - genetic (V26.3)
      - on behalf of third party (V65.1)
      - procreative management (V26.4)
    - **V65.40 Counseling NOS**
    - **V65.41 Excercise counseling**
    - **V65.42 Counseling on substance use and abuse**
    - **V65.43 Counseling on injury prevention**
    - **V65.44 Human immunodeficiency virus [HIV] counseling**
    - **V65.45 Counseling on other sexually transmitted diseases**
    - **V65.49 Other specified counseling**
  - **V65.5 Person with feared complaint in whom no diagnosis was made**
    - Feared condition not demonstrated
    - Problem was normal state
    - "Worried well"
  - **V65.8 Other reasons for seeking consultation**
    - EXCLUDES: specified symptoms
  - **V65.9 Unspecified reason for consultation**
- **V66 Convalescence**
  - **V66.0 Following surgery**
  - **V66.1 Following radiotherapy**
  - **V66.2 Following chemotherapy**
  - **V66.3 Following psychotherapy and other treatment for mental disorder**
  - **V66.4 Following treatment of fracture**
  - **V66.5 Following other treatment**
  - **V66.6 Following combined treatment**
  - **V66.9 Unspecified convalescence**
- **V67 Follow-up examination**
  - INCLUDES: surveillance only following completed treatment
  - EXCLUDES: surveillance of contraception (V25.40-V25.49)
  - **V67.0 Following surgery**
  - **V67.1 Following radiotherapy**
  - **V67.2 Following chemotherapy**
    - Cancer chemotherapy follow-up
  - **V67.3 Following psychotherapy and other treatment for mental disorder**
  - **V67.4 Following treatment of fracture**
  - **V67.5 Following other treatment**
    - **V67.51 Following treatment with high-risk medication, not elsewhere classified**
    - **V67.59 Other**
  - **V67.6 Following combined treatment**
  - **V67.9 Unspecified follow-up examination**
- **V68 Encounters for administrative purposes**
  - **V68.0 Issue of medical certificates**
    - Issue of medical certificate of:
      - cause of death
      - fitness
      - incapacity
    - EXCLUDES: encounter for general medical examination (V70.0-V70.9)
  - **V68.1 Issue of repeat prescriptions**
    - Issue of repeat prescription for:
      - appliance
      - glasses
      - medications
    - EXCLUDES: repeat prescription for contraceptives (V25.41-V25.49)
  - **V68.2 Request for expert evidence**
  - **V68.8 Other specified administrative purpose**
    - **V68.81 Referral of patient without examination or treatment**
    - **V68.89 Other**
  - **V68.9 Unspecified administrative purpose**

- **V69 Problems related to lifestyle** ▼
  - **V69.0** Lack of physical excercise
  - **V69.1** Inappropriate diet and eating habits
    - EXCLUDES: anorexia nervosa (307.1)
      bulimia (783.6)
      malnutrition and other nutritional deficiencies (260-269.9)
      other and unspecified eating disorders (307.50-307.59)
  - **V69.2** High-risk sexual behavior
  - **V69.3** Gambling and betting
    - EXCLUDES: pathological gambling (312.31)
  - ◆ **V69.8** Other problems related to lifestyle
    - Self-damaging behavior
  - ◆ **V69.9** Problem related to lifestyle, unspecified ▲

PERSONS WITHOUT REPORTED DIAGNOSIS ENCOUNTERED DURING EXAMINATION AND INVESTIGATION OF INDIVIDUALS AND POPULATIONS (V70-V82)

Note: Nonspecific abnormal findings disclosed at the time of these examinations are classifiable to categories 790-796.

- **V70 General medical examination**
  - Use additional code(s) to identify any special screening examination(s) performed (V73.0-V82.9) ◆
  - **V70.0** Routine general medical examination at a health care facility
    - Health checkup
    - EXCLUDES: health checkup of infant or child (V20.2)
  - **V70.1** General psychiatric examination, requested by the authority
  - ◆ **V70.2** General psychiatric examination, other and unspecified
  - ◆ **V70.3** Other medical examination for administrative purposes
    - General medical examination for:
      - admission to old age home
      - adoption
      - camp
      - driving license
      - immigration and naturalization
      - insurance certification
      - marriage
      - prison
      - school admission
      - sports competition
    - EXCLUDES: attendance for issue of medical certificates (V68.0)
      pre-employment screening (V70.5)
  - **V70.4** Examination for medicolegal reasons
    - Blood-alcohol tests
    - Blood-drug tests
    - EXCLUDES: examination and observation following:
      accidents (V71.3, V71.4)
      assault (V71.6)
      rape (V71.5)
  - **V70.5** Health examination of defined subpopulations
    - Armed forces personnel
    - Inhabitants of institutions
    - Occupational health examinations
    - Pre-employment screening
    - Preschool children
    - Prisoners
    - Prostitutes
    - Refugees
    - School children
    - Students
  - **V70.6** Health examination in population surveys
    - EXCLUDES: special screening (V73.0-V82.9)
  - **V70.7** Examination for normal comparison or control in clinical research
  - ◆ **V70.8** Other specified general medical examinations
    - Examination of potential donor of organ or tissue
  - ◆ **V70.9** Unspecified general medical examination

- **V71 Observation and evaluation for suspected conditions not found** ▼
  - INCLUDES: This category is to be used when persons without a diagnosis are suspected of having an abnormal condition, without signs or symptoms, which requires study, but after examination and observation, is found not to exist. This category is also for use for administrative and legal observation status. ▲
  - **V71.0** Observation for suspected mental condition
    - **V71.01** Adult antisocial behavior
      - Dyssocial behavior or gang activity in adult without manifest psychiatric disorder
    - **V71.02** Childhood or adolescent antisocial behavior
      - Dyssocial behavior or gang activity in child or adolescent without manifest psychiatric disorder
    - ◆ **V71.09** Other suspected mental condition
  - **V71.1** Observation for suspected malignant neoplasm
  - **V71.2** Observation for suspected tuberculosis
  - **V71.3** Observation following accident at work
  - ◆ **V71.4** Observation following other accident
    - Examination of individual involved in motor vehicle traffic accident
  - **V71.5** Observation following alleged rape or seduction
    - Examination of victim or culprit
  - ◆ **V71.6** Observation following other inflicted injury
    - Examination of victim or culprit
  - **V71.7** Observation for suspected cardiovascular disease
  - ◆ **V71.8** Observation for other specified suspected conditions
  - ◆ **V71.9** Observation for unspecified suspected condition

- **V72 Special investigations and examinations**
  - INCLUDES: routine examination of specific system
  - EXCLUDES: general medical examination (V70.0-V70.4)
    general screening examination of defined population groups (V70.5, V70.6, V70.7)
    routine examination of infant or child (V20.2) ▼
  - Use additional code(s) to identify any special screening examination(s) performed (V73.0-V82.9) ▲
  - **V72.0** Examination of eyes and vision
  - **V72.1** Examination of ears and hearing
  - **V72.2** Dental examination
  - **V72.3** Gynecological examination
    - Papanicolaou smear as part of general gynecological examination
    - Pelvic examination (annual) (periodic)
    - EXCLUDES: cervical Papanicolaou smear without general gynecological examination (V76.2)
      routine examination in contraceptive management (V25.40-V25.49)
  - **V72.4** Pregnancy examination or test, pregnancy unconfirmed
    - Possible pregnancy, not (yet) confirmed
    - EXCLUDES: pregnancy examination with immediate confirmation (V22.0-V22.1)
  - **V72.5** Radiological examination, not elsewhere classified
    - Routine chest x-ray
    - EXCLUDES: examination for suspected tuberculosis (V71.2)
  - **V72.6** Laboratory examination
    - EXCLUDES: that for suspected disorder (V71.0-V71.9)
  - **V72.7** Diagnostic skin and sensitization tests
    - Allergy tests
    - Skin tests for hypersensitivity
    - EXCLUDES: diagnostic skin tests for bacterial diseases (V74.0-V74.9)
  - **V72.8** Other specified examinations
    - **V72.81** Pre-operative cardiovascular examination
    - **V72.82** Pre-operative respiratory examination
    - ◆ **V72.83** Other specified pre-operative examination
    - ◆ **V72.84** Pre-operative examination, unspecified
    - ◆ **V72.85** Other specified examination
  - ◆ **V72.9** Unspecified examination

- **V73 Special screening examination for viral and chlamydial diseases**
  - V73.0 Poliomyelitis
  - V73.1 Smallpox
  - V73.2 Measles
  - V73.3 Rubella
  - V73.4 Yellow fever
  - ◆ V73.5 Other arthropod-borne viral diseases
    - Dengue fever
    - Hemorrhagic fever
    - Viral encephalitis:
      - mosquito-borne
      - tick-borne
  - V73.6 Trachoma
  - ● V73.8 Other specified viral and chlamydial diseases
    - ◆ V73.88 Other specified chlamydial diseases
    - ◆ V73.89 Other specified viral diseases
  - ● V73.9 Unspecified viral and chlamydial disease
    - ◆ V73.98 Unspecified chlamydial disease
    - ◆ V73.99 Unspecified viral disease
- ● **V74 Special screening examination for bacterial and spirochetal diseases**
  - **INCLUDES** diagnostic skin tests for these diseases
  - V74.0 Cholera
  - V74.1 Pulmonary tuberculosis
  - V74.2 Leprosy [Hansen's disease]
  - V74.3 Diphtheria
  - V74.4 Bacterial conjunctivitis
  - V74.5 Venereal disease
  - V74.6 Yaws
  - ◆ V74.8 Other specified bacterial and spirochetal diseases
    - Brucellosis
    - Leptospirosis
    - Plague
    - Tetanus
    - Whooping cough
  - ◆ V74.9 Unspecified bacterial and spirochetal disease
- ● **V75 Special screening examination for other infectious diseases**
  - V75.0 Rickettsial diseases
  - V75.1 Malaria
  - V75.2 Leishmaniasis
  - V75.3 Trypanosomiasis
    - Chagas' disease
    - Sleeping sickness
  - V75.4 Mycotic infections
  - V75.5 Schistosomiasis
  - V75.6 Filariasis
  - V75.7 Intestinal helminthiasis
  - ◆ V75.8 Other specified parasitic infections
  - ◆ V75.9 Unspecified infectious disease
- ● **V76 Special screening for malignant neoplasms**
  - V76.0 Respiratory organs
  - V76.1 Breast
  - V76.2 Cervix
    - Routine cervical Papanicolaou smear
    - **EXCLUDES** that as part of a general gynecological examination (V72.3)
  - V76.3 Bladder
  - ● V76.4 Other sites
    - V76.41 Rectum
    - V76.42 Oral cavity
    - V76.43 Skin
    - ◆ V76.49 Other
  - ◆ V76.8 Other neoplasm
  - ◆ V76.9 Unspecified
- ● **V77 Special screening for endocrine, nutritional, metabolic, and immunity disorders**
  - V77.0 Thyroid disorders
  - V77.1 Diabetes mellitus
  - V77.2 Malnutrition
  - V77.3 Phenylketonuria [PKU]
  - V77.4 Galactosemia
  - V77.5 Gout
  - V77.6 Cystic fibrosis
    - Screening for mucoviscidosis
  - ◆ V77.7 Other inborn errors of metabolism
  - V77.8 Obesity
  - ◆ V77.9 Other and unspecified endocrine, nutritional, metabolic, and immunity disorders
- ● **V78 Special screening for disorders of blood and blood-forming organs**
  - V78.0 Iron deficiency anemia
  - ◆ V78.1 Other and unspecified deficiency anemia
  - V78.2 Sickle cell disease or trait
  - ◆ V78.3 Other hemoglobinopathies
  - ◆ V78.8 Other disorders of blood and blood-forming organs
  - ◆ V78.9 Unspecified disorder of blood and blood-forming organs
- ● **V79 Special screening for mental disorders and developmental handicaps**
  - V79.0 Depression
  - V79.1 Alcoholism
  - V79.2 Mental retardation
  - V79.3 Developmental handicaps in early childhood
  - ◆ V79.8 Other specified mental disorders and developmental handicaps
  - ◆ V79.9 Unspecified mental disorder and developmental handicap
- ● **V80 Special screening for neurological, eye, and ear diseases**
  - V80.0 Neurological conditions
  - V80.1 Glaucoma
  - ◆ V80.2 Other eye conditions
    - Screening for:
      - cataract
      - congenital anomaly of eye
      - senile macular lesions
    - **EXCLUDES** general vision examination (V72.0)
  - V80.3 Ear diseases
    - **EXCLUDES** general hearing examination (V72.1)
- ● **V81 Special screening for cardiovascular, respiratory, and genitourinary diseases**
  - V81.0 Ischemic heart disease
  - V81.1 Hypertension
  - ◆ V81.2 Other and unspecified cardiovascular conditions
  - V81.3 Chronic bronchitis and emphysema
  - ◆ V81.4 Other and unspecified respiratory conditions
    - **EXCLUDES** screening for:
      - lung neoplasm (V76.0)
      - pulmonary tuberculosis (V74.1)
  - V81.5 Nephropathy
    - Screening for asymptomatic bacteriuria
  - ◆ V81.6 Other and unspecified genitourinary conditions
- ● **V82 Special screening for other conditions**
  - V82.0 Skin conditions
  - V82.1 Rheumatoid arthritis
  - ◆ V82.2 Other rheumatic disorders
  - V82.3 Congenital dislocation of hip
  - V82.4 Postnatal screening for chromosomal anomalies
    - **EXCLUDES** antenatal screening by amniocentesis (V28.0)
  - V82.5 Chemical poisoning and other contamination
    - Screening for:
      - heavy metal poisoning
      - ingestion of radioactive substance
      - poisoning from contaminated water supply
      - radiation exposure
  - V82.6 Multiphasic screening
  - ◆ V82.8 Other specified conditions
  - ◆ V82.9 Unspecified condition

E CODES

SUPPLEMENTARY CLASSIFICATION OF EXTERNAL CAUSES OF INJURY AND POISONING (E800-E999)

This section is provided to permit the classification of environmental events, circumstances, and conditions as the cause of injury, poisoning, and other adverse effects. Where a code from this section is applicable, it is intended that it shall be used in addition to a code from one of the main chapters of ICD-9-CM, indicating the nature of the condition. Certain other conditions which may be stated to be due to external causes are classified in Chapters 1 to 16 of ICD-9-CM. For these, the "E" code classification should be used as an additional code for more detailed analysis.

Machinery accidents [other than those connected with transport] are classifiable to category E919, in which the fourth-digit allows a broad classification of the type of machinery involved. If a more detailed classification of type of machinery is required, it is suggested that the "Classification of Industrial Accidents according to Agency," prepared by the International Labor Office, be used in addition. This is reproduced on page 307 for optional use.

Categories for "late effects" of accidents and other external causes are to be found at E929, E959, E969, E977, E989, and E999.

Definitions and examples related to transport accidents

(a) A **transport accident** (E800-E848) is any accident involving a device designed primarily for, or being used at the time primarily for, conveying persons or goods from one place to another.

> **INCLUDES** accidents involving:
> aircraft and spacecraft (E840-E845)
> watercraft (E830-E838)
> motor vehicle (E810-E825)
> railway (E800-E807)
> other road vehicles (E826-E829)

In classifying accidents which involve more than one kind of transport, the above order of precedence of transport accidents should be used.

Accidents involving agricultural and construction machines, such as tractors, cranes, and bulldozers, are regarded as transport accidents only when these vehicles are under their own power on a highway [otherwise the vehicles are regarded as machinery]. Vehicles which can travel on land or water, such as hovercraft and other amphibious vehicles, are regarded as watercraft when on the water, as motor vehicles when on the highway, and as off-road motor vehicles when on land, but off the highway.

> **EXCLUDES** accidents:
> in sports which involve the use of transport but where the transport vehicle itself was not involved in the accident
> involving vehicles which are part of industrial equipment used entirely on industrial premises
> occurring during transportation but unrelated to the hazards associated with the means of transportation [e.g., injuries received in a fight on board ship; transport vehicle involved in a cataclysm such as an earthquake]
> to persons engaged in the maintenance or repair of transport equipment or vehicle not in motion, unlesss injured by another vehicle in motion

(b) A **railway accident** is a transport accident involving a railway train or other railway vehicle operated on rails, whether in motion or not.

> **EXCLUDES** accidents:
> in repair shops
> in roundhouse or on turntable
> on railway premises but not involving a train or other railway vehicle

(c) A **railway train** or **railway vehicle** is any device with or without cars coupled to it, desiged for traffic on a railway.

> **INCLUDES** interurban:
> electric car } (operated chiefly on its own
> streetcar } right-of-way, not open to other traffic)
> railway train, any power [diesel] [electric] [steam]
> funicular
> monorail or two-rail
> subterranean or elevated
> other vehicle designed to run on a railway track

> **EXCLUDES** interurban electric cars [streetcars] specified to be operating on a right-of-way that forms part of the public street or highway [definition (n)]

(d) A **railway** or **railroad** is a right-of-way designed for traffic on rails, which is used by carriages or wagons transporting passengers or freight, and by other rolling stock, and which is not open to other public vehicular traffic.

(e) A **motor vehicle accident** is a transport accident involving a motor vehicle. It is defined as a motor vehicle traffic accident or as a motor vehicle nontraffic accident according to whether the accident occurs on a public highway or elsewhere.

> **EXCLUDES** injury or damage due to cataclysm
> injury or damage while a motor vehicle, not under its own power, is being loaded on, or unloaded from, another conveyance

(f) A **motor vehicle traffic accident** is any motor vehicle accident occurring on a public highway [i.e., originating, terminating, or involving a vehicle partially on the highway]. A motor vehicle accident is assumed to have occurred on the highway unless another place is specified, except in the case of accidents involving only off-road motor vehicles which are classified as nontraffic accidents unless the contrary is stated.

(g) A **motor vehicle nontraffic accident** is any motor vehicle accident which occurs entirely in any place other than a public highway.

(h) A **public highway [trafficway]** or **street** is the entire width between property lines [or other boundary lines] of every way or place, of which any part is open to the use of the public for purposes of vehicular traffic as a matter of right or custom. A roadway is that part of the public highway designed, improved, and ordinarily used, for vehicular travel.

> **INCLUDES** approaches (public) to:
> docks
> public building
> station

> **EXCLUDES** driveway (private)   roads in:
> parking lot   industrial premises
> ramp   mine
> roads in: private grounds
> airfield   quarry
> farm

(i) A **motor vehicle** is any mechanically or electrically powered device, not operated on rails, upon which any person or property may be transported or drawn upon a highway. Any object such as a trailer, coaster, sled, or wagon being towed by a motor vehicle is considerd a part of the motor vehicle.

> **INCLUDES** automobile [any type]
> bus
> construction machinery, farm and industrial machinery, steam roller, tractor, army tank, highway grader, or similar vehicle on wheels or treads, while in transport under own power
> fire engine (motorized)
> motorcycle
> motorized bicycle [moped] or scooter
> trolley bus not operating on rails
> truck
> van

> **EXCLUDES** devices used solely to move persons or materials within the confines of a building and its premises, such as:
> building elevator
> coal car in mine
> electric baggage or mail truck used solely within a railroad station
> electric truck used solely within an industrial plant
> moving overhead crane

(j) A **motorcycle** is a two-wheeled motor vehicle having one or two riding saddles and sometimes having a third wheel for the support of a sidecar. The sidecar is considered part of the motorcycle.

> **INCLUDES** motorized:
> bicycle [moped]
> scooter
> tricycle

(k) An **off-road motor vehicle** is a motor vehicle of special design, to enable it to negotiate rough or soft terrain or snow. Examples of special design are high construction, special wheels and tires, driven by treads, or support on a cushion of air.

> **INCLUDES** all terrain vehicle [ATV]
> army tank
> hovercraft, on land or swamp
> snowmobile

(l) A **driver** of a motor vehicle is the occupant of the motor vehicle operating it or intending to operate it. A **motorcyclist** is the driver of a motorcycle. Other authorized occupants of a motor vehicle are **passengers.**

(m) An **other road vehicle** is any device, except a motor vehicle, in, on, or by which any person or property may be transported on a highway.

> **INCLUDES** animal carrying a person or goods
> animal-drawn vehicles
> animal harnessed to conveyance
> bicycle [pedal cycle]
> streetcar
> tricycle (pedal)
>
> **EXCLUDES** pedestrian conveyance [definition (q)]

(n) A **streetcar** is a device designed and used primarily for transporting persons within a municipality, running on rails, usually subject to normal traffic control signals, and operated principally on a right-of-way that forms part of the traffic way. A trailer being towed by a streetcar is considered a part of the streetcar.

> **INCLUDES** interurban or intraurban electric or streetcar, when specified to be operating on a street or public highway
> tram (car)
> trolley (car)

(o) A **pedal cycle** is any road transport vehicle operated solely by pedals.

> **INCLUDES** bicycle   tricycle
> pedal cycle
>
> **EXCLUDES** motorized bicycle [definition (i)]

(p) A **pedal cyclist** is any person riding on a pedal cycle or in a sidecar attached to such a vehicle.

(q) A **pedestrian conveyance** is any human powered device by which a pedestrian may move other than by walking or by which a walking person may move another pedestrian.

> **INCLUDES** baby carriage   roller skates
> coaster wagon   scooter
> ice skates   skateboard
> perambulator   skis
> pushcart   sled
> pushchair   wheelchair

(r) A **pedestrian** is any person involved in an accident who was not at the time of the accident riding in or on a motor vehicle, railroad train, streetcar, animal-drawn or other vehicle, or on a bicycle or animal.

> **INCLUDES** person:
> changing tire of vehicle
> in or operating a pedestrian conveyance
> making adjustment to motor of vehicle
> on foot

(s) A **watercraft** is any device for transporting passengers or goods on the water.

(t) A **small boat** is any watercraft propelled by paddle, oars, or small motor, with a passenger capacity of less than ten.

> **INCLUDES** boat NOS   raft
> canoe   rowboat
> coble scull   rowing shell
> dinghy   skiff
> punt   small motorboat
>
> **EXCLUDES** barge
> lifeboat (used after abandoning ship)
> raft (anchored) being used as a diving platform
> yacht

(u) An **aircraft** is any device for transporting passengers or goods in the air.

> **INCLUDES** airplane [any type]   glider (hang)
> balloon   military aircraft
> bomber   parachute
> dirigible

(v) A **commercial transport aircraft** is any device for collective passenger or freight transportation by air, whether run on commercial lines for profit or by government authorities, with the exception of military craft.

RAILWAY ACCIDENTS (E800-E807)

Note: For definitions of railway accident and related terms see definitions (a) to (d).

> **EXCLUDES** accidents involving railway train and:
> aircraft (E840.0-E845.9)
> motor vehicle (E810.0-E825.9)
> watercraft (E830.0-E838.9)

The following fourth-digit subdivisions are for use with categories E800-E807 to identify the injured person:

.0 Railway employee
Any person who by virtue of his employment in connection with a railway, whether by the railway company or not, is at increased risk of involvement in a railway accident, such as:
catering staff of train
driver
guard
porter
postal staff on train
railway fireman
shunter
sleeping car attendant

.1 Passenger on railway
Any authorized person traveling on a train, except a railway employee.

> **EXCLUDES** intending passenger waiting at station (.8)
> unauthorized rider on railway vehicle (.8)

.2 Pedestrian
See definition (r)

.3 Pedal cyclist
See definition (p)

.8 Other specified person
Intending passenger or bystander waiting at station
Unauthorized rider on railway vehicle

.9 Unspecified person

● **E800 Railway accident involving collision with rolling stock**

> **INCLUDES** collision between railway trains or railway vehicles, any kind
> collision NOS on railway
> derailment with antecedent collision with rolling stock or NOS

● **E801 Railway accident involving collision with other object**

> **INCLUDES** collision of railway train with:
> buffers
> fallen tree on railway
> gates
> platform
> rock on railway
> streetcar
> other nonmotor vehicle
> other object
>
> **EXCLUDES** collision with:
> aircraft (E840.0-E842.9)
> motor vehicle (E810.0-E810.9, E820.0-E822.9)

● **E802 Railway accident involving derailment without antecedent collision**

● **E803 Railway accident involving explosion, fire, or burning**

> **EXCLUDES** explosion or fire, with antecedent derailment (E802.0-E802.9)
> explosion or fire, with mention of antecedent collision (E800.0-E801.9)

● **E804 Fall in, on, or from railway train**

> **INCLUDES** fall while alighting from or boarding railway train
>
> **EXCLUDES** fall related to collision, derailment, or explosion of railway train (E800.0-E803.9)

- **E805 Hit by rolling stock**
  - INCLUDES: crushed / injured / killed / knocked down / run over } by railway train or part
  - EXCLUDES: pedestrian hit by object set in motion by railway train (E806.0-E806.9)
- ◆ **E806 Other specified railway accident**
  - INCLUDES:
    - hit by object falling in railway train
    - injured by door or window on railway train
    - nonmotor road vehicle or pedestrian hit by object set in motion by railway train
    - railway train hit by falling:
      - earth NOS
      - rock
      - tree
      - other object
  - EXCLUDES: railway accident due to cataclysm (E908-E909)
- ◆ **E807 Railway accident of unspecified nature**
  - INCLUDES: found dead / injured } on railway right-of-way NOS
    - railway accident NOS

MOTOR VEHICLE TRAFFIC ACCIDENTS (E810-E819)

Note: For definitions of motor vehicle traffic accident, and related terms, see definitions (e) to (k).

EXCLUDES: accidents involving motor vehicle and aircraft (E840.0-E845.9)

The following fourth-digit subdivisions are for use with categories E810-E819 to identify the injured person:

- **.0 Driver of motor vehicle other than motorcycle**
  - See definition (1)
- **.1 Passenger in motor vehicle other than motorcycle**
  - See definition (1)
- **.2 Motorcyclist**
  - See definition (1)
- **.3 Passenger on motorcycle**
  - See definition (1)
- **.4 Occupant of streetcar**
- **.5 Rider of animal; occupant of animal-drawn vehicle**
- **.6 Pedal cyclist**
  - See definition (p)
- **.7 Pedestrian**
  - See definition (r)
- ◆ **.8 Other specified person**
  - Occupant of vehicle other than above
  - Person in railway train involved in accident
  - Unauthorized rider of motor vehicle
- ◆ **.9 Unspecified person**

- **E810 Motor vehicle traffic accident involving collision with train**
  - EXCLUDES:
    - motor vehicle collision with object set in motion by railway train (E815.0-E815.9)
    - railway train hit by object set in motion by motor vehicle (E818.0-E818.9)
- **E811 Motor vehicle traffic accident involving re-entrant collision with another motor vehicle**
  - INCLUDES: collision between motor vehicle which accidentally leaves the roadway then re-enters the same roadway, or the opposite roadway on a divided highway, and another motor vehicle
  - EXCLUDES: collision on the same roadway when none of the motor vehicles involved have left and re-entered the highway (E812.0-E812.9)
- ◆ **E812 Other motor vehicle traffic accident involving collision with motor vehicle**
  - INCLUDES:
    - collision with another motor vehicle parked, stopped, stalled, disabled, or abandoned on the highway
    - motor vehicle collision NOS
  - EXCLUDES:
    - collision with object set in motion by another motor vehicle (E815.0-E815.9)
    - re-entrant collision with another motor vehicle (E811.0-E811.9)
- **E813 Motor vehicle traffic accident involving collision with other vehicle**
  - INCLUDES: collision between motor vehicle, any kind, and:
    - other road (nonmotor transport) vehicle, such as:
      - animal carrying a person
      - animal-drawn vehicle
      - pedal cycle
      - streetcar
  - EXCLUDES: collision with:
    - object set in motion by nonmotor road vehicle (E815.0-E815.9)
    - pedestrian (E814.0-E814.9)
    - nonmotor road vehicle hit by object set in motion by motor vehicle (E818.0-E818.9)
- **E814 Motor vehicle traffic accident involving collision with pedestrian**
  - INCLUDES:
    - collision between motor vehicle, any kind, and pedestrian
    - pedestrian dragged, hit, or run over by motor vehicle, any kind
  - EXCLUDES: pedestrian hit by object set in motion by motor vehicle (E818.0-E818.9)
- ◆ **E815 Other motor vehicle traffic accident involving collision on the highway**
  - INCLUDES: collision (due to loss of control) (on highway) between motor vehicle, any kind, and:
    - abutment (bridge) (overpass)
    - animal (herded) (unattended)
    - fallen stone, traffic sign, tree, utility pole
    - guard rail or boundary fence
    - interhighway divider
    - landslide (not moving)
    - object set in motion by railway train or road vehicle (motor) (nonmotor)
    - object thrown in front of motor vehicle
    - safety island
    - temporary traffic sign or marker
    - wall of cut made for road
    - other object, fixed, movable, or moving
  - EXCLUDES: collision with:
    - any object off the highway (resulting from loss of control) (E816.0-E816.9)
    - any object which normally would have been off the highway and is not stated to have been on it (E816.0-E816.9)
    - motor vehicle parked, stopped, stalled, disabled, or abandoned on highway (E812.0-E812.9)
    - moving landslide (E909)
    - motor vehicle hit by object:
      - set in motion by railway train or road vehicle (motor) (nonmotor) (E818.0-E818.9)
      - thrown into or on vehicle (E818.0-E818.9)
- **E816 Motor vehicle traffic accident due to loss of control, without collision on the highway**
  - INCLUDES: motor vehicle: failing to make curve / going out of control (due to): blowout / burst tire / driver falling asleep / driver inattention / excessive speed / failure of mechanical part } and: colliding with object off the highway / overturning / stopping abruptly off the highway
  - EXCLUDES:
    - collision on highway following loss of control (E810.0-E815.9)
    - loss of control of motor vehicle following collision on the highway (E810.0-E815.9)

● **E817 Noncollision motor vehicle traffic accident while boarding or alighting**

INCLUDES: fall down stairs of motor bus
fall from car in street
injured by moving part of the vehicle
trapped by door of motor bus
} while boarding or alighting

◆ ● **E818 Other noncollision motor vehicle traffic accident**

INCLUDES: accidental poisoning from exhaust gas generated by
breakage of any part of
explosion of any part of
fall, jump, or being accidentally pushed from
fire starting in
hit by object thrown into or on
injured by being thrown against some part of, or object in
injury from moving part of
object falling in or on
object thrown on
} motor vehicle while in motion

collision of railway train or road vehicle except motor vehicle, with object set in motion by motor vehicle
motor vehicle hit by object set in motion by railway train or road vehicle (motor) (nonmotor)
pedestrian, railway train, or road vehicle (motor) (nonmotor) hit by object set in motion by motor vehicle

EXCLUDES: collision between motor vehicle and:
object set in motion by railway train or road vehicle (motor) (nonmotor) (E815.0-E815.9)
object thrown towards the motor vehicle (E815.0-E815.9)
person overcome by carbon monoxide generated by stationary motor vehicle off the roadway with motor running (E868.2)

◆ ● **E819 Motor vehicle traffic accident of unspecified nature**

INCLUDES: motor vehicle traffic accident NOS
traffic accident NOS

MOTOR VEHICLE NONTRAFFIC ACCIDENTS

Note: For definitions of motor vehicle nontraffic accident and related terms see definition (a) to (k).

INCLUDES: accidents involving motor vehicles being used in recreational or sporting activities off the highway
collision and noncollision motor vehicle accidents occurring entirely off the highway

EXCLUDES: accidents involving motor vehicle and:
aircraft (E840.0-E845.9)
watercraft (E830.0-E838.9)
accidents, not on the public highway, involving agricultural and construction machinery but not involving another motor vehicle (E919.0, E919.2, E919.7)

The following fourth-digit subdivisions are for use with categories E820-E825 to identify the injured person:

.0 Driver of motor vehicle other than motorcycle
See definition (l)
.1 Passenger in motor vehicle other than motorcycle
See definition (l)
.2 Motorcyclist
See definition (l)
.3 Passenger on motorcycle
See definition (l)
.4 Occupant of streetcar
.5 Rider of animal; occupant of animal-drawn vehicle
.6 Pedal cyclist
See definition (p)
.7 Pedestrian
See definition (r)
◆ .8 Other specified person
Occupant of vehicle other than above
Person on railway train involved in accident
Unauthorized rider of motor vehicle
◆ .9 Unspecified person

● **E820 Nontraffic accident involving motor-driven snow vehicle**

INCLUDES: breakage of part of
fall from
hit by
overturning of
run over or dragged by
} motor-driven snow vehicle (not on public highway)

collision of motor-driven snow vehicle with:
animal (being ridden) (-drawn vehicle)
another off-road motor vehicle
other motor vehicle, not on public highway
railway train
other object, fixed or movable
injury caused by rough landing of motor-driven snow vehicle (after leaving ground on rough terrain)

EXCLUDES: accident on the public highway involving motor driven snow vehicle (E810.0-E819.9)

◆ ● **E821 Nontraffic accident involving other off-road motor vehicle**

INCLUDES: breakage of part of
fall from
hit by
overturning of
run over or dragged by
thrown against some part of or object in
} off-road motor vehicle, except snow vehicle (not on public highway)

collision with:
animal (being ridden) (-drawn vehicle)
another off-road motor vehicle, except snow vehicle
other motor vehicle, not on public highway
other object, fixed or movable

EXCLUDES: accident on public highway involving off-road motor vehicle (E810.0-E819.9)
collision between motor driven snow vehicle and other off-road motor vehicle (E820.0-E820.9)
hovercraft accident on water (E830.0-E838.9)

◆ ● **E822 Other motor vehicle nontraffic accident involving collision with moving object**

INCLUDES: collision, not on public highway, between motor vehicle, except off-road motor vehicle and:
animal
nonmotor vehicle
other motor vehicle, except off-road motor vehicle
pedestrian
railway train
other moving object

EXCLUDES: collision with:
motor-driven snow vehicle (E820.0-E820.9)
other off-road motor vehicle (E821.0-E821.9)

◆● **E823 Other motor vehicle nontraffic accident involving collision with stationary object**
  INCLUDES: collision, not on public highway, between motor vehicle, except off-road motor vehicle, and any object, fixed or movable, but not in motion

◆● **E824 Other motor vehicle nontraffic accident while boarding and alighting**
  INCLUDES:
  - fall
  - injury from moving part of motor vehicle
  - trapped by door of motor vehicle

  while boarding or alighting from motor vehicle, except off-road motor vehicle, not on public highway

◆● **E825 Other motor vehicle nontraffic accident of other and unspecified nature**
  INCLUDES:
  - accidental poisoning from carbon monoxide generated by
  - breakage of any part of
  - explosion of any part of
  - fall, jump, or being accidentally pushed from
  - fire starting in
  - hit by object thrown into, towards, or on
  - injured by being thrown against some part of, or object in
  - injury from moving part of
  - object falling in or on

  motor vehicle while in motion, not on public highway

  motor vehicle nontraffic accident NOS

  EXCLUDES: fall from or in stationary motor vehicle (E884.9, E885)
  overcome by carbon monoxide or exhaust gas generated by stationary motor vehicle off the roadway with motor running (E868.2)
  struck by falling object from or in stationary motor vehicle (E916)

OTHER ROAD VEHICLE ACCIDENTS (E826-E829)

Note: Other road vehicle accidents are transport accidents involving road vehicles other than motor vehicles. For definitions of other road vehicle and related terms see definitions (m) to (o).

INCLUDES: accidents involving other road vehicles being used in recreational or sporting activities

EXCLUDES: collision of other road vehicle [any] with:
  aircraft (E840.0-E845.9)
  motor vehicle (E813.0-E813.9, E820.0-E822.9)
  railway train (E801.0-E801.9)

The following fourth-digit subdivisions are for use with categories E826-E829 to identify the injured person. Valid fourth digits are in [brackets] under each code.
  .0 Pedestrian
       See definition (r)
  .1 Pedal cyclist
       See definition (p)
  .2 Rider of animal
  .3 Occupant of animal-drawn vehicle
  .4 Occupant of streetcar
  ◆ .8 Other specified person
  ◆ .9 Unspecified person

●**E826 Pedal cycle accident**
  [0-9] INCLUDES: breakage of any part of pedal cycle
  collision between pedal cycle and:
    animal (being ridden) (herded) (unattended)
    another pedal cycle
    any pedestrian
    nonmotor road vehicle
    other object, fixed, movable, or moving, not set in motion by motor vehicle, railway train, or aircraft
  entanglement in wheel of pedal cycle
  fall from pedal cycle
  hit by object falling or thrown on the pedal cycle
  pedal cycle accident NOS
  pedal cycle overturned

●**E827 Animal-drawn vehicle accident**
  [0,2-4,8,9] INCLUDES: breakage of any part of vehicle
  collision between animal-drawn vehicle and:
    animal (being ridden) (herded) (unattended)
    nonmotor road vehicle, except pedal cycle
    pedestrian, pedestrian conveyance, or pedestrian vehicle
    other object, fixed, movable, or moving, not set in motion by motor vehicle, railway train, or aircraft

  - fall from
  - knocked down by
  - overturning of
  - run over by
  - thrown from

  animal-drawn vehicle

  EXCLUDES: collision of animal-drawn vehicle with pedal cycle (E826.0-E826.9)

●**E828 Accident involving animal being ridden**
  [0,2,4,8,9] INCLUDES: collision between animal being ridden and:
    another animal
    nonmotor road vehicle, except pedal cycle, and animal-drawn vehicle
    pedestrian, pedestrian conveyance, or pedestrian vehicle
    other object, fixed, movable, or moving, not set in motion by motor vehicle, railway train, or aircraft

  - fall from
  - knocked down by
  - thrown from
  - trampled by

  animal being ridden

  ridden animal stumbled and fell

  EXCLUDES: collision of animal being ridden with:
    animal-drawn vehicle (E827.0-E827.9)
    pedal cycle (E826.0-E826.9)

◆●**E829 Other road vehicle accidents**
  [0,4,8,9] INCLUDES:
  - accident while boarding or alighting from
  - blow from object in
  - breakage of any part of
  - caught in door of
  - derailment of
  - fall in, on, or from
  - fire in

  streetcar
  nonmotor road vehicle not classifiable to E826-E828

  collision between streetcar or nonmotor road vehicle, except as in E826-E828, and:
    animal (not being ridden)
    another nonmotor road vehicle not classifiable to E826-E828
    pedestrian
    other object, fixed, movable, or moving, not set in motion by motor vehicle, railway train, or aircraft
  nonmotor road vehicle accident NOS
  streetcar accident NOS

  EXCLUDES: collision with:
    animal being ridden (E828.0-E828.9)
    animal-drawn vehicle (E827.0-E827.9)
    pedal cycle (E826.0-E826.9)

WATER TRANSPORT ACCIDENTS (E830-E838)

Note: For definitions of water transport accident and related terms see definitions (a), (s), and (t).

INCLUDES watercraft accidents in the course of recreational activities

EXCLUDES accidents involving both aircraft, including objects set in motion by aircraft, and watercraft (E840.0-E845.9)

The following fourth-digit subdivisions are for use with categories E830-E838 to identify the injured person:

.0 Occupant of small boat, unpowered
.1 Occupant of small boat, powered
  See definition (t)
  EXCLUDES water skier (.4)
.2 Occupant of other watercraft crew
  Persons:
    engaged in operation of watercraft
    providing passenger services [cabin attendants, ship's physician, catering personnel]
    working on ship during voyage in other capacity [musician in band, operators of shops and beauty parlors]
.3 Occupant of other watercraft other than crew
  Passenger
  Occupant of lifeboat, other than crew, after abandoning ship
.4 Water skier
.5 Swimmer
.6 Dockers, stevedores
  Longshoreman employed on the dock in loading and unloading ships
.8 Other specified person
  Immigration and custom officials on board ship
  Person:
    accompanying passenger or member of crew visiting boat
  Pilot (guiding ship into port)
.9 Unspecified person

E830 Accident to watercraft causing submersion
INCLUDES submersion and drowning due to:
  boat overturning
  boat submerging
  falling or jumping from burning ship
  falling or jumping from crushed watercraft
  ship sinking
  other accident to watercraft

E831 Accident to watercraft causing other injury
INCLUDES any injury, except submersion and drowning, as a result of an accident to watercraft
  burned while ship on fire
  crushed between ships in collision
  crushed by lifeboat after abandoning ship
  fall due to collision or other accident to watercraft
  hit by falling object due to accident to watercraft
  injured in watercraft accident involving collision
  struck by boat or part thereof after fall or jump from damaged boat
EXCLUDES burns from localized fire or explosion on board ship (E837.0-E837.9)

E832 Other accidental submersion or drowning in water transport accident
INCLUDES submersion or drowning as a result of an accident other than accident to the watercraft, such as:
  fall:
    from gangplank
    from ship
    overboard
  thrown overboard by motion of ship
  washed overboard
EXCLUDES submersion or drowning of swimmer or diver who voluntarily jumps from boat not involved in an accident (E910.0-E910.9)

E833 Fall on stairs or ladders in water transport
EXCLUDES fall due to accident to watercraft (E831.0-E831.9)

E834 Other fall from one level to another in water transport
EXCLUDES fall due to accident to watercraft (E831.0-E831.9)

E835 Other and unspecified fall in water transport
EXCLUDES fall due to accident to watercraft (E831.0-E831.9)

E836 Machinery accident in water transport
INCLUDES injuries in water transport caused by:
  deck
  engine room
  galley } machinery
  laundry
  loading

E837 Explosion, fire, or burning in watercraft
INCLUDES explosion of boiler on steamship
  localized fire on ship
EXCLUDES burning ship (due to collision or explosion) resulting in:
  submersion or drowning (E830.0-E830.9)
  other injury (E831.0-E831.9)

E838 Other and unspecified water transport accident
INCLUDES accidental poisoning by gases or fumes on ship
  atomic power plant malfunction in watercraft
  crushed between ship and stationary object [wharf]
  crushed between ships without accident to watercraft
  crushed by falling object on ship or while loading or unloading
  hit by boat while water skiing
  struck by boat or part thereof (after fall from boat)
  watercraft accident NOS

AIR AND SPACE TRANSPORT ACCIDENTS (E840-E845)

Note: For definition of aircraft and related terms see definitions (u) and (v).

The following fourth-digit subdivisions are for use with categories E840-E845 to identify the injured person. Valid fourth digits are in [brackets] under codes E842-E845.

.0 Occupant of spacecraft
.1 Occupant of military aircraft, any
  Crew   } in military aircraft
  Passenger (civilian) [air force] [army]
    (military)   [national guard]
  Troops   [navy]
  EXCLUDES occupants of aircraft operated under jurisdiction of police departments (.5)
    parachutist (.7)
.2 Crew of commercial aircraft (powered) in surface to surface transport
.3 Other occupant of commercial aircraft (powered) in surface to surface transport
  Flight personnel:
    not part of crew
    on familiarization flight
  Passenger on aircraft (powered) NOS
.4 Occupant of commercial aircraft (powered) in surface to air transport
  Occupant [crew] [passenger] of aircraft (powered) engaged in activities, such as:
    aerial spraying (crops) (fire retardants)
    air drops of emergency supplies
    air drops of parachutists, except from military craft
    crop dusting
    lowering of construction material [bridge or telephone pole]
    sky writing
.5 Occupant of other powered aircraft
  Occupant [crew][passenger] of aircraft [powered] engaged in activities, such as:
    aerobatic flying
    aircraft racing
    rescue operation
    storm surveillance
    traffic surveillance
  Occupant of private plane NOS
.6 Occupant of unpowered aircraft, except parachutist
  Occupant of aircraft classifiable to E842

E CODES

.7 Parachutist (military) (other)
Person making voluntary descent
EXCLUDES: person making descent after accident to aircraft (.1-.6)

.8 Ground crew, airline employee
Persons employed at airfields (civil) (military) or launching pads, not occupants of aircraft

◆ **.9 Other person**

● **E840 Accident to powered aircraft at takeoff or landing**
INCLUDES: collision of aircraft with any object, fixed, movable, or moving
crash
explosion on aircraft
fire on aircraft
forced landing
} while taking off or landing

◆ ● **E841 Accident to powered aircraft, other and unspecified**
INCLUDES: aircraft accident NOS
aircraft crash or wreck NOS
any accident to powered aircraft while in transit or when not specified whether in transit, taking off, or landing
collision of aircraft with another aircraft, bird, or any object, while in transit
explosion on aircraft while in transit
fire on aircraft while in transit

● **E842 Accident to unpowered aircraft**
[6-9] INCLUDES: any accident, except collision with powered aircraft, to:
balloon
glider
hang glider
kite carrying a person
hit by object falling from unpowered aircraft

● **E843 Fall in, on, or from aircraft**
[0-9] INCLUDES: accident in boarding or alighting from aircraft, any kind
fall in, on, or from aircraft [any kind], while in transit, taking off, or landing, except when as a result of an accident to aircraft

◆ ● **E844 Other specified air transport accidents**
[0-9] INCLUDES: hit by:
aircraft
object falling from aircraft
injury by or from:
machinery on aircraft
rotating propeller
voluntary parachute descent
poisoning by carbon monoxide from aircraft while in transit
sucked into jet
} without accident to aircraft

any accident involving other transport vehicle (motor) (nonmotor) due to being hit by object set in motion by aircraft (powered)

EXCLUDES: air sickness (E903)
effects of:
high altitude (E902.0-E902.1)
pressure change (E902.0-E902.1)
injury in parachute descent due to accident to aircraft (E840.0-E842.9)

● **E845 Accident involving spacecraft**
[0,8,9] INCLUDES: launching pad accident
EXCLUDES: effects of weightlessness in spacecraft (E928.0)

VEHICLE ACCIDENTS NOT ELSEWHERE CLASSIFIABLE (E846-E848)

E846 Accidents involving powered vehicles used solely within the buildings and premises of industrial or commercial establishment
Accident to, on, or involving:
battery powered airport passenger vehicle
battery powered trucks (baggage) (mail)
coal car in mine
logging car
self propelled truck, industrial
station baggage truck (powered)
tram, truck, or tub (powered) in mine or quarry
Breakage of any part of vehicle
Collision with:
pedestrian
other vehicle or object within premises
Explosion of
Fall from
Overturning of
Struck by
} powered vehicle, industrial or commercial

EXCLUDES: accidental poisoning by exhaust gas from vehicle not elsewhere classifiable (E868.2)
injury by crane, lift (fork), or elevator (E919.2)

E847 Accidents involving cable cars not running on rails
Accident to, on, or involving:
cable car, not on rails
ski chair-lift
ski-lift with gondola
téléférique
Breakage of cable
Caught or dragged by
Fall or jump from
Object thrown from or in
} cable car, not on rails

◆ **E848 Accidents involving other vehicles, not elsewhere classifiable**
Accident to, on, or involving:
ice yacht
land yacht
nonmotor, nonroad vehicle NOS

● **E849 Place of occurrence**
The following category is for use with categories E850-E869 and E880-E928, to denote the place where the accident or poisoning occurred.

■ **E849.0 Home**
Apartment
Boarding house
Farm house
Home premises
House (residential)
Noninstitutional place of residence
Private:
driveway
garage
garden
home
Swimming pool in private house or garden
Yard of home

EXCLUDES: home under construction but not yet occupied (E849.3)
institutional place of residence (E849.7)

■ **E849.1 Farm**
Farm:
buildings
land under cultivation

EXCLUDES: farm house and home premises of farm (E849.0)

■ **E849.2 Mine and quarry**
Gravel pit
Sand pit
Tunnel under construction

■ **E849.3 Industrial place and premises**
Building under construction
Dockyard
Dry dock
Factory
building
premises
Garage (place of work)
Industrial yard
Loading platform (factory) (store)
Plant, industrial
Railway yard
Shop (place of work)
Warehouse
Workhouse

E849.4 Place for recreation and sport

Amusement park
Baseball field
Basketball court
Beach resort
Cricket ground
Fives court
Football field
Golf course
Gymnasium
Hockey field
Holiday camp
Ice palace
Lake resort
Mountain resort
Playground, including school playground
Public park
Racecourse
Resort NOS
Riding school
Rifle range
Seashore resort
Skating rink
Sports ground
Sports palace
Stadium
Swimming pool, public
Tennis court
Vacation resort

EXCLUDES that in private house or garden (E849.0)

E849.5 Street and highway

E849.6 Public building

Building (including adjacent grounds) used by the general public or by a particular group of the public, such as:

airport
bank
café
casino
church
cinema
clubhouse
courthouse
dance hall
garage building (for car storage)
hotel
market (grocery or other commodity)
movie house
music hall
nightclub
office
office building
opera house
post office
public hall
radio broadcasting station
restaurant
school (state) (public) (private)
shop, commercial
station (bus) (railway)
store
theater

EXCLUDES home garage (E849.0)
industrial building or workplace (E849.3)

E849.7 Residential institution

Children's home
Dormitory
Hospital
Jail
Old people's home
Orphanage
Prison
Reform school

E849.8 Other specified places

Beach NOS
Canal
Caravan site NOS
Derelict house
Desert
Dock
Forest
Harbor
Hill
Lake NOS
Mountain
Parking lot
Parking place
Pond or pool (natural)
Prairie
Public place NOS
Railway line
Reservoir
River
Sea
Seashore NOS
Stream
Swamp
Trailer court
Woods

E849.9 Unspecified place

ACCIDENTAL POISONING BY DRUGS, MEDICINAL SUBSTANCES, AND BIOLOGICALS (E850-E858)

INCLUDES accidental overdose of drug, wrong drug given or taken in error, and drug taken inadvertently
accidents in the use of drugs and biologicals in medical and surgical procedures

EXCLUDES administration with suicidal or homicidal intent or intent to harm, or in circumstances classifiable to E980-E989 (E950.0-E950.5, E962.0, E980.0-E980.5)
correct drug properly administered in therapeutic or prophylactic dosage, as the cause of adverse effect (E930.0-E949.9)

See Alphabetic Index for more complete list of specific drugs to be classified under the fourth-digit subdivisions. The American Hospital Formulary numbers can be used to classify new drugs listed by the American Hospital Formulary Service (AHFS). See appendix C.

E850 Accidental poisoning by analgesics, antipyretics, and antirheumatics

E850.0 Heroin
Diacetylmorphine

E850.1 Methadone

E850.2 Other opiates and related narcotics
Codeine [methylmorphine]   Morphine
Meperidine [pethidine]   Opium (alkaloids)

E850.3 Salicylates
Acetylsalicylic acid [aspirin]
Amino derivatives of salicylic acid
Salicylic acid salts

E850.4 Aromatic analgesics, not elsewhere classified
Acetanilid
Paracetamol [acetaminophen]
Phenacetin [acetophenetidin]

E850.5 Pyrazole derivatives
Aminophenazone [amidopyrine]
Phenylbutazone

E850.6 Antirheumatics [antiphlogistics]
Gold salts
Indomethacin

EXCLUDES salicylates (E850.3)
steroids (E858.0)

E850.7 Other non-narcotic analgesics
Pyrabital

E850.8 Other specified analgesics and antipyretics
Pentazocine

E850.9 Unspecified analgesic or antipyretic

E851 Accidental poisoning by barbiturates
Amobarbital [amylobarbitone]
Barbital [barbitone]
Butabarbital [butabarbitone]
Pentobarbital [pentobarbitone]
Phenobarbital [phenobarbitone]
Secobarbital [quinalbarbitone]

EXCLUDES thiobarbiturates (E855.1)

E852 Accidental poisoning by other sedatives and hypnotics

E852.0 Chloral hydrate group

E852.1 Paraldehyde

E852.2 Bromine compounds
Bromides
Carbromal (derivatives)

E852.3 Methaqualone compounds

E852.4 Glutethimide group

E852.5 Mixed sedatives, not elsewhere classified

E852.8 Other specified sedatives and hypnotics

E852.9 Unspecified sedative or hypnotic
Sleeping:
  drug
  pill   } NOS
  tablet

E853 Accidental poisoning by tranquilizers

E853.0 Phenothiazine-based tranquilizers
Chlorpromazine   Prochlorperazine
Fluphenazine   Promazine

E853.1 Butyrophenone-based tranquilizers
Haloperidol   Trifluperidol
Spiperone

E853.2 Benzodiazepine-based tranquilizers
Chlordiazepoxide   Lorazepam
Diazepam   Medazepam
Flurazepam   Nitrazepam

E853.8 Other specified tranquilizers
Hydroxyzine   Meprobamate

E853.9 Unspecified tranquilizer

E854 Accidental poisoning by other psychotropic agents

E854.0 Antidepressants
Amitriptyline
Imipramine
Monoamine oxidase [MAO] inhibitors

E854.1 Psychodysleptics [hallucinogens]
Cannabis derivatives   Mescaline
Lysergide [LSD]   Psilocin
Marihuana (derivatives)   Psilocybin

- E854.2 **Psychostimulants**
  - Amphetamine
  - Caffeine
  - EXCLUDES: central appetite depressants (E858.8)
- E854.3 **Central nervous system stimulants**
  - Analeptics
  - Opiate antagonists
- ● E855 **Accidental poisoning by other drugs acting on central and autonomic nervous system**
  - E855.0 **Anticonvulsant and anti-Parkinsonism drugs**
    - Amantadine
    - Hydantoin derivatives
    - Levodopa [L-dopa]
    - Oxazolidine derivatives [paramethadione] [trimethadione]
    - Succinimides
  - ◆ E855.1 **Other central nervous system depressants**
    - Ether
    - Gaseous anesthetics
    - Halogenated hydrocarbon derivatives
    - Intravenous anesthetics
    - Thiobarbiturates, such as thiopental sodium
  - E855.2 **Local anesthetics**
    - Cocaine
    - Procaine
    - Lidocaine [lignocaine]
    - Tetracaine
  - E855.3 **Parasympathomimetics [cholinergics]**
    - Acetylcholine
    - Pilocarpine
    - Anticholinesterase:
      - organophosphorus
      - reversible
  - E855.4 **Parasympatholytics [anticholinergics and antimuscarinics] and spasmolytics**
    - Atropine
    - Homatropine
    - Hyoscine [scopolamine]
    - Quaternary ammonium derivatives
  - E855.5 **Sympathomimetics [adrenergics]**
    - Epinephrine [adrenalin]
    - Levarterenol [noradrenalin]
  - E855.6 **Sympatholytics [antiadrenergics]**
    - Phenoxybenzamine
    - Tolazoline hydrochloride
  - ◆ E855.8 **Other specified drugs acting on central and autonomic nervous systems**
  - ◆ E855.9 **Unspecified drug acting on central and autonomic nervous systems**
- E856 **Accidental poisoning by antibiotics**
- ◆ E857 **Accidental poisoning by other anti-infectives**
- ● E858 **Accidental poisoning by other drugs**
  - E858.0 **Hormones and synthetic substitutes**
  - E858.1 **Primarily systemic agents**
  - E858.2 **Agents primarily affecting blood constituents**
  - E858.3 **Agents primarily affecting cardiovascular system**
  - E858.4 **Agents primarily affecting gastrointestinal system**
  - E858.5 **Water, mineral, and uric acid metabolism drugs**
  - E858.6 **Agents primarily acting on the smooth and skeletal muscles and respiratory system**
  - E858.7 **Agents primarily affecting skin and mucous membrane, ophthalmological, otorhinolaryngological, and dental drugs**
  - ◆ E858.8 **Other specified drugs**
    - Central appetite depressants
  - ◆ E858.9 **Unspecified drug**

ACCIDENTAL POISONING BY OTHER SOLID AND LIQUID SUBSTANCES, GASES, AND VAPORS

Note: Categories in this section are intended primarily to indicate the external cause of poisoning states classifiable to 980-989. They may also be used to indicate external causes of localized effects classifiable to 001-799.

- ● E860 **Accidental poisoning by alcohol, not elsewhere classified**
  - E860.0 **Alcoholic beverages**
    - Alcohol in preparations intended for consumption
  - ◆ E860.1 **Other and unspecified ethyl alcohol and its products**
    - Denatured alcohol
    - Grain alcohol NOS
    - Ethanol NOS
    - Methylated spirit
  - E860.2 **Methyl alcohol**
    - Methanol
    - Wood alcohol
  - E860.3 **Isopropyl alcohol**
    - Dimethyl carbinol
    - Rubbing alcohol subsitute
    - Isopropanol
    - Secondary propyl alcohol
  - E860.4 **Fusel oil**
    - Alcohol:
      - amyl
      - butyl
      - propyl
  - ◆ E860.8 **Other specified alcohols**
  - ◆ E860.9 **Unspecified alcohol**
- ● E861 **Accidental poisoning by cleansing and polishing agents, disinfectants, paints, and varnishes**
  - E861.0 **Synthetic detergents and shampoos**
  - E861.1 **Soap products**
  - E861.2 **Polishes**
  - ◆ E861.3 **Other cleansing and polishing agents**
    - Scouring powders
  - E861.4 **Disinfectants**
    - Household and other disinfectants not ordinarily used on the person
    - EXCLUDES: carbolic acid or phenol (E864.0)
  - E861.5 **Lead paints**
  - ◆ E861.6 **Other paints and varnishes**
    - Lacquers
    - Paints, other than lead
    - Oil colors
    - White washes
  - ◆ E861.9 **Unspecified**
- ● E862 **Accidental poisoning by petroleum products, other solvents and their vapors, not elsewhere classified**
  - E862.0 **Petroleum solvents**
    - Petroleum:
      - ether
      - benzine
      - naphtha
  - E862.1 **Petroleum fuels and cleaners**
    - Antiknock additives to petroleum fuels
    - Gas oils
    - Gasoline or petrol
    - Kerosene
    - EXCLUDES: kerosene insecticides (E863.4)
  - E862.2 **Lubricating oils**
  - E862.3 **Petroleum solids**
    - Paraffin wax
  - ◆ E862.4 **Other specified solvents**
    - Benzene
  - ◆ E862.9 **Unspecified solvent**
- ● E863 **Accidental poisoning by agricultural and horticultural chemical and pharmaceutical preparations other than plant foods and fertilizers**
  - EXCLUDES: plant foods and fertilizers (E866.5)
  - E863.0 **Insecticides of organochlorine compounds**
    - Benzene hexachloride
    - Dieldrin
    - Chlordane
    - Endrine
    - DDT
    - Toxaphene
  - E863.1 **Insecticides of organophosphorus compounds**
    - Demeton
    - Parathion
    - Diazinon
    - Phenylsulphthion
    - Dichlorvos
    - Phorate
    - Malathion
    - Phosdrin
    - Methyl parathion
  - E863.2 **Carbamates**
    - Aldicarb
    - Propoxur
    - Carbaryl
  - E863.3 **Mixtures of insecticides**
  - ◆ E863.4 **Other and unspecified insecticides**
    - Kerosene insecticides
  - E863.5 **Herbicides**
    - 2, 4-Dichlorophenoxyacetic acid [2, 4-D]
    - 2, 4, 5-Trichlorophenoxyacetic acid [2, 4, 5-T]
    - Chlorates
    - Diquat
    - Mixtures of plant foods and fertilizers with herbicides
    - Paraquat
  - E863.6 **Fungicides**
    - Organic mercurials (used in seed dressing)
    - Pentachlorophenols

- E863.7 **Rodenticides**
  - Fluoroacetates
  - Squill and derivatives
  - Thallium
  - Warfarin
  - Zinc phosphide
- E863.8 **Fumigants**
  - Cyanides
  - Methyl bromide
  - Phosphine
- ◆ E863.9 **Other and unspecified**

● **E864 Accidental poisoning by corrosives and caustics, not elsewhere classified**

> EXCLUDES   those as components of disinfectants (E861.4)

- E864.0 **Corrosive aromatics**
  - Carbolic acid or phenol
- E864.1 **Acids**
  - Acid:
    - hydrochloric
    - nitric
    - sulfuric
- E864.2 **Caustic alkalis**
  - Lye
- ◆ E864.3 **Other specified corrosives and caustics**
- ◆ E864.4 **Unspecified corrosives and caustics**

● **E865 Accidental poisoning from foodstuffs and poisonous plants**

> INCLUDES   any meat, fish, or shellfish
> plants, berries, and fungi eaten as, or in mistake for, food, or by a child

> EXCLUDES   food poisoning (bacterial) (005.0-005.9)
> poisoning and toxic reactions to venomous plants (E905.6-E905.7)

- E865.0 **Meat**
- E865.1 **Shellfish**
- ◆ E865.2 **Other fish**
- E865.3 **Berries and seeds**
- ◆ E865.4 **Other specified plants**
- E865.5 **Mushrooms and other fungi**
- ◆ E865.8 **Other specified foods**
- ◆ E865.9 **Unspecified foodstuff or poisonous plant**

● **E866 Accidental poisoning by other and unspecified solid and liquid substances**

> EXCLUDES   these substances as a component of:
> medicines (E850.0-E858.9)
> paints (E861.5-E861.6)
> pesticides (E863.0-E863.9)
> petroleum fuels (E862.1)

- E866.0 **Lead and its compounds and fumes**
- E866.1 **Mercury and its compounds and fumes**
- E866.2 **Antimony and its compounds and fumes**
- E866.3 **Arsenic and its compounds and fumes**
- ◆ E866.4 **Other metals and their compounds and fumes**
  - Beryllium (compounds)
  - Brass fumes
  - Cadmium (compounds)
  - Copper salts
  - Iron (compounds)
  - Manganese (compounds)
  - Nickel (compounds)
  - Thallium (compounds)
- E866.5 **Plant foods and fertilizers**

> EXCLUDES   mixtures with herbicides (E863.5)

- E866.6 **Glues and adhesives**
- E866.7 **Cosmetics**
- ◆ E866.8 **Other specified solid or liquid substances**
- ◆ E866.9 **Unspecified solid or liquid substance**

E867 Accidental poisoning by gas distributed by pipeline
- Carbon monoxide from incomplete combustion of piped gas
- Coal gas NOS
- Liquefied petroleum gas distributed through pipes (pure or mixed with air)
- Piped gas (natural) (manufactured)

● **E868 Accidental poisoning by other utility gas and other carbon monoxide**

- E868.0 **Liquefied petroleum gas distributed in mobile containers**
  - Butane
  - Liquefied hydrocarbon gas NOS
  - Propane
  } or carbon monoxide from incomplete conbustion of these gases

- ◆ E868.1 **Other and unspecified utility gas**
  - Acetylene
  - Gas NOS used for lighting, heating, or cooking
  - Water gas
  } or carbon monoxide from incomplete conbustion of these gases

- E868.2 **Motor vehicle exhaust gas**
  - Exhaust gas from:
    - farm tractor, not in transit
    - gas engine
    - motor pump
    - motor vehicle, not in transit
    - any type of combustion engine not in watercraft

> EXCLUDES   poisoning by carbon monoxide from:
> aircraft while in transit (E844.0-E844.9)
> motor vehicle while in transit (E818.0-E818.9)
> watercraft whether or not in transit (E838.0-E838.9)

- ◆ E868.3 **Carbon monoxide from incomplete combustion of other domestic fuels**
  - Carbon monoxide from incomplete combustion of:
    - coal
    - coke
    - kerosene
    - wood
  } in domestic stove or fireplace

> EXCLUDES   carbon monoxide from smoke and fumes due to conflagration (E890.0-E893.9)

- ◆ E868.8 **Carbon monoxide from other sources**
  - Carbon monoxide from:
    - blast furnace gas
    - incomplete combustion of fuels in industrial use
    - kiln vapor
- ◆ E868.9 **Unspecified carbon monoxide**

● **E869 Accidental poisoning by other gases and vapors**

> EXCLUDES   effects of gases used as anesthetics (E855.1, E938.2)
> fumes from heavy metals (E866.0-E866.4)
> smoke and fumes due to conflagration or explosion (E890.0-E899)

- E869.0 **Nitrogen oxides**
- E869.1 **Sulfur dioxide**
- E869.2 **Freon**
- E869.3 **Lacrimogenic gas [tear gas]**
  - Bromobenzyl cyanide
  - Chloroacetophenone
  - Ethyliodoacetate
- E869.4 **Second-hand tobacco smoke** ◆
- ◆ E869.8 **Other specified gases and vapors**
  - Chlorine
  - Hydrocyanic acid gas
- ◆ E869.9 **Unspecified gases and vapors**

MISADVENTURES TO PATIENTS DURING SURGICAL AND MEDICAL CARE (E870-E876)

> EXCLUDES   accidental overdose of drug and wrong drug given in error (E850.0-E858.9)
> surgical and medical procedures as the cause of abnormal reaction by the patient, without mention of misadventure at the time of procedure (E878.0-E879.9)

● **E870 Accidental cut, puncture, perforation, or hemorrhage during medical care**

- E870.0 **Surgical operation**
- E870.1 **Infusion or transfusion**
- E870.2 **Kidney dialysis or other perfusion**
- E870.3 **Injection or vaccination**
- E870.4 **Endoscopic examination**
- E870.5 **Aspiration of fluid or tissue, puncture, and catheterization**
  - Abdominal paracentesis
  - Aspirating needle biopsy
  - Blood sampling
  - Lumbar puncture
  - Thoracentesis

> EXCLUDES   heart catheterization (E870.6)

- E870.6 **Heart catheterization**
- E870.7 **Administration of enema**
- ◆ E870.8 **Other specified medical care**

- E870.9 Unspecified medical care
- ● E871 Foreign object left in body during procedure
  - E871.0 Surgical operation
  - E871.1 Infusion or transfusion
  - E871.2 Kidney dialysis or other perfusion
  - E871.3 Injection or vaccination
  - E871.4 Endoscopic examination
  - E871.5 Aspiration of fluid or tissue, puncture, and catheterization
    - Abdominal paracentesis
    - Aspiration needle biopsy
    - Blood sampling
    - Lumbar puncture
    - Thoracentesis
    - **EXCLUDES** *heart catheterization (E871.6)*
  - E871.6 Heart catheterization
  - E871.7 Removal of catheter or packing
  - ◆ E871.8 Other specified procedures
  - ◆ E871.9 Unspecified procedure
- ● E872 Failure of sterile precautions during procedure
  - E872.0 Surgical operation
  - E872.1 Infusion or transfusion
  - E872.2 Kidney dialysis and other perfusion
  - E872.3 Injection or vaccination
  - E872.4 Endoscopic examination
  - E872.5 Aspiration of fluid or tissue, puncture, and catheterization
    - Abdominal paracentesis
    - Aspiration needle biopsy
    - Blood sampling
    - Lumbar puncture
    - Thoracentesis
    - **EXCLUDES** *heart catheterization (E872.6)*
  - E872.6 Heart catheterization
  - ◆ E872.8 Other specified procedures
  - ◆ E872.9 Unspecified procedure
- ● E873 Failure in dosage
  - **EXCLUDES** *accidental overdose of drug, medicinal or biological substance (E850.0-E858.9)*
  - ◆ E873.0 Excessive amount of blood or other fluid during transfusion or infusion
  - E873.1 Incorrect dilution of fluid during infusion
  - E873.2 Overdose of radiation in therapy
  - E873.3 Inadvertent exposure of patient to radiation during medical care
  - E873.4 Failure in dosage in electroshock or insulin-shock therapy
  - E873.5 Inappropriate [too hot or too cold] temperature in local application and packing
  - E873.6 Nonadministration of necessary drug or medicinal substance
  - ◆ E873.8 Other specified failure in dosage
  - ◆ E873.9 Unspecified failure in dosage
- ● E874 Mechanical failure of instrument or apparatus during procedure
  - E874.0 Surgical operation
  - E874.1 Infusion and transfusion
    - Air in system
  - E874.2 Kidney dialysis and other perfusion
  - E874.3 Endoscopic examination
  - E874.4 Aspiration of fluid or tissue, puncture, and catheterization
    - Abdominal paracentesis
    - Aspiration needle biopsy
    - Blood sampling
    - Lumbar puncture
    - Thoracentesis
    - **EXCLUDES** *heart catheterization (E874.5)*
  - E874.5 Heart catheterization
  - ◆ E874.8 Other specified procedures
  - ◆ E874.9 Unspecified procedure
- ● E875 Contaminated or infected blood, other fluid, drug, or biological substance
  - **INCLUDES** presence of:
    - bacterial pyrogens
    - endotoxin-producing bacteria
    - serum hepatitis-producing agent
  - E875.0 Contaminated substance transfused or infused
  - E875.1 Contaminated substance injected or used for vaccination
  - ◆ E875.2 Contaminated drug or biological substance administered by other means
  - ◆ E875.8 Other
  - ◆ E875.9 Unspecified
- ● E876 Other and unspecified misadventures during medical care
  - E876.0 Mismatched blood in transfusion
  - E876.1 Wrong fluid in infusion
  - E876.2 Failure in suture and ligature during surgical operation
  - E876.3 Endotracheal tube wrongly placed during anesthetic procedure
  - ◆ E876.4 Failure to introduce or to remove other tube or instrument
    - **EXCLUDES** *foreign object left in body during procedure (E871.0-E871.9)*
  - E876.5 Performance of inappropriate operation
  - ◆ E876.8 Other specified misadventures during medical care
    - Performance of inappropriate treatment NEC
  - ◆ E876.9 Unspecified misadventure during medical care

SURGICAL AND MEDICAL PROCEDURES AS THE CAUSE OF ABNORMAL REACTION OF PATIENT OR LATER COMPLICATION, WITHOUT MENTION OF MISADVENTURE AT THE TIME OF PROCEDURE (E878-E879)

INCLUDES procedures as the cause of abnormal reaction, such as:
- displacement or malfunction of prosthetic device
- hepatorenal failure, postoperative
- malfunction of external stoma
- postoperative intestinal obstruction
- rejection of transplanted organ

EXCLUDES *anesthetic management properly carried out as the cause of adverse effect (E937.0-E938.9)*
infusion and transfusion, without mention of misadventure in the technique of procedure (E930.0-E949.9)

- ● E878 Surgical operation and other surgical procedures as the cause of abnormal reaction of patient, or of later complication, without mention of misadventure at the time of operation
  - E878.0 Surgical operation with transplant of whole organ
    - Transplantation of: heart kidney
    - Transplantation of: liver
  - E878.1 Surgical operation with implant of artificial internal device
    - Cardiac pacemaker
    - Electrodes implanted in brain
    - Heart valve prosthesis
    - Internal orthopedic device
  - E878.2 Surgical operation with anastomosis, bypass, or graft, with natural or artificial tissues used as implant
    - Anastomosis:
      - arteriovenous
      - gastrojejunal
    - Graft of blood vessel, tendon, or skin
    - **EXCLUDES** *external stoma (E878.3)*
  - E878.3 Surgical operation with formation of external stoma
    - Colostomy
    - Cystostomy
    - Duodenostomy
    - Gastrostomy
    - Ureterostomy
  - ◆ E878.4 Other restorative surgery
  - E878.5 Amputation of limb(s)
  - ◆ E878.6 Removal of other organ (partial) (total)
  - ◆ E878.8 Other specified surgical operations and procedures
  - ◆ E878.9 Unspecified surgical operations and procedures
- ● E879 Other procedures, without mention of misadventure at the time of procedure, as the cause of abnormal reaction of patient, or of later complication
  - E879.0 Cardiac catheterization
  - E879.1 Kidney dialysis
  - E879.2 Radiological procedure and radiotherapy
    - **EXCLUDES** *radio-opaque dyes for diagnostic x-ray procedures (E947.8)*
  - E879.3 Shock therapy
    - Electroshock therapy
    - Insulin-shock therapy
  - E879.4 Aspiration of fluid
    - Lumbar puncture
    - Thoracentesis
  - E879.5 Insertion of gastric or duodenal sound
  - E879.6 Urinary catheterization
  - E879.7 Blood sampling
  - ◆ E879.8 Other specified procedures
    - Blood transfusion
  - ◆ E879.9 Unspecified procedure

ACCIDENTAL FALLS (E880-E888)

EXCLUDES falls (in or from):
    burning building (E890.8, E891.8)
    into fire (E890.0-E899)
    into water (with submersion or drowning) (E910.0-E910.9)
    machinery (in operation) (E919.0-E919.9)
    on edged, pointed, or sharp object (E920.0-E920.9)
    transport vehicle (E800.0-E845.9)
    vehicle not elsewhere classifiable (E846-E848)

● **E880 Fall on or from stairs or steps**
    E880.0 Escalator
    ◆ **E880.9** Other stairs or steps
● **E881 Fall on or from ladders or scaffolding**
    E881.0 Fall from ladder
    E881.1 Fall from scaffolding
◆ **E882 Fall from or out of building or other structure**
    Fall from:
      balcony
      bridge
      building
      flagpole
      tower
    Fall from:
      turret
      viaduct
      wall
      window
      Fall through roof
    EXCLUDES collapse of a building or structure (E916)
      fall or jump from burning building (E890.8, E891.8)
● **E883 Fall into hole or other opening in surface**
    INCLUDES fall into:
      cavity
      dock
      hole
      pit
      quarry
    fall into:
      shaft
      swimming pool
      tank
      well
    EXCLUDES fall into water NOS (E910.9)
      that resulting in drowning or submersion without mention of injury (E910.0-E910.9)
    E883.0 Accident from diving or jumping into water [swimming pool]
      Strike or hit:
        against bottom when jumping or diving into water
        wall or board of swimming pool
        water surface
      EXCLUDES diving with insufficient air supply (E913.2)
        effects of air pressure from diving (E902.2)
    E883.1 Accidental fall into well
    E883.2 Accidental fall into storm drain or manhole
    ◆ **E883.9** Fall into other hole or other opening in surface
● **E884 Other fall from one level to another**
    E884.0 Fall from playground equipment
      EXCLUDES recreational machinery (E919.8)
    E884.1 Fall from cliff
    E884.2 Fall from chair or bed
    ◆ **E884.9** Other fall from one level to another
      Fall from:
        embankment
        haystack
      Fall from:
        stationary vehicle
        tree
    E885 Fall on same level from slipping, tripping, or stumbling
      Fall on moving sidewalk
● **E886 Fall on same level from collision, pushing, or shoving, by or with other person**
    EXCLUDES crushed or pushed by a crowd or human stampede (E917.1)
    E886.0 In sports
      Tackles in sports
      EXCLUDES kicked, stepped on, struck by object, in sports (E917.0)
    ◆ **E886.9** Other and unspecified
      Fall from collision of pedestrian (conveyance) with another pedestrian (conveyance)
◆ **E887 Fracture, cause unspecified**
◆ **E888 Other and unspecified fall**
    Accidental fall NOS
    Fall from bumping against object
    Fall on same level NOS

ACCIDENTS CAUSED BY FIRE AND FLAMES

INCLUDES asphyxia or poisoning due to conflagration or ignition
    burning by fire
    secondary fires resulting from explosion

EXCLUDES arson (E968.0)
    fire in or on:
      machinery (in operation) (E919.0-E919.9)
      transport vehicle other than stationary vehicle (E800.0-E845.9)
      vehicle not elsewhere classifiable (E846-E848)

● **E890 Conflagration in private dwelling**
    INCLUDES conflagration in:
      apartment
      boarding house
      camping place
      caravan
      farmhouse
      house
    conflagration in:
      lodging house
      mobile home
      private garage
      rooming house
      tenement
    conflagration originating from sources classifiable to E893-E898 in the above buildings
    E890.0 Explosion caused by conflagration
    E890.1 Fumes from combustion of polyvinylchloride [PVC] and similar material in conflagration
    ◆ **E890.2** Other smoke and fumes from conflagration
      Carbon monoxide } from conflagration in private building
      Fumes NOS
      Smoke NOS
    E890.3 Burning caused by conflagration
    ◆ **E890.8** Other accident resulting from conflagration
      Collapse of
      Fall from
      Hit by object falling from } burning private building
      Jump from
    ◆ **E890.9** Unspecified accident resulting from conflagration in private dwelling
● **E891 Conflagration in other and unspecified building or structure**
    Conflagration in:
      barn
      church
      convalescent and other residential home
      dormitory of educational institution
      factory
    Conflagration in:
      farm outbuildings
      hospital
      hotel
      school
      store
      theater
    Conflagration originating from sources classifiable to E893-E898, in the above buildings
    E891.0 Explosion caused by conflagration
    E891.1 Fumes from combustion of polyvinylchloride [PVC] and similar material in conflagration
    ◆ **E891.2** Other smoke and fumes from conflagration
      Carbon monoxide } from conflagration in building or structure
      Fumes NOS
      Smoke NOS
    E891.3 Burning caused by conflagration
    ◆ **E891.8** Other accident resulting from conflagration
      Collapse of
      Fall from
      Hit by object falling from } burning building or structure
      Jump from
    ◆ **E891.9** Unspecified accident resulting from conflagration of other and unspecified building or structure
    E892 Conflagration not in building or structure
    Fire (uncontrolled) (in) (of):
      forest
      grass
      hay
      lumber
      mine
    Fire (uncontrolled) (in) (of):
      prairie
      transport vehicle [any], except while in transit
● **E893 Accident caused by ignition of clothing**
    EXCLUDES ignition of clothing:
      from highly inflammable material (E894)
      with conflagration (E890.0-E892)

E893.0 **From controlled fire in private dwelling**
Ignition of clothing from:
normal fire (charcoal) (coal) (electric) (gas) (wood) in:
brazier
fireplace
furnace
stove
} in private dwelling (as listed in E80)

◆ E893.1 **From controlled fire in other building or structure**
Ignition of clothing from:
normal fire (charcoal) (coal) (electric) (gas) (wood) in:
brazier
fireplace
furnace
stove
} in other building or structure [as listed in E81]

E893.2 **From controlled fire not in building or structure**
Ignition of clothing from:
bonfire (controlled)
brazier fire (controlled), not in building or structure
trash fire (controlled)
EXCLUDES conflagration not in building (E892)
trash fire out of control (E892)

◆ E893.8 **From other specified sources**
Ignition of clothing from:
blowlamp
blowtorch
burning bedspread
candle
cigar

Ignition of clothing from:
cigarette
lighter
matches
pipe
welding torch

◆ E893.9 **Unspecified source**
Ignition of clothing (from controlled fire NOS) (in building NOS) NOS

E894 **Ignition of highly inflammable material**
Ignition of:
benzine
gasoline
fat
kerosene
paraffin
petrol
} (with ignition of clothing)

EXCLUDES ignition of highly inflammable material with:
conflagration (E890.0-E892)
explosion (E923.0-E923.9)

E895 **Accident caused by controlled fire in private dwelling**
Burning by (flame of) normal fire (charcoal) (coal) (electric) (gas) (wood) in:
brazier
fireplace
furnace
stove
} in private dwelling (as listed in E890)

EXCLUDES burning by hot objects not producing fire or flames (E924.0-E924.9)
ignition of clothing from these sources (E893.0)
poisoning by carbon monoxide from incomplete combustion of fuel (E867-E868.9)
that with conflagration (E890.0-E890.9)

◆ E896 **Accident caused by controlled fire in other and unspecified building or structure**
Burning by (flame of) normal fire (charcoal) (coal) (electric) (gas) (wood) in:
brazier
fireplace
furnace
stove
} in other building or structure (as listed in E891)

EXCLUDES burning by hot objects not producing fire or flames (E924.0-E924.9)
ignition of clothing from these sources (E893.1)
poisoning by carbon monoxide from incomplete combustion of fuel (E867-E868.9)
that with conflagration (E891.0-E891.9)

E897 **Accident caused by controlled fire not in building or structure**
Burns from flame of:
bonfire (controlled)
brazier fire (controlled), not in building or structure
trash fire (controlled)
EXCLUDES ignition of clothing from these sources (E893.2)
trash fire out of control (E892)
that with conflagration (E892)

● E898 **Accident caused by other specified fire and flames**
EXCLUDES conflagration (E890.0-E892)
that with ignition of:
clothing (E893.0-E893.9)
highly inflammable material (E894)

E898.0 **Burning bedclothes**
Bed set on fire NOS

◆ E898.1 **Other**
Burning by:
blowlamp
blowtorch
candle
cigar
fire in room NOS

Burning by:
lamp
lighter
matches
pipe

◆ E899 **Accident caused by unspecified fire**
Burning NOS

ACCIDENTS DUE TO NATURAL AND ENVIRONMENTAL FACTORS (E900-E909)

● E900 **Excessive heat**
E900.0 **Due to weather conditions**
Excessive heat as the external cause of:
ictus solaris
siriasis
sunstroke
E900.1 **Of man-made origin**
Heat (in):
boiler room
drying room
factory
furnace room

Heat (in):
generated in transport vehicle
kitchen

◆ E900.9 **Of unspecified origin**
● E901 **Excessive cold**
E901.0 **Due to weather conditions**
Excessive cold as the cause of:
chilblains NOS
immersion foot
E901.1 **Of man-made origin**
Contact with or inhalation of:
dry ice
liquid air
liquid hydrogen
liquid nitrogen
Prolonged exposure in:
deep freeze unit
refrigerator
◆ E901.8 **Other specified origin**
◆ E901.9 **Of unspecified origin**
● E902 **High and low air pressure and changes in air pressure**

E902.0 Residence or prolonged visit at high altitude
  Residence or prolonged visit at high altitude as the cause of:
  Acosta syndrome
  Alpine sickness
  altitude sickness
  Andes disease
  anoxia, hypoxia
  barotitis, barodontalgia, barosinusitis, otitic barotrauma
  hypobarism, hypobaropathy
  mountain sickness
  range disease

E902.1 In aircraft
  Sudden change in air pressure in aircraft during ascent or descent as the cause of:
  aeroneurosis
  aviators' disease

E902.2 Due to diving
  High air pressure from rapid descent in water
  Reduction in atmospheric pressure while surfacing from deep water diving
  } as the cause of:
  caisson disease
  divers' disease
  divers' palsy or paralysis

◆ **E902.8 Due to other specified causes**
  Reduction in atmospheric pressure while surfacing from underground

◆ **E902.9 Unspecified cause**

E903 Travel and motion

● **E904 Hunger, thirst, exposure, and neglect**
  EXCLUDES any condition resulting from homicidal intent (E968.0-E968.9)
  hunger, thirst, and exposure resulting from accidents connected with transport (E800.0-E848)

  E904.0 Abandonment or neglect of infants and helpless persons
  Exposure to weather conditions
  Hunger or thirst
  } resulting from abandonment or neglect
  Desertion of newborn
  Inattention at or after birth
  Lack of care (helpless person) (infant)
  EXCLUDES criminal [purposeful] neglect (E968.4)

  E904.1 Lack of food
  Lack of food as the cause of:
  inanition
  insufficient nourishment
  starvation
  EXCLUDES hunger resulting from abandonment or neglect (E904.0)

  E904.2 Lack of water
  Lack of water as the cause of:
  dehydration
  inanition
  EXCLUDES dehydration due to acute fluid loss (276.5)

  E904.3 Exposure (to weather conditions), not elsewhere classifiable
  Exposure NOS
  Humidity
  Struck by hailstones
  EXCLUDES struck by lightning (E907)

  E904.9 Privation, unqualified
  Destitution

● **E905 Venomous animals and plants as the cause of poisoning and toxic reactions**
  INCLUDES chemical released by animal
  insects
  release of venom through fangs, hairs, spines, tentacles, and other venom apparatus
  EXCLUDES eating of poisonous animals or plants (E865.0-E865.9)

E905.0 Venomous snakes and lizards
  Cobra   Mamba
  Copperhead snake   Rattlesnake
  Coral snake   Sea snake
  Fer de lance   Snake (venomous)
  Gila monster   Viper
  Krait   Water moccasin
  EXCLUDES bites of snakes and lizards known to be nonvenomous (E906.2)

E905.1 Venomous spiders
  Black widow spider   Tarantula (venomous)
  Brown spider

E905.2 Scorpion

E905.3 Hornets, wasps, and bees
  Yellow jacket

E905.4 Centipede and venomous millipede (tropical)

◆ **E905.5 Other venomous arthropods**
  Sting of:
    ant
    caterpillar

E905.6 Venomous marine animals and plants
  Puncture by sea urchin spine
  Sting of:
    coral
    jelly fish
    nematocysts
    sea anemone
    sea cucumber
    other marine animal or plant
  EXCLUDES bites and other injuries caused by nonvenomous marine animal (E906.2-E906.8)
  bite of sea snake (venomous) (E905.0)

◆ **E905.7 Poisoning and toxic reactions caused by other plants**
  Injection of poisons or toxins into or through skin by plant thorns, spines, or other mechanisms
  EXCLUDES puncture wound NOS by plant thorns or spines (E920.8)

◆ **E905.8 Other specified**

◆ **E905.9 Unspecified**
  Sting NOS
  Venomous bite NOS

● **E906 Other injury caused by animals**
  EXCLUDES poisoning and toxic reactions caused by venomous animals and insects (E905.0-E905.9)
  road vehicle accident involving animals (E827.0-E828.9)
  tripping or falling over an animal (E885)

E906.0 Dog bite
E906.1 Rat bite
E906.2 Bite of nonvenomous snakes and lizards

◆ **E906.3 Bite of other animal except arthropod**
  Cats   Rodents, except rats
  Moray eel   Shark

E906.4 Bite of nonvenomous arthropod
  Insect bite NOS

◆ **E906.8 Other specified injury caused by animal**
  Butted by animal
  Fallen on by horse or other animal, not being ridden
  Gored by animal
  Implantation of quills of porcupine
  Pecked by bird
  Run over by animal, not being ridden
  Stepped on by animal, not being ridden
  EXCLUDES injury by animal being ridden (E828.0-E828.9)

◆ **E906.9 Unspecified injury caused by animal**

E907 Lightning
  EXCLUDES injury from:
  fall of tree or other object caused by lightning (E916)
  fire caused by lightning (E890.0-E892)

E908 Cataclysmic storms, and floods resulting from storms
Blizzard
Cloudburst
Cyclone
Flood
  arising from remote storm
  of cataclysmic nature arising from melting snow
  resulting directly from storm
Hurricane
"Tidal wave" caused by storm action
Tornado
Torrential rain
Transport vehicle washed off road by storm

EXCLUDES *collapse of dam or man-made structure causing flood (E909)*
transport accident occurring after storm (E800.0-E848)

E909 Cataclysmic earth surface movements and eruptions
Avalanche
Collapse of dam or man-made structure causing flood
Earthquake
Landslide
Mud slide of cataclysmic nature
Tidal wave
Tsunami
Volcanic eruption

EXCLUDES *"tidal wave" caused by storm action (E908)*
transport accident involving collision with avalanche or landslide not in motion (E800.0-E848)

ACCIDENTS CAUSED BY SUBMERSION, SUFFOCATION, AND FOREIGN BODIES (E910-E915)

E910 Accidental drowning and submersion

INCLUDES immersion
swimmers' cramp

EXCLUDES *diving accident (NOS) (resulting in injury except drowning) (E883.0)*
diving with insufficient air supply (E913.2)
drowning and submersion due to:
  cataclysm (E908-E909)
  machinery accident (E919.0-E919.9)
  transport accident (E800.0-E845.9)
effect of high and low air pressure (E902.2)
injury from striking against objects while in running water (E917.2)

E910.0 While water-skiing
Fall from water skis with submersion or drowning

EXCLUDES *accident to water-skier involving a watercraft and resulting in submersion or other injury (E830.4, E831.4)*

E910.1 While engaged in other sport or recreational activity with diving equipment
Scuba diving NOS
Skin diving NOS
Underwater spear fishing NOS

E910.2 While engaged in other sport or recreational activity without diving equipment
Fishing or hunting, except from boat or with diving equipment
Ice skating
Playing in water
Surfboarding
Swimming NOS
Voluntarily jumping from boat, not involved in accident, for swim NOS
Wading in water

EXCLUDES *jumping into water to rescue another person (E910.3)*

E910.3 While swimming or diving for purposes other than recreation or sport
Marine salvage
Pearl diving
Placement of fishing nets
Rescue (attempt) of another person
Underwater construction or repairs
(with diving equipment)

E910.4 In bathtub

E910.8 Other accidental drowning or submersion
Drowning in:
  quenching tank
  swimming pool

E910.9 Unspecified accidental drowning or submersion
Accidental fall into water NOS
Drowning NOS

E911 Inhalation and ingestion of food causing obstruction of respiratory tract or suffocation
Aspiration and inhalation of food [any] (into respiratory tract) NOS

Asphyxia by
Choked on
Suffocation by
} food [including bone, seed in food, regurgitated food]

Compression of trachea
Interruption of respiration
Obstruction of respiration
} by food lodged in esophagus

Obstruction of pharynx by food (bolus)

EXCLUDES *injury, except asphyxia and obstruction of respiratory passage, caused by food (E915)*
obstruction of esophagus by food without mention of asphyxia or obstruction of respiratory passage (E915)

E912 Inhalation and ingestion of other object causing obstruction of respiratory tract or suffocation
Aspiration and inhalation of foreign body except food (into respiratory tract) NOS
Foreign object [bean] [marble] in nose
Obstruction of pharynx by foreign body

Compression
Interruption of respiration
Obstruction of respiration
} by foreign body in esophagus

EXCLUDES *injury, except asphyxia and obstruction of respiratory passage, caused by foreign body (E915)*
obstruction of esophagus by foreign body without mention of asphyxia or obstruction in respiratory passage (E915)

E913 Accidental mechanical suffocation

EXCLUDES *mechanical suffocation from or by:*
  accidental inhalation or ingestion of:
    food (E911)
    foreign object (E912)
  cataclysm (E908-E909)
  explosion (E921.0-E921.9, E923.0-E923.9)
  machinery accident (E919.0-E919.9)

E913.0 In bed or cradle

EXCLUDES *suffocation by plastic bag (E913.1)*

E913.1 By plastic bag

E913.2 Due to lack of air (in closed place)
Accidentally closed up in refrigerator or other airtight enclosed space
Diving with insufficient air supply

EXCLUDES *suffocation by plastic bag (E913.1)*

E913.3 By falling earth or other substance
Cave-in NOS

EXCLUDES *cave-in caused by cataclysmic earth surface movements and eruptions (E909)*
struck by cave-in without asphyxiation or suffocation (E916)

E913.8 Other specified means
Accidental hanging, except in bed or cradle

- **E913.9 Unspecified means**
  Asphyxia, mechanical NOS   Suffocation NOS
  Strangulation NOS

E914 Foreign body accidentally entering eye and adnexa
  EXCLUDES   corrosive liquid (E924.1)

- **E915 Foreign body accidentally entering other orifice**
  EXCLUDES   aspiration and inhalation of foreign body, any,
                    (into respiratory tract) NOS (E911-E912)

OTHER ACCIDENTS (E916-E928)

E916 Struck accidentally by falling object
  Collapse of building, except on fire
  Falling:
    rock
    snowslide NOS
    stone
    tree
  Object falling from:
    machine, not in operation
    stationary vehicle
  EXCLUDES   collapse of building on fire (E890.0-E891.9)
             falling object in:
               cataclysm (E908-E909)
               machinery accidents (E919.0-E919.9)
               transport accidents (E800.0-E845.9)
             object set in motion by:
               explosion (E921.0-E921.9, E923.0-E923.9)
               firearm (E922.0-E922.9)
               projected object (E917.0-E917.9)

● **E917 Striking against or struck accidentally by objects or persons**
  INCLUDES   bumping into or against   object (moving)
             colliding with   (projected)
             kicking against   (stationary)
             stepping on   pedestrian conveyance
             struck by   person
  EXCLUDES   fall from:
               bumping into or against object (E888)
               collision with another person, except when
                 caused by a crowd (E886.0-E886.9)
               stumbling over object (E885)
             injury caused by:
               assault (E960.0-E960.1, E967.0-E967.9)
               cutting or piercing instrument (E920.0-E920.9)
               explosion (E921.0-E921.9, E923.0-E923.9)
               firearm (E922.0-E922.9)
               machinery (E919.0-E919.9)
               transport vehicle (E800.0-E845.9)
               vehicle not elsewhere classifiable (E846-E848)

  E917.0 In sports
    Kicked or stepped on during game (football) (rugby)
    Knocked down while boxing
    Struck by hit or thrown ball
    Struck by hockey stick or puck

  E917.1 Caused by a crowd, by collective fear or panic
    Crushed
    Pushed   by crowd or human
    Stepped on   stampede

  E917.2 In running water
    EXCLUDES   drowning or submersion (E910.0-E910.9)
               that in sports (E917.0)

- **E917.9 Other**
    Accident caused by air rifle [BB gun]

E918 Caught accidentally in or between objects
  Caught, crushed, jammed, or pinched in or between moving or
    stationary objects, such as:
      escalator
      folding object
      hand tools, appliances, or implements
      sliding door and door frame
      under packing crate
      washing machine wringer
  EXCLUDES   injury caused by:
               cutting or piercing instrument (E920.0-E920.9)
               machinery (E919.0-E919.9)
               transport vehicle (E800.0-E845.9)
               vehicle not elsewhere classifiable (E846-E848)
             struck accidentally by:
               falling object (E916)
               object (moving) (projected) (E917.0-E917.9)

● **E919 Accidents caused by machinery**
  INCLUDES   burned by
             caught in (moving parts of)
             collapse of
             crushed by
             cut or pierced by
             drowning or submersion
               caused by
             explosion of, on, in
             fall from or into moving
               part of   } machinery
             fire starting in or on   accident
             mechanical suffocation
               caused by
             object falling from, on, in
               motion by
             overturning of
             pinned under
             run over by
             struck by
             thrown from

  caught between machinery and other object
  machinery accident NOS
  EXCLUDES   accidents involving machinery, not in operation
               (E884.9, E916-E918)
             injury caused by:
               electric current in connection with machinery
                 (E925.0-E925.9)
               escalator (E880.0, E918)
               explosion of pressure vessel in connection with
                 machinery (E921.0-E921.9)
               moving sidewalk (E885)
               powered hand tools, appliances, and
                 implements (E916-E918, E920.0-E921.9,
                 E923.0-E926.9)
               transport vehicle accidents involving machinery
                 (E800.0-E848.9)
               poisoning by carbon monoxide generated by
                 machine (E868.8)

  E919.0 Agricultural machines
    Animal-powered agricultural machine
    Combine
    Derrick, hay
    Farm machinery NOS
    Farm tractor
    Harvester
    Hay mower or rake
    Reaper
    Thresher
    EXCLUDES   that in transport under own power on the
                 highway (E810.0-E819.9)
               that being towed by another vehicle on
                 the highway (E810.0-E819.9,
                 E827.0-E827.9, E829.0-E829.9)
               that involved in accident classifiable to
                 E820-E829 (E820.0-E829.9)

E919.1 Mining and earth-drilling machinery
Bore or drill (land) (seabed) Shaft lift
Shaft hoist Under-cutter
EXCLUDES coal car, tram, truck, and tub in mine (E846)

E919.2 Lifting machines and appliances
Chain hoist
Crane
Derrick
Elevator (building) (grain) } except in agricultural or mining operations
Forklift truck
Lift
Pulley block
Winch

EXCLUDES that being towed by another vehicle on the highway (E810.0-E819.9, E827.0-E827.9, E829.0-829.9)
that in transport under own power on the highway (E810.0-E819.9)
that involved in accident classifiable to E820-E829 (E820.0-E829.9)

E919.3 Metalworking machines
Abrasive wheel Metal:
Forging machine   drilling machine
Lathe   milling machine
Mechanical shears   power press
  rolling-mill
  sawing machine

E919.4 Woodworking and forming machines
Band saw Overhead plane
Bench saw Powered saw
Circular saw Radial saw
Molding machine Sander
EXCLUDES hand saw (E920.1)

E919.5 Prime movers, except electrical motors
Gas turbine
Internal combustion engine
Steam engine
Water driven turbine
EXCLUDES that being towed by other vehicle on the highway (E810.0-E819.9, E827.0-E827.9, E829.0-E829.9)
that in transport under own power on the highway (E810.0-E819.9)

E919.6 Transmission machinery
Transmission: Transmission:
  belt   pinion
  cable   pulley
  chain   shaft
  gear

E919.7 Earth moving, scraping, and other excavating machines
Bulldozer Steam shovel
Road scraper
EXCLUDES that being towed by other vehicle on the highway (E810.0-E819.9, E827.0-E827.9, E829.0-E829.9)
that in transport under own power on the highway (E810.0-E819.9)

◆ E919.8 Other specified machinery
Machines for manufacture of:
  clothing
  foodstuffs and beverages
  paper
Printing machine
Recreational machinery
Spinning, weaving, and textile machines

◆ E919.9 Unspecified machinery

● E920 Accidents caused by cutting and piercing instruments or objects
INCLUDES accidental injury by fall on object: edged, pointed, sharp

E920.0 Powered lawn mower

E920.1 Other powered hand tools
Any powered hand tool [compressed air] [electric] [explosive cartridge] [hydraulic power], such as:
  drill
  hand saw
  hedge clipper
  rivet gun
  snow blower
  staple gun
EXCLUDES band saw (E919.4)
bench saw (E919.4)

E920.2 Powered household appliances and implements
Blender
Electric:
  beater or mixer
  can opener
  fan
  knife
  sewing machine
Garbage disposal appliance

E920.3 Knives, swords, and daggers

◆ E920.4 Other hand tools and implements
Axe Paper cutter
Can opener NOS Pitchfork
Chisel Rake
Fork Scissors
Hand saw Screwdriver
Hoe Sewing machine, not powered
Ice pick Shovel
Needle (hypodermic) (sewing)

◆ E920.8 Other specified cutting and piercing instruments or objects
Arrow Nail
Broken glass Plant thorn
Dart Splinter
Edge of stiff paper Tin can lid
Lathe turnings
EXCLUDES animal spines or quills (E906.8)
flying glass due to explosion (E921.0-E923.9)

◆ E920.9 Unspecified cutting and piercing instrument or object

● E921 Accident caused by explosion of pressure vessel
INCLUDES accidental explosion of pressure vessels, whether or not part of machinery
EXCLUDES explosion of pressure vessel on transport vehicle (E800.0-E845.9)

E921.0 Boilers
E921.1 Gas cylinders
Air tank
Pressure gas tank

◆ E921.8 Other specified pressure vessels
Aerosol can Pressure cooker
Automobile tire

◆ E921.9 Unspecified pressure vessel

● E922 Accident caused by firearm missile
E922.0 Handgun
Pistol Revolver
EXCLUDES Verey pistol (E922.8)
E922.1 Shotgun (automatic)
E922.2 Hunting rifle
EXCLUDES air rifle [BB gun] (E917.9)
E922.3 Military firearms
Army rifle Machine gun
◆ E922.8 Other specified firearm missile
Verey pistol [flare]
◆ E922.9 Unspecified firearm missile
Gunshot wound NOS Shot NOS

E923 Accident caused by explosive material

INCLUDES: flash burns and other injuries resulting from explosion of explosive material
ignition of highly explosive material with explosion

EXCLUDES: explosion:
in or on machinery (E919.0-E919.9)
on any transport vehicle, except stationary motor vehicle (E800.0-E848)
with conflagration (E890.0, E891.0, E892)
secondary fires resulting from explosion (E890.0-E899)

E923.0 Fireworks

E923.1 Blasting materials
Blasting cap
Detonator
Dynamite
Explosive [any] used in blasting operations

E923.2 Explosive gases
Acetylene
Butane
Coal gas
Explosion in mine NOS
Fire damp
Gasoline fumes
Methane
Propane

E923.8 Other explosive materials
Bomb
Explosive missile
Grenade
Mine
Shell
Torpedo
Explosion in munitions:
dump
factory

E923.9 Unspecified explosive material
Explosion NOS

E924 Accident caused by hot substance or object, caustic or corrosive material, and steam

EXCLUDES: burning NOS (E899)
chemical burn resulting from swallowing a corrosive substance (E860.0-E864.4)
fire caused by these substances and objects (E890.0-E894)
radiation burns (E926.0-E926.9)
therapeutic misadventures (E870.0-E876.9)

E924.0 Hot liquids and vapors, including steam
Burning or scalding by:
boiling water
hot or boiling liquids not primarily caustic or corrosive
liquid metal
steam
other hot vapor

E924.1 Caustic and corrosive substances
Burning by:
acid [any kind]
ammonia
caustic oven cleaner or other substance
corrosive substance
lye
vitriol

E924.8 Other
Burning by:
heat from electric heating appliance
hot object NOS
light bulb
steam pipe

E924.9 Unspecified

E925 Accident caused by electric current

INCLUDES: electric current from exposed wire, faulty appliance, high voltage cable, live rail, or open electric socket as the cause of:
burn
cardiac fibrillation
convulsion
electric shock
electrocution
puncture wound
respiratory paralysis

EXCLUDES: burn by heat from electrical appliance (E924.8)
lightning (E907)

E925.0 Domestic wiring and appliances

E925.1 Electric power generating plants, distribution stations, transmission lines
Broken power line

E925.2 Industrial wiring, appliances, and electrical machinery
Conductors
Control apparatus
Electrical equipment and machinery
Transformers

E925.8 Other electric current
Wiring and appliances in or on:
farm [not farmhouse]
outdoors
public building
residential institutions
schools

E925.9 Unspecified electric current
Burns or other injury from electric current NOS
Electric shock NOS
Electrocution NOS

E926 Exposure to radiation

EXCLUDES: abnormal reaction to or complication of treatment without mention of misadventure (E879.2)
atomic power plant malfunction in water transport (E838.0-E838.9)
misadventure to patient in surgical and medical procedures (E873.2-E873.3)
use of radiation in war operations (E996-E997.9)

E926.0 Radiofrequency radiation
Overexposure to:
microwave radiation
radar radiation
radiofrequency radiation [any]
from:
high-powered radio and television transmitters
industrial radiofrequency induction heaters
radar installations

E926.1 Infrared heaters and lamps
Exposure to infrared radiation from heaters and lamps as the cause of:
blistering
burning
charring
inflammatory change

EXCLUDES: physical contact with heater or lamp (E924.8)

E926.2 Visible and ultraviolet light sources
Arc lamps
Black light sources
Electrical welding arc
Oxygas welding torch
Sun rays

EXCLUDES: excessive heat from these sources (E900.1-E900.9)

E926.3 X-rays and other electromagnetic ionizing radiation
Gamma rays
X-rays (hard) (soft)

E926.4 Lasers

E926.5 Radioactive isotopes
Radiobiologicals
Radiopharmaceuticals

E926.8 Other specified radiation
Artificially accelerated beams of ionized particles generated by:
betatrons
synchrotrons

E926.9 Unspecified radiation
Radiation NOS

E927 Overexertion and strenuous movements
Excessive physical exercise
Overexertion (from):
lifting
pulling
pushing
Strenuous movements in:
recreational activities
other activities

E928 Other and unspecified environmental and accidental causes

E928.0 Prolonged stay in weightless environment
Weightlessness in spacecraft (simulator)

E928.1 Exposure to noise
Noise (pollution)
Sound waves
Supersonic waves

E928.2 Vibration

E928.8 Other

- ◆ **E928.9 Unspecified accident**
    Accident NOS
    Blow NOS
    Casualty (not due to war)
    Decapitation
    Injury [any part of body, or unspecified] } stated as accidentally inflicted, but not otherwise specified
    Killed
    Knocked down
    Mangled
    Wound

    EXCLUDES fracture, cause unspecified (E887)
    injuries undetermined whether accidentally or purposely inflicted (E980.0-E989)

LATE EFFECTS OF ACCIDENTAL INJURY (E929)

Note: This category is to be used to indicate accidental injury as the cause of death or disability from late effects, which are themselves classifiable elsewhere. The "late effects" include conditions reported as such or occurring as sequelae one year or more after accidental injury.

● **E929 Late effects of accidental injury**
    EXCLUDES late effects of:
    surgical and medical procedures (E870.0-E879.9)
    therapeutic use of drugs and medicines (E930.0-E949.9)

    E929.0 Late effects of motor vehicle accident
    Late effects of accidents classifiable to E810-E825

◆ **E929.1 Late effects of other transport accident**
    Late effects of accidents classifiable to E800-E807, E826-E838, E840-E848

E929.2 Late effects of accidental poisoning
    Late effects of accidents classifiable to E850-E858, E860-E869

E929.3 Late effects of accidental fall
    Late effects of accidents classifiable to E880-E888

E929.4 Late effects of accident caused by fire
    Late effects of accidents classifiable to E890-E899

E929.5 Late effects of accident due to natural and environmental factors
    Late effects of accidents classifiable to E900-E909

◆ **E929.8 Late effects of other accidents**
    Late effects of accidents classifiable to E910-E928.8

◆ **E929.9 Late effects of unspecified accident**
    Late effects of accidents classifiable to E928.9

DRUGS, MEDICINAL AND BIOLOGICAL SUBSTANCES CAUSING ADVERSE EFFECTS IN THERAPEUTIC USE (E930-E949)

INCLUDES correct drug properly administered in therapeutic or prophylactic dosage, as the cause of any adverse effect including allergic or hypersensitivity reactions

EXCLUDES accidental overdose of drug and wrong drug given or taken in error (E850.0-E858.9)
accidents in the technique of administration of drug or biological substance, such as accidental puncture during injection, or contamination of drug (E870.0-E876.9)
administration with suicidal or homicidal intent or intent to harm, or in circumstances classifiable to E980-E989 (E950.0-E950.5, E962.0, E980.0-E980.5)

See Alphabetic Index for more complete list of specific drugs to be classified under the fourth-digit subdivisions. The American Hospital Formulary numbers can be used to classify new drugs listed by the American Hospital Formulary Service (AHFS). See appendix C.

● **E930 Antibiotics**
    EXCLUDES that used as eye, ear, nose, and throat [ENT], and local anti-infectives (E946.0-E946.9)

E930.0 Penicillins
    Natural
    Synthetic
    Semisynthetic, such as:
        ampicillin
        cloxacillin
        nafcillin
        oxacillin

E930.1 Antifungal antibiotics
    Amphotericin B   Hachimycin [trichomycin]
    Griseofulvin   Nystatin

E930.2 Chloramphenicol group
    Chloramphenicol   Thiamphenicol

E930.3 Erythromycin and other macrolides
    Oleandomycin   Spiramycin

E930.4 Tetracycline group
    Doxycycline   Oxytetracycline
    Minocycline

E930.5 Cephalosporin group
    Cephalexin   Cephaloridine
    Cephaloglycin   Cephalothin

E930.6 Antimycobacterial antibiotics
    Cycloserine   Rifampin
    Kanamycin   Streptomycin

E930.7 Antineoplastic antibiotics
    Actinomycins, such as: Actinomycins, such as:
        Bleomycin   Daunorubicin
        Cactinomycin   Mitomycin
        Dactinomycin
    EXCLUDES other antineoplastic drugs (E933.1)

◆ **E930.8 Other specified antibiotics**
◆ **E930.9 Unspecified antibiotic**

● **E931 Other anti-infectives**
    EXCLUDES ENT, and local anti-infectives (E946.0-E946.9)

E931.0 Sulfonamides
    Sulfadiazine   Sulfamethoxazole
    Sulfafurazole

E931.1 Arsenical anti-infectives

E931.2 Heavy metal anti-infectives
    Compounds of: Compounds of:
        antimony   lead
        bismuth   mercury
    EXCLUDES mercurial diuretics (E944.0)

E931.3 Quinoline and hydroxyquinoline derivatives
    Chiniofon   Diiodohydroxyquin
    EXCLUDES antimalarial drugs (E931.4)

E931.4 Antimalarials and drugs acting on other blood protozoa
    Chloroquine phosphate   Proguanil [chloroguanide]
    Cycloguanil   Pyrimethamine
    Primaquine   Quinine (sulphate)

◆ **E931.5 Other antiprotozoal drugs**
    Emetine

E931.6 Anthelmintics
    Hexylresorcinol   Piperazine
    Male fern oleoresin   Thiabendazole

E931.7 Antiviral drugs
    Methisazone
    EXCLUDES amantadine (E936.4)
    cytarabine (E933.1)
    idoxuridine (E946.5)

E931.8 Other antimycobacterial drugs
    Ethambutol   Para-aminosalicylic
    Ethionamide   acid derivatives
    Isoniazid   Sulfones

◆ **E931.9 Other and unspecified anti-infectives**
    Flucytosine   Nitrofurand012derivatives

● **E932 Hormones and synthetic substitutes**

E932.0 Adrenal cortical steroids
    Cortisone derivatives
    Desoxycorticosterone derivatives
    Fluorinated corticosteroid

E932.1 Androgens and anabolic congeners
    Nandrolone phenpropionate
    Oxymetholone
    Testosterone and preparations

E932.2 Ovarian hormones and synthetic substitutes
    Contraceptives, oral
    Estrogens
    Estrogens and progestogens combined
    Progestogens

E932.3 Insulins and antidiabetic agents
    Acetohexamide
    Biguanide derivatives, oral
    Chlorpropamide
    Glucagon
    Insulin
    Phenformin
    Sulfonylurea derivatives, oral
    Tolbutamide
    EXCLUDES adverse effect of insulin administered for shock therapy (E879.3)

E932.4 Anterior pituitary hormones
    Corticotropin
    Gonadotropin
    Somatotropin [growth hormone]

E932.5 Posterior pituitary hormones
    Vasopressin
    EXCLUDES oxytocic agents (E945.0)

E932.6 Parathyroid and parathyroid derivatives

E932.7 Thyroid and thyroid derivatives
    Dextrothyroxine
    Levothyroxine sodium
    Liothyronine
    Thyroglobulin

E932.8 Antithyroid agents
    Iodides
    Thiouracil
    Thiourea

E932.9 Other and unspecified hormones and synthetic substitutes

● **E933 Primarily systemic agents**

E933.0 Antiallergic and antiemetic drugs
    Antihistamines
    Chlorpheniramine
    Diphenhydramine
    Diphenylpyraline
    Thonzylamine
    Tripelennamine
    EXCLUDES phenothiazine-based tranquilizers (E939.1)

E933.1 Antineoplastic and immunosuppressive drugs
    Azathioprine
    Busulfan
    Chlorambucil
    Cytarabine
    Fluorouracil
    Mechlorethamine hydrochloride
    Mercaptopurine
    Triethylenethiophosphoramide [thio-TEPA]
    EXCLUDES antineoplastic antibiotics (E930.7)

E933.2 Acidifying agents

E933.3 Alkalizing agents

E933.4 Enzymes, not elsewhere classified
    Penicillinase

E933.5 Vitamins, not elsewhere classified
    Vitamin A
    Vitamin D
    EXCLUDES nicotinic acid (E942.2)
              vitamin K (E934.3)

E933.8 Other systemic agents, not elsewhere classified
    Heavy metal antagonists

E933.9 Unspecified systemic agent

● **E934 Agents primarily affecting blood constituents**

E934.0 Iron and its compounds
    Ferric salts
    Ferrous sulphate and other ferrous salts

E934.1 Liver preparations and other antianemic agents
    Folic acid

E934.2 Anticoagulants
    Coumarin
    Heparin
    Phenindione
    Prothrombin synthesis inhibitor
    Warfarin sodium

E934.3 Vitamin K [phytonadione]

E934.4 Fibrinolysis-affecting drugs
    Aminocaproic acid
    Streptodornase
    Streptokinase
    Urokinase

E934.5 Anticoagulant antagonists and other coagulants
    Hexadimethrine bromide
    Protamine sulfate

E934.6 Gamma globulin

E934.7 Natural blood and blood products
    Blood plasma
    Human fibrinogen
    Packed red cells
    Whole blood

E934.8 Other agents affecting blood constituents
    Macromolecular blood substitutes

E934.9 Unspecified agent affecting blood constituents

● **E935 Analgesics, antipyretics, and antirheumatics**

E935.0 Heroin
    Diacetylmorphine

E935.1 Methadone

E935.2 Other opiates and related narcotics
    Codeine
    Meperidine [pethidine]
    Morphine
    Opium (alkaloids)

E935.3 Salicylates
    Acetylsalicylic acid [aspirin]
    Amino derivatives of salicylic acid
    Salicylic acid salts

E935.4 Aromatic analgesics, not elsewhere classified
    Acetanilid
    Paracetamol [acetaminophen]
    Phenacetin [acetophenetidin]

E935.5 Pyrazole derivatives
    Aminophenazone [aminopyrine]
    Phenylbutazone

E935.6 Antirheumatics [antiphlogistics]
    Gold salts
    Indomethacin
    EXCLUDES salicylates (E935.3)
              steroids (E932.0)

E935.7 Other non-narcotic analgesics
    Pyrabital

E935.8 Other specified analgesics and antipyretics
    Pentazocine

E935.9 Unspecified analgesic and antipyretic

● **E936 Anticonvulsants and anti-Parkinsonism drugs**

E936.0 Oxazolidine derivatives
    Paramethadione
    Trimethadione

E936.1 Hydantoin derivatives
    Phenytoin

E936.2 Succinimides
    Ethosuximide
    Phensuximide

E936.3 Other and unspecified anticonvulsants
    Beclamide
    Primidone

E936.4 Anti-Parkinsonism drugs
    Amantadine
    Ethopropazine [profenamine]
    Levodopa [L-dopa]

● **E937 Sedatives and hypnotics**

E937.0 Barbiturates
    Amobarbital [amylobarbitone]
    Barbital [barbitone]
    Butabarbital [butabarbitone]
    Pentobarbital [pentobarbitone]
    Phenobarbital [phenobarbitone]
    Secobarbital [quinalbarbitone]
    EXCLUDES thiobarbiturates (E938.3)

E937.1 Chloral hydrate group

E937.2 Paraldehyde

E937.3 Bromine compounds
    Bromide
    Carbromal (derivatives)

E937.4 Methaqualone compounds

E937.5 Glutethimide group

E937.6 Mixed sedatives, not elsewhere classified

E937.8 Other sedatives and hypnotics

E937.9 Unspecified
    Sleeping:
        drug
        pill   } NOS
        tablet

● **E938 Other central nervous system depressants and anesthetics**

E938.0 Central nervous system muscle-tone depressants
    Chlorphenesin (carbamate)
    Mephenesin
    Methocarbamol

E938.1 Halothane

E938.2 Other gaseous anesthetics
    Ether
    Halogenated hydrocarbon derivatives, except halothane
    Nitrous oxide

E938.3 Intravenous anesthetics
- Ketamine
- Methohexital [methohexitone]
- Thiobarbiturates, such as thiopental sodium

◆ E938.4 Other and unspecified general anesthetics

E938.5 Surface and infiltration anesthetics
- Cocaine
- Lidocaine [lignocaine]
- Procaine
- Tetracaine

E938.6 Peripheral nerve- and plexus-blocking anesthetics

E938.7 Spinal anesthetics

◆ E938.9 Other and unspecified local anesthetics

● E939 Psychotropic agents

E939.0 Antidepressants
- Amitriptyline
- Imipramine
- Monoamine oxidase [MAO] inhibitors

E939.1 Phenothiazine-based tranquilizers
- Chlorpromazine
- Fluphenazine
- Phenothiazine
- Prochlorperazine
- Promazine

E939.2 Butyrophenone-based tranquilizers
- Haloperidol
- Spiperone
- Trifluperidol

◆ E939.3 Other antipsychotics, neuroleptics, and major tranquilizers

E939.4 Benzodiazepine-based tranquilizers
- Chlordiazepoxide
- Diazepam
- Flurazepam
- Lorazepam
- Medazepam
- Nitrazepam

◆ E939.5 Other tranquilizers
- Hydroxyzine
- Meprobamate

E939.6 Psychodysleptics [hallucinogens]
- Cannabis (derivatives)
- Lysergide [LSD]
- Marihuana (derivatives)
- Mescaline
- Psilocin
- Psilocybin

E939.7 Psychostimulants
- Amphetamine
- Caffeine

EXCLUDES central appetite depressants (E947.0)

◆ E939.8 Other psychotropic agents
◆ E939.9 Unspecified psychotropic agent

● E940 Central nervous system stimulants

E940.0 Analeptics
- Lobeline
- Nikethamide

E940.1 Opiate antagonists
- Levallorphan
- Nalorphine
- Naloxone

◆ E940.8 Other specified central nervous system stimulants
◆ E940.9 Unspecified central nervous system stimulant

● E941 Drugs primarily affecting the autonomic nervous system

E941.0 Parasympathomimetics [cholinergics]
- Acetylcholine
- Anticholinesterase:
  - organophosphorus
  - reversible
- Pilocarpine

E941.1 Parasympatholytics [anticholinergics and antimuscarinics] and spasmolytics
- Atropine
- Homatropine
- Hyoscine [scopolamine]
- Quaternary ammonium derivatives

EXCLUDES papaverine (E942.5)

E941.2 Sympathomimetics [adrenergics]
- Epinephrine [adrenalin]
- Levarterenol [noradrenalin]

E941.3 Sympatholytics [antiadrenergics]
- Phenoxybenzamine
- Tolazolinehydrochloride

◆ E941.9 Unspecified drug primarily affecting the autonomic nervous system

● E942 Agents primarily affecting the cardiovascular system

E942.0 Cardiac rhythm regulators
- Practolol
- Procainamide
- Propranolol
- Quinidine

E942.1 Cardiotonic glycosides and drugs of similar action
- Digitalis glycosides
- Digoxin
- Strophantins

E942.2 Antilipemic and antiarteriosclerotic drugs
- Cholestyramine
- Clofibrate
- Nicotinic acid derivatives
- Sitosterols

EXCLUDES dextrothyroxine (E932.7)

E942.3 Ganglion-blocking agents
- Pentamethonium bromide

E942.4 Coronary vasodilators
- Dipyridamole
- Nitrates [nitroglycerin]
- Nitrites
- Prenylamine

◆ E942.5 Other vasodilators
- Cyclandelate
- Diazoxide
- Hydralazine
- Papaverine

◆ E942.6 Other antihypertensive agents
- Clonidine
- Guanethidine
- Rauwolfia alkaloids
- Reserpine

E942.7 Antivaricose drugs, including sclerosing agents
- Monoethanolamine
- Zinc salts

E942.8 Capillary-active drugs
- Adrenochrome derivatives
- Bioflavonoids
- Metaraminol

◆ E942.9 Other and unspecified agents primarily affecting the cardiovascular system

● E943 Agents primarily affecting gastrointestinal system

E943.0 Antacids and antigastric secretion drugs

E943.1 Irritant cathartics
- Bisacodyl
- Castor oil
- Phenolphthalein

E943.2 Emollient cathartics
- Sodium dioctyl sulfosuccinate

◆ E943.3 Other cathartics, including intestinal atonia drugs
- Magnesium sulfate

E943.4 Digestants
- Pancreatin
- Papain
- Pepsin

E943.5 Antidiarrheal drugs
- Bismuth subcarbonate
- Kaolin
- Pectin

EXCLUDES anti-infectives (E930.0-E931.9)

E943.6 Emetics

◆ E943.8 Other specified agents primarily affecting the gastrointestinal system

◆ E943.9 Unspecified agent primarily affecting the gastrointestinal system

● E944 Water, mineral, and uric acid metabolism drugs

E944.0 Mercurial diuretics
- Chlormerodrin
- Mercaptomerin
- Mercurophylline
- Mersalyl

E944.1 Purine derivative diuretics
- Theobromine
- Theophylline

EXCLUDES aminophylline [theophylline ethylenediamine] (E945.7)

E944.2 Carbonic acid anhydrase inhibitors
- Acetazolamide

E944.3 Saluretics
- Benzothiadiazides
- Chlorothiazide group

◆ E944.4 Other diuretics
- Ethacrynic acid
- Furosemide

E944.5 Electrolytic, caloric, and water-balance agents

◆ E944.6 Other mineral salts, not elsewhere classified

E944.7 Uric acid metabolism drugs
- Cinchophen and congeners
- Colchicine
- Phenoquin
- Probenecid

● E945 Agents primarily acting on the smooth and skeletal muscles and respiratory system

E945.0 Oxytocic agents
- Ergot alkaloids
- Prostaglandins

E945.1 Smooth muscle relaxants
- Adiphenine
- Metaproterenol [orciprenaline]

EXCLUDES papaverine (E942.5)

E945.2 Skeletal muscle relaxants
- Alcuronium chloride
- Suxamethonium chloride

◆ E945.3 Other and unspecified drugs acting on muscles

E945.4 Antitussives
- Dextromethorphan
- Pipazethate hydrochloride

E945.5 Expectorants
- Acetylcysteine
- Cocillana
- Guaifenesin [glyceryl guaiacolate]
- Ipecacuanha
- Terpin hydrate

E945.6 Anti-common cold drugs

● Additional digits required   ◆ Nonspecific code   ■ Not a primary diagnosis   Volume 1 — 203

- E945.7 Antiasthmatics
  - Aminophylline [theophylline ethylenediamine]
- ◆ E945.8 Other and unspecified respiratory drugs
- ● E946 Agents primarily affecting skin and mucous membrane, ophthalmological, otorhinolaryngological, and dental drugs
  - E946.0 Local anti-infectives and anti-inflammatory drugs
  - E946.1 Antipruritics
  - E946.2 Local astringents and local detergents
  - E946.3 Emollients, demulcents, and protectants
  - E946.4 Keratolytics, kerstoplastics, other hair treatment drugs and preparations
  - E946.5 Eye anti-infectives and other eye drugs
    - Idoxuridine
  - E946.6 Anti-infectives and other drugs and preparations for ear, nose, and throat
  - E946.7 Dental drugs topically applied
  - ◆ E946.8 Other agents primarily affecting skin and mucous membrane
    - Spermicides
  - ◆ E946.9 Unspecified agent primarily affecting skin and mucous membrane
- ● E947 Other and unspecified drugs and medicinal substances
  - E947.0 Dietetics
  - E947.1 Lipotropic drugs
  - E947.2 Antidotes and chelating agents, not elsewhere classified
  - E947.3 Alcohol deterrents
  - E947.4 Pharmaceutical excipients
  - ◆ E947.8 Other drugs and medicinal substances
    - Contrast media used for diagnostic x-ray procedures
    - Diagnostic agents and kits
  - ◆ E947.9 Unspecified drug or medicinal substance
- ● E948 Bacterial vaccines
  - E948.0 BCG vaccine
  - E948.1 Typhoid and paratyphoid
  - E948.2 Cholera
  - E948.3 Plague
  - E948.4 Tetanus
  - E948.5 Diphtheria
  - E948.6 Pertussis vaccine, including combinations with a pertussis component
  - ◆ E948.8 Other and unspecified bacterial vaccines
  - E948.9 Mixed bacterial vaccines, except combinations with a pertussis component
- ● E949 Other vaccines and biological substances
  - EXCLUDES gamma globulin (E934.6)
  - E949.0 Smallpox vaccine
  - E949.1 Rabies vaccine
  - E949.2 Typhus vaccine
  - E949.3 Yellow fever vaccine
  - E949.4 Measles vaccine
  - E949.5 Poliomyelitis vaccine
  - ◆ E949.6 Other and unspecified viral and rickettsial vaccines
    - Mumps vaccine
  - E949.7 Mixed viral-rickettsial and bacterial vaccines, except combinations with a pertussis component
    - EXCLUDES combinations with a pertussis component (E948.6)
  - ◆ E949.9 Other and unspecified vaccines and biological substances

SUICIDE AND SELF-INFLICTED INJURY (E950-E959)

INCLUDES injuries in suicide and attempted suicide
self-inflicted injuries specified as intentional

- ● E950 Suicide and self-inflicted poisoning by solid or liquid substances
  - E950.0 Analgesics, antipyretics, and antirheumatics
  - E950.1 Barbiturates
  - ◆ E950.2 Other sedatives and hypnotics
  - ◆ E950.3 Tranquilizers and other psychotropic agents
  - ◆ E950.4 Other specified drugs and medicinal substances
  - ◆ E950.5 Unspecified drug or medicinal substance
  - E950.6 Agricultural and horticultural chemical and pharmaceutical preparations other than plant foods and fertilizers
  - E950.7 Corrosive and caustic substances
    - Suicide and self-inflicted poisoning by substances classifiable to E864
  - E950.8 Arsenic and its compounds
  - ◆ E950.9 Other and unspecified solid and liquid substances
- ● E951 Suicide and self-inflicted poisoning by gases in domestic use
  - E951.0 Gas distributed by pipeline
  - E951.1 Liquefied petroleum gas distributed in mobile containers
  - ◆ E951.8 Other utility gas
- ● E952 Suicide and self-inflicted poisoning by other gases and vapors
  - E952.0 Motor vehicle exhaust gas
  - ◆ E952.1 Other carbon monoxide
  - ◆ E952.8 Other specified gases and vapors
  - ◆ E952.9 Unspecified gases and vapors
- ● E953 Suicide and self-inflicted injury by hanging, strangulation, and suffocation
  - E953.0 Hanging
  - E953.1 Suffocation by plastic bag
  - ◆ E953.8 Other specified means
  - ◆ E953.9 Unspecified means
- E954 Suicide and self-inflicted injury by submersion [drowning]
- ● E955 Suicide and self-inflicted injury by firearms and explosives
  - E955.0 Handgun
  - E955.1 Shotgun
  - E955.2 Hunting rifle
  - E955.3 Military firearms
  - ◆ E955.4 Other and unspecified firearm
    - Gunshot NOS   Shot NOS
  - E955.5 Explosives
  - ◆ E955.9 Unspecified
- E956 Suicide and self-inflicted injury by cutting and piercing instrument
- ● E957 Suicide and self-inflicted injuries by jumping from high place
  - E957.0 Residential premises
  - ◆ E957.1 Other man-made structures
  - ◆ E957.2 Natural sites
  - ◆ E957.9 Unspecified
- ● E958 Suicide and self-inflicted injury by other and unspecified means
  - E958.0 Jumping or lying before moving object
  - E958.1 Burns, fire
  - E958.2 Scald
  - E958.3 Extremes of cold
  - E958.4 Electrocution
  - E958.5 Crashing of motor vehicle
  - E958.6 Crashing of aircraft
  - E958.7 Caustic substances, except poisoning
    - EXCLUDES poisoning by caustic substance (E950.7)
  - ◆ E958.8 Other specified means
  - ◆ E958.9 Unspecified means
- E959 Late effects of self-inflicted injury
  - Note: This category is to be used to indicate circumstances classifiable to E950-E958 as the cause of death or disability from late effects, which are themselves classifiable elsewhere. The "late effects" include conditions reported as such or occurring as sequelae one year or more after attempted suicide or self-inflicted injury.

HOMICIDE AND INJURY PURPOSELY INFLICTED BY OTHER PERSONS (E960-E969)

INCLUDES injuries inflicted by another person with intent to injure or kill, by any means

EXCLUDES injuries due to:
legal intervention (E970-E978)
operations of war (E990-E999)

- ● E960 Fight, brawl, rape
  - E960.0 Unarmed fight or brawl
    - Beatings NOS
    - Brawl or fight with hands, fists, feet
    - Injured or killed in fight NOS
    - EXCLUDES homicidal:
      - injury by weapons (E965.0-E966, E969)
      - strangulation (E963)
      - submersion (E964)
  - E960.1 Rape
- E961 Assault by corrosive or caustic substance, except poisoning
  - Injury or death purposely caused by corrosive or caustic substance, such as:
    - acid [any]
    - corrosive substance
    - vitriol
  - EXCLUDES burns from hot liquid (E968.3)
  - chemical burns from swallowing a corrosive substance (E962.0-E962.9)
- ● E962 Assault by poisoning

E962.0 Drugs and medicinal substances
Homicidal poisoning by any drug or medicinal substance
- ◆ **E962.1** Other solid and liquid substances
- ◆ **E962.2** Other gases and vapors
- ◆ **E962.9** Unspecified poisoning

E963 Assault by hanging and strangulation
Homicidal (attempt):
  garrotting or ligature
  hanging
Homicidal (attempt):
  strangulation
  suffocation

E964 Assault by submersion [drowning]

● E965 Assault by firearms and explosives
- **E965.0** Handgun
  Pistol   Revolver
- **E965.1** Shotgun
- **E965.2** Hunting rifle
- **E965.3** Military firearms
- ◆ **E965.4** Other and unspecified firearm
- **E965.5** Antipersonnel bomb
- **E965.6** Gasoline bomb
- **E965.7** Letter bomb
- ◆ **E965.8** Other specified explosive
  Bomb NOS (placed in):
    car
    house
  Dynamite
- ◆ **E965.9** Unspecified explosive

E966 Assault by cutting and piercing instrument
Assassination (attempt), homicide (attempt) by any instrument classifiable under E920

Homicidal:
  cut
  puncture   } any part of body
  stab
  Stabbed

● E967 Child battering and other maltreatment
- **E967.0** By parent
- ◆ **E967.1** By other specified person
- ◆ **E967.9** By unspecified person

● E968 Assault by other and unspecified means
- **E968.0** Fire
  Arson
  Homicidal burns NOS
  EXCLUDES burns from hot liquid (E968.3)
- **E968.1** Pushing from a high place
- **E968.2** Striking by blunt or thrown object
- **E968.3** Hot liquid
  Homicidal burns by scalding
- **E968.4** Criminal neglect
  Abandonment of child, infant, or other helpless person with intent to injure or kill
- ◆ **E968.8** Other specified means
  Bite of human being
- ◆ **E968.9** Unspecified means
  Assassination (attempt) NOS
  Homicidal (attempt):
    injury NOS
    wound NOS
  Manslaughter (nonaccidental)
  Murder (attempt) NOS
  Violence, non-accidental

E969 Late effects of injury purposely inflicted by other person
Note: This category is to be used to indicate circumstances classifiable to E960-E968 as the cause of death or disability from late effects, which are themselves classifiable elsewhere. The "late effects" include conditions reported as such, or occurring as sequelae one year or more after injury purposely inflicted by another person.

LEGAL INTERVENTION (E970-E978)
INCLUDES injuries inflicted by the police or other law-enforcing agents, including military on duty, in the course of arresting or attempting to arrest lawbreakers, suppressing disturbances, maintaining order, and other legal action
  legal execution
EXCLUDES injuries caused by civil insurrections (E990.0-E999)

E970 Injury due to legal intervention by firearms
Gunshot wound
Injury by:
  machine gun
  revolver
  rifle pellet or rubber bullet
  shot NOS

E971 Injury due to legal intervention by explosives
Injury by:
  dynamite
  explosive shell
Injury by:
  grenade
  mortar bomb

E972 Injury due to legal intervention by gas
Asphyxiation by gas   Poisoning by gas
Injury by tear gas

E973 Injury due to legal intervention by blunt object
Hit, struck by:
  baton (nightstick)
  blunt object
  stave

E974 Injury due to legal intervention by cutting and piercing instrument
Cut   Injured by bayonet
Incised wound   Stab wound

◆ E975 Injury due to legal intervention by other specified means
Blow Manhandling

◆ E976 Injury due to legal intervention by unspecified means

E977 Late effects of injuries due to legal intervention
Note: This category is to be used to indicate circumstances classifiable to E970-E976 as the cause of death or disability from late effects, which are themselves classifiable elsewhere. The "late effects" include conditions reported as such, or occurring as sequelae one year or more after injury due to legal intervention.

E978 Legal execution
All executions performed at the behest of the judiciary or ruling authority [whether permanent or temporary] as:
  asphyxiation by gas
  beheading, decapitation (by guillotine)
  capital punishment
  electrocution
  hanging
  shooting
  other specified means

INJURY UNDETERMINED WHETHER ACCIDENTALLY OR PURPOSELY INFLICTED (E980-E989)
Note: Categories E980-E989 are for use when after a thorough investigation by the medical examiner, coroner, or other legal authority it cannot be determined whether the injuries are accidental, suicidal, or homicidal. They include self-inflicted injuries, but not poisoning, when not specified as accidental or as intentional.

● E980 Poisoning by solid or liquid substances, undetermined whether accidentally or purposely inflicted
- **E980.0** Analgesics, antipyretics, and antirheumatics
- **E980.1** Barbiturates
- ◆ **E980.2** Other sedatives and hypnotics
- **E980.3** Tranquilizers and other psychotropic agents
- ◆ **E980.4** Other specified drugs and medicinal substances
- ◆ **E980.5** Unspecified drug or medicinal substance
- **E980.6** Corrosive and caustic substances
  Poisoning, undetermined whether accidental or purposeful, by substances classifiable to E864
- **E980.7** Agricultural and horticultural chemical and pharmaceutical preparations other than plant foods and fertilizers
- **E980.8** Arsenic and its compounds
- ◆ **E980.9** Other and unspecified solid and liquid substances

● E981 Poisoning by gases in domestic use, undetermined whether accidentally or purposely inflicted
- **E981.0** Gas distributed by pipeline
- **E981.1** Liquefied petroleum gas distributed in mobile containers
- ◆ **E981.8** Other utility gas

● E982 Poisoning by other gases, undetermined whether accidentally or purposely inflicted
- **E982.0** Motor vehicle exhaust gas
- ◆ **E982.1** Other carbon monoxide
- ◆ **E982.8** Other specified gases and vapors
- ◆ **E982.9** Unspecified gases and vapors

- **E983 Hanging, strangulation, or suffocation, undetermined whether accidentally or purposely inflicted**
  - E983.0 Hanging
  - E983.1 Suffocation by plastic bag
  - ◆ E983.8 Other specified means
  - ◆ E983.9 Unspecified means
- E984 Submersion [drowning], undetermined whether accidentally or purposely inflicted
- **E985 Injury by firearms and explosives, undetermined whether accidentally or purposely inflicted**
  - E985.0 Handgun
  - E985.1 Shotgun
  - E985.2 Hunting rifle
  - E985.3 Military firearms
  - ◆ E985.4 Other and unspecified firearm
  - E985.5 Explosives
- E986 Injury by cutting and piercing instruments, undetermined whether accidentally or purposely inflicted
- **E987 Falling from high place, undetermined whether accidentally or purposely inflicted**
  - E987.0 Residential premises
  - ◆ E987.1 Other man-made structures
  - E987.2 Natural sites
  - ◆ E987.9 Unspecified site
- **E988 Injury by other and unspecified means, undetermined whether accidentally or purposely inflicted**
  - E988.0 Jumping or lying before moving object
  - E988.1 Burns, fire
  - E988.2 Scald
  - E988.3 Extremes of cold
  - E988.4 Electrocution
  - E988.5 Crashing of motor vehicle
  - E988.6 Crashing of aircraft
  - E988.7 Caustic substances, except poisoning
  - ◆ E988.8 Other specified means
  - ◆ E988.9 Unspecified means
- E989 Late effects of injury, undetermined whether accidentally or purposely inflicted

  Note: This category is to be used to indicate circumstances classifiable to E980-E988 as the cause of death or disability from late effects, which are themselves classifiable elsewhere. The "late effects" include conditions reported as such or occurring as sequelae one year or more after injury, undetermined whether accidentally or purposely inflicted.

INJURY RESULTING FROM OPERATIONS OF WAR (E990-E999)

INCLUDES injuries to military personnel and civilians caused by war and civil insurrections and occurring during the time of war and insurrection

EXCLUDES accidents during training of military personnel manufacture of war material and transport, unless attributable to enemy action

- **E990 Injury due to war operations by fires and conflagrations**

  INCLUDES asphyxia, burns, or other injury originating from fire caused by a fire-producing device or indirectly by any conventional weapon

  - E990.0 From gasoline bomb
  - ◆ E990.9 From other and unspecified source
- **E991 Injury due to war operations by bullets and fragments**
  - E991.0 Rubber bullets (rifle)
  - E991.1 Pellets (rifle)
  - ◆ E991.2 Other bullets

    Bullet [any, except rubber bullets and pellets]
    - carbine
    - machine gun
    - pistol
    - rifle
    - shotgun
  - E991.3 Antipersonnel bomb (fragments)
  - ◆ E991.9 Other and unspecified fragments

    Fragments from:
    - artillery shell
    - bombs, except anti-personnel
    - grenade
    - guided missile

    Fragments from:
    - land mine
    - rockets
    - shell
    - Shrapnel

- E992 Injury due to war operations by explosion of marine weapons
  - Depth charge
  - Marine mines
  - Mine NOS, at sea or in harbor
  - Sea-based artillery shell
  - Torpedo
  - Underwater blast
- ◆ E993 Injury due to war operations by other explosion
  - Accidental explosion of munitions being used in war
  - Accidental explosion of own weapons
  - Air blast NOS
  - Blast NOS
  - Explosion NOS
  - Explosion of:
    - artillery shell
    - breech block
    - cannon block
    - mortar bomb
  - Injury by weapon burst
- E994 Injury due to war operations by destruction of aircraft
  - Airplane:
    - burned
    - exploded
    - shot down
  - Crushed by falling airplane
- ◆ E995 Injury due to war operations by other and unspecified forms of conventional warfare
  - Battle wounds
  - Bayonet injury
  - Drowned in war operations
- E996 Injury due to war operations by nuclear weapons
  - Blast effects
  - Exposure to ionizing radiation from nuclear weapons
  - Fireball effects
  - Heat
  - Other direct and secondary effects of nuclear weapons
- **E997 Injury due to war operations by other forms of unconventional warfare**
  - E997.0 Lasers
  - E997.1 Biological warfare
  - E997.2 Gases, fumes, and chemicals
  - ◆ E997.8 Other specified forms of unconventional warfare
  - ◆ E997.9 Unspecified form of unconventional warfare
- E998 Injury due to war operations but occurring after cessation of hostilities

  Injuries due to operations of war but occurring after cessation of hostilities by any means classifiable under E990-E997
  Injuries by explosion of bombs or mines placed in the course of operations of war, if the explosion occurred after cessation of hostilities
- E999 Late effect of injury due to war operations

  Note: This category is to be used to indicate circumstances classifiable to E990-E998 as the cause of death or disability from late effects, which are themselves classifiable elsewhere. The "late effects" include conditions reported as such or occurring as sequelae one year or more after injury resulting from operations of war.

APPENDIX A: MORPHOLOGY OF NEOPLASMS

MORPHOLOGY OF NEOPLASMS

The World Health Organization has published an adaptation of the International Classification of Diseases for oncology (ICD-O). It contains a coded nomenclature for the morphology of neoplasms, which is reproduced here for those who wish to use it in conjunction with Chapter 2 of the *International Classification of Diseases, 9th Revision, Clinical Modification*.

The morphology code numbers consist of five digits; the first four identify the histological type of the neoplasm and the fifth indicates its behavior. The one-digit behavior code is as follows:

/0	Benign
/1	Uncertain whether benign or malignant Borderline malignancy
/2	Carcinoma in situ Intraepithelial Noninfiltrating Noninvasive
/3	Malignant, primary site
/6	Malignant, metastatic site Secondary site
/9	Malignant, uncertain whether primary or metastatic site

In the nomenclature below, the morphology code numbers include the behavior code appropriate to the histological type of neoplasm, but this behavior code should be changed if other reported information makes this necessary. For example, "chordoma (M9370/3)" is assumed to be malignant; the term "benign chordoma" should be coded M9370/0. Similarly, "superficial spreading adenocarcinoma (M8143/3)" described as "noninvasive" should be coded M8143/2 and "melanoma (M8720/3)" described as "secondary" should be coded M8720/6.

The following table shows the correspondence between the morphology code and the different sections of Chapter 2:

Morphology Code Histology/Behavior		ICD-9-CM Chapter 2	
Any	0	210-229	Benign neoplasms
M8000-M8004	1	239	Neoplasms of unspecified nature
M8010+	1	235-238	Neoplasms of uncertain behavior
Any	2	230-234	Carcinoma in situ
Any	3	140-195 200-208	Malignant neoplasms, stated or presumed to be primary
Any	6	196-198	Malignant neoplasms, stated or presumed to be secondary

The ICD-O behavior digit /9 is inapplicable in an ICD context, since all malignant neoplasms are presumed to be primary (/3) or secondary (/6) according to other information on the medical record.

Only the first-listed term of the full ICD-O morphology nomenclature appears against each code number in the list below. The ICD-9-CM Alphabetical Index (Volume 2), however, includes all the ICD-O synonyms as well as a number of other morphological names still likely to be encountered on medical records but omitted from ICD-O as outdated or otherwise undesirable.

A coding difficulty sometimes arises where a morphological diagnosis contains two qualifying adjectives that have different code numbers. An example is "transitional cell epidermoid carcinoma." "Transitional cell carcinoma NOS" is M8120/3 and "epidermoid carcinoma NOS" is M8070/3. In such circumstances, the higher number (M8120/3 in this example) should be used, as it is usually more specific.

CODED NOMENCLATURE FOR MORPHOLOGY OF NEOPLASMS

M800	**Neoplasms NOS**
M8000/0	Neoplasm, benign
M8000/1	Neoplasm, uncertain whether benign or malignant
M8000/3	Neoplasm, malignant
M8000/6	Neoplasm, metastatic
M8000/9	Neoplasm, malignant, uncertain whether primary or metastatic
M8001/0	Tumor cells, benign
M8001/1	Tumor cells, uncertain whether benign or malignant
M8001/3	Tumor cells, malignant
M8002/3	Malignant tumor, small cell type
M8003/3	Malignant tumor, giant cell type
M8004/3	Malignant tumor, fusiform cell type
M801-M804	**Epithelial neoplasms NOS**
M8010/0	Epithelial tumor, benign
M8010/2	Carcinoma in situ NOS
M8010/3	Carcinoma NOS
M8010/6	Carcinoma, metastatic NOS
M8010/9	Carcinomatosis
M8011/0	Epithelioma, benign
M8011/3	Epithelioma, malignant
M8012/3	Large cell carcinoma NOS
M8020/3	Carcinoma, undifferentiated type NOS
M8021/3	Carcinoma, anaplastic type NOS
M8022/3	Pleomorphic carcinoma
M8030/3	Giant cell and spindle cell carcinoma
M8031/3	Giant cell carcinoma
M8032/3	Spindle cell carcinoma
M8033/3	Pseudosarcomatous carcinoma
M8034/3	Polygonal cell carcinoma
M8035/3	Spheroidal cell carcinoma
M8040/1	Tumorlet
M8041/3	Small cell carcinoma NOS
M8042/3	Oat cell carcinoma
M8043/3	Small cell carcinoma, fusiform cell type
M805-M808	**Papillary and squamous cell neoplasms**
M8050/0	Papilloma NOS (except Papilloma of urinary bladder M8120/1)
M8050/2	Papillary carcinoma in situ
M8050/3	Papillary carcinoma NOS
M8051/0	Verrucous papilloma
M8051/3	Verrucous carcinoma NOS
M8052/0	Squamous cell papilloma
M8052/3	Papillary squamous cell carcinoma
M8053/0	Inverted papilloma
M8060/0	Papillomatosis NOS
M8070/2	Squamous cell carcinoma in situ NOS
M8070/3	Squamous cell carcinoma NOS
M8070/6	Squamous cell carcinoma, metastatic NOS
M8071/3	Squamous cell carcinoma, keratinizing type NOS
M8072/3	Squamous cell carcinoma, large cell, nonkeratinizing type
M8073/3	Squamous cell carcinoma, small cell, nonkeratinizing type
M8074/3	Squamous cell carcinoma, spindle cell type
M8075/3	Adenoid squamous cell carcinoma
M8076/2	Squamous cell carcinoma in situ with questionable stromal invasion
M8076/3	Squamous cell carcinoma, microinvasive
M8080/2	Queyrat's erythroplasia
M8081/2	Bowen's disease
M8082/3	Lymphoepithelial carcinoma
M809-M811	**Basal cell neoplasms**
M8090/1	Basal cell tumor
M8090/3	Basal cell carcinoma NOS
M8091/3	Multicentric basal cell carcinoma
M8092/3	Basal cell carcinoma, morphea type
M8093/3	Basal cell carcinoma, fibroepithelial type
M8094/3	Basosquamous carcinoma
M8095/3	Metatypical carcinoma
M8096/0	Intraepidermal epithelioma of Jadassohn
M8100/0	Trichoepithelioma
M8101/0	Trichofolliculoma
M8102/0	Tricholemmoma
M8110/0	Pilomatrixoma
M812-M813	**Transitional cell papillomas and carcinomas**
M8120/0	Transitional cell papilloma NOS
M8120/1	Urothelial papilloma
M8120/2	Transitional cell carcinoma in situ
M8120/3	Transitional cell carcinoma NOS
M8121/0	Schneiderian papilloma
M8121/1	Transitional cell papilloma, inverted type
M8121/3	Schneiderian carcinoma
M8122/3	Transitional cell carcinoma, spindle cell type
M8123/3	Basaloid carcinoma
M8124/3	Cloacogenic carcinoma
M8130/3	Papillary transitional cell carcinoma
M814-M838	**Adenomas and adenocarcinomas**
M8140/0	Adenoma NOS
M8140/1	Bronchial adenoma NOS
M8140/2	Adenocarcinoma in situ
M8140/3	Adenocarcinoma NOS
M8140/6	Adenocarcinoma, metastatic NOS
M8141/3	Scirrhous adenocarcinoma
M8142/3	Linitis plastica
M8143/3	Superficial spreading adenocarcinoma
M8144/3	Adenocarcinoma, intestinal type
M8145/3	Carcinoma, diffuse type
M8146/3	Monomorphic adenoma
M8147/3	Basal cell adenoma
M8150/0	Islet cell adenoma
M8150/3	Islet cell carcinoma
M8151/0	Insulinoma NOS
M8151/3	Insulinoma, malignant
M8152/0	Glucagonoma NOS
M8152/3	Glucagonoma, malignant
M8153/1	Gastrinoma NOS
M8153/3	Gastrinoma, malignant
M8154/3	Mixed islet cell and exocrine adenocarcinoma
M8160/0	Bile duct adenoma
M8160/3	Cholangiocarcinoma
M8161/0	Bile duct cystadenoma
M8161/3	Bile duct cystadenocarcinoma
M8170/0	Liver cell adenoma
M8170/3	Hepatocellular carcinoma NOS
M8180/0	Hepatocholangioma, benign
M8180/3	Combined hepatocellular carcinoma and cholangiocarcinoma
M8190/0	Trabecular adenoma
M8190/3	Trabecular adenocarcinoma
M8191/0	Embryonal adenoma
M8200/0	Eccrine dermal cylindroma
M8200/3	Adenoid cystic carcinoma
M8201/3	Cribriform carcinoma
M8210/0	Adenomatous polyp NOS
M8210/3	Adenocarcinoma in adenomatous polyp
M8211/0	Tubular adenoma NOS
M8211/3	Tubular adenocarcinoma
M8220/0	Adenomatous polyposis coli
M8220/3	Adenocarcinoma in adenomatous polyposis coli
M8221/0	Multiple adenomatous polyps
M8230/3	Solid carcinoma NOS
M8231/3	Carcinoma simplex
M8240/1	Carcinoid tumor NOS
M8240/3	Carcinoid tumor, malignant
M8241/1	Carcinoid tumor, argentaffin NOS
M8241/3	Carcinoid tumor, argentaffin, malignant
M8242/1	Carcinoid tumor, nonargentaffin NOS
M8242/3	Carcinoid tumor, nonargentaffin, malignant
M8243/3	Mucocarcinoid tumor, malignant
M8244/3	Composite carcinoid
M8250/1	Pulmonary adenomatosis
M8250/3	Bronchiolo-alveolar adenocarcinoma
M8251/0	Alveolar adenoma
M8251/3	Alveolar adenocarcinoma
M8260/0	Papillary adenoma NOS
M8260/3	Papillary adenocarcinoma NOS
M8261/1	Villous adenoma NOS

APPENDIX A

M8261/3	Adenocarcinoma in villous adenoma	M8440/3	Cystadenocarcinoma NOS	M8610/0	Luteoma NOS
M8262/3	Villous adenocarcinoma	M8441/0	Serous cystadenoma NOS	M8620/1	Granulosa cell tumor NOS
M8263/0	Tubulovillous adenoma	M8441/1	Serous cystadenoma, borderline malignancy	M8620/3	Granulosa cell tumor, malignant
M8270/0	Chromophobe adenoma			M8621/1	Granulosa cell-theca cell tumor
M8270/3	Chromophobe carcinoma	M8441/3	Serous cystadenocarcinoma NOS	M8630/0	Androblastoma, benign
M8280/0	Acidophil adenoma	M8450/0	Papillary cystadenoma NOS	M8630/1	Androblastoma NOS
M8280/3	Acidophil carcinoma	M8450/1	Papillary cystadenoma, borderline malignancy	M8630/3	Androblastoma, malignant
M8281/0	Mixed acidophil-basophil adenoma			M8631/0	Sertoli-Leydig cell tumor
M8281/3	Mixed acidophil-basophil carcinoma	M8450/3	Papillary cystadenocarcinoma NOS	M8632/1	Gynandroblastoma
		M8460/0	Papillary serous cystadenoma NOS	M8640/0	Tubular androblastoma NOS
M8290/0	Oxyphilic adenoma	M8460/1	Papillary serous cystadenoma, borderline malignancy	M8640/3	Sertoli cell carcinoma
M8290/3	Oxyphilic adenocarcinoma			M8641/0	Tubular androblastoma with lipid storage
M8300/0	Basophil adenoma	M8460/3	Papillary serous cystadenocarcinoma		
M8300/3	Basophil carcinoma			M8650/0	Leydig cell tumor, benign
M8310/0	Clear cell adenoma	M8461/0	Serous surface papilloma NOS	M8650/1	Leydig cell tumor NOS
M8310/3	Clear cell adenocarcinoma NOS	M8461/1	Serous surface papilloma, borderline malignancy	M8650/3	Leydig cell tumor, malignant
M8311/1	Hypernephroid tumor			M8660/0	Hilar cell tumor
M8312/3	Renal cell carcinoma	M8461/3	Serous surface papillary carcinoma	M8670/0	Lipid cell tumor of ovary
M8313/0	Clear cell adenofibroma	M8470/0	Mucinous cystadenoma NOS	M8671/0	Adrenal rest tumor
M8320/3	Granular cell carcinoma	M8470/1	Mucinous cystadenoma, borderline malignancy	**M868-M871**	**Paragangliomas and glomus tumors**
M8321/0	Chief cell adenoma			M8680/1	Paraganglioma NOS
M8322/0	Water-clear cell adenoma	M8470/3	Mucinous cystadenocarcinoma NOS	M8680/3	Paraganglioma, malignant
M8322/3	Water-clear cell adenocarcinoma			M8681/1	Sympathetic paraganglioma
M8323/0	Mixed cell adenoma	M8471/0	Papillary mucinous cystadenoma NOS	M8682/1	Parasympathetic paraganglioma
M8323/3	Mixed cell adenocarcinoma			M8690/1	Glomus jugulare tumor
M8324/0	Lipoadenoma	M8471/1	Papillary mucinous cystadenoma, borderline malignancy	M8691/1	Aortic body tumor
M8330/0	Follicular adenoma			M8692/1	Carotid body tumor
M8330/3	Follicular adenocarcinoma NOS	M8471/3	Papillary mucinous cystadenocarcinoma	M8693/1	Extra-adrenal paraganglioma NOS
M8331/3	Follicular adenocarcinoma, well differentiated type			M8693/3	Extra-adrenal paraganglioma, malignant
		M8480/0	Mucinous adenoma		
M8332/3	Follicular adenocarcinoma, trabecular type	M8480/3	Mucinous adenocarcinoma	M8700/0	Pheochromocytoma NOS
		M8480/6	Pseudomyxoma peritonei	M8700/3	Pheochromocytoma, malignant
M8333/3	Microfollicular adenoma	M8481/3	Mucin-producing adenocarcinoma	M8710/3	Glomangiosarcoma
M8334/0	Macrofollicular adenoma	M8490/3	Signet ring cell carcinoma	M8711/0	Glomus tumor
M8340/3	Papillary and follicular adenocarcinoma	M8490/6	Metastatic signet ring cell carcinoma	M8712/0	Glomangioma
				M872-M879	**Nevi and melanomas**
M8350/3	Nonencapsulated sclerosing carcinoma	**M850-M854**	**Ductal, lobular, and medullary neoplasms**	M8720/0	Pigmented nevus NOS
				M8720/3	Malignant melanoma NOS
M8360/1	Multiple endocrine adenomas	M8500/2	Intraductal carcinoma, noninfiltrating NOS	M8721/3	Nodular melanoma
M8361/1	Juxtaglomerular tumor			M8722/0	Balloon cell nevus
M8370/0	Adrenal cortical adenoma NOS	M8500/3	Infiltrating duct carcinoma	M8722/3	Balloon cell melanoma
M8370/3	Adrenal cortical carcinoma	M8501/2	Comedocarcinoma, noninfiltrating	M8723/0	Halo nevus
M8371/0	Adrenal cortical adenoma, compact cell type	M8501/3	Comedocarcinoma NOS	M8724/0	Fibrous papule of the nose
		M8502/3	Juvenile carcinoma of the breast	M8725/0	Neuronevus
M8372/0	Adrenal cortical adenoma, heavily pigmented variant	M8503/0	Intraductal papilloma	M8726/0	Magnocellular nevus
		M8503/2	Noninfiltrating intraductal papillary adenocarcinoma	M8730/0	Nonpigmented nevus
M8373/0	Adrenal cortical adenoma, clear cell type			M8730/3	Amelanotic melanoma
		M8504/0	Intracystic papillary adenoma	M8740/0	Junctional nevus
M8374/0	Adrenal cortical adenoma, glomerulosa cell type	M8504/2	Noninfiltrating intracystic carcinoma	M8740/3	Malignant melanoma in junctional nevus
		M8505/0	Intraductal papillomatosis NOS	M8741/2	Precancerous melanosis NOS
M8375/0	Adrenal cortical adenoma, mixed cell type	M8506/0	Subareolar duct papillomatosis	M8741/3	Malignant melanoma in precancerous melanosis
		M8510/3	Medullary carcinoma NOS		
M8380/0	Endometrioid adenoma NOS	M8511/3	Medullary carcinoma with amyloid stroma	M8742/2	Hutchinson's melanotic freckle
M8380/1	Endometrioid adenoma, borderline malignancy			M8742/3	Malignant melanoma in Hutchinson's melanotic freckle
		M8512/3	Medullary carcinoma with lymphoid stroma		
M8380/3	Endometrioid carcinoma			M8743/3	Superficial spreading melanoma
M8381/0	Endometrioid adenofibroma NOS	M8520/2	Lobular carcinoma in situ	M8750/0	Intradermal nevus
M8381/1	Endometrioid adenofibroma, borderline malignancy	M8520/3	Lobular carcinoma NOS	M8760/0	Compound nevus
		M8521/3	Infiltrating ductular carcinoma	M8761/1	Giant pigmented nevus
M8381/3	Endometrioid adenofibroma, malignant	M8530/3	Inflammatory carcinoma	M8761/3	Malignant melanoma in giant pigmented nevus
		M8540/3	Paget's disease, mammary		
M839-M842	**Adnexal and skin appendage neoplasms**	M8541/3	Paget's disease and infiltrating duct carcinoma of breast	M8770/3	Epithelioid and spindle cell nevus
				M8771/3	Epithelioid cell melanoma
M8390/0	Skin appendage adenoma	M8542/3	Paget's disease, extramammary (except Paget's disease of bone)	M8772/3	Spindle cell melanoma NOS
M8390/3	Skin appendage carcinoma			M8773/3	Spindle cell melanoma, type A
M8400/0	Sweat gland adenoma	**M855**	**Acinar cell neoplasms**	M8774/3	Spindle cell melanoma, type B
M8400/1	Sweat gland tumor NOS	M8550/0	Acinar cell adenoma	M8775/3	Mixed epithelioid and spindle cell melanoma
M8400/3	Sweat gland adenocarcinoma	M8550/1	Acinar cell tumor		
M8401/0	Apocrine adenoma	M8550/3	Acinar cell carcinoma	M8780/0	Blue nevus NOS
M8401/3	Apocrine adenocarcinoma	**M856-M858**	**Complex epithelial neoplasms**	M8780/3	Blue nevus, malignant
M8402/0	Eccrine acrospiroma	M8560/3	Adenosquamous carcinoma	M8790/0	Cellular blue nevus
M8403/0	Eccrine spiradenoma	M8561/0	Adenolymphoma	**M880**	**Soft tissue tumors and sarcomas NOS**
M8404/0	Hidrocystoma	M8570/3	Adenocarcinoma with squamous metaplasia		
M8405/0	Papillary hydradenoma			M8800/0	Soft tissue tumor, benign
M8406/0	Papillary syringadenoma	M8571/3	Adenocarcinoma with cartilaginous and osseous metaplasia	M8800/3	Sarcoma NOS
M8407/0	Syringoma NOS			M8800/9	Sarcomatosis NOS
M8410/0	Sebaceous adenoma	M8572/3	Adenocarcinoma with spindle cell metaplasia	M8801/3	Spindle cell sarcoma
M8410/3	Sebaceous adenocarcinoma			M8802/3	Giant cell sarcoma (except of bone M9250/3)
M8420/0	Ceruminous adenoma	M8573/3	Adenocarcinoma with apocrine metaplasia		
M8420/3	Ceruminous adenocarcinoma			M8803/3	Small cell sarcoma
M843	**Mucoepidermoid neoplasms**	M8580/0	Thymoma, benign	M8804/3	Epithelioid cell sarcoma
M8430/1	Mucoepidermoid tumor	M8580/3	Thymoma, malignant	**M881-M883**	**Fibromatous neoplasms**
M8430/3	Mucoepidermoid carcinoma	**M859-M867**	**Specialized gonadal neoplasms**	M8810/0	Fibroma NOS
M844-M849	**Cystic, mucinous, and serous neoplasms**	M8590/1	Sex cord-stromal tumor	M8810/3	Fibrosarcoma NOS
		M8600/0	Thecoma NOS	M8811/0	Fibromyxoma
M8440/0	Cystadenoma NOS	M8600/3	Theca cell carcinoma	M8811/3	Fibromyxosarcoma

MORPHOLOGY OF NEOPLASMS

M8812/0	Periosteal fibroma	M9010/0	Fibroadenoma NOS	M9160/0	Angiofibroma NOS
M8812/3	Periosteal fibrosarcoma	M9011/0	Intracanalicular fibroadenoma NOS	M9161/1	Hemangioblastoma
M8813/0	Fascial fibroma	M9012/0	Pericanalicular fibroadenoma NOS	**M917**	**Lymphatic vessel tumors**
M8813/3	Fascial fibrosarcoma	M9013/0	Adenofibroma NOS	M9170/0	Lymphangioma NOS
M8814/3	Infantile fibrosarcoma	M9014/0	Serous adenofibroma	M9170/3	Lymphangiosarcoma
M8820/0	Elastofibroma	M9015/0	Mucinous adenofibroma	M9171/0	Capillary lymphangioma
M8821/1	Aggressive fibromatosis	M9020/0	Cellular intracanalicular fibroadenoma	M9172/0	Cavernous lymphangioma
M8822/1	Abdominal fibromatosis			M9173/0	Cystic lymphangioma
M8823/1	Desmoplastic fibroma	M9020/1	Cystosarcoma phyllodes NOS	M9174/0	Lymphangiomyoma
M8830/0	Fibrous histiocytoma NOS	M9020/3	Cystosarcoma phyllodes, malignant	M9174/1	Lymphangiomyomatosis
M8830/1	Atypical fibrous histiocytoma	M9030/0	Juvenile fibroadenoma	M9175/0	Hemolymphangioma
M8830/3	Fibrous histiocytoma, malignant	**M904**	**Synovial neoplasms**	**M918-M920**	**Osteomas and osteosarcomas**
M8831/0	Fibroxanthoma NOS	M9040/0	Synovioma, benign	M9180/0	Osteoma NOS
M8831/1	Atypical fibroxanthoma	M9040/3	Synovial sarcoma NOS	M9180/3	Osteosarcoma NOS
M8831/3	Fibroxanthoma, malignant	M9041/3	Synovial sarcoma, spindle cell type	M9181/3	Chondroblastic osteosarcoma
M8832/0	Dermatofibroma	M9042/3	Synovial sarcoma, epithelioid cell type	M9182/3	Fibroblastic osteosarcoma
M8832/1	Dermatofibroma protuberans			M9183/3	Telangiectatic osteosarcoma
M8832/3	Dermatofibrosarcoma NOS	M9043/3	Synovial sarcoma, biphasic type	M9184/3	Osteosarcoma in Paget's disease of bone
M884	**Myxomatous neoplasms**	M9044/3	Clear cell sarcoma of tendons and aponeuroses		
M8840/0	Myxoma NOS			M9190/0	Juxtacortical osteosarcoma
M8840/3	Myxosarcoma	**M905**	**Mesothelial neoplasms**	M9191/0	Osteoid osteoma NOS
M885-M888	**Lipomatous neoplasms**	M9050/0	Mesothelioma, benign	M9200/0	Osteoblastoma
M8850/0	Lipoma NOS	M9050/3	Mesothelioma, malignant	**M921-M924**	**Chondromatous neoplasms**
M8850/3	Liposarcoma NOS	M9051/0	Fibrous mesothelioma, benign	M9210/0	Osteochondroma
M8851/0	Fibrolipoma	M9051/3	Fibrous mesothelioma, malignant	M9210/1	Osteochondromatosis NOS
M8851/3	Liposarcoma, well differentiated type	M9052/0	Epithelioid mesothelioma, benign	M9220/0	Chondroma NOS
		M9052/3	Epithelioid mesothelioma, malignant	M9220/1	Chondromatosis NOS
M8852/0	Fibromyxolipoma			M9220/3	Chondrosarcoma NOS
M8852/3	Myxoid liposarcoma	M9053/0	Mesothelioma, biphasic type, benign	M9221/0	Juxtacortical chondroma
M8853/3	Round cell liposarcoma			M9221/3	Juxtacortical chondrosarcoma
M8854/3	Pleomorphic liposarcoma	M9053/3	Mesothelioma, biphasic type, malignant	M9230/0	Chondroblastoma NOS
M8855/3	Mixed type liposarcoma			M9230/3	Chondroblastoma, malignant
M8856/0	Intramuscular lipoma	M9054/0	Adenomatoid tumor NOS	M9240/3	Mesenchymal chondrosarcoma
M8857/0	Spindle cell lipoma	**M906-M909**	**Germ cell neoplasms**	M9241/0	Chondromyxoid fibroma
M8860/0	Angiomyolipoma	M9060/3	Dysgerminoma	**M925**	**Giant cell tumors**
M8860/3	Angiomyoliposarcoma	M9061/3	Seminoma NOS	M9250/1	Giant cell tumor of bone NOS
M8861/0	Angiolipoma NOS	M9062/3	Seminoma, anaplastic type	M9250/3	Giant cell tumor of bone, malignant
M8861/1	Angiolipoma, infiltrating	M9063/3	Spermatocytic seminoma	M9251/1	Giant cell tumor of soft parts NOS
M8870/0	Myelolipoma	M9064/3	Germinoma	M9251/3	Malignant giant cell tumor of soft parts
M8880/0	Hibernoma	M9070/3	Embryonal carcinoma NOS		
M8881/0	Lipoblastomatosis	M9071/3	Endodermal sinus tumor	**M926**	**Miscellaneous bone tumors**
M889-M892	**Myomatous neoplasms**	M9072/3	Polyembryoma	M9260/3	Ewing's sarcoma
M8890/0	Leiomyoma NOS	M9073/1	Gonadoblastoma	M9261/3	Adamantinoma of long bones
M8890/1	Intravascular leiomyomatosis	M9080/0	Teratoma, benign	M9262/0	Ossifying fibroma
M8890/3	Leiomyosarcoma NOS	M9080/1	Teratoma NOS	**M927-M934**	**Odontogenic tumors**
M8891/1	Epithelioid leiomyoma	M9080/3	Teratoma, malignant NOS	M9270/0	Odontogenic tumor, benign
M8891/3	Epithelioid leiomyosarcoma	M9081/3	Teratocarcinoma	M9270/1	Odontogenic tumor NOS
M8892/1	Cellular leiomyoma	M9082/3	Malignant teratoma, undifferentiated type	M9270/3	Odontogenic tumor, malignant
M8893/0	Bizarre leiomyoma			M9271/0	Dentinoma
M8894/0	Angiomyoma	M9083/3	Malignant teratoma, intermediate type	M9272/0	Cementoma NOS
M8894/3	Angiomyosarcoma			M9273/0	Cementoblastoma, benign
M8895/0	Myoma	M9084/0	Dermoid cyst	M9274/0	Cementifying fibroma
M8895/3	Myosarcoma	M9084/3	Dermoid cyst with malignant transformation	M9275/0	Gigantiform cementoma
M8900/0	Rhabdomyoma NOS			M9280/0	Odontoma NOS
M8900/3	Rhabdomyosarcoma NOS	M9090/0	Struma ovarii NOS	M9281/0	Compound odontoma
M8901/3	Pleomorphic rhabdomyosarcoma	M9090/3	Struma ovarii, malignant	M9282/0	Complex odontoma
M8902/3	Mixed type rhabdomyosarcoma	M9091/1	Strumal carcinoid	M9290/0	Ameloblastic fibro-odontoma
M8903/0	Fetal rhabdomyoma	**M910**	**Trophoblastic neoplasms**	M9290/3	Ameloblastic odontosarcoma
M8904/0	Adult rhabdomyoma	M9100/0	Hydatidiform mole NOS	M9300/0	Adenomatoid odontogenic tumor
M8910/3	Embryonal rhabdomyosarcoma	M9100/1	Invasive hydatidiform mole	M9301/0	Calcifying odontogenic cyst
M8920/3	Alveolar rhabdomyosarcoma	M9100/3	Choriocarcinoma	M9310/0	Ameloblastoma NOS
M893-M899	**Complex mixed and stromal neoplasms**	M9101/3	Choriocarcinoma combined with teratoma	M9310/3	Ameloblastoma, malignant
				M9311/0	Odontoameloblastoma
M8930/3	Endometrial stromal sarcoma	M9102/3	Malignant teratoma, trophoblastic	M9312/0	Squamous odontogenic tumor
M8931/1	Endolymphatic stromal myosis	**M911**	**Mesonephromas**	M9320/0	Odontogenic myxoma
M8932/0	Adenomyoma	M9110/0	Mesonephroma, benign	M9321/0	Odontogenic fibroma NOS
M8940/0	Pleomorphic adenoma	M9110/1	Mesonephric tumor	M9330/0	Ameloblastic fibroma
M8940/3	Mixed tumor, malignant NOS	M9110/3	Mesonephroma, malignant	M9330/3	Ameloblastic fibrosarcoma
M8950/3	Mullerian mixed tumor	M9111/1	Endosalpingioma	M9340/0	Calcifying epithelial odontogenic tumor
M8951/3	Mesodermal mixed tumor	**M912-M916**	**Blood vessel tumors**		
M8960/1	Mesoblastic nephroma	M9120/0	Hemangioma NOS	**M935-M937**	**Miscellaneous tumors**
M8960/3	Nephroblastoma NOS	M9120/3	Hemangiosarcoma	M9350/1	Craniopharyngioma
M8961/3	Epithelial nephroblastoma	M9121/0	Cavernous hemangioma	M9360/1	Pinealoma
M8962/3	Mesenchymal nephroblastoma	M9122/0	Venous hemangioma	M9361/1	Pineocytoma
M8970/3	Hepatoblastoma	M9123/0	Racemose hemangioma	M9362/3	Pineoblastoma
M8980/3	Carcinosarcoma NOS	M9124/3	Kupffer cell sarcoma	M9363/0	Melanotic neuroectodermal tumor
M8981/3	Carcinosarcoma, embryonal type	M9130/0	Hemangioendothelioma, benign	M9370/3	Chordoma
M8982/0	Myoepithelioma	M9130/1	Hemangioendothelioma NOS	**M938-M948**	**Gliomas**
M8990/0	Mesenchymoma, benign	M9130/3	Hemangioendothelioma, malignant	M9380/3	Glioma, malignant
M8990/1	Mesenchymoma NOS	M9131/0	Capillary hemangioma	M9381/3	Gliomatosis cerebri
M8990/3	Mesenchymoma, malignant	M9132/0	Intramuscular hemangioma	M9382/3	Mixed glioma
M8991/3	Embryonal sarcoma	M9140/3	Kaposi's sarcoma	M9383/1	Subependymal glioma
M900-M903	**Fibroepithelial neoplasms**	M9141/0	Angiokeratoma	M9384/1	Subependymal giant cell astrocytoma
M9000/0	Brenner tumor NOS	M9142/0	Verrucous keratotic hemangioma		
M9000/1	Brenner tumor, borderline malignancy	M9150/0	Hemangiopericytoma, benign	M9390/0	Choroid plexus papilloma NOS
		M9150/1	Hemangiopericytoma NOS	M9390/3	Choroid plexus papilloma, malignant
M9000/3	Brenner tumor, malignant	M9150/3	Hemangiopericytoma, malignant		

APPENDIX A

M9391/3	Ependymoma NOS
M9392/3	Ependymoma, anaplastic type
M9393/1	Papillary ependymoma
M9394/1	Myxopapillary ependymoma
M9400/3	Astrocytoma NOS
M9401/3	Astrocytoma, anaplastic type
M9410/3	Protoplasmic astrocytoma
M9411/3	Gemistocytic astrocytoma
M9420/3	Fibrillary astrocytoma
M9421/3	Pilocytic astrocytoma
M9422/3	Spongioblastoma NOS
M9423/3	Spongioblastoma polare
M9430/3	Astroblastoma
M9440/3	Glioblastoma NOS
M9441/3	Giant cell glioblastoma
M9442/3	Glioblastoma with sarcomatous component
M9443/3	Primitive polar spongioblastoma
M9450/3	Oligodendroglioma NOS
M9451/3	Oligodendroglioma, anaplastic type
M9460/3	Oligodendroblastoma
M9470/3	Medulloblastoma NOS
M9471/3	Desmoplastic medulloblastoma
M9472/3	Medullomyoblastoma
M9480/3	Cerebellar sarcoma NOS
M9481/3	Monstrocellular sarcoma
M949-M952	**Neuroepitheliomatous neoplasms**
M9490/0	Ganglioneuroma
M9490/3	Ganglioneuroblastoma
M9491/0	Ganglioneuromatosis
M9500/3	Neuroblastoma NOS
M9501/3	Medulloepithelioma NOS
M9502/3	Teratoid medulloepithelioma
M9503/3	Neuroepithelioma NOS
M9504/3	Spongioneuroblastoma
M9505/1	Ganglioglioma
M9506/0	Neurocytoma
M9507/0	Pacinian tumor
M9510/3	Retinoblastoma NOS
M9511/3	Retinoblastoma, differentiated type
M9512/3	Retinoblastoma, undifferentiated type
M9520/3	Olfactory neurogenic tumor
M9521/3	Esthesioneurocytoma
M9522/3	Esthesioneuroblastoma
M9523/3	Esthesioneuroepithelioma
M953	**Meningiomas**
M9530/0	Meningioma NOS
M9530/1	Meningiomatosis NOS
M9530/3	Meningioma, malignant
M9531/0	Meningotheliomatous meningioma
M9532/0	Fibrous meningioma
M9533/0	Psammomatous meningioma
M9534/0	Angiomatous meningioma
M9535/0	Hemangioblastic meningioma
M9536/0	Hemangiopericytic meningioma
M9537/0	Transitional meningioma
M9538/1	Papillary meningioma
M9539/3	Meningeal sarcomatosis
M954-M957	**Nerve sheath tumor**
M9540/0	Neurofibroma NOS
M9540/1	Neurofibromatosis NOS
M9540/3	Neurofibrosarcoma
M9541/0	Melanotic neurofibroma
M9550/0	Plexiform neurofibroma
M9560/0	Neurilemmoma NOS
M9560/1	Neurinomatosis
M9560/3	Neurilemmoma, malignant
M9570/0	Neuroma NOS
M958	**Granular cell tumors and alveolar soft part sarcoma**
M9580/0	Granular cell tumor NOS
M9580/3	Granular cell tumor, malignant
M9581/3	Alveolar soft part sarcoma
M959-M963	**Lymphomas, NOS or diffuse**
M9590/0	Lymphomatous tumor, benign
M9590/3	Malignant lymphoma NOS
M9591/3	Malignant lymphoma, non Hodgkin's type
M9600/3	Malignant lymphoma, undifferentiated cell type NOS
M9601/3	Malignant lymphoma, stem cell type
M9602/3	Malignant lymphoma, convoluted cell type NOS
M9610/3	Lymphosarcoma NOS
M9611/3	Malignant lymphoma, lymphoplasmacytoid type
M9612/3	Malignant lymphoma, immunoblastic type
M9613/3	Malignant lymphoma, mixed lymphocytic-histiocytic NOS
M9614/3	Malignant lymphoma, centroblastic-centrocytic, diffuse
M9615/3	Malignant lymphoma, follicular center cell NOS
M9620/3	Malignant lymphoma, lymphocytic, well differentiated NOS
M9621/3	Malignant lymphoma, lymphocytic, intermediate differentiation NOS
M9622/3	Malignant lymphoma, centrocytic
M9623/3	Malignant lymphoma, follicular center cell, cleaved NOS
M9630/3	Malignant lymphoma, lymphocytic, poorly differentiated NOS
M9631/3	Prolymphocytic lymphosarcoma
M9632/3	Malignant lymphoma, centroblastic type NOS
M9633/3	Malignant lymphoma, follicular center cell, noncleaved NOS
M964	**Reticulosarcomas**
M9640/3	Reticulosarcoma NOS
M9641/3	Reticulosarcoma, pleomorphic cell type
M9642/3	Reticulosarcoma, nodular
M965-M966	**Hodgkin's disease**
M9650/3	Hodgkin's disease NOS
M9651/3	Hodgkin's disease, lymphocytic predominance
M9652/3	Hodgkin's disease, mixed cellularity
M9653/3	Hodgkin's disease, lymphocytic depletion NOS
M9654/3	Hodgkin's disease, lymphocytic depletion, diffuse fibrosis
M9655/3	Hodgkin's disease, lymphocytic depletion, reticular type
M9656/3	Hodgkin's disease, nodular sclerosis NOS
M9657/3	Hodgkin's disease, nodular sclerosis, cellular phase
M9660/3	Hodgkin's paragranuloma
M9661/3	Hodgkin's granuloma
M9662/3	Hodgkin's sarcoma
M969	**Lymphomas, nodular or follicular**
M9690/3	Malignant lymphoma, nodular NOS
M9691/3	Malignant lymphoma, mixed lymphocytic-histiocytic, nodular
M9692/3	Malignant lymphoma, centroblastic-centrocytic, follicular
M9693/3	Malignant lymphoma, lymphocytic, well differentiated, nodular
M9694/3	Malignant lymphoma, lymphocytic, intermediate differentiation, nodular
M9695/3	Malignant lymphoma, follicular center cell, cleaved, follicular
M9696/3	Malignant lymphoma, lymphocytic, poorly differentiated, nodular
M9697/3	Malignant lymphoma, centroblastic type, follicular
M9698/3	Malignant lymphoma, follicular center cell, noncleaved, follicular
M970	**Mycosis fungoides**
M9700/3	Mycosis fungoides
M9701/3	Sezary's disease
M971-M972	**Miscellaneous reticuloendothelial neoplasms**
M9710/3	Microglioma
M9720/3	Malignant histiocytosis
M9721/3	Histiocytic medullary reticulosis
M9722/3	Letterer-Siwe's disease
M973	**Plasma cell tumors**
M9730/3	Plasma cell myeloma
M9731/0	Plasma cell tumor, benign
M9731/1	Plasmacytoma NOS
M9731/3	Plasma cell tumor, malignant
M974	**Mast cell tumors**
M9740/1	Mastocytoma NOS
M9740/3	Mast cell sarcoma
M9741/3	Malignant mastocytosis
M975	**Burkitt's tumor**
M9750/3	Burkitt's tumor
M980-M994	**Leukemias**
M980	**Leukemias NOS**
M9800/3	Leukemia NOS
M9801/3	Acute leukemia NOS
M9802/3	Subacute leukemia NOS
M9803/3	Chronic leukemia NOS
M9804/3	Aleukemic leukemia NOS
M981	**Compound leukemias**
M9810/3	Compound leukemia
M982	**Lymphoid leukemias**
M9820/3	Lymphoid leukemia NOS
M9821/3	Acute lymphoid leukemia
M9822/3	Subacute lymphoid leukemia
M9823/3	Chronic lymphoid leukemia
M9824/3	Aleukemic lymphoid leukemia
M9825/3	Prolymphocytic leukemia
M983	**Plasma cell leukemias**
M9830/3	Plasma cell leukemia
M984	**Erythroleukemias**
M9840/3	Erythroleukemia
M9841/3	Acute erythremia
M9842/3	Chronic erythremia
M985	**Lymphosarcoma cell leukemias**
M9850/3	Lymphosarcoma cell leukemia
M986	**Myeloid leukemias**
M9860/3	Myeloid leukemia NOS
M9861/3	Acute myeloid leukemia
M9862/3	Subacute myeloid leukemia
M9863/3	Chronic myeloid leukemia
M9864/3	Aleukemic myeloid leukemia
M9865/3	Neutrophilic leukemia
M9866/3	Acute promyelocytic leukemia
M987	**Basophilic leukemias**
M9870/3	Basophilic leukemia
M988	**Eosinophilic leukemias**
M9880/3	Eosinophilic leukemia
M989	**Monocytic leukemias**
M9890/3	Monocytic leukemia NOS
M9891/3	Acute monocytic leukemia
M9892/3	Subacute monocytic leukemia
M9893/3	Chronic monocytic leukemia
M9894/3	Aleukemic monocytic leukemia
M990-M994	**Miscellaneous leukemias**
M9900/3	Mast cell leukemia
M9910/3	Megakaryocytic leukemia
M9920/3	Megakaryocytic myelosis
M9930/3	Myeloid sarcoma
M9940/3	Hairy cell leukemia
M995-M997	**Miscellaneous myeloproliferative and lymphoproliferative disorders**
M9950/1	Polycythemia vera
M9951/1	Acute panmyelosis
M9960/1	Chronic myeloproliferative disease
M9961/1	Myelosclerosis with myeloid metaplasia
M9962/1	Idiopathic thrombocythemia
M9970/1	Chronic lymphoproliferative disease

APPENDIX B: GLOSSARY OF MENTAL DISORDERS

GLOSSARY OF MENTAL DISORDERS
The psychiatric terms which appear in Chapter 5, "Mental Disorders," are listed here in alphabetic sequence. Many of the glossary descriptions originally appeared in the section on Mental Disorders in the *International Classification of Diseases, 9th Revision,*[1] and others are included to define the psychiatric conditions added to ICD-9-CM. The additional definitions are based on material furnished by the American Psychiatric Association's Task Force on Nomenclature and Statistics[2] and from *A Psychiatric Glossary.*[3] In a few instances definitions were obtained from *Dorland's Illustrated Medical Dictionary*[4] and from *Stedman's Medical Dictionary, Illustrated.*[5]

1. Manual of the *International Classification of Diseases, Injuries, and Causes of Death,* 9th Revision, World Health Organization, Geneva, Switzerland, 1975.

2. American Psychiatric Association, Task Force on Nomenclature and Statistics, Robert L. Spitzer, Chairman.

3. *A Psychiatric Glossary,* Fourth Edition, American Psychiatric Association, Washington, D.C., 1975.

4. *Dorland's Illustrated Medical Dictionary,* Twenty-fifth Edition, W. B. Saunders Company, Philadelphia, 1974.

5. *Stedman's Medical Dictionary,* Illustrated, Twenty-third Edition, the Williams and Williams Company, Baltimore, 1976.

Academic underachievement disorder: Failure to achieve in most school tasks despite adequate intellectual capacity, a supportive and encouraging social environment, and apparent effort. The failure occurs in the absence of a demonstrable specific learning disability and is caused by emotional conflict not clearly associated with any other mental disorder.[2]

Adaptation reaction — *see* Adjustment reaction

Adjustment reaction or disorder: Mild or transient disorders lasting longer than acute stress reactions which occur in individuals of any age without any apparent pre-existing mental disorder. Such disorders are often relatively circumscribed or situation-specific, are generally reversible, and usually last only a few months. They are usually closely related in time and content to stresses such as bereavement, migration, or other experiences. Reactions to major stress that last longer than a few days are also included. In children such disorders are associated with no significant distortion of development.[1]

    conduct disturbance: Mild or transient disorders in which the main disturbance predominantly involves a disturbance of conduct (e.g., an adolescent grief reaction resulting in aggressive or antisocial disorder).[1]

    depressive reaction: States of depression, not specifiable as manic-depressive, psychotic, or neurotic.[1]

        brief: Generally transient, in which the depressive symptoms are usually closely related in time and content to some stressful event.[1]

        prolonged: Generally long-lasting, usually developing in association with prolonged exposure to a stressful situation.[1]

    emotional disturbance: An adjustment disorder in which the main symptoms are emotional in type (e.g., anxiety, fear, worry) but not specifically depressive.[1]

    mixed conduct and emotional disturbance: An adjustment reaction in which both emotional disturbance and disturbance of conduct are prominent features.[1]

Affective psychoses: Mental disorders, usually recurrent, in which there is a severe disturbance of mood (mostly compounded of depression and anxiety but also manifested as elation, and excitement) which is accompanied by one or more of the following: delusions, perplexity, disturbed attitude to self, disorder of perception and behavior; these are all in keeping with the individual's prevailing mood (as are hallucinations when they occur). There is a strong tendency to suicide. For practical reasons, mild disorders of mood may also be included here if the symptoms match closely the descriptions given; this applies particularly to mild hypomania.[1]

bipolar: A manic-depressive psychosis which has appeared in both the depressive and manic form, either alternating or separated by an interval of normality.[1]

    atypical: An episode of affective psychosis with some, but not all, of the features of the one form of the disorder in individuals who have had a previous episode of the other form of the disorder.[2]

    depressed: A manic-depressive psychosis, circular type, in which the depressive form is currently present.[1]

    manic: A manic-depressive psychosis, circular type, in which the manic form is currently present.[1]

    mixed: A manic-depressive psychosis, circular type, in which both manic and depressive symptoms are present at the same time.[1]

depressed type: A manic-depressive psychosis in which there is a widespread depressed mood of gloom and wretchedness with some degree of anxiety. There is often reduced activity but there may be restlessness and agitation. There is marked tendency to recurrence; in a few cases this may be at regular intervals.[1]

    atypical: An affective depressive disorder that cannot be classified as a manic-depressive psychosis, depressed type, or chronic depressive personality disorder, or as an adjustment disorder.[2]

manic type: A manic-depressive psychosis characterized by states of elation or excitement out of keeping with the individual's circumstances and varying from enhanced liveliness (hypomania) to violent, almost uncontrollable, excitement. Aggression and anger, flight of ideas, distractibility, impaired judgment, and grandiose ideas are common.[1]

mixed type: Manic-depressive psychosis syndromes corresponding to both the manic and depressed types, but which for other reasons cannot be classified more specifically.[1]

Aggressive personality — *see* Personality disorder, explosive type

Agoraphobia — *see* agoraphobia under Phobia

Alcohol dependence syndrome: A state, psychic and usually also physical, resulting from taking alcohol, characterized by behavioral and other responses that always include a compulsion to take alcohol on a continuous or periodic basis in order to experience its psychic effects, and sometimes to avoid the discomfort of its absence; tolerance may or may not be present. A person may be dependent on alcohol and other drugs; if so, also record the diagnosis of drug dependence to identify the agent. If alcohol dependence is associated with alcoholic psychosis or with physical complications, *both* diagnoses should be recorded.[1]

Alcohol intoxication

    acute: A psychic and physical state resulting from alcohol ingestion characterized by slurred speech, unsteady gait, poor coordination, flushed facies, nystagmus, sluggish reflexes, fetor alcoholica, loud speech, emotional instability (e.g., jollity followed by lugubriousness), excessive conviviality, loquacity, and poorly inhibited sexual and aggressive behavior.[2]

    idiosyncratic: Acute psychotic episodes induced by relatively small amounts of alcohol. These are regarded as individual idiosyncratic reactions to alcohol, not due to excessive consumption and without conspicuous neurological signs of intoxication.[1]

    pathological — *see* Alcohol intoxication, idiosyncratic

Alcoholic psychoses: Organic psychotic states due mainly to excessive consumption of alcohol; defects of nutrition are thought to play an important role.[1]

    alcohol abstinence syndrome — *see* alcohol withdrawal syndrome below

    alcohol amnestic syndrome: A syndrome of prominent and lasting reduction of memory span, including striking loss of recent memory, disordered time appreciation and confabulation, occurring in alcoholics as the sequel to an acute alcoholic psychosis (especially delirium tremens) or, more rarely, in the course of chronic alcoholism. It is usually accompanied by peripheral neuritis and may be associated with Wernicke's encephalopathy.[1]

    alcohol withdrawal delirium [delirium tremens]: Acute or subacute organic psychotic states in alcoholics, characterized by clouded consciousness, disorientation, fear, illusions, delusions, hallucinations of any kind, notably visual and tactile, and restlessness, tremor and sometimes fever.[1]

    alcohol withdrawal hallucinosis: A psychosis usually of less than six months' duration, with slight or no clouding of consciousness and much anxious restlessness in which auditory hallucinations, mostly of voices uttering insults and threats, predominate.[1]

    alcohol withdrawal syndrome: Tremor of hands, tongue, and eyelids following cessation of prolonged heavy drinking of alcohol. Nausea and vomiting, dry mouth, headache, heavy perspiration, fitful sleep, acute anxiety attacks, mood depression, feelings of guilt and remorse, and irritability are associated features.[2]

    alcohol delirium — *see* alcohol withdrawal delirium above

    alcoholic dementia: Nonhallucinatory dementias occurring in association with alcoholism, but not characterized by the features of either alcohol withdrawal delirium [delirium tremens] or alcohol amnestic syndrome [Korsakoff's alcoholic psychosis].[1]

    alcoholic hallucinosis — *see* alcohol withdrawal hallucinosis above

    alcoholic jealousy: Chronic paranoid psychosis characterized by delusional jealousy and associated with alcoholism.[1]

    alcoholic paranoia — *see* Alcoholic jealousy

    alcoholic polyneuritic psychosis — *see* alcohol amnestic syndrome above

Alcoholism

    acute — *see* Alcohol intoxication, acute

    chronic — *see* Alcohol dependence syndrome

Alexia: Loss of a previously possessed reading facility that cannot be explained by defective visual acuity.[3]

Amnesia, psychogenic: A form of dissociative hysteria in which there is a temporary disturbance in the ability to recall important personal information which has already been registered and stored in memory. The sudden onset of this disturbance in the absence of an underlying organic mental disorder, and the extent of the disturbance being too great to be explained by ordinary forgetfulness, are the essential features.[2]

Amnestic syndrome: A syndrome of prominent and lasting reduction of memory span, including striking loss of recent memory, disordered time appreciation, and confabulation. The commonest causes are chronic alcoholism [alcohol amnestic syndrome; Korsakoff's alcoholic psychosis], chronic barbiturate dependence, and malnutrition. An amnestic syndrome may be the predominating disturbance in the early states of presenile and senile dementia, arteriosclerotic dementia, and in encephalitis and other inflammatory and degenerative diseases in which there is particular bilateral involvement of the temporal lobes, and certain temporal lobe tumors.[2]

APPENDIX B

alcoholic — *see* alcohol amnestic syndrome under Alcoholic psychoses
Amoral personality — *see* Personality disorder, antisocial type
Anancastic [anankastic] neurosis — *see* Neurotic disorder, obsessive-compulsive
Anancastic [anankastic] personality — *see* Personality disorder, compulsive type
Anorexia nervosa: A disorder in which the main features are persistent active refusal to eat and marked loss of weight. The level of activity and alertness is characteristically high in relation to the degree of emaciation. Typically the disorder begins in teenage girls but it may sometimes begin before puberty and rarely it occurs in males. Amenorrhea is usual and there may be a variety of other physiological changes including slow pulse and respiration, low body temperature, and dependent edema. Unusual eating habits and attitudes toward food are typical and sometimes starvation follows or alternates with periods of overeating. The accompanying psychiatric symptoms are diverse.[1]
Anxiety hysteria — *see* phobia under Neurotic disorders
Anxiety state (neurotic): Apprehension, tension, or uneasiness that stems from the anticipation of danger, the source of which is largely unknown or unrecognized.[1]
   atypical: An anxiety disorder that does not fulfill the criteria of generalized or panic attack anxiety. An example might be an individual with a single morbid fear.[2]
   generalized: A disorder of at least six months' duration in which the predominant feature is limited to diffuse and persistent anxiety without the specific symptoms that characterize phobic disorders, panic disorder, or obsessive-compulsive disorder.[2]
   panic attack: An episodic and often chronic, recurrent disorder in which the predominant features are anxiety attacks and nervousness. The anxiety attacks are manifested by discrete periods of sudden onset of intense apprehension, fearfulness, or terror often associated with feelings of impending doom.[2]
Aphasia, developmental: A delay in the production of spoken language. Rarely, there is also a developmental delay in the comprehension of speech sounds.[1]
Arteriosclerotic dementia: Dementia attributable, because of physical signs (on examination of the central nervous system), to degenerative arterial disease of the brain. Symptoms suggesting a focal lesion in the brain are common. There may be a fluctuating or patchy intellectual defect with insight, and an intermittent course is common. Clinical differentiation from senile or presenile dementia, which may coexist with it, may be very difficult or impossible. The diagnosis of cerebral atherosclerosis should also be recorded.[1]
Asocial personality — *see* Personality disorder, antisocial type
Astasia-abasia, hysterical: A form of conversion hysteria in which the individual is unable to stand or walk although the legs are otherwise under control.[4]
Asthenia, psychogenic — *see* neurasthenia under Neurotic disorders
Asthenic personality — *see* Personality disorder, dependent type
Attention deficit disorder — *see* attention deficit disorder under Hyperkinetic syndrome of childhood.
Autism, infantile: A syndrome present from birth or beginning almost invariably in the first 30 months. Responses to auditory and sometimes to visual stimuli are abnormal, and there are usually severe problems in the understanding of spoken language. Speech is delayed and, if it develops, is characterized by echolalia, the reversal of pronouns, immature grammatical structure, and inability to use abstract terms. There is generally an impairment in the social use of both verbal and gestural language. Problems in social relationships are most severe before the age of five years and include an impairment in the development of eye-to-eye gaze, social attachments, and cooperative play. Ritualistic behavior is usual and may include abnormal routines, resistance to change, attachment to odd objects, and stereotyped patterns of play. The capacity for abstract or symbolic thought and for imaginative play is diminished. Intelligence ranges from severely subnormal to normal or above. Performance is usually better on tasks involving rote memory or visuospatial skills than on those requiring symbolic or linguistic skills.[1]
Avoidant personality — *see* Personality disorder, avoidant type
"Bad trips": Acute intoxication from hallucinogen abuse, manifested by hallucinatory states lasting only a few days or less.[1]
Barbiturate abuse: Cases where an individual has taken the drug to the detriment of his health or social functioning, in doses above or for periods beyond those normally regarded as therapeutic.[1]
Bestiality — *see* Zoophilia
Bipolar disorder — *see* Affective psychosis, bipolar
   atypical — *see* Affective psychosis, bipolar, atypical
Body-rocking — *see* Stereotyped repetitive movements
Borderline personality — *see* Personality disorder, borderline type
Borderline psychosis of childhood — *see* Psychosis, atypical childhood
Borderline schizophrenia — *see* Schizophrenia, latent
Bouffée délirante — *see* Paranoid reaction, acute
Briquet's disorder — *see* somatization disorder under Neurotic disorders
Bulimia: An episodic pattern of overeating [binge eating] accompanied by an awareness of the disordered eating pattern with a fear of not being able to stop eating voluntarily. Depressive moods and self-deprecating thoughts follow the episodes of binge eating.[2]
Catalepsy schizophrenia — *see* Schizophrenia, catatonic type
Catastrophic stress — *see* Gross stress reaction
Catatonia (schizophrenic) — *see* Schizophrenia, catatonic type
Character neurosis — *see* Personality disorders
Childhood autism — *see* Autism, infantile
Childhood type schizophrenia — *see* Psychosis, child
Chronic alcoholic brain syndrome — *see* alcoholic dementia under Alcoholic psychoses
Clay-eating — *see* Pica
Clumsiness syndrome — *see* coordination disorder under Developmental delay disorders, specific
Combat fatigue — *see* Posttraumatic disorder, acute
Compensation neurosis — *see* compensation neurosis under Neurotic disorders
Compulsive conduct disorder — *see* impulse control disorders under Conduct disorders
Compulsive neurosis — *see* Neurotic disorder, obsessive-compulsive
Compulsive personality — *see* Personality disorder, compulsive type
Concentration camp syndrome — *see* Posttraumatic stress disorder, prolonged
Conduct disorders: Disorders mainly involving aggressive and destructive behavior and disorders involving delinquency. It should be used for abnormal behavior, in individuals of any age, which gives rise to social disapproval but which is not part of any other psychiatric condition. Minor emotional disturbances may also be present. To be included, the behavior, as judged by its frequency, severity, and type of associations with other symptoms, must be abnormal in its context. Disturbances of conduct are distinguished from an adjustment reaction by a longer duration and by a lack of close relationship in time and content to some stress. They differ from a personality disorder by the absence of deeply ingrained maladaptive patterns of behavior present from adolescence or earlier.[1]
   impulse control disorders: A failure to resist an impulse, drive, or temptation to perform some action which is harmful to the individual or to others. The impulse may or may not be consciously resisted, and the act may or may not be premeditated or planned. Prior to committing the act, there is an increasing sense of tension, and at the time of committing the act, there is an experience of either pleasure, gratification, or release. Immediately following the act, there may or may not be genuine regret, self-reproach, or guilt.[2] *See also* Intermittent explosive disorder, Isolated explosive disorder, Kleptomania, Pathological gambling, and Pyromania.
   mixed disturbance of conduct and emotions: A disorder characterized by features of undersocialized and socialized disturbance of conduct, but in which there is also considerable emotional disturbance as shown, for example, by anxiety, misery, or obsessive manifestations.[1]
   socialized conduct disorder: Conduct disorders in individuals who have acquired the values or behavior of a delinquent peer group to whom they are loyal and with whom they characteristically steal, play truant, and stay out late at night. There may also be sexual promiscuity.[1]
   undersocialized conduct disturbance
      aggressive type: A disorder characterized by a persistent pattern of disrespect for the feelings and well-being of others (bullying, physical aggression, cruel behavior, hostility, verbal abusiveness, impudence, defiance, negativism), aggressive antisocial behavior (destructiveness, stealing, persistent lying, frequent truancy, and vandalism), and failure to develop close and stable relationships with others.[2]
      unaggressive type: A disorder in which there is a lack of concern for the rights and feelings of others to a degree which indicates a failure to establish a normal degree of affection, empathy, or bond with others. There are two patterns of behavior found. In one, the child is fearful and timid, lacking self-assertiveness, resorts to self-protective and manipulative lying, indulges in whining demandingness and temper tantrums, feels rejected and unfairly treated, and is mistrustful of others. In the other pattern of the disorder, the child approaches others strictly for his own gains and acts exclusively because of exploitative and extractive goals. The child lies brazenly and steals, appearing to feel no guilt, and forms no social bonds to other individuals.[2]
Confusion, psychogenic — *see* Psychosis, reactive confusion
Confusion, reactive — *see* Psychosis, reactive confusion
Confusional state
   acute — *see* Delirium, acute
   epileptic — *see* Delirium, acute
   subacute — *see* Delirium, subacute
Conversion hysteria — *see* hysteria, conversion type under Neurotic disorders
Coordination disorder — *see* coordination disorder under Developmental delay disorders, specific
Culture shock: A form of stress reaction associated with an individual's assimilation into a new culture which is vastly different from that in which he was raised.[5]
Cyclic schizophrenia — *see* Schizophrenia, schizo-affective type
Cyclothymic personality or disorder — *see* Personality disorder, cyclothymic type
Delirium: Transient organic psychotic conditions with a short course in which there is a rapidly developing onset of disorganization of higher mental processes manifested by some degree of impairment of information processing, impaired

GLOSSARY OF MENTAL DISORDERS

or abnormal attention, perception, memory, and thinking. Clouded consciousness, confusion, disorientation, delusions, illusions, and often vivid hallucinations predominate in the clinical picture.[1,2]

acute: short-lived states, lasting hours or days, of the above type.[1]

subacute: states of the above type in which the symptoms, usually less florid, last for several weeks or longer, during which they may show marked fluctuations in intensity.[1]

Delirium tremens — *see* alcohol withdrawal delirium under Alcoholic psychoses

Delusions, systematized — *see* Paranoia

Dementia: A decrement in intellectual functioning of sufficient severity to interfere with occupational or social performance, or both. There is impairment of memory and abstract thinking, the ability to learn new skills, problem solving, and judgment. There is often also personality change or impairment in impulse control. Dementia in organic psychoses may be of a chronic or progressive nature, which if untreated are usually irreversible and terminal.[1,2]

alcoholic — *see* alcoholic dementia under Alcoholic psychoses

arteriosclerotic — *see* Arteriosclerotic dementia

multi-infarct — *see* Arteriosclerotic dementia

presenile — *see* Presenile dementia

repeated infarct — *see* Arteriosclerotic dementia

senile — *see* Senile dementia

Depersonalization syndrome — *see* depersonalization syndrome under Neurotic disorders

Depression: States of depression, usually of moderate but occasionally of marked intensity, which have no specifically manic-depressive or other psychotic depressive features, and which do not appear to be associated with stressful events or other features specified under neurotic depression.[1]

anxiety — *see* depression under Neurotic disorders

endogenous — *see* Affective psychosis, depressed type

monopolar — *see* Affective psychosis, depressed type

neurotic — *see* depression under Neurotic disorders

psychotic — *see* Affective psychosis, depressed type

psychotic reactive — *see* Psychosis, depressive

reactive — *see* depression under Neurotic disorders

reactive psychotic — *see* Psychosis, depressive

Depressive personality or character — *see* Personality disorder, chronic depressive type

Depressive reaction — *see* depressive reaction under Adjustment reaction

Depressive psychosis — *see* Affective psychosis, depressed type

Derealization (neurotic) — *see* depersonalization syndrome under Neurotic disorders

Developmental delay disorders, specific: A group of disorders in which a specific delay in development is the main feature. For many the delay is not explicable in terms of general intellectual retardation or of inadequate schooling. In each case development is related to biological maturation, but it is also influenced by nonbiological factors. A diagnosis of a specific developmental delay carries no etiological implications. A diagnosis of specific delay in development should not be made if it is due to a known neurological disorder.[1]

arithmetical disorder: Disorders in which the main feature is a serious impairment in the development of arithmetical skills.[1]

articulation disorder: A delay in the development of normal word-sound production resulting in defects of articulation. Omissions or substitutions of consonants are most frequent.[1]

coordination disorder: Disorders in which the main feature is a serious impairment in the development of motor coordination which is not explicable in terms of general intellectual retardation. The clumsiness is commonly associated with perceptual difficulties.[1]

mixed development disorder: A delay in the development of one specific skill (e.g., reading, arithmetic, speech, or coordination) is frequently associated with lesser delays in other skills. When this occurs, the diagnosis should be made according to the skill most seriously impaired. The mixed category should be used only where the mixture of delayed skills is such that no one skill is preponderantly affected.[1]

motor retardation — *see* coordination disorder above

reading disorder or retardation: Disorders in which the main feature is a serious impairment in the development of reading or spelling skills which is not explicable in terms of general intellectual retardation or of inadequate schooling. Speech or language difficulties, impaired right-left differentiation, perceptuo-motor problems, and coding difficulties are frequently associated. Similar problems are often present in other members of the family. Adverse psychosocial factors may be present.[1]

speech or language disorder: Disorders in which the main feature is a serious impairment in the development of speech or language (syntax or semantic) which is not explicable in terms of general intellectual retardation. Most commonly there is a delay in the development of normal word-sound production resulting in defects of articulation. Omissions or substitutions of consonants are most frequent. There may also be a delay in the production of spoken language. Rarely, there is also a developmental delay in the comprehension of sounds. Includes cases in which delay is largely due to environmental privation.[1]

Dipsomania — *see* Alcohol dependence syndrome

Disorganized schizophrenia — *see* Schizophrenia, disorganized type

Dissociative hysteria — *see* hysteria, dissociative type under Neurotic disorders

Drug abuse: Includes cases where an individual, for whom no other diagnosis is possible, has come under medical care because of the maladaptive effect of a drug on which he is not dependent (*see* Drug dependence) and that he has taken on his own initiative to the detriment of his health or social functioning. When drug abuse is secondary to a psychiatric disorder, record the disorder as an additional diagnosis.[1]

Drug dependence: A state, psychic and sometimes also physical, resulting from taking a drug, characterized by behavioral and other responses that always include a compulsion to take a drug on a continuous or periodic basis in order to experience its psychic effects, and sometimes to avoid the discomfort of its absence. Tolerance may or may not be present. A person may be dependent on more than one drug.[1]

Drug psychoses: Organic mental syndromes which are due to consumption of drugs (notably amphetamines, barbiturates, and opiate and LSD groups) and solvents. Some of the syndromes in this group are not as severe as most conditions labeled "psychotic," but they are included here for practical reasons. The drug should be identified, and also a diagnosis of drug dependence should be recorded, if present.[1]

drug-induced hallucinosis: Hallucinatory states of more than a few days, but not more than a few months' duration, associated with large or prolonged intake of drugs, notably of the amphetamine and LSD groups. Auditory hallucinations usually predominate and there may be anxiety or restlessness. States following LSD or other hallucinogens lasting only a few days or less ["bad trips"] are not included.[1]

drug-induced organic delusional syndrome: Paranoid states of more than a few days, but not more than a few months' duration, associated with large or prolonged intake of drugs, notably of the amphetamine and LSD groups.[1]

drug withdrawal syndrome: States associated with drug withdrawal ranging from severe, as specified for alcohol withdrawal delirium [delirium tremens], to less severe states characterized by one or more symptoms such as convulsions, tremor, anxiety, restlessness, gastrointestinal and muscular complaints, and mild disorientation and memory disturbance.[1]

Drunkenness

acute — *see* Alcohol intoxication, acute

pathologic — *see* Alcohol intoxication, idiosyncratic

simple: A state of inebriation due to alcohol consumption without conspicuous neurological signs of intoxication.[2]

sleep: An inability to fully arouse from the sleep state characterized by failure to attain full consciousness after arousal.[2]

Dyscalculia — *see* arithmetical disorder under Developmental delay disorders, specific

Dyslalia — *see* articulation disorder under Developmental delay disorders, specific

Dyslexia, developmental: A disorder in which the main feature is a serious impairment of reading skills which is not explicable in terms of general intellectual retardation or of inadequate schooling. Word-blindness and strephosymbolia (tendency to reverse letters and words in reading) are included.[1,3]

Dysmenorrhea, psychogenic: Painful menstruation due to disturbance of psychic control.[4]

Dyspareunia, functional — *see* functional dyspareunia under Psychosexual dysfunctions

Dyspraxia syndrome — *see* coordination disorder under Developmental delay disorders, specific

Dyssocial personality — *see* Personality disorder, antisocial type

Dysuria, psychogenic: Difficulty in passing urine due to psychic factors.[4]

Eating disorders: A group of disorders characterized by a conspicuous disturbance in eating behavior.[2] *See also* Bulimia, Pica, and Rumination, psychogenic.

Eccentric personality — *see* Personality disorder, eccentric type

Elective mutism: A pervasive and persistent refusal to speak in situations not attributable to a mental disorder. In some cases the behavior may manifest a form of withdrawal reaction to a specific stressful situation, or as a predominant feature in children exhibiting shyness or social withdrawal disorders.[2]

Emancipation disorder: An adjustment reaction in adolescents or young adults in which there is symptomatic expression (e.g., difficulty in making independent decisions, increased dependence on parental advice, adoption of values deliberately oppositional to parents) of a conflict over independence following the recent assumption of a status in which the individual is more independent of parental control or supervision.[2]

Emotional disturbances specific to childhood and adolescence: Less well-differentiated emotional disorders characteristic of the childhood period. When the emotional disorder takes the form of a neurosis, the appropriate diagnosis should be made. These disorders differ from adjustment reactions in terms of longer duration and by the lack of close relationship in time and content to some stress.[1] *See also* Academic underachievement disorder, Elective mutism, Identity disorder, Introverted disorder of childhood, Misery and unhappiness disorder, Oppositional disorder, Overanxious disorder, and Shyness disorder of childhood.

Encopresis: A disorder in which the main manifestation is the persistent voluntary or involuntary passage of formed stools of normal or near-normal consistency into places not intended for that purpose in the individual's own sociocultural setting. Sometimes the child has failed to gain bowel control, and sometimes he has gained control but then later again became encopretic. There may be a variety of associated psychiatric symptoms and there may be smearing of feces. The condition would not usually be diagnosed under the age of four years.[1]

Endogenous depression — see Affective psychosis, depressed type

Enuresis: A disorder in which the main manifestation is a persistent involuntary voiding of urine by day or night which is considered abnormal for the age of the individual. Sometimes the child will have failed to gain bladder control and in other cases he will have gained control and then lost it. Episodic or fluctuating enuresis should be included. The disorder would not usually be diagnosed under the age of four years.[1]

Epileptic confusional or twilight state — see Delirium, acute

Excitation
  catatonic — see Schizophrenia, catatonic type
  psychogenic — see Psychosis, excitative type
  reactive — see Psychosis, excitative type

Exhaustion delirium — see Stress reaction, acute

Exhibitionism: Sexual deviation in which the main sexual pleasure and gratification is derived from exposure of the genitals to a person of the opposite sex.[1]

Explosive personality disorder — see Personality disorder, explosive type

Factitious illness: A form of hysterical neurosis in which there are physical or psychological symptoms that are not real, genuine, or natural, which are produced by the individual and are under his voluntary control.[2]
  physical symptom type: The presentation of physical symptoms that may be total fabrication, self-inflicted, an exaggeration or exacerbation of a pre-existing physical condition, or any combination or variation of these.[2]
  psychological symptom type: The voluntary production of symptoms suggestive of a mental disorder. Behavior may mimic psychosis or, rather, the individual's idea of psychosis.[2]

Fanatic personality — see Personality disorder, paranoid type

Fatigue neurosis — see neurasthenia under Neurotic disorders

Feeble-minded — see Mental retardation, mild

Fetishism: A sexual deviation in which nonliving objects are utilized as a preferred or exclusive method of stimulating erotic arousal.[2]

Finger-flicking — see Stereotyped repetitive movements

Folie à deux — see Shared paranoid disorder

Frigidity: A psychosexual dysfunction in which there is partial or complete failure to attain or maintain the lubrication-swelling response of sexual excitement until completion of the sexual act.[2]

Frontal lobe syndrome: Changes in behavior following damage to the frontal areas of the brain or following interference with the connections of those areas. There is a general diminution of self-control, foresight, creativity, and spontaneity, which may be manifest as increased irritability, selfishness, restlessness and lack of concern for others. Conscientiousness and powers of concentration are often diminished, but measurable deterioration of intellect or memory is not necessarily present. The overall picture is often one of emotional dullness, lack of drive, and slowness; but, particularly in persons previously with energetic, restless, or aggressive characteristics, there may be a change towards impulsiveness, boastfulness, temper outbursts, silly fatuous humor, and the development of unrealistic ambitions; the direction of change usually depends upon the previous personality. A considerable degree of recovery is possible and may continue over the course of several years.[1]

Fugue, psychogenic: A form of dissociative hysteria characterized by an episode of wandering with inability to recall one's prior identity. Both onset and recovery are rapid. Following recovery there is no recollection of events which took place during the fugue state.[2]

Ganser's syndrome (hysterical): A form of factitious illness in which the patient voluntarily produces symptoms suggestive of a mental disorder.[2]

Gender identity disorder — see gender identity disorder under Psychosexual identity disorders

Gilles de la Tourette's disorder or syndrome — see Gilles de la Tourette's disorder under Tics

Grief reaction — see depressive reaction, brief under Adjustment reaction

Gross stress reaction — see Stress reaction, acute

Group delinquency — see socialized conduct disorder under Conduct disorders

Habit spasm — see chronic motor tic disorder under Tics

Hangover (alcohol) — see Drunkenness, simple

Head-banging — see Stereotyped repetitive movements

Hebephrenia — see Schizophrenia, disorganized type

Heller's syndrome — see Psychosis, disintegrative

High grade defect — see Mental retardation, mild

Homosexuality: Exclusive or predominant sexual attraction for persons of the same sex with or without physical relationship. Record homosexuality as a diagnosis whether or not it is considered as a mental disorder.[1]

Hospital addiction syndrome — see Munchausen syndrome

Hospital hoboes — see Munchausen syndrome

Hospitalism: A mild or transient adjustment reaction characterized by withdrawal seen in hospitalized patients. In young children this may be manifested by elective mutism.[1]

Hyperkinetic syndrome of childhood: Disorders in which the essential features are short attention span and distractibility. In early childhood the most striking symptom is disinhibited, poorly organized and poorly regulated extreme overactivity but in adolescence this may be replaced by underactivity. Impulsiveness, marked mood fluctuations, and aggression are also common symptoms. Delays in the development of specific skills are often present and disturbed, poor relationships are common. If the hyperkinesis is symptomatic of an underlying disorder, the diagnosis of the underlying disorder is recorded instead.[1]
  attention deficit disorder: Cases of hyperkinetic syndrome in which short attention span, distractibility, and overactivity are the main manifestations without significant disturbance of conduct or delay in specific skills.[1]
  hyperkinesis with developmental delay: Cases in which the hyperkinetic syndrome is associated with speech delay, clumsiness, reading difficulties, or other delays of specific skills.[1]
  hyperkinetic conduct disorder: Cases in which the hyperkinetic syndrome is associated with marked conduct disturbance but not developmental delay.[1]

Hypersomnia: A disorder of initiating arousal from sleep or maintaining wakefulness.[2]
  persistent: Chronic difficulty in initiating arousal from sleep or maintaining wakefulness associated with major or minor depressive mental disorders.[2]
  transient: Episodes of difficulty in arousal from sleep or maintaining wakefulness associated with acute or intermittent emotional reactions or conflicts.[2]

Hypochondriasis — see hypochondriasis under Neurotic disorders

Hypomania — see Affective psychosis, manic type

Hypomanic personality — see Personality disorder, chronic hypomanic type

Hyposomnia — see Insomnia

Hysteria — see hysteria under Neurotic disorders
  anxiety — see phobia under Neurotic disorders
  psychosis — see Psychosis, reactive
    acute — see Psychosis, excitative type

Hysterical personality — see Personality disorder, histrionic type

Identity disorder: An emotional disorder caused by distress over the inability to reconcile aspects of the self into a relatively coherent and acceptable sense of self, not secondary to another mental disorder. The disturbance is manifested by intense subjective distress regarding uncertainty about a variety of issues relating to identity, including long-term goals, career choice, friendship patterns, values, and loyalties.[2]

Idiocy — see Mental retardation, profound

Imbecile — see Mental retardation, moderate

Impotence: A psychosexual dysfunction in which there is partial or complete failure to attain or maintain erection until completion of the sexual act.[2]

Impulse control disorder — see impulse control disorders under Conduct disorders

Inadequate personality — see Personality disorder, dependent type

Induced paranoid disorder — see Shared paranoid disorder

Inebriety — see Drunkenness, simple

Infantile autism — see Autism, infantile

Insomnia: A disorder of initiating or maintaining sleep.[2]
  persistent: A chronic state of sleeplessness associated with chronic anxiety, major or minor depressive disorders, or psychoses.[2]
  transient: Episodes of sleeplessness associated with acute or intermittent emotional reactions or conflicts.[2]

Intermittent explosive disorder: Recurrent episodes of sudden and significant loss of control of aggressive impulses, not accounted for by any other mental disorder, which results in serious assault or destruction of property. The magnitude of the behavior during an episode is grossly out of proportion to any psychosocial stressors which may have played a role in eliciting the episode of lack of control. Following each episode there is genuine regret or self-reproach at the consequences of the action and the inability to control the aggressive impulse.[2]

Introverted disorder of childhood: An emotional disturbance in children chiefly manifested by a lack of interest in social relationships and indifference to social praise or criticism.[1]

Introverted personality — see Personality disorder, introverted type

Involutional melancholia — see Affective psychosis, depressed type

Involutional paranoid state — see Paraphrenia

Isolated explosive disorder: A disorder of impulse control in which there is a single discrete episode characterized by failure to resist an impulse which leads to a single, violent externally-directed act, which has a catastrophic impact on others, and for which the available information does not justify the diagnosis of another mental disorder.[2]

Isolated phobia — see simple phobia under Phobia

Jet lag syndrome: A phase-shift disruption of the 24-hour sleep-wake cycle due to rapid time-zone changes experienced in long-distance travel.[2]

Kanner's syndrome — see Autism, infantile

Kleptomania: A disorder of impulse control characterized by a recurrent failure to resist impulses to steal objects not for immediate use or their monetary value. An increasing sense of tension is experienced prior to committing the act, with an intense experience of gratification at the time of committing the theft.[2]

Korsakoff's psychosis
  alcoholic — see alcohol amnestic syndrome under Alcoholic psychoses
  nonalcoholic — see Amnestic syndrome

Latent schizophrenia — see Schizophrenia, latent

Lesbianism — see Homosexuality

Lobotomy syndrome — see Frontal lobe syndrome

LSD reaction: Acute intoxication from hallucinogen abuse, manifested by hallucinatory states lasting only a few days or less.[1]

GLOSSARY OF MENTAL DISORDERS

Major depressive disorder — *see* Affective psychosis, depressed type

Malingering: A clinical picture in which the predominant feature is the presentation of fake or grossly exaggerated physical or psychiatric illness apparently under voluntary control. In contrast to factitious illness, the symptoms produced in malingering are in pursuit of a goal which, when known, is recognizable and obviously understandable in light of knowledge of the individual's circumstances. Examples of understandable goals include, but are not limited to, becoming a "patient" in order to avoid conscription or military duty, avoid work, obtain financial compensation, evade criminal prosecution, and obtain drugs.[2]

Mania (monopolar) — *see* Affective psychosis, manic type

Manic-depressive psychosis
   circular type — *see* Affective psychosis, bipolar
   depressed type — *see* Affective psychosis, depressed type
   manic type — *see* Affective psychosis, manic type
   mixed type — *see* Affective psychosis, mixed type

Manic disorder — *see* Affective psychosis, manic type
   atypical — *see* Affective psychosis, manic type, atypical

Masochistic personality — *see* Personality disorder, masochistic type

Melancholia — *see* Affective psychoses
   involutional — *see* Affective psychosis, depressed type

Mental retardation: A condition of arrested or incomplete development of mind which is especially characterized by subnormality of intelligence. The coding should be made on the individual's *current* level of functioning *without regard to its nature* or causation, such as psychosis, cultural deprivation, Down's syndrome, etc. Where there is a specific cognitive handicap — such as in speech — the diagnosis of mental retardation should be based on assessments of cognition *outside the area of specific handicap*. The assessment of intellectual level should be based on whatever information is available, including clinical evidence, adaptive behavior, and psychometric findings. The IQ levels given are based on a test with a mean of 100 and a standard deviation of 15, such as the Wechsler scales. They are provided only as a guide and should not be applied rigidly. Mental retardation often involves psychiatric disturbances and may often develop as a result of some physical disease or injury. In these cases, an additional diagnosis should be recorded to identify any associated condition, psychiatric or physical.[1]

   mild mental retardation: IQ criteria 50–70. Individuals with this level of retardation are usually educable. During the preschool period they can develop social and communication skills, have minimal retardation in sensorimotor areas, and often are not distinguished from normal children until a later age. During the school age period they can learn academic skills up to approximately the sixth-grade level. During the adult years they can usually achieve social and vocational skills adequate for minimum self-support, but may need guidance and assistance when under social or economic stress.[1]

   moderate mental retardation: IQ criteria 35–49. Individuals with this level of retardation are usually trainable. During the preschool period they can talk or learn to communicate. They have poor social awareness and fair motor development. During the school age period they can profit from training in social and occupational skills, but they are unlikely to progress beyond the second-grade level in academic subjects. During their adult years they may achieve self-maintenance in unskilled or semi-skilled work under sheltered conditions. They need supervision and guidance when under mild social or economic stress.[2]

   severe mental retardation: IQ criteria 20–34. Individuals with this level of retardation evidence poor motor development, minimal speech, and are generally unable to profit from training and self-help during the preschool period. During the school age period they can talk or learn to communicate, can be trained in elementary health habits, and may profit from systematic habit training. During the adult years they may contribute partially to self-maintenance under complete supervision.[2]

   profound mental retardation: IQ criteria under 20. Individuals with this level of retardation evidence minimal capacity for sensorimotor functioning and need nursing care during the preschool period. During the school age period some further motor development may occur, and they may respond to minimal or limited training in self-help. During the adult years some motor and speech development may occur, and they may achieve very limited self-care and need nursing care.[2]

Merycism — *see* Rumination, psychogenic

Minimal brain dysfunction [MBD] — *see* Hyperkinetic syndrome of childhood

Misery and unhappiness disorder: An emotional disorder characteristic of childhood in which the main symptoms involve misery and unhappiness. There may also be eating and sleep disturbances.

Mood swings (brief compensatory) (rebound): Mild disorders of mood (depression and anxiety or elation and excitement, occurring alternately or episodically) seen in affective psychosis.[1]

Motor tic disorders — *see* Tics

Motor-verbal tic disorder — *see* Gilles de la Tourette's disorder under Tics

Multi-infarct dementia or psychosis — *see* Arteriosclerotic dementia

Multiple operations syndrome — *see* Munchausen syndrome

Multiple personality: A form of dissociative hysteria in which there is the domination of the individual at any one time by one of two or more distinct personalities. Each personality is a fully-integrated and complex unit with memories, behavior patterns, and social friendships which determine the nature of the individual's acts when uppermost in consciousness.[2]

Munchausen syndrome: A chronic form of factitious illness in which the individual demonstrates a plausible presentation of voluntarily produced physical symptomatology of such a degree that he is able to obtain and sustain multiple hospitalizations.[2]

Narcissistic personality — *see* Personality disorder, narcissistic type

Nervous debility — *see* neurasthenia under Neurotic disorders

Neurasthenia — *see* neurasthenia under Neurotic disorders

Neurotic delinquency — *see* mixed disturbance of conduct and emotions under Conduct disorders

Neurotic disorders: Neurotic disorders are mental disorders without any demonstrable organic basis in which the individual may have considerable insight and has unimpaired reality testing, in that he usually does not confuse his morbid subjective experiences and fantasies with external reality. Behavior may be greatly affected although usually remaining within socially acceptable limits, but personality is not disorganized. The principal manifestations include excessive anxiety, hysterical symptoms, phobias, obsessional and compulsive symptoms, and depression.[1]

   anxiety states: Various combinations of physical and mental manifestations of anxiety, not attributable to real danger and occurring either in attacks [*see* Anxiety state, panic attacks] or as a persisting state [*see* Anxiety state, generalized]. The anxiety is usually diffuse and may extend to panic. Other neurotic features such as obsessional or hysterical symptoms may be present but do not dominate the clinical picture.[1]

   compensation neurosis: Certain unconscious neurotic reactions in which features of secondary gain, such as a situational or financial advantage, are prominent.[3]

   depersonalization: A neurotic disorder with an unpleasant state of disturbed perception in which external objects or parts of one's own body are experienced as changed in their quality, unreal, remote, or automatized. The patient is aware of the subjective nature of the change he experiences. If depersonalization occurs as a feature of anxiety, schizophrenia, or other mental disorder, the condition is classified according to the major psychiatric disorder.[1]

   depression: A neurotic disorder characterized by disproportionate depression which has usually recognizably ensued on a distressing experience; it does not include among its features delusions or hallucinations, and there is often preoccupation with the psychic trauma which preceded the illness, e.g., loss of a cherished person or possession. Anxiety is also frequently present and mixed states of anxiety and depression should be included here. The distinction between depressive neurosis and psychosis should be made not only upon the degree of depression but also on the presence or absence of other neurotic and psychotic characteristics, and upon the degree of disturbance of the individual's behavior.[1]

   hypochondriasis: A neurotic disorder in which the conspicuous features are excessive concern with one's health in general or the integrity and functioning of some part of one's body, or less frequently, one's mind. It is usually associated with anxiety and depression. It may occur as a feature of some other severe mental disorder (e.g., manic-depressive psychosis, depressed type, schizophrenia, hysteria) and in that case should be classified according to the corresponding major disorder.[1]

   hysteria: A neurotic mental disorder in which motives, of which the patient seems unaware, produce either a restriction of the field of consciousness or disturbances of motor or sensory function which may seem to have psychological advantage or symbolic value.[1] There are three subtypes:

     conversion type: The chief or only symptoms of the hysterical neurosis consist of psychogenic disturbance of function in some part of the body, e.g., paralysis, tremor, blindness, deafness, seizures.[1]

     dissociative type: The most prominent feature of the hysterical neurosis is a narrowing of the field of consciousness which seems to serve an unconscious purpose and is commonly accompanied or followed by a selective amnesia. There may be dramatic but essentially superficial changes of personality [multiple personality], or sometimes the patient enters into a wandering state [fugue].[1]

   factitious illness: Physical or psychological symptoms that are not real, genuine, or natural, which are produced by the individual and are under his voluntary control.[2]

   neurasthenia: A neurotic disorder characterized by fatigue, irritability, headache, depression, insomnia, difficulty in concentration, and lack of capacity for enjoyment [anhedonia]. It may follow or accompany an infection or exhaustion, or arise from continued emotional stress. If neurasthenia is associated with a physical disorder, the latter should also be recorded as a diagnosis.[1]

obsessive-compulsive: States in which the outstanding symptom is a feeling of subjective compulsion, which must be resisted, to carry out some action, to dwell on an idea, to recall an experience, or to ruminate on an abstract topic. Unwanted thoughts which intrude, the insistency of words or ideas, ruminations or trains of thought are perceived by the individual to be inappropriate or nonsensical. The obsessional urge or idea is recognized as alien to the personality but as coming from within the self. Obsessional actions may be quasi-ritual performances designed to relieve anxiety, e.g., washing the hands to cope with contamination. Attempts to dispel the unwelcome thoughts or urges may lead to a severe inner struggle, with intense anxiety.[1]

occupational: A neurosis characterized by a functional disorder of a group of muscles used chiefly in one's occupation, marked by the occurrence of spasm, paresis, or incoordination on attempt to repeat the habitual movements (e.g., writer's cramp).[5]

phobic disorders: Neurotic states with abnormally intense dread of certain objects or specific situations which would not normally have that effect. If the anxiety tends to spread from a specified situation or object to a wider range of circumstances, it becomes akin to or identical with anxiety state and should be classified as such.[1] See also Phobia.

somatization disorder: A chronic, but fluctuating, neurotic disorder which begins early in life and is characterized by recurrent and multiple somatic complaints for which medical attention is sought but which are not apparently due to any physical illness. Complaints are presented in a dramatic, vague, or exaggerated way, or are part of a complicated medical history in which often many specific diagnoses have allegedly been made by other physicians. Complaints invariably refer to many organ systems (headache, fatigue, palpitations, fainting, nausea and vomiting, abdominal pains, bowel trouble, allergies, menstrual and sexual difficulties), and the individual frequently receives medical care from a number of physicians, sometimes simultaneously.[2]

Neurosis — see Neurotic disorders

Nightmares: Anxiety attacks occurring in dreams during REM sleep.[2]

Night terrors: A pathology of arousal from stage 4 sleep in which the individual experiences excessive terror and extreme panic (screaming, verbalizations), symptoms of autonomic activity, confusion, and poor recall for event.[2]

Nymphomania: Abnormal and excessive need or desire in the woman for sexual intercourse.[5]

Obsessional personality — see Personality disorder, compulsive type

Occupational neurosis — see Neurotic disorder, occupational

Oneirophrenia — see Schizophrenia, acute episode

Oppositional disorder of childhood or adolescence: A disorder characterized by pervasive opposition to all in authority regardless of self-interest, a continuous argumentativeness, and an unwillingness to respond to reasonable persuasion, not accounted for by a conduct disorder, adjustment disorder, or a psychosis of childhood. The oppositional behavior in this disorder is evoked by any demand, rule, suggestion, request, or admonishment placed on the individual.[2]

Organic affective syndrome: A clinical picture in which the predominating symptoms closely resemble those seen in either the depressive or manic affective disorders, occurring in the presence of evidence or history of a specific organic factor which is etiologically related to the disturbance, such as head trauma, endocranial tumors, and exocranial tumors secreting neurotoxic diatheses (e.g., pancreatic carcinoma). Excessive use of steroids, Cushing's syndrome, and other endocrine disorders may lead to an organic affective syndrome.[2]

Organic personality syndrome: Chronic, mild states of memory disturbance and intellectual deterioration, of nonpsychotic nature, often accompanied by increased irritability, querulousness, lassitude, and complaints of physical weakness. These states are often associated with old age, and may precede more severe states due to brain damage classifiable under senile or presenile dementia, dementia associated with other chronic organic psychotic brain syndromes, or delirium, delusions, hallucinosis, and depression in transient organic psychotic conditions.[1]

Organic psychosyndrome, focal (partial): A nonpsychotic organic mental disorder resembling the postcommotion syndrome associated with localized diseases of the brain or surrounding tissues.1

Organic psychotic conditions: Syndromes in which there is impairment of orientation, memory, comprehension, calculation, learning capacity, and judgment. These are the essential features but there may also be shallowness or lability of affect, or a more persistent disturbance of mood, lowering of ethical standards and exaggeration or emergence of personality traits, and diminished capacity for independent decision.[1] See also Alcohol psychoses, Arteriosclerotic dementia, Drug psychoses, Presenile dementia, and Senile dementia.

mixed paranoid and affective: Organic psychosis in which depressive and paranoid symptoms are the main features.[1]

transient: States characterized by clouded consciousness, confusion, disorientation, illusions, and often vivid hallucinations. They are usually due to some intra- or extracerebral toxic, infectious, metabolic or other systemic disturbance and are generally reversible. Depressive and paranoid symptoms may also be present but are not the main feature. The diagnosis of the associated physical or neurological condition should also be recorded.[1]

acute delirium: Short-lived states, lasting hours or days, of the above type.[1]

subacute delirium: States of the above type in which the symptoms, usually less florid, last for several weeks or longer during which they may show marked fluctuations in intensity.[1]

Organic reaction — see Organic psychotic conditions, transient

Overanxious disorder: An ill-defined emotional disorder characteristic of childhood in which the main symptoms involve anxiety and fearfulness.[1]

Panic disorder — see panic attack under Anxiety state

Paranoia: A rare chronic psychosis in which logically constructed systematized delusions have developed gradually without concomitant hallucinations or the schizophrenic type of disordered thinking. The delusions are mostly of grandeur (the paranoiac prophet or inventor), persecution, or somatic abnormality.[1]

alcoholic — see alcoholic jealousy under Alcoholic psychoses

querulans: A paranoid state which, though in many ways akin to schizophrenic or affective states, differs from other paranoid states and psychogenic paranoid psychosis.[1]

senile — see Paraphrenia

Paranoid personality — see Personality disorder, paranoid type

Paranoid reaction, acute: Paranoid states apparently provoked by some emotional stress. The stress is often misconstrued as an attack or threat. Such states are particularly prone to occur in prisoners or as acute reactions to a strange and threatening environment, e.g., in immigrants.[1]

Paranoid schizophrenia — see Schizophrenia, paranoid type

Paranoid state

involutional — see Paraphrenia

senile — see Paraphrenia

simple: A psychosis, acute or chronic, not classifiable as schizophrenia or affective psychosis, in which delusions, especially of being influenced, persecuted, or treated in some special way, are the main symptoms. The delusions are of a fairly fixed, elaborate, and systematized kind.[1]

Paranoid traits — see Personality disorder, paranoid type

Paraphilia — see Sexual deviations

Paraphrenia: Paranoid psychosis in which there are conspicuous hallucinations, often in several modalities. Affective symptoms and disordered thinking, if present, do not dominate the clinical picture, and the personality is well preserved.[1]

Paraphrenic schizophrenia — see Schizophrenia, paranoid type

Passive-aggressive personality — see Personality disorder, passive-aggressive type

Passive personality — see Personality disorder, dependent type

Pathological

alcohol intoxication — see Alcohol intoxication, idiosyncratic

drug intoxication: Individual idiosyncratic reactions to comparatively small quantities of a drug, which take the form of acute, brief psychotic states of any type.[1]

drunkenness — see Alcohol intoxication, idiosyncratic

gambling: A disorder of impulse control characterized by a chronic and progressive preoccupation with gambling and urge to gamble, with subsequent gambling behavior that compromises, disrupts, or damages personal, family, and vocational pursuits.[2]

personality — see Personality disorder

Pedophilia: Sexual deviations in which an adult engages in sexual activity with a child of the same or opposite sex.[1]

Peregrinating patient — see Malingering

Personality disorders: Deeply ingrained maladaptive patterns of behavior generally recognizable by the time of adolescence or earlier and continuing throughout most of adult life, although often becoming less obvious in middle or old age. The personality is abnormal either in the balance of its components, their quality and expression, or in its total aspect. Because of this deviation or psychopathy the patient suffers or others have to suffer, and there is an adverse effect upon the individual or on society. It includes what is sometimes called psychopathic personality, but if this is determined primarily by malfunctioning of the brain, it should be classified as one of the nonpsychotic organic brain syndromes. When the patient exhibits an anomaly of personality directly related to his neurosis or psychosis, e.g., schizoid personality and schizophrenia or anancastic personality and obsessive compulsive neurosis, the relevant neurosis or psychosis which is in evidence should be diagnosed in addition.[1]

affective type: A chronic personality disorder characterized by lifelong predominance of a pronounced mood. The illness does not have a clear onset, and there may be intermittent periods of disturbed mood separated by periods of normal mood.[1]

anancastic [anankastic] type — see Personality disorder, compulsive type

antisocial type: A personality disorder characterized by disregard for social obligations, lack of feeling for others, and impetuous violence or callous unconcern. There is a gross disparity between behavior and the prevailing social norms. Behavior is not readily modifiable by experience, including punishment. People with this personality are often affectively cold, and may be abnormally aggressive or

GLOSSARY OF MENTAL DISORDERS

irresponsible. Their tolerance to frustration is low; they blame others or offer plausible rationalizations for the behavior which brings them into conflict with society.[1]

asthenic type — *see* Personality disorder, dependent type

avoidant type: Individuals with this disorder exhibit excessive social inhibitions and shyness, a tendency to withdraw from opportunities for developing close relationships, and a fearful expectation that they will be belittled and humiliated. Desires for affection and acceptance are strong, but they are unwilling to enter relationships unless given unusually strong guarantees that they will be uncritically accepted. Therefore, they have few close relationships and suffer from feelings of loneliness and isolation.[2]

borderline type: Individuals with this disorder are characterized by instability in a variety of areas, including interpersonal relationships, behavior, mood, and self image. Interpersonal relationships are often intense and unstable with marked shifts of attitude over time. Frequently there is impulsive and unpredictable behavior which is potentially physically self-damaging. There may be problems tolerating being alone, and chronic feelings of emptiness or boredom.[2]

chronic depressive type: An affective personality disorder characterized by lifelong predominance of a chronic nonpsychotic disturbance involving either intermittent or sustained periods of depressed mood (marked by worry, pessimism, low output of energy, and a sense of futility).[2]

chronic hypomanic type: An affective personality disorder characterized by lifelong predominance of a chronic nonpsychotic disturbance involving either intermittent or sustained periods of abnormally elevated mood (unshakable optimism and an enhanced zest for life and activity).[2]

compulsive type: A personality disorder characterized by feelings of personal insecurity, doubt, and incompleteness leading to excessive conscientiousness, checking, stubbornness, and caution. There may be insistent and unwelcome thoughts or impulses which do not attain the severity of an obsessional neurosis. There is perfectionism and meticulous accuracy and a need to check repeatedly in an attempt to ensure this. Rigidity and excessive doubt may be conspicuous.[1]

cyclothymic type: A chronic nonpsychotic disturbance involving depressed and elevated mood, lasting at least two years, separated by periods of normal mood.[2]

dependent type: A personality disorder characterized by passive compliance with the wishes of elders and others and a weak inadequate response to the demands of daily life. Lack of vigor may show itself in the intellectual or emotional spheres; there is little capacity for enjoyment.[2]

eccentric type: A personality disorder characterized by oddities of behavior which do not conform to the clinical syndromes of personality disorders described elsewhere.[2]

explosive type: A personality disorder characterized by instability of mood with liability to intemperate outbursts of anger, hate, violence, or affection. Aggression may be expressed in words or in physical violence. The outbursts cannot readily be controlled by the affected persons, who are not otherwise prone to antisocial behavior.[1]

histrionic type: A personality disorder characterized by shallow, labile affectivity, dependence on others, craving for appreciation and attention, suggestibility, and theatricality. There is often sexual immaturity, e.g., frigidity and over-responsiveness to stimuli. Under stress hysterical symptoms [neurosis] may develop.[1]

hysterical type — *see* Personality disorder, histrionic type

inadequate type — *see* Personality disorder, dependent type

introverted type: A form of schizoid personality in which the essential features are a profound defect in the ability to form social relationships and to respond to the usual forms of social reinforcements. Such patients are characteristically "loners" who do not appear distressed by their social distance and are not interested in greater social involvement.[2]

masochistic type: A personality disorder in which the individual appears to arrange life situations so as to be defeated and humiliated.[2]

narcissistic type: A personality disorder in which interpersonal difficulties are caused by an inflated sense of self-worth, and indifference to the welfare of others. Achievement deficits and social irresponsibilities are justified and sustained by a boastful arrogance, expansive fantasies, facile rationalization, and frank prevarication.[2]

paranoid type: A personality disorder in which there is excessive sensitiveness to setbacks or to what are taken to be humiliations and rebuffs, a tendency to distort experience by misconstruing the neutral or friendly actions of others as hostile or contemptuous, and a combative and tenacious sense of personal rights. There may be a proneness to jealousy or excessive self-importance. Such persons may feel helplessly humiliated and put upon; others, likewise excessively sensitive, are aggressive and insistent. In all cases there is excessive self-reference.[1]

passive-aggressive type: A personality disorder characterized by aggressive behavior manifested in passive ways, such as obstructionism, pouting, procrastination, intentional inefficiency, or stubbornness. The *aggression* often arises from resentment at failing to find gratification in a relationship with an individual or institution upon which the individual is overdependent.[3]

passive type — *see* Personality disorder, dependent type

schizoid type: A personality disorder in which there is withdrawal from affectional, social, and other contacts with autistic preference for fantasy and introspective reserve. Behavior may be slightly eccentric or indicate avoidance of competitive situations. Apparent coolness and detachment may mask an incapacity to express feeling.[1]

schizotypal type: A form of schizoid personality in which individuals with this disorder manifest various oddities of thinking, perception, communication, and behavior. The disturbance in thinking may be expressed as magical thinking, ideas of reference, or paranoid ideation. Perceptual disturbances may include recurrent illusions and derealization [depersonalization]. Frequently, but not invariably, the behavioral manifestations include social isolation and constricted or inappropriate affect which interferes with rapport in face-to-face interaction without any of the frank psychotic features which characterize schizophrenia.[2]

Phobia: Neurotic states with abnormally intense dread of certain objects or specific situations which would not normally have that effect. If the anxiety tends to spread from a specified situation or object to a wider range of circumstances, it becomes akin to or identical with anxiety state, and should be classified as such.[1]

acrophobia: Fear of heights[3]

agoraphobia: Fear of leaving the familiar setting of the home, and is almost always preceded by a phase during which there are recurrent panic attacks. Because of the anticipatory fear of helplessness when having a panic attack, the patient is reluctant or refuses to be alone, travel or walk alone, or to be in situations where there is no ready access to help, such as in crowds, closed or open spaces, or crowded stores.[2]

ailurophobia: Fear of cats[3]

algophobia: Fear of pain[3]

claustrophobia: Fear of closed spaces[3]

isolated phobia — *see* simple phobia below

mysophobia: Fear of dirt or germs[3]

obsessional — *see* Neurotic disorder, obsessive-compulsive

panphobia: Fear of everything[3]

simple phobia: Fear of a discrete object or situation which is neither fear of leaving the familiar setting of the home [agoraphobia], or of being observed by others in certain situations [social phobia]. Examples of simple phobia are fear of animals, acrophobia, and claustrophobia.[2]

social phobia: Fear of situations in which the subject is exposed to possible scrutiny by others, and the possibility exists that he may act in a fashion that will be considered shameful. The most common social phobias are fears of public speaking, blushing, eating in public, writing in front of others, or using public lavatories.[2]

xenophobia: Fear of strangers[3]

Pica: Perverted appetite of nonorganic origin in which there is persistent eating of non-nutritional substances. Typically, infants ingest paint, plaster, string, hair, or cloth. Older children may have access to animal droppings, sand, bugs, leaves, or pebbles. In the adult, eating of starch or clay-earth has been observed.[2]

Postconcussion syndrome: States occurring after generalized contusion of the brain, in which the symptom picture may resemble that of the frontal lobe syndrome or that of any of the neurotic disorders, but in which in addition, headache, giddiness, fatigue, insomnia, and a subjective feeling of impaired intellectual ability are usually prominent. Mood may fluctuate, and quite ordinary stress may produce exaggerated fear and apprehension. There may be marked intolerance of mental and physical exertion, undue sensitivity to noise, and hypochondriacal preoccupation. The symptoms are more common in persons who have previously suffered from neurotic or personality disorders, or when there is a possibility of compensation. This syndrome is particularly associated with the closed type of head injury when signs of localized brain damage are slight or absent, but it may also occur in other conditions.[1]

Postcontusion syndrome or encephalopathy — *see* Postconcussion syndrome

Postencephalitic syndrome: A nonpsychotic organic mental disorder resembling the postconcussion syndrome associated with central nervous system infections.[1]

Postleucotomy syndrome — *see* Frontal lobe syndrome

Posttraumatic brain syndrome, nonpsychotic — *see* Postconcussion syndrome

Posttraumatic organic psychosis — *see* Organic psychotic conditions, transient

Posttraumatic stress disorder: The development of characteristic symptoms (re-experiencing the traumatic event, numbing of responsiveness to or involvement with the external world, and a variety of other autonomic, dysphoric, or cognitive symptoms) after experiencing a psychologically traumatic event or events outside the normal range of human experience (e.g., rape or assault, military combat, natural catastrophes such as flood or earthquake, or other disaster, such as airplane crash, fires, bombings).[2]

acute: Brief, episodic, or recurrent disorders lasting less than six months' duration after the onset of trauma.[2]

prolonged: Chronic disorders of the above type lasting six months or more following the trauma.[2]

Premature ejaculation — *see* premature ejaculation under Psychosexual dysfunctions

Prepsychotic schizophrenia — *see* Schizophrenia, latent

Presbyophrenia — *see* Organic personality syndrome

Presenile dementia: Dementia occurring usually before the age of 65 in patients with the relatively rare forms of diffuse or lobar cerebral atrophy. The associated neurological condition (e.g., Alzheimer's disease, Pick's disease, Jakob-Creutzfeldt disease) should also be recorded as a diagnosis.[1]

Prodromal schizophrenia — *see* Schizophrenia, latent

Pseudoneurotic schizophrenia — *see* Schizophrenia, latent

Psychalgia: Pains of mental origin, e.g., headache or backache, for which a more precise medical or psychiatric diagnosis cannot be made.[1]

Psychasthenia: A functioning neurosis marked by stages of pathological fear or anxiety, obsessions, fixed ideas, tics, feelings of inadequacy, self-accusation, and peculiar feelings of strangeness, unreality, and depersonalization.[4]

Psychic shock: A sudden disturbance of mental equilibrium produced by strong emotion in response to physical or mental stress.[4]

Psychic factors associated with physical diseases: Mental disturbances or psychic factors of any type thought to have played a major part in the etiology of physical conditions, usually involving tissue damage, classified elsewhere. The mental disturbance is usually mild and nonspecific, and the psychic factors (worry, fear, conflict, etc.) may be present without any overt psychiatric disorder. Examples of these conditions are asthma, dermatitis, eczema, duodenal ulcer, ulcerative colitis, and urticaria, specified as due to psychogenic factors. Use an additional diagnosis to identify the physical condition. In the rare instance that an overt psychiatric disorder is thought to have caused the physical condition, the psychiatric diagnosis should be recorded in addition.[1]

Psychoneurosis — *see* Neurotic disorders

Psycho-organic syndrome — *see* Organic psychotic conditions, transient

Psychopathic constitutional state — *see* Personality disorders

Psychopathic personality — *see* Personality disorders

Psychophysiological disorders: A variety of physical symptoms or types of physiological malfunctions of mental origin, not involving tissue damage, and usually mediated through the autonomic nervous system. The disorders are classified according to the body system involved. If the physical symptom is secondary to a psychiatric disorder classifiable elsewhere, the physical symptom is not classified as a psychophysiological disorder. If tissue damage is involved, then the diagnosis is classified as a *Psychic factor associated with diseases classified elsewhere.*[1]

Psychosexual dysfunctions: A group of disorders in which there is recurrent and persistent dysfunction encountered during sexual activity. The dysfunction may be lifelong or acquired, generalized or situational, and total or partial.[2]

functional dyspareunia: Recurrent and persistent genital pain associated with coitus.[2]

functional vaginismus: A history of recurrent and persistent involuntary spasm of the musculature of the outer one-third of the vagina that interferes with sexual activity.[2]

inhibited female orgasm: Recurrent and persistent inhibition of the female orgasm as manifested by a delay or absence of orgasm following a normal sexual excitement phase during sexual activity.[2]

inhibited male orgasm: Recurrent and persistent inhibition of the male orgasm as manifested by a delay or absence of either the emission or ejaculation phases, or more usually, both following an adequate phase of sexual excitement.[2]

inhibited sexual desire: Persistent inhibition of desire for engaging in a particular form of sexual activity.[2]

inhibited sexual excitement: Recurrent and persistent inhibition of sexual excitement during sexual activity, manifested either by partial or complete failure to attain or maintain erection until completion of the sexual act [impotence], or partial or complete failure to attain or maintain the lubrication-swelling response of sexual excitement until completion of the sexual act [frigidity].[2]

premature ejaculation: Ejaculation occurs before the individual wishes it, because of recurrent and persistent absence of reasonable voluntary control of ejaculation and orgasm during sexual activity.[2]

Psychosexual gender identity disorders: Behavior occurring in preadolescents of immature psychosexuality, or in adults, in which there is an incongruence between the individual's anatomic sex and gender identity.[2]

gender identity disorder: In children or in adults a condition in which the individual would prefer to be of the other sex, and strongly prefers the clothes, toys, activities, and companionship of the other sex. Cross-dressing is intermittent, although it may be frequent. In children the commonest form is feminism in boys.[2]

trans-sexualism: A psychosexual identity disorder centered around fixed beliefs that the overt bodily sex is wrong. The resulting behavior is directed towards either changing the sexual organs by operation, or completely concealing the bodily sex by adopting both the dress and behavior of the opposite sex.[1]

Psychosomatic disorders — *see* Psychophysiological disorders

Psychosis: Mental disorders in which impairment of mental function has developed to a degree that interferes grossly with insight, ability to meet some ordinary demands of life or to maintain adequate contact with reality. It is not an exact or well defined term. Mental retardation is excluded.[1]

affective — *see* Affective psychoses

alcoholic — *see* Alcoholic psychoses

atypical childhood: A variety of atypical infantile psychoses which may show some, but not all, of the features of infantile autism. Symptoms may include stereotyped repetitive movements, hyperkinesis, self-injury, retarded speech development, echolalia, and impaired social relationships. Such disorders may occur in children of any level of intelligence but are particularly common in those with mental retardation.[1]

borderline, of childhood — *see* Psychosis, atypical childhood

child: A group of disorders in children, characterized by distortions in the timing, rate, and sequence of many psychological functions involving language development and social relations in which the severe qualitative abnormalities are not normal for any stage of development.[2] *See also* Autism, infantile, Psychosis, disintegrative, Psychosis, atypical childhood.

depressive — *see* Affective psychosis, depressed type

depressive type: A depressive psychosis which can be similar in its symptoms to manic-depressive psychosis, depressed type but is apparently provoked by saddening stress such as a bereavement, or a severe disappointment or frustration. There may be less diurnal variation of symptoms than in manic-depressive psychosis, depressed type, and the delusions are more often understandable in the context of the life experiences. There is usually a serious disturbance of behavior, e.g., major suicidal attempt.[1]

disintegrative: A disorder in which normal or near-normal development for the first few years is followed by a loss of social skills and of speech, together with a severe disorder of emotions, behavior, and relationships. Usually this loss of speech and of social competence takes place over a period of a few months and is accompanied by the emergence of overactivity and of stereotypies. In most cases there is intellectual impairment, but this is not a necessary part of the disorder. The condition may follow overt brain disease, such as measles encephalitis, but it may also occur in the absence of any known organic brain disease or damage. Any associated neurological disorder should also be recorded.[1]

epileptic: An organic psychotic condition associated with epilepsy.[1]

excitative type: An affective psychosis similar in its symptoms to manic-depressive psychosis, manic type, but apparently provoked by emotional stress.[1]

hypomanic — *see* Affective psychosis, manic type

hysterical — *see* Psychosis, reactive

acute — *see* Psychosis, excitative type

induced — *see* Shared paranoid disorder

infantile — *see* Autism, infantile

infective — *see* Organic psychotic conditions, transient

Korsakoff's

alcoholic — *see* alcohol amnestic syndrome under Alcoholic psychoses

nonalcoholic — *see* Amnestic syndrome

manic-depressive — *see* Affective psychoses

multi-infarct — *see* Arteriosclerotic dementia

paranoid

chronic — *see* Paranoia

protracted reactive — *see* Psychosis, paranoid, psychogenic

psychogenic: Psychogenic or reactive paranoid psychosis of any type which is more protracted than the reactions described under Paranoid reaction, acute.[1]

acute — *see* Paranoid reaction, acute

postpartum — *see* Psychosis, puerperal

psychogenic — *see* Psychosis, reactive

depressive — *see* Psychosis, depressive type

puerperal: Any psychosis occurring within a fixed period (approximately 90 days) after childbirth.[3] The diagnosis should be classified according to the predominant symptoms or characteristics, such as schizophrenia, affective psychosis, paranoid states, or other specified psychosis.

reactive: A psychotic condition which is largely or entirely attributable to a recent life experience. This diagnosis is not used for the wider range of psychoses in which environmental factors play some, but not the *major,* part in etiology.[1]

brief: A florid psychosis of at least a few hours' duration but lasting no more than two weeks, with sudden onset immediately following a severe environmental stress and eventually terminating in complete recovery to the pre-psychotic state.[2]

confusion: Mental disorders with clouded consciousness, disorientation (though less marked than in organic confusion), and diminished accessibility often accompanied by excessive activity and apparently provoked by emotional stress.[1]

depressive — *see* Psychosis, depressive type

schizo-affective — *see* Schizophrenia, schizo-affective type

schizophrenic — *see* Schizophrenia

schizophreniform — *see* Schizophrenia

affective type — *see* Schizophrenia, schizo-affective type

confusional type — *see* Schizophrenia, acute episode

GLOSSARY OF MENTAL DISORDERS

senile — *see* Senile dementia, delusional type

Pyromania: A disorder of impulse control characterized by a recurrent failure to resist impulses to set fires without regard for the consequences, or with deliberate destructive intent. Invariably there is intense fascination with the setting of fires, seeing fires burn, and a satisfaction with the resultant destruction.[2]

Relationship problems of childhood: Emotional disorders characteristic of childhood in which the main symptoms involve relationship problems.[1]

Repeated infarct dementia — *see* Arteriosclerotic dementia

Residual schizophrenia — *see* Schizophrenia, residual type

Restzustand (schizophrenia) — *see* Schizophrenia, residual type

Rumination
   obsessional: The constant preoccupation with certain thoughts, with inability to dismiss them from the mind.[4] *See* Neurotic disorder, obsessive-compulsive.
   psychogenic: In children the regurgitation of food, with failure to thrive or weight loss developing after a period of normal functioning. Food is brought up without nausea, retching, or disgust. The food is then ejected from the mouth, or chewed and reswallowed.[2]

Sander's disease — *see* Paranoia

Satyriasis: Pathologic or exaggerated sexual desire or excitement in the man.[3]

Schizoid personality disorder — *see* Personality disorder, schizoid type

Schizophrenia: A group of psychoses in which there is a fundamental disturbance of personality, a characteristic distortion of thinking, often a sense of being controlled by alien forces, delusions which may be bizarre, disturbed perception, abnormal affect out of keeping with the real situation, and autism. Nevertheless, clear consciousness and intellectual capacity are usually maintained. The disturbance of personality involves its most basic functions which give the normal person his feeling of individuality, uniqueness, and self-direction. The most intimate thoughts, feelings, and acts are often felt to be known to or shared by others and explanatory delusions may develop, to the effect that natural or supernatural forces are at work to influence the schizophrenic person's thoughts and actions in ways that are often bizarre. He may see himself as the pivot of all that happens. Hallucinations, especially of hearing, are common and may comment on the patient or address him. Perception is frequently disturbed in other ways; there may be perplexity, irrelevant features may become all-important and accompanied by passivity feelings, may lead the patient to believe that everyday objects and situations possess a special, usually sinister, meaning intended for him. In the characteristic schizophrenic disturbance of thinking, peripheral and irrelevant features of a total concept, which are inhibited in normal directed mental activity, are brought to the forefront and utilized in place of the elements relevant and appropriate to the situation. Thus, thinking becomes vague, elliptical and obscure, and its expression in speech sometimes incomprehensible. Breaks and interpolations in the flow of consecutive thought are frequent, and the patient may be convinced that his thoughts are being withdrawn by some outside agency. Mood may be shallow, capricious, or incongruous. Ambivalence and disturbance of volition may appear as inertia, negativism, or stupor. Catatonia may be present. The diagnosis "schizophrenia" should not be made unless there is, or has been evident during the same illness, characteristic disturbance of thought, perception, mood, conduct, or personality — preferably in at least two of these areas. The diagnosis should not be restricted to conditions running a protracted, deteriorating, or chronic course. In addition to making the diagnosis on the criteria just given, effort should be made to specify one of the following subtypes of schizophrenia, according to the predominant symptoms.[1]

   acute (undifferentiated): Schizophrenia of florid nature which cannot be classified as simple, catatonic, hebephrenic, paranoid, or any other types.[1]

   acute episode: Schizophrenic disorders, other than simple, hebephrenic, catatonic, and paranoid, in which there is a dream-like state with slight clouding of consciousness and perplexity. External things, people, and events may become charged with personal significance for the patient. There may be ideas of reference and emotional turmoil. In many such cases remission occurs within a few weeks or months, even without treatment.[1]

   atypical — *see* Schizophrenia, acute (undifferentiated)

   borderline — *see* Schizophrenia, latent

   catatonic type: Includes as an essential feature prominent psychomotor disturbances often alternating between extremes such as hyperkinesis and stupor, or automatic obedience and negativism. Constrained attitudes may be maintained for long periods: if the patient's limbs are put in some unnatural position, they may be held there for some time after the external force has been removed. Severe excitement may be a striking feature of the condition. Depressive or hypomanic concomitants may be present.[1]

   cenesthopathic — *see* Schizophrenia, acute (undifferentiated)

   childhood type — *see* Psychosis, child

   chronic undifferentiated — *see* Schizophrenia, residual

   cyclic — *see* Schizophrenia, schizo-affective type

   disorganized type: A form of schizophrenia in which affective changes are prominent, delusions and hallucinations fleeting and fragmentary, behavior irresponsible and unpredictable, and mannerisms common. The mood is shallow and inappropriate, accompanied by giggling or self-satisfied, self-absorbed smiling, or by a lofty manner, grimaces, mannerisms, pranks, hypochondriacal complaints, and reiterated phrases. Thought is disorganized. There is a tendency to remain solitary, and behavior seems empty of purpose and feeling. This form of schizophrenia usually starts between the ages of 15 and 25 years.[1]

   hebephrenic type — *see* Schizophrenia, disorganized type

   latent: It has not been possible to produce a generally acceptable description for this condition. It is not recommended for general use, but a description is provided for those who believe it to be useful: a condition of eccentric or inconsequent behavior and anomalies of affect which give the impression of schizophrenia though no definite and characteristic schizophrenic anomalies, present or past, have been manifest.[1]

   paranoid type: The form of schizophrenia in which relatively stable delusions, which may be accompanied by hallucinations, dominate the clinical picture. The delusions are frequently of persecution, but may take other forms (for example, of jealousy, exalted birth, Messianic mission, or bodily change). Hallucinations and erratic behavior may occur; in some cases conduct is seriously disturbed from the outset, thought disorder may be gross, and affective flattening with fragmentary delusions and hallucinations may develop.[1]

   prepsychotic — *see* Schizophrenia, latent

   prodromal — *see* Schizophrenia, latent

   pseudoneurotic — *see* Schizophrenia, latent

   pseudopsychopathic — *see* Schizophrenia, latent

   residual: A chronic form of schizophrenia in which the symptoms that persist from the acute phase have mostly lost their sharpness. Emotional response is blunted and thought disorder, even when gross, does not prevent the accomplishment of routine work.[1]

   schizo-affective type: A psychosis in which pronounced manic or depressive features are intermingled with schizophrenic features and which tends towards remission without permanent defect, but which is prone to recur. The diagnosis should be made only when both the affective and schizophrenic symptoms are pronounced.[1]

   simple type: A psychosis in which there is insidious development of oddities of conduct, inability to meet the demands of society, and decline in total performance. Delusions and hallucinations are not in evidence and the condition is less obviously psychotic than are the hebephrenic, catatonic, and paranoid types of schizophrenia. With increasing social impoverishment vagrancy may ensue and the patient becomes self-absorbed, idle, and aimless. Because the schizophrenic symptoms are not clear-cut, diagnosis of this form should be made sparingly, if at all.[1]

   simplex — *see* Schizophrenia, simple type

Schizophrenic syndrome of childhood — *see* Psychosis, child

Schizophreniform
   attack — *see* Schizophrenia, acute episode
   disorder — *see* Schizophrenia, acute episode
   psychosis — *see* Schizophrenia
      affective — *see* Schizophrenia, schizo-affective type
      confusional type — *see* Schizophrenia, acute episode

Schizotypal personality — *see* Personality disorder, schizotypal type

Senile dementia: Dementia occurring usually after the age of 65 in which any cerebral pathology other than that of senile atrophic change can be reasonably excluded.[1]

   delirium: Senile dementia with a superimposed reversible episode of acute confusional state.[1]

   delusional type: A type of senile dementia characterized by development in advanced old age, progressive in nature, in which delusions, varying from simple poorly formed paranoid delusions to highly formed paranoid delusional states, and hallucinations are also present.[1,2]

   depressed type: A type of senile dementia characterized by development in advanced old age, progressive in nature, in which depressive features, ranging from mild to severe forms of manic-depressive affective psychosis, are also present. Disturbance of the sleep-waking cycle and preoccupation with dead people are often particularly prominent.[1,2]

   paranoid type — *see* Senile dementia, delusional type

   simple type — *see* Senile dementia

Sensitiver Beziehungswahn: A paranoid state which, though in many ways akin to schizophrenic or affective states, differs from paranoia, simple paranoid state, shared paranoid disorder, or psychogenic psychosis.[1]

Sensitivity reaction of childhood or adolescence — *see* Shyness disorder of childhood

Separation anxiety disorder: A clinical disorder in children in which the predominant disturbance is exaggerated distress at separation from parents, home, or other familial surroundings. When separation is instituted, the child may experience anxiety to the point of panic. In adults a similar disorder is seen in agoraphobic reactions.[2]

Sexual deviations: Abnormal sexual inclinations or behavior which are part of a referral problem. The limits and features of normal sexual behavior have not been stated absolutely in

APPENDIX B

different societies and cultures, but are broadly such as serve approved social and biological purposes. The sexual activity of affected persons is directed primarily either towards people not of the opposite sex, or towards sexual acts not associated with coitus normally, or towards coitus performed under abnormal circumstances. If the anomalous behavior becomes manifest only during psychosis or other mental illness the condition should be classified under the major illness. It is common for more than one anomaly to occur together in the same individual; in that case the predominant deviation is classified. It is preferable not to diagnose sexual deviation in individuals who perform deviant sexual acts when normal sexual outlets are not available to them.[1] *See also* Exhibitionism, Fetishism, Homosexuality, Nymphomania, Pedophilia, Satyriasis, Sexual masochism, Sexual sadism, Transvestism, Voyeurism, and Zoophilia. Gender identity disorder and trans-sexualism are considered to be psychosexual gender identity disorders and are not included here.

Sexual masochism: A sexual deviation in which sexual arousal and pleasure is produced in an individual by his own physical or psychological suffering, and in which there are insistent and persistent fantasies wherein sexual excitement is produced as a result of suffering.[2]

Sexual sadism: A sexual deviation in which physical or psychological suffering inflicted on another person is utilized as a method of stimulating erotic excitement and orgasm, and in which there are insistent and persistent fantasies wherein sexual excitement is produced as a result of suffering inflicted on the partner.[2]

Shared paranoid disorder: Mainly delusional psychosis, usually chronic and often without florid features, which appears to have developed as a result of a close, if not dependent, relationship with another person who already has an established similar psychosis. The delusions are at least partly shared. The rare cases in which several persons are affected should also be included here.[1]

Shifting sleep-work schedule: A sleep disorder in which the phase-shift disruption of the 24-hour sleep-wake cycle occurs due to rapid changes in the individual's work schedule.[2]

Short sleeper: Individuals who typically need only 4–6 hours of sleep within the 24-hour cycle.[2]

Shyness disorder of childhood: A persistent and excessive shrinking from familiarity or contact with all strangers of sufficient severity as to interfere with peer functioning, yet there are warm and satisfying relationships with family members. A critical feature of this disorder is that the avoidant behavior with strangers persists even after prolonged exposure or contact.[2]

Sibling jealousy or rivalry: An emotional disorder related to competition between siblings for the love of a parent or for other recognition or gain.[3]

Simple phobia — *see* simple phobia under Phobia

Situational disturbance, acute — *see* Stress reaction, acute

Social phobia — *see* social phobia under Phobia

Social withdrawal of childhood — *see* Introverted disorder of childhood

Socialized conduct disorder — *see* socialized conduct disorder under Conduct disorders

Somatization disorder — *see* somatization disorder under Neurotic disorders

Somatoform disorder, atypical — *see* hypochondriasis under Neurotic disorders

Spasmus nutans — *see* Stereotyped repetitive movements

Specific academic or work inhibition: An adjustment reaction in which a specific academic or work inhibition occurs in an individual whose intellectual capacity, skills, and previous academic or work performance have been at least adequate, and in which the inhibition occurs despite apparent effort and is not due to any other mental disorder.[2]

Stammering — *see* Stuttering

Starch-eating — *see* Pica

Status postcommotio cerebri — *see* Postconcussion syndrome

Stereotyped repetitive movements: Disorders in which voluntary repetitive stereotyped movements, which are not due to any psychiatric or neurological condition, constitute the main feature. Includes head-banging, spasmus nutans, rocking, twirling, finger-flicking mannerisms, and eye poking. Such movements are particularly common in cases of mental retardation with sensory impairment or with environmental monotony.[1]

Stereotypies — *see* Stereotyped repetitive movements

Stress reaction
  acute: Acute transient disorders of any severity and nature of emotions, consciousness, and psychomotor states (singly or in combination) which occur in individuals, without any apparent pre-existing mental disorder, in response to exceptional physical or mental stress, such as natural catastrophe or battle, and which usually subside within hours or days.[1]
  chronic — *see* Adjustment reaction

Stupor
  catatonic — *see* Schizophrenia, catatonic type
  psychogenic — *see* Psychosis, reactive

Stuttering: Disorders in the rhythm of speech, in which the individual knows precisely what he wishes to say, but at the time is unable to say it because of an involuntary, repetitive prolongation or cessation of a sound.[1]

Subjective insomnia complaint: A complaint of insomnia made by the individual, which has not been investigated or proven.[2]

Tension headache: Headache of mental origin for which a more precise medical or psychiatric diagnosis cannot be made.[1]

Systematized delusions — *see* Paranoia

Tics: Disorders of no known organic origin in which the outstanding feature consists of quick, involuntary, apparently purposeless, and frequently repeated movements which are not due to any neurological condition. Any part of the body may be involved but the face is most frequently affected. Only one form of tic may be present, or there may be a combination of tics which are carried out simultaneously, alternatively, or consecutively.[1]

  chronic motor tic disorder: A tic disorder starting in childhood and persisting into adult life. The tic is limited to no more than three motor areas, and rarely has a verbal component.[2]

  Gilles de la Tourette's disorder [motor-verbal tic disorder]: A rare disorder occurring in individuals of any level of intelligence in which facial tics and tic-like throat noises become more marked and more generalized, and in which later whole words or short sentences (often with obscene content) are ejaculated spasmodically and involuntarily. There is some overlap with other varieties of tic.[1]

  transient tic disorder of childhood: Facial or other tics beginning in childhood, but limited to one year in duration.[2]

Tobacco use disorder: Cases in which tobacco is used to the detriment of a person's health or social functioning or in which there is tobacco dependence. Dependence is included here rather than under drug dependence because tobacco differs from other drugs of dependence in its psychotoxic effects.[1]

Tranquilizer abuse: Cases where an individual has taken the drug to the detriment of his health or social functioning, in doses above or for periods beyond those normally regarded as therapeutic.[1]

Transient organic psychotic condition — *see* Organic psychotic conditions, transient

Trans-sexualism — *see* trans-sexualism under Psychosexual identity disorders

Transvestism: Sexual deviation in which there is recurrent and persistent dressing in clothes of the opposite sex, and initially in the early stage of the illness, for the purpose of sexual arousal.[2]

Twilight state
  confusional — *see* Delirium, acute
  psychogenic — *see* Psychosis, reactive confusion

Undersocialized conduct disorder — *see* undersocialized conduct disorder under Conduct disorders

Unsocialized aggressive disorder — *see* undersocialized conduct disorder, aggressive type under Conduct disorders

Vaginismus, functional — *see* functional vaginismus under Psychosexual dysfunctions

Vorbeireden: The symptom of the approximate answer or talking past the point, seen in the Ganser syndrome, a form of factitious illness.[2]

Voyeurism: A sexual deviation in which the individual repetitively seeks out situations in which he engages in looking at unsuspecting women who are either naked, in the act of disrobing, or engaging in sexual activity. The act of looking is accompanied by sexual excitement, frequently with orgasm. In its severe form, the act of peeping constitutes the preferred to exclusive sexual activity of the individual.[2]

Wernicke-Korsakoff syndrome — *see* alcohol amnestic syndrome under Alcoholic psychoses

Withdrawal reaction of childhood or adolescence — *see* Introverted disorder of childhood

Word-deafness: A developmental delay in the comprehension of speech sounds.[1]

Zoophilia: Sexual or anal intercourse with animals.[1]

1. Manual of the *International Classification of Diseases, Injuries, and Causes of Death*, 9th Revision, World Health Organization, Geneva, Switzerland, 1975.
2. American Psychiatric Association, Task Force on Nomenclature and Statistics, Robert L. Spitzer, Chairman.
3. *A Psychiatric Glossary*, Fourth Edition, American Psychiatric Association, Washington, D.C., 1975.
4. *Dorland's Illustrated Medical Dictionary*, Twenty-fifth Edition, W. B. Saunders Company, Philadelphia, 1974.
5. *Stedman's Medical Dictionary*, Illustrated, Twenty-third Edition, the Williams and Williams Company, Baltimore, 1976.

APPENDIX C: CLASSIFICATION OF DRUGS BY AHFS LIST

CLASSIFICATION OF DRUGS BY AMERICAN HOSPITAL FORMULARY SERVICE LIST NUMBER AND THEIR ICD-9-CM EQUIVALENTS

The coding of adverse effects of drugs is keyed to the continually revised Hospital Formulary of the American Hospital Formulary Service (AHFS) published under the direction of the American Society of Hospital Pharmacists. The following section gives the ICD-9-CM diagnosis code for each AHFS list.

	AHFS* List	ICD-9-CM Diagnosis Code
4:00	ANTIHISTAMINE DRUGS	963.0
8:00	ANTI-INFECTIVE AGENTS	
8:04	Amebacides	961.5
	hydroxyquinoline derivatives	961.3
	arsenical anti-infectives	961.1
8:08	Anthelmintics	961.6
	quinoline derivatives	961.3
8:12.04	Antifungal Antibiotics	960.1
	nonantibiotics	961.9
8:12.06	Cephalosporins	960.5
8:12.08	Chloramphenicol	960.2
8:12.12	The Erythromycins	960.3
8:12.16	The Penicillins	960.0
8:12.20	The Streptomycins	960.6
8:12.24	The Tetracyclines	960.4
8:12.28	Other Antibiotics	960.8
	antimycobacterial antibiotics	960.6
	macrolides	960.3
8:16	Antituberculars	961.8
	antibiotics	960.6
8:18	Antivirals	961.7
8:20	Plasmodicides (antimalarials)	961.4
8:24	Sulfonamides	961.0
8:26	The Sulfones	961.8
8:28	Treponemicides	961.2
8:32	Trichomonacides	961.5
	hydroxyquinoline derivatives	961.3
	nitrofuran derivatives	961.9
8:36	Urinary Germicides	961.9
	quinoline derivatives	961.3
8:40	Other Anti-Infectives	961.9
10:00	ANTINEOPLASTIC AGENTS	963.1
	antibiotics	960.7
	progestogens	962.2
12:00	AUTONOMIC DRUGS	
12:04	Parasympathomimetic (Cholinergic) Agents	971.0
12:08	Parasympatholytic (Cholinergic Blocking) Agents	971.1
12:12	Sympathomimetic (Adrenergic) Agents	971.2
12:16	Sympatholytic (Adrenergic Blocking) Agents	971.3
12:20	Skeletal Muscle Relaxants	975.2
	central nervous system muscle-tone depressants	968.0
16:00	BLOOD DERIVATIVES	964.7
20:00	BLOOD FORMATION AND COAGULATION	
20:04	Antianemia Drugs	964.1
20:04.04	Iron Preparations	964.0
20:04.08	Liver and Stomach Preparations	964.1
20:12.04	Anticoagulants	964.2
20:12.08	Antiheparin Agents	964.5
20:12.12	Coagulants	964.5
20:12.16	Hemostatics	964.5
	capillary-active drugs	972.8
	fibrinolysis-affecting agents	964.4
	natural products	964.7
24:00	CARDIOVASCULAR DRUGS	
24:04	Cardiac Drugs	972.9
	cardiotonic agents	972.1
	rhythm regulators	972.0
24:06	Antilipemic Agents	972.2
	thyroid derivatives	962.7
24:08	Hypotensive Agents	972.6
	adrenergic blocking agents	971.3
	ganglion-blocking agents	972.3
	vasodilators	972.5
24:12	Vasodilating Agents	972.5
	coronary	972.4
	nicotinic acid derivatives	972.2
24:16	Sclerosing Agents	972.7
28:00	CENTRAL NERVOUS SYSTEM DRUGS	
28:04	General Anesthetics	968.4
	gaseous anesthetics	968.2
	halothane	968.1
	intravenous anesthetics	968.3
28:08	Analgesics and Antipyretics	965.9
	antirheumatics	965.6
	aromatic analgesics	965.4
	non-narcotics NEC	965.7
	opium alkaloids	965.00
	heroin	965.01
	methadone	965.02

	AHFS* List	ICD-9-CM Diagnosis Code
28:08	Analgesics and Antipyretics—*continued*	
	opium alkaloids—*continued*	
	specified type NEC	965.09
	pyrazole derivatives	965.5
	salicylates	965.1
	specified type NEC	965.8
28:10	Narcotic Antagonists	970.1
28:12	Anticonvulsants	966.3
	barbiturates	967.0
	benzodiazepine-based tranquilizers	969.4
	bromides	967.3
	hydantoin derivatives	966.1
	oxazolidine derivative	966.0
	succinimides	966.2
28:16.04	Antidepressants	969.0
28:16.08	Tranquilizers	969.5
	benzodiazepine-based	969.4
	butyrophenone-based	969.2
	major NEC	969.3
	phenothiazine-based	969.1
28:16.12	Other Psychotherapeutic Agents	969.8
28:20	Respiratory and Cerebral Stimulants	970.9
	analeptics	970.0
	anorexigenic agents	977.0
	psychostimulants	969.7
	specified type NEC	970.8
28:24	Sedatives and Hypnotics	967.9
	barbiturates	967.0
	benzodiazepine-based tranquilizers	969.4
	chloral hydrate group	967.1
	glutethamide group	967.5
	intravenous anesthetics	968.3
	methaqualone	967.4
	paraldehyde	967.2
	phenothiazine-based tranquilizers	969.1
	specified type NEC	967.8
	thiobarbiturates	968.3
	tranquilizer NEC	969.5
36:00	DIAGNOSTIC AGENTS	977.8
40:00	ELECTROLYTE, CALORIC, AND WATER BALANCE AGENTS NEC	974.5
40:04	Acidifying Agents	963.2
40:08	Alkalinizing Agents	963.3
40:10	Ammonia Detoxicants	974.5
40:12	Replacement Solutions NEC	974.5
	plasma volume expanders	964.8
40:16	Sodium-Removing Resins	974.5
40:18	Potassium-Removing Resins	974.5
40:20	Caloric Agents	974.5
40:24	Salt and Sugar Substitutes	974.5
40:28	Diuretics NEC	974.4
	carbonic acid anhydrase inhibitors	974.2
	mercurials	974.0
	purine derivatives	974.1
	saluretics	974.3
40:36	Irrigating Solutions	974.5
40:40	Uricosuric Agents	974.7
44:00	ENZYMES NEC	963.4
	fibrinolysis-affecting agents	964.4
	gastric agents	973.4
48:00	EXPECTORANTS AND COUGH PREPARATIONS	
	antihistamine agents	963.0
	antitussives	975.4
	codeine derivatives	965.09
	expectorants	975.5
	narcotic agents NEC	965.09
52:00	EYE, EAR, NOSE, AND THROAT PREPARATIONS	
52:04	Anti-Infectives	
	ENT	976.6
	ophthalmic	976.5
52:04.04	Antibiotics	
	ENT	976.6
	ophthalmic	976.5
52:04.06	Antivirals	
	ENT	976.6
	ophthalmic	976.5
52:04.08	Sulfonamides	
	ENT	976.6
	ophthalmic	976.5
52:04.12	Miscellaneous Anti-Infectives	
	ENT	976.6
	ophthalmic	976.5
52:08	Anti-Inflammatory Agents	
	ENT	976.6
	ophthalmic	976.5

APPENDIX C

	AHFS* List	ICD-9-CM Diagnosis Code
52:10	Carbonic Anhydrase Inhibitors	974.2
52:12	Contact Lens Solutions	976.5
52:16	Local Anesthetics	968.5
52:20	Miotics	971.0
52:24	Mydriatics	
	adrenergics	971.2
	anticholinergics	971.1
	antimuscarinics	971.1
	parasympatholytics	971.1
	spasmolytics	971.1
	sympathomimetics	971.2
52:28	Mouth Washes and Gargles	976.6
52:32	Vasoconstrictors	971.2
52:36	Unclassified Agents	
	ENT	976.6
	ophthalmic	976.5
56:00	GASTROINTESTINAL DRUGS	
56:04	Antacids and Absorbents	973.0
56:08	Anti-Diarrhea Agents	973.5
56:10	Antiflatulents	973.8
56:12	Cathartics NEC	973.3
	emollients	973.2
	irritants	973.1
56:16	Digestants	973.4
56:20	Emetics and Antiemetics	
	antiemetics	963.0
	emetics	973.6
56:24	Lipotropic Agents	977.1
60:00	GOLD COMPOUNDS	965.6
64:00	HEAVY METAL ANTAGONISTS	963.8
68:00	HORMONES AND SYNTHETIC SUBSTITUTES	
68:04	Adrenals	962.0
68:08	Androgens	962.1
68:12	Contraceptives	962.2
68:16	Estrogens	962.2
68:18	Gonadotropins	962.4
68:20	Insulins and Antidiabetic Agents	962.3
68:20.08	Insulins	962.3
68:24	Parathyroid	962.6
68:28	Pituitary	
	anterior	962.4
	posterior	962.5
68:32	Progestogens	962.2
68:34	Other Corpus Luteum Hormones	962.2
68:36	Thyroid and Antithyroid	
	antithyroid	962.8
	thyroid	962.7
72:00	LOCAL ANESTHETICS NEC	968.9
	topical (surface) agents	968.5
	infiltrating agents (intradermal) (subcutaneous) (submucosal)	968.5
	nerve blocking agents (peripheral) (plexus) (regional)	968.6
	spinal	968.7
76:00	OXYTOCICS	975.0
78:00	RADIOACTIVE AGENTS	990
80:00	SERUMS, TOXOIDS, AND VACCINES	
80:04	Serums	979.9
	immune globulin (gamma) (human)	964.6
80:08	Toxoids NEC	978.8
	diphtheria	978.5
	and tetanus	978.9
	with pertussis component	978.6
	tetanus	978.4
	and diphtheria	978.9
	with pertussis component	978.6
80:12	Vaccines NEC	979.9
	bacterial NEC	978.8
	with	
	other bacterial component	978.9
	pertussis component	978.6
	viral and rickettsial component	979.7
	rickettsial NEC	979.6
	with	
	bacterial component	979.7
	pertussis component	978.6
	viral component	979.7
	viral NEC	979.6
	with	
	bacterial component	979.7
	pertussis component	978.6
	rickettsial component	979.7
84:00	SKIN AND MUCOUS MEMBRANE PREPARATIONS	
84:04	Anti-Infectives	976.0
84:04.04	Antibiotics	976.0
84:04.08	Fungicides	976.0
84:04.12	Scabicides and Pediculicides	976.0
84:04.16	Miscellaneous Local Anti-Infectives	976.0
84:06	Anti-Inflammatory Agents	976.0
84:08	Antipruritics and Local Anesthetics	
	antipruritics	976.1
	local anesthetics	968.5
84:12	Astringents	976.2
84:16	Cell Stimulants and Proliferants	976.8
84:20	Detergents	976.2
84:24	Emollients, Demulcents, and Protectants	976.3
84:28	Keratolytic Agents	976.4
84:32	Keratoplastic Agents	976.4
84:36	Miscellaneous Agents	976.8
86:00	SPASMOLYTIC AGENTS	975.1
	antiasthmatics	975.7
	papaverine	972.5
	theophyllin	974.1
88:00	VITAMINS	
88:04	Vitamin A	963.5
88:08	Vitamin B Complex	963.5
	hematopoietic vitamin	964.1
	nicotinic acid derivatives	972.2
88:12	Vitamin C	963.5
88:16	Vitamin D	963.5
88:20	Vitamin E	963.5
88:24	Vitamin K Activity	964.3
88:28	Multivitamin Preparations	963.5
92:00	UNCLASSIFIED THERAPEUTIC AGENTS	977.8

* American Hospital Formulary Service

APPENDIX D: INDUSTRIAL ACCIDENTS ACCORDING TO AGENCY

CLASSIFICATION OF INDUSTRIAL ACCIDENTS ACCORDING TO AGENCY
Annex B to the Resolution concerning Statistics of Employment Injuries adopted by the Tenth International Conference of Labor Statisticians on 12 October 1962

1 MACHINES

11	**Prime-Movers, except Electrical Motors**
111	*Steam engines*
112	*Internal combustion engines*
119	*Others*
12	**Transmission Machinery**
121	*Transmission shafts*
122	*Transmission belts, cables, pulleys, pinions, chains, gears*
129	*Others*
13	**Metalworking Machines**
131	*Power presses*
132	*Lathes*
133	*Milling machines*
134	*Abrasive wheels*
135	*Mechanical shears*
136	*Forging machines*
137	*Rolling-mills*
139	*Others*
14	**Wood and Assimilated Machines**
141	*Circular saws*
142	*Other saws*
143	*Molding machines*
144	*Overhand planes*
149	*Others*
15	**Agricultural Machines**
151	*Reapers (including combine reapers)*
152	*Threshers*
159	*Others*
16	**Mining Machinery**
161	*Under-cutters*
169	*Others*
19	**Other Machines Not Elsewhere Classified**
191	*Earth-moving machines, excavating and scraping machines, except means of transport*
192	*Spinning, weaving and other textile machines*
193	*Machines for the manufacture of foodstuffs and beverages*
194	*Machines for the manufacture of paper*
195	*Printing machines*
199	*Others*

2 MEANS OF TRANSPORT AND LIFTING EQUIPMENT

21	**Lifting Machines and Appliances**
211	*Cranes*
212	*Lifts and elevators*
213	*Winches*
214	*Pulley blocks*
219	*Others*
22	**Means of Rail Transport**
221	*Inter-urban railways*
222	*Rail transport in mines, tunnels, quarries, industrial establishments, docks, etc.*
229	*Others*
23	**Other Wheeled Means of Transport, Excluding Rail Transport**
231	*Tractors*
232	*Lorries*
233	*Trucks*
234	*Motor vehicles, not elsewhere classified*
235	*Animal-drawn vehicles*
236	*Hand-drawn vehicles*
239	*Others*
24	**Means of Air Transport**
25	**Means of Water Transport**
251	*Motorized means of water transport*
252	*Non-motorized means of water transport*
26	**Other Means of Transport**
261	*Cable-cars*
262	*Mechanical conveyors, except cable-cars*
269	*Others*

3 OTHER EQUIPMENT

31	**Pressure Vessels**
311	*Boilers*
312	*Pressurized containers*
313	*Pressurized piping and accessories*
314	*Gas cylinders*
315	*Caissons, diving equipment*
319	*Others*
32	**Furnaces, Ovens, Kilns**
321	*Blast furnaces*
322	*Refining furnaces*
323	*Other furnaces*
324	*Kilns*
325	*Ovens*
33	**Refrigerating Plants**
34	**Electrical Installations, Including Electric Motors, but Excluding Electric Hand Tools**
341	*Rotating machines*
342	*Conductors*
343	*Transformers*
344	*Control apparatus*
349	*Others*
35	**Electric Hand Tools**
36	**Tools, Implements, and Appliances, Except Electric Hand Tools**
361	*Power-driven hand tools, except electric hand tools*
362	*Hand tools, not power-driven*
369	*Others*
37	**Ladders, Mobile Ramps**
38	**Scaffolding**
39	**Other Equipment, Not Elsewhere Classified**

4 MATERIALS, SUBSTANCES AND RADIATIONS

41	**Explosives**
42	**Dusts, Gases, Liquids and Chemicals, Excluding Explosives**
421	*Dusts*
422	*Gases, vapors, fumes*
423	*Liquids, not elsewhere classified*
424	*Chemicals, not elsewhere classified*
43	**Flying Fragments**
44	**Radiations**
441	*Ionizing radiations*
449	*Others*
49	**Other Materials and Substances Not Elsewhere Classified**

5 WORKING ENVIRONMENT

51	**Outdoor**
511	*Weather*
512	*Traffic and working surfaces*
513	*Water*
519	*Others*
52	**Indoor**
521	*Floors*
522	*Confined quarters*
523	*Stairs*
524	*Other traffic and working surfaces*
525	*Floor openings and wall openings*
526	*Environmental factors (lighting, ventilation, temperature, noise, etc.)*
529	*Others*
53	**Underground**
531	*Roofs and faces of mine roads and tunnels, etc.*
532	*Floors of mine roads and tunnels, etc.*
533	*Working-faces of mines, tunnels, etc.*
534	*Mine shafts*
535	*Fire*
536	*Water*
539	*Others*

6 OTHER AGENCIES, NOT ELSEWHERE CLASSIFIED

61	**Animals**
611	*Live animals*
612	*Animal products*
69	**Other Agencies, Not Elsewhere Classified**

7 AGENCIES NOT CLASSIFIED FOR LACK OF SUFFICIENT DATA

APPENDIX E: LIST OF THREE-DIGIT CATEGORIES

LIST OF THREE-DIGIT CATEGORIES

1. INFECTIOUS AND PARASITIC DISEASES

Intestinal infectious diseases (001-009)
- 001 Cholera
- 002 Typhoid and paratyphoid fevers
- 003 Other salmonella infections
- 004 Shigellosis
- 005 Other food poisoning (bacterial)
- 006 Amebiasis
- 007 Other protozoal intestinal diseases
- 008 Intestinal infections due to other organisms
- 009 Ill-defined intestinal infections

Tuberculosis (010-018)
- 010 Primary tuberculous infection
- 011 Pulmonary tuberculosis
- 012 Other respiratory tuberculosis
- 013 Tuberculosis of meninges and central nervous system
- 014 Tuberculosis of intestines, peritoneum, and mesenteric glands
- 015 Tuberculosis of bones and joints
- 016 Tuberculosis of genitourinary system
- 017 Tuberculosis of other organs
- 018 Miliary tuberculosis

Zoonotic bacterial diseases (020-027)
- 020 Plague
- 021 Tularemia
- 022 Anthrax
- 023 Brucellosis
- 024 Glanders
- 025 Melioidosis
- 026 Rat-bite fever
- 027 Other zoonotic bacterial diseases

Other bacterial diseases (030-042)
- 030 Leprosy
- 031 Diseases due to other mycobacteria
- 032 Diphtheria
- 033 Whooping cough
- 034 Streptococcal sore throat and scarlatina
- 035 Erysipelas
- 036 Meningococcal infection
- 037 Tetanus
- 038 Septicemia
- 039 Actinomycotic infections
- 040 Other bacterial diseases
- 041 Bacterial infection in conditions classified elsewhere and of unspecified site
- 042 Human immunodeficiency virus [HIV] disease

Poliomyelitis and other non-arthropod-borne viral diseases of central nervous system (045-049)
- 045 Acute poliomyelitis
- 046 Slow virus infection of central nervous system
- 047 Meningitis due to enterovirus
- 048 Other enterovirus diseases of central nervous system
- 049 Other non-arthropod-borne viral diseases of central nervous system

Viral diseases accompanied by exanthem (050-057)
- 050 Smallpox
- 051 Cowpox and paravaccinia
- 052 Chickenpox
- 053 Herpes zoster
- 054 Herpes simplex
- 055 Measles
- 056 Rubella
- 057 Other viral exanthemata

Arthropod-borne viral diseases (060-066)
- 060 Yellow fever
- 061 Dengue
- 062 Mosquito-borne viral encephalitis
- 063 Tick-borne viral encephalitis
- 064 Viral encephalitis transmitted by other and unspecified arthropods
- 065 Arthropod-borne hemorrhagic fever
- 066 Other arthropod-borne viral diseases

Other diseases due to viruses and Chlamydiae (070-079)
- 070 Viral hepatitis
- 071 Rabies
- 072 Mumps
- 073 Ornithosis
- 074 Specific diseases due to Coxsackievirus
- 075 Infectious mononucleosis
- 076 Trachoma
- 077 Other diseases of conjunctiva due to viruses and Chlamydiae
- 078 Other diseases due to viruses and Chlamydiae
- 079 Viral infection in conditions classified elsewhere and of unspecified site

Rickettsioses and other arthropod-borne diseases (080-088)
- 080 Louse-borne [epidemic] typhus
- 081 Other typhus
- 082 Tick-borne rickettsioses
- 083 Other rickettsioses
- 084 Malaria
- 085 Leishmaniasis
- 086 Trypanosomiasis
- 087 Relapsing fever
- 088 Other arthropod-borne diseases

Syphilis and other venereal diseases (090-099)
- 090 Congenital syphilis
- 091 Early syphilis, symptomatic
- 092 Early syphilis, latent
- 093 Cardiovascular syphilis
- 094 Neurosyphilis
- 095 Other forms of late syphilis, with symptoms
- 096 Late syphilis, latent
- 097 Other and unspecified syphilis
- 098 Gonococcal infections
- 099 Other venereal diseases

Other spirochetal diseases (100-104)
- 100 Leptospirosis
- 101 Vincent's angina
- 102 Yaws
- 103 Pinta
- 104 Other spirochetal infection

Mycoses (110-118)
- 110 Dermatophytosis
- 111 Dermatomycosis, other and unspecified
- 112 Candidiasis
- 114 Coccidioidomycosis
- 115 Histoplasmosis
- 116 Blastomycotic infection
- 117 Other mycoses
- 118 Opportunistic mycoses

Helminthiases (120-129)
- 120 Schistosomiasis [bilharziasis]
- 121 Other trematode infections
- 122 Echinococcosis
- 123 Other cestode infection
- 124 Trichinosis
- 125 Filarial infection and dracontiasis
- 126 Ancylostomiasis and necatoriasis
- 127 Other intestinal helminthiases
- 128 Other and unspecified helminthiases
- 129 Intestinal parasitism, unspecified

Other infectious and parasitic diseases (130-136)
- 130 Toxoplasmosis
- 131 Trichomoniasis
- 132 Pediculosis and phthirus infestation
- 133 Acariasis
- 134 Other infestation
- 135 Sarcoidosis
- 136 Other and unspecified infectious and parasitic diseases

Late effects of infectious and parasitic diseases (137-139)
- 137 Late effects of tuberculosis
- 138 Late effects of acute poliomyelitis
- 139 Late effects of other infectious and parasitic diseases

2. NEOPLASMS

Malignant neoplasm of lip, oral cavity, and pharynx (140-149)
- 140 Malignant neoplasm of lip
- 141 Malignant neoplasm of tongue
- 142 Malignant neoplasm of major salivary glands
- 143 Malignant neoplasm of gum
- 144 Malignant neoplasm of floor of mouth
- 145 Malignant neoplasm of other and unspecified parts of mouth
- 146 Malignant neoplasm of oropharynx
- 147 Malignant neoplasm of nasopharynx
- 148 Malignant neoplasm of hypopharynx
- 149 Malignant neoplasm of other and ill-defined sites within the lip, oral cavity, and pharynx

Malignant neoplasm of digestive organs and peritoneum (150-159)
- 150 Malignant neoplasm of esophagus
- 151 Malignant neoplasm of stomach
- 152 Malignant neoplasm of small intestine, including duodenum
- 153 Malignant neoplasm of colon
- 154 Malignant neoplasm of rectum, rectosigmoid junction, and anus
- 155 Malignant neoplasm of liver and intrahepatic bile ducts
- 156 Malignant neoplasm of gallbladder and extrahepatic bile ducts
- 157 Malignant neoplasm of pancreas
- 158 Malignant neoplasm of retroperitoneum and peritoneum
- 159 Malignant neoplasm of other and ill-defined sites within the digestive organs and peritoneum

Malignant neoplasm of respiratory and intrathoracic organs (160-165)
- 160 Malignant neoplasm of nasal cavities, middle ear, and accessory sinuses
- 161 Malignant neoplasm of larynx
- 162 Malignant neoplasm of trachea, bronchus, and lung
- 163 Malignant neoplasm of pleura
- 164 Malignant neoplasm of thymus, heart, and mediastinum
- 165 Malignant neoplasm of other and ill-defined sites within the respiratory system and intrathoracic organs

Malignant neoplasm of bone, connective tissue, skin, and breast (170-175)
- 170 Malignant neoplasm of bone and articular cartilage
- 171 Malignant neoplasm of connective and other soft tissue
- 172 Malignant melanoma of skin
- 173 Other malignant neoplasm of skin
- 174 Malignant neoplasm of female breast
- 175 Malignant neoplasm of male breast

Malignant neoplasm of genitourinary organs (179-189)
- 179 Malignant neoplasm of uterus, part unspecified
- 180 Malignant neoplasm of cervix uteri
- 181 Malignant neoplasm of placenta
- 182 Malignant neoplasm of body of uterus
- 183 Malignant neoplasm of ovary and other uterine adnexa
- 184 Malignant neoplasm of other and unspecified female genital organs
- 185 Malignant neoplasm of prostate
- 186 Malignant neoplasm of testis
- 187 Malignant neoplasm of penis and other male genital organs
- 188 Malignant neoplasm of bladder
- 189 Malignant neoplasm of kidney and other unspecified urinary organs

Malignant neoplasm of other and unspecified sites (190-199)
- 190 Malignant neoplasm of eye
- 191 Malignant neoplasm of brain
- 192 Malignant neoplasm of other and unspecified parts of nervous system
- 193 Malignant neoplasm of thyroid gland
- 194 Malignant neoplasm of other endocrine glands and related structures
- 195 Malignant neoplasm of other and ill-defined sites
- 196 Secondary and unspecified malignant neoplasm of lymph nodes
- 197 Secondary malignant neoplasm of respiratory and digestive systems
- 198 Secondary malignant neoplasm of other specified sites

199 Malignant neoplasm without specification of site

Malignant neoplasm of lymphatic and hematopoietic tissue (200-208)
200 Lymphosarcoma and reticulosarcoma
201 Hodgkin's disease
202 Other malignant neoplasm of lymphoid and histiocytic tissue
203 Multiple myeloma and immunoproliferative neoplasms
204 Lymphoid leukemia
205 Myeloid leukemia
206 Monocytic leukemia
207 Other specified leukemia
208 Leukemia of unspecified cell type

Benign neoplasms (210-229)
210 Benign neoplasm of lip, oral cavity, and pharynx
211 Benign neoplasm of other parts of digestive system
212 Benign neoplasm of respiratory and intrathoracic organs
213 Benign neoplasm of bone and articular cartilage
214 Lipoma
215 Other benign neoplasm of connective and other soft tissue
216 Benign neoplasm of skin
217 Benign neoplasm of breast
218 Uterine leiomyoma
219 Other benign neoplasm of uterus
220 Benign neoplasm of ovary
221 Benign neoplasm of other female genital organs
222 Benign neoplasm of male genital organs
223 Benign neoplasm of kidney and other urinary organs
224 Benign neoplasm of eye
225 Benign neoplasm of brain and other parts of nervous system
226 Benign neoplasm of thyroid gland
227 Benign neoplasm of other endocrine glands and related structures
228 Hemangioma and lymphangioma, any site
229 Benign neoplasm of other and unspecified sites

Carcinoma in situ (230-234)
230 Carcinoma in situ of digestive organs
231 Carcinoma in situ of respiratory system
232 Carcinoma in situ of skin
233 Carcinoma in situ of breast and genitourinary system
234 Carcinoma in situ of other and unspecified sites

Neoplasms of uncertain behavior (235-238)
235 Neoplasm of uncertain behavior of digestive and respiratory systems
236 Neoplasm of uncertain behavior of genitourinary organs
237 Neoplasm of uncertain behavior of endocrine glands and nervous system
238 Neoplasm of uncertain behavior of other and unspecified sites and tissues

Neoplasms of unspecified nature (239)
239 Neoplasm of unspecified nature

3. ENDOCRINE, NUTRITIONAL AND METABOLIC DISEASES, AND IMMUNITY DISORDERS

Disorders of thyroid gland (240-246)
240 Simple and unspecified goiter
241 Nontoxic nodular goiter
242 Thyrotoxicosis with or without goiter
243 Congenital hypothyroidism
244 Acquired hypothyroidism
245 Thyroiditis
246 Other disorders of thyroid

Diseases of other endocrine glands (250-259)
250 Diabetes mellitus
251 Other disorders of pancreatic internal secretion
252 Disorders of parathyroid gland
253 Disorders of the pituitary gland and its hypothalamic control
254 Diseases of thymus gland
255 Disorders of adrenal glands
256 Ovarian dysfunction
257 Testicular dysfunction
258 Polyglandular dysfunction and related disorders
259 Other endocrine disorders

Nutritional deficiencies (260-269)
260 Kwashiorkor
261 Nutritional marasmus
262 Other severe protein-calorie malnutrition
263 Other and unspecified protein-calorie malnutrition
264 Vitamin A deficiency
265 Thiamine and niacin deficiency states
266 Deficiency of B-complex components
267 Ascorbic acid deficiency
268 Vitamin D deficiency
269 Other nutritional deficiencies

Other metabolic disorders and immunity disorders (270-279)
270 Disorders of amino-acid transport and metabolism
271 Disorders of carbohydrate transport and metabolism
272 Disorders of lipoid metabolism
273 Disorders of plasma protein metabolism
274 Gout
275 Disorders of mineral metabolism
276 Disorders of fluid, electrolyte, and acid-base balance
277 Other and unspecified disorders of metabolism
278 Obesity and other hyperalimentation
279 Disorders involving the immune mechanism

Diseases of blood and blood-forming organs (280-289)
280 Iron deficiency anemias
281 Other deficiency anemias
282 Hereditary hemolytic anemias
283 Acquired hemolytic anemias
284 Aplastic anemia
285 Other and unspecified anemias
286 Coagulation defects
287 Purpura and other hemorrhagic conditions
288 Diseases of white blood cells
289 Other diseases of blood and blood-forming organs

5. MENTAL DISORDERS

Organic psychotic conditions (290-294)
290 Senile and presenile organic psychotic conditions
291 Alcoholic psychoses
292 Drug psychoses
293 Transient organic psychotic conditions
294 Other organic psychotic conditions (chronic)

Other psychoses (295-299)
295 Schizophrenic psychoses
296 Affective psychoses
297 Paranoid states
298 Other nonorganic psychoses
299 Psychoses with origin specific to childhood

Neurotic disorders, personality disorders, and other nonpsychotic mental disorders (300-316)
300 Neurotic disorders
301 Personality disorders
302 Sexual deviations and disorders
303 Alcohol dependence syndrome
304 Drug dependence
305 Nondependent abuse of drugs
306 Physiological malfunction arising from mental factors
307 Special symptoms or syndromes, not elsewhere classified
308 Acute reaction to stress
309 Adjustment reaction
310 Specific nonpsychotic mental disorders following organic brain damage
311 Depressive disorder, not elsewhere classified
312 Disturbance of conduct, not elsewhere classified
313 Disturbance of emotions specific to childhood and adolescence
314 Hyperkinetic syndrome of childhood
315 Specific delays in development
316 Psychic factors associated with diseases classified elsewhere

Mental retardation (317-319)
317 Mild mental retardation
318 Other specified mental retardation
319 Unspecified mental retardation

6. DISEASES OF THE NERVOUS SYSTEM AND SENSE ORGANS

Inflammatory diseases of the central nervous system (320-326)
320 Bacterial meningitis
321 Meningitis due to other organisms
322 Meningitis of unspecified cause
323 Encephalitis, myelitis, and encephalomyelitis
324 Intracranial and intraspinal abscess
325 Phlebitis and thrombophlebitis of intracranial venous sinuses
326 Late effects of intracranial abscess or pyogenic infection

Hereditary and degenerative diseases of the central nervous system (330-337)
330 Cerebral degenerations usually manifest in childhood
331 Other cerebral degenerations
332 Parkinson's disease
333 Other extrapyramidal diseases and abnormal movement disorders
334 Spinocerebellar disease
335 Anterior horn cell disease
336 Other diseases of spinal cord
337 Disorders of the autonomic nervous system

Other disorders of the central nervous system (340-349)
340 Multiple sclerosis
341 Other demyelinating diseases of central nervous system
342 Hemiplegia
343 Infantile cerebral palsy
344 Other paralytic syndromes
345 Epilepsy
346 Migraine
347 Cataplexy and narcolepsy
348 Other conditions of brain
349 Other and unspecified disorders of the nervous system

Disorders of the peripheral nervous system (350-359)
350 Trigeminal nerve disorders
351 Facial nerve disorders
352 Disorders of other cranial nerves
353 Nerve root and plexus disorders
354 Mononeuritis of upper limb and mononeuritis multiplex
355 Mononeuritis of lower limb
356 Hereditary and idiopathic peripheral neuropathy
357 Inflammatory and toxic neuropathy
358 Myoneural disorders
359 Muscular dystrophies and other myopathies

Disorders of the eye and adnexa (360-379)
360 Disorders of the globe
361 Retinal detachments and defects
362 Other retinal disorders
363 Chorioretinal inflammations and scars and other disorders of choroid
364 Disorders of iris and ciliary body
365 Glaucoma
366 Cataract
367 Disorders of refraction and accommodation
368 Visual disturbances
369 Blindness and low vision
370 Keratitis
371 Corneal opacity and other disorders of cornea
372 Disorders of conjunctiva
373 Inflammation of eyelids
374 Other disorders of eyelids
375 Disorders of lacrimal system
376 Disorders of the orbit
377 Disorders of optic nerve and visual pathways

LIST OF THREE-DIGIT CATEGORIES

378 Strabismus and other disorders of binocular eye movements
379 Other disorders of eye

Diseases of the ear and mastoid process (380-389)
380 Disorders of external ear
381 Nonsuppurative otitis media and Eustachian tube disorders
382 Suppurative and unspecified otitis media
383 Mastoiditis and related conditions
384 Other disorders of tympanic membrane
385 Other disorders of middle ear and mastoid
386 Vertiginous syndromes and other disorders of vestibular system
387 Otosclerosis
388 Other disorders of ear
389 Deafness

7. DISEASES OF THE CIRCULATORY SYSTEM

Acute rheumatic fever (390-392)
390 Rheumatic fever without mention of heart involvement
391 Rheumatic fever with heart involvement
392 Rheumatic chorea

Chronic rheumatic heart disease (393-398)
393 Chronic rheumatic pericarditis
394 Diseases of mitral valve
395 Diseases of aortic valve
396 Diseases of mitral and aortic valves
397 Diseases of other endocardial structures
398 Other rheumatic heart disease

Hypertensive disease (401-405)
401 Essential hypertension
402 Hypertensive heart disease
403 Hypertensive renal disease
404 Hypertensive heart and renal disease
405 Secondary hypertension

Ischemic heart disease (410-414)
410 Acute myocardial infarction
411 Other acute and subacute form of ischemic heart disease
412 Old myocardial infarction
413 Angina pectoris
414 Other forms of chronic ischemic heart disease

Diseases of pulmonary circulation (415-417)
415 Acute pulmonary heart disease
416 Chronic pulmonary heart disease
417 Other diseases of pulmonary circulation

Other forms of heart disease (420-429)
420 Acute pericarditis
421 Acute and subacute endocarditis
422 Acute myocarditis
423 Other diseases of pericardium
424 Other diseases of endocardium
425 Cardiomyopathy
426 Conduction disorders
427 Cardiac dysrhythmias
428 Heart failure
429 Ill-defined descriptions and complications of heart disease

Cerebrovascular disease (430-438)
430 Subarachnoid hemorrhage
431 Intracerebral hemorrhage
432 Other and unspecified intracranial hemorrhage
433 Occlusion and stenosis of precerebral arteries
434 Occlusion of cerebral arteries
435 Transient cerebral ischemia
436 Acute but ill-defined cerebrovascular disease
437 Other and ill-defined cerebrovascular disease
438 Late effects of cerebrovascular disease

Diseases of arteries, arterioles, and capillaries (440-448)
440 Atherosclerosis
441 Aortic aneurysm
442 Other aneurysm
443 Other peripheral vascular disease
444 Arterial embolism and thrombosis
446 Polyarteritis nodosa and allied conditions
447 Other disorders of arteries and arterioles
448 Diseases of capillaries

Diseases of veins and lymphatics, and other diseases of circulatory system (451-459)
451 Phlebitis and thrombophlebitis
452 Portal vein thrombosis
453 Other venous embolism and thrombosis
454 Varicose veins of lower extremities
455 Hemorrhoids
456 Varicose veins of other sites
457 Noninfective disorders of lymphatic channels
458 Hypotension
459 Other disorders of circulatory system

8. DISEASES OF THE RESPIRATORY SYSTEM

Acute respiratory infections (460-466)
460 Acute nasopharyngitis [common cold]
461 Acute sinusitis
462 Acute pharyngitis
463 Acute tonsillitis
464 Acute laryngitis and tracheitis
465 Acute upper respiratory infections of multiple or unspecified sites
466 Acute bronchitis and bronchiolitis

Other diseases of upper respiratory tract (470-478)
470 Deviated nasal septum
471 Nasal polyps
472 Chronic pharyngitis and nasopharyngitis
473 Chronic sinusitis
474 Chronic disease of tonsils and adenoids
475 Peritonsillar abscess
476 Chronic laryngitis and laryngotracheitis
477 Allergic rhinitis
478 Other diseases of upper respiratory tract

Pneumonia and influenza (480-487)
480 Viral pneumonia
481 Pneumococcal pneumonia
482 Other bacterial pneumonia
483 Pneumonia due to other specified organism
484 Pneumonia in infectious diseases classified elsewhere
485 Bronchopneumonia, organism unspecified
486 Pneumonia, organism unspecified
487 Influenza

Chronic obstructive pulmonary disease and allied conditions (490-496)
490 Bronchitis, not specified as acute or chronic
491 Chronic bronchitis
492 Emphysema
493 Asthma
494 Bronchiectasis
495 Extrinsic allergic alveolitis
496 Chronic airways obstruction, not elsewhere classified

Pneumoconioses and other lung diseases due to external agents (500-508)
500 Coal workers' pneumoconiosis
501 Asbestosis
502 Pneumoconiosis due to other silica or silicates
503 Pneumoconiosis due to other inorganic dust
504 Pneumopathy due to inhalation of other dust
505 Pneumoconiosis, unspecified
506 Respiratory conditions due to chemical fumes and vapors
507 Pneumonitis due to solids and liquids
508 Respiratory conditions due to other and unspecified external agents

Other diseases of respiratory system (510-519)
510 Empyema
511 Pleurisy
512 Pneumothorax
513 Abscess of lung and mediastinum
514 Pulmonary congestion and hypostasis
515 Postinflammatory pulmonary fibrosis
516 Other alveolar and parietoalveolar pneumopathy
517 Lung involvement in conditions classified elsewhere
518 Other diseases of lung
519 Other diseases of respiratory system

9. DISEASES OF THE DIGESTIVE SYSTEM

Diseases of oral cavity, salivary glands, and jaws (520-529)
520 Disorders of tooth development and eruption
521 Diseases of hard tissues of teeth
522 Diseases of pulp and periapical tissues
523 Gingival and periodontal diseases
524 Dentofacial anomalies, including malocclusion
525 Other diseases and conditions of the teeth and supporting structures
526 Diseases of the jaws
527 Diseases of the salivary glands
528 Diseases of the oral soft tissues, excluding lesions specific for gingiva and tongue
529 Diseases and other conditions of the tongue

Diseases of esophagus, stomach, and duodenum (530-537)
530 Diseases of esophagus
531 Gastric ulcer
532 Duodenal ulcer
533 Peptic ulcer, site unspecified
534 Gastrojejunal ulcer
535 Gastritis and duodenitis
536 Disorders of function of stomach
537 Other disorders of stomach and duodenum

Appendicitis (540-543)
540 Acute appendicitis
541 Appendicitis, unqualified
542 Other appendicitis
543 Other diseases of appendix

Hernia of abdominal cavity (550-553)
550 Inguinal hernia
551 Other hernia of abdominal cavity, with gangrene
552 Other hernia of abdominal cavity, with obstruction, but without mention of gangrene
553 Other hernia of abdominal cavity without mention of obstruction or gangrene

Noninfective enteritis and colitis (555-558)
555 Regional enteritis
556 Ulcerative colitis
557 Vascular insufficiency of intestine
558 Other noninfective gastroenteritis and colitis

Other diseases of intestines and peritoneum (560-569)
560 Intestinal obstruction without mention of hernia
562 Diverticula of intestine
564 Functional digestive disorders, not elsewhere classified
565 Anal fissure and fistula
566 Abscess of anal and rectal regions
567 Peritonitis
568 Other disorders of peritoneum
569 Other disorders of intestine

Other diseases of digestive system (570-579)
570 Acute and subacute necrosis of liver
571 Chronic liver disease and cirrhosis
572 Liver abscess and sequelae of chronic liver disease
573 Other disorders of liver
574 Cholelithiasis
575 Other disorders of gallbladder
576 Other disorders of biliary tract
577 Diseases of pancreas
578 Gastrointestinal hemorrhage
579 Intestinal malabsorption

10. DISEASES OF THE GENITOURINARY SYSTEM

Nephritis, nephrotic syndrome, and nephrosis (580-589)
580 Acute glomerulonephritis
581 Nephrotic syndrome
582 Chronic glomerulonephritis
583 Nephritis and nephropathy, not specified as acute or chronic
584 Acute renal failure
585 Chronic renal failure
586 Renal failure, unspecified
587 Renal sclerosis, unspecified
588 Disorders resulting from impaired renal function
589 Small kidney of unknown cause

Other diseases of urinary system (590-599)
590 Infections of kidney

591 Hydronephrosis
592 Calculus of kidney and ureter
593 Other disorders of kidney and ureter
594 Calculus of lower urinary tract
595 Cystitis
596 Other disorders of bladder
597 Urethritis, not sexually transmitted, and urethral syndrome
598 Urethral stricture
599 Other disorders of urethra and urinary tract

Diseases of male genital organs (600-608)
600 Hyperplasia of prostate
601 Inflammatory diseases of prostate
602 Other disorders of prostate
603 Hydrocele
604 Orchitis and epididymitis
605 Redundant prepuce and phimosis
606 Infertility, male
607 Disorders of penis
608 Other disorders of male genital organs

Disorders of breast (610-611)
610 Benign mammary dysplasias
611 Other disorders of breast

Inflammatory disease of female pelvic organs (614-616)
614 Inflammatory disease of ovary, fallopian tube, pelvic cellular tissue, and peritoneum
615 Inflammatory diseases of uterus, except cervix
616 Inflammatory disease of cervix, vagina, and vulva

Other disorders of female genital tract (617-629)
617 Endometriosis
618 Genital prolapse
619 Fistula involving female genital tract
620 Noninflammatory disorders of ovary, fallopian tube, and broad ligament
621 Disorders of uterus, not elsewhere classified
622 Noninflammatory disorders of cervix
623 Noninflammatory disorders of vagina
624 Noninflammatory disorders of vulva and perineum
625 Pain and other symptoms associated with female genital organs
626 Disorders of menstruation and other abnormal bleeding from female genital tract
627 Menopausal and postmenopausal disorders
628 Infertility, female
629 Other disorders of female genital organs

11. COMPLICATIONS OF PREGNANCY, CHILDBIRTH AND THE PUERPERIUM

Ectopic and molar pregnancy and other pregnancy with abortive outcome (630-639)
630 Hydatidiform mole
631 Other abnormal product of conception
632 Missed abortion
633 Ectopic pregnancy
634 Spontaneous abortion
635 Legally induced abortion
636 Illegally induced abortion
637 Unspecified abortion
638 Failed attempted abortion
639 Complications following abortion and ectopic and molar pregnancies

Complications mainly related to pregnancy (640-648)
640 Hemorrhage in early pregnancy
641 Antepartum hemorrhage, abruptio placentae, and placenta previa
642 Hypertension complicating pregnancy, childbirth, and the puerperium
643 Excessive vomiting in pregnancy
644 Early or threatened labor
645 Prolonged pregnancy
646 Other complications of pregnancy, not elsewhere classified
647 Infective and parasitic conditions in the mother classifiable elsewhere but complicating pregnancy, childbirth, and the puerperium
648 Other current conditions in the mother classifiable elsewhere but complicating pregnancy, childbirth, and the puerperium

Normal delivery, and other indications for care in pregnancy, labor, and delivery (650-659)
650 Delivery in a completely normal case
651 Multiple gestation
652 Malposition and malpresentation of fetus
653 Disproportion
654 Abnormality of organs and soft tissues of pelvis
655 Known or suspected fetal abnormality affecting management of mother
656 Other fetal and placental problems affecting management of mother
657 Polyhydramnios
658 Other problems associated with amniotic cavity and membranes
659 Other indications for care or intervention related to labor and delivery and not elsewhere classified

Complications occurring mainly in the course of labor and delivery (660-669)
660 Obstructed labor
661 Abnormality of forces of labor
662 Long labor
663 Umbilical cord complications
664 Trauma to perineum and vulva during delivery
665 Other obstetrical trauma
666 Postpartum hemorrhage
667 Retained placenta or membranes, without hemorrhage
668 Complications of the administration of anesthetic or other sedation in labor and delivery
669 Other complications of labor and delivery, not elsewhere classified

Complications of the puerperium (670-677)
670 Major puerperal infection
671 Venous complications in pregnancy and the puerperium
672 Pyrexia of unknown origin during the puerperium
673 Obstetrical pulmonary embolism
674 Other and unspecified complications of the puerperium, not elsewhere classified
675 Infections of the breast and nipple associated with childbirth
676 Other disorders of the breast associated with childbirth, and disorders of lactation
677 Late effect of complication of pregnancy, childbirth, and the puerperium

12. DISEASES OF THE SKIN AND SUBCUTANEOUS TISSUE

Infections of skin and subcutaneous tissue (680-686)
680 Carbuncle and furuncle
681 Cellulitis and abscess of finger and toe
682 Other cellulitis and abscess
683 Acute lymphadenitis
684 Impetigo
685 Pilonidal cyst
686 Other local infections of skin and subcutaneous tissue

Other inflammatory conditions of skin and subcutaneous tissue (690-698)
690 Erythematosquamous dermatosis
691 Atopic dermatitis and related conditions
692 Contact dermatitis and other eczema
693 Dermatitis due to substances taken internally
694 Bullous dermatoses
695 Erythematous conditions
696 Psoriasis and similar disorders
697 Lichen
698 Pruritus and related conditions

Other diseases of skin and subcutaneous tissue (700-709)
700 Corns and callosities
701 Other hypertrophic and atrophic conditions of skin
702 Other dermatoses
703 Diseases of nail
704 Diseases of hair and hair follicles
705 Disorders of sweat glands
706 Diseases of sebaceous glands
707 Chronic ulcer of skin
708 Urticaria
709 Other disorders of skin and subcutaneous tissue

13. DISEASES OF THE MUSCULOSKELETAL SYSTEM AND CONNECTIVE TISSUE

Arthropathies and related disorders (710-719)
710 Diffuse diseases of connective tissue
711 Arthropathy associated with infections
712 Crystal arthropathies
713 Arthropathy associated with other disorders classified elsewhere
714 Rheumatoid arthritis and other inflammatory polyarthropathies
715 Osteoarthrosis and allied disorders
716 Other and unspecified arthropathies
717 Internal derangement of knee
718 Other derangement of joint
719 Other and unspecified disorder of joint

Dorsopathies (720-724)
720 Ankylosing spondylitis and other inflammatory spondylopathies
721 Spondylosis and allied disorders
722 Intervertebral disc disorders
723 Other disorders of cervical region
724 Other and unspecified disorders of back

Rheumatism, excluding the back (725-729)
725 Polymyalgia rheumatica
726 Peripheral enthesopathies and allied syndromes
727 Other disorders of synovium, tendon, and bursa
728 Disorders of muscle, ligament, and fascia
729 Other disorders of soft tissues

Osteopathies, chondropathies, and acquired musculoskeletal deformities (730-739)
730 Osteomyelitis, periostitis, and other infections involving bone
731 Osteitis deformans and osteopathies associated with other disorders classified elsewhere
732 Osteochondropathies
733 Other disorders of bone and cartilage
734 Flat foot
735 Acquired deformities of toe
736 Other acquired deformities of limbs
737 Curvature of spine
738 Other acquired deformity
739 Nonallopathic lesions, not elsewhere classified

14. CONGENITAL ANOMALIES
740 Anencephalus and similar anomalies
741 Spina bifida
742 Other congenital anomalies of nervous system
743 Congenital anomalies of eye
744 Congenital anomalies of ear, face, and neck
745 Bulbus cordis anomalies and anomalies of cardiac septal closure
746 Other congenital anomalies of heart
747 Other congenital anomalies of circulatory system
748 Congenital anomalies of respiratory system
749 Cleft palate and cleft lip
750 Other congenital anomalies of upper alimentary tract
751 Other congenital anomalies of digestive system
752 Congenital anomalies of genital organs
753 Congenital anomalies of urinary system
754 Certain congenital musculoskeletal deformities
755 Other congenital anomalies of limbs
756 Other congenital musculoskeletal anomalies
757 Congenital anomalies of the integument
758 Chromosomal anomalies
759 Other and unspecified congenital anomalies

15. CERTAIN CONDITIONS ORIGINATING IN THE PERINATAL PERIOD

Maternal causes of perinatal morbidity and mortality (760-763)
760 Fetus or newborn affected by maternal conditions which may be unrelated to present pregnancy

LIST OF THREE-DIGIT CATEGORIES

761 Fetus or newborn affected by maternal complications of pregnancy
762 Fetus or newborn affected by complications of placenta, cord, and membranes
763 Fetus or newborn affected by other complications of labor and delivery

Other conditions originating in the perinatal period (764-779)
764 Slow fetal growth and fetal malnutrition
765 Disorders relating to short gestation and unspecified low birthweight
766 Disorders relating to long gestation and high birthweight
767 Birth trauma
768 Intrauterine hypoxia and birth asphyxia
769 Respiratory distress syndrome
770 Other respiratory conditions of fetus and newborn
771 Infections specific to the perinatal period
772 Fetal and neonatal hemorrhage
773 Hemolytic disease of fetus or newborn, due to isoimmunization
774 Other perinatal jaundice
775 Endocrine and metabolic disturbances specific to the fetus and newborn
776 Hematological disorders of fetus and newborn
777 Perinatal disorders of digestive system
778 Conditions involving the integument and temperature regulation of fetus and newborn
779 Other and ill-defined conditions originating in the perinatal period

16. SYMPTOMS, SIGNS, AND ILL-DEFINED CONDITIONS

Symptoms (780-789)
780 General symptoms
781 Symptoms involving nervous and musculoskeletal systems
782 Symptoms involving skin and other integumentary tissue
783 Symptoms concerning nutrition, metabolism, and development
784 Symptoms involving head and neck
785 Symptoms involving cardiovascular system
786 Symptoms involving respiratory system and other chest symptoms
787 Symptoms involving digestive system
788 Symptoms involving urinary system
789 Other symptoms involving abdomen and pelvis

Nonspecific abnormal findings (790-796)
790 Nonspecific findings on examination of blood
791 Nonspecific findings on examination of urine
792 Nonspecific abnormal findings in other body substances
793 Nonspecific abnormal findings on radiological and other examination of body structure
794 Nonspecific abnormal results of function studies
795 Nonspecific abnormal histological and immunological findings
796 Other nonspecific abnormal findings

Ill-defined and unknown causes of morbidity and mortality (797-799)
797 Senility without mention of psychosis
798 Sudden death, cause unknown
799 Other ill-defined and unknown causes of morbidity and mortality

17. INJURY AND POISONING

Fracture of skull (800-804)
800 Fracture of vault of skull
801 Fracture of base of skull
802 Fracture of face bones
803 Other and unqualified skull fractures
804 Multiple fractures involving skull or face with other bones

Fracture of spine and trunk (805-809)
805 Fracture of vertebral column without mention of spinal cord lesion
806 Fracture of vertebral column with spinal cord lesion
807 Fracture of rib(s), sternum, larynx, and trachea
808 Fracture of pelvis
809 Ill-defined fractures of bones of trunk

Fracture of upper limb (810-819)
810 Fracture of clavicle
811 Fracture of scapula
812 Fracture of humerus
813 Fracture of radius and ulna
814 Fracture of carpal bone(s)
815 Fracture of metacarpal bone(s)
816 Fracture of one or more phalanges of hand
817 Multiple fractures of hand bones
818 Ill-defined fractures of upper limb
819 Multiple fractures involving both upper limbs, and upper limb with rib(s) and sternum

Fracture of lower limb (820-829)
820 Fracture of neck of femur
821 Fracture of other and unspecified parts of femur
822 Fracture of patella
823 Fracture of tibia and fibula
824 Fracture of ankle
825 Fracture of one or more tarsal and metatarsal bones
826 Fracture of one or more phalanges of foot
827 Other, multiple, and ill-defined fractures of lower limb
828 Multiple fractures involving both lower limbs, lower with upper limb, and lower limb(s) with rib(s) and sternum
829 Fracture of unspecified bones

Dislocation (830-839)
830 Dislocation of jaw
831 Dislocation of shoulder
832 Dislocation of elbow
833 Dislocation of wrist
834 Dislocation of finger
835 Dislocation of hip
836 Dislocation of knee
837 Dislocation of ankle
838 Dislocation of foot
839 Other, multiple, and ill-defined dislocations

Sprains and strains of joints and adjacent muscles (840-848)
840 Sprains and strains of shoulder and upper arm
841 Sprains and strains of elbow and forearm
842 Sprains and strains of wrist and hand
843 Sprains and strains of hip and thigh
844 Sprains and strains of knee and leg
845 Sprains and strains of ankle and foot
846 Sprains and strains of sacroiliac region
847 Sprains and strains of other and unspecified parts of back
848 Other and ill-defined sprains and strains

Intracranial injury, excluding those with skull fracture (850-854)
850 Concussion
851 Cerebral laceration and contusion
852 Subarachnoid, subdural, and extradural hemorrhage, following injury
853 Other and unspecified intracranial hemorrhage following injury
854 Intracranial injury of other and unspecified nature

Internal injury of chest, abdomen, and pelvis (860-869)
860 Traumatic pneumothorax and hemothorax
861 Injury to heart and lung
862 Injury to other and unspecified intrathoracic organs
863 Injury to gastrointestinal tract
864 Injury to liver
865 Injury to spleen
866 Injury to kidney
867 Injury to pelvic organs
868 Injury to other intra-abdominal organs
869 Internal injury to unspecified or ill-defined organs

Open wound of head, neck, and trunk (870-879)
870 Open wound of ocular adnexa
871 Open wound of eyeball
872 Open wound of ear
873 Other open wound of head
874 Open wound of neck
875 Open wound of chest (wall)
876 Open wound of back
877 Open wound of buttock
878 Open wound of genital organs (external), including traumatic amputation
879 Open wound of other and unspecified sites, except limbs

Open wound of upper limb (880-887)
880 Open wound of shoulder and upper arm
881 Open wound of elbow, forearm, and wrist
882 Open wound of hand except finger(s) alone
883 Open wound of finger(s)
884 Multiple and unspecified open wound of upper limb
885 Traumatic amputation of thumb (complete) (partial)
886 Traumatic amputation of other finger(s) (complete) (partial)
887 Traumatic amputation of arm and hand (complete) (partial)

Open wound of lower limb (890-897)
890 Open wound of hip and thigh
891 Open wound of knee, leg [except thigh], and ankle
892 Open wound of foot except toe(s) alone
893 Open wound of toe(s)
894 Multiple and unspecified open wound of lower limb
895 Traumatic amputation of toe(s) (complete) (partial)
896 Traumatic amputation of foot (complete) (partial)
897 Traumatic amputation of leg(s) (complete) (partial)

Injury to blood vessels (900-904)
900 Injury to blood vessels of head and neck
901 Injury to blood vessels of thorax
902 Injury to blood vessels of abdomen and pelvis
903 Injury to blood vessels of upper extremity
904 Injury to blood vessels of lower extremity and unspecified sites

Late effects of injuries, poisonings, toxic effects, and other external causes (905-909)
905 Late effects of musculoskeletal and connective tissue injuries
906 Late effects of injuries to skin and subcutaneous tissues
907 Late effects of injuries to the nervous system
908 Late effects of other and unspecified injuries
909 Late effects of other and unspecified external causes

Superficial injury (910-919)
910 Superficial injury of face, neck, and scalp except eye
911 Superficial injury of trunk
912 Superficial injury of shoulder and upper arm
913 Superficial injury of elbow, forearm, and wrist
914 Superficial injury of hand(s) except finger(s) alone
915 Superficial injury of finger(s)
916 Superficial injury of hip, thigh, leg, and ankle
917 Superficial injury of foot and toe(s)
918 Superficial injury of eye and adnexa
919 Superficial injury of other, multiple, and unspecified sites

Contusion with intact skin surface (920-924)
920 Contusion of face, scalp, and neck except eye(s)
921 Contusion of eye and adnexa
922 Contusion of trunk
923 Contusion of upper limb
924 Contusion of lower limb and of other and unspecified sites

APPENDIX E

Crushing injury (925-929)
925 Crushing injury of face, scalp, and neck
926 Crushing injury of trunk
927 Crushing injury of upper limb
928 Crushing injury of lower limb
929 Crushing injury of multiple and unspecified sites

Effects of foreign body entering through orifice (930-939)
930 Foreign body on external eye
931 Foreign body in ear
932 Foreign body in nose
933 Foreign body in pharynx and larynx
934 Foreign body in trachea, bronchus, and lung
935 Foreign body in mouth, esophagus, and stomach
936 Foreign body in intestine and colon
937 Foreign body in anus and rectum
938 Foreign body in digestive system, unspecified
939 Foreign body in genitourinary tract

Burns (940-949)
940 Burn confined to eye and adnexa
941 Burn of face, head, and neck
942 Burn of trunk
943 Burn of upper limb, except wrist and hand
944 Burn of wrist(s) and hand(s)
945 Burn of lower limb(s)
946 Burns of multiple specified sites
947 Burn of internal organs
948 Burns classified according to extent of body surface involved
949 Burn, unspecified

Injury to nerves and spinal cord (950-957)
950 Injury to optic nerve and pathways
951 Injury to other cranial nerve(s)
952 Spinal cord injury without evidence of spinal bone injury
953 Injury to nerve roots and spinal plexus
954 Injury to other nerve(s) of trunk excluding shoulder and pelvic girdles
955 Injury to peripheral nerve(s) of shoulder girdle and upper limb
956 Injury to peripheral nerve(s) of pelvic girdle and lower limb
957 Injury to other and unspecified nerves

Certain traumatic complications and unspecified injuries (958-959)
958 Certain early complications of trauma
959 Injury, other and unspecified

Poisoning by drugs, medicinals and biological substances (960-979)
960 Poisoning by antibiotics
961 Poisoning by other anti-infectives
962 Poisoning by hormones and synthetic substitutes
963 Poisoning by primarily systemic agents
964 Poisoning by agents primarily affecting blood constituents
965 Poisoning by analgesics, antipyretics, and antirheumatics
966 Poisoning by anticonvulsants and anti-Parkinsonism drugs
967 Poisoning by sedatives and hypnotics
968 Poisoning by other central nervous system depressants and anesthetics
969 Poisoning by psychotropic agents
970 Poisoning by central nervous system stimulants
971 Poisoning by drugs primarily affecting the autonomic nervous system
972 Poisoning by agents primarily affecting the cardiovascular system
973 Poisoning by agents primarily affecting the gastrointestinal system
974 Poisoning by water, mineral, and uric acid metabolism drugs
975 Poisoning by agents primarily acting on the smooth and skeletal muscles and respiratory system
976 Poisoning by agents primarily affecting skin and mucous membrane, ophthalmological, otorhinolaryngological, and dental drugs
977 Poisoning by other and unspecified drugs and medicinals
978 Poisoning by bacterial vaccines
979 Poisoning by other vaccines and biological substances

Toxic effects of substances chiefly nonmedicinal as to source (980-989)
980 Toxic effect of alcohol
981 Toxic effect of petroleum products
982 Toxic effect of solvents other than petroleum-based
983 Toxic effect of corrosive aromatics, acids, and caustic alkalis
984 Toxic effect of lead and its compounds (including fumes)
985 Toxic effect of other metals
986 Toxic effect of carbon monoxide
987 Toxic effect of other gases, fumes, or vapors
988 Toxic effect of noxious substances eaten as food
989 Toxic effect of other substances, chiefly nonmedicinal as to source

Other and unspecified effects of external causes (990-995)
990 Effects of radiation, unspecified
991 Effects of reduced temperature
992 Effects of heat and light
993 Effects of air pressure
994 Effects of other external causes
995 Certain adverse effects, not elsewhere classified

Complications of surgical and medical care, not elsewhere classified (996-999)
996 Complications peculiar to certain specified procedures
997 Complications affecting specified body systems, not elsewhere classified
998 Other complications of procedures, not elsewhere classified
999 Complications of medical care, not elsewhere classified

SUPPLEMENTARY CLASSIFICATION OF FACTORS INFLUENCING HEALTH STATUS AND CONTACT WITH HEALTH SERVICES

Persons with potential health hazards related to communicable diseases (V01-V08)
V01 Contact with or exposure to communicable diseases
V02 Carrier or suspected carrier of infectious diseases
V03 Need for prophylactic vaccination and inoculation against bacterial diseases
V04 Need for prophylactic vaccination and inoculation against certain viral diseases
V05 Need for other prophylactic vaccination and inoculation against single diseases
V06 Need for prophylactic vaccination and inoculation against combinations of diseases
V07 Need for isolation and other prophylactic measures
V08 Asymptomatic human immunodeficiency virus [HIV] infection status

Persons with potential health hazards related to personal and family history (V10-V19)
V10 Personal history of malignant neoplasm
V11 Personal history of mental disorder
V12 Personal history of certain other diseases
V13 Personal history of other diseases
V14 Personal history of allergy to medicinal agents
V15 Other personal history presenting hazards to health
V16 Family history of malignant neoplasm
V17 Family history of certain chronic disabling diseases
V18 Family history of certain other specific conditions
V19 Family history of other conditions

Persons encountering health services in circumstances related to reproduction and development (V20-V29)
V20 Health supervision of infant or child
V21 Constitutional states in development
V22 Normal pregnancy
V23 Supervision of high-risk pregnancy
V24 Postpartum care and examination
V25 Contraceptive management
V26 Procreative management
V27 Outcome of delivery
V28 Antenatal screening
V29 Observation and evaluation of newborn for suspected condition not found

Liveborn infants according to type of birth (V30-V39)
V30 Singleton
V31 Twin, mate liveborn
V32 Twin, mate stillborn
V33 Twin, unspecified
V34 Other multiple, mates all liveborn
V35 Other multiple, mates all stillborn
V36 Other multiple, mates live- and stillborn
V37 Other multiple, unspecified
V39 Unspecified

Persons with a condition influencing their health status (V40-V49)
V40 Mental and behavioral problems
V41 Problems with special senses and other special functions
V42 Organ or tissue replaced by transplant
V43 Organ or tissue replaced by other means
V44 Artificial opening status
V45 Other postsurgical states
V46 Other dependence on machines
V47 Other problems with internal organs
V48 Problems with head, neck, and trunk
V49 Problems with limbs and other problems

Persons encountering health services for specific procedures and aftercare (V50-V59)
V50 Elective surgery for purposes other than remedying health states
V51 Aftercare involving the use of plastic surgery
V52 Fitting and adjustment of prosthetic device
V53 Fitting and adjustment of other device
V54 Other orthopedic aftercare
V55 Attention to artificial openings
V56 Aftercare involving intermittent dialysis
V57 Care involving use of rehabilitation procedures
V58 Encounter for other and unspecified procedures and aftercare
V59 Donors

Persons encountering health services in other circumstances (V60-V69)
V60 Housing, household, and economic circumstances
V61 Other family circumstances
V62 Other psychosocial circumstances
V63 Unavailability of other medical facilities for care
V64 Persons encountering health services for specific procedures, not carried out
V65 Other persons seeking consultation without complaint or sickness
V66 Convalescence
V67 Follow-up examination
V68 Encounters for administrative purposes
V69 Problems related to lifestyle

Persons without reported diagnosis encountered during examination and investigation of individuals and populations (V70-V82)
V70 General medical examination
V71 Observation and evaluation for suspected conditions not found
V72 Special investigations and examinations
V73 Special screening examination for viral diseases
V74 Special screening examination for bacterial and spirochetal diseases
V75 Special screening examination for other infectious diseases
V76 Special screening for malignant neoplasms
V77 Special screening for endocrine, nutritional, metabolic, and immunity disorders
V78 Special screening for disorders of blood and blood-forming organs
V79 Special screening for mental disorders and developmental handicaps
V80 Special screening for neurological, eye, and ear diseases

LIST OF THREE-DIGIT CATEGORIES

V81 Special screening for cardiovascular, respiratory, and genitourinary diseases
V82 Special screening for other conditions

SUPPLEMENTARY CLASSIFICATION OF EXTERNAL CAUSES OF INJURY AND POISONING

Railway accidents (E800-E807)
E800 Railway accident involving collision with rolling stock
E801 Railway accident involving collision with other object
E802 Railway accident involving derailment without antecedent collision
E803 Railway accident involving explosion, fire, or burning
E804 Fall in, on, or from railway train
E805 Hit by rolling stock
E806 Other specified railway accident
E807 Railway accident of unspecified nature

Motor vehicle traffic accidents (E810-E819)
E810 Motor vehicle traffic accident involving collision with train
E811 Motor vehicle traffic accident involving re-entrant collision with another motor vehicle
E812 Other motor vehicle traffic accident involving collision with another motor vehicle
E813 Motor vehicle traffic accident involving collision with other vehicle
E814 Motor vehicle traffic accident involving collision with pedestrian
E815 Other motor vehicle traffic accident involving collision on the highway
E816 Motor vehicle traffic accident due to loss of control, without collision on the highway
E817 Noncollision motor vehicle traffic accident while boarding or alighting
E818 Other noncollision motor vehicle traffic accident
E819 Motor vehicle traffic accident of unspecified nature

Motor vehicle nontraffic accidents (E820-E825)
E820 Nontraffic accident involving motor-driven snow vehicle
E821 Nontraffic accident involving other off-road motor vehicle
E822 Other motor vehicle nontraffic accident involving collision with moving object
E823 Other motor vehicle nontraffic accident involving collision with stationary object
E824 Other motor vehicle nontraffic accident while boarding and alighting
E825 Other motor vehicle nontraffic accident of other and unspecified nature

Other road vehicle accidents (E826-E829)
E826 Pedal cycle accident
E827 Animal-drawn vehicle accident
E828 Accident involving animal being ridden
E829 Other road vehicle accidents

Water transport accidents (E830-E838)
E830 Accident to watercraft causing submersion
E831 Accident to watercraft causing other injury
E832 Other accidental submersion or drowning in water transport accident
E833 Fall on stairs or ladders in water transport
E834 Other fall from one level to another in water transport
E835 Other and unspecified fall in water transport
E836 Machinery accident in water transport
E837 Explosion, fire, or burning in watercraft
E838 Other and unspecified water transport accident

Air and space transport accidents (E840-E845)
E840 Accident to powered aircraft at takeoff or landing
E841 Accident to powered aircraft, other and unspecified
E842 Accident to unpowered aircraft
E843 Fall in, on, or from aircraft
E844 Other specified air transport accidents
E845 Accident involving spacecraft

Vehicle accidents, not elsewhere classifiable (E846-E849)
E846 Accidents involving powered vehicles used solely within the buildings and premises of an industrial or commercial establishment
E847 Accidents involving cable cars not running on rails
E848 Accidents involving other vehicles, not elsewhere classifiable
E849 Place of occurrence

Accidental poisoning by drugs, medicinal substances, and biologicals (E850-E858)
E850 Accidental poisoning by analgesics, antipyretics, and antirheumatics
E851 Accidental poisoning by barbiturates
E852 Accidental poisoning by other sedatives and hypnotics
E853 Accidental poisoning by tranquilizers
E854 Accidental poisoning by other psychotropic agents
E855 Accidental poisoning by other drugs acting on central and autonomic nervous systems
E856 Accidental poisoning by antibiotics
E857 Accidental poisoning by anti-infectives
E858 Accidental poisoning by other drugs

Accidental poisoning by other solid and liquid substances, gases, and vapors (E860-E869)
E860 Accidental poisoning by alcohol, not elsewhere classified
E861 Accidental poisoning by cleansing and polishing agents, disinfectants, paints, and varnishes
E862 Accidental poisoning by petroleum products, other solvents and their vapors, not elsewhere classified
E863 Accidental poisoning by agricultural and horticultural chemical and pharmaceutical preparations other than plant foods and fertilizers
E864 Accidental poisoning by corrosives and caustics, not elsewhere classified
E865 Accidental poisoning from foodstuffs and poisonous plants
E866 Accidental poisoning by other and unspecified solid and liquid substances
E867 Accidental poisoning by gas distributed by pipeline
E868 Accidental poisoning by other utility gas and other carbon monoxide
E869 Accidental poisoning by other gases and vapors

Misadventures to patients during surgical and medical care (E870-E876)
E870 Accidental cut, puncture, perforation, or hemorrhage during medical care
E871 Foreign object left in body during procedure
E872 Failure of sterile precautions during procedure
E873 Failure in dosage
E874 Mechanical failure of instrument or apparatus during procedure
E875 Contaminated or infected blood, other fluid, drug, or biological substance
E876 Other and unspecified misadventures during medical care

Surgical and medical procedures as the cause of abnormal reaction of patient or later complication, without mention of misadventure at the time of procedure (E878-E879)
E878 Surgical operation and other surgical procedures as the cause of abnormal reaction of patient, or of later complication, without mention of misadventure at the time of operation
E879 Other procedures, without mention of misadventure at the time of procedure, as the cause of abnormal reaction of patient, or of later complication

Accidental falls (E880-E888)
E880 Fall on or from stairs or steps
E881 Fall on or from ladders or scaffolding
E882 Fall from or out of building or other structure
E883 Fall into hole or other opening in surface
E884 Other fall from one level to another
E885 Fall on same level from slipping, tripping, or stumbling
E886 Fall on same level from collision, pushing or shoving, by or with other person
E887 Fracture, cause unspecified
E888 Other and unspecified fall

Accidents caused by fire and flames (E890-E899)
E890 Conflagration in private dwelling
E891 Conflagration in other and unspecified building or structure
E892 Conflagration not in building or structure
E893 Accident caused by ignition of clothing
E894 Ignition of highly inflammable material
E895 Accident caused by controlled fire in private dwelling
E896 Accident caused by controlled fire in other and unspecified building or structure
E897 Accident caused by controlled fire not in building or structure
E898 Accident caused by other specified fire and flames
E899 Accident caused by unspecified fire

Accidents due to natural and environmental factors (E900-E909)
E900 Excessive heat
E901 Excessive cold
E902 High and low air pressure and changes in air pressure
E903 Travel and motion
E904 Hunger, thirst, exposure, and neglect
E905 Venomous animals and plants as the cause of poisoning and toxic reactions
E906 Other injury caused by animals
E907 Lightning
E908 Cataclysmic storms, and floods resulting from storms
E909 Cataclysmic earth surface movements and eruptions

Accidents caused by submersion, suffocation, and foreign bodies (E910-E915)
E910 Accidental drowning and submersion
E911 Inhalation and ingestion of food causing obstruction of respiratory tract or suffocation
E912 Inhalation and ingestion of other object causing obstruction of respiratory tract or suffocation
E913 Accidental mechanical suffocation
E914 Foreign body accidentally entering eye and adnexa
E915 Foreign body accidentally entering other orifice

Other accidents (E916-E928)
E916 Struck accidentally by falling object
E917 Striking against or struck accidentally by objects or persons
E918 Caught accidentally in or between objects
E919 Accidents caused by machinery
E920 Accidents caused by cutting and piercing instruments or objects
E921 Accident caused by explosion of pressure vessel
E922 Accident caused by firearm missile
E923 Accident caused by explosive material
E924 Accident caused by hot substance or object, caustic or corrosive material, and steam
E925 Accident caused by electric current
E926 Exposure to radiation
E927 Overexertion and strenuous movements
E928 Other and unspecified environmental and accidental causes

Late effects of accidental injury (E929)
E929 Late effects of accidental injury

Drugs, medicinal and biological substances causing adverse effects in therapeutic use (E930-E949)
E930 Antibiotics
E931 Other anti-infectives
E932 Hormones and synthetic substitutes
E933 Primarily systemic agents
E934 Agents primarily affecting blood constituents
E935 Analgesics, antipyretics, and antirheumatics
E936 Anticonvulsants and anti-Parkinsonism drugs
E937 Sedatives and hypnotics
E938 Other central nervous system depressants and anesthetics
E939 Psychotropic agents

E940 Central nervous system stimulants
E941 Drugs primarily affecting the autonomic nervous system
E942 Agents primarily affecting the cardiovascular system
E943 Agents primarily affecting gastrointestinal system
E944 Water, mineral, and uric acid metabolism drugs
E945 Agents primarily acting on the smooth and skeletal muscles and respiratory system
E946 Agents primarily affecting skin and mucous membrane, ophthalmological, otorhinolaryngological, and dental drugs
E947 Other and unspecified drugs and medicinal substances
E948 Bacterial vaccines
E949 Other vaccines and biological substances

Suicide and self-inflicted injury (E950-E959)
E950 Suicide and self-inflicted poisoning by solid or liquid substances
E951 Suicide and self-inflicted poisoning by gases in domestic use
E952 Suicide and self-inflicted poisoning by other gases and vapors
E953 Suicide and self-inflicted injury by hanging, strangulation, and suffocation
E954 Suicide and self-inflicted injury by submersion [drowning]
E955 Suicide and self-inflicted injury by firearms and explosives
E956 Suicide and self-inflicted injury by cutting and piercing instruments
E957 Suicide and self-inflicted injuries by jumping from high place
E958 Suicide and self-inflicted injury by other and unspecified means
E959 Late effects of self-inflicted injury

Homicide and injury purposely inflicted by other persons (E960-E969)
E960 Fight, brawl, and rape
E961 Assault by corrosive or caustic substance, except poisoning
E962 Assault by poisoning
E963 Assault by hanging and strangulation
E964 Assault by submersion [drowning]
E965 Assault by firearms and explosives
E966 Assault by cutting and piercing instrument
E967 Child battering and other maltreatment
E968 Assault by other and unspecified means
E969 Late effects of injury purposely inflicted by other person

Legal intervention (E970-E978)
E970 Injury due to legal intervention by firearms
E971 Injury due to legal intervention by explosives
E972 Injury due to legal intervention by gas
E973 Injury due to legal intervention by blunt object
E974 Injury due to legal intervention by cutting and piercing instruments
E975 Injury due to legal intervention by other specified means
E976 Injury due to legal intervention by unspecified means
E977 Late effects of injuries due to legal intervention
E978 Legal execution

Injury undetermined whether accidentally or purposely inflicted (E980-E989)
E980 Poisoning by solid or liquid substances, undetermined whether accidentally or purposely inflicted
E981 Poisoning by gases in domestic use, undetermined whether accidentally or purposely inflicted
E982 Poisoning by other gases, undetermined whether accidentally or purposely inflicted
E983 Hanging, strangulation, or suffocation, undetermined whether accidentally or purposely inflicted
E984 Submersion [drowning], undetermined whether accidentally or purposely inflicted
E985 Injury by firearms and explosives, undetermined whether accidentally or purposely inflicted
E986 Injury by cutting and piercing instruments, undetermined whether accidentally or purposely inflicted
E987 Falling from high place, undetermined whether accidentally or purposely inflicted
E988 Injury by other and unspecified means, undetermined whether accidentally or purposely inflicted
E989 Late effects of injury, undetermined whether accidentally or purposely inflicted

Injury resulting from operations of war (E990-E999)
E990 Injury due to war operations by fires and conflagrations
E991 Injury due to war operations by bullets and fragments
E992 Injury due to war operations by explosion of marine weapons
E993 Injury due to war operations by other explosion
E994 Injury due to war operations by destruction of aircraft
E995 Injury due to war operations by other and unspecified forms of conventional warfare
E996 Injury due to war operations by nuclear weapons
E997 Injury due to war operations by other forms of unconventional warfare
E998 Injury due to war operations but occurring after cessation of hostilities
E999 Late effects of injury due to war operations